SIXTH EDITION

DENTAL ASSISTING

A Comprehensive Approach

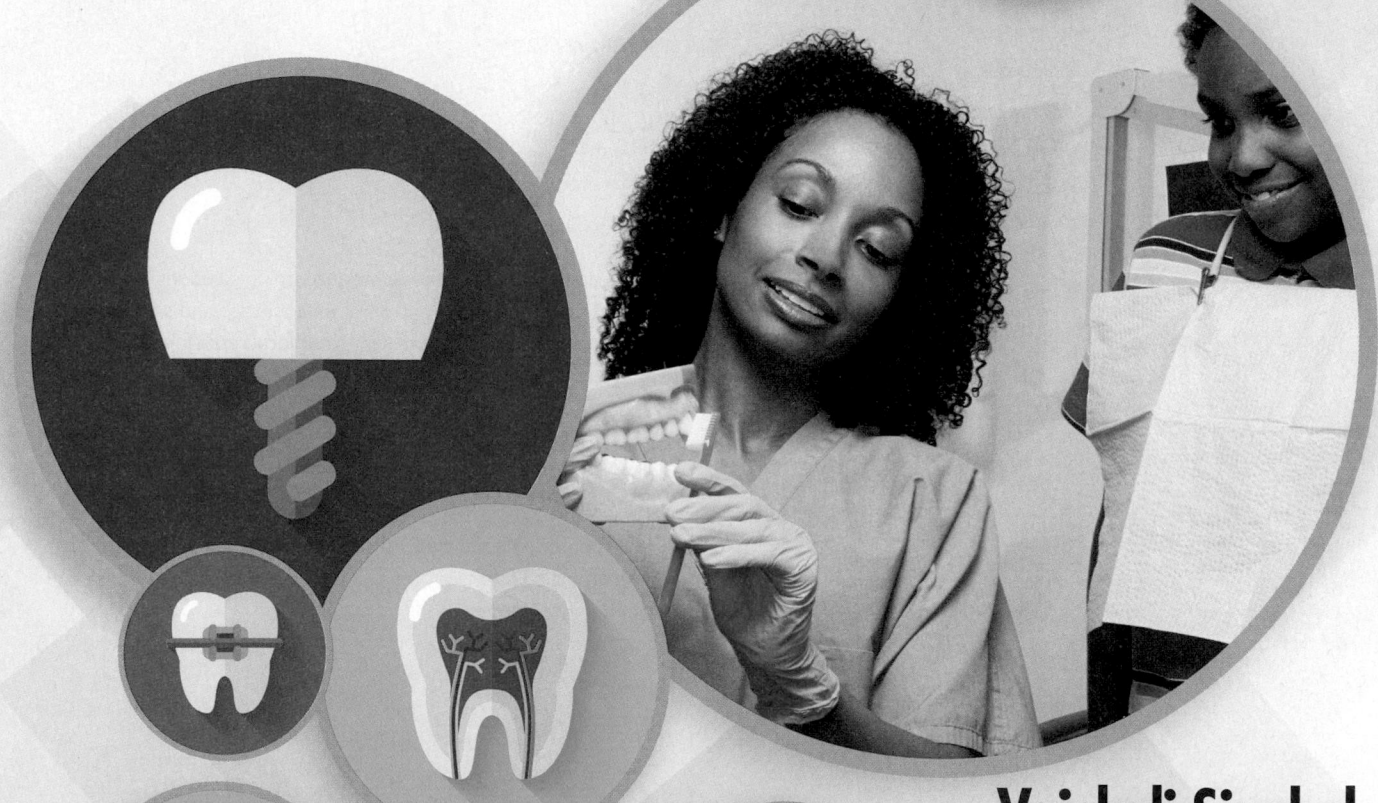

Vaishali Singhal
Susan Kantz
Melissa Damatta
Donna Phinney
Judy Halstead

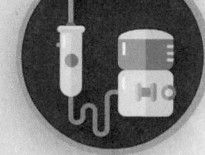

CENGAGE

Australia • Brazil • Mexico • Singapore • United Kingdom • United States

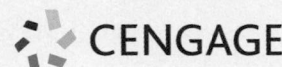

Dental Assisting, A Comprehensive Approach,
6th Edition
Vaishali Singhal, Susan Kantz, Melissa Damatta

SVP, Higher Education & Skills Product: Erin Joyner

VP, Higher Education & Skills Product: Thais Alencar

Product Director: Jason Fremder

Product Manager: Lauren Whalen

Product Assistant: Dallas Wilkes

Learning Designer: Mary Convertino

Senior Content Manager: Thomas Heffernan

Digital Delivery Lead: David O'Connor

Director, Marketing: Neena Bali

Marketing Manager: Courtney Cozzy

IP Analyst: Ashley Maynard

IP Project Manager: Kelli Besse

Production Service: Lumina Datamatics, Inc.

Designer: Felicia Bennett

Cover Image(s): istockphoto.com/XiXinXing

For product information and technology assistance, contact us at
**Cengage Customer & Sales Support, 1-800-354-9706
or support.cengage.com.**

For permission to use material from this text or product, submit all requests online at **www.cengage.com/permissions.**

Library of Congress Control Number: 2021914839

ISBN: 978-0-357-45652-1

Cengage
20 Channel Street
Boston, MA 02210
USA

Cengage is a leading provider of customized learning solutions with employees residing in nearly 40 different countries and sales in more than 125 countries around the world. Find your local representative at: **www.cengage.com.**

Cengage products are represented in Canada by
Nelson Education, Ltd.

To learn more about Cengage platforms and services, register or access your online learning solution, or purchase materials for your course, visit **www.cengage.com.**

Printed in the United States of America
Print Number: 02   Print Year: 2022

Dedication

This book is dedicated to Judy Halstead and the memory of Donna Phinney. Donna and Judy's professionalism, expertise, and dedication to their students were the backbone of the first five editions. Their shared passion for Dental Assisting education created and sustained this text over the years, and we are proud to continue their legacy.

BRIEF CONTENTS

LIST OF PROCEDURES

CONTENTS

SECTION VI Dental Radiography

SECTION VII Assist with Restorative Procedures and Dental Materials

SECTION VIII Assist with Comprehensive Patient Care

NEW TO THIS EDITION

General Updates

- Key Terms feature has been updated throughout the text to include phonetic pronunciation, the meaning of root and word parts, and the definition for each key term
- Dental operator steps were added to each step-by-step procedure, as applicable
- New images have been added throughout the text, including new step-by-step procedure photos, to enhance the topics discussed

Chapter 2

- Added/expanded discussion of:
  - Several health behavior theories in addition to Maslow's and how each can be utilized to improve the oral health of the patient
  - Characteristics of children, older adults, and Generation Alpha
  - Preparing dental presentations
- Expanded on the topic of written communication to include office letters and other forms of written communication, including electronic communication

Chapter 3

- Added/expanded discussion of:
  - Ethical principles
  - Ethical dilemmas
  - The differences between criminal law and tort law
  - Regulatory and nonregulatory agencies involved in dentistry
  - HIPAA responsibilities in various areas of dentistry, including technology
- Added image of a sample patient consent
- Added image of a sample acknowledgement of HIPAA policy
- Moved CDT codes to Chapter 44

Chapter 4

- Formerly Chapter 6
- Added/expanded discussion of:
  - Information on the cell and organization of the human body
  - The urinary system
  - The brain
  - The interrelationship between oral health and the various systems
- Added anatomical images including on the cell

Chapter 5

- Removed the section "Landmarks of the Face and Oral Cavity" and moved it to a new Chapter 6
- Added a new table that includes descriptions of all the cranial nerves

- Added several tables to provide concise information about nerves, arteries and veins, as well as their branches that supply the head and neck

Chapter 6

- This is a newly added chapter
- Added/expanded discussion of:
  - Regions of the face
  - Healthy and unhealthy gingiva

Chapter 7

- Reduced the Stages of Pregnancy topic/content
- Added histological images of tooth development
- Added several images to enhance the topics discussed in the chapter

Chapter 8

- Formerly Chapter 9
- Added/expanded discussion of:
  - Tooth landmarks from each aspect
  - Tooth characteristics and distinguishing features to assist in identifying teeth
  - Primary and permanent teeth
  - Universal Numbering System
- Added color images of tooth landmarks from each aspect

Chapter 9

- Moved chapter from Dental Specialties section to Dental Sciences section
- Added/expanded discussion of:
  - Tools available for oral cancer detection
  - Educating patients to perform an oral cancer screening on themselves
- Added tables that provide standard terms used to describe lesions
- Moved dental caries topic to this chapter and added detailed information in a table format regarding stages of decay
- Added step-by-step procedure for performing an intraoral and extraoral exam

Chapter 11

- Added/expanded discussion of:
  - Covid-related infection control procedures
  - Different surfaces in the dental office, with new images
  - Sanitizing surfaces, with new images
  - The Bloodborne Pathogens Standard and Hazard Communication Standard
- Additional images added for procedure related to handwashing

- Added new step-by-step procedures for:
  - Alcohol-based hand hygiene
  - Surgical hand scrub
  - Donning surgical gloves
  - Operating an ultrasonic cleaner
  - Operating an autoclave
- Expanded procedure related to treating a contaminated tray, with new images

Chapter 14

- Added/expanded discussion of:
  - Importance of knowing about drugs and how drugs are tested
  - Drug names
  - Routes of administration
  - Administration, distribution, metabolism, and excretion
  - Substance use disorder, including preventing drug diversion, identifying the patient with a substance use disorder, and medications used to treat substance use disorders
  - Adverse drug reactions
  - Commonly used drugs administered in a dental office or prescribed by a dentist
  - 2007 American Heart Association (AHA) guidelines for prophylactic antibiotics
  - American Society of Anesthesiologists (ASA) Classification of Risk Assessment
- Added new figures to include expanded information related to common abbreviations
- Added new tables detailing conversions for prescriptions, potential teratogenic effects of drugs, dental local anesthetics available for use in the United States, comparisons of over-the-counter analgesic medications, and comparisons of prescription pain medications
- Removed content related to caffeine, herbal and alternative medications

Chapter 15

- Added/expanded discussion of:
  - The importance of the medical history in preventing a medical emergency
  - The importance of vital signs
  - The most recent AHA blood pressure classifications and dental management protocol
  - Identification and management of the apprehensive patient
  - Stress reduction protocol
  - American Society of Anesthesiologist (ASA) classification
  - Medical consultation
  - The emergency kit

  - Each emergency that may occur in a dental office including prevention, management, medical history questions, predisposing factors, signs and symptoms, and ASA classifications
- Added new step-by-step procedures for:
  - Taking blood pressure
  - Obtaining pulse and respiration
- Added a sample medical history form
- Added a sample medical consultation
- Added tables that describe the drugs in the emergency kit along with images of drugs
- Categorized emergencies into syncope, respiratory disorders, adrenal disorders, thyroid disorders, diabetes, angina and MI, congestive heart failure, seizures, cerebrovascular accident, allergies, and airway obstruction
- Added several images to enhance the topics discussed in the chapter
- Moved discussion of dental emergencies to a separate chapter
- Removed CPR/BLS section

Chapter 23

- Added/expanded discussion of:
  - Noninjectable anesthetics
  - Complications related to local anesthesia
  - Postexposure management
- Added tables that provide coverage of:
  - Short, intermediate, and long-acting local anesthetics
  - Injection name, area anesthetized, needle insertion site, length and gauge of needle used, and depth of insertion
  - Prevention of dental local anesthetic related emergencies
  - Systemic adverse reactions of dental local anesthetics

Chapter 24

- This is a new Chapter highlighting preventative dental treatment
- Includes three new step-by-step procedures relating to preventative care: periodontal charting, oral prophylaxis, and scaling and root planning
- Formatted to focus on the ADHA standards for clinical dental hygiene practice

Chapter 25

- Added/expanded discussion of:
  - Silver Diamine Fluoride
  - Ergonomics during preventative care
  - Air-powder polishing
  - Stain
- Added a step-by-step procedure on air-powder polishing

Chapter 27

- Added/expanded discussion of:
  - Direct and indirect damage by an x-ray photon, including images
  - Shadow casting and the principles of shadow casting
  - Inverse square law
  - Linear nonthreshold curve, including image
- Added description and table with images of types of interactions with radiation
- Added table with information related to radioresistant and radiosensitive cells
- Included use of term "image receptor" to be inclusive of films and digital sensors unless specifically referring to traditional film

Chapter 28

- Updated the title for this chapter
- Added/expanded discussion of:
  - Infection control as it specifically relates to dental radiology equipment, digital systems, image receptors, supplies and processing for traditional films
  - Infection control before, during, and after exposures
  - Standard exposure sequence for paralleling and bisecting techniques
  - Anatomical landmarks to be used for bisecting technique
  - Object localization using SLOB rule and the right angle technique
- Included use of term "image receptor" to be inclusive of films and digital sensors unless specifically referring to traditional film
- Moved digital imaging from Chapter 23 to this chapter
- Added table and diagrams that specify maxillary and mandibular entry points for primary beam when using the bisecting technique
- Added step-by-step procedure for bisecting the angle technique

Chapter 29

- Updated the title for this chapter
- Added/expanded discussion of:
  - The coronal, axial and sagittal views of 3D imaging
  - Radiographic appearance of decay, with images
  - Radiographic pulpal and periapical lesions, with images
  - Radiographic appearance of periodontal disease, with images
  - Radiographic appearance of dental anomalies, with images
    Radiographic appearance of dental materials, with images
- Added direct and indirect digital panoramic options to the panoramic exposure procedure

- Added tables that summarize radiopaque and radiolucent maxillary landmarks and radiopaque and radiolucent mandibular landmarks

Chapter 33

- Updated step-by-step procedures to include automix cartridges with extruder guns
- Due to the eradication of polysulfide impressions, this step-by-step procedure was updated with taking a polyether impression

Chapter 38

- Added/expanded discussion of:
  - The classifications of periodontal disease based on the most recent American Academy of Periodontology guidelines
  - Periodontal risk assessment
  - Adjunctive periodontal therapies
  - Peridex®
- Added tables that cover:
  - The risk factors for periodontal disease
  - Glickman's classification of furcation involvement
  - Healthy gingiva and changes that take place related to periodontal disease
  - Locally applied antimicrobial agents

Chapter 39

- Added/expanded discussion of:
  - Indications and contraindications to dental implants
  - Patient selection for dental implants
  - The role of the implant coordinator

Chapter 40

- Added/expanded discussion of:
  - Clinical considerations for bridges
  - Shade selection
  - Digital communication
- Added table covering symbols and abbreviations used in fixed prosthodontics
- Added image of digital patient charting with fixed prosthodontic procedures

Chapter 41

- Added discussion on advantages and disadvantages of CAD/CAM technology

Chapter 42

- Added/expanded discussion of:
  - Transitional partial dentures as a type of partial denture
  - Nesbit partial denture as a type of partial denture
  - Kennedy classification for edentulous arches, with image

- Patient instructions for care of partial dentures
- Surfaces of a full denture
- Post palatal seal of a maxillary denture
- Xerostomia and impact on dentures
- Denture adhesives
- Denture sore spots
● Added image of an electronic patient charting record with removable procedures charted
● Added table covering abbreviations and symbols used in removable prosthodontics

Chapter 44

● Reorganized the chapter content for a better learning experience
● Added/expanded discussion of:
  - Language barriers
  - Teledentistry visits
  - CDT codes

PREFACE

The world of health care changes rapidly. The twenty-first century presents health care professionals with more challenges than ever before—but with challenge comes opportunity. Job prospects for dental assistants have never been better. The Bureau of Labor Statistics expects employment in our field to grow faster than the average for all occupations through the year 2030. Population growth, an increase in the aging population, and greater retention of natural teeth will fuel demands for dental services. As the health care industry requires more services to be completed by dentists, the dental assistant will be more valuable and needed than ever before. Many states are passing legislation allowing for an expansion in the skills that dental assistants can provide—with additional training. Placing restorations, obtaining virtual impressions, and monitoring general sedation are a few examples. As a dental assistant, you'll be expected to take on an increasing number of clinical and administrative responsibilities to stay competitive. Now is the time to equip yourselves with the range of skills and competencies you'll need to excel in the field. Now is the time to maximize your potential, to expand your base of knowledge, and to dedicate yourself to becoming the multifaceted dental assistant required in the twenty-first century. This text and complete learning system, *Dental Assisting: A Comprehensive Approach*, sixth edition, will guide you as a dental assisting student on this journey. The result of years of research, writing, and testing, this system is designed to prepare you for the Dental Assisting National Board (DANB) certification examination, some state credentialing, and the workplace. It presents information in a unique manner, using a variety of formats that account for the diverse ways in which today's students learn. To receive the full value of *Dental Assisting: A Comprehensive Approach*, sixth edition, it is important to understand the structure of the text, chapters, MindTap, and accompanying workbook as well as other supplements, and how they are all integrated into a complete learning system. Together, these materials will make your dental assisting education comprehensive and meaningful, providing you with the skills, knowledge, principles, values, and understanding needed to excel in your chosen profession.

Why We Wrote This Book Three dental educators, Vaishali Singhal, Susan Kantz, and Melissa Damatta, are the lead authors who developed the sixth edition of this textbook. Additionally, the book includes a team of contributing authors that includes notable educators and practitioners with expertise and national involvement in all phases and levels of dental assisting. We developed this edition according to the Commission on Dental Accreditation (CODA) Standards for Dental Assisting as well as the American Dental Association (ADA) content areas. The expansive table of contents for this textbook addresses some of the problems we identified with other dental assisting textbooks currently on the market; for example, educators have complained, "we were still fervently shopping for supplemental texts and media to improve our programs; most available videos were outdated and expensive, and often did not match the text; the chapters of the existing texts were extremely large and were often not in a sequence suitable for our programs; and as a result the texts inhibited the flexibility of instruction." Thus, the goal of this text is to provide all inclusive text and supporting materials for dental assisting program instructors—to provide a comprehensive educational program rather than simply a text. This comprehensive program is structured to provide built-in flexibility to support the individual academic freedom of faculty. The chapters are ordered to allow for performance-based sequencing of procedures arranged from basic to complex and from general to specialty practice.

The Learning System

The components of the learning system were developed with today's learner in mind. The authors and Cengage recognize that students learn in different ways—they read, write, listen, watch, interact, and practice. For this reason, we've created a variety of products learners can use to fully comprehend and retain what they are taught. An instructor's manual ties the components together, making classroom integration easy and fun.

- **The Text**

  This text delivers comprehensive coverage of dental assisting theory and practice, supported by full-color illustrations and photographs throughout with 169 step-by-step procedures in nine sections. Section I, *Dentistry as a Profession*, introduces learners to the profession and its history as well as communication and legal issues. Section II, *Dental Sciences*, covers the basics of general anatomy, head and neck anatomy, embryology, histology, tooth anatomy, and oral pathology, creating a foundation on which learners can move forward in skills training. Section III, *Preclinical Dental Sciences,* covers microbiology and infection control in dentistry, managing hazardous materials that may be found in a dental office, managing patients who are medically compromised or have special needs, preventing and managing common medical emergencies that may occur in a dental office, and pharmacology, all of which are critical elements to the profession. This textbook contains the latest and most up-to-date infection control protocol related to the recent COVID-19 pandemic. Section IV, *Prevention and Nutrition,* discusses general techniques to maintain health and wellness of the oral cavity and the dentition. Section V, *Assist with Diagnosis and Prevention*, introduces the learner to the dental office and equipment, chairside assisting, instruments, management of pain and anxiety, and preventive techniques in dentistry. This section also includes information on advanced functions such as coronal polish and dental sealants. Section VI, *Dental Radiography*, provides updated information on radiographic techniques and procedures, including the latest on digital and three-dimensional radiography. Section VII, *Assist with Restorative Procedures and Dental Materials*, introduces the learner to commonly used dental materials, assisting in procedures related to amalgam, dental cements, and composite as well as the management of dental emergencies. Section VIII, *Assist with Comprehensive Patient Care*, introduces learners to the specialized areas of dentistry and the importance of comprehensive care, as well as advanced skills of retraction cord placement and tooth whitening. Section IX, *Dental Practice Management*, contains coverage of dental office management, dental computer software, dental insurance, employment portfolios, and legal and ethical considerations, which are important components for managing a dental practice properly. New features such as patient dialogues and professional encounters have been added to the sixth edition. The professional encounter feature provides real-life scenarios regarding communication with a patient, offering the learner professional experiences of those in the field. Each chapter includes the following pedagogical features as applicable:

- Specific instructional objectives
- New feature: Comprehensive approach to building medical and dental terminology using root words along with key terms
- Introduction
- Step-by-step procedures with icons indicating handwashing, gloves, masks, protective clothing and protective eyewear, basic setup, and expanded functions (see icons below)
- In-text icons identifying legal and safety areas (see icons below)
- Boxed information containing tips and summaries
- New feature: Special features in online Instructor Manual that include documentation, patient dialogue, and professional encounters
- Chapter summary
- Case studies
- Review questions, including critical thinking questions
- New feature: Most up-to-date infection control protocol related to the COVID-19 pandemic

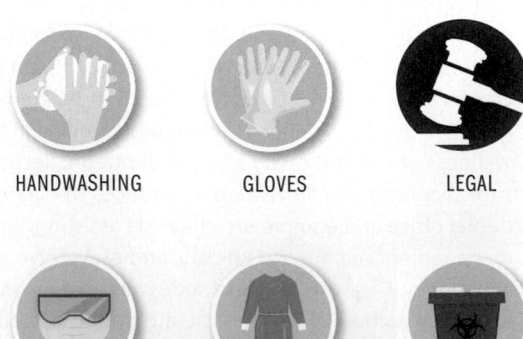

HANDWASHING   GLOVES   LEGAL

MASK AND PROTECTIVE EYEWEAR   CLOTHING   SAFETY

MindTap

It's 1 A.M. There are 20 tabs open on your computer. You lost your flashcards for the test, and you're so tired you can't even read. It would be nice if someone came up with a more efficient way of studying. Luckily, someone did. With a single login for MindTap® for *Dental Assisting: A Comprehensive Approach*, sixth edition, you can connect with your instructor, organize coursework, and have access to a range of study tools, including the ebook and apps, all in one place!

- **Manage your time and workload without the hassle of heavy books!** The MindTap Reader keeps all your notes together, lets you print the material, and will even read text out loud.
- **Want to know where you stand?** Use the Progress app to track your performance in relation to other students.
- **Engage with the material.** Videos and animations help your understanding of key concepts while simulations and quizzing help you bridge the gap from learning to real-world application.
- The **MindTap eReader** takes the textbook experience to a whole new level with the ability to have the material read to you with **Readspeaker**, print the material and take it with you for on-the-go preparation, and take notes or highlights within the eReader, which feeds to the StudyHub App for easy study guide creation.
- The **New MindTap Mobile App** not only includes access to the e-book both online and offline, but keeps you connected to your instructor and your course with alerts and notifications. It also arms you with on-the-go study tools like flashcards and quizzing, helping you to manage your limited time efficiently.
- **Flashcards** are prepopulated to provide a jump-start on your course preparation and studying. You can also create your own customized cards as you move through the course material, with theability to go directly to definitions by clicking on colored key terms within the text.

Instructor Resources

Additional instructor resources for this product are available online. Instructor assets include an Instructor's Manual, Educator's Guide, PowerPoint® slides, and a test bank powered by Cognero®. Sign up or sign in at **www.cengage.com** to search for and access this product and its online resources.

Components available on the Instructor Resource Center include:

- A computerized test bank, with questions geared to text chapters and mapped to CODA accreditation standards; available for download in many different LMS options
- Instructor presentations on PowerPoint™ with talking points, designed to support and facilitate classroom instruction
- An electronic version of the *Instructor's Manual* so that notes and ideas can be customized
- assisting materials to create a dynamic learning system

○ A transition guide to help make a smooth transition from the fifth to the sixth edition

○ Skill checklists to use for student evaluation.

○ Resources guide containing books, articles, and useful links, sorted by chapter.

● **Student Workbook**

The workbook, which corresponds to the text, contains chapter objectives and exercises in a variety of formats. Each workbook chapter was standardized to include a variety of activities such as matching, true/false, fill in the blank, multiple choice, certification review, critical thinking questions, and case studies to allow each student to learn the concepts in a manner that is best suited to their individual learning style. The questions are mapped to the objectives, providing a holistic exposure to the content of each chapter.

When you use all of these components together, you'll discover an innovative, comprehensive system of teaching and learning that prepares students for success in the twenty-first century.

About the Authors

Vaishali Singhal is an associate professor at Rutgers University's School of Health Professions (SHP) and Rutgers School of Dental Medicine (RSDM) in Newark, New Jersey. Teaching at the university since 2001, she currently serves as program director of the Bachelor of Sciences in Health Sciences Program as well as course director for Practice Management and Ethics and Jurisprudence at the RSDM. At the faculty practice of RSDM, Dr. Singhal specializes in treating patients with serious mental illness. In 2019 she completed her doctoral thesis at SHP, evaluating ways to improve the oral health of patients with serious mental illness. She completed a Master of Science in Health Sciences at Rutgers University in 2011 and received her DMD from the RSDM in 1993. Her PhD and MS programs included specialized courses in education, which is Dr. Singhal's passion.

Susan Kantz is the former Dental Assisting Program Director for a private college and a high school career center. During her career as an educator, Ms. Kantz was dedicated to helping each student achieve their greatest potential. She was an active HOSA (Health Occupations Students of America) local advisor, and her students consistently placed in the top 10, with a sound record of placing in the top 3 at National HOSA Leadership Conference. Ms. Kantz received Teacher of the Year and Indiana HOSA Advisor of the Year during her career as a high school instructor at a career center. Prior to teaching, she worked as an EFDA in pediatric and general dentistry private practice, at the Indiana University School of Dentistry in endodontics and Riley Children's Hospital Dental Clinic in pediatrics, orthodontics and as an operating room dental surgical assistant. Ms. Kantz was the curriculum developer for the Indianapolis Public Schools Health Professions Center. She was a member of the Indiana Department of Education cadre to teach writing duties/task lists and articulation agreements to vocational instructors throughout the state. After retirement, she worked as a dental assisting/dental hygiene adjunct instructor

at Ivy Tech Community College. Ms. Kantz completed her dental assisting and expanded dental assistant program at Indiana University School of Dentistry, earned a MS in allied health education from Indiana University and attended Indiana Wesleyan University Education Leadership Program.

Melissa Damatta began her career as a dental assistant at a young age. Her love of dentistry motivated her to return to school and pursue dental hygiene. Upon graduation, she immediately returned to school to pursue her second love: education. She began her education career at Rutgers School of Health Professions as an adjunct in the department of Allied Dental Education, where she taught both clinical and didactic courses. During that time she sought out her Certified Dental Assistant (CDA) certification. Ms. Damatta went on to teach in the dental hygiene program for Burlington County College in New Jersey. Currently, she is an associate professor for the dental hygiene program at Community College of Philadelphia, where she serves as clinic coordinator for second-year students and teaches radiology and a preclinical course to first-year students. Ms. Damatta has practiced dental hygiene for 18 years, with experiences in periodontal, pediatric, and general dentistry. A former president of Central New Jersey Dental Hygiene Association (CNDHA), she holds memberships in the American Dental Hygiene Association (ADHA) and the American Dental Education Association (ADEA). She continues to practice as a clinical dental hygienist for a private practice in New Jersey. Ms. Damatta completed her associate's degree in applied science in dental hygiene from Middlesex County College in New Jersey, her Bachelors of Science in Health Science–education track from The University of Medicine and Dentistry of New Jersey (now part of Rutgers University), and her Masters of Science in Dental Hygiene with an education concentration from the University of Bridgeport in Connecticut.

Donna J. Phinney was the program director for Spokane Community College's Dental Assisting Program. She spent more than 25 years in the dental field as a dental assistant, a dental office consultant, an office manager, and an educator. Ms. Phinney held a bachelor of arts from Eastern Washington University, a master's degree in education from Whitworth College, and an associate of science and certificate in dental assisting from Spokane Community College. A certified dental assistant, she was active in the Washington State Dental Assisting Association, where she served as president from 1992 to 1993. She obtained her fellowship from the American Dental Assisting Association in 2002. Donna was a consultant for the American Dental Association, was commissioner on dental accreditation for 17 years, was on the Dental Assisting Review Committee, and was a commissioner for the American Dental Association, appointed by the American Dental Assistants Association.

Judy H. Halstead is professor emeritus at Spokane Community College. She has more than 25 years' experience teaching and more than 10 years' experience as a dental assistant. She was a program director for dental assisting in a private college and for a high school skills center. Ms. Halstead holds a bachelor of arts from

Eastern Washington University, is a certified dental assistant, and has an expanded functions certificate. She has been a member of local, state, and national dental assistants associations for the past 25 years. She served as president of the Washington State Dental Assisting Association from 1994 to 1995. Ms. Halstead has presented lectures and workshops at local, state, and regional dental conferences.

Acknowledgments

The authors would like to thank the following individuals and institutions for providing valuable assistance in the development and production of the sixth edition:

Amy Mangan MS, BS, RDH

Amy Palagano, BS, RDH, CDA

Beatriz Fernandez, DMD

Caitlin LaFonte, BA, RDH

Cathy Alexander, CDA

Christine Casile MS, RDH, CDA

Cindy Schroeder MA, RDH, CDA

Damian Funke, MS, science instructor

Debbie Bordeaux

Gail Vasilenko MA, RDH, CDA

Jennifer Morelli MS, BS, RDH

Karen Finnerty MS, RDH, CDA

Keith Turner, CDT

Kim McMahon MS, RDH, RDA

Lawrence Schneider, DDS

Lucia Gonzales, CDA

Maxine Feinberg, DDS

Myke Carey AS, 3D Design and Animation

Rishi Singhal, BS, medical student

Rutgers School of Dental Medicine

Rutgers School of Health Professions

Steven R. Fink, DMD

Tracy Djani, RDH, MAED/e-Education, MH, ND

Usha Rana, DMD

Contributors

Michelle Ashley, RDH
Chapter 1: Introduction to the Dental Profession
Chapter 31: Amalgam Procedures and Materials

Dr. Cynthia Baker, DDS
Chapter 14: Pharmacology

Kathleen Baleno, RDH
Chapter 10: Microbiology
Chapter 11: Infection Control

Darci Barr, CDA
Chapter 3: Ethics, Jurisprudence, and the Health Information Portability and Accountability Act

Dr. Sabiha Bunek, DDS
Chapter 30: Dental Emergency Procedures and Dental Cements
Chapter 31: Amalgam Procedures and Materials
Chapter 32: Composite Procedures and Materials
Chapter 41: Computerized Impression and Restorative Systems
Chapter 43: Cosmetic Dentistry and Teeth Whitening

Joyce Hudson
Chapter 22: New Patient Examination
Chapter 24: Oral Prophylaxis and Recare Appointment
Chapter 25: Coronal Polishing and Topical Fluoride Application

Janet Jaccarino, CDA, RDH, MA
Chapter 2: Psychology, Communication, and Multicultural Interaction
Chapter 13: The Special Needs and Medically Compromised Patient
Chapter 16: Oral Health and Preventive Techniques
Chapter 17: Nutrition

Carrie Jacques
Chapter 4: General Anatomy and Physiology

Donna Kempf
Chapter 37: Endodontics
Chapter 44: Dental Practice Management

Jennifer Maggard
Chapter 27: Introduction to Dental Radiography, Radiographic Equipment, and Radiation Safety
Chapter 28: Dental Radiology Infection Control, Exposure, Processing and Evaluation of Dental Radiographs, and Mounting of Dental Radiographs
Chapter 29: Extraoral Radiography, Digital Radiography, and Radiographic Interpretation

Dr. Rebecca Poling, DDS, MSD
Dr. Rebecca Poling is the Primary Author for www.OrthoTraining.com, an online Orthodontic Education company. Dr. Poling wrote the content and provided the images for Chapter 35: Orthodontics. All Chapter 35 procedures were written by co-author Susan Kantz.

Dr. John Powers, PhD
Chapter 30: Dental Emergency Procedures and Dental Cements
Chapter 31: Amalgam Procedures and Materials
Chapter 32: Composite Procedures and Materials
Chapter 41: Computerized Impression and Restorative Systems
Chapter 43: Cosmetic Dentistry and Teeth Whitening

Shelley Rice, RDH
Chapter 27: Introduction to Dental Radiography, Radiographic Equipment, and Radiation Safety
Chapter 28: Dental Radiology Infection Control, Exposure, Processing and Evaluation of Dental Radiographs, and Mounting of Dental Radiographs
Chapter 29: Extraoral Radiography, Digital Radiography, and Radiographic Interpretation

Cathy Roberts, MADAA, EFDA, AGS
Chapter 34: Pediatric Dentistry

Christy Ross
Chapter 18: The Dental Office
Chapter 19: Dental Instruments and Tray Systems
Chapter 20: Ergonomics and Instrument Transfer
Chapter 22: New Patient Examination
Chapter 23: Anesthesia and Sedation
Chapter 26: Dental Sealants
Chapter 32: Composite Procedures and Materials

Minas Sarakinakis, CDA
Chapter 36: Oral and Maxillofacial Surgery

Cathy Sykes
Chapter 38: Periodontics

Dr. Janette Whisenhunt, CDA, RDH, BS, MEd, PhD
Chapter 5: Head and Neck Anatomy
Chapter 6: Landmarks of the Face and Oral Cavity
Chapter 7: Embryology and Histology
Chapter 8: Dental Anatomy
Chapter 9: Oral Pathology

Dr. Stacey Young, DC
Chapter 4: General Anatomy and Physiology

REVIEWERS

Reviewers of the Sixth Edition

Kathy Coy, CDA, RDH, BS
Wallace State Community College

Lindsey Evans, CDA, RDH, BS
Central Georgia Technical College

Gloria Pacheco, CDA, MA
Luna Community College

Teresa Ray-Connell
Lawson State Community College

Lori Scribner
ATA Career Education

Reviewers of the Fifth Edition

Terri Bannor
Northwest Technical College

Miriam Chacon
Passaic County Technical Institute

Cindy Cronick, BS, CDA
Metro Community College in Omaha

Cynthia Gasparik, CDA
Institute of Medical Careers

Robin Givens, CDA
Westwood College

Carol Hall-Pace
Martin Luther King Jr. Career Center

Tija Hunter, CDA, EFDA, CDIA, FADAA
Dental Careers Institute

Yolanda Johnson Gray
Fortis College

Shauna Phillips
Fortis College

Judith Shannon, CDA, RDH
Massasoit Community College

Donna Zagame, AS
Milwaukee Career College

Reviewers of the First, Second, Third and Fourth Editions

Robert Bennett, DMD
Texas State Technical College

Michelle Bissonette, CDA, EFDA, BS
Indiana University School of Dentistry

Valerie Blackenship, CDA, RDA
Simi Valley Adult School and Career Institute

Jill Brunson, CDA, RDA
Texas State Technical College Harlingen

Denis Campopiano, CDA, RDH, BS
Ogeechee Technical College

Robin Caplan, CDA
Medsafe, Inc.

Cynthia S. Cronick, CDA, AAS, BS
Southeast Community College

Terry R. Dean, DMD
Western Kentucky University

Jan DeBell, CDA, EFDA, BS
Front Range Community College

Heidi Denson
Ogden Weber Applied Technology

Marie Desmarais Cecil, CDA, MA
Central Community College

Sharon K. Dickinson, CDA, CDPMA, RDA
El Paso Community College

Jennifer Dumdei, LDARF, CDA
South Central College

Kerri H. Friel, RDH, COA, CDA, MA
Community College of Rhode Island

Kathy Foust, CDA, MS
Western Wisconsin Technical College

Dennis Garcia, DMD, RDA
Corinthian Colleges, Inc.

Lea Anna Harding, CDA, B.S.Ed
Gwinnett Technical College

Linda Kay Hughes, RDA, NRDA
PDE/Excelle College

Paulette Kehm-Yelton, CDA, EFDA, MPA
Northeast State Community College

Vivian Koistinen, ASDA
High Tech Institute, Inc.

Betty Ladley Finkbeiner, CDA, RDA, BS, MS
Washtenaw Community College

Deborah K. LeBeau, AACOM, CDA
Fortis College

Sandra Lo, DDS
Sacramento City College

Professor Teresa A. Macauley, CDA, EFDA, MS
Ivy Tech Community College of Indiana

Rebecca Mattney, CDA, RDA
Vatterott College

Judith A. McCauley, RDH, MA
Palm Beach State College

Connie Myers Kracher, PhD, MSD
Indiana University-Purdue University Fort Wayne

Stephanie Olson, BA, CDA
University of Alaska Anchorage

Krista M. Rodriguez, RDH, CDA, BA, NYCDA, FADAA
Monroe Community College

Stephanie Joyce Schmidt, CDA, CPFDA, CDT, RDAEF2, MS
Pasadena City College

Le Ann Schoelne, CDA, RDA, RF, BS
Central Lakes College

Jenny Schuler, CDA, BS
Bellingham Technical College

Bobby A. Sconyers, BA, CDA, CPFDA
South Florida State College

Annette Scranton, EFDA
Remington College/West Campus

Sheila Semler, CDA, RDH, MS, PhD
San Juan College

Lynette Sickelbaugh, CDA
Washington Local Adult Education

Karen F. Sperry, CDA, RDA, BVE
College of the Redwoods

Diana M. Sullivan
Dakota County Technical College

Kelly Svanda, CDA
Southeast Community College

Susan Thaemert, CDA, RDA, BS
Hennepin Technical College

Lynn Tyler
The American Institute of Medical-Dental Technology

Joyce T. Uyeda Yamada, CDA, RDH, MS
University of Hawaii Maui College

Tracie E. West
Remington College-Cleveland West

Janet Wilburn, BS, CDA
Phoenix College

Pamela G. Zarb, CDA, RDA, RDH, MA
Wayne County Community College

Language of Dentistry

Specific Instructional Objectives

At the completion of this section, you will be able to meet these objectives:

1. Defend the importance of being fluent in dental/medical terminology.
2. Analyze the structure of the dental terms.
3. Define dental terms.
4. Pronounce dental terms.
5. Apply rules in making words plural.
6. Recognize acronyms, eponyms, and homonyms.
7. Use terms presented in this chapter.

Dental Terminology

If you were going to a foreign country, you would need to learn its language to be able to communicate. In dentistry, you may find the words to be as foreign as another country's language. If you looked at some of the terms and said, "This looks like Greek to me," you would be right! Many of the terms used in **dentistry** and medicine come from Greek and Latin. Before you can study dentistry, you need to learn the dental language.

Every occupation uses a special language that has its own unique slang and technical terms. Computer programmers, for example, speak of "bits" and "bytes" and "megs" and "gigs." For someone unfamiliar with computers, those professional terms seem arcane and meaningless. Similarly, for the person unfamiliar with dentistry, the terms used in dentistry can be cryptic.

Dental **terminology** is the professional language used in dentistry. Dentistry uses medical and dental terminology in describing anatomy, pathology, treatment, procedures, and many other important facts needed to communicate dental care. It is important for the dental assistant to learn the dental language to communicate with other dental professionals and to read and understand dental communications.

Dental assistants have many responsibilities that relate to the proper use of dental terminology. For example, patient records are legal documents, and the assistant must complete them using acceptable terminology. In addition, dentistry uses a very precise and scientific language that may be difficult for the patient to understand. The dental assistant needs to translate these scientific and technical terms and procedures into terms the patient can comprehend. Accomplishing this requires mastery of dental terminology. In this chapter, you will be given the tools needed to build your dental vocabulary and converse as a dental professional.

Some dental terms may seem strange and impossible to understand at first, but learning them will be much easier if you remember a simple fact: *There are no big words; all big words consist of several small words linked together.* Much like working a jigsaw puzzle, you need to be able to understand the individual pieces and then put them together to form a complete picture. As with learning any language, it will take time to master. With dedicated effort and practice, you will find speaking and interpreting dental terminology enjoyable and a rewarding experience (Figure I-1).

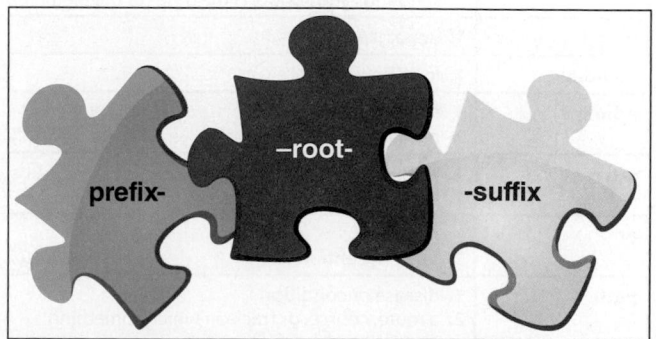

FIGURE I-1
Terminology is like pieces of a jigsaw puzzle fitting together.

Word Parts

Most words have three parts: a **root word**, a **suffix**, and a **prefix**. Some words might consist of only a root; others have several roots, or even several prefixes or suffixes. Learning how to identify roots, suffixes, and prefixes is the first step in mastering terminology in any field.

Root Words

The root is the main body or stem of the word; it is the foundation upon which all terminology is built. All words have a root word. For example, "term" is the root in the word *terminology*. The dictionary defines "term" as: "limit in time, place, set, or appointed period" and as "a word or group of words designating something, especially in a particular field." Many times you will find more than one definition and use of the term. Some common dental root words are *dent, odont, gingiv, mandible, dens, oral, cavity, path, odyn, coron, radic, maxill*, and *alveoli*. (Refer to Table I-1 for their meanings and Table I-2 for how they are pronounced.)

Compound Words A compound word is a word composed of two or more root words. For example, the word *toothbrush* is a compound word made from the words *tooth* and *brush*.

TABLE I-1 Meaning of Root Terms

Root Word	Meaning of Root Term
alveol	1. a little cavity, pit, or cell 2. any of the sockets in which the roots of the teeth are embedded; tooth socket 3. any of the tiny air sacs in the lungs
cavity	1. a hollow space within the body, an organ, a bone 2. a hollow space or a pit in a tooth, most commonly produced by caries; a cavity may be artificially made to support dental restorations
coron	1. a crown 2. part of a tooth above the gum
dent	1. a tooth 2. toothlike part
gingiv	1. technical name for gum 2. epithelial tissue attached to the bones of the jaw; surrounds and supports the bases of the teeth
maxill	1. upper jaw
mandibl	1. lower jaw
odont	1. tooth 2. having teeth
odyn	1. pain 2. painful
or	1. mouth 2. opening, entrance
path	1. disease or condition 2. a route, course, or track on which something moves
radic	1. part of a tooth within the tooth socket 2. the rootlike beginning or appearance
stoma	1. surgery, an artificial opening 2. anatomy, a mouth or mouthlike part

TABLE I-2 Pronunciation of Root Words

Dental/Medical Term	Pronunciation of Root Term
alveol	(al-**vee**-ohl)
cavity	(**kav**-i-tee)
coron	(*kuh*-**rohn**)
dent	(dent)
gingiv	(jin-**jahy**-v)
maxill	(mak-**sil**)
mandibl	(**man**-d*uh*-b*uh*l)
odont	(oh-**dohnt**)
odyn	(oh-**din**)
or	(ohr)
path	(pahth)
radic	(**rad**-ik)
stoma	(**stoh**-m*uh*)

Affixes

A root word can take on different meanings by adding word attachments to it called **affixes**. Affixes can modify, describe, and change the meaning of root words. They can also give direction and tell what is happening or when it is happening. When a word part is affixed (added) to the end of the word, it is called a suffix. A word part affixed to the beginning of the word is called a prefix.

Combining Forms Sometimes when combining roots and affixes, the word parts have to change to make the term easier to read and pronounce. The new, changed form of the word is called a combining form.

No combining form is needed when combining two words parts in which the second word part begins with a vowel. For example, the word *gingivitis* (meaning inflammation of the gums) is formed by combining the root word *gingiv* (meaning gum) with the suffix *itis* (meaning inflammation). Since the second word part, *itis*, begins in a vowel, no combining form is needed.

When a word part that follows another word part begins with a consonant, you must add a **vowel** (a, e, i, o, u, and y) to make a **combining form**. For example, the word *thermometer* combines the prefix *therm* (meaning heat) with the root word, *meter*, which is an instrument used for measuring. To make the combining form, we add "o" to make "thermometer"—an instrument used to measure a patient's body heat; "o" is the most commonly used combining vowel.

Suffixes

Suffixes are attachments added to the end of the root word to modify, change, or add to the meaning to form another word. Although prefixes are added to the beginnings of words and suffixes are added to the end, we will discuss suffixes first because they show how a word is used in a sentence and what part of speech the word represents. In dental terminology, suffixes are used to identify diseases, conditions, and diagnostic, operative, and surgical procedures. A dental term will have only one suffix.

Let's see how suffixes change the meaning of words by adding suffixes to the word defined previously: *term*. You learned that the word *term* has two meanings; limit in time, place, set, or period, and a word descriptive in a particular field. The combining form is *termin*. Here are some suffixes that can be attached: -al, -ate, -ology. The new words are the following:

- *Terminal*: an adjective meaning "leading to an ultimate end, or death." A terminal illness would be an illness that is ultimately fatal. Terminal can also be a noun that means "either end of a transportation line" such as a bus terminal.

- *Terminate*: a verb meaning "to dismiss from a job, to end, to come to an end of time, or to kill."

- *Terminology*: a noun meaning "the study of specialized words related to a particular subject."

When a suffix is written alone, it is usually preceded by a hyphen (for example, "-ed") indicating that a word part precedes it to form a complete word. Tables I-3 through Table I-6 define common suffixes indicating parts of speech. Table I-7 and Table I-8 list some common suffixes used in dental diagnosis and treatment.

Prefixes

Prefixes are attachments added before the root word to make the meaning more precise. Most prefixes can be added to the root word without changing the form of the prefix or the root word. When a prefix is written alone, it is usually followed by a hyphen indicating that a word part is added after the prefix (pre-) to form a complete word. A dental term may have more than one prefix to describe it.

Prefixes Describing Diagnosis Anatomical structures, diseases, and conditions are examined for diagnostic findings. They are often described by color and comparison to what is normal. The most common colors used in dentistry are listed in Table I-9, and Table I-10 describes findings from diagnosis.

Prefixes Describing Location When describing anatomy, diseases, and conditions, the exact location must be recorded.

TABLE I-3 Suffixes Used to Form Nouns

-a = singular ending of noun	**-acy** = like, state, **-cy** or quality, pertaining to	**-ine** = belonging to	**-ness** = condition
-age = belonging to, related to	**-dom** = place or state of being	**-ist** = doer	**-on** = chemical substance
-ance = state or **-ence** quality of	**-er** = a person or thing	**-ism** = state, belief, condition	**-or** = a person or thing
-ase = names enzymes	**-hood** = state or condition of being	**-ity** = state, quality	**-tion** = act of **-sion**
-ation = act of	**-ia** = condition or quality	**-ium** = membrane **-eum**	**-ure** = action, result
-ax = anatomical structure ending	**-ion** = action state	**-ment** = state, act	**-y** = to form familiar names

TABLE I-4 Suffixes Used to Form Adjectives

-able = capable of **-ble** being	**-eal** = pertaining to	**-ible** = capable of being	**-oid** = resembling, like
-ac, -al, -an, -ar, -ary, -eal, -ic, -ive, -tic = pertaining to; having quality of	**-en** = resembling, made of	**-ic** = pertaining to; **-ical** having quality of	**-ous** = like, full of **-ious**
-an = belonging to **-ian**	**-ent** = full of	**-il** = pertaining to, **-ile** capable of	**-tic** = pertaining to
-ant = full of	**-eous** = composed of	**-ish** = like	**-y** = characterized by
-ar = pertaining to; having quality of	**-form** = having the shape or form	**-ive** = having the nature of	
-ary = like, connected with	**-ful** = characterized	**-less** = without	

TABLE I-5 Suffixes Used to Form Adverbs

-ably = capable of	**-less** = lacking	**-ward** = indication direction
-acious = full of **-icious**	**-like** = similar to	**-wide** = a given space
-fold = having so many parts	**-ly** = in a certain manner	**-wise** = direction, manner
-ily = in a certain manner	**-most** = quality, order	
-ive = tendency, inclination	**-ular** = relating to, resembling	

TABLE I-6 Suffixes Used to Form Verbs

-ate = process	**-ify** = to make, create
-ed = past action	**-ing** = action of
-en = to be, to become	**-ise** = to become, to agree with
-fy = to make, cause to be	**-ize** = to affect, resemble
-iate = to begin, process	**-lyse** = loose, dissolve, break into

TABLE I-7 Suffixes Used in Diagnosis

-algia = pain	**-ology** = study of
-dynia = pain	**-oma** = tumor
-edema = swelling	**-opsy** = view
-gnosis = able to discern, come to know	**-osis** = abnormal condition
-ia = condition	**-path** = disease
-iasis = pathological condition	**-phylaxis** = watching, guarding
-itis = inflammation	**-rrhage** = excessive bleeding, hemorrhage **-rrhagia**

TABLE I-8 Suffixes Used in Dental Procedures

-centesis = surgical fixation	**-plasty** = surgical repair
-ectomy = excision, surgical removal, cutting out	**-rrhaphy** = suture
-ive = function	**-stomy** = formation of an opening
-pexy = surgical fixation	**-tomy** = incision, cutting into

TABLE I-9 Prefixes Describing Color

alb-, albin- = white, referring to lack of pigment	**erythr-** = red
chlor- = green	**leuk-** = white
chrom- = color **chromat-**	**melan-** = black
cyan- = blue	**xantho-** = yellow

Common prefixes used to describe specific location, position, and direction are listed in Table I-11.

Prefixes Describing Amounts In describing anatomical structures, diseases, and conditions, the dental professional has to know and explain how many, how much, and what size. Prefixes can describe numbers, quantity, size, and degree of change. See how many of these prefixes you already know in Table I-12.

Strategy for Building Dental Vocabulary

After what you've just read, do you think you would be more or less likely to suffer from *hippopotomonstrosesquipedaliophobia*? You may be thinking, "What does that mean and how do you expect me to answer the question?" Remember, however, there are no big words, just combinations of several smaller word parts. This is the first place to start when determining the meaning of a word.

TABLE I-10 Prefixes Describing Findings

brady- = slow movement	**gloss-** = tongue (referring to condition)	**onc-** = tumor, mass swelling
cheil- = lips (referring to condition)	**hemo-** = blood	**pharyn-** = throat, windpipe
dia- = thorough, complete knowledge	**labi-** = lips (referring to location) **lingual-** = tongue (referring to location)	**prog-** = probable outcome, course
dys = bad, abnormal, impaired	**lymph-** = clear fluid that bathes and nourishes tissues of body; lymphatic system	**sial-** = saliva, salivary gland
eu- = normal	**mal-** = bad, wrongful, ill **mis-** = bad, wrong,	**tachy-** = rapid, accelerated

TABLE I-11 Prefixes Describing Location

ab- = away from **abs-**	**ex-** = beyond	**post-** after, behind
ad- = toward	**infra-** = beneath, below	**pre-** = before, in front of
ante- = before, forward **anter-** = front	**inter-** = between	**proxim-** = near, adjacent
dextr- = right side	**intra-** = within	**sub-** = under
de- = away from, ending	**later-** = toward the side	**super-** = above **supra-**
dist- = directed away from midline	**mes-** = middle **med-**	**sy-, syl-, sym-, syn-** **sys-** = together
en- = inside, within, inner **end-** **ent-**	**peri-** = around	**trans-** = across, through

TABLE I-12 Prefixes Describing Amounts

a- = without, not **an-**	**iso-** = equal, like	**poly-** = many, excessive
bi- = two	**macro-** = large, long, big	**quad-** = four **quadr-**
di- = two **diplo-** = double	**meg-** = great, large **mega-** **megal-**	**semi-** = half
hemi- = half	**micro-** = small	**tetra-** = four
homo- = same	**mon-** = one	**tri-** three
hyper- = above, beyond, excessive	**multi-** = many	**uni-** one
hypo- = under, deficient	**non-** = not, lack of	**sext-** = six

Break the Word into Its Parts

To break the word into its various word parts, first identify any affixes (prefixes and suffixes) as well as any combing vowels, remembering that the most common combining vowel is "o." For example, this word (*hippopotomonstrosesquipedaliophobia*) contains no prefixes and one suffix (-ia). It also has four combining vowels—three "o's" and one "i." From this information, we can identify five root words: *hippo-poto-*, *monstro-*, *sesqui-*, *pedalio-*, and *phob-*, as well as the suffix *-ia*.

Define the Meaning of Each Word Part

Next define the meaning of each root word and affix. If you are not sure of the meaning, look it up in a dictionary:

hippopoto = hippopotamus; very large, massive mammal; second-largest land mammal

monstro = monstrous; abnormal, hideous, or unnatural in size, frightful in appearance

sesqui = one and a half; half as much again; many syllables

pedalio = relating to foot

phob = an intense, abnormal, or illogical fear of a specified thing; irrational fear of a specific object, activity, or situation that leads to a compelling desire to avoid it

-ia = disease; pathological, abnormal condition or mental disorder

Try to define the word.

Put the Parts Together

Now put the word parts together. Remember that the root word attached to the suffix is the stem upon which the word is built and is therefore the key to its meaning. In this case, the key to this word is *phobia*, which means a mental disorder caused by an intense fear of something. The rest of the word parts tell what that something is.

You have the meaning of the word parts. Can you define it now?

Assemble the Meaning

The term will not make sense until you put together the meanings of each of the word parts that compose it. Generally, you start with the suffix and key root word, and then you return to the start of the word and define the meanings of the rest of the word parts in order. In this case, that would produce: *A mental disorder, caused by irrational fear of something large and monstrous, with many syllables, a foot and a half long*. Or, as the dictionary defines *hippopotomonstrosesquipedaliophobia*: a fear of long words (words a foot and a half long with many syllables).

Use Your Senses

Cognitive research has proven that the best way to learn is to involve as many senses as possible. A popular quote says, "We learn 10% of what we read, 20% of what we hear, 30% of what we see, 50% of what we see and hear, 70% of what we discuss with others, 80% of what we experience, and 95% of what we teach to someone." Try to involve as many senses as possible in learning a new term.

For example, try to make a mental picture of what the word means. Imagine a person's reaction to a phobia: shortness of breath, smothering sensations, pounding heart, shaking, sweating, and nausea. Studying models or diagrams of technical terms, or drawing pictures, can help you commit terminology to memory models or diagrams and you can draw a picture of it.

Saying new words aloud also will help you retain new information. Dictionaries list the phonetic spelling of every word before defining it and usually provide a guide to the less familiar symbols often used in phonetic spellings. There are also online "talking dictionaries" that will pronounce any word aloud for you.

Make It Meaningful

Whenever possible, find the item you are learning and handle it; nothing can substitute for hands-on learning. This kind of "effortful processing" leads to more stable learning. According to the Association for Psychological Science, we encode based on meaning—we remember what is meaningful to us.

Meaningful repetition is the key to long-term memory, so make reviewing terms a part of your daily studies. However, do not simply memorize words; interact with and use them actively. Start a log of vocabulary words and practice using dental language every day. Take advantage of your learning environment and offer to peer-tutor a classmate who is struggling to learn the information. Explain to your friends and family what you are learning. This is good practice for teaching your patients in

the dental office. Remember, we learn 95% of what we teach to someone. Think that might be why your teachers remember so much detail?

Pronunciation

When you look up a word in the dictionary to find its meaning, you will notice that the word's **pronunciation** is also provided. It is important to learn how to say the word correctly (pronounce) to understand and remember what you have read. Your memory improves with the more senses you use. By pronouncing the word, you use your ears and mouth to speak the word. It is also important to pronounce words correctly so other dental professionals will know what you are saying.

Pronunciation is defined as the act of producing sounds of speech within the reference of a standard of correctness or acceptability. There is supposedly a correct manner of pronouncing sounds in any given language. In medical/dental terminology, there is often more than one correct way to pronounce the term. The most accepted pronunciation is generally listed first in the dictionary. However, certain terms do have more than one acceptable pronunciation. This is often due to different parts of the country and even the world. But, there is only one proper spelling of a term. Any change or error in spelling can totally change the meaning of a word; it may have an entirely different meaning that may result in improper diagnosis or treatment.

In this chapter, you will study how to pronounce a word using the **phonetic** transcription of a word. Dental term pronunciations are spelled out within parentheses and are broken into phonetic syllables. A syllable is a basic unit of speech generally containing only one vowel sound. For example, the word *base* contains one **syllable** and *basic* contains two syllables. Phonetics is what the term sounds like by an accepted standard of the human speech sounds and stress patterns of a syllable. Each term is broken into "sounds-like" syllables. The word *base* is phonetically translated as "beys" written as one syllable. Basic is phonetically translated into two syllables "**bey**-sik." Notice that the syllables are separated by a dash and the first syllable is in bold font. The bold font is used to show stress patterns of the syllables.

Syllables in bold font receive the most stress (emphasis, spoken louder) than the other syllables. If another syllable has intermediate stress (slightly louder), quotation marks follow the syllable. Otherwise, all syllables are equally stressed. Can you pronounce pronunciation (pr*uh*-nuhn'-see-**ey**-sh*uh* n)? Just say it as it is spelled out.

In Table I-2, the root words defined now have the phonetic pronunciation. Practice saying these words.

Some combinations of letters are misleading in figuring out how to pronounce them. These combinations include *ps* (psych—only the s is pronounced); *pn* (pneum—only the n is pronounced); *gn* (gnath—only the n is pronounced); and *ph* (physio—ph sounds like f). Be aware of these misleading pronunciations as you study terms.

Plurals

There are several basic rules for creating the plural forms of words. Add *es* for nouns that end in *s, ch,* or *sh.* If the word ends in *y* and has a preceding consonant (such as allergy), change the *y* to *i* and add *es* (allergies). When looking up terms, the plural form is often provided. It will be indicated by the abbreviation *pl* before the plural form. To learn more about the rules for forming more plurals, study Table I-13.

Acronyms/Eponyms/Homonyms

Not all dental language consists of word parts. Some of the terms are composed of letters representing a phrase. Others may be named after a person or place. There are even words that are spelled differently, but sound the same. As a dental professional, you need to know how to interpret all forms of dental terminology.

Acronyms

An **acronym** is a word formed from the initial letter or groups of letters or words in a set phrase or series. In the technology and health industry, there is always some new acronym. In making an acronym, the industry tries to choose a catchy, pronounceable series of letters and make a name out of it. Some of the more common acronyms that are related to dentistry are listed in Table I-14.

Eponyms

Eponyms are terms used in medicine and dentistry that are named after people, places, or things. Because of the nature of medicine, new discoveries are often attached to the people who made the discovery. The names of drugs, diseases, and treatments are named after scientists and doctors who discovered or invented them. Sometimes the name is derived from the proper name of a real or mythical person or place. Since eponyms are named after proper names, the term needs to be capitalized.

It usually involves a lot of research and publishing an article in a respected medical journal to have a medical eponym awarded. Down's syndrome is an eponym for the English physician, John Down, who described the syndrome. Down's syndrome is a genetic condition that is characterized by the presence of an extra copy of genetic material on the twenty-first chromosome. The syndrome may have some impairment of cognitive ability and physical growth and specific facial characteristics.

On occasion, an eponymous disease is named after a famous patient. Lou Gehrig's disease was named after Lou Gehrig, who was an American Major League Baseball player nicknamed "The Iron Horse" for his durability. Many eponymic diseases also have a more descriptive name. Lou Gehrig's disease is also called ALS (amyotrophic lateral sclerosis). ALS is a progressive neurodegenerative disease that affects nerve cells in the brain and the spinal cord. This disease's progressive degeneration of the motor neurons eventually leads to paralysis and to the patient's death.

Legionnaires' disease was given the name when an outbreak of pneumonia occurred among people attending an American Legion convention. Some famous medical signs and drugs are eponyms. The sounds heard when checking blood pressure called the Korotkoff sounds were discovered by Nikolai Korotkov, a cardiologist. Charles Mantoux, physician, is the developer of the eponymous serological test for tuberculosis, known as the Mantoux test.

TABLE I-13 Rules of Making Plurals

Singular Ending	Plural Ending	Examples
a	ae	gingiva, *pl* gingivae
ax	aces	thorax, *pl* thoraces
ex	ices	apex, *pl* apices
itis	ides	pulpitis, *pl* pulpitides
ix	ices	cervix, *pl* cervices
ma	s or mata	stoma, *pl* stomas / stoma, *pl* stomata
nx	nges	pharynx, *pl* pharnges
oma	s	odontoma, *pl* odontomas
on	a	protozoon, *pl* protozoa
sis	oses	diagnosis, *pl* diagnoses
um	a	bacterium, *pl* bacteria
us	i	alveolus, *pl* alveoli
y	ies	biopsy, *pl* biopsies

TABLE I-14 Acronyms

Acronym	Translation
ADA	American Dental Association
ADAA	American Dental Assistants Association
ADHA	American Dental Hygiene Association
ALARA	As Low As Reasonably Achievable
CDA	Certified Dental Assistant
CDC	Centers for Disease Control
CODA	Commission on Dental Accreditation
DANB	Dental Assisting National Board
DDS / DMD	Doctor of Dental Surgery / Doctor of Dental Medicine
BA / BS / MS / MA	Bachelor of Arts / Bachelor of Science / Master of Science / Master of Arts
OSHA	Occupational Safety and Health Administration
PPE	Personal Protection Equipment
RDA / EFDA	Registered Dental Assistant / Expanded Function Dental Assistant
RDH / LDH	Registered Dental Hygienist / Licensed Dental Hygienist

Many human anatomical parts are named after people. One of the founders of the science of human anatomy, Bartolomeo Eustachi, gained the reputation of having created the science of human anatomy because of the number of anatomical structures he discovered and wrote about. One of such structures, named after him, is the eustachian tube. The Achilles tendon was named after the Greek mythological character, Achilles.

Homonyms

Homonyms are words that sound the same, but the spelling is different and so is the meaning. These words can cause confusion in understanding the spoken word. Care should be taken to check the spelling and meaning of such words to prevent making this mistake. Some of the more common homonyms are listed in Table I-15.

Word Usage Reflects on the Dentist

Patient records are legal documents and can be the dentist's best defense in court if an incident results in litigation. All office records must be completed in detail using acceptable terminology and proper grammar.

Following is an example of an assistant's documentation of a patient's reaction after anesthetic. See if you can identify where the assistant had problems with homonyms.

The patient had sweet poring down her forehead. When asked if she had ever experienced this before, she said she felt she had a blood sugar problem and ate a very rich, sweat desert before coming for her appointment. The dentist told her she should follow up with her physician and eat well balanced meals especially on daze of her appointment. Unprofessional patient records can be the offense's best evidence.

Have you ever heard that a person's grammar reflects a person's level of education? Mastering dental terminology mirrors the assistant's knowledge of dentistry and reflects on the dentist.

TABLE I-15 Homonyms

Homonyms	Definitions
auxiliary axillary	a person that helps near the armpit
bite byte	a mouthful 8 bits
die die dye	exact replication of a structure; used as pattern to make dental appliance cease to live to color or stain
elicit illicit	to draw unlawful
esthetics aesthesia	concept of beauty; also spelled aesthetics ability to feel
facial fascial	relating to the face a band of tissue supporting internal parts of the body
heal heel	to cure of disease hind part of foot
know no	to be fully aware of meaning and implications denial or refusal
oral aural aural	pertaining to the mouth pertaining to the ear pertaining to an aura; sensation preceding a migraine or epileptic attack *two different meanings for same spelling*
pain pane	it hurts a single panel of glass
palpation palpitation	examine by touch abnormally rapid and violent beating of the heart
plural pleural	more than one related to lung
pore pore pour poor	minute opening to read or study carefully to cause flow of liquid to have little or no money
right right write rite	what is good, proper, and just side opposite location of the heart form letters with pen, pencil, etc formal act or ceremony
site cite sight	location to refer vision
suture suture	line of junction of two bones joining edges of open by stitches
week weak	a period of successive days not strong

Key Terms: Definitions and Pronunciation

Each chapter will end with a Key Terms feature. New terms introduced in the chapter appear in the first (far-left) column of the Key Terms table. Below each term is the phonetic spelling to help with the pronunciation. The middle column breaks the term into word parts along with the definition of each part. The last column lists the dictionary definition of the term. The terms in the Key Terms chart appear in blue font within each chapter. Key Terms features and charts help you learn the meanings of the terms in each chapter before you start reading, so you can more easily build your dental and medical terminology.

It will be helpful to learn a few word parts at a time and recognize them when you see them in a term. It is much better to understand the meaning of the word parts and learn how to build words than to try to memorize, look up, or skip over every new word you encounter.

Review Questions

Multiple Choice

1. What word part is the foundation and main meaning of the word?
   a. prefix
   b. root
   c. suffix
   d. combining vowel

2. What word part is *sub* in the word *submandibular*?
   a. prefix
   b. root
   c. suffix
   d. combining vowel

3. What word part is *ular* in the word *submandibular*?
   a. prefix
   b. root
   c. suffix
   d. combining vowel

4. Which dental term means "below the lower jaw"?
   a. alveolectomy
   b. gingivitis
   c. submandibular
   d. supramaxilla

5. Which dental term means "inflammation of the gums"?
   a. alveolectomy
   b. gingivitis
   c. periodontitis
   d. supramaxilla

6. A _____ is the basic unit of speech generally having only one vowel sound.
   a. pronunciation
   b. phonetic
   c. syllable
   d. simple term

7. What is the descriptive word for "sounds like" that is used to help the reader say the word correctly?
   a. pronunciation
   b. phonetic
   c. syllable
   d. simple term

8. Which is the plural for prognosis?
   a. prognosex
   b. prognosises
   c. prognoses
   d. prognosisies

9. Which is the plural for maxilla?
   a. maxillas
   b. maxillamata
   c. maxillae
   d. maxillaces

10. For what is the following sentence an example?
    The dental auxiliary was requested to take the patient's axillary. The patient told the dentist about their heart palpitations during the palpation examination.
    a. acronym
    b. eponym
    c. homonym
    d. compound

Critical Thinking

1. Why does the assistant need to know terminology when talking to the patient?

2. How will lack of knowledge of dental terminology affect the assistant's ability to communicate?

3. Place a slash (/) between the word parts for the following terms. Which term has a combining vowel?
   a. periodontal   c. alveolectomy
   b. gingivitis   d. supramaxillary

4. Why is it important to say a word correctly?

5. Referring to the sentence below, what is the acronym and what is the eponym?
   A patient was diagnosed with Vincent's disease, which is also referred to as ANUG.

Key Terms

Term and Pronunciation	Meaning of Root and Word Parts	Definition
acronym (**ak**-ruh-nim)	**acro-** = denoting something -**nym** = name, word	a word formed by combining the beginning letters of a name or phrase
affix (uh-**fiks**)	**af-** = to add, addition **fix-** = fasten, secure	a letter or a group of letters added to a word to change its meaning
combining vowel (kuhm-**bahyn-ing**) (**vou**-uhl)	**combine** = to unite for a common purpose -**ing** = to unite for a common purpose **vowel** = vocal letter (a, e, I, o, and y)	a vowel connects roots to suffixes and roots to other roots
dentistry (**den**-tuh-stree)	**dent** = relating to the teeth -**ist** = person who practices -**ry** = indicating place of business	the branch of medical science concerned with diagnosis and treatment of diseases/disorders of the teeth and gums
eponym (**ep**-uh-nim)	**epi-** = after **nym** = name, word	the person for whom something (such as a disease) is to be named
homonym (**hom**-uh-nim)	**homo-** = same **nym** = name, word	a word the same as another in sound and spelling but different in meaning
phonetic (fuh-**net**-ik)	**phon** = sound, voice -**tic** = pertaining to	pertaining to speech sounds in pronouncing words
prefix (**pree**-fiks)	**pre-** = before, in front of **fix-** = fasten, secure	a letter or a group of letters added to the front of a word to change its meaning
pronunciation (pruh-nuhn-see-**ey**-shuhn)	**pronounce** = to speak in correct way -**ate** = product of a process -**ion** =action state	the act of producing sounds of speech using an accepted standard of sound and stress patterns of a syllable or word
root word (root) (wurd)	**root** = essential, fundamental **word** = a unit of language; functions as carrier of meaning	the form of a word after all affixes are removed, main body or stem of the word; foundation for word building
suffix (**suhf**-iks)	**suf-** = secondary part of **fix-** = fasten, secure	a letter or a group of letters added to the end of a word to change its meaning
syllable (**sil**-uh-buhl)	**syl-** = together, with **lab** = shorten -**le** = denoting repeated or continuous action	a basic unit of speech generally containing only one vowel sound
terminology (tur-muh-**nol**-uh-jee)	**term** = a word designating something in a particular field -**ology** = to study, branch of knowledge	the body of specialized word relating to a particular subject, field, science, art

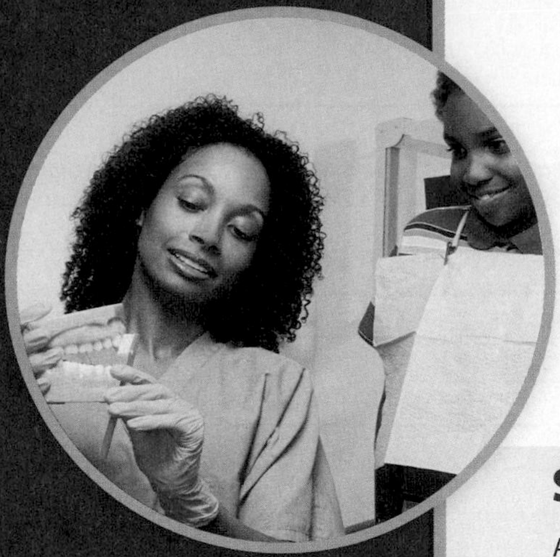

CHAPTER 1

Introduction to the Dental Profession

SECTION I
Dentistry as a Profession

Specific Instructional Objectives

At the completion of this chapter, you will be able to meet these objectives:

1. Use terms presented in this chapter.
2. Identify the major milestones in dental history from ancient times to present day.
3. Name the individuals who had a great impact on the profession of dentistry.
4. Identify the people who promoted education and organized dentistry.
5. State the nine specialties of dentistry.
6. Describe career skills of the direct and indirect care dental team members .
7. List the education required for each dental career path.
8. List the professional organizations that represent each dental career path.
9. Explain the importance of being cross-trained.
10. Discuss the advances in dentistry.
11. Identify career opportunities for a dental assistant.

Introduction

Humans have been plagued with dental problems from the very beginning of time. It is important to be familiar with the historic struggles that took place and contributions that were made to advance the dentistry profession into what it is today.

History of Dentistry

Beginning in ancient times, dental work was done by physicians. Often, each physician specialized in only one area of care for one part of the body. In fact, during the fifth century BC, a Greek historian named Herodotus wrote, "all the country is full of physicians, some of the eyes, some of the teeth, some of what pertains to the belly, and some of the hidden diseases." The earliest recognized figure in dentistry is Hesi-Re. Hesi-Re practiced in 3000 BC. Excavations of the Egyptian pyramids have shown that the Egyptians paid great attention to teeth cleaning, relieving toothaches, and restoring teeth. Also discovered in the burial remains of Egyptian mummies of that time were teeth filled with gold **restorations**. Table 1-1 provides a history of major developments in dentistry.

During these early times, dentistry primarily consisted of removing teeth when pain occurred. Some evidence has been found on human skulls that holes were drilled near the roots to allow infection to drain so that pressure in an abscessed tooth could be relieved. Other dental problems that date from ancient times derived from food preparation techniques. Grains were ground in stone bowls with stone pestles. During this process, particles of stone mixed with the

TABLE 1-1 Timeline of Dental History

Era	Events
Beginning of time	Tooth decay is noted.
3000 BC	First dentist, Hesi-Re, is recorded.
460–322 BC	Written information about tooth decay is recorded by Aristotle and Hippocrates.
460–377 BC	Oath of Hippocrates.
384–322 BC	Attention to oral hygiene (Diocles of Carystus).
1300–1368	Hygienic rules (Guy de Chauliac).
1452–1519	Tooth morphology identified (Leonardo da Vinci).
1678–1761	Founder of modern dentistry (Pierre Fauchard).
1760–1819	Josiah Flagg develops the dental chair.
1768–1770	Paul Revere places advertisements in a Boston newspaper offering his services as a dentist.
1790	James B. Morrison constructs the first known dental foot engine, which he adapted from his mother's spinning-wheel foot treadle.
1832	James Snell invents the first reclining dental chair.
1840	Horace Hayden and Chapin Harris establish the Baltimore College of Dental Surgery.
1840	American Society of Dental Surgeons established.
1841	Alabama enacts the first dental practice act to regulate dentistry.
1844	Horace Wells, a Connecticut dentist, discovers that nitrous oxide can be used for dental pain relief.
1859	American Dental Association (ADA) created.
1866	Lucy Beaman Hobbs Taylor, the first woman to earn a dental degree, graduates from Ohio College of Dental Surgery.
1869	Dr. Robert Tanner Freeman, the first African American to earn a dental degree, graduates from Harvard University Dental School.
1871	First commercially manufactured foot-treadle dental engine is patented by James B. Morrison.
1885	First "lady in attendance" employed by Dr. C. Edmund Kells.
1890	Dr. Ida Gray, the first African American woman to earn a dental degree, graduates from University of Michigan School of Dentistry.
1895	X-rays discovered (Wilhelm Conrad Roentgen).
1907	"Lost wax" casting machine is invented by William Taggart.
1913	Fones School of Dental Hygiene established.
1923	American Dental Hygienists' Association (ADHA) created.
1924	American Dental Assistants Association (ADAA) established; first president was Juliette Southard.
1930	First dental specialty board is founded, the American Board of Orthodontics.
1938	First synthetic bristle (nylon) toothbrush appears on the market.
1945	Water fluoridation era begins in the cities of Newburgh, New York, and Grand Rapids, Michigan.
1947	Dental Assisting National Board, Inc. (DANB) is established.
1950	First fluoride toothpastes are marketed.
1960	Four-handed, sit-down dentistry is utilized.
1970	The Occupational Safety and Health Administration is created by the U.S. Congress.
1980	Per-Ingvar Branemark introduced the technique for the osseointegration of implants.
1982	Hepatitis B vaccine becomes available.
1987	First digital radiography system invented by Dr. Francis Mouyen.
1988	DIAGNOdent invented by Kavo for digital detection of dental decay
1990	Tooth-whitening commercial products are marketed.
1992	Occupational Safety and Health Administration's Bloodborne Pathogens Standard becomes effective.
1997	The YAG laser, approved by the Food and Drug Administration, is used to treat tooth decay.
2000	Invisalign braces made available to public.
2006	VELscope fluorescent device to detect oral cancer became commercially available.

grain. This grit in the food caused severe wear of the biting (occlusal) surfaces of the teeth and possible pulp exposure.

Hippocrates (460–377 BC), the father of medicine, attempted to explain health and disease. Hippocrates was a pivotal figure in the history of dentistry. At the time, the theory that magic, demons, and spirits caused illnesses was an accepted notion. Hippocrates did not agree with those theories and started to teach a more educated method of medical care and medicine. Due to his advancements in the medical field, he was given the title "Father of Medicine." Hippocrates was not just interested in medicine, he also had opinions pertaining specifically to dentistry. He felt it was extremely important that teeth be kept in good condition, and he even developed his own toothpaste and mouth rinse to aid in oral health. He wrote about formation, eruption, diseases of teeth, and methods of dental treatment. He designed and invented some extraction instruments to make the removal of teeth easier and safer. Hippocrates felt strongly that physicians have an obligation to their patients to not allow any wrongdoing and adhere to confidentiality when treating all patients. From this belief, the establishment of the Hippocratic Oath was founded. To this day, the Hippocratic Oath is still a basic code of ethics for medical and dental professionals to "do no harm." An Athenian physician and pupil of Aristotle (384–322 BC), Diocles of Carystus, stated that oral hygiene should get proper attention, and he even gave instructions to this end. During the next couple of centuries, more importance was placed on good oral hygiene. A number of cleaning powders were made from crushed bones, oysters, and egg shells. At times, these substances were mixed with honey to make a paste to use in cleaning.

Later Progress of Dentistry

In France, a surgeon named Guy de Chauliac (1300–1368) became one of the fourteenth century's most influential authors on surgery. He also wrote the "Hygienic Rules for Oral Hygiene."

It is now known that the information given by de Chauliac was not entirely accurate. However, because it was based on sound logic, much of it is used today. For example, it is well known that

Hygienic Rules for Oral Hygiene
Written by Guy de Chauliac

1. Avoid food that putrefies readily.
2. Avoid food or drink that is too hot or too cold, and especially avoid swallowing extremely cold food after extremely hot food, and vice versa.
3. Do not bite into things that are too hard.
4. Avoid foods that stick to the teeth, such as figs and confections made with honey.
5. Avoid certain foods known to be bad for the teeth (his example was leeks).
6. Clean the teeth gently with a mixture of honey and burnt salt to which some vinegar has been added.

sticky, sweet foods increase dental decay. During the fifteenth and sixteenth centuries, artists became more interested in human anatomy to enhance the accuracy of their artwork. Leonardo da Vinci (1452–1519) painstakingly dissected the human skull and then drew his discoveries. He was the first to make a distinction between premolars and molars. His writings further define the morphology of teeth.

Pierre Fauchard (1678–1761), a French dentist, organized all known information about dentistry in a manuscript titled "Le Chirurgien Dentiste," relating to a title he used to refer to himself as a surgical dentist. It was clearly written and had step-by-step pictures that depicted easy-to-follow procedures. He rejected the idea that a tooth worm caused decay and noted that "caries" (his term for decay) were a result of a "hormonal imbalance" and was an early advocate of treating diseased gingival tissue. He combined early information and operative methods for replacing or transplanting teeth. He even noticed that he could straighten teeth by using gold braces that were fastened by waxed linen or silk threads and allowed the teeth to follow a pattern of wires. Pierre Fauchard developed a manual drill for use in dentistry that was powered by a catgut twisted around a cylinder. Fauchard believed that once the decay had been removed, something should replace the missing tooth structure. He would use tin or lead as the replacement. If the decay was too deep and the nerve was disturbed, he utilized oil of cloves to calm down the nerve. This technique is still used today. He believed that the use of urine as a mouthwash could maintain good oral hygiene. Fauchard also believed that in the event a tooth became avulsed (knocked out), the tooth should be reimplanted. Pierre Fauchard's findings were so highly admired and beneficial in dentistry that they were used for over a hundred years. Many refer to Pierre Fauchard as the "Founder of Modern Dentistry."

Wilhelm Conrad Roentgen (1845–1923), a German physicist, discovered x-rays in 1895. This discovery allowed dentists to further their knowledge of the diseases and structures of the mouth.

Progress of Dentistry in the United States

One of the first dentists to arrive in the United States from England was Robert Woofendale. Woofendale placed an advertisement in the *New York Mercury* on November 17, 1766, stating that he "performs all operations upon the teeth, sockets, gums, and palate, likewise fixes artificial teeth, so as to escape discernment." Soon after Woofendale arrived, John Baker came and started advertising in the Boston area. He spoke and wrote about fillings and artificial teeth. Baker was well known and was one of the dentists who treated George Washington. John Greenwood (1760–1819) was said to be the first president's favorite dentist (Figure 1-1). Greenwood had very little formal education but was a proficient practitioner in the eighteenth century. He thought children should care for their teeth and offered parents reduced rates for children's dental care. He also thought that tartar came from bad breath and was adamant about the regular removal of it for good oral health.

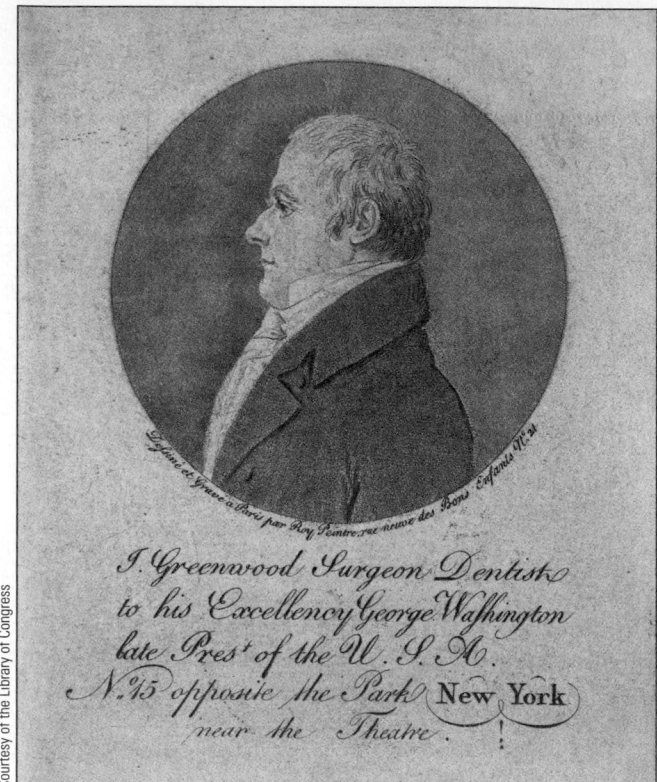

FIGURE 1-1
John Greenwood.

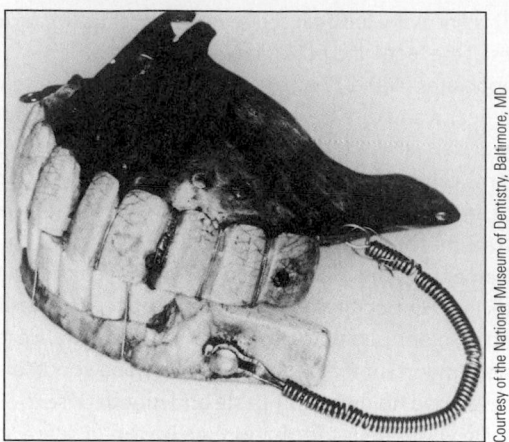

FIGURE 1-2
The last dental prosthesis worn by George Washington was made for him by John Greenwood. It is made of gold and ivory and is held together with springs.

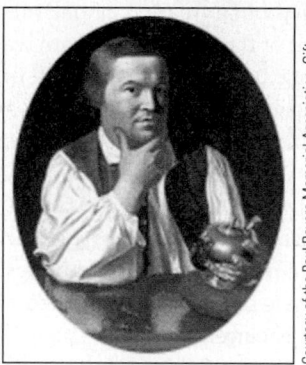

FIGURE 1-3
Paul Revere, shown as a silversmith.

At one time or another, George Washington was probably treated by every notable dentist of the time. A number of references in his diary note continual pain and discomfort from his teeth. At the time the picture that is currently on the one-dollar bill was painted, the president had only one tooth left, a lower-left bicuspid (premolar). In fact, the artist had to pad out the cheeks and lips with cotton to give the president's sunken face a more normal appearance. Washington's last set of **dentures**, made by Greenwood, were composed of ivory and gold and had two springs holding them together (Figure 1-2). A number of dentures were made for the president; however, contrary to popular belief, they were not made of wood.

Paul Revere (1735–1818), a silversmith (Figure 1-3), was a dentist for several years, but his greatest contribution to dentistry was making surgical instruments and artificial teeth. Paul Revere is also the first dentist documented to use **forensics** to identify the remains of a soldier from the Revolutionary War by an artificial tooth he had made for him. He may have had a part in training a notable dentist of the late 1700s, Josiah Flagg. Flagg's father was a partner to Revere. Flagg, a skilled surgeon, was accomplished in corrective procedures on cleft lips, orthodontics, **endodontics**, and operative dentistry. However, one of his major contributions to dentistry was the construction of a dental chair. It had an extension on the arm to hold dental instruments and an adjustable headrest.

In the early 1800s, U.S. dentistry took a giant leap forward. The establishment of a popular democracy—with the opportunity for personal financial gain, free public school education, and population growth—prompted some of the most notable dentists in the world to relocate to America. The literature and knowledge base expanded a great deal during this time. Most large cities now had resident dentists rather than traveling barbers who extracted teeth and sold tooth powders. The dentists of the time were better educated and involved in the communities they served. The profession was progressing far beyond massive tooth removals and occasional cleanings. Additionally, as dental techniques improved and developed, so did dental materials. The first dental engine with a functioning handpiece, motor, and foot treadle was manufactured and patented by James B. Morrison in 1871. This apparatus allowed dentists to restore teeth much more quickly. Organized dentistry was rapidly approaching.

Education and Organized Dentistry

Horace H. Hayden (1769–1844) (Figure 1-4) sought dental care from John Greenwood, the dentist who cared for George Washington. Hayden was inspired and encouraged to take up dentistry as a vocation. He became very active in the dental profession, writing for journals and lecturing on medical and dental topics. Hayden practiced dentistry in Baltimore,

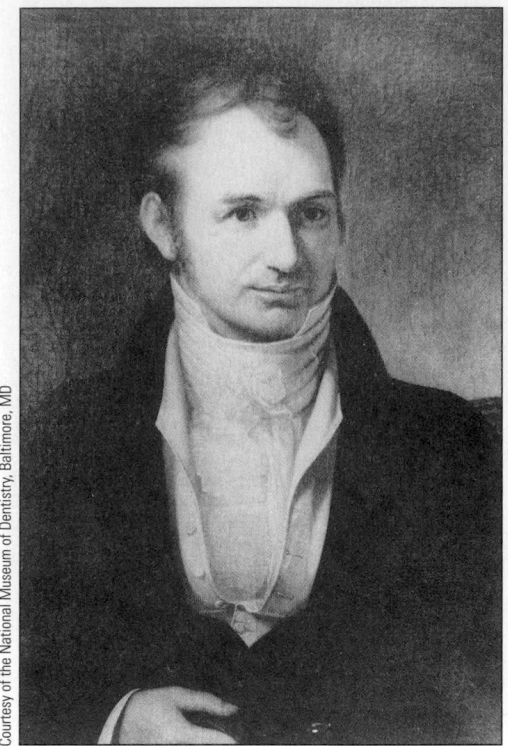

Courtesy of the National Museum of Dentistry, Baltimore, MD

FIGURE 1-4
Horace Hayden, one of the founders of professional dentistry in the United States, helped establish the world's first dental college.

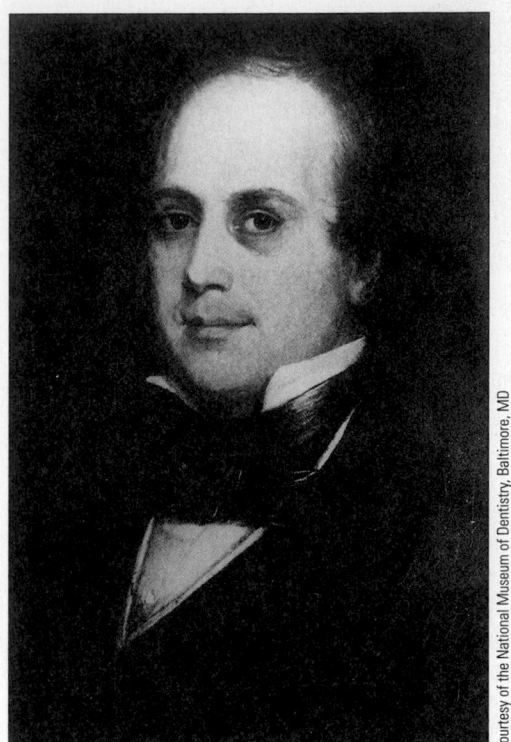

Courtesy of the National Museum of Dentistry, Baltimore, MD

FIGURE 1-5
Chapin Harris, one of the founders of professional dentistry in America, helped establish the first dental college in the world and the first national association representing dentistry.

Maryland, while concurrently attending medical school. He felt it was important that the field of dentistry require more formal education and scientific research and he is regarded as a leader in establishing a formal system of dental education.

One of the students who studied with Hayden was Chapin A. Harris (1806–1860) (Figure 1-5). Harris believed in education and built an extensive library of dental literature, including his own work, *The Dental Art: A Practical Treatise on Dental Surgery*. Due to the efforts of Hayden and Harris, the first dental college in the world, the Baltimore College of Dental Surgery, was founded on March 6, 1840. It is now called the School of Dentistry at the University of Maryland and is the home of the Dr. Samuel Harris National Museum of Dentistry.

Chapin Harris was a main founder and the first president of the American Society of Dental Surgeons in 1840, which was later to become the American Dental Association. He continued to pursue the advancement of dentistry in the United States until he died in 1844. The efforts of Horace Hayden and Chapin Harris took dentistry out of the association with medicine and hands of **preceptorship** to professional independence and one step closer to the modern world. Harris is considered one of the founding members of the profession of dentistry and a pioneer of dental journalism. He was the founder and chief editor of the first dental periodical, the *American Journal of Dental Science*, and published the first dental dictionary in the English language.

Dr. Samuel D. Harris, after whom the museum was named, was instrumental in founding the museum. It is the largest and most complete museum of dental artifacts and history. Visitors can learn about the heritage of dentistry and how to maintain their oral health. They can learn if President George Washington's teeth were really made of wood, engage in interactive exhibits, and partake in educational programs.

Dr. Greene Vardiman Black (1836–1915), known as G.V. Black (Figure 1-6), taught in dental schools such as the University of Iowa and the Northwestern University Dental School in Chicago. As the dean, he increased the library holdings and authored more than 500 articles and several books. He invented numerous machines for testing alloys and instruments to refine cavity preparations. Black later enlarged these instruments for demonstrations to students in the classroom. Many refer to him as the "grand old man of dentistry" or as one of the "founders of modern dentistry in the United States." His goal was to make dentistry independent from medicine. He wrote a number of books and articles, coining the term *extension for* **prevention** in **cavity preparation**. He conducted vast research, especially in the formulation of silver **amalgam**. His contributions are still being used today in his classification of instruments and restorations. His son, Arthur D. Black, followed in his footsteps, becoming dean of the Northwestern University Dental School in Chicago. In 1921, he developed the *Index to Dental Periodical Literature in the English Language*. Not only did this allow researchers to access the literature, but it also provided access to general practicing dentists who wanted to improve their knowledge and skills.

Lucy Beaman Hobbs Taylor, the first woman to graduate from a recognized dental college, earned her dental degree in 1866 (Figure 1-7). She was a teacher who became interested

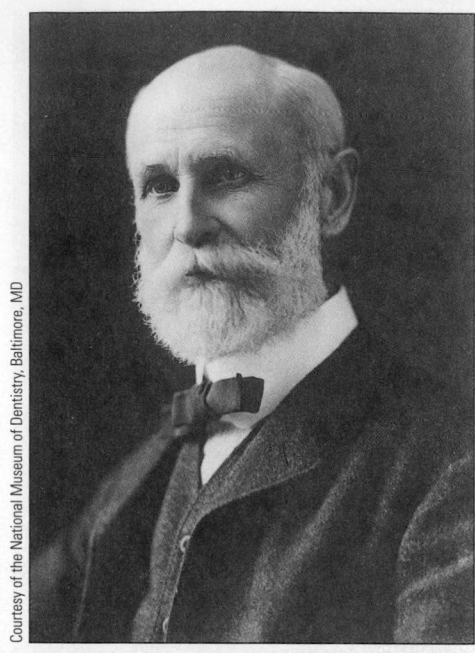

Courtesy of the National Museum of Dentistry, Baltimore, MD

FIGURE 1-6
Dr. Greene Vardiman Black (1836–1915), known as the "grand old man of dentistry" or as one of the "founders of modern dentistry in the United States."

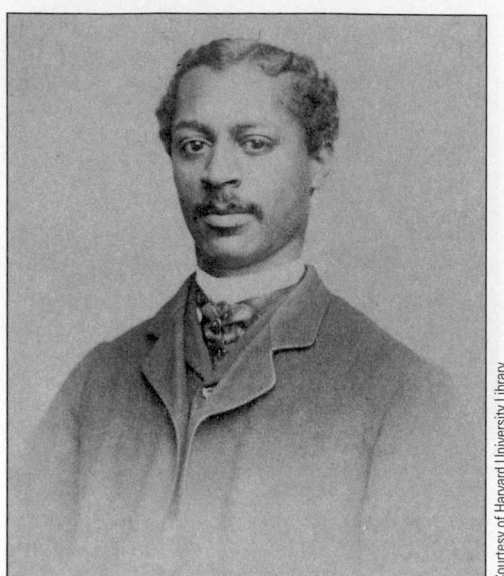

Courtesy of Harvard University Library

FIGURE 1-8
The first African American to earn a DMD, Dr. Robert Tanner Freeman graduated from the Harvard School of Dental Medicine in 1869.

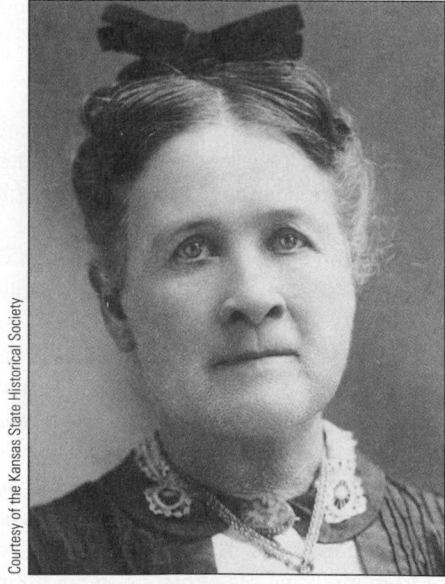

Courtesy of the Kansas State Historical Society

FIGURE 1-7
Lucy Beaman Hobbs Taylor.

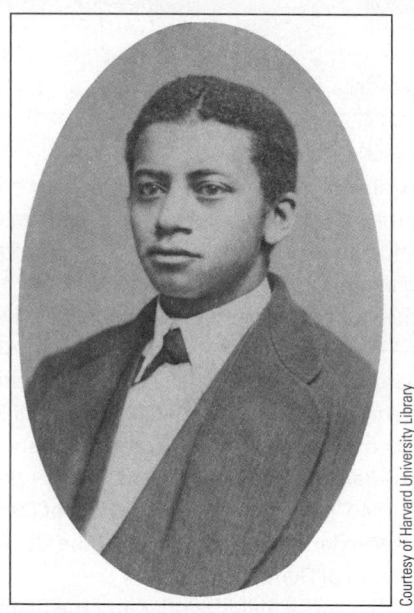

Courtesy of Harvard University Library

FIGURE 1-9
Dr. George Franklin Grant graduated from the second class of Harvard School of Dental Medicine.

in medicine and then pursued further education. She met with resistance, but after the Iowa State Dental Society amended its constitution and bylaws, she was admitted into the dental college.

Dr. Robert Tanner Freeman (Figure 1-8), the first African American to earn a dental degree, graduated from Harvard University Dental School in 1869. Eleven years later in 1890, Ida Gray became the first African American woman to earn a dental degree upon graduation from the University of Michigan School of Dentistry. George Franklin Grant (Figure 1-9), an African American,

graduated from the second class in dentistry in 1870 at Harvard University. He is credited as an authority on the cleft palate.

American Dental Association

At a time when dentistry education and literature were developing, it was thought that organizing dentists would promote sharing of information concerned with excellence in dentistry. Horace Hayden and Chapin Harris collaborated on endeavors such as forming the first nationwide association of dentists.

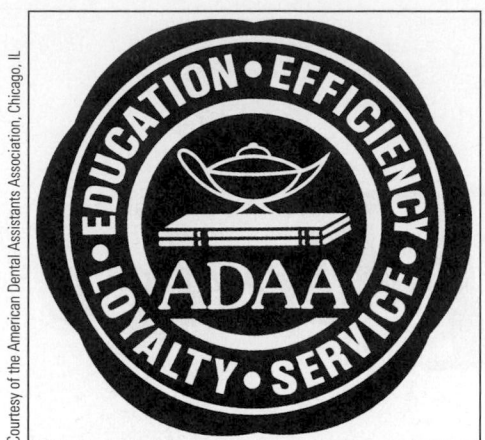

FIGURE 1-10
Logo for the American Dental Assistants Association.

Courtesy of the American Dental Assistants Association, Chicago, IL

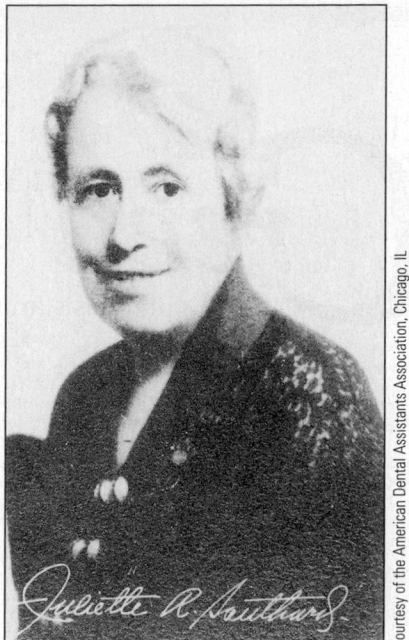

FIGURE 1-11
Juliette Southard, founder and first president of the American Dental Assistants Association.

Courtesy of the American Dental Assistants Association, Chicago, IL

The American Society of Dental Surgeons was formed in 1840, but was dissolved in 1856. Harris had long believed in the need for an informative dental periodical and was instrumental in its founding in 1839. This journal was called the *American Journal of Dental Science (AJDS)*. Later, in 1859, 25 delegates gathered in Niagara Falls, New York, and organized the American Dental Association (ADA). The association was small at first, but after grouping all local associations according to states and then giving all states representation in the national organization, membership began to increase. Today, each state has its own organization with bylaws approved by the ADA, and each local (regional) organization has ADA-approved bylaws that are sent to each state organization. For example, Texas is represented in the ADA by the Texas State Dental Association, and the Texas State Dental Association comprises individual local dental associations. The official publication of the ADA is the *Journal of the American Dental Association (JADA)*. The ADA also has a website, https://www.ada.org/en, which provides a link to the ADA for dental professionals and dental consumers.

Some offices/clinics are hiring a dental assistant called a **sterilization assistant** to do all the disinfecting/sterilizing of treatment rooms and instruments. This individual is responsible for monitoring all sterilizers, water lines, ultrasonic units, cold chemical solutions, and biohazard materials. They stay informed regarding updates on chemicals and the personal protective equipment required when using them.

American Dental Assistants Association The early 1900s became the groundbreaking period of the American dental assistants. The American Dental Assistants Association (ADAA) was founded in 1924 by Juliette Southard, its first president (Figure 1-10 and Figure 1-11). It was founded on four principles: education, efficiency, service, and loyalty. Membership offers a voice in national affairs regarding the career of dental assisting, opportunities in continuing education, professional liability insurance, and interaction with other professionals in the field. ADAA members can remain current in their knowledge through the ADAA publication *The Dental Assistant, Journal of the*

American Dental Assistants Association, or by accessing the ADAA website (http://www.adaausa.org/).

When pursuing a career in dental assisting, it is beneficial to use the "Creed for Dental Assistants" (Figure 1-12) and the "Dental Assistants Pledge" (Figure 1-13) as guidelines for professional behavior.

Advances in Equipment and Pharmaceuticals

During the nineteenth and twentieth centuries, many advances were made in science and technology, some of which were accelerated in the 1930s to help win the Second World War. New ideas, materials, and concepts resulted in the development of new dental techniques, medicines, instruments, equipment, and procedures. By the early 1960s, the practice of dentistry was in transition.

High-Speed Handpiece

Many types of drills, such as the bow drill, were developed over the years, even as far back as during the Mayan civilization. Hand drills with long handles spun by hand were attempted, but they were very cumbersome and inefficient. John Greenwood even attempted to construct a dental engine in the 1790s. The first foot treadle dental engine was developed by James Morrison. He received a patent for the machine in 1871. By the late 1800s, electricity was developed and the electric drill was invented. By 1915, the foot treadle drill was being surpassed by an early version of the electric drill.

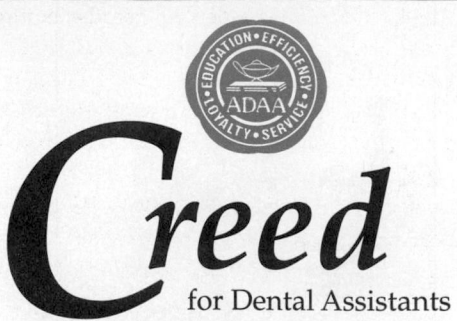

Creed
for Dental Assistants

"To be loyal to my employer, my calling, and myself.

To develop initiative–having the courage to assume responsibility and the imagination to create ideas and develop them.

To be prepared to visualize, take advantage of, and fulfill the opportunities of my calling.

To be a co-worker–creating a spirit of co-operation and friendliness rather than one of fault-finding and criticism.

To be enthusiastic–for therein lies the easiest way to accomplishment.

To be generous, not alone of my name but of my praise and my time.

To be tolerant with my associates, for at times I too make mistakes.

To be friendly, realizing that friendship bestows and receives happiness.

To be respectful of the other person's viewpoint and condition.

To be systematic, believing that system makes for efficiency.

To know the value of time for both my employer and myself.

To safeguard my health, for good health is necessary for the achievement of a successful career.

To be tactful–always doing the right thing at the right time.

To be courteous–for this is the badge of good breeding.

To walk on the sunny side of the street, seeing the beautiful things in life rather than fearing the shadows.

To keep smiling always."

– Juliette A. Southard

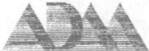

American Dental Assistants Association

FIGURE 1-12
The "Creed for Dental Assistants" by Juliette A. Southard.

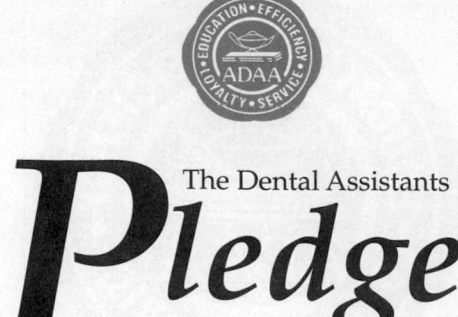

Pledge
The Dental Assistants

"I solemnly pledge that,
in the practice of my profession, I will always be loyal
to the welfare of the patients who come under my care,
and to the interest of the practitioner whom I serve.

I will be just and generous to the members of my profession,
aiding them and lending them encouragement to be loyal,
to be just, to be studious.

I hereby pledge to devote my best energies to the service
of humanity in that relationship of Life to which I consecrated
myself when I elected to become a Dental Assistant."

- Dr. C.N. Johnson

Printed and Distributed through the American Dental Assistants Association

FIGURE 1-13
"The Dental Assistants Pledge" by Dr. C. N. Johnson.

early 1960s, new delivery systems and cabinetry were designed to accommodate sit-down dentistry. Dentists began four-handed dentistry, but it was several years before this became standard.

Infection Control and Prevention

Can you imagine not washing your hands before performing surgery? Up until the 1850s, physicians and dentists did not wash their hands prior to surgery. In the late 1840s, the need for health care workers to participate in routine handwashing to prevent the spread of infectious disease was finally explored. Dr. Ignaz Semmelweis, a Vienna physician, recognized that maternity patients were dying at an alarming rate from hospital deliveries. He researched and demonstrated that routine handwashing could prevent the spread of disease. Dr. Semmelweis later discovered that disinfecting hands could further decrease the spread of disease for maternity patients. In 1847, he had all medical students wash their hands with chlorinated lime before assisting in deliveries. Oliver Wendell Holmes Sr. made similar discoveries in early 1837. He wrote about the moral obligation of physicians to purify their instruments to prevent the spread of contagious diseases, a practice his peers ridiculed.

A number of other prototypes were developed, but none compared to the Airotor **handpiece** developed by John Borden in 1957. The Airotor high-speed handpiece had rotational speeds up to 200,000 rpm (rotations per minute) and operated by air compression. This allowed the dentist to provide a more detailed, accurate preparation of a tooth for a restoration. This method was much safer and quicker. Newer versions of the high-speed handpiece now surpass speeds over 300,000 rpm.

Sit-Down Dentistry

Originally dentists worked standing up with the patient in an upright position. This was difficult and uncomfortable for the dentist and the assistant. With the use of the high-speed handpieces and their attachments, dentists began sitting down on stools and placing the patient into a reclined position. In the

Infection control and prevention were introduced to health care in England by Florence Nightingale (1820–1910), an English nurse. Although she did not have a scientific understanding of disease transmission, her research into hospital sanitary problems during the Crimean War (1853–1856) made her a believer in the need for pure air, pure water, and cleanliness. She was born into a rich upper-class, well-connected family with a lot of influence. With this influence, she was able to formalize standard cleanliness and sanitation in hospitals and the military.

There were no standards for infection control in health care until 1867 when Joseph Lister advocated disinfection with chemicals. He reasoned that Louis Pasteur's "germ theory" introduced in 1861 may also infect wounds, so he introduced disinfection in the operating rooms and gloves to prevent dermatitis from the disinfecting solutions. Up until then it was common practice that most dental instruments only had to be as clean as knives and forks. Dentists sterilized their needles and surgical instruments in boiling water. The primary means of disinfection by chemicals continued into the 1950s. The early 1960s was a new era of sterility as the use of sterilizers increased and cold disinfectants became commonplace. Infection control was not upgraded for more than a decade when the CDC began infection control training in the 1970s. The mission of the CDC expanded in the 1970s from a center of **epidemiology** to include the application of principles to prevent and control the spread of infection. The name was changed from Communicable Disease Center to Centers for Disease Control. In 1987, universal precautions were developed by the CDC to prevent the transmission of bloodborne infectious disease. The CDC published guidelines that included the use of protective barriers such as gloves, protective clothing, eyewear, and masks.

Up until the early 1980s, dentists did not routinely wear gloves while working in the patient's mouth despite the direct contact with blood. In 1988, the CDC recommended specific infection control practices for dentistry. Congress directed the Occupational Safety and Health Administration (OSHA) to finalize the **Bloodborne Pathogens Standard** by 1991 to protect the nation's health care workers from exposure to infectious pathogens. The standard included an exposure control plan and the use of personal protective equipment (PPE). Dental health care workers now wash their hands between patients and the use of gloves, eyes protection, protective clothing, and surgical masks has become the standard.

Nitrous Oxide

Pain during dental procedures deterred many patients from receiving any type of dental treatment. Dentists were searching for something to relieve that pain and make the patients less anxious. In 1844, Horace Wells, a dentist, heard a lecture on the effects of nitrous oxide. He learned that a patient under the influence of nitrous oxide did not remember being injured or the pain involved with the injury. Wells had the revelation that nitrous oxide could be used effectively for dental treatment. In order to research the use of nitrous oxide, Wells allowed his preceptor dentist to remove one of his teeth. Wells felt no pain from the procedure. With this discovery, the use of nitrous oxide was inducted into dental treatment. Nitrous oxide is still commonly used today to reduce patient anxiety associated with dental care.

Local Anesthesia

Nitrous oxide was a major advancement in making patients more comfortable during dental treatment, but some type of localized medicine was still being sought. In 1884, the **analgesic** property of cocaine was discovered by Carl Koller, an ophthalmic surgeon. Cocaine is highly addictive and ultimately was not the best product to use. In 1904, the synthetic analgesic *procaine* (Novocaine®) was developed in Germany. By 1950, an even safer version of analgesic, *lidocaine* (Xylocaine®), was introduced. Lidocaine was much safer than Novocaine and became the analgesic of choice for dentists. Lidocaine is currently the most commonly used local anesthetic.

Advances in Imaging

Although not a dentist, Wilhelm Conrad Roentgen was another great contributor to the dental field (Figure 1-14). Trained in the field of mechanical engineering, Roentgen later became a faculty member teaching physics. In 1895, he performed an experiment by passing an electrical current through gas in a tube. Roentgen discovered that by working in darkness and not allowing light in the tube, the rays coming out the other end would leave an image on paper plating. He placed a photographic plate with his wife's hand on the area and found that the rays permeated her soft tissues, leaving an outline of her skeletal bones and ring on the plate. The name of *x-ray* was given because the makeup of these rays was unknown.

Dr. C. Edmund Kells has been given credit for utilizing x-rays in the dental field after reading Roentgen's works. Kells developed a film and holder to fit in the patient's mouth. Even though the process of taking an intraoral dental film took 15 minutes and was tedious, the use of dental x-rays was born in 1895. Dental x-rays allowed the dentist to view inside the hard tissues of the mouth on a **radiograph**. This allowed dentists to see areas of decay and bone loss that was not visible before. The amount of radiation, speed of the dental film, and technique for traditional x-rays have evolved and improved and

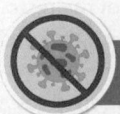

Infection Control

At a minimum the CDC recommended that, "gloves must be used where there is reasonable anticipation of employee hand contact with blood or other potentially infectious materials (OPIM), or non-intact skin (MMWR, 1988; 37:379). OSHA used the research of the CDC in developing it Bloodborne Pathogen Standard.

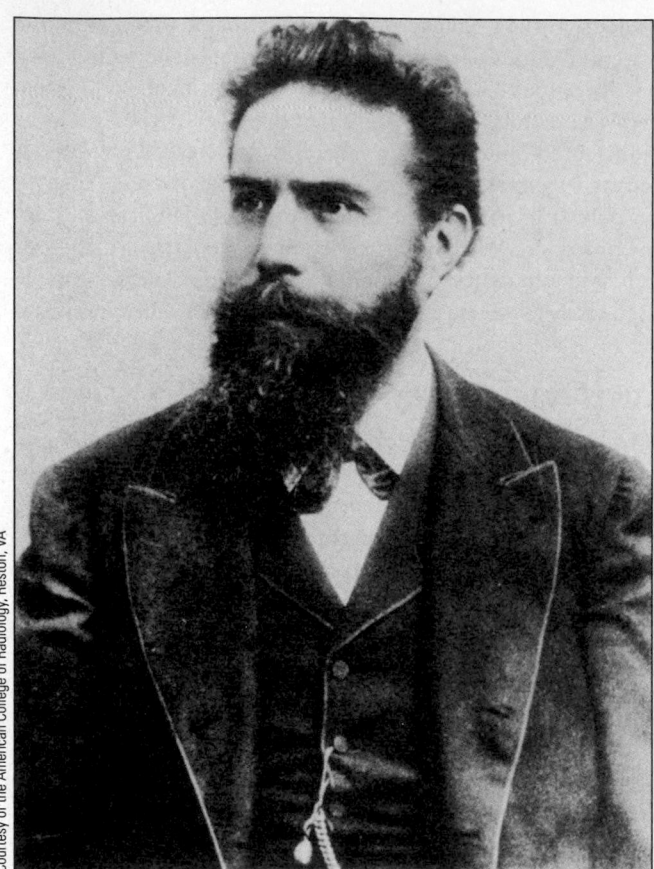

Courtesy of the American College of Radiology, Reston, VA

FIGURE 1-14
Wilhelm Conrad Roentgen.

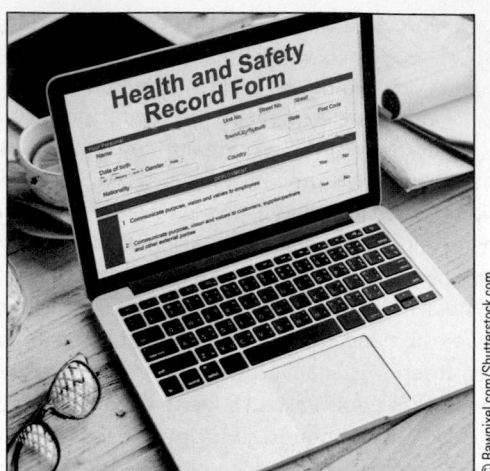

© Rawpixel.com/Shutterstock.com

FIGURE 1-15
Digital imaging system.

x-rays are currently still used today. In the late 1980s, digital radiography was introduced to dentistry. The use of digital radiographs did not take off quickly as it relies on computer systems and software to manage and view the x-rays. Eventually, computer use increased in dental offices, and an increase was seen in digital radiography. Sensors small enough to fit in the patient's mouth are connected to the computer. Once the radiation is exposed, the image is sent to the computer and viewed on the computer monitor. Advantages to using digital **radiology** surpassed the use of traditional x-rays: The dose of radiation is greatly decreased; the size of the x-ray can be manipulated to view it larger and more clearly; and storage of the films is much easier in a digital format. The cost of digital x-rays is becoming lower as improvements in technology are increasing. Hence, the use of digital x-rays in dentistry is also increasing (Figure 1-15).

Advances in Techniques

In the twentieth and twenty-first centuries, there have been many advances in techniques that allow for enhanced restorative and esthetic procedures. In 1980, Branemark introduced the technique for the osseointegration of implants, and in 1989 the first commercial home tooth whitening kit became

available. In 1990, new and improved tooth-colored restorative materials became available. These new materials as well as greater use of dental whitening kits and veneers led to an era of esthetic dentistry. In 1997, the Food and Drug Administration (FDA) approved the YAG laser for use in treating decay in dentin.

Dental Specialties

During the first half of the 1900s, a dentist performed most of the duties. It was realized that one person could not know everything or do all procedures. In the early 1960s, the age of dental specialty began to take hold. With the advent of specialists and general dentists furthering their education, the quality of dentistry being practiced in America continued to increase. General dentists began referring their patients to specialists.

Advances in Restorative Options

Although the use of **silver amalgam** dates back to the time of the Chinese Tang Dynasty in 659, Dr. G.V. Black perfected the use of silver amalgam in 1895. Amalgam has remained very similar for over a hundred years and is still used today. The use of gold as a restoration was used and is much more expensive than amalgam. If a patient needed a front tooth repaired, the options to restore that tooth were limited and not very esthetic. The need for a tooth-colored restoration was necessary. **Silicate cement** was first used in 1908 as a type of esthetic restorative material for anterior teeth. Solubility of the material in the oral cavity was high, resulting in the life span of the restoration to be very short. **Methyl methacrylate resin**, introduced in 1947, was not soluble in the mouth. Instead there was too much shrinkage of the restoration, which caused the margins to leak. Neither product proved to be a good **esthetic** option.

The system of **etching** a tooth prior to the application of resin for a greater mechanical retention was discovered in 1955. By 1962, self-cure **composite resins** were introduced to dentists. Because their properties were so much more advanced, the use of the cements and resins diminished. In 1973, **ultraviolet light curing** was introduced. The ability to cure a composite resin on demand versus waiting for it to cure on its own changed how esthetic dentistry was performed. Dentists now had the ability to place restorations in layers, curing from the inside out. In 1977, microfilled resins were introduced. Microfilled resins, when utilized with an acid-etch system, polished more esthetically and resisted stains.

Roles and Duties of the Dental Team Members

Many people working together make up the dental health team: dentists, dental assistants, dental hygienists, and dental lab technicians, as well as other members of the dental team (Figure 1-16). Each member of the team has specific skills, roles, and responsibilities. This team approach to dentistry improves efficiency and the overall patient experience. Dental team members often attend continued education together. All members of the dental team need to keep current on the knowledge and skills required for dentistry. Each member of the team must commit to being a lifelong learner within the ever-changing field of dentistry.

It has been said that dentistry is part art and part science, however, modern dentistry is both of these and part business. As a dental assistant, the more skilled you become in these three areas of dentistry, the more valuable your services will be. This is referred to as **cross-training**. The career path you choose will be guided by your strengths, and areas of interest may direct your career path. Are you artistic? If so, eventually you may be able to fabricate a temporary crown that is as beautiful and lifelike as those created by the dentist you assist. Are you interested in science? You may develop expertise in teaching patients who don't understand the science and importance of oral health care. Do you have a good business sense? You may become an office manager working your magic with

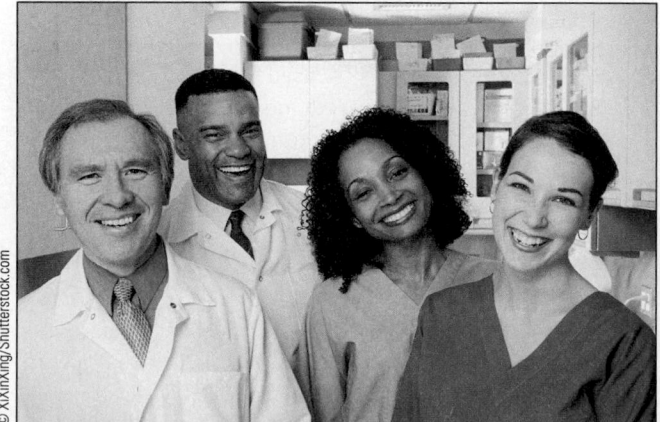

FIGURE 1-16
Dental team.

billing and coding. These career specialties describe both direct and indirect patient care. We will first discuss direct care, and then we will explore indirect care.

Direct Care Dental Team

Direct patient care is hands-on, working with the patient sitting in the dental chair. In other words, direct care requires the patient to be present.

Dentist (DDS or DMD)

The dentist is the leader of the dental team. The dentist is the only dental team member who can **diagnose** oral disease. As a rule, the dentist is also the only dental team member who can perform **irreversible** or permanent procedures. A dentist must provide legal supervision over the rest of the dental team. He or she is ultimately responsible under the law for everything that happens to patients during their treatment—even procedures performed by other members of the dental team.

After completing an undergraduate degree (three to four years), which includes dental prerequisite coursework, the aspiring dentist applies for acceptance at an accredited dental school. This requires a minimum of an additional four years of study (five years at Harvard) in a dental program accredited by the Commission on Dental Accreditation (CODA). The dentist must also pass both the national written and state-recognized clinical skill examinations to earn a Doctor of Dental Medicine (DMD) or Doctor of Dental Surgery (DDS) degree. These degrees are equivalent and both allow the holder to practice the full scope of general dentistry as permitted under each state's license. With a DMD or DDS degree, the dentist can continue in graduate studies for two to four years to become a dental specialist.

General dentists may encounter cases for which treatment is required that goes beyond the scope of their training. The general dentist would refer these cases to a dental specialist. There are nine dental specialties recognized by the ADA. Refer to Table 1-2 for a list describing the dental specialties. Specialist training includes two or more additional years of postgraduate

TABLE 1-2 The Nine Dental Specialties Recognized by the American Dental Association (ADA)

A general dentist can further specialize in:
Public Health
Periodontics
Endodontics
Prosthodontics
Orthodontics
Pediatric Dentistry
Oral and Maxillofacial Radiology
Oral and Maxillofacial Pathology
Oral and Maxillofacial Surgery

Source: Table created by Melissa Damatta

education in an approved, specialized training area. The specialist works with the general dentist to provide the optimum oral health and patient care. During and once the specialty treatment is completed, the patient continues regular visits with the general dentist.

Another area that requires additional training but is not regarded as a specialty of dentistry is **forensic** dentistry. This is a relatively new area that deals with a wide range of services, such as the identification of bite marks on the body and/or the identification of an individual through tooth restorations and morphology using dental records.

Dental Hygienist (RDH or LDH)

Early in the 1900s in Bridgeport, Connecticut, several dentists, along with a leader named Dr. Alfred Civilon Fones, stated that the dentists would not be able to both be surgeons and give preventive treatments. It was suggested that women be trained to clean teeth because "they have smaller and gentler hands." At that time, it was uncommon for women to work outside the home. A dental assistant, Irene Newman, was the first to be trained by Dr. Fones in dental hygiene. Dr. Fones established a school in 1913, and it exists today as the Fones School of Dental Hygiene, University of Bridgeport. The president, Elma Platt, presented the American Dental Association with a resolution to create a national hygienist association and it was accepted. The American Dental Hygiene Association (ADHA) was formed in 1923.

The dental hygienist is not just "the person who cleans your teeth." In the offices where hygienists are employed, they focus on preventive treatment, which allows the dentist to treat the surgical or restorative needs of the patients. Dental hygienists are trained to evaluate the **periodontal** health of their patients, perform **scaling** and **root planing** to remove **calculus**, and provide clean tooth surfaces below the gingiva. They clean and polish the teeth by performing a **dental prophylaxis** or **prophy** to remove **plaque** also called *biofilm*, calculus, and stains. Dental hygienists also provide oral care education to the patient. A career as a dental hygienist offers a variety of challenges and opportunities. Since each state has its own specific regulations regarding their responsibilities (as you will see with all dental team auxiliaries), the duties performed by hygienists vary from state to state. For example, many state practice acts allow licensed hygienists to apply **dental sealants**; to expose, process, and mount dental radiographs; and to chart conditions in the oral cavity. In some states, the licensed dental hygienist can inject local anesthetics or administer nitrous oxide after completing a course approved by the state's licensing board. These are functions that only a dentist can do in certain states. Depending on the state, the dental hygienist can do everything a dental assistant can do and more.

A dental hygienist must have at least one year of dental hygiene prerequisites prior to being accepted to a CODA-accredited dental hygiene program. As graduates of an accredited two- or four-year dental hygiene program, dental hygienists must pass the national written and state-recognized clinical skill exams before applying to obtain a state license to practice their profession. Dental hygienists use the credential of Registered Dental Hygienist (RDH) or Licensed Dental Hygienist (LDH).

Dental Assistant

Before the early twentieth century, dentists hired men and boys to assist them in their dental practices. Dr. C. Edmund Kells, who practiced in New Orleans, at first used his wife as his office assistant. He later employed Malvina Cueria (1893–1991) as another woman in attendance in his office. She was acknowledged as the first dental assistant in modern dental history. By 1911, it was commonplace for dentists to employ dental assistants.

Dr. Kells hired a female to replace a male assistant in 1885. He wanted this "lady assistant" to be "quick, quiet, gentle, and attentive." A number of dentists were unsure about a female in the dental office, but the public accepted it quickly. This change allowed a woman to go to a dental office without being accompanied by her husband or maiden aunt. Due to the popularity of "ladies in attendance," dentists advertised the fact that they had hired female dental assistants by displaying signs in their windows. Today, the educationally qualified dental assistant normally graduates from an institution accredited by the ADA Commission on Dental Accreditation. Training is approximately one academic year in length, and it includes didactic, laboratory, and clinical content. Each state has a dental practice act that governs which duties dental assistants can perform. This varies from performing intraoral procedures, such as placing a **retraction cord** and **dental dams**, to **extraoral** procedures, such as patient education. The dental assistant functions as a much-needed extra pair of hands and enables dentists to care for many more patients and to produce more dentistry than they could alone. Almost all dental offices employ one or more dental assistants. In the office, the person working directly with the dentist during patient procedures is the dental assistant (Figure 1-17).

In a dental assistant role, you may find yourself circulating around the dental office performing a variety of duties, preparing instrument setups and treatment rooms, or seating and dismissing patients. In a busy dental facility, you may find yourself

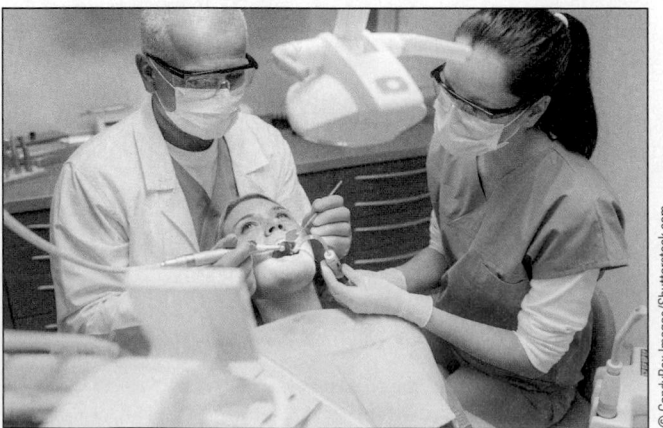

FIGURE 1-17
Expanded function dental assistant with patient.

performing a single task. For example, an entry-level assistant may be primarily responsible for preparing the treatment area and seating the patient.

Unlike other members of the dental team, entry-level dental assistants have no mandatory education requirements and do not have one national credential. However, their activities are limited by the statutes that govern the practice of dentistry in each state. In order to perform dental procedures on patients in most states, the dental assistant needs further training and credentialing.

Dental Assisting Career Opportunities

Dental assisting is an exciting career with many possibilities. Dental assistants help the dentist perform what is called four-handed dentistry, which is exactly as it sounds: A dentist has only two hands, and with a trained dental assistant sitting on the other side of the patient, two more hands now meet over the patient.

Working under the supervision of a licensed dentist, a dental assistant's responsibilities might include the following:

- Setting up and breaking down the treatment room
- Performing infection control procedures
- Maintaining and organizing tray setups for general and specialty procedures
- Assisting the dentist using four-handed instrumentation
- Preparing and delivering dental materials
- Providing postoperative instructions to patients
- Performing radiographic procedures (exposure, processing traditional films, digital images)
- Performing laboratory procedures such as pouring up diagnostic models and fabricating custom trays, whitening trays, and mouth guards
- Maintaining a quality assurance program

Passing instruments, mixing and handing materials, and keeping the mouth dry for visibility are just some of the duties that require the two important hands of a trained dental assistant. There are more than 300,000 dental assistants working in the United States— making it the largest oral health care profession. Dental assisting is one of the fastest-growing careers. In fact, the U.S. Bureau of Labor Statistics predicts a 7% growth in dental assisting jobs from 2019 to 2029.

Each state has its own requirements for dental assistants, which means there are more than 40 different job titles for dental assistants! Dental assistants who are just entering the field should consider looking into the dental assisting job titles and requirements in their state to figure out what type of education, experience, and credentials they might need to advance in their careers.

Earning DANB Certification

The Dental Assisting National Board, Inc. (DANB) is the national certification board for dental assistants. DANB exams and certifications are recognized or required by 39 states, the District of Columbia, the U.S. Air Force, and the Department of Veterans

Affairs. Although each state has different dental assisting requirements, earning DANB certification can make it easier if you plan to work in another state.

Some of the other benefits of earning DANB certification include personal pride, increased confidence, and a way to stand out in the field when applying for a job. Additionally, dental assistants who hold DANB certification earn nearly $2 more per hour, according to DANB's Salary Survey.

DANB offers five national certifications:

- National Entry Level Dental Assistant (NELDA®)
- Certified Dental Assistant™ (CDA®)
- Certified Orthodontic Assistant (COA®)
- Certified Preventive Functions Dental Assistant (CPFDA®)
- Certified Restorative Functions Dental Assistant (CRFDA®)

DANB's NELDA certification is intended for entry-level dental assistants who have less than two years of work experience or have met certain education requirements. DANB's NELDA certification is made up of three component exams: Radiation Health and Safety (RHS®), Infection Control (ICE®), and Anatomy, Morphology, and Physiology (AMP).

There are no requirements to take DANB's RHS, ICE, and AMP exams. These component exams can be taken together or separately. Dental assistants have three years to pass all three component exams to earn certification. After passing the exams, DANB will send information on the eligibility requirements and how to apply for NELDA certification. Dental assistants who plan on earning DANB certification can look at each component exam as a stepping-stone to earning certification.

DANB's CDA certification is made up of three component exams: RHS, ICE, and General Chairside Assisting (GC). To take DANB's GC exam or earn CDA certification, dental assistants must have at least two years of full-time or four years of part-time work experience, or they must have graduated from a dental assisting program that is accredited by the Commission on Dental Accreditation (CODA).

Dental assistants have five years to pass all three component exams and earn CDA certification. Dental assistants who have already earned NELDA certification do not need to retake the RHS and ICE exams if they are within the five-year window.

DANB's CPFDA certification covers several important preventive functions, including coronal polish, sealants, topical fluoride, and topical anesthetic. DANB's CRFDA certification focuses on restorative duties such as impressions, temporaries, isolation, and more. To learn more about earning DANB certification and meeting eligibility requirements, download an application packet from DANB's website at http://www.danb.org.

Duties of the Expanded Functions Dental Assistant (EFDA)

Dental assistants who are qualified to perform expanded functions go by many different titles, depending on the state. Some states might call this level Expanded Functions Dental Assistant (EFDA), while other states may refer to this type of dental assistant as a Registered Dental Assistant (RDA), Licensed Dental Assistant (LDA), or dental assistant qualified in expanded duties. Additionally, some states might require dental assistants to earn a state-specific permit or certificate to perform certain functions.

Being able to perform expanded functions is a goal for many dental assistants. Because each state is so different, it is best to check with the state dental board about specific job titles and requirements. This information is also available at the search-by-state map on DANB's website; visit http://www.danb.org and click on the "Meet State Requirements" tab to learn more.

Depending on the state in which they practice, Expanded Functions Dental Assistants may perform the following duties after meeting state requirements:

- Perform restorative dentistry procedures
- Place pit and fissure sealants
- Perform coronal polishing procedures
- Apply fluoride or anticaries agents
- Monitor nitrous oxide administration
- Remove sutures
- Place and remove periodontal dressing
- Place retraction cord
- Take primary and/or secondary impressions for dental **prosthesis**
- Perform orthodontic procedures such as replacing elastics, placing brackets and bands, and wire bending

The EFDAs' knowledge and advanced skills make them a dentist's most valuable assistants and the most desirable applicants for dental assistant positions.

Indirect Care Dental Team

If getting your gloves dirty is not your thing, no problem. There are career paths in dentistry that provide indirect care such as business administrator, dental laboratory technician, or even dental sales. More important, cross-trained dental team members (able to perform important tasks from another job) add value to an office. Just imagine how much more valuable you will become when the dentist knows they can count on you to jump right in to cover for another team member when needed!

Dental Business Assistant

This position does not require wearing surgical gloves or sterilizing instruments. The dental business assistant works in the business (front) office of a dental practice. The business assistant is often the first person a patient contacts. You will find the business assistant behind a desk (sometimes behind a sliding-glass window) with the appointment scheduler, the telephone, and a computer as their instruments. Primary duties include scheduling appointments, communicating with patients via phone, email and text messages. as well as handling financial and insurance issues. In a busy office there may be an office manager who may be responsible for overseeing the individuals working at the front desk, such as a business assistant, finance administrator, or receptionist. The office manager may be responsible for additional responsibilities such as accounts payable and receivable, staff evaluations, staff meetings, and other administrative tasks.

While direct care often involves four-handed dentistry (the dentist plus an assistant), the office manager can require the eight arms of an octopus on some days. Whether answering the phone or going through files, they remain the dental concierge, the person who provides the answers and explains the office policies that allow the patient to obtain the direct care they need. This is a career opportunity for a dental assistant who wishes for a change of scenery from the dental operatory and can be a place to shine if you have good business sense. ADA does not recognize separate business office training—it is included in CODA Dental Assisting Programs.

Certified Dental Laboratory Technician (CDT)

Fortunately, we can take dental impressions and pour replica models of a patient's dentition to work on any time of day without the patient there. Indirect care at its finest! Working with accurate models representing the patient's mouth and following detailed lab prescriptions written by a dentist, the dental laboratory technician is the artist who creates **prostheses** such as crowns, **bridges**, and veneers (Figure 1-18). The technician can also fabricate orthodontic appliances such as retainers or partial or full dentures. While they can make transitional (temporary) appliances, most of what they make is built to last. A dental assistant can do many indirect lab procedures, but a lab technician works with strong precious metals such as gold or lifelike materials such as porcelain to create dental masterpieces that look great and feel great. Some dental laboratory technicians are employed by the dentist, while others work in privately owned dental laboratories; they are essential members of the dental team.

In most states, a dental laboratory technician is not required to have formal training and may be trained on the job. Many technicians have graduated from two-year, CODA-accredited dental laboratory technician programs. These programs require extensive knowledge of dental anatomy and dental materials and the development of detailed mechanical skills. Individuals seeking credentials must pass an examination to become certified dental technicians (CDTs). The examination evaluates their technical

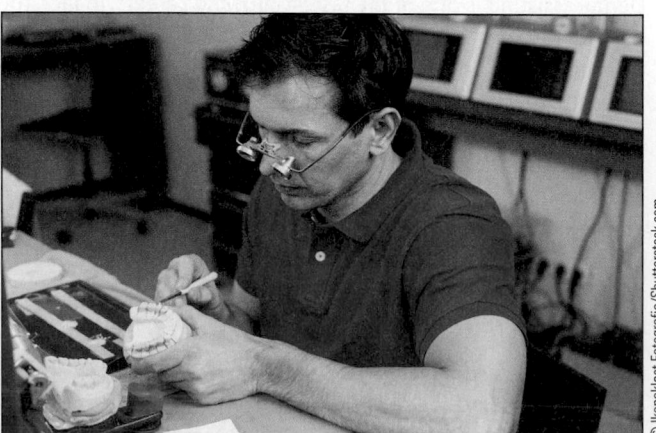

FIGURE 1-18
Dental lab technicians.

skills and knowledge and is administered by the National Board for Certification in Dental Laboratory Technology. Membership in the American Dental Laboratory Technician Association (ADLTA) is also offered to dental technicians.

Dental Products Salesperson

With knowledge gained from one of the positions detailed earlier, or training from a dental supply company or manufacturer, the dental salesperson brings product expertise and potential cost savings to the practice. While not involved directly in patient care, the dental salesperson must be aware of the latest dental products that allow dentists to provide the optimal patient experience.

Dental Educator

Unless you are reading this book for fun, you have already met a dental educator who is using this textbook to help teach you. Your instructor is a professional who has real-world experience. Faculty at CODA-accredited dental assisting programs providing didactic instruction must have earned at least a baccalaureate degree or be currently enrolled in a baccalaureate degree program. Laboratory, preclinical, and clinical faculty must be CDA certified by DANB.

Responsible for training the next generation of dental professionals, the dental educator focuses on two levels. First is ensuring the students have a thorough understanding of the material to successfully pass the course and credentialing examinations. Second, but no less important, is instilling the skills and knowledge that students will need day after day in the "real world" of their careers. Witnessing the professional growth and career advancement of their students is the great reward of being a dental educator. Not all educators have to be in front of students to teach—some create educational content for the Internet and some write books like this!

Other Members of the Dental Team

Additional members of the dental team are dental service technicians, dental representatives, and dental supply companies and representatives. The dental service technicians maintain dental equipment. The dental assistant works with the technicians and identifies equipment problems. The technicians may be required to make service calls, or they will direct the assistant to rectify a problem. Dental representatives demonstrate how to use new materials. Normally, they are trained in the materials they represent. Dental supply companies and representatives also give information on new materials and help the dental assistant order supplies for the dental office. They normally make weekly calls to the dental office. Dental supply companies could be mail order companies through which the assistant can order office supplies.

Chapter Summary

It is important to know the historic struggles that took place and contributions that were made to advance the dentistry profession into what it is today. Organized dentistry was formed with the intent to promote the sharing of information concerned with excellence in dentistry. To provide excellence in dentistry, additional dental team members (such as dental assistants, dental receptionists, dental hygienists, and dental laboratory technicians) would become recognized and add contributing roles to the field. Therefore, the dental assistant will need to be able to identify and define those who contribute to the dental profession and look forward to the future of dentistry.

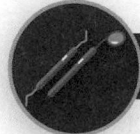

CASE STUDY

Lori Ann Smith was 18 years old in 1880 and was seeking a position in a dental office. The opinion of the dentists was to not allow women access to the profession. Lori's career dreams were denied. Over 100 years later, her great-great-granddaughter, Traci Lynd, was seeking a position in a dental office and found a very different environment. What changes and advancements took place for dental assistants during that time frame to allow Traci to reach her goal?

Case Study Review

1. When were gender barriers eliminated for dental assistants?

2. What career changes for dental assistants took place over four generations?

3. With the current educational advancements in the profession, what credentials are available to dental assistants today?

Review Questions

Multiple Choice

1. The basic code of ethics used by the medical and dental professions originated with
   a. Aristotle.
   b. Leonardo da Vinci.
   c. Pierre Fauchard.
   d. Hippocrates.

2. Who is the teacher and inventor recognized as the "grand old man" of dentistry?
   a. Chapin A. Harris
   b. G.V. Black
   c. John Greenwood
   d. Josiah Flagg

3. Which of the following is not an ADA-recognized dental specialty?
   a. endodontics
   b. oral and maxillofacial surgery
   c. forensic dentistry
   d. pediatric dentistry

4. The first president of the ADAA was
   a. Juliette Southard.
   b. Dr. Lucy Hobbs Taylor.
   c. Dr. C. Edmund Kells.
   d. Dr. Alfred Fones.

5. Whose greatest contribution to early dentistry was the creation of artificial teeth and surgical dental instruments?
   a. George Washington
   b. Robert Woofendale
   c. Paul Revere
   d. John Greenwood

6. What is the first recorded name of a practicing dentist?
   a. Hesi-Re
   b. Paul Revere
   c. Diocles of Carystus
   d. Hippocrates

7. Which dental specialty is concerned with the replacement of missing teeth through artificial means?
   a. periodontics
   b. prosthodontics
   c. pedodontics
   d. endodontics

8. Which dental team member allows the dentist to care for more patients and increase productivity?
   a. dental assistant
   b. dental laboratory technician
   c. dental practice management assistant
   d. dental products salesperson

9. Who was an early advocate for treating diseased gingival tissue?
   a. Aristotle
   b. Pierre Fauchard
   c. Robert Woofendale
   d. Guy de Chauliac

10. Who is believed to be George Washington's favorite dentist?
    a. John Baker
    b. Robert Woofendale
    c. John Greenwood
    d. Paul Revere

Critical Thinking

1. If a patient fell and fractured a front tooth, and it seemed to have pulpal involvement (nerve damage), what specialists could the general dentist refer the patient to?

2. Who would you contact for information about dental assisting organizations?

3. Which dental team members besides the dentist require a license?

4. Why does a dentist prefer an assistant who is cross-trained?

Key Terms

Term and Pronunciation	Meaning of Root and Word Parts	Definition
amalgam (uh-**mal**-guh m)	**amalgam** = soft mass formed by mechanical manipulation; a blend or combination	mixture of metals such as silver and mercury into a soft mass to repair a decayed tooth; used as a filling
analgesic (an-l-**jee**-zik, -sik)	**an-** = without **algia** = to feel pain **-ic** = pertaining to	an agent that relieves or removes pain

Term and Pronunciation	Meaning of Root and Word Parts	Definition
Bloodborne Pathogen Standard (bluhd-bawrn) (**path**-uh-juhn) (**stan**-derd)	**bloodborne** = carried or transmitted by blood **pathogen** = any disease-producing agent; microorganism **standard** = a rule or principle that is used as a basis for judgment	resource and regulations developed to help prevent health care workers from contracting infectious diseases
bridge (brij)	**bridge** = a structure that spans, joins two other structures	replacement of a missing tooth by placing an artificial tooth in its place that is attached to the teeth on either side of the space
calculus (tartar) (**tahr**-ter)	**tartar** = calcified buildup	a hard yellowish deposit on the teeth, consisting of organic secretions and food particles deposited in various salts, such as calcium carbonate; also called *dental calculus*
cavity preparation (**kav**-i-tee) (prep-uh-**rey**-shuhn)	**cavity** = a hollow place, empty space **prepare** = to put in proper condition or readiness **-tion** = expressing an action	a hollow space in a tooth produced to support a dental restoration
composite resin (kuhm-**poz**-it) (**rez**-in)	**composite** = made up of separate parts or elements **resin** = substance obtained from plant secretions; used in medicine in making varnishes and plastics	also referred to as tooth-colored filling; made from mixes of resins and fillers to give the filling strength and translucency for better color match and esthetics
confidentiality (kon-fi-**den**-shuh l-itee)	**confide** = trustful; to impart secrets trustfully **-ality** = indicating state or condition	strict privacy or secrecy; limited to persons authorized to use information
cross-training (kraws-**treyn**-ing)	**cross** = extend from one side to another **training** = to make proficient by instruction and practice for a profession or work	training that covers several tasks within a department or office; proficient at different yet related skills
dental dam (**den**-tl) (dam)	**dental** = pertaining to teeth **dam** = barrier preventing the flow of water	a rubber sheet used to keep saliva from the teeth during dental procedures
dental sealant (**den**-tl) (**see**-luh nt)	**dental** = pertaining to teeth **seal** = to securely cover **-ant** = agent that performs an action	transparent synthetic resin applied to the chewing surfaces of molars and premolars, usually in children as a preventive measure against tooth decay in the occlusal pits and fissures
denture (**den**-cher)	**dent** = tooth **-ure** = indicating act, process, result or instrument	replacement of one or more missing teeth; appliance is removable and sits on the gingival tissue covering the jawbone; laymen's term is dental plate, false teeth
diagnose (**dahy**-uh g-nohs)	**dia-** = through **gnosis** = knowledge	to recognize (as a disease) by signs and symptoms; to diagnose a disease or condition
endodontics (en-doh-**don**-tiks)	**endo-** = within, inside **odont** = tooth **-ics** = denotes body of knowledge	study, diagnosis, and treatment of diseases of the dental pulp; root canal therapy; endodontist
epidemiology (ep-i-dee-mee-**ol**-uh-jee)	**epidemic** = a disease affecting many persons at the same time; spreading from person to person **-ology** = study of	study of the distribution determinants of health-related states or events in specified populations and the application of this study to the control of health problems
esthetic (es-**thet**-ik)	**esthet** = relating to beauty **-ic** = related to	relating to the consideration of beauty
etching (**ech**-ing)	**etch** = to cut with an acid **-ing** = expressing action	used to make microscopic pores for better retention of the restoration by eating away the surface of enamel with acids
extraction (ik-**strak**-shuh n)	**extract** = to pull out **-tion** = indicating state, condition, action	the removal of a tooth from its socket of bone

(Continues)

Term and Pronunciation	Meaning of Root and Word Parts	Definition
extraoral (**ex**-tra-**aw**-ruhl)	**extra** = outside **oral** = involving the mouth	situated or occurring outside the mouth
forensics (f*uh*-**ren**-siks)	**forum** = a court of law, public debate **ensis** = pertaining to **-ics** = naming field of study	relating to or dealing with the application of scientific knowledge to legal problems
gingiva (jin-**jahy**-v*uh*)	**gingiv** = gums **-a** = ending of nouns	part of oral mucous membrane that covers and is attached to necks of the teeth and alveolar process of the jaws
handpiece (hand-**pees**)	**hand** = anatomical part of the upper limb consisting of fingers and thumb **piece** = a part of an object	dental equipment that is used by holding in the hand to remove tooth tissue and dental decay in preparation to replace structure with dental materials
irreversible (ir-i-**vur**-s*uh*-b*uh*l)	**ir-** = not **reversible** = capable to returning to its original shape	not reversible; once something is done, it cannot be changed
methyl methacrylate resin (**meth**-*uh*l) (meth-**ak**-r*uh*-leyt) (**rez**-in)	**methyl** = simplest hydrocarbon derived from methane **methacrylate** = common monomer in plastics **resin** = acrylic resin plastic used chiefly for its transparency	main component of dental tooth-colored restorations and tissue-colored prosthetics
oath (ohth)	**oath** = solemn truth or promise	promise to take care of or treat patient in their best medical interest
oral and maxillo-facial pathology (**ohr**- *uh*l) (mak-**sil**-oh) (**fey**-sh*uh*l) (p*uh*-**thol**-*uh*-jee)	**or-** = mouth **-al** = pertaining to **maxill** = upper jaw bone **facial** = pertaining to the face **path** = disease **-ology** = study of	the study, diagnosis, and sometimes the treatment of oral- and maxillofacial-related diseases; pathologist
oral and maxillo-facial radiology (**ohr**- *uh*l) (mak-**sil**-oh) (**fey**-sh*uh*l) (rey-dee-**ol**-*uh*-jee)	**or-** = mouth **-al** = pertaining to **maxill** = upper jaw bone **facial** = pertaining to the face **rad** = imaging techniques including x-rays, CAT scans, MRIs **-ology** = study of	the study and radiologic interpretation of oral and maxillofacial diseases; radiologist
oral and maxillo-facial surgery (**ohr**- *uh*l) (mak-**sil**-oh) (**fey**-sh*uh*l) (**sur**-j*uh*-ree)	**or-** = mouth **-al** = pertaining to **maxill** = upper jaw bone **facial** = pertaining to the face **surgery** = treating diseases, injuries, or deformities by manual or operative procedures	study, diagnosis, and surgery to correct a wide spectrum of diseases, injuries, and defects in the head, neck, face, jaws, and the hard and soft tissues of the oral and maxillofacial region; surgeon
orthodontics (awr-th*uh*-**don**-tiks)	**ortho-** = correct or right **odont** = tooth **-ics** = denotes body of knowledge	the straightening of teeth and modification of midface and mandibular growth; orthodontist
pediatric dentistry (pee-dee-**a**-trik) (**den**-t*uh*-stree)	**pedo-** = child **-iatric** = healing or medical treatment **dent-** = dentition, teeth **-ist** = a person who practices **-ry** = indicating a practice or occupation	study, diagnosis, and treatment of children and patients with special needs; pediatric dentist (formerly pedodontics)
periodontal (per-ee-*uh*-**don**-tl)	**peri-** = around **odont** = tooth **-al** = pertaining to	pertaining to the area around the tooth

Term and Pronunciation	Meaning of Root and Word Parts	Definition
periodontics (per-ee-*uh*-**don**-tiks)	**peri-** = around, about **odont** = tooth **-ics** = denotes body of knowledge	study and treatment of diseases of the periodontium (non-surgical and surgical) as well as placement and maintenance of dental implants; periodontist
plaque (plak)	**plaque** = soft bacterial buildup	a sticky, usually colorless biofilm on teeth that is formed by and harbors bacteria
preceptorship (pri-**sep**-ter-ship)	**precept** = guide, instruct **-or** = a person or thing that does what is expressed by the verb **ship** = to craft, skill	a practicing health care professional gives personal instruction, training, and supervision to a student
prevention (pri-**ven**-sh*uh* n)	**prevent** = to keep from occurring **-tion** = indicating action	the act of stopping an action prior to its start
prophylaxis (prophy) (proh-f*uh*-**lak**-sis)	**pro-** = in favor of **phylaxis** = watching, guarding	preventing of dental disease by means of cleaning and polishing the teeth by a dentist or dental hygienist
prosthesis (pros-**thee**-sis)	**pros** = to **thesis** = a placing **prostheses** = plural form	an artificial device to replace or augment a missing or impaired part of the body
prosthodontics (pros-th*uh*-**don**-tiks)	**prosth** = replacement of missing structures by artificial devices **odont** = tooth **-ics** = denotes body of knowledge	study and treatment of the replacement of lost oral structures; dentures, bridges and the restoration of implants; prosthodontist; some prosthodontists further their training in oral and maxillofacial prosthodontics, replacement of missing facial structures, such as ears, eyes, noses, etc.; prosthodontist
public health (**puhb**-lik) (helth)	**pub** = community as a whole **-ic** = pertaining to **health** = general condition of the body and mind	the study of dental epidemiology (study of disease affecting large populations) and social health policies; specialist
radiographs (**rey**-dee-oh-grafs, -grahfs)	**radio** = using radiation **graphs** = photographic image	image produced on a sensitive film by the action of x-ray radiation used in dental examination
radiology (rei-dee-**aa**-luh-jee)	**radio** = connected with rays, radiation, or radioactivity **logy** = denoting a subject of study or interest	a branch of medicine concerned with the use of radiant energy (such as x-rays)
restoration (res-t*uh*-**rey**-sh*uh* n)	**restore** = to build up, repair **-tion** = indicating state, condition, action	replacement of missing tooth structure by placing filling material in its place
retraction cord (ree-**trak**-shn)	**retraction** = the action of drawing something back or back in **cord** = thin, flexible string or rope made from several twisted strands	cord primarily used to push the gingival tissue away from the prepared margins of the tooth in order to obtain an accurate impression of the teeth
root planing (smoothing) (root) (pleyn-ing)	**root** = the part of a tooth normally within the socket **plane** = to smooth **-ing** = the action of	scraping away a bacteria-impregnated layer of cementum from the surface of a tooth root while smoothing the root surface to prevent or treat periodontitis
scaling (scraping) (*skey*-ling)	**scale** = to remove scales from **-ing** = the action of	to remove dental biofilm, its products, and calculus (tartar) on the teeth by means of instruments
silicate cement (**sil**-i-kit) (si-**ment**)	**silicate** = constitutes over 90% of rock-forming minerals of earth's crust **cement** = a hardening, adhesive, plastic substance	first tooth-colored filling material; modified over years and used as a utility cement for attaching dental fixed prostheses
silver amalgam (**sil**-ver) (*uh*-**mal**-g*uh*m)	**silver** = a very moldable grayish-white element **amalgam** = a mixture of mercury with other metals	a mixture of mercury, silver, tin, copper, and zinc used for dental fillings

(*Continues*)

Term and Pronunciation	Meaning of Root and Word Parts	Definition
specialty (**speh**-shuhl-tee)	**special** = a specific subject of study, line or work, area of interest; excelling beyond the ordinary **-ty** = denoting quality	a branch of medicine or dentistry in which a doctor specializes; the field or practice of a specialist; nine dental specialties
sterilization assistant (steh-ruh-luh-**zei**-shn) (uh-**si**-stnt)	**sterilize** = to free from living microorganisms **assist** = to help	one who collects, prepares, and organizes surgical tools and environmental protection—such as surgical drapes—for scheduled medical and dental procedures
ultraviolet light curing (uhl-tr*uh*-**vahy**-*uh*-lit) (lahyt) (**kyoor**-ing)	**ultraviolet** = beyond the violet end of the visible spectrum; part of the electromagnetic spectrum with wavelength shorter than light **light** = electromagnetic radiation wavelength perceived by the human eye **curing** = to promote hardening of a material	a photochemical process using high-intensity ultraviolet light to instantly harden/set a material

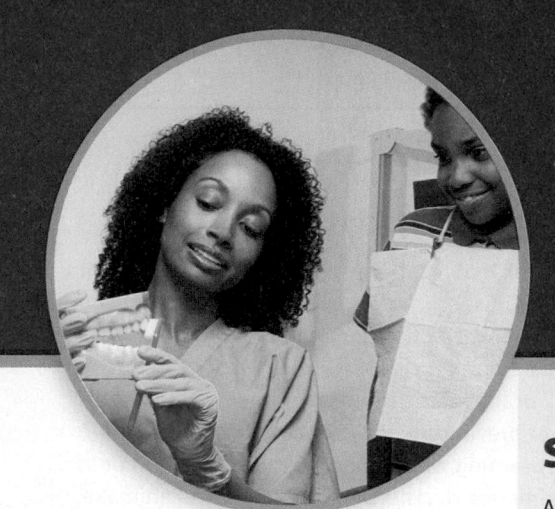

Psychology, Communication, and Multicultural Interaction

Specific Instructional Objectives

At the completion of this chapter, you will be able to meet these objectives:

1. Use terms presented in this chapter.
2. Define psychology.
3. Compare and contrast the learning theories discussed in this chapter.
4. Discuss how Maslow's hierarchy of needs relates to communication in today's dental office.
5. Describe how defense mechanisms can inhibit communication.
6. Describe the components of the communication process.
7. Discuss dental phobias.
8. Define the factors that can affect communication.
9. Discuss how to achieve resolution in conflicts related to office stress.
10. Define cultural competency.
11. Compare and contrast culture, ethnicity, and race.
12. Discuss techniques to communicate with people from different cultures.
13. Identify the advantages and disadvantages of written communication.
14. Discuss ways to create effective written materials.
15. Discuss the steps involved in preparing for a dental presentation.
16. Design visuals that will enhance a presentation.
17. Develop strategies to communicate effectively during a presentation.

Introduction

Communication is the process of sending and receiving messages from one person to another or to a group of people to achieve shared understanding. Forms of communication include writing, speaking, and nonverbal gestures or body language.

Words have power; they have the ability to arouse feelings, move people to action, and even change history. The writing and speeches of good communicators define moments in time; December 7 will always be "a date which will live in infamy" (President Franklin D. Roosevelt). The words "I have a dream" (Martin Luther King Jr.) and "one small step for man" (Neil Armstrong) have touched millions.

What you say and write may not be as inspirational as these figures in history; nonetheless, it is essential that as a dental professional, you are completely understood. Good written and verbal communication skills are one of the top factors for being offered employment. Writing an effective cover letter and resume may be enough to secure employment; however, once employed, you will interact with the dental team, patients, their families, and other health care professionals.

Communication also takes place through body language; regardless of the mode of communication, the message must be transmitted clearly. Communication is beneficial as it helps the dental assistant overcome the patient's defense mechanisms and fears, as well as understand how people from other cultures and generations interact. Employee stress will be encountered in the dental office, and it is important to recognize it and be able to effectively achieve conflict resolution through good communication. To be successful in the dental professions it is essential to use all forms of communication effectively.

Psychology

Every dental team member is responsible for communicating well and treating each patient and coworker respectfully. Employees can do many things to enhance the mental and physical comfort of patients, but they must first have a positive attitude toward patients and their treatment. The dental assistant must understand patients and how to meet patient needs during dental treatment.

The science of the mind and the reasons people think and act as they do is **psychology**. Historically, individuals have associated dental treatment with discomfort. Patients may think and react using past reasoning. Today the dental professional works diligently to make treatment comfortable for the patient. It is critical to listen to a patient's view about their dental experiences in order to better understand their attitude toward dentistry. With this information, the dental assistant can better help patients overcome fears they may have.

A person's **paradigm**, or acquired belief system, may also be a factor in attitudes toward dental care. Individuals have different life experiences that have contributed to their personal belief systems or paradigms. For example, a patient who always used a hard toothbrush and never had any cavities may believe that a toothbrush with hard bristles is better at cleaning their teeth. Through good communication, the dental assistant can make an assessment. If the teeth are indeed clean in all areas, and it does not appear that damage is being done to the tooth or tissue, then the dental assistant can encourage the patient to continue the existing practice. If the hard-bristled brush is damaging the teeth or gums, or failing to clean the entire tooth surface, then the dental assistant will have to begin educating the patient and changing the patient's paradigm. However, it may be difficult for the patient to associate clean teeth with a soft-bristled brush. Good communication skills, such as listening, are essential to understanding the patient's viewpoint and introducing new information that may challenge it. Listen first, and tell the patient what to expect when trying the new toothbrush. For instance, the brush is going to feel different in the mouth. Continue to listen to the patient's concerns, such as feeling the need to brush harder, or that the brush may wear more quickly. Acknowledge and address each of the patient's concerns. Watch the patient's nonverbal behavior and work with the patient to understand necessary changes in behavior. The patient's behavior may not change immediately. Share with the patient that it may take a while before the change feels comfortable, and that this is normal. Motivate the patient to continue the changed behavior.

Psychology in Dentistry

It is a mistake to think that just because we educate the patient about dental health, disease, and prevention, the patient will automatically adapt and practice good dental behaviors. Reality may be quite different, especially if you use a **directive** tone to preach a stock oral hygiene message. Patient education is an essential part of prevention, but it does not always result in behavior change. Learning, accepting, and practicing new ideas over a period of time are decisions only the patient can make. Clear communication, mutual respect, a tailored message, and a partnership in the patient's oral health will enable the dental assistant to provide effective counseling. Understanding and applying health behavior theories developed in psychology can provide insight into a patient's motivation level as well as their readiness to change.

Health Behavior Theories

There have been many theories developed through research in sociology, education, and psychology that attempt to explain behavior; several can be used with oral health education. It is always more effective to offer information to those who are ready to hear the message and change their behavior accordingly. Some behavior theories provide a model to help you assess a patient's readiness to change.

Choose a theory or theories that will work for your patient. However, keep in mind that there is no one way to use a theory and that more than one theory can be used at the same time for better insight into a problem. Apply the concepts of the theories you have chosen and use **evidence-based** facts to match your education efforts to your patient's needs. One tool that may lead to success is to apply theories that have been effective in similar prior circumstances. Dental assistants must use various tools available to them, in combination with their knowledge and skill, to work with the patient to develop strategies leading to better health outcomes (Table 2-1).

TABLE 2-1 Using Theories to Develop Interventions

- Use clinical data and careful communication techniques to identify a health problem or undesired behavior.
- Select or combine one or more theory-based intervention methods to initiate behavior change.
- Use evidenced based decision making to develop the best strategies for change.
- Evaluate and measure success of health outcome.

Courtesy of Janet Jaccarino

Stages of Change Theory (Transtheoretical Model)

The stages of change theory grew from work with smoking cessation and has expanded to include areas such as alcohol addiction, drug abuse, anxiety and eating disorders, and weight loss. The theory views change as a process of stages over time rather than a single event. People are at varying stages or levels of motivation or readiness to change at any point in time. Once a person's stage of readiness is identified, the dental assistant can match education efforts to that level.

Relapse is common when making a lifestyle change; the stages of change theory recognizes this fact. If relapse occurs, it is important to remain positive and shift from failure to encouragement. Focus on the patient's success and what made the intervention work. Remember that even though there may be failure at this time, the patient has learned something new and may fall back into a better level at any time. Key concepts for the stages of change theory and suggested interventions are outlined in Table 2-2.

Social Learning Theory (Social Cognitive Theory)

Social learning theory, also known as social cognitive theory, suggests that people and their environment are continually interacting. People learn from their own experience, by observing the actions of others, and by the results of those actions. Changes take place because the environment, information, and behavior all affect one another. The theory places emphasis on self-confidence or one's ability to attain success; the greater the success, the greater the motivation to overcome obstacles, change, and continue the behavior over time.

Modeling is another important characteristic of the theory. Observing others, sharing their experience and success, or having a role model all act to build confidence. Key concepts for social learning theory and suggested interventions are outlined in Table 2-3.

Health Belief Model

The health belief model has been used since the 1950s to explain why people will take action to prevent and/or control illness. It is

TABLE 2-2 Using the Stages of Change Theory

Stage	Definition	Intervention
Precontemplation	The patient is unaware of a problem or the need for behavior change.	Increase knowledge of the problem and risks. Help the patient learn new ideas and facts.
Contemplation	The patient is thinking about change and is aware of the pros and cons.	Motivate thinking. Recognize fear and emotion connected with change. Recognize procrastination.
Preparation	The patient intends to take positive action.	Take action to provide information and encourage realistic, gradual goals.
Action	The patient is acting toward change. Change is observable.	Provide support, positive reinforcement, and feedback. Patient may not have achieved total success.
Maintenance	Behavior change is successful. Patient is more confident, continues desired action, and works to prevent relapse.	Avoid relapse. Offer positive reinforcement, reminders, and alternatives. Solve any problems. Offer suggestions to cope with any difficulties that occur.

Courtesy of Janet Jaccarino

TABLE 2-3 Using the Social Learning Theory

Concept	Definition	Intervention
Shared interaction of people and environment	Behavior changes result from interaction with people and environment.	Share the experience of others. Cite knowledge of experts. Change environment if necessary.
Outcome expectations	Beliefs about likely benefits or results of action. Value of the consequences of the behavioral choices.	Provide information about the results of behavior change in advance. Change expectations through education.
Self-confidence	Beliefs about personal ability to perform action for behavior change.	Provide praise, rewards, and incentives as reinforcements. Reward may be toothbrush; incentive may be less expense in treatment.
Observational learning	Learning to perform new behaviors by observing others.	Involve observation of others. Use of demonstration, video, or presentation. Act as a role model for the patient by providing instruction, tools, and resources to help continue behavior.

Courtesy of Janet Jaccarino

useful to predict whether a person will comply with your recommendations over a period of time. This model is based on a person's beliefs and perceptions that they are susceptible to a disease, that the disease is severe enough to cause harm, that actions to prevent or reduce a disease are effective, and that the benefits of action will outweigh any barriers to taking action. The stronger the beliefs, the more likely the person will be to take action. Most recently, cues to action and self-confidence have been included in the model. Key concepts for the health belief model and suggested interventions are outlined in Table 2-4.

Learning Ladder

The learning ladder, also known as the decision-making continuum, is based on the theory that learning occurs in a series of sequential steps from being unaware of something to practicing a learned habit. The learner moves through the steps, gaining knowledge leading to making a commitment to a new behavior. By knowing where on the ladder the learner is, you can develop strategies that will enable them to move up the ladder finally making a habit of practicing good health behaviors. The steps in the learning ladder sequence are unawareness, awareness, interest, involvement, action, and habit. Key concepts for the learning ladder are outlined in Table 2-5.

Maslow's Hierarchy of Needs

Abraham Maslow (1908–1970), an American psychologist, is considered the founder of a movement called *humanistic psychology*. Abraham Maslow proposed that human behavior is motivated

TABLE 2-4 Using the Health Belief Model

Concept	Definition	Intervention
Perceived susceptibility	Beliefs about the risk or likelihood of getting a disease	Personalize risk and susceptibility if the patient continues current behavior. Discuss disease based on the patient's signs and symptoms after dentist has documented signs.
Perceived severity	Beliefs about how serious a disease is and how it will affect their life	Be specific about the severity of the disease and the medical, clinical, and social consequences of non-treatment. This information should be presented by the person discussing treatment plans and options.
Perceived benefits	Beliefs about the efficacy of action to reduce risk or seriousness of the disease	Define action to take. (how, where, when). Clarify the positive effects of the action.
Perceived barriers	Beliefs about the negative aspects of the action, psychological, physical, and financial side effects—it could be inconvenient or time consuming	Identify and reduce perceived barriers through reassurance, correction of misinformation, incentives, and assistance.
Cues to action	Strategies to achieve readiness and stimulate action	Provide how-to information, promote awareness, use reminders.
Self-confidence	Beliefs about personal ability to perform action for behavior change	Provide guidance and demonstration in performing action, set realistic goals, and give positive reinforcement.

Courtesy of Janet Jaccarino

TABLE 2-5 Using the Learning Ladder

Concept	Definition	Intervention
Unawareness	The learner lacks information or is misinformed about the problem.	Use questioning techniques to find out where the patient is on the ladder.
Awareness	The learner receives information that a problem exists.	Provide information and encouragement, tolerate mistakes, and help learner improve.
Interest	The learner recognizes the problem, information becomes meaningful, and the learner shows interest.	Focus on performance and give opportunities to practice.
Involvement	The learner has desire to act.	Provide encouragement, set realistic goals, troubleshoot problems, and offer alternatives.
Action	The learner is ready to act and accept new concepts and practices. Desire for knowledge increases.	Provide guidance and demonstration in performing action, refine skills, and give positive reinforcement.
Habit	Learner practices behavior and makes a permanent change.	Provide positive reinforcement and use reminders.

Courtesy of Janet Jaccarino

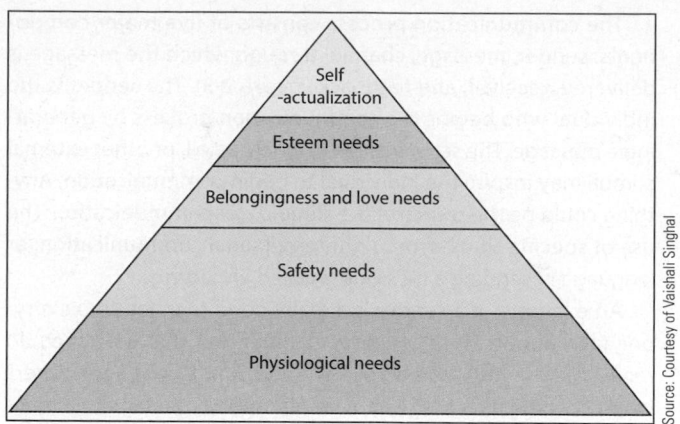

FIGURE 2-1
Maslow's hierarchy of needs.

Source: Courtesy of Vaishali Singhal

by certain needs that drive a person to action. Some needs are more important than others and have more power than others to motivate a person. According to Maslow, a person will not be concerned with higher level needs until lower level needs are satisfied. Needs are arranged in a pyramid diagram with the strongest need at the bottom of the pyramid. The importance of each of the needs is represented by its size in the pyramid. Additionally, when a lower level need reappears, any higher need will not be important to a person until that lower level need is met (Figure 2-1).

Maslow's hierarchy helps you understand the patient by understanding his or her environment and helps you design strategies that address specific needs. For example, if a patient is in pain, brushing and flossing become less important until the reason for the pain is addressed. To motivate a patient, the dental assistant must figure out where a patient is on the model. Key concepts and the relationship to dentistry with suggested interventions are outlined below:

- **Physiological Needs**—Basic human needs such as food, sleep, shelter, and physical health.
  Dental Implication—This level is the most powerful. If these needs are not satisfied, then all the other needs become unimportant.
  Dental Interaction—Dental professionals need to be aware of certain aspects of a person's environment and life outside of the dental office, as well as the importance of what a person needs at any one time during dental treatment.

- **Safety and Security Needs**—This level represents the need for stability, security, protection, structure, and freedom from fear and anxiety.
  Dental Implication—Patients may be in pain, anxious, or frightened. The patient may be worried about disease transmission or infection control practices. Introduction of new tasks such as brushing and flossing techniques, or new treatments can be threatening to the patient.
  Dental Interaction—At each visit, office staff and office policy do not change. A familiar environment creates a sense of stability and gives structure to the patient's visit. Create an ordered, stress free environment, fully explain each

procedure, involve the patient in the visit, and show **empathy** and respect for the patient's feelings and opinions.

- ***Social Needs***—The need for love and a sense of belonging is fulfilled with a place within one's own culture or society, being accepted, being part of a group, and contact with others.
  Dental Implication—Adolescents and teens are often affected by this level. Peer pressure, smoking, use of drugs and alcohol, risky health behaviors, and oral piercing and oral jewelry may be used to gain acceptance. Cultural behavior, diet, and family interventions may play a part in patient behavior.
  Dental Interaction—All encounters with the patient should be face to face. Make them feel they are welcomed and part of your office environment. Show concern and listen to what they have to say and that their opinion is valued. The patient's dental appearance may be important in getting a job and making friends.

- **Esteem or Ego Needs**—This level refers to feelings of self-worth, usefulness, competency, achievement, approval, respect from others, and mastery or independence. Meeting these needs leads to feelings of capability and a willingness to contribute to society. Not having these needs met results in feelings of inferiority, discouragement, and helplessness.
  Dental Implications—The patient needs to feel competency in new tasks, control over their own health, and self-worth in being healthy.
  Dental Interactions—Respect the patient for gaining new knowledge and their ability to follow recommendations. Give positive reinforcement and praise for accomplishments. Make the patient feel their opinion is important and worthy; give them options and let them decide on treatment modalities. By planning together, the patient feels in control of their own health; they are responsible and feel they have a stake in the outcome. Show sensitivity if a patient does not have a feeling of self-worth or if they fear rejection. Adults are highly motivated by this level.

- **Self-Actualization**—At this level, the person has fully achieved their potential, and they are able to cope realistically with life. Persons at this level have a need to problem solve, achieve goals, and master tasks.
  Dental Implications—The patient may be ready to fully achieve total oral health and have an understanding of the relationship between oral health and systemic health.
  Dental Interactions—Appeal to the patient's sense of self-care; solve problems and plan together. Setting goals and deciding on options can be accomplished by involving the patient because they understand their own health. Patients who reach this level may cope better with any serious oral or systemic health problems.

Dental professionals are in a unique position to address dental health as part of a patient's total health and wellness. We see patients on a regular basis for preventive oral health services, which includes patient education. Therefore, it is our responsibility to help the patient achieve lasting behavior changes that support oral health. Applying health behavior theories is one way the dental assistant can fulfill that responsibility.

Components of the Communication Process

Understanding how individuals think and feel is only part of interacting successfully with patients. A dental assistant must also have excellent communication skills. These skills can be learned and developed and are very important in patient care. The act of passing along information (the message), transmitting an idea (or receiving the message), or connecting with another individual (providing feedback) is communication. Transmitting thoughts, ideas, feelings, facts, and other information is done through verbal and nonverbal behavior. Every time a person communicates with another person, even if no verbal comments are taking place, information is being transmitted. In fact, people cannot avoid communicating with each other. In dental assisting, this communication is essential in establishing a relationship with the patient. This method of connecting with patients allows for patient comfort and safety so that the treatment can take place. The quality of the communication, and the way the patient feels connected to the dental assistant and dentist, directly relate to the patient's total experience while in the dental office. Listening is also very important. The adage, "You have two ears and one mouth so you can listen twice as much," is true. Often, people begin formulating their responses before they hear the entire question. In the dental office, pay special attention to what the person is saying, and then give the correct response.

When a staff member is going over the case presentation, a patient may say something like, "I just want to fix my front teeth." This may communicate a message to the dentist or **auxiliary** staff that appearance is important to this individual. Further communication with the patient will help determine why the patient wants the front teeth restored. If staff members listen carefully, they may find that this individual is applying for new employment, or that the patient is going to be in a daughter's wedding and wants to look good in the pictures. Once an understanding is reached as to where patients are coming from and what their desires and needs are, then a treatment plan can be established to help meet these needs (Figure 2-2).

The communication process consists of five major components: sender, message, channel through which the message is delivered, receiver, and feedback (Figure 2-3). The sender is the individual who begins the communication process by generating a message. The senses of taste, touch, smell, or other external stimuli may inspire the individual to begin communication. Anything could be the source of the stimulus for communication. The use of specific signs, symbols, interpersonal communication, or language in sending a message is called **encoding**.

An example of a sender is a really good teacher who everyone talks about. Most people remember that the teacher could really get the message across. A good sender engages others when sending a message and can transmit a message in a manner that is clear and concise. It may be beneficial to evaluate what an admired person in your life did to enhance their message. Use those qualities to become a better sender.

An individual starts with an idea, and then formulates that idea and sends it through a message to another individual. The sender must shape the idea, which often starts as an image the sender visualizes, into a message by translating the image into words that others can understand. This complicated process happens so routinely during the day that most people are unaware of it. The message is the stimuli—written, verbal, or nonverbal communication—produced by the sender to which the receiver will respond. Reception of the message could occur through visual, auditory, or **kinesthetic** channels. The message may be received by different individuals in different ways, depending on each individual's paradigm (Figure 2-3).

The channel is the communication medium through which a message is delivered. Dental assistants use each of these channels during a clinical procedure. It is critical to be a good listener. Patients may feel comfortable because of the connection they

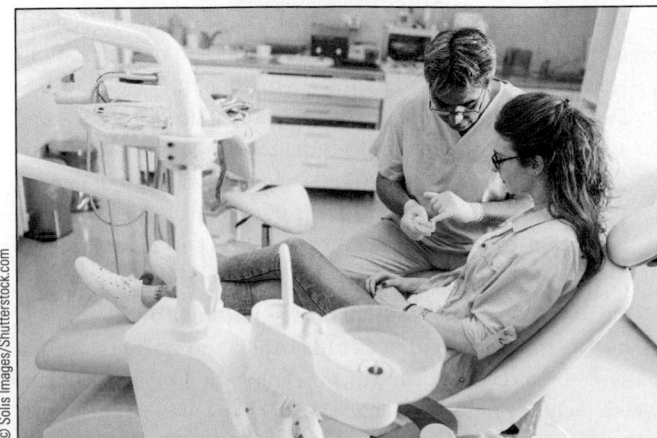

FIGURE 2-2
Dentist communicating with patient.

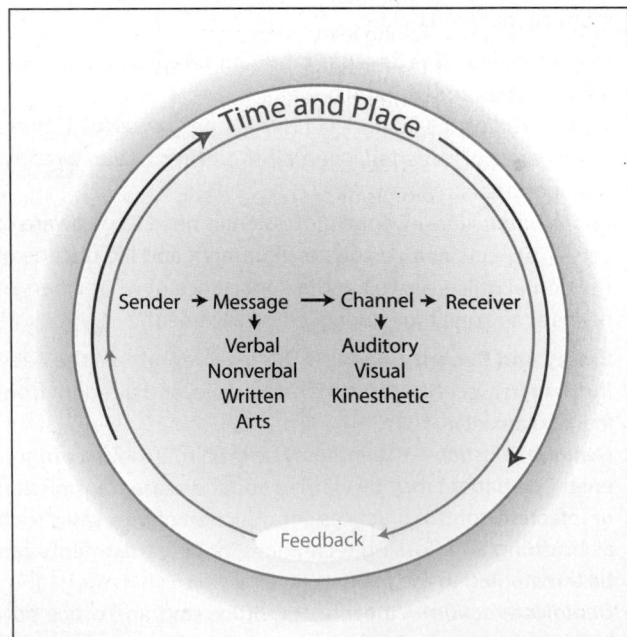

FIGURE 2-3
A communication model.

have with the auxiliary, and they may share more information with the auxiliary than they would with the dentist. In addition, when the dentist arrives, items are placed into the mouth, and it is more difficult for the patient to communicate verbally. Dental assistants also observe the patient during the procedure. Are the eyes of the patient closed tightly? Are the knuckles of the patient white because the patient's hands are tightly clutching the arms of the chair? The dentist is focusing on the procedure at hand, but the assistant can view the entire situation. Many dentists count on assistants to be their eyes and to notify them if the patient is uncomfortable. Dental assistants normally possess the quality of empathy for patients. They also have the ability to communicate through the kinesthetic channel, by using the procedural touch, and by asking the patient, "How does that feel?" The dental assistant may also use the caring touch by touching a patient's arm during the anesthesia process, or any other procedure that appears to make the patient fearful or uncomfortable. This reassuring touch shows the auxiliary to be compassionate, concerned, and empathetic.

It is important to note that, in the dental office, the channel can be lost due to the pressure of time. Often a dental assistant or dentist does not follow up on the channel method in which the message is being sent. The dental assistant may read the signs and ignore them due to lack of time and the fact that the next patient is waiting for treatment. Often, in such a rushed atmosphere, patients may feel that it is not worth going into what is bothering them, and they hold back because they feel that they cannot share how they feel about something. The dental assistant needs to develop skills to identify when the time should be taken to ensure that the patient's needs are met. These skills are developed over time, after the assistant understands the entire operation of the office, as well as when time can be made up and when more time is needed with a patient. Understanding how communication is channeled and how to read the signs that individuals are transmitting is a lifelong learning process.

The receiver takes the message and must make sense of it. This process uses feelings, intentions, and thoughts from a person's paradigm. Much of the message encoding comes from all the nonverbal clues the sender used to transmit the message. It is critical that the message is decoded correctly before providing feedback. Is the intent of the message clear? If not, state it back to the sender for correct interpretation. After making sure the message is clear, the individual formulates a response, much like the initial sender did. An idea is given shape and words are selected to express the idea to the other person. This interchange occurs until both people feel their ideas are expressed in the manner in which they intended, or they continue to another area of discussion.

Oral Communication

Some people are able to carry on conversations and be easily understood. Others may have difficulty with this process. Dental professionals must be able to communicate effectively in order to establish good patient relationships. The sender of the message needs to be clear, and the receiver needs to listen actively. Effective communication between the patient and the dental professional decreases the chances that a message is misunderstood. The benefits of good communication include patient involvement in treatment decisions, which often leads to increased compliance with care regimens; increased patient satisfaction; and a reduced potential for complaints and malpractice litigation.

Listening Skills

Listening skills are an important part of communication. Good listening skills allow the patient to see that we are paying attention to their feelings and thoughts. We spend more time listening than performing any other type of communication. Most college students spend about 50 percent of their time listening, 35 percent reading and writing, and about 15 percent talking. Some of the barriers to listening are preoccupation, message overload, and external noise. The external noise may come from others speaking, telephones ringing, or music. People are often preoccupied with concerns that are more important to them, which therefore diminish their ability to listen. We experience overload because the quantity of messages we encounter each day is tremendous. It is important for the dental assistant to have good listening skills as part of overall communication.

Attitude If you are speaking with a patient in the *operatory* or treatment room, sit at eye level, face the patient, and remove your mask as circumstances allow (currently under Covid-19 requirements, the mask must be worn at all times). Looking in another direction, being distracted, or multitasking, for example filling out the chart while in conversation, gives the impression that you are not listening or are not interested; this behavior may even be considered rude. You may miss parts of the message if you change the subject abruptly or are busy planning your response rather than listening. Carefully pay attention and give the patient time to speak. When you put yourself in someone else's place, you begin to understand why they feel the way they do. Respecting the feelings and opinion of others allows you to listen without judging. You do not have to agree with everything the other person says, but a hasty reaction of disapproval can create the feeling of rejection and quickly break down communication. Offering reassurance will often put a patient at ease, especially if they are anxious. However, do not promise something that is not possible, such as complete lack of discomfort during difficult procedures. Remember you are partners with the patient in their care; empathy, support, reassurance, and respect will only strengthen that partnership.

Active Listening Skills See the patient as a whole person. Messages that patients receive are filtered through their values, beliefs, and preferences. For successful patient interactions, you must actively listen. Active listening enables you to be sensitive to every issue that may have an effect on patient care. Active listening is a very important skill that involves more than just hearing the words that are spoken. Give the patient your undivided attention and concentration. This will enable you to understand both the patient's words as well as their body language.

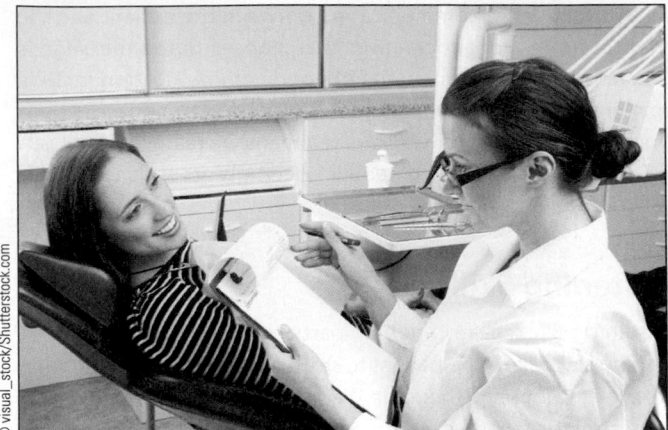

FIGURE 2-4
The operator's posture and correct positioning makes patients feel more comfortable and that the dental assistant is interested in them.

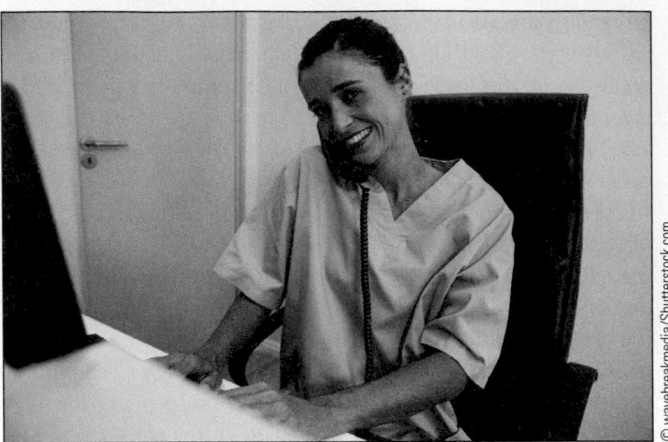

FIGURE 2-5
Dental assistant engaged while speaking on phone with patient.

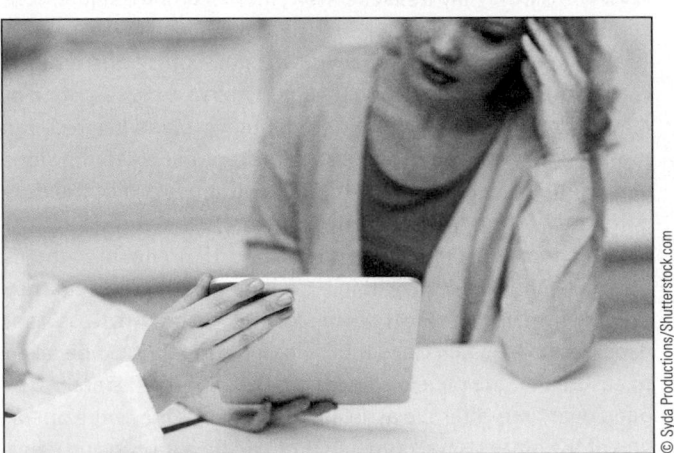

FIGURE 2-6
Body language and gestures often say more than the spoken word.

Because we spend half our time listening, it is impossible to stay focused and listen actively. The mind wanders and listening stops. Each person identifies when to actively listen to a message of great importance. When active listening takes place, the receiver **encodes** the message and responds during two-way communication. People can tell if the other person is listening actively, because the other person understands what has been said (Figure 2-4). In a dental office, it is critical to train your mind to listen to the patient so that you can understand other people more often and with greater clarity. The dental assistant may be required to listen to the concerns of the patient and respond accordingly, or to chart medical and dental patient history correctly. The dental assistant may need to listen to the directions of the dentist in carrying out patient treatment. Often, listening in the dental office is accompanied with analyzing and interpreting information. It may help to repeat the content back to the patient. For example, "I understand that you said the discomfort started several days ago in the upper left side of your face, close to this tooth." The dental assistant should spend time developing and becoming more adept at active listening skills.

Telephone Listening Skills It is often said that the telephone is where the patient derives his or her first impression of the office, and that the telephone is the office's lifeline. That being said, a telephone conversation is often like a conversation between two blindfolded individuals. The inflections in the auxiliary's voice, along with the verbal communication dialogue, give the message to the patient. Speaking in short sentences with a hard tone to the voice may not sound inviting to the patient. Patients may interpret this communication to mean that the auxiliary does not want them in the office. The message itself could say something like, "I am looking forward to seeing you in our office on May twenty-fifth," but the tone and perceived attitude may reflect a different message. The dental assistant will need to concentrate and obtain feedback from others on how the message is coming across. When listening on the telephone, sit in the correct posture and respond with the correct facial expression. These actions will have an effect on the message sent to the caller and will convey the message that you want to listen (Figure 2-5).

Nonverbal Communication (Body Language) It is often said that communication is less than 20 percent verbal or oral (speaking words) and 80 percent nonverbal. Communication without using words is defined as nonverbal communication. Body language can communicate more than spoken words (Figure 2-6). Body language includes the unconscious way we move our bodies, the physical distance between individuals, posture and position, facial expressions, gestures, and perceptions.

Nonverbal communication is first learned when we are infants. The tone of a voice and the presence or absence of a smile are picked up readily by an infant through nonverbal means. The infant adapts learned behaviors that bring positive responses from the caregiver. In the dental office, much of the communication with the patient is nonverbal. Sometimes, the patient cannot respond verbally due to the placement of the dental dam or other items in the oral cavity. The dental assistant should become aware of a patient's nonverbal communications, which could be a tightening of the hands on the chair arms, a look that indicates a need the patient may have, or posture or movement in the chair. Watch for this nonverbal communication and try to identify, with the patient's help, which feelings and emotions are being communicated nonverbally.

Nonverbal communication, or body language, enhances words, quickly conveys emotion, and provides important information. The simple gesture of pointing a finger can let someone know direction without anyone speaking a word. Facial expressions, such as eye contact and smiling, when used during patient interactions, help send a positive message. The face can also tell you if the person is happy, sad, confused, or in pain. Head nodding signals agreement and leaning forward expresses full attention. Being relaxed with uncrossed arms and legs or sitting with your hands in your lap sends the message of an accepting, open attitude. On the other hand, when a patient is speaking, the dental professional may deliver a stern message of disapproval by simply shaking their head. Therefore, it is important to be aware of your own facial expression and body language when talking to patients.

Careful observation of a person's body language reveals if there is a conflict between what a person is saying and how they really feel. Mixed messages can occur during treatment. Consider the following interaction. The dental assistant says, "Mrs. Garcia, are you comfortable?" and Mrs. Garcia replies, "Yes, I'm fine." However, the assistant notices that Mrs. Garcia is grasping the chair arm so tightly that her fingers are white, and there is a grimace on her face. Mrs. Garcia is physically showing signs of stress, but what she is saying is not how she really feels. By simply touching Mrs. Garcia's hand, arm, or shoulder, the dental assistant can offer warmth, understanding, caring, and reassurance. Be aware that some people may not like being touched and may pull away when you try to comfort them. Use touch cautiously to avoid misinterpretation.

Emotions such as anger, defensiveness, or unhappiness can be expressed through body language. Signs for these emotions are crossed arms, clenched fists, or sitting in a tight manner with legs and arms crossed. In many cases, the patient's body language will reveal true feelings. Close observation of nonverbal cues is part of active listening and can reveal the patient's hidden feelings or what is left unsaid.

 **HIPAA—Remember, these records are confidential. By law, information in patient records is considered "privileged information" and must not be shared outside of the office.**

Territoriality or spatial relation indicates the amount of space an individual needs to feel comfortable with others. This distance changes with the group we are in. Intimate touching, normally within six inches, is usually encountered with close family members or close friends. In the dental office, sometimes the procedures the dental assistants are doing require the assistants to invade the patient's space. It is best that the dental assistant tells the patient about the procedure so that it will not be perceived as threatening. The patient can then feel empowered by deciding

to allow the treatment to proceed. This interaction helps to build a sense of trust with the patient. After informing the patient, sit and perform procedures, if possible, from the side of the patient. When working straight toward a patient, the spatial distance required for comfort is much greater. Individuals are normally much more comfortable sharing the space to their side.

Patient posture indicates how patients are responding. If the patient is tense, it may indicate that the patient feels threatened. The patient may be seated with the arms and legs crossed, which is a message of closure or resistance. Slumped shoulders may indicate the patient is depressed or discouraged. The patient who sits with legs uncrossed, hands loose on the chair arms, and a slightly laid-back posture in the chair may be open to suggestions. The manner in which dental assistants position themselves is also important. Standing over the patient may indicate superiority. Sitting close to the patient and leaning toward the patient expresses interest, warmth, acceptance, and caring (Figure 2-7). This arrangement allows the patient to feel valued, listened to, and cared for.

Facial expression is one of the most observed and critical components of nonverbal communication. The sender's eyes give the receiver great insight; emotions such as happiness, sadness, and anger are reflected in the eyes. The eyebrows also indicate such nonverbal clues as puzzlement, worry, questioning, and surprise. The dental assistant should check the patient's eyes during the procedure and watch for nonverbal communication. Dental practitioners should be mindful of their facial expressions (e.g., eye expressions) behind the treatment masks (Figure 2-7).

Like facial expressions, gestures are a common form of nonverbal communication, and one of the most observed. Even while in a car at a stoplight, nonverbal communication can be observed inside the cars close to us. Gestures make it fairly easy to see if someone is angry, happy, or just trying to make a point to another individual. When we talk, we often use our hands to communicate. It enhances the spoken word by emphasizing the content and holding the attention of the receiver.

It is critical that dental assistants develop good perception skills as they relate to patient communication. The dental

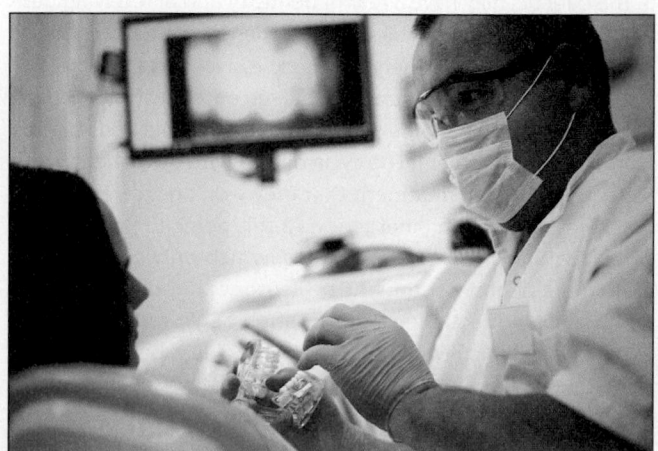

FIGURE 2-7
Dental assistant with attentive and friendly facial expression under mask.

assistant must be aware of the feelings of others and be able to sense patients' moods and their attitudes toward the dental treatment. Initially, the dental assistant can watch and observe other health care workers using good perception skills, and then emulate the others' examples.

Defense Mechanisms

Individuals often use defense mechanisms to block communication. The individual may feel ashamed, guilty, or threatened and therefore respond with defense mechanisms. It becomes difficult to go forward when the patient may be unintentionally defensive in order to gain control. For instance, when talking to the patient about the course of treatment to care for an area of decay, the patient may say, "The last dentist didn't find decay there!" or "You said that if I brushed and flossed, I wouldn't get cavities!"

In order to go forward, the dental assistant must recognize common defense mechanisms, and work with patients so that communication can be more effective. Denial is a common defense mechanism in health care. When patients do not brush and floss, and believe they will never get decay because they have not had it in the past, they are in denial. Patients may respond with regression, moving back to a former time to escape the fear, a tactic that creates temporary amnesia and an inability to cope with a situation. Often in the dental office, the patient uses rationalization to justify a situation. For instance, a patient may say, "My father has soft teeth and had a lot of cavities. I have inherited his soft teeth."

Understanding and recognizing patients' defense mechanisms helps the dental assistant get to the truth. This, in turn, helps patients improve communication and get beyond their defenses to achieve better outcomes. Dental assistants must constantly observe nonverbal behaviors and look for cues, as well as listen intently to verbal messages. Give patients your full attention so that communication has every opportunity to succeed.

Dental Phobias

Some patients may have a fear of dentistry and of receiving dental care; this is called dental phobia. Patients with dental phobias have fear and severe anxiety that is excessive, unreasonable, and irrational; they are often unable to overcome it without professional help. These patients often create a cycle that adds to their fear of dental treatment. The cycle begins with the patient being so fearful of dental treatment that they won't get care until the problem becomes an emergency. At this point, their treatment often requires invasive procedures, which only adds to their fear, so the phobia continues. The causes of dental phobias can be direct or indirect. Direct causes often begin with the patient experiencing difficult or painful treatment. The experience can be more traumatic if the dentist's behavior is not personable, understanding, and caring toward the patient. The indirect causes may be from several sources including the following:

- Hearing about another person's traumatic experience, or their negative views on dentistry and dental treatment.

- The media, which often portrays dentistry and dental treatment in a negative way, such as portraying dental treatment as painful.
- Negative experiences with medical doctors or hospitals may lead people to fear any type of treatment.
- People who have experienced sexual, physical, or emotional abuse may also transfer their fear to dental treatment.
- Fear of needles and injections.
- Embarrassment at the condition of their teeth and oral hygiene.
- Lack of control, feeling of helplessness, and loss of personal space.

Treatment of a patient with dental phobia often includes behavior and **pharmacological** techniques. Some patients are treated in the dental office, while others require specialized treatment where psychologists and dentists work together to help patients decrease and manage their fears. Behavior techniques include taking more time to explain procedures using visual aids, such as models and photos that are not too graphic; use of the "look, see, then do" approach to relax the patient; listening to their concerns and making sure they understand; or allowing the patient some control by giving them a sign when they want the dentist to stop. Pharmacological techniques include the provision of sedative medications in pill form or delivered intravenously, or use of **nitrous oxide**. The dentist can also use slow, careful injection techniques with the anesthetic in order to make the injection more comfortable. The dentist and dental assistant can aid dental phobia patients by being understanding and using gentle dental techniques.

Communicating with Patients, Staff, and Other Professionals

In the office, the dental assistant will encounter a wide variety of people, spanning all ages and from different cultural backgrounds. It is important to be aware of the differences among generations and to have cultural awareness in order communicate effectively.

The Different Generations

Individuals of different ages can be grouped by generation. It helps to have a basic understanding of the primary concerns of each generation. This will help the dental office aid the patient in getting their needs and wants met. It should be stated that this discussion is only a general description of the generations, and, certainly, individuality abounds within each characterization.

Children With a child's first dental experience, we have a great opportunity to create a positive attitude for a lifetime of good oral health. Infants, toddlers, and preschool children will be under the supervision of their parents, so do not forget to include them in the visit. However, it is important to recognize that it is the child's dental visit, so speak directly to the child and address them by

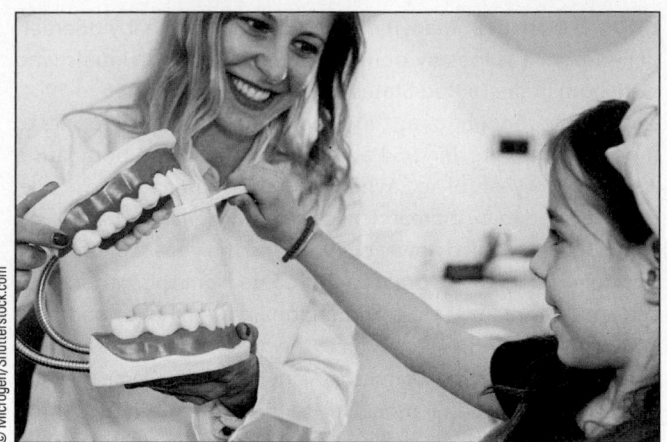

FIGURE 2-8
Dental assistant with child. Dental assistant teaches child about oral home care.

name. For toddlers and preschoolers, use a booster seat or make the dental chair smaller by removing the headrest. When speaking, use simple, short sentences with familiar words. Tell the child exactly what to expect and what is expected of them. Children this age learn through play, so make everything a fun experience. The dental chair is the rocket ship, the suction/evacuator is Mr. Thirsty, and the dental handpiece is Buzzy Bee (Figure 2-8).

Speak in the language the child can relate to; for example, instead of telling a child "this will take a half hour," they will be able to better understand "this will take one cartoon." Another approach is to use a timer. Be sure to praise good behavior. Do not speak down to the child, and have a consistent tone of voice. If cooperation is a problem, use voice tone and volume to gain attention. When behavior is an issue, it may be best to reschedule the visit. Once again, timing is important. It is best not to schedule dental visits during mealtimes, naptime, or when a child is ill.

Generation Alpha Generation Alpha was born beginning 2010 thru 2024. This generation is the children of the millennials and is extremely comfortable with electronic devices and with swiping a screen. Generation Alpha is influential in helping parents choose electronics for their homes. This newest generation will include many children of foreign born parents as well as children who are foreign born. This generation represents many countries across the globe and is the most diverse generation.

Generation Z Generation Z was born in the mid-1990s to early 2000s. In American culture specifically this group is a more diverse mix of ethnicities than the generations before them. As a generation growing up at the peak of technology advancement, they are technologically proficient, using, on average, five devices and communicating across a variety of devices. Technology has given them opportunities to engage with people all over the world, preparing them for global communication and interaction. As a group they are mature, fast learners, curious, driven, tolerant, and open-minded. They often feel they can't depend on the advice of older adults as they have watched the economy decline and seen the mistakes other generations have made. This generation wants to be heard and have input, which has led them to be active in their communities, and they care about the world and each other because they have always been connected through technology. They believe in investigating, experiencing, and creating things they love, which has led many to be mini entrepreneurs. Generation Z has taken hobbies and turned them into jobs, and then into businesses. These businesses become their own reality. To appeal to this generation, create communication that they relate to, using various technologies. Be authentic and appeal in a human sense, while listening to them and getting them involved.

Generation Y Most refer to Generation Y (those born between 1980 and 1994) as the generation following Generation X; they are also referred to as the *echo generation* (children of the baby boomers). This generation varies greatly in their social and economic conditions. It is known that this generation is delaying adulthood longer than prior generations, and staying in their parents' homes longer. This may be due to the housing crisis and high unemployment levels facing this generation. This generation communicates through texting and email, and follows websites such as YouTube and especially social networking sites such as Facebook and Twitter (Figure 2-9). Most individuals in this group are fascinated with communication and the latest

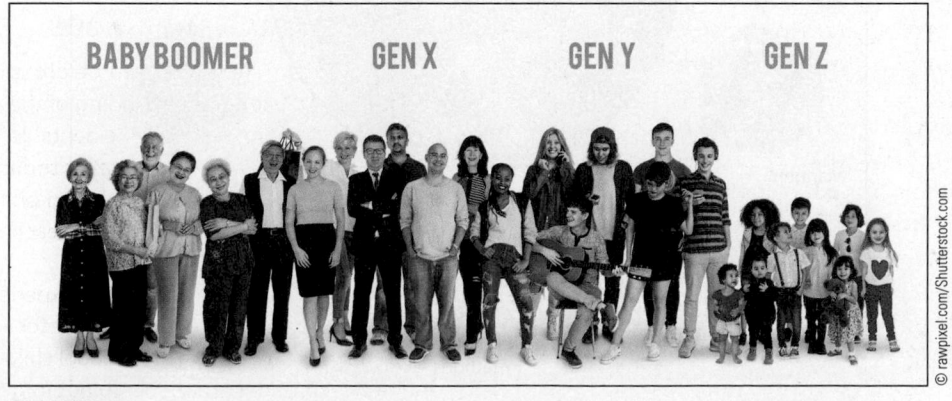

FIGURE 2-9
The different generations.

gadgets in technology. Knowing this helps us to communicate with them as patients in the dental office. This individual is going to check out websites and choose an office that uses the latest in digital technology. They may also want to have digital images of their braces or teeth sent to their phones. This age group wants responsibility, so take the opportunity to lead them toward care of their own oral health.

Generation X Generation X (also called the *MTV generation*) is thought to be those born during the 1960s and 1970s, and some consider it to include the 1980s. According to the U.S. Census Bureau, this generation statistically holds the highest education level when looking at age groups. They are a very diverse group in aspects such as race, ethnicity, sexual orientation, politics, and religion. They were influenced by heavy metal and disco music, the recession in the 1980s, and the oil and energy crisis. This generation is unsure about their future due to the savings and loan crisis and the overall economy. This generation has grown up with video games, cable television, and the Internet. When working with this group of individuals in dentistry, note that they may search out offices on the Internet and may want to be contacted by texting versus phone interaction. Adults know that oral health is important and are willing to be active partners in their care. All adults have had many life experiences that have shaped their values and beliefs; therefore, any of the strategies discussed in this chapter will help identify their wants and needs. Be sure to pace interactions to knowledge and differences in learning style.

Baby Boomers Many have heard about the "baby boomer" generation. It is loosely defined as the set of individuals who were born in the United States between the years 1946 to 1964, and is often thought of as those born after World War II. Due to the high birth rate, in 1964 about one-third of the population was under 19 years of age. When the baby boomers came of age, there seemed to be a great deal of parental defiance that played out with the so-called flower children and the impact of drugs on this generation. Many great minds came from this generation, and currently many large corporations are run by baby boomers, who will be passing the torch on to the next generation. The baby boomers are often in two-income families and have been often tagged as the me generation. Due to their parents, they grew up as one of the healthiest and wealthiest generations. Most of the individuals in this generation saw a president assassinated, people walk on the moon, and the birth of personal computers. This generation is interested in cosmetic dentistry, teeth whitening, and keeping their teeth for a lifetime (Figure 2-9).

Older Adults This age group, often called "traditionalists," is one of the fastest growing segments of the United States population. They also have a lifetime of dentistry and dental encounters. This generation may have experienced the Great Depression and lived through World War II. They believe in hard work and paying their dues. They value privacy and may feel that sharing intimate details of their life is not appropriate. Health history information may span 40–50 years. The patient may be taking multiple

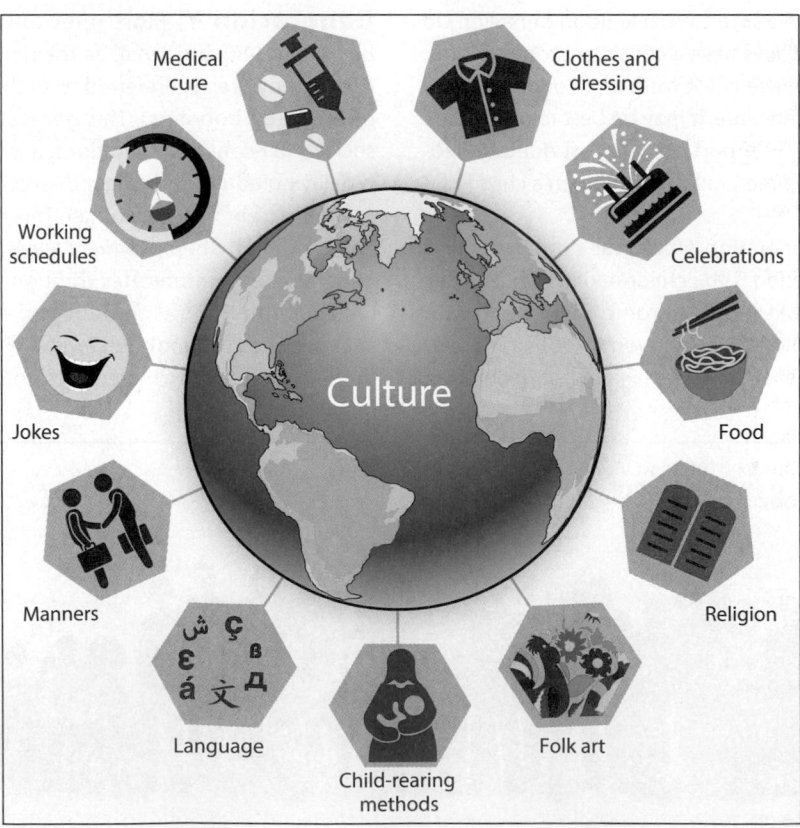

FIGURE 2-10
Things are done differently with each culture.

medications, some of which may have oral effects. These patients may be under the care of several physicians at one time. Medicare generally does not cover dental expenses, and many of these older adults live on a limited, fixed income, so they expect the best value for their dollar. Older adults will have the time to talk and value being respected in a "youth conscious" world.

Stress in the Dental Office

Working closely with other employees, waiting patients, and procedure change are all issues occurring in the dental office that cause stress. Stress is the body's method of reacting to specific conditions or stimuli. The manner in which each member of the dental team handles stress is an important aspect of how the dental office functions. Even with the best dental team members, the office is a stressful environment. The dental assistant is not only the greeter of the patients but is also the right hand of the dentist in a fast-paced environment. The dental assistant is expected to keep the room in top shape and always be prepared for the next procedure. Over time, the work environment can take a toll on the dental assistant, leading to back pain and carpal tunnel problems. The stress comes from the sources noted previously, along with overbooking appointments, being understaffed, equipment malfunctioning, and unavailable supplies, along with all of the tasks that have to be done in a timely manner. Things that often cause the most problems with stress are employees unhappy with their jobs, lack of advancement, salary, and poor communication. Stress can cause conflicts with patients and team members. An office that has staff that is cross trained will experience less stress as there will always be a backup staff member who can take address a particular task.

Learning to deal with stress and conflict will enable you to be able to make sound decisions at work and home. Maintaining a healthy lifestyle, eating properly, exercising regularly, setting realistic goals and expectations, and communicating well with others will aid in reducing stress.

Conflict A disagreement or power struggle between individuals or groups is defined as conflict. This may result from being contradictory or having a difference of opinion. Conflicts in the dental office with the employer or other colleagues create an atmosphere of stress. Conflicts continue to fester when ignored; they stay with us until we face them or resolve them. Conflicts trigger strong emotions. Gaining the conflict resolution skills that can turn conflicts into opportunities is a normal part of any healthy relationship.

Conflict Resolution The act of finding an answer or a solution to a problem is defined as resolution. An individual must first understand that a response to a conflict is based on individual perceptions of the situation, and not always on the facts. Good communication will aid in finding a method to resolve the conflict. If the problem or conflict is too out of control for the parties to resolve on their own, use of a mediator should be considered. This could be the office manager or dentist. If involved in a conflict, it is important to understand that it is not all about you. For example, your perception may be that a coworker is angry

with you when in fact something has happened in their life and they are having a bad day, and it has nothing to do with you. Try to depersonalize the conflict from "me versus you," and work on the situation. Be specific about the conflict and try to not bring in any other complaints. Be open and listen to the other person's point of view. Seeing it from an opposing side may help to understand the issue better. Try to resolve the dispute or conflict to allow for less stress in the working environment and, therefore, allow for better communication and patient care in the office.

Culture, Ethnicity, and Race

Culture is defined as a common set of behaviors such as language and customs, beliefs, values, and attitudes shared by a group of people. Understanding the concepts of culture, ethnicity, and race is necessary to gain insight into people of different backgrounds. A culture's belief about health and sickness affects the delivery of care. Therefore, it is vital that dental professionals recognize the influence of a patient's culture on their treatment decisions. Barriers between the professional and the patient occur when differences are not understood or accepted. This may lead to misunderstandings that can turn into serious mistakes. In addition, the patient who has an unpleasant experience will not want to return to your office.

It is important that dental assistants avoid stereotyping individuals according to their cultures, customs, traditions, or beliefs. Each patient is to be treated with respect and care. Make no assumptions about the behaviors and paradigms of the multicultural patient populations you serve. According to the U.S. Census Bureau, vast numbers of immigrants have relocated to the United States and Canada in recent years; many speak English as their second language. It would benefit any dental assistant to study the geographical data, cultural beliefs, and practices that have shaped the paradigms for the patients in the region where employment is sought.

Treating everyone in the manner in which you would like to be treated may not work across cultures. Eye contact, for example, may be disrespectful in some cultures; a person may instead show respect by looking down and away. In Western culture, because doing so may be viewed as disinterest, some communication difficulties may occur. When calling a patient back for treatment, it may be appropriate in Western culture to use a patient's first name to put the patient at ease. In other cultures, it may be appropriate to use the formal name to address the patient. Mistakes can be made, and therefore, inappropriate messages can be inadvertently given to the patient. Speak with patients and discover how to give them the best care. Individuals may come to the dental office having used culturally appropriate care in the past, or they may be using it currently. Find out what is working for the patient, and then inform the doctors so they can design treatments that will achieve the best results.

Cultural competence in health care is the ability to provide care to patients with diverse values, beliefs, and behaviors. The first step in gaining skill in cultural competence is to examine and understand how your own culture affects how you feel about the world around you. Empathy, curiosity, and respect, along with awareness and acceptance of the differences in all people, is a good place to start.

Diversity means understanding that each individual has their unique identity. These differences may be culture, race, religion, ethnicity, gender, sexual orientation, sexual identity, socioeconomic status, age, physical ability, or political beliefs. Acceptance of diversity means that differences are viewed as a positive and not a negative. Diversity means that everyone contributes in a positive manner to society. Lack of acceptance of diversity leads to misunderstandings and conflicts. These conflicts can occur in the work environment. Employees who accept diversity are better able to communicate, collaborate, and share ideas.

Ethnicity is a subgroup's shared ancestry, history, linguistic characteristics, religion, and culture. Ethnicity is made relevant through ongoing social situations and encounters, as well as through people's ways of coping with the demands and challenges of life. Typically, members of an ethnic group share a sense of solidarity and a desire to preserve their culture, traditions, religion, language, or some combination of these. People usually do not become members of an ethnic group voluntarily; they are born into it. By choice or necessity, members of an ethnic group tend to marry within the group (Figure 2-11).

A race is a subgroup that is believed to be distinct in some way from other groups based on real or imagined *physical* differences (Figure 2-12). Racial classifications are rooted in the idea of biological classification of humans according to morphological features, such as skin color or facial characteristics. Individuals are usually externally classified (meaning someone else makes the classification) into a racial group, rather than choosing where they belong as part of their identity (as occurs with ethnic identity).

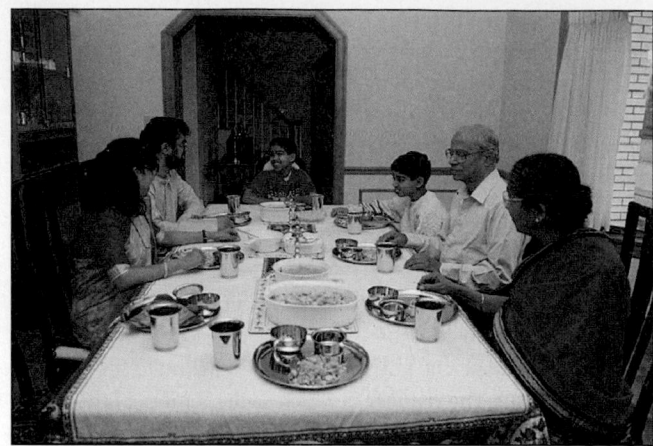

FIGURE 2-11
Mealtimes are often opportunities for families to share traditions and cultural customs.

Conceptions of race, as well as specific racial groupings, are often controversial due to their impact on social identity and how those identities influence an individual's position in social hierarchies.

Cultural subgroups are also based on other individual differences such as gender, age, profession and occupation, political/ideological beliefs and attitudes, nationality, socioeconomic status, skills, education, residence, geographic location, and family structure. One or more of these (or other distinctions) may be more salient or important to an individual than ethnicity (Figure 2-12).

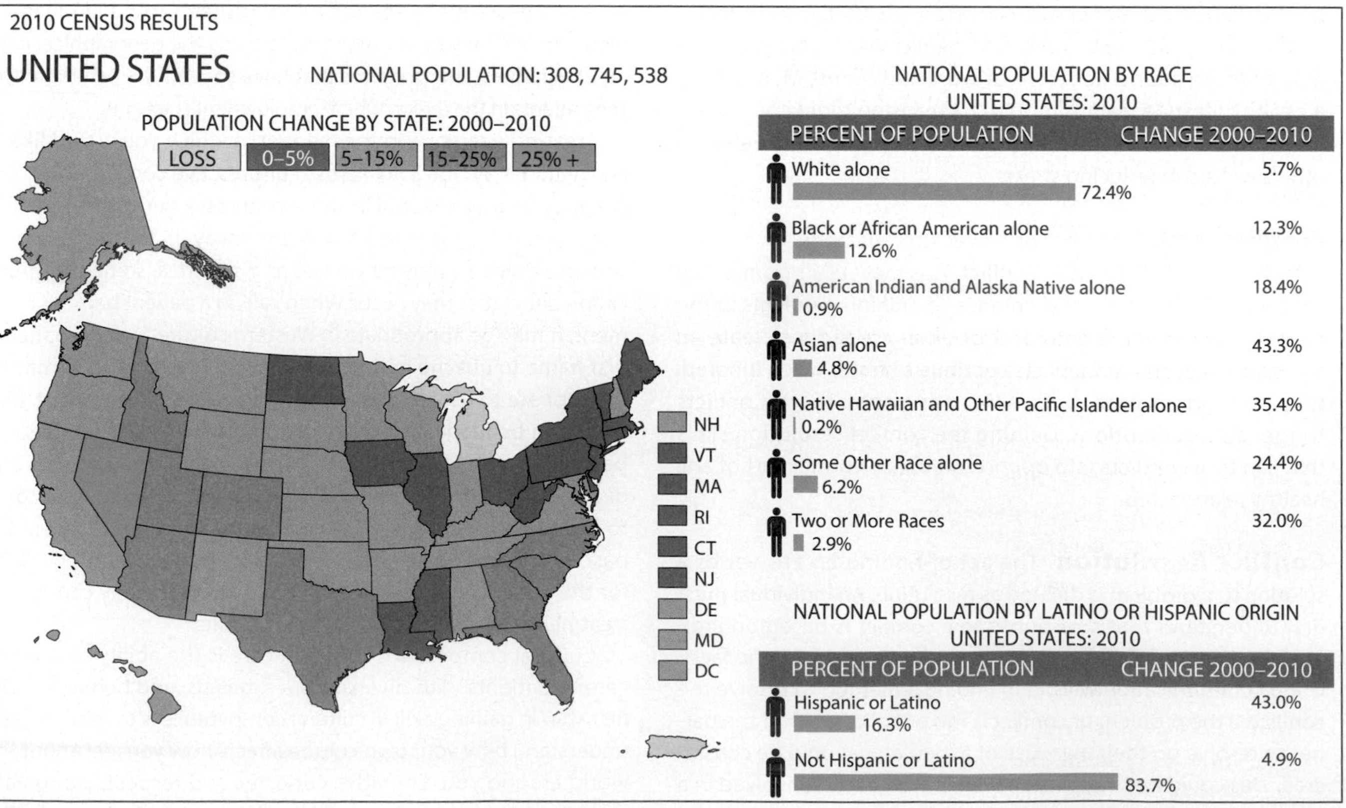

2010 CENSUS RESULTS

UNITED STATES

NATIONAL POPULATION: 308, 745, 538

POPULATION CHANGE BY STATE: 2000–2010

| LOSS | 0–5% | 5–15% | 15–25% | 25% + |

NH
VT
MA
RI
CT
NJ
DE
MD
DC

Courtesy of U.S. Census Bureau, July 1, 2010

NATIONAL POPULATION BY RACE
UNITED STATES: 2010

PERCENT OF POPULATION	CHANGE 2000–2010
White alone	5.7%
72.4%	
Black or African American alone	12.3%
12.6%	
American Indian and Alaska Native alone	18.4%
0.9%	
Asian alone	43.3%
4.8%	
Native Hawaiian and Other Pacific Islander alone	35.4%
0.2%	
Some Other Race alone	24.4%
6.2%	
Two or More Races	32.0%
2.9%	

NATIONAL POPULATION BY LATINO OR HISPANIC ORIGIN
UNITED STATES: 2010

PERCENT OF POPULATION	CHANGE 2000–2010
Hispanic or Latino	43.0%
16.3%	
Not Hispanic or Latino	4.9%
83.7%	

FIGURE 2-12
United States population of 308,745,538 divided into racial/ethnic categories, with the population changes by state noted (from U.S. Census Bureau, July 1, 2010).

Multicultural Interaction

Learn as much as you can about your patient's culture. During interactions, consider how family and social networks, dietary patterns, body image, and beliefs about the origins of disease will affect the outcome of care. Find out if there is a specific illness that affects your patient's population. For example, Native Americans and Hispanics are at higher risk for the development of diabetes.

Gender plays an important role in many cultures. Female patients in some cultures may want to be treated only by a female practitioner. Some cultures practice culturally competent forms of health care. Does the patient practice folk medicine? If so, encourage dialogue about the patient's self-treatment strategies because they may be using harmful home remedies.

Be aware of body language, and follow the patient's lead. Many cultures regard direct eye contact as disrespectful, while in others it shows attentiveness or concern. The same is true for smiling. In America, the smile is an expression of happiness, while in China, a smile may mean sadness or that one is uncomfortable. The Japanese may smile to hide emotion.

When interacting with culturally diverse patients, avoid the use of gestures. For example, the hand signal for OK (thumb and index finger forming a circle) has different meanings in different countries. In the United States, the gesture means everything is fine; in France, it is the symbol for the number zero, and in Japan it is the symbol for money. Americans think nothing if they see someone with their hands in their pockets, while in Germany, Indonesia, and Austria, this is considered a rude gesture. In Western culture, the belief is that the caregiver is to tell us everything, and that the informed patient should be included in the health care decisions. Many other cultures rely on the caregiver to make decisions without consulting the patient.

Patients who speak limited English present a challenge. A family member or friend may be asked to interpret, but be aware that the patient may avoid speaking freely with family or friends. By following a few simple guidelines, you will be able to communicate more effectively with your patient:

- Face the patient directly and speak slowly but not loudly; in some cultures, loudness means you are angry.

- Use appropriate gestures, pictures, and facial expressions. Watch the patient's response and body language for indications that they understood what was said.

- Avoid slang expressions. They may make sense to you but will only confuse the patient.

- Do not clutter the conversation with unnecessary words. Keep it simple, but get your point across.

- Paraphrase and summarize often; try to say the same thing at least two different ways.

- Avoid closed ended questions which require a simple yes or no from the patient. The patient may say yes when asked something but in reality may not understand.

- Ask open-ended questions which require the patient to summarize what you said and state it back to you.

TABLE 2-6 Resources for Communicating with Patients from Different Cultures

ALTA Language Services, *http://www.altalang.com/*
CAL Center for Applied Linguistics, *http://www.cal.org/*
Cross Cultural Health Care Program (CCHCP), *http://www.xculture.org/*
Indian Health Service, *http://www.ihs.gov/*
Hispanic Dental Association (HAD), *http://www.hdassoc.org/*
Massachusetts General Hospital—Working with an Interpreter: Tips for Stronger Outcomes, *http://www2.massgeneral.org/interpreters/working.asp*
National Center for Cultural Competence, *http://nccc.georgetown.edu/*
NMA Cultural Competence Primer, *http://www.npsf.org/askme3/pdfs/NMAPrimer.pdf*
Office of Minority Health, *http://minorityhealth.hhs.gov/*
Proctor and Gamble (several courses and resources for patient education and language), *http://www.dentalcare.com/*

Courtesy of Janet Jaccarino

The use of a professional interpreter may be necessary, especially if the dialogue concerns a serious issue. Make sure that the interpreter is trained specifically in your patient's language; someone from Spain may have trouble with subtleties spoken by someone from Puerto Rico. Follow these simple guidelines even if you have the advantage of an interpreter:

- Everyone in a conversation should face each other.

- Look directly at the person to whom you are speaking, not the interpreter.

- Before the translation, brief the interpreter. Try not to talk for more than two minutes without stopping to give the interpreter time to translate.

- Allow the interpreter time to think in their language before they translate.

- As the interpreter is speaking, observe the patient for signs of confusion, comprehension, agreement, or disagreement.

Table 2-6 lists several of the many resources available to help you interact more effectively with your patients from other cultures.

Written Communication

Written communication is used on a daily basis. One advantage written communication has over verbal communication is that the reader has control over how slow or quickly the information is read and understood; the material can be reviewed as many times as necessary. On the other hand, spoken communication allows you to enhance the message by the tone of your voice, body language, and facial expression. Writing does not allow for face-to-face interaction, so you must rely on word choice, punctuation, and sentence construction to convey your message.

Dental offices use both formal and informal writing depending on the message and the audience. Be sure to use the proper format for the message and audience. For instance, a referral letter to a specialist should be formal and set up like a business letter, while a thank you letter to a patient for a referral can be informal. Remember, whatever the format, your correspondence should be professional, clear, and easy to read.

Letters

Letters may be sent to patients, insurance companies, or other professionals. Letters such as referrals to specialists, postoperative reports, and narrative reports to insurance companies are considered legal documents serving as proof that the standard of care was followed. Your practice may write letters to patients to welcome them to the office, to introduce new staff, to thank them for a referral, to remind them of recare, or to collect delinquent or unpaid accounts.

Newsletters

Newsletters and fliers are a form of marketing sent to the community as well as potential patients. Information in the newsletter can promote your practice by introducing staff and office activities, providing educational articles about dental health, or reporting on new trends in dentistry. This type of advertising is subject to legal and ethical regulations by the American Dental Association and your state's dental practice act.

Patient Records

Good record keeping allows the office to remind patients of dental treatment needs. Should there be any question about treatment, records may be held up to judgment in court. The patient chart is considered a legal document and is owned by the dentist, not the patient. The patient paid for the diagnosis of the dentist, not the content of the chart. It is essential that all patient records be written in pen and kept organized, consistent, and complete. Sloppy, disorganized, and illegible records are a major issue in risk management. The following list is part of the patient record:

- **Personal Information**— includes the patient's name, address, phone number, social security number, credit card numbers, and insurance company. Medical history includes physician information, medical conditions and diseases, medications the patient is taking, and lifestyle habits. Dental history consists of chief complaint, risk assessment, and previous treatment. The Health Insurance Portability and Accountability Act (HIPAA) ensures protection and security of all personal information.

- **Treatment Plan**—lists recommendations and options for proposed treatment written in a sequence of appointments. After the patient accepts the treatment plan, the patient, or if necessary a legal guardian, and a representative of the dental practice both sign their acceptance.

- **Clinical Record**—consists of the progress notes of services provided at each patient visit. The clinical record documents all treatment including recommendations as well as patient failure to follow instructions. It is necessary to record all contact with the patient, including cancellations and any missed appointments. Employee name or number should be included after every notation entered.

Office Policy Manual

The office policy manual provides information and guidelines to employees on the practice's operations. The manual may include a mission statement, office policy, protocol(s), and job descriptions. As a new employee of a dental office, you may be asked to sign a document stating that you have read the policy manual and that you understand what the office's policies are.

Electronic Messaging

E-mail, texting, and any other forms of electronic messaging are brief memos that can be sent quickly within the office or to others who have a computer or electronic device. Because this type of communication is not secure, confidential information should not be sent in this manner.

Script Development

There are standard scripts that occur in every practice. For clarity, what you say should be logical, concise, and well organized. A written script ensures that no important information is omitted and all questions are asked. Scripts are used when scheduling appointments by phone or direct patient interaction, such as case presentation and making financial arrangements.

 **HIPAA—Remember, these records are confidential. By law, information in patient records is considered "privileged information" and must not be shared outside of the office.**

Effective Writing

Effective writing will result in a message that is well organized, clear, and easily understood. Being concise, or as brief as possible, ensures that the main idea does not get lost in the words. Use the following rules to ensure your writing is effective.

- **Organization**—Planning is part of the process. Your writing should be specific for your audience and their level of education, understanding, and attitude about the subject. Decide what your main theme will be, gather all of your facts, and make sure they are accurate. Create an outline to provide a logical framework for your writing. The first sentence should set the tone, introduce the topic, and gain the attention of the reader. In the body, continue to make your point with well-developed dialogue. Close by clearly restating your opening point and include contact information. If presenting in front of an audience, ask if there are any questions.

- **Clarity**— Say what you want to say as simply as possible using short, familiar words that are easy to read and understand. Use dental terminology sparingly unless you are writing to another dental professional who will understand the terms. Construct your sentences carefully: *This morning I ate pancakes in my pajamas* as opposed to *In my pajamas this morning, I ate pancakes.* This line illustrates how the placement of words in a sentence can lead to a misunderstanding.

- **Tone**— Tone should reflect your intent, your attitude toward the reader, the subject of the message, and the professionalism of the office. Tone will also affect how the reader takes in the meaning of a message. Match the tone to the subject and audience. "Hey Dude" may not be the proper opening for a letter of referral, but it may perfectly acceptable for an e-mail to a friend.

- **Length**— You do not want the reader to work hard to get your message. Your point can be lost in a sentence that is too long; use punctuation or make two sentences. On the other hand, too many short sentences can make reading choppy and disconnected. Alternate long and short sentences to make reading smooth and interesting; short sentences can work effectively to accentuate or stress a point. Extra words and phrases distract the reader and encourage skimming, which may lead to misinterpretation of the message.

- **Review**—Proofread to make sure your work is complete, brief, accurate, and neat. Check for grammar, punctuation, spelling, and use of capital letters. When writing electronically, even if you use spell check, look it over again. A good idea is to have someone else read it. If you have trouble with certain words such as *affect* and *effect*, or *their* and *there*, use the dictionary or a grammar check.

Preparing a Dental Presentation

The American Dental Education Association (ADEA) Core Competencies for Entrance into the Allied Dental Professions suggests that our responsibility as professionals is to share the latest information found through research with our peers and the public. Sharing information increases the knowledge base with the community and allows dentistry to evolve and benefit other professionals and the public they serve. One of the best ways to communicate the scientific information we learn is through the oral presentation.

Types of Oral Presentations

An oral presentation is ideal for sharing a large amount of scientific information with many people in a small amount of time. Round table discussions, poster sessions, and table clinics are three types of oral presentations. Keep in mind that the sponsor for your presentation, such as your state's dental assistants association, may specify guidelines for each type of presentation. If you are presenting at a professional association meeting, it is critical that you follow the rules and format the association requires; otherwise your presentation may be disqualified.

Round Table Discussion A round table discussion is an informal exchange of ideas with other professionals about a particular topic. This format is limited to the number of people that can fit around a table, usually 8–10 participants. When preparing a round table discussion, consider the following: time allotment, the facilitator, the role of the participants, and the format of any handouts or visual aids.

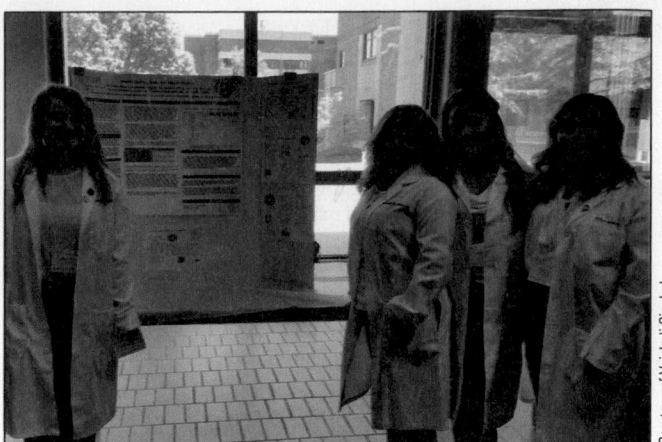

FIGURE 2-13
Poster presentation.

Courtesy of Vaishali Singhal

Poster Session Poster sessions last 1–3 hours and are usually presented at professional meetings using a visual format that includes artwork such as photos, graphs, and bullet lists displayed on a poster board representing your topic (Figure 2-13). No audio and/or video is allowed during a poster session presentation. Presenters discuss the visual display and answer any questions. The size of the audience can vary as those attending the meeting might only stop at presentations covering topics that are of interest to them.

Table Clinic A table clinic is a verbal and visual presentation on a specific topic limited to one or two presenters with a time limit of 5–7 minutes. Table clinics are often presented at professional association meetings or health fairs. Visuals that aid the presentation include slides, graphs, and pictures fastened to a tri-fold display board set atop a table; audio is not allowed. Samples, models, products, and materials are permitted, but the product manufacturer and name must be covered to avoid possible promotion of a specific product.

Preparing a Table Clinic Presentation

Table clinic presentations are the most common method of presentation at conferences and community events. Preparation is a big part of success, and the concepts discussed here can be applied to any of the ways you communicate information.

Topic Selection The first step in preparing a table clinic is to choose a topic. If you are presenting for a specific sponsor, the topic may have already been chosen for you. If not, be sure to pick one that interests you as well as your audience. It is hard to be excited about something that is not relevant. However, the most important factor is to tailor your topic to your audience: their needs, interests, and knowledge. For example, use of sealants may not be an ideal choice for an audience at an elder facility where most of the residents wear dentures. If your message is not specific for your listeners, then your talk will have little meaning. Any choice of topic should be current and useful. Topics

TABLE 2-7 Examples of Table Clinic Topics

1. PUBLIC AND COMMUNITY HEALTH

Dental health education, fluoridation, community projects, holistic health

2. CLINICAL PROCEDURES

Aspects of patient education and management, clinical skills, expanded functions, office emergencies, oral physiotherapy, prevention tactics, practice management, or interior design

3. BASIC and/or DENTAL SCIENCE

Periodontics, oral pathology, radiology, physiology, head and neck anatomy, pharmacology and therapeutics, morphology and occlusion, nutrition

4. RESEARCH

Utilization and/or interpretation of project design, microbacterial analysis, statistics and methodologies related to dentistry

5. ALTERNATIVE CAREER OPPORTUNITIES

Utilization of services in hospitals or extended care facilities for the physically or mentally challenged or the aged; in office settings dedicated to educating patients and providing preventive services; in the school setting; in the education setting as administrator, instructors, formulators of curricular aids and activities; in the industrial setting planning and helping to implement preventive dental programs

6. FOREIGN AND INTERNATIONAL HEALTH CARE SYSTEMS

Comparison among various health care systems and agencies regarding dental health and preventive care, analysis of the varying needs of specific groups, descriptions of educational levels and designated functions of dental health professionals and personnel

Adopted from ADHA Annual Session Table Clinic Categories

Courtesy of Janet Jaccarino

may include a new product, material, technique, or procedure. Ideas for topics can be found in journals, textbooks, magazines and newspapers, the library, or a bookstore. Some topic suggestions are listed in Table 2-7.

Finding and Organizing the Information Remember 5–7 minutes is not a long time. If your subject is broad, you may need to select only one or two ideas to refine and narrow the focus to make your presentation as direct as possible. You will need to prioritize the most important and beneficial information. For example, "Nutritional Medicine in Dentistry" is a broad topic, but you can narrow your focus by concentrating on just one part of nutrition such as the use of vitamin C in the prevention of periodontal disease. A good way to narrow down a topic is to form a question.

The best way to search for information on your topic is to use evidence-based decision making. Remember, the process of searching involves forming clinical questions using the PICO method. In some cases, you will just be searching for information and not comparing treatment of products. In this case you can eliminate the C in PICO to form the question.

P Patient problem (periodontal disease)

I Intervention being considered (vitamin C)

C Compare—is there another product that your first choice can be? (in this case there is no comparison)

O Outcome—What do you want to happen? (prevent periodontal disease)

Example—Will the use of vitamin C contribute to the prevention of periodontal disease?

Key words for searching—vitamin C, prevention and periodontal disease.

If your topic is too new or if there is not enough information available, you may need to broaden your topic. Broadening is easier than narrowing; just think about your topic in a broader sense. Examine a parallel association, or other issues that relate to the topic.

Example—What are the effects of vitamin C deficiency to gingival tissue?

You could also look at public opinions or legislation involving your topic.

When searching for scientific information, remember to use evidenced based decision making (EBDM) principles and reliable websites such as the National Library of Medicine database or Pub Med. You may be able to contact an agency and/or a company directly. Dental associations are dependable sources for information. The American Dental Association (ADA) and any of the other dental specialty associations, like the American Academy of Periodontology (AAP), the American Dental Assistants Association (ADAA), and the American Dental Hygienists' Association (ADHA), are just a few. If your presentation is required to express a point of view, consider interviewing an expert such as another dental professional or a government official.

Planning and Organization Planning is a major part of being prepared and organized. It will help prioritize the most important information, ensure that nothing is left out, and make your presentation effective and successful. Establish goals and deadlines, and if you are working with another person, divide the tasks. Planning may even decrease nervousness when you present.

Once your research is complete, you will need to organize the information. Start with a written outline of a detailed script including an introduction, body, and conclusion. Write out exactly what you will say and make sure to reference all your sources for information and artwork. Putting the words on paper allows you look over the speech and revise if necessary. Check for wording that may be confusing or that jumps from one topic to another. Choose the most effective way to explain difficult ideas. As you create your detailed script, question yourself to make sure nothing is left out and the presentation is easy for your audience to follow (Table 2-8).

Practice to be an expert with the information, memorize your speech, and be ready to answer any questions the audience may have. Practice in front of others and ask for their feedback. Videotape your speech, self-evaluate, and be sure to stay within the allotted time. It may be a good idea to watch someone else present a table clinic before presenting your own (Table 2-9).

Creating Good Visuals

When you are satisfied with your speech, you will need to create visuals that will complement your presentation. You will explain most of what the topic is about in your speech; visuals are meant

TABLE 2-8 Creating a Detailed Script

Introduction • Used to gain attention and establish a rapport with the audience • Create an overview, main ideas	1. Does my introduction relate to my presentation? 2. Will my intro motivate and interest the audience about the topic?
Body • Main ideas should flow in a sensible sequence • Keep to a minimum—three ideas may be all that people can remember	1. Is the pace of the lesson correct? 2. Have I covered the major points of the lesson? 3. Have I allowed time for pausing between major points and for student thinking and note taking? 4. Have I planned with clarity, organization, and variety in mind? 5. Does the lecture flow, and are the transitions placed appropriately?
Conclusion • No new material • Do not reteach material • Restate main ideas	1. Have I planned for a few minutes for a wrap-up of the lesson? 2. Did I allow time for audience questions? 3. Does the lesson fit the time allotted? 4. Did I practice?

Courtesy of Janet Jaccarino

TABLE 2-9 Planning for the Table Clinic

- Establish goals and deadlines, divide the tasks.
- Research the topic.
- Write outline (Introduction, Body, Conclusion).
- Reference all sources including any artwork used for display.
- Edit the information.
- Build interesting visuals to complement the information.
- Create interesting handouts.
- Know the information and be prepared to answer questions from the audience.
- Memorize and practice.
- Use carefully structured wording so that your presentation is spontaneous.
- Practice in front of others to decrease nervousness, keep to 5–7 minutes, ask for feedback.
- Videotape practice sessions and critique yourself.
- Attend other table clinic presentations.

Courtesy of Janet Jaccarino

to highlight the major point(s) of your presentation. There are a wide variety of ways you can add to your words. You can incorporate things such as photographs, diagrams, symbols, graphs, flowcharts, tables, and art. All visuals should be large enough to be seen at a distance and be of the highest quality. You want your audience listening to what you are saying instead of struggling to figure out the meaning of a blurry picture.

Backdrop

Selection of your **backdrop** is important for the overall appearance of your presentation. A tri-fold board may be the best choice as it can display a lot of information and is easily transported (Figure 2-13). Before setting anything on the board, first design your visuals on paper. If you are traveling, be sure to protect your board with a plastic covering or a portfolio case.

Title

Place the title (theme) of the presentation at the top and in the center of the board. The title should be short and get the attention of your audience, such as *Going Green in Dentistry*. Each supporting graphic should have title descriptors below the image. Think of the title of each graphic as a newspaper headline. It

should be simple, short, less than 10 words, and on target to inform the audience about the presentation. Cute or funny titles do not appear professional and may even detract or take away from the presentation. Some of the best titles ask or answer questions.

Content

Use clear, concise language and avoid slang expressions and jargon. Too many words give the visual a cluttered, overcrowded look. It is easier for the audience to read a bulleted format with key words or phrases instead of full sentences. Place the most important elements at eye level. Balance the visual weight of text and graphics so that everything is even; for example, a top heavy or lopsided display can be distracting. Balance will enable the eye to travel from one point to another as you speak. Most people read from left to right and top to bottom, so it is best to set information and graphics in this logical order. Consider using numbers, letters, or arrows, to make the sequence of information obvious. Keep your visual simple, clean, and readable. Remember to proofread to avoid embarrassment.

Design

Use of lettering, color, and space are design characteristics that create visual impact.

- **Lettering**—The audience should be able to read from a distance. Start with 14-point type and work your way up. If there is not enough room to fit all the text, then shorten the content rather than change the type size. Be consistent with your lettering. Choose uniform, straight letters, without curls. Arial or Times New Roman are the preferred fonts. Use headings and subheadings to guide the reader. Capital letters are difficult to read and should only be used in headings. Width, texture, color, boldface, and underlining are other ways to distinguish words.

- **Color**—Color is known to have an effect on emotion. Red and yellow are stimulating while blue and green create calm. Wise use of color can emphasize major points, show differences, and indicate changes. Black and white or dark on light and vice versa create interest. While adding a great deal to your visuals, color can also be distracting. Use of overly bright colors attracts attention but can wear out the reader's eye. Neon and rainbow are inappropriate for a professional presentation. Use only two or three colors and keep a consistent pattern. Otherwise, the viewer may spend time trying to figure out the pattern rather than absorbing the information. When thinking about color, remember that some people may have a problem distinguishing one color from another, most commonly, an inability to distinguish green from red.

- **Space**—The use of "white space" or open space between the elements of your poster creates balance. Space can be used to separate and emphasize information. A few large areas divided into smaller sections are easier to read. Cautious use of white space is important. Too much white space causes the eye to wander. Too little looks crowded and may cause confusion. For example, too little space between words or lines makes text difficult to read, and too much space disconnects the text. A caption placed too close to an image looks cluttered and makes the words hard to read. If the words are too far from each other or pictures, the design flow is lost and the idea becomes disconnected. Be creative, be consistent, and check your design with a smaller version of your work.

Handouts

Handouts will make your presentation complete. A good quality handout will serve to outline, summarize, and reinforce your presentation. It is important that a handout match the presentation. Include your name and affiliation, if any. Add the title, the date, and a brief summary of the presentation. Do not forget references for all of the information and the visuals that you used. It is also important to include your contact information in case the audience would like to ask questions or would like additional information about the topic. All of the design characteristics discussed earlier in this lesson can be applied to your handout.

Wait to distribute the handout until the end of your presentation to avoid audience members reading instead of listening. Finally, it is often difficult to know the number of people in your audience, but if possible, try to have enough handouts for everyone that will be attending your presentation. If the group is small, you will have more opportunity to interact and you may want to give a short pretest or ask questions in the handout to determine the audience's knowledge about the topic. If the audience is large, interaction may not be possible.

Delivering the Presentation

Once you have prepared your speech and created good visuals to compliment the message, it is time to present the information. As discussed before, being prepared is the key to a successful presentation. Get enough sleep the night before the presentation,

and the next day eat a healthy breakfast. Try to avoid caffeinated beverages because they may make you hyperactive and add to nervousness.

Dress

How you dress sends a message as clear as your words. To make a good impression, it is important to look professional. Dress comfortably but appropriately and use a nametag so people know who you are. Business professional attire is considered appropriate for professional presentations. Business professional attire includes dress pants or business skirts that are at or below the knee in navy, black, gray, or brown. Trouser socks or stockings and conservative matching pumps with heels of 1.5 inches in height are considered appropriate business attire. A light-colored blouse or shirt with sleeves and a simple collar should be paired with the pants or skirt. A suit jacket may be worn if considered appropriate for the presentation environment. Jewelry should be minimal. Earrings, if worn, should be small studs. Nose rings and tongue rings are not considered appropriate for a business presentation.

Body Language

Being nervous is normal, but remember that the audience has come to hear you speak and they are on your side. Accept how you feel and know that being prepared will decrease this feeling. Try to relax, be natural, and avoid staged or planned gestures. Avoid placing your hands in your pockets and keep them by your side Speak directly to the audience and use eye contact to create a relationship. Instead of trying to look at the entire audience, pick several faces around the room and imagine that you are talking to them. Remember when speaking stand to one side of your board so you do not block the visual.

Speaking

Just like a stage performer, rehearse your delivery so you do not mumble your words. Use voice control and voice projection to be sure you are reaching those in the back of the audience. Pace your delivery: speaking too slowly gives the impression you are nervous and not sure of the material, while speaking too quickly does not allow the listener time to digest the information. Pause to give your listeners time to make notes. Unlike reading, the listener cannot go back to clarify what was said. If they are confused at the start of the presentation, then they may be confused for the rest of the talk. Repeating what was said using different words and the use of visuals will reinforce what you say. Although interaction with the audience is ideal, too much can be disruptive; for example, save questions and answers until the end so as not to disrupt the flow of the presentation. Avoid wrapping up your talk with the expression "in conclusion." Such expressions may signal to the audience that it is time to get ready to leave instead of paying attention to your final points.

Chapter Summary

The role of the dental assistant includes making dental treatment comfortable for patients of any culture or generation by understanding those patients' psychological backgrounds and their paradigms concerning dentistry. Appropriate communication is the key to successful interaction. A dental assistant should have skills in listening and in verbal and nonverbal communication, and should know how to overcome defense mechanisms to meet patient needs. Stress is a part of life in the dental office; however, recognizing its causes, and being able to acknowledge and resolve conflict, will aid in keeping the office running smoothly.

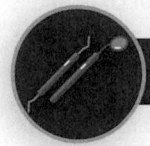

CASE STUDY

Li Min is a dental assistant in Dr. Velez's office. The office is currently working on dental teamwork, and Li cannot stay focused. In the past, Li was involved and ready to accomplish the task at hand, but now everyone has noticed that Li is no longer acting as part of the team. What the rest of the dental team members do not know is that Li's husband has left her and she is about to have her home repossessed. Li has not shared this with anyone at the office. According to Maslow's hierarchy of needs, what must happen in Li's life before she can be emotionally present in the discussions and seek to become part of the team again at the office?

Case Study Review

1. What levels of Maslow's hierarchy of needs are addressed in this scenario?

2. According to Maslow, is it true that the basic levels of need must be met before seeking a higher level?

3. At what level in the hierarchy of needs does dental office teamwork belong?

Review Questions

Multiple Choice

1. The science of the mind and the reasons people think and act as they do is _____.
   a. communication
   b. psychology
   c. paradigm
   d. encoding

2. A person's acquired belief system is their _____.
   a. communication
   b. psychology
   c. paradigm
   d. encoding

3. The level on Maslow's hierarchy at which a person has fully achieved their potential is which of the following?
   a. Esteem or Ego
   b. Social
   c. Self-Actualization
   d. All of these

4. Which of the following are the correct sequence of steps in the learning ladder?
   a. unawareness, awareness, interest, involvement, action, and habit
   b. interest, unawareness, awareness, involvement, action, and habit
   c. involvement, unawareness, awareness, interest, action, and habit
   d. interest, involvement, awareness, unawareness, action, and habit

5. That people learn from their own experience, by observing the actions of others, and by the results of those actions, and that changes take place because the environment, information, and behavior all affect one another, are the main concepts of which of the following?
   a. transtheoretical model
   b. social learning theory
   c. health belief model
   d. Both a and b

6. The stages of change theory recognizes that a person may relapse into undesirable health behaviors. If relapse occurs, it is important to remain positive and shift from failure to encouragement.
   a. Both statements are true.
   b. Both statements are false.
   c. The first statement is true; the second statement is false.
   d. The first statement is false; the second statement is true.

7. Health behavior theories can be used during oral health education to do which of the following?
   a. Assess a patient's readiness to change behavior
   b. Provide a standard way to determine health messages
   c. Explain the benefits of oral self-care
   d. Determine which type of toothbrush method to teach the patient

8. Which of the following is an example of how adolescents and teens may be affected by social needs on Maslow's hierarchy?
   a. Peer pressure and practicing unhealthy behaviors
   b. Exhibiting dental fear
   c. Feelings of competency
   d. None of these

9. Which of the following is not a commonly used communication channel?
   a. auditory
   b. visual
   c. kinesthetic
   d. All of the these are commonly used communication channels.

10. Intimate spatial relationships with family members or close friends is normally within _____ inches.
    a. 3
    b. 6
    c. 10
    d. 24

11. Which of the following is correct about oral communication?
    a. It is not important for the dental professional to be able to communicate effectively with patients.
    b. Effective oral communication between the patient and the dental professional increases the chance of being understood.
    c. Good oral communication results in decreased chances of litigation.
    d. Good oral communication results in a poor patient to dental professional relationship.

12. Most college students spend about _____ percent of their time listening.
    a. 25
    b. 35
    c. 50
    d. 70

13. Communication is said to be _____ percent verbal and_____ percent nonverbal.
    a. 50; 50
    b. 30; 70
    c. 70; 30
    d. 20; 80

14. What is the term used to describe communication that takes place without words?
    a. gestures
    b. expressions
    c. nonverbal communication
    d. perceptions

15. A patient who is not comfortable in the dental chair and is not verbally expressing it may exhibit physical signs such as a_____.
    a. relaxed look on their face
    b. smile on their face
    c. grimace on their face
    d. relaxed grip on the arms of the dental chair

16. Which of the following is correct regarding work related conflicts?
    a. When a work related conflict arises, it is best to ignore the conflict as it will usually resolve itself.
    b. Good communication is not important in order to resolve a work related conflict.
    c. Conflicts in the office do not cause stress since everyone goes home at the end of the day.
    d. Unhappy employees are one of the reasons that stress can occur in the dental office

17. Which of the following is correct regarding the Baby Boomer generation?
    a. Also known as Generation X
    b. Born in the mid 1990 to early 2000s
    c. Also known as the echo generation
    d. Born after World War II

18. Culture is defined as a set of values and beliefs that are the same across a group of people; culture does not affect the delivery of healthcare.
    Select the correct response based on the statements above.
    a. Both statements are true.
    b. Both statements are false.
    c. The first statement is true; the second statement is false.
    d. The first statement is false; the second statement is true.

19. Written communication can be advantageous as compared to verbal communication because written communication can be reviewed multiple times by the readers. The voice, tone, and body language of the sender of the message are clear in the written document.

    Select the correct response based on the statements above.
    a. Both statements are true.
    b. Both statements are false.
    c. The first statement is true; the second statement is false.
    d. The first statement is false; the second statement is true.

20. The visuals for a table clinic presentation may include a backdrop. The visuals should be large enough so they can be viewed from a distance.

    Select the correct response based on the statements above.
    a. Both statements are true.
    b. Both statements are false.
    c. The first statement is true; the second statement is false.
    d. The first statement is false; the second statement is true.

Critical Thinking

1. What are some treatment management techniques for patients with dental phobias?

2. What are the advantage of verbal communication and nonverbal communication?

3. Why is it important for a dental office to have standard scripts? What are some topics that may require a script?

Key Terms

Term and Pronunciation	Meaning of Root and Word Parts	Definition
auxiliary (awg-**zil**-y*uh*-ree)	**auxilium** = help	someone who provides additional help or support
backdrop (bak-drop)	**back** = situated at or in the rear **drop** = pass in conversation	provide background for setting for an event or presentation
cognitive (kog-ni-tiv)	**cognition** = process of knowing; understanding; perceiving **-ive** = expressing function, tendency	mental processes such as reasoning, memory, perception, and judgment
directive (dih-rek-tiv)	**direct** = to manage or guide by advice **-ive** = expressing tendency, disposition, function, connection	instruction that serves to direct, guide toward an action or goal
empathy (em-puh-thee)	**em-** = to cause to be in a certain condition **pathos** = evoking a feeling of compassion, pity	understanding of another's feelings
encode (en-**kohd**)	**en** = within **code** = convert	to convert a message
evidence-based (**ev**-i-d*uh*ns) (beysd)	**evidence** = that which tends to prove or disprove an idea **based** = support	an approach that stresses the practical application of the findings of the best available current research
kinesthetic (kin-*uh*s-**the**-tic)	**kin** = to put in motion **esthetic** = perception by the senses	information received through movement such as facial expressions or gestures or lack of movement
litigation (lit-i-gey-shuh n)	**litigate** = to dispute **-tion** = indicating result	a lawsuit

(Continues)

Term and Pronunciation	Meaning of Root and Word Parts	Definition
nitrous oxide (**nahy**-tru*uh* s) (**ok**-sahyd, -sid)	**nitrosus** = containing nitrogen **oxygene** = oxygen	a colorless, sweet smelling gas that produces a feeling of euphoria when inhaled
paradigm (**par**-*uh*-dahym)	**para** = beside **digm** = to show	widely accepted belief
pharmacological (fahr-m*uh*-**kol**-*uh*-j-ic-al)	**pharmaco** = medications **logy** = study of	related to medications
psychology (sahy-**kol**-*uh*-jee)	**psych** = related to the mind **ology** = subject of study	science of the mind

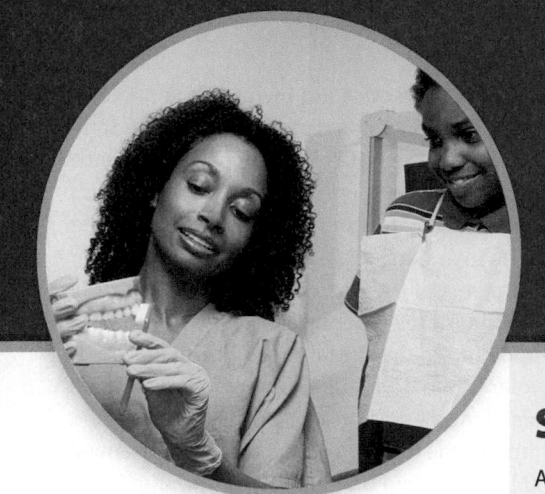

CHAPTER 3

Ethics, Jurisprudence, and the Health Information Portability and Accountability Act

Specific Instructional Objectives

At the completion of this chapter, you will be able to meet these objectives:

1. Use terms presented in this chapter.
2. Define the ethical principles.
3. Determine approaches with possible outcomes to different ethical dilemmas.
4. Summarize the Professional Code of Conduct.
5. State what is covered by the Dental Practice Act.
6. Explain how jurisprudence is related to the dental assistant.
7. Discuss jurisprudence as it relates to civil law.
8. Discuss violations of the law in a dental setting.
9. Identify the agencies that influence dental practice.
10. Explain the individual roles of OSHA, EPA, FDA, CDC, OSAP, NIOSH.
11. Discuss HIPAA law.
12. Recall HIPAA practices in the dental office.
13. Relate HIPAA compliancy practices relative to third party requests.
14. Identify the responsibilities of the dental team in relation to HIPAA.
15. Explain under what conditions HIPAA information should be shared.
16. Recall HIPAA policies and practices in technology.

Introduction

Each dental team member is faced with daily decisions that require judgments regarding legal and **ethical principles**. Maintaining professional ethical standards at all times is essential. The area of dental **jurisprudence**, the law(s) that governs dentistry, is more clearly defined than dental ethics or moral judgment(s). At a minimum, ethical behavior in the dental office must follow the letter of the law or dental jurisprudence. The consequences of not doing what should be legally done or doing what should not be done can be imposed on an individual in the form of fines or imprisonment.

Ethics for the Dental Assistant

Many discussions on the topic of ethics occur in society; particularly in professional fields such as health care. The dental assistant must understand ethics as it relates to dental practices. Ethics are often defined as the rules of conduct recognized in respect to a particular class of human actions or a particular group or culture. Each person determines their own personal **code** of ethics, one that only they can decide based upon their values. The dental professional also follows an established code of ethics such as the one defined by the American Dental Association (ADA) or the American Dental Assistants Association (ADAA). Both the personal and professional ethical standards should coincide, providing a strong foundation for which to build confidence and trust from patients, coworkers, and employers.

Personal ethics may be defined from a number of factors, each of varying importance. For some individuals, ethics are strongly formed by family values or those values which have been definite throughout childhood. Personal experiences tend to have the most influence on shaping personal ethics. Religious and political views are also key factors in individual ethical standards. The best way situations should be handled reflect professional ethics. Often, the professional code of ethics includes the standard duty of care, performing one's duties within the perimeters of legalities set by regulating agencies, contracting and accrediting bodies, and state/providence acts for the best interest of the patient.

Ethics are also shaped from cultural, societal, and environmental influences. The discussion of ethics includes issues of morality as it relates to society. From a societal viewpoint, demographics play into the overall creation of ethical standards; various places around the world carry a combination of social norms that impact ethical philosophies for that particular area. Health care ethics are not uniform in every part of the world. Ethical standards may be defined culturally, causing decisions made in one country or part of a country to differ vastly from another. These differences often surface across health care professions. Separate professions may agree on similar ethical standards; however, they may prioritize the standards differently, especially in an ethical **dilemma**.

The subjects of ethics and legalities are interrelated; however, the relationship is often confused. For some, ethical standards include acting within the perimeters of legal boundaries. Most of the time, this is true for the dental professional; however, it is important to realize that some behaviors may be legal yet not necessarily ethical. Situations such as this are termed "ethical dilemmas," discussed later in this lesson. The first step to separating ethical standards from legal standards is becoming knowledgeable (and continually educated) on the legalities of dentistry, and more importantly, specific job duties. Within the United States, the legalities change between states and are dependent upon the laws approved by each state. Dentists, hygienists, and dental assistants all have specific lists of allowable duties that can be performed in patient care, which are determined by the State Dental Practice Act (each state has its own). For example, the duties of an expanded dental assistant (EFDA) often vary among states, and if one is not carefully educated, they may easily violate

TABLE 3-1 State Dental Boards

The Laws and Regulations pertaining to dentistry are different for each state, and the information may change. It is important to learn the laws and regulations pertaining to dentistry of the state of which you are employed. Dental assistants should visit the respective state board's website for the most up-to-date information annually. Contact information for each state dental board within the United States is cited at www.ada.org/...dental.../state-dental-boards.

a state **statute**. The dental practice act includes the name of the administrative board that supervises the act, such as the State Board of Dental Examiners or the state's Dental Quality Assurance Board. The members of this board are appointed by the state's governor, normally from a list of recommendations from the state dental association. The membership usually has one lay member from the state, and the rest of the board members are normally licensed dentists. In some states, a dental assistant and/or a dental hygienist are appointed to the dental board. The dental assistant and dental hygienist are normally appointed to participate and bring their profession's viewpoints into discussions but often are nonvoting members. One function of this board is to examine applicants for dental licenses and grant licenses if the criteria are met. Another function of the board is to set guidelines for advertising for dental offices. Table 3-1 provides additional information regarding dental state board laws and regulations.

License to Practice

Each state's board grants a license to a dentist if they have met all the minimum requirements. The license is to protect the public from unqualified individuals providing dental treatment. Each state also requires the dental hygienist to become licensed. Some of the states require dental assistants to become licensed or registered in order to perform specific dental tasks. To obtain a license, an individual must meet educational and ethical requirements as well as successfully pass a written examination and a clinical practice examination as specified by the administrative board of that state or region. The requirements may vary from state to state, so if the individual wants to practice in another state, an additional license may be required. In some states, an individual who has passed the requirements for one state may apply for a **reciprocity** agreement in another state. Reciprocity is an agreement between two or more states that allows an individual licensed in one state to receive, without further examination, a similar license in the other state(s) identified in the reciprocity agreement. The reciprocity agreement normally takes place in states with adjoining borders and similar testing requirements.

The factors for revoking, suspending, or denying renewal of a license vary from state to state. Most states take action if the licensed person has a felony conviction or misdemeanors of drug addiction, moral corruption, or incompetence, or a mental or physical disability that may cause harm to patients under his or her dental care.

Dental assistants can become nationally certified by the Dental Assisting National Board, Inc. (DANB). Some states require dental assistants to be certified, licensed, or registered to perform specific functions in the dental office. The first state to grant licensure to dental assistants was Minnesota. Certification from DANB is granted after education or work requirements have been met and a written test covering general chair-side skills, radiology, and infection control has been passed. Continuing education is required to maintain current certification from DANB, and many states require continuing education to maintain registration or licensure.

Once the professional thoroughly understands their legal parameters, they can begin to understand the ethical standards. An excellent reference is the code of conduct written for dentists and auxiliaries established by the ADA. Table 3-2 provides information about the five sections of the Code of Professional Conduct. The DANB Professional Code of Conduct is outlined in Table 3-3. More references may be found on the DANB website (www.danb.org) or the ADAA website (www.dentalassistant.org).

The codes of conduct are lists of ethical responsibilities. While legal compliance is always the dental assistant's concern, remaining ethical and upholding one's responsibility with pride and consistency is the true professional standard. This concept may be understood further when discussing ethical principles. Often, a situation may call for an ethical action, one that goes

beyond "staying legal." Dental assistants must be prepared to act ethically as well as professionally in *all* situations the moment they decide to pursue dentistry as a career.

Societal Trust

As with most professions, the public will seek treatment trusting that the professionals will act legally and ethically throughout patient care. Societal trust should never be taken lightly and must be valued by the dental assistant always. When the patient seeks care from your dental office for themselves or for a loved one, that patient is looking for advice. Consciously, the dental assistant must approach advisements ethically and legally, furthering the trust of that patient. Patients appreciate professionals who value their business and have proved to be trustworthy with pleasant outcomes. Gaining societal trust is not always easy and is at times greatly affected by outside reputations or stereotypes of health care practices, people, or communities. Societal trust must not be taken for granted as the dental assistant cannot afford a negative reputation. While the dental profession is ever growing, the communities are often small. The professional dental assistant must demonstrate high standards at all times (Figure 3-1).

Confidentiality

Perhaps the most vital principal introduced in this lesson is that of confidentiality. Health care professionals cannot stress enough the importance of remaining private when handling, discussing, or documenting patient information. In fact, confidentiality is not just an ethical responsibility but also a very important legal standard. The dental assistant must make a conscious effort at all times to follow the HIPAA policy so as to consistently remain compliant and avoid violations. A breach in confidentiality will harm individual and societal trust and introduce liability to the dental office in which it occurs.

 Violations of confidentiality may not always be apparent; therefore, the dental assistant must avoid discussing patients' cases and information even when sharing stories with other

TABLE 3-2 ADA Code of Professional Conduct

"The Code of Professional Conduct is organized into five sections. Each section falls under the Principle of Ethics that predominately applies to it."
SECTION 1—PRINCIPLE: PATIENT AUTONOMY ("self-governance")
SECTION 2—PRINCIPLE: NONMALEFICENCE ("do no harm")
SECTION 3—PRINCIPLE: BENEFICENCE ("do good")
SECTION 4—PRINCIPLE: JUSTICE ("fairness")
SECTION 5—PRINCIPLE: VERACITY ("truthfulness")

Excerpted from American Dental Association Principles of Ethics and Code of Professional Conduct. Refer to www.ada.org for more details.

TABLE 3-3 Excerpted from DANB Code of Professional Conduct

"To promote quality and ethical practice and to assist DANB Individuals in understanding their ethical responsibilities to patients; employers; professional colleagues, including fellow DANB Individuals; the dental assisting profession; and the public, DANB has established the following *DANB Code of Professional Conduct*. The *DANB Code of Professional Conduct* includes a DANB Individual's responsibilities to patients, employers, colleagues, the profession, the public and DANB."

- Individual Autonomy and Respect for Human Beings
- Health and Well-Being of Patients and Colleagues
- Justice and Fairness
- Truth
- Confidentiality
- Responsibility to Profession
- Community, Society, and DANB

Refer to www.danb.org for more details.

FIGURE 3-1
Patient trust in a dental professional.

professionals. Societal trust takes time to build and one instant to demolish. Confidentiality is a critically significant ethical and legal principal.

Ethical Principles

The dental assistant must understand and remember the principles of ethics in order for him or her to perform their duties with a level of excellence each day. The ethical principles include *justice*, **veracity**, **autonomy**, **beneficence**, and **nonmaleficence**. These five principles provide a foundation consistent with the dental assistant's code of conduct and when implemented, serve as an avenue of direction in ethical situations.

Justice The dentist has a duty to treat patients in a fair and just manner. Treatment must be delivered in a manner free of prejudice. Patients may be selected based on ability to pay but may not be selected based on race, religion, creed, color, gender or gender identity, sexual orientation, national origin, or disability.

Veracity Veracity means telling the truth. Trust is established through the honesty of the dental professional. An examples of this include, providing information (including risks) to patients seeking surgical, restorative, or cosmetic care. This information includes the risks of performing or denying treatment, pain management symptoms or side effects, as well as the risks of improper oral hygiene. The patient must be informed in words that can be understood. If the patient is a minor child, the parent or legal guardian must give consent. If the parents are separated and share custody, both parents must provide authorizing consent and ability to provide emergency treatment if needed. If the parents live separately, the custodial parent must provide authorizing consent. This should be noted on the child's record. In order to give an **informed consent**, a patient or the parent/legal guardian of a patient must understand the truthful risk of having a procedure and the truthful risk of denying the procedure.

Autonomy The dental assistant must recognize the patient's right of autonomy. Patients trust the dental professional to act honestly and privately in the treatment process; however, they also expect that they have a right to determine any course of action which may affect their lives. This means that a patient, no matter how much the dental assistant has stressed the risks of denying treatment, may choose to neglect treating oral conditions; they have the ultimate right to do so.

Beneficence Beneficence is acting for the benefit of the patient. The professional dental assistant must be careful to remain legally compliant and ethically trustworthy while offering patient care, advice, or education. The dental assistant should seek to care for patients in ways that most benefit the patient. This act may be as simple as providing additional information on a procedure, assisting the patient's decisions.

Nonmaleficence As supported by the Hippocratic Oath, it is the healthcare worker's responsibility to "do no harm" to a patient. Nonmaleficence includes avoiding situations which may cause unnecessary harm to a patient. By avoiding situations that may cause physical, psychological, or physiological harm, the dental assistant is exercising nonmaleficence.

Ethical Dilemmas

A situation may arise in which the professional dental assistant must decide on what actions *should* be taken, especially when all options include remaining legal. An ethical dilemma may be defined as a situation that causes an individual to have to choose among two moral obligations of which either decision will have negative outcomes, leaving the individual to decide between the "lesser of two evils." In some cases, moral obligations require a prioritization of moral values; which value is more important than another?

How to approach an ethical dilemma may seem overwhelming initially. Which decision is the right one? What is the right choice of words? How does one avoid conflict with the dentist while fulfilling their role in patient care? Remember, keeping an open mind and slowing down the emotions enough to really contemplate the situation will allow for a good decision (Table 3-4).

TABLE 3-4 Problem Solving for an Ethical Dilemma

Determine	**Is there a dilemma?**	**Assess the situation. Are all legalities being followed; is there more than one possible option? If so, you may really have an ethical dilemma.**
Identify	What are the key values and principles involved?	Consider the situation and how it relates to ethical principles; which one(s) will you have to sacrifice?
Rank	Which values and principles are most important?	Think about which principle is prioritized over another. This will set the stage for your approach to the situation.
Develop	What action plan will you implement?	Think about a possible way or two of handling the situation; what actions will take place, and who will they affect?
Implement	Are you prepared to implement your action with professionalism?	Once you have made your decision, it is time to follow through. Remain professional and choose your words and actions carefully for a successful outcome.
Reflect	How did the plan of action go?	Assess the situation again. What steps could have been in place to prevent the dilemma? Was your action plan successful? Is there anything you could have done differently for a better outcome?

Dental Jurisprudence for the Dental Assistant

The establishment, regulation, and enforcement of laws may be collectively discussed as a science or philosophy known as jurisprudence. The role of jurisprudence in dentistry is as equally important as the ethical responsibility of a dental assistant. One should be conscious and continuously aware of the legalities associated with everyday dental practices. Jurisprudence may be compartmentalized into topic areas such as criminal law (punishment of the offender) and civil law (compensation of the victim), which further includes tort, contract, and administrative law.

Criminal Law Criminal law involves the laws written to penalize offenders who commit wrongful acts against society. Criminal law is different from civil law in that the crimes committed negatively affect the public; civil law affects an individual.

Civil Law Civil law concerns crimes which have been committed by an individual or group of individuals on another. Legal action is often initiated by an individual seeking nominal, compensatory or punitive damages. If a civil charge is brought against a dentist, he or she becomes the defendant. The *plaintiff*, the person who is bringing the charges against the defendant, must prove that a civil wrong was committed. If able to prove wrongdoing, restitution is awarded to the plaintiff in a monetary amount for any pain, suffering, and loss of wages that the dentist or dental treatment has caused. The statute of limitations defines law that sets the maximum allowable time the plaintiff has to initiate legal action from the date of an alleged offense. The law varies from state to state; some time limits run from the beginning of treatment, some from the time the accused neglect took place, and others from the time the treatment was completed.

Only 51% (majority) of jurors need to agree that the offender is responsible for the crime to pass a guilty verdict. Civil law encompasses three areas of law, which specifically address contract law, tort law, and administrative law. Each of these areas of law are discussed individually as they all three pertain to the dental assistant.

Contract Laws Contract laws have been written to protect individuals or groups such as corporations or organizations. A contract is considered to be a statement of promise between two competent persons of mutual agreement. Contracts may be implied or expressed. Implied contracts do not require a stated purpose, but rather the intentions are implied when services are sought. For example, a new patient arriving at a dental office shows that the patient wants to enter into a contract with the dentist to receive due care. An expressed contract involves some type of statement made, whether as a written statement or a verbal agreement including a telephone conversation. Through either method, a contract is legally binding and must not be breached in any way unless by mutual agreement. Professional dental assistants will be conscious of this fact and careful

to not make any promises on behalf of the dental practice and its employees while in conversation. A breach of contract involves many situations including but not limited to failure to:

- uphold confidentiality
- uphold a financial agreement
- uphold agreed services
- provide services within agreed time frame
- provide services within legal compliance
- maintain legal credentials

A contract can be terminated when one of the parties does not meet contractual obligation. Until the contract is broken, or a breach of contract occurs, the dentist is legally bound to treat the patient. The contract can be terminated if:

- The patient discharges the dentist or fails to return to the office. This can occur if the patient does not does not return for completion of care. Legally, the dentist should send a letter to the patient to document the termination of contract. The letter should be sent via certified mail with a return receipt request which should be maintained in the patient's chart.

- The patient fails to follow instructions given by the dentist. For example, a patient who had implants placed, was advised by the dentist that routine prophylaxis appointments would be necessary to maintain the implants. Despite multiple attempts, the patient does not return for the appointments.

- The dentist formally withdraws from patient care. This may occur if the dentist feels that they can no longer provide appropriate treatment to the patient or if the patient is non-compliant. In order to avoid charges of abandonment, the dentist should send a letter via certified mail with return receipt to the patient notifying the patient that the dentist is withdrawing from the case.

- The patient no longer needs treatment/all requirements agreed upon have been met. The dentist is responsible for providing treatment until the patient no longer needs treatment or the dentist has formally withdrawn from the case. For example, if an oral surgeon has seen a patient to remove four wisdom teeth and this service has been completed, and the patient has healed accordingly and therefore no longer needs this treatment, the contract would be terminated.

Tort Law Tort law concerns civil wrong doings that may have been intentional or unintentional acts of omission or commission. An example of an intentional violation would be purposefully breaching confidentiality by sharing private information of an individual outside of reasonable allowances. Unintentional wrongdoings may or may not result in a legal punishment according to whether harm had occurred or not. An example of an unintentional wrongdoing is accidentally misidentifying a patient (calling them by the wrong name or believing they are someone else). If the misstep is corrected and no harm results, then the act is considered unintentional. Should the misstep not be identified, resulting in unnecessary treatment of the individual, then the wrongdoing may result in a legal punishment.

Omission and Commission   Civil wrong doings may result from acts of omission (failure to do something that should have been done) or commission (doing something that should not have been done). The dental assistant should be cautious to avoid performing either of these wrongdoings. An example of an act of omission is a situation of when a dental assistant neglects to update a medical history, resulting in injury to the patient. An example of commission is a situation of which a dental assistant performs expanded functions without the adequate knowledge and/or the proper credentialing to perform the procedure. It is important that each dental professional understands their parameters, only performing tasks as defined by the state.

Expanded functions dental assistants work under the direct supervision of the dentist, which means the dentist must first delegate the tasks as well as remain physically present in the office at the time the procedures are performed. All functions of the dental assistant fall under the responsibility of the employer legally referred to as *respondeat superior* ("let the master answer"). As with every situation, the dental assistant must remain conscious of the legal and ethical risks involved in patient care. However, this does not mean that the dental assistant is not held responsible and cannot be sued. It merely means that a suit can be filed against either the employee or the dentist, or both. The dental assistant should be cautious because his or her actions and words at work may become binding on the employer, the dentist. Any statements either pro or con made spontaneously at the time of an alleged act can be admissible as evidence in a court of law. This is true because the principle of res gestae, which means that any events or statements related to an event are admissible as evidence in a case.

Dental assistants who perform expanded functions are advised to carry their own **malpractice**/liability insurance. The dental assistant who is a current member of the ADAA has a $50,000 professional liability insurance policy that is included as part of ADAA dues. Other organizations and professional groups offer medical malpractice/professional liability insurance and risk management information. The Health Providers Service Organization and many others are available to provide this coverage. Often, the dentist is sued because the plaintiff anticipates greater recovery in financial damages from the dentist. Additionally, dentist has the right to direct and control the employees; therefore, along with the right comes the responsibility for the consequences of their actions. If the patient suffers harm, it is due to the employer exposing the patient to his or her employee. Therefore, the dentist is required to compensate the patient for any harm that was caused.

Malpractice   Malpractice is determined when negligence results in harm to a patient due to lack of standard of care. In litigation, the accuracy of the dental record directly relates to the credibility of the professionals. If necessary, an expert witness may be called to verify malpractice litigation (Table 3-5). In other

TABLE 3-5 The Four Ds of a Malpractice Lawsuit

- *Duty*—There must be an established relationship between the dentist and the patient.
- *Derelict*—The dentist must have truly neglected patient care in some way.
- *Direct cause*—Injury has resulted from the dentist's negligent act.
- *Damages*—Damages include emotional and/or physical loss, income loss, or an accruement of medical bills.

cases, the evidence is clear, also referred to as *res ipsa loquitur* ("the act speaks for itself"). In most situations, malpractice may be avoided with adequate and effective communication between the provider and the patient.

The most prominent mistakes are lack of:

- beneficence
- professional conduct
- competence
- appropriate skill level
- legal compliancy

Abuse   Other torts or civil wrongs include abuse, assaults and defamations. Abuse is the physical or psychological harm to a person by an individual or group of individuals. There are several different types of abuse, many with differing symptoms. In instances involving children, 65%–75% of reported cases involve injury to the head and neck area. Only 1 in 14 abuse incidents of the elderly is ever brought forward to the authorities.

Abuse is not always easy to determine or recognize; however, the dental assistant should be aware of the legal and ethical responsibilities concerning abuse. An individual is expected to report suspected abuse in accordance with regulations. A situation may arise throughout one's career of which abuse is suspected, leaving the dental assistant with conflicting decisions. For example, a dental assistant may suspect abuse, but is not certain and is afraid of the implications if reported falsely or not reported at all. This situation may also present itself if a parent refuses to obtain needed dental care for their child. When the dentist and staff examine a patient, any injuries should be documented and photographs placed in the patient's files. Every state requires certain professionals and institutions to report suspected abuse. Included are providers of medical, dental, and mental health care; teachers and other education personnel; social workers; and law enforcement personnel. Reporters of abuse are immune from criminal liability provided they make the report in good faith and do so in accordance with state law.

Emotional Abuse, Domestic Violence, and Elder Abuse   Behaviors used by one person in a relationship to control the other person in the relationship are defined as emotional abuse or domestic violence. More and more individuals live in a situation where they are abused and controlled. Often they are afraid to tell anyone for fear of retaliation or losing the only security they have. In the dental office, the staff may see signs of abuse and have conversations with the patient indicating abuse. The patient may

Documentation

05/06/2019: Emergency extraction #9; patient (Samuel Scott, age 9) presents in office with partial avulsion (dislodged) of upper right central incisor. Patient accompanied by school nurse (Ms. Johnson) who was unable to contact parents. Nurse has no guardianship, but is required to seek proper care for the child if necessary during school hours. Periapical images of #8, #9, #10 were taken; fracture on cervical third of #8 is evident. Rampant caries evident in intraoral exam; noted in extraoral exam were multiple lacerations surrounding the upper lip and left temple, yellow/blue contusion evident near left eye and lower left mandible. Patient will not speak with dental staff; sensitivity of the maxilla is evident by the nonverbal behavior of the patient 200mg. Ibuprofen is given to patient for pain control; lacerations were cleaned with antiseptic and a sterile package of gauze given to the nurse, Ms. Johnson. Patient is referred to a pediatric dentist w/ recommendation of endodontic treatment Ms. Johnson indicates that abuse is suspected and requests a copy of documented findings. It was explained to Ms. Johnson that patient records could not be released without the consent of legal guardian or court order, but given the suspicious nature of the injuries a report to the child abuse hotline will be made. Ms. Johnson indicated that she understood and thanked the staff for treating the patient. Samuel Scott left the dental office escorted by Ms. Johnson.

appear withdrawn, have physical bruising, broken teeth, and other signs of injury. Abuse of persons 65 and older is defined as elder abuse and may come from care takers or family. They find it difficult to speak up for themselves, especially if the abuse comes from their family. The dental office staff should be aware of the signs of abuse and violence and be prepared to refer or assist the patient in obtaining help with the situation (Figure 3-2).

Assault and Battery Assaults are not as common in dentistry compared to other professions; however, it is important that the dental professional understand the parameters of assault and battery and how to avoid an altercation. Assault is threatening to harm another individual. Battery is physically touching an individual with the intention to harm. Technical assault and battery involves touching without the permission to do so; thus, the dental assistant should be careful when assisting the dentist. For example, a dentist assigns the dental assistant to remove stitches, but the assistant fails to obtain consent form. Should an injury result (even if minor) during the procedure, the patient may pursue assault and battery charges against the assistant! A consent form must be obtained for in dentistry prior to the start

of treatment. The obtained consent is legally required and is a standard general consent. However, some procedures that are considered to be more invasive than others, require a separate consent to be signed by the patient every time that particular procedure is performed. For example, anytime a patient requires an extraction, a separate new consent must be signed each time prior to the start of that procedure (Figure 3-3).

Defamation Defamation (also known as **slander**) is another tort law offense occurring more often than people realize. Defamation involves making false and opinionated statements about another individual or professional to a third party, harming that individual's reputation. Dental assistants must be very cautious to avoid committing defamation. Dentists are especially prone to be victims of defamation; dental workers must be careful to remain professional while in discussions concerning dentistry!

Administrative Law Administrative law involves offenses related to government agencies who have been appointed to establish, enforce, and evaluate violations of regulations such as compliancy with Occupational Safety and Health **Administration** (OSHA) standards. Administrative law also applies to state agencies with enforcement authority such as violations of the State Dental Practice Act or the State Board of Certifications (regulates credentials). Administrative laws apply to everyone, employers and employees alike. Many individuals are not careful enough and assume that the employer (e.g., a dentist) is the responsible party. In some cases, this is true; however, each and every person is responsible for knowing and following the law.

Regulatory versus Nonregulatory Agencies

It is the responsibility of the entire dental team to ensure the safety of patients and employees through compliant and ethical practices. To avoid potential confusion or misinterpretations of legal standards, the dental team must understand the differences

FIGURE 3-2
Elder abuse.

I authorize Dr. Smith and staff to perform routine and/or emergency procedures.

I further consent to the administration of medications including local anesthesia that may be deemed necessary in my treatment plan, and understand that there is an element of risk inherent in the administration of any medication.

An explanation of all complications is available upon my request from the doctor. I have had an opportunity to ask any questions I have, and have had them sufficiently answered.

I realize that regardless of possible complications, my proposed treatment is necessary and chosen by me.

I am aware that the practice of dentistry and surgery is not exact science and I acknowledge that there are no guarantees have been made to me concerning the results of the treatment.

I realize that it is mandatory to give accurate and complete medical and personal history as possible, follow any and all instructions as directed and permit prescribed diagnostic procedures.

I hereby permit photographs of me during my dental treatment, and /or to make and maintain audio, electronic and written records of said treatment. I have been informed that this is policy for all patients treated in this facility and, therefore, I hereby agree to permit my medical, dental and personal information to be entered and maintained in the facility's database. I have also been informed that any photographs of me or records for me will be considered strictly confidential

I acknowledge that payment is due at the 1st visit and only check or credit card is accepted.

All patients must allow at least two (2) weeks lead time when requesting radiographs. Radiographs will be provided as a hard copy and must be picked up and signed out by patient or provide the name and address of the dentist to whom the radiographs should be sent. By having my signature in my chart, I am adhering to all statements listed in this document.

Signed this _____ day of _____ 20_____
Patient Signature _____
Patient Printed Name _____
Witness Signature _____
Witness Printed Name _____
Date _____

FIGURE 3-3
Sample patient consent.

between **regulatory** agencies and nonregulatory (**consultative**) agencies and organizations.

Regulatory Agencies Regulatory agencies are government funded organizations given authority by Congress to identify, write, research, and implement **mandatory** requirements applicable to state and local governments. Regulatory agencies clearly define the rules and requirements corporations, businesses and individuals are expected to follow. Failure of compliance may result in legal actions of varying severities, such as fines, suspensions, licensure **revocation**, or imprisonment. Depending on the institution or business, regulatory agencies may conduct a site visit for a routine inspection or investigation. To ensure compliance, each dental office should provide a training and reference manual to facilitate the employees' understanding and expectations of conduct based on the regulated standards. The training should take place within a reasonable time frame after hiring of the new employee. Retraining should take place when duties change or privacy policies change. Many offices provide annual training to refresh all employees regarding HIPAA policies and other office policies. If an employee appears not to follow the office's privacy policies, then discussion should occur

and additional training should be provided. Continued violation of office privacy policies can be grounds for dismissal. Dentists must develop a policy for disciplining employees who violate and continue to violate the office privacy policy. This policy should be part of the office HIPAA manual.

Occupational Safety and Health Administration (OSHA) On December 30, 1970, the U.S. Department of Labor created the Occupational Safety and Health Administration (OSHA) as a result of the Occupational Safety and Health Act.

OSHA's mission is to ensure the health and safety of American workers through the prevention and management of work-related practices. Numerous regulations have been created to support the OSHA mission. Among the top 10 most referenced standards are those addressing blood-borne pathogens, hazard communications, **hazardous** wastes operations and emergency response, and personal protective equipment (PPE). In addition to mandating federal standards for the protection of working Americans, OSHA also provides employer and employees with outreach programs, training and educational resources, which are accessible through the website: www.osha.org. While all states are federally regulated by OSHA, there are 22 states and territories that maintain individually approved and federally funded state-specific OSHA plans for **implementation** by all businesses in that state. The dental assistant is expected to perform his or her duties according to OSHA standards and should not assume that only the dentist is required to do so. Compliance is the responsibility of the entire dental team, ensuring the safety of themselves as well as their patients.

United States Food and Drug Administration (FDA)
As a division of the U.S. Department of Health and Human Services, the United States Food and Drug Administration (FDA) is a large agency designed to protect and promote public health through vigorous regulation processes.

The FDA regulates human and veterinary drugs, vaccinations and biological products, food supplies, dietary supplements, cosmetics, and medical devices. In 2008, the FDA added international offices in addition to the 223 field offices and 13 laboratories located throughout the United States. Most dental equipment is FDA approved including dental instruments, laboratory equipment, and patient chairs. Only FDA approved equipment should be considered for use.

United States Environmental Protection Agency (EPA)
The Environmental Protection Agency (EPA) is another regulatory agency given authority by Congress to regulate and enforce laws designed to protect the environment and its habitants.

Created by President Nixon in 1970, the EPA initiates a great deal of research, assessments, and education in support of their mission. The EPA has most recently conducted research regarding the disposal of mercury amalgam scraps and extracted teeth. The dental assistant must be fully aware and educated on standards regulated by the EPA as it is their duty to maintain safe conditions, which will impact patient care and community health. Many patients ask questions related to fluoride and fluoride ingestion, which is also regulated by the EPA. Answering the patient's questions or concerns with accuracy and assurance will enhance societal trust.

State Regulations
Each state has the authority to regulate work practices that fall within the parameters of federal regulations. Through statutes and administrative code, states have the ability to strictly enforce regulations and define penalties. Federal standards serve as a minimum for work practices; each state has the authority to "tighten" the regulations within reason. For example, the state of Indiana has a state-approved OSHA program as well as its own EPA procedures. These may be stricter guidelines than found in neighboring states; although, both would be acting within federal guidelines. Additionally, each state has a code to regulate and define the duties, conducts and practices of various professions. The dental assistant is responsible for knowing the parameters of the state they are working in and should refer to their state's *Dental Practice Act*. Not every state defines the dental assistant's duties the same. Some functions in one state may require a credential in expanded functions and in another state performance of the same skills may be illegal. Each and every working citizen, including all members of the dental team, must adhere to the administrative code and statutes of their state.

Nonregulatory Agencies
Nonregulatory agencies often referred to as advisory or consultative agencies do not have the authority to mandate legal regulations. These organizations are most respected as an education resource, offering guidance and consultation to relevant businesses. To support and enhance public knowledge, nonregulatory agencies often conduct scientific research. There are many "advisory" organizations. It is important to understand that these agencies are for reference and planning purposes, recommending ways to maintain compliancy. Each of these organizations serve as a great resource for the dental assistant and the entire dental team committed to conducting a safe and compliant environment.

Centers for Disease Control and Prevention (CDC)
The Center for Disease Control (CDC) is a government agency and a division of the Department of Health and Human Services. The CDC is *not* a regulatory agency, but rather an *advisory* agency, making recommendations for public health safety and management. Consistent with their mission to create expertise, information, and tools for the protection of community health, the CDC is known globally for their research and scientific investigations. In addition to the 47 state health departments, the CDC has personnel in over 40 countries. The CDC provides active education supporting a wide range of health-related research; however, they are most respected for their prevention and control programs regarding infectious and **chronic** diseases. Information on the trends and research gathered from various health departments is published by CDC in the *Morbidity and Mortality Weekly Report* (MMWR). Many federal, state, and local agencies refer to the CDC guidelines as a trustworthy source to ensure updated research for which to build stronger healthcare management and disease prevention programs. In 2003, the *Guidelines for Infection Control in Dental Healthcare Settings* was released. It now serves as the foundation of acceptable infection control practices in dentistry. Currently, the CDC is involved in ensuring the safety of the public during the ongoing Covid-19 pandemic. The CDC is also responsible for setting pandemic-related infection control guidelines for the dental office setting.

Organization for Safety, Asepsis, and Prevention (OSAP)
The Organization for Safety and Asepsis Procedures (OSAP) is a not-for-profit organization founded in 1984 and dedicated to becoming the nation's leading resource for infection control and safety information in the dentistry.

OSAP is a unique team of scientists, dentists, educators, manufacturers, distributors, and other dental professionals who work together to support the guidelines as defined by the CDC standards. OSAP is a well-respected organization in the dental community, offering accessible information through publications such as newsletters highlighting the latest topic interests, training guides to facilitate infection control plans, and workbooks to provide education on how to approach the CDC guidelines. Many dental professionals become official members of OSAP, staying alerted to any new developments **relative** to dentistry.

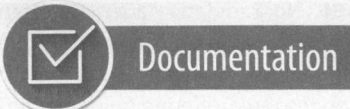

Date of incident: <u>06/27/XX</u>
Injury type: <u>Needle stick –percutaneous injury</u>
Incident location: <u>Sterilization center, near sharps container, Brand X; 25 gauge anesthetic dental needle</u>
Description of incident: <u>While attempting to clean a contaminated surgical tray, Sara Keener, a dental assistant, attempted to discard</u>
<u>a capped needle into the sharps container using one gloved hand. The needle cap caught the edge of the container and Ms. Keener</u>
<u>lost grip of the needle, which fell towards the counter top. Ms. Keener attempted to catch the needle with her left hand and the</u>
<u>cartridge penetration end perforated Ms. Keener's glove and skin on left inside palm. A small amount of blood was drawn due to</u>
<u>injury. Ms. Keener immediately de-gloved and washed the injury site thoroughly. She immediately notified Dr. Smith, the dentist on</u>
<u>staff at the time of the incident.</u>
Actions taken: <u>The Bloodborne Pathogens Exposure Plan was implemented. Ms. Keener was directed to the nearest medical center,</u>
<u>ReadyMed. Appropriate information to support adequate lab testing and results has been submitted to the advising physician by</u>
<u>Dr. Smith.</u>
Reporting Signature: Amy Johnson, CDA, EFDA - Business Manager
Date: June 27, 20XX

National Institute for Occupational Safety and Health (NIOSH)

The National Institute of Occupational Safety and Health (NIOSH) was created around the same time as OSHA. Like OSHA, NIOSH was a result of the National Occupation and Health Safety ACT of 1970 and is an affiliation of the CDC.

NIOSH is a federal institute without regulatory authority, conducting research to provide new knowledge and making recommendations in the field of occupation and health safety. NIOSH provides a great deal of information resulting from their **conduction** of research and study. The *Health Hazard Evaluation Program* is designed to assist workers by conducting workplace assessments to determine if workers are exposed to harmful and health hazardous chemicals. In dentistry, NIOSH is a great resource in matters that have dental implications such as research developments in nitrous oxide or the needle-stick injury management of anesthetic syringes, which includes proper documentation of every needle-stick incident.

American Dental Association (ADA)

With over 157,000 members, the ADA is the oldest dental society in the world. First founded in New York by 26 dentists in 1859, the ADA's mission is *"to advance oral health in the United States and abroad"* as well as advance science in dentistry. The ADA is **tripartite** with national, state, and local organizations. Dentists may become members at the national level and serve as advocates through state and local memberships. The ADA has a wide range of educational resources to support their mission and continue their dedication to dental public health. Operating under the **auspices** of the ADA, the Commission on Dental Accreditation (CODA) is the national accrediting body for various dental and allied dental education programs as recognized by the U.S. Department of Education. The ADA seal of acceptance has been given to over 300 dental products, which are determined to be safe and effective for public use. Dental assistants may talk to their patients about choosing over-the-counter dental aids having the ADA seal.

The dentist and the dental team members must be responsible to maintain accurate, up-to-date patient records. Accurate records of all transactions must be kept by the dental office for quality assurance and validity. The dental office personnel must never forget to deliver and obtain the signed HIPAA form *before* the initial exam is implemented. Doing so protects the dentist and the business from potential legal liability. It is required by law that all dental records including any images be maintained by the office and are a property of the practice. Offices should follow the requirements for record maintenance as outlined by their state's board. For example, in the state of New Jersey, the Board of Dentistry requires that adult records be maintained for seven years from the last date of treatment.

Each patient, including minors and legal guardians of minors, has the right to view and copy their health information, such as the dental chart. The patient also has the right to request alternative forms of communication with their dentist as well as the right to dispute a suspected breach of HIPAA policies. For example, a patient may request to be contacted through postal service only and may formally complain if the request is not honored. The patient is entitled to the knowledge and record of any transactions or release of PHI that have been made for reasons *other than* the exchange of treatment, payment, or healthcare operations (known as TPO).

A patient who is of record in the office may call to ask questions about their treatment or about finances. It is important

TABLE 3-6 Additional HIPAA Policy and Security Resources

- www.hhs.gov
- www.privacyrights.org
- www.osha.gov
- www.hipaastore.com
- www.hedonline.com
- www.aapcps.com

**ACKNOWLEDGEMENT OF RECEIPT OF
HIPAA NOTICE OF PRIVACY PRACTICES**

<<date>>
<<patient_full_name>>

I do hereby acknowledge that I have received a copy of **<Insert dental office name> HIPAA Notice of Privacy Practices**.

By signing this document, I understand and acknowledge all statements in the HIPAA Privacy Practices in the **<insert office name>** handout, as given to me prior to signing. The office staff are a witness to me signing.

Sign name: Print name:

Please Note: It is your right to refuse to sign this Acknowledgement. However, as per office policy, all patient information must be entered and saved electronically. Failure to do so can be cause for dismissal from dental services.

FIGURE 3-4
Acknowledgement of receipt of HIPAA Notice of Privacy Practices.

---

that the office employee speaking with the patient confirm the patient's identity prior to providing any information. This may accomplished by asking the patient for information such as full name, social security number, date of birth, street address, and designated password (Figure 3-4).

Patient Relations HIPAA is intended to protect the patient's right of privacy (Table 3-6). Dental assistants must be careful when in conversation regarding a patient's private health information. Consistent with the code of ethics, the dental assistant has a duty to provide the best care while respecting the patient's right of autonomy and privacy of information. There are many opportunities throughout the patient's treatment plan for the disclosure and transmission of PHI. The dental assistant must be prepared to act according to the HIPAA laws from the new patient exam to the completion of the treatment plan. For most routine dental care and processing situations, permission from the patient to disclose PHI to professional(s) involved in their treatment is not necessary (Table 3-7).

Referrals Because some verbal communication is necessary in patient care, HIPAA regulations address the disclosure of PHI between individuals and businesses. There are times when a dental office may need to refer a patient to a specialty practice for appropriate treatment. All dental personnel should be prepared to answer the patient's questions surrounding the referral, which

TABLE 3-7 Permitted Use and Disclosure of PHI

- The individual requests information.
- Treatment, payment, and health care operations are involved.
- The patient has opportunity to agree or object to information.
- Information is important for public interest and benefit activities.
- There is an incident PHI may be shared for permitted use and disclosure.
- Limited data is used for the purpose of research, public health, or health care operations.

often includes the financial commitment and billing transactions. Whoever is designated as the financial communicator of the office should discuss sensitive information with the patient to avoid misinterpretation of the referral process. Because patients usually confide in the dental assistant, it is important that the assistant encourage the patient to speak with the *right* personnel and do not offer advice on matters assigned to someone else.

To ensure the confidentiality of the patient's healthcare information, the dentist will have a specific process in place for electronic exchanges. Dental personnel must be careful to follow the processes *exactly* as it is designed, to remain compliant with HIPAA regulations. The dental assistant should be cautious about discussions regarding the patient's treatment plan, revealing only which is necessary to the office the patient will be referred to.

Team Discussions It is common practice among dental offices to have "team meetings" at the beginning of each day. During the discussions, dentists, hygienists, dental assistants, and other dental personnel will converse about the schedule for the day. For adequate preparation, the team will conduct a "plan of approach," deciding what steps will be taken for each patient case. At times, the patient may require a referral or a receipt of payment before further treatment can be provided. Any member of the dental team may have to engage in conversation with other entities such as another dental office, an insurance company, or legal guardians. HIPAA standards must be upheld during each conversation.

Dental team members should exercise sound judgment during conversations regarding the dental patients. It is likely that patients know various members of the dental team from outside contact, such as a neighbor or school teacher. Dental assistants (and other personnel) must not confuse familiarity with responsibility. Knowing a patient on a personal level does not authorize a dental assistant to release PHI for reasons outside the designated HIPAA allowance! There are times that many dental workers unintentionally breach confidentiality through personal conversation. Personal information should be discussed at a minimum,

TABLE 3-8 Four Ways Information May Be Shared in the Dental
Setting

Seeing	Patient records should be kept away from direct viewing, including information on computer screens.
Speaking	All employees must remain away of bystanders when discussing patient's cases.
Hearing	Employees of a dental team must be careful to avoid eavesdropping on patient information outside the scope of their specific job duty.
Open records	All patient records must remain private and only viewed by those authorized to do so.

revealing only what information is necessary . . . even in team discussions! Comments and private information that do not pertain to the patient's treatment for the day should be omitted from team discussions (Table 3-8).

Insurance Relations

Title I of HIPAA addresses medical/dental insurance exchange and transfers. Dental Insurance can be a tricky field to maintain; the dental personnel must be very knowledgeable of the HIPAA administrative policies and regulations. Only information which is necessary for the implementation of treatment and the transaction of associated financial responsibilities should be exchanged. It is not uncommon for a patient to experience a change in dental insurance coverage; the patient may have lost a job, changed jobs, gained new coverage or switched from a current plan. HIPAA protects the patient's right to transfer insurance coverage *without* regard to preexisting conditions; therefore, the dental personnel must be fully aware of the established transfer and reporting process of the dental office. Not only will all information be kept at a minimum and private, but also reported through specific safeguard methods. The requirement of identifying medical codes for each patient procedure as well as utilizing the provider's identification number (PIN) is an example of the methods used during insurance transactions. The dentist will have a specific **protocol** for handling insurance relations, often located in the office procedural manual. Proper charting and coding is very important and should be approached carefully.

Legal Relations

It is very important that dental personnel understand the legalities associated with PHI of patients. Not every situation, no matter how "legal" it seems, **warrants** a release of information. Should a dental office receive a third-party request for a patient's health and/or financial information, the dental worker must **validate** the request. HIPAA policy requires covered entities to develop reasonable policies and practices for the verified identity of the requesting individual as well as the patient's authority to release the information. **Verification** may be obtained in writing or by verbal confirmation as long as the requisite documentation is within the HIPAA policies for release. Each dental office will have

a set policy and procedure for the verification of PHI requests and the method of exchange to satisfy those requests. The dental assistant must document information requests and/or exchanges as HIPAA policy indicates.

There are special situations of which a dental office may receive a request from "authorities" such as an attorney or a social worker. An individual's credentials are not always a sufficient reason for PHI exchange and should not be considered above the patient's right to privacy. The patient must be made aware of the request and authorize the release of information. If the patient does not authorize the exchange of information, then a legally binding request is necessary, such as a court-ordered **subpoena**. Verification of an individual's credentials is necessary to obtain, even if the patient consents to the release of information. Verification practices are set by the dental office, including the recording of the individual's state-issued licensing number. For example, if a patient would like the dental office to release a copy of their treatment chart to their lawyer or physician, then the office personnel will obtain the accepting individual's licensing number as verification of validity before releasing the information.

HIPAA in Public Health

While the HIPAA laws remain consistent among healthcare environments, there are a few situations which require a slightly different approach in management. For instance, there are responsibilities attached to providing short term care such as during an emergency. Other special situations include correctional dentistry or educational facilities conducting service learning projects.

Emergency Care

There are special considerations regarding the HIPAA policy in emergency situations. If a true emergency is underway and private information is necessary for adequate care, then the healthcare provider is expected to release that information. For instance: A long term patient with a history of heart disease arrives to your office for routine care. Just before treatment has begun the patient experiences a **myocardial infarction** (heart attack). The emergency response team is summoned and the patient is immediately treated by way of an automated external defibrillator (AED). A paramedic asks the dentist for an account of the incident as well as any health information available. During this situation, the dentist should give whatever information is necessary for the proper assessment of the patient and the successful contact of a spouse or family member.

HIPAA states that healthcare providers/responders are exempt from the requirement of first obtaining consent before the transferring of PHI in emergency situations; however, they are to obtain the consent at the first reasonable chance. A health care provider is also excused from normal protocol if a communication barrier exists and the circumstances infer the patient's consent. Additionally, a healthcare provider who attempts to obtain a consent form, but the patient refuses to sign, may still transfer information if required by law to treat the individual. The dental assistant should be prepared to act accordingly in an emergency situation, assisting the dentist and /or emergency responders in any way possible to facilitate proper immediate care for dental patients.

Correctional Dentistry

HIPAA states that individuals have the right to receive notice from a covered entity of privacy practices, except in special circumstances. Dental assistants who work in correctional dentistry may experience a slightly different routine during the "new patient" exam. Correctional institutions that only use or disclose PHI for business purposes do not have to produce a privacy practice notices to incarcerated individuals as they are under the custodial care of the state. There are times when a healthcare provider may share the inmate's (minimal) PHI with a correctional officer for the purposes of providing adequate care. For example, a physician or a dentist may inform/authorize specific medication an inmate should be receiving and administering for treatment.

Most healthcare professionals uphold the patient's requests for privacy, even in correctional healthcare. The dental assistant should caution against "privacy requests" that challenge safety. In most cases, it is appropriate for a correctional officer to remain present and/or nearby while a potentially dangerous inmate receives dental care. Medical ethics are not intended to create unsafe environments; if the presence of an officer is required, the dentist and dental assistant are expected to comply. At such times, the officer may learn of personal health information and should exercise sound ethics, avoiding the sharing of PHI with other inmates or officers.

Additionally, an inmate's healthcare record must be kept separate from the inmate's personal charts. Each inmate will have a separate "health record," which may include psychological evaluations, physician's treatment plans, dentist's treatment plans, and so on. The medical record will be stored in a specially designated place, away from institution's records containing legal information. Dental assistants working in the correctional setting must be thoroughly aware of the legal boundaries associated with the disclosure of health information to the requesting individual. If ever unsure, the dental assistant should consult the dentist or healthcare administrator for guidance. It is important for a dental professional to remember that correctional healthcare is slightly different than private practice and that the patient approach must be handled carefully. Inmates, like all patients, have the right to understand and approve or decline healthcare; however, copies of their health records must be approved by the responsible health authority. Legal authorities are determined by state statute or, for privatized correctional healthcare, the existing contract agreement. The dental assistant must remain cognizant of the state's dental practice act and the legalities associated with the ethical responsibilities and expectations.

Education

Covered by the HIPAA laws, PHI includes all individually identified information that may be communicated or transferred through various methods. There are exceptions to PHI, such as the "education records" governed by the *Family Education Rights and Privacy Act* (FERPA) and only applies to federally funded schools. If the school provides a nurse, that nurse becomes a healthcare provider (covered entity). Records held by post-secondary educational institutions of students 18 or older may be disclosed for medical treatment only and only if authorized by the student.

The HIPAA privacy rule defines specific guidelines regarding the de-identification of health information in efforts of protecting PHI. All identifiers such as the individual's relatives, employer, household members or geographic codes (address, zip codes, township, etc.) must be removed from records if the record is being viewed for purposes other than healthcare treatment of the specific individual. An example in an educational facility could be viewing a person's radiographs for learning purposes. A full mouth set of radiographic images will include the patient's personal information; this information must be removed or made unidentifiable to respect the privacy rights of the patient.

HIPAA in Technology

Appropriate for technological advances, HIPAA also addresses and enforces security laws for electronic data. HIPAA requires that all healthcare information be stored and/or converted to electronic format by 2014. Many offices are now utilizing software that allows for paperless charting. The dental record, radiographs, medical and dental history, and all other aspects of the chart are maintained through a computer backup system. These electronic files constitute a legal record that must be securely maintained. All paper-based HIPAA documents should be copied and scanned into the electronic record. Any prescriptions used in patient care would also be saved as part of the record, and a copy printed for the patient.

Other online/electronic information must be protected including conversations through email or text. Electronic media encompasses a number of devices such as memory storage cards and magnetic or optical disks and transmission media such as the internet, dial-up lines, and private networks.

Electronic Medical Records As previously noted, protected health information must meet a number of security requirements, particularly if the health information is in an electronic format. The majority of dental offices use some type of an electronic practice management system for production and office flow optimization. HIPAA policy regulates the security practices of electronic protected health information. The dentist or the designated security manager will evaluate and confirm that the chosen software is designed to facilitate HIPAA compliance. If a third-party business (e.g., clearinghouse) is assisting the dental office with the administrative tasks involving PHI, then that business will have to provide evidence of their security practices as well. The Health Insurance Portability and Accountability Act requires that all health plans, health care clearinghouses, and dentists who transmit health information in an electronic transaction use a standard format.

Electronic managements systems as well as all other computer practices in the dental office must use safe guarded passwords to identify the user and to protect from unauthorized access. The HIPAA policy still applies to the transmission of the electronic medical record. Should the dental assistant be asked to share PHI with a third party or another office, he or she must be certain to remain compliant with the HIPAA practices, only sharing information relevant to the request (Table 3-9).

Email Accounts and Social Media

Email being used for business purposes must be accompanied with a statement notifying the reader that the email contains private information only to be used for the purpose of providing adequate patient care. Emails generated from the dental office should not serve as personal email as well. Careful attention must be given to the protected content being shared. For instance, if a mass email is being sent to all of the patients of the dental office, then privacy settings must be in placed so that patients may not see the personal addresses of the other recipients. This can be accomplished by adding recipients to the BCC address line. Their address will not be visible to other recipients.

Many businesses have moved toward establishing a "virtual presence," utilizing the many options available for creating an identity in the social media world. At times, the business's social media site may be managed by the dentist or a designated assistant. A health care provider must be extremely carefully regarding the content displayed on the business' webpage, Facebook, Twitter, or similar applications. If confidentiality is breached, litigation could result. No private information should be shared, including patient cases of which identifiable information is given, such as names, locations, photos or even appointment dates. Monitoring of "friends" comments must also occur to avoid the disclosure and misrepresentation of protected health information.

TABLE 3-9 Privacy Protocol for Electronic Records

Employees of the dental office should be careful to protect computer information; the following practices will help to ensure confidentiality:

- Turn the screen away from easy vision of others.
- Click out of the screen prior to leaving the computer.
- Use a screen shield.
- Assign different passwords to different employees for differing tasks.
- Do not share passwords.
- If using a chairside computer, be certain that the previous patient's information has been closed out *before* seating another patient.

The dental assistant should also use extreme care when using their own social media sites. Posting inappropriate pictures or using inappropriate language that may be seen by patients of the office may impact the image of the office in a negative manner. It is also a violation of HIPAA to discuss patient treatment on social media. We use social media as an extension of our personalities. When looking for a job, many employers look at the candidate's social media site to get a better idea of the personality of the candidate. A site that is considered unacceptable in terms of imagery and language may result in loss of a position that has been applied for. The dental assistant should also refrain from using social media during working hours. A patient and an employer who sees the dental assistant using social media during working hours may be viewed as unprofessional and less productive. This may negatively impact annual performance reviews and eventually employment.

Mobile Applications

Cell phones are being used more frequently than ever before in today's healthcare practices. As technology advances, cell phones are serving more purposes than just for casual conversations. Physicians are often contacted through text messages rather than a pager system. In the dental setting, patients are often given a cell number to contact the dentist should an emergency occur outside normal business hours. The advantages of using cell phones to accomplish adequate patient response and care are many; however, the risks are just as abundant. Most healthcare workers using cell phones are not communicating through **encrypted** messages due to the extra costs. In other words, the potential for a security breach is high. The National Institute of Standards and Technology states that special risks apply to cell phones and have identified these risks in their "Guidelines for Cell Phone and PDA Security." The risks associated with cell phones include theft, loss, or disposal and unauthorized access.

Dental assistants should be cautious when using mobile healthcare applications. There are some dental offices that use a third-party recall system to text to remind patients of their appointments. Such systems are designed to originate from a computer program and transmit to cell phones. Dental assistants should not use their personal cell phones to text patients. They will not have the necessary and required protections in place to comply with HIPAA regulations.

Since many cell phones being used for businesses purpose are not encrypted, HIPAA violations occur frequently. The healthcare provider does not have to notify the patient of the use of PHI in most circumstances; however, they do have to provide the patient with a copy of their security practices, which should include information regarding all methods of transmission of PHI. Because of the associated risks with cell phone usage, it is not advisable for healthcare workers to repeat PHI through mobile applications unless necessary during a telephone conversation. If a cell phone or a similar mobile device is going to be use, additional encryption applications should be installed.

Chapter Summary

Each dental team member is faced with daily decisions that require judgments regarding legal and ethical principles. Maintaining professional ethical standards at all times is essential. The consequences for not doing what should be legally done or doing what should not be done can include fines or imprisonment. A license is granted to protect the public from unqualified individuals providing dental treatment. Some states require dental assistants to become licensed to perform specific dental tasks. The expanded functions are most often specified in the Dental Practice Act according to how they are to be delegated. The dental assistant must thoroughly understand the law in order to protect the patient, the dentist, and the profession. Dental health care continues to change, and the assistant must understand how the law affects these changes and must stay within the law. HIPAA regulations are required to protect patient information. It is the responsibility of the dental team members to stay informed and comply with the standards.

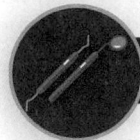

CASE STUDY

Desiree is a dental assistant for Dr. Wyatt. Jack, her best friend Kendra's boyfriend, came in as a patient. When Jack filled out the health history, Desiree learned that he is HIV positive. He asked that she not share that with Kendra.

Case Study Review

1. Should Desiree discuss this with her best friend?

2. Can she discuss this with her friend legally?

3. How should she handle this information?

4. Should she discuss this with her dentist?

Review Questions

Multiple Choice

1. Which of the following is the correct sequence of steps in approaching an ethical dilemma?
   a. determine, identify, rank, develop, implement, reflect.
   b. identify, determine, rank, develop, implement, reflect.
   c. rank, identify, determine, develop, implement, reflect.
   d. develop, rank, identify, determine, implement, reflect.

2. Which of the following is part of the American Dental Assistants' Association (ADAA) Code of Conduct?
   a. Cause no harm.
   b. Create and maintain a safe work environment.
   c. Strive for self-improvement through continuing education.
   d. Never misrepresent professional credentials or education.
   e. All of these are part of the ADAA Code of Conduct.

3. The Dental Practice Act is state specific and outlines allowable duties for the dental assistant.
   Select the correct response based on the statement above.
   a. Both statements are true.
   b. Both statements are false.
   c. The first statement is true; the second statement is false.
   d. The second statement is true; the first statement is false.

4. Which of the following is correct regarding expanded functions?
   a. Expanded functions for the dental assistant are outlined in the Dental Practice Act.
   b. Expanded functions do not require additional education.
   c. Expanded function must be performed under direct supervision by the dentist.
   d. The expanded functions dental assistant would not be sued by a patient since the dentist is responsible.

5. Select the correct answer regarding the relationship between jurisprudence and the dental assistant.
   a. The establishment, regulation, and enforcement of laws may be known as jurisprudence.
   b. Jurisprudence is more important than ethics in the responsibilities of the dental assistant.
   c. Jurisprudence includes only civil law, which is subdivided into tort, contract, and administrative law.
   d. All of the statements above are correct.

6. Select the two correct statement regarding omission and commission.
   a. Civil wrong doings may result from acts of commission such as failure to do something that should have been done.
   b. Civil wrong doing may result from an act of omission or doing something that should not have been done.
   c. An example of commission is a situation of which a dental assistant performs expanded functions without the adequate knowledge and/or the proper credentialing to perform the procedure.
   d. An example of an act of omission is a situation of when a dental assistant neglects to update a medical history, resulting in injury to the patient.

7. A binding agreement between two or more people is a(n)
   a. agent.
   b. reciprocity.
   c. contract.
   d. breach.

8. Fraud is defined as deliberate deception to secure unfair or unlawful gain. An example of fraud in the dental office is sending incorrect information to dental insurance companies for payment.
   a. Both statements are true.
   b. Both statements are false.
   c. The first statement is true; the second statement is false.
   d. The second statement is true; the first statement is false.

9. A wrongful act that results in injury to one person by another is a(n)
   a. tort.
   b. contract.
   c. omission.
   d. commission.

10. Which three of the following are regulatory agencies?
    a. Occupational Safety and Health Administration (OSHA)
    b. United States Food and Drug Administration (FDA)
    c. United States Environmental Protection Agency (EPA)
    d. Centers for Disease Control (CDC)

11. Which three of the following are nonregulatory agencies?
    a. Center for Disease Control (CDC)
    b. United States Food and Drug Administration (FDA)
    c. Organization for Safety and Asepsis Procedures (OSAP)
    d. National Institute of Occupational Safety and Health (NIOSH)

12. Violation of HIPAA may result in:
    a. monetary fines and jail time.
    b. monetary fines and community service.
    c. jail time and community service.
    d. There is no punishment for HIPAA violations.

13. Select the correct statement regarding HIPAA practices related to the new patient exam and referral process.
    a. The new patient does not need to receive the HIPAA policy at the initial visit.
    b. According to HIPAA, the patient is not allowed to see their own chart.
    c. If the patient wishes to share health information, the patient must sign a form.
    d. When referring to a specialist, sharing the dental record is a violation of HIPAA.

14. Which of the following is not a violation of HIPAA following a team discussion about a patient?
    a. If the dental assistant is a friend of a patient in the office, it is allowable to share the patient's information with other people the patient may know.
    b. It is acceptable for the dental assistant to discuss personal information related to a patient during team discussions.
    c. The dental assistant must uphold HIPAA standards during team discussions.
    d. It is acceptable for the dental assistant to discuss a patient with a colleague so that patients in the waiting room can hear the conversation.

15. Based on HIPAA law, a patient is allowed to request alternative modes of communication from the dental office and has a right to dispute suspected breaches of HIPAA policies.
    Based on the statements above, which of the following choices is correct?
    a. Both statements are true.
    b. Both statements are false.
    c. The first statement is true; the second statement is false.
    d. The second statement is true; the first statement is false.

16. Title I of HIPAA addresses medical/dental insurance exchange and transfers. Only information which is necessary for the implementation of treatment and the transaction of associated financial responsibilities should be exchanged.
    Based on the statements above, which of the following choices is correct?
    a. Both statements are true.
    b. Both statements are false.
    c. The first statement is true; the second statement is false.
    d. The second statement is true; the first statement is false.

17. You are a dental assistant working in an office. You have received a verbal request from a social worker for one of the patients in the office. What is the correct course of action that you should take?
    a. Release the records immediately as this is an authoritative request and you should not delay.
    b. You do not need to verify that the request for records is valid since the person stated that they were a social worker.
    c. You should speak to the patient; if the patient does not authorize the release of records, a court subpoena may be necessary.
    d. It is not important for the office to have a standard verification protocol in the event that such records requests are received.

18. The informed consent provides truthful information to the patient about the risks and benefits of the dental procedure that will be performed. The informed consent does not need to include the risks to the patient if the patient denies treatment.
   Based on the statements above, which of the following choices is correct?
   a. Both statements are true.
   b. Both statements are false.
   c. The first statement is true; the second statement is false.
   d. The second statement is true; the first statement is false.

19. Select the correct answer regarding statute of limitation.
   a. The time limit for a patient to file a lawsuit is the same in all states in the United States.
   b. Generally, an injured patient may file a lawsuit within five years of the last date of treatment or within three years of the date that the injury was discovered.
   c. A patient can file a lawsuit at anytime after the injury was discovered and a statute of limitation does not apply.
   d. A statute of limitation is defined as the period of limitation for bringing forth certain types of legal action.

20. Select the correct response regarding HIPAA policies and practices related to technology.
   a. Online electronic transmission of personal health information must be protected under HIPAA.
   b. HIPAA does not mandate electronic storage of medical records; paper format is acceptable under HIPAA.
   c. Use of non-encrypted personal cell phones for personal health information transmission may lead to HIPAA violations.
   d. Posting before and after treatment pictures of patents of the office is acceptable and does not violate HIPAA.

Critical Thinking

1. What is the definition of ethics?
2. How does autonomy relate to patient care?
3. In what ways do the core ethical principles interrelate and support each other?

Key Terms

Term and Pronunciation	Meaning of Root and Word Parts	Definition
administration (ad-min-*uh*-**strey**-*shuh'n*)	**administrate** = to administer **-ion** = action, condition of	the process or activity of running a business, organization
auspices (**aw**-spuh-siz)	**auspex** = benevolent influence of greater power **-ices** = plural form	patronage; support; sponsorship
autonomy (aw-**ton**-uh-mee)	**auto-** = self **nomos-** = custom law	independence, freedom from external control or influence
beneficence (buh-**nef**-uh-suh ns)	**benefic-** = doing something good; kind **-ence** = equivalent to	action that is done for the benefit of others; charitable
breach (breech)	**bhreg** = to break	a violation of a law or trust or promise
clearinghouse (**kleer**-ing-hous)	**clearing** = reciprocal exchange between institutions **house** = building for any purpose	an agency or organization that collects and distributes something, especially information
chronic (**kron**-ik)	**chron** = time **-ic** = pertaining to	continuing a long time or recurring frequently
code (kohd)	**code** = authoritative written statement of legal rules	a set of laws or regulations; a set of ideas or rules about how to behave

(Continues)

Term and Pronunciation	Meaning of Root and Word Parts	Definition
defendant (dih-**fen**-d*uh* nt)	**de** = away **fend** = protect **ant** = serving in the capacity of	an individual or organization who is accused or sued in a court of law
commission (k*uh*-**mish**-*uh* n)	**com** = together **mission** = an important assignment	the act of entrusting a group with supervisory powers
compensatory (k*uh* m-**pen**-s*uh*-tawr-ee)	**compentence** = make up, make amends **-ory** = something having a specified use	serving as a payment to someone who has experienced loss, suffering, injury
competence (**komp**-pi-t*uh* ns)	**competen**t =having suitable or sufficient skill, knowledge **-ence** = equivalent to	ability to do something successfully or efficiently
compliance (kuh m-**plahy**-uh ns)	**comply** = in accordance with **-ance** = state or condition of	the action or fact of complying with a wish or command
conduction (kuh n-**duhk**-sh*uh* n)	**conduct** = a bringing together **-ion** = action, condition of	the transmission or conveying of something through a medium or passage
consultative (*kuh* n-**suhl**-*tuh*-tiv)	**consult** = seek advice or information from **-ative** = being of	giving advice or assistance
converse (kuh'n-**vurs**)	**con** = with **verse** = speak	to engage in an exchange of thoughts and feelings by means of speech
defendant (dih-**fen**-d*uh* nt)	**de** = away **fend** = protect **ant** = serving in the capacity of	an individual or organization who is accused or sued in a court of law
dilemma (dih-**lem**-uh)	**di-** = two **-lemma** = an assumption, premise	a situation in which a difficult choice has to be made between two or more alternative; especially equally undesirable one
disclosure (dih-**skloh**-zehr)	**disclose** = to make known **ure** = act, process, result	the action of making new or secret information known
encrypt (en-**kript**)	**en** =in) **crypt** = secret location	convert information or data into a code; especially to prevent unauthorized access
enforcement (en-**fawrs**-m*uh*'nt)	**enforce** = to put or keep in place **-ment** = an action or state	to make sure that people do what is required by law or rule
entities (**en**-ti-tee)	**enti** = present **-ty** = quality or state	things with distinct and independent existence
ethical (**eth**-i-kuhl)	**ethic-** = moral **-al** = relationship, concern of	being in accordance with the accepted principles of right and wrong that govern the conduct of a profession
expressed (uhk-**sprest**)	**ex** = squeeze out **press** = push against	convey a thought or feeling through gestures or words.
hazardous (**haz**-er-d*uh* s)	**hazard** = danger or risk **-ous** = possessing, full of	something dangerous or risky
implied (im-**plahyd**)	**imply** = infer **-ed** = past tense	suggested but not directly expressed; to hint at
incarcerate (in-**kahr**-suh-reyt)	**in** = in with force **-carcer** = prison **-ate** = state of	to put in prison, confinement; constrict closely
implementation (im-pluh-men-**ta**-shuhn)	**implement** = to put into effect **-ation** = condition of	the process of putting a decision or plan into effect to achieve a goal; execution

Term and Pronunciation	Meaning of Root and Word Parts	Definition
informed consent (in-**fawrmd**) (ku*h*n-**sent**)	**informed** = prepared with information **consent** = to approve or give permission	a patient's consent to a health care procedure or to participation in a clinical study after being fully advised of the benefits and the risks involved
jurisprudence (joor-is-**prood**-ns)	**juris-** = right of law **-prudentia** = knowledge, a foreseeing **-ence** = indicating a quality	the study and philosophy of law
malpractice (mal-**prak**-tis)	**mal-** = bad, wrongful **practice** = observe or do repeatedly	improper, illegal, or negligent professional activity or treatment; especially by a medical practitioner, lawyer, or public official
mandatory (**man**-d*uh*-tawr-ee)	**mandate** = to order or require **-ory** = having the effect of	required by law or rules
myocardial infarction (mahy-*uh*-**kahr**-dee-*uh*-l in-**fahrkt**, in-**fahrkt**)	**myo** = muscle **cardio** = heart **infarct** = localized area of tissue that has been deprived of blood and is dying or dead	heart attack
nonmaleficence (non-m*uh*-**lef**-*uh*-s*uh* ns)	**non** = not **malefic** = doing harm **-ence** = indicating an action; condition	ethical principle of doing no harm
omission (oh-**mish**-*uh* n)	**omit** = fail to	something not done or left out
optimization (op-tuh-muh-**zey**-shuh'n)	**optimize** = to make perfect, better **-ation** = equivalent to; action, process, state	an act, process of making a system or decision as fully perfect, functional, or effective as possible
philosophy (fi-**los**-uh-fee)	**philo-** = like, love **-sophy** = knowledge, wisdom	the study of ideas about knowledge, truth, the nature and meaning of life
principles (**prin**-suh-puhl)	**principia** = beginning, first part	a fundamental truth that serves as the foundation for a system of belief or behavior or reasoning
protocol (**proh**-t*uh*-kawl)	**proto** = first; foremost **-col** = between, join	a system of rules that explain the correct conduct and procedures to be followed in formal situations
punitive (**pyoo**-ni-tiv)	**punish** = to inflict a penalty **-ive** = expressing disposition	inflicting or intended as punishment or sanction
reciprocity (res-*uh*-**pros**-i-tee)	**re** = back **procus** = forward	mutual exchange
regulatory (**reg**-*yuh*-luh-t*awr*-ee)	**regulate** = to control or direct by rule **-ory** = place for; specific of	governing; supervisory to control or direct according to rule, principle, or law
relative (**rel**-uh-*tiv*)	**relate** = reference or relation to **-ive** = to subject to	considered in relation to something else; comparative; connection to
restitution (res-ti-**too**-sh*uh*n)	**re** = again **statuere** = restore	reparation by giving compensation for damages or injury
revocation (rev-uh-**key**-shuh n)	**revoke** = taking away **-ion** = action, condition of	the act of cancelling of something by some authority
slander (**slan**-der)	**slander** = malicious, false, statement	the action or crime of making a false, negative spoken statement damaging a person's reputation

(Continues)

Term and Pronunciation	Meaning of Root and Word Parts	Definition
statute (**stach**-oot)	**statute** = a law, decree	a written law passed by a legislative body
subpoena (suh-**pee**-*nuh*)	**sub-** = under **poena** = penalty	a document that requires its recipient to appear in court as a witness
transmission (trans-**mi** sh-uh'n)	**transmiss** = across **-ion** = action of	the act or process by which something is spread or passed from one person or thing to another
tripartite (trahy-**pahr**-tahyt)	**tri-** = three **part** = divide **-ite** = involving	shared by or involving three parties
validate (**val**-i-deyt)	**valid** = sound **-ate** = function	to check or prove the validity or accuracy of something, to confirm
veracity (vuh-**ras**-i-tee)	**verac-** = true **-ity** = quality or condition of	conformity to facts; accuracy, truth
verification (ver-*uh*-fi-**key**-shuh'n)	**verify** = to prove **-cation** = being of	the process of establishing the truth, accuracy, or validity of something
violations (vahy-*uh*-**ley**-shuh'n)	**violate** = break; infringement **-ion** = being of	an action that breaks or acts against something, especially a law, agreement, principle
warrant (**wawr**-uh'nt)	**warrant** = authorize	document giving authority to do something

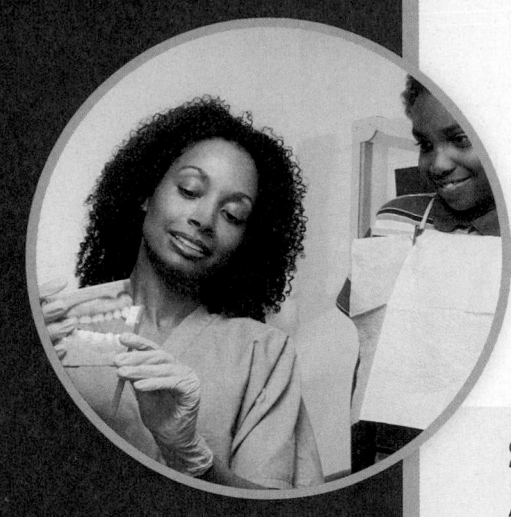

General Anatomy and Physiology

Specific Instructional Objectives

At the completion of this chapter, you will be able to meet these objectives:

1. Use terms presented in this chapter.
2. List the body systems, body planes and directions, and cavities of the body, and describe the structure and function of the cell.
3. Explain the functions and divisions of the skeletal system, list the composition of the bone, and identify the types of joints.
4. List the functions and structure of the muscular system.
5. List the functions and structure of the nervous system.
6. List the functions and structure of the endocrine system.
7. Explain dental concerns related to the reproductive system.
8. List the functions and structure of the circulatory system.
9. List the functions and structure of the digestive system.
10. List the functions and structure of the respiratory system.
11. List the functions and structure of the lymphatic system and the immune system.
12. List the functions and structure of the integumentary system.
13. List the functions and structure of the urinary system.

Introduction to Anatomy and Physiology

The study of the human body allows the dental assistant to gain an understanding of the body and how it operates. **Anatomy** is the study of the structures and organs of the body, including size and shape. **Physiology** is the study of how the body functions and includes the relationship between bodily functions and how they work together. This chapter will present each body system. At the end of each body system discussion, the interrelationship between oral health and overall health will be discussed.

Organization of the Human Body

Prior to looking at the entire human body, the organization of its parts needs to be examined. *Atoms* are the smallest components of elements (e.g., carbon, hydrogen, and oxygen). *Molecules* are formed when two or more atoms combine through a chemical bond to form units such as a carbohydrate (1 carbon, 2 hydrogens, and 1 oxygen atom). At the most basic level, the body is composed of cells that come together to form tissues. These tissues come together to form organs, and organs come together to form systems that comprise the entire human body (Figure 4-1).

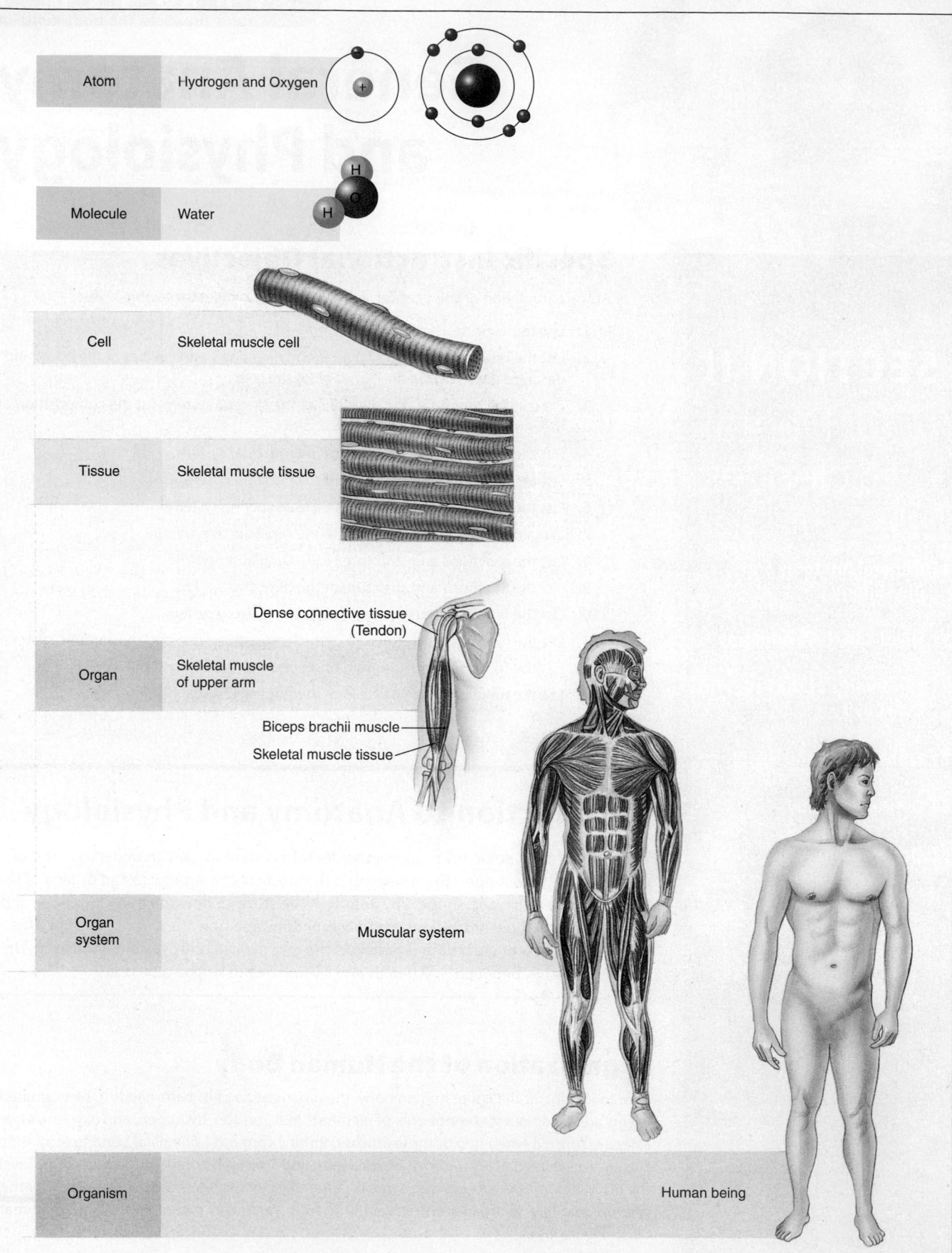

Atom — Hydrogen and Oxygen

Molecule — Water

Cell — Skeletal muscle cell

Tissue — Skeletal muscle tissue

Organ — Skeletal muscle of upper arm

Dense connective tissue (Tendon)

Biceps brachii muscle

Skeletal muscle tissue

Organ system — Muscular system

Organism — Human being

FIGURE 4-1
The structural levels of organization of the body.

Cell

The *cell* is the basic foundation of all living things. *Protoplasm* is the content of the cell, including the cell membrane and nucleus. Every tiny cell in the body has the ability to reproduce, produce energy, grow, and excrete waste products. The body contains many types of cells that have their own specific purposes depending on the body systems in which they are contained. Cells differ in appearance, function, and structure according to what they do. The study of cells is called **cytology**. Regardless of their shape, size, or location, all cells consists of the same basic components—a cell membrane, cytoplasm, and a nucleus (Figure 4-2).

The *cell membrane* is a very thin covering that surrounds the cell. It has two specific functions: It helps the cell maintain its shape and allows for the passage of nutrients and waste in and out of the cell.

The *cytoplasm* of the cell is a gel-like fluid inside the cell that is made up of mostly water. Two-thirds of the body's water is found here. This water contains minerals, gases, and organic molecules necessary to perform chemical reactions within the cell. This gel suspends the cell structures so they can perform their functions of transporting nutrients and proteins and disposing of cellular wastes.

The **nucleus** is a large cell **organelle** that acts as the control center of the cell. The **chromosomes** are in the nucleus and contain **deoxyribonucleic acid** (DNA), which transmits **genetic** information. The nucleus controls the **metabolic** activity, growth, and reproduction of the cell using the DNA's genetic information. Within the nucleus is the **nucleolus** that produces ribosomes for the cell and houses **ribonucleic acid** (RNA).

The cell contains many organ-like structures inside the cell called cell-organelles (Figure 4-3). Each has a specific structural makeup and function. (Refer to the feature Common Cell Organelles for details about the most common.)

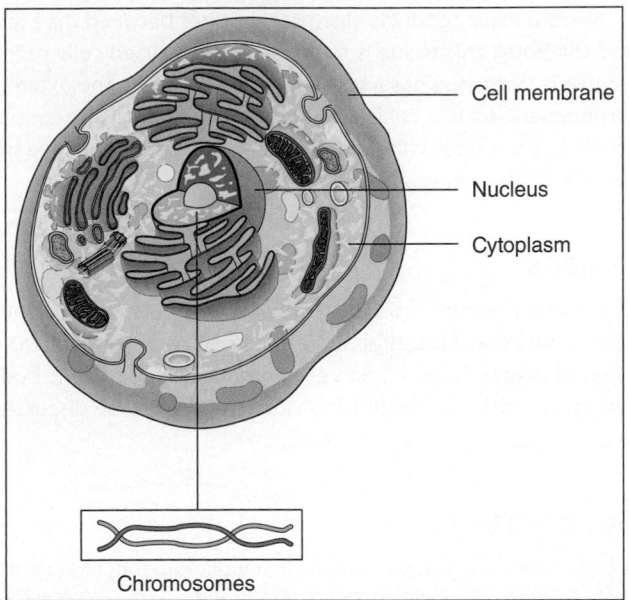

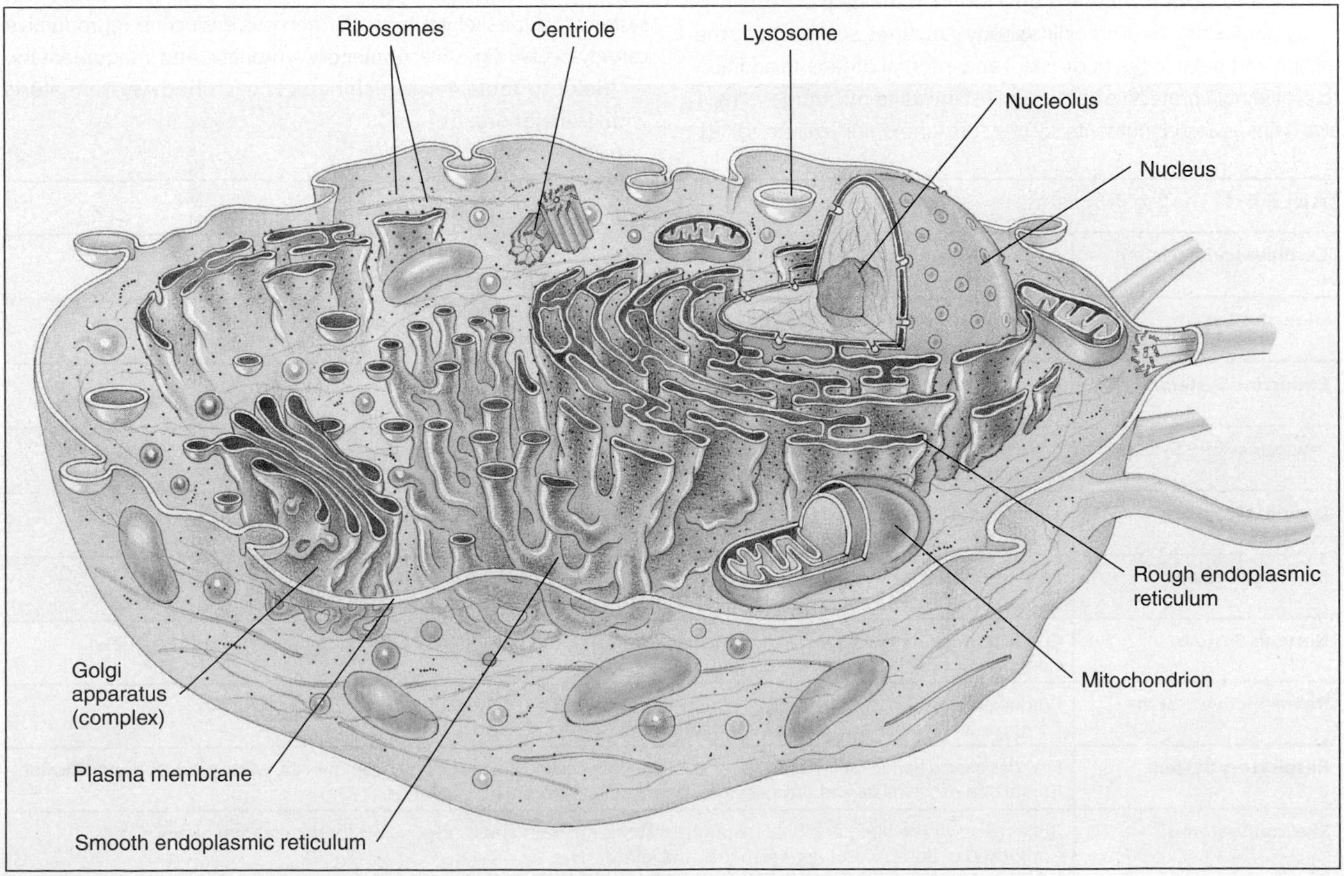

Cell membrane

Nucleus

Cytoplasm

Chromosomes

FIGURE 4-2
Basic cell structures

Ribosomes   Centriole   Lysosome

Nucleolus

Nucleus

Rough endoplasmic reticulum

Mitochondrion

Golgi apparatus (complex)

Plasma membrane

Smooth endoplasmic reticulum

FIGURE 4-3
A diagram of a typical animal cell illustrating a three-dimensional view of cell ultrastructure.

Common Cell Organelles

Ribosomes—nicknamed the protein factories of the cell, they synthesize a variety of proteins that are essential for the survival of the cell.

Endoplasmic reticulum—part of it is lined with ribosomes and is involved with manufacturing protein; the rest of the organelle produces vital fats.

Golgi apparatus—modifies and transports proteins within the cell.

Lysosome—contains digestive enzymes and is nicknamed the stomach of the cell; digests excess or worn out organelles, food particles, viruses, and bacteria.

Mitochondrion—referred as the powerhouses of the cell; their functions include cellular respiration, transforming glucose into energy, and fueling the cellular process by breaking high-energy chemical bonds.

Tissue

Tissue is formed when a group of similar cells function together to perform a specific task. There are four main types of tissues in the human body: muscle tissue, epithelial tissue, connective tissue, and nervous tissue.

Muscle tissue controls movement of the body, or movement of substances through the body, by contracting individual muscle cells. There are three types of muscle tissue: Skeletal muscle is attached to our bones, smooth muscle is found in internal organs, and **cardiac** muscle is only found in the heart.

Epithelial tissue covers or lines body structures, such as inside the mouth and outside the body (skin) and internal organs. In addition to providing a protective barrier against invading microorganisms, it also helps to absorb nutrients, secrete substances, and excrete wastes.

Connective tissue supports, protects, and connects the tissues of the body structures. Depending on the location, connective tissue may perform many different functions. For example, blood is a connective tissue that transports oxygen to the cells and tendons, and ligaments are fibrous connective tissues that connect muscle to bone in order to provide movement.

Nervous tissue conducts electrical impulses between the brain and the body. This tissue is made up of specialized cells called **neurons**. This tissue has a special ability to react to the external environment, such as cold, heat, light, and pressure. For example, touching a hot stove will send a signal to the brain to remove the hand from the heat source.

Organs

Organs are a group of tissues that work together to perform a specific function. Most organs are composed of several different types of tissues. Table 4-1 lists each organ and the specific body system in which it is located. Individual organs will be discussed in each upcoming body system section.

Body Systems

A *body system* is a group of organs that work together to keep the body healthy and functional. The human body is composed of eleven organ body systems that all function together to maintain **homeostasis**. Although each of these systems has a unique function, each organ system depends directly or indirectly on all the others. These systems include skeletal, muscular, nervous, endocrine, reproductive, cardiovascular, digestive, respiratory, lymphatic, and integumentary.

(Refer to Table 4-1, which depicts each body system along with its major organs.)

TABLE 4-1 The Organ Systems

Cardiovascular System	Responsible for pumping blood throughout the body. Composed of the heart along with the blood vessels; brings oxygen and nutrients to the cells.
Digestive System	Breaks down food into its basic forms called nutrients that can be absorbed and used by the body. Composed of the esophagus, stomach, small intestines, and large intestines.
Endocrine System	Uses hormones to control the functions of the body systems. Composed of pituitary gland, thyroid gland, ovaries, and testes.
Integumentary System	Protects the body from various kinds of damage, including loss of water or abrasion from the outside. Composed of the skin and its appendages, including hair and nails.
Lymphatic System	Cleanses the blood and aids in protection from foreign substances. Composed of lymph nodes, thymus, spleen, and tonsils.
Muscular System	Responsible for the movement of the body. Composed of skeletal muscle tissue, cardiac muscles, smooth muscles, blood vessels, tendons, and nerves
Nervous System	Conducts and interprets sensory information from inside and outside the body, which then responds as needed. Composed of the brain, spinal cord, and connecting nerves.
Reproductive System	Produces cells that carry the genetic material for the purpose of creating a new organism. Composed of ovaries and uterus in the female and testes and penis in the male.
Respiratory System	Provides gas exchange for the body. It constantly supplies oxygen to the cells and removes the waste product carbon dioxide. Composed of the nasal and oral passages, larynx, trachea, bronchi, and lungs.
Skeletal System	Bones support the body and hold it upright. It stores minerals and is responsible for the creation of blood cells. Composed of bones, cartilage, ligaments, and joints.
Urinary System	Removes liquid wastes from the blood and regulates blood pressure. Composed of the kidneys and bladder.

Source: Courtesy of Stacey Young and Carrie Jacques

Body Locations and Directions

When discussing and naming anatomical structures, specific body locations and directions, including anatomical position, body planes, and cavities, are referenced.

Anatomical Position

In order to correctly identify and discuss specific locations and directions of the body, it is important to have a starting point known as the *anatomical position*. The anatomical position is standing upright with arms at the sides, palms facing forward, and eyes straight ahead. The legs are parallel, with the feet and toes facing forward and shoulder width apart (Figure 4-4).

Body Planes

One way to describe the body and its parts is to use planes to divide the body into different sections or portions. The **sagittal plane**, also known as the median plane, divides the body into right and left portions. The *frontal plane*, also known as the **coronal** plane, divides the body into front and back portions.

The **transverse** *plane*, also known as the horizontal plane, divides the body into upper and lower portions. (Refer back to Figure 4-4.)

Body Cavities

The body is not a solid structure; it has many open spaces or cavities. There are four major cavities in the body: The **cranial cavity** surrounds the brain; the *spinal cavity* surrounds the spinal cord; the **thoracic** (chest) cavity encompasses the lungs, heart, and accessory organs; and the **abdominopelvic cavity** includes the digestive, urinary, and reproductive organs. Between the thoracic and the abdominopelvic cavity lies the **diaphragm,** which separates the two cavities and is a muscle used for breathing (Figure 4-5).

Directional Terms of the Body

Directional terms assist health care professionals in discussing the position or location of a patient's complaint, as well as help to describe a procedure, organ, or system and how it is related to the body. Table 4-2 lists the terms commonly used to describe the position of the body. Note that most terms are in pairs and have opposite meanings.

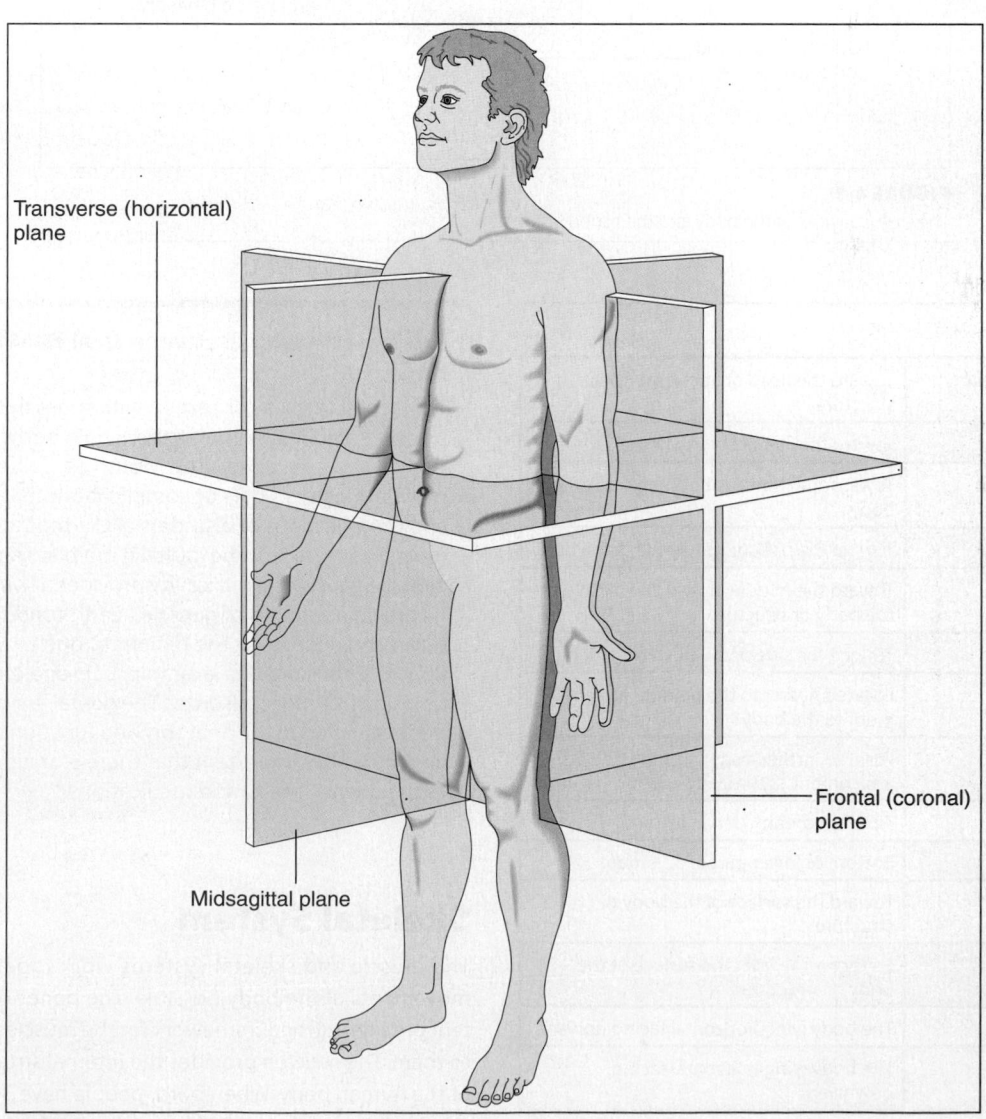

FIGURE 4-4
The human body in correct anatomic position, illustrating the planes of the body.

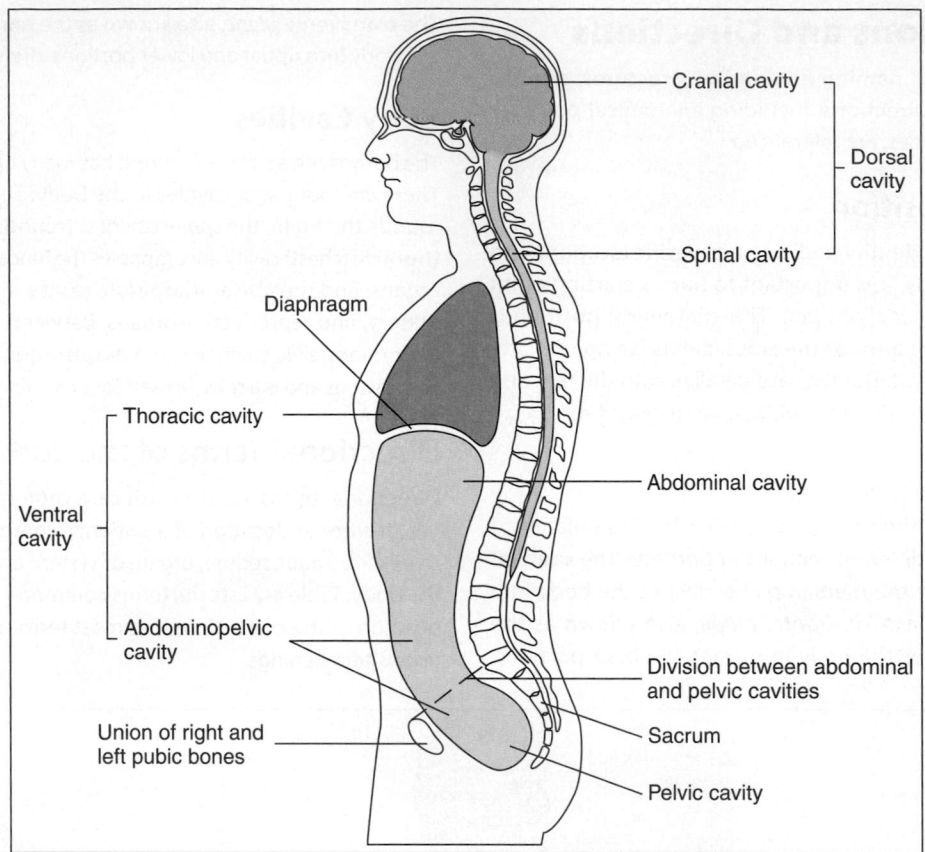

FIGURE 4-5
The major cavities of the body and their subdivisions.

TABLE 4-2 Directional Terms

Superior or cephalic	Toward the head or above another structure
Inferior or caudal	Toward the feet or below another structure
Anterior or ventral	Toward the front or abdomen side of the body
Posterior or dorsal	Toward the back or spinal side of the body
Medial	Toward the middle or near the middle of the body or structure
Lateral	Toward the side of the body or structure
Proximal	Located nearer to the point of attachment to the body
Distal	Located farther away from the point of attachment to the body
Apex	Tip of an organ
Base	Bottom or lower part of an organ
Superficial	Toward the surface of the body or structure
Deep	Farther away from the surface of the body or structure
Supine	The body lying horizontal facing upward
Prone	The body lying horizontal facing downward

Source: Courtesy of Stacey Young and Carrie Jacques

Interrelationship Between Oral Health and the Body

The dental team is concerned with more than just oral health, because oral health affects the whole body. The health of the body as a whole affects the mouth as well. Each body system may develop disorders or complications that affect the mouth, and complications or disorders of the mouth may affect one or more body systems. The dental team plays an important role in early diagnosis. The oral cavity provides a "window" to the body by providing signals of general health condition. Both the physician and dentist ask the patient to open wide and say "Ah" as they look for signs. For example, pale and bleeding gums may be a sign of a blood disorder. The dental assistant must have an understanding of the anatomy and function of the whole body in general. It is important that there is an up-to-date record of each patient's health and medications.

Skeletal System

The muscle and skeletal systems work together to make the movements of the body possible. The bones of the skeletal system provide a strong framework for the muscles that are attached to them. The *skeleton* provides the internal structure and support of the human body. When born, people have 300 bones that will eventually fuse into the 206 bones found in adults.

Anatomy of Bones

Each *bone* in the human body is unique and carries its own blood supply, lymph vessels, and nerves (Figure 4-6). Bone or **osseous tissue** is made up of connective tissue consisting mainly of **collagen fibers** and an **inorganic** bone material tissue that is one of the strongest materials in the body. The bone tissue is 20% water, and of the remaining 80%, two-thirds consist of minerals and inorganic matter, and one-third is organic matter, including blood cells, lymphatic vessels, and nerves. A dense layer of vascular tissue that covers many of the bones (except at the joints) is called the **periosteum.** It serves as protection and as a channel for the blood supply and nutrients for bone tissue and bone-building cells called **osteoblasts.** Each bone end is called an epiphysis. The area running through the two ends is called the diaphysis or shaft. The two types of bone tissue are compact and spongy. Compact (or **cortical**) bone is a dense, hard tissue that makes up the outer layers of bone. **Osteoblast** cells are found in the compact. When bone is damaged or stressed, the osteoclast dissolves and reabsorbs the calcium salts of the bone matrix. Spongy (or **cancellous**) bone is found inside the bones and has a sponge-like appearance (**trabeculae**). Trabeculae provide strength without adding weight (Figure 4-7).

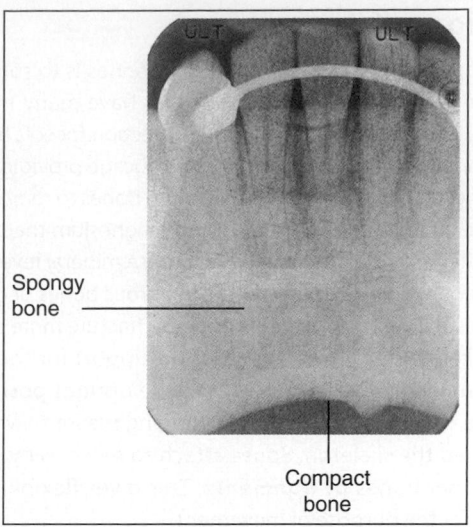

FIGURE 4-7
Dental radiograph showing compact and spongy bone.

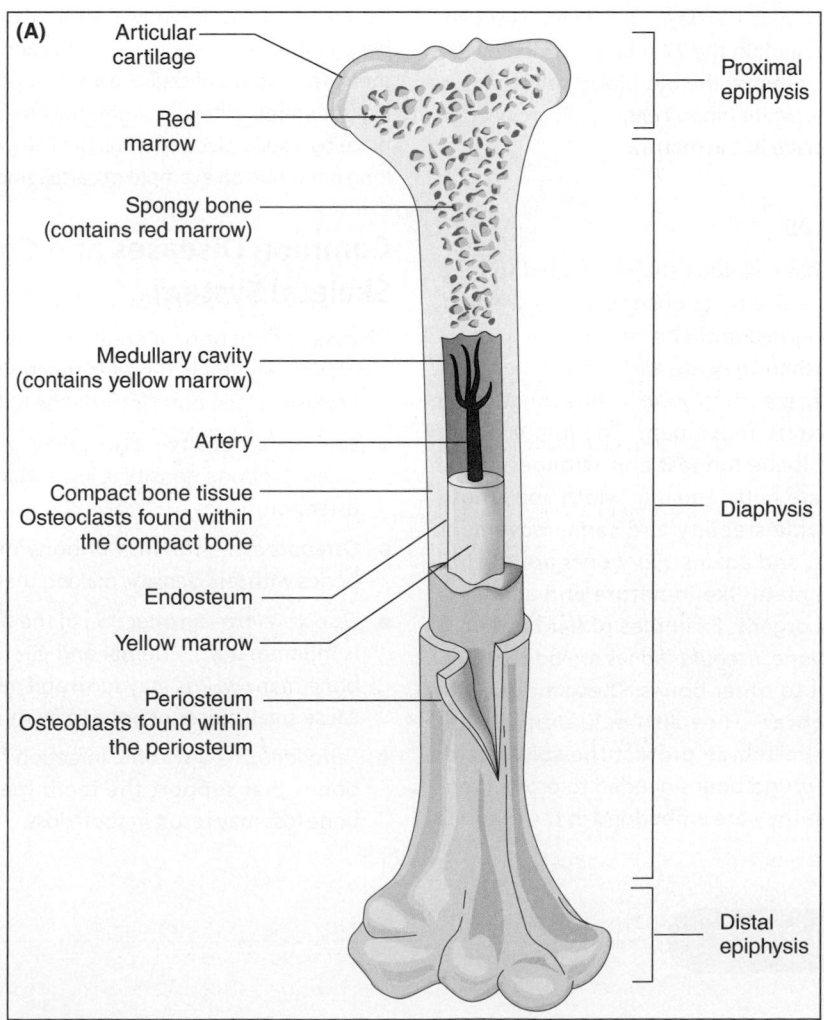

FIGURE 4-6
Anatomic feature of a long bone.

Functions of Bones

Most people know the basic function of bones is to support the body and to allow for movement. Bones have many more vital functions. They provide strength and protection for soft tissue and internal organs. An example of this is the ribcage providing protection for the heart and lungs. In order for the bones to remain strong, they store minerals such as calcium and magnesium that help provide for their strength and hardness. If these mineral levels are too low and not replenished, it can result in porous bones or **osteoporosis**. These conditions can cause bones to fracture more easily.

The skeleton provides the physical support for the body. It allows humans to be able to walk in the upright position. The bones are connected to each other, forming the framework of the body called the skeleton. Bones attach to muscles by **tendons** and to other bones by **ligaments**. This gives flexibility to the skeleton for the purpose of movement.

Each bone in the body is unique and carries its own blood supply, **lymph** vessels, and nerves. Blood cells are produced within the **bone marrow**. There are two types of bone marrow in the body. The red marrow manufactures most of the blood cells and the yellow bone marrow is made up mainly of fat cells. The production of red blood cells is truly an incredible process. The blood cells only have a lifespan of about 120 days, so red blood cells are in constant production to maintain the 27 trillion needed by the body. The *spleen* is able to remove the old blood cells that are worn out and damaged. The white blood cells, which are needed to fight infection, are also made in the marrow.

Categories of Bones

Different types of bones have various shapes related to their particular function. There are five types of bones in the skeleton: long, short, flat, irregular, and **sesamoid** bones.

Long bones are longer than they are wide. The majority of bones in the human body are long bones. They function to support weight and facilitate movement. The femur (thigh bone) is an example and is the longest and strongest bone in the body. *Short bones* are fairly equal in width and length (cube-shaped). They provide stability and some movement and are found in the wrist and ankles. *Flat bones* are thinner flattened bones that are plate-like in nature and act like a shield to protect internal organs. Examples of flat bones are the skull, ribs, and breastbone. *Irregular bones* are odd-shaped bones needed to connect to other bones. These include the hip bones and the **vertebrae**. They also help protect vital organs; for example, the vertebrae protect the spinal cord. *Sesamoid bones* are small, round bones needed to protect tendons from stress and wear. They are embedded in the tendons of the hands, knees, and feet. The patella (kneecap) is an example of a sesamoid bone.

Divisions of the Skeleton

The skeleton is divided into two main sections: the *axial skeleton* and the *appendicular skeleton*. The axial skeleton includes bones of the head, neck, spine, chest, and trunk of the body. These bones form the central axis for the whole body and protect many of the internal organs. The appendicular skeleton consists of the upper and lower extremities and the pelvis. These bones, along with the muscles attached to them, are responsible for body movement (Figure 4-8).

Types of Joints

Joints (**articulations**) are formed when two or more bones meet. There are three types of joints in the human body based on the amount of movement allowed between the bones: **synovial** joints, **fibrous** joints, and **cartilaginous** joints. Table 4-3 illustrates the three types of joints. Synovial joints are free-moving joints lined by synovial fluid. This fluid helps reduce friction in the joints and provides flexibility. Ball-and-socket joints such as in the hip and shoulder are examples of synovial joints (Figure 4-9). Fibrous joints are held together by thick fibrous tissue and allow for almost no movement. The sutures of skull are an example of this type of joint. Cartilaginous joints allow for slight movement but hold bones firmly in place by a solid piece of cartilage. The growth regions of immature long bones are an example of cartilaginous joints.

Common Diseases and Conditions of the Skeletal System

Diseases of the bone increase the risk for breaking bones and interfering with their intended function.

Diseases of the bone include the following:

- Low bone density—also called osteopenia—is diagnosed when the bone density is lower than normal. This can lead to osteoporosis.

- *Osteoporosis*—the loss of bony material, thus leaving the bones with less density, making them brittle and soft.

- *Osteomyelitis*—an infection of the bone-forming tissue. There is inflammation, edema, and circulatory congestion in the bone marrow. Pus may form and inflammatory pressure may cause small pieces of bone to fracture.

- *Periodontitis*—a chronic infection that affects the gums and bones that support the teeth (periodontium). Significant bone loss may result in tooth loss.

 Documentation

A very important responsibility of the dental assistant is to complete or assist the patient in the completion of their medical history. The assistant's knowledge of anatomy and physiology, along with disease, will help the assistant to understand the process and ask pertinent questions. Accurate documentation is critical for proper treatment.

- *Osteoarthritis*—the most common type of arthritis; it is chronic, degenerative disease in which the cartilage that acts like a cushion breaks down and the bones rub together, causing pain, inflammation, and stiffness.
- *Cleft palate*—the failure of the palate (roof of the mouth) to form and join correctly.
- *Fractures*—breaks of the bone or cartilage.
- *Temporomandibular joint disorder (TMD)*—degeneration or disease of the joint where the mandible (lower jaw) articulates with the temporal bone.

Muscular System

The muscular system makes up 30% to 40% of total body weight. The muscles contract and relax to provide for all movements of the body, both internally and externally.

Anatomy of Muscles

Muscles are bundles of tissue fibers that contract to produce movement within the body. The human body has over 600 muscles, of which 400 are skeletal muscles that account for

Interrelationship Between Oral Health and the Skeletal System

The skeletal system contains the cranium, facial bones, maxilla (upper jaw), mandible (lower jaw), and the temporomandibular joint (joint that connects the maxilla and mandible). These bones support the teeth and surrounding tissues and are the primary focus of dentistry. It is important for the dental assistant to recognize and understand how the muscles and bones work together to properly chew food (process of mastication). The digestive process begins with the muscles of mastication that attach to the bones. Proper **occlusal function** and mastication are vital for a healthy body.

One of the responsibilities of the assistant is to mount dental radiographs. The ability to identify bones by their appearance and location makes mounting easier. Many oral diseases and injuries change the appearance of the normal jawbone structure and when recognized during a routine dental examination can result in early diagnosis. Diseases such as Paget's disease will appear as abnormal bone resorption of the mandible, and osteoporosis can cause loss of bone of the jaws, resulting in lack of tooth support and eventual loss. The assistant acts as the dentist's "second pair of eyes" in recognizing abnormalities on the radiograph and in the patient's mouth.

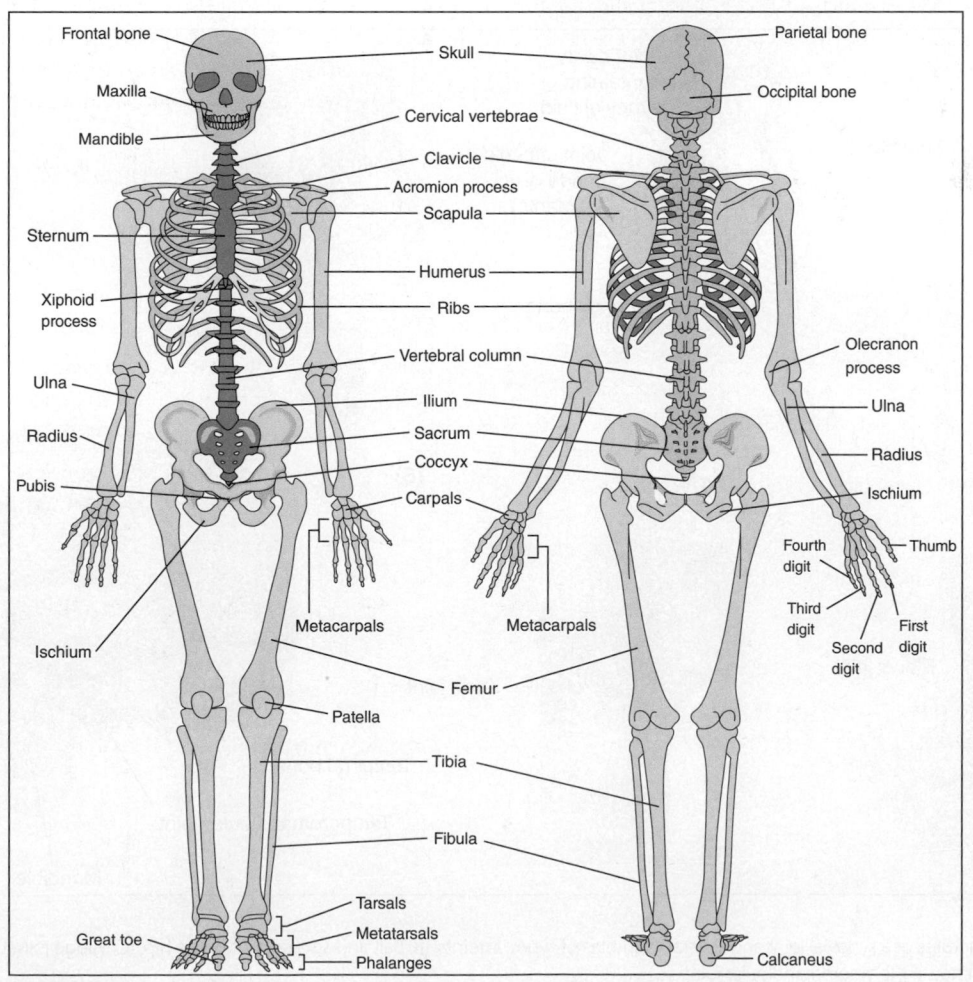

FIGURE 4-8
Axial (highlighted in blue) and appendicular (highlighted in gray) skeleton.

TABLE 4-3 Joints

Name of Joint	Description of Joint	Type of Movement	Example
Fibrous joint	Fibrous connective tissue	Immovable or fixed	Sutures found between the bones of the cranium.
Cartilaginous joint	Connective tissue, cartilage	Slightly movable	Joints found between bones of the vertebrae.
Synovial joint	Fluid within the joint (synovial fluid)	Considerable or free movement	There are six types of synovial joints: ball and socket, hinge, pivot, gliding, saddle, and condyloid. The temporomandibular joint is a synovial joint.

almost 50% of the body weight. The size of the muscles depends on how much they are used and how big the person is. Muscles serve three important functions for the body: support, heat production, and movement. Muscles work with the bones to hold the body erect. The muscles control the internal temperature by shivering when the core temperature drops too low and sweating when it gets too hot. Movement may take the form of pushing food through the digestive system, pumping blood through the blood vessels, or bringing two bones closer together. (Refer to Figure 4-10 and Figure 4-11 to view the muscles of the muscular system.)

Types of Muscles

There are three types of muscles: skeletal, smooth, and cardiac. Muscle tissue may be either voluntary or involuntary (Figure 4-12). Voluntary muscle movement means that a person consciously chooses to move a muscle, and involuntary muscle movement is under the subconscious regions of the brain and works automatically. The heart would be an example of an involuntary muscle, and the extremities are under voluntary control. All muscles have the ability to be stretched.

Skeletal muscles are attached to bones and produce voluntary movement of the skeleton. These muscles have the largest

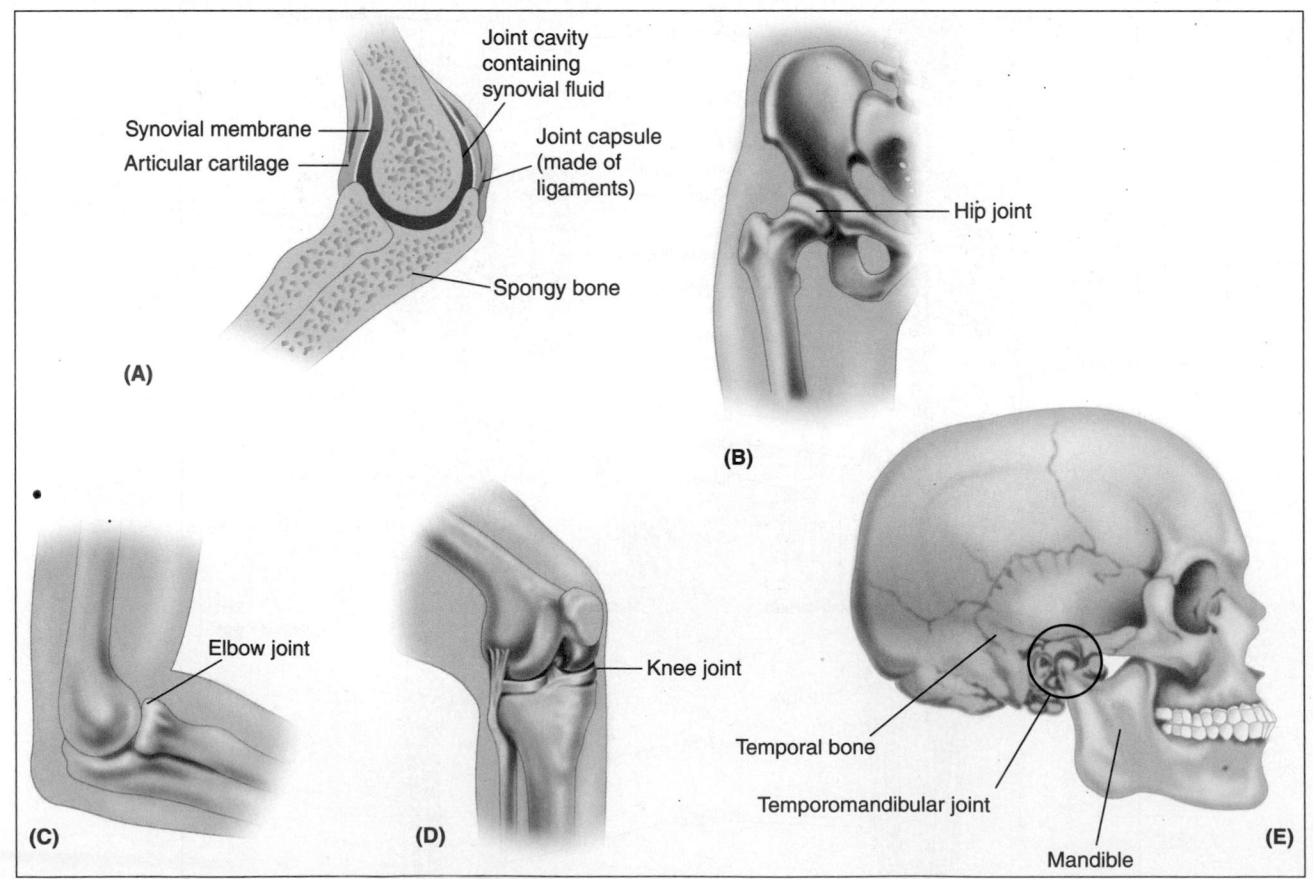

FIGURE 4-9
Skeletal joints: (A) Structures of a synovial joint and several examples of synovial joints. (B) Ball-and-socket joint of the hip. (C) Hinge joint of the elbow. (D) Hinge joint of the knee. (E) Temporomandibular joint.

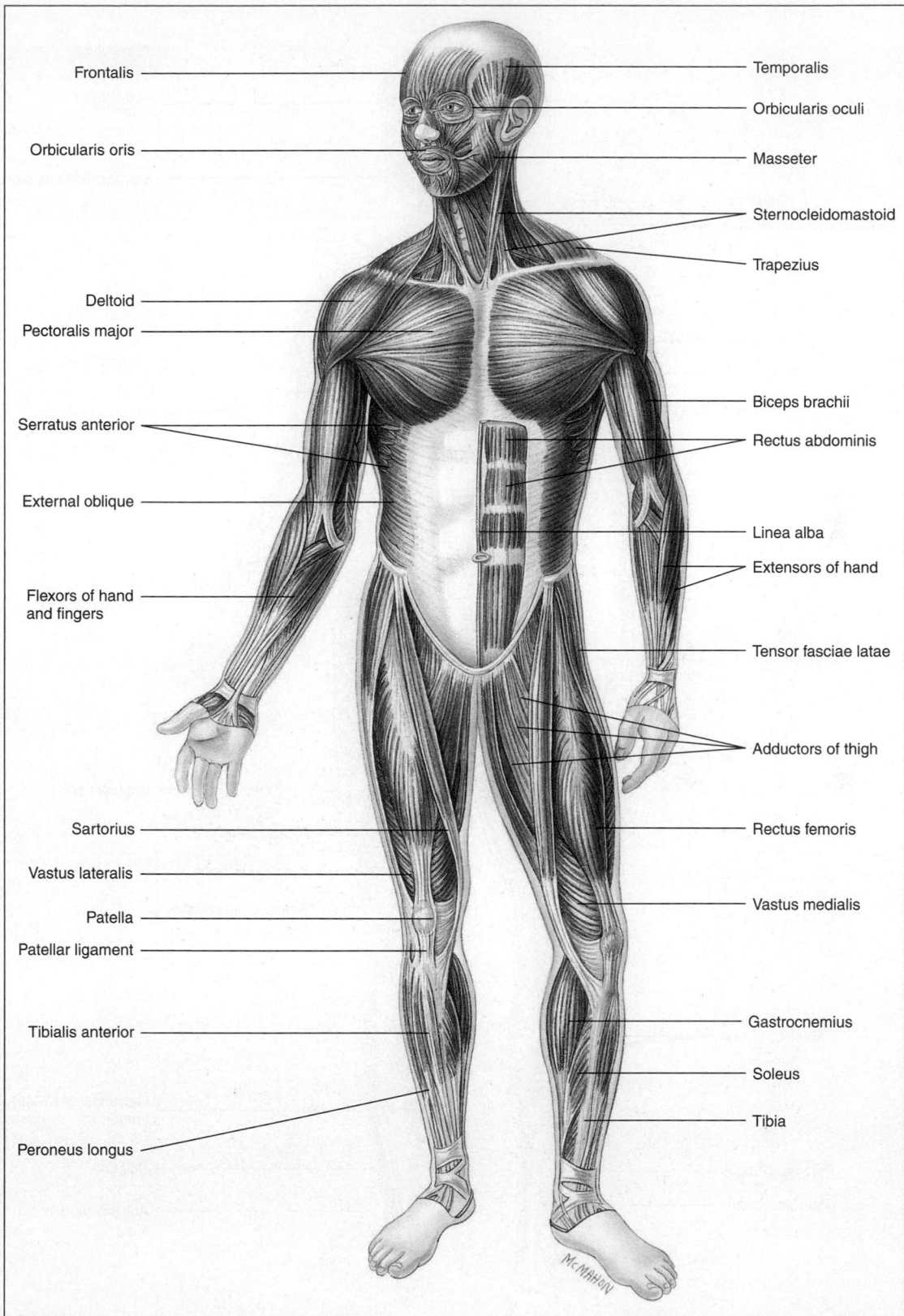

Frontalis

Orbicularis oris

Deltoid

Pectoralis major

Serratus anterior

External oblique

Flexors of hand
and fingers

Sartorius

Vastus lateralis

Patella

Patellar ligament

Tibialis anterior

Peroneus longus

Temporalis

Orbicularis oculi

Masseter

Sternocleidomastoid

Trapezius

Biceps brachii

Rectus abdominis

Linea alba

Extensors of hand

Tensor fasciae latae

Adductors of thigh

Rectus femoris

Vastus medialis

Gastrocnemius

Soleus

Tibia

FIGURE 4-10
The superficial muscles of the body (anterior view).

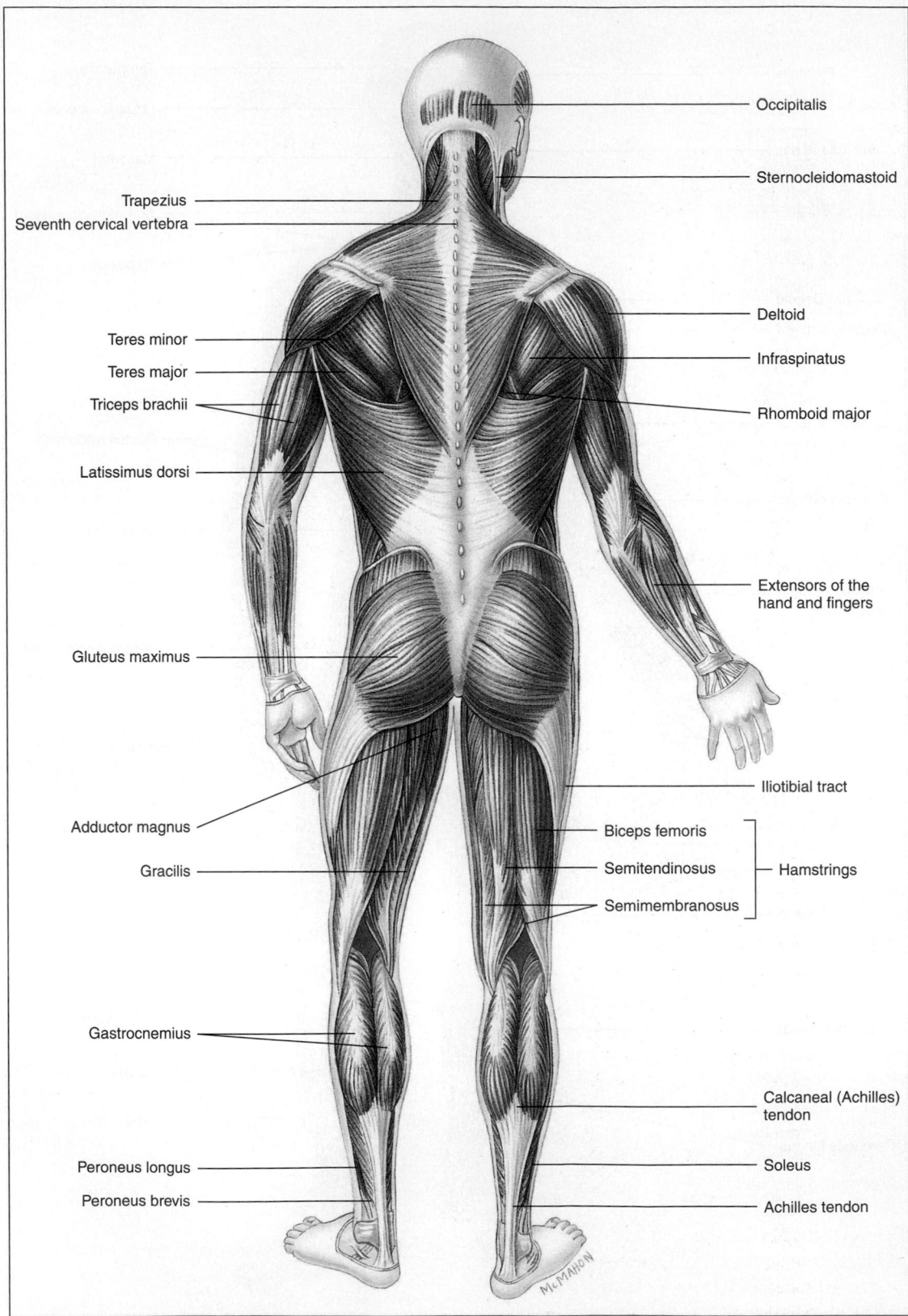

FIGURE 4-11
The superficial muscles of the body (posterior view).

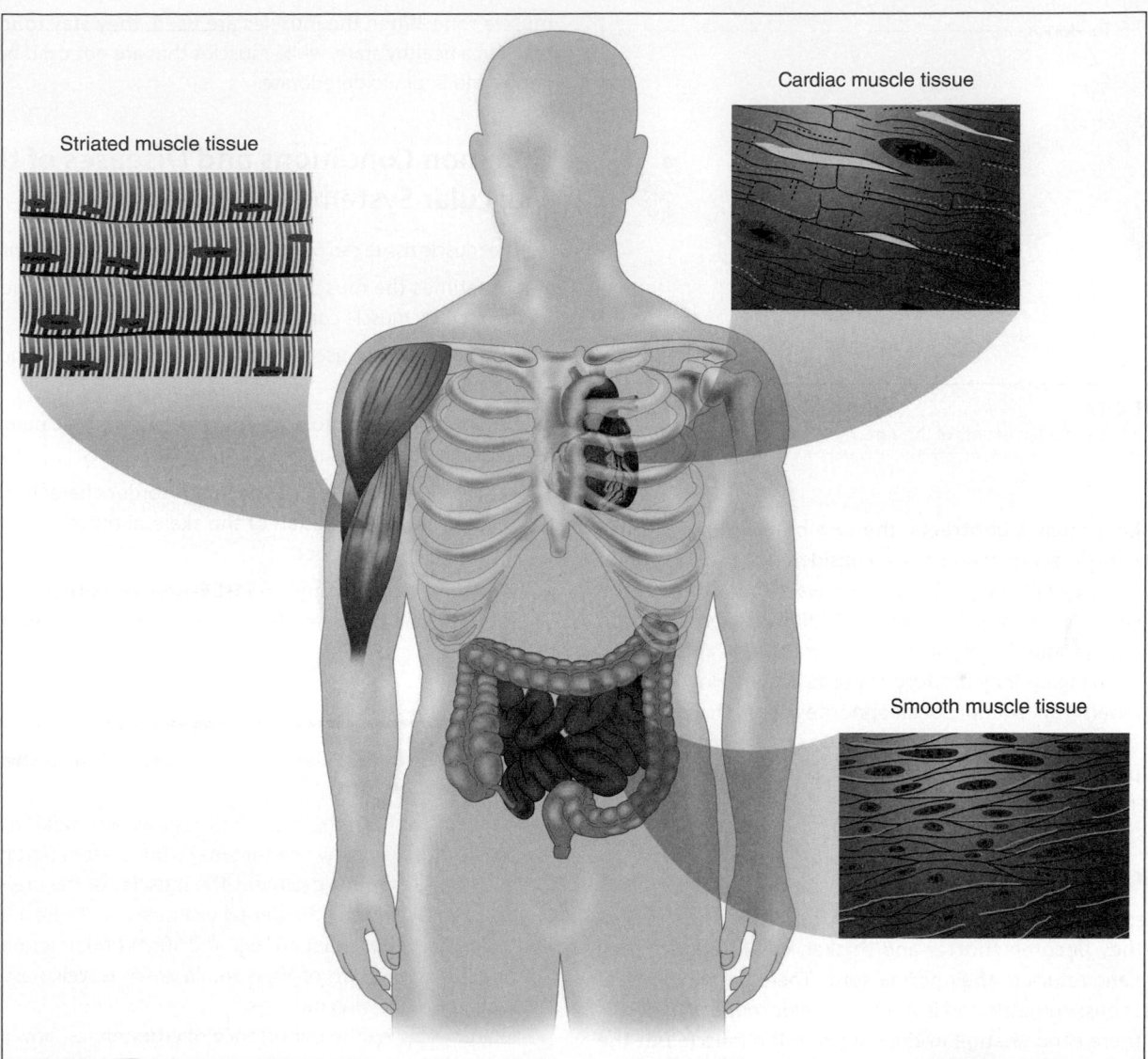

FIGURE 4-12
Types of muscles: (A) striated muscle. (B) Cardiac muscle. (C) Smooth muscle.

amount of muscle tissue of the three and allow the body to do things such as running, lifting, masticating, talking, and making facial expressions. Skeletal muscles are made of long, thin cells that have stripes or bands across them (striated).

Smooth muscles are nonstriated and are found within the internal organs (except the heart). They are responsible for the involuntary muscle action controlled by the **autonomic** nervous system and are not consciously controlled. Smooth muscles are associated with constriction of blood vessels, uterine contractions, and churning of food in the digestive tract.

Cardiac *muscles* make up the wall of the heart and have the same striated or striped appearance as the skeletal muscle. This type of muscle is found only in the heart and is under involuntary control. The involuntary contraction of the heart sends circulation through the body. The cardiac muscles receive approximately 75 **stimuli** per minute. These muscle cells are specially designed in a chain-like arrangement and are able to receive an impulse, respond, and relax very rapidly, thereby keeping the heart beating in an even rhythm.

Physiology of Skeletal Muscles

Each muscle is made of cells in various shapes and sizes depending on muscle function. Groups of muscle cells are often called fibers. Each fiber is about the size of a human hair and can support 1,000 times its own weight. Humans have over a trillion fibers in over 600 muscles in their bodies. Each fiber has nerves and a blood supply; it also has a fibrous sheet of connective tissue that covers, supports, and separates the muscle fibers. This sheet is called the **fascia**.

The skeletal muscles are overlapped by a joint and attached to two different bones. Muscles are attached to bones by strong bands of fibrous connective tissue known as tendons (Figure 4-13). Certain muscles require a broad, flattened extension called an *aponeurosis*. The aponeurosis attaches muscle to bone and binds muscle to muscle. Ligaments are composed of bands or sheets of fibrous tissue and act to connect or support two or more bones.

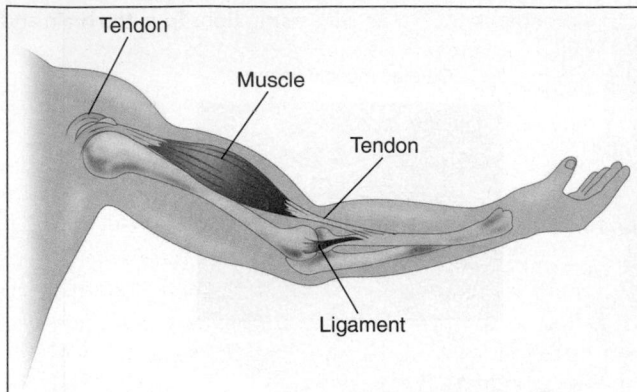

FIGURE 4-13
Muscle tissue and attachments of the arm.

When a muscle contracts, the two bones move but not equally. The lesser moving bone is considered the starting point for the muscle or the origin. The more movable bone is where the muscle ends or the insertion. This production is called the action of the muscle. Muscles of the body are arranged in antagonistic pairs, which means they produce opposite actions. How the forearm is raised is an example of an opposite action. The biceps are on the front of the upper arm, and the triceps are on the back of the upper arm. To raise the forearm, the biceps contract and the triceps relax to lower the forearm.

Muscle Function

Muscles work by contracting and relaxing. When muscles contract, they become shorter and thicker. When relaxed, they release and return to their normal form. There are two types of contractions: isometric and isotonic. *Isometric contraction* occurs when there is no change in the length of the muscle but the muscle tension is increased. Pushing against a solid object is an example of isometric contraction. Lifting weights is an example of *isotonic* contractions—the muscle tension remains the same but the muscles shorten.

It takes energy for muscles to function. Energy is received in the form of oxygen and **glucose**. Oxygen comes to the muscle through the circulating blood, and glucose is stored as a substance called **glycogen**. Muscles go through chemical changes to provide energy for body functions. Sometimes, when the activity is too rapid, there is not enough oxygen and an incomplete breakdown of glycogen occurs, resulting in a waste product called **lactic acid**. When the activity stops, the normal metabolic process readjusts and sufficient oxygen is restored.

Muscle tissue has the capacity, called excitability or irritability, to respond to stimuli. This response puts the muscle into motion or activity. The ability of the muscle to stretch or spread in order to perform tasks is **extensibility**. Muscle tone is the tension of the muscular system. The brain and spinal cord continually send stimuli to the muscles on a subconscious level. The increase or decrease of the constant stimuli from the nervous system affects muscle tone. When the muscles are used, they stay toned and ready in a healthy state, while muscles that are not used become flabby and begin to deteriorate.

Common Conditions and Diseases of the Muscular System

- The muscle tissue can be *strained, sprained, cramped,* or *inflamed.*
- Sometimes the muscles go into *spasm,* which is a sudden, involuntary muscle contraction.
- If muscles are not used, they begin to deteriorate, known as *atrophy.*
- *Fibromyalgia* (figh-broh-my-**AL**-jee-ah) is chronic pain in the muscles and soft tissues surrounding the joints.
- *Muscular dystrophy* is a congenital disorder characterized by progressive degeneration of the skeletal muscles. It usually strikes in early childhood.
- *Myasthenia gravis* (my-as-**THEE**-nee-ah **GRAH**-vis) is an autoimmune disorder that leaves the muscles weak and fatigued.

Interrelationship Between Oral Health and the Muscular System

Chewing, swallowing, facial expressions, and talking are all specific muscular activities that make this system pertinent to dentistry. The dentist evaluates the muscles of the oral cavity, neck, and face during the dental examination. There are many medical conditions that appear and affect oral functions. One of the first symptoms of Myasthenia gravis is weakness in the facial and swallowing muscles.

In Chapter 20, the importance of ergonomics (how people work in their environment and work-related injuries) in chairside assisting is discussed. When the assistant sits and moves improperly, the muscles in the lower back and the neck can become strained when assisting the dentist and performing procedures directly on the patient. The assistant needs to recognize these muscles and to learn how to strengthen them to maintain good posture and positioning to avoid work-related injuries. Seating the patient in the dental chair also requires proper positioning to avoid muscle strain and provide comfort for the patient.

Nervous System

The *nervous system* is responsible for all communication throughout the body. The body receives external and internal information (stimuli) and uses that information to control the actions made by the body. The nervous system can be subdivided into two parts: the central nervous system (CNS) and the peripheral nervous system (PNS). The CNS consists of the brain and the spinal cord, and the PNS consists of all the cranial and spinal nerves (Figure 4-14).

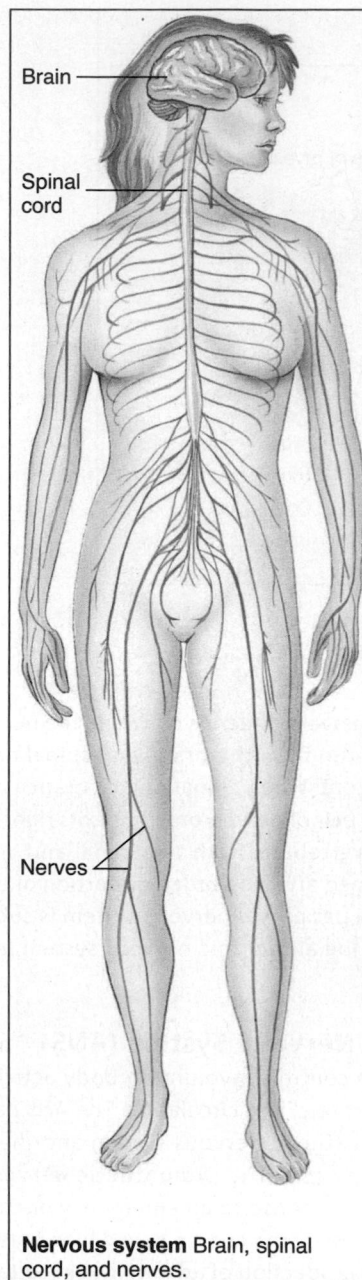

Brain

Spinal cord

Nerves

Nervous system Brain, spinal cord, and nerves.

FIGURE 4-14
Nervous system: brain, spinal cord, and nerves.

Structure of the Nervous System

There are two basic types of cells found in nervous tissue: neuroglial cells and neurons. **Neuroglial cells** do not carry electrical impulses or information as do **neurons**; their main function is to support the neurons. Neurons are individual nerve cells and are responsible for the conduction of electrical impulses in response to a stimulus.

The three different kinds of neurons are named according to their function:

1. Sensory neurons originate from the skin or a sensory organ and carry information to the brain and spinal cord.

2. Motor neurons carry activity instructions from the brain and spinal cord to the muscles or glands in the body.

3. Associative neurons (interneurons) carry information between two neurons in the CNS.

The neuron structure includes a nucleus surrounded by a cell membrane with thread-like projections called nerve fibers. The nerve fibers that conduct impulses toward the cell body are called dendrites (Figure 4-15). Axons are nerve fibers that conduct impulses away from the cell body. Some dendrites and axons can be up to two feet long. Nerve fibers move impulses from one cell body to another through a synapse. This is a junction where chemicals are released from the ends of axons to allow the stimuli to jump to the next dendrite. Some nerves in the PNS are covered with layers of Schwann cells. These layers insulate and protect nerves and are known as the myelin sheath.

Central Nervous System (CNS)

Since the *central nervous system* is a combination of the brain and the spinal cord, it has the ability to receive information, process this information, and act as found necessary to all parts of the body. The brain and spinal cord are protected by a watery substance that surrounds the area called *cerebrospinal fluid* (CSF). The CSF protects the nervous system from sudden motion and shock.

Brain and Cranial Nerves The *brain* is responsible for coordination of most of the body's activities. The brain receives incoming stimuli and interprets and processes the information. Stimuli are directed to various parts of the brain, depending on which area of the body the stimuli is coming from.

Each section of the brain is responsible for a specific body function. There are four sections of the brain: cerebrum, cerebellum, diencephalon, and the brain stem (Figure 4-16).

The *cerebrum* is located in the upper part of the brain and is the largest section of the brain. This area controls thoughts, memory, problem solving, judgment, and language. The cerebrum is divided into the left and right hemisphere and each contains four lobes:

- The *frontal lobe* is located in the front or anterior portion of the brain. This area controls speech, motor function, and personality.

- The *parietal lobe* is in the top or the superior portion of the brain. This area controls the ability to interpret language, as well as receives and interprets nerve impulses from the body.

- The *occipital lobe* is the back or the posterior portion of the brain. This area controls vision.

- The *temporal lobe* is on the right and left side or lateral portion of the brain. This area controls hearing and smell.

The *cerebellum* is located in the bottom portion of the brain, underneath the cerebrum. This area of the brain controls voluntary movements of the body, as well as **equilibrium** and balance.

The *diencephalon* is located between the cerebellum and the cerebrum. This area contains the *thalamus* and the *hypothalamus*. The thalamus controls pain receptors and relays messages from the eyes, ears, and skin to the cerebrum. The hypothalamus

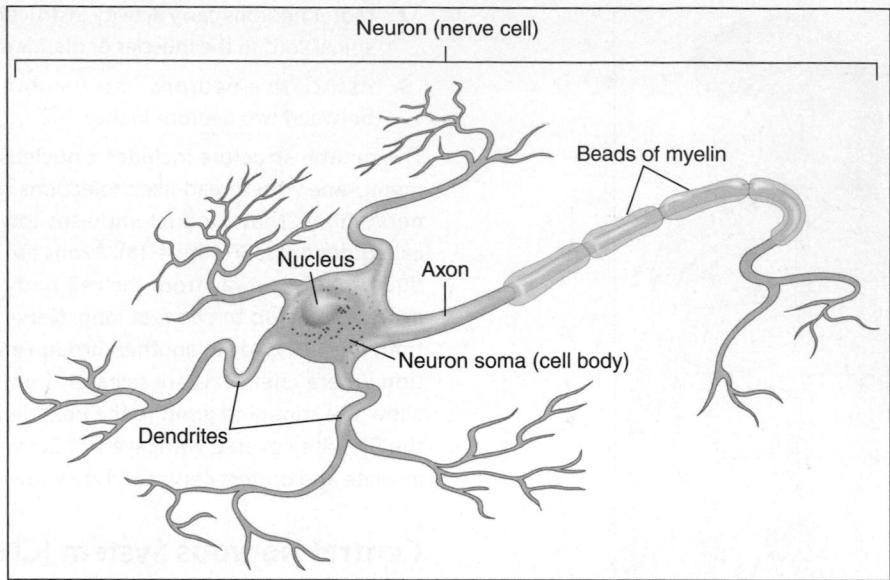

FIGURE 4-15
Structure of a neuron.

controls body temperature, emotions, sexual responses, appetite, and sleep. It also controls the release of hormones, the cardiovascular system, and the digestive system, as well as the autonomic nervous system (ANS).

The *brainstem* is the pathway between the brain and spinal cord and is located below the brain. This area is extremely important because it controls respirations, heart rate, temperature, and blood pressure. Also, this is the area of the brain where the nerve tracts cross from one side to the other; in other words, the left side of the brain controls the right side and vice versa, with few exceptions.

There are 12 pairs of *cranial* nerves that mainly involve the head. They are numbered with Roman numerals beginning in the front of the brain and moving toward the back (Table 4-4).

Spinal Cord and Spinal Nerves The *spinal cord* is the pathway for electrical impulses to travel to and from the brain. It is a column of nervous tissue where spinal nerves emerge through openings in the **vertebrae**. The activity of the spinal cord is twofold. First, it is a center for reflex or involuntary responses. When a stimulus is sent through the sensory neurons into the spinal cord and a response is automatically processed and sent back through motor neurons for an action, a reflex arc occurs (Figure 4-17).

Second, the spinal cord transmits stimuli from the body to the brain, where the message is interpreted, and then a response is sent back to an organ or a muscle.

The body has 33 vertebral bones that form the backbone of the body. This canal, or vertebral cavity, serves as protection of the spinal cord and spinal nerves. The nerves are named and numbered according to the closest vertebrae.

Peripheral Nervous System (PNS)

The *peripheral nervous system* consists of 12 pairs of cranial nerves and 31 pairs of spinal nerves. The determination of

what type the nerve is depends on where the nerve originates. Cranial nerves run from the brain, and spinal nerves branch off the spinal cord. When spinal nerves branch off the spinal cord, it forms a pair of nerves, one that exits right and one that exits left of a vertebrae. Both the spinal and cranial nerves are usually named after the organ or portion of the body that they serve. The peripheral nervous system is subdivided into two divisions: the autonomic nervous system (ANS) and the somatic nerves.

Autonomic Nervous System (ANS) The *autonomic nervous system* controls involuntary body activities, such as breathing, heart rate, and circulation. The ANS had two major parts: the sympathetic nervous system and the parasympathetic nervous system. The **sympathetic nerves** control our "fight-or-flight" response to an emergency or crisis situation. These nerves increase the heart rate and blood pressure, as well as increase the production of **adrenaline** in certain situations. The **parasympathetic nerves** control the everyday functions and balance the body system to normal functioning after a crisis situation. These nerves decrease the heart rate and blood pressure, as well as function to stimulate digestion and elimination.

Somatic Nerves The **somatic nerves** control the voluntary body activities, such as skeletal muscles and sensory information found in the skin, including touch, temperature, and pain.

Common Diseases of the Nervous System

The nervous system is vulnerable to various diseases. It can be damaged by the following: trauma, infections, degeneration, structural defects, tumors, blood flow disruption, and autoimmune disorders.

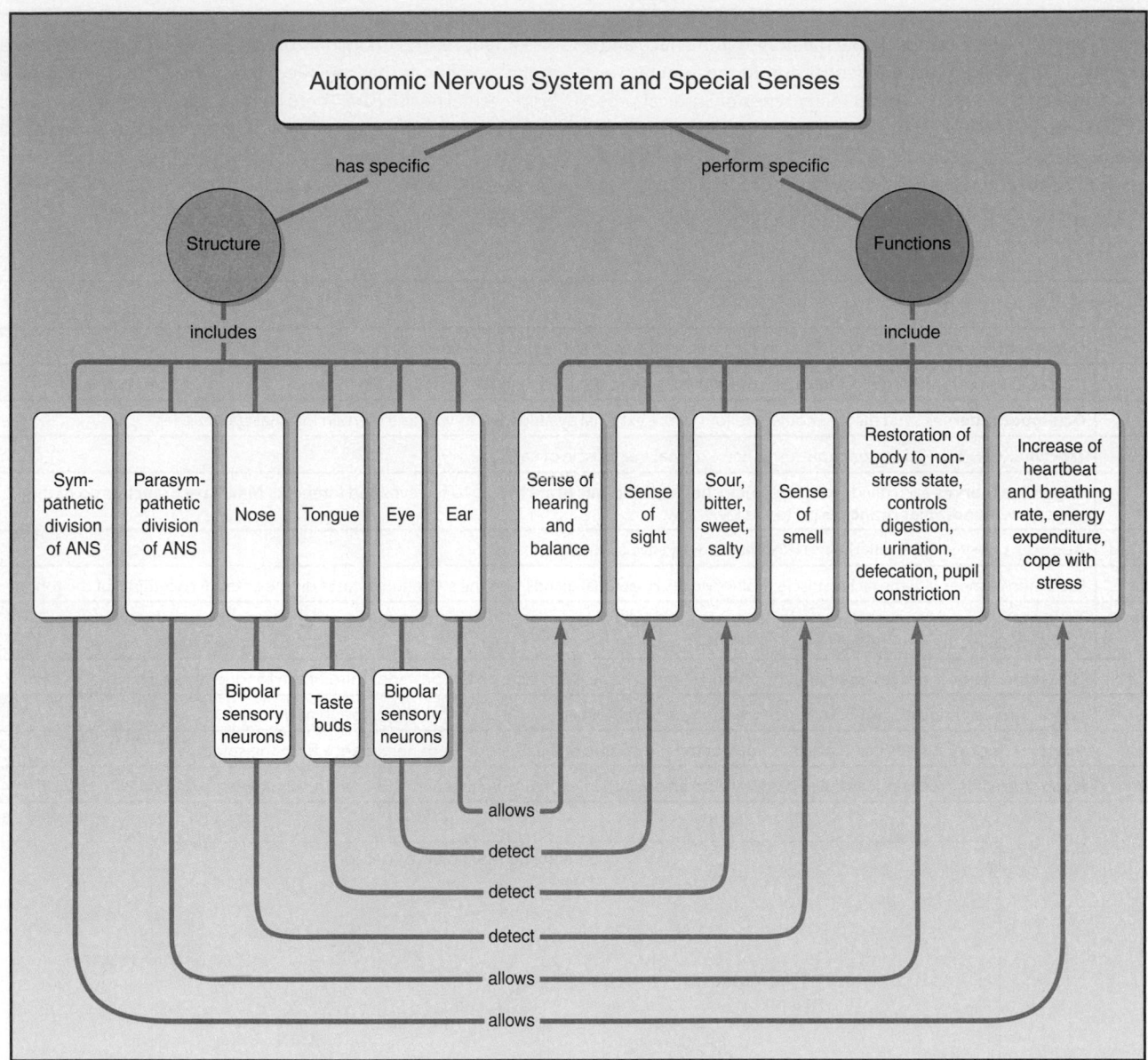

FIGURE 4-16
The principal parts of the brain.

- *Neuritis* is the inflammation of nerves. It may be the result of a fall or blow and can affect one or more nerves in the body. The term *neuritis* is also used when describing nerve tissue degeneration.

- *Multiple sclerosis (MS)* is a disease that usually appears in people aged 20 to 40. This disease destroys the myelin sheath of neurons in the CNS. When this happens, impulses cannot be transmitted to their destinations.

- *Parkinson's disease* is a chronic nervous system disease characterized by slowly spreading tremors, muscular weakness, and a peculiar gait.

- *Bell's palsy* is a sudden onset of facial paralysis.

Interrelationship Between Oral Health and the Nervous System

The mouth is the most sensitive part of the body and houses 30% to 40% of the body's sensory and motor nerves. The cranial nerves regulate swallowing, taste, and mucous and saliva secretions. Understanding its structure and how the nervous system works will help the dental assistant work with the dentist and the patient.

Patients often fear going to the dentist because they assume it will be a physically painful experience. The dentist uses a local anesthetic that blocks the nerves that sense or transmit pain, thus making the area numb and the dental procedures

(Continues)

possible. Dental assistants must know the nerves in the face and oral cavity to effectively assist the dentist during the administration of anesthetic, as well as during many types of surgical procedures. Dental team members sometimes experience physical problems themselves, especially with the sciatic nerve located in the lower back and traveling down the back of the thigh. This is due to the positions they must hold for long periods of time.

Patients with Parkinson's disease have uncontrollable shaking of their hands that can affect the patient's ability to complete home dental health care. There is also a risk of aspirating (choking) during procedures due to a weakened swallowing capability. Patients who have been on certain prescription medications for an extended time often develop teeth grinding and a decrease in saliva flow, which results in an increase in dental decay.

TABLE 4-4 Cranial Nerves and Their Functions

I.	**Olfactory nerves** conduct impulses from receptors in the nose to the brain and are sensory in function.
II.	**Optic nerves** conduct impulses from receptors in the eyes to the brain and are sensory in function.
III.	**Oculomotor nerves** send motor impulses to four of the external eye muscles, as well as to certain internal eye muscles.
IV.	**Trochlear nerves** send motor impulses to one external eye muscle of each eye.
V.	**Trigeminal nerves** each divide into three branches: **Ophthalmic branches** go to the eyes and forehead. **Maxillary branches** go to the upper jaw. **Mandibular branches** go to the lower jaw.
VI.	**Abducens nerves** innervate the muscles that turn the eye to the side.
VII.	Facial nerves innervate the facial muscles, salivary glands, lacrimal glands, and the sensation of taste on the anterior two-thirds of the tongue.
VIII.	**Acoustic nerves** each divide into two branches: **Cochlear branches** are concerned with the sense of hearing. **Vestibular branches** are concerned with the sense of balance.
IX.	**Glossopharyngeal nerves** innervate the parotid glands, the sense of taste on the posterior third of the tongue, and part of the pharynx.
X.	**Vagus nerves** innervate part of the pharynx, larynx, and vocal cords, and parts of the thoracic and abdominal viscera.
XI.	**Spinal accessory nerves** innervate the shoulder muscles. Some of the fibers of these nerves arise from the spinal cord.
XII.	**Hypoglossal nerves** primarily innervate the muscles concerned with movements of the tongue.

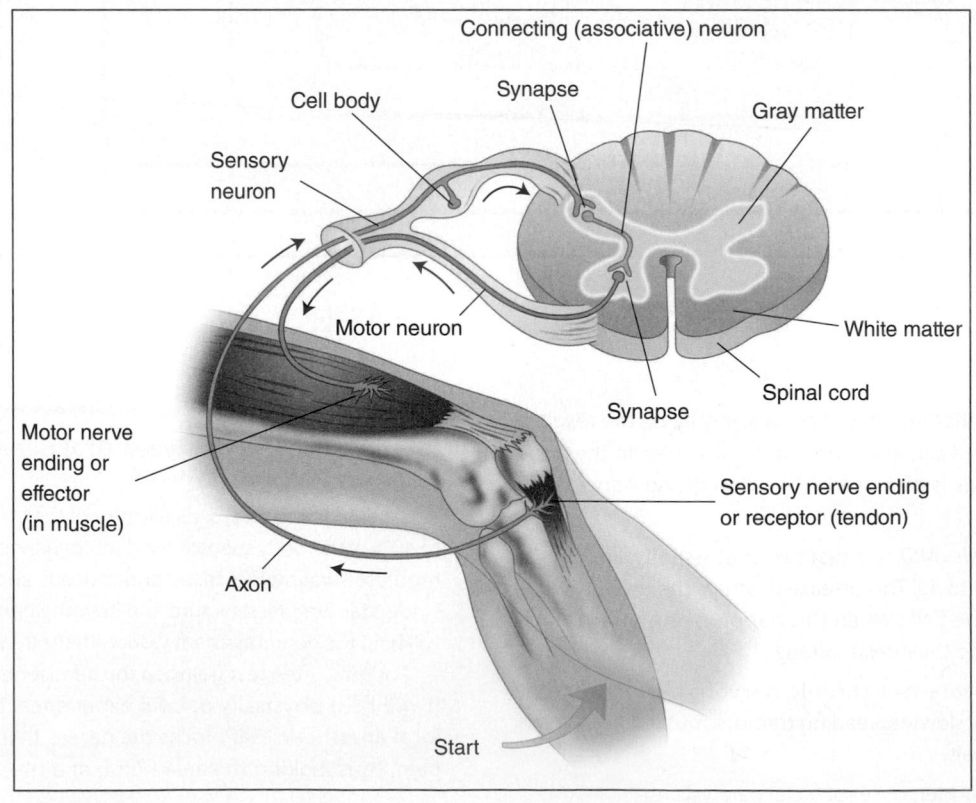

FIGURE 4-17
Simple reflex arc.

Endocrine System

The **endocrine system**, like the nervous system, is a control and communication system. The nervous system acts rapidly to transmit stimuli, whereas the endocrine system is much slower and the results are longer lasting. The nervous system and the endocrine system are connected because the nervous system controls the pituitary gland and this gland controls the other glands. The endocrine system generally controls the body's growth; protects the body in stressful situations; controls development of sex characteristics; regulates utilization of calcium; aids in regulating the body's water balance; and produces insulin, which aids in the transport of glucose into cells.

Function of the Endocrine System

The endocrine system is made of glands spread throughout the body (Figure 4-18). They are grouped according to structures and interrelated functions. The endocrine glands produce secretions called **hormones** and are ductless—there is no tube for secretions from the glands to pass through, so the hormones empty directly into the bloodstream and circulate throughout the body. Hormones are chemicals that are made specifically to work with cells, an organ, or system to increase or decrease its activity level depending on the need of the body at that time. They control the internal environment of the body from the cellular to the organ level. They are analogous to the furnaces and thermostats in our homes. We set the thermostat to a particular temperature, and when the temperature falls below that temperature, the thermostat causes the furnace to turn on. Once the temperature reaches the set temperature on the thermostat, the furnace turns off. The hormonal system functions in a similar manner. When the concentration of a particular hormone reaches a certain level in the body, the endocrine gland that secretes that hormone is inhibited and secretion of the hormone ceases or decreases. Later, when the concentration of that gland's hormone falls below normal levels, the inhibition of the gland stops and it begins to produce and secrete the hormone once again.

Endocrine Glands

The endocrine system consists of the following glands: two adrenal glands, two ovaries (female), two testes (male), thyroid gland, four parathyroid glands, pituitary gland, pancreas, pineal gland, and the thymus gland.

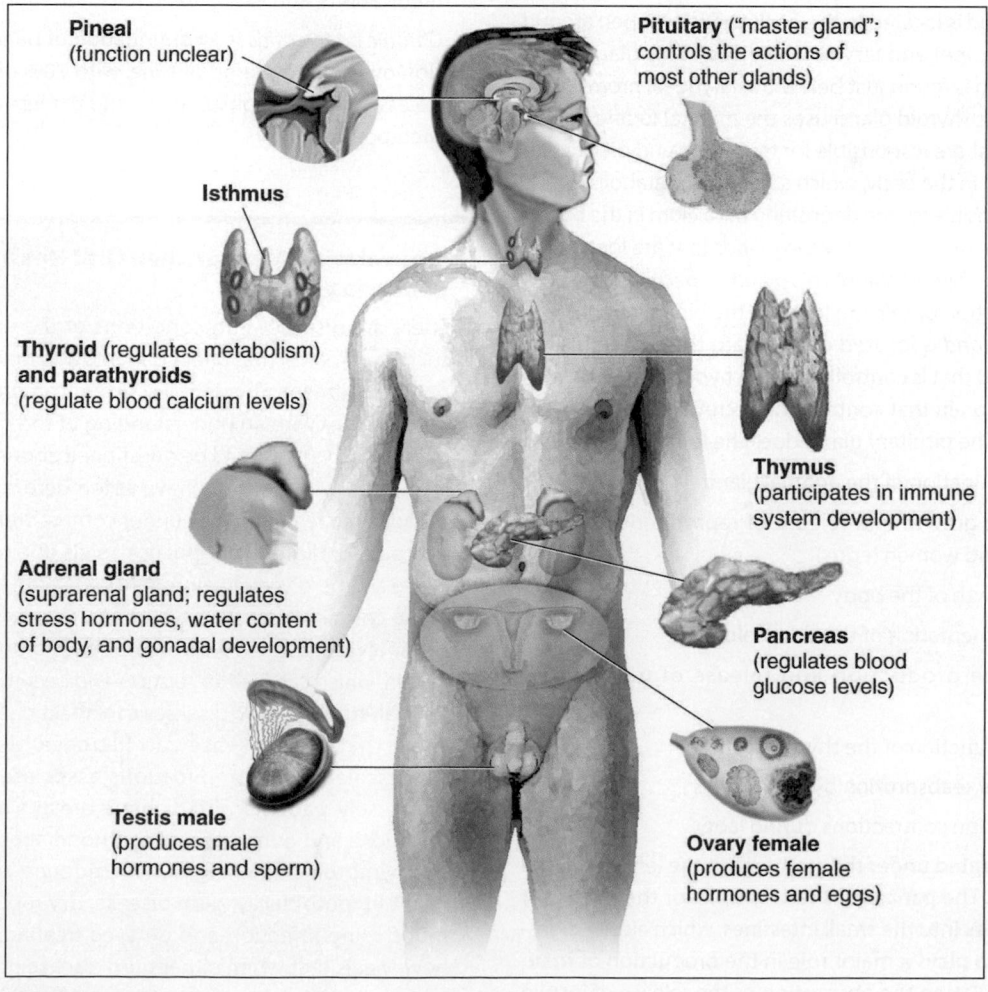

FIGURE 4-18
Structures of the endocrine system.

The body contains two **adrenal glands,** which are located above each kidney. The adrenal glands are responsible for the following:

- The regulation of carbohydrate (source of energy) levels in the body
- The regulation of sodium and potassium levels in the body
- The production of sex hormones that are necessary for reproduction and secondary sexual characteristics
- Critical body responses in emergency situations that increase the body's blood pressure, heart rate, and respiration levels that will increase levels of performance due to secretion of a hormone called **epinephrine** or **adrenaline**

The body contains two *ovaries*, which are located in the lower abdominopelvic cavity of a female. The ovaries are responsible for the production and secretion of the female sex hormones that regulate the menstrual cycle, the appearance of secondary sexual characteristics, such as breast development and hair growth, and they maintain a healthy environment for pregnancy.

The body contains two *testes*, which are located in the scrotum sac that extends externally between the legs of a male. The testes are responsible for the production and secretion of the male sex hormone, which regulates sperm production and the appearance of secondary sexual characteristics.

The *thyroid gland* is located in the neck and is wrapped around the trachea (windpipe) and larynx (voice box). This gland has a butterfly shape and is found just below the laryngeal prominence (Adam's apple). The thyroid gland uses the mineral iodine to produce hormones that are responsible for regulation and production of energy and heat in the body, which stimulates metabolism. This gland is also responsible for the depositing of calcium in the bones.

The body contains four *parathyroid glands* that are located on the back side of the thyroid gland. This gland is specifically responsible for the regulation of calcium levels in the bloodstream.

The *pituitary gland* is located underneath the brain. This is a marble-sized gland that is controlled by the hypothalamus, which is a section of the brain that controls the secretion and release of many hormones. The pituitary gland does the following:

- Regulates the function of the adrenal gland
- Stimulates the growth and release of reproductive cells, of men (sperm) and women (eggs)
- Stimulates growth of the body
- Stimulates pigmentation of the skin (color)
- Stimulates the production and release of milk during lactation
- Regulates the function of the thyroid gland
- Promotes water reabsorption by the kidneys
- Stimulates uterine contractions during labor

The *pancreas* is located under the stomach on the left side of the abdominal cavity. The pancreas is responsible for the release of **digestive enzymes** into the small intestines, which aids in digestion of food. It also plays a major role in the production of **insulin**, as well as regulating the absorption or the release of insulin into the bloodstream depending on what our body needs.

The *pineal gland* is located inside the thalamus, which is a section of the brain. This gland is responsible for the regulation of the sleep-and-wake cycles, our internal body clock.

The *thymus gland* is located above and in front of the heart in the thoracic (chest) cavity. This gland is unique in that it is present at birth and continues to grow larger through puberty; at that time, it begins to shrink in size and eventually turns into tissue. The thymus gland is responsible for the development of cells in the immune system, the body's defense system. This is most crucial in the growth and development of a newborn's immune system.

Common Diseases and Conditions of the Endocrine and Reproductive Systems

- *Diabetes mellitus* is the most common endocrine disorder that occurs when the pancreas produces an insufficient amount of insulin.
- *Hypothyroidism* is an underactive thyroid gland.
- *Hyperthyroidism* is an overactive thyroid gland with excessive secretion of hormones.
- *Acute pancreatitis* develops over a short period of time and may be caused by gallstones, excessive alcohol consumption, medications, and exposure to infections and injuries.
- *Chronic pancreatitis* is a continuation of pancreatic inflammation over a long period of time, with 70% of the cases due to excessive alcohol consumption and the less common cause of metabolic disorders.

Interrelationship Between Oral Health and the Endocrine System

There are diseases and conditions of the endocrine system, such as diabetes, that affect patients and how they respond to dental treatment. The dental assistant can prepare for possible emergencies with an understanding of the patient's needs. All diabetic patients should be questioned about their blood sugar levels and whether they have eaten before treatment. If the blood sugar levels are not under control, treatment should be postponed. High blood glucose levels due to low insulin may cause a hyperglycemic emergency that can lead to life-threatening complications. Hypoglycemia happens when the blood sugar levels are too low from not eating or taking too much insulin, which can lead to seizures and become life-threatening.

Diabetes and gum diseases can affect one another. Reports show that gum disease can increase blood sugar levels and escalate the complications associated with diabetes. Conversely, patients with diabetes are at a greater risk of oral infections and gum disease than nondiabetic patients. These oral symptoms have a greater incidence with diabetes and result in tooth decay, gum disease, dry mouth, lesions in the mouth, and infection and delayed healing. The good news, however, is that when either gum disease or diabetes is properly treated, improvements in the other condition can result.

Reproductive System

The *reproductive* system includes the male reproductive organs and the female reproductive organs. The male and female reproductive systems' main function is the creation of life. In both sexes, primary and accessory organs must be protected in certain procedures used in dentistry. For example, when exposing radiographs, using a lead apron is required to protect the male and female reproductive organs and to protect the developing child during pregnancy from radiation. The male sperm and female ovaries can be permanently damaged by radiation (may result in difficulty in becoming pregnant). Radiation exposure to unborn babies may increase the risk of birth defects and cancer. Safety guidelines are routinely followed in the dental office to protect the patient and the dental staff.

Female Reproductive System

The female reproductive system consists of the internal and external **genitalia** or reproductive organs. The internal organs are located in the lower **pelvic** cavity and consist of the uterus, two ovaries, two fallopian tubes, and the vagina. The vagina leads to the external organs, which are collectively called the vulva (Figure 4-19).

The *uterus* is a hollow, upside-down, pear-shaped organ that sits in the center of the lower pelvic cavity between the bladder and the rectum. The inner lining of the uterus, called the *endometrium*, contains a very rich blood supply and reacts to hormonal changes of the female body. The endometrium will thicken throughout the month and if a fertilized egg is not implanted, will slough off, resulting in *menstruation*. If a fertilized egg is received, the thickened endometrium will serve as a place of nourishment and protection as a fetus develops and grows inside the uterus.

The ovaries are small, almond-shaped organs that sit bilaterally on each side of the uterus. These organs are responsible for the production of the female sex hormones (estrogen and progesterone) and the *ova* or female reproductive cell (egg). Approximately every 28 days, the anterior pituitary gland (located in the brain) will release specific hormones that will trigger ovulation, or the release of the ova from one of the ovaries. Depending on whether *sperm,* or the male reproductive cell, is present in the female system, fertilization will occur and a pregnancy will begin. If fertilization does not occur, the female will eventually menstruate. As females age, hormones that are secreted by the ovaries will decrease in production, which will cause the cessation of the menses, also known as menopause.

The *fallopian tubes*, also known as the uterine tubes, are bilateral extensions off the upper part of the uterus and are the pathway for an ovum (egg) to enter the uterus. The open end, which sits directly next to each ovary, has finger-like projections called *fimbriae*. Fimbriae catch the ovum after ovulation and direct the ovum into the fallopian tube. If fertilization of the ovum takes place, it usually occurs in the upper one-half of the fallopian tube and then the ovum is directed into the uterus for implantation inside the uterus.

The *vagina* is the muscular tube that connects the uterus to the outside of the body. The opening between the uterus and the vaginal canal is called the cervix. The vagina is the passageway for menstrual blood to exit the body as well as the passageway that receives sperm from the male penis during sexual intercourse. In addition, the vagina also serves as the birth canal the fetus passes through during a vaginal birth.

The *vulva* is a group of structures that make up the external female reproductive organs. The vaginal external skin folds are called the labia majora and the labia minora, and both serve as protection for the genitalia. They are also the external openings

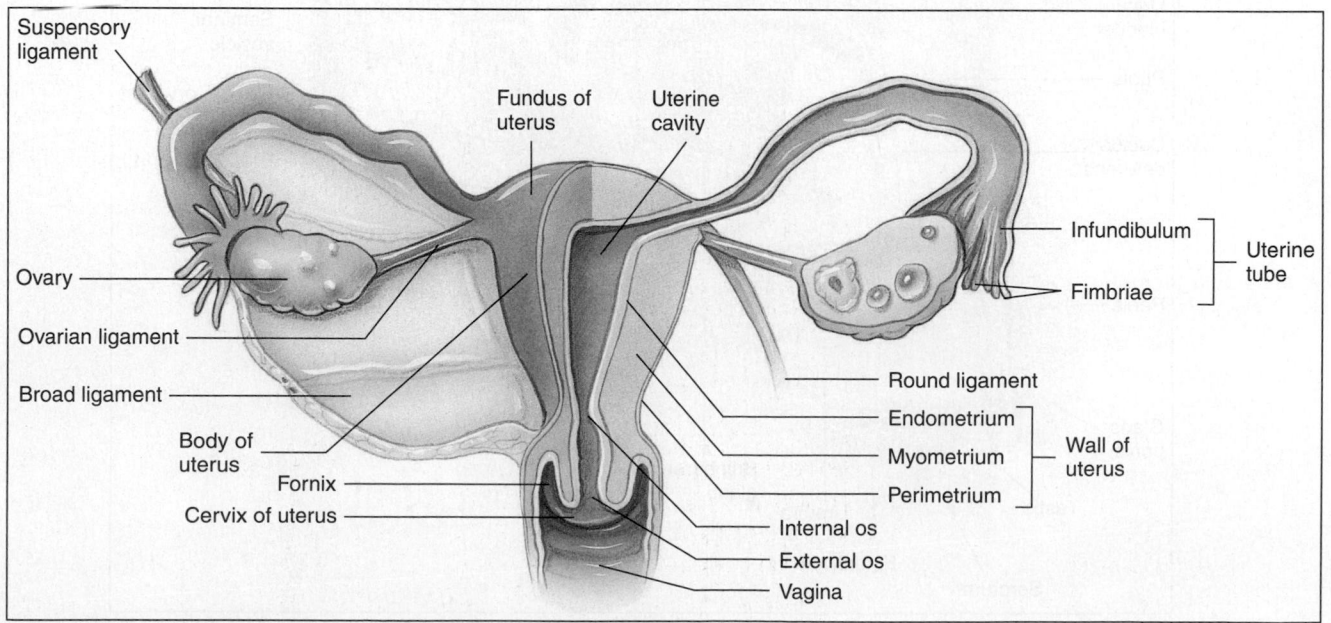

FIGURE 4-19
The position of the ovaries, uterine tubes, uterus, and vagina of the female reproductive system.

of the urinary system. The *clitoris* is a very small organ that is covered by the labia minora and contains sensitive tissues that are aroused during sexual stimulation.

The breasts, or the mammary glands, play a major role in the female reproductive system. They have the ability to produce milk (a process called lactation) to nourish the infant after birth. Milk is produced by glands located inside the breast called lactiferous glands. Lactation is caused by hormonal changes and stimulation from the suckling infant. The pigmented or darkened part of the breast around the nipple is called the areola, and the nipple has external openings through which the infant will receive milk.

Male Reproductive System

The male reproductive system is a combination of the organs of reproduction and the urinary tract. The major reproduction organs, the penis and the scrotum, are located outside the male body (Figure 4-20).

The *penis* is the male sex organ that delivers the sperm (the male reproductive cell) into the vagina during sexual intercourse. The penis is a cylindrical-shaped organ that is externally suspended in the lower pelvic region. At the tip of the penis is an opening called the urinary meatus. The urinary meatus is the ending of the **urethra**, which is the tube that

is connected to the urinary bladder and expels the urine. This opening is used for the elimination of urine as well as the release of sperm.

The *scrotum* is the external sac that lies between the legs and behind the penis. This sac, which is divided by a septum, contains two testicles (testes).

Testes are organs that are oval in shape and are suspended in the external scrotum sac. This is where *sperm*, the male reproductive cell, is produced, as well as testosterone. Testosterone is the male hormone that is responsible for the growth and development of the male reproductive organs and sperm. It is important that the testes maintain a proper temperature for the sperm to survive. This is why the scrotum and testes are stored outside the body.

The *epididymis* is a coiled tube that is located on top of both testes inside the scrotum. These tubes store sperm as they are produced until they are released. The sperm are held here until they reach full maturation and then are released into the vas deferens.

The internal reproductive organs consist of two tubes called the *vas deferens* that carry mature sperm from the epididymis to the pelvic cavity. There are two small glands, *seminal vesicles*, which sit at the base of the urinary bladder just before it empties into the urethra. These glands are connected to the vas deferens and secrete a fluid that nourishes or feeds the sperm and which is also released with the sperm.

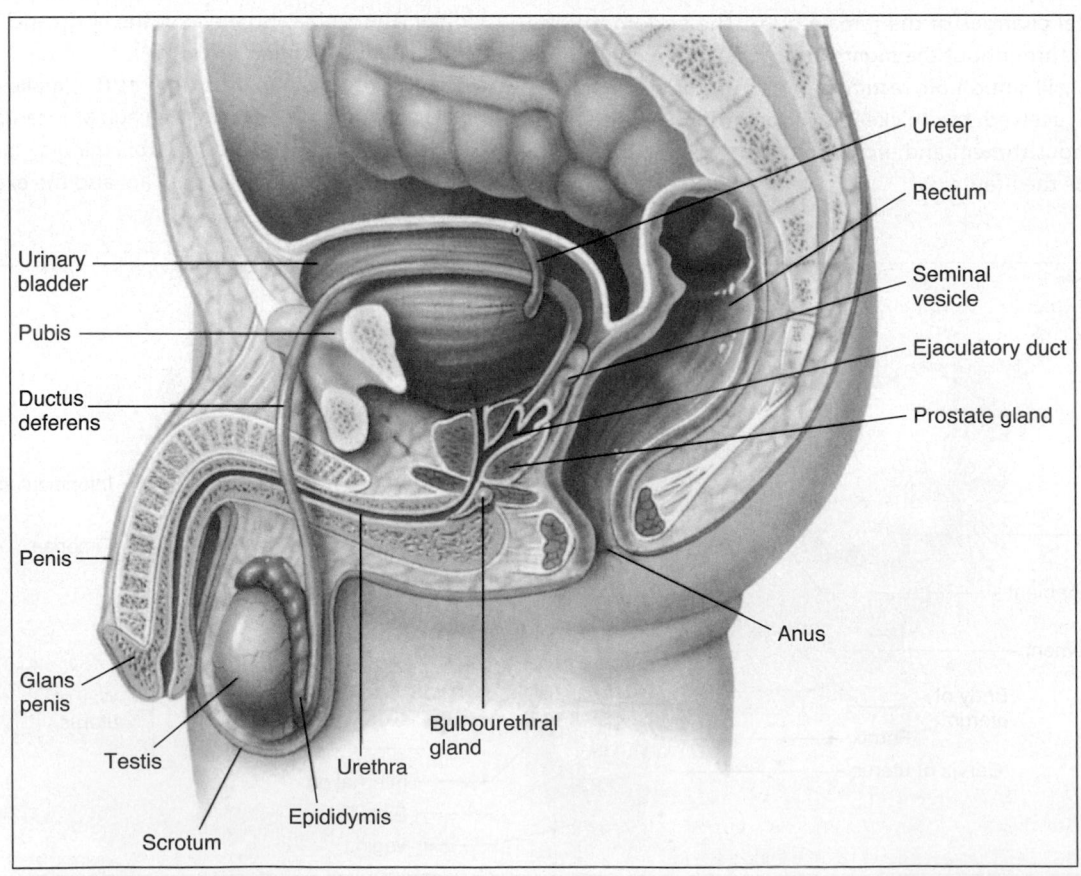

FIGURE 4-20
The organs and ducts of the male reproductive system.

The **prostate gland** is a single gland located below the urinary bladder and secretes a fluid with the sperm that keeps the pH neutralized in the vagina and urethra in order to keep sperm alive. This gland surrounds the urethra, and if it enlarges, it can cause difficulty with urination.

Common Diseases and Conditions of the Reproductive Systems

Fibrocystic mastopathy is one of the main diseases that occurs in premenopausal women and affects the woman's breasts. It is characterized by benign, small, painful cysts that vary in size.

Endometriosis is a problem affecting a woman's uterus. In this condition, the uterine tissue grows somewhere else and causes pain in the abdomen, lower back, or pelvic area.

Testosterone deficiency is a condition in which a man's body does not produce the primary male hormone and can lead to abnormalities in muscle and bone development, underdeveloped genitalia, decreased motivation, and depression.

Prostate cancer is the most common cancer among men with symptoms of lower back pain, urge of frequent urination, painful urination, and blood in the urine.

Interrelationship Between Oral Health and the Reproductive System

Oral health during pregnancy should be an important part of prenatal care. Approximately 60% to 75% of pregnant mothers have gingivitis (inflammation of the gums). Hormones change during pregnancy, and hormones have a negative effect on the gingiva (pregnancy gingivitis). If the gingivitis is neglected, it can lead to the loss of the bone that supports the teeth, infection of the gums, and eventually the loss of teeth. Pregnant mothers are also at a greater risk for developing cavities due to lack of good oral hygiene and the increase of sweets in their diet. Research shows that mother who have high levels of untreated cavities are three times more likely to have children with cavities and has correlated that a mother with periodontitis has a risk of pre-term births and low-weight babies.

The developing fetus is also very sensitive to radiation and nitrous oxide. The dental assistant is responsible for knowing and following all precautions and standards regarding radiation and the use of nitrous oxide in the treatment area. The dental assistant needs to ask all women if there is a possibility of their being pregnant. Female dental assistants must also take precautions in the event of a pregnancy.

Cardiovascular System

The *cardiovascular system* is the body's means of transporting a continuous supply of oxygen, nutrients, hormones, and antibodies throughout the body while carbon dioxide and other cellular wastes are being removed from the body. This system maintains a balance between intracellular and extracellular fluids. The cardiovascular system is composed of the heart and blood vessels that carry blood throughout the body. The cardiovascular system consists of the **pulmonary** circulation and the systemic circulation (Figure 4-21). The pulmonary circulation transports **deoxygenated** blood to the lungs to get oxygen and remove waste products. The *systemic circulation* carries oxygenated blood away from the heart and delivers it to cells and tissues of the body. Main components of the cardiovascular system include the heart, blood vessels (arteries, veins, and capillaries), and blood.

The Heart

The *heart* is a muscle that pumps blood throughout the body at an average rate of 60–100 beats per minute. The heart is located to the left of the sternum (breastbone) in the center of the thoracic (chest) cavity. It is the approximate size of a fist and shaped

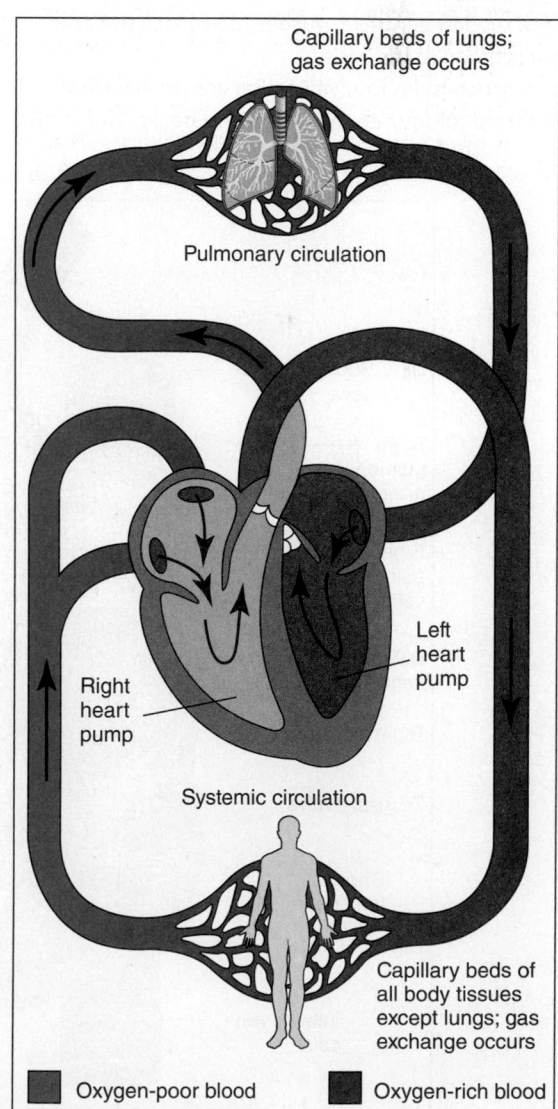

FIGURE 4-21
Systemic and pulmonary circulation.

like an upside-down pear. The tip at the inferior edge is called the *apex*. The wall of the heart is composed of three layers. The inner layer, called the *endocardium*, helps reduce friction as the blood passes through each heart chamber. The middle layer is the *myocardium* and is muscle tissue that provides the pumping action of the heart. The outer layer called the *epicardium* is considered the sac that cushions the heart and reduces friction as the heart beats (Figure 4-22).

Chambers and Valves

A **septum** divides the heart into right and left halves. Each half is divided again into upper chambers called the **atria** and lower chambers called **ventricles**. The heart is composed of four **chambers** and basically works as two different pumps. The right upper chamber, also referred to as the right atrium, receives deoxygenated blood from the *superior* and *inferior vena cava*. The right lower chamber, the right ventricle, pushes blood into the lungs to receive oxygen and remove waste products. The left upper chamber, also referred to as the left atrium, receives oxygenated blood from the lungs. The left lower chamber, the left ventricle, pushes blood into the aorta, which distributes blood to the body.

The heart contains four *valves* that control backflow of blood and separate all four chambers of the heart. These one-way valves open and close with each heartbeat. The tricuspid valve is located between the right atrium and right ventricle. The **pulmonary** valve is located between the right ventricle and the *pulmonary artery*, which takes blood to the lungs for oxygenation. The mitral valve is located between the left atrium and left ventricle. The aortic valve is located between the left ventricle and the *aorta*, which distributes blood throughout the body.

Blood Flow Pattern The blood flows through the heart in a very basic pattern. Deoxygenated blood is pumped from the right side of the heart to the lungs to receive oxygen and then to the left side of the heart to be distributed throughout the body (Figure 4-23).

The process is as follows:

1. Deoxygenated blood enters the right atrium via two large veins: the superior vena cava from the upper half of the body and the inferior vena cava from the bottom half of the body.

2. The right atrium contracts and pushes blood through the tricuspid valve into the right ventricle.

3. The right ventricle then contracts and pushes blood through the pulmonary valve into the pulmonary artery. This blood gets carried to the lungs for oxygenation.

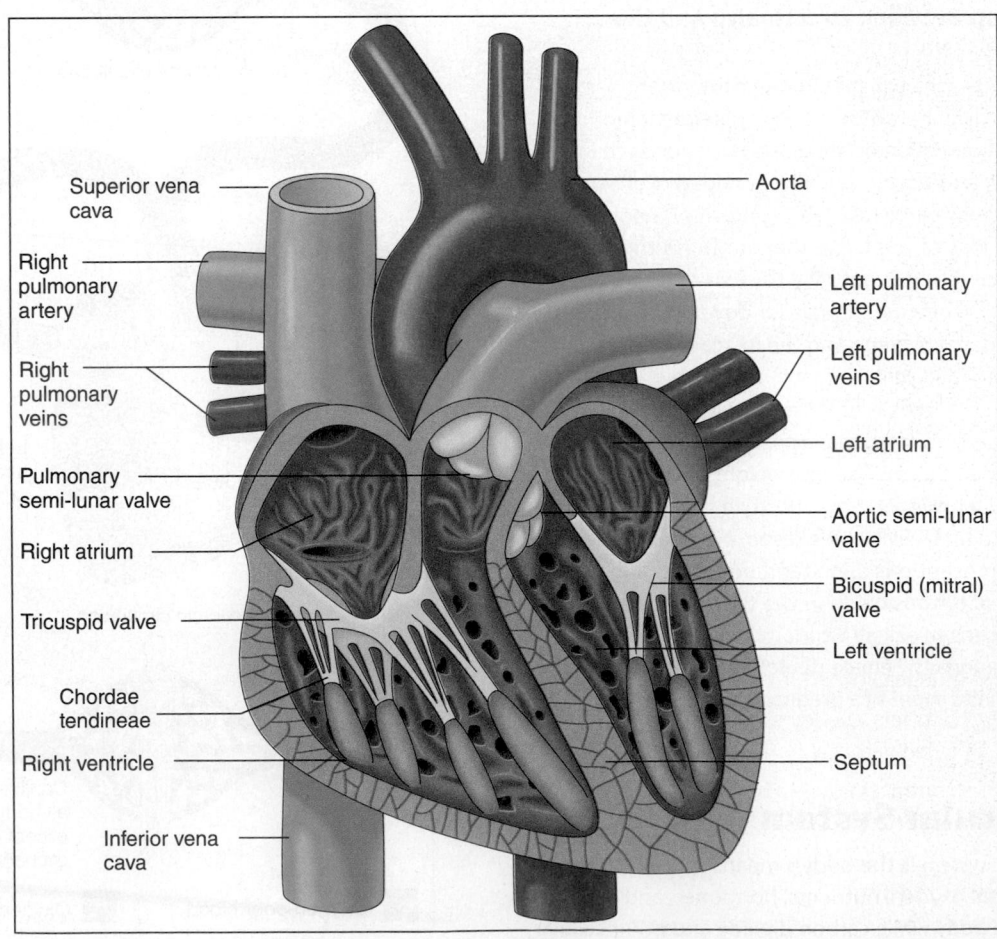

FIGURE 4-22
Structures of the heart.

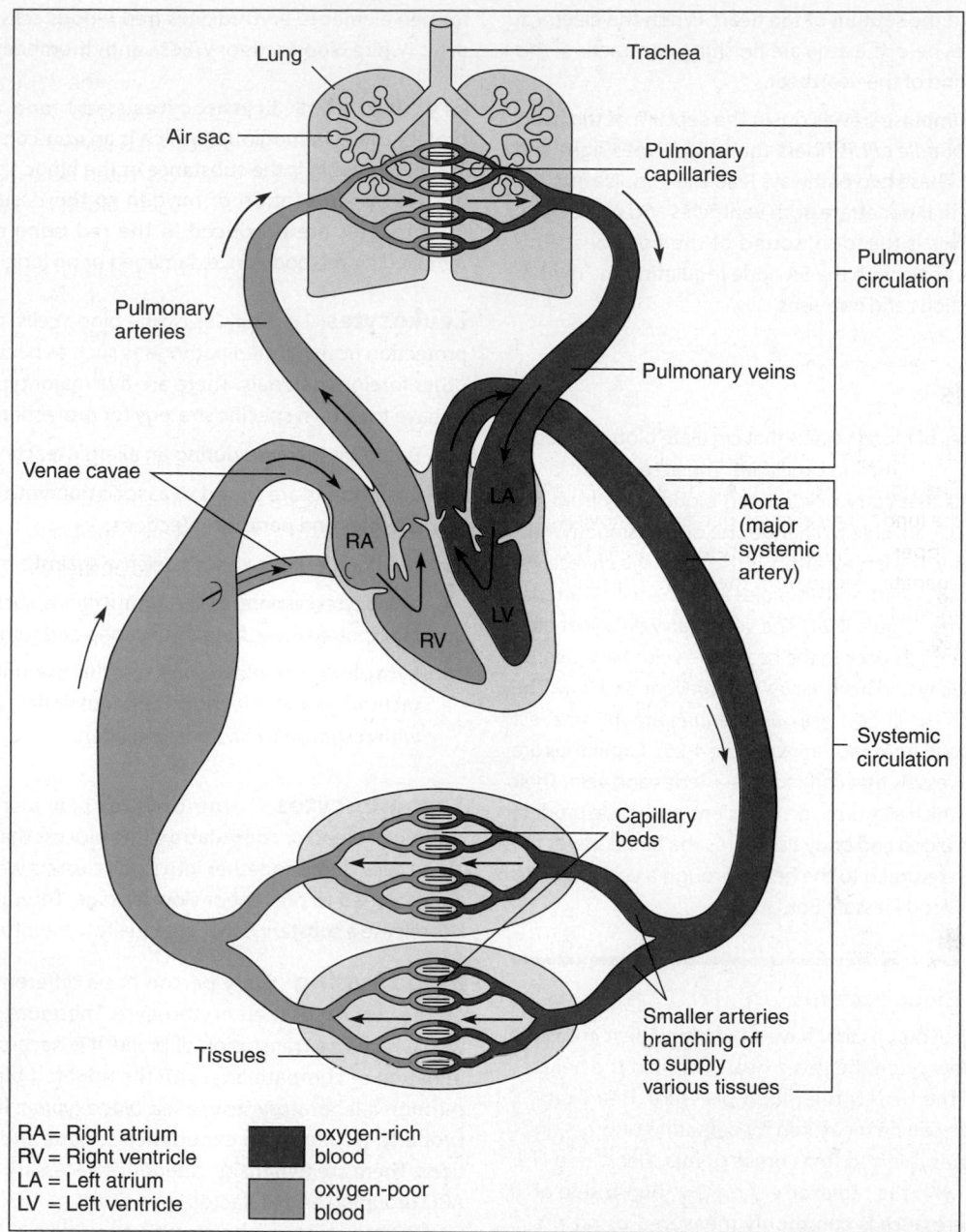

FIGURE 4-23
Schematic drawing of blood flow through the heart showing pulmonary and systemic circulation.

4. The left atrium receives oxygenated blood from the pulmonary veins after leaving the lungs.

5. The left atrium contracts and pushes blood through the mitral valve into the left ventricle.

6. The left ventricle contracts and pushes blood through the aortic valve into the aorta for distribution to all parts of the body.

7. Deoxygenated blood then returns to enter the right atrium via the superior vena cava and inferior vena cava to continue the cycle of circulation of blood throughout the body.

Electrical System of the Heart The heart contains an electrical system that is responsible for the contracting of heart muscles that force blood to be pumped throughout the heart and out to the body. The force of blood through the heart produces the sound of the heart: lub-dub. The path that the electrical impulse travels is as follows:

1. The *sinoatrial (SA) node*, also known as the pacemaker of the heart, is where the electrical impulse begins. It is located in the right atrium and initiates the heart contraction.

2. The impulse travels down the right atrium into the *atrioventricular (AV) node*. This node is located between the right

and left atria in the septum of the heart. When the electrical impulse arrives here, the atria are finishing contracting; this is the "lub" sound of the heartbeat.

3. The electrical impulse travels down the septum of the heart through the *bundle of His* fibers that divide into right and left pathways. These two pathways lead the impulse into the *Purkinje fibers* that penetrate both ventricles and cause them to contract. This is the "dub" sound of the heartbeat. This cycle will start again with the SA node regulating the rhythm of the contractions and impulses.

Blood Vessels

There are three types of blood vessels that circulate blood throughout the body: arteries, veins, and capillaries. The **arteries** are large, thick-walled vessels that carry oxygenated blood away from the heart. The artery walls are able to change size due to smooth muscle and their elasticity. The largest artery is the aorta, which receives blood directly from the heart, and arterioles are the smallest arteries leading into capillaries (Figure 4-24). The **veins** carry deoxygenated blood and waste products back to the heart. The veins have thinner walls with less elasticity and have valves that prevent backflow. The inferior vena cava is the largest vein, and *venules* are the smallest veins and collect blood from capillaries (Figure 4-25). **Capillaries** are a network of small vessels that connect the arteries and vein. Their walls are very thin, which allows oxygen, nutrient, and waste product exchange between blood and body tissues. As the blood leaves the capillaries, it is then returned to the heart through a vein. (Refer to the Heart Rate and Blood Pressure Box.)

Heart Rate and Blood Pressure

Arteries are like small pumps that have a pulse and beat in time with the artery. How often the heart beats is called the heart rate. The force of the beat is the blood pressure. Heart rate and blood pressure can be measured by palpating or pressing the different arteries referred to as pulse points. Heart rate is most often taken with the radial artery on the thumb side of the wrist. Blood pressure is commonly measured using the brachial artery on the little finger side of the upper arm. When doing cardiopulmonary resuscitation (CPR), the carotid artery in the neck is preferred for counting heart rate.

Components of Blood

Blood is a thick fluid that varies in color from bright red to a darker, brownish red. An average adult has about 5 liters of blood, which is equal to about 10 to 12 pints, that circulate throughout the body. Blood is transported throughout the cardiovascular system through the blood vessels. Blood has three main functions: transportation of nutrients, gases, waste products, and hormones; regulation of the amount of body fluids, pH balance, and body temperature; and protection against **pathogens** and blood loss after injury through the clotting mechanism. About 45% of the blood is made up of formed elements and about 55% is made up of a watery substance called plasma. There are three types of

formed elements: erythrocytes (red bloods cells or RBCs), leukocytes (white blood cells or WBCs), and thrombocytes (platelets).

Erythrocytes   **Erythrocytes** (red blood cells) contain a protein called hemoglobin, which is an iron-containing pigment. The hemoglobin is the substance of the blood that is responsible for the transportation of oxygen to the tissues of the body. Erythrocytes are produced in the red bone marrow and are removed by the body once damaged or no longer useful.

Leukocytes   **Leukocytes** (white blood cells) provide the body protection from harmful pathogens such as bacteria, viruses, and other foreign materials. There are five major types of WBCs, and all have their own specific strategy for protecting our body:

1. Basophils increase during an allergic reaction.
2. Eosinophils are found in association with defense against allergies and parasitic infections.
3. Neutrophils are the body's defense against a bacterial infection.
4. Monocytes respond to certain infections, such as Rocky Mountain spotted fever, fungal infections, and some leukemias.
5. Lymphocytes play many roles in the immune response, including viral infections and leukemias, and occasionally with response to bacterial infections.

Thrombocytes   **Thrombocytes** play a critical role in the clotting of blood or **coagulation** (the process that stops bleeding). These cells clump together into small clusters when blood vessels are damaged to prevent or slow leakage. Thrombocytes or platelets release a substance that eventually turns into a blood clot.

Blood Typing   Every person has a different marker protein on the surface of their erythrocyte. Therefore, before a person would receive a transfusion of blood, it is necessary for the determination of compatibility with the donated blood. This is done through a laboratory test called *blood typing*. If this is not done properly, patients can experience serious and even fatal reactions. There are two major categories necessary for blood typing: ABO grouping and Rh factor.

ABO grouping can be classified as either A, B, AB, or O blood type. There are two possible erythrocyte or red blood cell markers that can identify the type of blood, A and B. The presence of an A marker is said to mean a person has type A blood and produces anti-B antibodies that will attack type B blood. The presence of a B marker is said to mean a person has type B blood and produces an anti-A antibody that will attack type A blood. If both A and B markers are present, the blood is type AB and does not contain any antibodies. This means that a person's type AB blood will not attack any other blood type and is said to be a universal recipient, meaning in emergency situations, the person may receive any blood type without complications. The absence of marker A or B results in blood type O, which contains anti-A and anti-B antibodies. Due to the presence of anti-A and anti-B antibodies, type O blood will attack any other types of blood; therefore, people with this blood type are only able to receive type O blood. However, because type O blood does not have a marker A or marker B, it will not react with anti-A or anti-B antibodies, therefore it is considered to be a

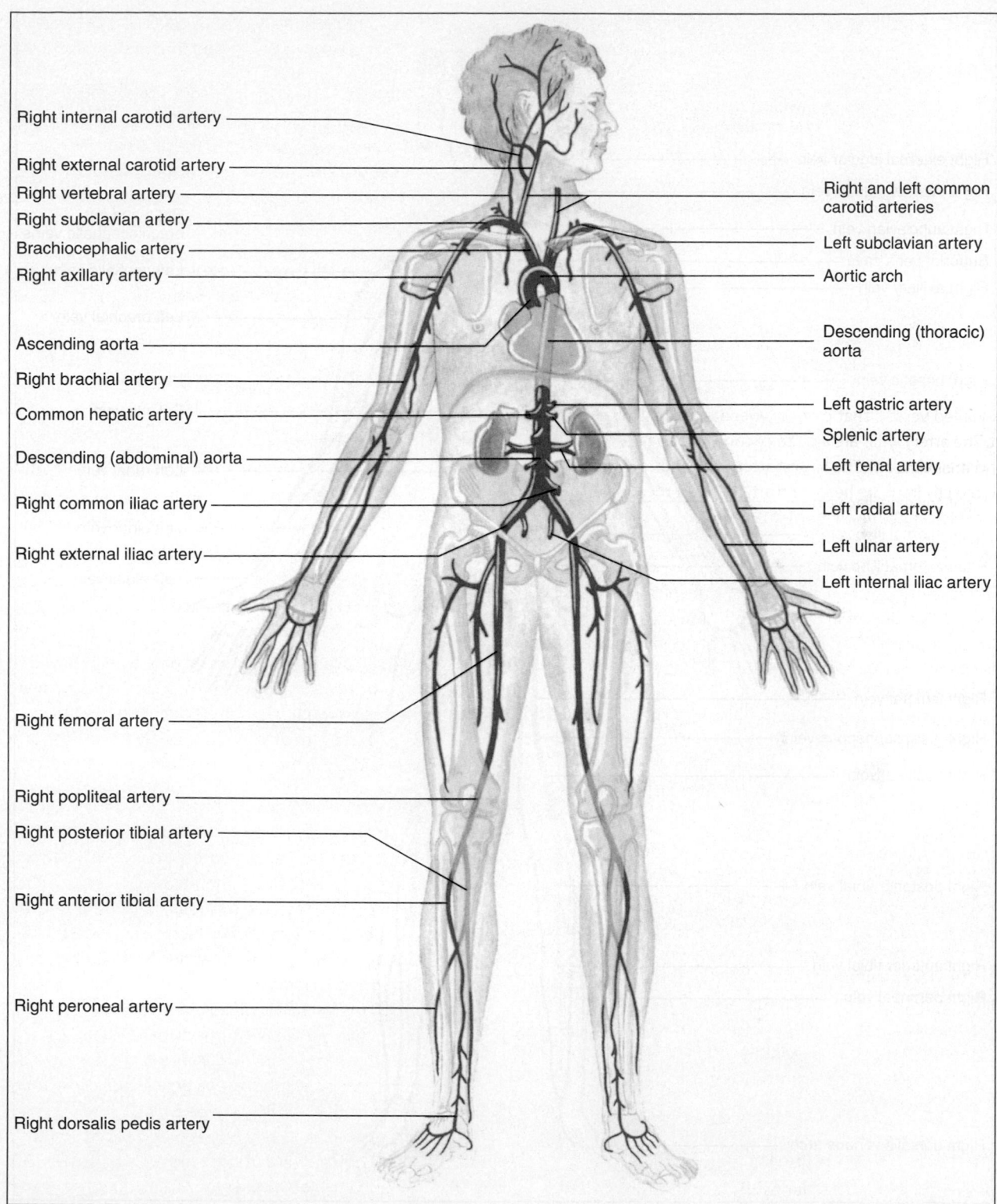

FIGURE 4-24
The major arteries of the systemic circulation.

Right internal carotid artery

Right external carotid artery

Right vertebral artery

Right subclavian artery

Brachiocephalic artery

Right axillary artery

Ascending aorta

Right brachial artery

Common hepatic artery

Descending (abdominal) aorta

Right common iliac artery

Right external iliac artery

Right femoral artery

Right popliteal artery

Right posterior tibial artery

Right anterior tibial artery

Right peroneal artery

Right dorsalis pedis artery

Right and left common carotid arteries

Left subclavian artery

Aortic arch

Descending (thoracic) aorta

Left gastric artery

Splenic artery

Left renal artery

Left radial artery

Left ulnar artery

Left internal iliac artery

universal donor. This means that in an emergency situation anyone with any blood type may receive type O blood (Table 4-5).

Rh factor is an additional antigen, which is a protein on the surface of a cell that identifies the type of cell, which is found on the surface of the erythrocyte. It is important not only to know the type of blood a person has but to also know if this additional antigen is present. If it is present, the person is considered to be Rh positive and they will not make anti-Rh antibodies. If this antigen is not present, the person is considered to be Rh negative and will produce anti-Rh antibodies. Therefore, a person who is Rh positive may receive blood with Rh positive or Rh negative antigen, but a Rh negative person may only receive Rh negative blood.

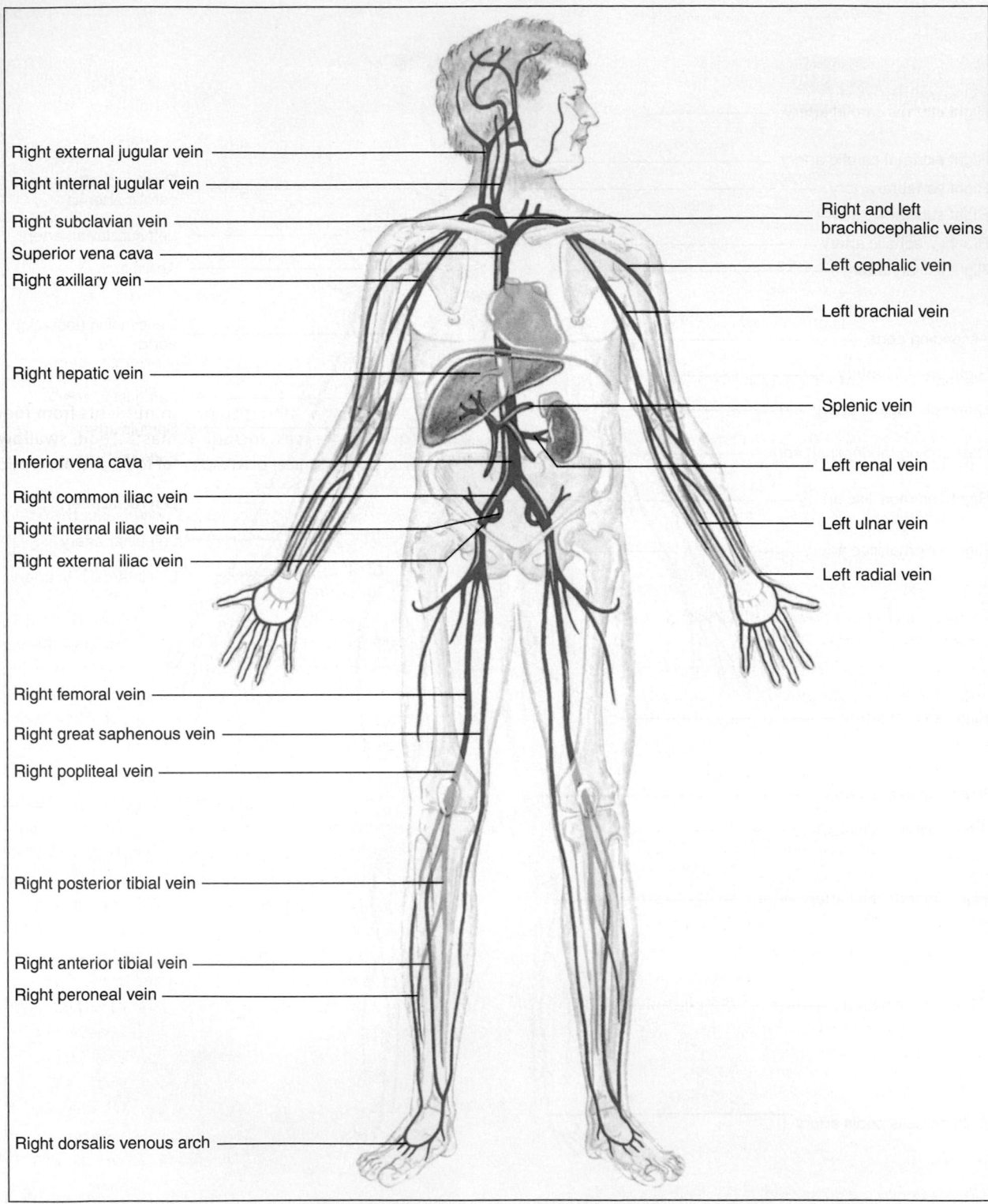

Right external jugular vein

Right internal jugular vein

Right subclavian vein

Superior vena cava

Right axillary vein

Right hepatic vein

Inferior vena cava

Right common iliac vein

Right internal iliac vein

Right external iliac vein

Right femoral vein

Right great saphenous vein

Right popliteal vein

Right posterior tibial vein

Right anterior tibial vein

Right peroneal vein

Right dorsalis venous arch

Right and left brachiocephalic veins

Left cephalic vein

Left brachial vein

Splenic vein

Left renal vein

Left ulnar vein

Left radial vein

FIGURE 4-25
The major veins of the body.

Common Diseases and Conditions of the Cardiovascular System

- *Heart disease* refers to any disorders and deformities of the heart. Heart disease may be treated by medication or surgery. Coronary heart disease (narrowing of coronary arteries), arrhythmia (irregular heartbeat), and myocardial infarction (heart attack) are some examples of heart disease.

- *Bacterial endocarditis* is an inflammation of the lining of the heart. Patients who have a history of rheumatic fever, congenital heart disease, open-heart surgery, organ transplants,

TABLE 4-5 Blood Types, Donors, and Recipients

Blood Group/ Type	Percent of Population	Antigen/Agglutinogen on Red Blood Cells	Antibody/ Agglutinin in Plasma	Can Receive	Can Donate to
A	41	A	Anti-B	A or O only	A or AB only
B	12	B	Anti-A	B or O only	B or AB only
AB	3	A and B	None	A, B, AB, O (Universal recipient)	AB only
O	44	None	Anti-A and Anti-B	O only	A, B, AB, O (Universal donor)

or dental implants should always be treated with antibiotics before dental treatment.

● *Hemophilia* is a disorder in which the blood fails to form a clot.

● *Leukemia* is a malignant, progressive disease of the blood-forming organs that is marked by unrestrained growth of abnormal leukocytes. Leukemia cells infiltrate the bone marrow and lymph tissue. These cells then advance to the bloodstream and various body organs.

Interrelationship Between Oral Health and the Cardiovascular System

The population is aging and geriatric dentistry is growing and so is the prevalence of cardiovascular disease. Understanding heart disease and frequently prescribed medications helps the assistant to be alert for possible complications; dry mouth is a common complication. Heart disease is the leading cause of death for both men and women; therefore, another consideration is to be prepared for an emergency—dental treatment can present a stressful situation to an already compromised patient.

Periodontitis has been associated with an increased risk of heart disease, stroke, and cardiovascular disease. Poor dental health has been linked to bacterial infection of the bloodstream that can damage the heart valves, especially in patients who have artificial valves. The dental assistant can play a role in educating the patient that treating their gum disease is vital in reducing vascular heart problems.

Digestive System

The *digestive system*, also known as the gastrointestinal (GI) system, contains 30 feet of continuous muscular tube that stretches between the mouth and **anus**. This digestive system has three main functions: digestion, absorbing nutrients, and elimination of waste. Digestion includes the physical and chemical breakdown of food into small nutrient molecules that cells can use. Food is then absorbed by the intestines and circulated through the body by the cardiovascular system. Any food that the body cannot digest or absorb is eliminated from the body as solid waste.

Route of Digestion

The digestive system consists of approximately 30 feet of winding tube starting from the oral cavity and ending at the anus (Figure 4-26). Its function is to obtain nutrients from food by a number of processes, including mastication, swallowing, mechanical and chemical breakdown of food, and absorption of nutrients and elimination of waste.

The digestive system is divided into two groups: the *alimentary canal* and *accessory organs*. The alimentary canal forms a canal or tube from the mouth to the anus. The canal includes the mouth (oral cavity), pharynx, esophagus, stomach, small intestine, and large intestine. Accessory organs aid in the process of digestion. Included are the teeth, tongue, salivary glands and ducts, liver, gallbladder, and pancreas. Even before food is ingested, the sight, smell, and thought of food stimulate the saliva glands to produce saliva, and stomach secretions begin to flow. Then the process of digestion begins as outlined in Table 4-6.

Oral Cavity The digestive system begins when food enters the mouth, also called the **oral cavity**, and is broken up by chewing. The food is mixed with *saliva*, which contains enzymes that break it down and make it easier to swallow. The teeth are an important part of the body's first stage of digestion. The anterior teeth known as *incisors* and *cuspids* bite and tear the food into small pieces. The posterior teeth, which include *bicuspids* and *molars*, grind and crush the food into finer pieces. The tongue moves food from the anterior teeth to the posterior teeth and gathers the food before it is swallowed. Since the oral cavity is the place where digestion begins, it is very important to have good oral care. Problems in the mouth such as gum disease and tooth decay can indicate a gastrointestinal problem. The teeth, tongue, lips, cheeks, and salivary glands all work together to mechanically break food into small pieces and then move the food to the throat area (pharynx).

Pharynx The **pharynx** connects the oral cavity to the esophagus, which is where food is swallowed. The pharynx also functions as part of the respiratory system. Therefore, sometimes during swallowing, food may go into the larynx instead of the esophagus. To prevent this from occurring, the **epiglottis** (a small, leaf-shaped cartilage) covers the larynx. Swallowing is a complex, multistepped process that is controlled by the medulla part of the brain. Swallowing, or deglutition, provides movement for the food to proceed from the mouth to the stomach.

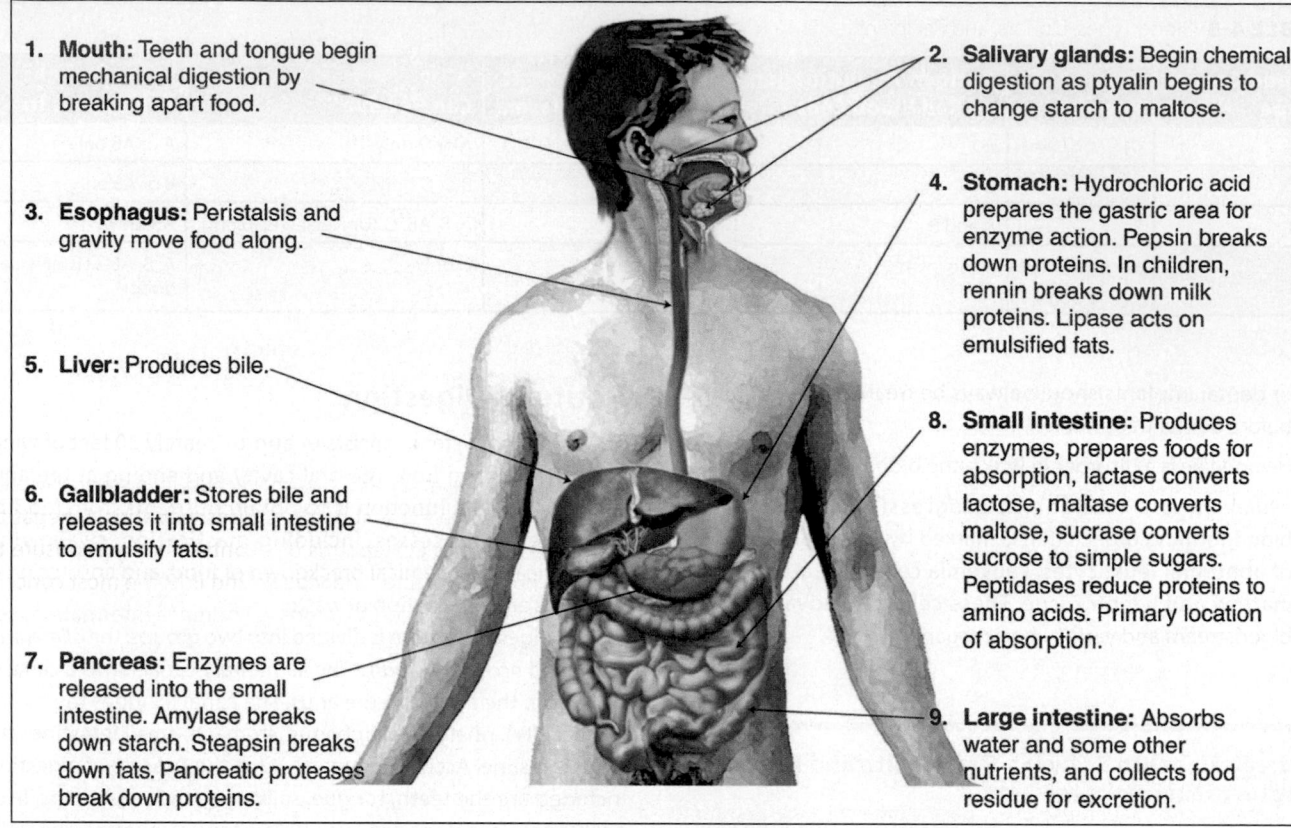

1. **Mouth:** Teeth and tongue begin mechanical digestion by breaking apart food.

2. **Salivary glands:** Begin chemical digestion as ptyalin begins to change starch to maltose.

3. **Esophagus:** Peristalsis and gravity move food along.

4. **Stomach:** Hydrochloric acid prepares the gastric area for enzyme action. Pepsin breaks down proteins. In children, rennin breaks down milk proteins. Lipase acts on emulsified fats.

5. **Liver:** Produces bile.

6. **Gallbladder:** Stores bile and releases it into small intestine to emulsify fats.

7. **Pancreas:** Enzymes are released into the small intestine. Amylase breaks down starch. Steapsin breaks down fats. Pancreatic proteases break down proteins.

8. **Small intestine:** Produces enzymes, prepares foods for absorption, lactase converts lactose, maltase converts maltose, sucrase converts sucrose to simple sugars. Peptidases reduce proteins to amino acids. Primary location of absorption.

9. **Large intestine:** Absorbs water and some other nutrients, and collects food residue for excretion.

FIGURE 4-26
Structures of the digestive system.

TABLE 4-6 Mechanism of Digestion

Organ	Process	Description of Process
Oral cavity (mouth, teeth, tongue, and saliva)	Taste Mastication Swallowing or deglutition	Receives the food, tastes Mechanical breakdown of food Saliva glands produce enzymes to start chemical digestion
Pharynx	Deglutition	Movement of food as a result of swallowing Passageway for food and air
Esophagus	Deglutition Peristalsis	Mucus is secreted as food is transported in waves toward the stomach
Stomach	Churning Peristalsis	Chemical breakdown continues as stomach enzymes are released and mechanical movements churn the contents
Small intestine	Absorption Peristalsis	Absorption of digested food Move contents along intestinal track
Large intestine	Peristalsis Defecation	Mechanical movements occur Emptying of the rectum

Esophagus Food is carried down the **esophagus** to the stomach. The esophagus is a muscular tube that is about 10 inches long in an adult. It takes approximately 10 seconds for swallowed food to reach the stomach. Food is propelled along the esophagus by wavelike contractions called **peristalsis**. The lower esophageal sphincter (**SFINK**-ter) muscle, at the end of the esophagus, relaxes to allow food into the stomach, and then contracts to prevent it from flowing backward.

Stomach The *stomach* is a muscular organ that acts as a sac to collect, churn, digest, and store food. It is about 12 inches long and can hold about a quart of food. Food mixes with **digestive enzymes** in the stomach to form a liquid mixture called *chyme*. This mixture passes through the remaining portion of the digestive system. After about three hours, chyme leaves the stomach in spurts and enters the small intestine.

Small Intestine The *small intestine* is the next stop and the major site for digestion and absorption of nutrients from food. The small intestine is the longest portion of the digestive system with an average length of 20 feet. It is divided into three sections called the duodenum, ileum, and jejunum. The first section of the small intestine is called the duodenum. Here, other digestive juices enter and the breakdown process continues. In the walls of the small intestine are finger-like projections called villi. Here, the digested food is absorbed into the bloodstream. It can take up to four hours for chyme to pass through the small intestine.

Large Intestine After absorption of nutrients is completed in the small intestine, the fluid that remains enters the *large intestine*. The large intestine is approximately five feet long and extends down to the anus. This is where the water that is left is absorbed by the body. The large intestine contains 400 different species of bacteria. The material that remains is solid waste called *feces*. This waste is expelled through the anus by bowel movements.

Accessory Organs

There are four accessory organs to the digestive system. These organs produce enzymes and digestive fluids that are necessary for the breakdown of food. Digestion would not be possible without these organs. All of these organs are attached to the digestive system by a **duct**.

Salivary Glands The *salivary glands* located in the oral cavity produce saliva. Saliva is a sticky fluid that allows food to be swallowed in a smooth manner without choking. The enzymes present in saliva start the digestive process: amylase is an enzyme to begin the digestive process of starches; sodium bicarbonate increases pH, which accelerates amylase function; and water dilutes and facilitates food mixing. Three salivary glands surround the mouth: the parotid gland, the submandibular gland, and the sublingual gland. More information on the tongue and salivary glands is found in Chapter 7, Head and Neck Anatomy.

Liver The *liver* is one of the largest organs and works by processing nutrients and detoxifying harmful substances. It is on the right side of the body, just below the diaphragm. The liver weighs about four pounds and is able to regenerate itself. It produces *bile*, which breaks up fat molecules, making them easier to digest.

Gallbladder The *gallbladder* is a small organ located behind the liver. The bile produced in the liver is stored in the gallbladder. The gallbladder sends bile to the small intestine where it aides in digesting fat.

Pancreas The *pancreas* produces secretions that are emptied into the duodenum to aid digestion and produce **insulin**. The pancreas produces two important secretions that aide in digestion: buffers that help neutralize acids and pancreatic enzymes that help in digestion of carbohydrates, fats, and proteins.

Common Diseases and Conditions of the Digestive System

- *Irritable bowel syndrome (IBS)* has symptoms of stomach discomfort and abdominal bloating; some experience diarrhea, while others are constipated.
- *Gastroesophageal reflux disease (GERD)* happens when stomach acids back up and flow into the esophagus. This is usually followed by a burning sensation and chest pain after meals or at night at least twice a week.
- *Diverticulitis* happens when small pouches lining the large intestines become infected and inflamed. This disorder causes severe lower-left-side abdominal pain, constipation, fever, and nausea.
- *Hepatitis* is inflammation of the liver caused by several viruses. There are three main hepatitis viruses: hepatitis A, hepatitis B, and hepatitis C. Hepatitis B is contracted by exposure to body fluids of infected individuals and is of the most concern because of its serious prognosis. For more information, see Chapter 12, Microbiology.

Oral Health and the Digestive System Interrelationship

The digestive system begins with the oral cavity, which is the focus in dentistry. Knowing the components of this system and how each contributes to the processing of food enables the dental assistant to detect disease and communicate with the patient. Common causes of digestive problems include eating too quickly and not chewing food well enough. Dental problems such as infected, missing, and misaligned teeth affect the ability for the patient to adequately chew their food, which can lead to digestive problems. There is also a link between digestive disorders and oral health. Gastroesophageal reflux (heartburn) causes stomach acids to enter the mouth, which can erode the tooth enamel. The dentist may prescribe an oral rinse or fluoride treatment to strengthen the enamel and remineralization treatment for wearing of enamel. Inflammatory bowel disease can present with oral signs and symptoms (mouth sores, infections, bleeding, or swollen gums), which often lead to early diagnosis during the dental examination.

Respiratory System

The *respiratory system* is responsible for bringing fresh air into the lungs, the gas exchange of oxygen to **carbon dioxide**, and the removal of waste from the lungs. The cells of the body require continuous delivery of oxygen and removal of carbon dioxide. The respiratory system works in conjunction with the cardiovascular system to carry out this task. This process must be continuous, and if interrupted for even a few minutes can result in brain damage or even death (Figure 4-27).

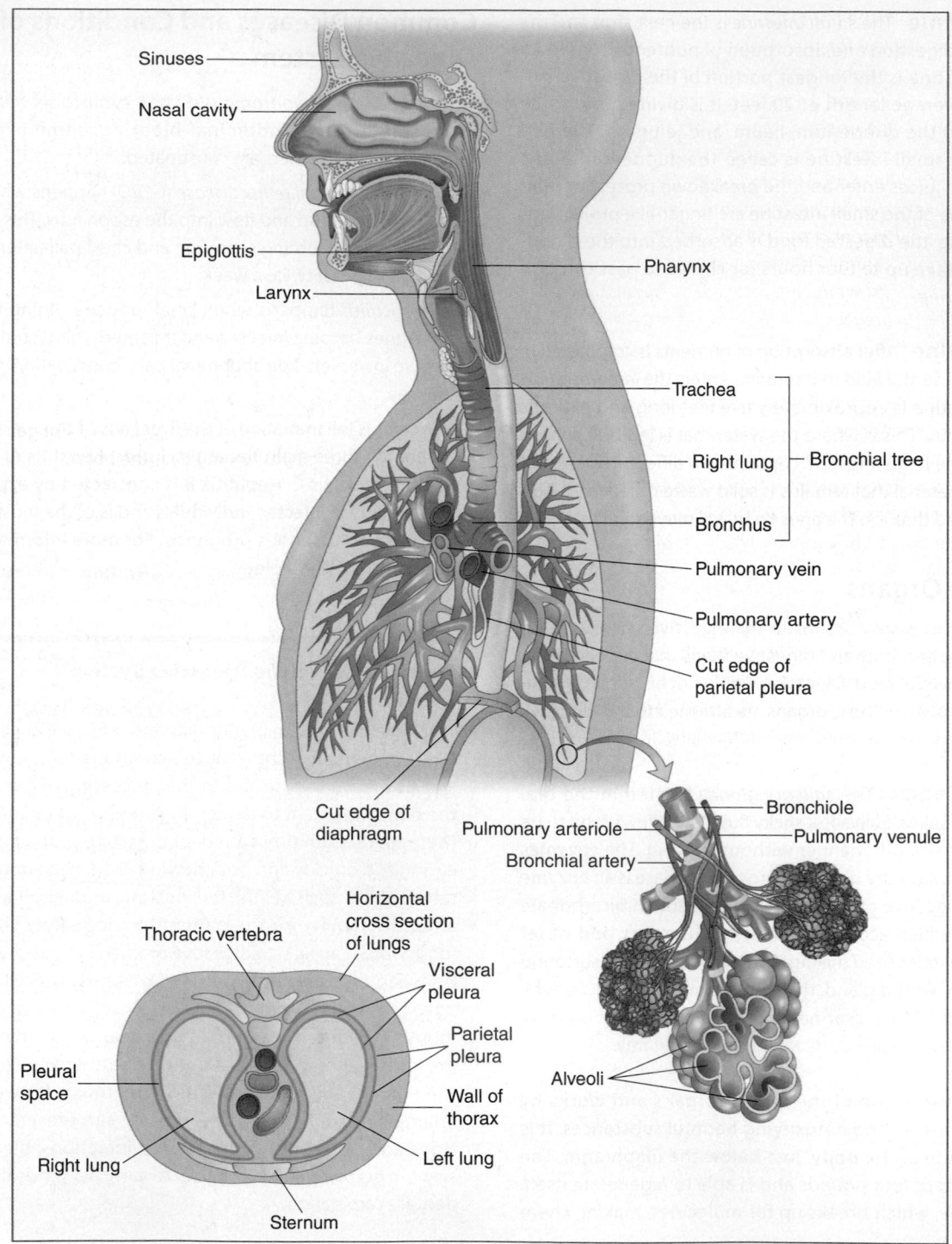

FIGURE 4-27
Structures of the respiratory system.

Anatomy and Physiology of the Respiratory System

The respiratory system consists of the nasal cavity, pharynx, larynx, trachea, bronchi, and lungs.

Nasal Cavity Breathing starts with the *nasal cavity* as outside air enters the body. The nose contains two *nasal cavities*, which are divided by the *nasal septum*. Air enters the nose and is filtered by **cilia** or very small hairs that trap large dirt particles before they can enter the lungs. The wall of the nasal cavity is covered by a **mucous membrane** that secretes **mucus**, which helps cleanse the air by removing dirt and bacteria. There are numerous blood vessels in the nose that help warm and humidify the inhaled air as it passes through. This is why nosebleeds are very common in some people. The nose also contains the *olfactory receptors*, which facilitate the sense of smell.

Pharynx Air enters the *pharynx,* also called the throat, which serves as a passageway for the respiratory and digestive systems. The pharynx is about five inches long, shaped like a tube for air and food passage, and divided into three sections. The first is the *nasopharynx,* the upper section behind the nasal cavity. The *eustachian (auditory) tubes* open into the pharynx. The *oropharynx,* the middle section, is the portion behind the mouth. It is lined with the same mucosa as found in the oral cavity. The lower section, the *laryngopharynx,* divides and has an opening in the front to the larynx and in the back to the esophagus. There are three sets of *tonsils,* which are located in strategic places in the throat. They help prevent **pathogens** from entering the body through air or food (Figure 4-28).

Larynx The **larynx** or voice box contains the vocal cords and is located above the trachea. The vocal cords produce sound by vibrating as air passes through the *glottis,* the opening between the two vocal cords. The *epiglottis* is a flap of tissue that sits above the glottis and provides a barrier against food and liquids being inhaled into the lungs. The larynx is made up of cartilage and is supported by muscles.

Trachea The **trachea** or windpipe is the passageway for air to move down to the bronchi. The trachea is about four inches long and composed of smooth muscle that is lined by cilia and a mucous membrane. This helps in warming, moisturizing, and cleansing air as it continues to travel to the lungs.

Bronchi The *bronchial tubes* are located at the end of the trachea. They are the two branches that form at the end of the trachea and enter the lungs. The bronchi continue to branch out into smaller and smaller branches (bronchioles) in the lungs. At the end of the bronchioles are alveolar sacs, which resemble clusters of grapes. These alveolar sacs consist of individual air sacs called *alveoli.* Each of the lungs has approximately 150 million alveoli. This is where the exchange of oxygen and carbon dioxide takes place. The thin walls of the alveoli make for easy passage of air entering and leaving the blood capillaries.

Lungs The *lungs* are located within the thoracic (chest) cavity and are protected from external damage by the ribs. There is a double membrane covering the lungs called the *pleura,* and fluid between the layers helps reduce friction when the lungs repeatedly expand and contract. The two lungs are divided into lobes. The right lung has three lobes, and the left has two. The right lung is larger and accounts for about 60% of the gas exchange due to the left lung's positioning over the heart.

Respiratory Process

Oxygen is essential for human life. The process of respiration is divided into three distinct parts: ventilation, internal respiration, and external respiration. Most of the time breathing is an unconscious act, but in some circumstances we can hold our breath or take extra-large breaths.

Ventilation is defined as the flow of air between the lungs and the outside environment. *Inhalation* is the flow of air into the lungs, which delivers oxygen to the alveoli. *Exhalation* is the flow of air out of the lungs, which removes **carbon dioxide** from the body.

Internal respiration is the process that allows gas exchange at the cellular level. This occurs when oxygen leaves the bloodstream and is delivered to the tissues. The waste product carbon dioxide then enters the bloodstream from the tissues and is transported back to the lungs for disposal.

External respiration refers to the gas exchange that takes place in the lungs. Oxygen enters the blood from the alveoli and is delivered to the body. Carbon dioxide leaves the blood and enters the alveoli to be exhaled from the body.

Respiratory Muscles

The *diaphragm* is a muscle that separates the abdomen from the thoracic (chest) cavity. The air moves in and out of the lungs due to pressure within the chest cavity. The diaphragm contracts and air then flows into the lungs with inhalation. The *intercostal muscles* lay between the ribs and aid in inhalation by raising the ribcage to further enlarge the thoracic cavity. When these muscles relax, the thoracic cavity becomes smaller and exhalation occurs.

Respiration Rate

Respiratory rate is the measure of breaths per minute. The respiratory rate is regulated by the carbon dioxide levels in the blood. When carbon dioxide levels are high, we breathe more rapidly to expel the excess. If levels drop, the rate will also drop. If the respiratory rate falls outside its normal rate, it may indicate an illness

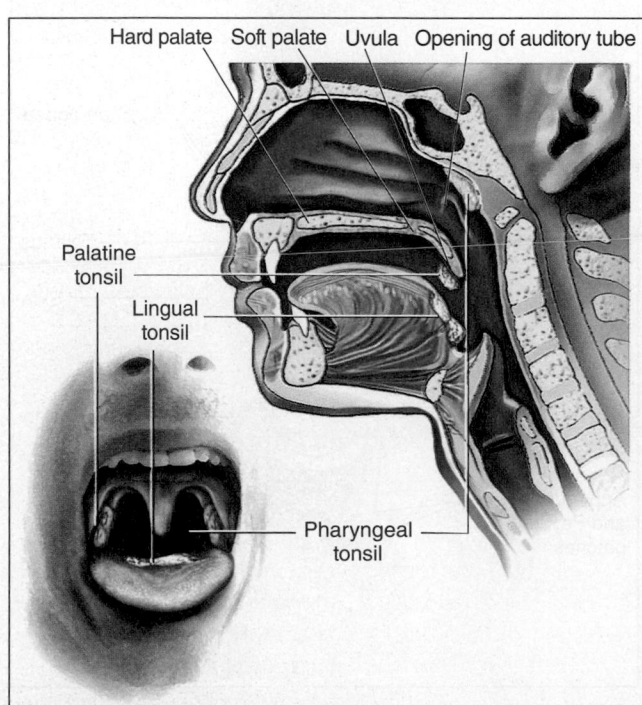

Hard palate Soft palate Uvula Opening of auditory tube

Palatine tonsil

Lingual tonsil

Pharyngeal tonsil

FIGURE 4-28
Tonsils.

TABLE 4-7 Respiratory Rates for Different Age Groups

Age	Respirations Per Minute
Newborn	30–60
1-year-old	18–30
16-year-old	16–20
Adult	12–20

Source: Courtesy of Stacey Young and Carrie Jacques

or medical condition. For example, if someone is running a temperature or has pneumonia, it may cause a dramatic increase in respiratory rate. In contrast, certain medications or brain injuries may cause a decrease in the respiratory rate. (See Table 4-7 for normal respiratory rate ranges).

Common Diseases of the Respiratory System

- *Asthma* is the muscular spasm of the walls of the bronchi. The air passages are constricted so the person cannot easily exhale.

- *Tuberculosis* is a highly contagious disease of the respiratory system. Tuberculosis is transmitted by breathing or swallowing droplets contaminated by the TB bacillus.

- *Lung cancer* is a malignancy of the lung tissue. It is a very common form of cancer and is often caused by cigarette smoking.

- Other conditions include the common cold, pneumonia, and bronchitis. Following standard precautions protects the office staff and the patient when treatment is required during times of infection.

Interrelationship Between Oral Health and the Respiratory System

Good oral hygiene and periodontal health play an important role in the prevention of respiratory diseases. Epidemiological studies have shown a link between oral pathogens from poor oral hygiene and periodontitis to respiratory illnesses like aspiration pneumonia. As you just studied, there is an anatomical continuity between the oral cavity and the lungs (air enters through the nose and mouth, to the airway and into the lungs). It has been discovered that the bacteria from oral infections also pass through the airway and into the lungs. Patients with an existing respiratory condition are normally vulnerable to respiratory infections and need to be encouraged to be diligent in their oral hygiene program.

The dental assistant should watch the patient for signs of discomfort or problems with breathing. The use of nitrous oxide may be contraindicated when a patient has respiratory disease. Allergic reactions can and do occur in the dental office. A patient could choke on materials that fall to the back of the throat, and respiratory diseases or conditions can make treatment difficult. Understanding the respiratory system could save a patient's life.

Lymphatic System

The *lymphatic system* works with the body's *immune system* to serve as the primary defense mechanism against the invasion of **pathogens**. This system is also responsible for collecting and returning extra fluids (**lymph**) back from the tissues to the *cardiovascular system*. Additionally, the lymphatic system is able to transport absorbed fats around the body for use and is able to remove cells of the body that have become diseased.

Anatomy and Physiology of the Lymphatic System

The lymphatic system is composed of lymph vessels, lymph nodes, the spleen, the thymus gland, and the tonsils. Lymph, also called *tissue fluid*, is a clear liquid formed in tissue spaces. The lymph enters the lymphatic capillary system and drains away excess fluid and carries proteins back to the bloodstream. Lymph is transported through a specialized network of vessels called lymphatic capillaries. These capillaries are very thin-walled and only allow lymph to travel in one direction on the way back to the general circulation system (Figure 4-29).

Lymphatic Vessels The *lymph vessels* carry fluids to the lymph nodes for filtering and then carry the extra fluids from the tissues back to the circulatory system. The lymph vessels run alongside the vessels of the circulatory system. However, the lymph vessels are not in a closed loop like the circulatory system. Instead, the lymph vessels are only one-way vessels for the tissues that dump all extra fluids into the thoracic cavity. These

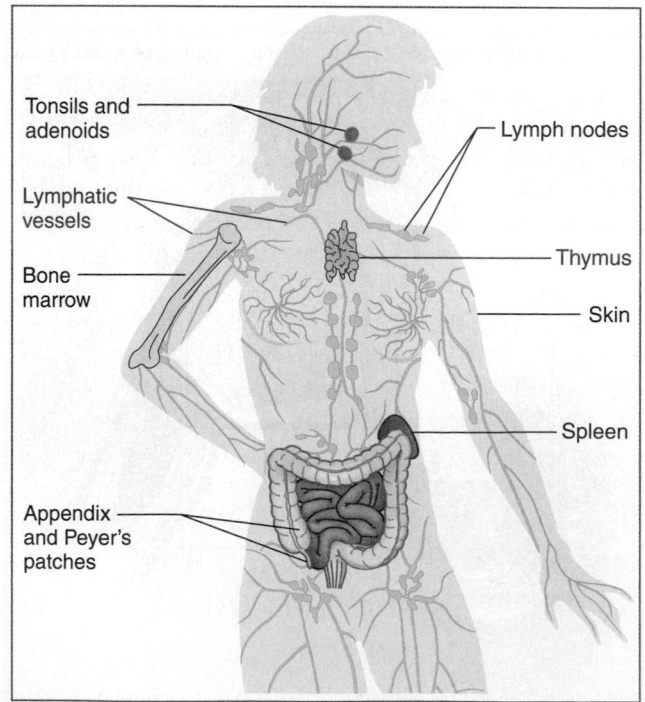

FIGURE 4-29
Organs and vessels from other body systems involved in the immune system.

vessels start out very small and get larger as they get closer to the duct that empties into the circulatory system. Lymph vessels contain one-way *valves* that prevent backflow of fluids.

Lymph Nodes *Lymph nodes* are located throughout the route of the lymphatic vessels. They are small, round masses that vary in size and location. The lymph nodes most commonly known are the ones in the armpit, neck, and groin. The purpose of the lymph nodes is to filter the lymph as it journeys back to the bloodstream and to manufacture antibodies and other active materials of the immunity process.

The lymph fluid, which is primarily made of water and white blood cells, runs through the lymph vessels and filters through the lymph nodes. This is where pathogens and cell debris are trapped, destroyed, and removed from the body by the white blood cells and antibodies inside the lymph nodes. **Macrophages** and lymphocytes are cells in the sinuses that detect and destroy foreign substances. Macrophages engulf foreign substances and cell debris. Lymphocytes assist the macrophages in detecting foreign substances.

Tonsils *Tonsils* are located on each side of the pharynx or throat and make a protective circle around the inside of the oral cavity. These glands are a collection of lymph tissue that filters pathogens that attempt to pass through the digestive or respiratory system. Tonsils contain a large quantity of white blood cells that will trap and destroy pathogens. However, the tonsils are not considered a vital organ and can be removed if they become a constant source of infection.

Spleen The *spleen* is a large lymphoid organ located at the upper-left side of the abdomen, close to the stomach. This organ has a large blood supply (vascular), and the blood filtered through it moves very slowly. This gives time for the spleen to filter out and destroy old red blood cells and pathogens, recycle iron, and store blood for future use. Humans can live without the spleen because other lymphoid tissues take over its functions. However, without the spleen, a person may be more susceptible to certain bacterial infections.

Thymus Gland The *thymus gland* is located above and in front of the heart in the thoracic (chest) cavity. This gland is responsible for the proper development of the immune system, especially during the newborn and adolescent stage of life. It is large and active from before birth through puberty, but then shrinks and almost disappears in adults.

Common Diseases and Conditions of the Lymphatic and Immune Systems

- *Tonsillitis* is a chronic infection of the tonsil tissue.
- *Hodgkin's disease* is a malignant disorder that causes enlargement of the lymph nodes.
- *Allergies* are a hypersensitivity to certain substances. These are often common substances such as pollen, pet dander, or

cigarette smoke and are referred to as allergens. The reaction to allergens can cause an inflammatory response or a severe allergic reaction.

- *Immune deficiency disease* is a failure in some part of the immune system.
- Bacterial and viral infections, fungi, parasites, cancer cells, and foreign tissue implants are all conditions that the immune system protects and fights against.

Interrelationship Between Oral Health and the Lymphatic System

Patients with a weakened immune system are more prone to developing gum and periodontal disease. Conversely, bacteria in the mouth can cause infection in other parts of the body when the immune system has been compromised by disease or medical treatment. A substance (C-reactive protein CRP) is an immune response and is released from the liver whenever there is inflammation in the body. CRP is a natural response and causes no harm; however, when CRP is released constantly, as with chronic periodontal disease, it can lead to other health conditions (stiffening, clotting of arteries, and heart attacks).

The dental assistant is constantly exposed to disease and infection. A major responsibility of each dental team member is to maintain a safe environment. Continuing education on prevention of and protection from health risks is necessary for all dental professionals.

Integumentary System

The *integumentary system* is an organ system consisting of the skin, hair, nails, and exocrine glands. The skin is only a few millimeters thick, yet it is by far the largest organ in the body. In an average person, the skin comprises 16% of the body's weight and has a surface area of approximately 20 square feet.

Functions of the Integumentary System

The skin is considered the body's first line of defense, helping in ways such as protection, the housing of sensory receptors, secretion of fluids, and temperature regulation.

The primary function of the skin is *protection*. The skin forms a two-way barrier that helps keep pathogens and harmful chemicals out of the body. It also keeps vital fluids in the body, such as blood, and it protects the internal organs from injury.

The body's *sensory receptors* are located in the middle layer of the skin. These sensory receptors detect pain, touch, pressure, and temperature by working with the nervous system to send messages to the brain. The purpose of these receptors is to provide the central nervous system with information about the external environment such as heat and cold. This information will stimulate responses such as scratching an insect bite that itches.

There are two types of fluids secreted in the skin. *Sweat* is produced in the sweat glands and helps to maintain the internal body temperature through evaporation, which causes a cooling effect. The *sebaceous glands* secrete oil that helps give the skin moisture.

The body regulates temperature in several ways. If the *internal temperature* needs to be lowered, the blood vessels in the skin dilate, or open, which causes blood to rise to the surface. This allows the release of heat. In opposition, if the body needs to raise its temperature, the blood vessels constrict, keeping warm blood away from the surface. As previously noted, when sweat evaporates, it cools the body down. The third layer of our skin, or subcutaneous layer, also has a continuous layer of fat that serves as insulation.

Layers of the Skin

The skin consists of three layers: the epidermis, the dermis, and the subcutaneous (Figure 4-30).

Epidermis The *epidermis*, or top layer of the skin, consists of flat cells that overlap and are arranged in layers. The epidermis is composed of **epithelial** tissue and does not have a blood supply, so it depends on the deeper layers for its nourishment. This is why a wound such as a paper cut does not bleed. The cells of this layer continually grow and multiply and then shrink and die. The epithelial cells are shed from the skin's surface and replaced with new cells from the base of the epidermis. This process allows the skin to act as a protective barrier and makes it waterproof. This seal keeps the body hydrated by preventing water loss. This layer

also contains melanocytes, specialized cells that produce a black pigment called **melanin**. Melanin is responsible for our skin color and protection from the sun. Damage of this layer can result in permanent DNA damage and skin cancer. Darker-skinned people have more melanin and fewer wrinkles and occurrences of skin cancer.

Dermis The middle layer of the skin is the *dermis*. The name means true skin because of its rich blood supply. The dermis supports the epidermis and consists of connective tissue. This living layer contains all the accessory organs, including hair follicles, sweat glands, sebaceous glands, lymph vessels, sensory receptors, muscles fibers, and blood vessels. Fingerprints are also formed in this layer. Fingerprints do not change throughout a lifetime and are unique to each individual. An individual fingerprint forms on the skin surface during fetal development; therefore, genetic makeup plays a role in the formation, but it is not the only factor. This is evident because identical twins with identical genetic makeup will have unique fingerprints. It is unknown exactly what other factors play a role in the development of fingerprints. This layer gives our skin its strength and elasticity. With age the skin loses this ability, resulting in wrinkles.

Subcutaneous The deepest layer of the skin is called the *subcutaneous* layer. This layer contains fat cells called *lipocytes*. These cells protect the deeper organs, provide a cushion for bones, and act as an insulator for heat and cold.

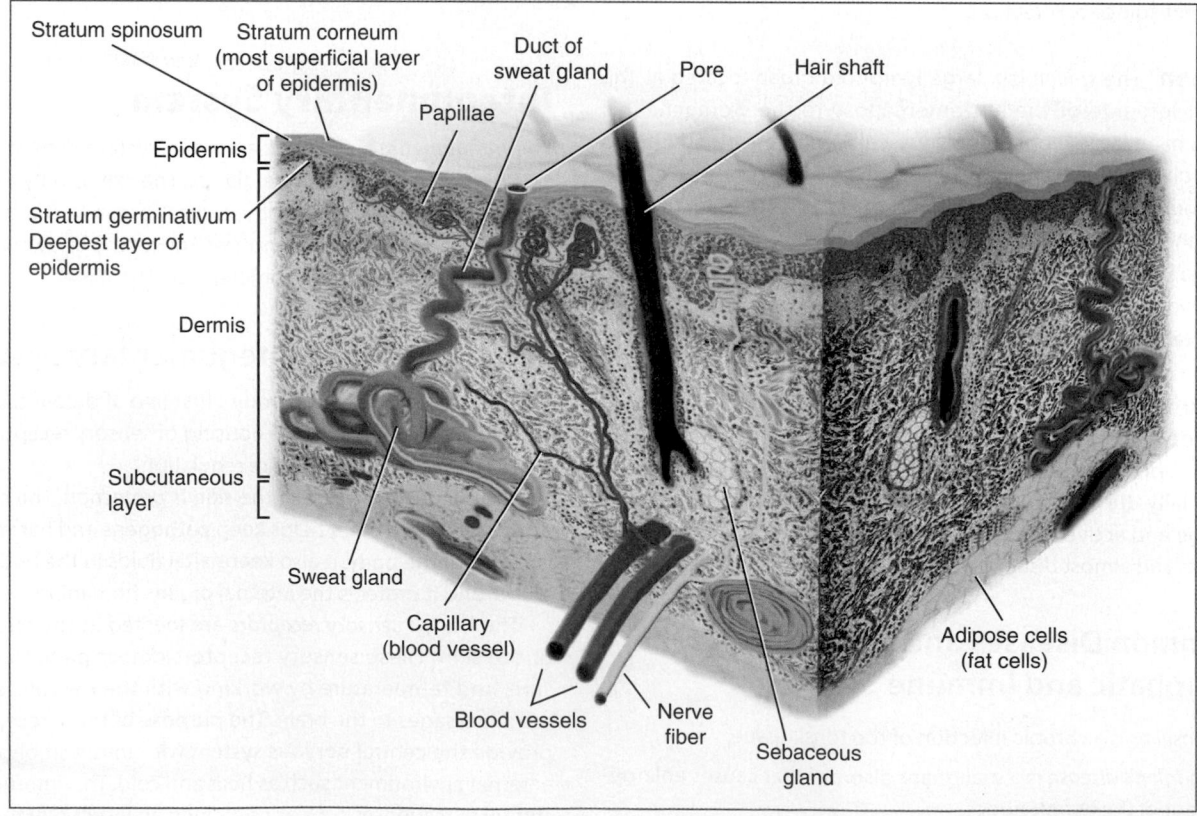

FIGURE 4-30
Parts of the integumentary system, including the different sections of the skin and hair follicles.

Abnormal skin colorations that may be seen in the dental office include:

- Albinism—a patient with pale skin, white hair, and pink coloration of the iris.
- Cyanosis—the skin appears bluish as a result of oxygen deficiency in the circulating blood.
- Erythema—the skin appears reddish.
- Hematoma—bruising of the skin; skin color may appear reddish to purple.
- Jaundice—the skin and sclera (white of the eyes) appear yellowish.
- Pallor—the skin is ashen and pale due to white collagen fibers in the dermis.

Accessory Organs

The accessory organs of the skin are located in the dermis or middle layer. These anatomical structures include the hair, nails, sweat glands, and sebaceous glands.

Hair is found all over the body, excluding the lips, palms of the hands, and soles of the feet. The hair is composed of a protein called keratin. Each hair consists of a root portion and a thin, flexible shaft. The hair shaft grows from hair follicles found in the dermis and sometimes the subcutaneous tissue. Melanin gives hair its color. As part of the normal aging process, hair turns gray or white due to a decrease in production of melanin. Hairs such as eyelashes and nose hairs have a protective function that keeps particles out of the eyes and respiratory tract. Each hair has a tiny muscle called the *arrector pili muscle* attached to it. These muscles contract in response to cold or fright, which causes what is commonly known as "goose bumps."

Nails are also made of keratin and help protect the fingers and toes. Nutrients for the nails come from blood vessels located in the dermis. Nerves are also located here, which explains why it is so painful when the nail gets pulled away from the skin. If a fingernail is lost, it takes approximately 150 days to grow a new one. The nail bed is an excellent place to check a patient's oxygen level because of its rich blood supply. Fingernails and toenails are composed of two parts: the body and the root. Both portions lay on the nail bed, or matrix. The body is the exposed section, and the root is hidden under a fold of skin called the *cuticle*.

There are about two million *sweat glands*, also called sudoriferous glands, throughout the body. As mentioned previously, sweat cools the body. There are specialized sweat glands called *apocrine glands* that are located in the pubic and underarm areas. These glands produce odor by a process that occurs when bacteria on the skin come in contact with this thicker sweat.

Sebaceous glands produce oil that lubricates the skin and prevents drying and cracking. Oil secretions from the sebaceous glands increase during adolescence, which causes the development of acne. These secretions diminish with age. This, along with sun exposure, can account for wrinkles and dry skin.

Diseases and Conditions of the Integumentary System

- *Carcinoma* is a cancerous tumor in the mucous membrane, skin, or similar body tissue. Basal cell carcinoma is the most common form of skin cancer. It begins as a small elevated area of the skin like a pimple, ulcer, or mole. It may be red, brown, black, or white in color and it may occur singly or in a group (Figure 4-31). One in five Americans will experience some type of skin cancer in their lifetime.
- *Malignant melanoma* is associated with exposure to the sun. The lesion is characterized by an irregular border and uneven color.
- *Dermatitis* is an inflammation of the skin. The skin is pink to red in color and forms an itchy rash. There are many causes of dermatitis, including systemic conditions, local irritants, and hypersusceptibility by the patient.
- *Acne* is the most common skin disorder in which the sebaceous glands and the hair follicles of the skin become infected and clogged, causing pimples and blackheads.
- *Cellulitis* is a bacterial infection of the skin that spreads through the tissues.
- *Warts* are small growths caused by viral infections of the skin.

Interrelationship Between Oral Health and the Integumentary System

Poor oral health and acne may be linked! Studies have shown that if the bacteria from gum disease or an abscessed (infected) tooth get on the face, skin irritation and breakouts can result. Breakouts around the chin, lips, and lower cheeks indicate poor dental hygiene. These areas need to be washed thoroughly after brushing teeth as the bacteria can drip onto these areas. There is a chance that the patient is allergic to ingredients in their toothpaste. Have them switch brands to see if there is an improvement and again remind them that washing their face after brushing is important.

The dental assistant works very closely with a patient and should always perform a quick visual exam of the patient's face and neck areas while the patient is seated. The assistant should take note of any discolorations, lesions, sores, and/or rashes found on the skin and inform the dentist. Many dental offices have discovered a suspicious lesion on a patient's face and referred the patient to another doctor for further examination. With the increase in skin cancer, early detection often contributes to successful treatment.

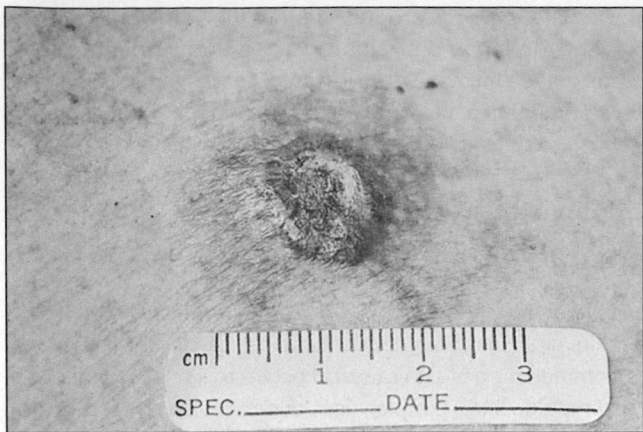

FIGURE 4-31
Basal cell carcinoma.

Urinary System

The urinary system, also known as the **renal** system or **genitourinary** system, is the body's most efficient **regulatory system**, and it keeps the body chemically balanced. It works with the skin, intestines, and lungs to maintain the balance of chemicals and water in the body.

Functions of the Urinary System

The urinary system is continually adjusting the chemical condition in the body that allows for survival. There are four major ways that the urinary system maintains a healthy status and balance:

1. Disposal of toxic waste products produced normally in the body's **metabolic** processes
2. Maintaining a constant **blood pH**, making sure that our body does not become too **acidic** or too **alkaline** by selecting or disposing of certain **ions**
3. Reabsorbing vital nutrients
4. Maintaining a constant blood pressure through regulation of water absorption or excretion and stimulation of blood cell production when needed

Organs of the Urinary System

There are multiple organs that work together to maintain proper functioning of the urinary system. The organs of the urinary system include two kidneys, two ureters, the bladder, and the urethra (Figure 4-32).

Kidneys   The **kidneys** are two bean-shaped organs that are located bilaterally in the rear of the abdominal cavity underneath the lower part of the ribcage. Due to the liver on the right side, the right kidney is usually slightly lower than the left kidney. The kidneys are very closely connected to the body's main artery, the aorta, due to the necessity of the large amount of blood that enters the kidneys: over one liter per minute. This is important because the kidneys' main function is to filter waste products from the blood and to form urine for excretion from the body. The kidneys are able to selectively reabsorb or eliminate water,

oxygen, waste products, vitamins, hormones, and vital nutrients to keep the body at a constant level.

Accessory Organs   The urinary system has accessory organs that serve to transport, store, and eliminate urine.

Ureters   Once urine is formed in the kidneys, it is drained through very narrow cylindrical tubes, known as **ureters**. Each kidney has its own ureter and both drain directly into the bladder.

Urinary Bladder   The **bladder** serves as a storage unit for urine that is dumped out of the ureters until it is able to be emptied to the outside. The bladder is made of smooth muscle and sits on the pelvic floor. It is able to expand and contract as needed to hold up to approximately 350 ml of urine before the body signals the need to empty. At the base of the bladder is a **sphincter** muscle, which is a voluntary muscle movement to expel urine.

Urethra   The tube that carries the urine to the outside is called the **urethra**. A male urethra is approximately 8 inches in length and extends from the bladder into the shaft of the penis. A female urethra is much shorter, about 1.5 inches long, and extends into the vagina. This is a major reason why women are more prone to bacterial infections of the bladder.

Composition of Urine

Normal **urine** is usually straw colored to clear and **sterile**. Urine is usually a sterile liquid until it reaches the end of the urethra, when it could come into contact with outside microorganisms. It is usually composed of approximately 95% water and 5% solutes. The 5% of solutes consists of all of the eliminated products that were selected by the kidneys for removal. Normally, during a 24 hours period, the output of urine will be 1,000 to 2,000 ml, equivalent to 2 liters of soda. This can vary depending on the general health of the person as well as their consumption of fluids. Urine is able to give health care providers many clues to how the body is functioning. There are multiple different urine tests that can easily detect abnormalities. A urinalysis can detect dehydration, bacterial infections, signs of diabetes, or signs of kidney failure, to name just a few.

Common Diseases and Conditions of the Urinary System

- *Cystitis* is a bladder infection usually caused by bacteria.
- *Kidney infection* is when a bladder infection backs up the ureters to the kidneys.
- *Incontinence* (in-**kon**-tn-*uhns*) is the inability to control urine flow, and urine leaks out of the urethra.
- *Enlarged prostate* occurs in men and can make it difficult to empty the bladder.
- *Chronic kidney disease* occurs when the kidneys are damaged and unable to filter blood properly. This can lead to a buildup of waste substances. Most common causes include diabetes, heart disease, and high blood pressure.

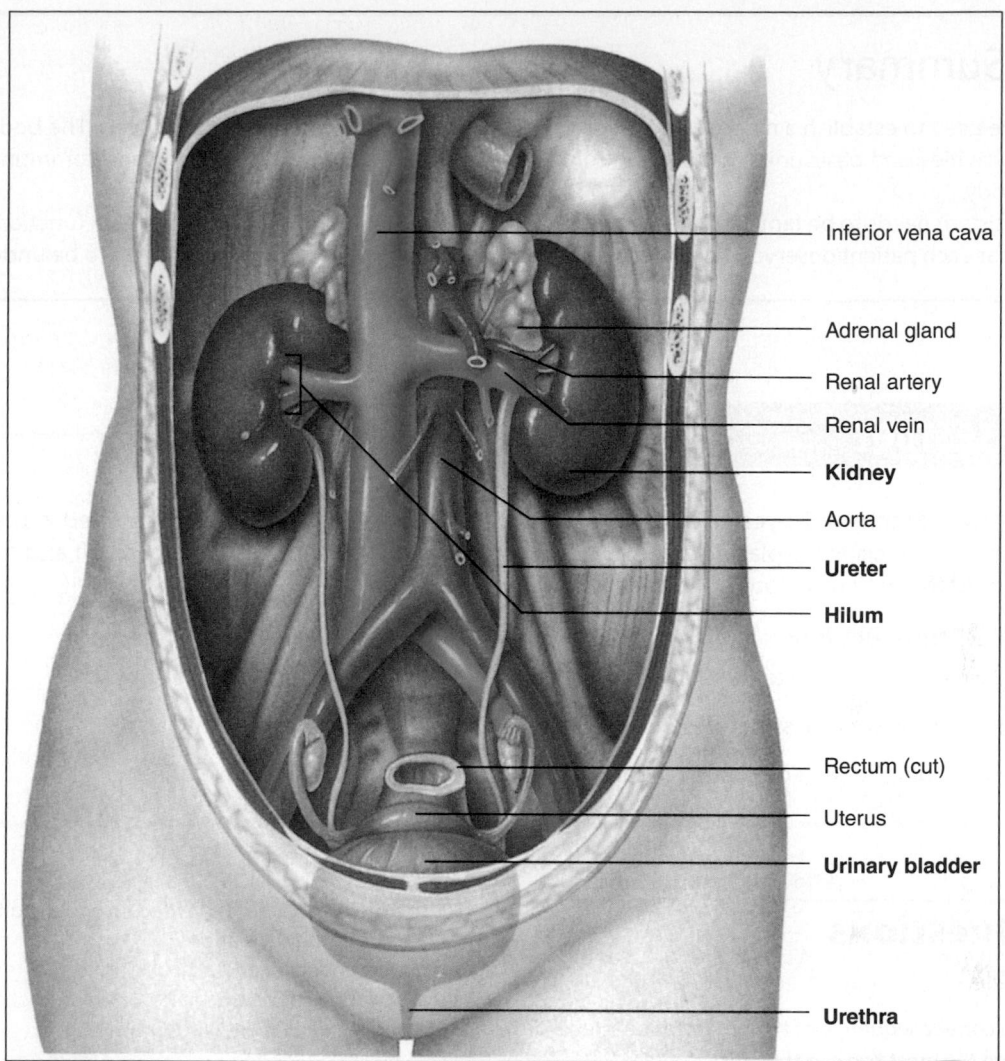

FIGURE 4-32
The organs of the urinary system of a female.

- Inferior vena cava
- Adrenal gland
- Renal artery
- Renal vein
- **Kidney**
- Aorta
- **Ureter**
- **Hilum**
- Rectum (cut)
- Uterus
- **Urinary bladder**
- **Urethra**

Interrelationship Between Oral Health and the Urinary System

Good oral health isn't just about preventing dental decay and gum disease; both conditions can lead to problems for people with kidney disease. Studies have reported that patients with kidney disease who are on dialysis are more likely to have periodontal disease than the general population. One of the side effects of some drugs used to treat kidney disease is dry mouth, which makes it easier for dental decay and gum disease to develop. The dental team needs to work with the patient to increase saliva. Biotene is a saliva substitute that can be recommended, and the need to increase chewing to stimulate saliva production and increase water intake can be discussed with the patient.

When a patient's medical records show they are on dialysis, they may also be on blood-thinning medicine that prevents clotting. It is important to schedule dental treatment on non-dialysis days. With serious kidney disease, the patient may need a kidney transplant. The patient receives medications to prevent rejection of the transplant, but these medications also weaken the immune system. Prior to being approved for a kidney transplant, the patient is evaluated for serious infections, including dental infections (tooth decay and periodontal disease), which need to be treated to prevent post-transplant complications.

Chapter Summary

Specific terms are used to establish a means for health professionals to communicate more effectively. The body is divided into systems, planes, cavities, and basic units that provide common references and terms for studying and communicating information about the body.

The dental assistant needs to be familiar with the terminology of body systems and how each system functions to provide the quality of care that each patient deserves. Both the anatomy and physiology of all body systems need to be understood.

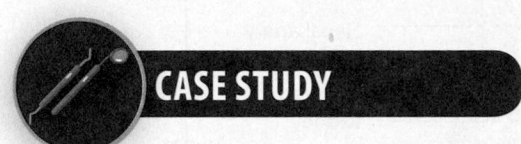

CASE STUDY

Charlie T. Smith is a 23-year-old patient with a history of diabetes. The patient is reclined in the dental chair. The dental assistant is placing a dental dam clamp on a tooth when the clamp pops off and drops to the back of the patient's mouth. The patient swallows the clamp.

Case Study Review

1. List the body systems affected.

2. List the specific structures of the primary system that could become involved.

3. Would the patient's age or medical condition impact the situation? If so, how?

Review Questions

Multiple Choice

1. Which is the correct sequence of the organizational level of the body from the most basic to the most complex?
   a. systems, organs, tissues, and cells
   b. organs, tissues, cells, and systems
   c. cells, tissues, organs, and systems
   d. tissues, cells, systems, and organs

2. Which part of the cell controls the function of the cell?
   a. chromosomes
   b. ribosomes
   c. mitochondria
   d. nucleus

3. Which of the following divides the body into left and right halves?
   a. horizontal plane
   b. transverse plane
   c. sagittal plane
   d. frontal plane

4. What body cavity includes the lungs and heart?
   a. abdominopelvic
   b. cranial
   c. thoracic
   d. spinal

5. The skeletal system is divided into two main divisions:
   a. axial and articulations
   b. appendicular and articulations
   c. axial and appendicular
   d. appendicular and vertebral

6. Which joint(s) is(are) lined by fluid and is(are) free moving?
   a. cartilaginous
   b. fibrous
   c. synovial
   d. fibrous and synovial

7. The skeletal muscles consist of what type of muscle tissue?
   a. striated muscle
   b. cardiac muscle
   c. smooth muscle
   d. involuntary muscle

8. The neurons that carry messages away from the spinal cord and brain are:
   a. sensory neurons.
   b. motor neurons.
   c. associative neurons.
   d. interneurons.

9. What nerves control the voluntary body activities of the skeletal muscles and sensory information?
   a. sympathetic
   b. parasympathetic
   c. spinal
   d. somatic

10. Which glands regulate carbohydrate levels and secrete epi-nephrine as the body responds in an emergency situation?
    a. thyroid
    b. parathyroid
    c. adrenal
    d. pituitary

11. The release of digestive enzymes and the production of insulin are a function of the _____.
    a. thymus gland
    b. pancreas
    c. pineal gland
    d. pituitary gland

12. What serves as a place of nourishment and protection for a fetus as it develops and grows?
    a. ovaries
    b. uterus
    c. fallopian tubes
    d. vagina

13. Which is located below the urinary bladder, surrounds the urethra, and if enlarged may cause difficulty with urination?
    a. urinary meatus
    b. prostate
    c. vas deferens
    d. epididymis

14. What type of blood vessel carries oxygenated blood away from the heart?
    a. arteries
    b. veins
    c. capillaries
    d. fibrous

15. The muscular tube that carries food from the mouth to the stomach is the _____.
    a. larynx
    b. esophagus
    c. throat
    d. food tract

16. What is the name of the passageway for air to the bronchial tubes?
    a. pharynx
    b. trachea
    c. alveoli
    d. larynx

17. Where does the actual exchange of oxygen and carbon dioxide occur?
    a. pharynx
    b. trachea
    c. alveoli
    d. larynx

18. Where are pathogens and cell debris trapped and destroyed?
    a. lymph nodes
    b. lymph vessels
    c. tonsils
    d. thymus

19. What is the name of the top layer of skin?
    a. dermis
    b. epidermis
    c. subcutaneous
    d. keratin

20. The _____ stores urine until it needs to be emptied.
    a. ureter
    b. bladder
    c. urethra
    d. kidney

Critical Thinking

1. Why it is important for the dental assistant to study anatomy and physiology? How is this necessary in taking medical histories?

2. Explain the significance of the muscular system to oral health.

3. Explain why the pulmonary arteries are called arteries even though they carry deoxygenated blood and why the pulmonary veins are called veins even though they carry oxygenated blood.

4. Why is it harder to replace lost blood in elderly patients?

Key Terms

Term and Pronunciation	Meaning of Root and Word Parts	Definition
abdominopelvic cavity (ab-**dom**-*uh*-noh- **pel**-vik) (**kav**-i-tee)	**abdomen** = belly; cavity encloses stomach, liver, spleen, and pancreas **pelvis** = cavity formed by hipbones and sacrum and encloses intestines, bladder, and internal reproductive organs **-ic** = pertaining to **cavity** = hollow space within body	pertaining to the abdomen and the pelvic cavity
acidic (*uh*-**sid**-ik)	**acid** = pH less than 7; chemical capable of dissolving and burning structures; caustic **-ic** = indicating state	a substance that contains a pH less than 7
adrenal gland (*uh*-**dreen**-l) (gland)	**ad-** = near or next to **renal** = descriptive term for kidney **gland** = an organ or group of specialized cells in the body that produces and secretes a specific substance	gland located on top of each kidney that secretes hormones that help control heart rate, blood pressure, the way the body uses food and minerals, and reproduction
adrenaline (*uh*-**dren**-l-in)	**adrenal** = pertaining to the adrenal gland **-ine** = indicating a chemical substance produced	a hormone secreted by the adrenal glands that helps the body meet physical or emotional stress
alkaline (**al**-*kuh*-lahyn)	**alkali** = pH greater than 7; base capable of neutralizing acid **-ine** = having the properties of	a substance that contains a pH greater than 7
anatomy (*uh*-**nat**-*uh*-mee)	**anatomy** = study of the structure of living bodies	the branch of science that studies the structures of organisms
anus (**ey**-nuhs)	**anus** = opening at lower end of the digestive tract	the outlet of the rectum lying in the fold between the buttocks
artery (**ahr**-*tuh*-ree)	**artery** = vessel that carries blood from heart through the body	a thick-walled vessel that carries oxygenated blood away from the heart
articulation (ahr-tik-*yuh*-**ley**-sh*uh*n)	**articulate** = join or connect together **-ion** = denoting action or condition	to join a joint, bones, or movable parts; connect together loosely to allow motion between the structures
atrium (**ey**-tree-*uhm*)	**atrium** = main or central room; a cavity or chamber	the two upper chambers of the heart; atria plural form
autonomic (aw-t*uh*-**nom**-ik)	**autonomy(y)** = functioning as an independent organism **-ic** = having characteristics	involuntary or unconscious functions
bladder (**blad**-er)	**bladder** = a membranous sac or organ serving as a receptacle for a fluid or air; cyst	a storage unit for urine until it is able to be emptied to the outside
blood pH (bluhd) (ph)	**blood** = fluid circulating in vascular system **pH** = potential hydrogen; acid and base (alkaline) balance in blood; measure of hydrogen ion concentration; 7 is neutral	a measure of hydrogen ion concentration in the blood
bone marrow (bohn) (**mar**-oh)	**bone** = hard connective tissue forming the substance of the skeleton **marrow** = soft, fatty, vascular tissue in the cavities of bones	soft tissue in the marrow cavities of long bones where blood cell production occurs
cancellous (**kan**-s*uh*-luhs)	**cancellate** = of spongy or porous structure **-ous** = possessing a given quality	bone tissue with a lattice-like structure containing many pores; found in interior of mature bones
capillary (**kap**-*uh*-ler-ee)	**capillary** = thin tube, narrow passage, hairlike	network of small vessels that connect arteries and veins
carbon dioxide (**kahr**-b*uh*n) (dahy-**ok**-sahyd)	**carbon** = element occurring in all known forms of life **dioxide** = two atoms of oxygen	a colorless gas that is eliminated through the lungs

Term and Pronunciation	Meaning of Root and Word Parts	Definition
cardiac (**kahr**-dee-ak)	**card** = heart **-ic** = pertaining to	referring to the heart
cartilaginous joint (kahr-tl-**aj**-uh-nuhs) (joint)	**cartilage** = a firm, elastic, flexible type of connective tissue **-ous** = of or resembling **joint** = the movable or fixed part where two bones of a skeleton join	a joint in which there is cartilage between the bones
chamber (**cheym**-ber)	**chamber** = a room	a compartment or a closed space
chromosomes (**kroh**-m*uh*-sohm)	**chromo-** = color origin **-some** = body	a threadlike structure of nucleic acids and protein found in the nucleus of most cells; single chain of DNA carrying genetic information
cilia (**sil**-ee-*uh*)	**cilia** = minute hairlike organelles lining surfaces that provide movement of liquids	threadlike projections lining the trachea and bronchi
coagulation (koh-**ag**-y*uh*-ley-sh*uh*n)	**coagulum** = clot, curd **-ate** = denoting functions	the change from a fluid into a thickened mass; process of forming a clot
collagen fibers (**kol**-*uh*-j*uh*n)	**collagen** = most abundant protein in the human body **fiber** = a slender thread or filament	a long fibrous structural protein that supports tissues and gives structure to individual cells; major building block of bones, skin, muscles, tendons, and ligaments
coronal (**kawr**-*uh*-nl)	**coron** = crown; head **-al** = of or relating to	relating to the crown of the head; vertical plane from head to foot and parallel to the shoulders
cortical (**kawr**-ti-k*uh*l)	**cortex** = the outer layer of any organ or part **-al** = of or relating to	hard outer shell of most bones in the body
cranial cavity (**krey**-nee-*uh*l) (**kav**-i-tee)	**cranium** = skull **cavity** = hollow space within body	pertaining to the skull or brain
cytology (sahy-**tol**-*uh*-jee)	**cyte** = cell **-ology** = study of	the branch of science that studies the formation, structure, and function of cells
deoxygenate (dee-**ok**-si-j*uh*-neyt)	**de-** = removal, separation **oxygen** = natural gas essential for life in most organisms **ate** = denote function	blood that does not contain oxygen
deoxyribonucleic acid (dee-**ok**-si-**rahy**-boh-noo-**klee**-ik) (**as**-id)	**deoxy-** = presence of less oxygen than in a specified related compound **ribose** = a pentose sugar (monosaccharide with 5 carbon atoms) that is a component of RNA **nucle(i)** = central part about which other parts are grouped **-ic** = having characteristics of **acid** = chemical species that donates protons or hydrogen ions and/or accepts electrons	DNA, main component of chromosomes; material that transfers genetic characteristics in all life forms; transmission of hereditary characteristics from parents to offspring
dialysis (dahy-**al**-uh-sis)	**dia-** = going apart **-lysis** = breaking down	the process by which uric acid and urea circulating in blood are remove by a dialyzer machine; a substitute for normal kidney function
diaphragm (**dahy**-*uh*-fram)	**diaphragm** = muscular wall separating two cavities	a skeletal muscle that separates the abdomen and the thoracic cavity; contracts and relaxes, which promotes proper breathing
digestive enzymes (dih-**jes**-tiv) (**en**-sahym)	**digest** = to convert food into simpler chemical compounds; absorbable **-ive** = expressing function **enzymes** = proteins from living cells capable of producing chemical changes	proteins that chemically break down food to facilitate the absorption of nutrients by the body
duct (duhkt)	**duct** = tube conveying a body fluid	a narrow vessel or channel

(Continues)

Term and Pronunciation	Meaning of Root and Word Parts	Definition
endocrine system (**en**-d*uh*-krin)	**endo-** = inside, within **endocrine** = secreting internally into the blood or lymph **system** = a group of bodily organs with similar structures or that work together to perform some function	group of glands that produce and secrete hormones in the body in order for the body to function properly
epidermis (ep-i-**dur**-mis)	**epi-** = on, upon **dermis** = dense inner layer; true skin	the outermost layer of the skin
epiglottis (ep-i-**glot**-is)	**epi-** = upon, on, over **glottis** = opening at the upper part of the larynx; mouth of the windpipe	the cartilage of the larynx that prevents food from entering the lungs
epinephrine (ep-*uh*-**nef**-rin)	**epi-** = close to, near **nephro-** = kidney-like structure **-ine** = indicating a chemical substance produced	a hormone secreted by the adrenal glands that helps the body meet physical or emotional stress; also referred to as adrenaline
epithelial tissue (ep-*uh*-**thee**-lee-*uhl*) (**tish**-oo)	**epithelium** = layer of cells closely bound to one another to form continuous sheets covering surfaces **-al** = pertaining to **tissue** = large number of cells of similar structure and function forming a structural material	tissue that covers and lines body structures
erythrocyte (ih-**rith**-*ruh*-sahyt)	**erythro-** = red **-cyte** = cell	red blood cell; contains hemoglobin, which is responsible for the transportation of oxygen to the tissues
esophagus (ih-**sof**-*uh*-g*uh*s)	**esophagus** = muscular passage connecting pharynx with stomach, gullet	the muscular tube that carries swallowed food from the pharynx to the stomach
equilibrium (ee-kwuh-**lib**-ree-*uh*m)	**equi-** = equal **libra** = balance **-ium** = associating status	a state of balance between opposing forces or influences; may be chemical or physical between opposite forces of actions that are static or will have small changes
extensibility (ik-**sten**-s*uh*-**bil**-i-tee)	**extens** = extend, enlarge the scope, lengthen **-ibility** = capable of	ability for a muscle to be stretched
fascia (**fash**-ee-*uh*)	**fasces** = bundle, pack **-ia** = denoting condition or quality	a sheet or band of fibrous connective tissue that envelops, separates, or binds muscles, organs, and other soft structures of the body
fibrous joint (**fahy**-br*uh*s) (joint)	**fiber** = an elongated threadlike cell **-ous** = containing **joint** = the movable or fixed part where two bones of a skeleton join	a joint in which there is fibrous tissue between the bones
genetic (j*uh*-**net**-ik)	**genes** = basic physical unit of heredity; DNA codes for the production of proteins **-tic** = relating to or produced by	tending to occur among family members due to heredity; the sum of characteristics transmitted from parents to their offspring
genitalia (jen-i-**tey**-lee-*uh*)	**genital** = sexual organs, reproduction **-ia** = pertaining to	another term for the reproductive organs
genitourinary (jen-i-toh-**yoor**-*uh*-ner-ee)	**genital** = reproductive (sex) organs **urine** = matter excreted by kidneys **-ary** = pertaining to	another term used for the urinary system, the genitals, and urinary organs
glucose (**gloo**-kohs)	**glucose** = sugar found in plants	a monosaccharide sugar in the blood that serves as the major source of energy for the body
glycogen (**glahy**-k*uh*-j*uh*n)	**glyco-** = sugar **-gen** = that which produces	carbohydrate consisting of a long chain of many glucose molecules; stored form of glucose
homeostasis (hoh-mee-*uh*-**stey**-sis)	**homeo-** = similar **stasis** = stable; state of equilibrium or no progression (static)	the process of maintaining a stable environment suitable for sustaining life; compensating for environmental changes
hormone (**hawr**-mohn)	**hormone** = that which sets in motion	chemicals that are formed in endocrine glands; made specifically to work with an organ or system to increase or decrease the activity level depending on the body's need

Term and Pronunciation	Meaning of Root and Word Parts	Definition
inorganic (in-awr-**gan**-ik)	**in-** = not **organic** = derived from living organisms	not having the structure or organization characteristic of living organisms; may be product of once-living organisms such as minerals
insulin (**in**-suh-lin)	**insulin** = hormone produced in the pancreas	hormone that controls the breakdown and uptake of sugars, proteins, and fats
ion (**ahy**-uhn)	**ion** = an electrically charged atom or group of atoms formed by the loss or gain of one or more electron	retaining or excreting minerals from the blood; potassium, magnesium, sodium, calcium, sulfur
keratin (**ker**-uh-tin)	**keratin** = fibrous proteins forming chemical basis of horny epidermal tissue (as hair and nails)	an extremely tough protein substance found in hair and nails
kidney (**kid**-nee)	**kidney** = organ named by its shape; kidney bean shape	the organ responsible for filtering waste products from the blood and for forming urine for excretion by the body
lactic acid (**lak**-tik) (**as**-id)	**lact** = milk **-ic** = derived from **acid** = any class of compounds that form hydrogen ions when dissolved in water; sharp or biting, sour	present normally in blood and muscle tissue; produced during muscle contraction as product of metabolism of glucose; abundant in sour milk by bacterial action on milk
larynx (**lar**-ingks)	**larynx** = upper part of the trachea containing vocal cords; muscular/cartilaginous structure lined with mucous membrane	the cartilaginous organ at the top of the trachea
leukocyte (**loo**-kuh-sahyt)	**leuko** = white **-cyte** = cell	white blood cell; responsible for protecting our body from harmful pathogens
ligament (**lig**-uh-muhnt)	**ligament** = fibrous connective tissue that ties bone or cartilage together	a band or sheet of strong fibrous connective tissue connecting the ends of bones
lymph (limf)	**lymph** = clear fluid containing white blood cells; removes bacteria from tissue	clear and colorless tissue fluid that has entered the lymph capillaries and vessels; it is mainly composed of white blood cells and water
lymphocyte (**lim**-fuh-sahyt)	**lymph(o)-** = fluid, chiefly white blood cells, collected from body tissues and transported in lymphatic system **-cyte** = indicating a cell	one of the subtypes of white blood cells; these cells have immunologic memory resulting in a more rapid, vigorous response to a second encounter with the same antigen
macrophage (**mak**-ruh-feyj)	**macro-** = large **-phage** = a thing that devours	a large white blood cell that engulfs and ingests foreign particles and infectious microorganisms by process called phagocytosis
mastication (**mas**-ti-key-shuhn)	**masticate** = to chew **-tion** = expressing action	to chew or grind something up; chewing food
melanin (**mel**-uh-nin)	**melanin** = group of naturally occurring black or dark brown pigments found in skin and hair	a pigment produced in the skin that gives color to hair and skin
metabolic (met-uh-**bol**-ik)	**metabolism** = chemical processes by which cells produce the substances and energy needed to sustain life **-ic** = indicating action of	physical and chemical changes that take place within the body; waste products of metabolism are filtered through the kidneys and excreted if needed
mucous membrane (**myoo**-kuhs) (**mem**-breyn)	**mucous** = containing, producing, or secreting mucus **membrane** = a thin layer of tissue covering surfaces	an epithelial tissue that secretes mucus; lines many body cavities and the respiratory passages, mouth, and stomach
mucus (**myoo**-kuhs)	**mucus** = slippery and somewhat sticky fluid secreted by glands in the mucous membranes	lubricates and protects the mucous membranes; composed of large glycoproteins (mucins) and inorganic salts in water
neuroglial cells (noo-**rog**-lee-uhl)	**neuro** = neuron, nerve cell **glia** = a delicate web of connective tissue that surrounds and support nerve cells **cells** = the smallest structural units of an organism	cells of the nervous system that support the neurons
neurons (**noor**-on)	**neuron** = nerve cells; impulse-conducting cells; functional unit of nervous system	individual nerve cells that initiate and transmit electrical impulses in response to a stimulus

(Continues)

Term and Pronunciation	Meaning of Root and Word Parts	Definition
nucleolus (noo-**klee**-uh-luhs)	**nucleus** = central region of the cell **-ole** = indicating something small	rounded body within the nucleus of a cell; regulates the interactions of proteins and every cellular function
nucleus (**noo**-klee-uhs)	**nucleus** = central region of the cell	structure within a cell that is responsible for the cell's metabolism, growth, and reproduction
occlusal function (uh-**kloo**-zhuhl) (**fuhngk**-shuhn)	**occlude** = to close with opposing teeth fitting together **-al** = pertaining to **function** = natural action or intended purpose; job	relationship between the upper and lower teeth when they approach each other; occurs during chewing or at rest
oral cavity (**ohr**-uhl) (**kav**-i-tee)	**or-** = mouth **-al** = pertaining to **cavity** = hollow space within body	concerning the part of the mouth behind the gums and teeth
organelle (awr-guh-**nel**)	**organ** = part of an organism that performs one or more specialized functions **-elle** = indicating smallness	a cell organ; one small part of a cell that has a very specific function or job
osseous tissue (**os**-ee-uhs) (**tish**-oo)	**oss-** = bone **-eous** = composed of or containing **tissue** = part of an organism consisting of a large number of cells having similar structure and function	major structural supportive connective tissue of the body that forms the rigid part of the bone organs
osteoblasts (**os**-tee-uh-blast)	**osteo-** = indicating bone or bones **blast** = formative cells or cell layer	bone-forming cell
osteoporosis (os-tee-oh-puh-**roh**-sis)	**osteo-** = indicating bone or bones **pore** = small hole **-osis** = denoting condition	disorder caused by loss of calcium and other minerals from bones; bones become porous, brittle, and subject to fracture
parasympathetic nerves (par-uh-sim-puh-**thet**-ik) (nurvs)	**para** = against, in opposition **sympathy** = relation between parts or organs in which one induces an effect in the other **-ic** = relating to **nerves** = bundle of fibers made of neurons that carry sensory and motor information throughout body	part of the autonomic nervous system that controls our daily bodily functions (stimulate digestion and elimination) as well as returning the body system to normal after a crisis situation (lowers blood pressure and pulse)
pathogen (**path**-uh-juhn)	**patho-** = disease **gen** = producing agent	a microorganism that is capable of causing disease
pelvic (**pel**-vik)	**pelvis** = wide curved group of bones at the level of the hips **-ic** = or of relating to	bowl-shaped group of bones connecting the trunk of the body to the legs; provides for movement and protection for reproductive organs and bladder
periosteum (per-ee-**os**-tee-uhm)	**peri-** = around **oste** = bone **-um** = indicating structure	dense, fibrous two-layered membrane covering of the surface of bones to which muscles attach
peristalsis (per-uh-**stawl**-sis)	**peri-** = around, about **stal** = compress **-sis** = denoting action, process	the involuntary progressive wave of contraction and relaxation of a tubular muscle; forces contents through the system
pharynx (**far**-ingks)	**pharynx** = passage leading from the nose and mouth to the larynx; throat	the passageway for air from the nasal cavity to the larynx
physiology (fiz-ee-**ol**-uh-jee)	**physical** = relating to the body **-ology** = study of	the branch of science that studies the functions of an organism and the chemical and physical processes involved
prostate gland (**pros**-teyt) (gland)	**prostate** = male gland that secretes semen and controls release of urine **gland** = organ producing a secretion	a gland that is located at the bottom of the bladder that secretes an alkaline fluid that is mixed with the sperm and which assists with keeping sperm alive during ejaculation and placement in the female reproductive system
pulmonary (**puhl**-muh-ner-ee)	**pulmo** = a lung **-ary** = pertaining to	referring to the lungs

Term and Pronunciation	Meaning of Root and Word Parts	Definition
regulatory system (**reg**-yuh-ley-tohr-ee) (**sis**-tuhm)	**regulate** = mechanism for accurate and proper functioning **-ory** = having the effect of **system** = group of bodily organs that have similar structures or work together to perform some function	keeping the body at a constant chemical balance needed to sustain life
renal (**reen**-l)	**renal** = descriptive term for kidneys	pertaining to the kidney
ribonucleic acid (**rahy**-boh-noo-**klee**-ik) (**as**-id)	**ribose** = a pentose sugar (monosaccharide with 5 carbon atoms) that is a component of RNA **nucle(i)** = central part about which other parts are grouped **-ic** = having characteristics of **acid** = chemical species that donates protons or hydrogen ions and/or accepts electrons	RNA, directly codes for amino acids and acts as a messenger between ribosomes in the cell to make protein; is a copy of genetic information stored in a DNA strand, identical to and complements the DNA; except RNA has sugar ribose instead of deoxyribose of the DNA that has one more OH (oxygen atom bonded to a hydrogen atom)
sagittal plane (**saj**-i-tl) (pleyn)	**sagittal** = of or relating to the suture (sagittal suture) uniting the two parietal bones of the skull **plane** = an imaginary line used to identify parts of the body	a descriptive term used that divides the body into right and left portions
septum (**sep**-tuhm)	**septum** = a dividing wall	a thin membrane dividing two cavities or soft tissue of an organism
somatic nerves (soh-**mat**-ik) (nurvs)	**soma** = cells of the body with the exception of the reproductive cells **-ic** = pertaining to **nerves** = bundle of fibers made of neurons that carry sensory and motor information throughout body	part of the autonomic nervous system that controls the voluntary body activities, such as skeletal muscles and sensory information, such as touch, temperature, and pain
sphincter (**sfingk**-ter)	**sphincter** = band, anything that binds tight; ringlike muscle	a circular muscle constricting an opening
sterile (**ster**-il)	**sterile** = free from living germs	free from living microorganisms
stimuli (**stim**-yuh-lahy)	**stimulus** = to cause a response in an organism **stimuli** = plural form	Something that can elicit or evoke a physiological response in a cell, tissue, or an organism; sense organs in ear and skin are sensitive to sound and touch
sympathetic nerves (sim-puh-**thet**-ik) (nurvs)	**sympathy** = relation between parts or organs in which one induces an effect in the other **-ic** = relating to **nerves** = bundle of fibers made of neurons that carry sensory and motor information throughout body	part of the autonomic nervous system that controls the body's fight-or-flight response to a crisis situation, increasing blood pressure and heart rate
synovial joint (si-**noh**-vee-uhl) (joint)	**synovia** = a lubricating fluid secreted by membranes in joints and cavities **-al** = pertaining to **joint** = the movable or fixed part where two bones of a skeleton	a joint in which the articulating surfaces are separated by synovial fluid
tendon (**ten**-duhn)	**tendon** = dense, inelastic fibrous tissue connecting muscle to bone	fibrous connective tissue that serves as the attachment of muscles to bones and other parts
thoracic cavity (thaw-**ras**-ik) (**kav**-i-tee)	**thorax** = part enclosed by ribs, chest **-ic** = of or pertaining to **cavity** = hollow space within body	pertaining to the chest cavity
thrombocyte (**throm**-buh-sahyt)	**thrombo** = another name for platelet; promotes blood clotting **-cyte** = cell	platelet; responsible for the clotting of blood
trabeculae (truh-**bek**-yuh-luh)	**trabecula** = resembling a little beam or crossbar **-ae** = plural form	rod-shaped structures that divide organs into separate chambers; e.g, network of bone tissue that makes up cancellous structure

(Continues)

Term and Pronunciation	Meaning of Root and Word Parts	Definition
trachea (**trey**-kee-*uh*)	**trachea** = principal passage for air to and from the lungs; the windpipe	the cartilaginous tube that extends from the larynx to the primary bronchi
transverse plane (trans-**vurs**)	**transverse** = in a cross direction; crossing from side to side	a descriptive term used that divides the body into upper and lower or superior and posterior portions
ureter (y*oo*-**ree**-ter)	**ureter** = duct that transmits urine from each kidney to the bladder	the muscular duct that carries urine from the kidneys to the bladder
urethra (y*oo*-**ree**-thr*uh*)	**urethra** = tube from bladder to outside; carries urine; in males also carries semen	the tube that carries urine from the bladder to the external opening in the body for removal; in males carries semen
urine (**y**o*o*r-in)	fluid waste material excreted by kidneys	sterile liquid that is formed by the kidneys by products that need to be eliminated from the body; waste products
vein (veyn)	**vein** = blood vessel carrying blood from body to heart	a vessel that carries deoxygenated blood and waste products back to the heart
ventricle (**ven**-tri-k*uh*l)	**ventricle** = lower cavities of the heart	the two lower chambers of the heart
vertebrae (**vur**-t*uh*-brey)	**vertebra** = one of the bony segments of the spinal column **vertebrae** = plural form	bones composing the spinal column; cylindrical in shape, forming an opening for the spinal cord passage

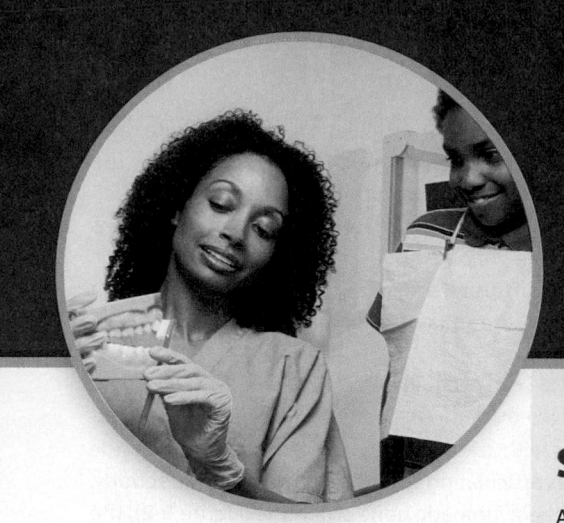

## CHAPTER 5

Head and Neck Anatomy

Specific Instructional Objectives

At the completion of this chapter, you will be able to meet these objectives:

1. Use terms presented in this chapter.
2. Identify the bones of the cranium.
3. Identify the landmarks of the face and the oral cavity, including the tongue, floor of the mouth, and salivary glands.
4. Label the landmarks that are important in dentistry of the following: maxilla, mandible, and sphenoid bone.
5. Describe how the parts of the TMJ are involved in the articulation and movement of the joint.
6. Discuss the possible problems associated with the TMJ.
7. Discuss the functions of the following: muscles of the head, muscles of mastication, muscles of facial expression, the floor of the mouth, the tongue, muscles of the neck.
8. Describe the structure of the tongue.
9. Discuss the salivary glands.
10. Discuss the salivary secretions.
11. Describe the major divisions of the nervous system.
12. Identify the nerves of the maxilla and the mandible.
13. List the areas innervated by each cranial nerve in order by name and Roman numeral.
14. Explain in detail the innervation of the major divisions of the trigeminal nerve.
15. Discuss the pathway of blood in the body.
16. Discuss in detail, the arteries and veins of the head, neck, tongue, teeth, and face.
17. Discuss the location of the important lymph nodes in dentistry.
18. Explain why a patient head and neck exam is important during a dental visit.

Introduction

This chapter will focus on the anatomy of the head, neck, and oral cavity, particularly those of importance to the dental assistant. The structures that are of importance to the dental assistant are the bones of the skull as well as the muscles of the head, neck, oral cavity as well as the arteries, **veins**, and **lymph nodes** in these areas.

Bones of the Cranium

The human skull is composed of 22 bones, each with its own characteristics and function. The neurocranial bones of the skull serve to surround and protect the brain. The viscerocranial bones make up the **facial** structure (Figure 5-1).

Bones of the Neurocranium

There are eight bones—two paired sets of bones and four single bones—of the **neurocranium**. These bones are designed to protect the brain (Figure 5-2).

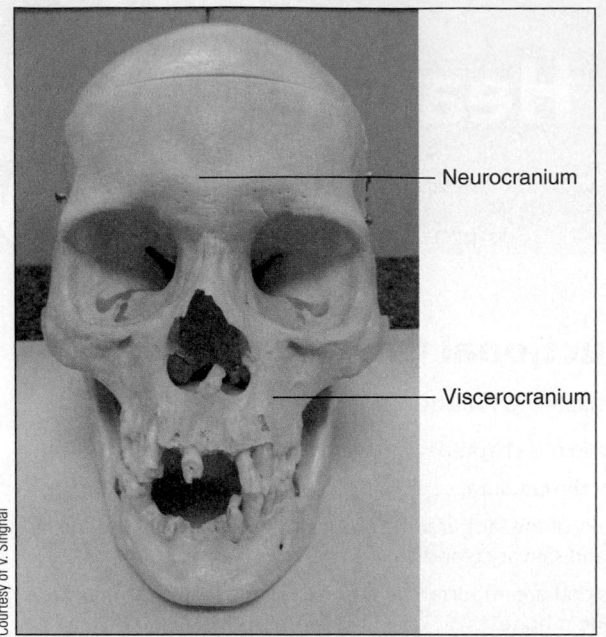

- Neurocranium
- Viscerocranium

FIGURE 5-1
Skull bones with landmarks: neurocranium and viscerocranium.

Frontal Bone (Single) The single frontal bone forms the forehead, upper areas of the eye orbit, and the anterior superior portion of the skull. The frontal bone has a few characteristics to note. The supraorbital **foramen** is found on the anterior view and superior to the eye orbit portion of the bone. Below each of these you will find the curved elevations of bone called the supraorbital ridges. This is the prominent portion of bone where the eyebrows would be found. Between these supraorbital ridges, or between the eyes, is an area called the **glabella** (Figure 5-3).

Parietal Bones (Paired) The paired parietal bones make up the superior lateral sides of the skull (Figure 5-2). The right and left parietal bones touch each other or articulate at the midsagittal plane along the sagittal suture. These bones fit directly behind

the frontal bone. The suture or articulation of the parietal and frontal bone is called the *coronal suture*. In a newborn baby, the junction of the coronal and midsagittal suture is not fully calcified and is termed the bregma or the soft spot. The parietal bones also articulate with the *occipital* bone (Figure 5-2) in the posterior, along the lambdoidal suture, and along the lateral surface with the temporal bones at the squamosal sutures.

Temporal Bones (Paired) The lateral sides of the skull, under the parietal bones, are the temporal bones (Figure 5-2). The temporal bone articulates with several other bones to help form the side of the skull. Besides articulating with the parietal bone superiorly, it articulates with the zygomatic bone anteriorly (Figure 5-2), the occipital bone posteriorly, and the sphenoid bone also anteriorly. There is an **articular eminence** and the glenoid **fossa** on the inferior surface of the temporal bone that articulates with the mandible and forms the temporomandibular joint or TMJ (Figure 5-2).

The temporal bone has several important **processes**. The **styloid process** is a thin, spine-like process that extends downward from the inferior surface of the bone (Figure 5-4). There are several muscles, tendons, and ligaments that attach to this process. Directly behind the styloid process is the *mastoid* process (Figure 5-4), which is a large bulbous, boney process that is also right behind the external auditory meatus (ear canal). The external auditory meatus is a foramen where the ear canal and *tympanic* portion of the temporal bone is found (Figure 5-4).

The *zygomatic* process extends anteriorly from the temporal bone and articulates with the *zygoma* at the side of the skull to form the zygomatic arch. This arch has a bridge-like appearance at the lateral side of the skull. Several muscles attach to this zygomatic arch (Figure 5-2).

Occipital Bone (Single) The occipital bone is found at the most posterior portion of the skull, behind the parietal bones and helps form the back and inferior surface of the skull (Figure 5-2). The occipital bone is a large bone that articulates with the sphenoid bone anteriorly, the temporal bones laterally, and the parietal bones posteriorly. At the base of the skull, in the occipital

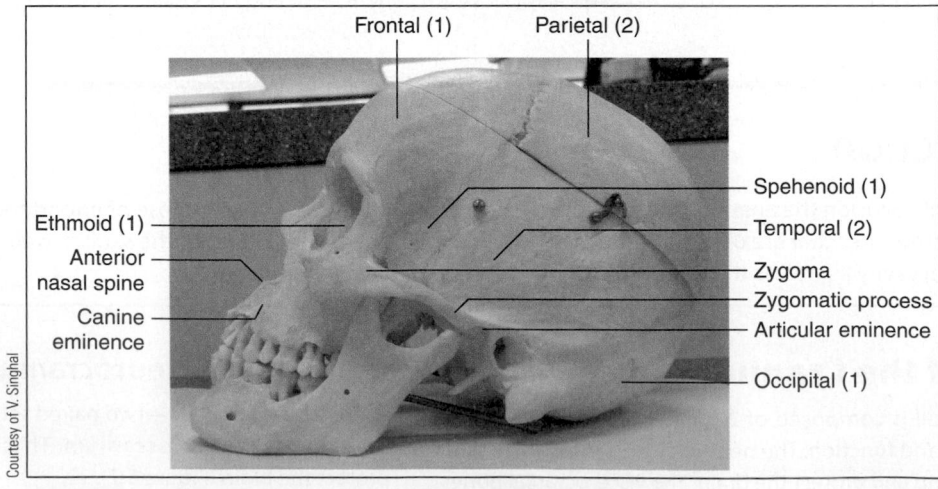

- Frontal (1)
- Parietal (2)
- Ethmoid (1)
- Anterior nasal spine
- Canine eminence
- Spehenoid (1)
- Temporal (2)
- Zygoma
- Zygomatic process
- Articular eminence
- Occipital (1)

FIGURE 5-2
Skull: Eight bones of the neurocranium.

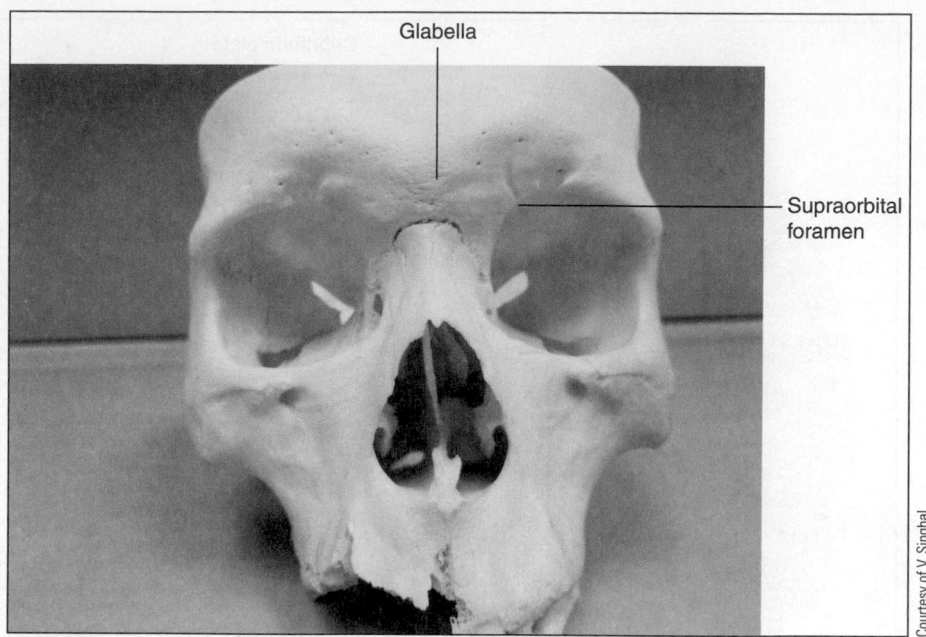

FIGURE 5-3
Glabella and infraorbital foramen.

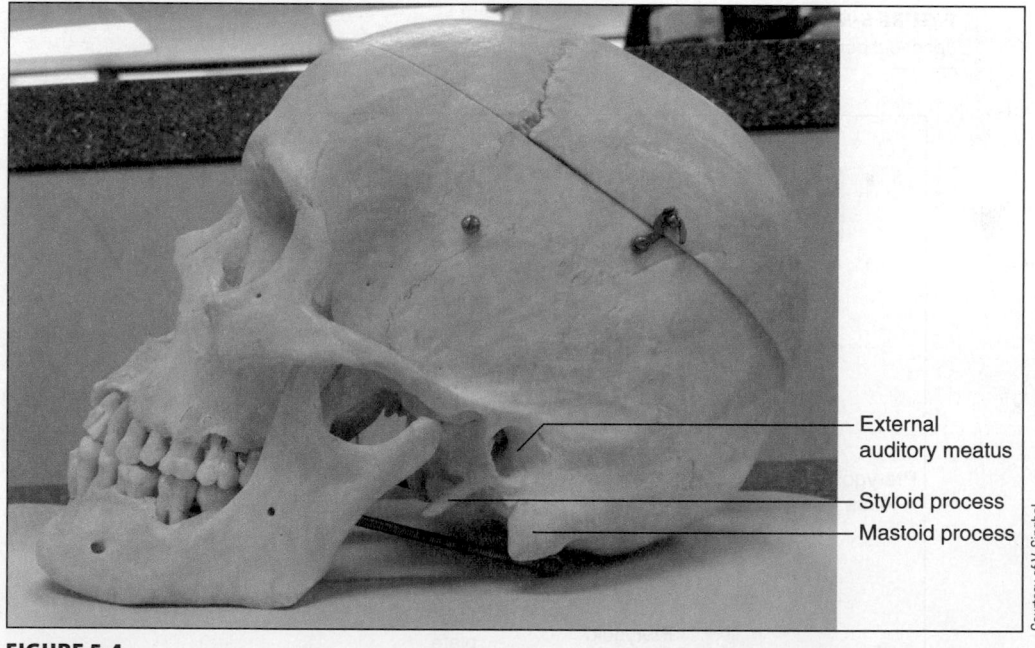

FIGURE 5-4
Skull with styloid process, tympanic area, and mastoid process.

bone, is the largest foramen or opening in the skull. This is known as the foramen *magnum* and is the opening through which the spinal cord exits the skull (Figure 5-5A).

Sphenoid Bone (Single) The *sphenoid* bone is the only neurocranial bone that articulates with every other neurocranial bone. It is probably the most oddly shaped bone of the skull. It looks as if it has a body and two sets of wings with legs that hang downward. The larger set of wings is called the greater wings, and

the smaller set is called the lesser wings. The right and left legs that extend downward are the **pterygoid** processes. The body of the sphenoid has a saddle-shaped depression called the *sella tursica* (Latin for Turkish saddle). The most inferior part of the sella tursica is known as the *hypophyseal* fossa (seat of the saddle). This depression is where the important *pituitary* gland sits.

The greater wings articulate with the frontal, parietal and temporal bones on the lateral sides of the skull. The lesser wings are much smaller and help form a portion of the back of

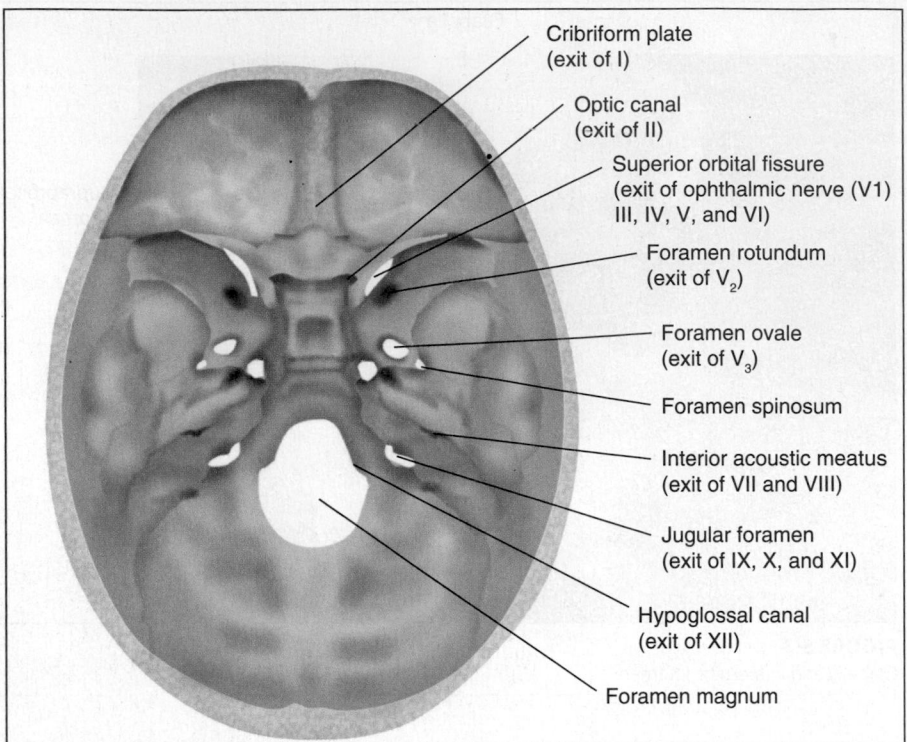

FIGURE 5-5A
Sphenoid bone with foramen spinosum, rotundum and ovale, and foramen magnum.

Labels in figure:
- Cribriform plate (exit of I)
- Optic canal (exit of II)
- Superior orbital fissure (exit of ophthalmic nerve (V1) III, IV, V, and VI)
- Foramen rotundum (exit of V_2)
- Foramen ovale (exit of V_3)
- Foramen spinosum
- Interior acoustic meatus (exit of VII and VIII)
- Jugular foramen (exit of IX, X, and XI)
- Hypoglossal canal (exit of XII)
- Foramen magnum

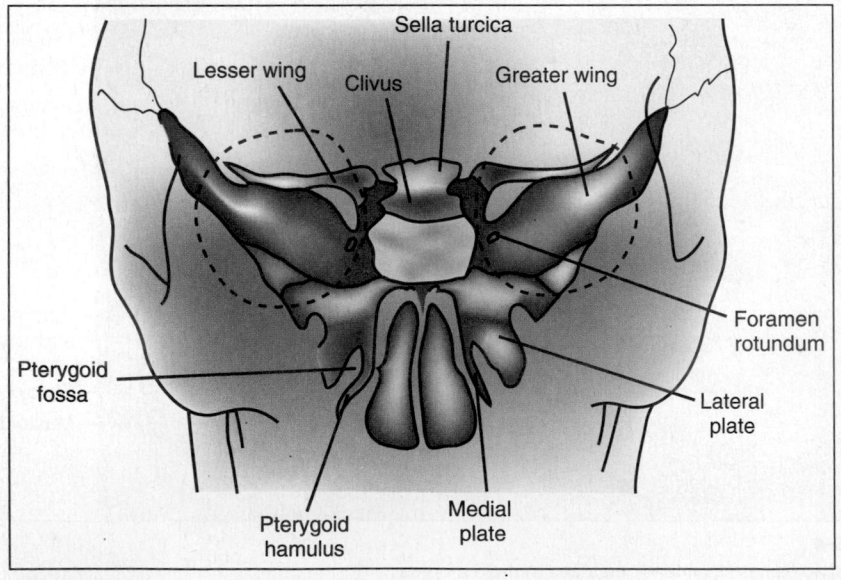

FIGURE 5-5B
Sphenoid bone.

Labels in figure:
- Sella turcica
- Lesser wing
- Clivus
- Greater wing
- Foramen rotundum
- Lateral plate
- Medial plate
- Pterygoid hamulus
- Pterygoid fossa

the eye orbit, which includes the superior orbital **fissure**, fora-men *spinosum*, foramen *ovale*, and foramen *rotundum*, which are important pathways for cranial nerves and blood vessels. The pterygoid processes are found behind the **palatine** bones. Each process consists of a lateral pterygoid plate, a pterygoid fossa, and a medial pterygoid plate, which are muscle attach-ment sites (Figure 5-5A). The *hamular* process or *pterygoid hamulus* is a small, rounded end to the medial plate of the pterygoid

process that can often be seen in a maxillary molar radiograph (Figure 5-5B).

Ethmoid Bone (Single)
The ethmoid bone is found behind and between the orbits at the base of the nose and separates the nasal cavity from the brain (Figure 5-2). The ethmoid bone con-tains sinus cavities, and its perpendicular plate helps form the superior portion of the nasal septum that divides the nasal cavity

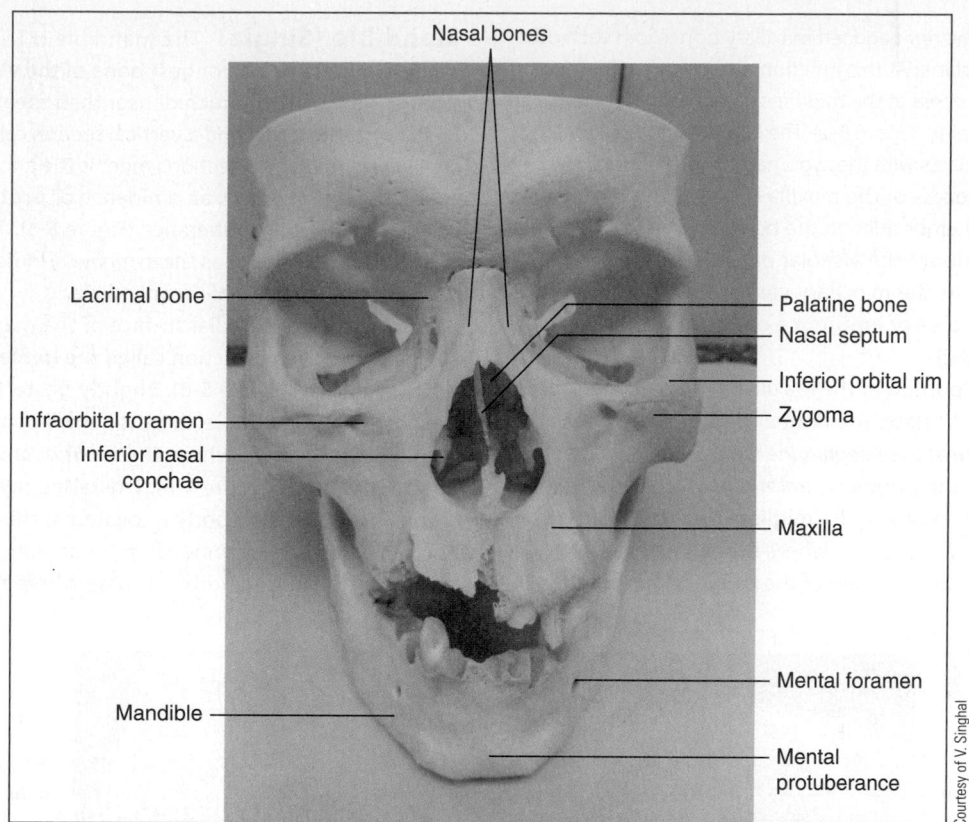

Courtesy of V. Singhal

FIGURE 5-6
Bones and landmarks of the viscerocranium.

into a right and left side. The lateral portion of the ethmoid bone contains the superior nasal conchae and the middle nasal concha. The inferior nasal conchae are considered to be a separate pair of facial bones (Figure 5-6).

Bones of the Viscerocranium

There are six pairs and two single bones that make up the facial structure of a skull. They create an individual's personal appearance and also provide the **alveolar** bone for the **dentition**.

Vomer (Single) The vomer is a small plow-shaped bone that sits at the midsagittal plane in the nose and helps form the inferior portion of the nasal septum (Figure 5-6). It articulates with the perpendicular plate of the ethmoid bone to form the nasal septum. The nasal septum separates the right and left side of the nasal cavity.

Lacrimal Bones (Paired), Inferior Nasal Conchae (Paired), and Nasal Bones (Paired) The *lacrimal* bones are found in the medial wall of the orbit (Figure 5-6). The lacrimal duct and foramen are found in this bone and are where tears exit. The paired inferior nasal conchae are found inside the nasal cavity along the lateral walls below the middle nasal conchae (Figure 5-6). The small, rectangular, paired nasal bones are found on the outside of the nose below the frontal bone. The nasal bones articulate with the frontal bone and with each other (Figure 5-6).

Zygomatic Bones (Paired) The zygomatic bones can also be called the *malar* bones, and they form the cheek bones (Figure 5-6). They articulate posteriorly with the temporal bones and help form the zygomatic arch with the temporal bone. One process articulates superiorly with the frontal bone, while the anterior portion of the bone articulates with the maxilla. A small portion of the zygomatic bones helps to form the lateral, inferior rim of the orbit (Figure 5-6).

Palatine Bones (Paired) Vertical and horizontal plates help form this L-shaped bone found at the posterior of the hard palate, which articulates with the palatine process of the maxilla bones. The *greater palatine foramen* and *lesser palatine foramen* are two openings found in the horizontal plate portion of the palatine bone or the posterior portion of the hard palate. These two foramen allow for the exit of the greater and lesser palatine nerves, which will be discussed later in this chapter. The vertical plate portion of the bone goes up into the nasal cavity and helps form the posterior, inferior, lateral wall of the nasal cavity (Figure 5-7).

Maxilla Bones (Paired) The **maxilla** is the second largest of the bones of the **viscerocranium** and makes up the upper jaw (Figure 5-6). The maxilla has a frontal process that extends up alongside the nasal cavity and next to the orbit. The **infraorbital** foramen is located in the maxillary bone and is where nerves and blood vessels exit onto the face (Figure 5-6). There is also a large maxillary sinus in the body portion. The right and left maxillary bones join each other at the midsagittal plane. At this junction, the two maxillary bones form a spine-like process at the midline of the nasal septum called the anterior nasal spine (Figure 5-2). The lateral surface of the body of the maxilla articulates with the zygomatic bone (Figure 5-6).

The alveolar process of the maxilla is where the roots of the maxillary teeth are embedded in the bone (Figure 5-7). The area at the most posterior of the alveolar process is called the maxillary **tuberosity**. At the maxillary canine area of the alveolar process is a raised area or **eminence** of bone called the canine eminence (Figure 5-2).

On the inferior portion of the maxilla is the palatine process that forms the hard palate. The right and left maxillary palatine processes articulate at the *midpalatine* suture, and also meet the palatine bones at the *transverse palatine* suture. On the anterior portion of the palate, at the midline, behind the maxillary incisors, is the incisive foramen where blood vessels and **nerve fibers** exit onto the anterior part of the palate (Figure 5-7).

Mandible (Single) The mandible is U-shaped and is the longest, largest, and strongest bone of the viscerocranial bones (Figure 5-6). It is also much denser than the maxillary bone and has a horizontal body and a vertical section called the **ramus**. The area where these two sections meet is the angle of the mandible. At the chin or midline is an eminence or **protuberance** of bone called the mental protuberance (Figure 5-6). The midline area of the mandible is known as the *symphysis*, indicating the fusion of the right and left sides of the mandible.

On the anterior medial surface of the mandibular midline is a small spine-like projection called the **genial tubercles** where muscles attach (Figure 5-8). Slightly posterior and medial, on the body of the mandible, there is a small bony depression called the sublingual fossa, where the *sublingual salivary gland* rests against the bone (Figure 5-8). The raised mylohyoid line in the medial portion of the body is located in the area of the molars and serves as an attachment for the mylohyoid muscle. Below this line is the submandibular fossa where the submandibular

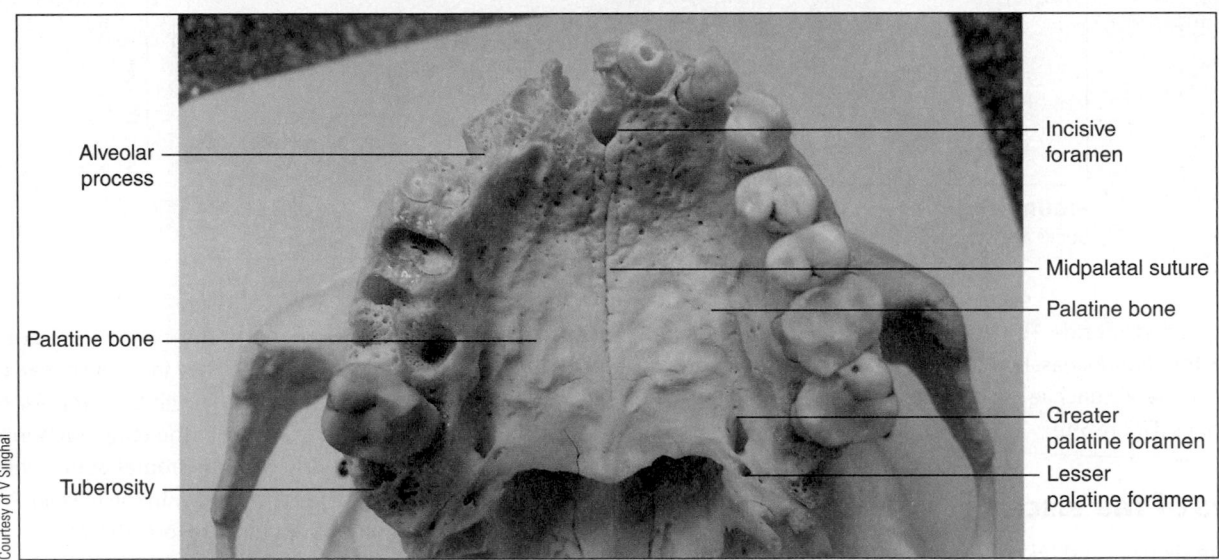

Courtesy of V Singhal

Alveolar process

Palatine bone

Tuberosity

Incisive foramen

Midpalatal suture

Palatine bone

Greater palatine foramen

Lesser palatine foramen

FIGURE 5-7
Palatal bones and landmarks.

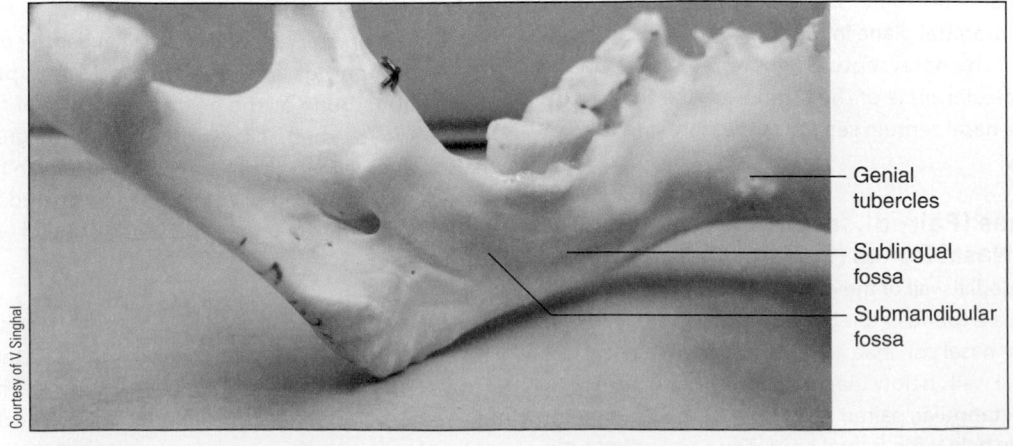

Courtesy of V Singhal

Genial tubercles

Sublingual fossa

Submandibular fossa

FIGURE 5-8
Genial tubercles, sublingual fossa, and submandibular fossa.

gland sits (Figure 5-8). In the mandible, the alveolar process houses the roots of the mandibular teeth. On the lateral surface of the body of the mandible is a landmark known as the mental foramen which is found at the apex of the mandibular second premolar area (Figure 5-6). This foramen can be mistaken for an abscess on a radiograph but is a normal anatomical landmark.

The vertical ramus of the mandible has the mandibular foramen which has a spine-like projection of bone above it termed the **lingula**. The mandibular foramen is the entrance to the inferior alveolar canal, through which nerves and blood vessels travel to reach the apices of each tooth (Figure 5-9).

The ramus of the mandible also has two distinct processes on it. The coronoid process is a shark-fin-like projection of bone where several muscles attach. A shadow of this can often be seen on a radiographic maxillary molar image. The other process is the *condylar process* or condyle, and it is involved with the temporomandibular joint (TMJ) and the movement of the mandible. It has a ball-like structure that fits into the mandibular fossa of the temporal bone and forms the joint. Between these two processes is a depression called the *sigmoid* (mandibular) notch where muscles attach (Figure 5-10).

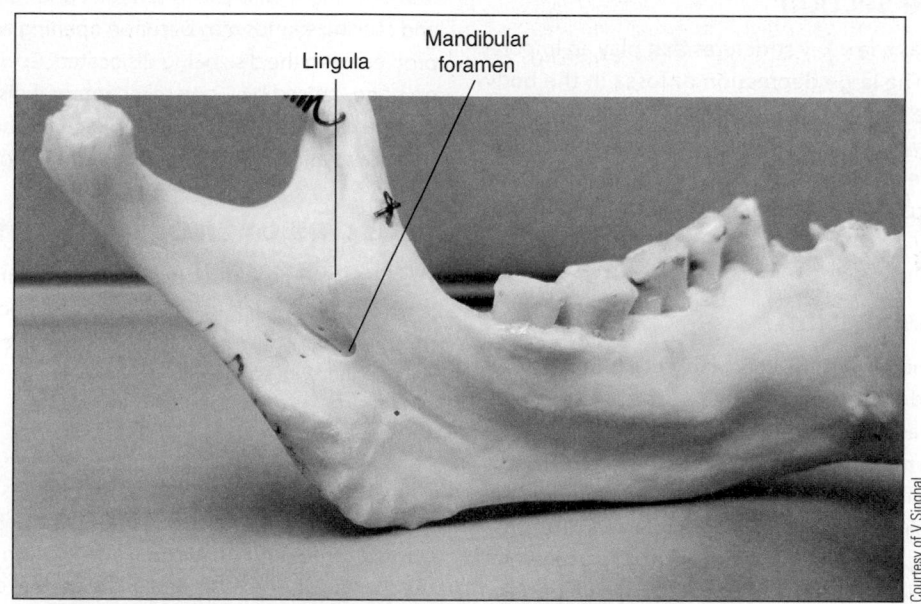

Courtesy of V Singhal

FIGURE 5-9
Mandibular foramen and lingula.

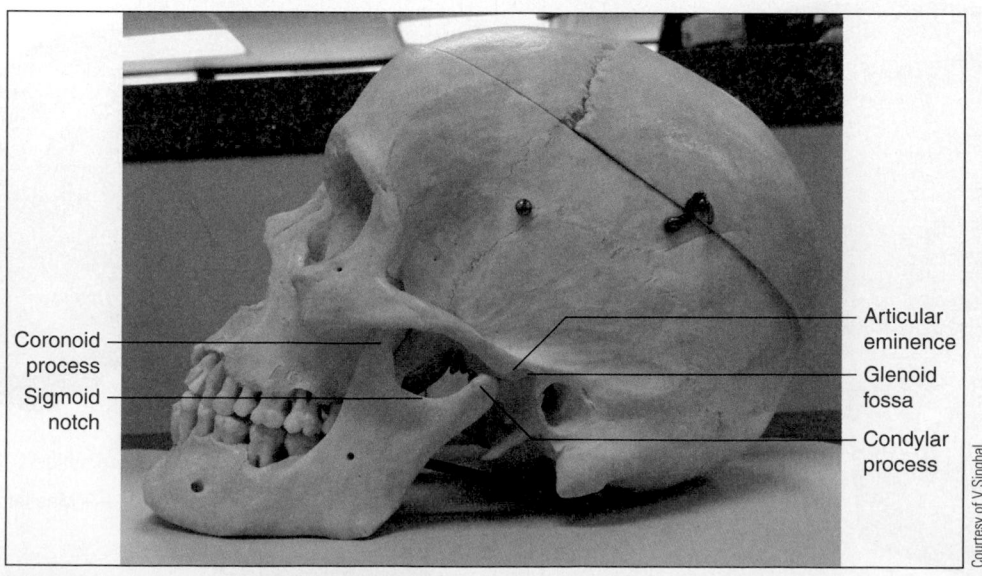

Courtesy of V Singhal

FIGURE 5-10
TMJ: Joint major parts and temporal bone landmarks.

Temporomandibular Joint (TMJ)

There is only one moveable bone in the skull, which is the mandible. It moves freely when talking or chewing because of a joint called the temporomandibular joint (TMJ) located between the mandible and the temporal bone of the maxilla. The joint is named for the two bones involved. The TMJ is composed of three parts (Figure 5-10):

1. Glenoid fossa of the temporal bone
2. Articular eminence of the temporal bone
3. Condyloid process of the mandible

Temporal Bone Section

The temporal bone has a few key structures that play an important role in the TMJ. The large depression or fossa in the body of the temporal bone is called the glenoid fossa. In front of the fossa is a bulged area of bone called the *articular eminence*. The glenoid fossa is where the condylar process of the mandible sits and moves; the articular eminence helps keep the condyle in place (Figure 5-10).

Mandible Bone Section

The ramus of the mandible has the condylar process that is a ball portion of the ball and socket type of joint. As in most joints, there is not a bone on bone articulation between the condyle and the glenoid fossa. In between the boney parts is a disc or *meniscus* of fibrous cartilage tissue. The joint is surrounded by synovial fluid in synovial cavities to allow the joint to move freely. The whole joint is covered in fibrous tissue or a **capsule** structure. There are also ligaments that hold the mandible in place. The muscles, ligaments, and fibrous capsule that encircle the joint help open and close the mouth, as well as allow for lateral *excursion*, *retrusion* or movement of the mandible posteriorly, and *protrusion* or movement of the mandible anteriorly.

The articulation between the bones in the TMJ has two types of movement. When the mandible is starting to open, there is a basic hinge movement at the joint. As the mandible opens wider, there is a gliding movement where the mandible glides forward and downward. In this gliding movement the meniscus slides along the articulating surface or the anterior superior portion of the condyle. There can also be problems associated with the TMJ. If the articular eminence of the temporal bone is flatter, then the mandible can slide too far forward, and get "locked" open or *subluxation* can occur. If this happens the dentist has to push down and back on the jaw to snap the condyle back into the socket of the glenoid fossa. The opposite problem can occur where the patient has a limited opening. This is called **trismus** and can be painful. Popping and clicking sounds may occur on opening and closing if there is a problem with the disc being dislocated. **Crepitus** is bone rubbing on bone, caused by a severely damaged disc. Severe grinding or *bruxism* can cause TMJ problems. Because the TMJ is a joint, arthritis can also affect this joint, as it does other joints in the body.

Muscles of the Head and Neck

The head and neck muscles are skeletal muscles that are voluntary muscles. Muscles of the head and neck include muscles of mastication, facial expression, floor of the mouth, tongue, soft palate, pharynx, and neck.

Muscles of Mastication

There are four pairs of muscles that make up the group of muscles known as the muscles of mastication. This group of muscles is responsible for chewing or mastication and is comprised of the **masseter**, the temporalis, the medial or internal pterygoid, and the lateral or external pterygoid (Figure 5-11). They are also responsible for opening, closing, protrusion, retraction, and lateral excursion of the mandible. These muscles work closely

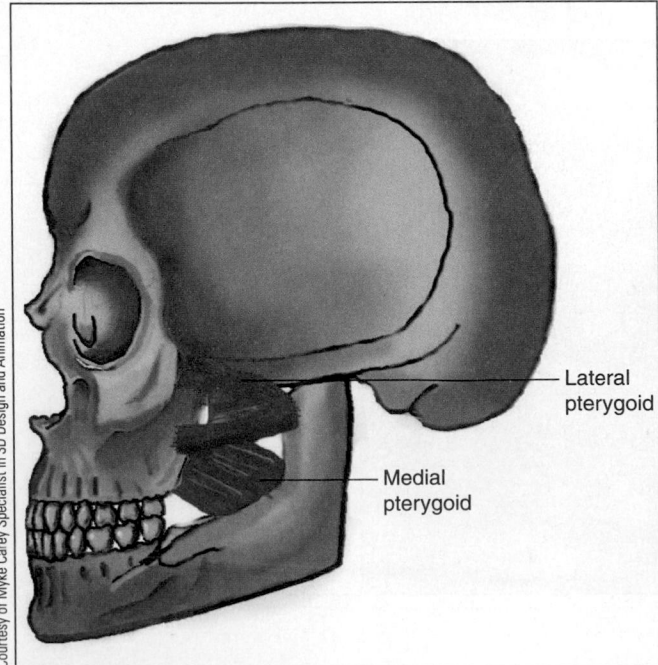

Courtesy of Myke Carey Specialist in 3D Design and Animation

FIGURE 5-11
Muscles of mastication.

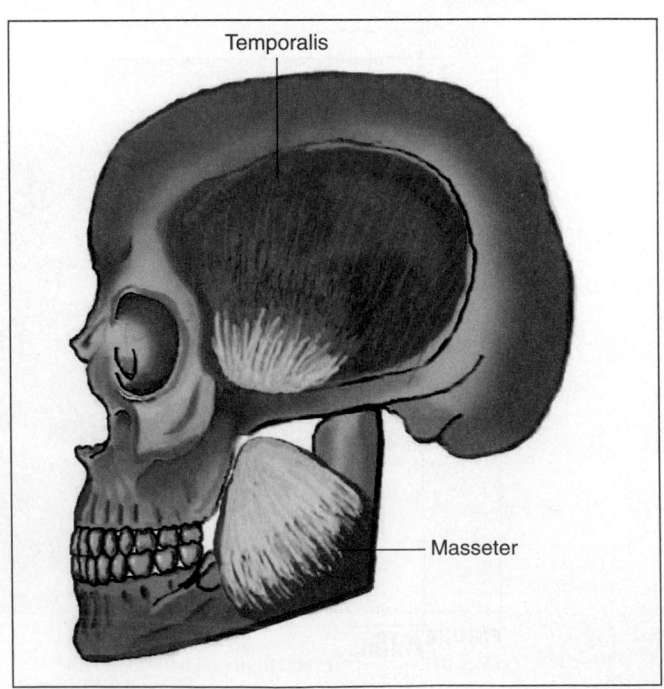

with the TMJ or temporomandibular joint because they work to open and close the mouth.

Temporalis The temporalis is the largest of the muscles of mastication. It is a fan-shaped muscle that originates at the temporal fossa on the side of the skull. The fibers run down and insert into the coronoid process and anterior border of the ramus of the mandible and help close or elevate the mandible. Some of the fibers of the temporalis muscle run horizontally at the temple area; when these are contracted, they can retract the mandible (Figure 5-11).

Masseter The masseter is the strongest of the muscles of mastication and is found running vertically from its origin at the zygomatic arch to the insertion at the lateral surface of the angle of the mandible. When it contracts it closes the mouth by elevating the mandible to deliver a powerful bite (Figure 5-11).

External (Lateral) Pterygoid The lateral or external pterygoid muscle is the only one of the four muscles of mastication that is involved in opening the mouth (Figure 5-11). This small muscle has two heads and runs horizontally originating at the inferior surface of the greater wing of sphenoid bone and the lateral surface of the lateral pterygoid plate of the pterygoid process of the sphenoid bone. Both of these heads merge and continue posteriorly until inserting at the anterior surface of the neck of the condylar process of the mandible. Some of the superficial fibers insert into the capsule of the TMJ. When this short muscle is contracted, it pulls the condyle forward and depresses the mandible or opens the mouth. It can also work to protrude the mandible and cause the mandible to move from side to side.

Internal (Medial) Pterygoid The medial or internal pterygoid muscle runs vertically like the masseter (Figure 5-11). However, this muscle is found on the internal surface of the mandible. It originates at the pterygoid fossa and the medial surface of the lateral pterygoid plate of the pterygoid process of the sphenoid bone. It inserts at the medial surface of the angle of the mandible, and when it contracts it elevates or closes the mandible (Figure 5-11).

Muscles of Facial Expression

There are many muscles of the face, but only the facial muscles that are specific to the oral cavity will be discussed in this text.

Orbicularis Oris The orbicularis oris is a muscle that encircles the mouth and does not have a skeletal attachment or origin as most muscles do (Figure 5-12). The function of this muscle is to pucker the lips and aid in speaking and chewing. The facial expression that this muscle produces when contracted is the pucker.

Levator Anguli Oris The levator anguli oris is one of the major muscles that make a person smile when contracted. The origin of the muscle is at the canine fossa, and it inserts into the angle of the orbicularis oris. The facial expression produced when contracted is a smile.

Levator Labii Superioris The levator labii superioris is a broader flat muscle that originates at the infraorbital rim of the maxilla and inserts into the middle area of skin in the upper lip (Figure 5-12). The function of this muscle is to pull the upper lip upwards. The facial expression that this muscle produces when contracted is to aid in a smile.

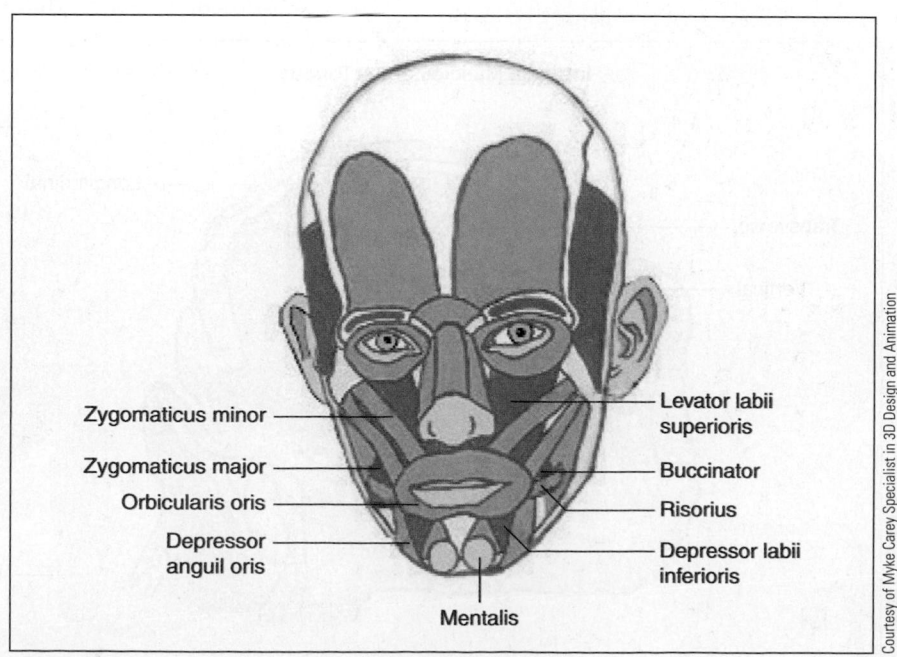

FIGURE 5-12
Facial muscles.

Courtesy of Myke Carey Specialist in 3D Design and Animation

Zygomaticus Major   The zygomaticus major is the lateral and larger of a pair of muscles: zygomaticus major and minor (Figure 5-12). The origin of this muscle is the zygomatic bone, and it inserts in the angle of the orbicularis oris. The function of this muscle is to pull the corners of the mouth up when contracted, and the facial expression produced is a smile. It is considered one of the other major smiling muscles.

Zygomaticus Minor   The zygomaticus minor is the more medial and smaller of the pair of muscles: zygomaticus major and minor (Figure 5-12). The origin of this muscle is the zygomatic bone located medial to the zygomaticus major, and it inserts more medial to the angle of the orbicularis oris. This muscle works with the zygomaticus major and pulls the corners of the mouth up. When contracted, the facial expression produced is a smile.

Depressor Anguli Oris   The depressor anguli oris is a triangular muscle that originates at the lower border of the mandible and inserts into the angle of the orbicularis lower lip (Figure 5-12). The main function of this muscle is to pull the corners of the lip downward, and the facial expression produced is a frown. This muscle is considered the major frown muscle.

Depressor Labii Inferioris   The depressor labii inferioris is a small muscle that originates at the lower border of the mandible and inserts into the middle area of the skin of the lower lip (Figure 5-12). When this muscle is contracted it produces a pout by pulling the lower lip downward.

Mentalis   The mentalis is a small muscle below the lower lip that originates at the midline of the mandible and inserts into the skin of the chin (Figure 5-12). The function of this muscle is to raise the chin and narrow the mandibular vestibule in that area

of the mouth. The facial expression that is produced when this muscle is contracted is doubt.

Buccinator   The buccinator is a facial expression muscle that aids in mastication (Figure 5-12). It makes up the bulk of the cheeks and helps hold food on the occlusal surfaces of the teeth during chewing or mastication. It runs horizontally in the cheek and has an origin at three different areas that include the alveolar process of the maxilla, mandible, and a fibrous connective tissue band called the *pterygomandibular raphe*. The muscle runs forward and inserts into the skin at the angle of the mouth. When it is contracted, it helps pull the cheek back laterally and presses the cheek against the teeth.

Risorius   The risorius is a small, thin muscle that originates from fascia tissue on top of the masseter and goes forward to insert at the skin at the angle of the mouth (Figure 5-12). When it is compressed, it produces the facial expression of a grimace. It also stretches the lips and widens the opening of the mouth.

Muscles of the Tongue and Floor of the Mouth

There are two sets of tongue muscles. One set of muscles is the fibers that make up the actual tongue muscle. The other set of muscles originate in various areas on the skull and insert into the tongue to hold the tongue in the oral cavity. The floor of the mouth is made up of two main muscles that will be discussed: the mylohyoid and the digastric muscles.

Intrinsic Muscles of Tongue   There are four pairs of *intrinsic* muscles of the tongue that have fibers that begin and end in the tongue muscle itself. These are the superior and inferior longitudinal muscles, vertical muscles, and transverse muscles (Figure 5-13).

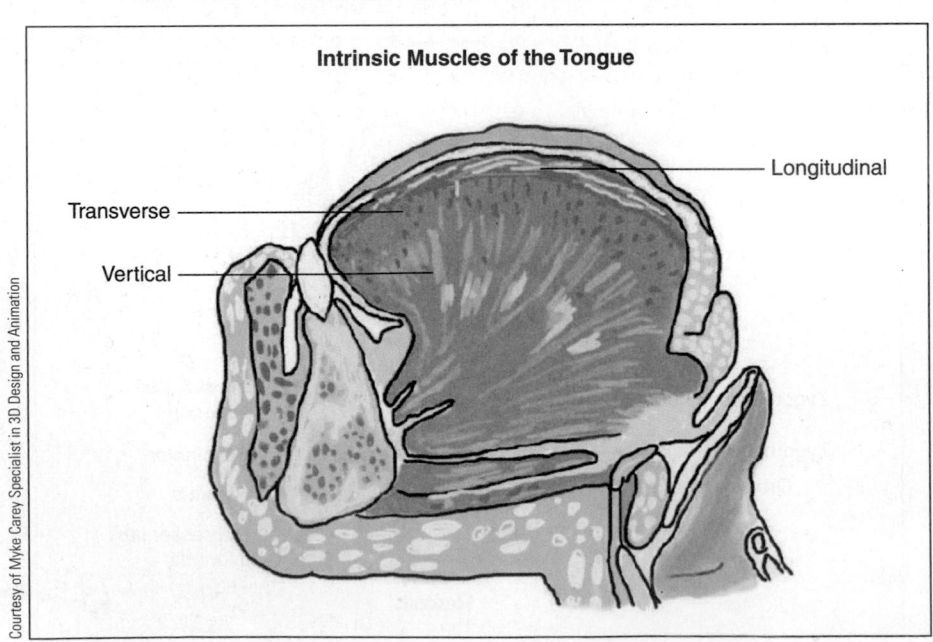

Courtesy of Myke Carey Specialist in 3D Design and Animation

Intrinsic Muscles of the Tongue

Transverse

Vertical

Longitudinal

FIGURE 5-13
Intrinsic muscles of the tongue.

Extrinsic Muscles of Tongue The *extrinsic* muscles originate outside of the tongue in different areas located on-the skull and end with insertion into the tongue muscle. These muscles function as a group to hold the tongue into the floor of the mouth and aid in swallowing (Figure 5-14).

Styloglossus The *styloglossus* muscle originates at the spine-like styloid process of the temporal bone behind the ear (Figure 5-14). The fibers run forward and insert into the back portions of the lateral surface of the tongue. When contracted, the styloglossus helps pull the tongue back into the mouth and helps it move superiorly and posteriorly.

Hyoglossus The hyoglossus muscle originates on the hyoid bone in the neck and runs superiorly into the base of the tongue. When contracted it helps retract and pull down the sides of the tongue. It also aids in swallowing (Figure 5-14).

Palatoglossus The *palatoglossus* muscle can also fall into the category of muscles of the soft palate in some texts. It originates at the anterior arch at the side of the throat and inserts along the side of the tongue most posteriorly. When contracted it helps elevate the tongue and depresses the soft palate toward the tongue (Figure 5-14).

Genioglossus The *genioglossus* originates at the genial tubercles at the medial surface at the midline of the mandible and inserts into the front inferior surface of the tongue. This small muscle has an important job, as it helps hold the tongue into the floor of the mouth. When the chin is tilted up during cardiopulmonary resuscitation (CPR), it pulls the tongue up to keep it from blocking the airway (Figure 5-14).

Muscles of the Floor of the Mouth The floor of the mouth is formed predominantly by a pair of flat triangular muscles called the mylohyoid muscles.

Mylohyoid The mylohyoid muscles originate in the mylohyoid ridge and insert into the hyoid bone. The hyoid bone is located in the neck and is an attachment for many muscles and ligaments.

Its main function is to form the floor of the mouth and help raise the tongue, depress or open the mandible, and raise the hyoid bone (Figure 5-15).

Digastric The digastric is located inferior to the mylohyoid muscle. It has an anterior and posterior belly with a tendon-like structure between them. The anterior belly originates at the lower border of the mandible and inserts at the hyoid bone by a tendon loop. The posterior belly originates at the mastoid process of the temporal bone and inserts in the tendon that joins the bellies. The main function of the digastric muscle is to support the mylohyoid and aid in swallowing (Figure 5-15).

Muscles of the Soft Palate

There are five muscles of the soft palate that are involved in deglutition and breathing. The palatoglossus, tensor veli palatini, and levator veli palatine muscles are involved in swallowing. The *musculus uvulae* (Figure 5-16) is involved in movement of the uvula (Figure 5-17). The palatopharyngeal muscles are involved in breathing and raise the soft palate during deglutition.

Muscles of the Neck

There are three main neck muscles that will be discussed in this text, although there are several other neck muscles deeper in the neck. The ones presented here are the larger, more superficial muscles that can be palpated during an extraoral examination. These three include the *sternocleidomastoid*, the *platysma*, and the *trapezius* (Figure 5-18).

Sternocleidomastoid (SCM) The sternocleidomastoid neck muscle originates in two areas: at the *clavicle* or collarbone and the lateral surface of the sternum. It travels superiorly up the neck and makes a diagonal pathway to insert at the mastoid process of the temporal bone behind the ear. This long, thick muscle is very important in the extraoral examination. It has a long chain of lymph nodes in front and behind it that have to be palpated

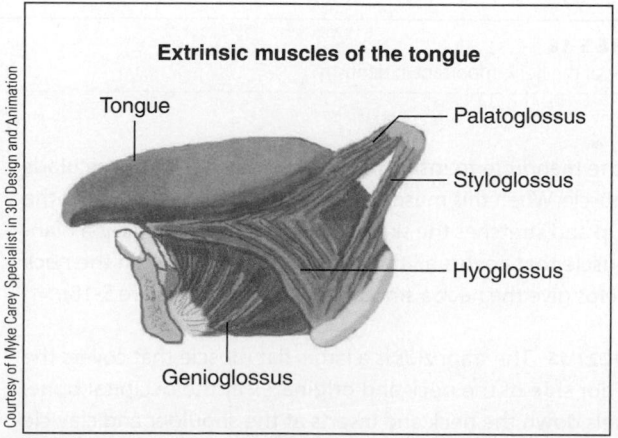

FIGURE 5-14
Extrinsic muscles of the tongue.

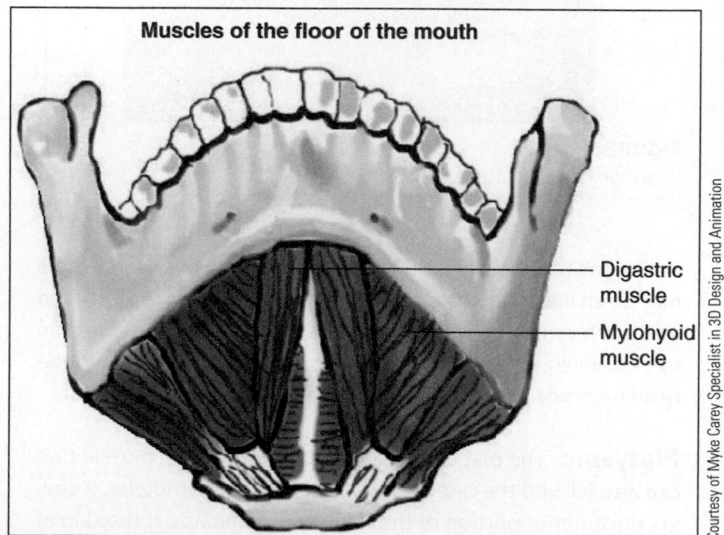

FIGURE 5-15
Muscles of the floor of the mouth.

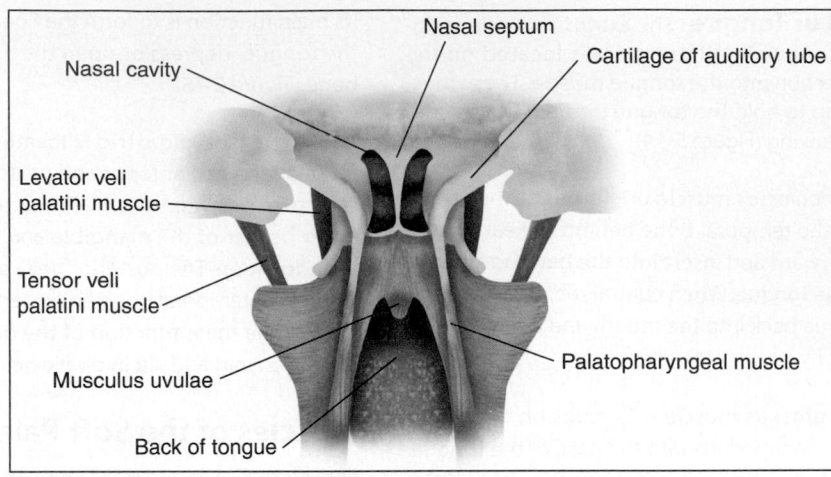

FIGURE 5-16
Muscles of the soft palate.

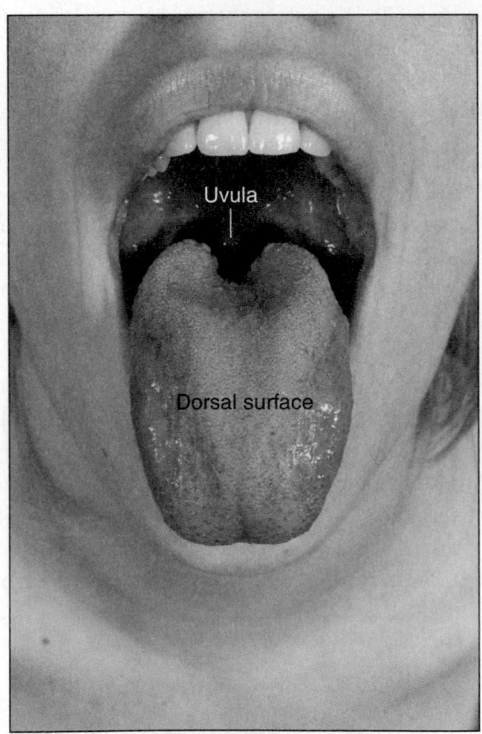

FIGURE 5-17
Uvula and dorsal surface of tongue.

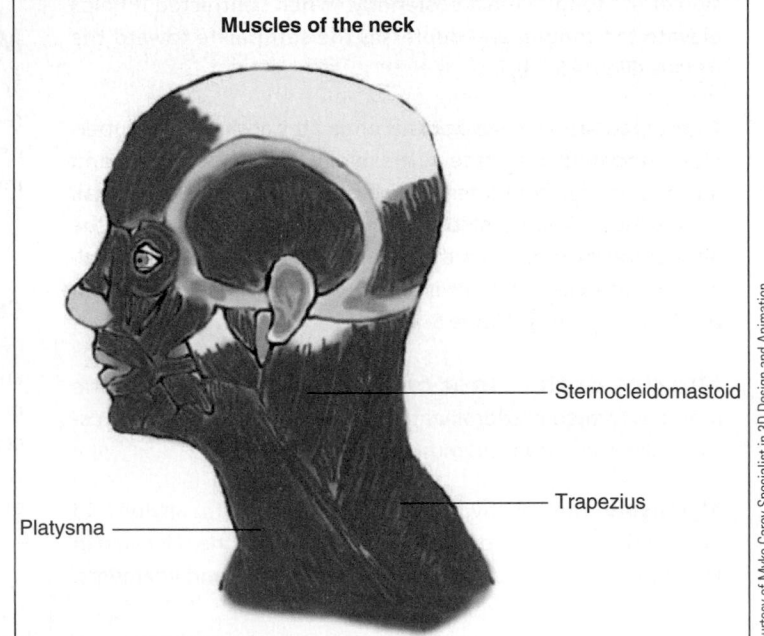

Courtesy of Myke Carey Specialist in 3D Design and Animation

FIGURE 5-18
Muscles of the neck important in dentistry.

during the patient exam. If a lymph node is hard or swollen, there may be an infection in the body that needs attention. An infection in a tooth can cause lymph nodes in the neck or under the chin to be swollen, sore, or hardened. This neck muscle helps turn the head from side to side and tilt the head on its axis (Figure 5-18).

Platysma The platysma is a large, flat, sheet-like muscle that can also fall into the category of facial expression muscles. It covers the anterior portion of the neck and originates at the skin at the clavicle and shoulder and travels up the neck to insert into the lower border of the mandible. A small portion of it also travels

over the mandible to insert in the lower lip and the orbicularis oris muscle. When this muscle is contracted it pulls the skin of the neck up and stretches the skin on the neck. It functions as a blanket muscle that covers all the other muscles deeper in the neck and helps give the neck a smoother appearance (Figure 5-18).

Trapezius The trapezius is a large, flat muscle that covers the posterior side of the neck and originates at the occipital bone. It travels down the neck and inserts at the shoulder and clavicle bones and helps to turn the head from side to side and extend it backwards (Figure 5-18).

Tongue and Salivary Glands

The tongue is an important muscle as it aids in mastication of food and also allows us to speak. The salivary glands are **exocrine** glands that produce saliva. Saliva plays in important role in mastication as well as in cleansing the oral cavity. This section will discuss the tongue as well as the salivary glands and saliva.

Body: Dorsal Surface: Tongue Structure

The tongue is a broad, flattened muscle in the mouth where the top surface is called the **dorsum** or dorsal surface. The dorsum is the surface you see when you stick out your tongue (Figure 5-17). The dorsum of the tongue is covered with papilla, which will be discussed in detail later (Figure 5-19A). The structure of the tongue is divided into the anterior two-thirds and the posterior one-third. The anterior two-thirds is the part that is found inside the oral cavity when you look in the mouth. The posterior one-third is located in the throat area and is not visible.

The posterior one-third is known as the pharyngeal part and is attached in the throat and back of the oral cavity. It also contains specialized tissue called the *lingual* tonsils (Figure 5-19B). The posterior of the tongue is divided by the *sulcus terminalis*. It is an inverted V-shaped line that extends horizontally from the right to the left side of the tongue where the posterior one-third meets the anterior two-thirds (Figure 5-19B). This central area has an indented pit that is called the **foramen cecum** or **caecum** (Figure 5-19B). This pit area is the **embryonic** origin of part of the thyroid gland. As the neck develops, the thyroid tissue slides

down to its natural place in the middle of the neck. The only remnant left that the thyroid was there is the small pinpoint indentation in the middle of the sulcus terminalis. The term *foramen cecum* indicates that it is a hole, but this is not the case.

Another line that is found on the dorsum of the tongue is the *median lingual sulcus* or median sulcus (Figure 5-19B). This line divides the tongue into right and left halves extending along the middle of the tongue from posterior to anterior. Sometimes this line is easy to see because it is slightly depressed, but it varies from patient to patient.

Papillae   The whole dorsum of the tongue is covered in mucous membrane and raised specialized tissue called **papillae** (Figure 5-19A). There are four types of papillae that cover the dorsum of the tongue.

The *fungiform* papillae can be found on the anterior two-thirds of the dorsum of the tongue and are shaped like a mushroom with a base and rounded top. They are brighter red in color than the rest of the tongue and look like small, round, raised dots on the tongue. They are the second most numerous in number and do contain a taste bud in the center (Figure 5-19A). Taste buds are the small cells that help you differentiate different flavors on your tongue like sweet, salty, sour, and bitter (Figure 5-20). There are 2,000–8,000 taste buds embedded in the papilla of the upper surface of the tongue, soft palate, upper esophagus, cheek, and epiglottis. This great span in number of taste buds contributes to the difference in taste sensations experienced by individuals. Each taste bud contains receptor cells that respond to distinct chemical stimuli.

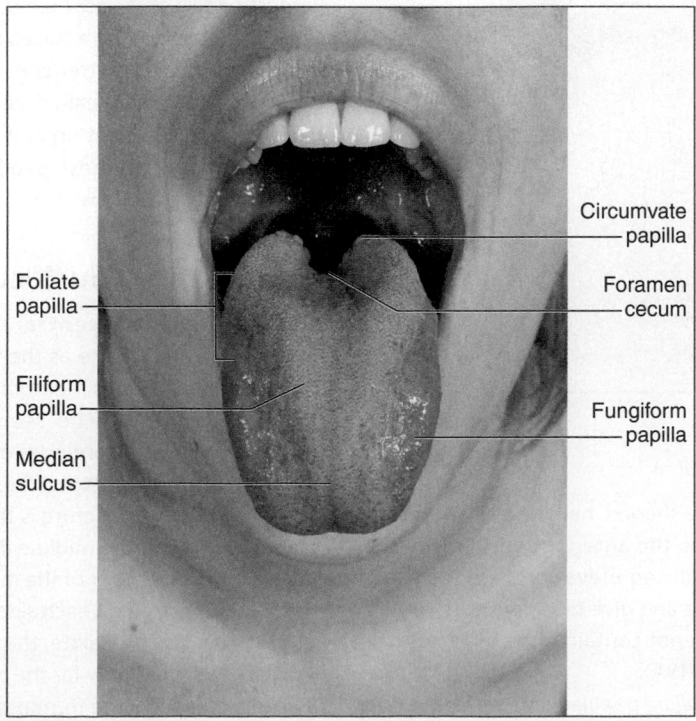

FIGURE 5-19A
Dorsum of the tongue.

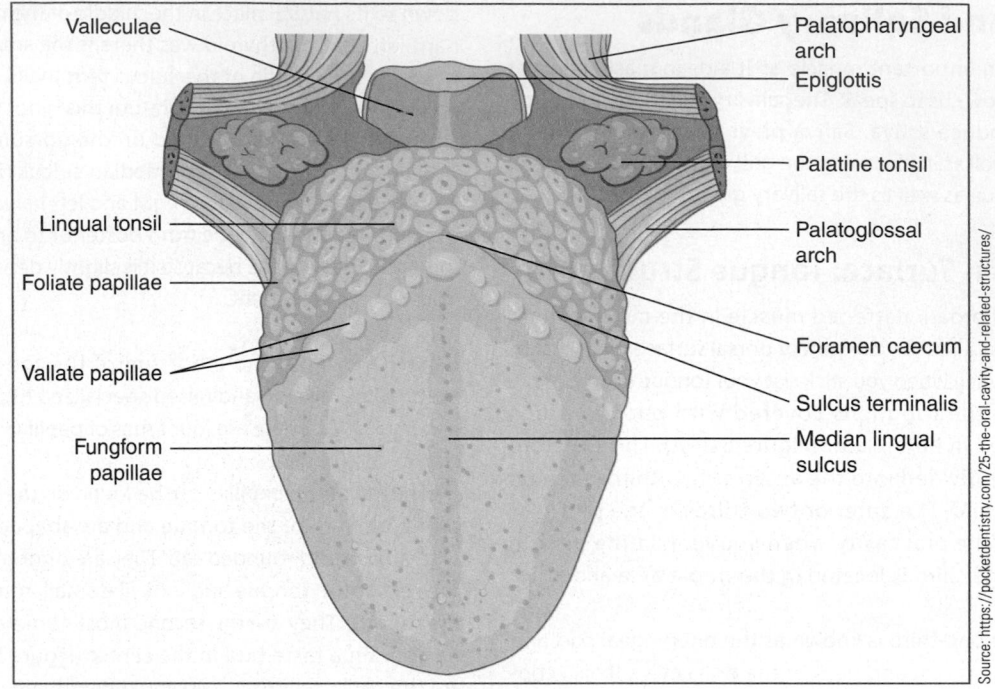

FIGURE 5-19B
Structures of the tongue.

Source: https://pocketdentistry.com/25-the-oral-cavity-and-related-structures/

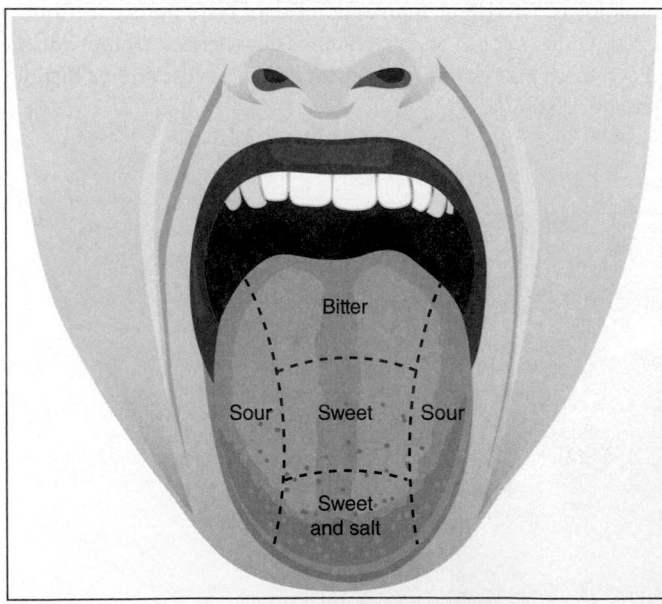

FIGURE 5-20
Location of taste buds.

The *filiform* papillae are spike shaped, hairlike papilla located around the fungiform papilla on the anterior two-thirds of the dorsum tongue. These tiny pointed elevations are the most numerous of the lingual papillae and give the tongue its velvety texture. The filiform papillae do not contain taste buds, so they have no taste function (Figure 5-19A).

The third type is called the *foliate* papillae and are located on the lateral posterior borders of tongue. These are only seen if the tongue is extended and turned to the side. These papillae look like folds and give the sides a roughened surface. These papillae contain taste buds (Figure 5-19A).

The largest papillae on the dorsum of the tongue are the *circumvallate papilla* or vallate papilla (Figure 5-19A). They are doughnut shaped and the fewest in number with only 8–12 elevations found anterior to the sulcus terminalis. These are the largest papilla and most elevated of all the lingual papilla, and each is surrounded by a sulcus containing taste buds and serous glands. In these tiny trenches surrounded by the papillae are small salivary glands called **von Ebner's salivary glands** that deposit a serous secretion into the sulci to keep them clean and free of food debris. These papillae are also harder to see unless the tongue is grasped with a gauze square and pulled forward.

Body: Ventral Surface: Tongue Structure

The covering of the **ventral** surface is significantly different from the dorsal surface as the tissue on the ventral surface is a much thinner mucous membrane. Because the tissue is thinner, the blood vessels may be seen under the tissue, and this same mucous membrane continues onto the floor of the mouth.

There are several structures to mention on this part of the tongue. The main structure is the *lingual frenum*, which is a long band-like tissue at the midline that attaches the ventral surface of the tongue to the floor of the mouth. The *sublingual folds* are soft tissue folds located on each side of the frenum. When the tongue is lifted toward the palate, the lingual frenum is pulled against itself and will limit how far the tongue can be lifted (Figure 5-21). Some people have the frenum attached closer to the tip or apex of the tongue, and it cannot be lifted very far (Figure 5-22). This is known as *ankyloglossia* or tongue tie.

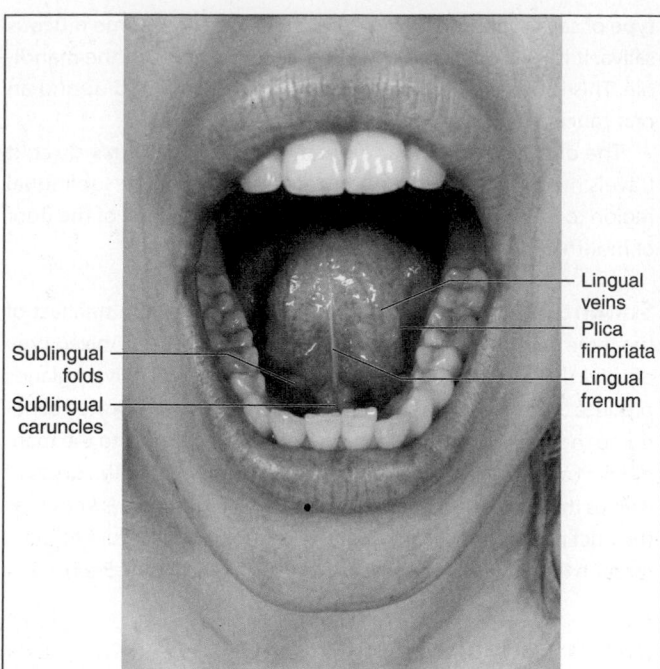

FIGURE 5-21
Ventral surface of tongue.

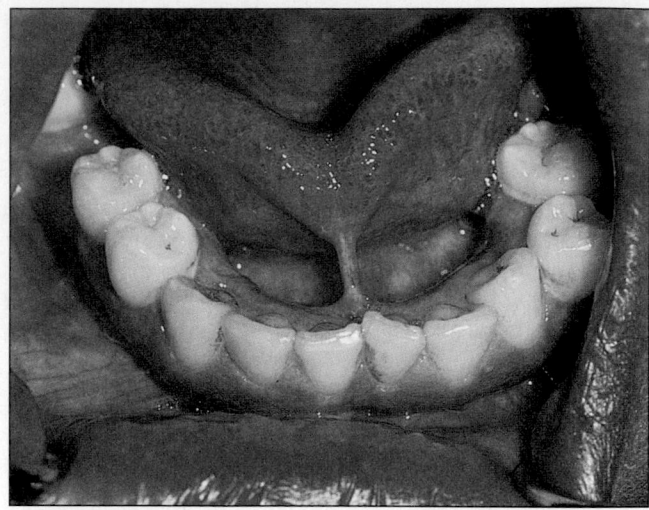

FIGURE 5-22
Ankyloglossia.

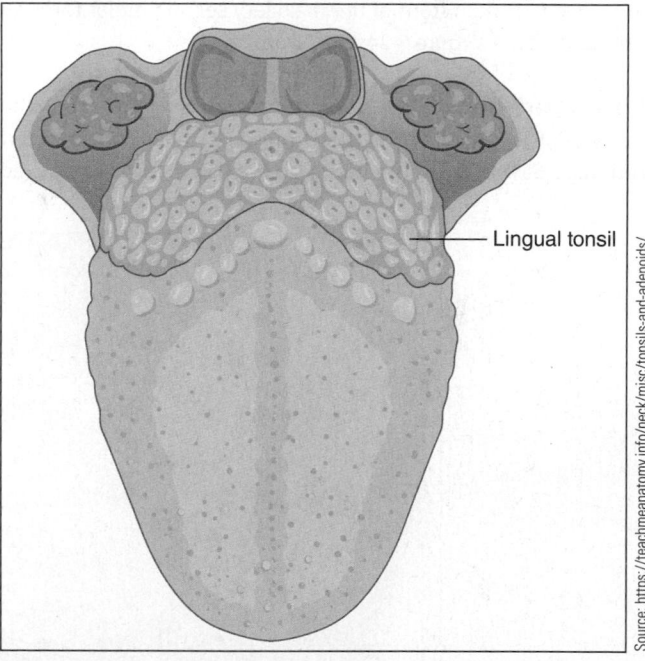

FIGURE 5-23
Lingual tonsils.

On each side of the lingual frenum are fringed folds that run parallel with the lingual frenum called **plica fimbriata** (Figure 5-21). Some people have exaggerated fringes of tissue on these folds that look like strands of tissue. Some people will not have the fringed areas that are so obvious. This is one of the structures under the tongue that is normal but may look unusual.

Lingual veins on the ventral surface of the tongue appear bluish and are sometimes raised structures alongside the lingual frenum and plica fimbriata (Figure 5-21). As the patient ages the lingual veins may become more prominent. The sublingual glands are drained via 8–20 **ducts of Rivinus**. The largest duct, known as the **Bartholin's duct**, joins with the submandibular duct and drains through the **sublingual caruncles** located in each side of the lingual frenum (Figure 5-21).

Base of Tongue

The most posterior and inferior part of the tongue is the base of the tongue. The dorsal surface of the base of the tongue in the throat is covered with a specialized tissue called lingual tonsils. These raised elevations are crinkled **lymphoid tissue** that helps filter foreign substances that may enter the oral cavity (Figure 5-23).

Function of Saliva

The most important function of the saliva is to moisten the mucous membranes of the mouth and wet food for tasting, chewing, and swallowing. Saliva helps cleanse the oral cavity. If a patient is taking medications that causes **xerostomia**, it can affect how much saliva is produced. A drier oral cavity can cause the bacterial biofilm to grow faster because the cleansing effect is decreased.

Saliva is 99.5% water, and the half of a percent that is left contains a few very important items. Several enzymes are found in saliva that help to break down food, particularly starches, by means of **amylase**. Another enzyme called *lysozyme* breaks down the cell walls of bacteria. Saliva also contains inorganic salts such as chlorides, sulfates, phosphates, and carbonates. It also contains various types of white blood cells and *antibodies*, particularly immunoglobulin A (IgA).

Even though the basic content of saliva is about the same, there are two main types of saliva that are produced: the *serous* and *mucous* types. Serous saliva is more of the thin, watery type while the mucous type is thicker, stickier, and ropey. Each of the major salivary glands that we will discuss next produces one of

Source: https://teachmeanatomy.info/neck/misc/tonsils-and-adenoids/

these types or a mixture of both. A typical person can produce 2–4 pints of saliva each day.

Major Salivary Glands

There are three major pairs of salivary glands, which are exocrine glands as their secretions reach an epithelial surface. An exocrine gland has a duct where the saliva empties on its way to a surface or the mucous membranes, as may be the case, in the oral cavity. Sometimes we say that our "mouth waters" when we smell good food or eat something flavorful, and these are the glands that can make that happen.

Parotid   The parotid glands are the largest of the major salivary glands and produce 20% of total saliva volume in the oral cavity. The type of saliva that it produces is only the serous type. The glands are located in front of the ear on the masseter muscle and surround the posterior surface of the ramus of the mandible. The duct leaves the gland and travels anteriorly across the masseter muscle. It then pierces the buccinator muscle in the cheek to enter the mouth in front of the maxillary second molar through Stensen's duct (Figure 5-24 and Figure 5-25).

Submandibular   The *submandibular salivary gland* is the second largest of the three pairs of major salivary glands but produces 65% of the saliva in the oral cavity. It secretes a mixed type of saliva solution which is mostly serous with some mucous saliva. It is located below and anterior to the angle of the mandible. This is one of the salivary glands that is palpated during an oral cancer screening (Figure 5-24 and Figure 5-25).

The duct of the submandibular gland is Wharton's duct; it travels medially forward and upward and ends in the sublingual region to open into the sublingual caruncle at midline of the floor of mouth (Figure 5-24 and Figure 5-25).

Sublingual   The sublingual salivary glands are the smallest of the three pairs of major salivary glands. They produce a mixed type of saliva that is mostly mucous in type. The sublingual salivary glands produce 5% of the overall saliva total volume. They are located superior to the mylohyoid muscle in the floor of mouth next to the mandibular canines. There are several small ducts known as the ducts of Rivinus that drain the sublingual glands. The largest duct is known as the duct of Bartholin, which joins the submandibular duct to drain through the sublingual caruncle (Figure 5-24 and Figure 5-25).

Minor Salivary Glands

The three pairs of major salivary glands are not the only source of saliva production in the mouth. These make up about 90% of the total production, but there is still about 10% that can be attributed to other minor or accessory salivary glands. The difference between minor and major salivary glands is the number of

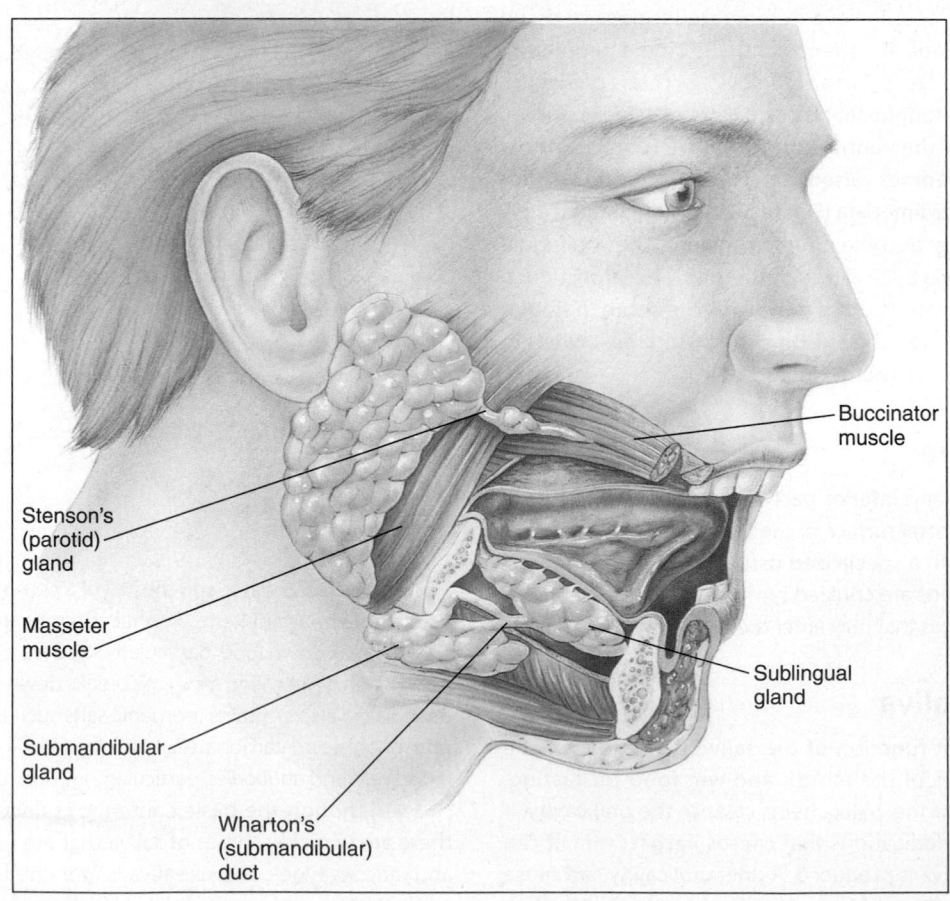

FIGURE 5-24
Locations and ducts of the major salivary glands.

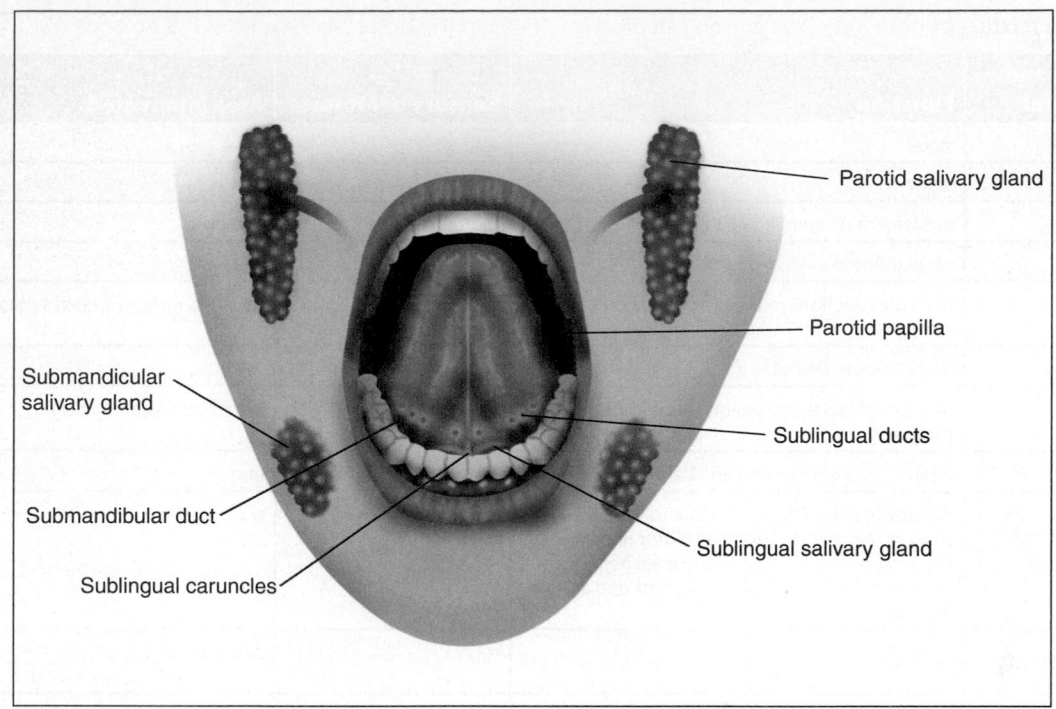

FIGURE 5-25
Major salivary glands and their ducts.

acini or secretory cells. There are about 300 to 500 minor salivary glands distributed throughout the oral cavity. Most of these are very small and only have a few acini. Table 5-1 provides a list of minor salivary glands and their locations.

Nerves of the Head and Neck

Cranial nerves are part of the peripheral nervous system and branch out to various parts of the head, neck, and body. Several of these nerve bundles are very important in dentistry because they supply the teeth, tongue, and muscles of the face with nerve sensation.

TABLE 5-1 Minor Salivary Glands

Minor Salivary Gland Groups	Area Supplied in Oral Cavity
Labial	Upper/lower lips
Buccal	Inner cheek
Palatine	Soft palate Posterior two-thirds of hard palate
Glossopalatini glands	Posterior lateral palate Tissue in front of palatine tonsils
Anterior lingual	Near tip of tongue Open onto ventral surface (also called glands of Blandin and Nuhn)
von Ebner's glands	Dorsum of the base of the tongue Associated with the circumvallate papillae

Cranial Nerves

The 12 pairs of cranial nerves leave the brain in a specific order from the front of the brain to the back. As would be expected, the areas that the first cranial nerve supplies are on the front of the face, and the last cranial nerve supplies the back of the neck and tongue deeper in the oral cavity. Each nerve branches off of the brain and goes through a foramen or fissure in the skull to reach its destination. The main bundle of each nerve then branches further and **innervates** its respective area as it travels. The nerve branches may supply sensory or **afferent** fibers, motor or **efferent** fibers, or both.

The 12 cranial nerves are summarized in Table 5-2 with a more in depth discussion about the nerves that are important to dentistry.

Branches of the Trigeminal Nerve

The *trigeminal* nerve is of great importance in dentistry and will be discussed in detail. This is the largest cranial nerve and it has three main divisions, all of which have several branches (Figure 5-26).

Ophthalmic (V1) The *ophthalmic* nerve or ophthalmic division is the first and most superior branch of the trigeminal nerve. It is also known as V1. This division exits the brain through the superior orbital fissure (Figure 5-5) and innervates the upper portion of the face in the eye and forehead area. The ophthalmic nerve is totally sensory and has three major branches that are not involved in dentistry (Table 5-3; Figure 5-26).

TABLE 5-2 Cranial Nerves

Cranial Nerve and Roman Numeral	Function	Sensory or Motor	Area Innervated
olfactory (I)	smell	sensory	nose
optic (II)	Sight	sensory	eye
oculomotor (III)	movement of eyeball and raises upper eyelid	motor	eye
trochlear (IV)	movement of eyeball downward	motor	eye
trigeminal (V)	multiple functions related to head and oral cavity	mixed	teeth, tongue, muscles of mastication, face
abducens (VI)	lateral movement of eyeball	motor	eye
facial (VII)	muscles of facial expression and part of the tongue	mixed	facial expression muscles
statoacoustic (VIII)	hearing and equilibrium and balance	sensory	ear
glossopharyngeal (IX)	Provides sensory fibers for taste to the posterior third of the tongue; provides motor nerves for the secretion of saliva, and provides general sensation to the mucosa of the pharynx and around the ear	mixed	tongue, pharynx
vagus (X)	Important in swallowing	mixed	pharynx, larynx, base of tongue, epiglottis, soft palate, and various other areas of body
accessory spinal (XI)	Motor control to sternocleidomastoid and trapezius	motor	sternocleidomastoid and trapezius
hypoglossal (XII)	Motor control of tongue	motor	intrinsic and extrinsic tongue muscles except palatoglossus

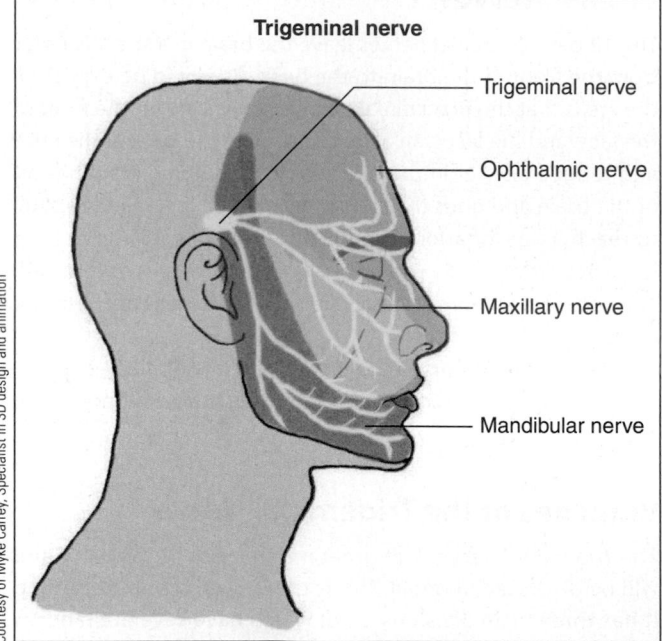

Trigeminal nerve

- Trigeminal nerve
- Ophthalmic nerve
- Maxillary nerve
- Mandibular nerve

Courtesy of Myke Carrey, Specialist in 3D design and animation

FIGURE 5-26
Branches of the trigeminal nerve.

TABLE 5-3 Branches of the Ophthalmic Division of the Trigeminal Nerve

Branch	Area Innervated
frontal	Divides into the supraorbital nerve and the supratrochlear nerve. This branch provides sensory innervation to the skin above the eye, forehead, and upper, medial corner of the eye.
lacrimal	Provides sensory innervation to the skin above the lateral eye area and the lacrimal gland, which supplies the tears to the eye
nasociliary	Divides into four branches: the anterior ethmoidal, posterior ethmoidal, infratrochlear, and external nasal nerves. All of these branches provide sensory innervation to the inferior, medial corner of eye, ethmoid area, and skin of the nose.

Maxillary (V2) The second major division of the trigeminal nerve is the maxillary division or maxillary nerve, also called V2. This sensory division exits the brain through the foramen rotundum (Figure 5-5) and enters the **pterygopalatine** fossa. The pterygopalatine fossa is a fossa deep in the skull below the apex of the orbit. The maxillary nerve is of major importance in dentistry because it provides innervations to the maxillary bone, maxillary sinus, nasal cavity, and all of the maxillary teeth. There are several important branches of the maxillary division of the trigeminal nerve while it is in the pterygopalatine fossa. These branches are detailed in Table 5-4.

Once the maxillary nerve enters the infraorbital canal through the infraorbital fissure, it becomes the infraorbital nerve. The infraorbital nerve is a continuation of the maxillary nerve. The infraorbital nerve continues in the canal until it emerges onto the face through the infraorbital foramen to provide innervation to the skin of the face under the eye, the side of the nose, and the upper lip. While the nerve is in the infraorbital canal it gives off two branches that are important in dentistry: the middle superior alveolar nerve and the anterior superior alveolar nerve (Table 5-4; Figure 5-27).

TABLE 5-4 Branches of the Maxillary Division of the Trigeminal Nerve

Sensory Branches of the Maxillary Division while in the Pterygopalatine Fossa	
Name of Nerve	**Areas Innervated**
zygomatic nerve	Enters the orbit through the inferior orbital fissure and divides into the zygomaticotemporal and zygomaticofacial nerves to provide sensory innervation to the skin of temple and skin of face over the cheek respectively
pharyngeal nerve	Provides sensory innervation to the nasopharynx
nasopalatine nerve	Enters the oral cavity through the incisive foramen to provide sensory innervation to the tissues surrounding the incisive papilla and the gingival margins of the maxillary anterior teeth
posterior superior alveolar nerve	Provides sensory innervation to the pulps and buccal gingiva of the maxillary molars with the exception of the pulp of the mesiobuccal root of the maxillary first molar as well as the maxillary sinus
greater palatine nerve	Provides sensory innervation to the palatal gingiva and soft tissues of the hard palate from the distal of the maxillary canine to the distal of the maxillary third molar
lesser palatine nerve	Provides sensory innervation to the soft tissues of the soft palate
Branches of the Maxillary Division while in the Infraorbital Canal	
Name of Nerve	**Areas Innervated**
infraorbital nerve	Provides sensory innervation to the lower eyelid, upper lip, nasal cavity and emerges onto the face through the infraorbital foramen
middle superior alveolar nerve	Provides sensory innervation to all of the pulps of the maxillary premolar teeth as well as the mesiobuccal root of the maxillary first molars. It also supplies the buccal gingiva of these teeth and part of the maxillary sinus.
anterior superior alveolar nerve	Provide sensory innervation to all of the pulps of the anterior teeth from canine to canine and the facial gingiva of these teeth

Mandibular (V3)   The last major division of the trigeminal nerve is the mandibular division or mandibular nerve. It is also known as V3. It exits the skull through the foramen ovale (Figure 5-5) and goes to the mandible. There are several branches of this important mixed nerve (Figure 5-28), and each is discussed in detail in Table 5-5.

Facial Nerve   The facial nerve is cranial nerve number seven (CN VII) and mainly innervates the muscles of facial expression and part of the tongue (Figure 5-29). This is a mixed nerve that has five motor branches and one sensory branch. This nerve is also very important in dentistry. The branches of the facial nerve and their areas of innervation are provided in detail in Table 5-6.

Circulation of the Head and Neck

The arteries and veins of the face and oral cavity are near each other. The arteries supply blood and nutrients to their specific areas. The veins drain deoxygenated blood and waste products from their specific areas.

Pathway of Blood to the Head

The pattern of blood flow through the heart and to the rest of the body via the aorta is discussed in Chapter 4 of this text. This chapter will focus on the continuing pathway of oxygenated blood to the oral cavity. It will start as the blood leaves the heart at the aorta and travels up the neck in to the common carotid arteries. Depending on the destination, there are only a few pathways that the arterial blood will travel.

Carotid Artery   The common carotid arteries go up towards the neck and at the area of the larynx divide further into the *internal carotid* and *external carotid arteries* (Figure 5-30). The internal carotid travels up the neck, and goes inside the skull and supplies blood to the inside of the brain. The external carotid is the main artery that is important to dentistry, because it goes to the outside of the face and oral cavity. Each branch of the external carotid will be discussed in more detail in Table 5-7. One important branch of the external carotid artery is the maxillary artery. The areas supplied by the maxillary artery and its branches are provided in detail in Table 5-8 and Figure 5-31.

Branches of Veins Important to Dentistry

There are several main branches of veins that will be discussed in detail that are important to dentistry (Figure 5-32). Many of them correspond to the artery that supplies that area. Most of the arteries and veins will have the same name and supply or drain the same areas. There are a few differences between the arteries and veins, and those will be discussed in the text where appropriate. Table 5-9 provides details on the veins important in dentistry.

Head and Neck Lymph Nodes

The lymph nodes of the head and neck are very important to dentistry and in detecting oral cancer (Figure 5-33 and Table 5-10). Palpation of the head and neck lymph nodes should be a common practice during an extra-oral examination. During this pressing and feeling of the nodes, a hardened lymph node that indicates an infection may be found. There are lymph nodes scattered all across the face and neck, and those will be discussed in this chapter.

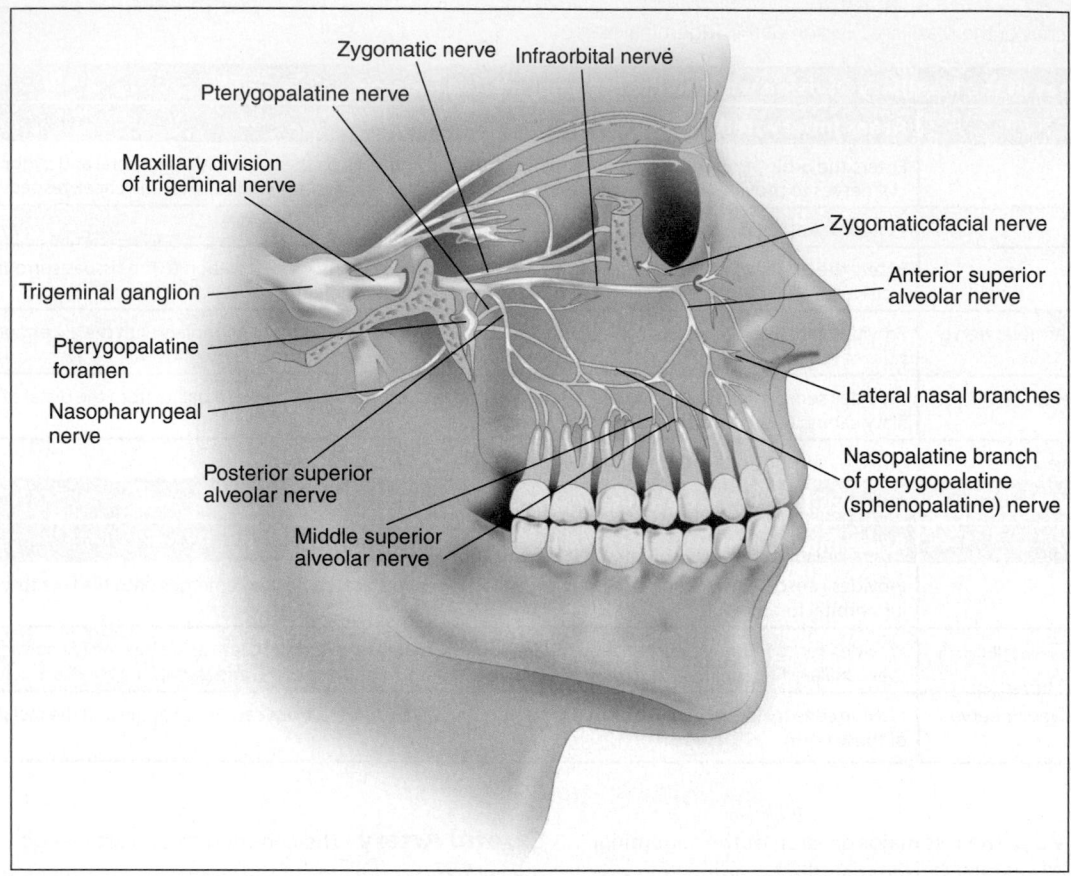

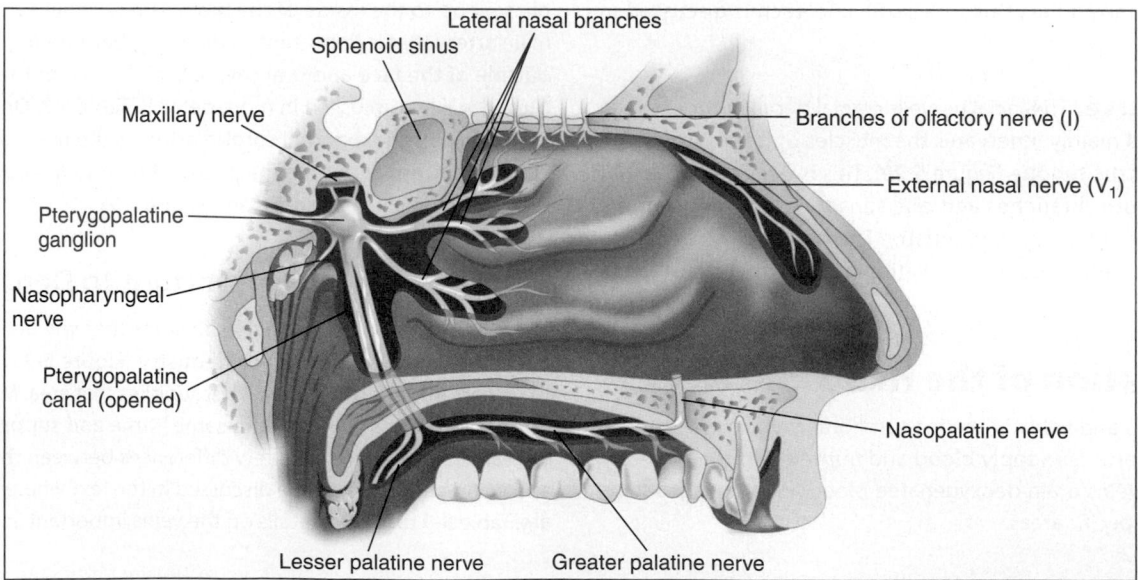

FIGURE 5-27
Branches of the maxillary nerve and areas innervated.

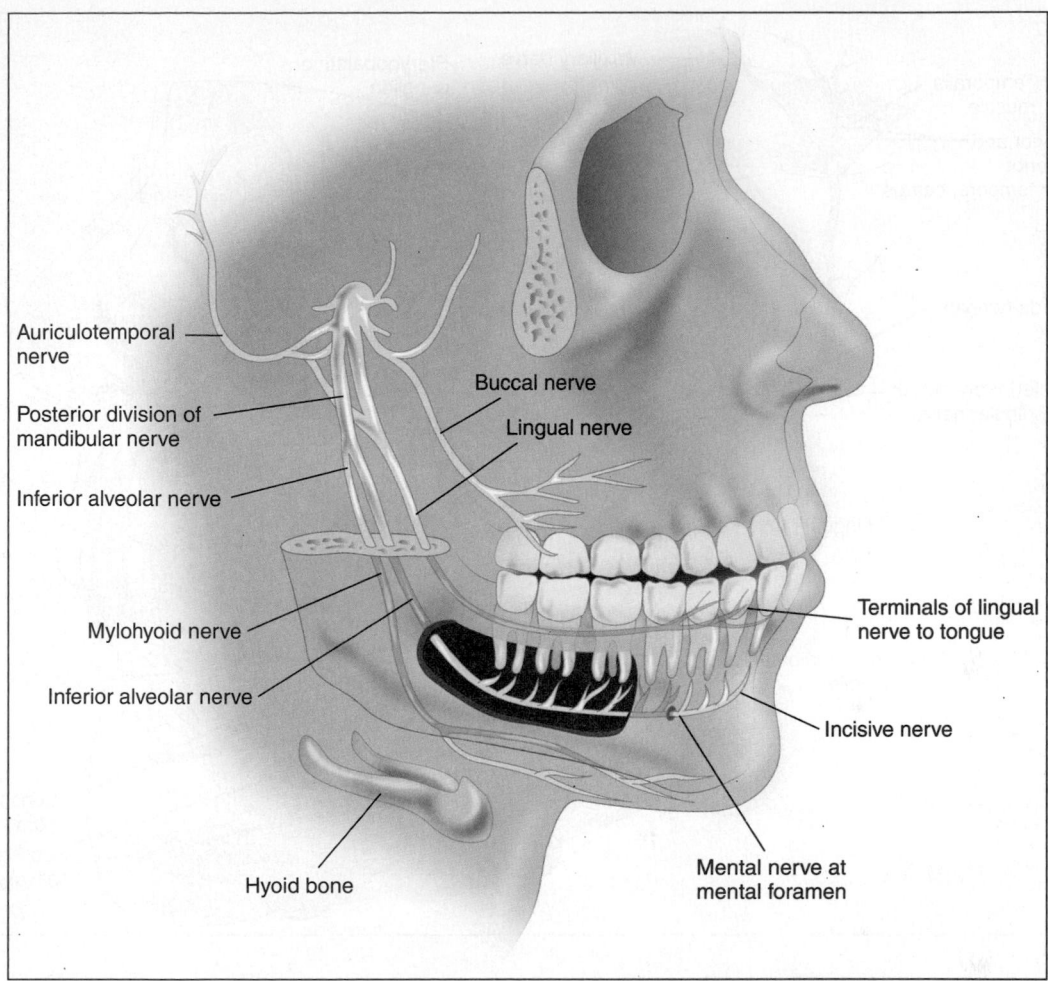

FIGURE 5-28
Branches of the mandibular nerve and areas innervated.

TABLE 5-5 Sensory Branches of the Mandibular Division of the Trigeminal Nerve

Name of Nerve	Areas Innervated
inferior alveolar nerve	The inferior alveolar nerve is a direct branch off the third division of the trigeminal nerve and travels down the ramus and enters into the mandibular foramen. The mandibular foramen is the entrance into the inferior alveolar canal. While in the canal this nerve will provide branches for sensory innervation to the pulps of each mandibular tooth from the third molar to the central incisor on each side. This nerve also provides sensory innervation to the buccal mucosa of the premolars and the anterior teeth. The inferior alveolar nerve ends at the mental foramen.
mental nerve	At the mental foramen, the inferior alveolar nerve divides into two branches. One branch is the mental nerve. This branch provides sensory innervation to the soft tissues of the chin.
incisive nerve	At the mental foramen, the inferior alveolar nerve divides into two branches. One branch is the incisive nerve. This branch provides sensory innervation to the mandibular incisors.
lingual nerve	The lingual nerve branches off the trigeminal nerve and runs parallel and inferior to the inferior alveolar nerve. It does not enter the inferior alveolar foramen but enters the tongue to provides sensory innervation. It also provides sensory innervation to the lingual gingiva of the mandibular teeth.
long buccal nerve	The long buccal nerve is a branch of the trigeminal nerve that provides sensory innervation to the buccal mucosa, buccinator muscle, and the facial gingiva of the three mandibular molars.
auriculotemporal nerve	The auriculotemporal nerve is a direct branch of the mandibular division of the trigeminal nerve. This branch provides sensory innervation to the area in front of the ear and the parotid gland.
mylohyoid nerve	The mylohyoid nerve travels along with the lingual nerve to provide sensory innervation to the anterior belly of the digastric and the mylohyoid muscle.

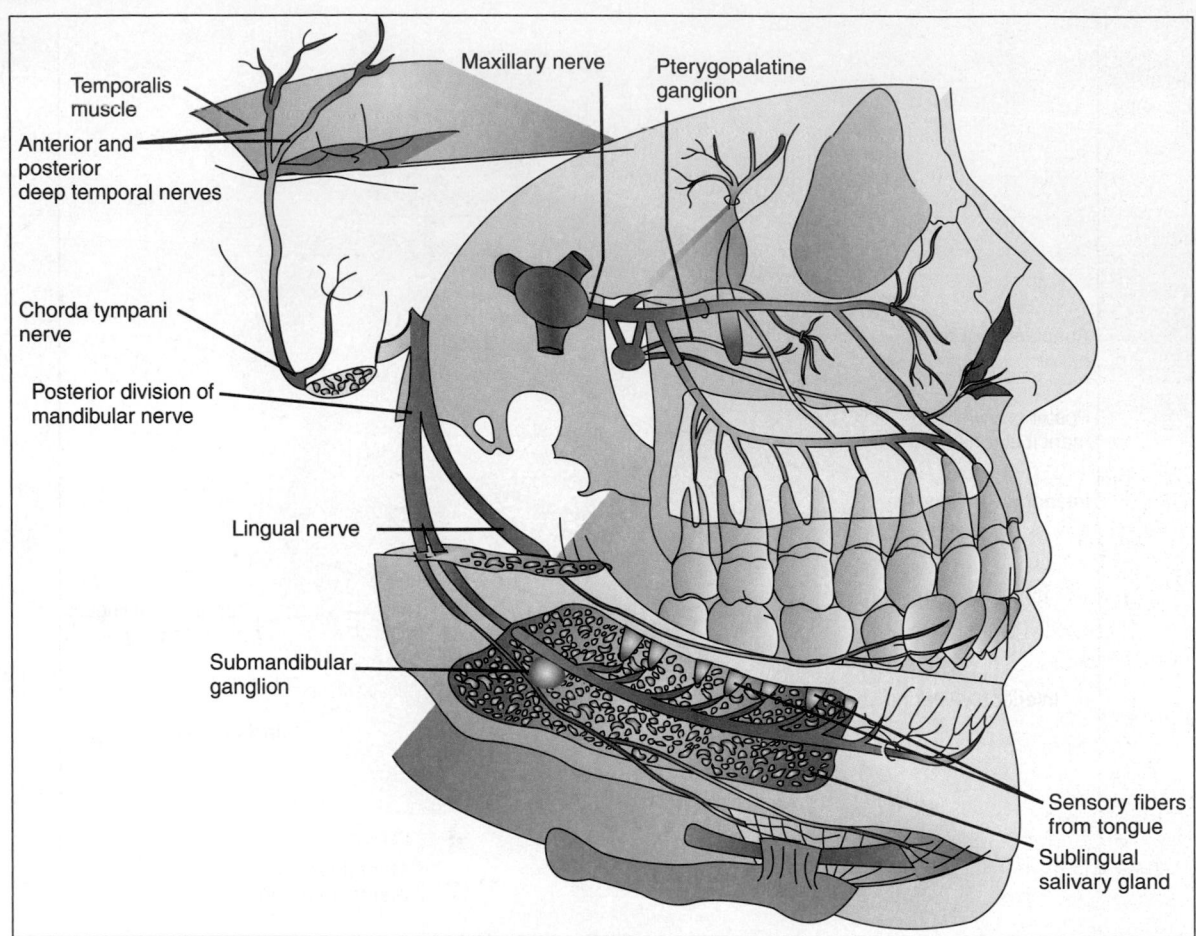

Temporalis muscle

Anterior and posterior deep temporal nerves

Chorda tympani nerve

Posterior division of mandibular nerve

Lingual nerve

Submandibular ganglion

Maxillary nerve

Pterygopalatine ganglion

Sensory fibers from tongue

Sublingual salivary gland

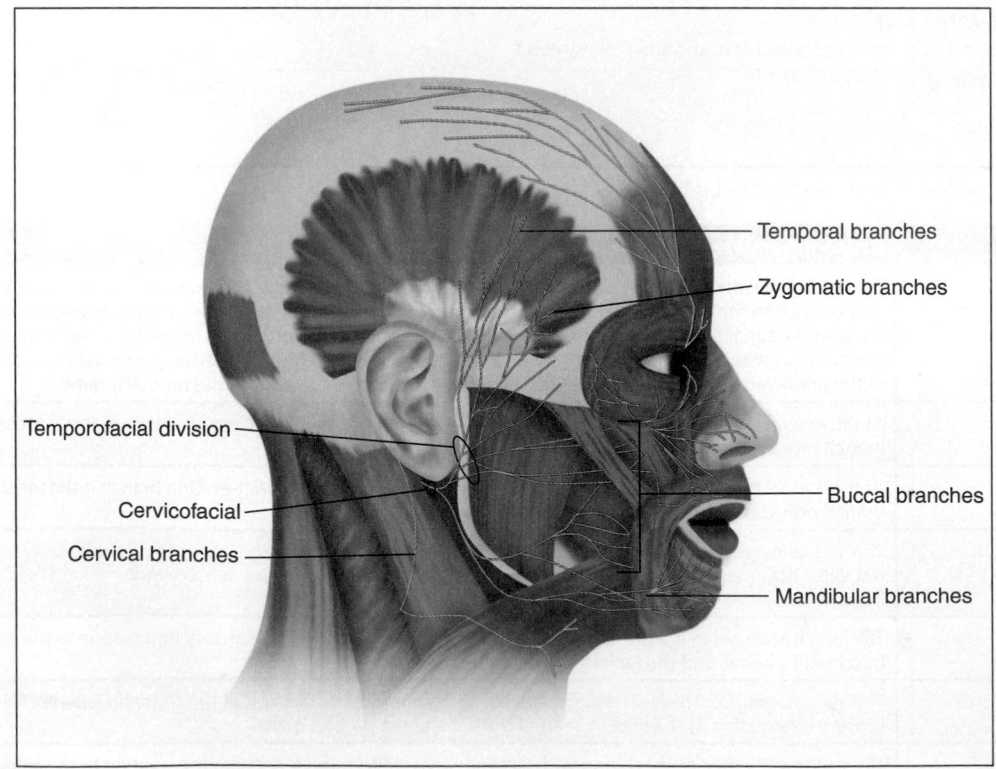

Temporal branches

Zygomatic branches

Temporofacial division

Cervicofacial

Cervical branches

Buccal branches

Mandibular branches

FIGURE 5-29
Branches of the facial nerve.

TABLE 5-6 Branches of the Facial Nerve

Name of Branch	Areas Innervated
chorda tympani	Only sensory branch of the facial nerve; travels to meet the lingual branch of the mandibular division of the trigeminal nerve and supplies the sensory innervations to the anterior two-thirds of the tongue. It also innervates the submandibular and sublingual salivary glands.
temporal	Provides motor innervation to the temporalis muscle and the temporal area of the lateral portion of the skull
zygomatic	Provides motor innervation to the muscles in the area of the zygomatic bone
buccal	Provides motor innervation to the buccinator muscle and area around the buccal mucosa and cheeks
mandibular	Branches off the cervicofacial trunk and provides motor innervation to the muscles of the face in the area of the mandible
cervical	Branches off the cervicofacial trunk and provides motor innervation to the muscles under the chin and side of the neck

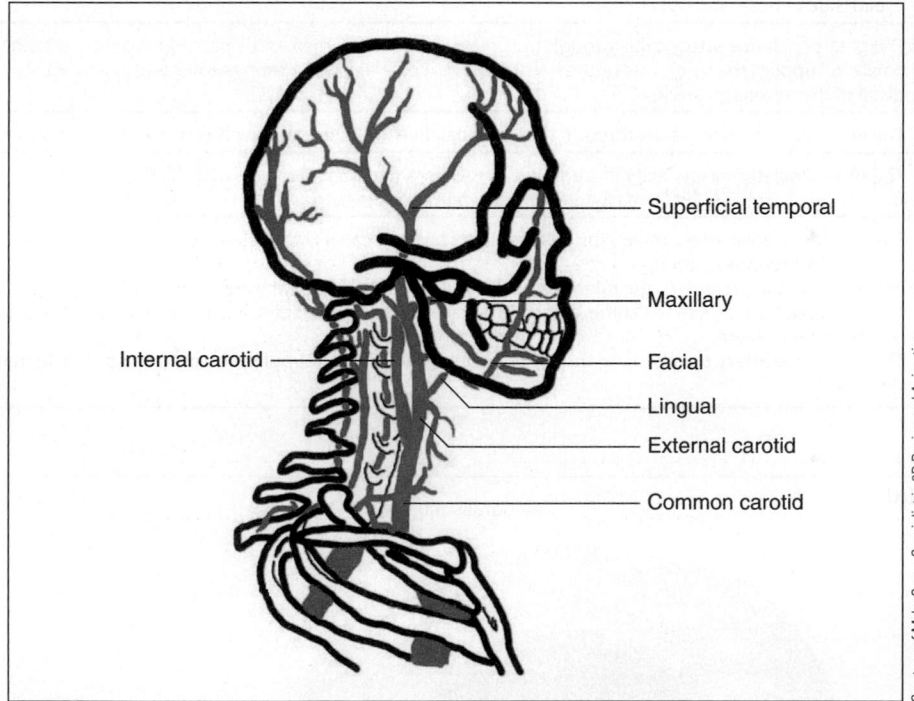

Courtesy of Myke Carey, Specialist in 3D Design and Animation

FIGURE 5-30
Branches of the external carotid arteries important in dentistry.

TABLE 5-7 Branches of the External Carotid Artery Important in Dentistry

Name	Areas Supplied
lingual artery	Branches off of the external carotid at the height of the hyoid bone in the neck. It travels forward into the posterior portion of the tongue. The artery travels all the way to the apex of the tongue and has several smaller branches. It supplies the base of the tongue, several suprahyoid muscles, the floor of the mouth, the sublingual salivary gland, and the body and tip of the tongue.
facial artery	Supplies the muscles of facial expression. It travels upward and over the edge of the angle of the mandible, spreads out over the side of the oral cavity, and continues toward the inner canthus of the eye where it ends. Along the way to the inner canthus of the eye, it splits into smaller branches that go to supply the buccal, zygomatic, infraorbital, orbital, and side of the nose areas of the face.
superficial temporal artery	This major branch of the external carotid supplies the upper and lateral parts of the scalp.
maxillary artery	This is the largest branch of the external carotid. The maxillary artery supplies the muscles of mastication and the oral cavity, which includes all of the teeth. Many of the arteries that supply the teeth have the same name as the corresponding nerves and veins. The maxillary artery has many branches that supply deep structures of the head and muscles in the face. These are discussed in detail in Table 5-8.

TABLE 5-8 Branches of the Maxillary Artery and Areas Supplied

Artery Name	Areas Supplied
middle meningeal artery	The middle meningeal nerve through the foramen spinosum into the brain. It supplies the **meninges** or the three layers of membranes that cover the brain.
masseteric, ptery-goid, and temporal arteries	The masseteric artery supplies the large masseter muscle of the cheek. The temporal artery goes upward and supplies the temporalis muscle at the lateral portion of the skull. The pterygoid artery supplies both the lateral pterygoid and medial pterygoid muscles.
buccal artery	The buccal artery supplies the buccinator muscle in the cheek and also supplies the buccal region of the oral cavity.
posterior superior alveolar artery	Posterior superior alveolar (PSA) artery supplies the posterior maxillary teeth and the maxillary sinus area. The posterior superior alveolar artery is slightly different from the PSA nerve in that it supplies all the molars and premolars of the maxillary arch.
infraorbital and anterior superior alveolar arteries	This infraorbital artery supplies a portion of the eye orbit. It travels in the infraorbital canal and drops a branch called the anterior superior alveolar (ASA) artery. The ASA artery supplies all of the maxillary anterior teeth and the facial gingiva in that area of the oral cavity. This area is slightly different from the ASA nerve because there is no middle superior alveolar artery. The infraorbital artery ends as it exits the infraorbital foramen under the orbit and spreads across the face to supply the lower eyelid, side of nose, and upper lip.
greater palatine artery	The greater palatine artery exits through the greater palatine foramen and emerges onto the posterior area of the hard palate. It supplies the soft tissue of the hard palate and palatal gingiva from the distal of the maxillary third molars up to the distal of the maxillary canines.
lesser palatine artery	The lesser palatine artery exits through the lesser palatine foramen and travels posteriorly to supply the soft palate.
sphenopalatine artery	The sphenopalatine artery exits through the incisive foramen behind the maxillary central incisors to supply the soft tissue from distal of canine to distal of canine of the *premaxilla* of the hard palate and palatal gingiva.
inferior alveolar, mylohyoid, mental, and incisive arteries	The inferior alveolar artery travels inside the inferior alveolar canal with the inferior alveolar nerve to supply the mandibular teeth and surrounding bone. In the area of the premolars, the inferior alveolar artery splits into the **incisive** artery, which supplies the anterior portion of the mandible from canine to canine, and the mental artery, which supplies the lower lip, chin, and facial gingiva of the mandibular anterior teeth. The mylohyoid artery travels along the mylohyoid ridge or line and supplies the mylohyoid muscle that makes up the floor of the mouth.

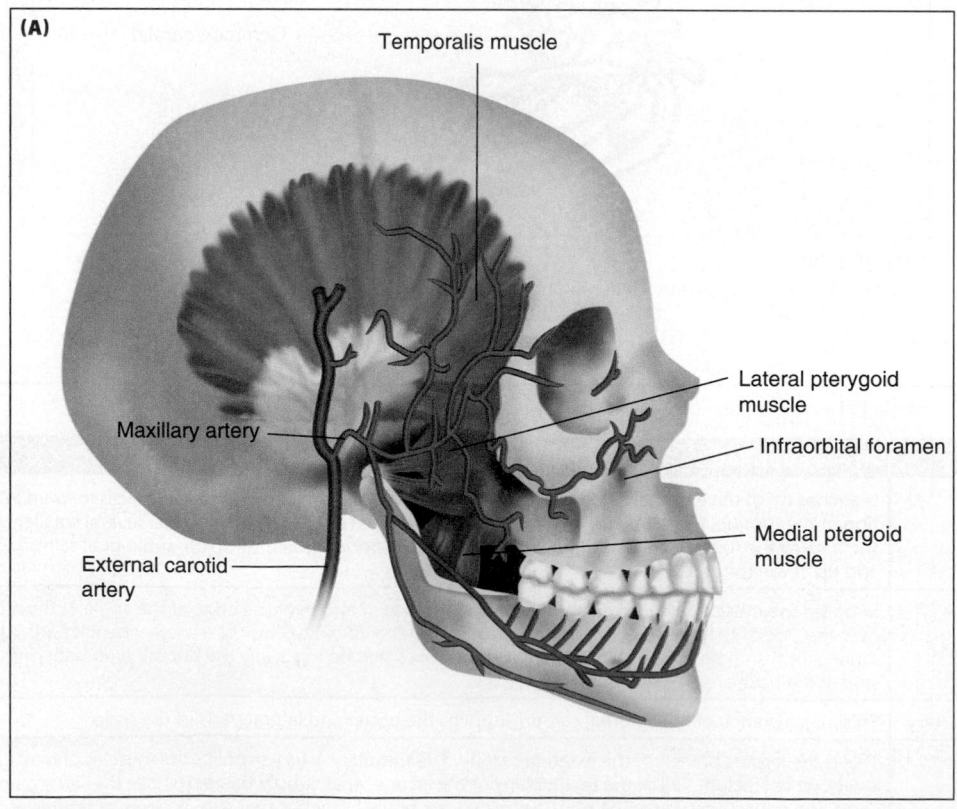

FIGURE 5-31
Branches of the maxillary arteries important in dentistry.

(B)

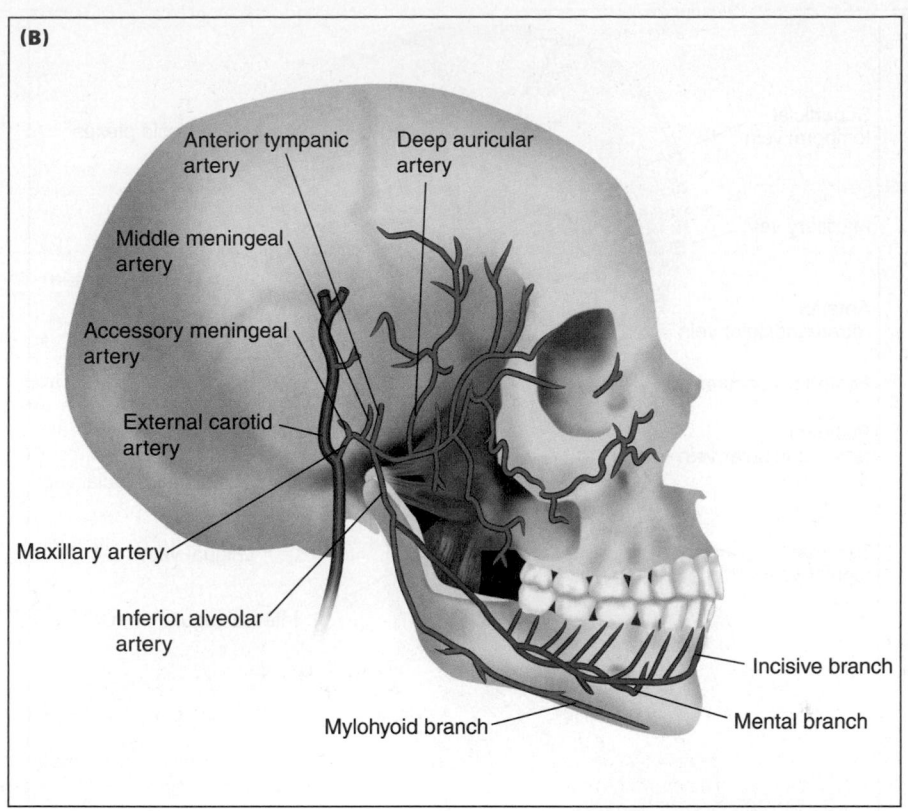

Anterior tympanic artery

Deep auricular artery

Middle meningeal artery

Accessory meningeal artery

External carotid artery

Maxillary artery

Inferior alveolar artery

Incisive branch

Mental branch

Mylohyoid branch

(C)

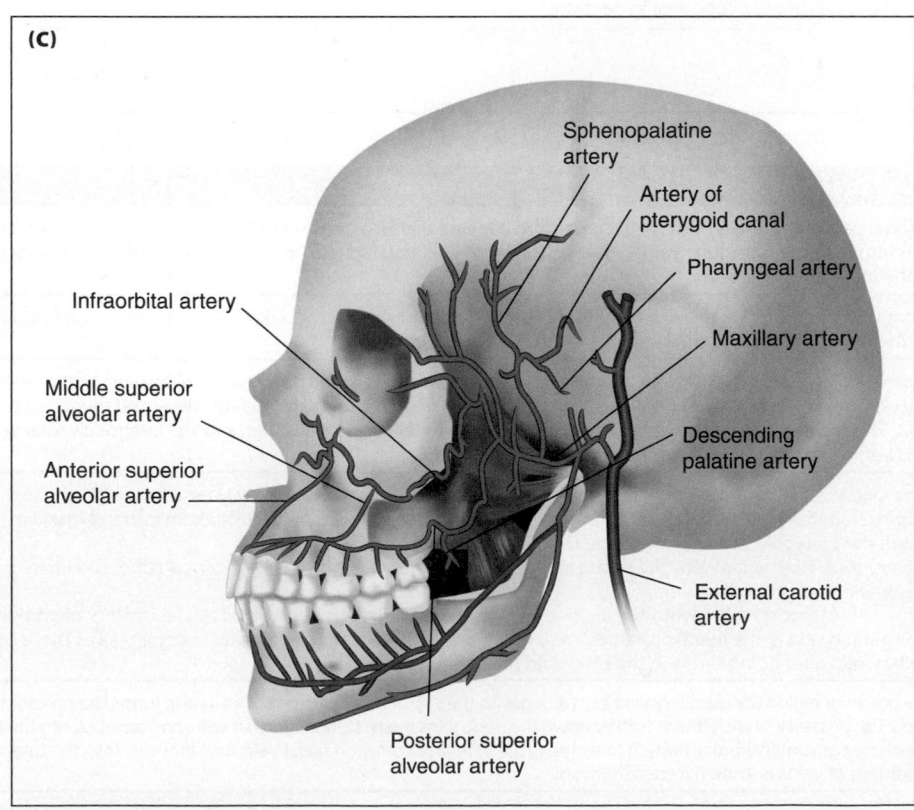

Sphenopalatine artery

Artery of pterygoid canal

Pharyngeal artery

Maxillary artery

Infraorbital artery

Middle superior alveolar artery

Anterior superior alveolar artery

Descending palatine artery

External carotid artery

Posterior superior alveolar artery

FIGURE 5-31 (Continued)

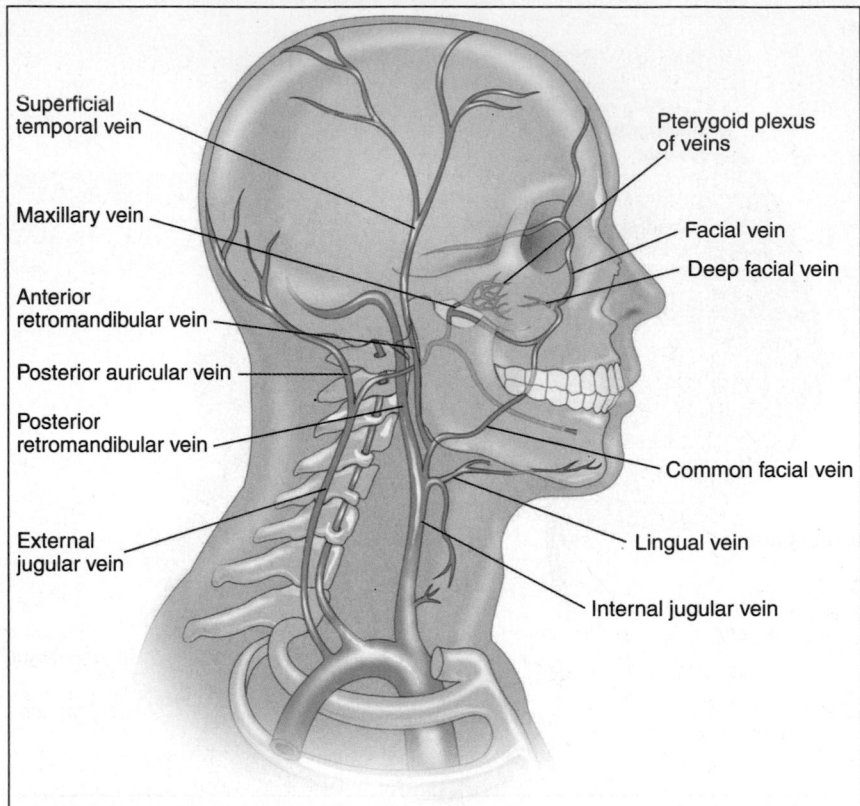

FIGURE 5-32
Branches of veins important in dentistry.

TABLE 5-9 Branches of Veins Important in Dentistry

Vein	Area of Drainage
facial vein	The facial vein drains the area of the face starting at the medial area of the eye and extending across the face and cheeks, and drains into the internal jugular vein in the neck. Most of the facial expression muscles are drained by the facial vein, which drains into the internal jugular vein.
lingual vein	The lingual vein has many small branches that drain all areas of the tongue. All of these branches will travel into the lingual vein until they eventually drain into the internal jugular vein.
pterygoid plexus	The **pterygoid plexus** is a network of interconnecting veins and is found near the maxillary vein at the lateral portion of the face. Many branches of veins, including those from the muscles of mastication and the maxillary and mandibular teeth, drain into the plexus. This includes the **posterior superior alveolar**, anterior superior alveolar, and the inferior alveolar veins. The plexus further drains into the maxillary vein and then into the internal jugular.
maxillary vein	The maxillary vein drains many smaller branches that correspond to the arteries discussed earlier in the text. The veins from the muscles of mastication, maxillary teeth, and mandibular teeth all drain into the maxillary vein after going through the pterygoid plexus in many areas. The pterygopalatine vein drains the palate along with the sphenopalatine, the greater palatine, and lesser palatine veins. All of these drain into the maxillary vein. The mandibular incisors drain into the incisive vein. The inferior alveolar vein drains the rest of the mandibular teeth. It is joined by the mental vein at the mental foramen area, which drains the skin of the chin and lower lip. All of these branches drain into the maxillary vein after going through the pterygoid plexus.
retromandibular vein: anterior and posterior branches	In the posterior region the maxillary vein joins along with the **superficial temporal vein** and forms the posterior retromandibular branch. The posterior branch drains further down the neck, joins the posterior auricular vein, and empties into the external **jugular** vein. The anterior retromandibular branch joins the facial vein and common facial vein and empties into the internal jugular vein. This joining of veins is known as *anastomosis*.
external jugular vein	The external jugular receives blood from the external parts of the skull and the deeper structures of the face. It drains the facial structures around the eye, nose, lips, tongue, maxilla, and mandible. The external jugular empties into the subclavian veins from the arms and then drains into the **brachiocephalic vein**, which will flow directly into the **superior vena cava** and into the right atrium of the heart.

TABLE 5-9 *(Continued)*

Vein	Area of Drainage
internal jugular	The internal jugular vein drains the brain, many areas of the face, the maxillary vein, pterygoid plexus, and anterior retromandibular vein. As the blood travels downward, it joins the brachiocephalic vein along with the external jugular vein. The blood will empty into the superior vena cava and end in the right atrium of the heart.
brachiocephalic vein	The brachiocephalic vein is a much larger vessel and is found in the area of the sternum and clavicle in the upper chest. It is formed by the union of the subclavian and the internal jugular veins. These larger vessels receive blood from the upper portion of the head, neck, and arms. There is a difference in the veins from the arteries here in that there are two brachiocephalic veins, with one on the right side and one of the left side of the body. However, there is only a brachiocephalic artery on the right side of the body and not the left side.
superior vena cava	The superior vena cava is the largest vein in the body, and it transports deoxygenated blood to its final destination. It travels down the chest into the right atrium of the heart. Here the blood will travel to the right ventricle and to the lungs for release of the carbon dioxide and to get oxygenated.

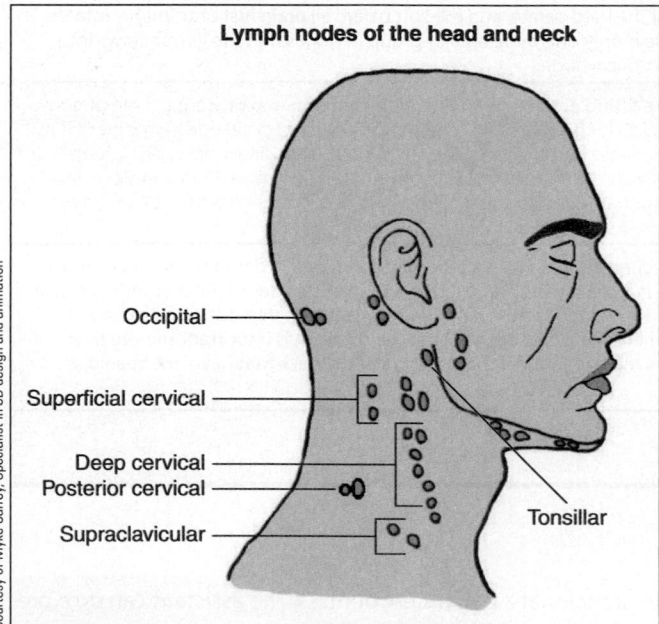

Courtesy of Myke Carrey, Specialist in 3D design and animation

FIGURE 5-33
Head and neck lymph nodes.

Lymph Nodes Important in Dentistry The area of the face and neck will determine which lymph nodes the infection will drain into first. The first set of lymph nodes are known as the **primary nodes**. There are four main groups of nodes that will be discussed that drain the oral cavity, face, and teeth (Figure 5-33). There is a specific pattern that is followed once the lymph enters these nodes in the head and neck. The basic pattern is the submental nodes to the submandibular nodes, to the superior (upper) deep **cervical nodes** to the inferior (lower) deep cervical nodes. Once the lymph flows out of this area, it goes to either the right **lymphatic duct** on the right side or the **thoracic duct** on the left side. If the infection is closer to the anterior of the oral cavity, then the infection will go through more of the groups of lymph nodes, but if the infection is in the third molar area, then the infection will only travel through two groups of these nodes. Table 5-11 provides details regarding the lymph nodes important in dentistry.

TABLE 5-10 Head and Neck Lymph Nodes

Lymph Node	Location
cervical	The cervical nodes are several groups of nodes that are on or around the neck and face. The parotid lymph nodes are on and around the parotid salivary gland in the cheek in front of the ear. There are also several groups of small nodes in front, below, and behind the ear. These are called the pre-auricular for those in front, the infra-auricular for those below, and the post-auricular for those behind the ear. These groups of nodes drain into the submandibular nodes that will be discussed later.
occipital	The occipital lymph nodes are at the back and base of the skull and neck. To palpate these, the patient needs to look downward and the assistant palpates at the base of the hairline at the middle of the neck.
clavicular	The clavicular lymph nodes are found in the front area of the base of the neck around the clavicle.
tonsils	The **tonsils** are masses of lymphoid tissue that are found in three separate areas in the neck. They form a ring of immunologically active tissue. The three types of tonsils are the palatine tonsils that are on the sides of the throat at the posterior end of the oral cavity, the lingual tonsils that are found on the surface of the base of the tongue, and the **pharyngeal tonsils** or adenoids that are found at the roof of the posterior wall of the nasopharynx. Tonsils are important groups of lymph tissue that help fight infections from the oral cavity of the nose. These three groups of tonsillar tissue form almost a complete ring that encircles the pharynx.

TABLE 5-11 Lymph Nodes Important in Dentistry

Lymph Nodes	Locations
submental	The submental lymph nodes are a small cluster of lymph nodes found under the chin in the floor of the oral cavity. When there is an infection in the mandibular incisors, the tip of the tongue, the floor of the mouth, or at the midline of the lower lip, it drains into this group of nodes as the primary nodes. The next group of nodes that the lymph will flow into are the submandibular nodes.
submandibular	The submandibular lymph nodes are located between the submandibular salivary glands and drain the majority of the areas of the oral cavity, teeth, anterior portion of the palate, and body of the tongue. All of the teeth drain into the submandibular nodes except the previously mentioned mandibular incisors, which drain into the submental nodes, and the third molars, which drain into the superior deep cervical nodes first. The next group of lymph nodes that this lymph will flow into is the superior deep cervical group of nodes.
superior (upper) deep cervical chain	The superior deep cervical nodes are the superior portion of the anterior and posterior cervical chain that is found along the sternocleidomastoid neck muscle. The areas further in the back of the oral cavity or throat are drained first. The maxillary and mandibular third molars, the base of the tongue, the palatine and lingual tonsils, the posterior of the hard palate, and the soft palate all drain first or primarily into the superior deep cervical nodes. There is only one more area or group of nodes that the lymph flows into after this group, the inferior deep cervical nodes.
inferior (lower) deep cervical chain	The inferior deep cervical nodes are found at the inferior end of the anterior and posterior chain of nodes along the sternocleidomastoid muscle in the neck. All of the superior deep cervical node lymph will flow here along with the lymph from the areas at the back of the neck and the occipital nodes. This group is found about 2 inches above the clavicle at the base of the neck muscle. The lymph then completes its journey and flows into the right lymphatic duct or the thoracic duct depending on what side of the head it is draining from.
anterior and posterior cervical chains	There is a long chain of interconnecting lymph nodes all the way down both sides of the sternocleido-mastoid muscle of the neck. There is a chain medial and lateral to the muscle termed the anterior cervical chain and the posterior cervical chain, respectively. When this muscle is palpated during an extraoral examination, it should be noted where the lymphadenopathy was found. It is important to note that there are hundreds of lymph nodes much deeper in the structure of the neck that have not been discussed in this text.

Chapter Summary

In many dental practices, the dental assistant is the first dental professional that a patient encounters. The assistant can do a preliminary examination of the patient and document any abnormalities in the chart to bring to the dentist's attention. It is important for the assistant to know how to do a thorough extraoral and intraoral examination and knowing what muscles that are involved is necessary. When describing any findings, the dental assistant would discuss them with the dentist using proper terminology.

When performing a thorough intraoral and extraoral examination of a patient, palpation must be applied to the muscles of the head and neck. Evidence of disease or abnormalities can often be discovered during this process. It is important for the dental assistant to understand and identify the normal structure of the muscles of the face and neck in order to observe an abnormality. Any malformation, abnormality, red area, or hardened area that is detected during the examination should be brought to the attention of the dentist.

A thorough examination of the lymph nodes should be completed at every examination in the dental office. When palpating during an extraoral examination, any of these lymph nodes may be hardened or swollen and tender. The term for swollen, hardened, or tender lymph nodes is **lymphadenopathy** and can be of serious concern. If that is noticed, then it needs to be brought to the dentist's attention. Many times there is a reason why these nodes may be swollen, so the patient should be questioned. If an area under the angle of the mandible is noticed as sore, and the patient states that he or she just got over a sore throat, then that swollen node makes sense.

There may be a time that a hardened node is discovered and that is when another consultation with an oral surgeon may be needed. The general treatment in this situation is that if the dentist is unable to find an area in the oral cavity that caused this node to be infected, then the patient is to come back in two weeks to see if there is a change. If no change is noted or if it has gotten larger, then a consultation to an oral surgeon for a closer look is in order. A more detailed description of how to perform an extraoral and intraoral examination or oral cancer screening will be discussed in Chapter 9.

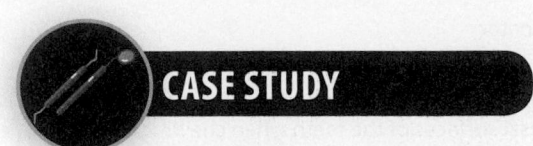

CASE STUDY

Olessia is a 35-year-old patient at Dr. Fleidener's office. Olessia has had a series of headaches and pain during mastication (chewing). She also experiences clicking and popping when opening her mouth. These symptoms have continued for 6 months and seem to be worsening.

Case Study Review

1. List the components of the head and neck affected, identifying the specific anatomy.

2. Identify the possible conditions.

3. How might the dental assistant be involved in this patient's care?

Review Questions

Multiple Choice

1. Which of the following bones makes up the forehead, upper areas of the eye orbit, and the anterior superior portion of the skull?
   a. frontal
   b. glabella
   c. parietal
   d. temporal

2. How many bones are in the human skull?
   a. 20
   b. 22
   c. 24
   d. 26

3. Which of the following muscles does not have a skeletal attachment or origin?
   a. levator anguli oris
   b. levator labii superioris
   c. orbicularis oris
   d. depressor anguli oris

4. The parotid gland is located behind the ear *and* on the masseter muscle. *Select the correct answer based on the statements above.*
   a. Both statements are true.
   b. Both statements are false.
   c. The first statement is true; the second statement is false.
   d. The first statement is false; the second statement is true.

5. On which bone are the mental foramen, genial tubercles, and lingual foramen found?
   a. maxilla
   b. mandible
   c. vomer
   d. frontal

6. The temporomandibular joint is composed of all of the following except the
   a. glenoid fossa of the temporal bone.
   b. greater wing of the zygomatic bone.
   c. articular eminence of the temporal bone.
   d. condyloid process of the mandible.

7. For each muscle of neck, match the correct muscle with its function.
   1. sternocleidomastoid
   2. trapezius
   3. platysma
   a. helps turn head side to side and tilt it on its axis
   b. functions as a blanket for the deeper muscles and gives the neck a smoother appearance
   c. helps turn head from side to side and pull it backwards

8. Which of the following is correct regarding the intrinsic muscles of the tongue?
   a. They originate at various locations on the skull and insert in the tongue.
   b. They function to hold the tongue in the floor of the mouth.
   c. The fibers of the intrinsic muscles are named according to the direction they run in.
   d. The styloglossus muscle is an intrinsic muscle of the tongue.

9. What percentage of total saliva volume is produced by the parotid glands?
   a. 30%
   b. 35%
   c. 25%
   d. 40%

10. Which of the following statements is correct regarding the minor salivary glands?
   a. They produce about 10% of the total volume of saliva.
   b. The secretory units of the minor salivary glands are called acini.
   c. There are approximately 100 minor salivary glands.
   d. Minor salivary glands are found only on the lips and buccal mucosa.

11. What is the function of saliva?
   a. help cleanse the oral cavity
   b. wet food to allow for better taste
   c. moisten the mucous membranes
   d. All of these are functions of saliva.

12. Which of the following cranial nerves are purely motor?
   a. oculomotor, trochlear, abducens, hypoglossal, accessory
   b. oculomotor, trochlear, abducens, hypoglossal, optic
   c. oculomotor, trochlear, abducens, facial, optic
   d. oculomotor, trochlear, vagus, facial, optic

13. Which of the following nerves supplies all the roots of the maxillary bicuspids (premolars)?
    a. zygomatic nerve branch
    b. anterior superior alveolar nerve
    c. middle superior alveolar nerve
    d. posterior superior alveolar nerve

14. Which division of the common carotid artery supplies the face and the oral cavity?
    a. external carotid artery
    b. internal carotid artery
    c. facial artery
    d. maxillary artery

15. Which of the following is correct regarding the pathway of deoxygenated blood from the head?
    a. internal jugular vein to brachiocephalic vein to superior vena cava to right atrium of heart to right ventricle of heart to lungs for oxygen
    b. internal jugular vein to brachiocephalic vein to superior vena cava to right ventricle of heart to right atrium of heart to lungs for oxygen
    c. internal jugular vein to superior vena cava to brachiocephalic vein to right atrium of heart to right ventricle of heart to lungs for oxygen
    d. internal jugular vein to brachiocephalic vein to superior vena cava to right atrium of heart to lungs right ventricle of heart for oxygen

16. Which of the following muscles works to pull the corners of the mouth up to produce a smile?
    a. zygomaticus major
    b. zygomaticus minor

    c. buccinator
    d. mentalis

17. Which of the following muscles helps to hold the food on the occlusal surfaces of the teeth when chewing?
    a. zygomaticus major
    b. zygomaticus minor
    c. buccinator
    d. mentalis

18. The first lymph node that encounters an infection is called the _____ node. If the infection is not destroyed and travels out of that node and into another node, that node is called the _____ node.
    a. primary, secondary
    b. secondary, primary
    c. primary, tertiary
    d. tertiary, secondary

19. Which of the following muscles works to pull the corners of the mouth up to produce a smile?
    a. zygomaticus major
    b. zygomaticus minor
    c. buccinator
    d. mentalis

20. A nerve fiber is also called a/an
    a. neuron
    b. dendrite
    c. axon
    d. soma

Critical Thinking

1. What are the two types of movement of the TMJ?
2. What are the types of problems that can occur with the TMJ?
3. What are the functions of the muscles of the floor of the mouth?
4. What are the nerves of the maxilla and the mandible?
5. Why is it important for the patient to have a head and neck exam?

Key Terms

Term and Pronunciation	Meaning of Root and Word Parts	Definition
afferent (**af**-er-*uh*nt)	**afferent** = carries sensory information toward a central organ or part	conducting toward the nerve or central nervous system
alveolar (al-**vee**-*uh*-ler)	**alveolus** = tooth socket -**ar** = pertaining to	pertaining to an alveolus, the bony socket of a tooth
amylase (**am**-*uh*-leys)	**amyl(o)** = indicating starch -**ase** = indicating an enzyme	enzyme in saliva that starts digestion process of carbohydrates
anguli (**ang**-g*uh*-lahy)	**angle** = a corner; a common point between two planes	at corner or angle of mouth

Term and Pronunciation	Meaning of Root and Word Parts	Definition
articular eminence (ahr-**tik**-*yuh*-ler) (**em**-*uh*-nuh ns)	**articular** = pertaining to joints **eminent** = stand out, project	a raised area located at the anterior of the temporal bone; assists in keeping condyle in the glenoid fossa
Bartholin's duct (bahr-th*uh*-lin) (duhkt)	**Bartholin** = Danish anatomist and physician who described the Bartholin glands **duct** = any tube, canal, vessel conveying body fluid	largest of all, the Bartholin duct joins the submandibular duct to drain through the sublingual caruncle
belly (bel-ee)	**belly** = bulging, central part	the fleshy, central portion of a muscle
brachiocephalic vein (**brey**-kee-*oh*- s*uh*-**fal**-ik) (veyn)	**brachi-** = upper arm **cephal-** = head **-ic** = of, relating to **vein** = blood vessels taking blood from part of the body to the heart	two large veins on each side of the neck formed by the union of the internal jugular and subclavian veins; receive blood from head and neck
buccinator (**buhk**-s*uh*-ney-ter)	**bucc** = cheek **-ator** = something that performs a certain action	a thin, flat muscle lining the cheek, the action of which contracts and compresses the cheek
canthus (**kan**-th*uh* s)	**canthus** = the angle of corner of each eye	the angular junction of the eyelids at either of the corners of the eyes
capsule (**kap**-s*uh* l)	**capsule** = cartilaginous membrane surrounding certain organs or parts	lymphoid cells enclosed with capsule such as lymph nodes, spleen and thymus
cervical nodes (**sur**-vi-k*uh* l) (nohd)	**cervix** = neck **-al** = pertaining to **node** = small mass of lymph tissue	lymph nodes found in the neck
crepitus (**krep**-i-t*uh* s)	**crepitus** = a rattling, creaking	the grating sound of two ends of bone rubbing together
dentition (den-**tish**-*uh* n)	**dentition** = to cut teeth	arrangement of teeth in a particular species
depressor (dih-**pres**-er)	**depress** = to put into a lower position; push down **-or** = a person or thing	an instrument for drawing down a body part
dorsum (**dawr**-s*uh* m)	**dorsum** = technical term for back	the upper, outer surface of an organ, an appendage, or a part
ducts of Rivinus (duhkt) (r*uh*-**vee**-n*uh* s)	**Augustus Rivinus** = German anatomist and botanist names glands **duct** = any tube, canal, vessel conveying body fluid	8–20 excretory duct openings from sublingual salivary gland
efferent (**ef**-er-*uh* nt)	**efferent** = carries motor impulses away from central organ or part	conducting or conducted away from something
embryonic (em-bree-**on**-ik)	**embryo** = earliest stage of development, before all the major body structures **-ic** = characteristics of	first eight weeks of pregnancy at the being of development
eminence (**em**-*uh*-nuh ns)	**eminent** = stand out, project **-ent** = existing condition	a prominence, bump, bulge, or projection, especially of bone
exocrine (**ek**-s*uh*-krin)	**exo-** = outside, external **-crine** = denoting secretions	gland with a duct that opens on a body surface
jugular (**juhg**-y*uh*-lahr)	**ex-** = out of; situated on or near outside **-al** = pertaining to **jugul-** = region of neck or throat **-ar** = of, relating to, or located	large vein of the neck

(Continues)

Term and Pronunciation	Meaning of Root and Word Parts	Definition
facial (**fey**-shuh l)	**face** = front part of the head **-al** = pertaining to	pertaining to the face
fiber (**fahy**-ber)	**fiber** = a fine, threadlike structure	any of various elongated cells or threadlike structures of a muscle or nerve fiber
fissure (**fish**-er)	**fissure** = a narrow opening produced by cleavage or separation of parts	a groove, natural division, deep furrow in various parts of the body
foramen/foramina (fuh-**rey**-muh n) (fuh -**ram**-uh-nuh) plural	**foramen** = natural opening, passage	a passage or opening, on orifice, a hole in a bone for the passage of nerves or blood vessels
foramen cecum (fuh-**rey**-muh n) (**see**-kuh m)	**foramen** = an opening, orifice, or short passage **cecum** = a saclike cavity	small, indented area at midline on dorsum of tongue at middle of sulcus terminalis V-shape; embryonic origin of thyroid
fossa (**fos**-uh)	**fossa** = depression; hollow area	a furrow or shallow depression
genial tubercles (**jeen**-yuh l) (**too**-ber-kuh l)	**gen(i)-** = chin **-al** = of or relating to **tuber** = oblong or rounded thickening or outgrowth **-cle** = indicating smallness	a slight projection in the middle line of the posterior surface of the body of the mandible, giving attachment to the geniohyoid muscle and the genioglossus
glabella (gluh-**bel**-uh)	**glabella** = the flat area of bone between the eyebrows	a smooth elevation of the frontal bone just above the bridge of the nose
hyoglossus (**hahy**-oh- glaws-uhs)	**hyoid** = a U-shaped bone at the root of the tongue **gloss** = tongue **-us** = possessing, full of	a muscle with origin from the hyoid bone, with insertion to the side of the tongue
hyoid (**hahy**-oid)	**hyoid** = a U-shaped bone at the root of the tongue	the horseshoe-shaped bone that lies at the base of the tongue and above the thyroid cartilage
incisive (in-**sahy**-siv)	**incise** = to cut into **-ive** = function	branch of the inferior alveolar nerve
infraorbital (**in**-fruh-**awr**-bi-tl)	**infra** = below, lower **orbit** = eye socket **-al** = pertaining to	below the orbit of the eyes
innervate (ih-**nur**-veyt)	**in** = into, within **nerve** = bundle(s) of fibers sending sensory and motor impulses **-ate** = product of a process	to supply an organ or a body part with nerves
labii (**ley**-bee)	**labi-** = lips	pertaining to the lips
levator (li-**vey**-ter)	**levitate** = lift or raise a part **-or** = a person or thing	a muscle that raises or elevates a part, opposite of depressor
lingual (**ling**-gwuh l)	**lingu-** = tongue **-al** = pertaining to	pertaining to the tongue
lymphadenopathy (lim-fad-n-**op**-uh-thee)	**lymph** = a clear, yellowish fluid containing white blood cells **aden-** = gland **path** = disease **-y** = characterized by	any disease affecting the lymph nodes; chronically swollen lymph nodes
lymph node (limf) (nohd)	**lymph** = a clear, yellowish fluid containing white blood cells **node** = a knot, circumscribed swelling	a number of small swellings in the lymphatic system where lymph is filtered and lymphocytes are formed

Term and Pronunciation	Meaning of Root and Word Parts	Definition
lymphatic duct (lim-**fat**-ik) (duhkt)	**lymph** = a clear, yellowish fluid containing white blood cells **-tic** = pertaining to	pertaining to a lymph vessel
lymphoid tissue (**lim**-foid) (**tish**-oo)	**lymph** = clear, watery, sometimes faintly yellowish fluid derived from body tissues that contains white blood cells and circulates throughout the lymphatic system **-oid** = of or relating to **tissue** = a part of an organism consisting of a large number of cells having a similar structure and function	part of the body's immune system that is important for the immune response and helps protect it from infection and foreign bodies; acts to remove bacteria and certain proteins from the tissues
masseter (ma-**see**-ter)	**masseter** = a muscle of the cheek used in moving the jaw, especially in chewing	a short, thick, masticatory muscle, the action of which assists in closing the jaws by raising the mandible or lower jaw
maxillary (**mak**-suh-ler-ee) (**ahr**-tuh-ree)	**maxilla** = upper jaw **-ary** = pertaining to	pertaining to upper arch of the oral cavity
meninges (mi-**nin**-jeez)	**meninges** = membranes that envelop the brain and spinal cord	three membranes (dura mater, arachnoid, and pia mater) that line the skull and enclose the brain and spinal cord
mylohyoid (mahy-loh-**hahy**-oid)	**myl-** = molar **hyoid** = a U-shaped bone at the root of the tongue	relating to the region of the molar teeth of the lower jaw and the hyoid bone; a flat, triangular muscle that forms the floor of the mouth
neurocranium (**nyoo** r-oh- **krey**-nee-uh m)	**neuro** = nerve **crani-** = part of skull that encloses the brain **-um** = indicating a structure	the portion of the skull that surrounds the brain, eyes, nose, and ears
nerve fibers (nurv) (**fahy**-ber)	**nerve** = bundle(s) of fibers sending sensory and motor impulses **fiber** = a fine, threadlike structure	a nerve is formed of a bundle of many nerve fibers with their sheaths
orbicularis oris (or-**bik**-ya-**lar**-is) (**or**-is)	**orbicule** = like an orbit; circular, ringlike **-ar** = denoting process **-is** = having to do with **or-** = mouth	circular muscle that encircles the mouth
palatine (**pal**-uh-tahyn)	**palate** = roof of the mouth **-ine** = of, near, or in	related to the roof of the oral cavity
palpate (**pal**-peyt)	**palpate** = to examine by touch **-ate** = expressing action	examination by application of the hands or fingers to the external surface of the body to detect evidence of disease or abnormalities
papillae (puh-**pil**-uh)	**pap** = nipple, nipple-like; small projection **-illa** = any of several	a small nipple-like projection or process
parotid gland (puh-**rot**-id) (gland)	**par-** = beside, at, or to one side of **oto-** = side **gland** = a cell, group of cells, or organ producing a secretion	largest of the major salivary glands located within cheek
pharyngeal tonsils (fuh-**rin**-jee-uhl) (**ton**-suh l)	**pharynx** = throat **-al** = pertaining to **tonsil** = mass of lymphoid tissue on each side of the throat	superior-most of the tonsils where the nose blends into the throat; also known as the adenoid
plica fimbriata (**plahy**-kuh) (**fim**-bree- **ah**-tuh)	**plica** = a fold or folding **fimbria** = a fringe or fringed border **-ata** = state of	a slight fold of the mucous membrane on the underside of the tongue; runs laterally on the side of the frenulum

(Continues)

Term and Pronunciation	Meaning of Root and Word Parts	Definition
posterior superior alveolar artery (po-**steer**-ee-er) (s*uh*-**peer**-ee-er) (al-**vee**-*uh*-ler) (**ahr**-t*uh*-ree)	**post-** = behind or at the rear **-or** = indicating state **super** = above, beyond **alveol** = a cavity; socket within jaw that holds tooth **-ar** = belonging to **artery** = blood vessel carrying oxygenated blood	part of maxillary artery that supplies molar and premolar teeth, gingiva, and mucous membrane of maxillary sinus
primary nodes (**prahy**-mer-ee) (nohd)	**primary** = being first; highest in importance **node** = small mass of lymph tissue	any of numerous bean-shaped masses of tissue; situated along the vessels of the lymphatic system
process (**pross**-ess)	**process** = a natural outgrowth	the projection or outgrowth of a bone or tissue
protuberance (proh-**too**-ber-*uh*ns)	**protuberant** = bulging out beyond the surrounding surface **-ant** = condition of	a part that is prominent beyond a surface, like a knob, a bony bump, or elevation
pterygoid (**tar**-ee-goid)	**ptery-** = winglike; region of the sphenoid bone **-oid** = of, relating to, located in	related to the sphenoid bone
pterygoid plexus (**tar**-ee-goid) (**plek**-s*uh*s)	**ptery-** = winglike; region of the sphenoid bone **-oid** = of, relating to, located in **plexus** = a network of nerve or blood vessels	a venous plexus of considerable size; situated between the temporalis muscle and pterygoid muscles
pterygopalatine (tari-ee-goh-**pal**-*uh*-tahyn)	**ptery-** = winglike; region of the sphenoid bone **-go** = of, relating to, located in **palate** = roof of the mouth **-ine** = of, near, or in	related to the region of the sphenoid bone and palatal bone
ramus (**rey**-m*uh*s)	**ramus** = any part or organ that branches from another part	a bony process extending like a branch from a larger bone, especially the ascending part of the lower jaw that makes a joint at the temple
Stensen's duct (sten-**senz**) (duhkt)	**Stensen Niels** = Danish anatomist who discovered duct **duct** = a tube conveying a body fluid	the route that saliva takes from the parotid salivary gland; opens from the cheek into the mouth; also called parotid duct
styloid process (**stahy**-loid) (pros-es)	**styl(o)-** = styloid; relating to any of several slender pointed bone processes, especially the spine that projects from the base of the temporal bone **process** = a natural outgrowth, projection, or appendage	a slender projection of bone, such as that from the lower surface of the temporal bone of the skull
sublingual caruncle (suhb-**ling**-gw*uh* l) (**kar**-uhng-k*uh* l)	**sub-** = under, below, beneath **lingua-** = tongue **-al** = of or relating to **caruncle** = a small, fleshy growth	small, fleshy protuberance at midline of floor of mouth at end of sublingual fold, submandibular gland duct empties from it
superficial temporal vein (soo-per-**fish**-*uh* l) (veyn) (tem-pr-uhl)	**super** = above, beyond **-ficial** = pertaining to the surface of **vein** = blood vessels taking blood from part of the body to the heart **temporal** = related to the temples	a network of veins that join across the scalp and then merge with the maxillary vein
superior vena cava (s*uh*-**peer**-ee-er) (**vee**-n*uh*) (**key**-v*uh*)	**super** = above, beyond **-or** = indicating state **vena** = a vein **cava** = hollow	a large vein carrying deoxygenated blood from the head, arm, and upper body into the heart
thoracic duct (thaw-**ras**-ik) (duhkt)	**thorax** = chest **-ic** = of or pertaining to **duct** = tube to conduct body fluid	the main vessel of the lymphatic system; passing upward in front of the spine and opens into the left subclavian vein
tonsils (**ton**-s*uh* l)	**tonsil** = mass of lymphoid tissue on each side of the throat	either of two small masses of lymphoid tissue in the throat; one on each side of the root of the tongue
trismus (**triz**-m*uh* s)	**trismus** = lockjaw; a spasm of the jaw muscles that makes it difficult to open the mouth	the state or condition of being unable to open the mouth because of sustained contractions of jaw muscles; it is usually associated with a form of tetanus

Term and Pronunciation	Meaning of Root and Word Parts	Definition
tuberosity (too-buh-**ros**-i-tee)	**tubercle** = small rounded projection **-ity** = expressing state	an elevated round process of a bone, a tubercle or nodule
ventral (**ven**-tr*uh* l)	**venter** = belly, abdominal **-al** = pertaining to	underside of tongue
vein (veyn)	**vein** = blood vessels taking blood from part of the body to the heart	vessels carrying oxygen-depleted blood toward the heart
viscerocranium (**vis**-er-*oh*- **krey**-nee-*uh* m)	**viscera** = internal organs **crani-** = part of skull that encloses the brain **-um** = indicating a structure	the portion of the skull derived from the pharyngeal arches
von Ebner's salivary glands (vawn) (**eb**-ner) (*suh*-**lahy-ver**-ee)	**Von Ebner** = Austrian anatomist and histologist who discovered glands **saliva** = a viscid, watery fluid, secreted into the mouth by the salivary glands, functions in the tasting, chewing, and swallowing of food, moistens the mouth, and starts the digestion of starches **-ary** = pertaining to, connected with **glands** = a cell, group of cells, or organ producing a secretion	salivary glands just anterior to the posterior third of the tongue
Wharton's duct (**hwawr**-tn) (duhkt)	**Thomas Wharton** = English physician and anatomist who rediscovered duct **duct** = a tube conveying a body fluid	duct from submandibular gland, opens at sublingual caruncle in floor of mouth
xerostomia (zeer-*uh*-**stoh**-mee-*uh*)	**xero-** = dry **-stome** = mouth **-ia** = disease; pathological or abnormal condition	dryness of mouth; caused by diminished function of the salivary glands due to aging, disease, drug reaction

## CHAPTER 6

Landmarks of the Face and Oral Cavity

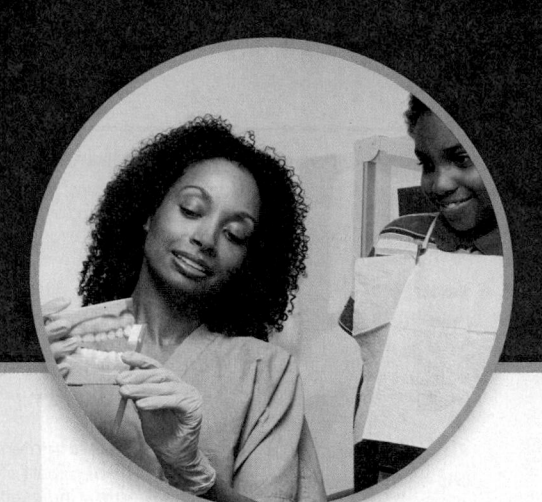

Specific Instructional Objectives

At the completion of this chapter, you will be able to meet these objectives:

1. Use terms presented in this chapter.
2. Identify landmarks in each region of the face.
3. Identify landmarks in the oral cavity.
4. Discuss the boundaries of each division of the oral cavity.
5. List the structures in each division of the oral cavity.
6. Discuss the soft tissues that surround the dentition.

Introduction

The landmarks of the face and oral cavity are usually skeletal or soft tissue structures that are easily recognizable. They are used as reference points in describing the locations of anatomical structures or for taking measurements.

Landmarks of the Face and Oral Cavity

It is important for the dental assistant to be familiar with all the normal structures and areas of the patient's face and oral cavity. It helps to know what is normal in order to identify any abnormal problem areas. Many structures found on the face and in the oral cavity that are normal can vary in appearance from patient to patient. Knowing that structures can vary but still be considered normal is important in the identification of abnormalities.

Landmarks of the Face

There are common landmarks that can be found on every face. Most of the time, the anatomical lines and grooves on the face will get deeper and more prominent. One of the most prominent grooves is the *nasolabial sulcus* or groove. This groove is the line that goes from the side of the nose to the labial *commissure* or corner of the mouth (Figure 6-1A).

The second common groove on the face is the **labiomental groove** that extends from the right to the left under the lower lip and above the chin. This groove is usually not as deep and is not seen in some facial expressions. The **alae (ala)** are the fleshy, flared-out portion of the outside of the nostrils of the nose.

The prominent knob-like boney projection of the chin is called the *mental protuberance*. This can be slight or exaggerated, depending on the person (Figure 6-1A).

The lips or *labia* are an important landmark of the face. Above the upper lip is an indented area that is called the **philtrum**. The transition area around the upper and lower lips where the skin of the face stops and mucosa of the lip starts

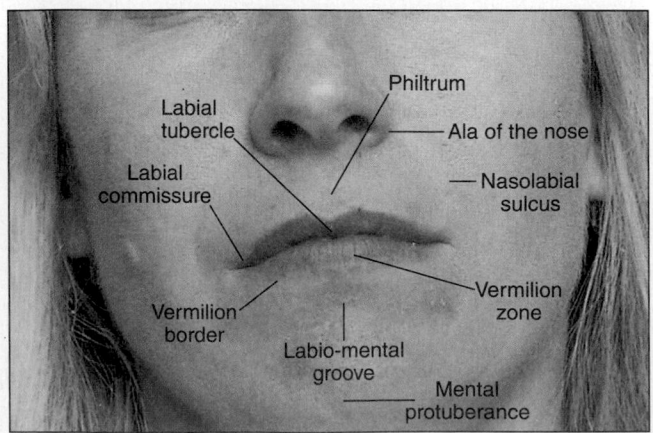

FIGURE 6-1A
Landmarks of the face.

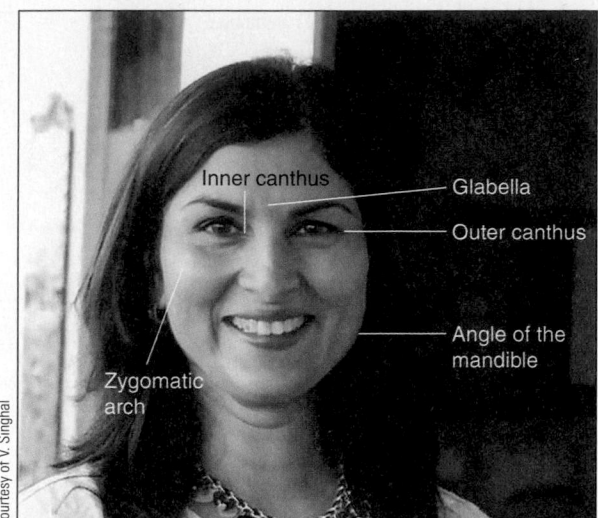

FIGURE 6-1B
Landmarks of the face.

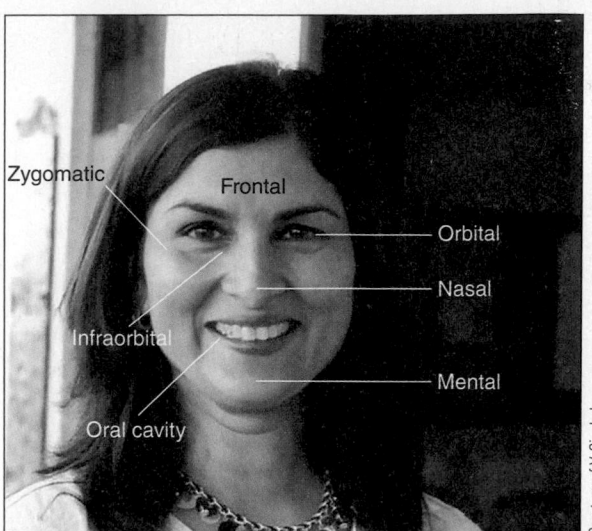

FIGURE 6-2
Regions of the face.

is called the **vermillion border**. The pinkish–red part of the lips is called the vermillion zone and is where you would apply lip balm (Figure 6-1A).

The glabella is the area of the forehead between and above the eyebrows. The inner canthus (inner corner) of the eye and the outer canthus (outer corner of the eye) and naris (nostrils) are three additional important landmarks found on every face. The junction of the lower border of the ramus of the mandible and the body of the mandible is known as the angle of the mandible. The cheekbone or the zygomatic arch is a prominent landmark of the face (Figure 6-1B).

Regions of the Face A few areas or regions of the face can be found on the soft tissues of the face. The area of the forehead termed the *frontal region* is located above the eyes. The area around the eyes is known as the *orbital region*. The area below the eyes is the *infraorbital* region. The *nasal* region is around and including the nose. The *zygomatic* region is over the cheekbone. The oral cavity is centrally located in the oral region, and beneath that is the mental region, which contains the chin or mental protuberance (Figure 6-2).

Structures of the Oral Cavity and Pharynx In order to discuss structures in a professional manner with other dental professionals, it is important to be able to define and identify all structures of the oral cavity. One way to do this is to put them in categories based on location. Before we divide the oral cavity into sections, we need to make sure we have our boundaries identified well. If we think of the mouth as a box with six sides—top, front, back, right side, left side, and bottom—then we can visualize where the boundaries are located. The top boundary is formed by both the hard and soft palates, and the front boundary is formed by the lips. The right and left sides of the box are the

cheeks. The inferior or bottom border is the floor of the mouth. The posterior or back boundary is the pharynx at the throat.

Divisions of the Oral Cavity

The mouth can be divided into two main sections, the **vestibule** and the oral cavity proper.

Vestibule

The vestibule is the area between the cheeks, lips, and teeth. The *vestibular fornix* forms the inferior and superior margins of the oral vestibule (Figure 6-3A).

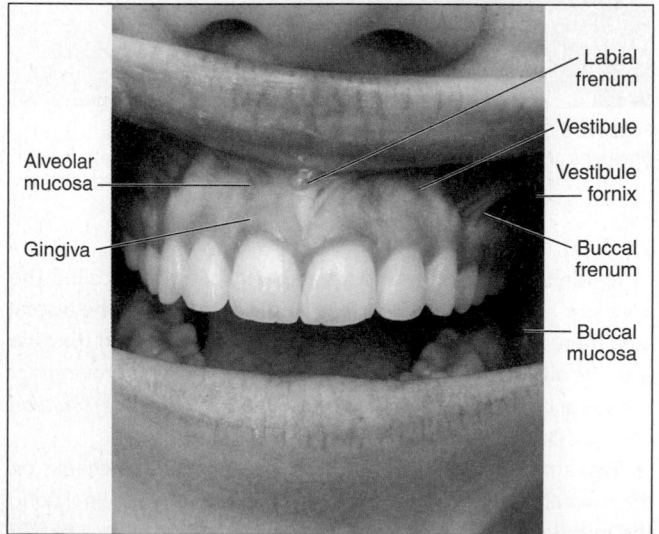

FIGURE 6-3A
Oral vestibule.

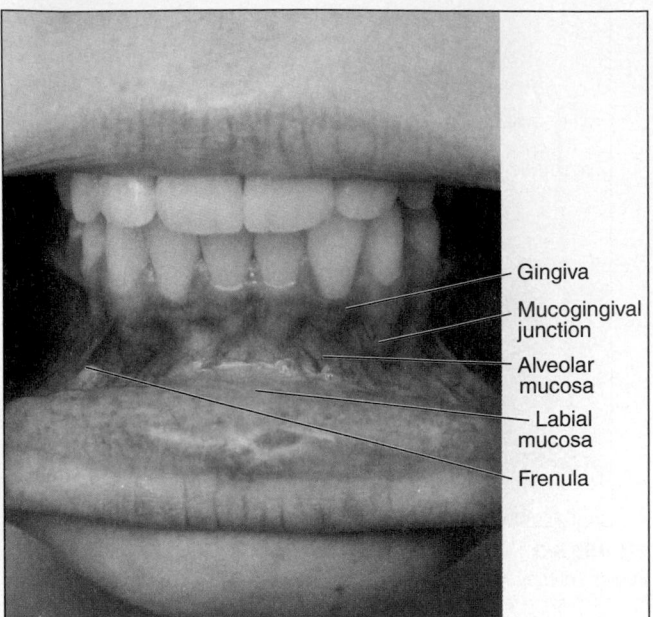

FIGURE 6-3B
Oral vestibule.

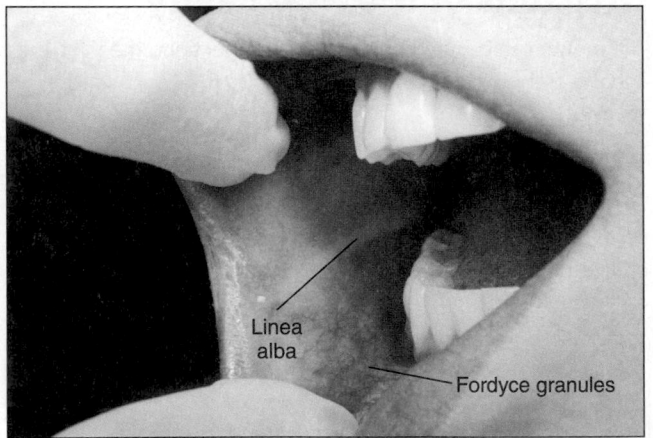

FIGURE 6-3C
Linea alba and Fordyce granules.

Inside the cheeks and lips is a specialized tissue called the **alveolar mucosa**. In the midline and a few areas in the buccal area there are folds of tissue that connect the attached **gingiva** with the alveolar mucosa. These folds are visible when you retract the lips or cheeks and are called *frenula (plural)* or *frenum (singular)* (Figure 6-3a and 6-3B).

Two structures can be found on the inside of the cheeks on the **buccal mucosa** (Figure 6-3A). A thin, raised white line along the middle of the cheek is called **linea alba**. It can be a partial line, full line, appear **bilaterally**, or *unilaterally* (only on one side and not the other). Another common finding that can be seen on the labial and/or buccal mucosa are small yellowish granules. These are trapped **sebaceous glands** close to the outer layer of mucosal tissue, and they are called **Fordyce granules**. The linea

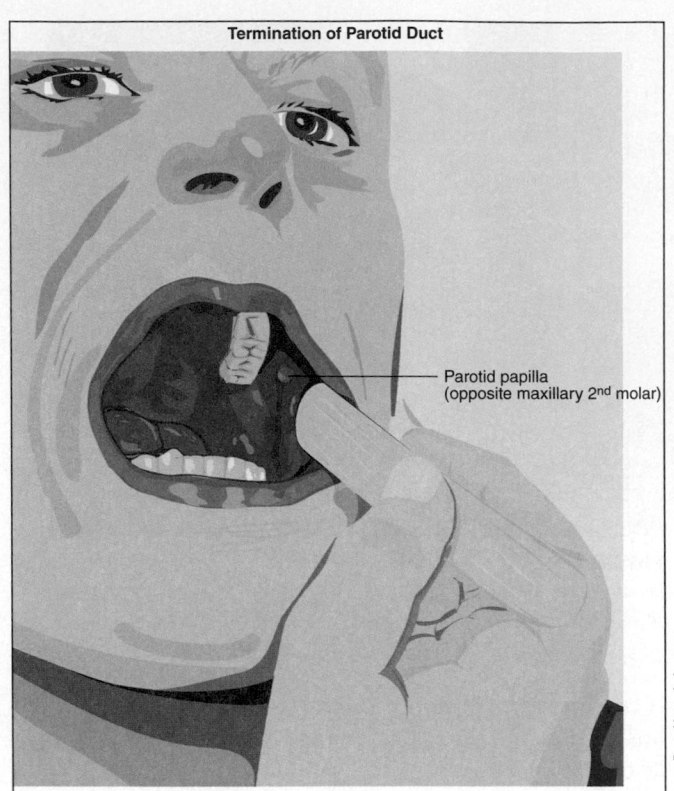

Termination of Parotid Duct

Parotid papilla
(opposite maxillary 2nd molar)

Source: From Netter's Anatomy

FIGURE 6-4
Parotid papilla and Stensen's duct.

alba and Fordyce granules are both typical but may not be present in everyone (Figure 6-3C).

Inside the buccal mucosa in the posterior near the maxillary second molar is the parotid papilla. The papilla is a small bump that has an opening through which saliva from the parotid gland empties into the oral cavity. The duct through which the saliva from the parotid gland travels is known as Stensen's duct. The duct varies in size from patient to patient. In some patients the papilla may be flat and in others it may be more prominent (Figure 6-4).

Oral Cavity Proper

The oral cavity proper is the rest of the mouth excluding the vestibule. If you close your mouth with teeth together and slide your tongue around inside, this is the oral cavity proper. Your tongue is inside the oral cavity proper and as you move and touch the inside of the teeth, the floor of the mouth, and the roof of the mouth, then you can feel the borders of the oral cavity proper. The following sections describe the structures of the oral cavity proper.

Posterior Boundary: Pharynx   There are several structures to identify in the pharynx. The *palatine tonsils* are rounded masses of lymphatic tissue with crypts or deep folds in them and are found on the right and left sides of the opening of the throat (Figure 6-5). The tonsils are part of the lymphatic system of the body. They help filter out toxins and protect the body against disease processes.

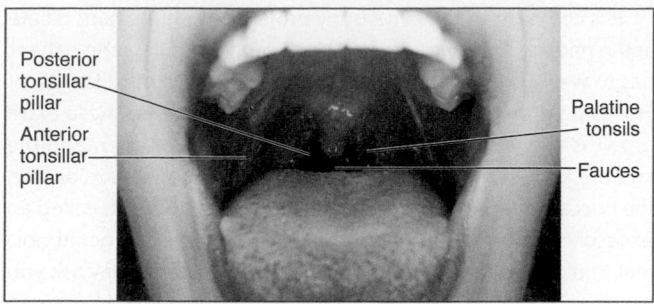

FIGURE 6-5
Landmarks of the oropharynx area.

The palatine tonsils are found embedded between these two folds of tissue (Figure 6-5).

The **retromolar pad** (Figure 6-7) is the triangular area of soft tissue found behind the last mandibular molar on each side of the mandibular dental arch. This area is palpated during an intraoral exam to determine if wisdom teeth are erupting, or after

There is another pair of tonsils above the palatine tonsils in the nasopharynx above the throat area where you cannot clinically see. These are the pharyngeal tonsils, also called the **adenoids**. Usually when someone has to have their palatine tonsils surgically removed, they may have their adenoids or pharyngeal tonsils removed as well. When we include these two sets of tonsils along with the lingual tonsils that are located on the posterior third of the dorsum of the tongue, we have a ring of tonsillar tissue called **Waldeyer's ring**. These three sets of tonsils work together to protect us from toxins and pathogens that are ingested (Figure 6-6).

In the pharynx or posterior part of the oral cavity are two structures known as the anterior and posterior pillars of **fauces**. The anterior pillars (*palatoglossal arches*) extend laterally, downward and forward to the lateral portion of the base of the tongue. The posterior pillars (*palatopharyngeal arches*) are larger and extend laterally, down and back to the lateral area of the pharynx.

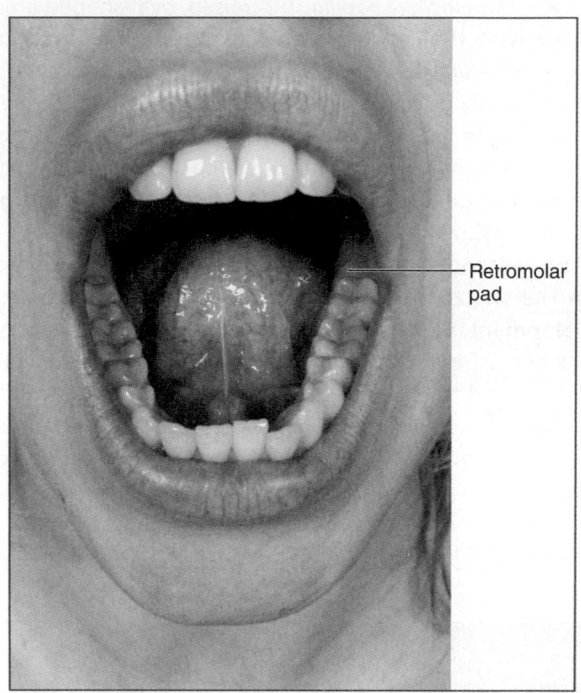

FIGURE 6-7
Retromolar pad.

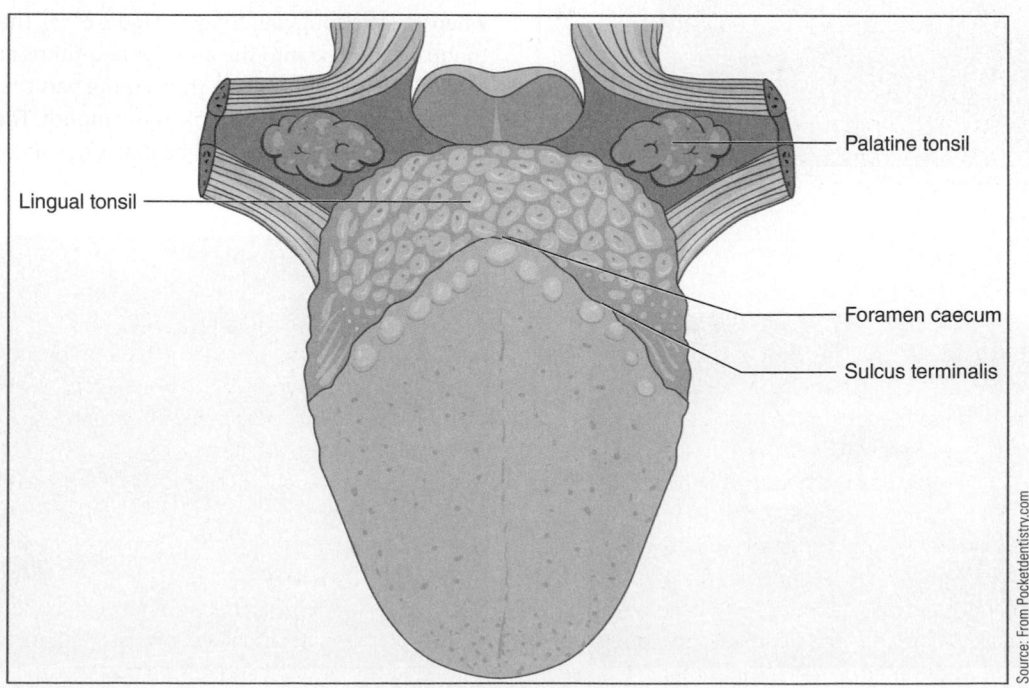

FIGURE 6-6
Lingual and palatine tonsils.

an extraction to ensure that there are no root fragments remaining. A similar area exists on the maxillary arch, but it is called the **maxillary tuberosity** and is a dense bony area (Figure 6-8).

Superior Boundary: Hard Palate

There are several structures to identify on the hard and soft palate. Behind the central incisors on the maxilla is a raised area of soft tissue called the *incisive papilla*. This raised, oval-shaped area of tissue covers the incisive foramen where blood vessels and nerves exit from the anterior portion of the palate. Near the incisive papilla but closer to the laterals and canines are small, raised, wrinkle-like folds of tissue that are called **palatal rugae**. These give the anterior portion of the palate a roughened texture and can be slightly raised or exaggerated depending on the patient (Figure 6-8).

The center of the palate has a line or **midpalatine raphe** over the two halves of the palate that were joined during development. Sometimes this line is raised and very easy to see, while other times the raphe is a barely visible small line. It will extend from behind the palatal rugae at the midline and extend to where the soft palate starts down the center of the palate (Figure 6-8). At the location of the **posterior nasal spine** and soft palate border are two small indentations called **fovea palatini** (Figure 6-9). These two indentations are the openings of ducts to the minor palatine salivary glands.

It is common to see extra bony projections on the hard palate at the midline. This extra bone is not a problem unless the patient has to wear a partial or full denture made for the maxillary arch. This extra growth of bone is called a **palatal torus**. These extra growths may also occur on the lingual aspect of the mandible and are known as **mandibular tori**. If extra bone develops on the buccal surface of the maxilla (or mandible), then it is called an **exostosis**. These are both examples of extra bone and not abnormal. You will not find this on everyone, but patients may ask you what the structure is (Figures 6-10 to 6-12).

Superior Boundary: Soft Palate

As we move farther back on the palate from the hard palate to the soft palate, we will see a definite color change. The soft palate does not have any bone under it, so it will be flexible and more red or more pink in color as compared to the hard palate. The shorter soft palate goes toward the posterior boundary where it blends in with the structures in the back of the mouth. At the midline of the soft palate is a structure that hangs down into the area of the fauces. This hanging structure is the *uvula*, and it aids in swallowing (Figure 6-5). If there is a disruption in the development of the palate later during fusion, the uvula can be split into two pieces called a *bifid* uvula.

Inferior Boundary: Tongue

The tongue and floor of the mouth are in the bottom of the mouth and considered the inferior boundary. The tongue is a fleshy, strong muscular organ attached to the floor of the mouth. The tongue is an important muscle as it aids in mastication of food and also allows us to speak. The salivary glands are exocrine glands that produce saliva.

Body: Dorsal Surface: Tongue Structure

The tongue is a broad flattened muscle in the mouth. The top surface is called the dorsum or *dorsal surface*. The dorsum is the surface you see when you stick out your tongue (Figure 6-13). The structure of the tongue is divided into the anterior two-thirds and the posterior one-third. The anterior two-thirds is the part that is found inside the oral cavity when you look in the mouth. The posterior one-third is located in the throat area that is not visible.

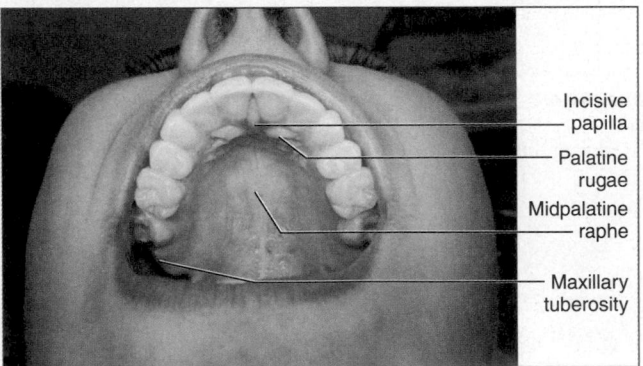

Incisive papilla
Palatine rugae
Midpalatine raphe
Maxillary tuberosity

FIGURE 6-8
Maxillary tuberosity.

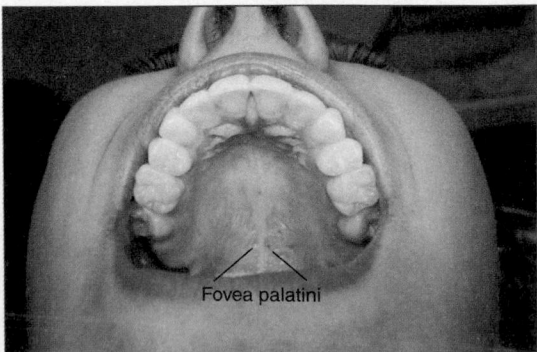

Fovea palatini

FIGURE 6-9
Fovea palatini.

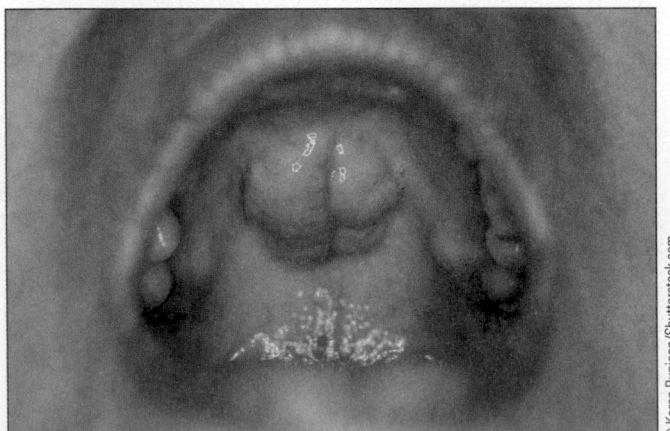

© Karan Bunjean/Shutterstock.com

FIGURE 6-10
Palatal torus.

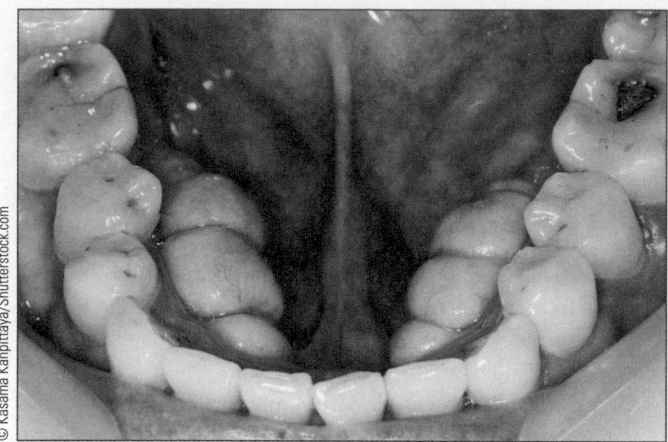

FIGURE 6-11
Mandibular tori.

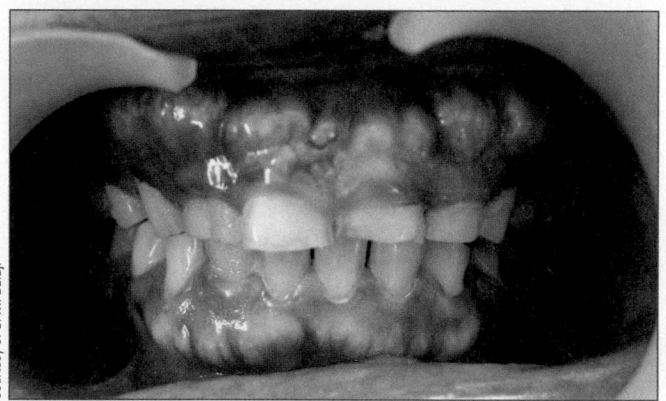

FIGURE 6-12
Buccal exostoses.

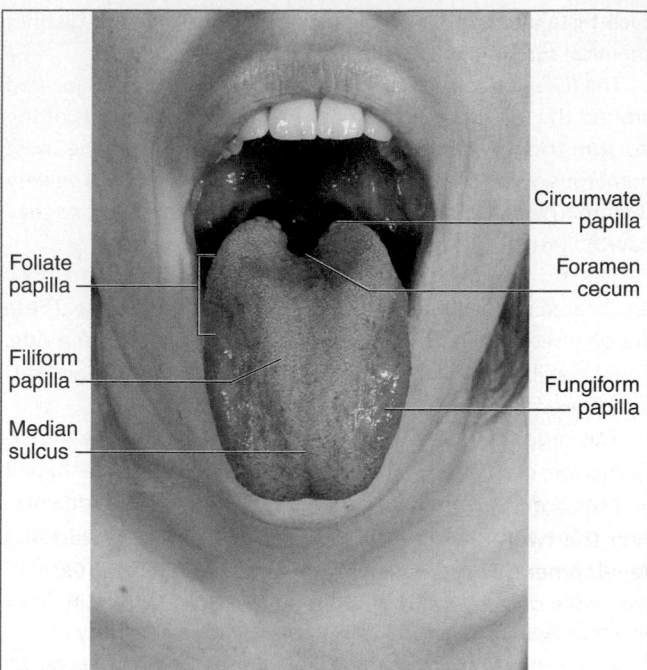

FIGURE 6-13
Dorsum of tongue.

The posterior one-third is known as the pharyngeal part and is attached in the throat and back of the oral cavity. It also contains specialized tissue called the *lingual tonsils*. The posterior of the tongue is divided by the *sulcus terminalis* (Figure 6-6). It is an inverted V-shaped line that extends horizontally from the right to the left side of the tongue where the posterior one-third meets the anterior two-thirds. This central area has an indented pit that is called the *foramen cecum*. This pit area is the embryonic origin of part of the thyroid gland. As the neck develops, the thyroid tissue slides down to its natural place in the middle of the neck. The only remnant left that the thyroid was there is the small pinpoint indentation in the middle of the sulcus terminalis. The term *foramen cecum* indicates that it is a hole, but not in this case (Figure 6-13).

Another line that is found on the dorsum of the tongue is the *median lingual sulcus*. This line divides the tongue into right and left halves extending along the middle of the tongue from posterior to anterior. Sometimes this line is easy to see because it is slightly depressed, but it varies from patient to patient (Figure 6-13).

Papillae The whole dorsum of the tongue is covered with mucous membrane and raised specialized tissue called **papillae**. Four types of papillae cover the dorsum of the tongue.

The *fungiform* papillae can be found on the anterior two-thirds of the dorsum of the tongue and are shaped like a mushroom with a base and rounded top. They are brighter red in color than the rest of the tongue and look like small round, raised dots on the tongue. They are the second-most numerous in number and do contain taste buds in the center (Figure 6-13). Taste buds are the small cells that help you differentiate different flavors on your tongue like sweet, salty, sour, and bitter (Figure 6-14). There are 2,000–8,000 taste buds embedded in the papilla of the upper surface of the tongue, soft palate, upper esophagus, cheek, and epiglottis. This great span in number of taste buds contributes to the difference in taste sensations experienced by individuals.

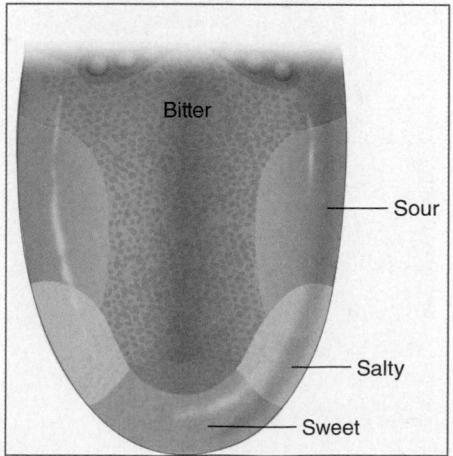

FIGURE 6-14
Location of taste buds.

Each taste bud contains receptor cells that respond to distinct chemical stimuli.

The *filiform* papillae are spike-shaped, hairlike papilla located around the fungiform papilla on the anterior two-thirds of the dorsum tongue. These tiny, pointed elevations are the most numerous of the lingual papillae and give the tongue its velvety texture. The filiform papillae do not contain taste buds, so they have no taste function (Figure 6-13).

The third type is called the *foliate* papillae, and they are located on the lateral posterior borders of the tongue. These are only seen if the tongue is extended and turned to the side. These papillae look like folds and give the sides a roughened surface. These papillae contain taste buds (Figure 6-14).

The largest papillae on the dorsum of the tongue are the *circumvallate papilla* or *vallate papilla*. They are doughnut-shaped and the fewest in number with only 8–12 elevations found anterior to the sulcus terminalis. These are the largest papilla and most elevated of all the lingual papilla, and each is surrounded by a sulcus that contains taste buds and serous glands. In these tiny trenches surrounded by the papillae are small salivary glands called *Von Ebner's salivary glands* that deposit a serous secretion into the sulci to keep them clean and free of food debris. The circumvallate papilla are also harder to see unless the tongue is grasped with a gauze square and pulled forward (Figure 6-13).

Body: Ventral Surface: Tongue Structure The *ventral* surface of the tongue is the underside of the tongue. The covering of the ventral surface is significantly different from the dorsal surface because the tissue on the ventral surface is a much thinner mucous membrane. Because the tissue is thinner, the

blood vessels may be able to be seen under the tissue, and this same mucous membrane continues onto the floor of the mouth.

There are several structures to mention on this part of the tongue. The main structure is the *lingual frenum*, which is a long band-like tissue at the midline that attaches the ventral surface of the tongue to the floor of the mouth. The *sublingual folds* are soft tissue folds located on each side of the frenum. When the tongue is lifted toward the palate, the lingual frenum is pulled against itself and will limit how far the tongue can be lifted. Some people have the frenum attached closer to the tip or apex of the tongue and it cannot be lifted very far. This is known as *ankyloglossia* or tongue-tied (Figure 6-15).

On each side of the lingual frenum are fringed folds called *plica fimbriata* that run parallel with the lingual frenum. Some people have exaggerated fringes of tissue on these folds that look like strands of tissue. Some people will not have the fringed areas that are so obvious. This is one of the structures under the tongue that is normal but may look unusual (Figure 6-15).

Lingual veins on the ventral surface of the tongue appear bluish and are sometimes raised structures alongside the lingual frenum and plica fimbriata. As the patient ages, the lingual veins may become more prominent. The sublingual glands are drained via 8–20 ducts of Rivinus. The largest duct, known as the duct of Bartholin, joins with the submandibular duct and drains through the sublingual caruncles located in each side of the lingual frenum (Figure 6-15).

Inferior Boundary: Soft Tissues Under the Tongue As we continue on the inferior boundary of the mouth, we will identify the appearance of this area. The tissue is lighter in color and thinner, and blood vessels may be more visible in this area. The vessels will appear as thin blue lines within the tissues (Figure 6-15).

The Teeth There are two primary parts of a tooth: the crown and the root.

Crown of the Tooth The part of the tooth that you can see when you smile is called the *crown* of the tooth. The crowns are shaped differently depending on the type of tooth. They are covered on the outside by the strongest tissue of the body called **enamel**, which protects the tooth (Figure 6-16).

Root of the Tooth The roots of the teeth are covered in **cementum** and are not visible in most cases because they are embedded in the alveolar bone of the maxilla and the mandible. The line where the enamel of the crown meets the cementum of the root is called the *cementoenamel* junction or the CEJ (Figure 6-17). The roots of the teeth may become visible in the presence of periodontal disease. Periodontal disease results in gingival recession leading to exposure of the surfaces of the roots of the teeth. Periodontal disease will be discussed in detail in Chapter 38.

Soft Tissues of the Dentition Healthy gingivae are usually coral pink, but may contain **melanin** pigmentation (Figure 6-18A and Figure 6-18B). The gingival tissue is divided into sections that we will identify as free gingiva and attached gingiva.

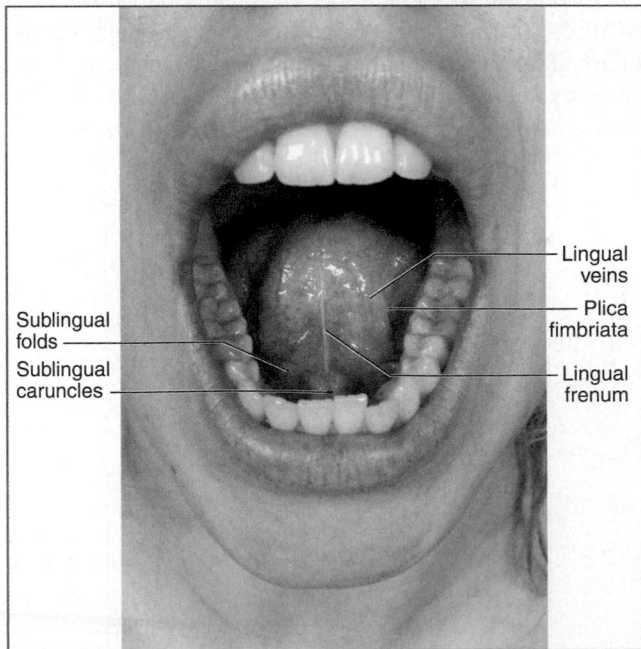

Sublingual folds
Sublingual caruncles
Lingual veins
Plica fimbriata
Lingual frenum

FIGURE 6-15
Ventral surface of tongue.

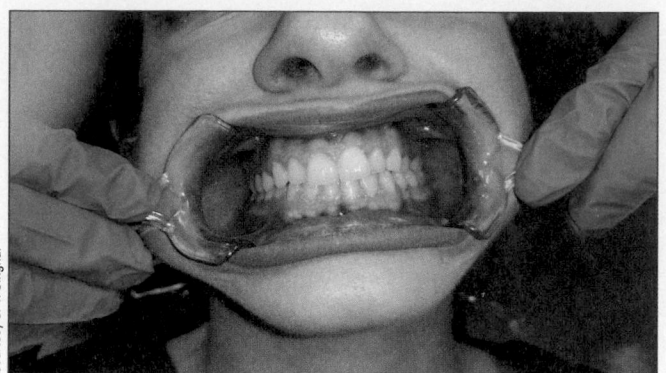

FIGURE 6-16
Crown of tooth with enamel.

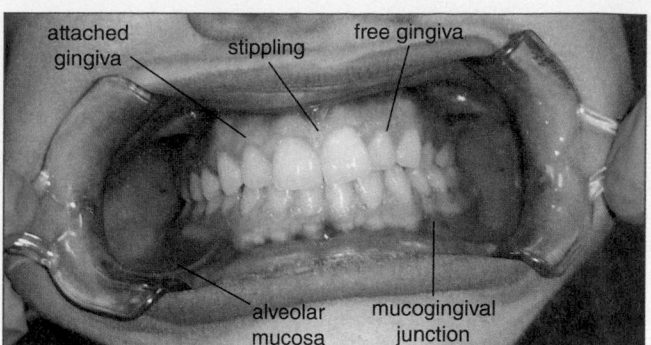

FIGURE 6-18A
Healthy gingiva.

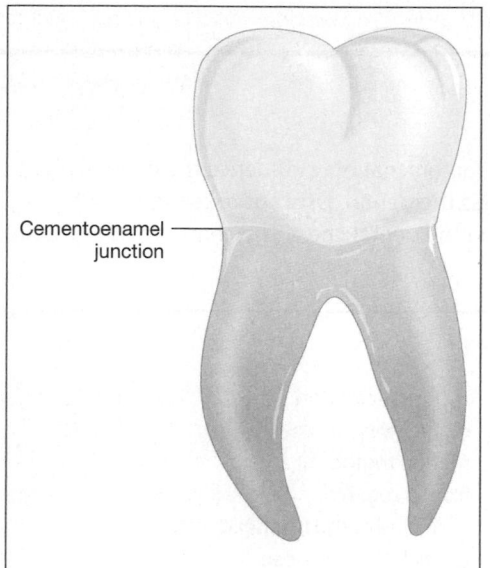

FIGURE 6-17
Cementoenamel junction (CEJ).

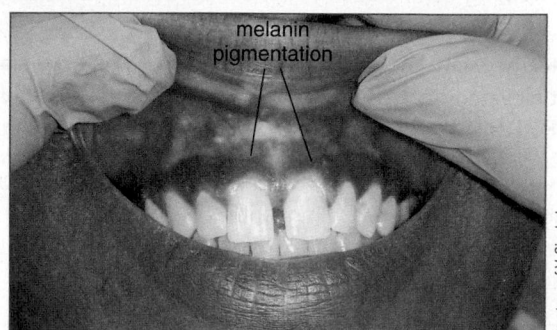

FIGURE 6-18B
Healthy gingiva with melanin pigmentation.

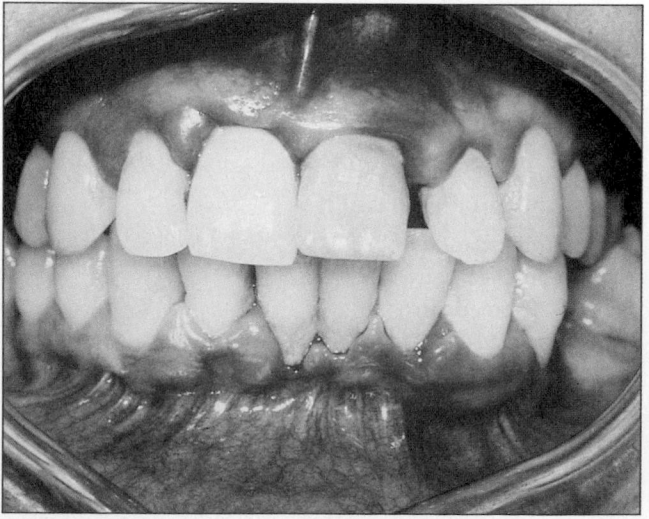

FIGURE 6-19
Unhealthy gingiva.

Free Gingiva The free gingiva (marginal gingiva) is the first type of gingival tissue that starts where the gingiva is in contact with the tooth (Figure 6-18A). The edge or highest area of the tissue is called the gingival margin. This margin can be located at different levels of the tooth. Normal healthy tissue has a margin that is slightly above the CEJ of the crown of the tooth or *coronally* (Figure 6-18A).

The free gingiva is unattached from the alveolar bone and it is normally one to three millimeters of tissue starting at the margin. This is the tissue into which you can place the tip of a periodontal probe or under which you can floss. The space between the free gingiva and the tooth that the periodontal probe or floss slides into is called the *gingival sulcus*. The sulcus is the natural space between the tooth and the cuff of soft tissue that surrounds the tooth. In health, the sulcus is between one to three millimeters deep. The base of the sulcus is the *epithelial attachment* to the alveolar bone. The free gingiva tissue is movable and also fills in the triangular area between adjacent teeth. This triangular area

of soft tissue is called the *interdental papilla*. In healthy gingiva, the free gingiva is flat and knife-edged or pointed between the teeth, but when disease is present, the free gingiva can become enlarged, swollen, and red, or the interdental papilla can become blunted or flat (Figure 6-19). As we move away from the margin and free gingiva we go across a structure on the gingiva called the *free gingival groove* or marginal groove. This marks where the free gingiva stops and the attached gingiva begins. It is a very slight depressed line or indentation that can be difficult to see (Figure 6-18A).

Attached Gingiva The attached gingiva is the tissue that is attached to the bones of the maxilla or mandible. Healthy attached gingiva is thicker and more keratinized than the lining mucosa, which covers the ventral surface of the tongue, floor of the mouth, and inside of the cheeks and lips as well as the soft palate and the alveolar bone. The keratinization helps resist the friction of food while chewing. This tissue has a *stippled* or orange peel appearance (Figure 6-18A). This stippling is caused by the fibers attaching the tissue to the bone beneath it. In health, this stippling can be seen when the tissue is dried and gives the appearance of an orange peel. In disease, the stippling can disappear because of swelling, and the tissue will look smooth, red, and shiny. As we move away from the attached gingiva, we go across another boundary that marks where the attached gingiva meets the next type of tissue called the alveolar mucosa. The junction of these tissues is called the **mucogingival junction** or MGJ. This line is scalloped and can be seen where these two tissues meet. It marks the end of the gingiva and beginning of the mucous membrane type of tissue that lines the cheeks and lips (Figure 6-18A).

The alveolar mucosa is a thinner and less keratinized tissue that lines the maxillary and mandibular lips and inside the cheeks. This tissue is found inside the vestibules along the maxilla and mandible and on both sides of the mouth and in the front along the lips.

Chapter Summary

As a vital team member, the dental assistant needs to be able to recognize factors that may influence the general physical health of the patient. Understanding landmarks of the face and oral cavity enables the dental assistant to recognize what is abnormal and what is normal. For this reason, accuracy is important when completing the dental chart. The chart provides a point of comparison for future visits.

Review Questions

1. Match the landmark with the description.
   1. nasolabial sulcus
   2. commissure
   3. labiomental groove
   4. ala
   5. philtrum
   6. vermillion border
   7. glabella
   8. inner canthus
   9. outer canthus
   10. zygomatic arch
       a. Goes right to left under the lower lip and above the chin
       b. Goes from side of nose to corner of lip
       c. Corner of lip
       d. Fleshy part of nostrils
       e. Pinkish-red part of lips
       f. Indented area above the center of the upper lip
       g. Inner corner of eye
       h. Area between and above the eyebrows
       i. Outer corner of eye
       j. Cheekbone

2. Match the region of the face with the correct description.
   1. orbital region
   2. nasal region
   3. zygomatic region
   4. oral region
   5. mental region
   6. frontal region
      a. Includes the forehead
      b. Includes the nose
      c. Includes the eyes
      d. Includes the cheekbones
      e. Includes the mouth
      f. Includes the chin

3. What are the two main division of the oral cavity?
   a. vestibule and oral cavity proper
   b. vestibule and pharynx
   c. oral cavity proper and pharynx
   d. pharynx and hard palate

4. Which of the following is not correct regarding linea alba?
   a. It is found on the buccal mucosa.
   b. It is always bilateral.
   c. It can be a partial line or a full line.
   d. All of these are correct.

5. Fordyce granules are trapped sebaceous glands *and* are visible on everyone.
   Select the correct response based on the preceding statements.
   a. Both statements are true.
   b. Both statements are false.
   c. The first statement is true; the second statement is false.
   d. The first statement is false; the second statement is true.

6. Which of the following is correct regarding the parotid papilla?
   a. The papilla is located on the buccal mucosa near the maxillary first premolar.
   b. The duct through which the saliva from the parotid gland travels is Stensen's duct.
   c. The papilla is quite prominent and visible in all patients.
   d. All of these are correct.

7. The anterior pillars are larger than the posterior pillars of fauces. The anterior pillars extend laterally, downward, and forward to the lateral portion of the base of the tongue.
   Select the correct response based on the preceding statements.
   a. Both statements are true.
   b. Both statements are false.
   c. The first statement is true; the second statement is false.
   d. The first statement is false; the second statement is true.

8. The retromolar pad is the triangular area of soft tissue found behind the last maxillary molar. A similar landmark exists in the mandibular arch and is known as the tuberosity.
   Select the correct response based on the preceding statements.
   a. Both statements are true.
   b. Both statements are false.
   c. The first statement is true; the second statement is false.
   d. The first statement is false; the second statement is true.

9. Which of the following landmarks are wrinkled folds of tissue that give the anterior portion of the palate its roughened texture?
   a. midpalatine raphe
   b. incisive papilla
   c. palatal rugae
   d. fovea palatini

10. A bony projection seen at the midline of the palate is known as a(n) _____.
    a. maxillary torus
    b. mandibular tori
    c. exostosis
    d. palatal rugae

11. Which of the following structures of the dorsum of the tongue is the embryonic origin of part of the thyroid gland?
    a. sulcus terminalis
    b. foramen cecum
    c. foliate papilla
    d. median lingual sulcus

12. The inverted V-shaped structure that extends horizontally from the right to the left side of the tongue where the posterior one-third meets the anterior two-thirds is called the_____.
    a. sulcus terminalis
    b. foramen cecum
    c. foliate papilla
    d. median lingual sulcus

13. Identify the papilla with the correct description.
    1. foliate
    2. filiform
    3. fungiform
    4. circumvallate
       a. Found on anterior two-third of tongue, second-most numerous in number, contains taste buds
       b. Located on anterior two-third of tongue and are most numerous in number; do not contain taste buds
       c. Located on lateral posterior border of tongue and contain taste buds
       d. Largest in size and fewest in number; each is surrounded by a sulcus with taste buds and serous glands

14. Which of the following structures are located on the ventral surface of the tongue?
    a. plica fimbriata
    b. circumvallate papilla
    c. median lingual sulcus
    d. foramen cecum

15. The crown portion of the teeth is covered in enamel, *and* the roots of the teeth are covered in cementum.
    Select the correct response based on the preceding statements.
    a. Both statements are true.
    b. Both statements are false.
    c. The first statement is true; the second statement is false.
    d. The first statement is false; the second statement is true.

16. The fringed folds that run parallel with the lingual frenum are called_____.
    a. sublingual caruncles
    b. sublingual veins
    c. plica fimbriata
    d. sulcus terminalis

17. Which of the following is correct regarding the free gingival margin?
    a. Healthy tissue has a margin that is slightly coronal to the CEJ.
    b. The free gingiva is attached to the alveolar bone.
    c. In health, the tissue is enlarged, swollen, and red.
    d. None of these are correct.

18. Which landmark denotes where the free gingiva stops and the attached gingiva begins?
    a. mucogingival junction
    b. sulcus
    c. free gingival groove
    d. epithelial attachment

19. Which of the following is false regarding the attached gingiva?
    a. It is keratinized.
    b. It has a stippled appearance.
    c. It is attached to the bone of the maxilla and the mandible.
    d. It covers the ventral surface of the tongue and the soft palate.

20. Which of the following structures is not considered to be part of the vestibule?
    a. tongue
    b. alveolar mucosa
    c. Fordyce granules
    d. linea alba

Critical Thinking

1. What structures make up the boundaries of the oral cavity?
2. What are the structures in the vestibule of the oral cavity?
3. What are the structures in the oral cavity proper?

Key Terms

Term and Pronunciation	Meaning of Root and Word Parts	Definition
adenoid (**ad**-n-oid)	**aden-** = gland **-oid** = resembling, like	an enlarged mass of lymphoid tissue in the upper pharynx
ala (**ey**-luh)	**ala** = a winglike part, process	flared-out portion of the outside of the nostrils
alveolar mucosa (al-**vee**-uh-ler) (myoo-**koh**-suh)	**alveol-** = alveolus; tooth socket **-ar** = belonging to **mucosa** = a mucus-secreting membrane that lines body cavities or passages	mucous membrane apical to attached gingiva
bilaterally (bahy-**lat**-er-uh-lee)	**bi-** = two **later** = side **-al** = pertaining to	affecting two or both sides
buccal mucosa (**buhk**-uh l) (myoo-**koh**-suh)	**bucc-** = cheek **-al** = pertaining to **mucosa** = a mucus-secreting membrane that lines body cavities or passages	inside lining of the cheeks
cementum (si-**men**-tuh m)	**cementum** = layer of calcified tissue that covers outside of root	a thin bone-like tissue that covers the dentin in the root of a tooth; forms the outer surface of the root of the tooth
enamel (ih-**nam**-uh l)	**enamel** = outer surface of the crown of the tooth	hard, glistening substance covering coronal (crown) dentin of tooth, made up of 90% hydroxyapatite and about 6% calcium carbonate, calcium fluoride, and magnesium carbonate, with 4% of organic matrix of protein
exostosis (ek-so-**stoh**-sis)	**ex-** = out, from **oste-** = bone **-osis** = denoting actions, conditions	the abnormal formation of a bony growth on a bone or tooth
fauces (**faw**-seez)	**fauces** = space between the cavity of the mouth and the pharynx	area between oral cavity and pharynx bounded by soft palate and lingual base
Fordyce granules (**fawr**- dahys) (**gran**-yool)	**John Addison Fordyce** = American dermatologist discovered granules **granule** = enclosed grainy (any small, hard) matter found in a cell	a normal condition marked by the presence of numerous small, yellowish-white bodies or granules on the inner surface of the cheek and vermilion border of the lips; visible sebaceous glands
fovea palatine (**foh**-vee-uh) (**pal**-uh-tahyn)	**fovea** = any small pit or depression in the surface of a bodily organ or part **palate** = the roof of the mouth **-ine** = of or pertaining to	two small depressions in the posterior aspect of the palate, one on each side of the midline, at or near the attachment of the soft palate to the hard palate

Term and Pronunciation	Meaning of Root and Word Parts	Definition
frenulum (frenula plural) (**fren**-y*uh*-l*uh* m)	**frenum** = a band of fibrous tissue that checks or restrains the motion of a part **-ule** = indicating smallness **-um** = used when describing single parts	fold of mucous membranes that attaches two areas; as the fold on the underside of the tongue
gingiva (gingivae *pl*) (jin-**jahy**-v*uh*)	**gingiv-** = technical name for gum **-a** = plural ending	portion of the oral mucous membrane that covers and is attached to the necks of the teeth and the alveolar process of the jaws
labiomental groove (**ley**-bee-*oh*- **men**-tl) (groov)	**labium** = lip or liplike part **mentum** = chin or chin-like part **-al** = pertaining to **groove** = narrow depression in a surface	a depression that passes between the lip and the chin
linea alba (**lee**-ne-ah) (**ahl**-b*uh*)	**linea** = a line **alba** = white matter	white horizontal line on the inner surface of the cheek level with the biting plane
mandibular tori (man-**dib**-y*uh*-ler) (**tawr**-ahy)	**mandible** = lower jaw **-ar** = pertaining to **torus** = a rounded ridge; protuberance	a bony growth in the mandible along the surface nearest to the tongue
maxillary tuberosity (**mak**-s*uh*-ler-ee) (too-b*uh*-**ros**-i-tee)	**maxilla** = upper jaw **-ary** = of or relating to **tuber** = a localized rounded projection, a knob **-ose** = full of **-ity** = expressing condition	bulging extremity of the posterior of the body of the maxilla behind the last molar tooth
melanin (**mel**-*uh*-nin)	**pingere** = to paint	natural coloring of hair, skin, and soft tissues of oral cavity
midpalatal raphe (**mid**) (**pal**-*uh*-tl) (**rey**-fee)	**mid-** = middle **palate** = the roof of the mouth **-al** = pertaining to **raphe** = a seamlike union between two parts or halves of an organ	the ridge of oral mucosa that marks the median line of the hard palate
mucogingival junction (myoo-**koh**- jin-**jahy**-v*uh* l) (**juhngk**-sh*uh* n)	**muco-** = mucous membrane; lubricating lining of the oral cavity **gingiv-** = technical name for gum **-al** = pertaining to **junction** = area where 2 or more things unite	where the boundaries of the freely movable mucosa of the cheeks and floor of the mouth join to the gingiva; recognized by where the darker-colored mucosa meet the lighter pink of the gingiva
palatal ruga (ae plural) (**pal**-*uh*-tl) (**roo**-g*uh*)	**palate** = the roof of the mouth **-al** = pertaining to **ruga** = a wrinkle, fold, or ridge	mucosal ridges on the anterior of the roof of the mouth
palatal torus (**pal**-*uh*-tl) (**tawr**-*uh* s)	**palate** = the roof of the mouth **-al** = pertaining to **torus** = a rounded ridge; protuberance	a bony growth in the roof of the mouth usually present on the midline of the hard palate
philtrum (**fil**-tr*uh* m)	**philtrum** = dimple in the middle of the upper lip	indentation or groove on upper lip directly below the tip of the nose; also referred to as infranasal depression
posterior nasal spine (po-**steer**-ee-er) (**ney**-z*uh* l) (spahyn)	**posterior** = situated behind or at the rear of **naso-** = nose **-al** = of, or relating to **spine** = any bone-like part	the medial end of the posterior border of the union of the palatal bones; is sharp and pointed
retromolar pad (re-troh- **moh**-ler) (pad)	**retro-** = behind, back, backward **molar** = any of the last three teeth in a quadrant **pad** = a cushion-like mass of tissue	a cushioned mass of tissue located on the alveolar process of the mandible behind the area of the last natural molar

(Continues)

Term and Pronunciation	Meaning of Root and Word Parts	Definition
sebaceous glands (si-**bey**-sh*uh* s) (gland)	**sebum** = oily, fatty secretion that acts as a lubricant **-aceous** = having the nature of **gland** = a cell, group of cells, or organ producing a secretion	microscopic exocrine glands in the skin that secrete an oily or waxy matter called sebum
vermillion border (ver-**mil**-y*uh* n) (**bawr**-der)	**vermilion** = a scarlet red **border** = a band or margin around or along the edge of something	sharp line of color change between the margin of the lip and normal skin
vestibule (**ves**-t*uh*-byool)	**vestibule** = entrance; cavities forming an approach to entrance to another cavity	small cavity or space, in dental area between cheeks, lips, and teeth
Waldeyer's ring (vawl-**dahy**-ur) (ring)	**Heinrich Waldeyer** = German anatomist named ring **ring** = a circular or surrounding line mark	the palatine, pharyngeal, and lingual tonsils encircle the pharynx

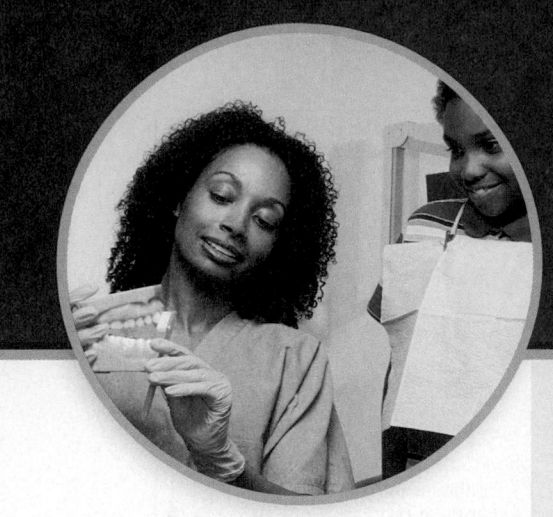

## CHAPTER 7

Embryology and Histology

Specific Instructional Objectives

At the completion of this chapter, you will be able to meet these objectives:

1. Use terms presented in this chapter.
2. Discuss the developmental stages of the human from fertilization to birth.
3. Describe the development of the human face.
4. Discuss the development of the following structures of the oral cavity: upper lip, palate, and tongue.
5. Discuss the role of the pharyngeal arches in the development of the structures of the face.
6. Identify the mechanism leading to development of a cleft palate.
7. Describe the various stages of tooth development.
8. Describe the function of the following in relation to tooth development: dental papilla, dental sacs, and enamel organ.
9. Describe changes that occur in the inner enamel epithelial cells as they mature to become ameloblasts.
10. Describe the structural properties of enamel.
11. Describe the structural properties of dentin.
12. Differentiate among the various types of dentin.
13. Discuss the formation of cementum.
14. Define artifacts that may occur in enamel, dentin, or cementum.
15. Describe each of the four tissues of a tooth.
16. State the components of the periodontium.
17. Describe the structure of the following: alveolar process, cementum, periodontal ligament, and gingiva.
18. Define the junctions of the tissues.

Introduction

Dental assistants should be familiar with the general embryological development of the face and the oral cavity and with general histology to understand the composition, formation, and eruption of the teeth. In addition to embryology and histology, this chapter covers the components of the periodontium and describes the structures of the gingiva.

As a dental assistant, you should be able to use proper terminology to describe embryology and development. The key terms highlighted in the chapter focus on the foundations. Additional terms are placed in italic and should be learned as well.

Development of the Orofacial Complex

The term *oro* means oral cavity or mouth and *facial* pertains to the face or structures that make up the face. When we put the two together, *orofacial* means the mouth and face. This lesson will discuss how the oral cavity and face of a human develop from the beginning to birth. Embryology is the study of the development of an **embryo**. The embryo development occurs in three stages from the time of fertilization until birth. We will be looking specifically at how the oral cavity, lips, tongue, and the face develop.

Prenatal Development: Stage 1 Germinal Stage

It all begins with fertilization when the male gamete or sperm fertilizes the female gamete or egg. After this occurs, the **zygote** begins to travel to the uterus to be implanted; this can take place 24–36 hours after conception. The first two weeks is called the germinal stage. The mass of cells divides over and over, multiplying and doubling with every division. The cells then differentiate and the mass of cells is now known as a *blastocyst*. The blastocyst attaches to the wall of the uterus. The blastocyst has three primary germ layers or tissue layers: **ectoderm**, **mesoderm**, and **endoderm**. At this time, the sphere shape starts changing shape into a disc shape with the same layers (Figure 7-1).

Prenatal Development: Stage 2 Embryonic Stage

At the start of the third week, the embryonic period begins and continues through week eight. The embryo divides into three layers that will develop into various body systems. At week four, the neural tube forms; this will become the nervous system. The tube will close to form the brain during this period. Around this same time, the head, eyes, ears, nose, and mouth form. During this stage, the embryo will grow from ⅛ inch to 1 inch in five weeks. The end of the neural tube will start closing and exhibit further growth by developing extensions called processes, or pharyngeal

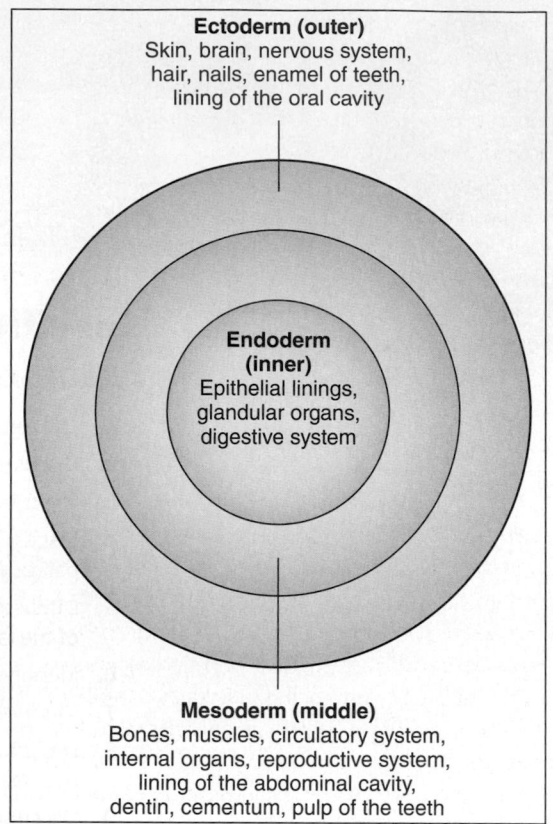

FIGURE 7-1
The three primary embryonic layers—ectoderm (outer), mesoderm (middle), and endoderm (inner)—and associated tissues.

arches. One end of the neural tube will eventually become the head and face and is called the *cephalic* end or cranial end, and the other end or tail end is called the *caudal* end (Figure 7-2).

Prenatal Development: Stage 3 Fetal Stage

From week nine through birth is considered the fetal period. At the beginning of this stage, the embryo is about 1 inch long, and by

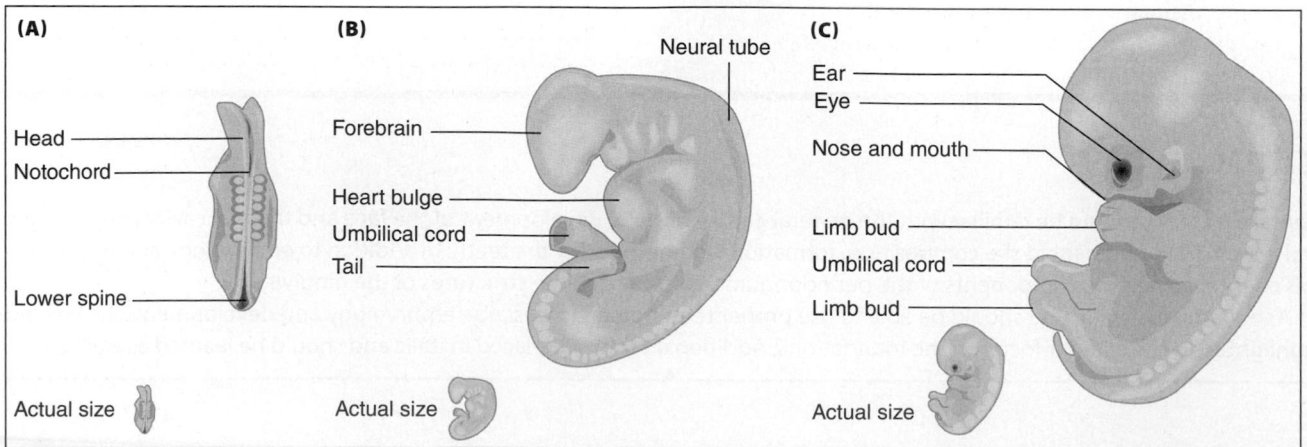

FIGURE 7-2
(A) At 3 weeks the embryo becomes pear shaped and has a rounded head and a rather pointed lower spine, and the notochord (a long flexible rod of cells that supports the body, referred to as a primitive backbone) runs along its back. (B) At 4 weeks the embryo becomes C-shaped and has a visible tail. The forebrain enlarges and an umbilical cord forms. There is also a bulge where the heart is located. (C) At 6 weeks the embryo has visible eyes, mouth, nose, and ears, and the arms and legs are growing from the limb buds. The umbilical cord has enlarged.

3 months, it is 2½ inches in length. At 4 months, the **fetus** is about 4 inches long. A full-term baby is usually approximately 20 inches at birth. Even though it is amazing how fast the cells multiply, it is even more amazing how small details are carried out like clockwork with great organization.

The development that takes place during weeks two through eight will be discussed first. The three primary germ layers mentioned earlier are continuously developing through all the stages. The ectoderm will always be on the outside of the layers, with the mesoderm in the middle and the endoderm on the inside. Every cell, every tissue, every organ in the human body will be made from these three primary germ layers.

Development of the Oral Cavity and Face

The development of each layer of the embryo as well as the development of the oral cavity and face will be covered in this section. The ectoderm forms the oral cavity, the **enamel** of the teeth, hair, skin, and nails, the oral mucosa of the oral cavity and nose, as well as the nervous tissue. The mesoderm, or middle layer, is extremely diverse and makes up the majority of the major portions of the body. It forms the tissues of the teeth other than the enamel, dermis of the skin, heart, muscles, urogenital system, bones, bone marrow, and blood. The endoderm is responsible for all the internal linings in the body. This thin layer lines the pharynx, lungs, gastrointestinal tract, stomach, vagina, and bladder (Figure 7-1).

At the beginning of the embryonic stage, the **cephalic** end forms a depression that deepens to an **invagination** to where the oral cavity will be located. This invagination of ectoderm pushes in and forms the primitive oral cavity and is also known as the **stomodeum**. The stomodeum becomes the main focal point for the development of the face. The face is formed from five bulges or prominences in the developing embryo (Figure 7-3).

Above the stomodeum is a larger bulge that becomes the *frontonasal prominence*, or process. The frontonasal prominence is singular and is a collection of tissue from which structures originate. In addition to the frontonasal process, there are two mandibular processes and two maxillary processes.

The frontonasal prominence starts growing thicker at the midline. The frontonasal prominence develops into the forehead

and bridge of the nose. A larger section splits off and migrates down the center of the face; this additional process is called the *median nasal prominence*. This section will become the main middle portion of the nose, **nasal septum**, and tip of nose. As this is growing downward, both sides of the median nasal process start to split off into another long section that grows downward as well. These right and left additional processes are called the right and left *lateral nasal prominences*. These are thinner and smaller than the median nasal process and are separated at the tip of the nose area by a depression that becomes the **olfactory pits** or nasal pits. These depressions invaginate further and will become the future nostrils of the nose, or nares. These two lateral nasal processes become the sides of the nose and the side of nostril or ala of the nose (Figure 7-4).

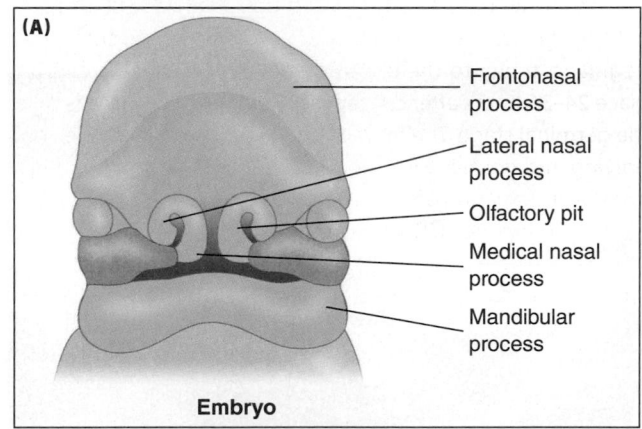

(A)
- Frontonasal process
- Lateral nasal process
- Olfactory pit
- Medical nasal process
- Mandibular process

Embryo

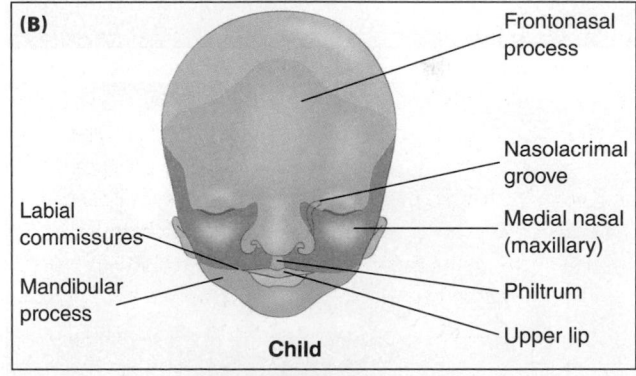

(B)
- Frontonasal process
- Nasolacrimal groove
- Medial nasal (maxillary)
- Philtrum
- Upper lip
- Labial commissures
- Mandibular process

Child

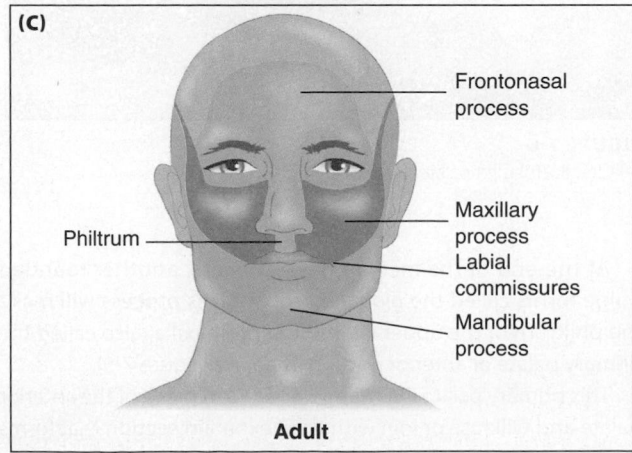

(C)
- Frontonasal process
- Maxillary process
- Labial commissures
- Mandibular process
- Philtrum

Adult

FIGURE 7-4
Embryonic facial processes shown on (A) embryo, (B) child, and (C) adult.

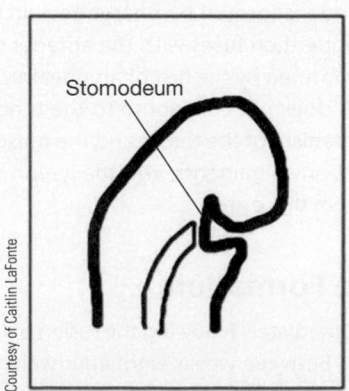

Stomodeum

Courtesy of Caitlin LaFonte

FIGURE 7-3
Stomodeum and development of the face.

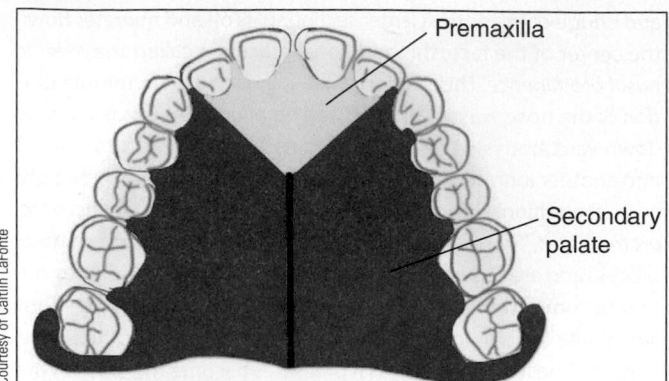

Courtesy of Caitlin LaFonte

FIGURE 7-5
Primary palate (premaxilla) and secondary palate.

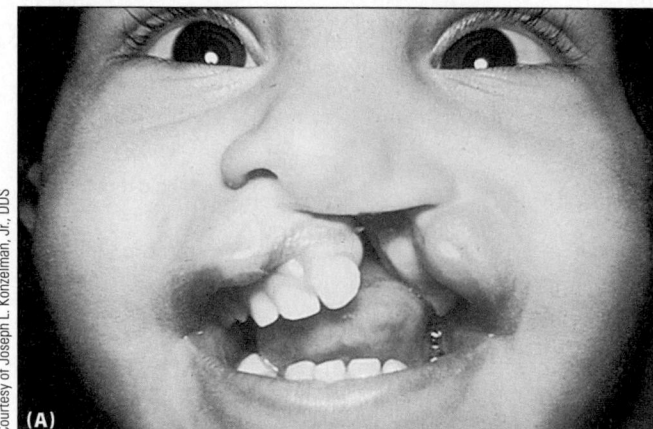

Courtesy of Joseph L. Konzelman, Jr., DDS

(A)

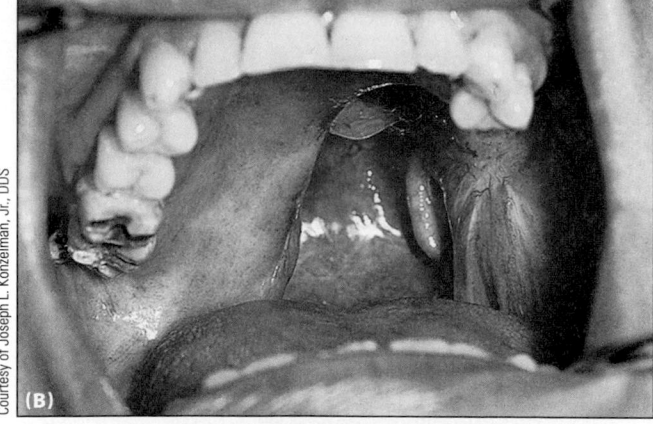

Courtesy of Joseph L. Konzelman, Jr., DDS

(B)

FIGURE 7-6
(A) Cleft lip. (B) Cleft palate.

At the end of the median nasal process, another rounded bulge forms called the *globular process*. This process will make the philtrum of the upper lip and the premaxilla, also called the primary palate or anterior portion of palate (Figure 7-5).

This primary palate is a triangular-shaped piece of the anterior palate and will fuse or join with the next main section that forms the rest of the palate. If this fusion does not happen in time, then a **cleft** of the palate will occur (Figures 7-6 and 7-7).

All of this growth from the frontal process happens by the seventh week. Week seven is when the philtrum area of the lip fuses with the other section of the upper lip, and if it does not occur then, there will be a cleft of the lip. Clefting can occur on one side (unilaterally), or it can occur on both sides (bilaterally). During this time, there are many other processes growing on the embryo, and two of them are very important in forming the rest of the face (Figures 7-6 and 7-7).

Pharyngeal Arches

The rest of the face is developed from other main processes called pharyngeal arches. Pharyngeal arch I is also called the mandibular arch. It is found immediately below the stomodeum and it begins developing at the third week (Figure 7-8).

Pharyngeal arch I will be responsible for forming the majority of the rest of the face and mouth. Soon after it forms, it will split into two distinct processes that are named the maxillary prominence (process) and the mandibular prominence (process). The maxillary prominence grows along on the sides of the face with the stomodeum separating the right and left sides. The mandibular prominence will form the mandible and all associated structures and tissues in that area. The mandibular bone, floor of the mouth, the chin, the anterior two-thirds of the tongue, and all glands in that area are developed from the mandibular process of the first pharyngeal arch (Figure 7-9).

In the same respect, the two parts of the maxillary prominence will develop above the mandible and form the maxillary bone, sides of the upper lip, sinuses, posterior sides of the hard palate, and all tissues and glands associated in that area of the face. The maxillary prominences will form the alveolar ridge of the maxilla where the teeth from the canine to the third molar will sit. This part of the palate is also called the secondary palate and it will fuse with the primary palate in the premaxilla that formed from the globular process (Figure 7-9).

Pharyngeal arch I will also form the four pairs of the muscles of mastication and the nerves and blood vessels to all these areas of the face. The posterior third of the base of the tongue and the muscles of facial expression are formed by pharyngeal arch II, also known as the hyoid arch, which is located beneath pharyngeal arch I. Pharyngeal arches III, IV, and VI are mainly involved in forming the neck and throat. A small portion of the base of the tongue is formed by pharyngeal arch III. The posterior of the tongue then fuses with the anterior portion of the tongue, which is formed by the first pharyngeal arch. The second pharyngeal arch does not contribute to the tongue. All of the swallowing mechanism of the throat and the muscles that move the neck, hyoid bone, ligaments, and the lymph glands in that area are made from these arches.

Hard Palate Formation

In week eight, immediately following the fusion of the lip, the palate starts to fuse. Between weeks eight and twelve, the fusion of the hard palate takes place. The maxillary process has two shelves, or lateral processes, that come off the side where the majority of

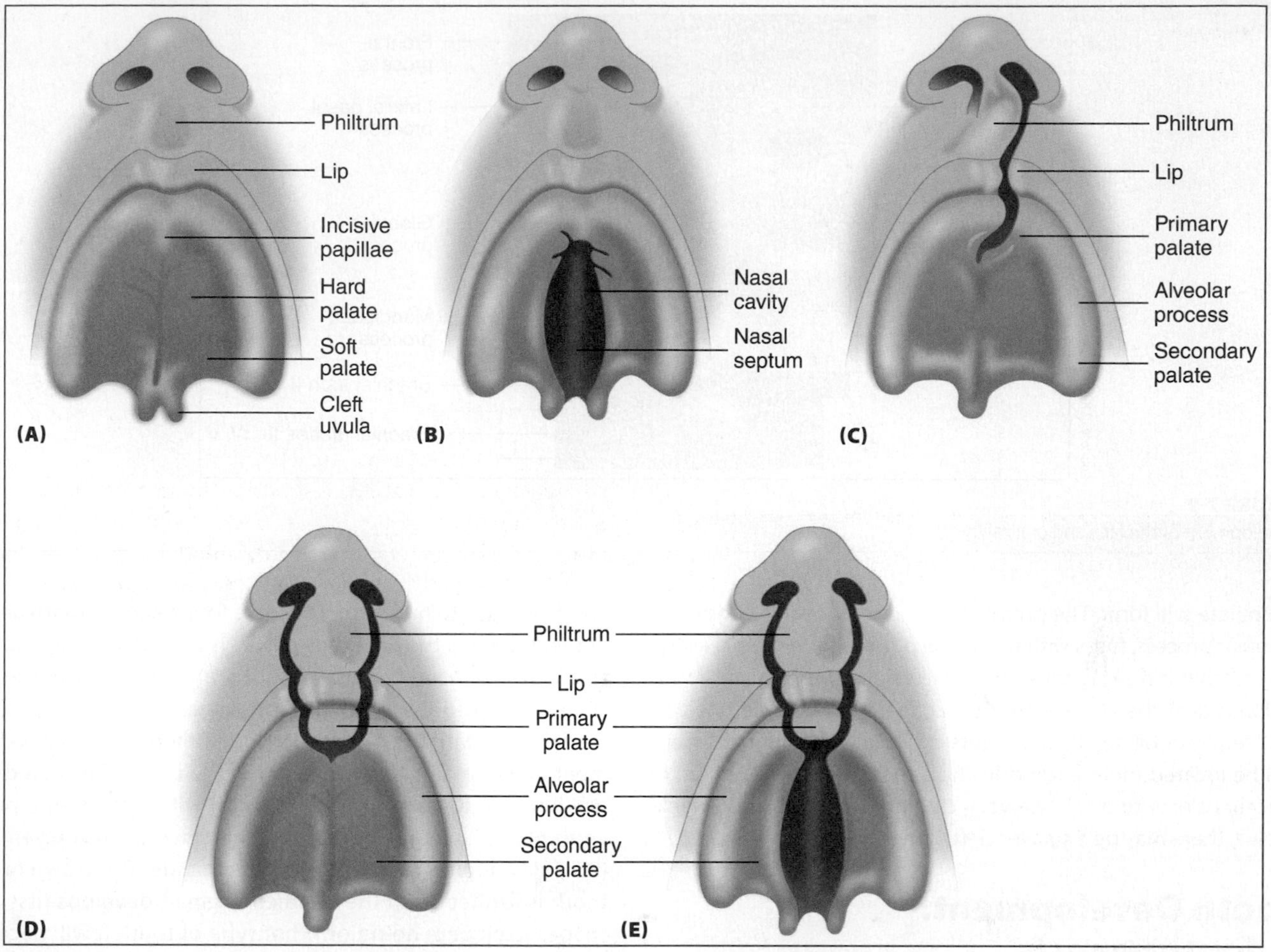

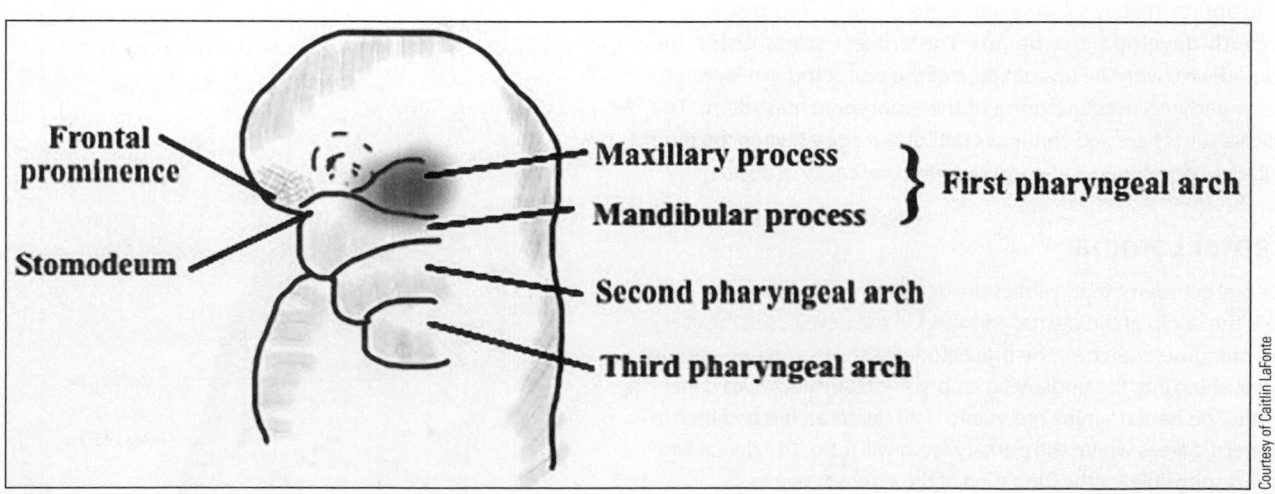

FIGURE 7-7
(A) Cleft uvula. (B) Bilateral cleft of the secondary palate. (C) Unilateral cleft lip, primary palate, and alveolar process. (D) Bilateral cleft of the lip, alveolar process, and primary palate. (E) Bilateral cleft of the lip, alveolar process, and primary and secondary palates.

Courtesy of Caitlin LaFonte

FIGURE 7-8
Pharyngeal arches.

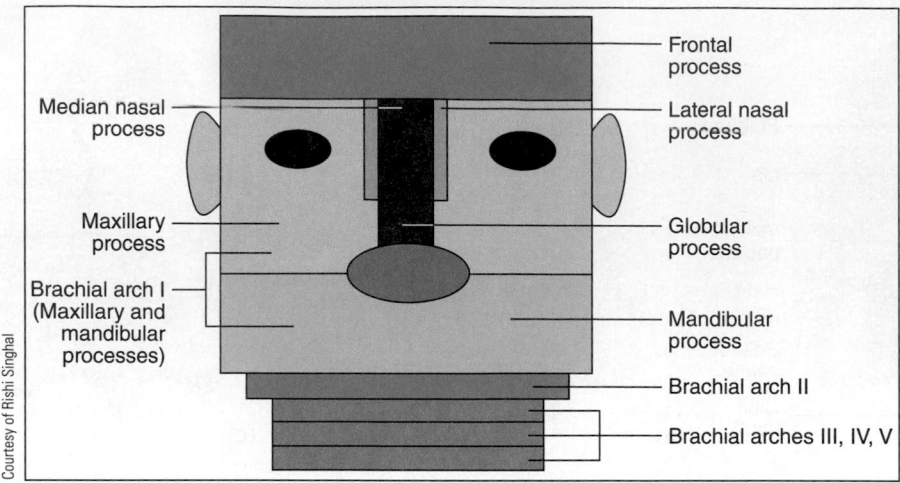

Courtesy of Rishi Singhal

FIGURE 7-9
Development of the face and oral cavity.

the palate will form. The premaxilla, or primary palate from the globular process, fuses with the lateral process from the maxillary process that is making the right and left sides of the palate. If this fusion is disturbed or does not occur, there will be a cleft palate unilaterally or bilaterally. If it occurs closer to week eight, the cleft will be located more anteriorly and appear more severe than if it occurs closer to week twelve. If clefting occurs closer to week twelve, there may be a smaller cleft of the soft palate or uvula.

Tooth Development: Odontogenesis

While the oral cavity and the alveolar bone are being formed and the palate is fusing in weeks eight through twelve, the developing bone of the maxilla and mandible are also forming **tooth germs**.

At approximately six to seven weeks in utero, **odontogenesis**, or tooth development, begins. The process starts inside the stomodeum, with the invagination of the oral ectoderm layer into the underlying **mesenchyme** of the embryonic mesoderm. The process starts here and continues until about age 21 when the third molar has developed and erupts into the oral cavity of an adult.

Dental Lamina

The oral ectoderm that overlies the developing maxilla and mandible is the origin of the **dental lamina**. On the developing maxillary and mandibular arches, the oral ectoderm starts growing rapidly and pushing into the underlying embryonic tissue known as *mesenchyme*. This dental lamina grows into both dental arches and then in 10 specific areas where the primary teeth will form. The dental lamina is responsible for the formation of the **enamel organ**.

Stages of Tooth Development

The primary teeth start to develop at weeks six though seven, and the permanent teeth start developing at about week 17 in utero. Both sets of teeth are developing simultaneously before the fetus

has developed to half-term. There are four stages in tooth development. Each of the first three stages is named according to the shape of the enamel organ (bud, cap, and bell stages). The last stage, **apposition**, is when the tooth tissues are being deposited.

It is important to note that the beginning of tooth development only pertains to the enamel of the crown. The ectoderm will become the enamel of the tooth with the **dentin**, **pulp**, **cementum**, alveolar bone, and the **periodontal ligament** (PDL) developing from mesenchymal tissue. The crown of the tooth is formed from the enamel organ. It develops first and shapes itself depending on what type of tooth it will become (Figure 7-10).

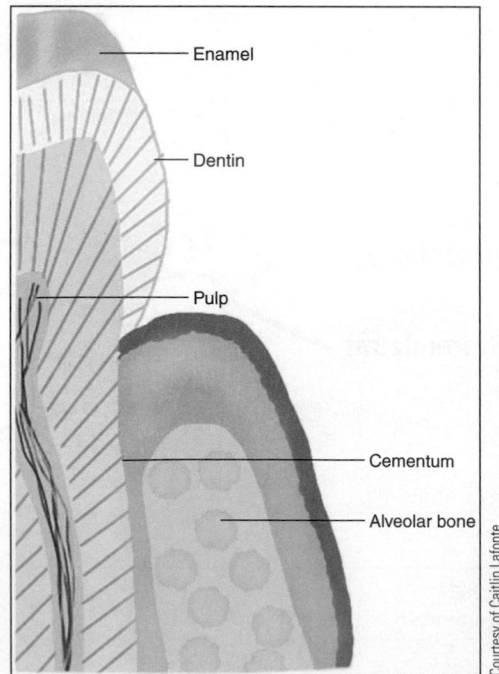

Courtesy of Caitlin Lafonte

FIGURE 7-10
Enamel, dentin, pulp.

Bud Stage

During the first stage of tooth development, the dental lamina begins to bulge out in areas in both arches. This is called the bud stage because it is very similar in appearance to a bud of a flower on the branch of a tree. Therefore, on a deciduous or primary dentition, 10 growths or buds on each arch are apparent; these later become the primary teeth. The permanent teeth develop in a similar manner. Each arch has 16 buds developing into one tooth each. The last three molars in each quadrant develop behind the primary dentition. The branch of the tree is the dental lamina that pushed into the mesenchyme with the bud stage of a tooth at the end. In this first stage, the cells are not differentiated but are *proliferating* or multiplying rapidly. This stage will continue until the shape of the bud starts to change (Figure 7-11).

Cap Stage

The second stage is the cap stage. This is named because the bud becomes shaped like a cap that is curved on top and concave underneath. This gives it the cap-like shape. The cells at this stage are still proliferating and are also beginning to **histodifferentiate** into certain cells that will make the enamel organ of the tooth. The cap-shaped enamel organ sits over the dental papilla. The dental papilla is the collection of mesenchymal cells discussed earlier. The cap-like shape will begin to grow into the size of the tooth it will become. The incisor will be smaller overall when compared to the size of a molar. At this point of development, there are three layers of cells that make up the framework of the enamel organ. The outside top two-thirds of the enamel organ are bordered with cells called the *outer enamel epithelium* (OEE). These cells will begin to shape the enamel organ. The bottom third of the enamel organ is a concave area and is layered with cells called the *inner enamel epithelium* (IEE). This layer will eventually become the **ameloblasts** that form the enamel of the tooth. The third layer of cells that are present in the cap stage is the **stellate reticulum** (SR). This layer helps hold the shape of the enamel organ and the crown of the developing tooth (Figure 7-12).

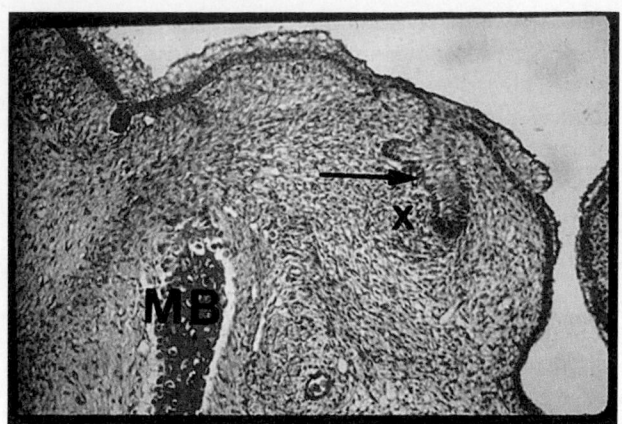

FIGURE 7-12
Cap stage of tooth development: X= mesenchyme, MB = alveolar bone.

Bell Stage

The third stage of tooth development is the *bell stage* and is so named because of the shape of the enamel organ. The cells inside the enamel organ become fully differentiated to be able to start the next stage of laying down enamel in the appositional stage. The laying down of enamel is known as *amelogenesis*. This is the last stage before the tooth tissues are laid down. There are four distinct layers in the bell stage. The **stratum intermedium** (SI) is the last developed layer. The SI layer is adjacent to the IEE and is not very thick, but plays an important role in nourishing the inner enamel epithelium (IEE). The SI layer appears around the fourteenth week in utero. When the IEE cells are maturing into ameloblasts and forming enamel, they need to have energy and nourishment. It is believed that the SI layer nourishes the ameloblasts, though the exact function of the cells in the SI layer is unknown. These four layers form the crown of the tooth and prepare the enamel organ for its final and most important stage, the appositional stage. It is in this stage that certain anomalies can occur. A supernumerary or extra tooth may form at this time. An odontoma or extra calcified tissue may form at this time as well (Figure 7-13).

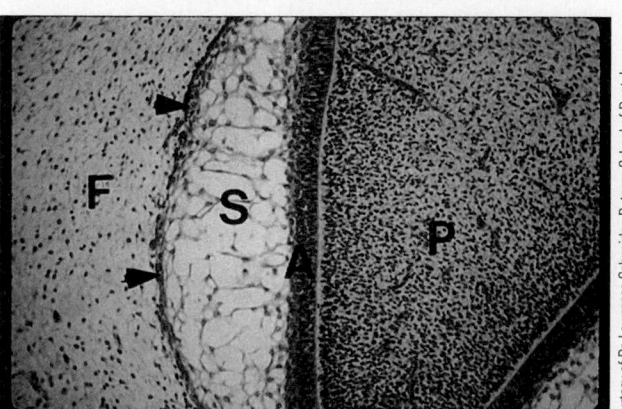

FIGURE 7-13
Bell stage of tooth development. Arrowheads = outer enamel epithelium, S= stellate reticulum, A=inner enamel epithelium and stratum intermedium, P = dental papilla, and F = dental follicle.

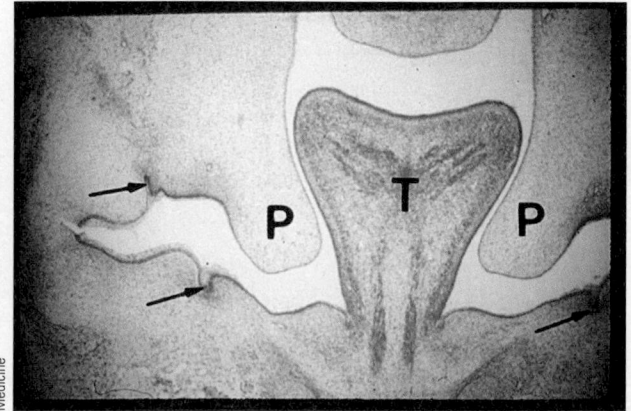

FIGURE 7-11
Bud stage of tooth development. Arrows demonstrate dental lamina. T is primitive tongue; P is right and left palatal bones.

The enamel organ now has four distinct layers of cells that have developed: the outer enamel epithelium, the inner enamel epithelium, the stellate reticulum, and the stratum intermedium. The four layers of the enamel organ are ready to make enamel and go into the final stage of tooth development (Figure 7-13).

Appositional Stage

The last stage of tooth development is called the appositional stage and begins when the tooth tissues start to be laid down (Figure 7-14). During this stage, enamel, dentin, and cementum are laid down in increments. **Predentin** is the first tissue laid down. This signals the ameloblasts to secrete the amelogenin from the Tome's process located at the **apical** side of the cell adjacent to the layer of predentin. Tome's process guides the enamel matrix into place. Next, hydroxyapatite crystals are deposited into the amelogenin, it becomes mineralized, and is now called enamel. Enamel is laid down in increments just like dentin. As each increment of amelogenin is produced, it then becomes mineralized and another layer of amelogenin is laid down. The enamel is deposited in layers that form keyhole-shaped cells that are called *enamel rods* or *prisms* once the enamel is hardened (Figure 7-15). These rods, which are not visible to the naked eye,

are four micrometers in diameter, have variable lengths, and are shaped in the pattern of a fish. Their location in the enamel is such that the head is surrounded by the tails of two other enamel rods. *Hunter Schreger* bands are visible in enamel under a microscope. These are alternating light and dark bands caused by the arrangement of enamel prisms at right angles to each other. This arrangement strengthens the enamel and prevents it from cracking. The substance surrounding the inner portion, the *rod core*, of each enamel rod is the **interprismatic substance**. Of these substances, the enamel rods are hardest, and the interprismatic substance is the weakest.

This repeating process creates lines, like rings of a tree called Striae of Retzius, and can be seen under a microscope (Figure 7-16). The **enamel rods** are keyhole shaped and can be compared to bricks. The mortar is the interprismatic substance (interred substance) that holds the enamel rods together. Both the enamel rods and the interprismatic substance make up the structure of the tooth enamel. As the enamel hardens to its 96% **inorganic** and 4% **organic** composition, it becomes the hardest substance in the body. It cannot repair itself, so once it is damaged, decayed, or worn down, it is gone. Enamel is thinner at the area on the tooth where the enamel and the cementum meet; this allows the yellower dentin under it to show through. Enamel is whiter at the chewing surfaces and cusp tips where it is thicker. Fluoride during development helps make enamel stronger; however, too much fluoride during development can make the enamel gray, brownish, or striped in bluish-gray colors. The strength and hardness of enamel make it resist wear; it is durable and smooth, which allows it to be self-cleansing.

All of these tissues are very vulnerable at this stage. If the pregnant female takes an antibiotic such as tetracycline, the enamel may be permanently stained. If the mother experiences an illness at this stage, the enamel may not form properly. Enamel *dysplasia* results in a reduction in the normal levels of enamel. Dysplasia usually is caused by enamel *hypoplasia* or enamel malformation or by enamel *hypocalcification*, which is a decrease in the hardness of the enamel. Both of these abnormalities can also take place during this stage of gestation.

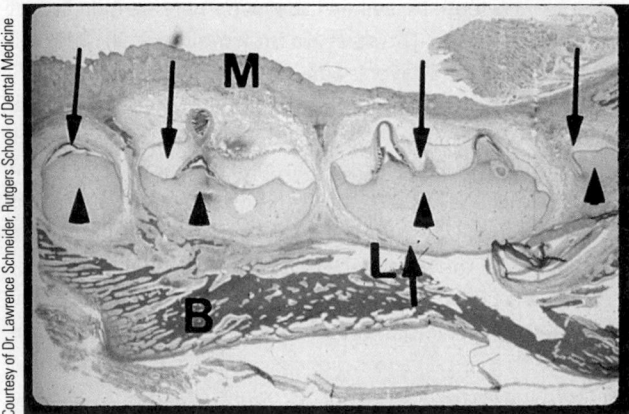

Courtesy of Dr. Lawrence Schneider, Rutgers School of Dental Medicine

FIGURE 7-14
Appositional stage. Long arrows point to enamel organ, arrowheads point to dental papilla, overlying oral mucosa M, underlying bone B, and L = cervical loop.

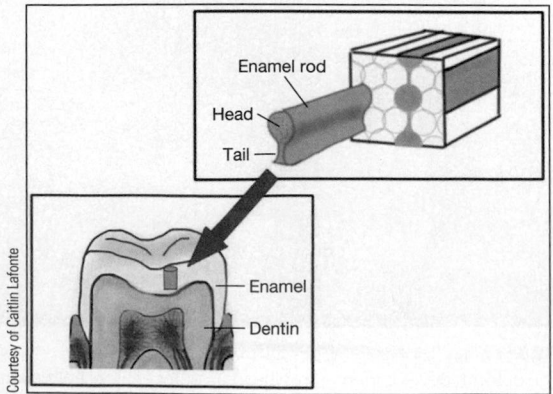

Courtesy of Caitlin Lafonte

FIGURE 7-15
Keyhole shape of enamel rods.

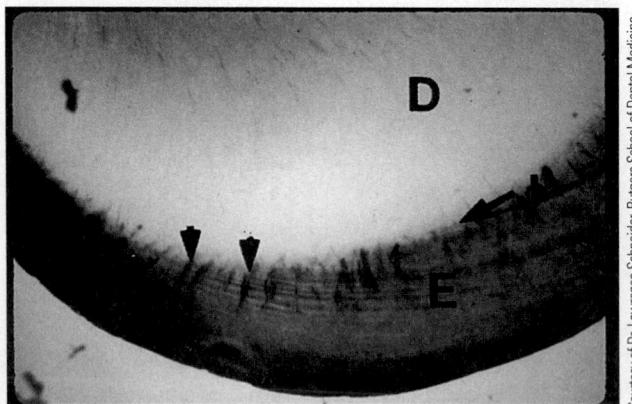

Courtesy of Dr. Lawrence Schneider, Rutgers School of Dental Medicine

FIGURE 7-16
Striae of retzius in enamel (E), DEJ (J), and dentin (D).

Dentinogenesis

The **dental papilla** develops adjacent to the lower half of the enamel organ at the same time that the enamel organ is forming. It starts out as a collection of mesenchyme that changes into specialized cells called *odontoblasts* that will secrete and mineralize the dentin of the tooth. Predentin is formed before the dentin. The formation of predentin sends a signal to the IEE to differentiate into ameloblasts that will secrete the enamel matrix. The predentin is laid down in increments and then hardened before the next layer of predentin is laid down. These layers can be identified under a microscope and look like rings on a tree; they are called *imbrication lines of von Ebner*. *Contour lines of Owen* are accentuated lines of von Ebner that demonstrate a disturbance in the formation of the matrix or **mineralization**.

The dentin will mineralize to its 70% inorganic and 30% organic level. The process of dentinogenesis continues until it fills the crown portion of the tooth and will continue into the root after the crown portion is almost complete. The odontoblasts migrate apically as they lay down dentin, and the ameloblasts migrate coronally as they lay down enamel in the crown of the tooth.

Dentin is the second-hardest substance in the body and the second-hardest tooth tissue. Dentin is more yellow in color than enamel. Dentin makes up the bulk of the tooth structure. It is located beneath the enamel in the crown and the **cementum** in the root. One of the major differences between dentin and enamel is that dentin can repair itself to a certain extent and continues to grow throughout the life of the tooth.

The structure of dentin is very different from enamel in that it has *odontoblasts* living inside the calcified tissue. These cells have long processes or tails that start out at the junction of the dentin and enamel (DEJ) or junction of the dentin and cementum (DCJ) when the pre-dentin is first laid down. As the dentin grows thicker, then the odontoblastic process grows longer and longer with the main body of the odontoblast located within the pulp cavity (Figure 7-17A and Figure 7-17B). These processes extend into the dentin and because they are living and not hardened tooth structure, they become encircled with the hard dentin and end up in tunnel-like channels called *dentinal tubules*, which contain dentinal fluid. These processes can conduct sensitivity into the tooth's pulp by way of these tubules. If the enamel or cementum is ever broken or worn away, it can expose the dentin and make the tooth very sensitive. This can be a very common problem, and dentistry has several remedies for covering up these tubules to decrease sensitivity.

Primary, Secondary, and Tertiary Dentin Dentinogenesis continues throughout the life of a tooth. The dentin that is laid down in different stages of a tooth's life is identified with different terms. Once the predentin is calcified, and before the tooth erupts into the oral cavity, this newly formed dentin is also called primary dentin. The layer of primary dentin closest to the enamel is known as *mantle* dentin. The amount of dentin that forms at this time is the bulk of the dentin for that tooth. The dentin that forms once a tooth erupts into the oral cavity after the root of a tooth has fully formed falls in the category of secondary dentin. Secondary dentin forms slowly throughout the life of the tooth at the expense of the pulp cavity. As a person gets older, the pulp chamber gets smaller and smaller until there is very little pulp tissue left in the tooth. This is one reason why many older patients do not have much dental sensitivity.

Another type of dentin, tertiary dentin, is called *reparative* dentin and it forms in response to trauma. This trauma can be caused by invading *decay*, a cavity, or **occlusal** pressures that can damage the tooth. When a tooth has a threat of decay, then the pulp lays down a thicker layer of dentin under that part of the tooth where the caries is advancing. The reparative dentin is less organized and laid down faster than the secondary dentin. This dentin can often give a tooth a little more time before the pulp is invaded with the carious lesion. Having radiographs and routine dental care can help the dental team discover decay earlier and remove it in a timely manner so the tooth can be restored.

Dentin also differs from area to area and is not uniform throughout. *Peritubular dentin* is the dentin that creates the wall

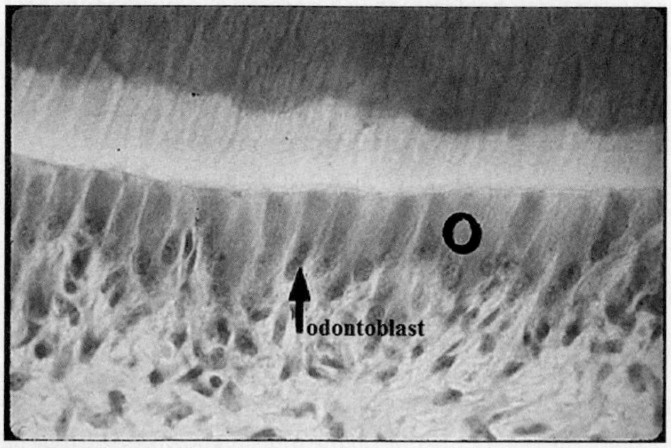

FIGURE 7-17A
Odontoblastic processes in dentin.

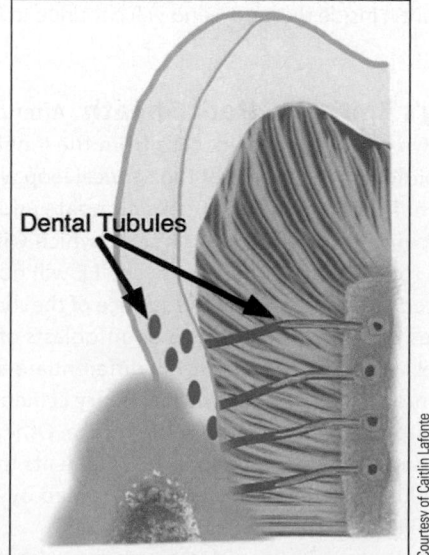

Courtesy of Caitlin Lafonte

FIGURE 7-17B
Dental tubules.

of the dentinal tubule. Dentin found between the tubules is called *intertubular dentin*. The first predentin that is formed and matures within the tooth is called *mantle dentin*. The layer of dentin that surrounds the pulp is called *circumpulpal dentin*.

Cementogenesis

Surrounding the dental papilla and the enamel organ is the *dental sac*, the third and final part of the tooth germ. This layer of cells is derived from the mesenchyme and encircles the dental papilla and enamel organ. The dental sac will eventually form the cementum that covers the root of the tooth. Cementum is formed by cells called *cementoblasts; cementoclasts* are involved in root **resorption**.

Cementum is a thin layer of hard tissue found only on the outside of the root. Cementum is 55% organic and 45% inorganic, which makes it slightly harder than alveolar bone. The main function of cementum is to serve as an attachment of the tooth to the alveolar bone by way of the PDL that surrounds the root. The dental sac is also responsible for the formation of the periodontal ligament or PDL surrounding the root of the tooth as well as the alveolar bone in which they sit. There are two types of cementum found on the root of the tooth. **Acellular** or primary cementum is a very thin layer that covers the entire root, and after it is laid down and mineralized, the cells, called cementoblasts, stop producing cementum. The second type, **cellular** cementum or secondary cementum, is found at the apical third of the root tip and will continue to slowly be deposited throughout the life of the tooth.

When we start to see how the rest of the tooth develops, we start at the edges of the enamel organ's inner enamel epithelium (IEE) and outer enamel epithelium (OEE) cells at the CEJ of the tooth. The OEE cells around the CEJ finish their role by becoming the epithelial attachment at the base of the sulcus. These two layers stop forming the crown of the tooth, but the tooth is not finished forming yet. The cells of the dental papilla have been forming dentin inside the crown and will continue to form dentin in the root.

Hertwig's Epithelial Root Sheath After the enamel of the crown has been formed, cells from the inner and outer enamel epithelium in the area of the cervical loop will continue to function. These two layers of cells elongate and now comprise **Hertwig's epithelial root sheath**, which will form and shape the roots. The cells that were the IEE will now produce the intermediate cementum on the surface of the root dentin as it continues to be deposited by the odontoblasts of the dental papilla. Cells from the dental sac will differentiate and change into cementoblasts that will form secondary cementum on the intermediate cementum on the root surface. Other cells from the dental sac will form the periodontal ligaments that suspend the root in the alveolar bone, which is formed by cells of the dental sac (Figure 7-18).

The two layers of cells of Hertwig's root sheath give the odontoblasts the matrix to start to lay down predentin. The IEE cells from Hertwig's root sheath lay down cementoid, and the DCJ

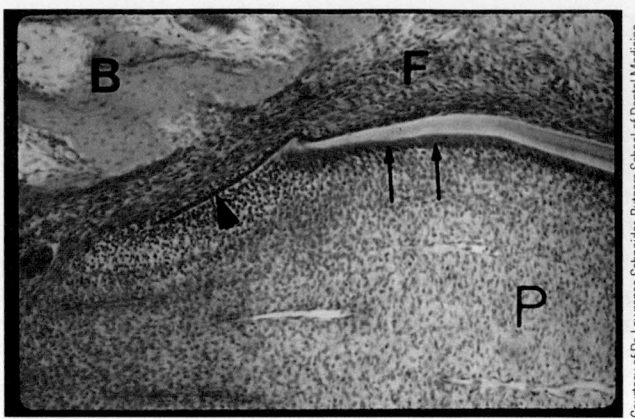

FIGURE 7-18
Hertwig's epithelial root sheath.

or dentinocemental junction is formed. The cementoid is then mineralized as hydroxyapatite crystals are added to the matrix in the same manner that the dentin and enamel were formed. Hertwig's epithelial root sheath continues to elongate and shape the roots through *cementogenesis*. The process of the root formation can take up to four years after a tooth has erupted into the oral cavity. The apex of the root is not completed until a few years after the tooth erupts.

Epithelial Rests of Malassez Once the tooth has erupted and the apex is completed a few years later, Hertwig's epithelial root sheath has completed its function. Normally these cells are resorbed by the body. Sometimes Hertwig's epithelial root sheath is not totally resorbed and cells can remain within the periodontal ligament space. These remaining cells can become trapped and are known as the **epithelial rests of Malassez**. It is believed that these cells can proliferate to form the lining of cysts or can become calcified within the PDL.

Successional Laminae The process of odontogenesis occurs for every tooth in both the primary and the permanent dentitions. After the primary tooth germs develop, there are successional laminae that form slightly **lingual** to the primary teeth. These successional laminae will become the permanent tooth germs to replace the primary teeth. These *succedaneous* or permanent tooth germs grow lingual to the primary tooth germ. The same process occurs with the non-succedaneous molars, but instead of the laminae extending from the primary tooth, it is a distal extension of the original dental lamina posterior to the primary molars.

The Pulp

The pulp of the tooth is the vital part of the tooth. It is located at the central portion of the tooth in the crown portions and in the roots of teeth. The part of the pulp in the crowns is known as the *coronal* pulp. The part of the pulp in the roots is known as the *radicular* pulp. The radicular pulp is continuous with the apical foramen. The part of the pulp that extends into the tips of each tooth is known

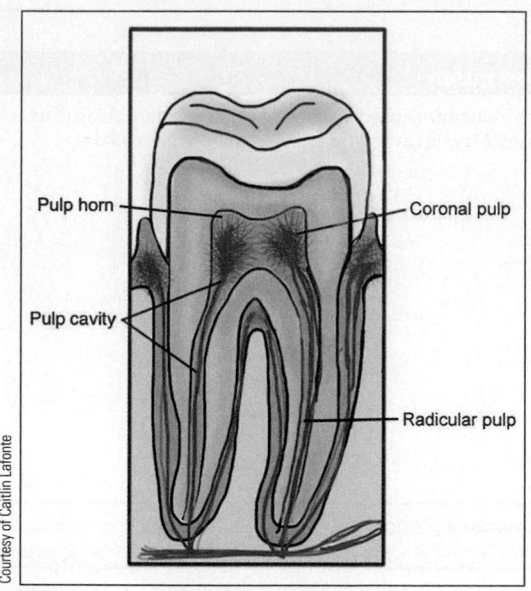

Courtesy of Caitlin Lafonte

Pulp horn

Pulp cavity

Coronal pulp

Radicular pulp

FIGURE 7-19
Pulp of tooth.

as a pulp horn. The pulp basically follows the shape of the tooth in which it is contained. The pulp is the nerve center of each tooth and contains living connective tissue as well as odontoblasts, fibroblasts, osteoblasts, and osteoclasts. The pulp also contains nerves and blood vessels that enter the pulp chamber through the apical foramen (Figure 7-19). Similar to dentin, the pulp is formed from the dental papilla. When the dentin forms around the dental papilla, the central tissues are the pulp of each tooth.

Artifacts of Enamel, Dentin, Cementum, and Pulp

As with any tissue development, there can be some types of variations that can occur. Sometimes these tissues do not mineralize completely and leave empty areas, or they may fill in too densely, and other times some cells can be found in the wrong areas. The last part of this section describes some of these artifacts that can be found in the enamel, dentin, or cementum. See Tables 7-1 and 7-2 regarding artifacts found during the development in enamel, dentin, cementum, and the pulp.

TABLE 7-1 Artifacts of Enamel

Artifact	Description
Enamel lamella	Linear areas of hypomineralized enamel that extend from the DEJ to the surface of the enamel.
Enamel pearl	Enamel projection that is found on the DEJ area of a tooth. Usually found during a routine exam and does not require treatment.
Enamel spindle Image legend: enamel = E, dentin = D, DEJ = J, enamel spindle = S.	Tubular projection of the end of odontoblastic process of dentin that extended into enamel from DEJ before the DEJ is fully calcified.
Enamel tuft Image legend: enamel tufts = T.	Brush-shaped areas of hypomineralized enamel that extend from the DEJ into the enamel.

TABLE 7-2 Artifacts of Dentin, Cementum, and Pulp

Artifact	Description
Dead tract Image legend: pulp chamber = P, enamel = E, dead tract = T, R = tertiary dentin. 	Area in dentin caused by degeneration of odontoblastic processes. May be caused by caries, attrition, or erosion.
Hypercementosis	Excessive deposition of secondary cementum on root; caused by trauma or inflammation.
Interglobular dentin 	Incomplete calcified dentinal matrix between calcified areas; caused by low levels of vitamin D.
Granular layer of Tomes Image legend: C = cementum, D = dentin, G = granular layer of Tomes. 	Narrow layer of interglobular dentin found in the dentin of the root just under the cementum. This gives the area a granular appearance.
Pulp stones	Calcified masses found in either the coronal portion of the pulp or the root portion of the pulp. Usually found during a routine exam and do not require treatment.

Parts of a Tooth

There are two primary parts of a tooth: the crown and the root. The next section will discuss both of these parts.

Crown of the Tooth The part of the tooth that you can see when you smile is called the *crown* of the tooth (Figure 7-20).

The crowns are shaped differently depending on the type of tooth. They are covered on the outside by the strongest tissue of the body—enamel—which protects the tooth.

Root of the Tooth The root is the part of the tooth that you cannot see located beneath the gingiva (Figure 7-20). The root

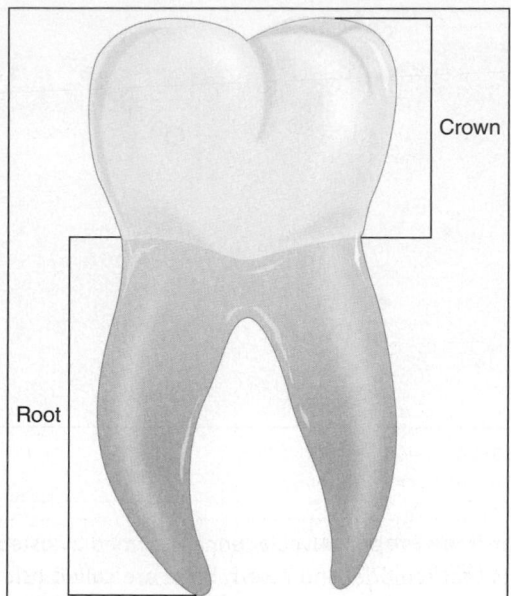

FIGURE 7-20

Mandibular first molar from the buccal side showing the furcation or dividing area where the roots fork off.

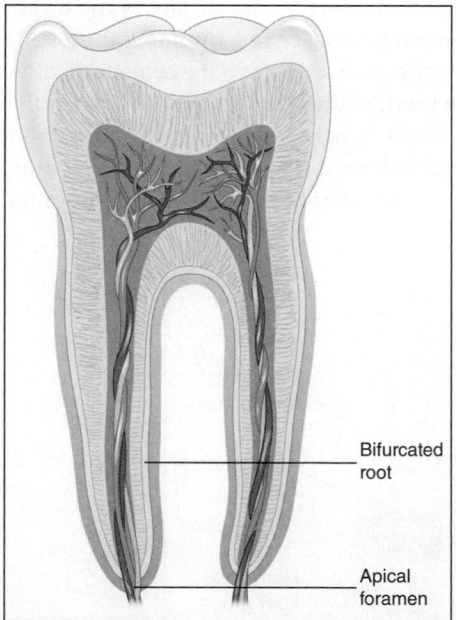

FIGURE 7-21

Tissues of the tooth.

is embedded in the bone of the maxilla and mandible, which securely holds the tooth in the jaw. A tooth can have a single, **bifurcated**, or **trifurcated** root. (Chapter 8, Dental Anatomy, provides details about each tooth and its specific characteristics.) The end of the root tip is called the **apex** or *apical* end. At the very end of the root apex is a hole or **foramen** where the blood vessels and nerves enter and exit the tooth and make it a vital, living part of our mouth (Figure 7-21).

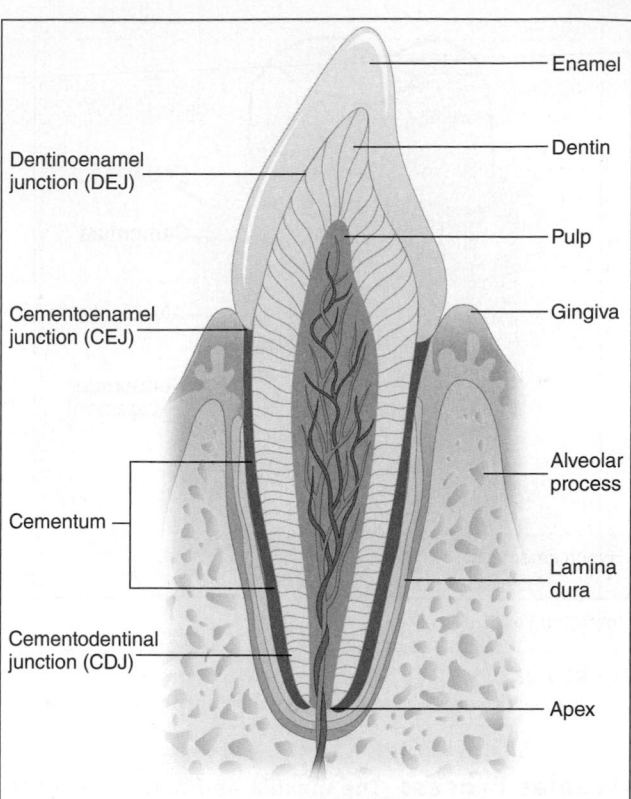

FIGURE 7-22

The tooth and surrounding tissues.

Tissue Junctions   Where the crown meets the root is the cervical area or cervix of the tooth. It is also where the enamel of the crown and the cementum of the root meet. This is known as the cementoenamel junction, or CEJ (Figure 7-22). There is usually a raised line here called the cervical line. When looking at the CEJ, there are three possibilities of a junction between the cementum and enamel. The cementum will overlap the enamel slightly 60% of the time and meet the enamel exactly 30% of the time. That leaves 10% of the time when there is a small gap between the enamel and cementum. When this gap occurs, exposed dentinal tubules in the area can be very sensitive since that area is not protected.

Inside the tooth's hard structure are two other junctions. Where the enamel meets the dentin on the inside of the crown is the dentoenamel junction, or the DEJ (Figure 7-22). In the root, the area where the cementum meets the dentin is called the dentocemental junction of CDJ (Figure 7-22).

Periodontium

The **periodontium** is composed of the structures that surround and support your teeth. It is made up of four major structures: the alveolar process, cementum, **periodontal ligament (PDL)**, and gingiva. There are two divisions of the periodontium: the attachment unit and gingival unit.

Attachment Unit

The attachment unit (apparatus) is composed of the alveolar process, cementum, and periodontal ligament (Figure 7-23).

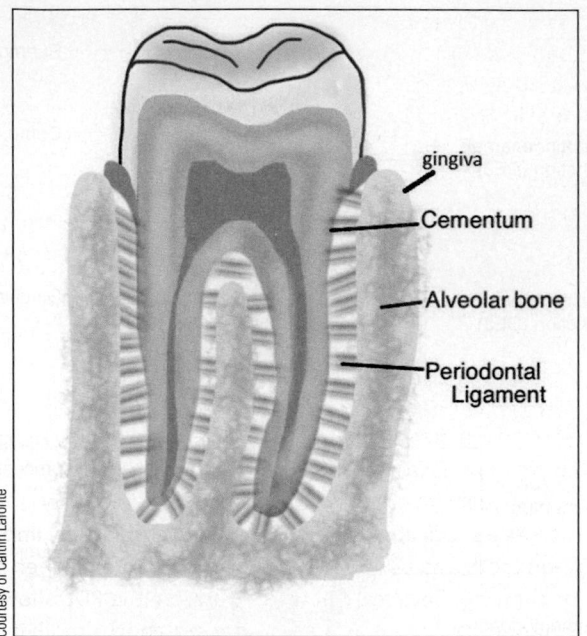

Courtesy of Caitlin Lafonte

FIGURE 7-23
Attachment unit apparatus (alveolar bone, cementum and periodontal ligament).

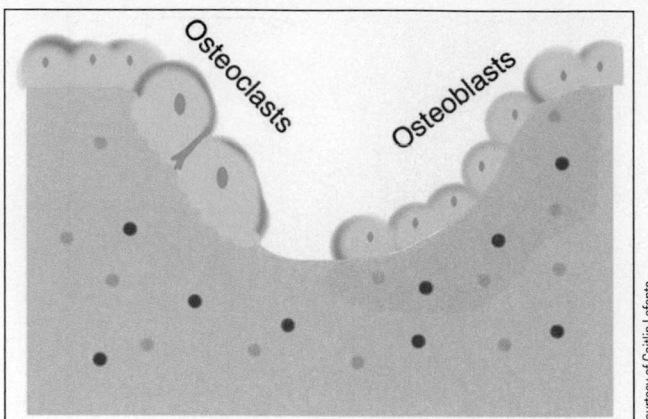

Courtesy of Caitlin Lafonte

FIGURE 7-24
Cells that remodel bone.

Alveolar Process The maxilla and mandible are the tooth-bearing bones of the alveolar process. The alveolar process provides the bony support for the roots of the teeth, attachment for the gums that protect the teeth and bone, and attachment points for muscles involved in jaw and tongue movement. The alveolar process is a thick ridge on the inferior surface of the maxilla and superior surface of the mandible called the **cortical plates**. It is divided into the alveolar bone proper and the supporting alveolar bone.

Alveolar Bone Proper Alveolar bone is formed by osteoblasts. The cells that remodel and resorb bone are called *osteoclasts* (Figure 7-24). The alveolar bone proper is composed of compact bone that lines the **alveolus** and makes up the **alveolar crests** and **interdental septum**. The interdental septum separates each tooth socket. If the tooth has multiple roots, the bone that separates the roots is identified as the *interradicular septum* (Figure 7-25).

The alveolus or alveolar socket, is a cavity within the alveolar process that holds the tooth. Lining the alveolus is very dense compact bone called the *lamina dura*. The PDL is attached to the lamina dura and the cementum of the tooth to secure the tooth in the jaw. The lamina dura contains numerous holes where canals pass from the alveolar bone into the periodontal ligament (Figure 7-25). The alveolus does not actually contact the root because the periodontal ligament suspends it in place.

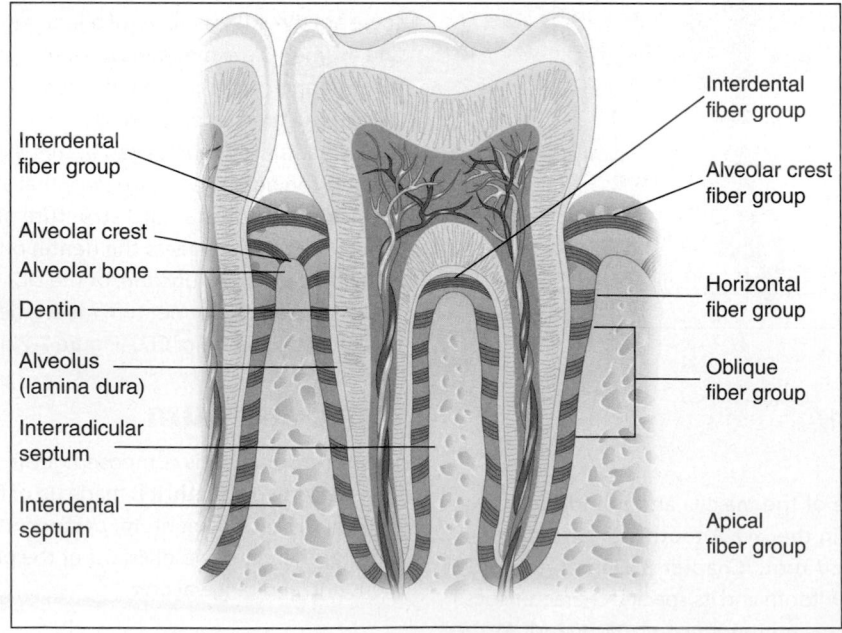

FIGURE 7-25
Interradicular septum and interdental septum and principal fiber groups.

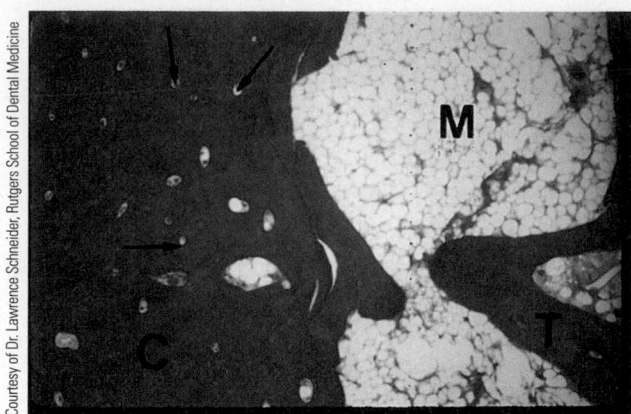

FIGURE 7-26
Cancellous bone and marrow (M) and cortical bone (C) and trabeculae
(T) histological appearance.

A healthy alveolar crest is the highest point of the *alveolar ridge* and joins the facial and lingual cortical plates (Figure 7-25). It is located approximately 1.5 to 2 mm apical to the CEJ. Interdental bone or septa are plates of bone that separate the individual alveolus, and the interradicular septum or bone separates roots of multi-rooted teeth (Figure 7-25).

Supporting Alveolar Bone The outer border of the supporting alveolar bone consists of plates of compact bone or cortical plates on both the facial and lingual surfaces of the alveolar bone. The cortical plates are 1.5 to 3 mm thick over the posterior teeth and are thinner over the anterior teeth. *Cancellous bone*, also referred to as trabecular bone or spongy bone, is located between the alveolar bone proper and the cortical plates (Figure 7-26).

Cancellous bone forms a lattice-like, spongy, porous bone tissue made of open spaces connected by flat planes of bone known as trabeculae. Red bone marrow, blood vessels, and connective tissue fill the spaces to carry out regenerative and regular functions of the bone. Inside the trabeculae are three types of bone cells: osteoblasts, osteocytes, and osteoclasts. Their function is formative, and they make new tissues for self-repair of damaged tissue. The alveolar bone function is to support, maintain, and retain the tooth in the arch. The alveolar process contains nerves to receive and transmit stimuli and blood supply to provide moisture and nutrients to nourish the bone and teeth.

Cementum

The PDL fibers are embedded into the cementum of the tooth and lamina dura of the alveolar bone, securely attaching the tooth in the alveolus. The periodontal ligament is also known as the periodontal membrane (Figure 7-23).

Periodontal Ligament (PDL) Components

The periodontal ligament occupies the space between the cementum of the root and the alveolar bone that lines the alveolus or tooth socket. This ligament is wider at the cervix (CEJ)

and at the apex and narrow between these points. The main components of the PDL include collagen fibers that create fiber bundles that help literally attach the tooth to the bone. The periodontal ligament also includes a variety of cells such as fibroblasts, cementoblasts, osteoblasts, nerves, blood vessels, and lymphatic vessels. It is derived from the dental sac in embryonic development.

PDL Functions The PDL is a layer of fibrous connective tissue that serves as a cushion between the tooth and the bone. Its main function is to have a supportive role and hold the tooth in the alveolus. It is composed of rubber band–like tissue of fibers that suspend the tooth in the alveolus or tooth socket. The periodontal ligament has a sensory function also that transmits tactile sense, pressure, and pain. It can act as a suspensory mechanism that keeps the root and bone from abrading away, and it also acts as a shock absorber. The PDL fibers cushion any impact between tooth and bone when pressure is exerted or when biting or chewing. Because it acts as a cushion, the PDL allows a slight movement of the tooth when chewing, and the tooth is not set directly against bone.

Other functions of the PDL are formative; it carries blood supply to the periodontium for nutrition and remodeling in which it provides cells involved in the formation and resorption of the cementum and bone and also of itself. It also allows some degree of movement of the tooth and allows it to slightly tip, rotate, or be compressed. It also helps keep a constant mesial drift of the tooth.

PDL Principal Fibers The PDL has what are called principal fibers that are groups of fibers which are orientated to give the tooth optimal resistance to all types of functional loading patterns. The PDL principal fiber groups are named according to their location in respect to the tooth's root or how they are oriented along the root surface. There are five groups of PDL fibers that belong to the *alveolodental* ligament fibers group, and one group that belongs to the interdental or *transseptal* fibers group (Figure 7-27). Table 7-3 provides a description of the principal fibers.

There are other fibers and unusual calcifications besides the principle fibers that can be found in the periodontal ligament. *Sharpey's fibers* are one of the other types of fibers found in the PDL. These are thicker, more fibrous, collagen-type fibers with sharper ends that embed into the cementum and bone across the PDL at right angles. *Cementicles* are small calcifications of cementum that are trapped within the PDL. They are not attached to the bone, but sometimes can be attached to the cementum of the tooth.

Gingival Unit

Gingiva is the part of the oral mucosa covering the alveolar bone that supports the teeth. Healthy gingival tissues are very important for a healthy mouth. The gingival unit is composed of epithelial tissue that is attached to the alveolar bone and surrounds the neck of the teeth, providing a seal around the base of the teeth to prevent the entry of bacteria carrying plaque and calculus.

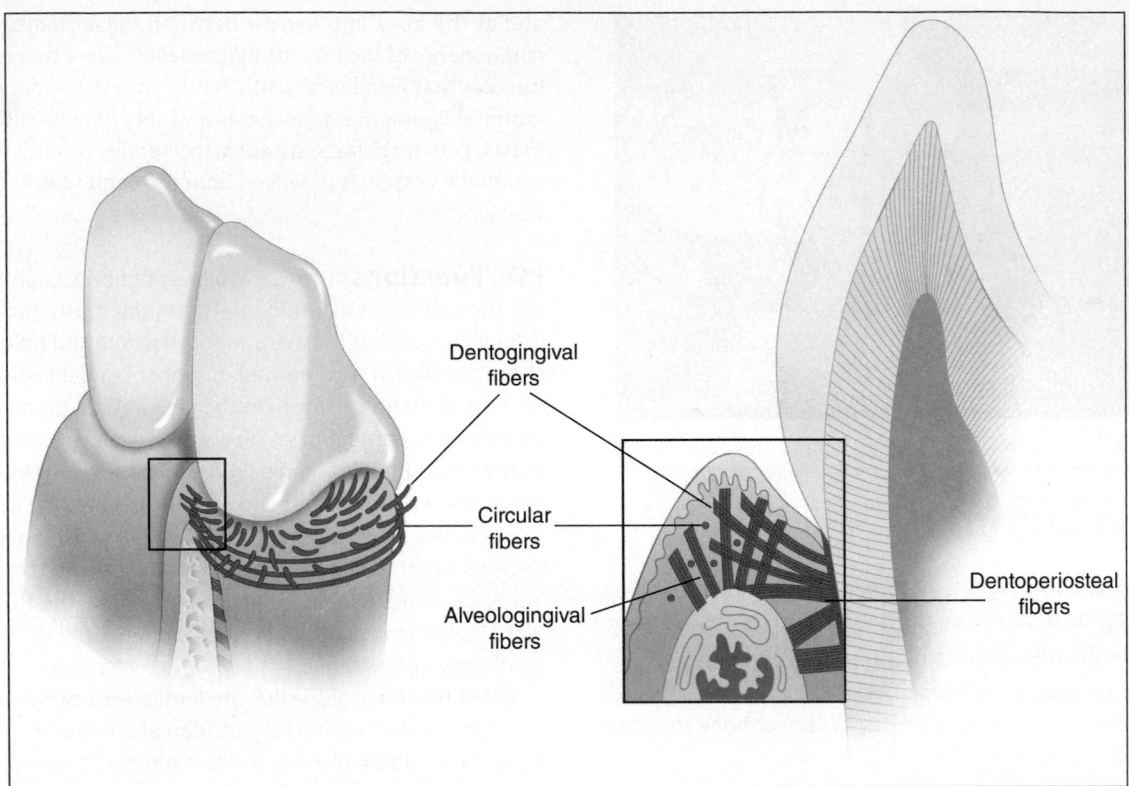

FIGURE 7-27
Gingival fiber groups: dentogingival, circular, alveologingival, and dentoperiosteal.

TABLE 7-3 Principal Fibers

Alveolodental Fibers	Location and Function
alveolar crest	Located closest to CEJ. Located at the cervical portion of the root, and goes from the cervical area to the alveolar crest of alveolar bone. The function of this group of fibers is to resist vertical and intrusive forces and help keep the tooth in the socket.
horizontal	Near CEJ; located at mid-root from cementum to alveolar bone. Their function is to resist horizontal and tipping forces of the tooth.
oblique	Locate in the middle of the root and are the largest group. Go from the middle one-third of root from cementum to bone. Their function is to resist vertical and intrusive forces, because of the angle of the fibers being slanted; they help keep the tooth from hitting against bone when biting down on something hard.
apical	They are located at the end of apex of root tips. They function to resist vertical forces of lifting, extracting, and tipping of the tooth.
interradicular	They are only found between roots of multi-rooted teeth. Their function is to resist vertical and lateral forces and forces of luxation.
transseptal fibers	They are found over the alveolar bone and extend into the cementum of adjacent teeth. They function to keep the teeth aligned. These can also be considered as gingival fibers since they have no bony connections.

Thus, when healthy, it presents an effective barrier to the barrage of periodontal insults to deeper periodontal tissue. When the gingiva is not healthy, it can provide a gateway for infection to advance into the deeper tissue of the periodontium, leading to periodontal disease and a loss of teeth. Gingiva is discussed in Chapter 6 (Landmarks of the Face and Oral Cavity).

Gingival Unit Fibers

If we could look inside the gingival tissues under a microscope, we would see that five fiber groups make up the gingival unit. The overall function of these fibers is to resist gingival displacement. Table 7-4 provides a description of the gingival unit fibers.

TABLE 7-4 Gingival Unit Fiber Groups

Gingival Unit Fiber Groups	Location and Function
circumferential or circular	Are found right at the CEJ at the neck of the tooth and encircle the tooth within the free gingiva. These fibers are above or coronal to alveolar crest of the bone and they are not attached to cementum, but exist only within the tissue. The function of this fiber group is to provide support and contour to the free gingiva and keep the tissue tight around the neck of the tooth.
dentogingival (attached gingival fibers)	Located near the CEJ and go from the cementum to the gingival tissues. They attach the gingiva to the teeth and provide support to the attached gingiva to resist displacement of the gingiva.
alveologingival (free gingival fibers)	These fibers go from the alveolar crest of bone up to the free gingiva. This group helps attach the gingiva to the alveolar bone that is right around the neck of the teeth.
dentoperiosteal	These fibers extend from the cementum in the cervical area of the tooth and insert into the alveolar bone.

Chapter Summary

It is vital for the entire dental team to be able to communicate about the structure and function of the oral cavity. Therefore, it is important for the dental assistant to understand the structure/function of tissue, the prenatal growth/development process of oral embryology, and the oral cavity that surrounds the teeth.

Review Questions

Multiple Choice

1. The embryonic layer that differentiates into enamel and the lining of the oral cavity is the
   a. ectoderm.
   b. mesoderm.
   c. endoderm.
   d. stomodeum.

2. An incremental line in the enamel indicating the trauma of birth, found in all primary teeth and several permanent teeth, is the
   a. line of Retzius.
   b. imbrication line.
   c. Tome's process.
   d. neonatal line.

3. The softest tooth structure is the
   a. alveolar bone.
   b. cementum.
   c. dentin.
   d. enamel.

4. The development of different tissues is
   a. cytodifferentiation.
   b. histodifferentiation.
   c. morphodifferentiation.
   d. proliferation.

5. Name the connective tissue that is formed by the fibroblast cells and which secures the tooth into the socket by a number of organized fiber groups.
   a. lamina dura
   b. periodontal ligaments
   c. gingiva
   d. epithelial attachment

6. Which of the following terms is used to identify the second prenatal phase of pregnancy from week two through week eight?
   a. fetus
   b. embryo
   c. zygote
   d. ovum

7. Which of the following terms describes the invagination of ectoderm, which pushes in and forms the primitive oral cavity?
   a. ectoderm
   b. mesoderm
   c. endoderm
   d. stomodeum

8. Which of the pharyngeal arches is responsible for the development of the muscles of facial expression?
   a. pharyngeal arch I
   b. pharyngeal arch II
   c. pharyngeal arch III
   d. pharyngeal arch IV

9. Between weeks eight and twelve, the primary palate of the globular process fuses with the lateral processes from the maxillary process. If this fusion is disturbed, the result is a cleft palate.

   Based on the preceding statements, select the correct response.
   a. Both statements are true.
   b. Both statements are false.
   c. The first statement is true; the second statement is false.
   d. The first statement is false; the second statement is true.

10. Which of the following layers of the cap stage will lead to formation of the ameloblasts?
    a. outer enamel epithelium
    b. inner enamel epithelium
    c. stellate reticulum
    d. dental laminae

11. Which of the following layers of the bell stage is responsible for nourishing the developing ameloblasts?
    a. outer enamel epithelium
    b. inner enamel epithelium
    c. stellate reticulum
    d. stratum intermedium

12. Which of the following is not correct regarding the structure of enamel?
    a. Enamel is laid down in increments, which results in the striae of Retzius.
    b. Hydroxyapatite crystals are deposited into amelogenin, causing mineralization.
    c. The enamel rod is shaped like a keyhole.
    d. Hardened enamel is 96% organic and 4% inorganic.

13. Some areas of enamel are naturally hypocalcified. Examples of a hypocalcified area of enamel are enamel tufts.

    Based on the preceding statements, select the correct response.
    a. Both statements are true.
    b. Both statements are false.
    c. The first statement is true; the second statement is false.
    d. The first statement is false; the second statement is true.

14. Hypocalcification is considered to be a normal formation of enamel. Hypocalcification of enamel can occur during tooth development or during later stages of life.

    Based on the preceding statements, select the correct response.
    a. Both statements are true.
    b. Both statements are false.
    c. The first statement is true; the second statement is false.
    d. The first statement is false; the second statement is true.

15. Which of the following is correct regarding dentin?
    a. Dentin formation begins after enamel formation.
    b. Odontoblasts within the dental papilla form dentin.

    c. Dentin is 30% organic and 70% inorganic material.
    d. The dentin of the tooth is laid down all at once and then calcified.

16. Which of the following structures is directly responsible for formation of the cementum?
    a. dental sac
    b. dental papilla
    c. enamel organ
    d. dental lamina

17. Which of the following statements regarding enamel is not correct?
    a. Enamel is the hardest substance in the body.
    b. Enamel has the ability to repair itself.
    c. Enamel is thinner at the cementoenamel junction (CEJ).
    d. Enamel is whiter at the chewing surface and cusp tips.

18. Which of the following is not correct regarding the periodontal ligament fibers?
    a. The periodontal ligament fibers embed into the cementum of the tooth and the lamina dura of the alveolar bone.
    b. The periodontal ligament is located in the space between the alveolar socket and the root of the tooth.
    c. The periodontal ligament is rigid, thus preventing any movement of the tooth during function.
    d. The periodontal ligament carries blood supply to the periodontium for nutrition and remodeling.

19. Which of the following structures marks where the free gingiva ends and the attached gingiva begins?
    a. free marginal groove
    b. epithelial attachment
    c. sulcus
    d. mucogingival junction

20. At the apex of each root, there is a tiny opening that allows nerve fibers and blood vessels to enter and nourish the tooth. This opening is called a(n) _____.
    a. apical foramen
    b. pulp cavity
    c. pulp chamber
    d. pulp canal

Critical Thinking

1. While in the hospital maternity ward, a dental assistant sees a newborn child with a severe unilateral cleft lip. At what stage of development did the cleft lip take place? What step in development did not take place?

2. If a child has enamel dysplasia, a dental assistant would assume that a disturbance took place during which stage of development?

3. What is the difference between primary, secondary, and tertiary dentin?

Key Terms

Term and Pronunciation	Meaning of Root and Word Parts	Definition
acellular (**ey**-sel-*yuh*-**ler**)	**a-** = without **cell** = basic structural unit of all organisms **-ular** = pertaining to or characterized by	without cells
alveolar crest (al-vee-uh-ler) (krest)	**alveol(o)** = alveolus; tooth socket **-ar** = pertaining to **crest** = the highest point of anything	highest point of alveolar bone between adjacent teeth

Term and Pronunciation	Meaning of Root and Word Parts	Definition
alveolus (al-**vee**-*uh*-luh s)	**alveol-** = a small cell, cavity, or socket; tooth socket **-us** = possessing, full of	the socket within the jawbone in which the root or roots of a tooth are set; tooth socket
ameloblast (**am**-*uh*-loh-blast)	**(en)amel-** = the hard, glossy, calcareous covering of the crown of a tooth, containing only a slight amount of organic substance **-o-** = used to connect compound word **blast** = indicating an embryonic cell or formative layer	a type of cell involved in forming dental enamel; one of a layer of enamel-secreting cells covering the dentin of a developing tooth
apical (**ey**-pi-k*uh* l)	**apex** = the pointed end or tip of something **-al** = pertaining to	the extremity of a conical or pyramidal structure as in root of a tooth/relating to the apex or tip of a root
apposition (ap-uh-zish-uh n)	**apposite** = suitable, well-adapted; well-placed or applies **-ion** = denoting action or condition	growth in the thickness of a cell wall by the deposition of successive layers of material
bifurcate (bahy-fer-keyt)	**bi-** = two **furcate** = to form a fork, branch	a forking, a division into two branches
cellular (sel-**yuh**-ler)	**cell** = basic structural unit of all organisms **-ular** = pertaining to or characterized by	contains cells
cleft (kleft)	**cleft** = a space or opening made by a cleavage; split	a fissure or elongated opening, divided or split
dental lamina (den-tl) (lam-uh-nuh)	**dent-** = teeth **-al** = pertaining to **lamina** = a layer or coat lying over another, as the plates of minerals or bones	band of ectodermal cells growing from oral epithelium into underlying mesenchyme that becomes the tooth buds and eventually the enamel organs
dentin (**den**-tn)	**dentin** = the main bulk of the tooth	second-hardest tooth tissue, in crown and root, surrounds pulp, and under enamel and cementum
ectoderm (ek-tuh-durm)	**ecto-** = outer, external **-derm** = indicating skin; layer of tissue	the outer layer of cells in an embryo
embryo (em-bree-oh)	**embryo** = early stages of development within the womb	the human product of conception up to approximately the end of the second month of pregnancy
enamel (ih-**nam**-*uh* l)	**enamel** = outer surface of the crown of the tooth	hard, glistening substance covering coronal (crown) dentin of tooth, made up of 90% hydroxyapatite and about 6% calcium carbonate, calcium fluoride, and magnesium carbonate, with 4% of organic matrix of protein
enamel organ (ih-nam-uh l) (awr-guh n)	**enamel** = the hard, glossy, calcareous covering of the crown of a tooth, containing only a slight amount of organic substance **organ** = a grouping of tissues into a distinct structure that performs a specialized task	part of tooth germ that forms enamel of crown of tooth; a cellular aggregation seen in histologic sections of a developing tooth
endoderm (en-duh-durm)	**endo-** = within; innermost **-derm** = indicating skin; layer of tissue	innermost of the three primary germ layers of a developing embryo
epithelial rests of Malassez (ep-uh-thee-lee-uh l) (rest) (mahl-ah-seyz)	**epithelium** = membranous tissue composed of one or more layers of cells separated by very little intercellular substance and forming the covering of most internal and external surfaces of the body and its organs **-al** = pertaining to **rest** = the part that is left or remains; remainder **Malassez, Louis-Charles** = French anatomist and histologist, named structure	discrete clusters of residual cells from Hertwig's epithelial root sheath (HERS) that didn't completely disappear; the epithelial cell rests of Malassez are part of the periodontal ligament cells around a tooth
fetus (fee-tuh s)	**fetus** = the young while in the womb	the human product at the end of second month of pregnancy; development of body structures are in recognizable form
Hertwig's epithelial root sheath (hur-twig) (ep-uh-thee-lee-uhl) (root) (sheeth)	**Hertwig, Oskar** = German zoologist, named sheath **epithelium** = membranous tissue composed of one or more layers of cells separated by very little intercellular substance and forming the covering of most internal and external surfaces of the body and its organs **-al** = pertaining to **root** = part of a **tooth** below the gum; the root anchors the tooth to the jawbone **sheath** = a closely enveloping, tubular part or structure	two layers of cells that guide the shape of root during its development
inorganic (in-awr-**gan**-ik)	**in-** = not, non **organic** = pertaining to, or derived from living organisms	not organic, not formed by living organisms, not containing carbon

(Continues)

Term and Pronunciation	Meaning of Root and Word Parts	Definition
invagination (in-vaj-uh-ney-shuh n)	**in-** = in, within **vaginate** = forming or enclosed in a sheath (close-fitting covering) **-ion** = denoting action or condition	to insert one part of a structure within a part of the same structure, to grow in from an ingrowth or in-pocketing
lingual (**ling**-gwuh l)	**lingua-** = the tongue **-al** = pertaining to	relating to the tongue, side of tooth closest to tongue
mesenchyme (mes-eng-kahym)	**mesenchyme** = part of the embryonic mesoderm that consists of loosely packed, unspecialized cells that are set in a gelatinous ground substance	cells of mesodermal origin that are capable of developing into connective tissues, blood, and lymphatic and blood vessels
mesoderm (mez-uh-durm)	**meso-** = middle **-derm** = indicating skin; layer of tissue	middle layer of the three primary germ layers of a developing embryo
mineralization (**min**-er-uh-lahy-**zey**-shuh n)	**mineral** = class of inorganic substances; usually of definite crystal structure **-ize** = to convert into **-ation** = indicating an action, process	introduction of minerals into a structure, such as bones and teeth
nasal septum (ney-zuh l) (sep-tuh m)	**naso-** = nose **-al** = pertaining to **septum** = a dividing wall, membrane in an animal structure	the membrane dividing the nasal cavity into halves
occlusal (uh-kloo-zhuh l)	**occlude** = to shut or close, with the cusps of the opposing teeth of the upper and lower jaws fitting together **-al** = pertaining to	pertaining to the occlusion or closure, pertaining to the contacting surfaces of opposing biting surfaces, masticating surfaces
olfactory (nasal) pits (ol-fak-tuh-ree) (pits)	**olfactory** = an organ or nerve concerned with the sense of smell **pits** = naturally formed holes or cavities	paired depressions formed when nasal placodes (local thickening of the endoderm in embryo) come to lie below general external contour of developing face at nose
organic (awr-**gan**-ik)	**organic** = pertaining to, or derived from living organisms	formed by living organisms, contains carbon
periodontal ligament (PDL) (per-ee-uh-**don**-tl) (**lig**-uh-muh nt)	**peri-** = around, about **odont** = tooth **-al** = pertaining to **lig-** = to tie **-ment** = denoting state	periodontal ligament, investing and supporting tissue by which the roots of a tooth are anchored within its alveolus, consists of bands of collagen fibers connecting the cementum to both gingiva and alveolar bone and to cementum and adjacent teeth
periodontium (per-ee-uh-don-shuh m)	**peri(o)** = surrounding, around **-odont** = having teeth **-ium** = indicating a biological structure	specialized tissues that surround and support the teeth
pulp (puhlp)	**pulp** = a soft, moist, shapeless mass of matter	the inner substance of the tooth, containing arteries, veins, and lymphatic and nerve tissue that communicate with their respective vascular, lymph, and nerve systems
resorption (ri-**sawrp**-shuh n)	**re-** = back, backward **sorption** = uptake of substances by a tissue	the destruction, disappearance, or dissolution of a tissue or part by biochemical activity, as the loss of bone or of tooth dentin
stellate reticulum (stel-it) (ri-tik-yuh-luh m)	**stellate** = arranged or shaped like a star; radiating from a center **reticulum** = a network of structures in the endoplasm or nucleus of certain cells	the bulk of enamel organ; it serves to shape the crown of the forming tooth and becomes nourishment for the stratum intermedium
stomodeum (stoh-muh-dee-uh m)	**stoma** = a mouth or ingestive opening **-ode** = like **-eum** = indicating a biological structure	a midline ectodermal depression surrounding by the mandibular arch, becomes continuous with foregut and forms mouth.
stratum intermedium (strey-tuh m) (mee-dee-uh m)	**stratum** = a layer of tissue **inter** = between **medium** = an intervening substance through which something else is transmitted or carried on	a layer of the enamel organ that is between the IEE and stellate reticulum; becomes nourishment for the IEE during amelogenesis
tooth germ (tooth) (jurm)	**tooth** = any of various bonelike structures set in the jaws for biting, tearing, or chewing **germ** = something that serves as a source or initial stage for subsequent development	includes the enamel organ, dental papilla, and dental sac
trifurcate (trahy-**fur**-keyt)	**tri-** = three **furcate** = to form a fork, branch	division of a root structure into three sections
zygote (zahy-goht)	**zygote** = a fertilized egg cell	the cell resulting from the union of an ovum and a spermatozoon; before cleavage

Dental Anatomy

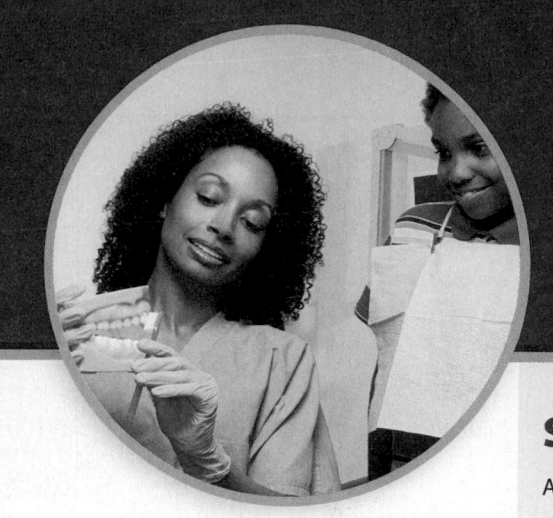

Introduction

Dental anatomy is the study of teeth. A human being has two sets of teeth, called **dentitions**, in a lifetime. As a child, the first dentition is called the primary dentition and consists of 20 teeth. As a child grows, by the age of 12 or 13 the primary dentition is replaced with an adult dentition consisting of 32 teeth. In this chapter, you will study the types, appearance, function, and location of teeth.

Types of Teeth and Their Functions

Healthy teeth are vital to oral health and play a major role in the ability to eat and speak and in self-esteem. Humans have four types of teeth: incisors, canines, premolars, and molars. Each type of tooth has a specific function in the process of mastication.

Incisors

Incisors are located in the front of the mouth and are visible when you smile. Their primary function is to cut (**incise**) and tear into food. Incisors are shaped like small chisels with sharp, flat edges (*incisal*

edge) to incise into food. The side of the tooth toward the tongue is shallow and scooped out like a shovel and aids in guiding food into the mouth. Incisors are also important in talking. The incisors work with the lips, tongue, and roof of the mouth to form different sounds.

Canines

Canines are located at the corners of the mouth, act as guideposts to the rest of the teeth, and help shape the face. Their primary function is to assist incisors in cutting. Canines have a sharp, pointed tip (called a **cusp** tip) and may also be referred to as cuspids. They are larger and stronger than incisors and have the added function of tearing tougher food like meat. They also work with the incisors to help form sounds.

Premolars

Premolars are found behind the canines. They have two or three sharp cusps and a broader surface than canines and are also called bicuspids. Premolars assist the canines in tearing and chewing and grinding food to a consistency that is easier to swallow and digest. There are no premolars in the primary dentition.

Molars

The final type of teeth are the molars, which are found behind the premolars. They have four to five cusps, a broader chewing surface than premolars, and are the largest teeth in the mouth. Molars sustain a great amount of force to chew and grind food into easily swallowed pieces.

Dental Arches

The dentition is the type, number, and arrangement of teeth in the arches of the mouth. The upper arch is the **maxillary arch**, because the teeth are set in the maxilla bone. The lower teeth are located in the mandible bone, and therefore are located in the **mandibular arch** (Figure 8-1). The maxillary arch is fixed to the skull and the mandibular arch is movable, bringing the biting force toward the maxillary arch. Each arch has an identical number of teeth, and the teeth are designed so that proper function and positioning can be maintained. Each arch contains one-half of the dentition: 10 primary teeth or 16 adult teeth. The teeth in the maxillary arch slightly overlap the mandibular teeth when in proper alignment. The teeth in each arch touch the teeth **adjacent** (next) to them, except for the last tooth in each arch. The teeth from the maxillary arch contact the teeth from the mandibular arch each time the mouth is closed. Each tooth supports the teeth beside it and the teeth in the **opposing arch** so that displacement does not occur.

Dental Quadrants

Each of the dental arches is divided in two halves by an imaginary line called the *midline* (**median line**), which creates two sections called **quadrants** (one-fourth of the dental arches). Thus, there are four quadrants, containing five primary teeth and eight permanent teeth each, found in the dentition. The arrangement of the teeth is identical in each quadrant (Figure 8-2). The primary teeth in sequence from the median line are the following:

- Two incisors (central incisor and lateral incisor)
- One canine (also referred to as cuspid)
- Two molars (first molar and second molar)

The adult teeth in sequence are the following:

- Two incisors (central incisor and lateral incisor)
- One canine (also referred to as cuspid)
- Two premolars (first premolar and second premolar; also referred to as bicuspids)
- Three molars (first molar, second molar, and third molar)

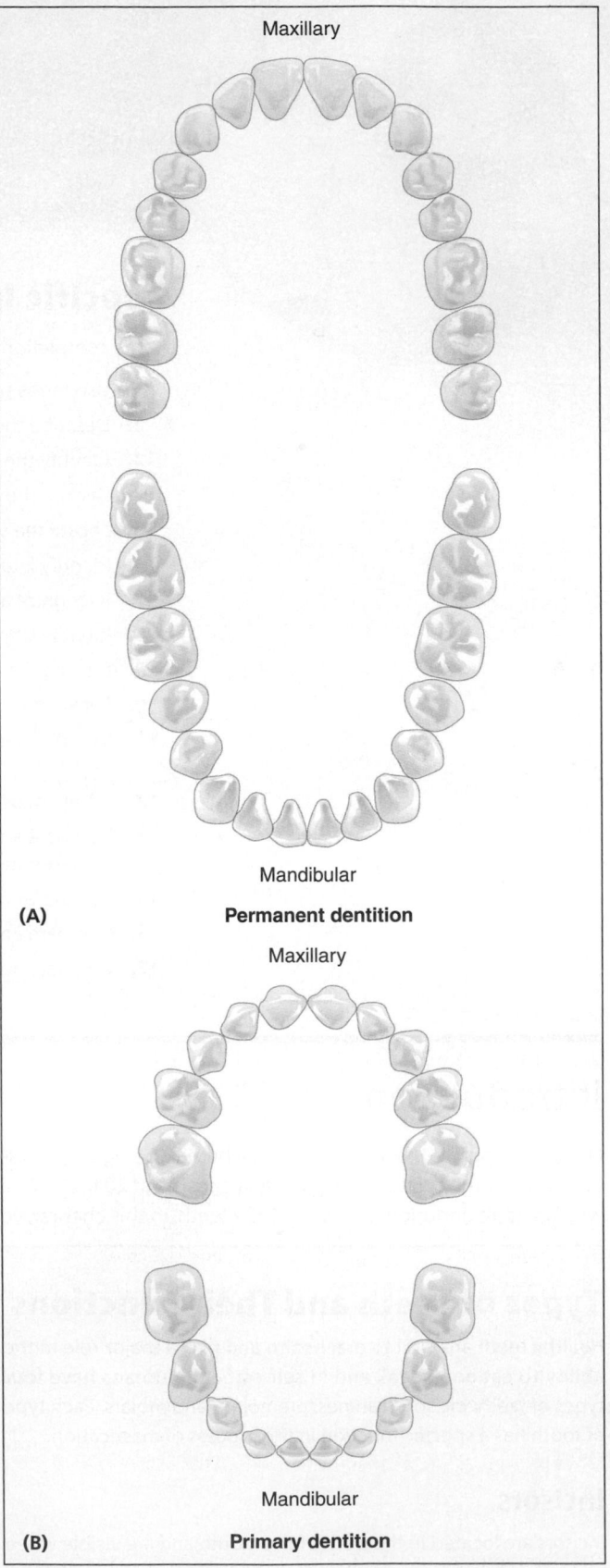

FIGURE 8-1

(A) Maxillary and mandibular dentition of an adult (permanent dentition).
(B) Maxillary and mandibular dentition of a child (primary dentition).

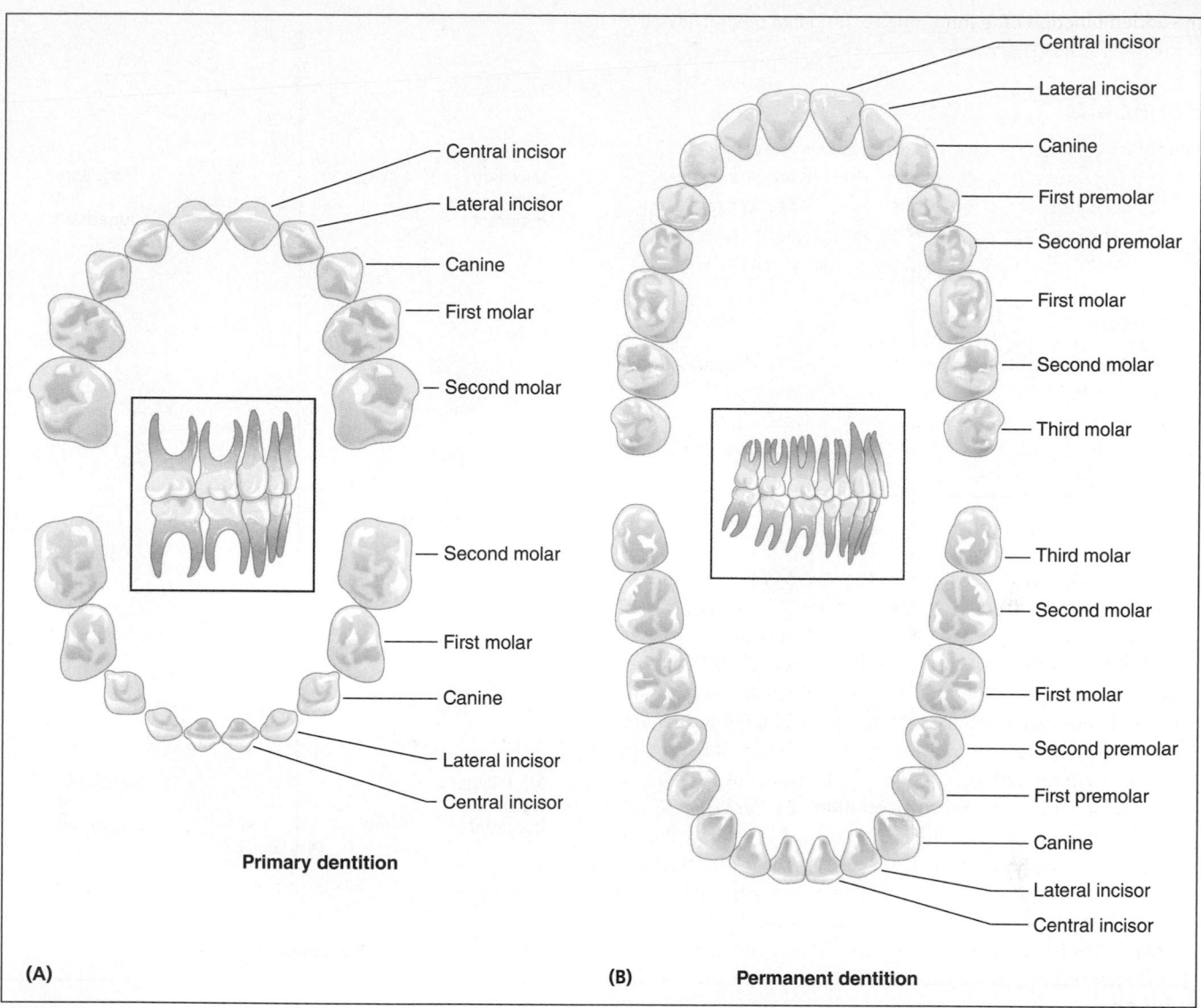

FIGURE 8-2
(A) Primary dentition, identifying each tooth by name. (B) Adult dentition, identifying each tooth by name.

Each quadrant is named according to its location in the dentition (Figure 8-3). The quadrants are labeled according to the patient's right or left. Looking into the oral cavity from the front of the patient makes the directions of right and left reversed to the dental assistant; the assistant's left is the patient's right and the assistant's right is the patient's left. This is very important to remember when naming and charting teeth. In order to identify a specific tooth, the quadrant must be named before the name of the tooth. For example, there are four total central incisors in the mouth, maxillary right central incisor, maxillary left central incisor, mandibular left central incisor, and mandibular right central incisor.

Dental Sextants

The dentition can also be divided into *sextants*, or sixths. There is one **anterior** sextant in each arch and two **posterior** sextants. There is an anterior and a right and left posterior sextant in each arch. The adult dentition anterior sextant consists of six front teeth,

and each posterior sextant has five teeth in each posterior sextant. (Figure 8-4).

Dentition Periods

Two dentitions have already been identified; however, there are three dentition periods. The primary teeth erupt first and are replaced by the adult dentition. The period of time while the primary teeth are being replaced is referred to as mixed dentition.

Primary Dentition

The primary dentition, which laypersons commonly refer to as baby teeth, begins with the **eruption** of the primary mandibular central incisors at approximately six months of age and is completed with the eruption of the maxillary second molars between 24–32 months (Table 8-1.) Between six and seven years of age, the central incisors **exfoliate**. The term *deciduous dentition*

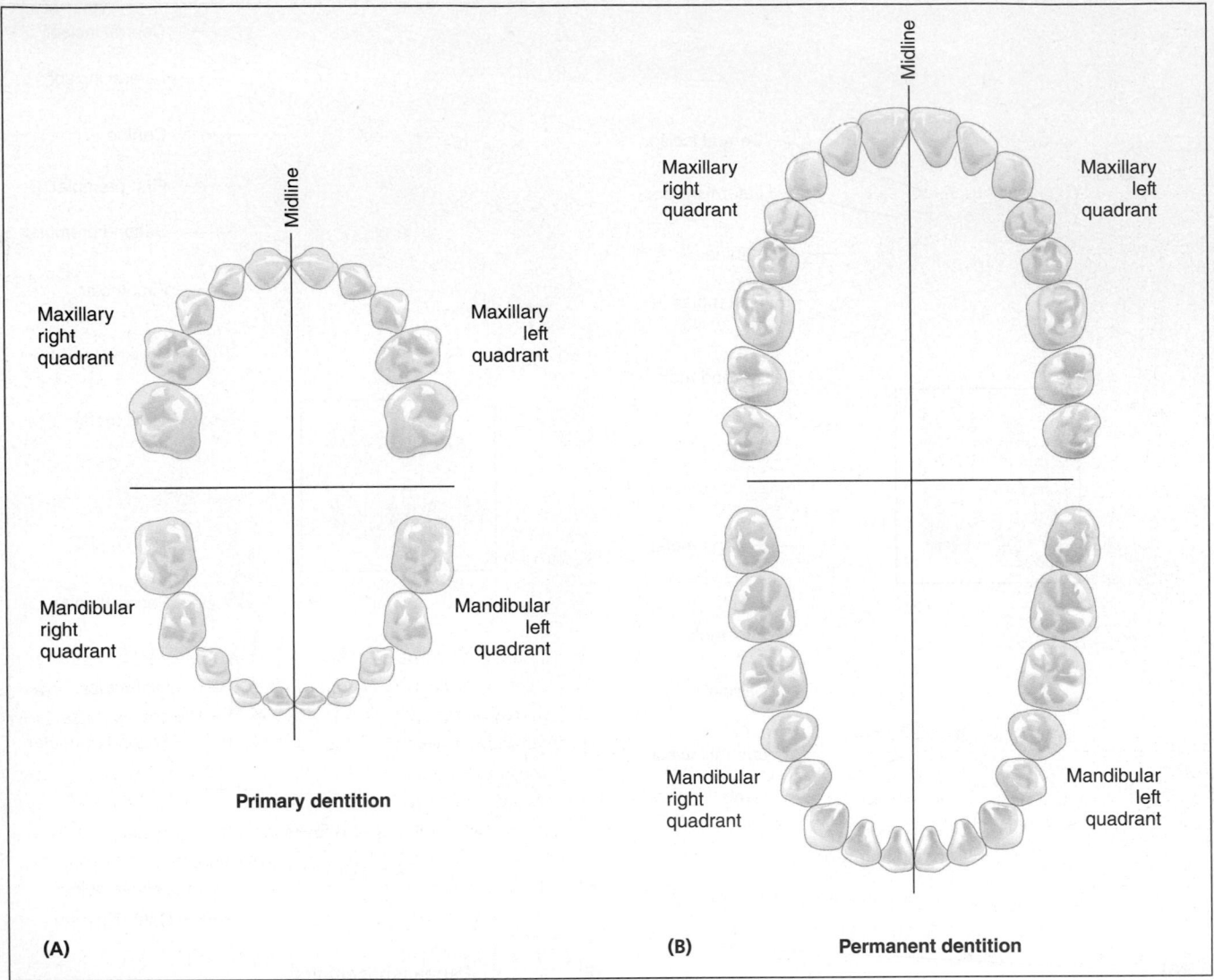

FIGURE 8-3
Dental arches of (A) primary dentition and (B) adult dentition divided into quadrants with the midline identified.

is an older dental term and is used less frequently to describe the primary dentition; it relates to the process of shedding the primary teeth as with deciduous trees.

Mixed Dentition

The period when both primary teeth and permanent teeth are in the dentition is called the *mixed dentition* period (Figure 8-5). This period lasts from approximately 6 to 12 years of age. After the age of 12, most of the primary teeth have exfoliated.

Permanent Dentition

The permanent dentition, also referred to as adult dentition, begins to erupt from about 6 years of age until around 17 to 21 years of age (Table 8-2). The permanent teeth that replace the primary teeth are called **succedaneous** teeth (Figure 8-6). The term refers to succeeding the primary teeth. Therefore, because there are 20 primary teeth, there are also 20 succedaneous teeth. In the anterior, the tooth of the same name is replaced by the succedaneous,

and the premolars replace the primary molars. **Nonsuccedaneous** teeth are the teeth that do not replace primary teeth. This would reference the permanent molars erupting in each quadrant behind the primary molars. Therefore, there could be up to 12 nonsuccedaneous teeth in the permanent dentition.

Surfaces of the Teeth

An easy way to understand the surfaces of the tooth is to view each tooth as if it were a box with five sides (surfaces): a top, front, back, and a right and left side (Figure 8-7).

The tooth's front surface is called the **facial** surface, is the surface that faces the lips and cheeks, and is the surface you see when you smile. Another name for the facial surface of anterior teeth can be the *labial surface* because it is close to the lips, and in the posterior, this same facial surface can be called *buccal* because it is next to the cheeks.

The opposite side from facial or the back side of the box is the **lingual** surface. This surface faces the tongue or inside of the

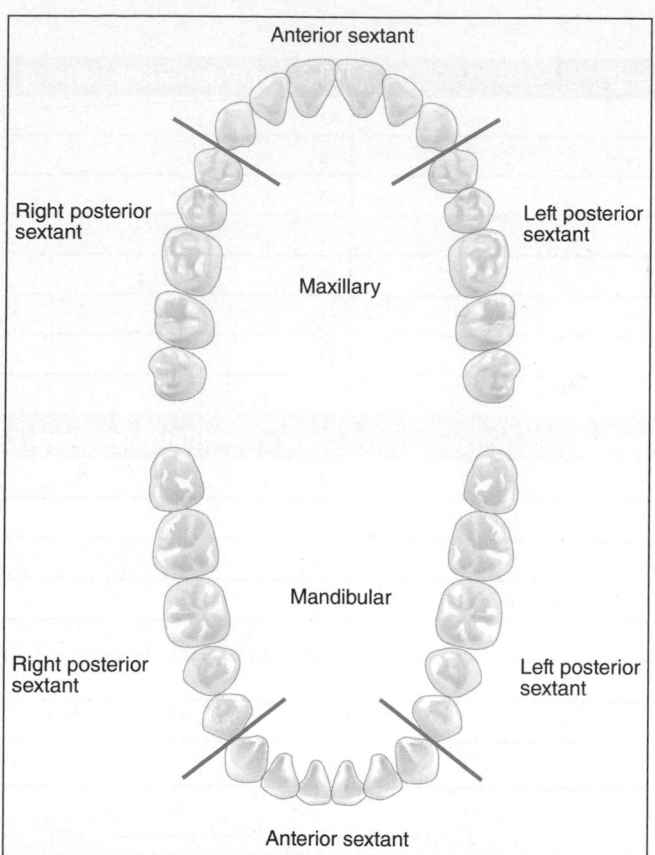

FIGURE 8-4
Adult dentition divided into sextants. The maxillary and mandibular arches each have two posterior sextants and one anterior sextant.

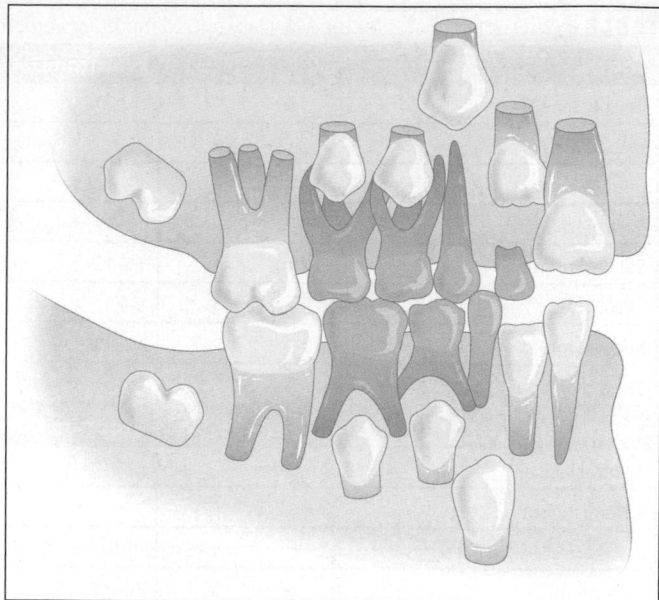

FIGURE 8-5
Mixed dentition of a seven- to eight-year-old.

mouth. Another name for the lingual surface on the maxillary arch is *palatal*, because it is the surface next to the palate. This surface is the only one that is different and separates the maxillary and mandibular instead of anterior or posterior.

Because the dental arches curve, the sides of the tooth are named by their relationship to the midline. The side that is closest to the midline is called the *mesial surface*, and the opposite side of the tooth that is farthest away from the midline is the *distal surface*. These two surfaces do not have any additional names.

The top side is the only one remaining. On anterior teeth, this is the biting or cutting surface called the *incisal surface*, and in the posterior the chewing surface where the top is flatter and wider is called the *occlusal surface*.

In naming the sides of the teeth, you will notice that four of the five sides of a tooth remained the same and it did not depend whether it is an anterior or posterior tooth. The only difference is the top surface that changes names from anterior to posterior. There are a few surfaces that have more than one name, but there is always a generic name for each one:

Anterior Teeth Surfaces	Posterior Teeth Surfaces
1. mesial	1. mesial
2. distal	2. distal
3. lingual (or palatal)	3. lingual
4. facial (labial)	4. facial (buccal)
5. incisal	5. occlusal

TABLE 8-1 Eruption and Exfoliation Dates for Primary Teeth

Tooth	Eruption Date (Months)	Exfoliation Date (Years)	Maxillary Order
Central incisor	6–10	6–7	#1
Lateral incisor	9–12	7–8	#2
Canine	16–22	10–12	#4
First molar	12–18	9–11	#3
Second molar	24–32	10–12	#5
Tooth	Eruption Date (Months)	Exfoliation Date (Years)	Mandibular Order
Central incisor	6–10	6–7	#1
Lateral incisor	7–10	7–8	#2
Canine	16–22	9–12	#4
First molar	12–18	9–11	#3
Second molar	20–32	10–12	#5

TABLE 8-2 Eruption Dates for the Maxillary and Mandibular Permanent Teeth

Tooth	Eruption Date (Years)	Order of Eruption (Maxillary)
Central incisor	7–8	#2
Lateral incisor	8–9	#3
Canine	11–12	#6
First premolar	10–11	#4
Second premolar	11–12	#5
First molar	6–7	#1
Second molar	12–13	#7
Third molar	17–21	#8
Tooth	**Eruption Date (Years)**	**Order of Eruption (Mandibular)**
Central incisor	6–7	#2
Lateral incisor	7–8	#3
Cuspid	9–10	#4
First premolar	10–11	#5
Second premolar	11–12	#6
First molar	6–7	#1
Second molar	11–13	#7
Third molar	17–21	#8

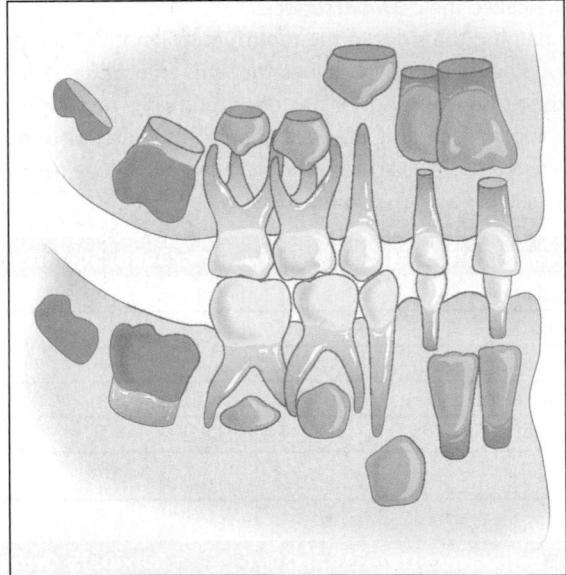

FIGURE 8-6
Mixed dentition of a five-year-old. Unerupted succedaneous teeth are shaded in blue, and nonsuccedaneous teeth are shaded in green.

Points of Reference

The dental team needs to communicate specific tooth locations in order to chart present conditions, facilitate better diagnosis, and allow the dentist to give detailed information about a tooth to the dental laboratory technician and patient's dental insurance. For the most precise description, angles and divisions of teeth are identified.

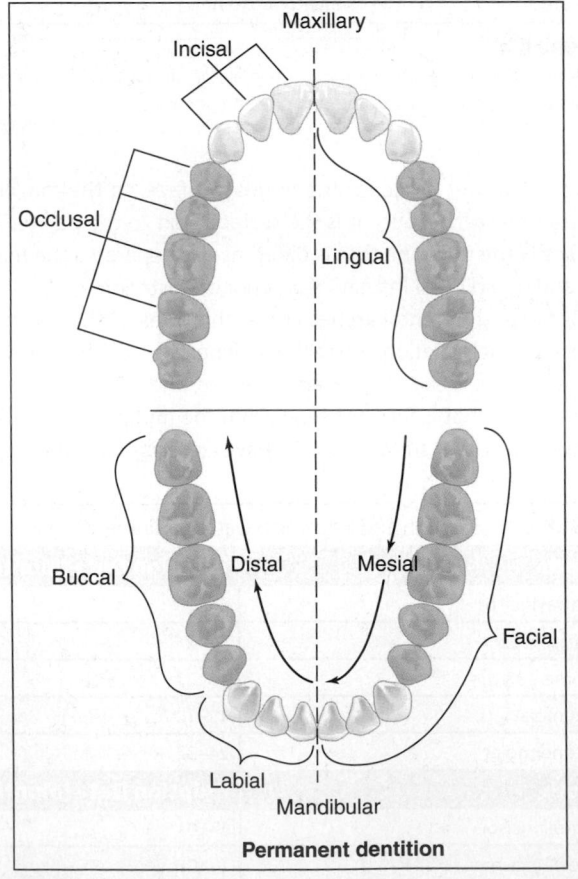

FIGURE 8-7
Surfaces of the teeth identified on the dental arches in a permanent dentition. Posterior teeth are colored in blue.

Line Angles and Point Angles

When two adjacent surfaces touch, they form a line angle (Figure 8-8). When three neighboring surfaces meet, they form a point angle, or a corner of the tooth. When naming these line or point angles, the two or three surfaces are put together by dropping the "al" off the end of the surface and adding an "o" to join the terms. (See Table 8-3.)

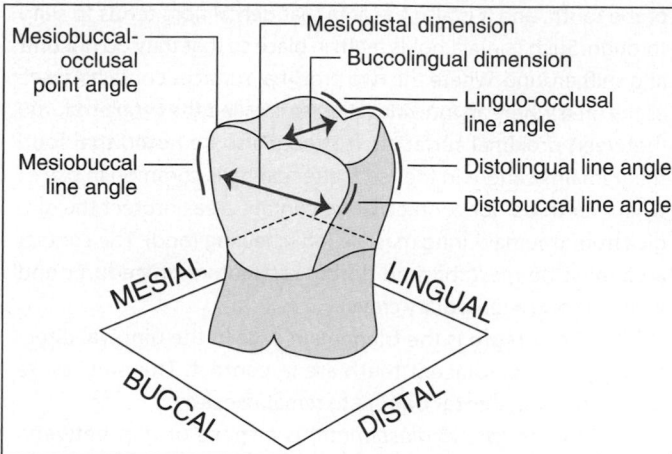

FIGURE 8-8
Line and point angles.

Divisions into Thirds

Tooth surfaces are further identified by dividing them into approximate thirds. This practice helps the dental team identify specific areas on each surface. Also identified are the spaces between the teeth and where the teeth are touching.

The crown of the tooth and the root of the tooth are divided into approximate thirds (Figure 8-9). The area on the crown of the tooth that is nearest the incisal edge on the anterior tooth is called the

TABLE 8-3 Name of Line Angles and Point Angles of Teeth

Line Angles (2 surfaces touch)	Point Angles (3 surfaces touch)
mesial + facial = mesiofacial	mesial + facial + incisal =mesiofacioincisal
mesial + lingual = mesiolingual	mesial + lingual + incisal = mesiolinguoincisal
distal + facial = distofacial	distal + facial + incisal = distofacioincisal
distal + lingual = distolingual	distal + lingual + incisal = distolinguoincisal
facial + incisal =facioincisal	
lingual + incisal = linguoincisal	
mesial + incisal = mesioincisal	
distal + incisal = distoincisal	

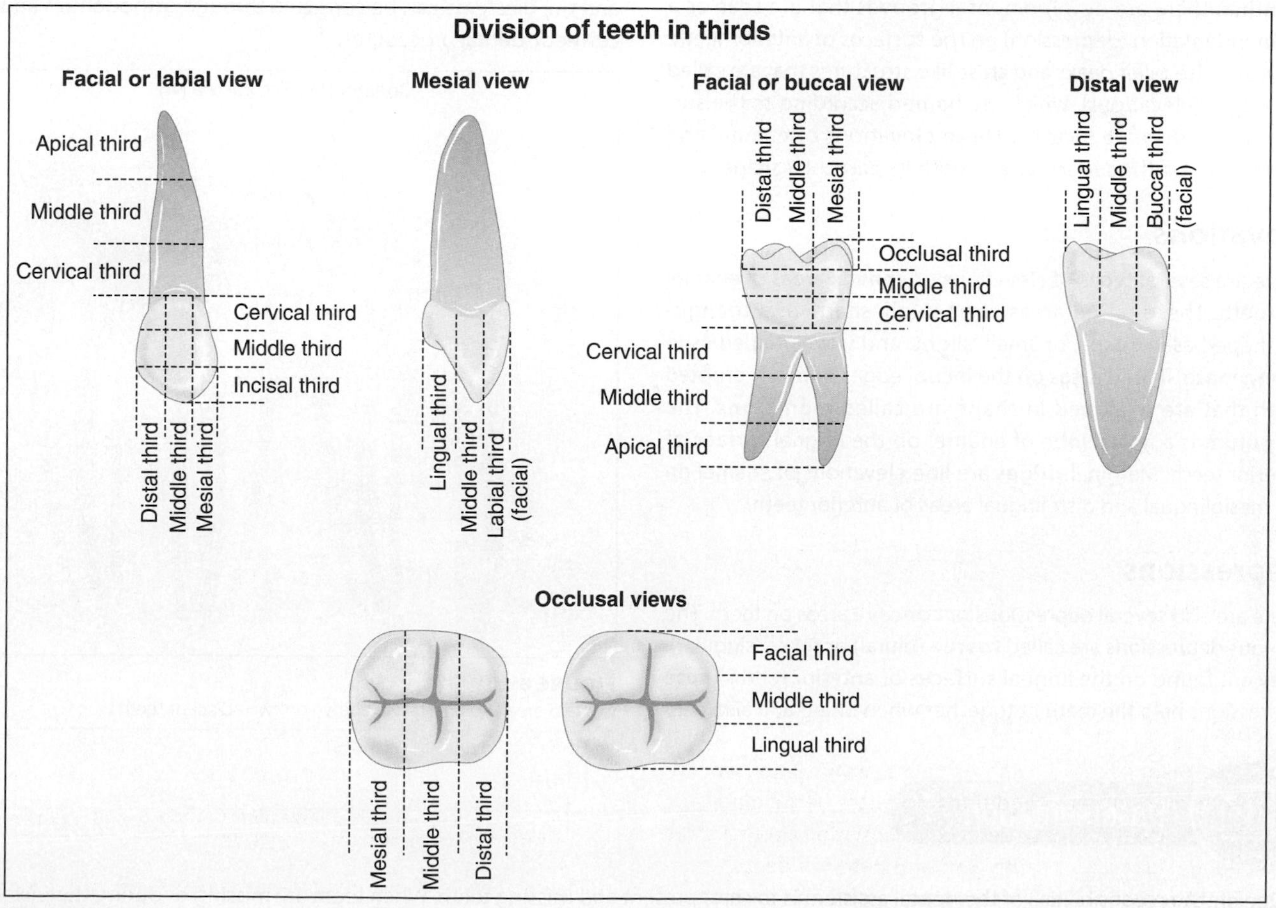

Division of teeth in thirds

Facial or labial view

Apical third
Middle third
Cervical third

Cervical third
Middle third
Incisal third

Distal third
Middle third
Mesial third

Mesial view

Lingual third
Middle third
Labial third (facial)

Facial or buccal view

Distal third
Middle third
Mesial third

Occlusal third
Middle third
Cervical third

Cervical third
Middle third
Apical third

Distal view

Lingual third
Middle third
Buccal third (facial)

Occlusal views

Mesial third
Middle third
Distal third

Facial third
Middle third
Lingual third

FIGURE 8-9
The crown and the root are divided into proximal thirds from all surfaces.

incisal third of the tooth, and the occlusal surface of the posterior tooth is called the *occlusal third* of the tooth. The area on the crown of the tooth that is closest to the **cervical** area (or to the gingiva) is called the *cervical third* of the tooth. The area between the incisal third and the cervical third is called the middle third. The root is also divided into imaginary thirds with the area nearest the **apex** as the *apical third* and the area nearest the crown of the tooth as the cervical third of the root. The area between the apical third of the root and the cervical third of the root is called the middle third of the root.

Tooth Morphology

Tooth **morphology** is the study of the form and shape of teeth. Knowledge of morphology helps the dental assistant identify and chart teeth present by their appearance. Morphology is necessary with restoring a tooth, making a temporary crown, and recognizing normal and abnormal tooth structures. To best understand tooth morphology, the assistant should know which landmarks are present of specific teeth and how the teeth contact with other teeth in the arch. Anterior tooth morphology will be discussed first, followed by the posterior teeth.

Anatomic Landmarks of Anterior Teeth

There are many specific landmarks or areas on the teeth that occur during development that are consistent with specific teeth. For example, when the four **lobes** that form a tooth join together, there are developmental grooves that are seen as a slight indentation (depression) on the surfaces of anterior teeth. There are also taller peaks and crest-like structures that are called the ridges (elevations), which are named according to the surface where they are located. These elevations of enamel and depressions on the surface give a tooth its particular shape.

Elevations

There are several types of elevations or **convex** areas of enamel on teeth. These raised areas can be tall, sharp, and triangular-shaped as in **cusps**, or small, slight, and wave-shaped as in **perikymata**. Raised areas on the incisal edges of newly erupted teeth that are scalloped in shape are called **mamelons**. The **cingulum** is a raised lobe of enamel on the lingual surface of anterior teeth. Marginal **ridges** are line elevations of enamel on the mesiolingual and distolingual areas of anterior teeth.

Depressions

There are also several depressions or **concave** areas on teeth. The obvious depressions are called **fossae** (plural) or **fossa** (singular). They are found on the lingual surfaces of anterior teeth. These depressions help the teeth fit together when biting and also help

with mastication. Shallow depressions can be found where the developmental lobes unite.

Contact Areas

Identifying the *contact area* on the tooth refers to where the **proximal** sides of two teeth come together and touch (Figure 8-10). This is normally the mesial of one tooth and the distal of another tooth, except where the two central incisors mesial surfaces touch at the midline in each arch. The area is generally in the middle third of the tooth, and it is also the area that dental floss tends to snap through. Such contact holds teeth in place so that they do not drift and shift around. Where the two proximal surfaces contact as well as the area where an individual flosses is called the *interproximal* (between proximal surfaces). It should also be noted that food that remains caught in the teeth after eating is common in places where teeth do not contact. Good contact areas protect the gingiva from trauma during mastication (chewing food). The contact area must be reestablished during restorative procedures and when making a temporary crown.

The **embrasure** is the triangular space in the gingival direction when two adjacent teeth are in contact. The embrasure allows the **interdental papilla** to remain healthy.

A *diastema* (plural *diastemata*) is a space or gap between teeth. The term *diastema* is most often used in reference to a gap between the "front teeth" maxillary central incisors. In most cases, it is caused by the **frenum** attachment, which can be removed, and the diastema can be corrected through orthodontics and/or cosmetic dental procedures.

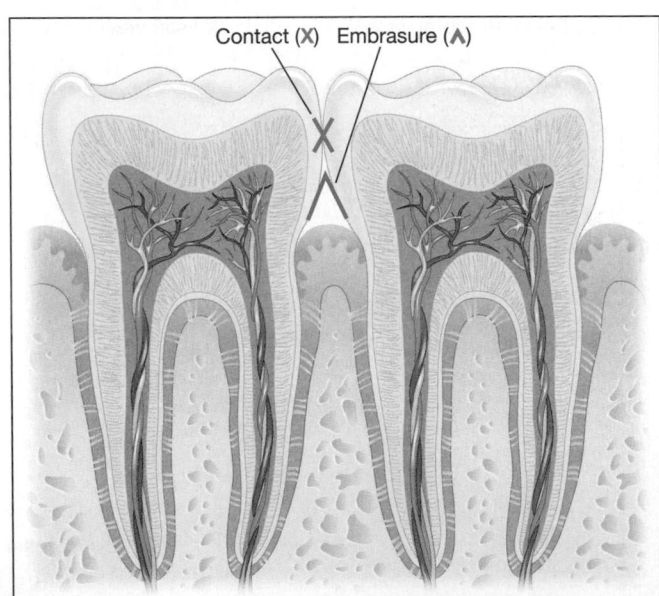

Contact (X)   Embrasure (∧)

FIGURE 8-10
Contact area and embrasure shown on two adjacent teeth.

Documentation

One of the responsibilities of the dental assistant is to chart present and missing teeth. When teeth are missing or during the mixed dentition period, it can be very challenging. The assistant must be able to identify teeth by the anatomic landmarks because the order of the teeth and eruption dates cannot be used alone.

Anterior Permanent Dentition

The anterior teeth include the central incisors, lateral incisors, and canines in both the maxillary and mandibular arches. These six teeth in each arch make up the anterior teeth or anterior sextants (maxillary anterior sextant and mandibular anterior sextant). The anterior teeth are very important for the patient's esthetics and self-esteem and are the first teeth that are seen when they smile or speak. When these teeth are broken, missing, or decayed, it can cause a person to be embarrassed, to not want to smile, or to cover their mouth when they talk. Over the course of your career in dentistry, you will see that a positive change in someone's smile can cause a person to change their disposition from being very shy and embarrassed to being happy, smiling, and outgoing! When a patient has their smile restored, they are proud to show their smiles. This is one of the things that make dentistry such a rewarding career. All anterior teeth are wedge-shaped when looking from the mesial and distal, which enables them to cut and bite into food.

In this portion of this chapter, each type of anterior tooth and its basic characteristic will be discussed, starting at the midline of the maxillary arch and then moving to the same type of tooth in the mandibular arch before moving posteriorly.

Maxillary Central Incisor

The maxillary central incisors (abbreviated Max CI) are the front teeth to the right and left of the midline of the maxillary arch. This tooth erupts at about eight years of age and succeeds the primary maxillary central incisor. They are the only teeth along with the mandibular centrals that have a mesial surface contacting another mesial surface. The proximal surface of every other tooth has a mesial surface touching the distal surface of the tooth next to it. The most distinguishing characteristic of the maxillary central incisor is that it is the largest and widest of the anterior incisors.

Facial Aspect The *facial* is the surface seen when the patient smiles. The mesial incisal (MI) line angle is almost 90 degrees, which is a distinguishing characteristic of this tooth. The distoincisal (DI) line angle is more curved than the mesial and is not as sharp. On all the incisors, as a general rule, the distoincisal angle is curved more than that of the mesial surfaces. Many times when these teeth erupt, the three facial lobes can be seen, and the incisal ridge is sharp and scalloped where the three lobes grew together. Eventually, during normal chewing these scalloped edges, called **mamelons**, are worn off. The ridge becomes flat across, and then instead of an incisal ridge, it is called an incisal edge.

The facial surface of the central incisor is not flat but is convex and has a slight curve. There are two depressed areas called developmental grooves where the three facial developmental lobes joined to form the bulk of the tooth. These two developmental grooves are located from the incisal third to the middle third of the crown (see Figure 8-11). The grooves run vertically from the incisal edge, which gives the facial surface three slight elevations separated by two depressions. There are

also small horizontal, wavelike ripples along the cervical third area on the facial surface of the anterior crowns. These horizontal indentations are called *perikymata*, and are also known as *imbrication lines* (Figure 8-12). These are usually only found on the cervical third of the tooth and are not on the entire facial surface. Along the cutting surface is a slight ridge called the *labioincisal ridge*.

Lingual Aspect The lingual surface of the crown looks quite different from the facial aspect. This surface is concave, and the concavity on the lingual has a fossa that looks shovel-shaped. The center of the fossa is deeper than the outer edges of the fossa. Bordering the fossa are the mesial and distal marginal ridges proximally. These proximal sides and incisal edge also have slightly raised ridges (the mamelons are along this ridge on newly erupted incisors). In the cervical third of the lingual surface is the fourth lobe that forms a large, convex protuberance of enamel called the *cingulum*. A lingual ridge extends from the cingulum into the fossa. As the result of the mamelons being worn off, a flat chewing surface called the incisal edge remains. On either side of the incisal edge ridges remain (labioincisal and linguoincisal ridges). The incisal edge slopes lingually as the maxillary incisors extend over and slide against the mandibular incisors during mastication.

Root Characteristics The maxillary central incisors have one root, which resembles the shape of an ice cream cone. It is fairly round at the crown cervical margin and gets smaller at the apex. The root itself is blunted, not sharp, on the end and tilts slightly to the distal. The apex of the root is not directly in line with the middle of the crown but is also slightly tilted to the distal.

Mandibular Central Incisor

The most distinguishing characteristic of the mandibular central incisor (Mand CI) is that it is the smallest tooth in the dental arch and entire mouth. It is very different from its maxillary counterpart. The Mand CI erupts at about seven years of age and succeeds the primary mandibular central incisor.

Facial Aspect The mesial and distal incisal angles are **symmetrical**, and it can be very difficult to distinguish the right from the left mandibular central incisors. Both angles are at almost 90 degrees. (See Figure 8-13.) The distoincisal angle is not more curved than the mesial surface as it is in the maxillary central incisors. About the only way to tell the mesial and distal apart is to look at how the root is slightly curved to the distal (provided the root developed normally). Mamelons also occur on the cutting surface on these newly erupted incisors. Ridges (labioincisal and linguoincisal ridges) remain on either side of the incisal edge. The incisal edge slopes labially instead of lingually as found with the maxillary incisors due to the overlapping and sliding against the mandibular incisors during mastication. The mamelons are located along the incisal ridge when the tooth is newly erupted.

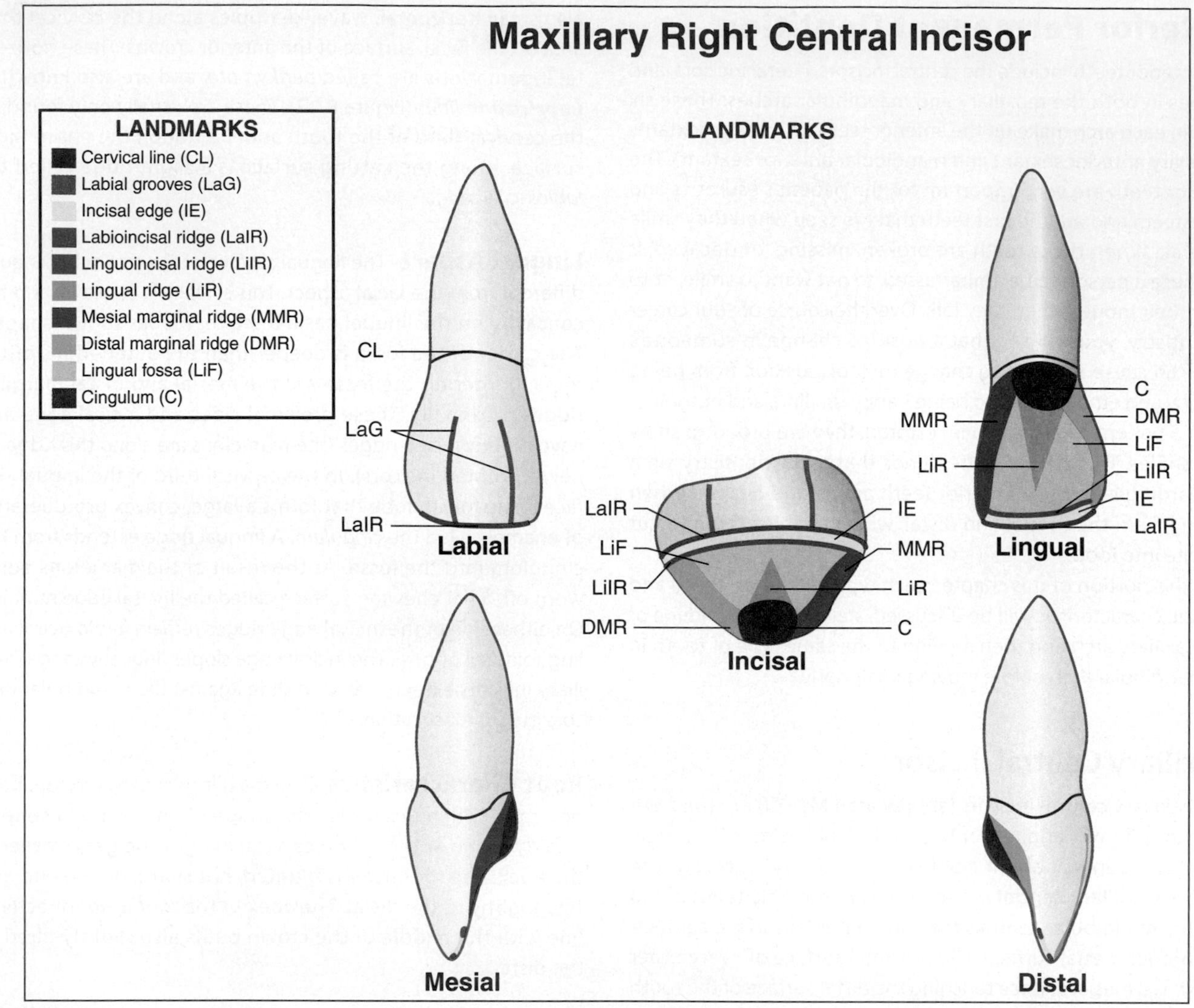

Maxillary Right Central Incisor

LANDMARKS

- ■ Cervical line (CL)
- ■ Labial grooves (LaG)
- □ Incisal edge (IE)
- ■ Labioincisal ridge (LaIR)
- ■ Linguoincisal ridge (LiIR)
- ■ Lingual ridge (LiR)
- ■ Mesial marginal ridge (MMR)
- ■ Distal marginal ridge (DMR)
- □ Lingual fossa (LiF)
- ■ Cingulum (C)

LANDMARKS

Labial

CL
LaG
LaIR

Incisal

LaIR
LiF
LiIR
DMR

IE
MMR
LiR
C

Lingual

C
DMR
LiF
LiIR
IE
LaIR

MMR
LiR

Mesial

Distal

FIGURE 8-11
Maxillary right central incisor landmarks. The labial diagram is viewing the tooth looking at it from in front of the mouth, and the lingual view is as if you were standing on the tongue looking out. The incisal is from the cutting surface, and the mesial and distal are looking at the teeth from the sides.

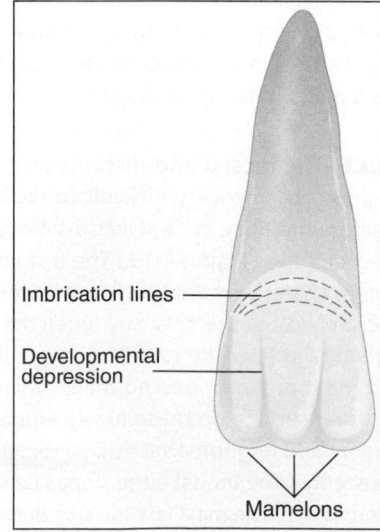

Imbrication lines

Developmental depression

Mamelons

FIGURE 8-12
Labial surface of the maxillary right central incisor with the mamelons, developmental depressions, and imbrication line identified.

Lingual Aspect The lingual surface of the mandibular central incisor looks similar to that of the maxillary central incisor. The lingual surface is somewhat concave instead of slightly convex as with the facial surface. The concavity is not as deep as that on the maxillary central incisor. Along the mesial and distal sides of the fossa are the mesial and distal marginal ridges. They are formed from a raised area of enamel that borders the sides of the fossa. The marginal ridges are not well defined on the mandibular central incisors, either. The cingulum is adjacent to the gingiva. It is the large raised area of the enamel formed from the fourth developmental lobe during tooth formation. A small lingual ridge extends from the cingulum into the fossa. Overall, on the mandibular incisors, the structures like the fossa and cingulum are much less pronounced than they are on the maxillary incisors.

Root Characteristics The root of the mandibular central incisor is much smaller because it is the smallest tooth in the

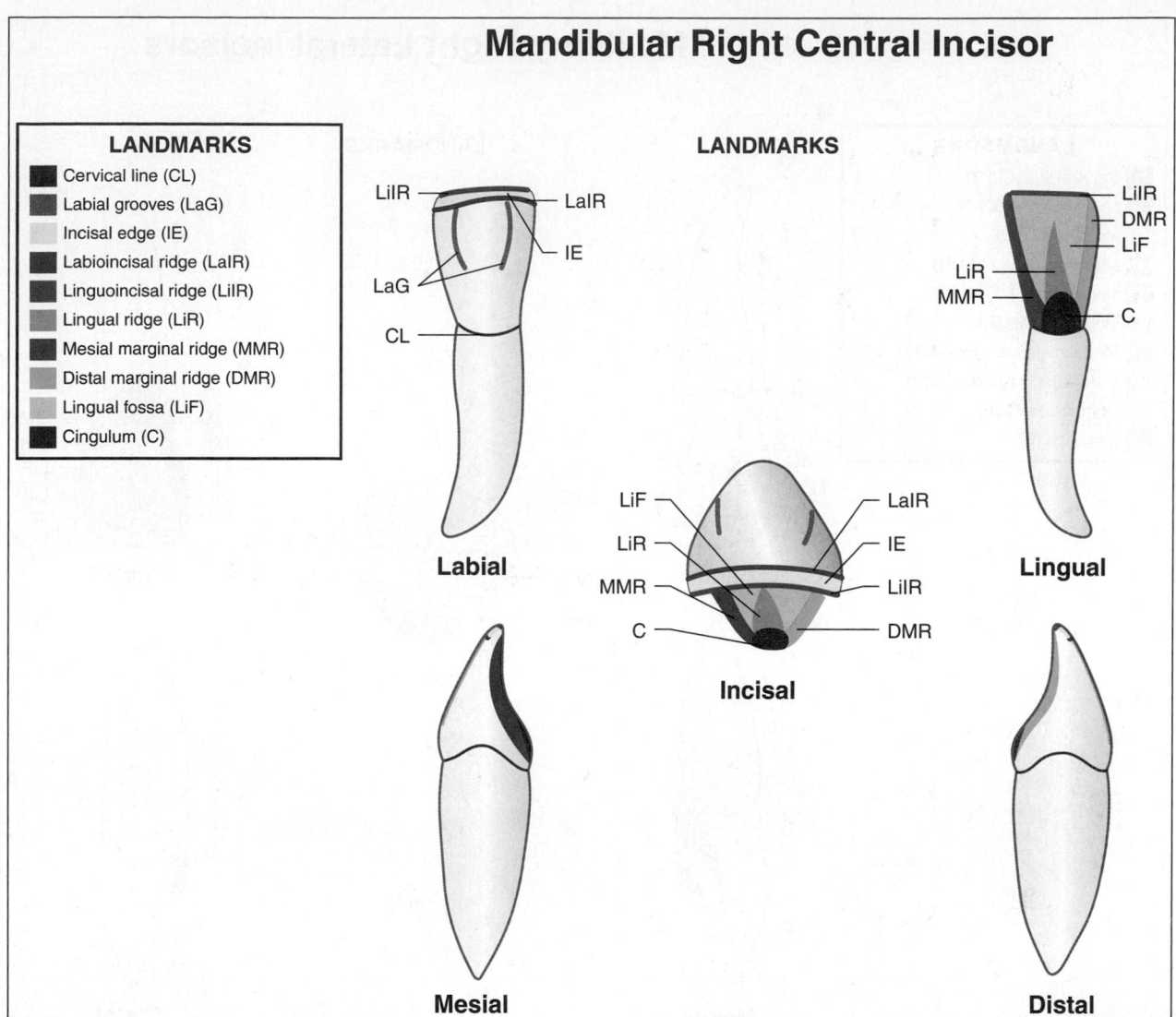

FIGURE 8-13
Mandibular right central incisor landmarks.

mouth, and the root is flattened mesio-distally. Along the sides of the root surface are depressions on the mesial and distal surfaces called *fluting*.

Maxillary Lateral Incisor

The maxillary lateral incisor (Max LI) is a smaller, thinner version of the maxillary central incisor. The landmarks apply to the lateral as with the central incisor (see Figure 8-14). This tooth erupts at about eight years of age and succeeds the primary maxillary lateral incisor.

Facial Aspect
The mesioincisal (MI) line angle is sharper than the distoincisal (DI) line angle, but not as sharp as the angle on the maxillary central incisor. The maxillary laterals are the second-most common tooth to be **congenitally missing**, next to the third molars. It is also very common for the lateral to be malformed with only two lobes instead of the normal four. The two-lobed tooth

forms from the lingual and facial central lobe and this then causes the crown to look like a peg, hence the term *peg lateral*. This causes the lateral incisor to be very small and pointed.

Lingual Aspect
The same developmental depressions, fossa and cingulum, apply for the lateral as on the central. The crown of the lateral is smaller than the central incisor. The lingual fossa is slightly different in that it can be deeper than that of the central incisor and can have a lingual **pit** where the cingulum and fossa meet. This is one characteristic where decay can form in the pit, as it can in any pit on other teeth.

Root Characteristics
The root characteristics of the lateral incisor are similar to those of the central incisor except the root is just as long as or longer than that of the central incisor. Like the central incisors, the root is also tilted toward the distal. Another anomaly with this tooth is that the roots may be curved in usual ways.

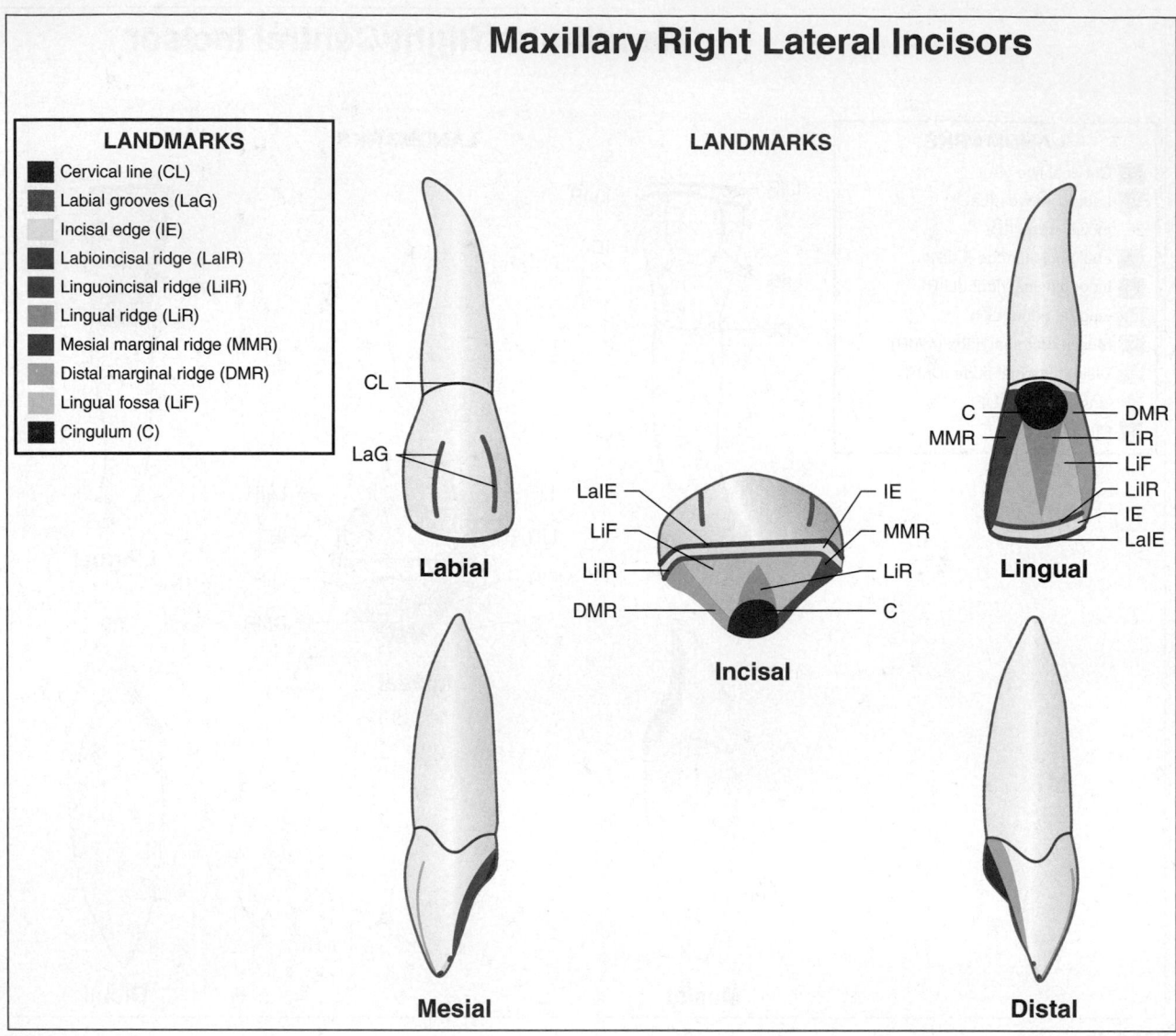

FIGURE 8-14
Maxillary right lateral incisors landmarks.

Mandibular Lateral Incisor

The mandibular lateral incisors (Mand LI) are very similar to the mandibular central incisors with a few distinct differences (see Figure 8-15). It erupts at about seven years of age and succeeds the primary mandibular lateral incisor.

Facial Aspect   One of the main differences is that the mandibular lateral incisor is actually slightly wider mesiodistally than the mandibular central incisor. The tooth is not symmetrical like the mandibular central incisor with the mesial slightly longer, and the mesial incisal line angle is almost 90 degrees. The distoincisal line angle is more curved than the mesial and is not as sharp. The crown of the mandibular incisor is twisted toward the distal, which makes it easier to tell the difference between the right and left mandibular lateral incisors.

Lingual Aspect   The main difference here is that instead of the cingulum being centered on the lingual as on the central, the

lateral has the cingulum set off toward the distal of the lingual surface. This gives the tooth the appearance of being twisted or sloped toward the distal. It is obvious from this view that the tooth is not symmetrical. The mesio-lingual surface is longer and straighter and the distal has a curve to it, because the cingulum is off center.

Root Characteristics   The root characteristics are very similar to those of the mandibular central incisors with the roots thinner and fluted along the mesial and distal surfaces. The root is tilted toward the distal.

Maxillary Canines

Canines are the anterior "cornerstones" of the mouth. They play an important role in holding the shape of the face and are very strong teeth in the mouth. The canines are also known as cuspids, have the longest roots, and can be used as anchor teeth for partials, bridges, or over-dentures. Because of the strength of these

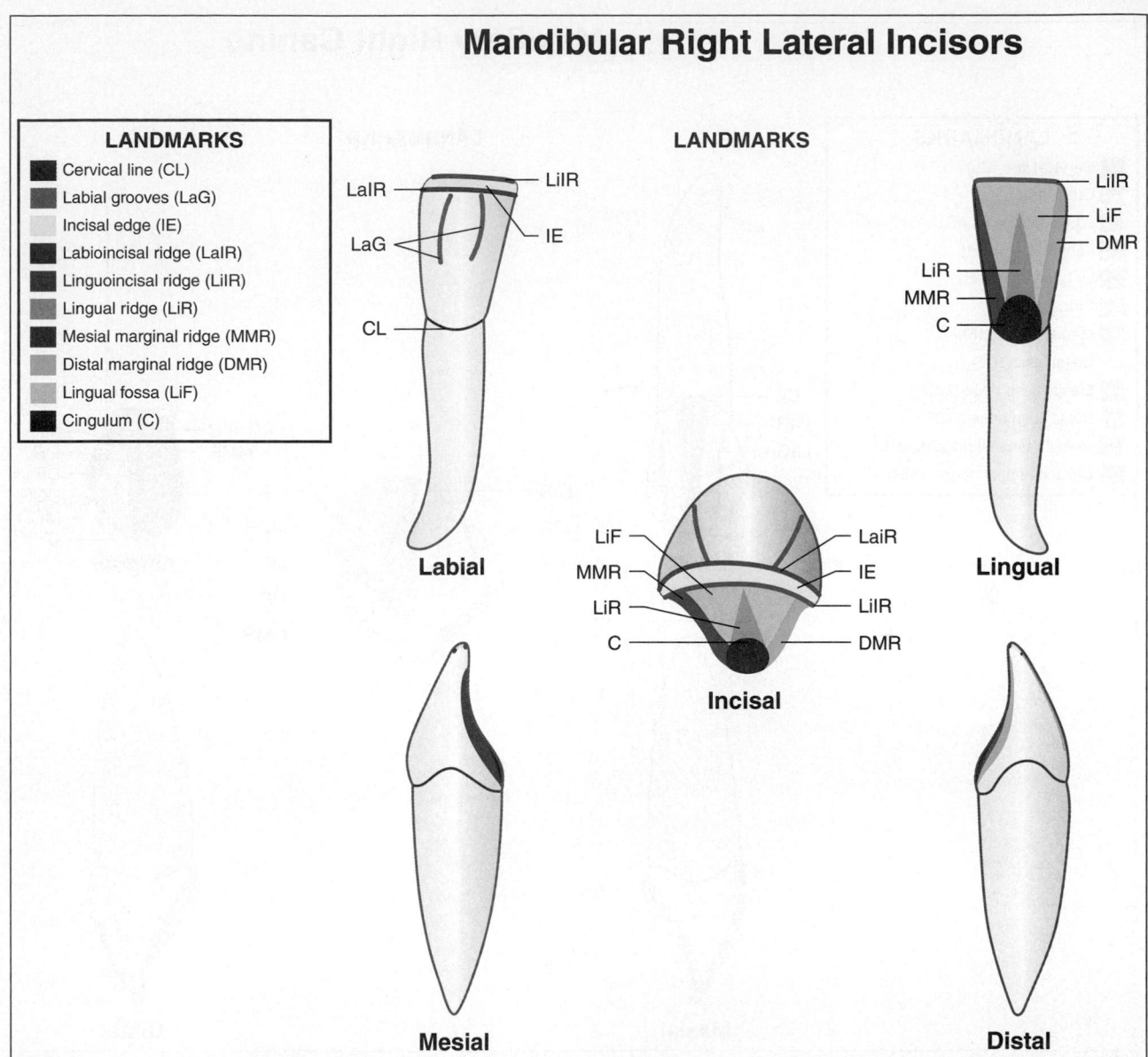

Mandibular Right Lateral Incisors

LANDMARKS
- Cervical line (CL)
- Labial grooves (LaG)
- Incisal edge (IE)
- Labioincisal ridge (LaIR)
- Linguoincisal ridge (LiIR)
- Lingual ridge (LiR)
- Mesial marginal ridge (MMR)
- Distal marginal ridge (DMR)
- Lingual fossa (LiF)
- Cingulum (C)

LANDMARKS

Labial

Lingual

Incisal

Mesial

Distal

FIGURE 8-15
Mandibular right lateral incisors landmarks.

teeth, a dentist will try to retain these teeth if at all possible. The canine appears darker than the incisors because of the bulk of the dentin.

The maxillary canine (Max C) erupts at about 11 years of age and succeeds the primary maxillary canine. The functions of the canines are to cut, pierce, and tear food. They are the longest of the maxillary teeth.

Facial Aspect The facial surface feature that is very obvious is the large central lobe that protrudes and gives the tooth its large facial bulge of enamel called the labial ridge and pointed cusp tip (see Figure 8-16). There is shallow **groove** on both sides of the labial ridge. On either side of the cusp tip are the cusp ridges, referred to as the mesial cusp ridge and distal cusp ridges. The mesial side of the tooth is straighter, and the mesial cusp ridge

is shorter than the distal, which is used to distinguish the mesial from the distal.

Lingual Aspect The lingual surface of the maxillary canine has a large, centrally located cingulum. From the cingulum, there is a lingual ridge that divides the lingual fossa into two fossae: the mesiolingual fossa and a distolingual fossa. The mesial and distal marginal ridges are also present bordering the two lingual fossae. There is a cusp tip instead of an incisal ridge that is pointed instead of flat.

Root Characteristics One characteristic of the root of the maxillary canine is that it is very long and triangular in shape. This long, triangular-shaped root makes this tooth very difficult to extract. It also contributes to the formation of the

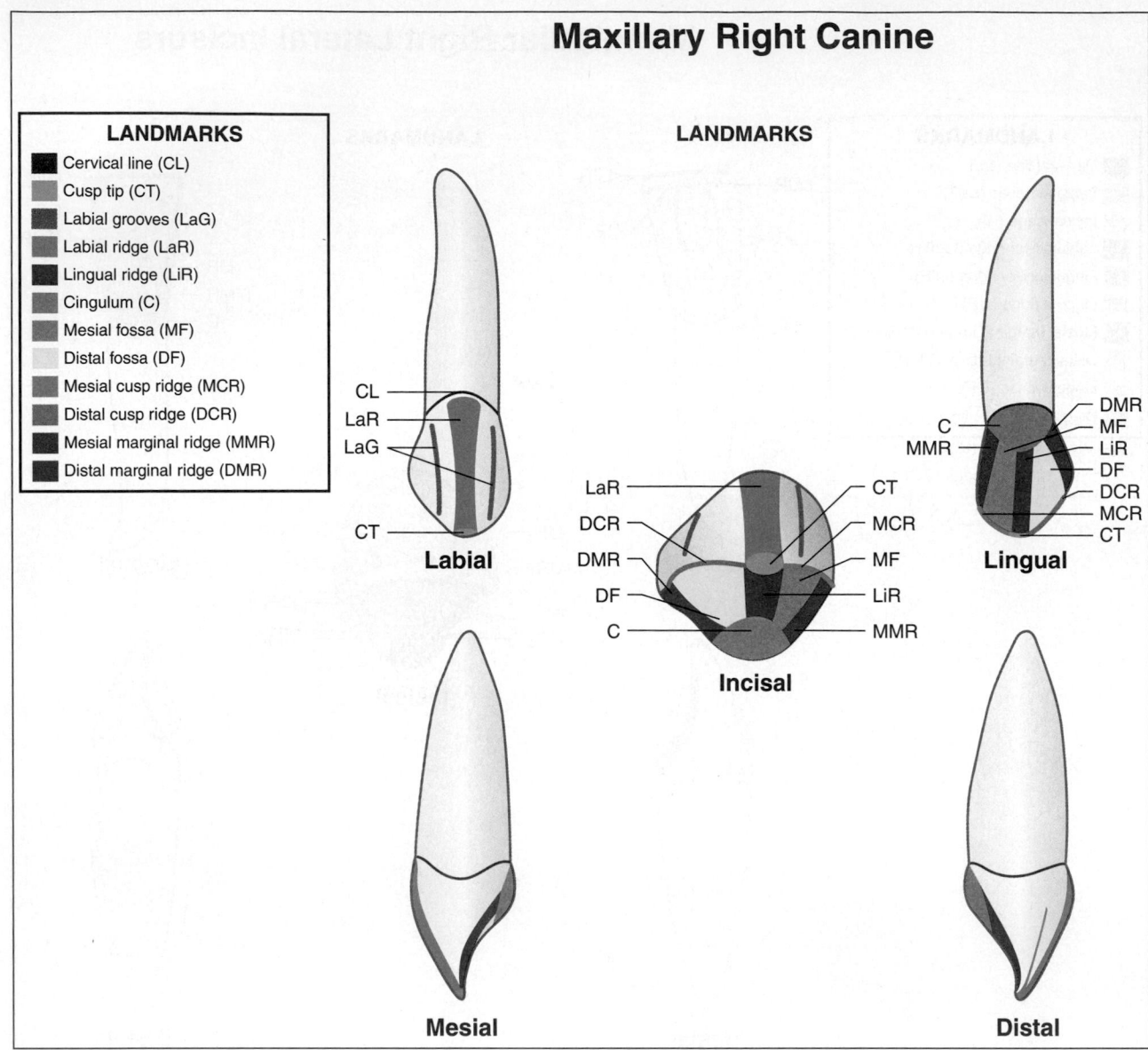

Maxillary Right Canine

LANDMARKS
- ■ Cervical line (CL)
- ■ Cusp tip (CT)
- ■ Labial grooves (LaG)
- ■ Labial ridge (LaR)
- ■ Lingual ridge (LiR)
- ■ Cingulum (C)
- ■ Mesial fossa (MF)
- ■ Distal fossa (DF)
- ■ Mesial cusp ridge (MCR)
- ■ Distal cusp ridge (DCR)
- ■ Mesial marginal ridge (MMR)
- ■ Distal marginal ridge (DMR)

LANDMARKS

Labial

Incisal

Lingual

Mesial

Distal

FIGURE 8-16
Maxillary right canine landmarks.

canine eminence in the maxillary arch. Due to the shape of the root, and the bone around the root surface, the canine eminence gives the middle third of the face some of its shape.

Mandibular Canine

The mandibular canine (Mand C) has similar features as the maxillary canine, but they are less pronounced. This tooth erupts at about 10 years of age and succeeds the primary mandibular canine.

Facial Aspect The middle facial lobe is more pronounced but not as much as the maxillary canine. The cusp tip on the middle lobe is not as pointed as on the maxillary canine. It is often smoother and slightly toward the distal instead of centered. (See Figure 8-17.) As with the maxillary canine, the

mesial side is straighter, and the mesial cusp ridge is shorter than the distal.

Lingual Aspect All of the general features found on the lingual surface of the maxillary canine are all less pronounced on the mandibular canine. The central lobe is slightly taller, and the overall crown is thinner mesiodistally than the maxillary canine.

Root Characteristics The mandibular canine root is a blend of the flatter, thinner incisor roots and the triangular shape of the maxillary canine. It is long, but not as long as the maxillary canine, and it is thinner and shorter than the maxillary canine root. The apex of the root may be mesially inclined. Although the root is slightly shorter, the crown is slightly longer than the maxillary, which makes both maxillary and mandibular canine teeth about the same overall length.

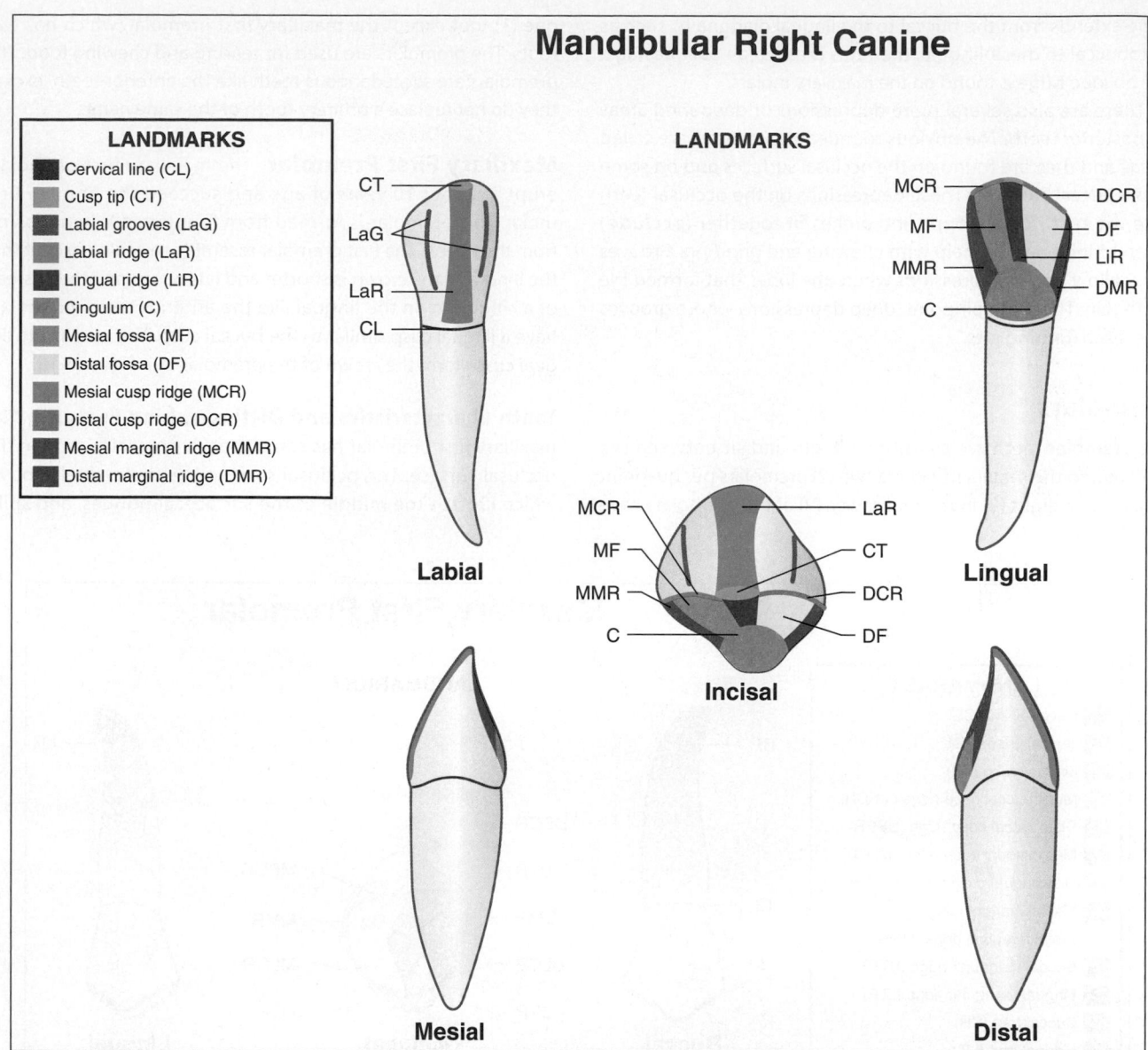

FIGURE 8-17
Mandibular right canine landmarks.

Posterior Permanent Dentition

The permanent posterior teeth include two premolars and three molars in each quadrant. As with the anterior teeth, each posterior has a distinct shape and landmarks. The posterior teeth are larger and have a greater number of lobes, elevations, and depressions.

There are several types of elevations of enamel on posterior teeth. These raised areas can be tall, sharp, and triangular-shaped as in cusps, or line elevations called ridges that connect cusps called ridges.

Marginal ridges are elevations along the mesial and distal proximal surfaces of the occlusal surface on the tooth. The marginal ridges on anterior teeth border the lingual fossa mesially and distally. On the posterior teeth, they are on the edge of the

occlusal surface adjacent to the fossae and pits. Some posterior teeth also have a groove that crosses the marginal ridge.

Triangular ridges are part of the cusps on posterior teeth. Cusps are the four-sided, pyramid-shaped peaks that are found on the occlusal surface. These triangular ridges can make a variety of sizes of cusps, but they all have a similar pyramid shape with four sides. When a triangular ridge on the buccal cusp is across from a triangular ridge on the lingual cusp, the two triangular ridges together form a transverse ridge. These ridges join in the valley of the occlusal and meet at a groove in the center of the occlusal (central groove), and the ridges continue from one side to the other. When this ridge continues from buccal to lingual on the same side of the tooth, such as the mesiobuccal half to mesiolingual, then it is called a *transverse ridge*. When a triangular ridge extends from the buccal to the lingual diagonally, such as distobuccal to mesiolingual, then this is called an *oblique ridge*. The oblique ridge is found on the maxillary molars.

There are also several more depressions or deepened areas on posterior teeth. The obvious rounded depressions are called *fossae* and they are found on the occlusal surfaces and on some of the buccal surfaces. These depressions on the occlusal teeth help the teeth of the opposing arches fit together (**occlude**) when biting and also help with chewing and grinding. Grooves are shallow, linear depressions where the lobes that formed the tooth join. There are pinpoint, deep depressions where grooves cross each forming pits.

Premolars

The premolar teeth are transitional teeth and sit between the canines and the molars. There are two (2) premolars per quadrant for a total of eight (8) in the oral cavity. All of the premolars have one (1) root except the maxillary first premolar, which has two roots. The premolars are used for tearing and chewing food. The premolars are succedaneous teeth like the anterior teeth, except they do not replace a primary tooth of the same name.

Maxillary First Premolar The maxillary first premolars erupt at about 10 years of age and succeed the primary first molar. This premolar is formed from four lobes. When looking from the buccal, the first premolar resembles a canine except that the length of the crown is shorter and it is not as pointed. Instead of a cingulum on the lingual like the anterior teeth, premolars have a lingual cusp similar to the buccal cusp. The buccal and lingual cusps form the crown of the premolar (see Figure 8-18).

Tooth Characteristics and Distinguishing Features The maxillary first premolar has some specific characteristics on the occlusal surface. The occlusal surface has the central groove, which crosses the middle of the surface, continues, and spills

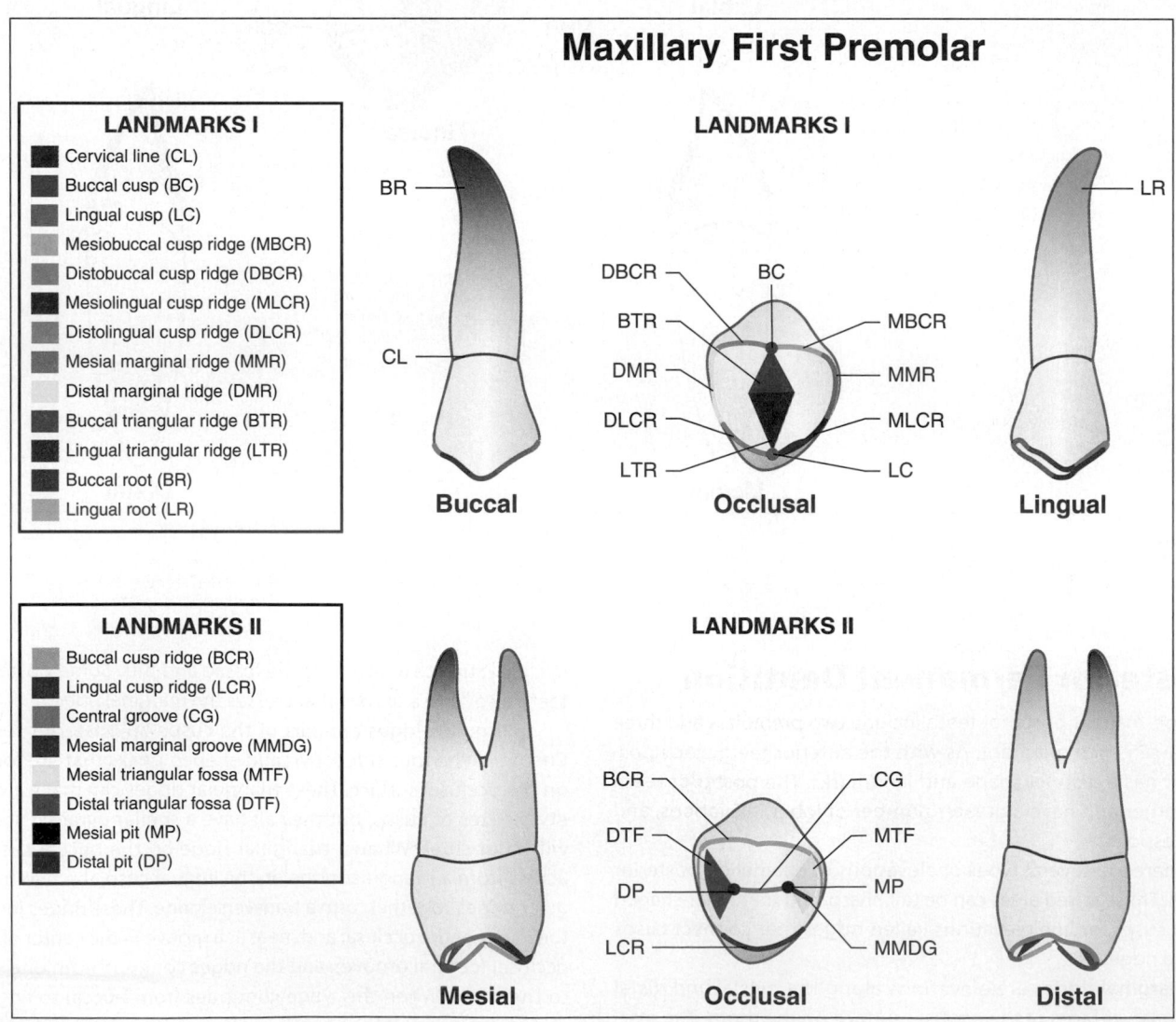

FIGURE 8-18
Maxillary right first premolar landmark views (I) and (II).

over the mesial marginal ridge called the *mesial marginal ridge groove*. There are two pits: a mesial pit and a distal pit, each surrounded by a fossa. They are named according to the proximal surface they are located near: mesial and distal fossa. There are two cusps: one taller buccal and one shorter lingual cusp. The buccal and lingual triangular ridges located on the cusps connect across the occlusal surface, forming a transverse ridge.

The most distinguished characteristic of the maxillary first premolar is the root. It is the only premolar that has a **bifurcated** root. There is a long **root trunk** that divides into a buccal and a lingual root, which each contain their root canals. There is a developmental depression on the mesial surface of the root trunk that extends to the crown.

Maxillary Second Premolar The maxillary second premolar erupts into the oral cavity about age 11 and succeeds the primary second molar. This premolar is formed by four lobes and resembles the maxillary first premolar from the buccal, except that

it is slightly smaller (see Figure 8-19). There is a buccal and similarly sized lingual cusp that makes up the crown of this premolar.

Tooth Characteristics and Distinguishing Features The major difference between the maxillary second premolar and the first is that this second premolar has a single root. The occlusal surface of the second premolar has a slightly wrinkled occlusal surface as compared to the first premolar because the cusp tips are closer together. The maxillary second premolar does not have a groove extending over the mesial marginal ridge as found on the maxillary first premolar.

Mandibular First Premolar The mandibular first premolars teeth erupt into the oral cavity at about age 10 and succeed the primary first molars. As with all premolars, this tooth develops from three facial lobes and one lingual lobe to make the two cusps (see Figure 8-20). This is a single-rooted tooth and has two uneven cusps on the crown; the buccal cusp is larger than the lingual.

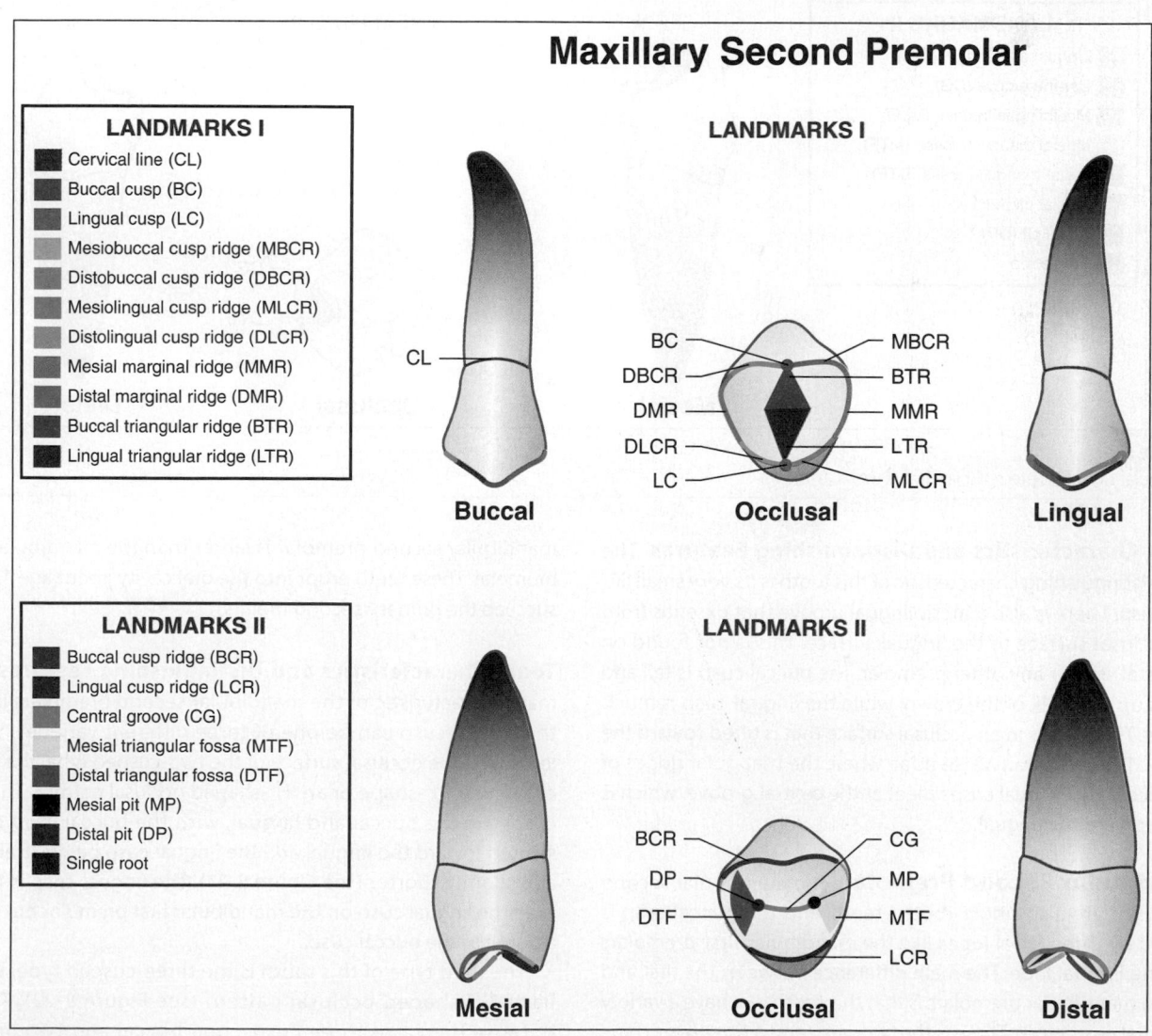

FIGURE 8-19
Maxillary right second premolar landmarks views (I) and (II).

Mandibular First Premolar

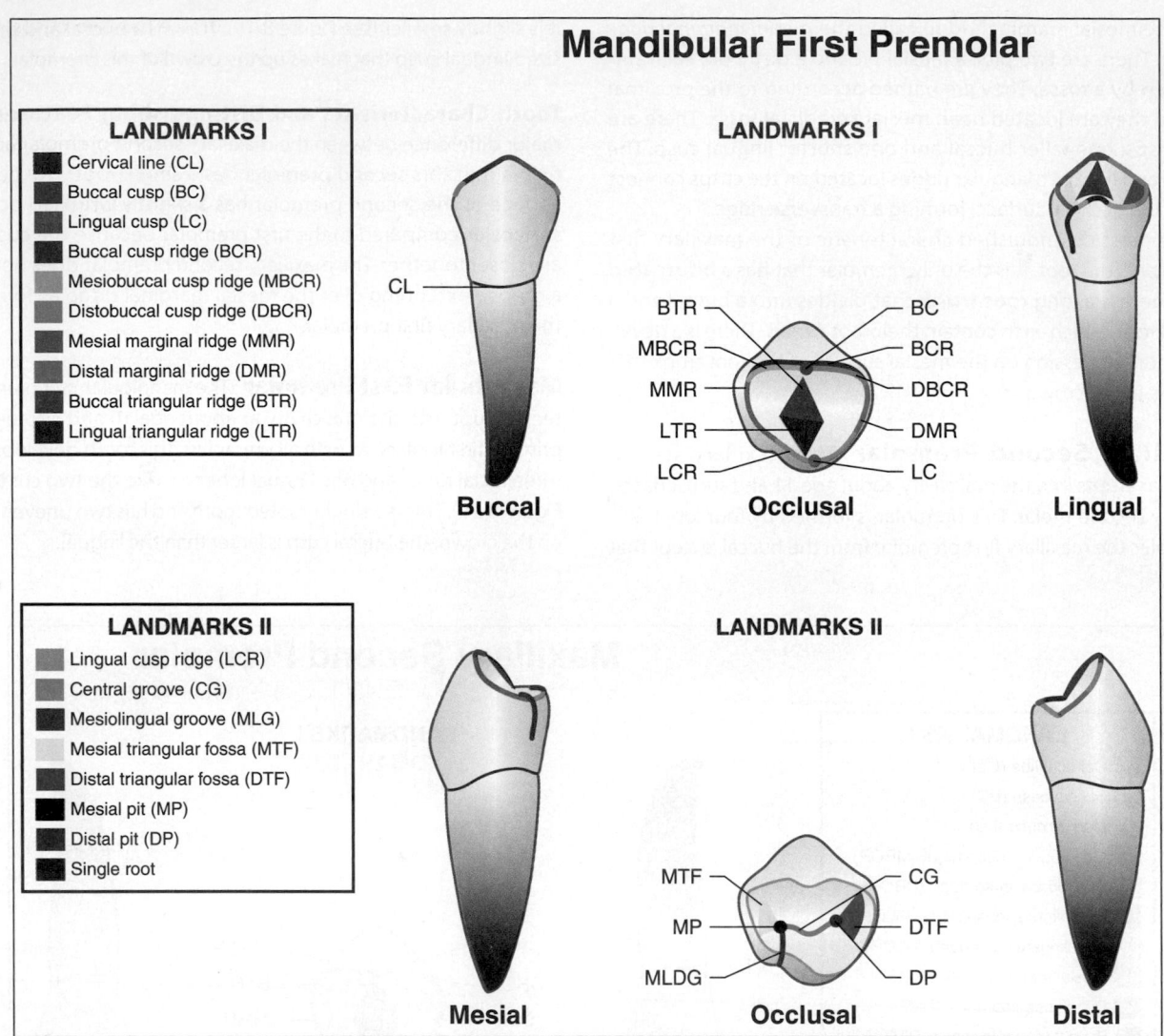

LANDMARKS I

- Cervical line (CL)
- Buccal cusp (BC)
- Lingual cusp (LC)
- Buccal cusp ridge (BCR)
- Mesiobuccal cusp ridge (MBCR)
- Distobuccal cusp ridge (DBCR)
- Mesial marginal ridge (MMR)
- Distal marginal ridge (DMR)
- Buccal triangular ridge (BTR)
- Lingual triangular ridge (LTR)

LANDMARKS II

- Lingual cusp ridge (LCR)
- Central groove (CG)
- Mesiolingual groove (MLG)
- Mesial triangular fossa (MTF)
- Distal triangular fossa (DTF)
- Mesial pit (MP)
- Distal pit (DP)
- Single root

Buccal

LANDMARKS I

Occlusal

BTR — BC
MBCR — BCR
MMR — DBCR
LTR — DMR
LCR — LC

Lingual

LANDMARKS II

Mesial

Occlusal

MTF — CG
MP — DTF
MLDG — DP

Distal

FIGURE 8-20
Mandibular right first premolar landmark views (I) and (II).

Tooth Characteristics and Distinguishing Features The most distinguishing characteristic of this tooth is its very small lingual cusp. There is also a mesiolingual groove that extends from the occlusal surface to the lingual surface. This is not found on the distal side or any other premolar. The buccal cusp is tall and makes up the bulk of the crown, while the lingual cusp is much smaller. This results in an occlusal surface that is tilted toward the lingual. There is a transverse ridge where the triangular ridges of the buccal and lingual cusps meet at the central groove, which is offset toward the lingual.

Mandibular Second Premolar The mandibular second premolars are also single-rooted teeth, and the buccal cusp is formed by three facial lobes like the mandibular first premolars and one lingual lobe. The main difference between the first and second mandibular premolars is that this tooth can have a variety of lingual cusp types. There is the two-cusp and a three-cusp type of mandibular second premolar; these variations are discussed in greater detail in the following sections. The overall size of the

mandibular second premolar is larger than the mandibular first premolar. These teeth erupt into the oral cavity about age 11 and succeed the primary second molars.

Tooth Characteristics and Distinguishing Features The main characteristic of the mandibular second premolars is that the lingual cusp can be one of three different varieties. When looking at the occlusal surface of the two-cusped type, the tooth can have a "U"-shape or an "H"-shaped occlusal pattern. The two cusps are the buccal and lingual, with the buccal cusp being slanted toward the lingual and the lingual cusp being straighter and slightly shorter (see Figure 8-21). The lingual cusp is larger than the lingual cusp on the mandibular first premolar but is not as large as the buccal cusp.

The third type of this tooth is the three-cusped type, which has a "Y"-shaped occlusal pattern (see Figure 8-22). This is because there are three cusps, one buccal and two lingual cusps, which form the "Y" shape. There are three occlusal pits, which makes this the only premolar that has three pits; all the others have two pits. The lingual surface has two cusps, which are the mesiolingual and distolingual cusps, divided by a short, lingual groove. The crown of the three-cusped version is more square-shaped than the two-cusped version. This is the most common version of this tooth overall, and is the only version of the mandibular second premolar formed by five lobes, with three lobes making the facial cusp and two lobes making the two lingual cusps.

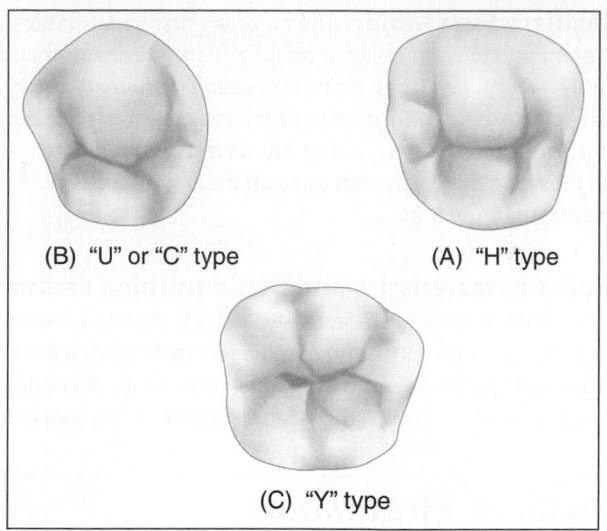

FIGURE 8-21
Different shapes of the occlusal surface of the permanent mandibular second premolar. (A) is the H-type shape. (B) is the "U" or "C" shape, and (C) is the "Y" shape.

TABLE 8-4 Summary of Distinguishing Characteristics of Premolars

Premolar	Distinguishing Characteristics
maxillary first premolar	Bifurcated root, M marginal ridge groove, M depression at CEJ, looks slightly bent
maxillary second premolar	M and D marginal ridge grooves, more symmetrical
mandibular first premolar	Poorly defined lingual cusp, ML groove
mandibular second premolar	Two-cusp or three-cusp variety, U-, H-, or Y-shaped occlusal

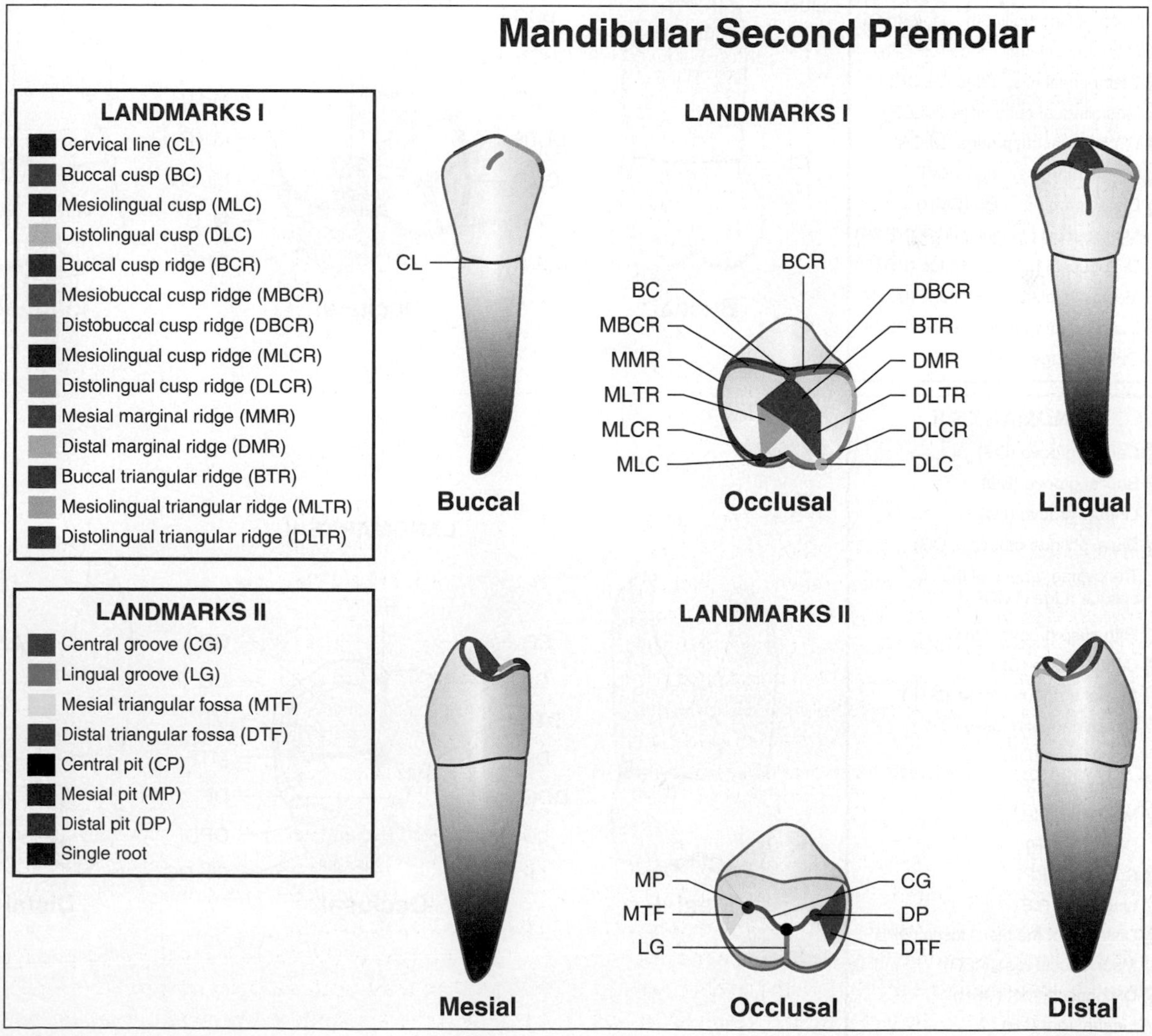

Mandibular Second Premolar

LANDMARKS I

- Cervical line (CL)
- Buccal cusp (BC)
- Mesiolingual cusp (MLC)
- Distolingual cusp (DLC)
- Buccal cusp ridge (BCR)
- Mesiobuccal cusp ridge (MBCR)
- Distobuccal cusp ridge (DBCR)
- Mesiolingual cusp ridge (MLCR)
- Distolingual cusp ridge (DLCR)
- Mesial marginal ridge (MMR)
- Distal marginal ridge (DMR)
- Buccal triangular ridge (BTR)
- Mesiolingual triangular ridge (MLTR)
- Distolingual triangular ridge (DLTR)

LANDMARKS II

- Central groove (CG)
- Lingual groove (LG)
- Mesial triangular fossa (MTF)
- Distal triangular fossa (DTF)
- Central pit (CP)
- Mesial pit (MP)
- Distal pit (DP)
- Single root

LANDMARKS I

CL — Buccal

Occlusal:
BC, MBCR, MMR, MLTR, MLCR, MLC
BCR, DBCR, BTR, DMR, DLTR, DLCR, DLC

Lingual

LANDMARKS II

Mesial

Occlusal:
MP, MTF, LG
CG, DP, DTF

Distal

FIGURE 8-22
Mandibular right second premolar landmarks views (I) and (II).

Molars

The molars are the largest permanent teeth in the dentition of an adult. All molars are developed from either four or five lobes, and thus either have four or five cusps. There are three molars in each quadrant, with the first molars being the largest and the most posterior third molars being the smallest. As we go posteriorly from first to third molars, overall the roots get shorter and closer together on both the maxillary and mandibular arches. The maxillary molars have three roots (**trifurcated**) with one lingual (also called palatal), and two on the buccal: mesiobuccal and distobuccal and with a long root trunk. The molars on the mandibular arch only have two roots (bifurcated), the mesial and distal roots and a shorter root trunk.

Maxillary First Molar The maxillary first molars (Max first M) erupt into the oral cavity at about age six and are nicknamed the six-year molars. They do not succeed any primary teeth, as the molars are the only nonsuccedaneous teeth in the permanent dentition. The first molars are developed from five lobes and thus form five cusps with three on the lingual and two on the buccal (see Figure 8-23).

Tooth Characteristics and Distinguishing Features

The most distinguishing characteristic of this tooth is that it has five cusps. With the maxillary first molar, the four main cusps are similar in size except for the largest mesiolingual cusp and its tiny, nonfunctioning **cusp of Carabelli** (also referred to as the fifth cusp) that is

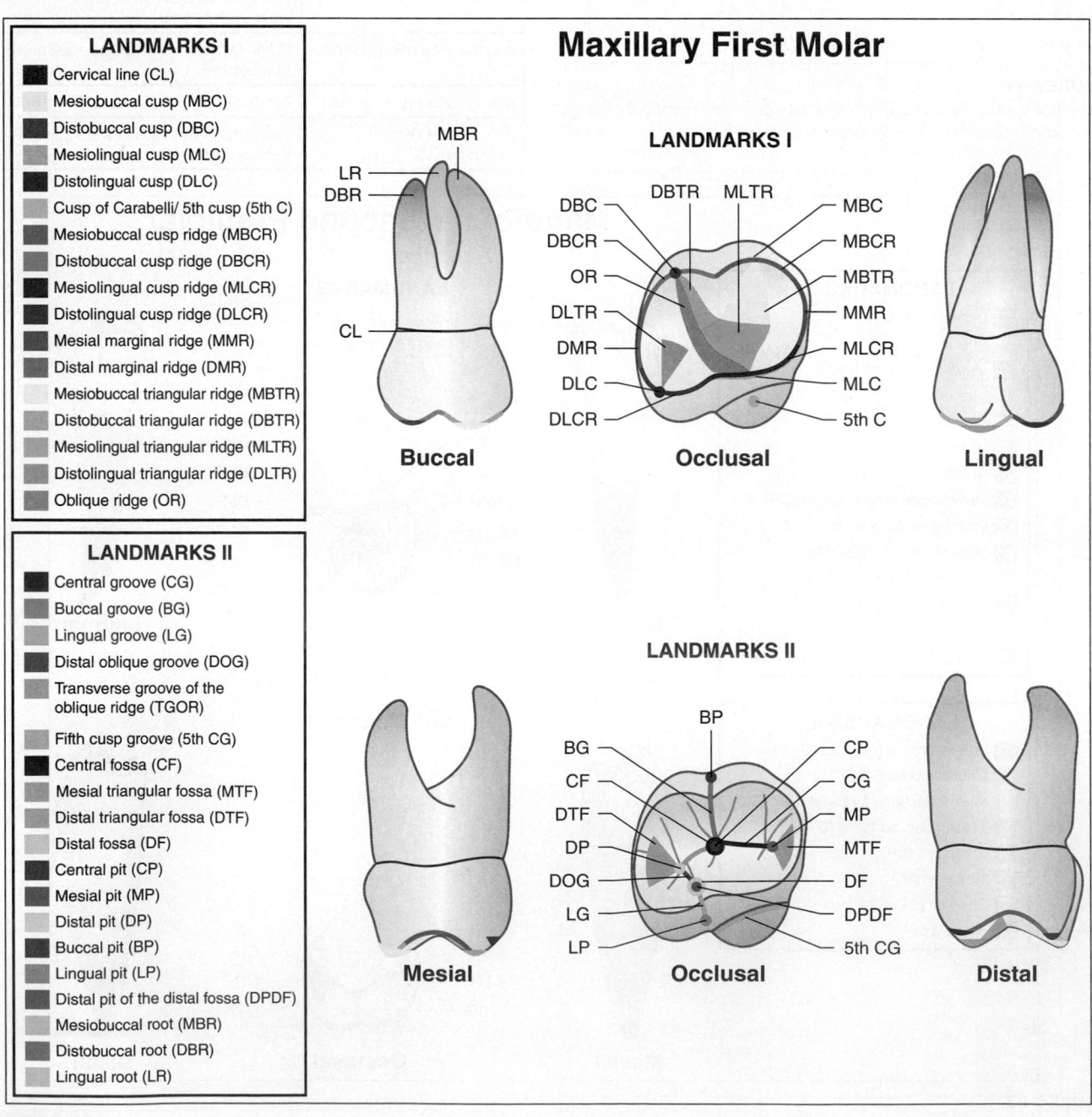

FIGURE 8-23

Maxillary first molar landmarks views (I) and (II).

found where it piggybacks on the lingual side of the mesiolingual (ML) cusp. Sometimes this small cusp is only a slight bump, but it can be larger and quite sharp. There is a small mesiolingual groove that separates the mesiolingual cusp from the smallest cusp of Carabelli.

The buccal and lingual cusps are separated by a central groove. The buccal cusps are divided by a buccal groove that has a buccal pit at the end of the groove. The lingual cusps are divided by a deep lingual groove. The first molar has four fossae—central, distal and mesial triangular fossa, and distal fossa—located mesial of the triangular fossa at the lingual groove. These is a pit at the bottom of each fossa.

There are two cusp ridges on the mesiolingual cusp, one angled toward the mesiobuccal and the other leaning toward the distobuccal. With this arrangement of cusp ridges, on the mesial side of the occlusal there is one transverse ridge extending from the mesiolingual to the mesiobuccal, and there is one oblique ridge extending from the second cusp ridge of the mesiolingual cusp to the triangular ridge distobuccal cusp. The maxillary molars are unique in that they are the only teeth that have this slanted oblique ridge on the occlusal. There are only transverse ridges on the mandibular molars.

The palatal root is the largest and longest root of the three roots on the maxillary molars. Often these roots are spread apart, making this tooth very difficult to extract.

Maxillary Second Molar The maxillary second molar (Max second M) is a shorter, smaller version of the maxillary first molar with a few exceptions. They erupt into the oral cavity at about age 12 and are also nonsuccedaneous because they do not replace any primary teeth. The maxillary second molars develop from four lobes and develop four cusps (see Figure 8-24). The roots are closer together and not spread out as far as those of the maxillary

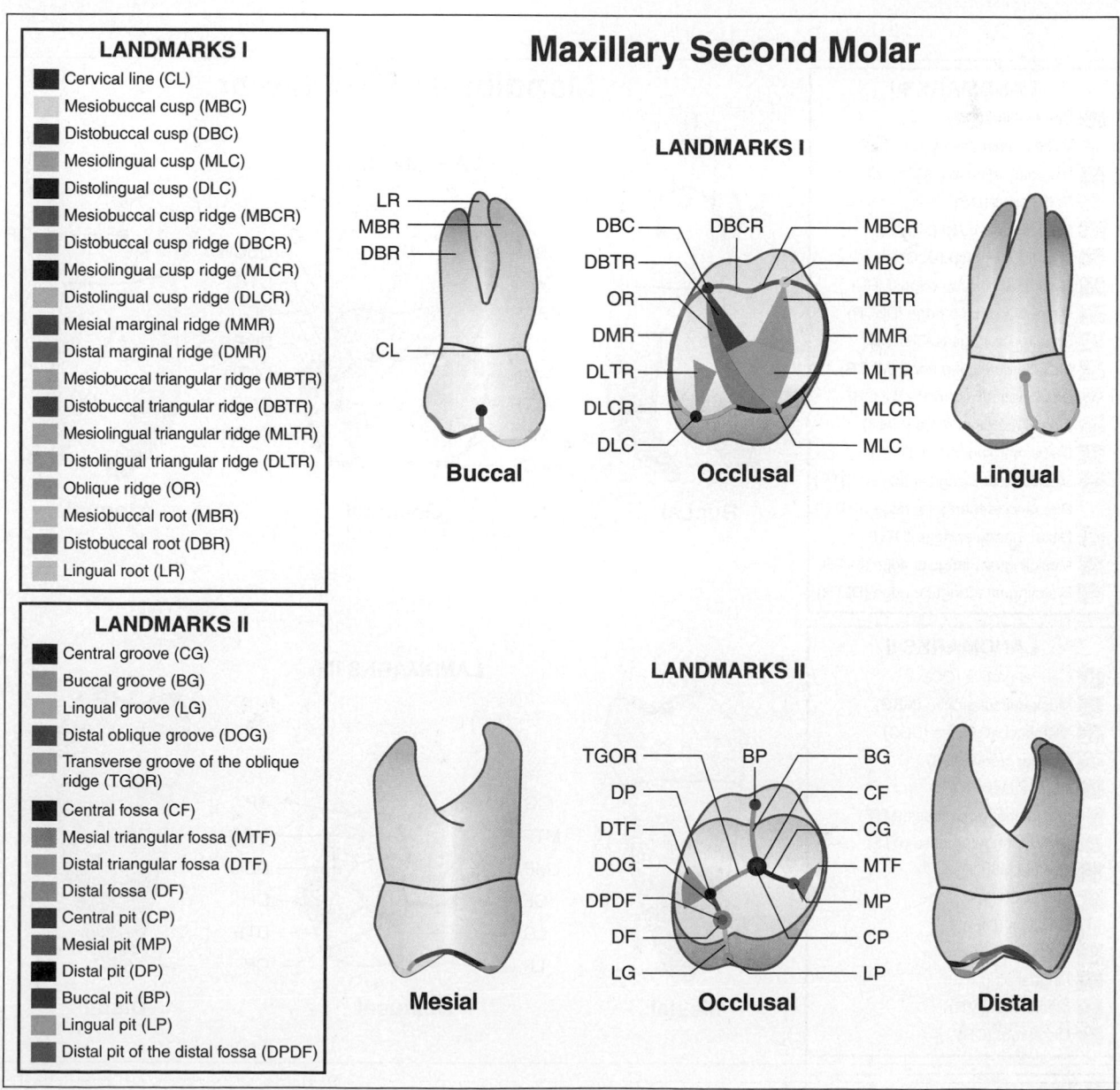

FIGURE 8-24
Maxillary second molar landmark views (I) and (II).

first molar. The roots are often almost fused with apices turned toward the distal.

Tooth Characteristics and Distinguishing Features The maxillary second molar is almost exactly like the maxillary first molar with all of the same features, except it does *not* have a cusp of Carabelli. Besides being slightly smaller, the crown of the tooth is not as square as the maxillary first molar with all the cusps being smaller and rounder. The mesiolingual cusp is still the largest of the four major cusps. The crown of the maxillary second molar is shorter in height occlusocervically than the first molar. The buccal groove is not as deep as on the first molar, and often this tooth does not have a buccal pit as on the first molar.

Mandibular First Molar The mandibular first molars (Mand first M) are the first permanent teeth to erupt before the

maxillary first molars. They erupt into the oral cavity at about age six, are nonsuccedaneous teeth, and erupt distal to the primary second molars. The mandibular molars only have two roots. They are the mesial and distal roots with both of them tilted toward the distal, and the mesial root is a little larger and longer than the distal root (see Figure 8-25). The root trunk is shorter than the root trunk of the maxillary molars because the root bifurcation area is closer to the CEJ than the trifurcation area is on the trifurcated maxillary molars.

Tooth Characteristics and Distinguishing Features The most distinguishing feature about the mandibular first molar, besides being the largest mandibular molar, is that it has three cusps on the buccal named *mesiobuccal*, *distobuccal*, and *distal*. They are separated by the mesiobuccal and the distobuccal grooves that separate the three developmental lobes. The distal cusp is the smallest and helps distinguish the distal surface

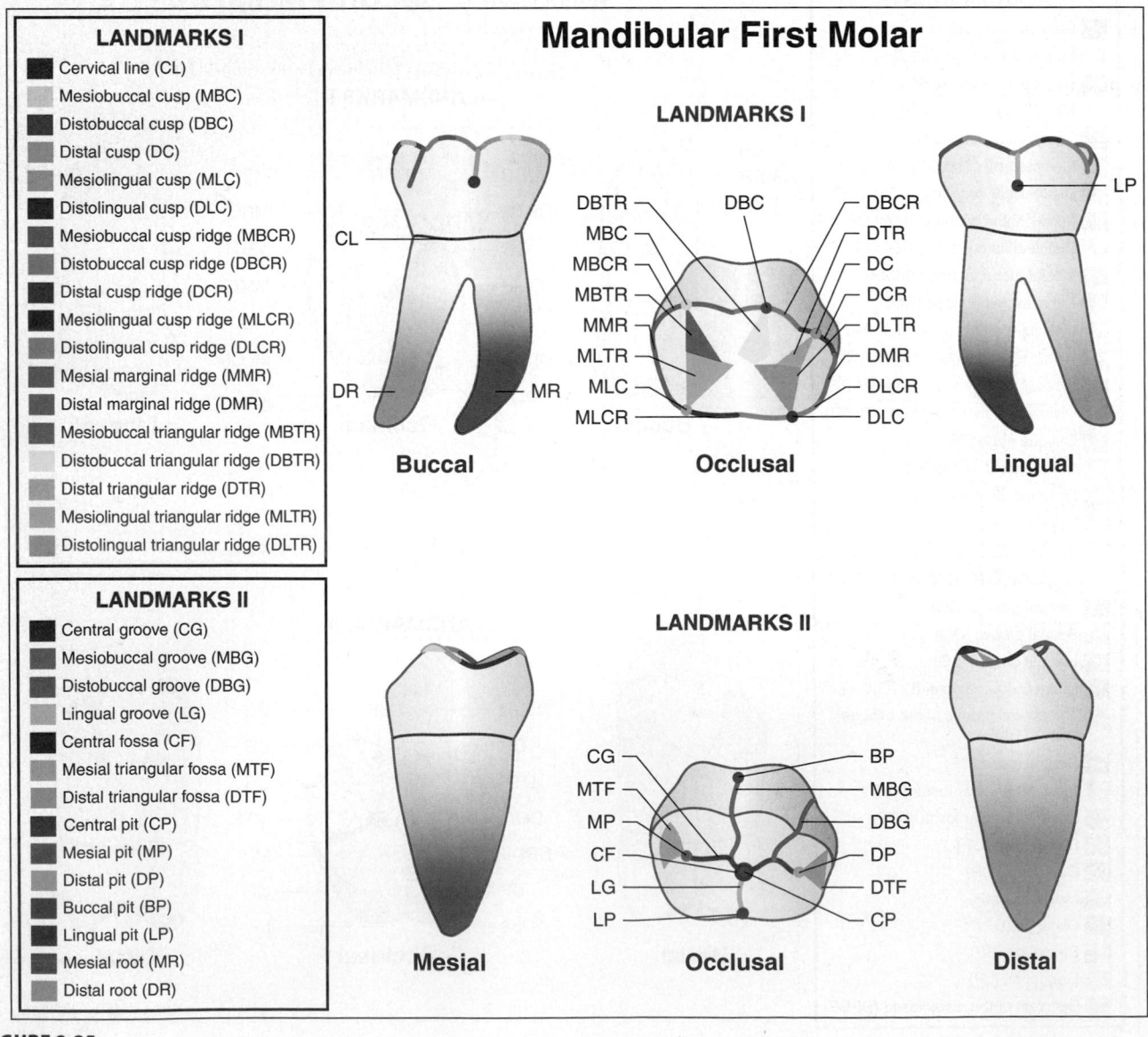

FIGURE 8-25
Mandibular first molar landmark views (I) and (II).

because it is set about at the line angle of the corner of the tooth. The two lingual cusps are about of the same size and are slightly taller and straighter than the buccal cusps.

Looking at the occlusal surface of this tooth, the five cusps are easily viewed and are separated by the central grooves. The occlusal surface has three occlusal pits (disto-occlusal [DO], central, and mesio-occlusal pits [MO]). The mesiobuccal and distobuccal grooves separate the three buccal cusps, and a lingual groove separates the two lingual cusps. Often the mesiobuccal groove is deeper and ends with a buccal pit, but the distobuccal groove is not as deep and often does not display a buccal pit.

Mandibular Second Molar
The mandibular second molars (Mand second M) are formed by four lobes and thus have four cusps. They erupt into the mouth at about age 12. This tooth is more rectangular in shape than the mandibular first molar. It also has the two roots situated on the mesial and distal with them both tilted toward the distal (Figure 8-26).

Tooth Characteristics and Distinguishing Features The most distinguishing feature of these teeth is that the occlusal

surface shows the four similarly sized cusps separated by a cross or "+" pattern. There are two transverse ridges that run from the mesiobuccal cusp to the mesiolingual cusp and the second one that runs from the distobuccal cusp to the distolingual cusp. The central groove separates the buccal from the lingual cusps, and the buccal and lingual grooves separate the mesial from the distal cusps. With the similar size of cusps and no particular groove that distinguishes one side over the other, this is a harder tooth to tell the right from the left when it is out of the mouth. Looking at how the roots tilt toward the distal is the way to tell the mesial apart from the distal side (Table 8-5).

TABLE 8-5 Summary of Distinguishing Characteristics of Molars

Molar	Distinguishing Characteristics
maxillary first molar	Cusp of Carabelli on ML cusp (fifth), oblique ridge from ML to DB cusps
maxillary second molar	Oblique ridge from ML to DB cusps, *no* cusp of Carabelli
mandibular first molar	Distal (fifth) cusp on facial
mandibular second molar	Cross or "X" mark in occlusal, no fifth cusp

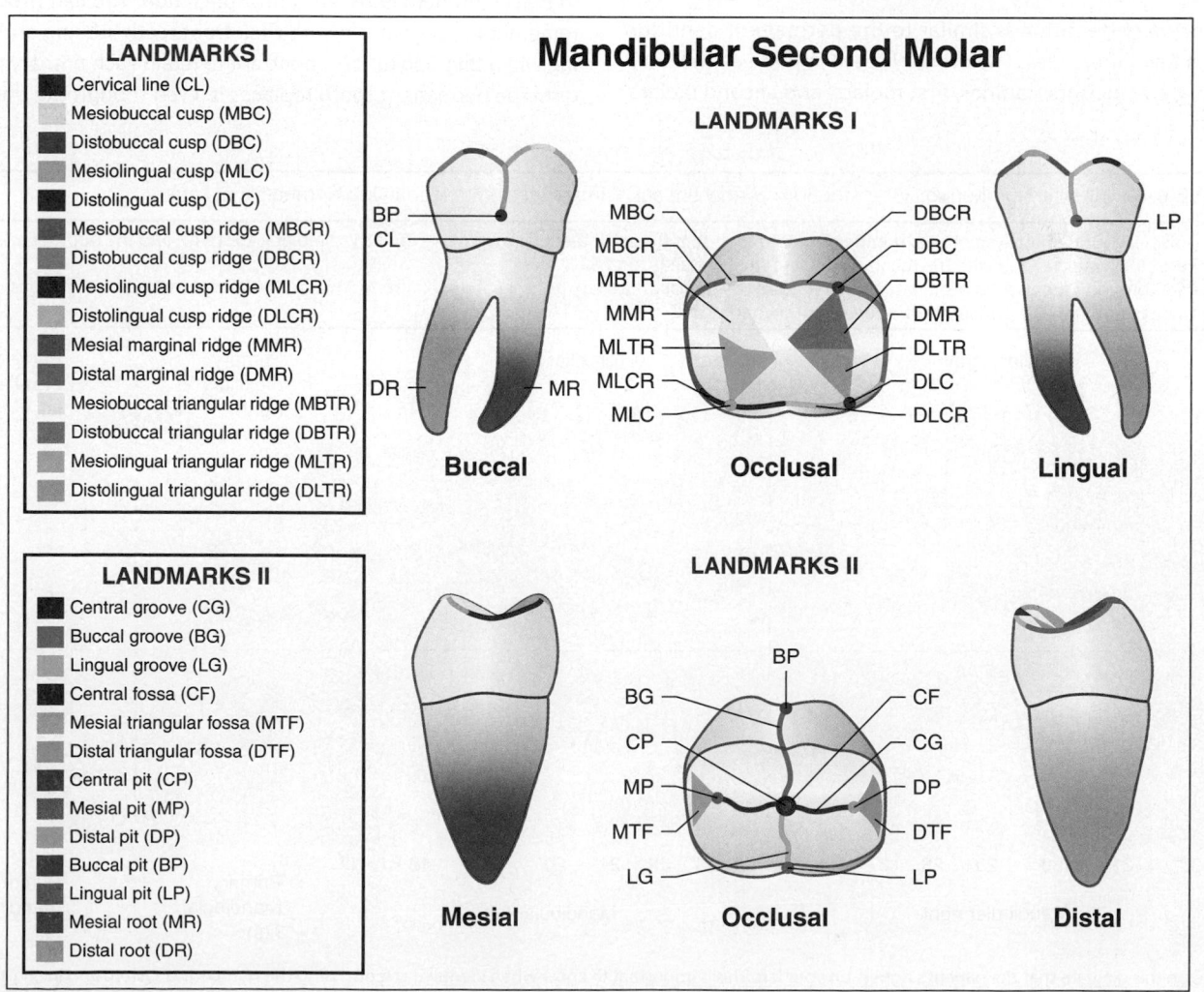

FIGURE 8-26
Mandibular second molar landmarks views (I) and (II).

Third Molars In general, all of the third molars (Max and Mand third M) are the smallest molars and have the most variations in shape. These teeth are the most often congenitally missing of any other teeth in the mouth. Sometimes these teeth only form from three lobes instead of the four or five as with the other molars. These teeth are often very small and vary in size more than any other molars, and the occlusal characteristics are often wrinkled, making it difficult to tell what cusp is where or if a transverse or an oblique ridge is even present. It is common for the roots to be poorly developed and they are often fused, shorter, and curved sharply or dilacerated toward the distal.

Universal Numbering System

Writing the complete name of a tooth is time-consuming and takes up a lot of space in the chart. Numbering systems are designed to represent the teeth. The Universal Numbering System is currently the most commonly used in the United States (Table 8-6).

Primary Dentition

The primary dentition is similar to the permanent dentition with a few differences. The primary teeth include central incisors, lateral incisors, canines, first molars, and second molars.

There are no premolars or third molars in the primary dentition. The primary teeth are referred to as the baby teeth, milk teeth, first teeth, or deciduous teeth, but the correct clinical term is primary teeth. They begin to erupt when the child is six months of age and finish erupting when the child is approximately two to three years of age. The quadrants are named and go in the same order as the permanent quadrants. To differentiate if it is a primary or permanent tooth, a capital "D" is written before the quadrant to designate that it is a deciduous tooth: D maxillary right, D maxillary left, D mandibular left, and D mandibular right.

Importance of Primary Teeth

Some people still think that primary or "baby" teeth are not important because they will eventually fall out or *exfoliate*. Nothing could be further from the truth. Primary teeth are important for several reasons besides chewing food. The primary teeth hold the space for the permanent teeth, help the child eat properly to get nourishment, are important in the development of speech, and play an important role in establishing a child's positive self-image (see Figure 8-27). The teeth help hold the tongue in place and help with word pronunciation. You can probably remember a six-year-old with their front teeth missing and lisping when they spoke. It is important to retain each primary tooth until the permanent tooth replaces it. Even though the primary

TABLE 8-6 Universal Numbering System for Both Permanent and Primary Teeth with Identifying Numbers and Letters

The Universal Numbering System uses numbers 1–32 to represent the adult teeth. The maxillary right third molar is tooth #1, and the numbers continue clockwise and end with the mandibular right third molar as tooth#32.
Letters A through T are used to designate primary teeth. The primary maxillary right second molar is designated "#A" and the lettering continues clockwise to end with the primary mandibular right second as "#T."

Note on this diagram that the patient's right is on your left. This is important to know when identifying teeth using the numbering system and in charting.

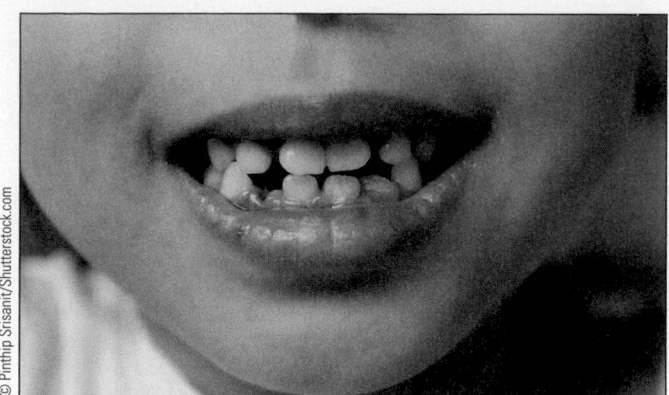

FIGURE 8-27
Mixed dentition begins with the mandibular permanent central incisors erupting. The mandibular left lateral incisor is erupting. A space is waiting for the eruption of the permanent right lateral incisor.

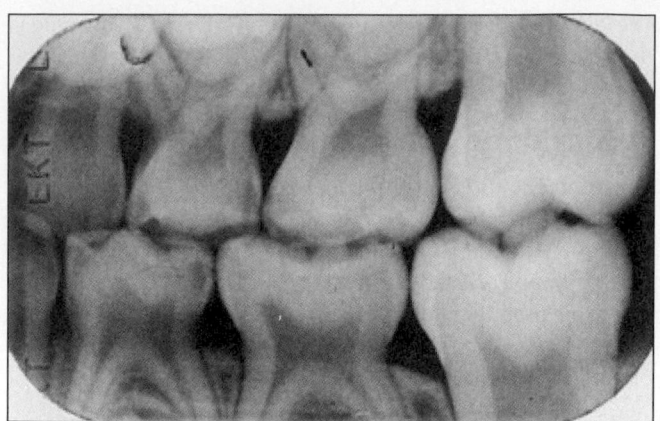

FIGURE 8-28
The radiograph shows erupting permanent premolars within the flared roots of the primary molars. The roots of the primary molar show the resorption that occurs during the exfoliation/eruption process.

teeth begin exfoliation by age six, they are still an important part of facial development.

When a primary tooth gets decayed, it is important to get it treated quickly because the **enamel** is much thinner in the primary dentition than it is in the permanent dentition. The decay can also spread much faster, which means an **abscess** can form; if it is not treated in time, it can become painful. An infected or abscessed tooth can be dangerous for a child, and the infection can spread to other areas in the mouth and head. An abscessed or decayed tooth should be treated because it may be in the mouth for four or five years before it exfoliates. If a primary tooth is prematurely lost or **extracted** too early, then it often allows the teeth beside the space to drift into the space, resulting in crowding when the permanent tooth tries to erupt. This makes it difficult for the permanent tooth to erupt into the proper location, which may result in **malocclusion** (crooked permanent teeth). These facts should be explained to the parents or caregivers so that they can understand that the primary teeth are important and worth saving.

Comparison of Primary and Permanent Teeth

When comparing a permanent tooth and primary tooth, there are some similarities and differences. Of course, the main difference is the overall size of the tooth; the primary teeth are much smaller than the permanent teeth and the crown portion is quite short in comparison to the root. The crowns of the primary teeth appear whiter or light bluish in color as compared to the yellow-gray color of the permanent teeth. This is because the enamel and dentin are much thinner. The **pulp chamber** is also much larger with especially large mesial **pulp horns** in primary teeth. Knowing that the pulp is larger and closer to the surface of the primary tooth, great care must be taken during the coronal polish procedure not to overheat the tooth and injure the pulp.

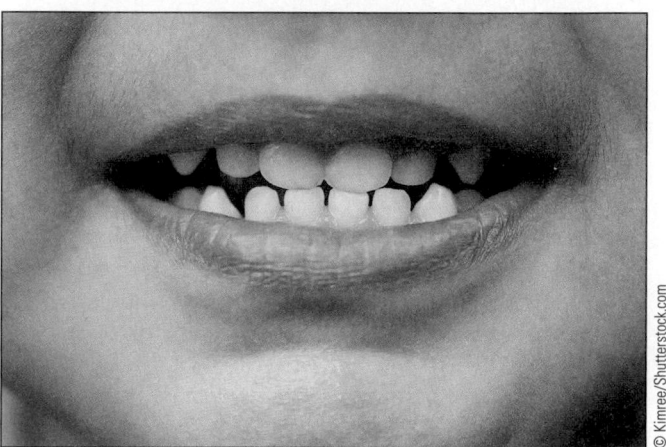

FIGURE 8-29
Anterior primate spacing.

The **neck** of the primary tooth also has a bulge at the **cervical margin**. The occlusal surface of it is also smoother, flatter, and does not have as many grooves as a permanent tooth does. The roots of the permanent molars are within the diameter of the crown, and the roots of the primary molars are flared (Figure 8-28). The number of cusps found on permanent and primary teeth are reversed. Whereas, the permanent first molar has five cusps, the primary first molar has four cusps. The permanent second and third molars have four cusps and the primary second molar has five cusps. It is important to not mischart during mixed dentition. The dental assistant needs to be able to recognize these differences and know the eruption patterns to make certain there are no errors in charting.

Unlike the permanent teeth, the primary teeth do not have tight contacts. Primary teeth have what is called **primate spacing** (Figure 8-29). The primate spaces are development spaces that provide extra room for the larger-sized permanent teeth to erupt.

The lack of primate spacing suggests a severe risk for crowding in the permanent dentition.

D. Maxillary Central Incisor

The primary maxillary central incisor (D. Max CI) resembles the permanent maxillary central in shape (Figure 8-30). It is much smaller in size than the permanent maxillary central and has a more pronounced cervical line. The crown is the only anterior tooth in either dentition to have a shorter inciso-cervical height than the mesio-distal width. This tooth erupts with no mamelons, and the labial surface is convex and smooth.

D. Maxillary Lateral Incisor

The primary maxillary lateral incisor (D. Max LI) is similar to the permanent lateral incisor except it is smaller (Figure 8-31). Another difference is that it is longer than it is wide. The incisal edge of the primary maxillary lateral incisor is more rounded on the mesial and distal sides than the straight incisal edge of the central incisor.

D. Maxillary Canine

The primary maxillary canine (D. Max C) appears to be wider than it is long; however, with the pointed incisal edge, it is slightly longer than it is wide (Figure 8-32). It is more convex than the permanent maxillary canine and constricts more at the cervix of the tooth. The mesioincisal slope has a

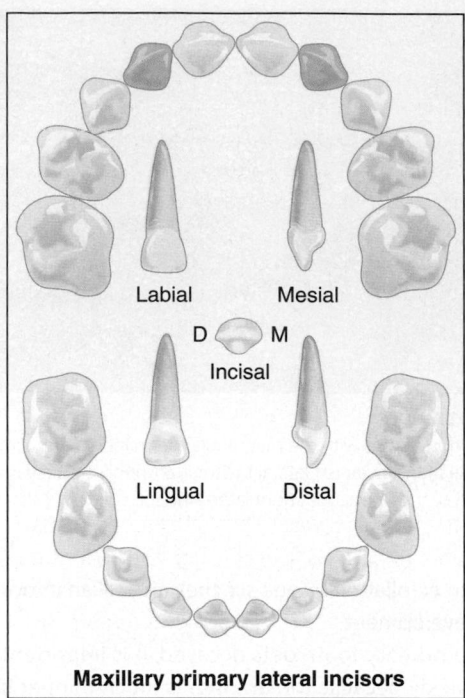

Maxillary primary lateral incisors

FIGURE 8-31
Primary dentition with D. maxillary lateral incisors identified.

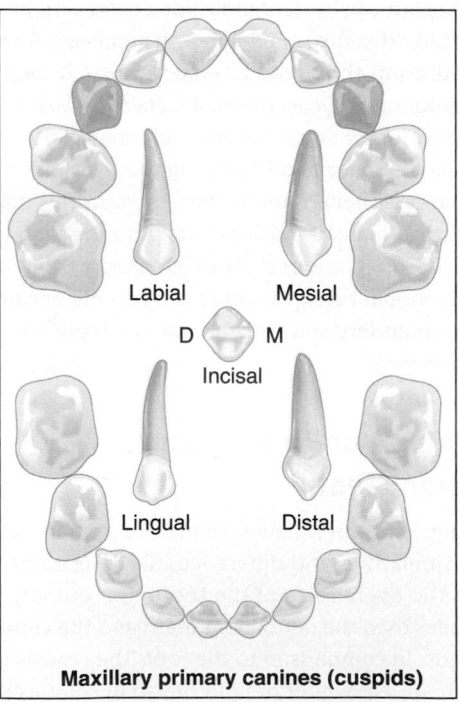

Maxillary primary canines (cuspids)

FIGURE 8-32
Primary dentition with D. maxillary canines identified.

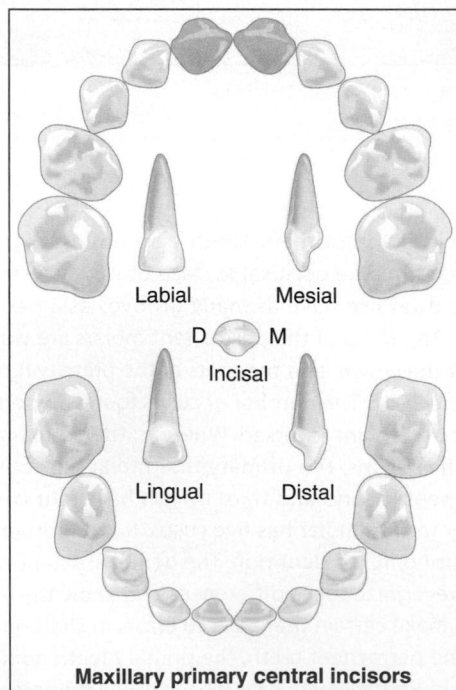

Maxillary primary central incisors

FIGURE 8-30
Primary dentition with D. maxillary central incisors identified.

pronounced cingulum and mesial and distal marginal ridges. The root is similar to the incisors but is longer (but nothing like the permanent canine).

D. Maxillary First Molar

The primary maxillary first molar (D. Max first M) resembles the permanent second molar in many respects (Figure 8-33). It has four cusps; the mesiobuccal and the mesiolingual are the most prominent. The mesiolingual is the longest and the largest. The distolingual is the smallest or may even be absent. The tooth has transverse and oblique ridges like the permanent maxillary second molar, but they are not as prominent. The roots, like those of all primary molars, spread out rapidly from the crown of the tooth and are widely spaced. The primary maxillary first molar has three roots, like its permanent counterparts.

D. Maxillary Second Molar

The primary maxillary second molar (D. Max second M) resembles the permanent maxillary first permanent molar because it has four primary cusps and may even have a cusp that resembles the cusp of Carabelli (Figure 8-34). It has three roots that are widely spaced.

D. Mandibular Central Incisor

The primary mandibular central incisor (D. Mand CI) more closely resembles the permanent mandibular lateral incisor than its central incisor counterpart (Figure 8-35). The crown of the tooth is slightly wider than the permanent lateral incisor. The shape and form of the incisal edge are almost exactly the same as that of the permanent lateral. The root is slender and rather long. Mesial and distal surfaces of the root are flat, while lingual and labial surfaces are convex.

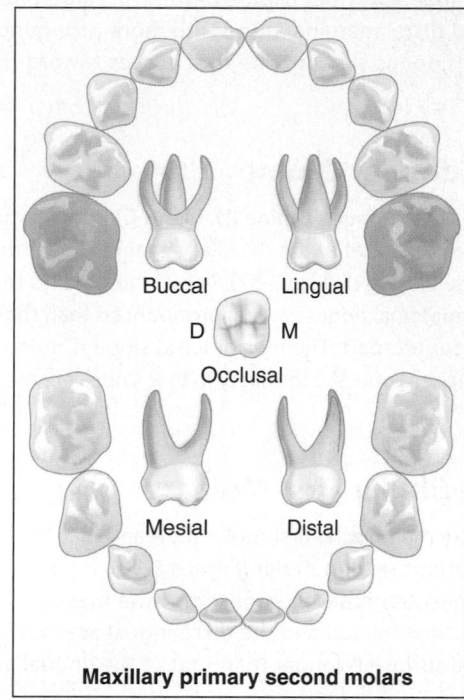

Maxillary primary second molars

FIGURE 8-34
Primary dentition with D. maxillary second molars identified.

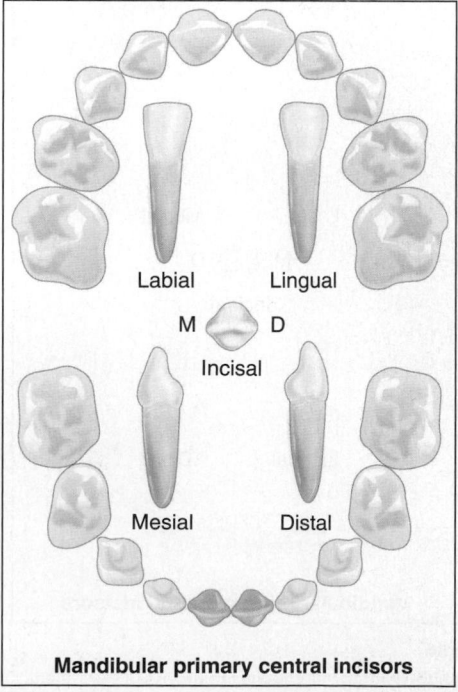

Mandibular primary central incisors

FIGURE 8-35
Primary dentition with D. mandibular central incisors identified.

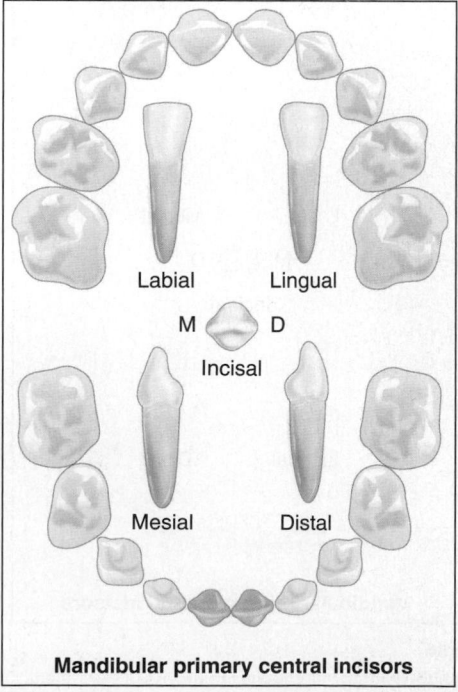

Maxillary primary first molars

FIGURE 8-33
Primary dentition with D. maxillary first molars identified.

D. Mandibular Lateral Incisor

The primary mandibular lateral incisor (D. Mand LI) resembles the mandibular primary central incisor except that it is slightly longer and wider (Figure 8-36). The cingulum and the mesial and distal marginal ridges are more pronounced, and the fossa is not as shallow. The root curves toward the distal at the apex.

D. Mandibular Canine

The primary mandibular canine (D. Mand C) is much more delicate in form than that of the maxillary canine—even the root is not as large or long (Figure 8-37). The cingulum and the mesial and distal marginal ridges are less pronounced than those of the maxillary counterpart. The mesioincisal slope is not as long as the distoincisal slope; the maxillary incisal slopes are more nearly equal in length.

D. Mandibular First Molar

The primary mandibular first molar (D. Mand first M) resembles the permanent second molar (Figure 8-38). It has four cusps, with the mesiobuccal the largest and the mesiolingual next in size. The distobuccal and the distolingual are much smaller. The buccal surface is longer than that of the lingual and has a

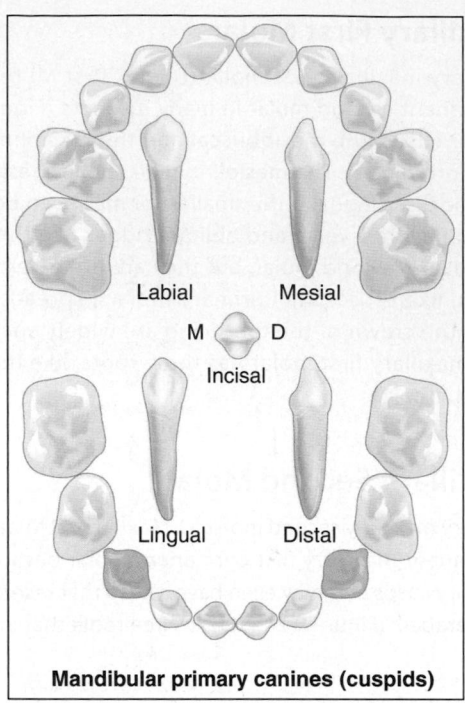

Mandibular primary canines (cuspids)

FIGURE 8-37
Primary dentition with D. mandibular canines identified.

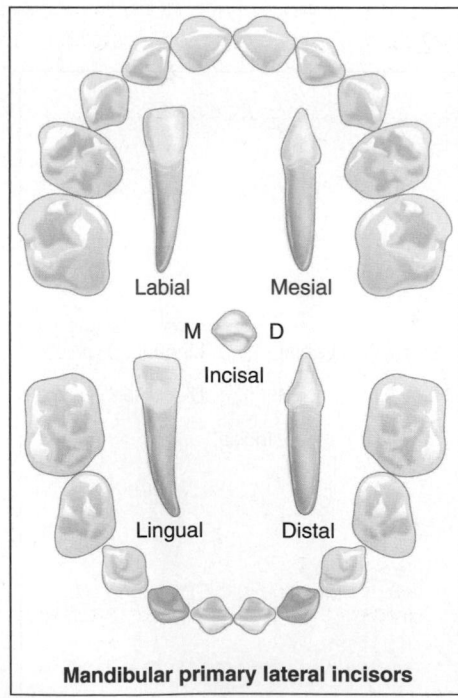

Mandibular primary lateral incisors

FIGURE 8-36
Primary dentition with D. mandibular lateral incisors identified.

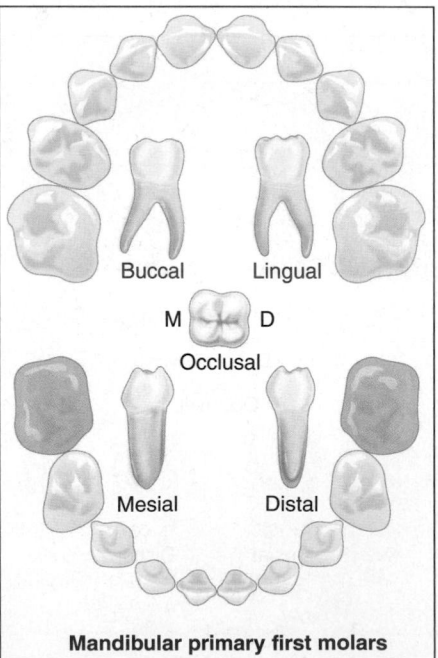

Mandibular primary first molars

FIGURE 8-38
Primary dentition with D. mandibular first molars identified.

very prominent cervical ridge across the gingival area, directly above where the tooth constricts at the cervix. The tooth has two roots, including a mesial root, which is much longer and wider, and a distal root. The apex of the mesial root is flattened or squared off.

D. Mandibular Second Molar

The primary mandibular second molar (D. Mand second M) closely resembles the permanent mandibular first molar (Figure 8-39). It is smaller in all dimensions, and the mesiobuccal and the distobuccal cusps are nearly equal in size, unlike the permanent mandibular first molar. The distal root is smaller, while the mesial root is longer and wider.

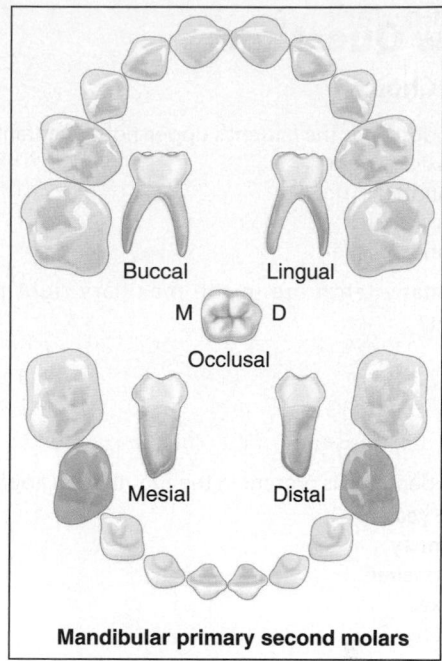

Mandibular primary second molars

FIGURE 8-39
Primary dentition with D. mandibular second molars identified.

Chapter Summary

Understanding tooth morphology prepares the assistant to record accurately for the dentist or hygienist, contributing in a vital way to help those team members make a more accurate diagnosis. Therefore, the dental assistant will need to be able to identify each tooth from its anatomical form.

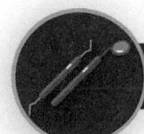

CASE STUDY

Travis Charles, age 12, complains of discomfort in the back of the mouth on both sides. The patient says it feels like the skin has broken open behind his teeth. Upon dental examination, it was noted that there was redness and edema.

Case Study Review

1. What probable condition is present?

2. Is the discomfort constant? Should Travis be concerned?

3. Does any one thing bring on the discomfort? Should Travis expect primary tooth loss in these areas?

Review Questions

Multiple Choice

1. Which describes the patient's upper-right quadrant?
   a. maxillary right
   b. mandibular right
   c. maxillary left
   d. mandibular left

2. How many teeth are in the maxillary right posterior sextant?
   a. 3
   b. 4
   c. 5
   d. 6

3. Which dentition is present in the mouth from approximately 6 to 12 years?
   a. primary
   b. permanent
   c. mixed
   d. adult

4. Which primary tooth erupts around 24 months and is often referred to as the two-year molar?
   a. first
   b. second
   c. third
   d. fourth

5. Which surfaces are only found on posterior teeth?
   a. incisal and labial
   b. occlusal and buccal
   c. lingual and incisal
   d. occlusal and labial

6. What is the name for the third of the tooth on the chewing surface of a posterior tooth?
   a. apical
   b. cervical
   c. middle
   d. occlusal

7. What is the junction of three surfaces of a tooth?
   a. line angle
   b. point angle
   c. embrasure
   d. proximal

8. Which of these landmarks are elevations?
   a. cusps, grooves, and fossae
   b. grooves, fossae, and pits
   c. cusps, ridges, and cingula
   d. cingula, ridges, and fossae

9. Which landmark appears as a shallow dip in places on the teeth?
   a. groove
   b. fossae
   c. mamelons
   d. cingula

10. A convex area on the lingual surface of the anterior teeth near the gingiva is called the _____.
    a. cusp
    b. fossa
    c. cingulum
    d. lobe

11. On what surface are mamelons found on newly erupted central incisors?
    a. mesial
    b. distal
    c. lingual
    d. incisal

12. Which are the largest to smallest of the anterior incisors?
    a. maxillary central, maxillary lateral, mandibular lateral, and mandibular central incisor
    b. maxillary lateral, maxillary central, mandibular central, and mandibular lateral incisor
    c. maxillary central, maxillary lateral, mandibular central, and mandibular lateral incisor
    d. mandibular lateral, maxillary central, maxillary lateral, and mandibular central incisor

13. Where can the marginal ridges be found on posterior teeth?
    a. from the cusp tips to the center
    b. from the facial directly to the lingual
    c. sides of the occlusal surface
    d. from the facial at an angle to the lingual

14. The cusp on the mesial lingual surface of the permanent maxillary first molar is the _____.
    a. oblique cusp
    b. cusp of Carabelli
    c. transverse cusp
    d. lobe cusp

15. Which teeth have the distinguishing feature of an oblique ridge?
    a. maxillary premolars
    b. mandibular premolars
    c. maxillary molars
    d. mandibular molars

16. Which teeth have five cusps?
    a. second premolars
    b. first molars
    c. second molars
    d. third molars

17. Which teeth have trifurcated roots?
    a. maxillary premolars
    b. mandibular premolars
    c. maxillary molars
    d. mandibular molars

18. All of these statements in comparing primary to permanent teeth are true *except* _____.
    a. primary teeth are smaller
    b. primary teeth are whiter
    c. primary teeth have thinner enamel
    d. primary teeth are better developed

19. Which teeth have five cusps?
    a. primary and permanent first molars
    b. primary second molars and permanent first molars
    c. primary and permanent second molars
    d. primary first molars and permanent second molars

20. Which teeth have four cusps?
    a. primary and permanent first molars
    b. primary second molars and permanent first molars
    c. primary and permanent second molars
    d. primary first molars and permanent second molars

Critical Thinking

1. If a patient has not formed a permanent mandibular first bicuspid on the left side, which primary tooth is retained in its place?

2. How does the tooth's morphology affect its function?

3. Defend the need for taking care of primary teeth.

Key Terms

Term and Pronunciation	Meaning of Root and Word Parts	Definition
abscess (**ab**-ses)	**abscess** = collection of pus	a localized collection of pus in the tissues of the body, often accompanied by swelling and inflammation and frequently caused by bacteria
adjacent (uh-**jey**-shuhnt)	**adjacent** = being near or close; touching	having a common boundary
anterior (an-**teer**-ee-er)	**ante-** = before **-ior** = denoting a certain characteristic	before, in front of
bifurcate (**bahy**-fer-keyt)	**bi-** = two **furcate** = forking, branching	to divide into two branches
buccal (**buhk**-uh l)	**bucc(o)** = cheek **-al** = pertaining to	surface on posterior teeth that is on the facial surface or next to the cheeks
canine eminence (**key**-nahyn) (**em**-uh-nuhns)	**canine** = doglike; pointed teeth located at four front corners of the mouth **eminent** = projecting, protruding **-ence** = indicating a condition or quality	a bulge on the surface of the jawbone where it covers the root of a canine
cervical (**sur**-vi-kuhl)	**cervix** = neck, constricted portion of an organ or part **-al** = pertaining to	of or relating to the neck of the tooth; area where the crown meets the root
cervical margin (**sur**-vi-kuh l) (**mahr**-jin)	**cervix** = neck, constricted portion of an organ or part **-al** = pertaining to **margin** = border or edge	the constricted part of the tooth connecting the crown to the root
cingulum (**sing**-gyuh-luh m)	**cingulum** = a girdle-like part, such as the ridge around the base of a tooth	elevation of enamel on lingual cervical surface of anterior teeth
concave (kon-**keyv**)	**con** = with or together **cave** = to hollow area	curved area like the interior of a circle
congenitally (kuh n-**jen**-i-tl-ee)	**con-** = with **gen-** = genetics; the science of heredity **-al** – pertaining to **-ly** = having the nature or qualities of	of or relating to a condition present at birth, whether inherited or caused by the environment, especially the uterine environment
convex (kon-**veks**)	**convex** = curved or rounded outward	having a surface that curves outward
cusp (kuhsp)	**cusp** = a point or pointed end	a point, projection, or elevation, as on the crown of a tooth
cusp of Carabelli (kuhsp) (**kar**-uh- **bel**-ee)	**cusp** = a point, projection, or elevation	fifth cusp on maxillary first molars, found on the side of the largest mesiolingual (ml) cusp
deciduous dentition (dih-**sij**-oo-uh s) (den-**tish**-uh n)	**deciduous** = falling off or shedding at stage of growth **dent-** = teeth **-tion** = denoting condition	deciduous teeth, also called primary teeth, are shed for the eruption of permanent teeth; the type, number, and arrangement of teeth in the dental arch
dentition (den-**tish**-uhn)	**dent-** = teeth **-tion** = denoting condition	the makeup of a set of teeth; their type, number, and position
dilacerated (roots) (dih-**las**-uh-reyt-ed)	**di-** = apart, two **lacerate** = mangled, torn	bent roots, not a normal flare or tilt, makes extraction very difficult

(Continues)

Term and Pronunciation	Meaning of Root and Word Parts	Definition
distal (**dis**-tl)	**dist(ant)** = far away; not near at hand -**al** = pertaining to	surface of tooth that is the farthest side away from midline
embrasure (em-**brey**-sher)	**embrace** = to take up -**ure** = indicating process or result	the space between adjacent teeth
enamel (ih-**nam**-uh l)	**enamel** = dental tissue covering the crown of the tooth	the hard, calcareous tissue covering the exposed portion of a tooth
eruption (ih-**ruhp**-shuh n)	**erupt** = to burst forth -**ion** = denoting action	a visible breaking out, the breaking of a tooth through the gum
exfoliate (eks-**foh**-lee-yet)	**ex-** = out of, from, without **foliate** = relating to, possessing, or resembling leaves	the shedding or casting off of a body surface, in this case, primary teeth
extract (ik-**strakt**)	**extract** = to withdraw, pull out, or uproot by force	pull tooth from the jawbone
facial (**fey**-shuh l)	**face** = the front part of the head -**al** = pertaining to	surface of tooth that is on front that faces lips and cheeks, generic term for this surface in anterior and posterior teeth
fossa (**fos**-uh)	**fossa** = a pit, cavity, or depression, as in a bone	depression or scooped-out area on tooth surface, found mainly on lingual surfaces of anterior and occlusal of posterior teeth
frenum (**free**-nuhm)	**frenum** = anatomical structure resembling a fold; limits movement of a part	small folds of tissue under the tongue, front upper and lower lips
groove (groov)	**groove** = a long, narrow cut or indentation in a surface	the fine lines found in the surface of a **tooth**; marks the junction of part during in its development; also called developmental line
imbrication (im-bri-**key**-shuhn)	**imbricate** = overlapping (like scales on a fish) in a regular arrangement -**ion** = denoting action or condition	slight, horizontal, scale-like ridges on the labial cervical third of some anterior teeth
incisal (in-**sahyz**-uhl)	**incise** = to cut into -**al** = pertaining to	biting edge of anterior teeth
incise (in-**sahyz**)	**incise** = to cut into	to cut into food by action of front teeth (incisors)
interdental papilla (in-ter-**dent**-tl) (puh-**pil**-uh)	**inter** = between **dent** = tooth -**al** = of or relating to **papilla** = a small projection of tissue	the triangular part of the gingiva that fills the area between adjacent teeth
interproximal (in-**tur-prok**-suh-muh l)	**inter** = between **proximal** = near or next to a point of reference or attachment	in between teeth, space in between two adjacent teeth
labial (**ley**-bee-uh l)	**labium** = lip -**al** = pertaining to	facial surface of anterior teeth next to lips
lingual (**ling**-gwuh l)	**lingu-** = tongue -**al** = pertaining to	surface of tooth that is inside, next to tongue; generic term for anterior and posterior teeth
lobe (lohb)	**lobe** = a roundish projection or division; any rounded projection forming part of a larger structure	a part or section of tooth that forms and fuses with adjacent lobes to form entire tooth; most teeth form from 4–5 lobes
malocclusion (mal-uh-**kloo**-shuhn)	**mal-** = faulty, bad **occlude** = to close; to bring upper and lower teeth together -**ion** = denoting action or condition	a condition in which the upper teeth and lower teeth are misaligned when they meet
mamelon (**meym**-uh-lon)	**mamelon** = nipple-like elevation	scalloped incisal edge of newly erupted anterior incisors; maxillary and mandibular anterior incisors where three lobes join to make crown
mandibular arch (man-**dib**-yuh-ler) (ahrch)	**mandible** = the bone of the lower jaw -**ar** = of or belonging to **arch** = something bowed or curved	the anatomical structure pertaining to the natural curvature of the lower jaw (mandible) of the mouth

Term and Pronunciation	Meaning of Root and Word Parts	Definition
maxillary arch (**mak**-*suh*-ler-ee) (ahrch)	**maxilla(a)** = the bone of the upper jaw **-ary** = pertaining to **arch** = something bowed or curved	the anatomical structure pertaining to the natural curvature of the upper jaw (maxilla) of the mouth
mesial (**mee**-zee-*uh* l)	**mes-** = middle **-al** = of, relating to	surface of side of tooth that is closest to midline
midline (**mid**-lahyn)	**mid-** = indicating middle point **line** = an indication of demarcation; boundary	any line that bisects a structure that is bilaterally symmetrical, divides body in right and left halves; also referred to as midsagittal plane and median line
morphology (mawr-**fol**-*uh*-jee)	**morph(o)** = form, structure **-ology** = used in the names of sciences or bodies of knowledge	the branch of biology dealing with the form and structure of organisms
neck (nek)	**neck** = any narrow, connecting, or projecting part	the constricted part of the tooth connecting the crown to the root; also referred to as cervix
nonsuccedaneous (non- suhk-si-**dey**-nee-*us*)	**non-** = not **suc-** = succeed, to follow or replace another **cede** = to yield or formally surrender to another **-an** = belonging to or relating to **-eous** = having the nature of	not following a substitute; pertaining to those permanent teeth that are not preceded by a primary tooth
oblique ridge (*uh*-**bleek**) (rij)	**oblique** = slanting, sloping; diverging from a given straight line or course **ridge** = a long elevation; upper edge or crest	triangular ridges that connect diagonally across the occlusal surface on a posterior tooth ml to distobuccal (DB)
occlude (*uh*-**klood**)	**occlude** = to close	to bring upper and lower teeth together
occlusal (*uh*-**kloo**-zh*uh* l)	**occlus-** = occlude; to close, shut **-al** = pertaining to	chewing surface on top of posterior teeth
opposing arch (*uh*-**pohz**-ing) (ahrch)	**oppose** = to act against; to place opposite **arch** = upper or lower jaw	the upper arch opposes the lower arch and vice versa; refers to the opposite arch
palatal (**pal**-*uh*-tl)	**palate** = roof of the mouth **-al** = pertaining to	lingual (tongue) surface of maxillary teeth, close to palate
perikymata (pair-ih-**kiy**-muh-tuh)	**peri-** = around, about **kymata** = wave motions	small waves of enamel found on facial surface of anterior teeth made during development, found on cervical third
pit (pit)	**pit** = a naturally formed hole; depression in the body	a sharp-pointed depression in the enamel surface of a tooth; caused by faulty or incomplete calcification or formed by the confluent point of two or more lobes of enamel
posterior (po-**steer**-ee-er)	**post-** = behind, after **-er** = having certain characteristics **-ior** = denoting comparatives	located at or toward the rear of the body
proximal (**prok**-*suh*-m*uh*l)	**proximal** = near or next to a point of reference or attachment	the surface of a tooth in relation to an adjacent tooth being nearer or farther from the median line
pulp chamber (puhlp) (**cheym**-ber)	**pulp** = soft, innermost part of a tooth; contains nerves and blood vessels **chamber** = cavity; enclosed space	cavity within the crown of a tooth that contains the pulp tissue
pulp horns (p*uh*lp) (hawrnz)	**pulp** = soft, innermost part of a tooth; contains nerves and blood vessels **horn** = curved, pointed projection	an elongation of the pulp that extends toward the incisal/occlusal surface
ridge (rij)	**ridge** = a long, narrow elevation; raise to a higher position	elevation of enamel of tooth that makes sharp mountain peak on occlusal surface; makes cusp ridges
quadrant (**kwod**-r*uh*h nt)	**quad-** = comprising four people or things **-ant** = exiting in a certain condition	any of the four sections of the mouth; each dental arch is divided in half
root trunk (root) (truhngk)	**root** = the embedded part of an organ or structure; serving as a base or support **trunk** = the body excluding head and limbs	section of root from CEJ to where root splits on bifurcated or trifurcated teeth

(Continues)

Term and Pronunciation	Meaning of Root and Word Parts	Definition
succedaneous (suhk-si-**dey**-nee-*us)*	**suc-** = succeed, to follow or replace another **cede** = to yield or formally surrender to another **-an** = belonging to or relating to **-eous** = having the nature of	following a substitute; pertaining to those permanent teeth that are preceded by a primary tooth
symmetrical (si-**me**-tri-k*uh* l)	**symmetr(y)** = relation of parts, proportion; an exact matching of form and arrangement of parts on opposite sides **-ical** = characterized by or exhibiting	similar and can be identical on right and left sides; same characteristics
trifurcate (trahy-**fur**-keyt)	**tri-** = three **furcate** = forking, branching	to divide into three branches

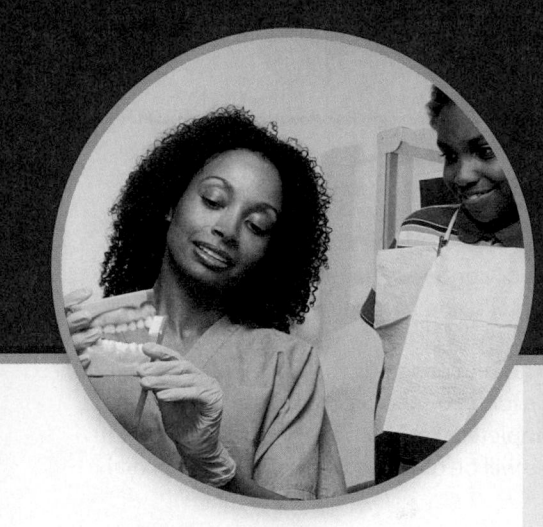

## CHAPTER 9

Oral Pathology

Specific Instructional Objectives

At the completion of this chapter, you will be able to meet these objectives:

1. Use terms presented in this chapter.
2. Define oral pathology.
3. Identify the role of the dental assistant in the area of oral pathology.
4. Discuss the methods used to identify a lesion.
5. Define the three phases of inflammation.
6. Identify various lesions based on location.
7. Discuss the dental caries process.
8. Explain the four stages of decay.
9. Summarize the causes of rampant caries.
10. Compare and contrast lesions of the oral cavity caused by biological agents.
11. Differentiate between amelogenesis imperfect and dentinogenesis imperfecta.
12. Compare and contrast anodontia and hypodontia.
13. Compare and contrast fusion and gemination.
14. Differentiate between macrodontia and microdontia.
15. Explain the various anomalies of the tongue.
16. Summarize the lesions produced by chemical agents.
17. Differentiate among the lesions produced by physical agents.
18. Identify the lesions that are caused by hormonal imbalances.
19. Differentiate among the lesions produced by nutritional deficiencies.
20. Compare and contrast between benign and malignant neoplasms.
21. List the common sites for oral cancer.
22. State the warning signs for oral cancer.
23. Compare and contrast leukoplakia and erythroplakia.
24. Discuss the two forms of lichen planus.
25. Discuss the oral lesions related to HIV and AIDS.
26. Explain the importance of oral cancer screening.
27. Outline the steps in a head and neck exam for oral cancer.
28. Outline the steps for a patient self-exam for oral cancer.
29. Compare and contrast the types of diagnostic tools available for oral cancer screening.
30. Compare and contrast patient treatment before, during and after radiation therapy.

Introduction to Oral Pathology

Pathology is a term that means the study of the nature and cause of disease. It usually involves changes in the structure of function of cells. An *oral pathologist* is a dentist who, after graduation from dental school, continues training in a three-year oral pathology residency program to specialize in the scientific examination of tissues, cells, and specimens of body fluids for evidence of oral disease.

The dental assistant is responsible for setting up for initial exam appointments. After the patient is seated, the dental assistant reviews the medical history and documents any concerns found. Any oral **lesions** found on the preliminary exam should be documented as well. Some questions come to mind as the preliminary exam is completed. For example, how long has the lesion been there? Could it be oral cancer? How do you know if it is or not? All of these will be discussed in this chapter on oral pathology.

Diagnosis of Lesions

Diseases present with signs and symptoms. A symptom is a deviation from normal function or feeling that is obvious to a patient. It is subjective, observed by the patient, and cannot be measured directly, whereas a sign is objectively observable by others.

To be able to see something that is not normal, the dental health care worker should be aware of what normal oral anatomy looks like. Keep in mind that there are variations of normal. Knowing normal anatomy will allow for identification of an abnormality. This section will focus on what is not considered to be *within normal limits* (WNL) as well as how to describe and document what is found using the proper terminology and procedures.

Identifying a lesion is a lot like putting together a puzzle. Each separate diagnosis provides another piece of the puzzle and helps the dentist gather more information. There are a variety of oral lesions that can be found in the oral cavity. By completing a preliminary diagnosis, the dentist can put these puzzle pieces together to identify the lesion exactly and treat it properly. There are several methods of diagnoses a dentist can perform in order to identify a lesion with certainty. Each of the ones listed below is discussed in this lesson.

Clinical Diagnosis

The clinical diagnosis is the first and most basic examination of the lesion. There are five phases to the clinical diagnosis, designed to identify five important physical characteristics of

the lesion: location, size, shape, color, and texture or consistency. The dental assistant aids the dentist with this routine procedure on a patient. If an area is discovered as not WNL, then it should be brought to the dentist's attention for further investigation. The area should always be documented in the patient's chart, measured, and photographed if possible. It is important to have a baseline exam and description recorded of a particular area because it provides a way to compare or contrast any differences that may be noted later.

Location The location of a lesion needs to be stated in detail. If appropriate, use the teeth numbers to designate the location, for example, "The lesion is located on the attached gingiva 2 mm above the gingival margin of tooth #8." In this example, the exact location of the lesion is not in question. If the lesion is on the face, indicate what side of the face it is on and what structure it is near. Always use professional terms covered in Chapters 5 and 6 for the oral cavity when documenting the location of a lesion.

Size One of the most important things that the dental assistant can do upon finding a lesion is to measure the size accurately. Use a clearly marked periodontal probe to measure the length and width of the lesion (Figure 9-1). Be careful to ensure how the probe is marked since they can be marked in a number of ways. Some probes have markings every 3 millimeters, others every millimeter, and some are color coded. When holding the probe to the lesion, be sure to measure from one margin of the lesion to the opposite margin as precisely as possible to get

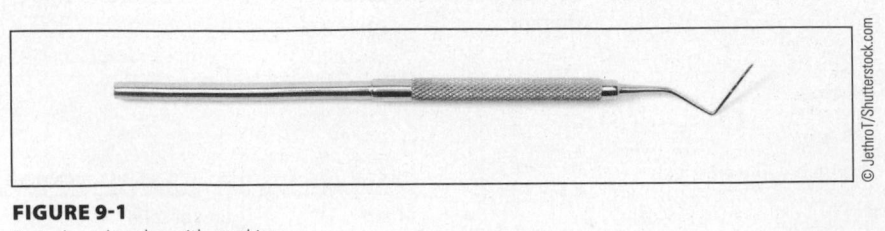

FIGURE 9-1
Periodontal probe with markings.

a correct measurement, expressed in millimeters. Accuracy is of extreme importance, and an inaccurate measurement of the initial lesion may render subsequent measurements invalid. Some lesions may be in several lobes or segmented parts, called *lobulated*; in such cases, each lobe of the lesion should be measured separately.

Photographing a lesion is a good way to track growth or change in the lesion over time. Hold the periodontal probe against the lesion when taking a photo to provide a baseline measurement for documentation. These photos can later be compared and contrasted to photos taken at subsequent appointments to identify any growth or change in the lesion.

Shape Many times the shape of a lesion will help determine what the lesion is or what category it belongs in. Table 9-1 lists terms that are appropriate for describing the shape of a lesion. If the shape does not fit into any of those categories, try to describe it as accurately as possible. A drawing or photograph of the lesion placed in the chart also can be helpful.

Color Lesions appear in a wide variety of colors, making color description challenging. For one thing, some lesions are very close in color to the surrounding tissues, while others are distinctly different. The margin around a lesion may also be a different color from the lesion itself. A lesion may also be *variegated* or have a mixture of colors inside it. If either of these is the case, then both colors should be differentiated from each other and all colors included in the description. It is important to be as accurate as possible when describing the color of the lesion and any surrounding margin or tissues. Table 9-2 provides terms for colors when describing a lesion.

TABLE 9-1 Shapes of Lesions and Appropriate Description

Lesion Shape	Description
round	circular
oval	oval shaped, not circular, slightly longer than wide
oblong	oblong shaped, much longer than wider
linear	lines, striped, streaked
striated	net like, striations that intermingle, spiderweb-like
lobulated	in sections or parts, bubble like
pedunculated	on a stalk like a mushroom
edematous	swollen, larger than usual
sessile	broad based
ulcer/erosion	depressed lesion
macule	flat lesion
plaque	slightly elevated and broad
vesicle	elevated lesion
pustule	pus filled
nodule	raised lesion without any fluid
papule	less than 5 mm and no fluid inside

TABLE 9-2 Descriptive Colors for Documentation of Oral Tissues and Oral Lesions

Black/Brown/Blue	Normal/Red	White
black	red (erythema)	white (leukoplakia)
brown	bright red	pale/pallor
purple/blue	dark pink	gray
magenta (blue red)	pink	yellow
pigmented (in darker color skin the gingival tissue will also be darker in areas)	coral pink	variegated (multicolor)

Consistency/Texture The final part of the clinical diagnosis involves describing the consistency and texture of the lesion to determine if it is flat, raised, with raised margins, or ill defined. The outer layer of the lesion can sometimes have a specific texture that should be included in the description. Table 9-3 provides terms that can be used to describe the consistency and texture of a lesion and surrounding tissues.

Radiographic Diagnosis

Taking and analyzing radiographs is a key part of the preliminary diagnosis. Radiographs are used when bone, teeth, or other hard tissues are involved or around the lesion. Many times a final diagnosis can be made from the image and no further investigation is needed. A common example of this occurs

TABLE 9-3 Terms to Describe Lesion Consistency and Texture

Lesion Consistency or Texture	Description
smooth	smooth with no bumps or irregularity
corrugated	wrinkled, rippled, layered appearance
shiny	wet look, as in a blister
stippled	orange-peel-like dimpling, as in healthy gingival tissue
edematous	swollen, enlarged, usually shiny, often causes shape of tissue to change
keratinized	thickened and covered with keratinized tissue
papillary	covered in multiple small bump-like areas
knife-edged	sharp, pointed, fills embrasure area in-between teeth, as in healthy gingiva
nonkeratinized	mucosa-like, smooth
denuded	raw, as in under a blister after it pops and peels, scraped, open wounds
fluctuant	fluid-filled and moveable
indurated	hardened
fissured	deep groves
soft	not firm upon touching
hard	firm or solid

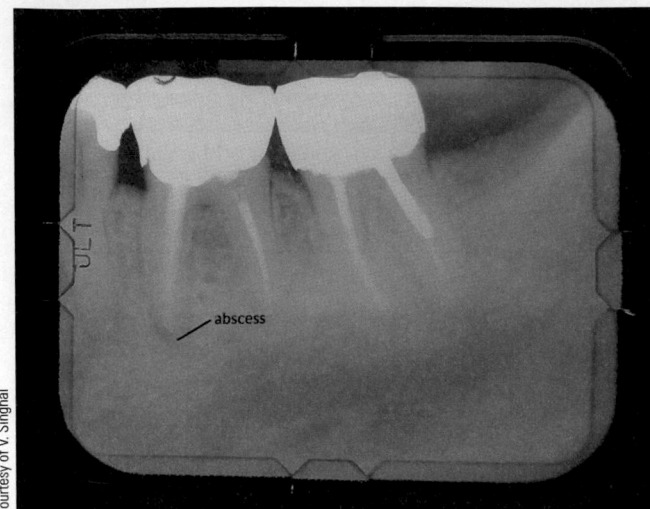

Courtesy of V. Singhal

abscess

FIGURE 9-2
Radiographic image of an abscess.

when a raised, red area is found in the vestibule and a subsequent radiograph reveals an **abscess** at the apex or root tip of a tooth (Figure 9-2). There is no longer any need for further diagnosis, because the image has revealed the cause of the lesion. Chapters 28 and 29 will discuss the radiographic appearance of structures in detail.

Historical Diagnosis

Another procedure that can be used to gather pieces to solve the puzzle is the historical diagnosis, which entails gathering information about the history of the lesion by asking the patients such questions as, Has it occurred before? Is there a family history of the same lesions? How long has the lesion been present? Has the lesion changed over time in size, shape, and/or color? The patient's full medical and dental history is included in this diagnosis, including any medication that the patient is taking. Many times by questioning the patient thoroughly about historical items, a crucial piece of information that aids in the diagnosis may be revealed.

Laboratory, Microscopic, and Surgical Diagnoses

A laboratory diagnosis is often performed on lesions that are difficult to identify using the methods described above. Lab tests including blood work, urinalysis, or **cultures** can add helpful information. For example, you can determine definitively whether a raw, red throat is strep throat by performing a throat culture.

In some cases, the dentist may need to conduct a microscopic diagnosis, which involves examining cells from a lesion under a microscope. In order to get cells from the lesion, the patient must undergo an *excisional* biopsy, in which the whole lesion is removed, or *incisional* biopsy, where only part of the lesion is removed. This is referred to as a surgical diagnosis.

Therapeutic Diagnosis

A therapeutic diagnosis involves supplementing nutritional deficiencies in the patient's diet in an attempt to diagnose the problem. For example, suppose a patient with red, crusty lesions at the corners of the mouth takes vitamin B complex and the lesions go away. In this case, we can diagnose the lesions as **angular cheilitis**, which was caused by a nutritional deficiency of vitamin B complex. Common fungal infections of the oral cavity such as *Candida albicans* can be diagnosed by administering antifungal agents and observing whether the fungus disappears.

Differential Diagnosis

Based on the methods discussed above, a differential diagnosis is conducted to narrow down the possibilities. This requires the dentist first to make a list of every possible lesion based on the information gained. Then the dentist systematically compares and contrasts every piece of information available to the symptoms and common characteristics of each possible cause for the lesion. The differential diagnosis can help eliminate possible answers and narrow down the possibilities of a final answer.

Final Diagnosis

A final diagnosis can be made by using all of the previous diagnoses and putting them together to get an appropriate and correct decision. Sometimes only one or two pieces of the puzzle are needed; sometimes several are required to positively diagnose a lesion. With any of the previous diagnoses, the proper documentation has to be included in the patient's chart. On the initial visit it is important to get as much information as possible and then refer the patient to an oral surgeon for other diagnoses to be completed as soon as possible. It is important that the dental healthcare worker explain thoroughly the reasoning behind the need for further treatment without alarming the patient. The patient needs to understand why a lesion may need to be checked by a biopsy or other means so that it can be treated correctly. The dental assistant can help the patient make an appointment at the oral surgeon and explain what the surgeon will do. It is always important to be considerate and truthful with patients and to let them know that your office will work to help them get the treatment they need.

If a lesion is questionable, it is important that the patient return in two (2) weeks to see if healing has progressed. If it has not, then a referral to an oral surgeon can be made. It is also important at a subsequent visit to take a second photo and to compare and contrast the clinical diagnoses with the data from the first visit.

Inflammatory Process

The acute inflammatory process plays a role in the development of many types of lesions. Thus, in order to understand how a lesion develops, it is important to understand the process of *inflammation*. Inflammation is a response that occurs when the

TABLE 9-4 Common Symptoms of Inflammation

redness/erythema	caused by vasodilation
heat	caused by vasodilation
edema/swelling	caused by vessel permeability
pain	chemicals and pressure from edema
acute inflammation	lasts less than 2 weeks
chronic inflammation	lasts longer than 2 weeks—if inflammation continues, more tissue damage will occur (as in periodontal disease in gingival tissues)

body becomes injured. It is the body's attempt to protect itself from foreign substances such as bacteria, viruses, trauma, and other irritants. *Edematous* or swollen tissues are the first indication that some injury has occurred and the body is responding. Table 9-4 provides common symptoms of inflammation. Tissue inflammation can be reversed in many cases by removing the irritant that caused it. The process of acute inflammation, no matter what the cause, consists of three phases: initiation, amplification, and termination.

Initiation Phase

Initiation of the body's response occurs when tissue is injured in any way. The body's *mast cells* release chemicals called *histamines* into the bloodstream that trigger *vasoconstriction* or narrowing of the blood vessels to control any bleeding. After this initial vasoconstriction, the vessels dilate, allowing blood to flow into the affected area, causing swelling. As the process continues, blood flowing to the site of the injury begins leaking into the tissues, increasing swelling and pressure on the nerve endings that can cause pain. Pain can also occur because of the chemicals that are stimulating this phase of the inflammatory process.

Amplification Phase

In the second phase of the inflammatory process, amplification, white blood cells (WBCs) start to fight off the infection using cells called *neutrophils* and *macrophages* to destroy the invading agents. These cells engulf the foreign substance in a process called *phagocytosis* and construct a layer of connective tissue around it to prevent the inflammation from spreading to other parts of the body.

Termination Phase

During phase three, the chemical processes start to slow down and eventually the inflammatory response stops. The lymphatic system filters out any toxins from the area and rids the body of the foreign invaders that triggered the inflammatory process. Following termination, cells in the affected area are either regenerated, or restored to normal, or repaired, which means that some damage was fixed but the cell has not returned to its original function.

Classification of Lesions by Location

Lesions typically are categorized by their location in regard to the surface of the oral mucosa. Thus, a lesion primarily is identified as being either above, below, or flat with the oral mucosa surface. Classifying lesions according to location relative to the oral mucosa surface can help with the differential or final diagnosis since most lesions are found specific to certain locations.

Lesions Classified above the Surface of the Oral Mucosa

Table 9-5 provides details about lesions that are above the soft tissue of the oral cavity and are visible during the clinical examination. These lesions vary in size, shape, and cause.

Lesions Classified below the Surface of the Oral Mucosa

Table 9-6 provides details about lesions that are found within the alveolar bone and in the tissue beneath the oral mucosa surface.

Lesions Classified as Flat or Even with the Surface of the Oral Mucosa

Table 9-7 provides details about lesions that are found even with the surface of the oral mucosa.

Infectious Diseases of the Tooth

The most common chronic childhood disease is dental **decay** or **caries**. Dental caries also impacts adults. It is a progressive bacterial disease that, if left untreated, will affect the dental pulp and periapical tissues and cause eventual loss of the tooth or teeth involved.

Dental Caries Process

Mutans streptococci (including both *Streptococcus mutans* and *Streptococcus sobrinus*) and *Lactobacillus species* are the acid-forming bacteria that grow on the teeth with the dental plaque biofilm. This biofilm makes metabolic acids when it is in the mouth with fermentable carbohydrates.

Development of dental caries can take months to years. It occurs when more minerals from the enamel are lost due to *demineralization* than are deposited through remineralization. Demineralization is the process in which the minerals of the tooth are dissolved out of the tooth, leaving the surface less densely packed with minerals. In *remineralization*, the minerals are deposited back into the enamel.

This cycle of demineralization and remineralization does not necessarily cause loss of tooth enamel. Instead, dental caries is a constant cycle of both processes and is accompanied by a diet of fermentable carbohydrates including sucrose, fructose, and starches. The biofilm *metabolize* the sugars and carbohydrates

TABLE 9-5 Lesions above the Surface of the Oral Mucosa

blister, vesicle, bulla

A *blister* is a raised, ovoid or circular, fluid filled lesion that often results from some form of trauma. The fluid consists of blood that leaks into the underlying layers of skin tissue. A small blister less than one centimeter is called a *vesicle* (Figure 9-7). Vesicles have a thin epithelial lining that breaks down, resulting in an ulcerated area. Vesicles are common in viral infections like herpes simplex or chicken pox. A blister greater than half an inch in diameter is called a *bulla*. In a bulla, the fluid accumulates in the epidermis and dermis junction. Bullae are often seen in mucosal burns and vesculobullous (characterized by vesicles and bullae) diseases like pemphigus.

hematoma

A *hematoma* is a slightly raised bruised area due to a collection of localized, clotted blood, commonly called a blood blister. It is caused by bleeding from a ruptured blood vessel that may appear after administration of dental local anesthetic (refer to Chapter 23). When this occurs in the oral cavity, the dental assistant should alert the dentist immediately. It usually appears fairly quickly after the injection is administered. If a hematoma does occur, the dentist should apply pressure and ice to the area to minimize enlargement of the hematoma. Hematomas related to administration of local anesthesia will be discussed further in Chapter 23.

papule, nodule, tumor

A *papule* is a circumscribed, solid elevation up to 1 cm in diameter on the skin. A papule may be pigmented and either smooth or bumpy in texture. It can be *pedunculated* (attached by a stalk) or *sessile* (broad based). Most papules are slow growing and benign.

A similar lesion up to 1.0 cm in diameter, solid, with palpable depth is called a *nodule* and can occur above, beneath, or level with the skin. It can be harder or softer than a papule. A nodule can be asymptomatic and cause no pain, or it can be painful. It can be found inside the edges of lips, corners of lips or commissures, and even on the tongue.

The term *tumor*, meaning a swelling, is often used as a synonym for the word *neoplasm*, which is a new growth that contains cells that exhibit uncontrolled proliferation or cell multiplication. Tumors may be benign or *malignant* (cancerous).

plaque

A plaque is also commonly known as an age spot. It is a raised, flat patch on the skin that is normally pigmented and less than one centimeter in diameter. It is normally seen in the elderly and also called *senile keratosis*. It is a benign skin discoloration and usually presents no medical problem.

pustule

A *pustule* is a small, raised, pus-containing vesicle or blister-like lesion. This is often seen on the skin in someone with severe acne. A pustule can also be found at the end of an irritated eyelash follicle, also known as a *sty* (stye). A pustule can also be found inside the oral cavity on the gingivae when a tooth has a draining *fistula*. This happens when a tooth's pulp is infected, and the infection goes out the end of the apex of the tooth, creating an abscess at the end of the root in the bone. The infection bores a hole through the bone to the inside of the mouth and drains out into the oral cavity. The *parulis*, found at the end of the drain, is an elevated nodule at the site of the abscess. This condition can also happen in the periodontium or gingiva in the form of a periodontal abscess. A pustule is different from an abscess. A pustule is above or on the oral mucosa, but the abscess is found in the bone and can only be detected through a radiograph.

granuloma

A granuloma is a lesion associated with chronic inflammation that may appear as a tumor filled with granulation tissue. It is often a hemorrhagic and ulcerated gingival mass that appears during pregnancy, thus earning it the names pregnancy tumor, pregnancy granuloma, or *pyogenic* granuloma.

A granuloma can grow large quickly but is typically not painful nor malignant. Because of its appearance, it can be alarming, and a patient may be afraid that it is cancerous. The dentist can explain to the patient that the hormones released during pregnancy cause the granuloma, and that it typically is removed after the pregnancy is over. Depending on where the granuloma occurs, it may be removed before childbirth (e.g., between teeth #8 and #9). However, the dentist would make this decision with the patient and the patient's obstetrician. If removed before the termination of the pregnancy, it usually returns.

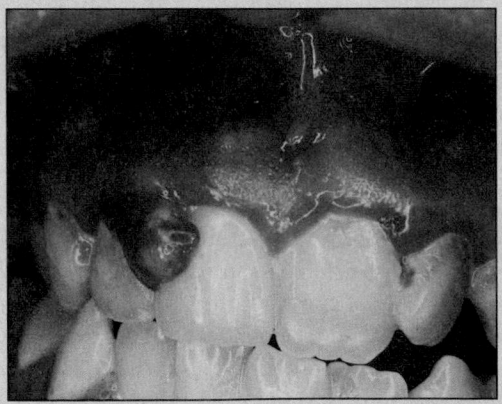

TABLE 9-6 Lesions below the Surface of the Oral Mucosa

abscess

There are two types of abscesses seen in dentistry. They both form as a result of infection by bacteria and can be differentiated by a radiograph of a tooth, showing up as a radiolucency in the bone. If the abscess is along the side of the periodontal ligament (PDL) of the root, then it is a periodontal abscess. If it is at the apex of the root of the tooth, then it is a periapical abscess (Figure 9-2). Dentists may prescribe antibiotics to take care of the infections that cause these lesions. The periodontal abscess usually requires deeper scaling to remove bacteria that caused the lesion. The periapical abscess usually requires a root canal to save the tooth. If the tooth cannot be treated with a good prognosis, the tooth may be extracted.

TABLE 9-6 *(Continued)*

cyst

A *cyst* is a fluid or semisolid filled sac found in the bone or in tissue beneath the oral mucosa surface. Often the epithelial cells become trapped and form a cavity that fills with fluid. Most dental cysts occur as a result of the blockage of a duct leading to a gland.

There are also cysts found around the crown of an unerupted tooth prior to eruption. This is called a dentigerous cyst, and it ruptures when the tooth erupts. A dentigerous cyst is often found around third molars and can stay around the impacted tooth if the tooth is unable to erupt due to lack of space in the maxilla or the mandible. Many times, the cyst is the reason that a dentist would recommend extraction of a third molar.

An eruption cyst can be found right under the gingival surface of a tooth that is getting ready to erupt.

A nasopalatine duct cyst is found along the canal at the nasopalatine foramen between teeth #8 and #9 and can often be misdiagnosed as the foramen.

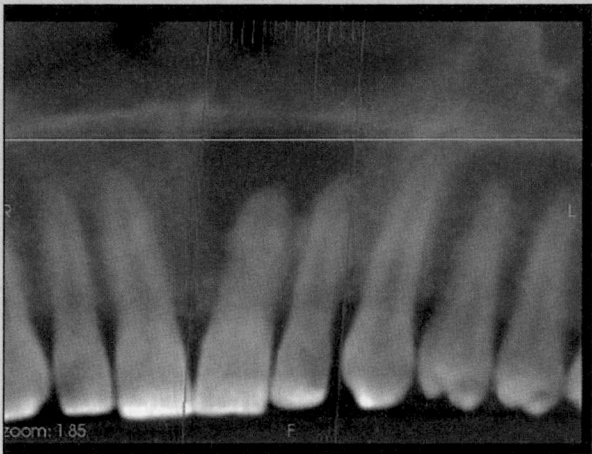

Courtesy of Dr. Ashish Kakar

ulcer

An *ulcer* is an open sore on tissue that extends below the basal layer of epithelium into the dermis. An ulcer is often red, inflamed, and painful and may cause a scar when it heals. It can be caused by destruction of the mucous membrane by trauma (Figure 9-9). The most common traumatic ulcer is self-induced when the patient bites the lip, mucosa, tongue, or repeatedly rubs the tissue with an object such as a pencil.

erosion

Erosion is a soft tissue lesion in which the epithelium above the basal layer is denuded or raw. It can be caused by a defect left from trauma or an injury and can be red, raw, and painful. Unlike an ulcer, it heals without scarring.

TABLE 9-7 Lesions Flat or Even with the Surface of the Skin Oral Mucosa

purpura, petechiae, ecchymosis

Purpura are red or purple spots that occur on the skin or mucosa and are caused by localized hemorrhage. They range in size from pinpoints, which are called petechiae, to larger ones called purpura, to the largest size named ecchymosis. The smallest petechiae can often be seen on the soft palate or any area of the skin. The middle-sized purpura can be seen on skin or mucosa, and the ecchymosis is often seen on the skin at the site of a large bruise. All of these lesions may appear as brown, purple, or pink spots, and all of them are caused by bleeding under the skin or tissue layer. Petechiae may also be visible in the oral cavity in patients who have leukemia. Many times this is the first sign of leukemia.

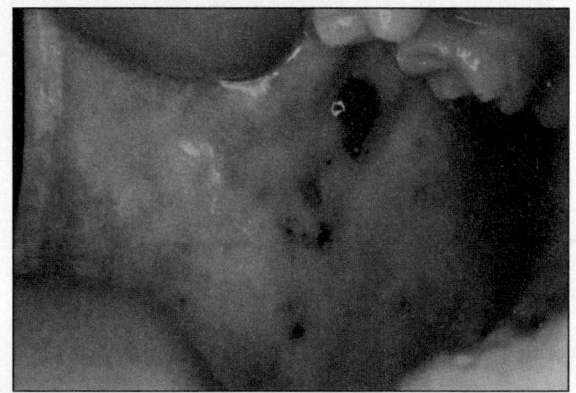

melanotic macule

A melanotic macule is a flat, pigmented, benign spot that can be found on the skin, lips, or inside mucosa and is commonly called a mole or a freckle. The color is usually brown, gray, or black. A common location on the lips is on the vermillion border. A mole or freckle is benign and is usually of no consequence, except that someone who has many moles needs to keep a check on them for any size, shape, or color changes. Some warning signs of skin cancer include moles that are irregular, vary in color, and change in texture. If this is the case, then the patient needs to have the lesion checked by a dermatologist.

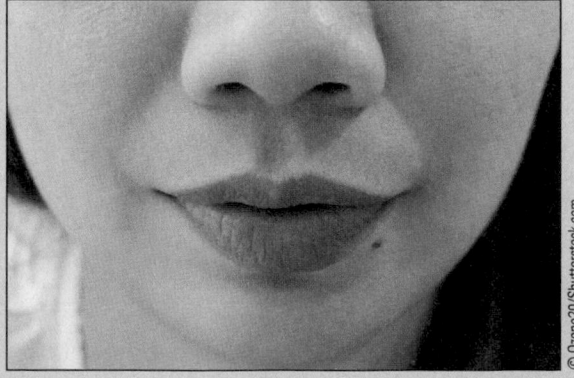

© Ozone20/Shutterstock.com

(Continues)

TABLE 9-7 *(Continued)*

ecchymosis Medical term for bruising of tissue.	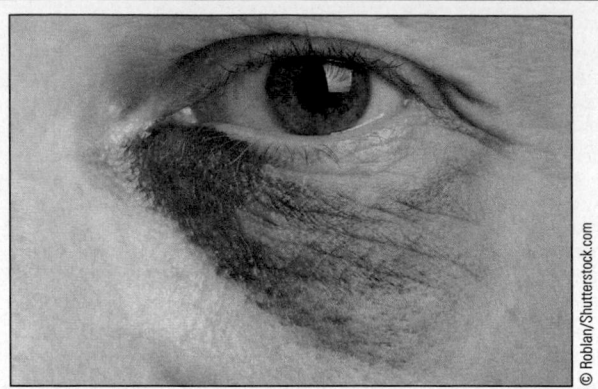
patch An area of skin that is a different color from the surrounding skin.	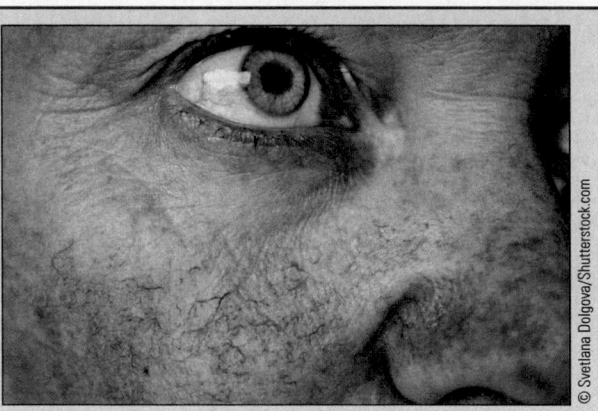

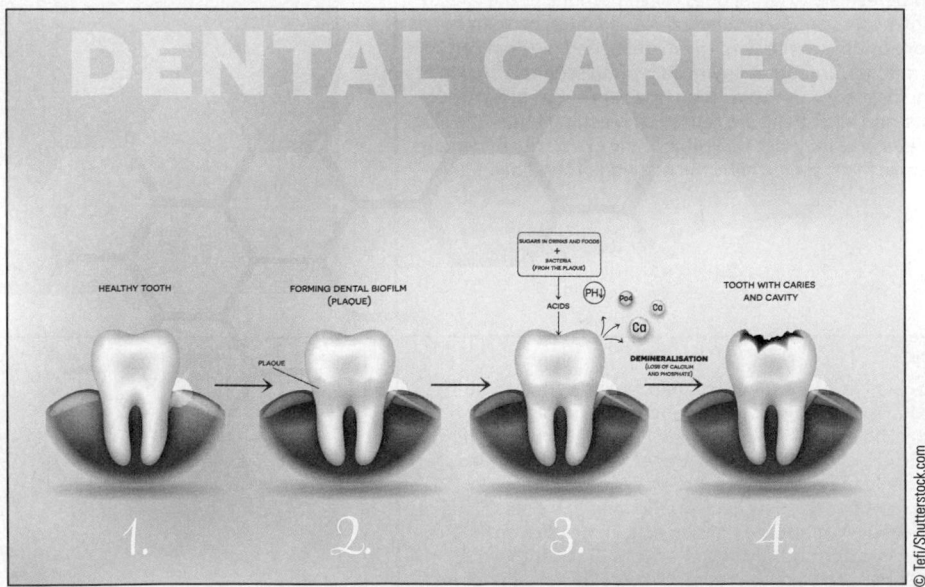

FIGURE 9-3
pH Levels and the process of demineralization and remineralization.

to produce acids. The acids demineralize the enamel or exposed cementum and dissolve the calcium and phosphorus. Thus, the alternating cycle of demineralization and remineralization begins.

The pH of the oral cavity becomes acidic after ingestion of sugary substances or carbohydrate rich substances (Figure 9-3). Because acid is produced every time fermentable carbohydrates are mixed with plaque, it is important to maintain a low sugar diet to decrease the risk of tooth decay. The dental assistant can help patients with a high decay rate to understand how their diet can cause a greater number of cavities in a short amount of time. Ingesting sugar of any type triggers acid production when plaque biofilm is present in the oral cavity. This acid remains on the tooth for 10 minutes or longer each time of the tooth is exposed to sugar before the pH returns to normal. This leaves the tooth vulnerable to decay. Making a few dietary changes can help the patient reduce acid production and decrease the decay rate significantly. Tooth decay is transmittable from a mother or caregiver to a young child by way of the specific bacteria that colonize on the teeth.

Stages of Decay There are several stages of dental decay that a tooth experiences as the decay progresses. Table 9-8 provides the stages of dental decay.

Rampant Caries

Rampant caries is a type of caries that appear suddenly and rapidly and results in early pulp involvement. There are several types of rampant caries.

Early childhood caries (ECC) is an infectious disease that can happen to any child. Older terms for ECC are nursing bottle caries and baby bottle caries. If a baby sleeps with a bottle, the chances

TABLE 9-8 Stages of Dental Decay

stage I, enamel decalcification

In stage I enamel decalcification, the enamel has a chalky white appearance. This takes place because *biofilm* or plaque increases and calcium in those areas decreases. These areas can be reversed with the use of fluoride and changes to low carbohydrate and low sugar diets.

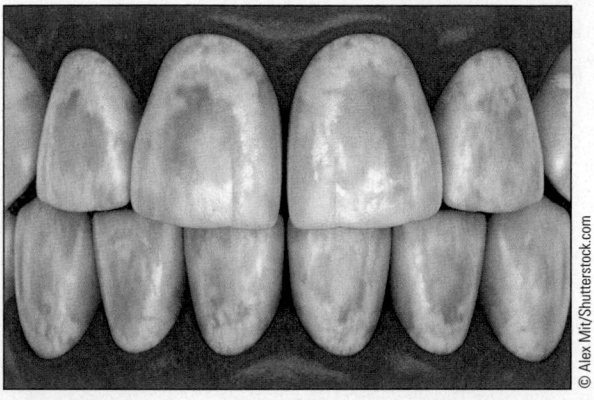

© Alex Mit/Shutterstock.com

stage II, enamel decay

In this stage, the decay breaks through the enamel. The remineralization process is not able to restore the mineral content. The area of the lesion becomes soft due to the decay process and may break.

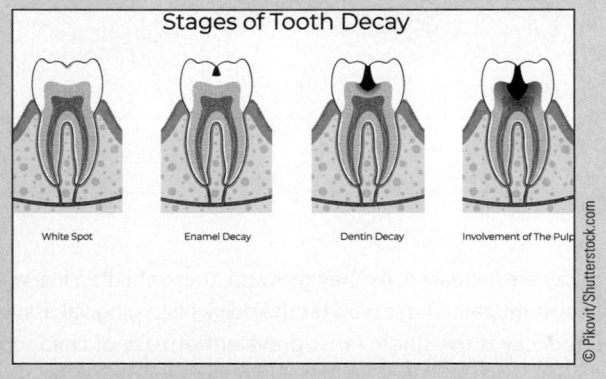

Stages of Tooth Decay

White Spot | Enamel Decay | Dentin Decay | Involvement of The Pulp

© Pikovit/Shutterstock.com

stage III, dentin decay

As the decay progresses, it enters the dentinal structure of the tooth. The patient may experience sensitivity or pain. Treatment includes removal of the decayed tooth structure and a restoration such as an amalgam or a composite. These materials will be discussed in detail in Chapters 31 and 32. Refer to figure shown under stage II enamel decay.

stage IV, pulpal invasion

The decay will proceed apically, destroying more tooth tissue until it enters and inflames the pulp of the tooth. This process is called *pulpitis*. There are two types of pulpitis. In reversible pulpitis, the pulp is irritated and pain is to thermal stimuli. The elimination of the irritant and placement of a sedative filling may save the pulp. In irreversible pulpitis, there are symptoms of lingering pain. Clinical diagnostic findings will show that the pulp is now infected and cannot heal. The only way to save a tooth with irreversible pulpitis is to remove the pulp from the tooth with root canal therapy. Root canal therapy will be discussed further in Chapter 37. The pulp's response to infection is to retreat and build reparative or tertiary dentin (refer to Chapter 7), which is denser than dentin, to protect itself. If the tooth is not treated, this pulp chamber may become sclerotic or pulp stones may develop. If this occurs, root canal treatment may be very difficult and the tooth may have to be extracted Refer to figure shown under stage II enamel decay.

stage V, tooth loss

If the patient does not seek treatment, eventually the tooth will become nonrestorable. This occurs because the decay is so extensive that a significant amount of natural tooth structure has been lost or the decay has affected the root of the tooth. The tooth must then be extracted.

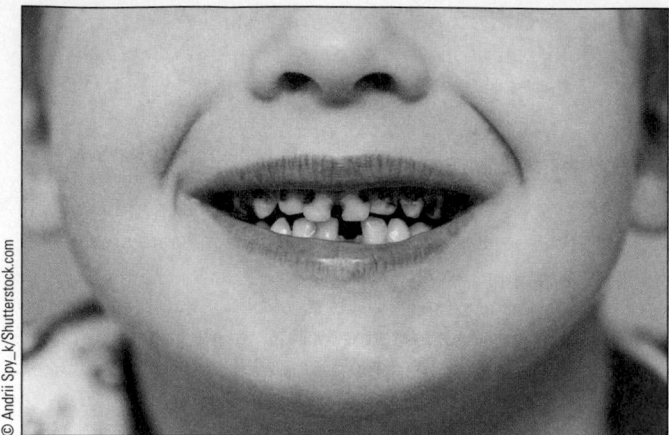

FIGURE 9-4
Early childhood caries.

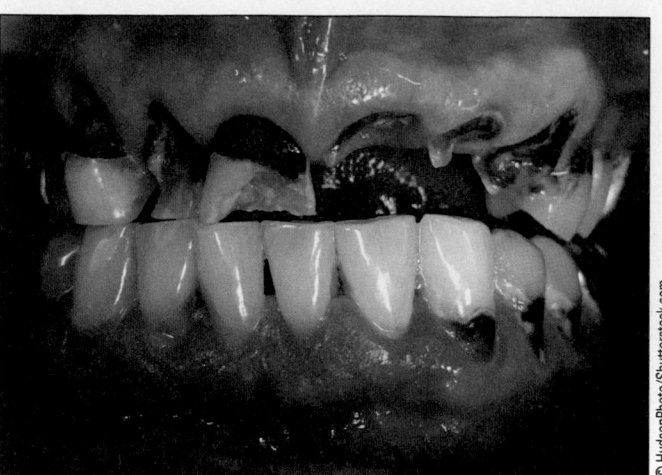

FIGURE 9-6
Destruction of teeth due to methamphetamine use.

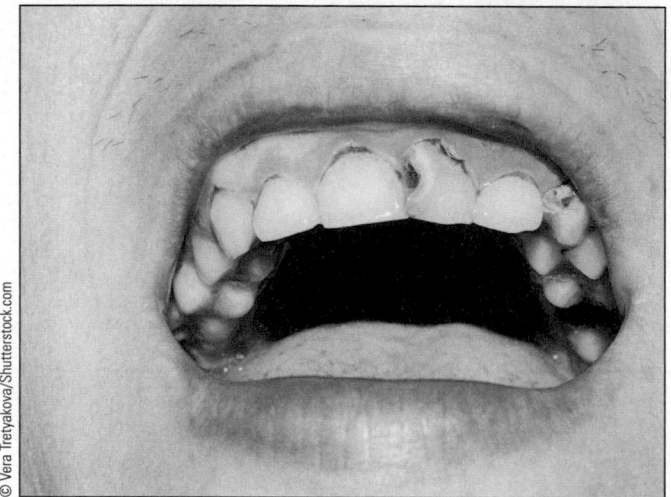

FIGURE 9-5
Rampant adult caries.

from the dental plaque. If salivary function is reduced for any reason, teeth are at increased risk for decay. Many medications can cause xerostomia. The effects of medications will be discussed in Chapter 14. Treatment of head and neck cancer with radiation therapy can lead to reduced function of the salivary glands and a reduction in salivary flow.

The condition known as "meth mouth" is caused by the illegal recreational use of methamphetamine. It is a potent central nervous system stimulant that can cause brain damage and severe oral health effects. The drug is cheap and easy to make, and the high lasts up to 12 hours—much longer than crack cocaine. Methamphetamines cause xerostomia, leading to caries and cracking of teeth (Figure 9-6). The pattern of rampant caries is most often seen on the buccal smooth surface of the teeth and the interproximal surfaces of the anterior teeth. Drug-related xerostomia (dry mouth), poor oral hygiene, frequent consumption of sugary soft drinks, and clenching and grinding of the teeth all contribute to rampant caries. Dental professionals must be aware of the signs and symptoms of methamphetamine use.

of decay are increased. As they grow up, these children live with the constant pain of decayed teeth and swollen gingival tissues. Tooth decay is the single most prevalent disease of childhood and if left untreated results in pain and infection. Contributing factors to ECC include lack of fluoride in the water supply, lack of appropriate education for parents and caregivers, and lack of oral health care for the child (Figure 9-4).

Another type of rampant caries is adolescent rampant caries. It has the same etiology and pattern as that of nursing bottle syndrome. During adolescence, some children habitually put chocolates, cookies, and other sweets in their mouth and go to sleep resulting in this type of caries.

The third type of rampant caries is **xerostomia**-induced rampant caries, which is often associated with illness, medication, or radiation therapy (Figure 9-5). A good flow of saliva is necessary to wash away food and debris from the teeth and to control caries. If a sufficient amount of saliva is present, it provides a cleansing effect, and the fluid dilutes and removes acid components

Prevention and Treatment of Dental Caries

Treatment of dental caries involves removing the infected tooth tissue and replacing it with a restoration (a filling) while the tooth can still be saved. Preventing decay is the most important factor in maintaining a decay free dentition. Using fluoridated water or fluoride treatments in the office are effective ways to harden the enamel and make the acid assault less effective. Excellent oral home care reduces the amount of plaque biofilm on the teeth so that fewer bacteria are present. A diet low in sugars helps to prevent the creation of an acidic environment in the oral cavity which leads to demineralization of the enamel. Chapter 16 will discuss fluoride and other oral preventive methods.

Lesions of the Oral Cavity Caused by Biological Agents

There are a number of lesions that are caused by biological agents such as bacteria and viruses. They are considered infectious because they are acquired by being exposed to a biological agent in some way. The term does not necessarily mean that all the lesions are infectious from person to person, although some of them are.

Actinomycosis

Actinomycosis is a rare bacterial disease that is caused by the *Actinomyces israelii*, a Gram positive anaerobic bacteria that normally is found in the GI tract and oral cavity. It can occur in any age group, but mostly is seen in adults. The disease usually starts with a tissue irritation that becomes a chronic infection and eventually forms an abscess that often drains outside of the oral cavity. Since actinomycosis is part of the normal oral flora, it can be transmitted from person to person. It often develops after a type of trauma, such as a tooth extraction, root canal, or deep caries. The mucosa in the mouth can be torn or irritated and infected with the bacteria.

The main lesion can be ulcerated and **indurated**. The most common characteristic of the infection is that it will have an abscess that forms a *fistula* or drain. Many times this fistula drains out through the skin and empties onto the face or neck. There is a great deal of exudate associated with the infection. While exudate is normally called pus, this exudate consists of a yellow pus-like fluid containing sulfur granules that can be identified under the microscope and diagnosed with cultures. The infection is treated with extended periods of penicillin in high doses. The prognosis is usually very good once the infection is taken care of.

Herpes Simplex Virus

Herpes simplex is caused by a strain of virus in the herpes family known as *Herpes viridae*. There are several strains of the virus, but the two main categories are HSV-1 (herpes simplex virus 1) and HSV-2 (herpes simplex virus 2). HSV-1 is associated with the herpetic **gingivostomatitis**, recurrent oral herpes, and herpes labialis. Herpes labialis is also known as the common cold sore (Figure 9-7) Lesions normally appears around the mouth and are found on the lips, tongue, or buccal mucosa. HSV-2 is associated with genital herpes lesions. The two are similar in structure and appearance, but they are from different versions of the virus. Each of the types can also be found in a small percentage in the opposite area, which means that HSV-1 can be found in the genital area and HSV-2 can be found orally as a result of oral–genital contact.

Approximately two-thirds of those under the age of 50 years carry the HSV-1 virus. Kissing, sharing beverages, or sharing utensils can cause this virus to be transferred to others through the saliva. It is important to diagnose the lesion, if present, before performing any dental treatment, which can cause the virus to spread further in the mouth, face, eyes, and other mucosal areas of the body. Because the virus is contagious, and because it can survive on a countertop for a few minutes to several hours, it is

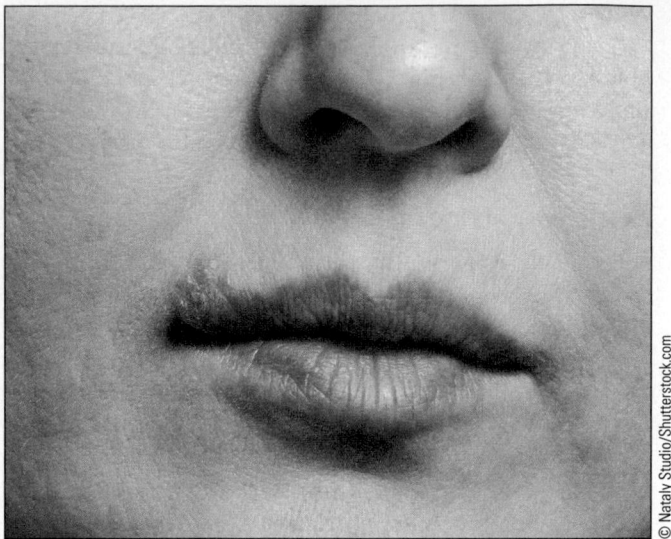

FIGURE 9-7
Herpes labialis blisters.

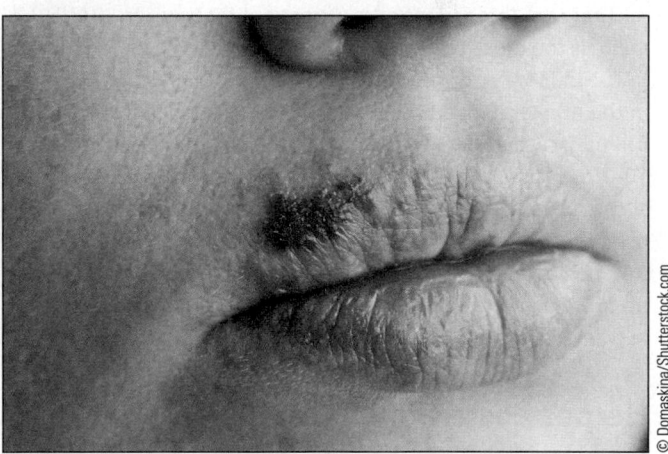

FIGURE 9-8
Herpes labialis in later stages of healing.

extremely important to maintain strict infection control practices in the operatory.

HSV-1 usually starts with a **prodromal** stage in which the patient experiences a burning or tingling sensation that is a precursor to the lesion breaking out. If antiviral medication is administered as soon as the tingling starts, often the severity and duration of the lesion's outbreak can be decreased. Early symptoms may include fever, swollen lymph nodes, and a feeling of being generally unwell. Once the lesion appears, it has the appearance of small *vesicles* or blisters that are clustered together (Figure 9-7). The lesion lasts about 7–10 days, and the blisters dry and form a scab as the skin heals underneath (Figure 9-8). The virus then enters a *latent phase* during which there are no symptoms but the virus can stay in the facial nerve tissues. When trauma, allergies, or an illness occurs, there may be a reoccurrence of the outbreak. Exposure to the sun can also result in an outbreak. Dental treatment should be postponed during the vesicular or blister stage of the lesion as it is highly contagious. For oral herpetic lesions, an over-the-counter antiviral such as Abreva® can shorten the duration of the lesions. Prescription antiviral medications such as acyclovir are also available. The dentist would determine which medication is best for the patient.

Aphthous Ulcers

Aphthous ulcers are circular, slightly cratered ulcers with yellowish centers and an **erythematous** halo or margins (Figure 9-9). They may be mistaken for herpetic lesions; the dental assistant should know the difference between the two. Unlike herpetic lesions, aphthous ulcers normally are found on nonkeratinized tissue in the oral cavity. They are seen more often in women and in younger people rather than in those over 40. Aphthous ulcers can be very painful and usually appear as a result of stress, hormonal changes, trauma, or vitamin deficiencies. Outbreaks last from 10 days to two weeks and can be treated by using over-the-counter topical anesthetics. Even though the aphthous ulcers are not contagious, dental treatment on a patient experiencing aphthous ulcers should be delayed as the ulcers are painful.

There are three types of recurrent aphthous ulcers (RAU): *RAU minor* is the most common of the three types, making up 80% of RAU. Ulcers vary from 8 to 10 mm in size. It is most commonly seen in the nonkeratinized mucosal surfaces like labial mucosa, buccal mucosa, and floor of the mouth. *RAU major* is found in about 10–15% of patients. Ulcers exceed 1 cm in diameter. Most common sites of involvement are the lips, soft palate, and throat. *RAU herpetiform* or herpetiform ulceration make up about 5–10% of RAU. RAU herpetiform is characterized by multiple ulcers that may add up to 100 in number. These are small in size and measure 2–3 mm in diameter. Lesions may combine to form large irregular ulcers.

Herpes Zoster (Shingles)

Herpes zoster is a recurrence of the virus that causes chicken pox (varicella) in children. The virus lays dormant in a nerve ganglion until the carrier is **immunocompromised**, at which time it may break out. The lesions appear as small, erupting pustules that break out along the nerve endings at the site of the dormant virus. Herpes zoster can last for up to 5 weeks and causes a painful, burning sensation where the lesions erupt. There is little in the way of treatment. A doctor may prescribe antiviral drugs for patients that are immunocompromised, and corticosteroids can be given to prevent some pain and numbness that may occur for weeks following an outbreak (Figure 9-10).

Syphilis

Syphilis is an infectious disease caused by the bacteria *Treponema pallidum*. It can be contracted through sexual contact or transferred from an infected mother to her fetus during birth. It progresses in three stages, each associated with the appearance of oral lesions.

Stages of Syphilis The first, or primary, stage begins when the bacterial spirochete enters the body. This is also where the first oral lesion, or **chancre**, may appear (Figure 9-11). The

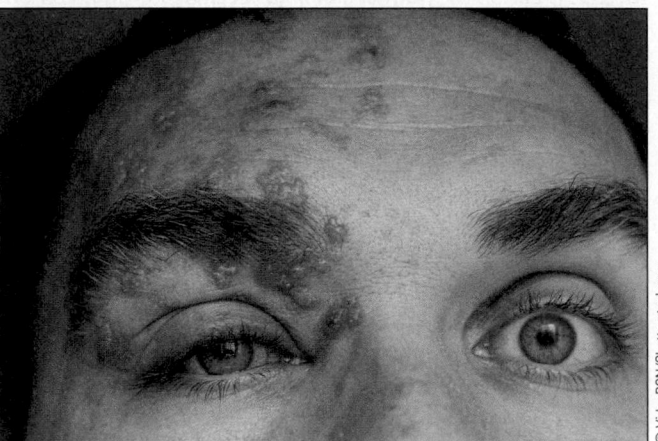

FIGURE 9-10
Patient with Herpes zoster.

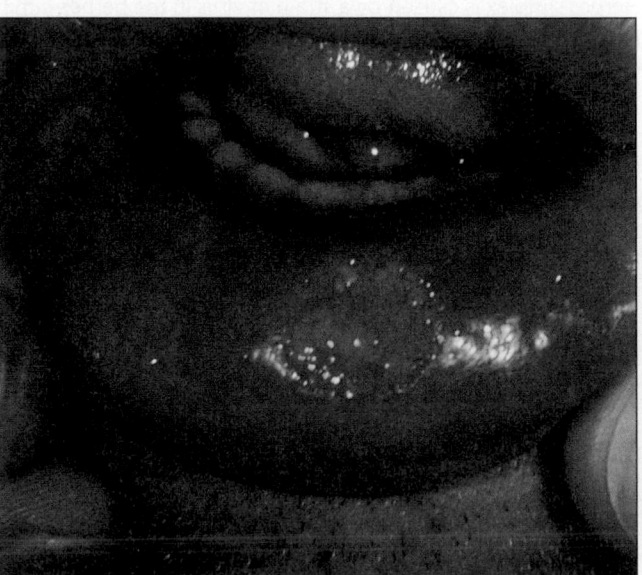

FIGURE 9-11
Lip chancre from primary syphilis.

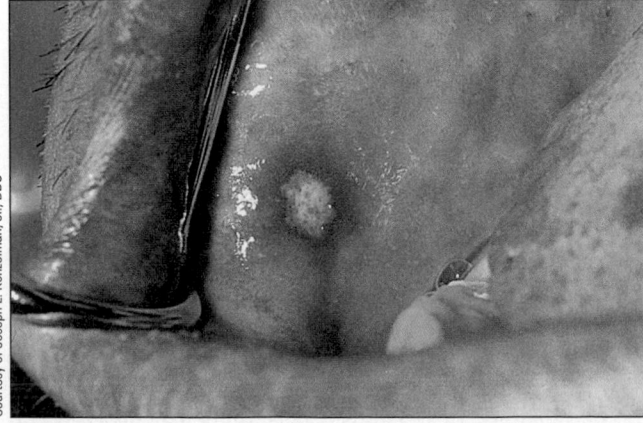

FIGURE 9-9
Recurrent aphthous ulcer on buccal mucosa.

primary stage of syphilis is highly contagious. Many times the lymph nodes in the area are swollen while this lesion appears. The chancre appears from 10–90 days after the spirochete infects the body. The lesion is a nonpurulent ulcer that is marginated and is painless and indurated. It ranges in size from 0.3 to 3 cm. It can be found on the genitals or on the lips, tongue, gingiva, or palate. Lesions will heal in 3–12 weeks with or without treatment. If there is no treatment at all, the disease will enter a latent period.

The secondary stage begins with flu-like symptoms. This stage begins about 2 to 8 weeks after the primary stage lesions appear. This stage is also highly contagious. During this stage other oral lesions manifest themselves. Covering ulcerated mucosa, mucous patches appear as moist, painless, grayish-white plaques. They can spontaneously resolve in 4–12 weeks, and the virus enters the latent phase. A second type of oral lesion found in the secondary stage is split papules, which are found at the lip commissures. The patient also may have skin eruptions of various types like rashes similar to measles and oozing sores (Figure 9-12). The lesions of this stage are the most infectious. Following this stage, the disease enters a period of latency that may last years and even decades. A blood test can be conducted to confirm a diagnosis of syphilis. Even though the rash has healed and the virus is latent, the patient can still be infectious. A female in the latent stage can pass the virus to her fetus during delivery. The child would then be born with congenital syphilis. Congenital syphilis is discussed later in this section.

The tertiary stage can occur years after the initial lesion and is much more likely to occur if the patient did not receive treatment earlier in the disease process. Not all people infected with syphilis will experience a tertiary phase. During this stage there can also be significant, irreversible cardiovascular and central nervous system damage. The oral lesion involved with this stage is a localized lesion called *gumma*, found most commonly on the tongue and palate. It presents as a firm, ulcerated mass that can be very destructive and large. If it is on the palate, it can destroy the bone of the maxilla.

Congenital Syphilis A woman can transmit syphilis to a developing fetus up to five years after initially contracting the disease, which is known as congenital syphilis. This condition can result in abortion, stillbirth, death soon after delivery, or numerous developmental disabilities. Children born with congenital syphilis also experience tooth development anomalies known as mulberry molars (Figure 9-13) and Hutchinson's incisors (Figure 9-14). In mulberry molars the first permanent molars' occlusal surface is composed of an aggregate of enamel nodules. In Hutchinson's incisors, the secondary lateral incisors are peg-shaped or screwdriver-shaped, widely spaced, and notched at the end, with a central crescent-shaped deformity.

Candida Albicans

Candida albicans is a fungal infection of the mouth and is often seen in children (where it is also known as thrush), patients who have the *human immunodeficiency virus (HIV)* or have AIDS, and

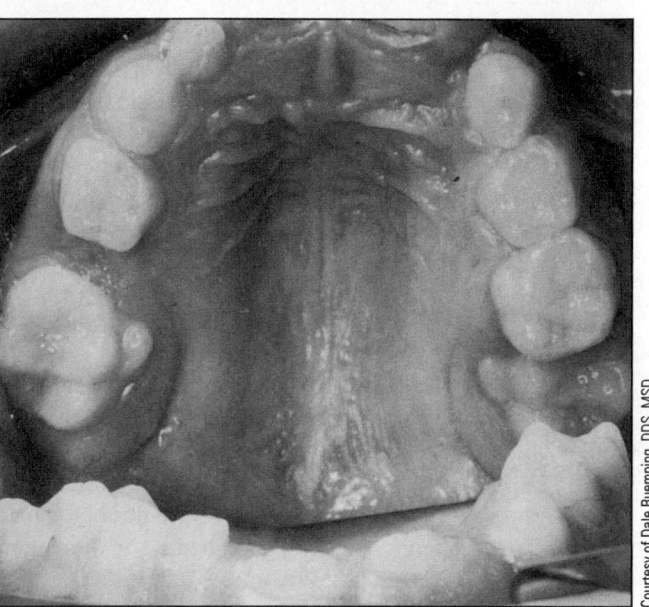

FIGURE 9-13
Mulberry molars from prenatal syphilis.

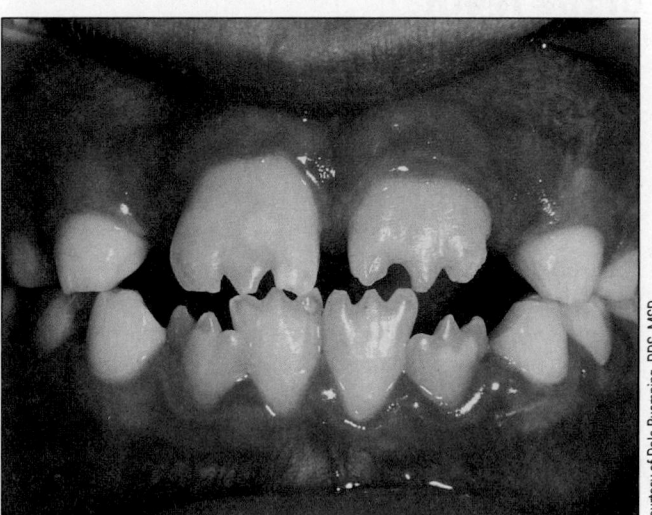

FIGURE 9-14
Hutchinson's incisors from prenatal syphilis.

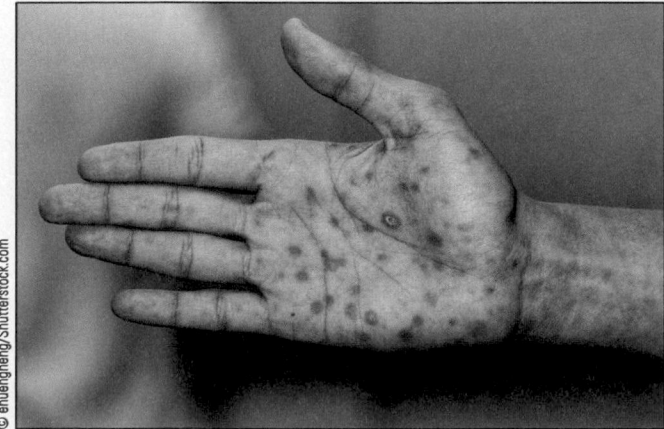

FIGURE 9-12
Skin rash on palm due to secondary stage of syphilis.

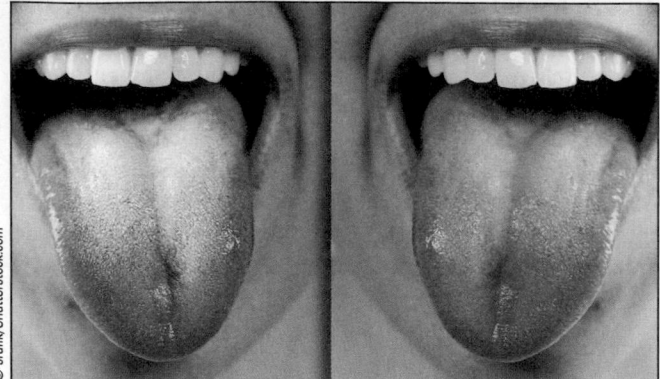

FIGURE 9-15
Oral candida before treatment and after treatment with antifungal agents.

in patients who are immunocompromised. HIV will be discussed later in this chapter. Candida albicans consists of a white, thick covering over the oral mucous membranes that can be removed by wiping with a 2×2 gauze (Figure 9-15). It is not painful and is treated with antifungal agents such as Nystatin or Ketoconazole (Figure 9-15). Antifungal agents are discussed in detail in Chapter 14. Newborns can acquire the fungus as they travel through the birth canal.

Cellulitis

Cellulitis is a bacterial skin infection in which there is uncontrolled inflammation in an area that is localized. It can occur anywhere on the body and can be caused by an abscessed tooth, resulting in cellulitis of the face (Figure 9-16). Among the symptoms are rapid swelling, high fever, red skin, and severe throbbing pain. Cellulitis can spread quickly to the lymph nodes and throughout the body, becoming life threatening.

Developmental Disturbances of the Teeth

Inherited and congenital disturbances of the tooth cause a variety of poor tooth development. They may result in discoloration, weakening of tooth structure, increased susceptibility to caries, and change in tooth shape and size.

Amelogenesis Imperfecta

Amelogenesis imperfecta is an inherited condition of the teeth in which the enamel is discolored, partially missing, or very thin (Figure 9-17). This condition usually affects both the primary and the permanent teeth. Enamel in this condition makes the teeth susceptible to dental caries. It is important that the dental assistant ensure that the patient with amelogenesis imperfecta has good oral hygiene to decrease the risk of decay.

There are a variety of levels of developmental issues, from the mildest form showing teeth with white snowcaps on the cusp ridges, to more severe levels with pitted surfaces or orange colored, chipped enamel. The most severe form shows brown to

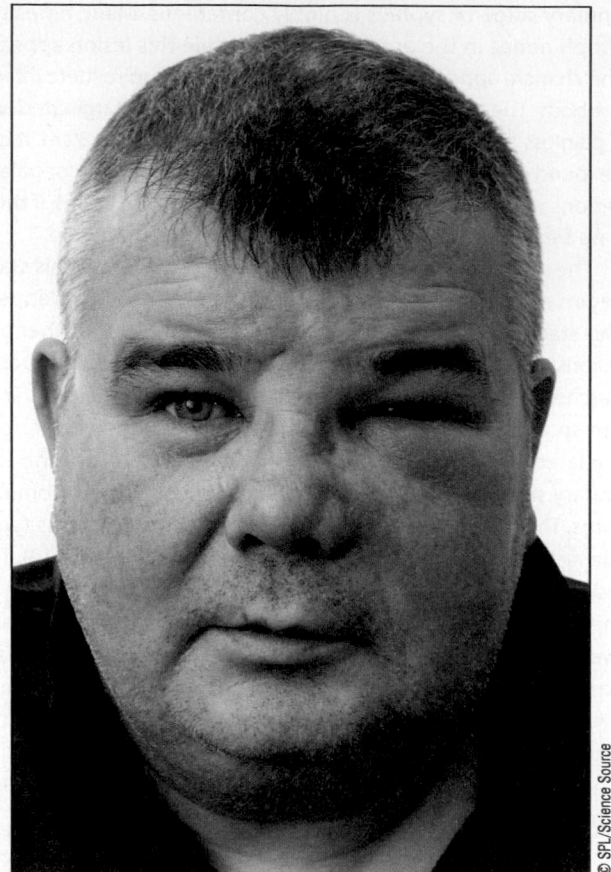

FIGURE 9-16
Patient with cellulitis from third molar infection.

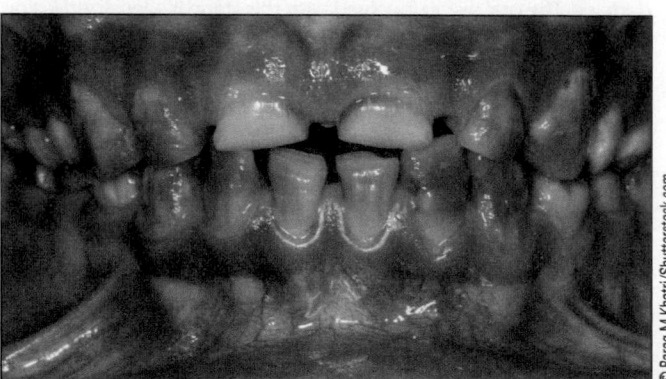

FIGURE 9-17
Amelogenesis imperfecta.

orange enamel, which can be chipped away with hand instruments, leaving sensitive dentin underneath. Treatment is usually with composite restorations or veneers or crowns that cover the entire tooth.

The enamel that does develop is thinner and can be hypocalcified, hypoplastic, or hypomatured. Radiographs show a similar radiopacity to dentin and a larger pulp chamber. Since there are several varieties of amelogenesis imperfecta and it is inherited, a thorough family medical history should be taken.

Dentinogenesis Imperfecta

Dentinogenesis imperfecta is another hereditary disease of tooth development. It is characterized by opalescent to brownish-blue tinted enamel that usually affects the primary teeth more than the permanent teeth. The dentin is not as calcified, and the pulp chambers are almost nonexistent. Since the dentin is so soft, the enamel chips off and leaves the softer dentin exposed. *Attrition* of the dentin is common, and sometimes the teeth are worn down all the way to the alveolar ridge. Radiographs demonstrate anterior teeth with premature closure of the pulp chambers and canals.

Ankylosis

Ankylosis is a term that is defined as a tooth where the root is fused to the alveolus or tooth socket. Ankylosis is rare but does have a genetic predisposition. The cementum or dentin of the deciduous or primary tooth is in contact with the bone in several places, and the periodontal ligament (PDL) is nonexistent in those areas. This restricts movement of the tooth as well as eruption. The tooth will not be exfoliated or lost as usual, because the erupting perma-nent tooth under it cannot push it out, but its pressure may cause some of the primary tooth root to resorb. The primary molars are the most common teeth to be ankylosed.

If the primary ankylosed tooth has a permanent tooth trying to erupt under it, the dentist may want to extract the ankylosed tooth to allow the permanent tooth to erupt. The primary anky-losed tooth can be very difficult to extract because of the tooth being fused to the socket (Figure 9-18).

Anodontia and Hypodontia

Anodontia means that all teeth are congenitally missing. It affects primary or permanent teeth or both. Total anodontia, where all the teeth do not develop, is very rare but possible and is usually caused by *ectodermal dysplasia*, a rare group of genetic disorders in which the ectoderm is affected.

Hypodontia is a condition in which one or two teeth (other than third molars) are congenitally missing. Hypodontia most commonly occurs with the maxillary laterals and second premolars.

Fusion

Tooth *fusion* takes place when two separate tooth germs join together. The fusion may be a complete fusion or incomplete fusion depending on the stage at which the fusion occurs. If it is a complete fusion earlier in tooth development, then the tooth will look like one giant tooth (Figure 9-19). The tooth is broader in appearance and often shows an indentation between the two crowns. This condition will cause a reduced number of teeth in the dental arch. For example, if a lower anterior tooth is fused, then instead of counting six teeth from canine to canine, there will only be five teeth present, and one of them would be larger than normal. Later fusion will result in only the root portions of both teeth being attached to each other. It is most often seen in the mandibular anterior primary teeth or permanent incisors.

Gemination

Gemination or twinning is when a single tooth bud attempts to divide but fails to do so. There is an indentation where the crown tried to divide. With fusion, a tooth is missing. With gemination, there is a full complement of teeth, but one of them looks wider than normal. A radiograph would verify that only one root is pres-ent with a wider crown.

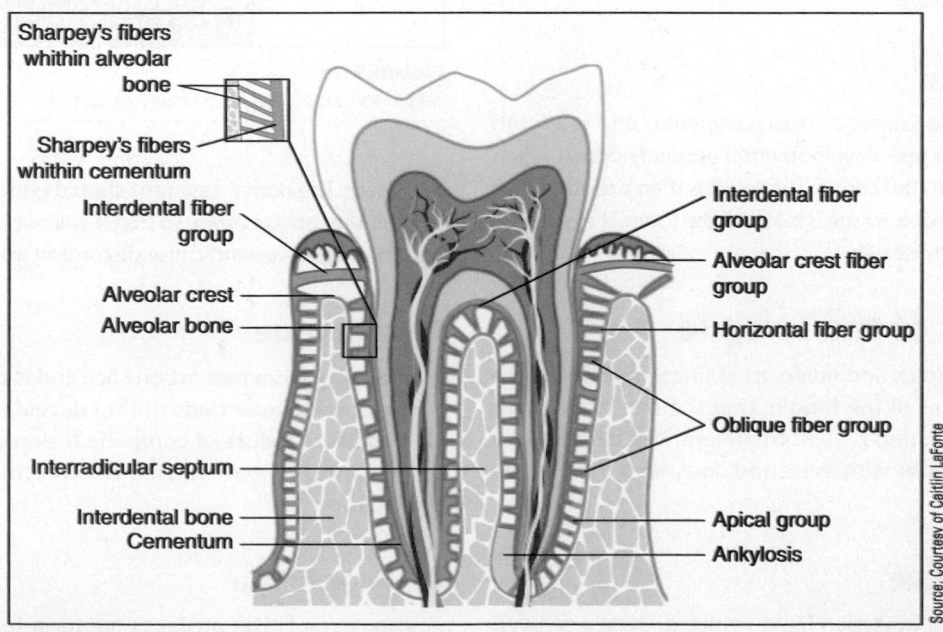

Sharpey's fibers whithin alveolar bone
Sharpey's fibers whithin cementum
Interdental fiber group
Alveolar crest
Alveolar bone
Interradicular septum
Interdental bone
Cementum

Interdental fiber group
Alveolar crest fiber group
Horizontal fiber group
Oblique fiber group
Apical group
Ankylosis

Source: Courtesy of Caitlin LaFonte

FIGURE 9-18
Ankylosis of a tooth.

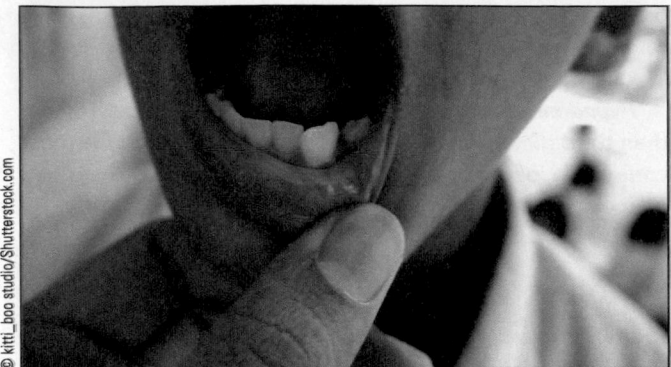

FIGURE 9-19
Tooth fusion.

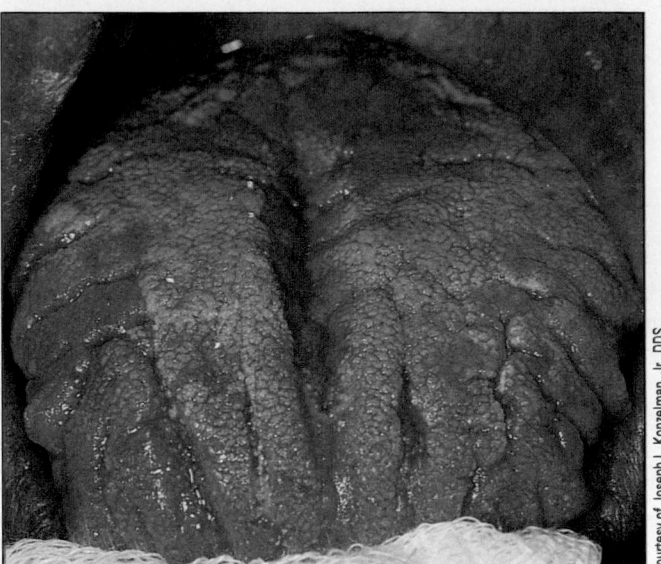

FIGURE 9-20
Fissured tongue.

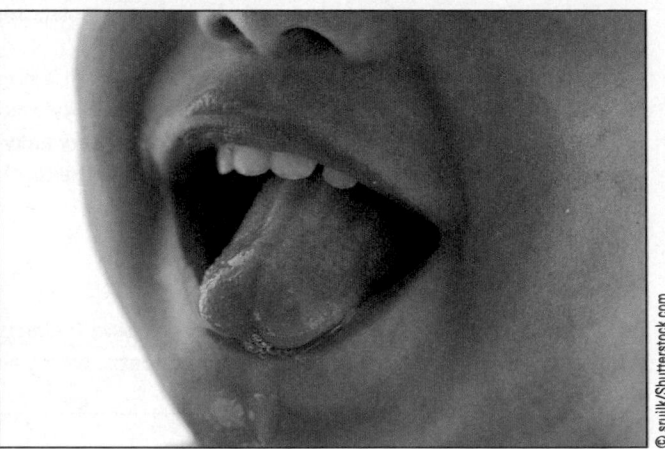

FIGURE 9-21
Bifid tongue due to failure of distal tongue buds.

Macrodontia/Microdontia

Macrodontia is defined as abnormally large teeth and can occur with one or two teeth, such as the maxillary incisors, or the entire dentition. The opposite can also occur and is called *microdontia*, which is abnormally small teeth. This is often seen in individuals with *Down's syndrome*, which is caused by an extra chromosome and impacts the entire dentition. It can also occur with one or two teeth. The most commonly affected tooth is the maxillary lateral incisors, which are often called peg laterals.

Supernumerary Teeth

Extra teeth, or supernumerary teeth, are usually dwarfed in size and shape but normal otherwise. The most common is a *mesiodens* and is seen in the maxillary anterior area between the two maxillary central incisors. The second most common supernumerary teeth are fourth and fifth molars, which are seen behind the third molars.

Dens in Dente

Dens in dente is also known as *dens invaginatus* and is a tooth within a tooth. This rare developmental anomaly occurs when the enamel folds into the dentin. The result is then a tooth within a tooth. If a radiographic image is taken of the tooth, it appears as if another tooth is inside of it.

Anomalies of the Tongue

The tongue is complex and made up of many muscles. There are some anomalies of the tongue that the dental assistant may come across during patient treatment. The dental assistant should be familiar with these and document them in the patient record.

Fissured Tongue

Five percent of the population has a wrinkled, deeply grooved surface of the dorsum of the tongue that is called fissured (Figure 9-20). It is a variant of normal, and no treatment is

necessary. The dental assistant should educate the patient how to keep the tongue clean, so that it will not harbor food and bacteria in the grooves and cause discomfort and odor.

Bifid Tongue

A bifid tongue is a rare occurrence and is due to partial fusion of the distal tongue buds during development (Figure 9-21). The result is a failure of complete fusion of the lateral halves of the anterior two thirds. No treatment is needed for bifid tongue.

Ankyloglossia

Ankyloglossia is the professional term for a tongue tie. It is when the lingual frenum is attached near the tip of the tongue (Figure 9-22). The short lingual frenum can also attach the tip

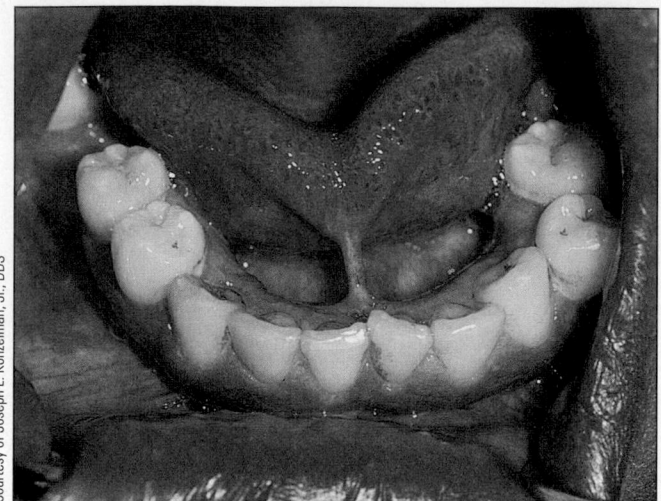

Courtesy of Joseph L. Konzelman, Jr., DDS

FIGURE 9-22
Ankyloglossia.

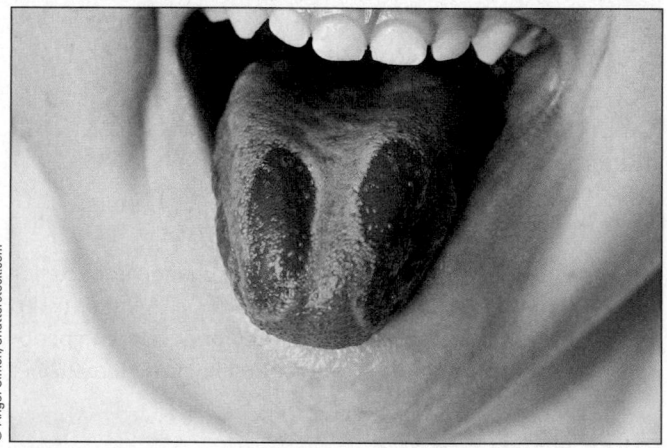

© Angel Simon/Shutterstock.com

FIGURE 9-23
Geographic tongue.

of tongue to floor of the mouth. This limits movements of the tongue and can on occasion result in speech disturbances. It is treated by a *frenectomy*, which is the surgical removal of a portion of the lingual frenum.

Geographic Tongue

Genetic factors may play a role in the development of a geographic tongue that affects about 3% of the population. The dorsal and lateral surfaces of the tongue have red, smooth patches where the filiform papillae are not present (Figure 9-23). It can resemble a map, and this is how the anomaly receives its name. It is also called benign migratory glossitis because it can change looks and other areas can become smooth as others are not. It is like a migrating map. Some think that it can flare up when one is under emotional stress. Spicy foods can cause the tongue to be irritated in some patients. Most of the time it is not painful, and no treatment is necessary.

Lesions Produced by Chemical Agents

Some materials used in dentistry are caustic and can cause chemical burns. The chemicals in tobacco also cause oral lesions. The most common chemical agents seen in patients' oral cavities are aspirin burns, nicotine stomatitis, and chewing tobacco lesions.

Aspirin Burns

Sometimes, when someone is experiencing a toothache, they may place aspirin over the area of the painful tooth. Since aspirin is an acid, it causes a tissue burn (Figure 9-24). This burn is characterized by a **necrotic**, white tissue that may slough off and result in a large, painful ulcer. Normally the area will heal in 7–14 days once aspirin use is discontinued.

The patient should always be told that aspirin should not be used this way again. They think that the aspirin took care of the pain locally, but it is because the aspirin slowly dissolved and was swallowed. It eventually works systemically to take care of the pain.

Nicotine Stomatitis

Another chemical induced lesion is caused by the heat and irritating effect of the chemicals in tobacco when it is smoked. Nicotine stomatitis is most often seen in pipe smokers or in those who practice reverse cigarette smoking. It is not seen as commonly in those who some cigars or cigarettes. The area first turns red, then white and red, or erythematous hyperkeratinized nodules form on the palate (Figure 9-25). The red spots form at the openings of the minor salivary glands on the palate and appear inflamed. These are not thought to be precancerous, but with increased use of tobacco there can be an increase in the risk of developing oral cancers.

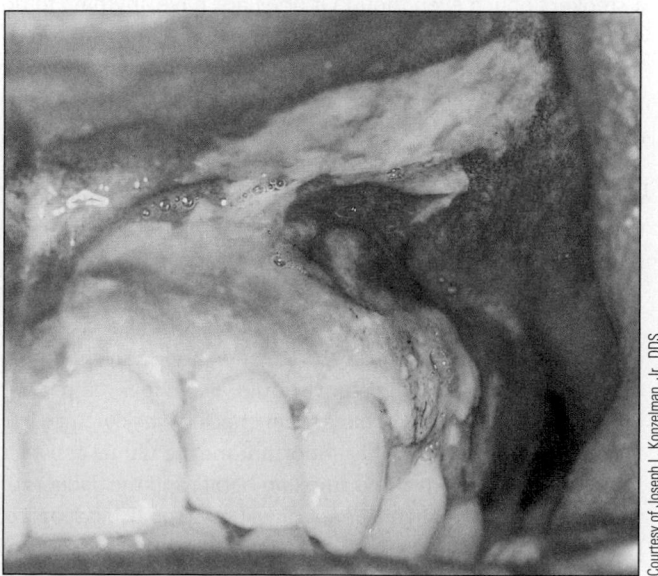

Courtesy of Joseph L. Konzelman, Jr., DDS

FIGURE 9-24
Aspirin burn.

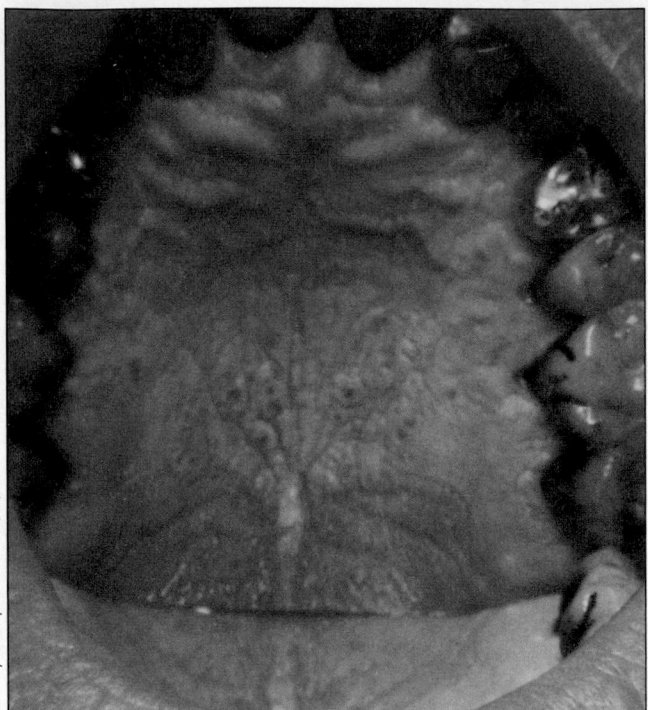

Courtesy of Joseph L. Konzelman, Jr., DDS

FIGURE 9-25
Nicotine stomatitis.

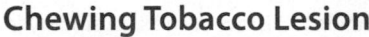

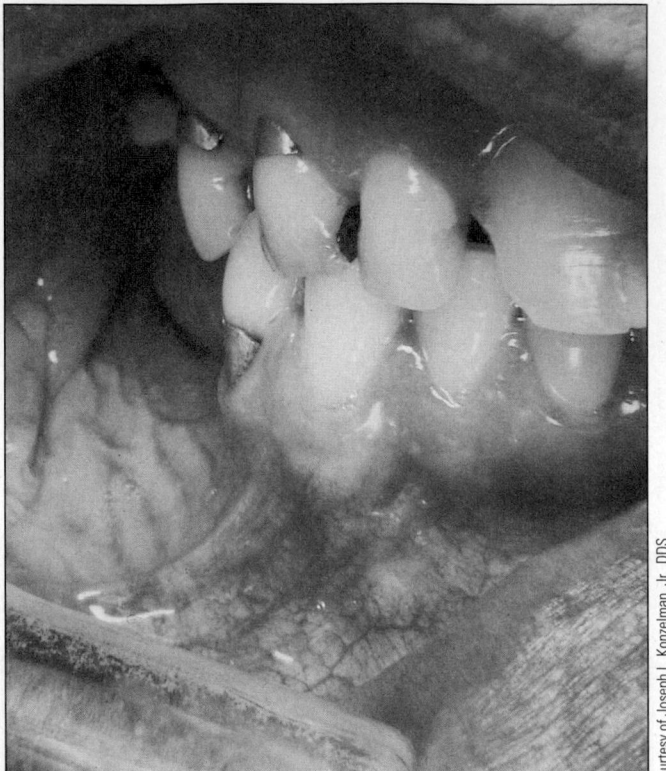

Courtesy of Joseph L. Konzelman, Jr., DDS

FIGURE 9-26
Chewing tobacco (snuff) lesion.

Chewing Tobacco Lesion

The use of all types of smokeless tobacco can cause a chemical induced lesion where the tobacco is held against the oral mucosa tissue. It appears in the oral vestibule, normally the lower anterior area between the lip and the teeth or in the mandibular vestibule in the premolar and molar region. The lesion appears as a *corrugated* or wrinkled, white, thickened, and hyperkeratinized area of tissue between the cheek and gingiva. It is often called a smokers pouch even though it does not have anything to do with actually smoking; it is called this because of the tobacco use. It stretches the tissue in the area where the tobacco is held; therefore the pouch appearance occurs. Due to the white color and texture change, this lesion can be considered premalignant. There are documented cases of squamous cell carcinoma developing from these tobacco pouches. A biopsy is recommended if the patient will not stop using the tobacco or if the area does not heal after usage has stopped.

If this kind of lesion is found on a patient, they should be shown the lesion. A picture of the lesion should be taken and maintained in the patient's records, and the lesion should be measured. The dental assistant should also show the patient how to find the lesion and have them check it weekly. Since this is a premalignant lesion, it is important for the dental assistant to educate the patient about smoking habits and the dangers of tobacco use. If the patient cannot or will not stop using tobacco, they should be asked to move the tobacco to a different area of the oral cavity and give the prior area time to heal. The amount and frequency of tobacco can be decreased over time. If the area starts returning to a pink color and the corrugation starts to go

away, then the area is healing. If it does not change or becomes worse or larger, then a biopsy should be done. A patient who uses smokeless tobacco has a greater risk for developing periodontal disease, decay, attrition, and tooth staining (Figure 9-26).

Black Hairy Tongue

Filiform papillae on the dorsum of the tongue can become elongated and appear like hairs because of a build-up of stain by food, tobacco, and **chromogenic** bacteria (Figure 9-27). These brown to black "hairs" can also be associated with mouth rinses and antibiotics. The best way to treat this is to stop using tobacco, use a tongue cleaner, and brush the tongue.

Gingival Hyperplasia

Gingival hyperplasia is a chemically induced condition that manifests as the connective fibrous gingival tissue overgrowing a normal size (Figure 9-28). It is not painful but can interfere with eating and alter the patient's appearance. Certain medications like Dilantin (phenytoin) and certain cardiovascular medications can cause the gingiva to overgrow. Dilantin is an anticonvulsant that is used to treat epilepsy, and it causes gingival enlargement in 50% of the patients. This is referred to as Dilantin hyperplasia, and there is excessive enlargement of the facial and lingual gingiva. Because the tissue is so large and bulbous, it can be very difficult to perform proper oral home care and remove plaque. If the patient has orthodontic braces, they can irritate the tissue

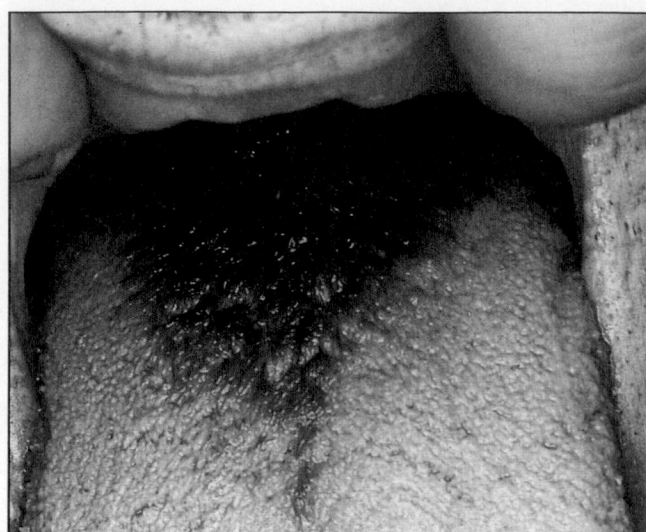

FIGURE 9-27
Hairy tongue.

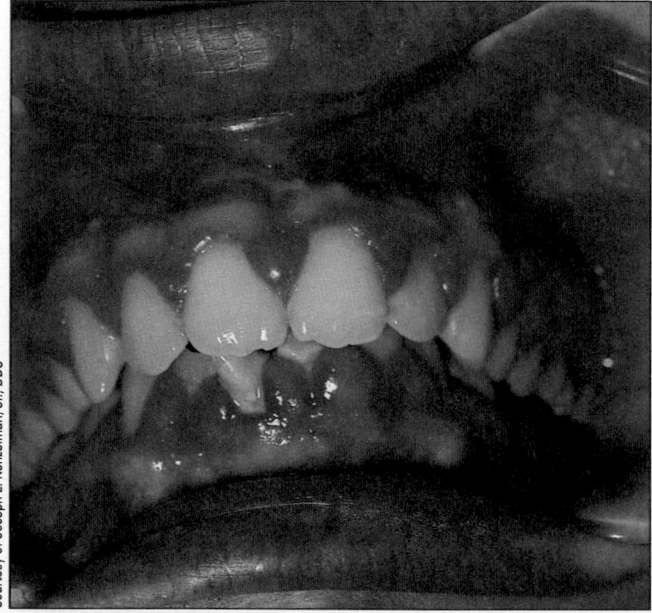

Courtesy of Joseph L. Konzelman, Jr., DDS

FIGURE 9-28
Gingival hyperplasia.

and make it more difficult to keep clean. In severe cases, surgical removal of the overgrown tissue can be completed, but the gingiva usually regrows due to the medication use. If possible, the treating physician may change medications to one that does not cause this side effect.

Lesions Produced by Physical Agents

Trauma induced ulcerations are most often self-induced like inadvertently biting the cheek or lips. Trauma-induced lesions can also result from dental instruments if not handled properly. These usually heal once the source of irritation is removed.

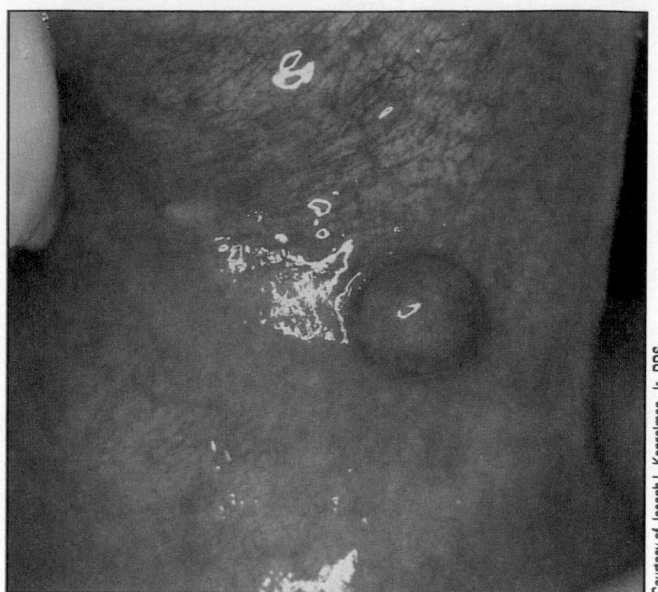

Courtesy of Joseph L. Konzelman, Jr., DDS

FIGURE 9-29
Mucocele.

Mucocele/Ranula

A *mucocele* or mucous cyst is a lesion caused by blockage of a salivary gland duct with mucous or a broken salivary gland duct that results in spillage of mucus into the soft tissue. As a result, a fluid filled lesion, related to minor salivary glands, appears (Figure 9-29). The most common site of occurrence is the lower labial mucosa. It usually resolves without any treatment within 3 to 6 weeks, but some may need surgical intervention. A similar lesion, a *ranula*, is caused by damage or disease of the sublingual salivary ducts. As a result, the saliva leaks out into the tissues surrounding the gland and forms a ranula. It forms unilaterally on the floor of the mouth. Surgery is usually needed to remove fluid from the tissues and to remove the damaged salivary gland.

Denture Induced Hyperplasia

An ill-fitting denture can cause the formation of small ulcers that after continued irritation become folds of excess connective tissue known as *denture hyperplasia* or *epulis fissuratum* (Figure 9-30). Denture hyperplasia is usually found in the maxilla and more commonly occurs in females. The lesion does not resolve even after prolonged removal of the denture. The folds of tissue must be removed surgically and then a soft tissue reline of the denture can be done. It may be necessary to remake the denture depending on the age of the denture and whether or not a reline will result in a better fit.

Amalgam Tattoo and Oral Piercings

When amalgam particles become trapped in the tissue during oral surgery or most often during an amalgam procedure, the gingival tissue in the immediate area appears blue-gray and looks like a tattoo (Figure 9-31A). There is no discomfort, and

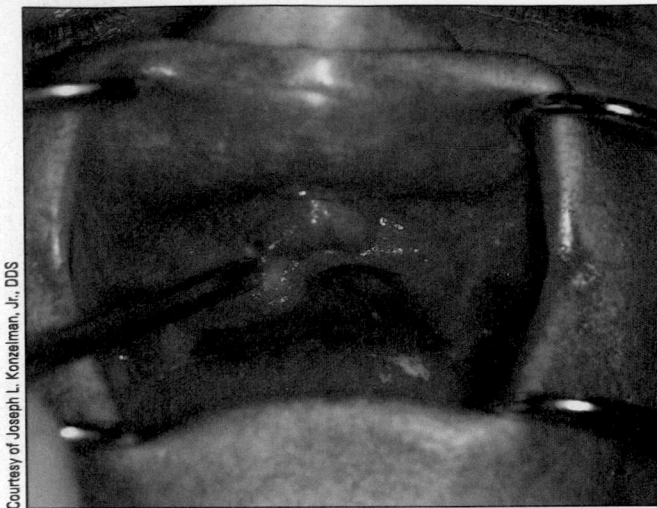

Courtesy of Joseph L. Konzelman, Jr., DDS

FIGURE 9-30
Hyperplasia from denture irritation.

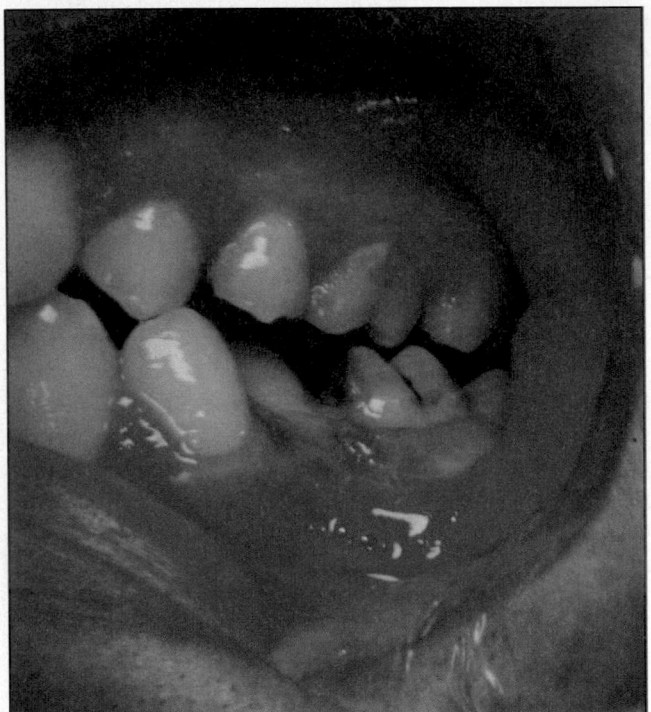

FIGURE 9-31A
An amalgam tattoo in the oral cavity.

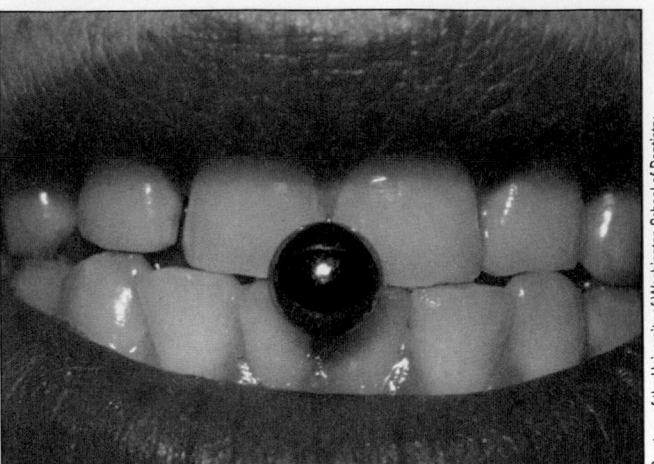

Courtesy of the University of Washington School of Dentistry

FIGURE 9-31B
Oral piercing.

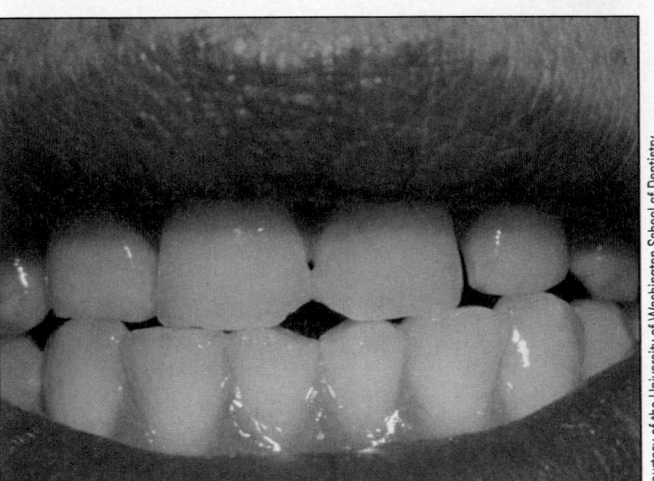

Courtesy of the University of Washington School of Dentistry

FIGURE 9-31C
Oral piercing with damage to the teeth and tissues.

no treatment is needed. To prevent these amalgam pieces from becoming imbedded in the tissue, a dental dam can be used during the procedure. The dental assistant should always be sure to suction out all the particles of amalgam after a procedure.

Oral piercings (Figure 9-31B) are a means of self-expression and body art, and the majority of them involve the tongue. A barbell-shaped piece of jewelry is placed in the midline of the tongue after a needle pierces the area. Often, a temporary device is placed so that it can be adjusted if swelling occurs. When the barbell is placed through the tongue a ball is screwed on the lower side of the tongue to secure it. If a blood vessel is punctured during the piercing, severe bleeding may occur. In some instances, blood poisoning or blood clots will develop. Other sites include cheeks, lips, uvula, and the side of the tongue; sometimes multiple sites are pierced. Healing in any of these areas takes a month or more.

Before a person chooses oral piercing, possible outcomes and related symptoms should be investigated. Tongue piercings are most commonly placed in the center of the tongue to minimize vesicle and neural damage. Keeping the site clean is essential. In dentistry this is another concern because, often, the piercing affects treatments such as radiographs. Side effects are common. The most serious side effect is tongue swelling, which can actually close off the airway and thus hamper breathing. Other symptoms include pain, infection, swelling, increased saliva flow, tooth and tissue damage (Figure 9-31C), metal hypersensitivity, scar tissue development, and problems with *mastication* (chewing). Speech is often affected as well. Piercing has been identified by the National Institutes of Health as a possible factor in transmission of hepatitis B, C, D, and G. (For more information see the American Dental Association's policies on oral piercing.)

Oral Conditions Related to Hormonal Imbalances

Oral conditions can be caused by a change in the individual's hormonal balance, especially during puberty or pregnancy. Whereas normally the patient may not be sensitive to the plaque that is present in their oral cavity, during pregnancy or puberty, the oral soft tissue may become inflamed. Pregnancy gingivitis may occur in some pregnant women. Due to the hormonal changes, the gingival tissues become red and inflamed and sometimes enlarged. There is redness and bleeding on brushing.

Patients with diabetes mellitus are also at a higher risk for developing periodontal disease, tooth mobility, and tooth loss. Because of the sensitivity to plaque for these patients, the dental assistant needs to explain how important good oral home care is to patients who have hormonal issues.

Lesions Caused by Nutritional Deficiencies

Some oral lesions may also be caused from a deficiency or malabsorption of vitamins and minerals.

Angular Cheilitis

Angular cheilitis in some cases may be caused by a deficiency of vitamin B. Angular cheilitis is characterized by ulcerations at the corners of the mouth (Figure 9-32). These are red and painful and may bleed. If it is found that there is a vitamin B deficiency, taking vitamin B supplements will help to correct the angular cheilitis. Because the cracking of the mucosa and skin at the corners is painful, the patient may lick their lips to provide moisture to that area. However, the warmth and moisture also can lead to candida albicans or a fungal growth. As a result, the patient may also need a topical antifungal ointment to eliminate the fungal infection and heal the lesion.

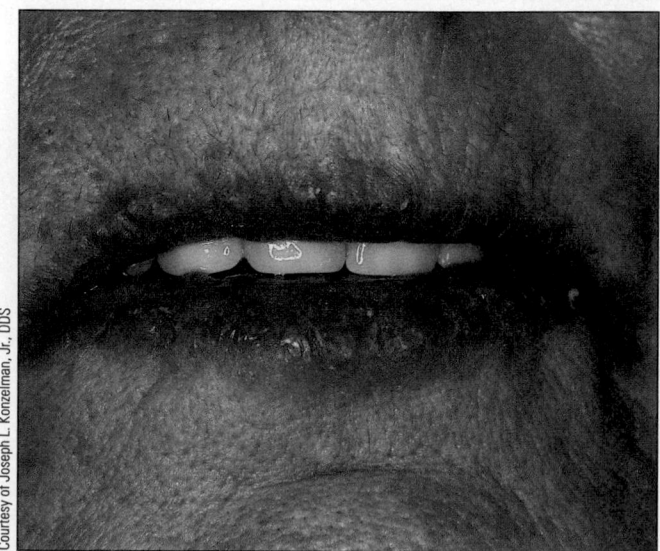

FIGURE 9-32
Angular cheilitis.

Glossitis

Glossitis or smooth tongue is basically an inflammation of the tongue. It occurs due to atrophy of the papilla to create a smooth, erythematous tongue. Glossitis is caused by a variety of reasons and may be painless or may cause some discomfort. These include allergic reactions, irritation from foods, or vitamin deficiencies. The treatment of the glossitis depends on the cause. If it is determined that a food is causing the problem, the patient will be asked to refrain from the food. If it is found that the cause is a vitamin deficiency, adding the vitamin to the diet will resolve the glossitis. The dentist or physician would determine the best course of treatment.

Anorexia Nervosa and Bulimia

Anorexia nervosa and bulimia are both eating disorders that affect the oral cavity. Anorexia nervosa is characterized by an abnormally low body weight and a distorted view of one's appearance. Patients may starve themselves and not eat a normal amount of food when they do eat. If this prolongs, it can cause a state of malnutrition and can be fatal.

Bulimic patients will go through bouts of binge eating and self-induced vomiting. The patient with this disorder often maintains normal weight but is very secretive of their eating habits. This vomiting has a direct effect on the oral cavity and the teeth. The lingual surfaces of anterior teeth become decalcified, and the enamel becomes eroded. Existing restorations deteriorate, and rampant caries and enlargement of the parotid gland can also be present. There is a loss of enamel and dentin on the maxillary teeth especially because of the acid from the stomach flowing across the teeth when vomiting. There may be traumatic lesions on the back of the fingers by their continual use to induce vomiting.

Both aneroxia nervosa and bulimia result in nutritional deficiencies that can further impact the oral cavity as discussed earlier. Treatment for both of these disorders involves counseling, working with a dietician and physician to get the patient back to a normal and healthy weight. The patient needs help to maintain good oral health until the condition can be reversed or better controlled.

Neoplasms

One of the most life-changing diagnoses that a patient may receive is that of oral cancer. It is very upsetting for the patient because they understand how life threatening any type of cancer can be. If a patient in your office is diagnosed with oral cancer, there are many things the dental assistant must understand about the treatment and how the patient can be supported. This section reviews several of the most common benign and **malignant** oral cancers, as well as common oral lesions of patients with human immunodeficiency virus (HIV) and **acquired immune deficiency syndrome (AIDS)**.

A new growth of tissue in which the cells divide more than they should is called a *neoplasm*, also known as a tumor. Many times when the term *tumor* is used, it indicates a potentially alarming diagnosis, but that is not always the case. Tumors or neoplasms can either be benign (noncancerous) or malignant (cancerous).

Benign Neoplasms

Benign lesions are not cancerous and are usually slow growing, **encapsulated**, not ulcerated, and not indurated (hard). A benign neoplasm usually displaces structures from their natural position. These neoplasms are not fatal, resemble normal cells, and, most importantly, are not *metastatic*. Metastatic means that the lesions spreads through the lymphatic system to other areas of the body and grow in those areas. Some examples of benign neoplasms are ameloblastoma, pleomorphic adenoma, papilloma, and fibroma.

Ameloblastoma An *ameloblastoma* is a tumor that can expand the mandible or maxilla and causes the jaw to have a large, radiolucent, multilocular or soap-bubble-like look in the radiograph (Figure 9-33). It is called an ameloblastoma because it is composed of ameloblast-like epithelial cells that surround the stellate reticulum in the enamel organ when a tooth is developing. An ameloblastoma usually occurs in association with a *dentigerous cyst* around an unerupted tooth. It is most commonly found associated with mandibular molars though it can occur in the area of maxillary molars. Most ameloblastomas occur in adults and are treated with surgical removal but can recur.

Pleomorphic Adenoma A *pleomorphic adenoma* is a tumor of the salivary glands and is most often associated with the parotid gland. Clinically, the cheek in front of the ear appears swollen as the tumor enlarges (Figure 9-34). Microscopically, it appears to be a mixture of epithelial and connective tissue and for this reason is also called a benign mixed tumor. Pleomorphic adenoma can be found in all age groups, but most often in patients aged 30–50 and more common in women than men.

They are slow growing, firm masses that can be compressed when subjected to pressure. Pleomorphic adenomas are removed surgically and can recur later. Even though these are considered benign neoplasms, if left to grow and not treated, they have the potential to transform into malignant tumors.

Papilloma A *papilloma* is a pink, red, or white exophytic growth of squamous epithelial cells that is caused by the human papilloma virus (HPV). It is normally 1–3 cm in diameter, has a cauliflower-like appearance, and is usually *pedunculated* or on a stalk (Figure 9-35). Papillomas can also have finger-like projections covering the surface of the lesion. The squamous cells are

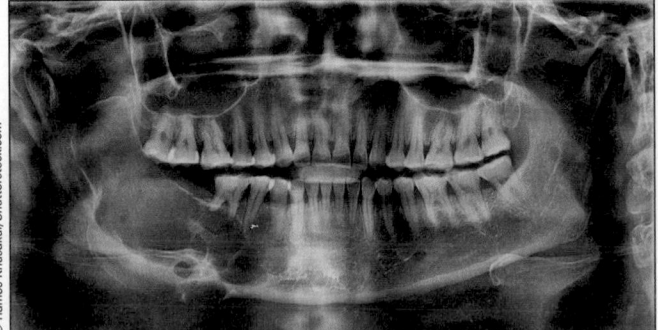

FIGURE 9-33
Ameloblastoma of right mandible.

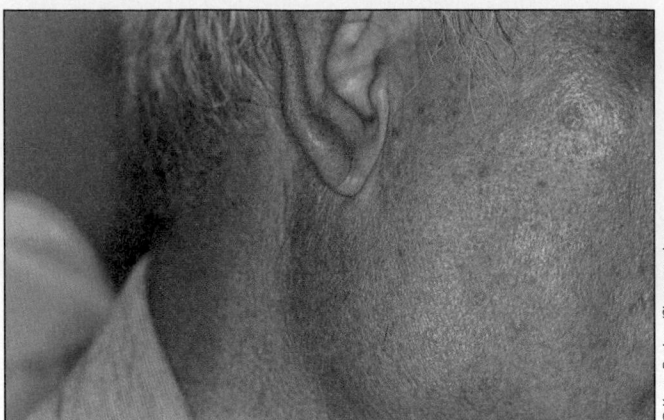

FIGURE 9-34
Pleomorphic adenoma of parotid.

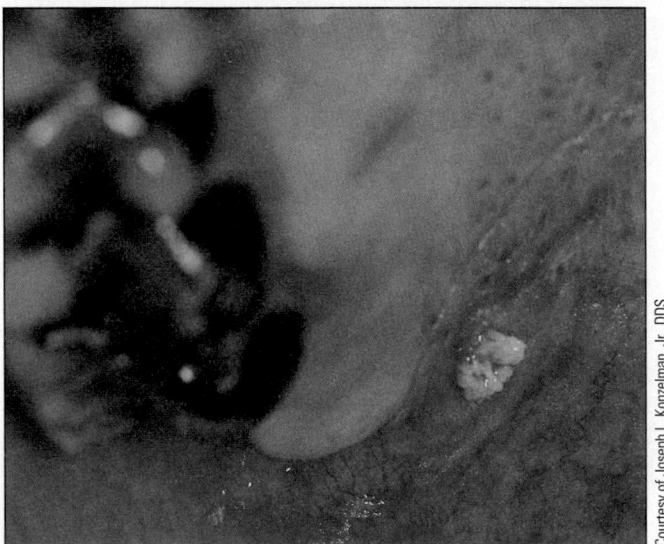

FIGURE 9-35
Papilloma.

involved, so you may see the term "oral squamous papilloma" or "squamous cell papilloma." A papilloma can be found anywhere in the oral cavity and is common on the soft palate or tongue. A papilloma of this type is usually painless, well circumscribed, and mostly pedunculated, but it can be also have a wider base. Treatment involves surgical removal, a procedure that is highly recommended because the virus can be transmitted to others.

Fibroma A *fibroma* is a benign tumor of connective tissue cells that is not a true neoplasm. The fibroma is the most common tumor found in the oral cavity. It is usually caused by continuous irritation to an area that causes the tissue to grow. For that reason, it is also called an irritation fibroma or traumatic fibroma. This tumor can grow anywhere in the oral cavity where irritation is a constant factor. A sharp tooth that is broken can rub and irritate the cheek, lip, or tongue and cause a fibroma to occur. A denture that does not fit properly and rubs the alveolar mucosa can cause a fibroma. A fibroma is usually less than 2 cm in size, dome shaped, pink, and smooth in texture (Figure 9-36).

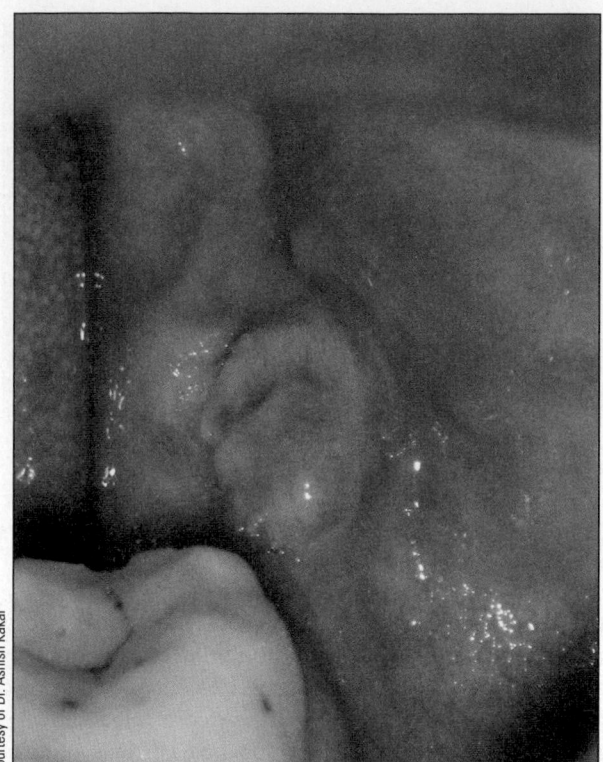

Courtesy of Dr. Ashish Kakar

FIGURE 9-36
Fibroma on third molar.

Fibromas are often seen in patients between the ages of 40 and 60 and more often in females than males. It is important for the dental team to find the origin of the irritation that is causing the fibroma and remove that irritation. Fibromas are normally removed easily with surgery. If they are not bothering the patient, they can be left alone, but it is a good idea to remove the cause of the irritation so that the fibroma does not get larger.

Malignant Neoplasms

Malignant neoplasms are usually fast growing, and the cells are multiplying uncontrollably. They can be fixed to tissues, indurated, and have an ulcerated surface. They are invasive and destructive and often metastasize into other areas in the body. They also tend to have very irregular cell arrangement and size.

There are two main types of malignant neoplasms, characterized by the type of tissue involved. *Carcinomas* involve lesions that originate from epithelial cells, and *sarcomas* originate from connective tissue cells. The dental clinician will need to screen every patient for them during an intraoral examination.

Carcinoma   A carcinoma is a type of cancer that has an epithelial origin. This section discusses the carcinomas that are of most concern in dentistry.

Squamous Cell Carcinoma   The two types of carcinoma that are of most concern in dentistry are *squamous cell carcinoma* and *basal cell carcinoma*. They differ principally in the layer of epithelium in which each lesion originates. Squamous cell carcinoma accounts for 90% of oral cancers, which make up approximately

3–5% of all types of cancer in the United States. It can metastasize and spread to other parts of the body through the lymph nodes of the lymphatic system. The cells are not well organized, and it is asymptomatic in early stages. When the first symptoms do appear, they most commonly include pain, soreness, irritation, numbness, or a burning sensation. Thus, screening in order to detect oral squamous cell carcinomas is important for early treatment once a diagnosis is made. The most common intraoral location for oral squamous cell carcinoma is on the posterior lateral surface of the tongue and the ventral surface of the tongue (Figure 9-37A). The second most common intraoral location for squamous cell carcinoma is the floor of the oral cavity. The most common extraoral location for squamous cell carcinoma is the lip (Figure 9-37B).

Several predisposing factors have been implicated in the development of squamous cell carcinoma. The most prevalent of these are tobacco and alcohol use and excessive sun exposure.

Squamous cell carcinoma is more common in individuals over 40 and affects males more than females. Treatment for squamous

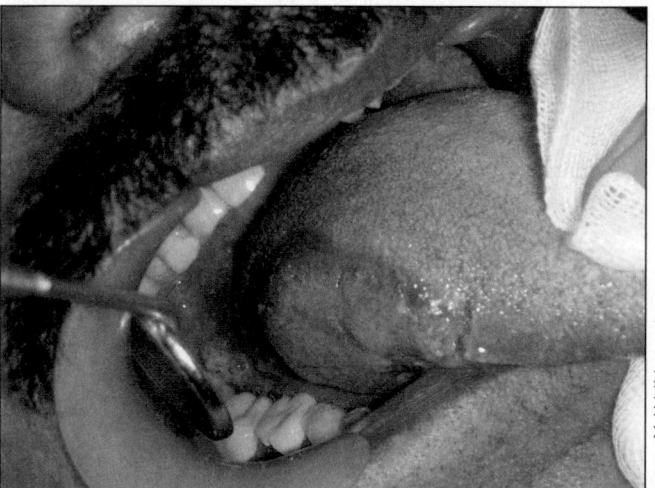

Courtesy of Ashish Kakar

FIGURE 9-37A
Carcinoma of tongue.

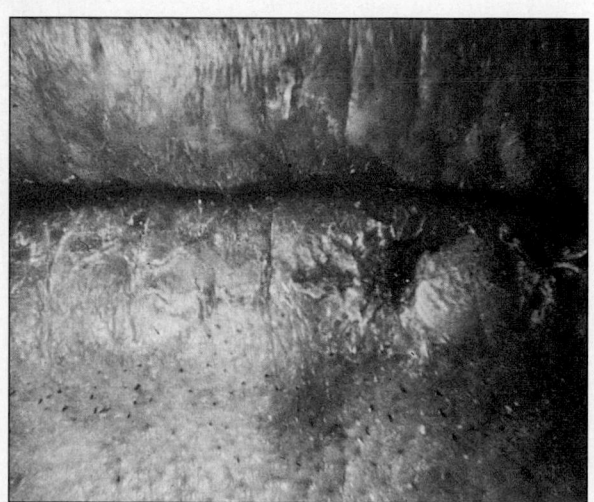

Courtesy of Joseph L. Konzelman, Jr., DDS

FIGURE 9-37B
Squamous cell carcinoma.

cell carcinoma can be surgery, chemotherapy, radiation therapy, or any combination of these three. However, squamous cell carcinoma has a poor survival rate. About half the time it metastasizes before it is even detected.

Basal Cell Carcinoma Basal cell carcinoma is the most common neoplasm of the skin and commonly is known as skin cancer. The etiology is usually unknown, but there are some common factors that put a person at a higher risk including fair colored skin, chronic sun exposure, being over 40 years old, and having a history of skin burns including sunburns.

Basal cell carcinomas commonly are found on areas of the skin that are most often exposed to the sun. The lesions often occur on the mid to upper face and the top of a balding head; they are not found on mucous membranes (Figure 9-38). They are more often found on males than on females and most often in those over 40 years of age. These lesions also can have a variety of shapes and sizes and can be very slight and hard to discover. It is important to look at a patient's face, carefully around the hairline, and on top of the head of a patient that is balding. If a male patient has a beard, be careful to check the neck around the margins of the beard or mustache.

Some early clinical signs of basal cell carcinoma include induration, an elevated nodule with a smooth center, ulceration, a crusted center, and **hyperkeratosis**. As the lesion grows it may develop larger nodules with or without ulceration, and it may become pigmented. Many times it has an ulcerated area that will not heal. These carcinomas typically are locally invasive, slow

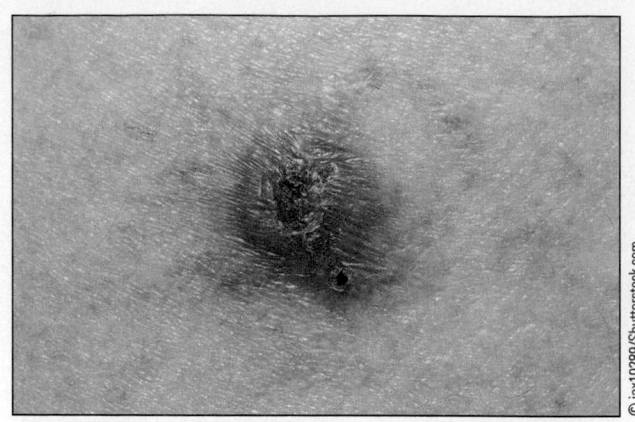

FIGURE 9-38
Basal cell carcinoma.

growing, and rare to metastasize. Treatment of basal cell carcinoma can include surgery and radiation.

Sarcoma *Sarcomas* are uncommon malignant tumors of connective tissue. They are named by their tissue of origin using a prefix. For example, a sarcoma of cartilage is called a chondrosarcoma, one that has invaded bone is an osteosarcoma, and one in the lymphatic vessels is called a lymphangiosarcoma. In the oral cavity, a sarcoma may start in the maxilla or mandible but may spread to surrounding tissues. Figure 9-39 provides the names of various types of sarcomas.

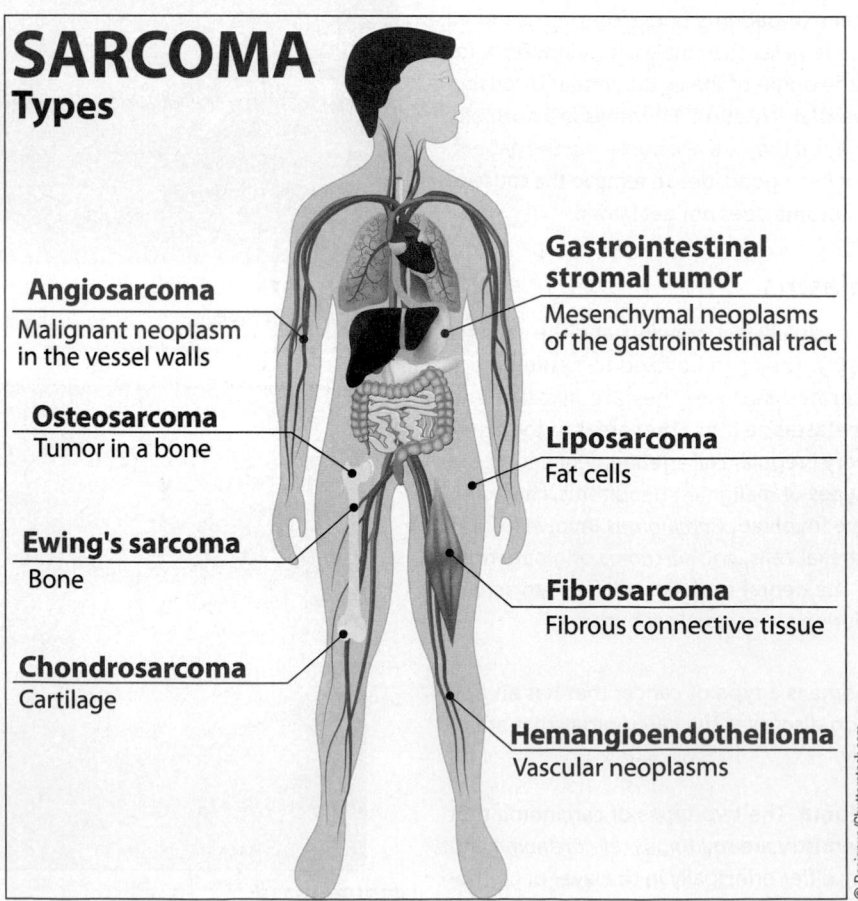

SARCOMA Types

Angiosarcoma
Malignant neoplasm in the vessel walls

Osteosarcoma
Tumor in a bone

Ewing's sarcoma
Bone

Chondrosarcoma
Cartilage

Gastrointestinal stromal tumor
Mesenchymal neoplasms of the gastrointestinal tract

Liposarcoma
Fat cells

Fibrosarcoma
Fibrous connective tissue

Hemangioendothelioma
Vascular neoplasms

FIGURE 9-39
Names of various types of sarcomas.

BOX 9-1 Common Sites for Oral Cancer

Approximately 50% of oral cancer is found on the tongue. Most of these are on the lateral posterior border of the tongue. Most cancers on the tongue are indurated, non-healing ulcerations, exophitic, and either white or reddish in color.

The second most common site for oral cancer is the floor of the oral cavity.

The third most common site is the buccal mucosa or gingiva. Lesions in this area often are caused by using smokeless tobacco and holding it in the vestibule. Most of the lesions here are white patches and nonhealing ulcerations that can invade the bone.

The fourth most common site is the palate, especially the soft palate. Lesions here are most often ulcerated and either red or white.

The last common site is the lips, most often the lower lip. The lesions are usually nonhealing ulcerations and exophitic. Causes for lesions in this area are excessive sun exposure and tobacco use. A common sign to look for with this area of lesion is a thinning or blurring of the vermillion border between the skin of the lips and that of the face. Patients who spend a lot of time in the sun should be advised to wear high SPF sunscreen on their lips.

BOX 9-2 Oral Cancer Warning Signs

- A sore in the oral cavity or on the face that bleeds easily and does not heal within 2 weeks
- Lumps or bumps, rough spots, or swelling in the oral cavity, on the lips, or on the neck
- White, red, or rash-like lesions in the oral cavity or on the lips
- Dryness in the mouth over a period of time for no apparent reason
- Hoarseness, chronic sore throat, change in the voice for no apparent reason
- Numbness, pain, tenderness in or around the oral cavity, ear, and neck
- Soreness or burning sensation in or around the oral cavity
- Feeling that something is caught in the back of the throat
- Difficulty speaking, chewing, or swallowing, or moving the jaw or the tongue
- Change in the way the teeth fit together or the way dentures fit
- Repeated bleeding in a specific area of the oral cavity for no apparent reason
- Significant weight lost for no known reason

Common Sites for Oral Cancer

There are some common sites for oral cancer. These are areas that should be carefully checked during a head and neck exam. Box 9-1 provides details on the most common areas for oral cancers.

Stages of Cancer

All cancers are classified according to a system of stages, ranging from stage I cancers that have the highest survival rate, up to stage IV with the lowest survival rate. A pathologist determines the classification based upon on how much tissue is involved and how deeply the lesion has progressed into the tissue. If a patient says that they have been diagnosed with cancer, the dental assistant should ask at what stage cancer was diagnosed, what the treatment is, and if the patient is currently undergoing treatment.

The dentist should consult with the treating oncologist before treatment. All elective treatment should be postponed until after treatment for cancer is completed. The patient should be monitored closely for dental infections, and the dentist should treat these after consultation with the oncologist.

Warning Signs of Oral Cancer

There are several warning signs of oral cancer of which the dental team needs to be aware. These signs can form the basis for questions to ask the patient during the medical history review. Box 9-2 provides the warning signs for oral and pharyngeal cancer. Usually when examining for oral cancer, the dental assistant should look for lesions that are red, white, or very dark in color like black, purple, or brown. Some lesions are precancerous, which means if they are found and caught early enough, they can be removed or treated before they become malignant. Whenever a normal cell starts to change color or texture, it is a sign that there is a high possibility of it being a precancerous lesion.

Precancerous Lesions

Precancerous lesions are tissues that are not like the usual tissues or do not have the normal form of a tissue under a microscopic examination. These cells have the potential to become cancerous.

Leukoplakia

A lesion called *leukoplakia* is a white, sometimes leathery patch that cannot be identified as any other white lesion (Figure 9-40). It can be found anywhere in the oral cavity and can be densely packed or diffuse (hard to tell where it stops and starts). The white cells cannot be wiped off and normally show hyperkeratinzation. A leukoplakia often has abnormally shaped or sized cells that are irregularly arranged. A biopsy is required to identify the lesion. Leukoplakias can be caused by the use of tobacco products.

Erythroplakia

An *erythroplakia* is a red patch of tissue that cannot be associated with any other specific lesion. It is often seen on the soft palate, tongue, or floor of the mouth, especially in patients over 60 years

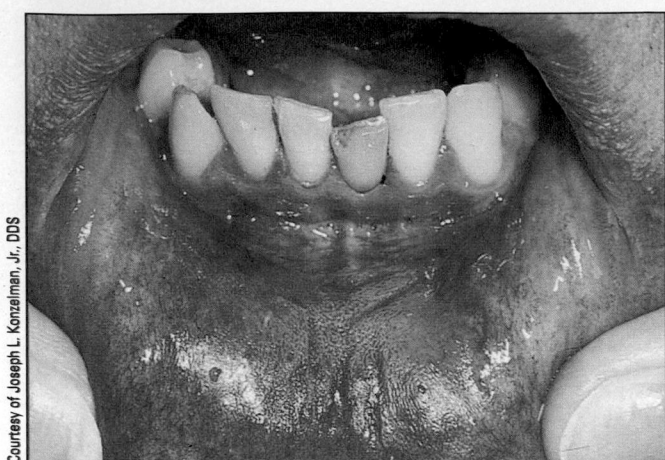

FIGURE 9-40
Leukoplakia.

of age or in those who use tobacco and alcohol. The lesions can appear with white and red specks. These are called speckled leukoplakia rather than erythroplakia. Though erythroplakia and speckled leukoplakia are not cancerous, they have a high potential to become cancerous.

An erythroplakia is not painful in the early stages, so the patient may not notice it. Because erythroplakias are precancerous, it is of the utmost importance to examine the oral cavity carefully for red lesions during an oral cancer screening. The treatment for erythroplakia depends on the extent of the lesion.

Lichen Planus

Lichen planus is an autoimmune system condition in which the body's immune system attacks its own skin and mucous membrane cells. On the skin, lichen planus appears as purple bumps

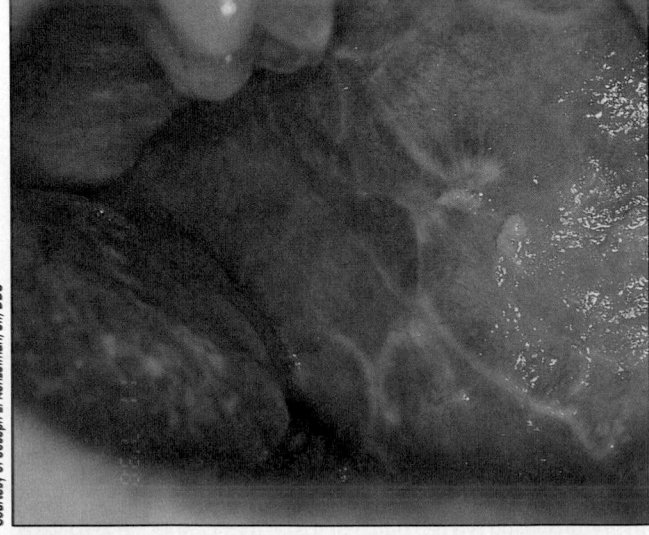

FIGURE 9-41
Lichen planus.

that are itchy. There are two manifestations of lichen planus in the oral cavity. Reticular lichen planus consists of small, white papules that grow together and form interlacing white lines called Wickham striae (Figure 9-41). These have a lacy appearance and cannot be rubbed off. These are commonly found along the buccal mucosa of the cheeks and usually are not painful.

The second type, erosive lichen planus, causes a loss of epithelium in areas and can be painful. These lesions can be found on mucosal tissue like the buccal area but can also occur on the lips. They can cause erosive lesions on the gingiva, can be called desquamative gingivitis, and can worsen with emotional stress. Lichen planus is treated with topical or oral steroid therapy and is considered precancerous.

Oral Lesions Related to HIV and AIDS

Often the dental care provider is the first to see lesions that are related to human immunodeficiency virus (HIV). This virus causes the body's own immune system to start killing its own helper T cells, which enable the body to fight off infection. If the viral load can be kept low and under control, the disease process can be managed with continued blood work and *antiretroviral* medications, which act against the retrovirus HIV. However, when the virus is allowed to progress, it will eventually lead to acquired immunodeficiency syndrome (AIDS). The helper T cells and the B cells produce antibodies against foreign bodies and also have the capacity to remember a previously encountered antigen. AIDS occurs when these cells are decreased to the point that the body cannot fight off opportunistic infections. Many of these infections include severe pneumonia and cancers that eventually take the person's life.

The following section discusses lesions in the oral cavity commonly found among HIV+ patients. They are discussed in order of most common to least common. If found, these must be noted and carefully examined in the dentist's office. In addition, HIV+ patients should always be given home care instructions for performing a self-screening for oral cancer in order to catch lesions as early as possible. Poor oral hygiene and smoking are two factors that will increase the risk of oral lesions in these patients.

Candida Albicans

Candida albicans is a fungal infection in the oral cavity that is characterized by a white to light yellow *pseudomembranous*, curd-like covering on the oral mucosa resembling cottage cheese (Figure 9-42). These white deposits can be wiped off leaving a red, or bleeding surface underneath. Other names for this condition are candidiasis, moniliasis, and thrush. It usually occurs in those who are immunocompromised, such as those with uncontrolled diabetes, those taking antibiotics or corticosteroids, or those who are HIV positive. This infection is common in HIV patients who wear dentures. The patient will sometimes complain of a burning sensation or a numb feeling and say they cannot taste things like they used to. Topical antifungal lozenges or rinses are used for treatment. Nystatin is the most common

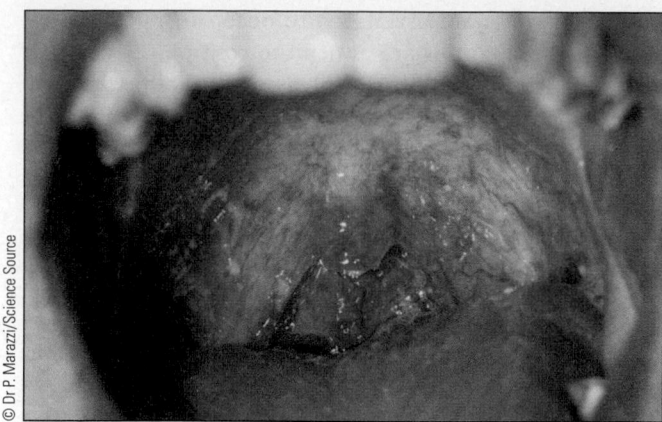

FIGURE 9-42
Candidiasis in an HIV patient.

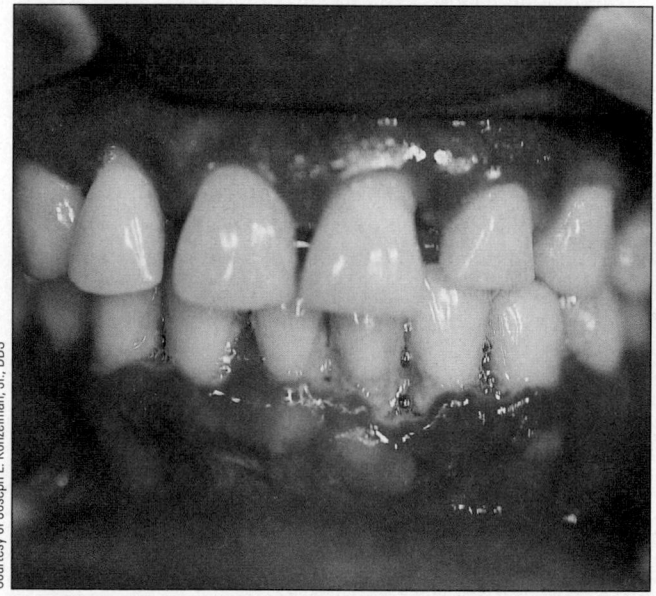

FIGURE 9-43
Acute necrotizing ulcerative gingivitis.

Herpetic Lesions

HIV positive patients may experience long extended periods of herpetic outbreaks which are more severe than those experienced by the general population. Sometimes, these lesions are the first sign that the patient is HIV positive. Refer to the discussion earlier in the chapter regarding herpetic lesions.

Hairy Leukoplakia

Hairy leukoplakia is a white lesion on the lateral border of the tongue that has a corrugated or wrinkled appearance. It also can enlarge and cover the dorsal and ventral surface of the tongue. Sometimes, the papilla on the tongue develops a shaggy or hair-like appearance. This lesion is associated with the Epstein-Barr virus, a part of the herpes virus family, and is often seen in patients that are immunocompromised. Hairy leukoplakia in those who are HIV+ can be resolved with use of antiviral medications that treat HIV (Figure 9-44).

Oral Ulcerations

A patient whose immune system is compromised will show an increase in ulcers in the oral cavity, typically aphthous ulcers or herpetic ulcers. Some of these can be large and painful. They can be irregular and have punched out borders and a pseudomembranous covering. As AIDS progresses in a patient, these ulcerations can be seen in increased numbers in the oral cavity as well as the oropharynx and esophagus.

Kaposi's Sarcoma

The most common malignant cancerous neoplasm found in AIDS patients is Kaposi's sarcoma. These lesions, which are associated with the Kaposi sarcoma herpes virus (KSHV), are not seen in other patients and have unique characteristics. They start as purple to red macules which are found under the skin, in the lining of the oral cavity, and various other organs. They progress into

topical antifungal; Ketoconazole and fluconazole are other common systemic antifungals used for treatment. Refer to Chapter 14 for details regarding antifungal agents.

Periodontal Disease

Chronic gingivitis and periodontal disease are very common in HIV positive and AIDS patients. With the immune system compromised, the bacteria that cause these diseases can multiply and make the disease progress rapidly. Necrotizing ulcerative gingivitis (NUG) and necrotizing ulcerative periodontitis (NUP) are commonly seen in patients who are immunocompromised (Figure 9-43). Both of these can be sudden and destructive to the periodontium. Periodontal diseases will be discussed in detail in Chapter 38.

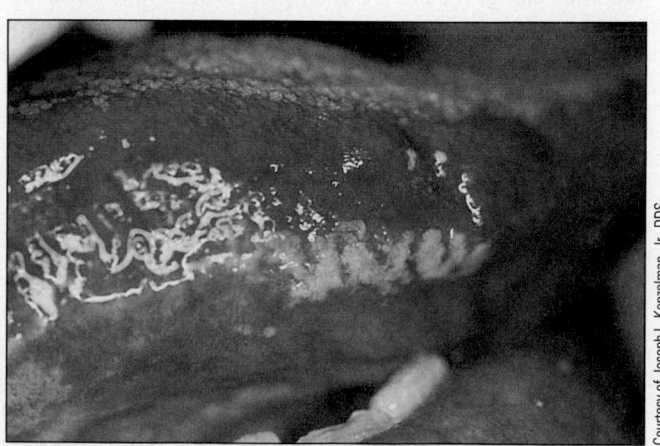

FIGURE 9-44
Hairy leukoplakia.

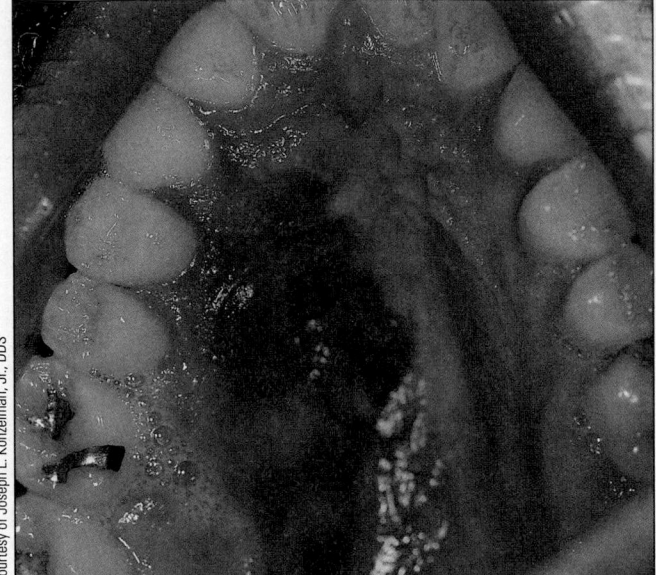

Courtesy of Joseph L. Konzelman, Jr., DDS

FIGURE 9-45
Kaposi's sarcoma.

nodule-like lesions and become *exophytic* or outwardly growing. The tumors may be found on the face, arms, and palate or gingiva and can spread to the lungs, liver, or gastrointestinal tract (Figure 9-45). They can be removed with *cryotherapy* (freezing) or laser excision, and are normally treated with surgery, chemotherapy, or radiation.

Lesions Caused by the Human Papilloma Virus

There are other human papilloma virus strains that manifest oral lesions in the HIV+ patient. These lesions are verruca vulgaris, condyloma acuminatum, and focal epithelial hyperplasia.

Verruca vulgaris is known as the common wart and is found in young people. The virus is spread by direct contact and may be transmitted from skin to oral mucosa through thumb sucking or fingernail biting. The lips are one of the most common intraoral sites for this lesion. The verruca vulgaris is usually a white, papillary lesion. HIV positive patients experience verruca vulgaris as well. Treatment is usually aggressive with the use of a variety of medications as it may be difficult to treat due to the compromised immune system.

Condyloma acuminatum is a small, benign wart on or around the genitals and anus also known as a genital wart. It is spread to the oral cavity through oral–genital contact or self-inoculation. Multifocal epithelial hyperplasia, or Heck disease, is characterized by the presence of multiple whitish to pale pink nodules distributed throughout the oral mucosa. These lesions, besides appearing wart-like, are nodular, not painful, irregular or cauliflower-like projections. They are commonly seen in the nonkeratinized tissue in the oral cavity, including the oral mucosa, palate, vestibules, and tongue.

These oral warts are estimated to occur in 1–4% of HIV+ patients. These lesions are difficult to control. Treatment of these oral wart-like lesions involves surgical removal, cryotherapy, **laser ablation**, or **electrocautery**. Sometimes the lesions reoccur and must be removed again. Recurrence and proliferation of HPV lesions in patients with HIV infection is common.

Oral Cancer Screening

Implementing regular and consistent oral cancer screenings would enable the dental clinician to find more oral lesions earlier and decrease the death rate. Statistics on oral cancer suggest that more than 50,000 Americans will be diagnosed with oral cancer this year, and about half will still be alive after 5 years. However, if caught early, about 90% of oral cancers are treatable.

Even though all patients should get an oral cancer screening, there are several characteristics of those who contract oral cancer that can be used to determine which patients are at a higher risk for oral cancer. It has been shown that about 75% of oral cancers are attributed to tobacco use and alcohol use. Oral cancer also is found twice as often in men than women and is more common in those over 40 years of age. Thus, it would make sense that the men over 40 who use tobacco and alcohol would be the most likely group of patients to experience a diagnosis of oral cancer.

There are some common signs and symptoms all dental personnel should be familiar with, and these should be looked for during examinations (Box 9-2). If any of these signs or symptoms are present, then further investigation and questioning should be completed.

It is also important to inform the patient what you are doing and why before you start the procedure. Let the patient know that you are going to perform an oral cancer screening and that you are looking for any lesions, sores, lumps, or bumps. Ask the patient if he or she has noticed any burning, soreness, numbness, or unusual bleeding in their mouth lately. If the patient answers "yes" to any question, the dental professional should investigate further. Ask more questions about the location of the problem, how long it has been since symptoms started, and when the symptoms are bothersome. All patient responses should be documented in the patient record.

Steps in Oral Cancer Screening Procedure

When a head and neck exam for oral cancer screening procedure is performed, it is important that it be consistent and thorough. It is best to follow a standard routine each time to be sure that all areas of the mouth are examined in a consistent and thorough manner. Always follow a standard sequence so that an area is not missed. Procedure 9-1 outlines the steps in the extraoral and intraoral components of a head and neck exam.

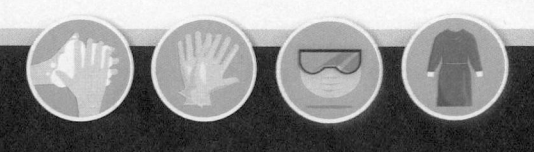

Procedure 9-1
The Extraoral and Intraoral Exams

Follow infection control guidelines. Operator should use protective eyewear, protective clothing, gloves, and mask. Cover gloves should be worn over examination gloves for the extraoral exam.

Equipment and Supplies
- Patient napkin and napkin clip
- Patient protective goggles
- Mouth mirror
- Gauze squares
- Cover gloves

Procedure Steps

The Extraoral Exam

1. Perform a visual extraoral exam by looking at the patient and observing for any changes in color or contour.

2. Perform a tactile extraoral exam.

3. Check for changes in color, contour, consistency, and function in all areas inspected. Also note asymmetrical areas (Figures 9-46 and 9-47).
   - Note pigmented areas and evaluate for irregular borders, diameters greater than 6 mm, history of lesion, and how it evolved over time.

4. Ask the patient to open and close slowly and check the TMJ for clicking or for asymmetry on closing or opening (Figure 9-48).

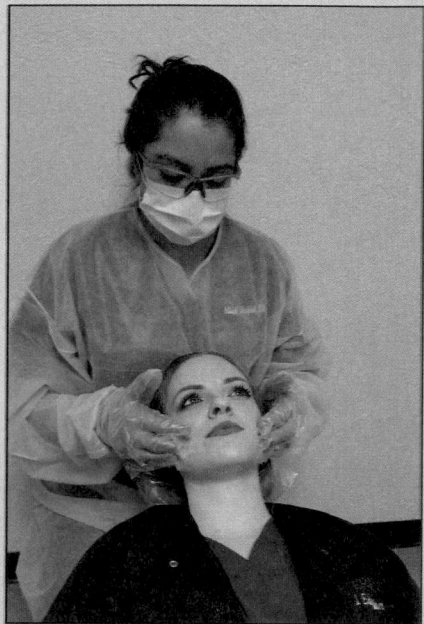

FIGURE 9-47

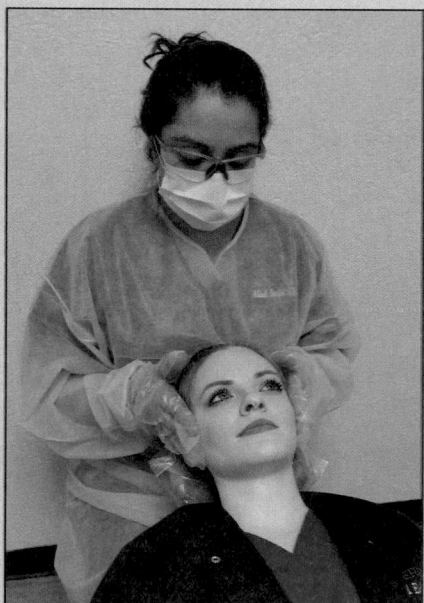

FIGURE 9-46

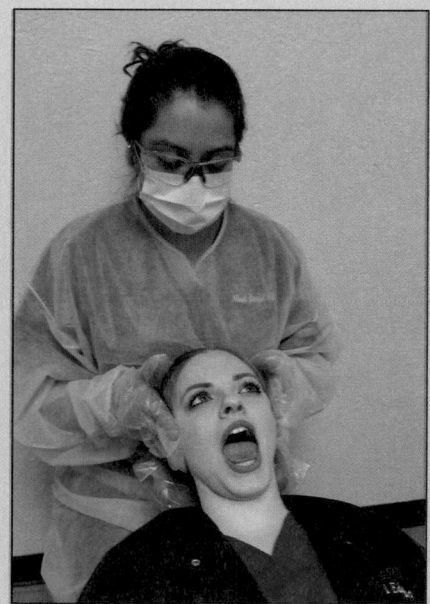

FIGURE 9-48

(Continues)

5. **Palpate** neck on both sides. If there are enlarged lymph nodes, examine for size, whether they are fixed or moveable, and whether or not they are painful (Figure 9-49).

6. Palpate the sternocleidomastoid on both sides.

7. Palpate the thyroid area and ask patient to swallow. The hyoid bone should move (Figure 9-50).

8. Evaluate lips for contour, color, consistency, and function. Look for abnormalities such as indurated areas or ulcerated areas.

Intraoral Exam

1. Wash hands and change gloves before intraoral exam (if cover gloves were not used for the extraoral exam).

2. Palpate the lips by retracting the lips and feel for any abnormalities or masses (Figure 9-51).

3. Examine the alveolar processes and gingiva. Look for color changes and changes in consistency. Look for any areas that are poorly healed (Figure 9-52).

4. Palpate the hard and soft palate and look for any abnormal areas.

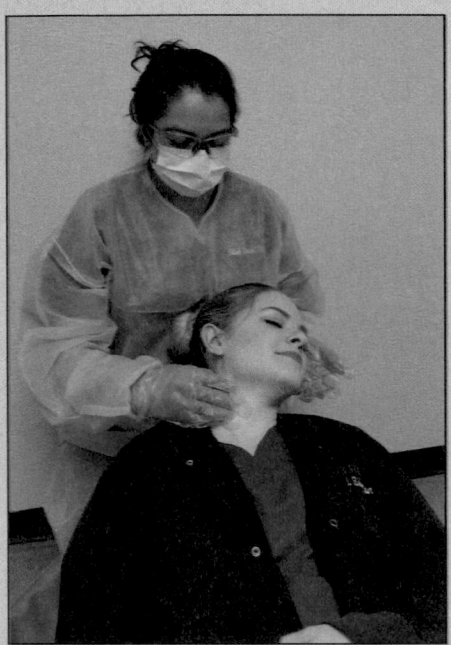

FIGURE 9-49

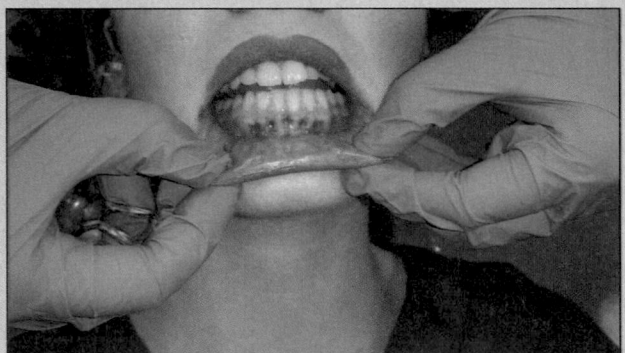

FIGURE 9-51

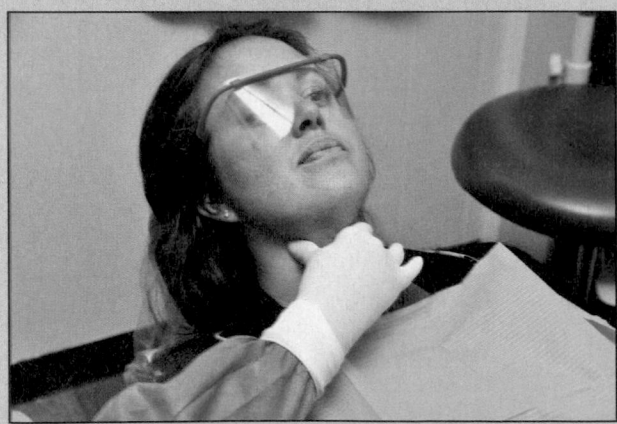

FIGURE 9-50

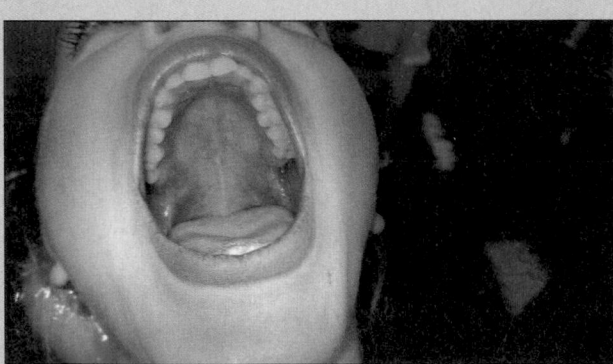

FIGURE 9-52

5. Use the mouth mirror to depress the tongue and ask patient to say "ahhh." Inspect the uvula, the posterior area of the oral pharynx, and the anterior and posterior fauces (Figure 9-53).

6. Use a gauze square to grasp tongue. Move to left and right to examine the lateral borders and dorsum of the tongue (Figures 9-54A, B, and C).

7. Palpate tongue and the salivary gland ducts (Figures 9-55A and B).

8. Ask patient to touch the roof of their mouth with the tip of their tongue (Figure 9-56).

9. Inspect and palpate the floor of the mouth using two hands (Figure 9-57).

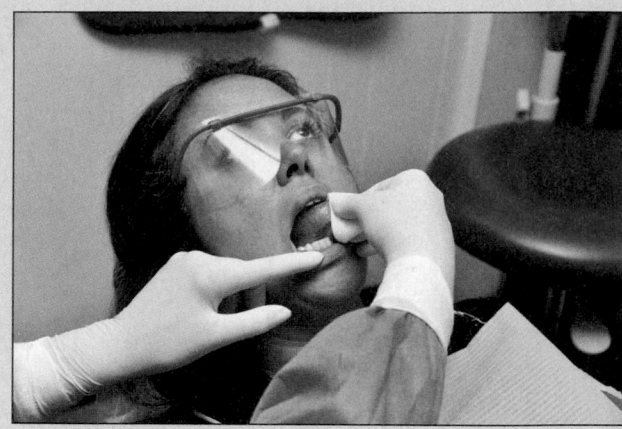

FIGURE 9-54B

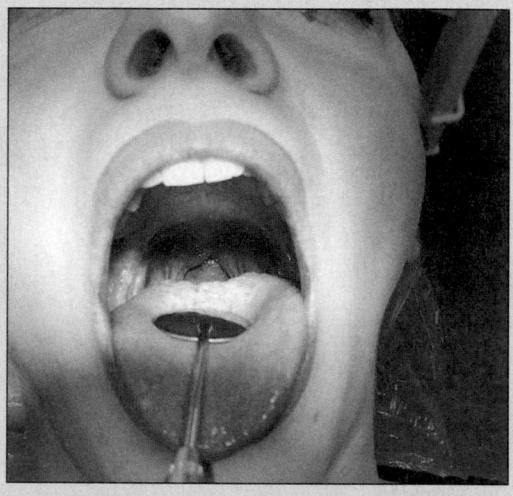

FIGURE 9-53

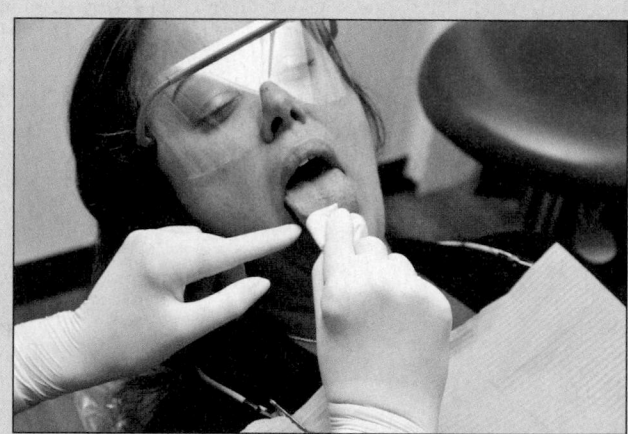

FIGURE 9-54C

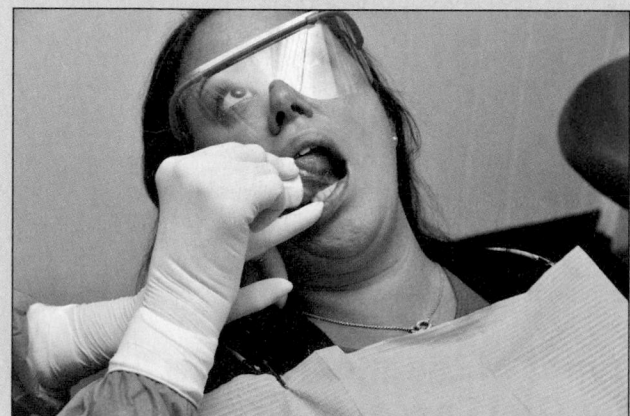

FIGURE 9-54A

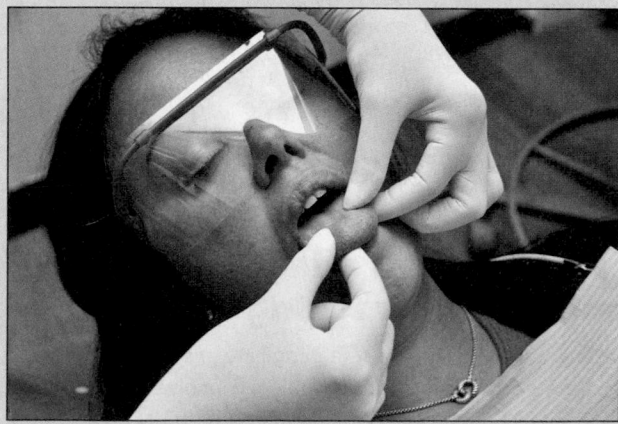

FIGURE 9-55A

(Continues)

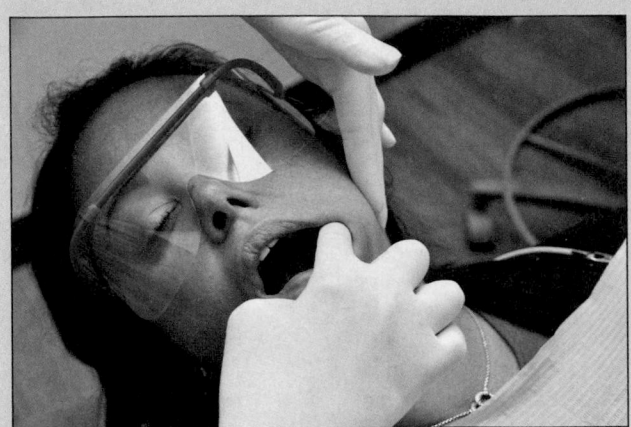

FIGURE 9-55B

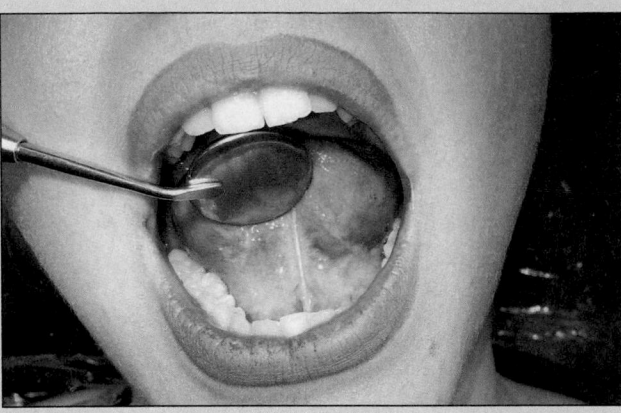

FIGURE 9-56

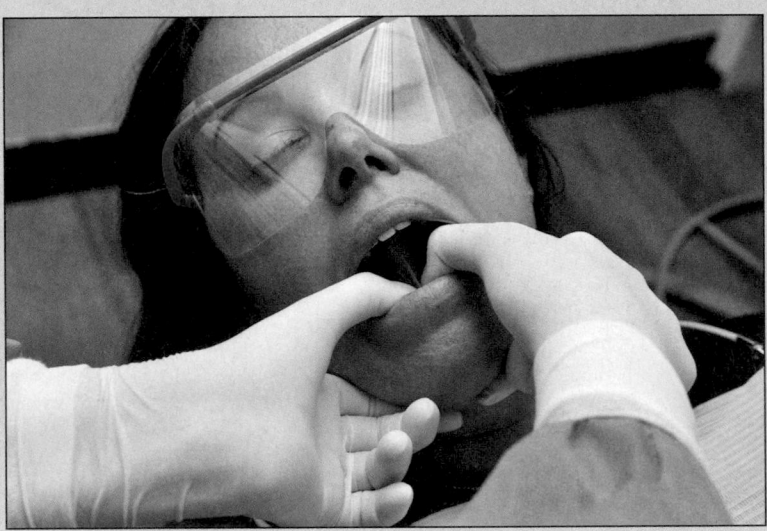

FIGURE 9-57

Teaching Your Patient to Do Oral Cancer Self-Screening

Monthly oral self-exams or screenings are easy to perform, and the benefits outweigh any inconvenience involved. They are just another healthy habit, like flossing, that the dental team should encourage a patient to do. The easiest way to teach a patient to do a self-screening is to give them a hand mirror and have them watch while you perform the screening. Explain to them what you are doing in each section you examine and what you are looking for. Box 9-3 provides the steps the patient can follow at home during a monthly self-exam for oral cancer. These steps can be provided to the patient.

Types of Diagnostic Tools Available for Oral Cancer Screening

There are a variety of diagnostic tools available to help identify abnormal tissue and enable the dental professional to know if the patient should be sent to an oral surgeon for a biopsy. We will discuss how these tools help diagnose abnormal tissue. It is up to the individual office to decide which, if any, of these tools would be useful for the practice and to get the appropriate training to use them properly.

OralCDx Brush Test®

Also known as a computer-assisted transepithelial oral brush, the OralCDx® is a specially designed brush that is used to painlessly obtain a sample of an oral lesion. The OralCDx brush obtains a complete transepithelial biopsy specimen, collecting cells from all three layers of the epithelium: the superficial, intermediate, and basal layer (Figure 9-58). OralCDx requires no anesthesia and causes no pain and minimal or no bleeding. The OralCDx sample is then analyzed by specially trained pathologists at a separate laboratory using highly sophisticated computers.

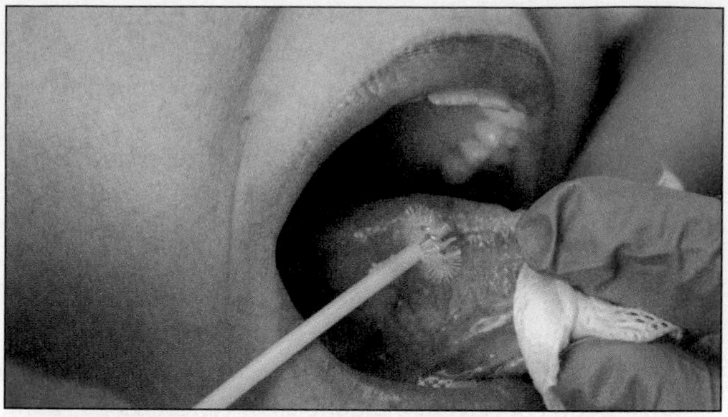

ViziLite® and Vizilite TBlue®

The ViziLite system is a *chemiluminescence* or reflective tissue fluorescence that uses a 1% acetic acid wash or 5% vinegar rinse. This rinse is applied for 30 seconds to remove debris and increase the visibility of the cells by mildly dehydrating the tissue. When a blue light stick is shone on the area, abnormal tissue will appear white and bright with sharp edges; normal tissue will look light blue. If well controlled, this technique can be a good tool for diagnosing oral cancer. However, it can be difficult to discriminate some lesions, and the solution causes highlights that can be distracting in normal lights. A second generation of this system uses a blue stain called Tblue.

FIGURE 9-58
Oral CDx Brush Test®

Courtesy of CDx Diagnostics

ViziLite TBlue® is used to help oral health care professionals identify, evaluate, monitor, and mark abnormal oral cell lesions, including precancerous and cancerous cells that may be difficult to see during a regular visual exam. The procedure only takes 2 minutes to complete.

VELscope®

The hand-held VELscope device is used to examine inside the oral cavity for suspicious-looking tissue. It emits a safe blue light into the oral cavity, which causes the tissue to fluoresce. Abnormal tissue typically appears as an irregular, dark area that stands out against the otherwise normal, green fluorescence pattern of surrounding healthy tissue. The patient wears protective glasses while the VELscope is being used. The VELscope has been shown to have high sensitivity and specificity in identifying areas of dysplasia and cancers.

Caring for Patients Undergoing Cancer Treatment

The education the dental team provides patients can make a difference before, during, and after treatment for oral cancer. Some basic things such as using fluoride gel daily may prevent the occurrence of rampant decay due to the side effects of cancer treatment. Once a patient has been diagnosed with any type of oral cancer, the dental team should be involved. The next section of text discusses the various types of cancer treatment, focusing on radiotherapy or radiation treatments.

Types of Treatment

Treatment for head and neck cancer can involve radiation, surgery, chemotherapy, or a combination of these treatments. The purpose of radiation treatment is to shrink tumors or kill

---

BOX 9-3 Steps for Self-Exam for Oral Cancer

1. Stand in front the mirror and view both sides of face and neck. The should both appear the same.

2. Examine skin on the neck and face for color and any changes in moles.

3. Feel the right and left sides of the neck for any lumps or soreness of changes.

4. Place your fingers over the front of the throat on your Adam's apple and swallow. You should feel an up-and-down movement when you swallow.

5. If you wear dentures, remove them and use a flashlight to check the inside of your mouth. Use a disposable mouth mirror if possible.

6. Feel the roof of the mouth for any lumps or sore areas.

7. Use a piece of gauze and grasp your tongue. Pull it out and move it to one side. Check that side for any changes in color or sore spots. Do the same with the other side.

8. Look at your gums for swollen areas or sore spots. Also feel your lips both inside and outside for any bumps or sore spots. Look for color changes in these areas.

9. Anything unusual or abnormal should be reported to your dentist.

cancer cells by damaging their DNA. Typically, patients receive external-beam radiation treatments five times a week for five to eight weeks. The regimen will vary per patient, situation, and modality used.

Radiation therapy, though an effective cancer fighter, poses numerous dental challenges during and after treatment. Because normal cells are also destroyed during the process, nearly all patients undergoing radiation therapy suffer from treatment related oral side effects. These effects can be acute or last for a lifetime and, most significantly, may manifest years after the actual completion of the radiation therapy.

Most people receiving a diagnosis of cancer do not think about seeing their dentist; however, the dentist and dental team play a crucial part in the overall treatment of a patient undergoing radiation therapy. One of the priorities is to complete a comprehensive evaluation prior to cancer treatment. One of the reasons is to prevent osteoradionecrosis.

The dental team provides care prior to treatments to minimize side effects, educate the patient as to what to expect, and provide **palliative** care during treatment, and is instrumental in maintaining a healthy oral cavity post treatment. As it is unlikely that many cancer treatment centers employ an onsite dental team, it is vitally important that area dentists and their team are trained to handle these patients and possess the knowledge to collaborate with the oncologist.

Patient Treatment Prior to Radiation Therapy

Patients should see a dentist at least four weeks prior to radiation therapy. Prophylaxis, a head and neck exam, patient specific oral hygiene instruction, and radiographs should be completed. Strict dental care is the most important preventive measure to minimize side effects. Treatment plans should be in collaboration with the radiation oncologist and even head and neck surgeons during all phases of dental care. Some general recommendations are outlined in Table 9-9.

Patient Treatment during Radiation Therapy

The intensity and incidence of the oral effects will vary among patients. Some patients may experience mild xerostomia where as others may experience more severe xerostomia and thus may develop **dysphagia**, **dysgeusia**, and pain. Since **mucositis** is most likely inevitable, the dental hygienist can provide palliative recommendations and act as a support to the patient. Instruct your patient to call their cancer team if they notice increased soreness, swelling, or bleeding, or notice a sticky white film in their mouth.

The dental assistant is a crucial health professional during the radiation therapy process since poor dental hygiene and lack of dental motivation are important risk factors for side effects. With that being said, poor home care could result in the delay of radiation treatment intervals or stall treatment altogether, resulting in detrimental outcomes. If a patient presents to your office who will be having radiation therapy for oral cancer, you should inform your patient of possible side effects and how to prevent or treat symptoms. Table 9-10 provides methods for palliative care of symptoms related to radiation therapy.

Patient Treatment after Radiation Therapy

In order to minimize prolonged oral side effects, a patient should see their dentist more often after the radiation therapy

---

TABLE 9-9 General Recommendations for Patient Care Prior to the Start of Radiation Therapy

- Request radiation oncologist phone numbers for collaboration.
- Take all dental radiographs needed, especially a panoramic (PAN).
- Complete comprehensive dental exam and prophylaxis with fluoride varnish application.
- Teach the patient how to complete a self-oral cancer exam. Educate them about normal versus abnormal findings and explain which findings should initiate a prompt phone call to the dental office.
- Evaluate entire dentition, extract any teeth that may be in the direct site of radiation beam that are nonrestorable, that have moderate to severe periodontal disease, or that are questionable in any way. This is to prevent the possible future threat of extraction induced osteonecrosis.
- Restore caries and replace faulty restorations to minimize risk of abscess; abscessed teeth should be treated endodontically or extracted.
- Remove rough surfaces of restorations or teeth to reduce trauma to mucosa.
- Consider advising patient to not wear dentures or partials during treatment time span due to high likelihood of *Candida albicans* infection.
- Fabricate radiation guard in collaboration with the radiation oncologist.
- Fabricate custom made fluoride trays.
- Provide patient with extensive home care instructions and nutritional counseling.
- Collaborate with a registered dietician who is part of the oral cancer treatment team when appropriate.
- Provide written instructions and pamphlets from reputable sources to the patient.

is completed and should continue to perform daily self-oral cancer exams. The reason for the short time intervals suggested in Table 9-11 is to help the patient with any salivary concerns, to prevent dental caries, and to discover any infections once treatment is over. Some side effects can manifest months to years afterwards, so more frequent dental visits and thorough oral cancer screenings at each visit are important. Late conditions such as radiation caries and osteonecrosis typically show up within three months to a year, respectively, following treatment. This reinforces the need for long-term follow up. The dental hygienist should be sure to encourage the patient to continue meticulous oral home care. The patient needs to be scrupulous about their oral home care in order to encourage symptoms to improve. A post treatment panoramic image may be considered.

Radiation therapy is effective against cancer but leaves the patient at risk for numerous oral side effects that have the potential to diminish quality of life. Oral tissues directly affected by head and neck radiation therapy include the salivary glands, mucosal membranes, jaw muscles, and bone. If side effects are extreme, patients may not be able to keep up with their treatment, or radiation therapy may be stopped altogether. The dental team plays a crucial role in preventing, minimizing, and managing oral side effects of radiation therapy in order to preserve dental health and contribute to successful treatment.

The *Dental Provider's Oncology Pocket Guide* and *Oncology Pocket Guide to Oral Health* from the National Institute of Dental and Craniofacial Research are helpful resources to keep on hand. A form that summarizes low to high risk areas of treatment may be helpful in decision making and provide smooth collaboration with the radiation oncologist and other members of the oncology team. The dental assistant should take the next step by further educating him- or herself about the impact he or she may have on patient quality of life after treatment.

One of the best services that dental professionals can provide for their patients is a thorough oral cancer screening and instruction of self oral cancer exams with every dental procedure. Taking the time to do this may save a life or eliminate the need for more aggressive treatments on already compromised patients. Early detection is an important "key" that dental assistants should not neglect to "turn."

TABLE 9-10 *Palliative Care Radiation Therapy Symptoms*

Symptoms	Treatment or Palliative Care Recommendations
xerostomia	<ul><li>crushed ice</li><li>sugarless gum, sugarless hard candy</li><li>saliva substitutes</li><li>nonalcoholic mouthwashes</li><li>Drink 8 glasses of water daily</li><li>Reduce sugar and carbohydrate intake</li><li>Avoid acidic foods</li></ul>
mucositis	<ul><li>Use a soft toothbrush</li><li>crushed ice</li><li>alcohol free products</li><li>avoid spicy foods</li></ul>
sense of taste change/loss	<ul><li>This may be permanent change</li><li>Foods that are high in nutritional value are important for successful healing of the body</li></ul>
difficulty swallowing/chewing	<ul><li>Physical therapist and speech language pathologist are often members of the oral cancer treatment team which can help restore function</li></ul>
thick saliva	<ul><li>Warm water rinses to help clean the oral cavity</li></ul>
radiation caries	<ul><li>At home and in office fluoride treatments</li></ul>
osteonecrosis	<ul><li>Postpone elective oral surgical procedures and elective treatment</li><li>Extract any questionable teeth prior to treatment to prevent osteonecrosis</li></ul>

TABLE 9-11 Treatment Considerations Post Radiation Therapy

	Treatment Considerations
Invasive dental procedures	• Postpone for six months if possible • Consult with oncologist before treatment
Noninvasive dental procedures	• Postpone for 3 months after completion of radiation therapy • Treat based on consultation with oncologist
osteonecrosis	• Avoid extractions post radiation therapy due to increased risk of necrosis • Refer to oral surgeon for any required extractions
Radiation caries and xerostomia induced caries	• Home and office fluoride treatments • Reduce intake of high carbohydrate foods • Drink 8 glasses of water daily
Preventive dental visits	• Dental exam monthly for first 6 months after completion of radiation therapy • Three month recall for prophylaxis and fluoride treatment application
xerostomia	• May be permanent • Drink 8 glasses of water daily and use crushed ice

Chapter Summary

It is important to know what to do, how to ask questions, what questions to ask, and how to get the information you need without alarming your patient. What lesions are common, and which ones belong to certain types of diseases? What should you as a dental assistant be familiar with, and after you find a lesion, what do you do to measure it and describe it?

The role of the dental assistant is important when dealing with pathology. There are many ways the assistant is a helpful and important member of the dental team when treating patients and identifying lesions that may be harmful. Many times the dental assistant has the opportunity to discuss health issues with the patient and go over their medical history. This gives the assistant the chance to ask appropriate questions. Many times the assistant is the first staff member to look in the oral cavity when preparing for a restoration or applying the topical anesthetic.

The dental assistant helps the dentist with a biopsy if a lesion is removed for further medical testing. The assistant is the one who usually documents in the patient's chart a description of what the dentist finds. The measurements and pictures of a lesion can also be taken by the assistant. If a cancerous lesion is found, the assistant can explain procedures to be followed before, during, and after treatments of chemotherapy or radiation.

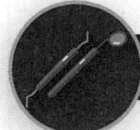

CASE STUDY

A patient presents to the office with pain in the area of tooth #30. You seat the patient and look at the area to let the dentist know what you find. You notice an ulcerated area on the buccal mucosa of #30. You ask the patient what they have been using to alleviate the pain. The patient states they have been using aspirin.

Case Study Review

1. What do you think has caused the ulcerated area?

2. What would you tell the dentist?

3. What would you advise the patient?

Review Questions

Multiple Choice

1. Pathology is a term that means the study of the nature and cause of disease. Oral pathology is the examination of tissues, cells, and specimens of body fluids for evidence of oral disease. *Select the correct response based on the statements above.*
   a. Both statements are true.
   b. Both statements are false.
   c. The first statement is true; the second statement is false.
   d. The first statement is false; the second statement is true.

2. Which of the following is not a role of the dental assistant in relation to oral pathology?
   a. Diagnosing oral lesions
   b. Setting for an initial exam appointment
   c. Documenting oral lesions found during exam
   d. Review of medical history once patient is seated

3. Which one of the following is not part of a clinical diagnosis?
   a. location
   b. size
   c. historical
   d. shape

4. A 55-year-old male patient presents to the office for a recare visit. You notice a white lesion on the corners of the oral cavity. You notify the dentist, who diagnoses it as angular cheilitis caused by a fungal infection as opposed to a bacterial infection. The dentist prescribes an antifungal medication and asks the patient to use as directed. The patient is to return in 1 week for evaluation and to determine if the medication helped to cure the lesion. What type of diagnosis is this?
   a. therapeutic
   b. clinical
   c. radiographic
   d. historical

5. Initiation, amplification, and termination are the three phases of acute inflammation. Match the term with the correct description.
   a. amplification
   b. initiation
   c. termination
      1. Mast cells release chemicals called histamines into the bloodstream that cause vasoconstriction followed by vasodilation and swelling.
      2. White blood cells fight off infection and prevent it from spreading to surrounding tissues.
      3. The inflammatory response stops and the lymphatic system filters out any toxins from the area and rids the body of the foreign invaders that triggered the inflammatory process.

6. Which of the following lesions are at the surface of the oral mucosa?
   a. papule
   b. pustule
   c. ecchymosis
   d. granuloma

7. Match each of the causes of rampant caries with the correct description.
   a. early childhood caries
   b. xerostomia induced
   c. adolescent
   d. methamphetamine mouth
      1. Caused by the illegal recreational use of methamphetamine
      2. Associated with illness, medication, or radiation therapy
      3. Also known as nursing bottle decay
      4. Associated with sleeping with sugary substances such as chocolates in the oral cavity

8. Which of the following is correct regarding amelogenesis imperfecta?
   a. The dentin is softer than normal in amelogenesis imperfecta.
   b. Amelogenesis imperfecta is not a genetic disorder.
   c. Radiographs show a large pulp chamber.
   d. The soft dentin causes the enamel to chip off.

9. Which of the following statements about anodontia is correct?
   a. Anodontia means that all teeth are congenitally missing.
   b. Anodontia may affect the primary or the permanent teeth.
   c. Ectodermal dysplasia is a rare genetic disorder that can cause total anodontia.
   d. All of these are correct.

10. Which of the following is correct regarding tooth fusion?
    a. Fusion occurs when a tooth bud attempts to divide into two but fails to do so.
    b. Fusion may be complete or incomplete depending on the stage in which it occurs.
    c. Fusion is also known as twinning.
    d. With fusion, all the teeth are present, but one looks wider than the others.

11. Which of the following is not correct regarding microdontia?
    a. Microdontia is defined as abnormally large teeth.
    b. Microdontia can impact either the entire dentition or just one or two teeth.
    c. The teeth most commonly affected are the maxillary lateral incisors.
    d. Those with Down syndrome experience microdontia.

12. Which of the following is correct regarding a mucocoele?
    a. It is a fluid filled lesion related to the major salivary glands.
    b. It is most commonly seen in the maxillary labial mucosa.
    c. It may be caused by medications such as Dilantin.
    d. It usually resolves within 3 to 6 weeks.

13. During pregnancy or puberty, hormonal changes may make the patient more sensitive to the plaque that is normally in the oral cavity. This sensitivity decreases the risk of gingival inflammation that may occur due to the plaque.
    Select the correct response regarding color of a lesion based on the statements above.
    a. Both statements are true.
    b. Both statements are false.
    c. The first statement is true; the second statement is false.
    d. The first statement is false; the second statement is true.

14. Which of the following is not correct regarding benign neoplasms?
    a. Benign neoplasms are encapsulated.
    b. Benign neoplasms are slow growing.
    c. Benign neoplasms can metastasize.
    d. Benign neoplasms have normal cells.

15. A 40-year-old female patient presents to the office because of concerns related to a recent swelling. You seat the patient and review the medical and dental history forms. The patient's chief complaint is a recent swelling in front of the right ear. The swelling has been enlarging over time. Upon palpation, you notice that the swelling is firm but is compressible. Which of the following do you suspect is causing the swelling?
    a. pleomorphic adenoma
    b. papilloma
    c. ameloblastoma
    d. fibroma

16. Malignant neoplasms are usually fast growing and may be indurated. Malignant neoplasms are invasive and can metastasize into other areas in the body.
    Select the correct response regarding color of a lesion based on the statements above.
    a. Both statements are true.
    b. Both statements are false.
    c. The first statement is true; the second statement is false.
    d. The first statement is false; the second statement is true.

17. Which of the following is the most common intraoral site for squamous cell carcinoma?
    a. tongue
    b. floor of the oral cavity
    c. lip
    d. exposed skin

18. Which of the following is not a warning sign for oral cancer?
    a. burning
    b. pain
    c. irritation
    d. comfort

19. Which of the following is correct regarding erythroplakia?
    a. An erythroplakia is a white patch of tissue that cannot be associated with any other specific lesion.
    b. Erythroplakias are usually found in those under the age of 50.
    c. Erythroplakias can appear white with red speckles.
    d. Erythroplakias are cancerous lesions.

20. Reticular lichen planus is commonly found on the buccal mucosa of the cheeks and consists of small, white papules that grow together and form Wickham striae. Erosive lichen planus is caused by loss of epithelium on mucosal tissue, the lips, and the gingiva.
    Select the correct response regarding color of a lesion based on the statements above.
    a. Both statements are true.
    b. Both statements are false.
    c. The first statement is true; the second statement is false.
    d. The first statement is false; the second statement is true.

Critical Thinking

1. Explain the signs and symptoms of the three stages of syphilis.

2. A patient presents to the office with the chief complaint of a recent growth on the palate. The patient is a 45-year-old male, and the medical history reveals that he is HIV positive.
    1. What do you suspect the lesion is?
    2. How would this lesion be managed?
    3. What is the cause of this lesion?

3. What are the steps that should be followed during a head and neck exam for oral cancers?

Key Terms

Term and Pronunciation	Meaning of Root and Word Parts	Definition
abscess (**ab**-ses)	**abscess** = an inflamed area in the body tissues that is filled with pus	collection of purulent exudate or pus
acquired immune deficiency syndrome (AIDS) (eydz) acronym for: A = **A**cquired I = **I**mmune D = **D**eficiency S = **S**yndrome	**acquired** = to get **immune** = protected from a disease **deficiency** = lack, insufficiency **syndrome** = group of symptoms together are characteristic of a specific disease or disorder	acquired immune deficiency syndrome: an infectious disease caused by the human immunodeficiency virus (HIV); there are two variants of the HIV virus, HIV-1 and HIV-2, both of which ultimately cause AIDS

Term and Pronunciation	Meaning of Root and Word Parts	Definition
angular cheilitis (**ang**-gyuh-ler) (kahy-**lahy**-tis)	**angular** = having an angle **cheil** = lip **-itis** = inflammation	inflammation or chapping of lips, especially at corners of mouth
caries (**kair**-eez)	**caries** = decay	a destructive process causing decalcification of the tooth enamel and leading to continued destruction of enamel and dentin, and cavitation of the tooth
chancre (**shang**-ker)	**chancre** = an ulcer arising from syphilitic poison	small hard nodular growth; first sign of syphilis
chromogenic (**kroh**-moh- **jen**-ik)	**chromo** = color **genic** = arising from genes	producing color or pigmentt
culture (**kuhl**-cher)	**culture** = cultivate	the growing of microorganisms in a controlled medium
decay (dih-**key**)	**decay** = to rot or cause to rot as a result of bacterial, fungal, or chemical action	the destruction or decomposition of organic matter as a result of bacterial or fungal action; rot
dysgeusia (dis-**gyoo**-zhuh)	**dys** = ill or bad **geusia** = sense of taste	impairment or perversion of the gustatory (taste) sense
dysphagia (dis-**fey**-juh, -jee-uh)	**dys** = ill or bad **phagia** = to eat	impairment of speech resulting from a brain lesion or neurodevelopmental disorder.
electrocautery (ih-lek-troh-**kaw**-tuh-ree)	**electro** = electric **cautery** = burning	a handheld, needle type of device which is heated by electricity
encapsulated (en-**kap**-suh-leyt)	**en** = within **capsulate** = formed into a capsule	enclosed by a protective coating or membrane
erythematous (er-uh-**thee**-muh)	**erythro-** = red **-emia** = denotes condition of the blood	reddening of the skin, common sign of irritation or inflammation
gingivostomatitis (jin-**jahy**-vuh- stoh-muh-**tahy**-tis)	**gingiva** = of the soft tissue of the mouth **stomatitis** = inflammation of the mouth	inflammation of the gingiva and oral mucosa
hyperkeratosis (hahy-per-ker-uh-**toh**-sis)	**hyper** = overstimulated **keratosis** = skin disease characterized by a growth	thickening of the stratum corneum, often associated with a quantitative abnormality of the keratin
immunocompromised (im-yuh-noh-**kom**-pruh-mahyzd)	**immune** = protected **compromised** = not functioning at an optimal level	incapable of developing a normal immune response, usually as a result of disease, malnutrition, or immunosuppressive therapy
indurated (**in**-doo-reyt-ed)	**indurat** = to harden	hardened, usually used with reference to soft tissues becoming extremely firm but not as hard as bone
laser ablation (**ley**-zer) (a-**bley**-shuhn)	**maser** = acronym for microwave amplification stimulated emission radiation **ab** = off **latus** = lengthened	the process of removing material from a solid (or occasionally liquid) surface by irradiating it with a laser beam
lesion (**lee**-zhuhn)	**lesion** = a wound or injury	an area of pathologically altered tissue, injury or wound, infected patch
malignant (muh-**lig**-nuhnt)	**malign** = bad effect **-ant** = characterized by	growing worse, resisting treatment, threatening to produce death
mucositis (myoo-kuh-**sai**-tuhs)	**muco** = relating to mucus **-itis** = inflammation	inflammation of a mucous membrane

(Continues)

Term and Pronunciation	Meaning of Root and Word Parts	Definition
necrotic (nuh-**kraa**-tuhk)	**nekros** = dead body **-ic** = having to do with	pathologic death of one or more cells, or of a portion of tissue or organ, resulting from irreversible damage
oncologist (aang-**kaa**-luh-juhst)	**onco** = tumor **logy** = study of	specialist in the branch of medicine dealing with cancer
osteonecrosis (aa-stee-ow-nuh-**krow**-suhs)	**osteo** = related to bone **nek** = death **rosis** = condition	death of bone
palliative (**pa**-lee-uh-tiv)	**palliate** = to cloak	relieving or alleviating without curing, an agent that alleviates or eases a painful or uncomfortable condition
palpate (**pal**-pey-t)	**palpate** = to examine by touch	examination by application of hands or fingers to body to detect abnormalities, to feel or rub and push on area to feel for consistency or any abnormalities
prodromal (prow-**drow**-muhl)	**prodrome** = running forward	early symptoms that signify the start of a disease
xerostomia (zee-ruh-**stow**-mee-uh)	**xero** = dry **stomia** = condition of oral cavity	decreased production of lack of saliva

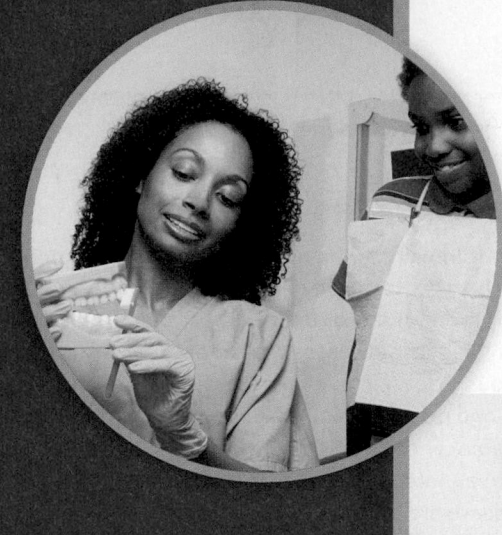

## CHAPTER 10

Microbiology

SECTION III
Preclinical Dental Skills

Specific Instructional Objectives

At the completion of this chapter, you will be able to meet these objectives:

1. Use terms presented in this chapter.
2. Explain why the study of microbiology is important to the dental assistant.
3. Identify the early pioneers in microbiology and their contributions to current understanding of microorganism.
4. Discuss the nature of the disease process.
5. Discuss the major groups of microorganism, prions, and normal flora.
6. Distinguish bacterial, viral, protozoal, fungal, rickettsial, algal, and prion diseases.
7. Discuss the harmful effects of normal flora.
8. Describe the body's resistance to disease.
9. Explain types of immunity and vaccines.
10. Discuss the role of epidemiology in controlling communicable diseases.

Introduction

It is important for the dental assistant to have a basic knowledge and understanding of **microbiology** and the nature of **pathogens**. This knowledge aids the dental assistant in making best-practice decisions regarding infection control products and procedures and methods of preventing **disease** transmission in the dental office.

Microbiology is the study of **microorganisms**. The study of microbiology and disease plays an integral role in oral health care delivery. Bacteria, viruses, prions, protozoa, and fungi will be explored in this chapter as well as some of the associated disease entities.

Microorganisms may be helpful or potentially harmful. More microorganisms are helpful than harmful. Some microorganisms, such as *Streptococcus and Lactobacillus*, are helpful and are used to make dairy foods. Bacteria such as *Actinomycetes* and fungi are used in fertilizers and for compost. Pharmaceutical companies use bacteria such as *Streptomyces* in the manufacturing of drugs to produce tetracycline. Bacterial products are used to produce vaccines such as those for diphtheria and tetanus.

Microorganisms generally become harmful when they are where they should not be or they grow out of control. These types of microscopic organisms are called **pathogenic microorganisms**. For example, microorganisms are capable of causing dental disease, including **dental caries** and **periodontitis**.

History of Microbiology

Prior to the development of the microscope, humans were unaware of the existence of pathogenic microorganisms and thus lacked knowledge of the true causes of diseases. Dutch scientist Antony van Leeuwenhoek (1632–1723), is considered the first true microbiologist because he was the first to use microscopes to observe microorganisms in a variety of substances, including water, blood, hay, and scrapings from teeth.

Microbiology advanced rapidly during the eighteenth century. In the 1850s, English physicist John Tyndall (1820–1893) discovered the existence of bacteria in the air. He found that bacteria could be destroyed by prolong and intermittent heat. Ferdinand Cohn (1828–1898), a German botanist, discovered that during the life cycle of specific bacteria, a heat-resistant form—**endospores**—existed. This led to the development of the germ theory of disease and the recognition of airborne disease. Joseph Lister (1827–1912), a British surgeon, later recognized the role of these airborne microorganisms in postsurgical infections and pioneered the practice of **antiseptic** surgery.

One of the most important figures in the field was French chemist Louis Pasteur (1822–1895), often known as the "Father of Microbiology." Pasteur discovered the pasteurization process that kills germs; he identified viruses; he discovered the rabies vaccination; and he introduced the medical world to practices aimed at minimizing the spread of disease. Working about the same time as Pasteur, German biologist Robert Koch (1843–1910) isolated the organisms that cause the deadly diseases anthrax, tuberculosis, and cholera. Koch's assistant, Julius Petri (1852–1921), designed shallow glass plates and dishes in which to isolate and grow cultures of microorganisms. Koch used these to isolate bacterial colonies. These are known as Petri plates and dishes and are still used in microbiology laboratories today (Figure 10-1). Koch's four postulates, or guidelines, are still used to prove particular diseases are caused by specific microorganisms.

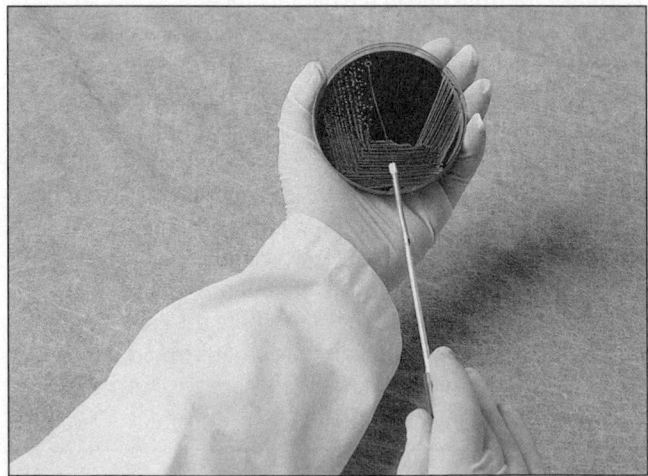

FIGURE 10-1
Microorganism being grown in a medium in a Petri dish.

These early pioneers provided the basis for current infection control products, procedures, and methods.

Infectious Diseases

Disease refers to the impairment of normal function, or an interruption in normal **homeostasis**. An **infectious** disease is caused by pathogenic microorganisms or their **toxic** products. There is a wide variety of infectious diseases that impact the health of patients. Infectious diseases may be **communicable** and be transferred from one person to another. Some are **contagious** (very communicable) and are spread rapidly from contact and close proximity to an infected person. It is important to know what kinds of disease are prevalent, what causes the diseases, and how the diseases are spread. Diseases are categorized and classified to help answer these questions. Classifications of diseases are important in studying the statistics on the cause of an illness (morbidity) and causes of death (mortality). The most widely used classifications of disease are the following:

- Pathological—nature of the disease process
- Etiological—cause of disease
- Epidemiological—how diseases are spread
- Physiological—effect on the function of body
- Anatomical—body system, regions of the body and organ or tissues affected
- Juristic—speed of the advent of death

Pathogenicity

A pathogen is a microorganism able to produce disease. **Pathogenicity** refers to the ability of the microorganism to produce disease in a host organism. The **host** organism is the one infected by the microorganism. Several factors such as **virulence**, **invasiveness**, and **toxigenesis** influence the pathogenicity of the microorganism.

Acute and Chronic Diseases

Diseases may be **acute**, of short duration, or **chronic**, of long duration. Acute diseases usually have a rapid onset of symptoms followed by recovery to a state of health comparable to that experienced before the disease. Examples of acute diseases are influenza and hepatitis A. Health conditions that are persistent or long lasting, such as cancer, diabetes, and heart disease are examples of chronic diseases. The term *chronic* is usually applied when the effects of the disease last more than three months. Furthermore, a disease may localize to a specific body part or organ, such as appendicitis or tonsillitis, or it may be systemic, affecting the entire body, such as arthritis or diabetes.

Latent Diseases

Latent disease refers to a persistent infection, such as cold sores (oral herpes simplex) that come and go. The microorganism responsible for causing the disease lies quiet and inactive or **dormant** until something triggers recurrence. The causes of recurrence of cold sores are unknown, but some triggers may be anxiety, stress, and sun exposure.

The herpes virus, *varicella zoster,* responsible for chickenpox, can cause another latent disease. The herpes virus may lie dormant in the body's nerve cells and later cause the disease shingles. The cause of the reactivation of this virus is unclear but seems to be related to the diminished capacity of the immune response during aging. Because most people who develop shingles are over the age of 60, the CDC recommends the shingles vaccine (Shringrix).

Opportunistic Diseases

Organisms that would normally not cause illness or disease are called nonpathogenic. People with healthy immune systems do not become ill when exposed to nonpathogenic organisms. However, if a person's immune system is weakened, these same nonpathogenic organisms can cause what are referred to as **opportunistic** infections (OI) or diseases. In other words, if the person's immune system is impaired, the microorganism takes the "opportunity" to cause disease. Microorganisms that are normally present in the mouth without causing disease can become opportunistic microorganisms. Examples of oral infectious diseases caused by opportunistic microorganisms include dental caries, pulpitis, and periodontal disease.

People living with human immunodeficiency virus (HIV) are especially susceptible to opportunistic disease-producing microorganisms. The Centers for Disease Control and Prevention (CDC) has compiled a list of over 20 opportunistic infections (OI) that are considered when diagnosing acquired immune deficiency syndrome (AIDS). If a person with HIV develops one or more of the OIs, they are diagnosed with AIDS.

Groups of Microorganisms

Specific microorganisms are associated with a variety of disease entities. The groups of microorganisms that may cause disease are bacteria, viruses, protozoa, and fungi.

Bacteria

Bacteria are a microscopic group of single-celled organisms that live on virtually every environmental surface from countertops to human digestive tracts; if 2,000 bacteria were lying side by side in a line, they would be about the width of the period at the end of this sentence. These unicellular life forms, which contain no nucleus, are referred to as **prokaryotes**. Bacteria divide by simple fission: they elongate and divide into two separate cells and then continuously repeat this cycle. In ideal conditions (warm, dark, nutrient-rich, and moist), they divide about every 20 minutes. Bacteria are often incorrectly called "germs."

They can represent **normal flora**, or non-disease-causing microorganisms, that exist in and on the healthy human body. Normal flora may exist on the skin, in the eyes, nose, throat, and intestinal tract. They can also be pathogenic, or disease-causing, microorganisms if the conditions under which they would normally thrive become compromised, such as with the elderly or a medically compromised patient. Bacteria may be rod-shaped, round, curved or spiral, representing the variation of size, shape, and arrangement of these one-celled microorganisms.

Bacteria Morphology The shape of bacteria (morphology) is unique to this group of microorganisms. Under a microscope, the types of microorganisms are *bacilli* (rod-shaped), *cocci* (round or bead-shaped), *spirilla/spirochetes* (S-shaped), and *vibrios* (curved like a comma). (Refer to Figure 10-2.)

When the bacteria are grown in colonies, or masses, they appear differently. The prefix *diplo,* as in *diplococci,* identifies pairs of bacteria; *staphylococci* grow in clusters much like grapes; and *streptococci* identifies chains of bacteria.

Bacteria Oxygen Needs **Aerobic** bacteria require oxygen, and **anaerobic** bacteria are actually destroyed by oxygen. An example of aerobic bacteria is *Staphylococcus aureus,* which is found as normal flora in the respiratory system. Anaerobic bacteria, such as *Clostridium,* reside as normal flora in the gastrointestinal tract. Bacteria that can grow in either the presence or absence of oxygen, such as *Salmonella,* are referred to as **facultative anaerobes** and are considered to be disease-producing microorganisms. Some types of bacteria form a capsule that provides a protective covering over the cell wall. An example of this is *Streptococcus mutans*. The capsule may prevent destruction of the bacteria by certain **antibiotics**. This type of bacteria is virulent, capable of causing serious disease. Bacteria can be spread through the air by coughing or sneezing, close contact, and through food and water.

Hans Christian Gram (1853–1938) developed a process for separating bacteria into two groups: gram-positive and gram-negative. *Gram staining* uses violet dye, iodine solution, alcohol solution, and safranin dye. Bacteria that are stained purple or blue by the dye are classified as *gram-positive;* those that stain pink or red are classified as *gram-negative.* This process aids in the diagnosis of bacterial infections and appropriate therapeutic intervention. For example, the antibiotic penicillin works best on gram-positive bacteria.

Bacterial Spores **Spores** are bacteria that have changed as a result of unfavorable conditions; these are highly resistant. Spores become enclosed in layers of protein (endospores) and are the most resistant form of bacteria. They can survive extremes of heat, dryness, radiation, disinfectants, and boiling. Spores are

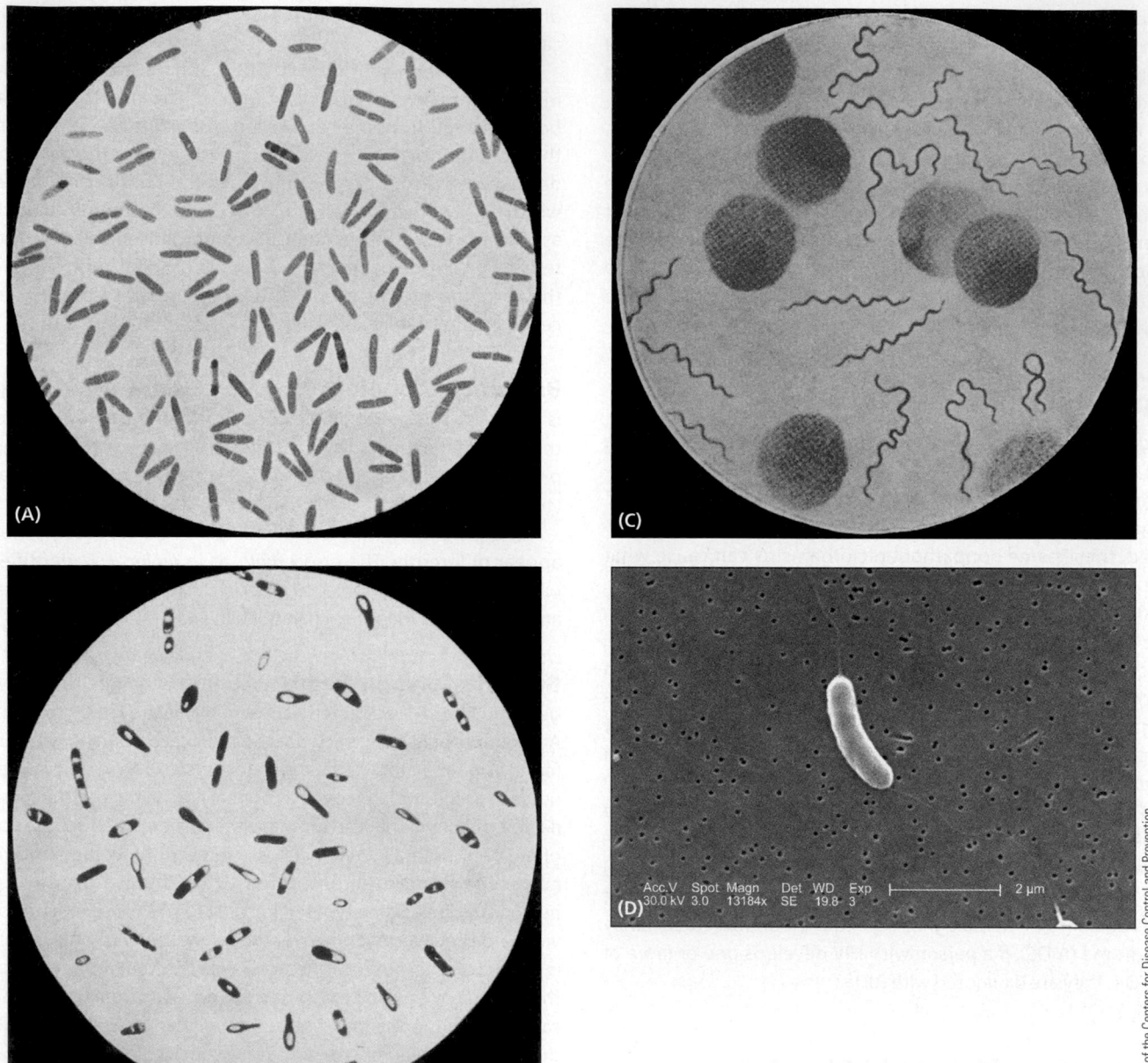

Courtesy of the Centers for Disease Control and Prevention

FIGURE 10-2
The unique shapes of bacteria. (A) Bacilli: rod shaped. (B) Cocci: round. (C) Spirilla: S-shaped. (D) Vibrios: curved.

Infection Control

Antibiotics are drugs that fight bacterial infections. According to the **CDC**, repeated and improper uses of antibiotics are primary causes of the increase in drug-resistant bacteria. Antibiotic resistance occurs when the bacteria change in some way, making the antibiotic ineffective. Antibiotic-resistant bacteria will actually multiply and cause more harm. This is one of the CDC's top concerns. Someone who is infected with a certain microorganism that has become resistant to antibiotics can then pass that resistant infection to another person.

Antibiotic use can promote the development of antibiotic-resistant bacteria. Every time a person takes antibiotics, sensitive bacteria are killed, but resistant germs may be left to grow and multiply.

While antibiotics should be used to treat bacterial infections, they are not effective against viral infections like the common cold, most sore throats, and the flu. Widespread use of antibiotics promotes the spread of antibiotic resistance. Smart use of antibiotics is the key to controlling the spread of resistance. If your health care provider does prescribe an antibiotic, it is essential that you take it exactly as it is prescribed. Do not skip doses. Complete the prescribed course of treatment even if you are feeling better. If treatment stops too soon, some bacteria may survive and cause reinfection.

used to test sterilization methods. Sporulating is a means of survival for bacteria, and bacteria have been known to survive for years in this state. Later, they may land on a surface that is moist and nutrient rich and reactivate. The process is much like a seed that floats and then lands on rich soil and begins growing. Examples of diseases caused by spore-forming bacteria are anthrax and tetanus.

Viruses

Viruses are much smaller than bacteria (one-hundredth the size) and can only be seen under an electron microscope. Unlike bacteria, viruses are **parasites** and must rely on a living *host* to survive and, therefore, represent the microorganism most responsible for diseases today.

Viruses can live inside cells and multiply very rapidly. Many cause fatal diseases such **HIV** and **hepatitis**. Some viruses are capable of crossing the placenta and infecting the fetus. Some viruses may lay dormant in host cells and become reactivated by stress, another infection, or exposure to ultraviolet light. Most are easy to kill by disinfecting or exposure to air, but the hepatitis B virus is very resistant. It can live on a dry surface for up to two weeks.

Viruses can be spread by direct contact, insect bites, blood transfusions, inhalation of droplets expelled by coughing or sneezing, or by contamination of food or water. It can be difficult to treat viral diseases due to their resistance to antibiotics and vaccines. There are antiviral drugs to treat viral diseases just as antibiotic drugs are used to treat bacterial diseases. Antiviral resistance can occur when the virus changes in some way, rendering the antiviral medication ineffective, in much the same way as antibacterial resistance occurs. The CDC, state public health departments, and the World Health Organization (WHO) study antiviral resistance patterns to make public health policy recommendations regarding antiviral medications.

Protozoa

Protozoa may be single-celled or multicelled animal life and, unlike bacteria, do contain a nucleus and genetic material. These microorganisms, or **eukaryotes**, are much larger than bacteria and are just below the visibility of the naked eye (about 100 microns in size). Often mistakenly called an amoeba (an amoeba is an organism within the class protozoa), they live in fluids in the bloodstream, mouth, and intestinal tract and survive in polluted water in pools and ponds. Some protozoa are able to move around with whiplike tails called flagella, some are sporulating, and most are aerobic.

Most protozoa do not cause disease but may live in hosts, causing damage. For example, the protozoa *Entamoeba gingivalis* is found in patients infected with periodontal disease. Protozoans enter the body through inhalation and aspiration into the respiratory tract. Some protozoa are responsible for intestinal infections, while others cause infection in the blood, lungs, liver, or brain.

Fungi

Fungi are aerobic eukaryotic, requiring oxygen and containing a nucleus. Their cell wall contains chitin, which makes fungi insensitive to antibiotics. Examples include molds, yeast, and mushrooms. Some are sporulating and they reproduce by **budding**. They may be used to make antibiotics, such as penicillin, or in the fermentation process of fruit juice and bread. Although penicillin is made from mold, it does not act upon the fungi from which it is made. These microorganisms are considered to be opportunistic when they become pathogenic, invading tissues of individuals with impaired resistance.

Although most fungal infections are mild, they can become life threatening in **immunosuppressed** patients and the elderly. *Candida albicans* is a common fungus or yeast found on the skin, in the oral cavity, gastrointestinal tract, and the female genital tract. In healthy individuals, this organism is a part of the normal flora. A change in the body can cause overpopulation of *candida albicans*. Change in the body may occur as a result of multiple rounds of antibiotics, a diet rich in carbohydrates or sugar, or even from prolonged periods of stress. Oral **candidiasis**, which is an overgrowth of *candida albicans*, is considered an opportunistic infection. It is characterized by a coating of white membranes on the surface of the oral mucosa and tongue.

Saprophytes and Parasites Fungi may be **saprophytes** or parasites. Parasitic fungi attach to other organisms and obtain their nutrients from the host. An example of a parasitic fungus is *candida albicans*. Saprophytic fungi feed on dead plant and animal remains. This is beneficial for breaking down organic material into humus, minerals, and nutrients that can be used by plants. Mold that grows on bread and cheese is saprophytic fungi. Visible spots of mold that can be seen on the surface of bread and cheese have poisonous root threads that run down through the food. These molds grow very fast and food products that have mold spots on them should be discarded. Fungal infection can be spread from person to person through contact with infected areas and occur in people with weak immune systems.

Rickettsiae

A parasitic form of bacteria is classified as **rickettsiae**. Lice, fleas, ticks, and mites are often hosts to rickettsiae. They multiply only by invading the cells of another life form. The hosts then transmit the disease to humans.

Algae

Algae are simple, nonflowering aquatic plants or plantlike organisms that are found in abundance in freshwater and marine habitats. They range from a microscopic single-cell organisms to larger multiple-cell organisms including seaweed and kelp. Human illness is associated through the consumption of contaminated seafood products containing toxic harmful algae.

Prions

Prions are a relatively new and separate class of infectious particles, unlike bacteria, fungi, viruses, and other known pathogens. Prions are not considered a major group but are unique due to their lack of both DNA and RNA, which are nucleic acids found in the nuclei of all other living organisms.

Prions convert normal protein molecules into dangerous ones simply by changing the shape of normal protein molecules. Prions are responsible for bovine spongiform encephalopathy, commonly called mad cow disease. There is no treatment or vaccine against prion diseases.

Current epidemiological evidence does not indicate a concern for the transmission of prion diseases in the dental health care setting. However, dental unit waterlines can become contaminated with prions. Therefore, it is recommended that the dental unit waterline and evacuation system not be used for patients with known prion disease. A disposable bowl should be provided for expectorate and a stand-alone suction unit utilized. As with all patients, infection control measures are diligently performed.

Normal Flora

In healthy human beings, internal tissues are typically free of microorganisms. However, the external tissues, such as the skin and mucous membranes of the nose, are exposed to and in contact with environmental bacteria. Normal flora refers to the microorganisms found at any anatomical site. Bacteria are the most common and numerous components of normal flora with fewer numbers of eukaryotic fungi, protozoa, and algae present as well.

It is important to understand normal flora in order to understand the possibility and consequences of microbial growth in areas normally free of microorganisms. Understanding will further increase knowledge and awareness of the immune response to migration of normal flora into these areas.

Benefits of Normal Flora

Healthy human beings benefit in many ways from the colonization of normal flora. This benefit is referred to as mutualistic because the microorganisms of normal flora also benefit by receiving their nutrition from the human host, an amicable environment in which to thrive, protection from the physiologic characteristics of the host, and a mode of transport on and in the human body.

Normal flora provides nutritional and digestive benefits to the human host by helping to break down food products and extracting the nutritional components for use by the human body. Bacterium of the normal flora also aid in building the human immune system, facilitating the actions of the immune system and fighting the invasion and growth of pathogenic bacteria.

Normal flora synthesizes and excretes vitamins, such as K and B_{12}, which are then absorbed by the body. Normal flora inhibits growth of pathogenic microorganisms by competing for attachments sites and essential nutrients required for colonization. The bacteria of normal flora also help to stimulate the production of natural antibodies against pathogenic bacteria, helping the human host fight infection and disease.

Diseases Caused by Microorganisms

The health and life of human beings are under constant threat by microorganisms. These microorganisms invade the tissue and cause infectious diseases. In this section of the chapter, the etiology of different diseases caused by microorganisms will be presented.

Bacterial Diseases

Pathogenic bacteria create toxic substances that cause disease symptoms. Infectious diseases caused by bacteria include anthrax, botulism, tetanus, tuberculosis, pneumonia, and dental decay.

Anthrax Anthrax is an acute infectious disease that most often occurs in animals and is caused by bacillus anthracis. It can occur in humans if they are exposed to an infected animal. It can also be contracted by inhalation of spores, cuts in the skin (cutaneous anthrax), or eating meat from an infected animal. Failure to treat the disease before symptoms are present normally results in death. It is not contagious, nor can it be spread from person to person. The disease can be prevented by a vaccination or an antibiotic treatment before symptoms manifest.

Diphtheria, Pertussis, and Tetanus Diphtheria, pertussis, and tetanus are serious diseases caused by bacterial infections. Diphtheria is an upper respiratory illness caused by *Corynebacterium diphtheria*. It is an infectious disease that can be

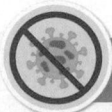

Infection Control

Prions are regarded as being highly resistant to the routine methods of decontamination and sterilization that are currently accepted for medical device reprocessing. It is important for the dental assistant to stay current with methods as diseases are evolving.

In 2001, the CDC and state and local health departments reported several confirmed cases of inhalation anthrax. These cases were related to bioterrorism acts in which the *Bacillus anthracis* spores were placed inside letters and packages. Anthrax is one of the most likely agents to be used as a weapon because the microscopic spores can be released into the air or put into food and water. These spores last for a long time in the environment and are 100,000 times more deadly than any other chemical. The CDC continues to work with other federal agencies, state and local health departments, hospitals, laboratories, emergency response teams, and health care providers to prepare for anthrax attacks.

caught from an infected person who coughs or sneezes. The symptoms include a sore throat, fever, swollen neck glands, and breathing difficulties. The distinguishing sign of diphtheria is a sheet of thick, gray material covering the back of the throat. If not treated properly, it produces a poison that can cause serious complications such as heart failure or paralysis. In the past, diphtheria was common, and due to the widespread use of vaccination only two cases have been reported in the twenty-first century.

Pertussis, often referred to as whooping cough, is a highly contagious respiratory disease caused by *Bordetella pertussis*. Symptoms include uncontrollable, violent coughing with difficulty in breathing followed by a need to take deep breaths that make a "whooping" sound. Infants and young children are most commonly affected and it can be fatal.

Tetanus, often referred to as lockjaw, also attacks the nervous system and is caused by *Clostridium tetani*, gram-positive, spores-forming bacteria. This organism is found in soil, dust, or animal or human feces and enters the body through a puncture wound. It can be prevented by vaccination, although booster doses every ten years must be administered for continued immunity. Because tetanus can be fatal, a tetanus vaccination is routinely ordered when puncture wounds occur.

A diphtheria-pertussis-tetanus (DTaP) vaccine is available. CDC states that diphtheria is rare due to widespread vaccination,

pertussis is the most vaccine preventable disease and tetanus is increasingly rare in the United States.

Tuberculosis Tuberculosis is a highly contagious bacterial infection involving the lungs. It is caused by *Mycobacterium tuberculosis* and is a leading cause of death worldwide. Tuberculosis is contracted through inhalation of aerosolized droplets from an infected individual during coughing, sneezing, speaking, or singing. Contraction through the inhalation of aerosolized droplets from an infected individual is referred to as primary tuberculosis. The infection may stay dormant for many years before symptoms appear, or symptoms may appear within just a few weeks following exposure. Symptoms include fatigue, low-grade fever, night sweats, loss of weight, and, finally, a persistent cough. The disease can be detected by a skin test and by a chest x-ray. Treatment for this disease includes antibiotics and other drugs.

Most patients who undergo treatment for primary tuberculosis will recover without further complications. However, some patients may experience a reactivated occurrence; this is referred to as secondary tuberculosis. It can be transmitted by TB carriers when there is the presence of chronic infection. It is important for the dental assistant to ask if the patient has ever had TB.

People at risk for contracting tuberculosis include the elderly, infants, and HIV-infected patients who have a weakened immune system, making them highly susceptible to contracting tuberculosis.

Streptococcal Infection Streptococcal infection is one of the most common bacterial diseases in humans. Strep throat (acute streptococcal pharyngitis) is the most common throat infection caused by bacteria (*streptococcus mutans*, group A strep). Symptoms include a red, painful sore throat, white patches on the tonsils, swollen lymph nodes, fever, and headache. Strep throat is treated with antibiotics. Scarlet fever is a rash that sometimes occurs in a person who has strep throat. Symptoms are a high fever, a rash, sore throat, and a strawberry-like appearance of the tongue. Scarlet fever is treated by antibiotics, rest, and a cool mist humidifier. If left untreated, it can result in conditions that affect the heart, kidneys, and other parts of the body.

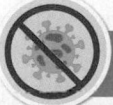 Infection Control

The CDC Advisory Committee on Immunization recommends a DTaP vaccine for all school-age children and tetanus vaccine boosters every 10 years.

 Infection Control

Treating a Patient with Active TB

The CDC and ADA state that standard precautions are insufficient to prevent transmission of TB in the dental office. They recommend using the "Dental Management Protocol for Active Tuberculosis Patient" described in detail on the ADA web page. It is recommended to defer elective dental treatment until the patient's physician declares that they are noninfectious. Urgent dental care should be provided in a facility with capacity for airborne infection isolation and that has a respiratory protection program in place (uses fitted, disposable N-95 respirators).

Strep infections are also the causative factor for pneumonia, rheumatic fever, dental decay, and endocarditis. The ADA recommends prophylactic antibiotic treatment prior to any dental procedures that may cause endocarditis in patients with underlying cardiac conditions.

Pneumonia Pneumonia is also an infection of the lungs. Bacteria, viruses, or fungi may cause pneumonia. The most common cause of bacterial pneumonia is *Streptococcus pneumoniae*. The most common cause of viral pneumonia is influenza; therefore, annual influenza vaccines are provided as a preventive measure. Fungal pneumonia is the type most often associated with **AIDS** patients.

Legionnaires' Disease Legionnaires' disease is a type of potentially fatal pneumonia caused by bacteria. It is usually contracted by breathing in a mist from water that contains *Legionella pneumophila*, an aerobic bacterium. The mist may come from hot tubs, showers, air-conditioning units, or biofilm found in dental unit waterlines. Dental office infection control includes monitoring and treatment of dental unit waterlines. Legionnaire's disease was named after an epidemic of the disease that occurred during the Philadelphia American Legion convention. The symptoms include high fever, chills, a cough, muscle pain, and headaches. Prompt treatment with antibiotics usually cures Legionnaire's disease. Older adults, smokers, and people with weakened immune systems are more at risk.

Methicillin-Resistant Staphylococcus Aureus (MRSA) MRSA is a strain of staph bacteria that is resistant to many antibiotics (penicillin, methicillin) that treat staph infections. Most MRSA infections begin as skin infections and develop into a painful skin boil (Figure 10-3). MRSA can spread, causing life-threatening bloodstream infections, pneumonia, and surgical site infections. It is transferred by skin-to-skin contact or by touching contaminated objects. The at-risk groups include high school wrestlers, child care workers, and people in crowded conditions. To help prevent the spread of MRSA infections, wash hands using soap and water or an alcohol-based sanitizer, shower immediately after exercise, don't share items that touch the bare skin, cover cuts and scrapes, and wash uniforms after each use.

Dental Caries The primary bacteria causing dental caries (tooth decay) are *Streptococcus mutans*. The initial breakdown, or demineralization, of the enamel surface of teeth is caused by the colonization of these bacteria, acid by-products of the bacteria, and loss of tooth structure. Once this initial breakdown occurs, other bacteria, such as *Lactobacilli* and *Actinomyces,* gain access to the inner regions of the tooth.

Current evidence-based research indicates that *Streptococcus mutans* can be transmitted from parent or caregiver to an infant or child by direct or indirect contact. Direct contact occurs through kissing or by a parent or other caregiver cleaning a pacifier or bottle nipple with their own saliva and then giving it back to the child. Indirect contact occurs through the sharing of eating utensils, cups, or toothbrushes.

Although dental decay is a preventable disease, the CDC reports it is the most common chronic disease among children and adolescents from 6 to 19 years of age. Research has shown that water fluoridation can reduce dental decay in children's teeth by up to 40%.

Viral Diseases

Viral diseases are widespread diseases caused by viruses. They are contagious and spread from person to person when a virus enters the body and begins to multiply. Viruses can enter the body in several ways: breathing in airborne droplets infected with a virus; eating food or drinking water contaminated with a virus; having an unprotected sexual relationship with a person infected with a sexually transmitted virus; touching surfaces or body fluids contaminated with a virus; and indirectly by a virus host, such as a mosquito.

Bloodborne diseases, or **bloodborne pathogens,** are of great concern. The Occupational Safety and Health Administration (OSHA) addresses this problem in the Bloodborne Pathogen Standard (see Chapter 11). Bloodborne diseases of concern to the dental assistant are viral hepatitis (HBV) and human immunodeficiency virus (HIV), which later might develop into acquired immunodeficiency syndrome (AIDS). These diseases are transmitted directly through contaminated blood and other body fluids.

Childhood Diseases Measles, mumps, and rubella are highly contagious childhood diseases caused by viruses. These

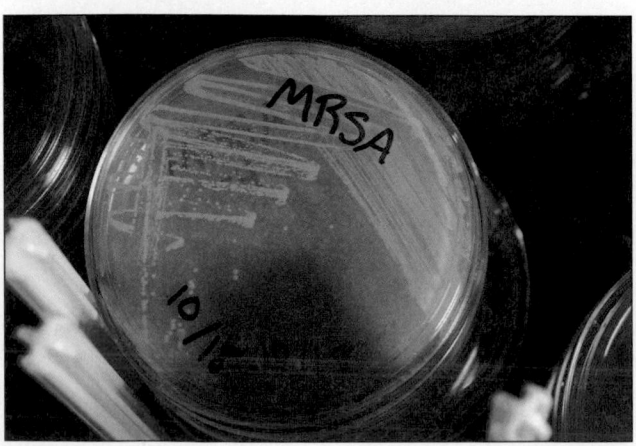

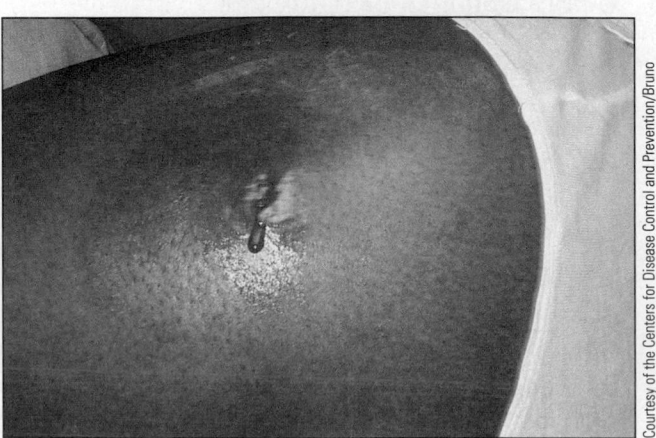

FIGURE 10-3
MRSA bacterium and an example of MRSA skin lesion.

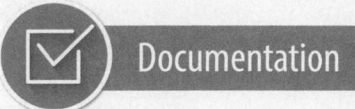
Documentation

Documentation for patients with an infectious disease should include the following information:

- Treatment for the condition, medications, oral implications
- Record of all consultations with specialists
- Results of specific laboratory tests that affect dental treatment

viruses are spread from person-to-person by respiratory droplets (sneezing and coughing) and by contact with objects contaminated with the virus. Before the development of vaccines, all of these childhood diseases were common illnesses in infants, children, and young adults, but now they can be prevented by the combination MMR (measles, mumps, and rubella) vaccine.

The *measles* virus causes fever, runny nose, cough, and a rash all over the body, and many children get an ear infection. Of the infected children, one out of 20 will contract pneumonia and one of every 1,000 will die. Measles is spread by sneezing and coughing. Small, bluish-white spots (Koplik spots) occur on reddish mucosa on the inside of the cheeks, palate, and throat two days before the measles skin rash appears.

Mumps is caused by the mumps virus. Infected persons have a few days of fever, headache, tiredness, muscle aches, and loss of appetite, which are followed by painful swelling of the parotid glands (salivary glands in front of the ear). Complications in teenage males and men may include infertility and subfertility.

Rubella, also called German measles, is caused by the rubella virus. It appears as a rash on the face and may spread to the trunk and limbs. If a mother is infected within the first trimester, the child may be born with congenital rubella syndrome (CRS). Common characteristics of CRS include deafness, eye abnormalities, and congenital heart disease.

Chickenpox is a highly contagious childhood disease caused by the *varicella zoster virus* (VZV), which is spread easily through coughing, sneezing, and contact with contaminated objects. Early symptoms include nausea, loss or appetite, and aching muscles followed by a rash of small read bumps that progress into blisters (200–500 itchy blisters) and pustules (blisters containing pus), oral sores, and fever. Complications with chickenpox may be shingles, arterial ischemic stroke (AIS), and dangers to the fetus of an infected mother. Effects on the fetus can range from underdeveloped toes and fingers to severe malformations of the bladder, brain, and eyes and other neurological disorders. A varicella vaccine is available to prevent the occurrence of chickenpox. Before the vaccine, about four million people would become infected and 100–150 died each year as a result of chickenpox.

Common Cold   The common cold (**nasopharyngitis, rhinopharyngitis**) is a viral infectious disease of the upper respiratory tract primarily affecting the nose. The cold is caused by over 200 virus strains, with rhinoviruses the most common, and affects over one billion people in the United States each year. The cold is spread by air droplets when a sick person sneezes, cough, or blows their nose. Symptoms include coughing, sneezing, sore throat, stuffy nose, runny nose, and fever that generally last 10 days. The cold may lead to pneumonia. There is no cure for the common cold.

Documentation

- Patients should be advised of the importance of keeping the medical history up-to-date. Informing dental health care professionals of all current health conditions, medications, and exposures to and immunizations to prevent communicable diseases assists in providing the most comprehensive oral health care to each patient.
- Appointments may need to be postponed based on infectious disease status to ensure respect for the health and safety of the patient and the dental team. Documentation of such postponement should include the rationale.
- Patients should be advised of the importance of thorough oral hygiene with toothbrush and dental floss to lower the bacterial count and decrease aerosol contamination in the treatment room.
- Patients should be educated about the possibility of transferring oral bacteria to children.

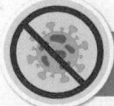
Infection Control

Experts from the **FDA, WHO, CDC,** and other institutions conduct research of virus samples collected from around the world to make annual recommendations for influenza vaccinations. Through this research, they identify the viruses most likely to cause illness during the upcoming influenza season, usually from October to May. The CDC recommends annual vaccination as the primary step in protecting against influenza illness.

Influenza *Influenza,* commonly referred to as the flu, is a serious respiratory illness caused by the influenza viruses; this includes influenza A (H1N1), influenza A (H3N2), and influenza B viruses. Common symptoms include fever, cough, sore throat, runny/stuffy nose, body aches, and headaches, and some may have vomiting and diarrhea. The flu is easily spread by coughs, sneezes, and touching an infected person or contaminated objects. It may lead to severe complications, especially for the very old and young. Persons with asthma and other lung diseases are at a higher risk of developing complications and even dying from the flu. The CDC recommends yearly flu vaccination.

Influenza A viruses that can cross between species are also called swine flu. Up until recently, it was not known to affect humans. Virus B influenza only infects humans. The best prevention against catching the flu is to receive the vaccine and frequently wash hands.

West Nile Virus. The *West Nile Virus (WNV)* can be very serious. It is often thought of as a seasonal virus that arrives in the spring and continues until the fall. It is transmitted by means of mosquito bites and, according to the CDC, can develop into a severe illness in about one in 150 infected people. The symptoms of severe illness can include extreme high fever, neck stiffness, disorientation, headache, convulsions, tremors, muscle weakness, vision loss, coma, numbness, and paralysis lasting several weeks; however, some symptoms can become permanent. Mild symptoms occur in about 20% of the people infected and include fever, head and body aches, nausea, vomiting, and lymph glands that are swollen, along with a skin rash on the back, chest, and stomach. The symptoms can last from a few days to several weeks. The majority of people who are infected with West Nile Virus will not have symptoms. The CDC states that "about four out of five who are infected with WNV will not show any symptoms at all." If symptoms occur, they will develop between three to fourteen days after the infected mosquito bite. No identified treatment is used to treat WNV, but symptoms are treated to make the patient comfortable.

Herpes Viruses Herpetic lesions present a significant problem for dental health care workers. **Herpes** simplex virus type 1 (HSV-1) is the most common type of herpetic infection and is characterized by distinct local symptoms such as blisters on the lips marked by a period of altered sensation and swelling. The initial infection of the herpes simplex virus is through close contact with an

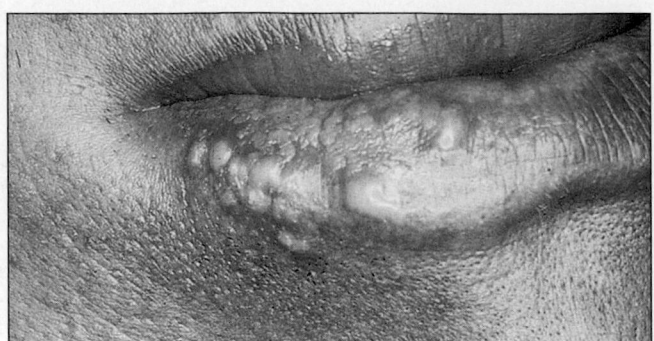

FIGURE 10-4
Herpeticlabialis lesion.

Courtesy of Joseph L. Konzelman, Jr., DDS

infected person. An infected person can pass the virus on through kissing, touching, or sharing objects such as toothbrushes, lip balm, razors, towels, and eating utensils. Once infected, the virus goes through periods of being dormant and active. Activation of the virus can be brought on by fatigue, stress, exposure to sunlight, trauma to the affected area, high-acid foods, or immunosuppression. The sores associated with HSV-1 frequently develop when the patient has a cold or fever and have become commonly referred to as fever blisters or cold sores (Figure 10-4). Lesions may also occur on the palate or gingiva. There is no cure for HSV-1; the sores will heal without treatment. Some people prefer treatment for the uncomfortable symptoms of burning, itching, and tingling associated with the lesions. Prescription antiviral medications such as Acyclovir, Famciclovir, and Valacyclovir can be applied topically or taken systemically.

Primary herpes is highly contagious and usually makes its initial appearance in children one to three years of age. The child may develop a fever and experience pain in the mouth, increased salivation, bad breath, and a general feeling of illness. Healing of the lesions occurs naturally within three days. After this initial infection, the virus lies dormant and may reappear later in life as fever blisters or cold sores. This is referred to as recurrent herpes labialis.

Herpes simplex virus type 2 (HSV-2) is also known as genital herpes. This is one of the most common sexually transmitted infections (STIs) in the United States. Once infected with the virus, outbreak may recur. This disease is highly transmissible, even before signs are evident. Microscopically, HSV-1 and HSV-2 are almost identical. The difference between them is their choice of location

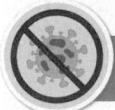

Infection Control

Herpes transmission occurs through direct contact with lesions. However, if there are no active lesions, there is the possibility of transmission through saliva or aerosol spray from a dental handpiece. Protective eyewear and gloves are particularly important in prohibiting infection.

Should patients who have active oral herpes be seen in the dental office?

According to the CDC, there are two treatments that should be provided: emergency treatment for dental conditions and treatment of the lesion. No other treatment should be rendered.

Should a dental health care profession with active herpes treat patients?

Because herpes is transmittable to patients from dental health care professionals who have active herpes, direct patient care should be restricted.

or site of latency. HSV-1 establishes its site of latency in the trigeminal nerve, the nerve associated with sensations in the face and the motor functions of biting and chewing. HSV-1 outbreaks typically occur on the face and lips. HSV-2 establishes its site of latency in the nerves at the base of the spine. HSV-2 outbreaks typically occur in the genital and anal regions. However, it should be understood that both viruses could occur in either or both parts of the body. Both HSV-1 and HSV-2 can be spread to other parts of the body and to other people. To avoid this, do not kiss when either you or your partner have a cold sore; avoid oral sex in the presence of lesions on either the lips or genitals; avoid sexual contact whenever sores are present; always use a condom for sexual intercourse, even when symptoms are not present; do not wet contact lenses with saliva.

Outbreaks can be stimulated by times of stress or illness or by the friction of sexual intercourse. Symptoms of HSV-2 outbreaks include cracked, raw, or red areas around the genitals; itching or tingling around the genital and/or anal region; small blisters around the genital and/or anal region; pain with urination from urine passing over the sores; headache; fatigue; lower backache, and flu-like symptoms, including fever and swollen glands. These symptoms are not unique to HSV-2; diagnosis by a health care provider will be based upon a physical examination and a swab test of a fresh sore or fluid from a blister.

There is no cure for HSV-2; the sores will heal without treatment. Some people prefer treatment for the uncomfortable symptoms of burning, itching, and tingling associated with the lesions. Prescription antiviral medications such as Acyclovir, Famciclovir, and Valacyclovir can be applied topically or taken systemically.

Additional herpetic infections include herpes zoster (chicken pox and shingles), Epstein-Barr (mononucleosis, pharyngeal cancer, and lymphoma), and herpetic whitlow, an infection affecting the fingers, usually distinguished by pain and fluid-containing vesicles.

HIV and AIDS

The human immunodeficiency virus (HIV) is a bloodborne viral disease infecting and killing special CD4 T-cells in the body. CD4 (cluster of differentiation 4) is found on the surface of immune cells like T-helper cells. CD4 T-cells are white blood cells that initiate the body's response to infection. In the case of HIV, the virus attaches to the CD4 cells, and then infects and damages the cell and aids HIV in replication. If CD4 cells become depleted, the body is left vulnerable to a wide range of infections. HIV is spread by sexual contact with infected persons, by infected needles, and by transfusions. It can also be passed from infected mother to child during pregnancy, labor, delivery, and breast-feeding. People who have HIV but are unaware that they carry it are called asymptomatic carriers. Some have vague complaints, such as fever, weight loss, or unexplained diarrhea. HIV attacks body organs such as the kidneys, heart, and brain.

The patient's immune system becomes unable to fight the HIV infection, causing serious illnesses that can lead to acquired immunodeficiency syndrome (AIDS). After much research, the virus was found to be transmitted via the semen and blood of infected individuals. "Casual" spreading of the disease does not seem to happen. For example, kissing does not spread the disease. A person with full-blown AIDS exhibits cancers, infections, diarrhea, or a number of other viral diseases. In most cases, the disease progresses and the infected individual develops some brain damage in the form of dementia. If the individual is in this state for a long period of time, more severe brain damage may occur; normally, the infected individual most likely succumbs to AIDS before this happens. The prognosis is often fatal, but life may be sustained for a number of years with appropriate diet and health measures. Current treatment focuses on symptoms and not the disease itself.

There is no cure for AIDS. The complications are treated accordingly. Several antiviral drugs are used, such as Zidovudine (AZT) and Acyclovir. AZT has a number of side effects but has been shown to slow progression of the disease. Research continues in an effort to find a vaccine for HIV, with several drugs showing promise.

Hepatitis

Hepatitis is a viral infection affecting the liver. The liver is responsible for processing everything an individual consumes and is, therefore, susceptible to injury, inflammation, and infection. At least five different types of hepatitis viruses, lettered A through E, are known. The most common types are Hepatitis A, B, and C (Table 10-1). Hepatitis is very contagious while the patient has symptoms. It can be transmitted by hepatitis carriers with the presence of chronic infection. It is important for the dental assistant to ask if the patient has ever had hepatitis. Carriers do not always develop symptoms and may never get sick, but they can pass the virus to other people in close personal contact.

Hepatitis A virus (HAV) is an acute infection contracted by consuming contaminated food. This is the least serious form of viral hepatitis and is vaccine-preventable. HAV is common in developing countries. In the United States, the risk factor is international travel.

Hepatitis B (HBV) can cause chronic infection. This virus is found in blood and certain body fluids, such as saliva, and is spread when a person comes in contact with infected blood or body fluids. The symptoms include loss of appetite, digestive upset, upper abdominal pain and tenderness, fever, weakness, muscle pain, and jaundice (yellowing of the skin). *Hepatitis B* is of major concern to dental personnel and is commonly referred to as serum hepatitis. A blood test may be taken from a person exposed to HBV. The presence of hepatitis B surface antigen (HBsAg) indicates the person is infectious.

Hepatitis C (HCV), often called non-A and non-B, reacts somewhat like hepatitis B. Symptoms include upper-right abdominal pain, dark urine, light-colored bowel movements, jaundice, and nausea. About 50 percent of the people infected become chronic carriers. Chronic HCV is usually curable with oral medications taken every day for two to six months.

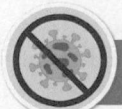

Infection Control

Personal protective equipment such as gloves, mask, and a face shield provide protection of the dental health care team from contracting diseases such as HIV and COVID-19.

TABLE 10-1 Types of Viral Hepatitis

Disease & Cause	Transmission	Symptoms	Prevention	Long-Term Effects
Viral Hepatitis A (HAV)	Human feces of persons with HAV being transmitted to oral cavity of other person. Example: not washing hands after using bathroom and then preparing food.	Fatigue, loss of appetite, fever, nausea, diarrhea, and jaundice.	• Hepatitis A vaccine recommended for people 12 months and older. • Wash hands. • Immune globulin can be taken within 2 weeks of contact.	• No chronic infection. • Have it only once.
Viral Hepatitis B (HBV)	• Blood from Infected person enters a person who is not infected. • Spread through contaminated needles, or other sharps. • Sex. • Infected mother to baby during birth.	Fatigue, loss of appetite, fever, nausea, vomiting, joint and abdominal pain, and jaundice. Approximately 1/3 of infected persons have no symptoms.	• Hepatitis B vaccine. • Use of latex condom during sexual activity. • Don't shoot drugs and share needles. • Don't share items that may have blood on them.	• 15–25% will die from chronic liver disease. • High rate of chronic liver disease in infants born to infected mothers.
Viral Hepatitis C (HCB)	• Blood from Infected person enters a person who is not infected. • Spread through contaminated needles, or other sharps. • From Infected mother to baby during birth. • It can be spread through sexual activity but that is rare.	Fatigue, loss of appetite, nausea, abdominal pain, dark urine, and jaundice.	• No vaccine. • Don't shoot drugs and share needles. • Don't share items that may have blood on them. • Wash hands.	• Chronic infection in 55–85% of infected individuals. • 1–5% may die. • Leading indication for liver transplant. • Leading indication for liver transplant. • Uncommon in the United States.
Viral Hepatitis D (HDV)	Same as viral hepatitis B: • Blood from Infected person enters a person who is not infected. • Spread through contaminated needles, or other sharps. • Sex. • Infected mother to baby during birth.	Fatigue, loss of appetite, nausea, vomiting, joint and abdominal pain, jaundice, and dark urine.	• Hepatitis B vaccine. • Education to reduce risk behaviors.	If co-infection with HBV, the individual may have more severe symptoms and is more likely to have chronic liver disease.
Viral Hepatitis E (HEV)	Same as HAV: Human feces of persons with HAV being transmitted to oral cavity of other person. Example: not washing hands after bathroom and then preparing food.	Fatigue, loss of appetite, nausea, vomiting, dark urine, and jaundice.	• No vaccine. • Wash hands.	• No long-term infection. • More severe in pregnant women in their third trimester.

This information was taken from the Centers for Disease Control Web site fact sheets for Viral Hepatitis A–E.

Vaccines are available to prevent HAV and HBV but not for HCV. These vaccines are administered in a series of three injections. The schedule is an initial injection, then one a month later, and then another three months after the first vaccine administration. After completing the three series of HBV vaccines, a blood test is performed to ensure that immunity has developed. A booster dosage is not recommended by the CDC unless an exposure incident has occurred or it is recommend by a physician after a blood test.

Hepatitis D virus (HDV) cannot occur without the presence of HBV. Symptoms include joint pain, abdominal pain, and jaundice.

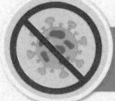 **Infection Control**

It should be noted that, according to OSHA standards, the employer is responsible for offering the HBV 3 series vaccination to new employees within 10 days of employment at no cost to the employee. The employee can refuse the vaccine by signing an informed refusal form that is to be kept in the employee's file. After completing the three series of HBV, a blood test is performed to ensure that immunity has developed. The employer is not responsible for the blood test, because it is not noted in the OSHA standard, but it is an important step for the dental assistant to take to ensure prevention of hepatitis B. If the dental assistant tests negative for seroconversion, the physician must make a determination about additional dosages of the HBV vaccine. (See Chapter 11, Infection Control, for more details).

Vaccination against HBV will prevent infection with HDV. Hepatitis E (HEV) is not transmitted through bloodborne contact. This disease is most often seen in developing countries in Africa, Asia, and Latin America. It is transmitted through contaminated food or water via the fecal–oral route.

Hepatitis E (HEV) is found in the feces of people and animals and is therefore spread through contaminated water and food. The symptoms are loss of appetite, dark urine, fatigue, and nausea. To prevent this disease, an individual should wash hands carefully when preparing food, and when traveling they should take special care in avoiding contaminated water.

Ebola

Ebola is a virus in which the symptoms appear anywhere from 2 to 21 days after exposure. The transmission is spread through bodily fluids of a person who is sick or has died from Ebola. The symptoms include fever greater than 101 degrees, diarrhea, sore throat, severe headache, vomiting, joint/muscle ache, abdominal pain, rash, and internal bleeding. Some individuals with the disease bleed from the eyes, nose, ears, and rectum. In 2014, Ebola affected multiple countries in West Africa where the largest incidence of infection in history took place. The highest risk is to friends and family of the infected individual and the health care workers taking care of the patient. Many new guidelines for caring for Ebola-infected individuals have been put in place. The Centers for Disease Control CDC is a good source for updated information.

Epstein-Barr Virus and Infectious Mononucleosis

Epstein-Barr Virus (EBV) is one of the most common viruses in humans. The Centers for Disease Control (CDC) reports that close to 95% of adults between the ages of 35 and 40 have been infected with EBV. When infants, children, or young adults are infected, about 35% to 50% (according to the CDC) develop infectious *mononucleosis*. Symptoms of EBV are not much different from any other childhood illness; mononucleosis symptoms are fever, sore throat, and swollen lymph glands. Other symptoms such as liver concerns, a swollen spleen, and heart or nervous system involvement rarely occur, and this disease is almost never fatal. Laboratory tests along with the reporting of the symptoms help determine if the individual is indeed infected with the disease. The patient may need rest, and the symptoms are gone in about one to two months. EBV transmission occurs with intimate contact with saliva, which is why this disease is referred to as the "kissing disease." The newly infected individual will experience symptoms within four to six weeks after contact.

Zika Virus

The *Zika* virus is transmitted by mosquitoes from Africa (named after the Zika forest in Uganda) and other tropical regions, including South America. It generally causes a mild illness that lasts for several days and has symptoms that include a fever, joint pain, rash, and conjunctivitis (painful, red eyes). The greatest concern is the increased incidence of microcephaly (small head), hearing deficits, defects of the eye, and impaired growth in infants born to pregnant women infected with the virus. There is no cure or antiviral treatment for the Zika virus and symptoms are treated with rest, fluids, and mild pain relievers.

Novel Coronavirus

There was an outbreak of the novel (new) coronavirus SARS-CoV-2 (also referred to as COVID-19) first identified in China in August of 2019 which quickly spread to other international locations (more than two dozen countries). The CDC closely monitored the new disease. The WHO declared COVID-19 as a pandemic on March 11, 2020. NIH states that the "COVID-19 pandemic is among the deadliest infectious diseases to have emerged in recent history." The virus is spread by respiratory droplets when in contact with an infected person, has four to five days of incubation, and symptoms appear 2-14 days after exposure to the virus. COVID-19 primarily affects the respiratory system and reports state that the heart, brain and kidney can also be affected. People at the greatest risk of severe illness or death are age 65 or older. 8 out of 10 COVID-19 deaths reported in the U.S. have been in people 65 years old and older, and those with underlying medical conditions (cancer, chronic kidney disease, chronic lung disease, diabetes, heart conditions, obesity, weakened immunocompromised, and pregnancy).

People with COVID-19 have a wide range of symptoms from mild symptoms to severe illness. The symptoms can include fever, cough, shortness of breath, fatigue, muscle or body aches, headache, new loss of taste or smell, sore throat, congestion or runny nose, nausea or vomiting, and diarrhea. When outbreaks occur, the CDC sends constant updates about the disease for health providers. The ADA issued an interim recommendation on April 1, 2020 that advised dentists to keep their offices closed to all but urgent and emergency procedures. The FDA issued an Emergency Use Authorization (EAU) allowing the use of vaccines to prevent COVID-19 in individuals 18 years of age and older.

Protozoal Diseases

Most protozoa do not cause disease but may live in hosts as parasites, causing damage. For example, protozoa are found in the periodontal tissues of some patients who have just completed radiation treatment. Some protozoa are responsible for intestinal infections, while others cause infection in the blood, lungs, liver, or brain.

Amebiasis

Amebiasis is most common to people living in tropical areas with poor sanitation. Symptoms include stomach cramping and pain, loose stools, and fever. Though rare, it can spread to the liver and the brain. It is recommended that travelers to areas outside the United States drink only bottled water and carbonated beverages, such as soda. Drug treatment is necessary to effectively kill the parasite.

Periodontal Disease

Periodontal disease, periodontitis, is caused by protozoa and bacteria. Both microorganisms are found in the inflamed tissue around the tooth. Protozoa are in the **biofilm** in the periodontal pockets around the tooth. Treatment includes a thorough cleaning around the area to remove any biofilm and diseased tissue and then impeccable oral hygiene maintenance. Periodontal disease is covered in more detail in Chapter 38.

Giardiasis

The parasite associated with this disease lives in the intestines of infected people or animals. It is passed through fecal contamination. Giardiasis can be contracted by drinking water from contaminated sources or touching surfaces contaminated with fecal matter. Symptoms include upset stomach, diarrhea, and dehydration. Those at risk for contracting giardiasis are childcare providers, hikers, campers, and international travelers. Prevention includes conscientious hand hygiene and not drinking or eating contaminated water or food.

Malaria Malaria and sleeping sickness are two other diseases caused by protozoa. Both are prevalent throughout the tropics and have symptoms during the first two weeks, such as fever and soreness at the point of entry. Malaria is spread via mosquito bites, and sleeping sickness is spread by the tsetse fly. Both require drug therapy to kill the parasites in the bites.

Fungal Diseases

Although most fungal infections are mild, they can become life threatening in immunosuppressed patients and the elderly. *Candida albicans* is a common fungus or yeast found in the oral cavity, gastrointestinal tract, and female genital tract and on the skin. Oral *candidiasis* is considered an opportunistic infection characterized by white membranes on the surface of the oral mucosa and tongue. The disease may cause raised patches that may become irritated and cause discomfort. It is commonly called thrush, or moniliasis (Figure 10-5). If antibiotics destroy too many of the "normal" bacteria, or if the body's immune system is impaired, such as is the case with acquired immunodeficiency syndrome (AIDS), then the fungi multiply and overgrow. Treatment includes topical antifungal medications such as clotrimazole lozenges (troches) and nystatin mouth swishes (suspension).

Candidemia This fungal infection occurs when *Candida* enters the bloodstream, where it can spread, causing infection in other parts of the body, such as the kidneys, liver, spleen, and eyes. Symptoms depend upon the organ affected. According to the CDC, people at risk for contracting *Candidemia* are surgical patients, intensive care patients, HIV/AIDS patients, and low-birth-weight infants. Diagnosis is by blood culture, and treatment is with antifungal medications.

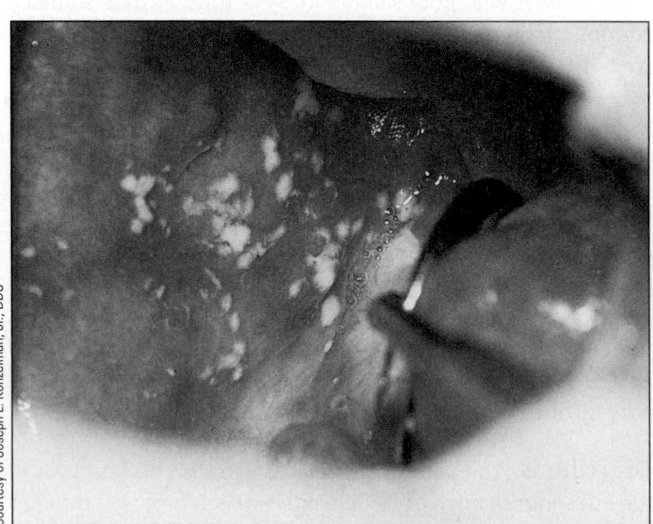

Courtesy of Joseph L. Konzelman, Jr., DDS

FIGURE 10-5
Patient presenting with thrush.

Coccidioidomycosis *Coccidioidomycosis* is commonly referred to as Valley Fever. It is contracted by inhalation of **fungal spores** disrupted from soil. This disease causes flu-like symptoms including fever, cough, muscle aches, and joint pain. Valley Fever is common in the southwest areas of the United States, with the majority of cases specific to Arizona. It is diagnosed by microscopic examination of the sputum or infected tissues and a chest x-ray. Though spontaneous resolution without treatment is most common, sometimes antifungal medications may be used.

Rickettsial Diseases

There are about 800 species of ticks in the world and fewer than 60 species transmit bacteria when they bite. One group of bacteria that ticks carry is rickettsiae, which causes Rocky Mountain spotted fever.

Rocky Mountain Spotted Fever Rocky Mountain spotted fever is a rare bacterial infection caused by the bite of an infected tick. Symptoms occur about a week to 10 days after transmission from the host and are much like those of the flu, consisting of fever, headache, nausea, vomiting, and muscle pain. Two to six days after the symptoms first occur, small pink spots appear on the ankles and wrists. The body is soon covered with these spots. Treatment with antibiotics normally cures the disease.

Typhus Typhus, also known as typhus fever, is another fairly rare disease, similar to Rocky Mountain spotted fever. The microorganism is spread by infected lice, mites, and fleas. Symptoms appear rapidly and include a severe headache, nausea, vomiting, back and limb pain, constipation, and high fever. A rash similar to measles appears, the heart beats weakly, and confusion is common. Typhus fever is treated with antibiotic drug therapy.

Algal Diseases One alga, *prothotheca*, causes the disease protothecosis, which is found principally among people living in the tropics. This disease occurs in populations with poor nutrition or poor sanitation and in persons with impaired immune systems. The primary symptom is the formation of skin ulcers. Treatment consists of antifungal therapy and surgical removal of isolated lesions.

Prion Diseases

Prions are a relatively new and separate class of infectious particles, unlike bacteria, fungi, viruses, and other known pathogens. Prions are not considered a major group but are unique due to their lack of both DNA and RNA, nucleic acids found in the nuclei of all other living organisms.

Animal Prion Disease Prion diseases affect a number of animal species, including cattle, sheep, goats, mink, and cats. Although the cause is not completely understood, it is thought that contaminated feed is the causative agent.

Bovine spongiform encephalopathy (BSE) is a progressive neurological disorder that affects cattle. BSE is commonly called mad cow disease. Eating the meat of affected cattle is responsible for acquiring vCJD.

Human Prion Disease Prion diseases are also known as transmissible spongiform encephalopathies (TSE). These diseases typically progress rapidly and are always fatal. Prions are not typically considered to be airborne; they enter the body by eating infected foods or are introduced directly to the brain via contaminated instruments during neurosurgery. The prion proteins invade the brain, resulting in severe brain damage. Signs and symptoms include impaired brain function, dementia, personality changes, and impaired motor control.

Variant Creutzfeldt-Jakob Disease Variant Creutzfeldt-Jakob disease (vCJD) is associated with mad cow disease; it is the human form of mad cow disease. This form is not inherited. It is acquired by eating beef from cattle affected with the disease. Signs and symptoms of this form are primarily psychological and behavioral in nature. The median duration of symptoms of illness is 13 to 14 months and the median age at death is 28. Great precautions are being taken by the Centers for Disease Control and Prevention and the United States Department of Agriculture to monitor the beef industry for this disease.

Creutzfeldt-Jakob Disease Creutzfeldt-Jakob disease (CJD) is not associated with mad cow disease. This disease is familial in origin, meaning that the altered gene was inherited from an affected parent. The median duration of symptoms of illness is four to five months, and the median age at death is sixty-eight. It presents with rapidly progressing dementia, memory loss, speech impairment, involuntary jerky movements, weakness, blindness, and then coma. The disease is fatal due to the neurological deterioration. CJD is rare; the worldwide rate is approximately one case per one million people.

There are several variants of this disease that affect individuals earlier in life. The cause of the disease is currently unknown. It is believed that this disease is related to the prion proteins, but some think that it is a slowly growing virus that is latent, suppressed, or dormant for a period of time.

Harmful Effects of Normal Flora

There are some harmful effects associated with normal flora. As mentioned previously, normal flora synthesizes and excretes certain vitamins that are helpful to the human host. These same vitamins can also serve as nutrition for potentially pathogenic bacteria, helping them to survive and grow.

Some members of the normal flora may become pathogenic if they travel to a distant site that is compromised or that cannot survive the host's defenses. Bacteria of the normal flora depend on the host for transmission to a compromised host in whom they can become pathogenic. For example, *Streptococcus pneumoniae* exists as normal flora in the pharynx and mouth of healthy individuals. However, if the individual should become compromised through lack of sleep, poor nutrition, or illness, this bacterium can become pathogenic, causing pneumonia. This can then be transmitted to others, spreading this infectious disease. See Table 10-2 for examples of other bacterium of normal flora capable of becoming pathogenic.

Normal Oral Flora Normal flora of the oral cavity includes *Streptococci, Lactobacilli, Staphylococci,* and *Corynebacteria,* as well as numerous anaerobes, especially *Bacteroides.* At birth, the oral cavity is sterile, but it becomes colonized through exposure to the environment. Until teeth erupt, the predominant bacterium is *Streptococcus salivarius.* As teeth erupt, the bacterial colonization includes *S. mutans* and *S. sanguis.* The diversity of the oral flora continues to increase over time, with Bacteroides and spirochetes colonizing around the time of puberty.

The normal oral flora provides the same benefits of normal flora elsewhere in the body, as described earlier. By occupying colonization sites, it makes it difficult for pathogenic bacteria to colonize. Normal flora also synthesizes and secretes vitamins for use by the host; contributes to immunity by introducing low-levels of antigens that stimulate the production of antibodies; and influences the oral environment with the secretion of peroxides and bacteriocins, which are toxic to other potentially pathogenic bacteria.

Conversely, bacteria of the oral cavity can induce various oral diseases, such as abscesses, gingivitis, periodontitis, and dental caries. If the oral bacteria gain entrance into the body system, they can cause destruction of the alveolar bone, lungs, brain, and heart valves. These can all result from actions of the normal oral flora.

TABLE 10-2 Normal Flora Capable of Becoming Pathogenic

Bacterium	Normal Flora	Potential Pathogen
Staphylococcus aureus	Skin, nose, pharynx, mouth, lower gastrointestinal tract, vagina	Yes; leading cause of bacterial infection in humans
Streptococcus mutans	Pharynx, mouth	Yes; involved in biofilm formation and initiation of caries
Streptococcus pneumoniae	Pharynx, mouth	Yes; leading cause of pneumonia
Streptococcus pyogenes	Pharynx, mouth	Yes; strep throat, pneumonia, endocarditis
Pseudomonas aeruginosa	Lower gastrointestinal tract	Yes; opportunistic pathogen capable of invading any tissue
Haemophilus influenzae	Nose, pharynx, mouth	Yes; influenza and meningitis

Components of Biofilm Microscopic examination of dental biofilm reveals colonies of bacteria embedded in an adhesive substance called the *pellicle*. Biofilm is composed of bacteria, extracellular products, and components of saliva, the pellicle, that adhere to the surfaces of the teeth.

The primary bacterial components are *Streptococcus sanguis* and *Streptococcus mutans*. The bacteria in biofilm produce enzymes and toxins that can cause inflammation of the gingival tissues. This is called gingivitis. Inflammation causes the gingival tissues to appear red and swollen and may cause the gums to bleed. Continued accumulation of biofilm can lead to destruction of the tissues that surround and support the teeth. This is called periodontal disease or periodontitis. The type of bacteria, length of time biofilm bacteria is left on the teeth, and the host's immune response are all factors that determine the extent of the inflammation and destructive processes.

Biofilm Formation Initial formation of biofilm is dependent on the pellicle, which is composed of salivary enzymes, proteins, and immunoglobulins. Once the tooth surface is covered by the pellicle, gram-positive bacteria such as *Streptococcus sanguis* and *Streptococcus mutans* begin to colonize. Protein molecules of these microorganisms interact with protein molecules of the pellicle to form an attachment mechanism. Biofilm formation begins on the exposed tooth surfaces above the gumline; this is called supragingival biofilm.

As the biofilm mass accumulates and matures, gram-negative anaerobic bacteria, such as *Actinobacillus* and *Porphyromonas*, begin to colonize. If supragingival biofilm is allowed to accumulate undisturbed by regular toothbrushing and flossing, the microbial flora continue to change, and migration of bacterial below the gumline occurs. Biofilm formation on tooth surfaces below the gumline is called subgingival biofilm. Subgingival bacterial biofilm colonies include *Prevotella nigrescens*, *Prevotella intermedia*, *Bacteroides forsythus*, and *Porphyromonas gingivalis*.

The Body's Resistance to Disease

The healthy human body is capable of self-defense against infectious diseases. These defenses may be general (nonspecific), providing protection from a wide variety of bacteria. Other defense mechanisms are specific to particular pathogens.

Nonspecific Defenses

The environment is laden with potentially pathogenic bacteria. Natural, general defenses against these bacteria help maintain health. Nonspecific defenses are the body's primary resistance to disease. These defenses include anatomical barriers, physiologic barriers, and the inflammatory response.

Anatomical Barriers The first line of defense prevents the entrance of the microorganisms to the body. The skin is a major barrier if it is not broken. Intact skin provides a barrier to internal invasion by disease-producing bacteria. Doctors are challenged with effective means of treating burn victims because these patients are severely compromised by the absence of skin. The nasal opening to the respiratory system is a good example of a natural barrier. The mucous membranes and nose hairs help to filter out potentially pathogenic airborne particles. The opening consists of a long, convoluted passage to the lungs covered by a slippery mucous membrane. The mucus continues the entrapment of airborne microorganisms and keeps most from reaching the lungs. The skull and spinal cord help to protect the central nervous system from potentially pathogenic bacteria.

Physiological Barriers Natural openings also are protected by a variety of physiological barriers. For example, the secretion of tears helps flush debris from the eye before it enters the tear ducts. After microorganisms are trapped by mucus in the respiratory tract, they are moved by cilia as well as by coughing and sneezing. The normal flora protects the host by competing with infectious organisms, preventing the organisms from invading the host tissues. For example, when the normal flora is suppressed by antibiotic treatment, opportunistic organisms are allowed to grow in numbers and are able to infect and cause disease such as oral candidiasis.

Antimicrobial elements on the body prevent most microorganisms from growing and multiplying. The nasal and oral openings are protected by nasal secretions and saliva that contain lysozymes. A lysozyme is an enzyme that breaks down the bacterial cell wall. The skin surface is composed of relatively dry, hardened cells; skin secretions are somewhat acidic, and as sweat evaporates it leaves salt on the skin. The skin's low moisture, low pH, and high salinity inhibit the growth of microorganisms.

Blood contains several protection factors, such as phagocytes and white blood cells, that kill disease-producing bacteria and infected host cells. Blood plasma provides a clotting mechanism that initiates formation of a clot to seal off the injured site, protecting from pathogenic invasion. The proteins in the blood trigger molecular events that result in inflammation.

Inflammatory Response The inflammatory response is a defense mechanism that helps prevent infectious agents from spreading further in the body, destroys the agent, and begins the healing process. The response (inflammation) is programmed in the cells and occurs when cells are damaged by microorganisms, trauma, and toxins. The characteristic signs of inflammation are swelling, redness, heat, and pain. Chemicals are released from the damaged cells and a biological response of the vascular tissues is initiated. The response signals local vasodilation to increase blood flow to the damaged area, then blood flows to the site of damage, which in turn causes redness and brings phagocytes to destroy the microorganisms and dead cells. The chemicals also cause the blood vessels to leak fluid (lymph) into the tissues and become swollen. The swelling helps to isolate the microorganisms from contact with body tissues. The heating effect during an inflammatory response is the rush of blood into the area, the body's attempt to destroy the agent and initiate the healing process. Inflammatory pain is associated with tissue damage, infiltration of immune cells, and pressure on nerve cells.

Fever or pyrexia is a process in which the body temperature rises above normal temperature values. A fever often occurs when an infection is caused by pathogens. A fever is a beneficial process as long as it does not persist or reach 39.4444° C or 103° F. Fevers act to inhibit and destabilize pathogens.

Specific Defenses

The specific immune response is activated when the general defenses are unable to prevent invasion by disease-producing bacteria. This second line of defense fights specific pathogens and pathogenic-infected host cells. Specialized white blood cells called *lymphocytes* provide this defense. These lymphocytes include T-cells, which are produced by the thymus gland, and B-cells, which are produced in the bone marrow. The thymus gland is located in the upper part of the chest behind the breastbone; it is part of both the immune system and the lymphatic system. Bone marrow is found in the hollow interior of the long bones.

Components of the specific immune response are cell **mediated** and antibody mediated. T-cells isolate or kill invading cells and make up the cell-mediated component. Together these comprise what is referred to as the **complement** system.

B-cells produce antibodies and make up the **antibody**-mediated component. When foreign substances, called antigens, enter the body, cells work at trying to recognize them and respond. This response triggers reaction from the B-cells to produce antibodies to lock onto the antigens. After this happens, whenever that same antigen enters the body, the circulating antibodies recognize it and react. This is why, for example, once a person has contracted the viral disease chickenpox, that person does not typically suffer illness from it a second time. However, this virus may lie dormant in the body's nerve cells and later cause the disease shingles. The cause of the reactivation of this virus is unclear but seems to be related to the diminished capacity of the immune response during aging. Because most people who develop shingles are over the age of 60, the CDC recommends the shingles vaccine (Shringrix).

Immunity

Immunity is the state of having sufficient biological defenses to resist the entry of harmful microbes and avoid infection and disease. Immunity involves nonspecific and specific defenses.

Innate Immunity

A person is born with the natural defense referred to as an **innate immunity** (nonspecific). Several physical, chemical, and cellular defenses work to prevent the entry, growth, and spread of microbes. Microorganisms are first encountered by the physical barriers of the skin and mucous membranes. Chemicals are signaled to attack and destroy microbes that break through the barrier. Antimicrobial substances, phagocytosis, and the inflammatory response work to prevent the occurrence of disease.

Adaptive Immunity

Adaptive immunity remembers previous encounters with specific pathogens and destroys them when they attack again. Naturally acquired immunity and artificially acquired immunity are the two major types of adaptive immunity.

Naturally acquired active immunity occurs from contact with a disease-causing agent (antigen). A person is exposed to a live pathogen and develops a primary immune response. This leads to immunological memory. When the body is encountered with an antigen, B-cells or T-cells are activated to destroy the antigen. Due to the activation, the cells have specificity for the antigen and react more swiftly in the next encounter. The body's immune system remembers the encounter with the specific antigen.

Naturally acquired passive immunity occurs when antibodies are transferred to the fetus by its mother during pregnancy. It is also provided to the newborn through breast milk containing *IgA antibodies* or *colostrum* to protect against bacterial infections. This helps protect newborns until they are able to produce their own antibodies.

Artificially acquired immunity develops through deliberate actions such as **gamma globulin** injections and **vaccines**. Artificial immunity can be acquired passively or actively. With passive immunity, antibodies or activated T-cells from an immune host are transferred to a susceptible person. This is a short-term immunization lasting only a few months. Passive immunity is used prophylactically for immunodeficiency diseases. Gamma globulin injections may be given in an attempt to temporarily boost a patient's immunity against a disease. Injections are most commonly used after exposure to hepatitis A or measles.

An antigen is induced into the host with artificially acquired active immunity. A vaccine is a substance that contains antigens that is injected into a host. It stimulates a primary response in the host against the antigen without causing symptoms of the disease. Artificially acquired active immunity sometimes lasts a lifetime.

Vaccines

Vaccinations stimulate the antibody-mediated response by introducing the body to a specific antigen without actually making the person ill. This causes the formation of the antibody so if that person should be exposed to that particular pathogen again, the circulating antibody would isolate it. B-cells cannot, however, destroy the antigens. This is the responsibility of the T-cells, which destroy the antigens marked with the antibodies produced by the B-cells.

There are five main types of vaccinations:

- Live, attenuated vaccines fight viruses. These vaccines contain viruses that have been weakened so they do not cause serious disease in people with a healthy immune system. Examples are the chickenpox vaccine and the measles, mumps, rubella (MMR) vaccine.

- Inactivated virus vaccines also fight viruses. These vaccines contain viruses that have been destroyed in the process of making the vaccine. Usually multiple doses are required to build up and maintain immunity. An example of an inactivated virus vaccine is the polio vaccine.

- Toxoid vaccines prevent disease caused by the poisons produced by bacteria. In the process of making the vaccine, the poisons (toxoids) are weakened so that they do not cause illness. An example of toxoid vaccination is the diphtheria, tetanus, and acellular pertussis (DTaP) vaccine.

- Subunit vaccinations contain only a part of the virus or bacteria, rather than the entire germ. The pertussis (whooping cough) portion of the DTaP is an example of a subunit vaccine.
- Conjugate vaccinations fight a specific type of bacteria, which have an outer coating of polysaccharides. This coating makes it difficult for the immune system to recognize the bacteria. An example of this type of vaccination is the *Haemophilus influenzae* type B (Hib) vaccine.

Recommended Vaccinations These recommendations are based on control and prevention of disease transmission. The following **immunizations** are highly recommended by the CDC for health care personnel: hepatitis B, influenza, measles, mumps, rubella, and varicella-zoster.

Vaccine Recommendations

Vaccine	Recommendations
hepatitis B	3 dose series (dose #1 now, #2 in 1 month, #3 5 months after #2 Obtain anti-HBS serologic testing 2 months after dose #3
influenza	1 dose annually
MMR (measles, mumps, rubella)	2 doses 4 weeks apart
varicella (chickenpox)	2 doses 4 weeks apart
DTaP (diphtheria, tetanus, acellular pertussis)	1 dose; boosters every 10 years

Although not a vaccination, it is important to mention here that tuberculosis testing for dental health care personnel (DHCP) is also a means of controlling and preventing disease transmission. As previously discussed, tuberculosis is caused by the resistant organism *Mycobacterium tuberculosis*. Aerosolized droplets of infected individuals during coughing, sneezing, and speaking spread this organism. Aerosols may also be created by the use of ultrasonic dental equipment and other handpieces. The Centers for Disease Control and Prevention recommends all newly hired DHCP be screened for tuberculosis and any DHCP with a persistent cough lasting more than three (3) weeks be evaluated by a medical physician.

Epidemiology

Epidemiology is the branch of medicine that studies of how disease spreads and can be controlled. Factors determining and influencing the frequency, distribution, and causes of disease in the human population are statistically examined and evaluated. The findings are reported to governmental agencies for the benefit of the public health. After identifying a communicable disease, the epidemiologist (disease detective) intervenes to end the health problem and prevent its recurrence. The benefit of epidemiology is witnessed every day when the news reports that a specific food is causing botulism and the items are removed from specific grocery stores, when specific locations are having a high incidence of a newly identified disease, or when there is an outbreak of giardiasis related to inadequate treatment of surface water.

The terms *outbreak*, *epidemic*, and *pandemic* are used to describe infectious disease situations. An outbreak exists when there are more cases of a disease than are expected in a limited location or a limited group of people. An epidemic involves a sudden situation involving large number of people over a wide geographic area. An epidemic implies a crisis situation. A pandemic refers to an epidemic that has spread over several countries affecting a large number of people.

Chapter Summary

To safeguard against pathogenic microorganism exposure in a dental office, dental assistants must understand how pathogens cause diseases in a susceptible person. Within this chapter, you have been given information about pathogenic microorganisms along with the diseases they cause and how the body can defend against them.

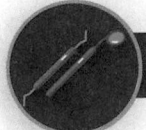

CASE STUDY

Darin Scott came down with a low-grade fever, night sweats, and weight loss. He exhibited fatigue and finally a persistent cough.

Case Study Review

1. What is one disease you would consider?
2. Is this disease common?
3. What treatment will most likely be prescribed?
4. What microorganism caused this disease?

Review Questions

Multiple Choice

1. Who discovered the germ theory of disease while studying endospores?
   a. Joseph Lister
   b. Louis Pasteur
   c. Ferdinand Cohn
   d. Robert Koch

2. Who is known as the Father of Microbiology because he discovered the process to kill germs, identified viruses, and developed the rabies vaccination and practices that minimized the spread of disease?
   a. Joseph Lister
   b. Lois Pasteur
   c. Ferdinand Cohn
   d. Robert Koch

3. Which is the study of how diseases are spread?
   a. pathology
   b. etiology
   c. epidemiology
   d. physiology

4. What term is used to describe a health condition that lasts a long time?
   a. acute
   b. pathogenic
   c. latent
   d. chronic

5. Which type of disease lies dormant and recurs when triggered?
   a. acute
   b. pathogenic
   c. latent
   d. chronic

6. Which type of bacteria requires air to survive?
   a. aerobic
   b. anaerobic
   c. facultative
   d. gram positive

7. Which form of bacteria is highly resistant to disinfectants and dying due to its enclosure in layers of protein?
   a. anaerobic
   b. spirochetes
   c. staphylococci
   d. spores

8. Which microorganism is parasitic and is responsible for most diseases?
   a. bacteria
   b. virus
   c. protozoa
   d. fungi

9. Which microorganism converts normal protein molecules into dangerous ones and is highly resistant to methods of decontamination and sterilization?
   a. bacteria
   b. algae
   c. rickettsia
   d. prions

10. Which bacterial disease may require that the patient's routine dental care be deferred until they are no longer in the active stage with symptoms?
    a. pneumonia
    b. tuberculosis
    c. streptococcal infection
    d. tetanus

11. Which bacteria has been implicated in dental caries?
    a. Staphylococcal
    b. *Mycobacterium tuberculosis*
    c. Bacillus *Corynebacterium diphtheria*
    d. *Streptococcus mutans*

12. Which viral disease forms blisters, is highly contagious, and when visible oral lesions are present, the patient may be asked to reschedule until the lesions have healed?
    a. primary herpes
    b. HIV
    c. hepatitis
    d. Epstein-Barr

13. Which viral disease is found in blood and body fluids, is a major concern, and for which OSHA requires a vaccination for dental personnel?
    a. HIV
    b. hepatitis B
    c. Epstein-Barr
    d. hepatitis C

14. What disease characterized by white membranes may be caused when a common fungus found in the oral cavity multiplies and overgrows after a patient has taken antibiotics for a long time?
    a. Candidemia
    b. Coccidiodomycosis
    c. Candidiasis
    d. thrush

15. All of these diseases can be induced by bacteria found in oral flora *except*:
    a. abscesses.
    b. gingivitis.
    c. dental caries.
    d. thrush.

16. When a person coughs, the microorganisms trapped in mucus are also moved by the hairlike organelles called _____.
    a. flagella
    b. cilia
    c. enzymes
    d. flora

17. When a patient is exposed to a live pathogen, becomes infected, and develops an immune response, it is called _____.
    a. innate immunity
    b. naturally acquired passive immunity
    c. artificially acquired immunity
    d. natural immunity

18. What term does the CDC use to describe when infectious disease occurs as a sudden situation that involves a large number of people infected over a wide geographic area?
    a. outbreak
    b. epidemic
    c. pandemic
    d. severely contagious

19. COVID-19 is an example of a(an) _____.
    a. outbreak
    b. epidemic
    c. pandemic
    d. severely contagious

20. The CDC recommends vaccines to control and prevent disease transmission. Hepatitis B, influenza, measles, mumps, rubella and varicella-zoster vaccines are recommended for healthcare personnel by the CDC.
    a. Both statements are true.
    b. Both statements are false.
    c. The 1st statement is true, the 2nd statement is false.
    d. The 1st statement is false, the 2nd statement is true.

Critical Thinking

1. Explain why the study of microbiology is important to the dental assistant.
2. What are the benefits of having healthy normal flora?
3. The CDC recommends immunizations and testing based on control and prevention of disease transmission. What vaccines and testing are recommended for the dental assistant?
4. Research the CDC web page (https://www.cdc.gov) for an outbreak, epidemic, or pandemic that is current today. Describe the area(s) that are involved along with its cause, symptoms, and how it is transmitted.

Key Terms

Term and Pronunciation	Meaning of Root and Word Parts	Definition
acute (*uh*-**kyoot**)	**acute** = sharp or severe in effect; intense	a disease or a condition with a rapid onset and a short, severe course
AIDS (**eydz**)	**A**(cquired) **I**(mmunodeficiency) **D**(efficiency) **S**(yndrome)	a disease of the immune system; transmitted primarily through blood or blood products that enter the body's bloodstream, especially through sexual contact or contact with contaminated hypodermic needles
aerobic (ai-**roh**-bik)	**aero** = air **-bios** = life	requiring the presence of air or free oxygen for life
algae (**al**-jee)	**algae** = seaweed	any of a variety of organisms that grown mostly in water; includes seaweed
anaerobic (an-*uh*-**roh**-bik)	**an-** = without **aero** = air **-bios** = life	living in the absence of air or free oxygen
antibiotic (an-ti-bahy-**ot**-ik)	**anti-** = against **biotic** = pertaining to life	a drug used to treat bacterial infections; derived from fungi and bacteria; such as penicillin and streptomycin
antibody (**an**-ti-bod-ee)	**anti-** = against **body** = referring to a physical organism	a protein produced mainly by plasma cells (a type of blood cell) used by the immune system to neutralize pathogenic bacteria and viruses

Term and Pronunciation	Meaning of Root and Word Parts	Definition
antigen (**an**-ti-j*uh* n)	**anti-** = against **-gen** = to produce	any substance capable of stimulating the production of an antibody
antimicrobial (an-tee-mahy-**kroh**-bee-*uh*l)	**anti-** = against **microbe** = a microorganism; especially a pathogenic bacterium **-al** = pertaining to	an agent that kills or inhibits the growth or reproduction of pathogenic microorganisms
antiseptic (an-t*uh*-**sep**-tik)	**anti-** = against **sepsis** = infected **-ic** = pertaining to or the nature of	a product the prevents the development of bacteria and viruses
artificially acquired immunity (ahr-t*uh*-**fish**-*uh*l-ee) (*uh*-**kwahyuhrd**) (ih-**myoo**-ni-tee)	**artificial** = not natural **acquired** = attained **immune** = protected from a disease **-ity** = expressing state or condition	protection from a disease produced by deliberate exposure to an antigen to help the body produce it's own antibodies; such as immunizations
bacteria (bak-t**eer**-ee-*uh*)	**bacteria** = group of microorganisms	one-celled organisms, spherical, spiral, or rod-shaped and appearing singly or in chains,
biofilm (**bahy**-oh-film)	**bio-** = life **film** = a thin layer or coating	a sticky mass that contains bacteria and grows in colonies on the teeth; also referred to as dental plaque
bloodborne pathogen (**bluhd**- bohrn) (**path**-*uh*-juhn)	**blood** = fluid that circulates through heart, arteries and veins; contains red blood cells, white blood cells and platelets **borne** = to be located or situated **patho-** = disease, suffering **-gen** = that which produces	a disease-producing microorganism carried or transmitted by blood; typically a disease or pathogen
budding (**buhd**-ing)	**bud** = to begin to develop **-ing** = expressing action	a small, rounded outgrowth produced from a fungus spore or cell by a process of asexual reproduction
candidiasis (kan-di-**dahy**-*uh*-sis)	**Candida** = an opportunistic pathogenic yeast located in the stomach; most common cause of fungal infections **-iasis** = combining form indicating disease	a fungal infection or disease caused by a species of *Candida*; occurs most often in the mouth, respiratory tract and vagina
carrier (**kar**-ee-er)	**carry** = to take from one place to another **-er** = a person or thing	person or thing that carries; person shows no symptoms but harbors infectious agent of a disease and capable of transmitting to others
CDC	**C**(enters) for **D**(Disease) **C**(ontrol)	Centers for Disease Control and Prevention is a US agency that publishes key health information; tracks and investigates public health trends; educates public on recognition and avoidance of contracting common infectious diseases; monitors outbreaks of chronic diseases
chronic (**kron**-ik)	**chronic** = continuing a long time or recurring frequently	a disease of slow progress and long continuance
cilia (**sil**-ee-*uh)*	**cilia** = short thread-like projections of the surface of a cell, organism	minute hair-like organelles that line the surface of cells providing movement of fluid along internal epithelial tissue
colonize (**kol**-*uh*-nahyz)	**colony** = group of organisms growing on a solid nutrient surface **-ize** = to establish	a group of microorganisms derived from one or a few spores
communicable (k*uh*-**myoo**-ni-k*uh*-b*uh* l)	**communicate** = transmitted; to give to another **-able** = capable of	a disease capable of being passed on readily

(*Continues*)

Term and Pronunciation	Meaning of Root and Word Parts	Definition
compromised (**kom**-pr*uh*-mahyzd)	**compromise** = to cause impairment, weakened by accepting standards that are lower than desirable	unable to function optimally; especially with regard to immune response due to underlying disease, harmful environment and side effect so treatment
contagious (k*uh* n-**tey**-j*uh* s)	**contagion** = an infectious disease transmitted by direct or indirect contact **-ous** = capable of	capable of being transmitted by bodily contact with an infected person or object
dental caries (**den**-tl) (**kair**-eez)	**dental** = pertaining to the teeth **caries** = decay	the formation of decay in tooth structure
diphtheria (dif-**theer**-ee-*uh*)	**diphtheria** = an acute bacterial infectious disease	characterized by the formation of a false membrane of the throat and other respiratory passages; causes difficulty in breathing, high fever and weakness; heart and nervous system inflammation
disease (dih-**zeez**)	**dis** = having a negative force **-ease** = freedom from pain or discomfort	illness, sickness or ailment
dormant (**dawr**-m*uh*nt)	**dormant** = inactive, sleeping or hibernating	in a state of minimal metabolic activity with cessation of growth,
endospore (**en**-d*uh*-spawr)	**endo** = inner **spore** = a walled cell; capable of giving rise to a new cell	an inactive, protective form taken by bacteria under conditions of extreme temperature, dryness and lack of food
enzyme (**en**-zahym)	**enzyme** = a substance that causes an alteration	a group of proteins produced by living cells that accelerate biochemical reactions; ie digestion
epidemic (ep-i-**dem**-ik)	**epi-** = among, upon **demo** = indicating people or population, district **-ic** = having characteristics	a rapid spread or increase of a disease affecting many persons at the same time where the disease is not permanently prevalent; incidence data of an attack rate in excess of 15 cases per 100,000 for two consecutive weeks
epidemiological (ep-i-dee-mee-**ol**-uh-jee-k*uh*l)	**epidemic** = disease affecting many persons at a time **-ology** = study of **-al** = pertaining to	adjective form of epidemiology; for example, epidemiological information about a disease
epidemiology (ep-i-dee-mee-**ol**-*uh*-jee)	**epidemic** = disease affecting many persons at a time **-ology** = study of	the branch of medicine that deals with the study of the causes, distribution and control of disease in populations
etiology (ee-tee-**ol**-*uh*-jee)	**etiology** = science of causes	the study of the causes or origins of disease
eukaryote (yoo-**kar**-ee-oht)	**eu-** = true or genuine **karyotype** = organized arrangement of chromosome pairs	a domain of organisms having cells with a distinct nucleus containing genetic DNA material; includes all organisms except bacteria
excrete (ik-**skreet**)	**ex-** = out of **-crete** = to sift or discharge	to eliminate waste material
expectorate (ik-**spek**-t*uh*-reyt)	**ex-** = out of or from **pectus** – the breast **-ate** = the act of	to eject or expel matter, as phlegm, from the throat or lungs by coughing or hawking and spitting; to spit
facultative anaerobe (**fak**-*uh*l-tey-tiv) (**an**-*uh*-rohb)	**faculty** = ability or power **-ative** = relating to **an-** = without **aero** = air **-bios** = life	having the capacity to live under more than one set of environmental circumstances; can survive with or without oxygen

Term and Pronunciation	Meaning of Root and Word Parts	Definition
FDA	**F**(ood) and **D**(rug) **A**(dministration)	US Food and Drug Administration is responsible for protecting and promoting public health by assuring safety of drugs, medical devices and food
flora (**flohr**-*uh*)	**flora** = plant life of a particular area/region	the formation of microorganisms normally occurring on or in the bodies
fungal spores (**fuhng**-*guhl*) (spohrz)	**fungus** = kingdom of organisms that includes molds, mildews, rusts, yeasts and mushrooms **-al** = pertaining to **spore** = reproductive body resistant to heat	microscopic cell(s) that disperse from parent fungus; can become dormant for a long time until conditions are favorable for growth
fungus (**fuhng**-*guhs*) **fungi** (**fuhn**-jahy)	**fungus** = kingdom of organisms that includes molds, mildews, rusts, yeasts and mushrooms **fungi** = plural of fungus	any of a diverse group of eukaryotic single-celled or multinucleate organisms that live by decomposing and absorbing the organic material in which they grow.
gamma globulin (**gam**-*uh*) (**glob**-*yuh*-lin)	**gamma** = a protein produced by T cells that regulates the immune response **globulin** = any of several groups of blood plasma proteins generally insoluble in water	a blood plasma protein that responds to stimulation of antigens (bacteria or viruses); therapeutic treatment of some viral disease
hepatitis (hep-*uh*-**tahy**-tis)	**hepat-** = liver **-itis** = inflammation	inflammation of the liver
herpes (**hur**-peez)	**Herpes** = any of several diseases caused by the herpesvirus	viral diseases characterized by eruption of blisters on the skin and mucous membranes; chickenpox, oral herpes, shingles, genital herpes
HIV	**H**(uman) **I**(mmunodeficiency) **V**(irus)	retrovirus responsible for AIDS and AIDS-related complex
homeostasis (hoh-mee-*uh*-**stey**-sis)	**homeo** = similar **-stasis** = state of equilibrium	the ability of the entire human body system to maintain internal stability
host (*ho*hst)	**host** = guest, stranger	a living animal or plant from which a parasite obtains nutrition
immunity (ih-**myoo**-ni-tee)	**immune** = protected from a disease **-ity** = expressing state or condition	inherited, acquired or induced resistance to infection by a specific pathogen
immunoglobulin (im-*yuh*-noh-**glob**-*yuh*-lin)	**immuno-** = indicates immunity **-globulin**: blood plasma proteins	any of several classes of proteins that function as antibodies; found in blood plasma
immunosuppressed (im-*yuh*-noh-*suh*-**pres** d)	**immune** = protected from a disease **suppress** = to restrain, inhibit, prohibit **-ion** = denoting action or condition	the blocking of the normal immune response because of disease; drugs or surgery
infectious (in-**fek**-shuh s)	**infect** = to affect or contaminate with disease-producing microorganisms **-ious** = characterized by or full of	tending to spread pathogenic microorganisms from one to another
inflammatory response (in-**flam**-*uh*-tawr-ee) (ri-**spons**)	**in-** = within **flame** = bright color; redness **-ory** = something having a specified use **response** = a reaction to a specific stimulus	redness, swelling, pain, tenderness, heat, and disturbed function of an area of the body, especially as a reaction of tissues to injurious agents

(Continues)

Term and Pronunciation	Meaning of Root and Word Parts	Definition
inhibit (in-**hib**-it)	**inhibit** = to restrain, hinder, arrest or check	to decrease, limit or block the action or function of a pathogenic microorganism
innate immunity (ih-**neyt**) (ih-**myoo**-ni-tee)	**innate** = possessed at birth; inborn; natural **immune** = protected from a disease **-ity** = expressing state or condition	natural immunity; resistance to disease that occurs as part of the individual's natural biologic makeup
invasiveness (in-**vey**-siv-ness)	**invasion** = entrance of something harmful **-ness** = a state or condition	ability to enter into a part of the body to cause harm or disease
latent (**leyt**-nt)	**late** = coming or arriving after a time **-ent** = existing in a certain condition	present but not visible or apparent
Legionnaires' disease (lee-juh-**nair** z) (dih-**zeez**)	**Legionnaire** = a member of a certain military force or association **dis** = having a negative force **-ease** = freedom from pain or discomfort	a form of bacterial pneumonia first identified after an outbreak at an American Legion meeting
lysozymes (**lahy**-suh-zahym)	**lyso-** = dissolving **-zyme** = a substance capable of causing alteration or change	a cell organelle containing enzymes that digests and destroys the cell after its death
lysozymes (**lahy**-suh-zahym)	**lyso-** = dissolving **-zyme** = a substance capable of causing alteration or change	a cell organelle containing enzymes that digests and destroys the cell after its death
microbiology (mahy-kroh-bahy-**ol**-uh-jee)	**micro** = very small **-bio** = living organisms **-ology** – the study of	the study of microscopic living organisms
microorganism (mahy-kroh-**awr**-guh-niz-uhm)	**micro** = very small **organism** = form of life	a very small form of life not visible to the human eye; must be viewed by a microscope to be visible
nasopharyngitis (nahy-zoh-**far**-in-jahy-tis)	**naso** = nose **pharynx** = tube or cavity that connects the mouth and nasal (nose) passages **-itis** = inflammation	inflammation of the nasal passages and upper part of pharynx; infectious, inflammatory condition
naturally acquired active immunity (**nach**-er-uh-lee) (uh-**kwahy**uhrd) (**ak**-tiv) (ih-**myoo**-ni-tee)	**nature** = fundamental qualities **-al** = pertaining to **acquired** = attained **active** = state of progress, involving action, motion **immune** = protected from a disease **-ity** = expressing state or condition	when the person is exposed to a live pathogen, develops the disease and becomes immune as a result of the primary immune response
normal flora (**nawr**-muhl) (**flawr**-uh)	**norm** = standard or common type, regular **-al** = pertaining to **flora** = plant life of a particular region	microorganisms that normally inhabit a bodily organ or part
opportunistic (op-er-too-**nis**-tik)	**opportunity** = a favorable time or occasion **-ist** = denoting a performing a certain action **-ic** = relating to	a microorganism causing disease only under certain conditions; as when a person's immune system is impaired
outbreak (**out**-breyk)	**out** = denoting a going beyond, surpassing a particular action indicated **break** = to weaken or overwhelm	happens when a disease occurs in greater numbers than expected in a community or during a season
pandemic (pan-**dem**-ik)	**pan** = all or every **demo** = indicating people or population, district **-ic** = having characteristics	is a global disease epidemic; involves an entire country, continent or the whole world

Term and Pronunciation	Meaning of Root and Word Parts	Definition
parasite (**par**-*uh*-sahyt)	**parasite** = something that lives on others	an organism that lives on or in an organism of another species, known as the host, from the body of which it obtains nutriment.
pathogen (**path**-*uh*-juhn)	**patho** = suffering or disease **-gen** = produces	a disease-producing agent
pathogenic microorganism (path-*uh*-**jen**-ik) (mahy-kroh-**awr**-g*uh*-niz-*uh*m)	**patho** = suffering or disease **-gen** = produces **-ic** = having characteristics **micro** = very small **organism** = form of life	any microorganism capable of injuring its host; infectious organism of a disease; disease causing microorganism
pathogenicity (path-oh-*juh*-**nis**-i-tee)	**patho** = suffering or disease **-gen** = produces **-ity** = expressing state or condition, capacity	the disease producing capacity of a pathogen
pellicle (**pel**-i-k*uh*l)	**pellicle** = coating or covering	a thin protein film that forms on the surface of enamel; protects tooth from acids produced by oral microoganisms
periodontitis (per-ee-oh-don-**tahy**-tis)	**peri-** = around **-odonto-** = the tooth **-itis** = inflammation	bacterial inflammation of the supporting structures around the teeth
pertussis (per-**tuhs**-is)	**pertussis** = technical term for whooping cough	a highly contagious airway infection that primarily affects children; severe hacking cough followed by a high-pitched intake of breath that can last several months or years
phagocyte (**fag**-*uh*-sahyt)	**phago-** = to eat, devour **-cyte** = cell	any cell that ingests and destroys foreign particles, bacteria, and cell debris
pneumonia (noo-**mohn**-*yuh*)	**pneumon-** = lungs, air or breath **-ia** = disease, pathological or abnormal condition	inflammation of the lungs with congestion
prion (**prahy**-on)	**prion** = tiny particle; **PR**otein infect**ION**	a tiny particle, likened to viruses, but having no genetic component, thought to be an infectious agent in bovine spongiform encephalopathy, Creutzfeldt-Jakob disease, and similar encephalopathies
prokaryote (proh-**kar**-ee-oht)	**pro-** = similar to **karyotype** = organized arrangement of chromosome pairs	a single-celled microorganism that has no distinct nucleus and no organelles and has its genetic material in the form of single continuous strands forming coils or loops; includes bacteria
protozoa (proh-t*uh*-**zoh**-*uh*)	**proto-** = similar to **-zoa** = organisms	any of a diverse group of microorganisms that are primarily unicellular, do not contain nucleus or organelles; includes bacteria
rhinopharyngitis (rahy-noh-far-in-**jahy**-tis)	**rhino** = nose **pharynx** = tube or cavity that connects the mouth and nasal (nose) passages **-itis** = inflammation	inflammation of mucous membranes of the nose and pharynx; also referred to as the common cold
rickettsia (ri-**ket**-see-*uh*)	**rickettsia** = a group of parasitic bacteria that are carried as parasites ticks, fleas, and lice	parasitic bacteria that is the cause of febrile (fever) diseases in humans such as typhus and Rocky Mountain Fever
saprophyte (**sap**-r*uh*-fahyt)	**sapro-** = dead or dying **-phyte** = plant	any organism that lives on dead organic matter, as certain fungi and bacteria
spores (spohr)	**spore** = seed; capable of growing into a new organism	a reproductive body produced by bacteria, fungi, plants and protozoa; also refers to a dormant, nonreproductive body formed by bacteria in response to unfavorable condition resistant to drying and heat

(Continues)

Term and Pronunciation	Meaning of Root and Word Parts	Definition
Streptococcus mutans (strep-tuh-**kok**-uhs) (**myoo**-tanz)	**strepto-** = twisted or spiral **coccus** = spherical bacterium **mutant** = a new type of organism	a species of bacteria responsible for dental caries
synthesize (**sin**-th*uh*-sahyz)	**syn-** = together **-thesis** = to make	to make or combine elements into a single or unified element
tetanus (**tet**-n-*uhs*)	**tetanus** = spasm of muscles	an infectious disease caused by bacteria that enters the body through wounds; causes spasms and rigidity
toxic (**tok**-sik)	**toxin** = poison or poisonous **-ic** = pertaining to	affected with or caused by poison
toxigenesis (tok-si-**jen**-ik)	**toxin** = poison or poisonous **genesis** = origin or source	the ability of a microorganism to produce a poison
tuberculosis (t*oo*-bur-ky*uh*-**loh**-sis)	**tubercle** = small, firm swelling **-osis** = denotes condition or state	an infectious bacterial disease, especially of the lungs, characterized by the growth of nodules (tubercles)
vaccine (vak-**seen**)	**vaccine** = a preparation of weakened or killed pathogen that stimulates immune cells	any preparation introduced into the body in order to induce immunity against a specific disease
virulent (**vir**-y*uh*-lu*h*nt)	**virulent** = poison	intensely poisonous; causing clinical symptoms
virus (**vahy**-*ruhs*)	**virus** = full of poison	an infectious agent that replicates in living cells
WHO	**W**(orld) **H**(ealth) **O**(rganization)	World Health Organization role is to direct international health within the United Nations and lead in global health responses

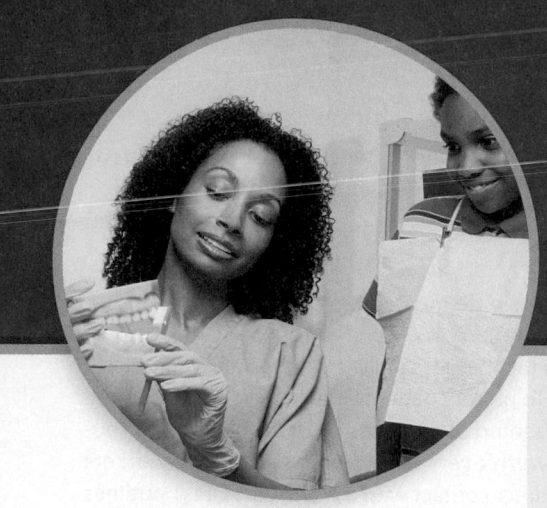

## CHAPTER 11

Infection Control

Specific Instructional Objectives

At the completion of this chapter, you will be able to meet these objectives:

1. Use terms presented in this chapter.
2. Describe the five steps to achieving asepsis in the dental office.
3. Identify when to perform hand hygiene.
4. Outline the steps in the three hand hygiene techniques used in dentistry.
5. State the purpose of each component of personal protective equipment (PPE).
6. Compare and contrast among the types of gloves used in dentistry.
7. Describe the steps in donning and doffing personal protective equipment (PPE).
8. Define sanitization.
9. Differentiate among housekeeping surfaces and clinical contact surfaces.
10. Compare and contrast precleaning and disinfecting of contaminated surfaces.
11. Discuss clinical surface barriers.
12. Discuss waste disposal.
13. Describe the recommended layout of the instrument processing area.
14. Describe the seven steps in instrument processing for contaminated instruments.
15. Discuss the purpose of the ultrasonic cleaner.
16. Outline the steps in operating an ultrasonic cleaner.
17. Discuss the steps in managing a contaminated patient tray in the sterilization area.
18. Define disinfection.
19. Compare and contrast the three categories of instruments.
20. Compare and contrast among the different levels of disinfectants.
21. Discuss the disinfection process of clinical contact surfaces.
22. Discuss the disinfection process of transfer surfaces.
23. Discuss the process of disinfecting contaminated instruments.
24. Identify the factors that can impact disinfectant efficiency.
25. Discuss the importance of disinfecting waterlines.
26. Discuss the importance of disinfecting dental vacuum hoses.
27. Discuss the importance of sterilization.
28. Compare and contrast among the various methods of sterilization.
29. Outline the steps in operating a steam autoclave.
30. Discuss the process of handpiece sterilization.
31. Describe the factors that can impact sterilization.
32. Compare and contrast the methods of monitoring sterilization.
33. Describe the roles of the various agencies in providing guidelines for infection control in dentistry.
34. Define standard precautions.
35. Discuss the Bloodborne Pathogens Standard.
36. Discuss the Hazard Communication Standards.

Aseptic Technique

Sepsis means presence of disease-producing microorganisms. **Asepsis** (a = without; absence of disease-producing microorganisms) is essential in minimizing the hazard of exposure to pathogenic microorganisms. Complete absence of microorganisms is not possible in the dental office; however, most cross-infection can be eliminated by using caution and following aseptic procedures. This chapter will cover aseptic methods and techniques to provide conditions free from pathogenic microorganisms. Asepsis awareness will ensure protection of the patient, doctor, and yourself from infection (Figure 11-1).

Asepsis Steps

There are five steps to achieve asepsis in the dental office. These steps include:

1. Dental team hand hygiene and use of personal protective equipment
2. Sanitization of surfaces, instruments, equipment, and items
3. Disinfection of surfaces, instruments, equipment, and items
4. Sterilization of instruments and items
5. Maintenance of an aseptic work area during patient treatment

Hand Hygiene

Hand hygiene is the single most important step in preventing the transfer of microorganisms— and thus in preventing infection. Handwashing technique is a basic yet essential clinical skill in dental assisting. To protect patients from health care–acquired infections, handwashing techniques must be performed routinely and gloves worn every time dental health care workers (DHCWs) come in direct contact with a patient. Box 11-1 outlines infection control guidelines for when to perform hand hygiene.

Hand Hygiene Techniques

In October 2002, the Centers for Disease Control (CDC) published a Guideline of Hand Hygiene in Health-Care Settings. It states that handwashing is one of the most important components of infection control. The DHCW harbors both resident and transient flora. The resident flora naturally occurs in the deeper layers of

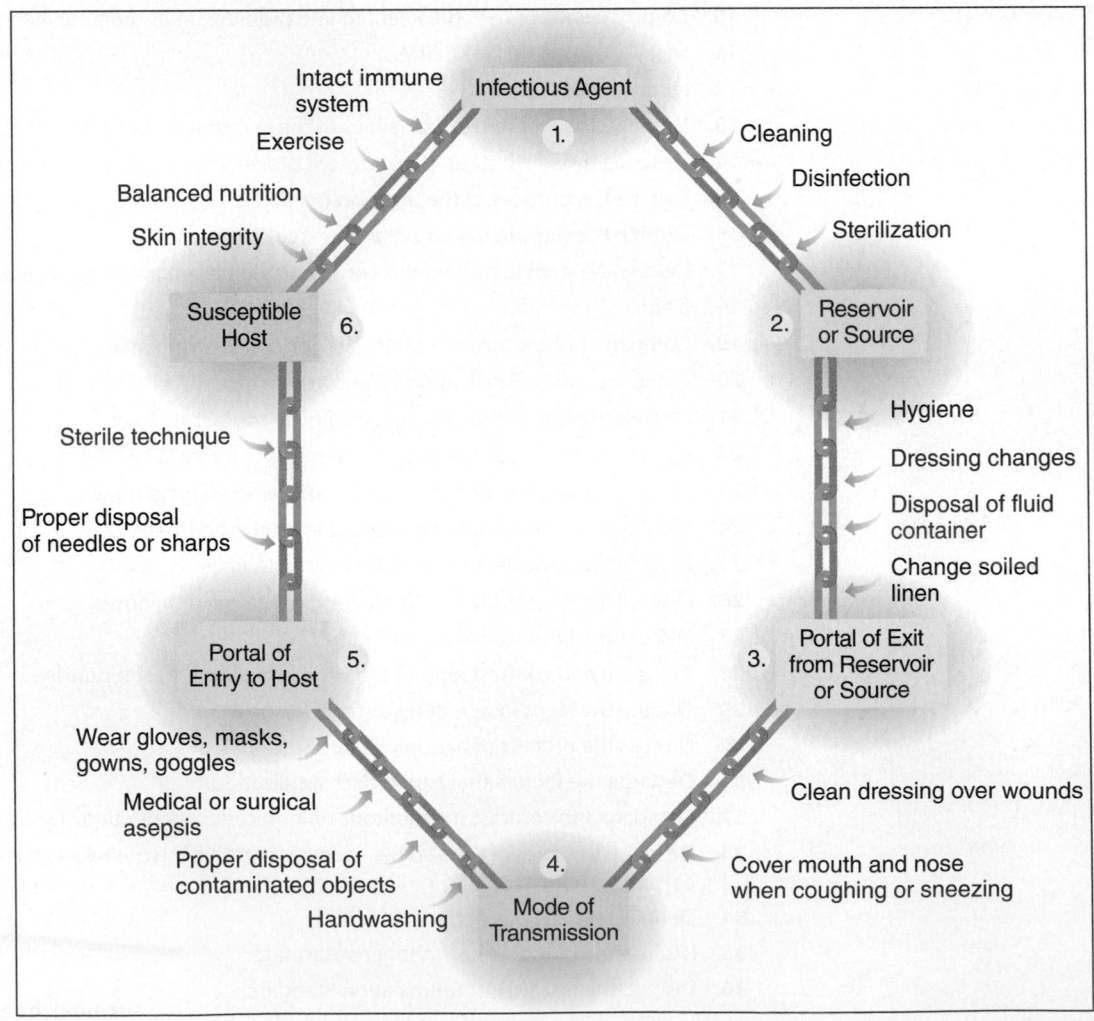

FIGURE 11-1
Chain of infection; preventive measures follow each link.

BOX 11-1 Infection Control Guidelines for Hand Hygiene

When to perform hand hygiene

- start and end of each day
- before and after each patient
- whenever disinfecting or sterilizing instruments or equipment
- before and after eating
- before and after restroom breaks
- when hands are visibly soiled
- before donning gloves and immediately after removing gloves

skin which carry a lower level threat of infectious disease transmission than the transient. Transient flora are picked up from environmental surfaces, reside on the outer layers of the skin, are most frequently associated with health care–acquired infections, and can be removed with proper handwashing techniques. There are three hand hygiene techniques used in the dental facility.

1. Clinical handwashing
2. Alcohol-based hand rub
3. Surgical handwashing

Clinical Handwashing Clinical handwashing is required when performing nonsurgical dental procedures, the hands are visibly soiled, there is a tear in gloves, or there is potential contamination from blood, saliva, and other potentially infectious material (OPIM). Bar soap harbors bacteria and should *never* be used in a health care facility. The DHCW should use recommended handwash products (soap) contained in hands free (activated electronically or

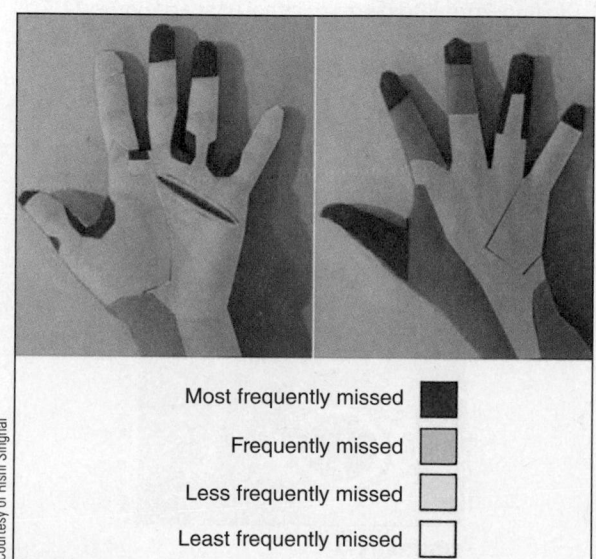

Most frequently missed ■
Frequently missed ▨
Less frequently missed ▢
Least frequently missed ▢

Courtesy of Rishi Singhal

FIGURE 11-2
Areas missed when handwashing.

with foot pedals) or pump containers. To maintain the asepsis of the soap container, the assistant should *never* top off the containers. The containers should be completely emptied, cleaned, and rinsed before refilling, or disposable containers should be used.

If DHCWs choose to wear jewelry, a fob watch and smooth rings are preferred. The rings must be smooth to prevent tearing gloves and be able to move up and down finger to clean beneath the ring. Before performing handwashing, all jewelry should be removed. Jewelry harbors dirt and skin microorganisms that can cause cross-infection.

Hands are rinsed under clean, running water, and approximately a quarter size amount of soap is placed in the palm of hand. A generous lather is produced by rubbing hands together vigorously for 10–15 seconds. Pay special attention to protected and overlooked areas under fingernails, thumbs, knuckles, palms, and sides of fingers and hands where bacteria are harbored (Figure 11-2). Soap and warm water reduce surface tension, and added friction loosens surface microorganisms and washes away in the lather.

Rinse hands and wrists well; running water flushes soil, soap, and microorganisms away. Avoid splashing water on yourself or the floor; microorganisms spread more easily on wet surfaces. Pat hands and wrists dry with a paper towel. Avoid rubbing, which can cause abrasion and chaffing of the hands, increasing crevices of damaged skin. Do not touch sink or faucets or potentially contaminated areas after cleaning hands. It is recommended to use a hands-free faucet. Turn faucets off using a paper towel or elbow when foot controls are not available. Refer to Procedure 11-1 for clinical handwashing steps.

Alcohol-based Hand Rub An alcohol-based hand rub, also referred to as hand sanitizing, has been proven to be more effective at reducing microbial count than handwashing with soap and water. It is the preferred routine hygienic hand antisepsis if hands are not visibly soiled or contaminated by blood. It is faster, more effective, more convenient, and better tolerated by hands than washing with soap and water. Hand sanitizing is gentler on the hands causing less hand dryness and damage. It has the highest residual activity, lasting after hands are cleaned.

Alcohol based hand rubs (hand sanitizers) are waterless agents that are available as gels, foams, or rinses. Products with 60 to 95% concentrations of ethanol or isopropanol-alcohol are the most effective. Both higher and lower concentrations of alcohol and amount of product used by the individual can affect effectiveness; therefore, manufacturer's directions should be carefully followed. Hand sanitizer is 10 times more effective than washing with 2% chlorhexidine hand wash for 30 seconds and 100 times more effective than washing with ordinary plain soap for 15 seconds.

The hand sanitizer is placed into the palm of the hand and vigorously rubbed between the hands for 10 to 15 seconds. It is crucial to contact all the surfaces of the hand as outlined in the clinical handwashing procedure. The sanitizer should be allowed to evaporate. Refer to Procedure 11-2 for alcohol-based hand rub steps.

Surgical Hand Scrub The surgical hand scrub is recommended whenever the procedure requires having the patient's tissue open and exposed during a surgical procedure.

Procedure 11-1
Clinical Handwashing

Equipment and Supplies
- Sink
- Disposable paper towels
- Soap
- Waste receptacle

Procedure Steps

1. Turn on faucet (hands free faucet or with towel) (Figure 11-3).

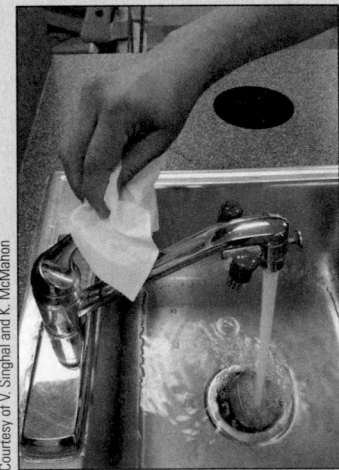

FIGURE 11-3

2. Wet hands and place adequate amount of soap into palm of hand (Figures 11-4 and 11-5).

3. Soap and rub hands for 15–20 seconds (approximately the length of time it takes to sing Happy Birthday) (Figure 11-6).

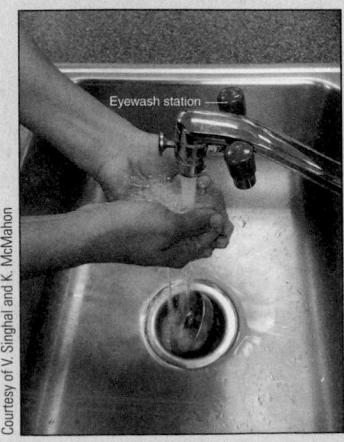

FIGURE 11-4

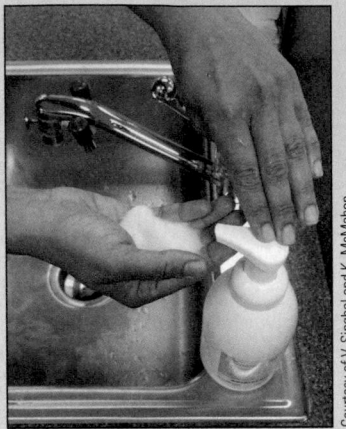

FIGURE 11-5

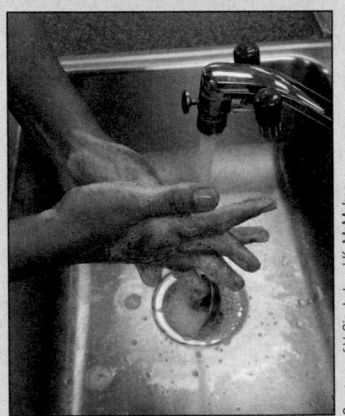

FIGURE 11-6

4. Dip fingertips into palms of lathered soap (Figure 11-7).

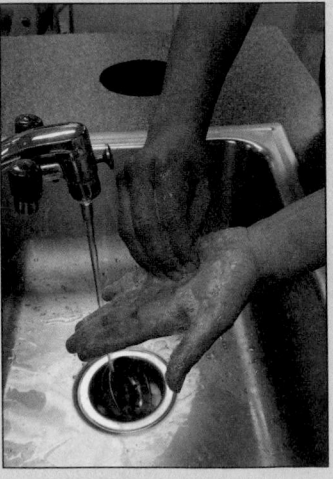

FIGURE 11-7

Courtesy of V. Singhal and K. McMahon

5. Rub hands palm to palm.

6. Rub back of both hands.

7. Rub hands palm to palm with fingers interlaced (Figure 11-8).

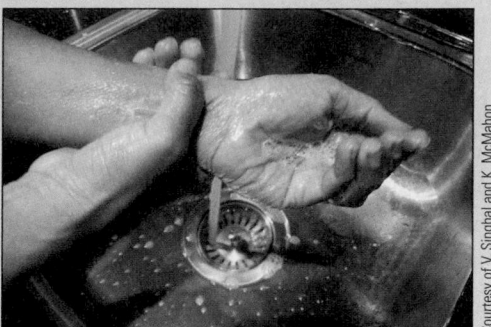

FIGURE 11-10

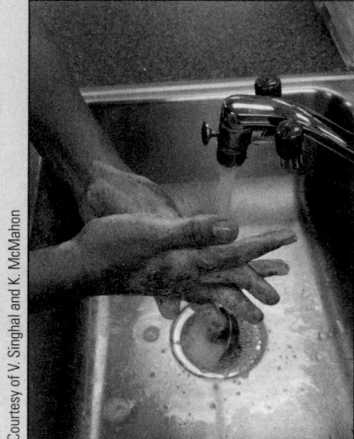

FIGURE 11-8

8. Place back of fingers to opposing palms with fingers interlocked.

9. Wash between each finger separately (Figure 11-9).

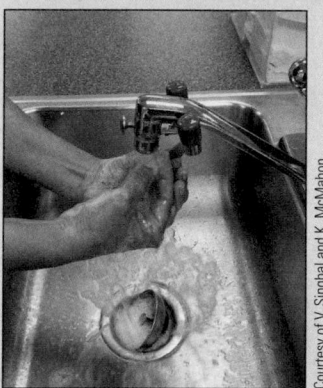

FIGURE 11-11

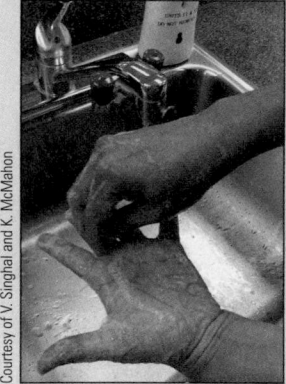

FIGURE 11-9

10. Wrap right hand over left wrist and rub back and forth, and vice versa for right wrist (Figure 11-10).

11. Rinse hands thoroughly from fingertips to wrist (Figure 11-11).

12. Pat hands dry (Figure 11-12).

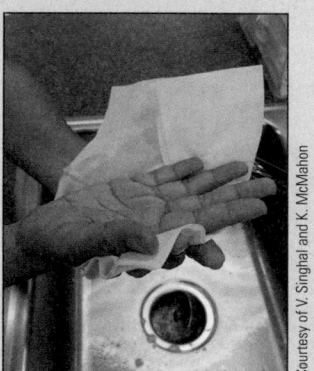

FIGURE 11-12

13. Turn off tap (hands free or with toweling).

14. Spray-wipe-spray to clean and dry sink with layers of paper toweling.

15. Dispose of paper towels in waste receptacle.

To reduce the risk of postoperative infections, more stringent hand hygiene and antimicrobial agents are used. Only antimicrobial soap (chlorhexidine 4% and povidone-iodine) is used during the surgical hand scrub, which helps prevent intra-operative infections. A surgical scrub requires that the hands are soaped two times or that the second time an alcohol rub is used. Disposable orange sticks or nailbrushes are used during the scrubbing to clean around the cuticles. The surgical

Procedure 11-2
Using Alcohol-based Hand Rubs

Equipment and Supplies
- Alcohol-based rub dispenser
- Disposable paper towels

Procedure Steps

1. Dispense rub into palm of hand using hands-free dispenser or using a towel on dispenser (Figure 11-13).

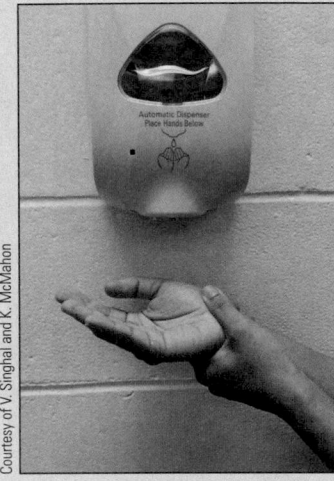

FIGURE 11-13

2. Rub hands together palm to palm (Figure 11-14).

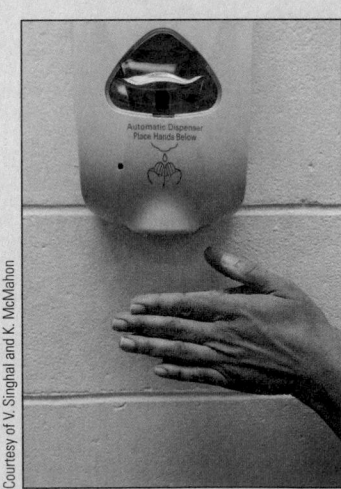

FIGURE 11-14

3. Rub between fingers, interlaced (Figure 11-15).

4. Rub back of each hand with palm of the other hand (Figure 11-16).

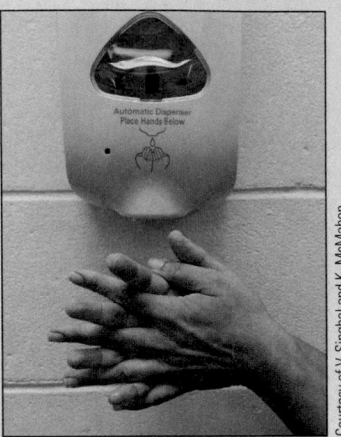

FIGURE 11-15

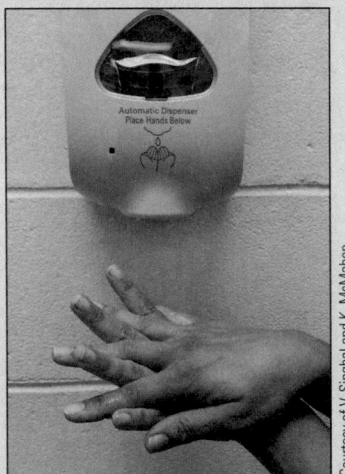

FIGURE 11-16

5. Rub fingers tips of each hand in palm of opposite hand (Figure 11-17).

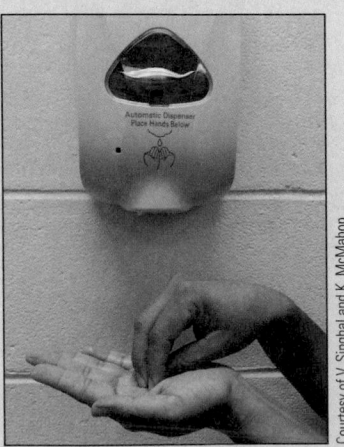

FIGURE 11-17

6. Rub each thumb clasped in opposite hand (Figures 11-18 and 11-19).

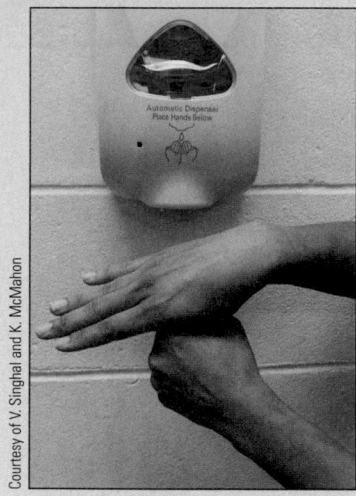

Courtesy of V. Singhal and K. McMahon

FIGURE 11-18

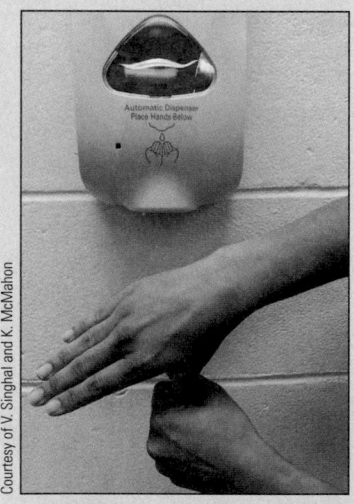

Courtesy of V. Singhal and K. McMahon

FIGURE 11-19

7. Rub each wrist clasped in opposite hand (Figure 11-20).

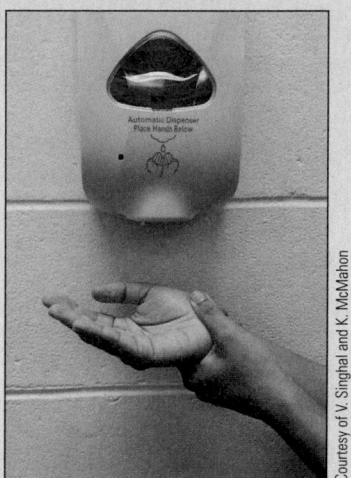

Courtesy of V. Singhal and K. McMahon

FIGURE 11-20

8. Continue rubbing until hands are dry (Figure 11-21).

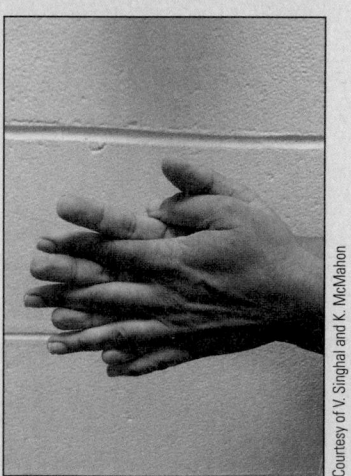

Courtesy of V. Singhal and K. McMahon

FIGURE 11-21

scrub is recommended to last 4–6 minutes, and the DHCW cleans from the fingertips to 2 inches above the elbow. Refer to Procedure 11-3 for steps in performing a surgical hand scrub and donning surgical gloves.

Hand Care

Hand care is especially important since intact skin is the most effective barrier to pathogenic microorganisms. DHCWs perform multiple hand hygiene procedures every day and must maintain healthy, intact skin to protect against microorganisms. Hands should be thoroughly dried before putting gloves on. Moisture inside the gloves promotes bacterial growth. Using skin cream

or lotion can help to alleviate dry, chapped hands and dermatitis caused by frequent handwashing and the wearing of gloves. Lotions containing mineral oil or petroleum will affect the integrity of gloves and should be avoided.

Fingernails should be kept trimmed to less than ¼ inch long to avoid puncturing gloves and filed smooth to inhibit microbial growth under the nails. Artificial fingernails should not be worn as they, too, promote microbial growth between the natural nail and the artificial nail. Rings, long nails, and artificial nails are all likely to puncture gloves and harbor pathogens. The CDC Guidelines recommend that rings, fingernail polish, and artificial nails should not be worn at work.

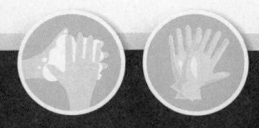

Procedure 11-3
Performing a Surgical Hand Scrub and Donning Surgical Gloves

Surgical Hand Scrub

Equipment and Supplies
- Sink
- Antimicrobial soap
- Hand brush
- Nail brush or orange stick
- Alcohol-based hand rub

Procedure Steps

1. Perform a prewash and rinse with an antimicrobial agent from the fingertips to 2 inches above the elbow.

2. Scrub hands from wrist to fingertips with a hand brush (Figure 11-22).

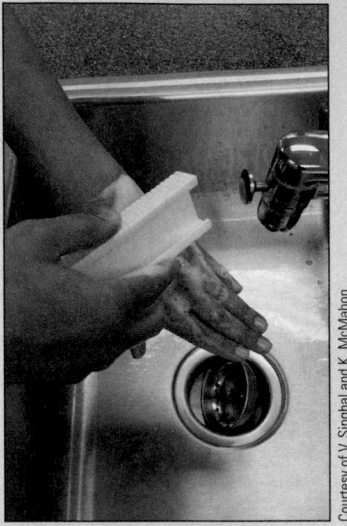

FIGURE 11-23

Courtesy of V. Singhal and K. McMahon

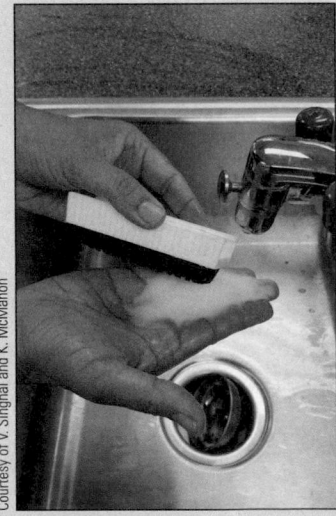

FIGURE 11-22

Courtesy of V. Singhal and K. McMahon

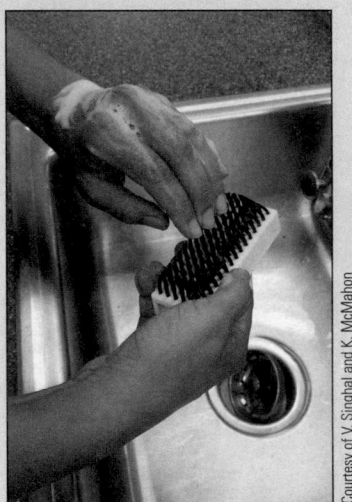

FIGURE 11-24

Courtesy of V. Singhal and K. McMahon

3. Always brush away from your body and into the sink (Figure 11-23).

4. Clean around cuticles using a nail brush or orange stick (Figure 11-24).

5. Scrub forearms with a hand brush (Figure 11-25).

6. Rinse from above elbows to fingertips. Hold fingertips up so the water runs off the elbows. This keeps the fingertips the cleanest part of the washed hands.

7. After prewash, perform a second wash on dry hands and then perform alcohol-based rub. Allow the hands to air-dry before donning a sterile gown and sterile gloves. The procedure to don sterile gloves is below.

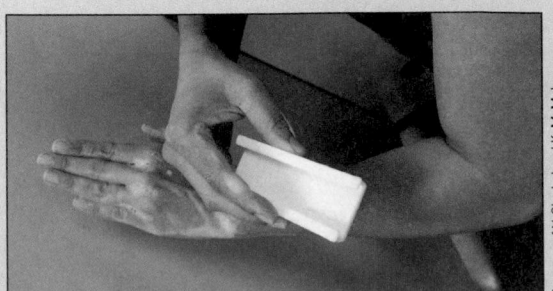

FIGURE 11-25

Courtesy of V. Singhal and K. McMahon

Donning Sterile Gloves

Equipment and Supplies

- Sterile gloves

Procedure Steps

1. Sterile gloves are specific to the right and left hands. The sterile glove package should be opened. The inner wrapping is sterile (Figure 11-26).

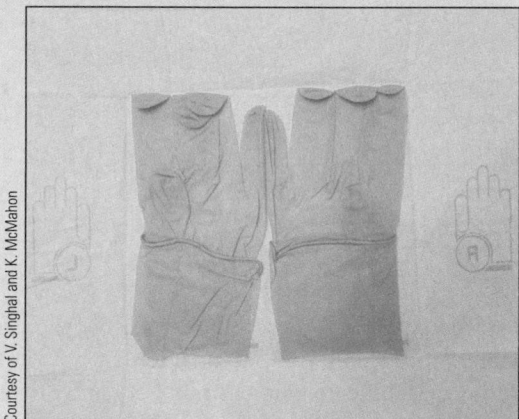

FIGURE 11-26

2. The gloves have a cuff. When donning sterile gloves, the operator should touch only the inner part of the cuff so the outer part does not get contaminated (Figure 11-27).

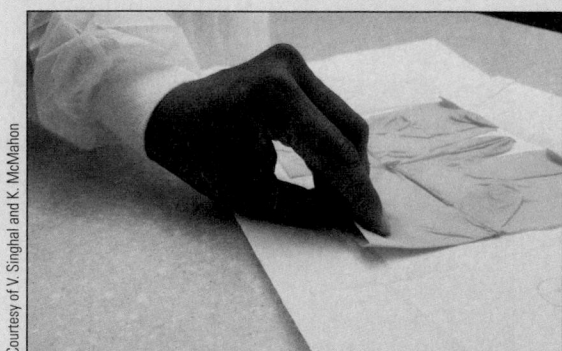

FIGURE 11-27

3. Always don first glove on the dominant hand. This will make it easier to glove the nondominant hand (Figure 11-28).

4. Once the glove on the dominant hand is on and over the cuff of the protective gown, insert gloved fingers on the outer part of the second glove. Touch only the sterile part of the second glove (Figure 11-29).

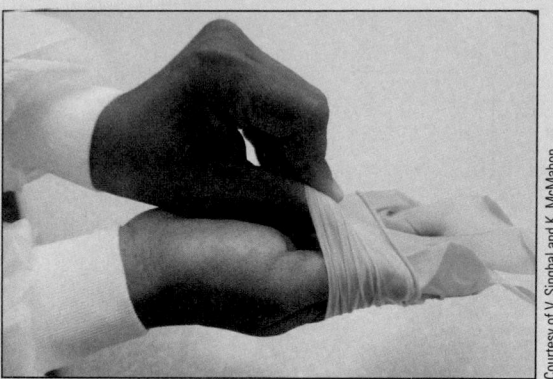

FIGURE 11-28

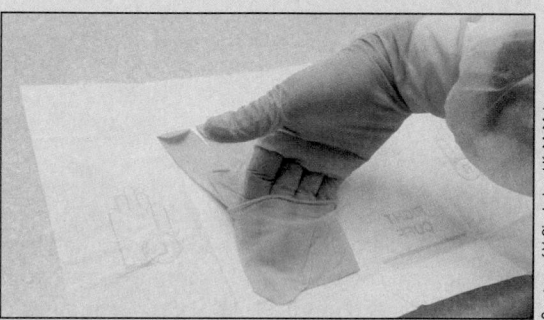

FIGURE 11-29

5. Place the second sterile glove on the nondominant hand (Figure 11-30).

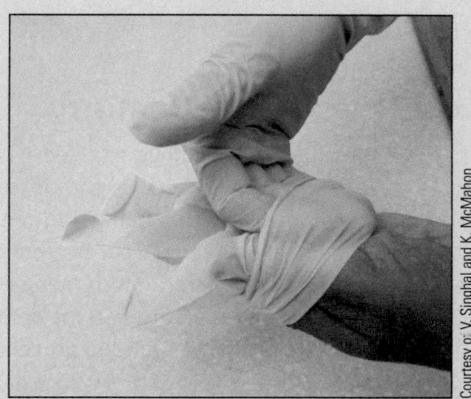

FIGURE 11-30

6. Pull over the hand using the cuff (Figure 11-31).

7. Both cuffs should be over the cuffs of the protective gown (Figure 11-32).

(Continues)

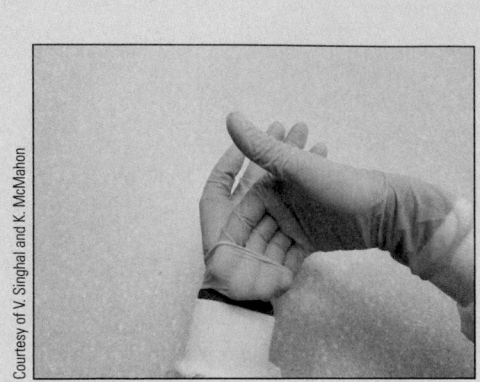

FIGURE 11-31

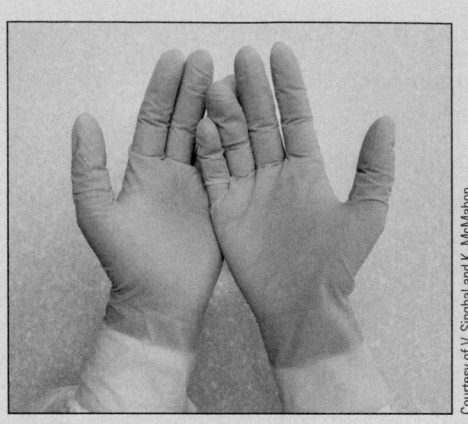

FIGURE 11-32

Personal Protective Equipment (PPE)

PPE is designed to protect the skin and mucous membranes of the eyes, nose, and mouth of DHCW from exposure to blood, OPIM, and chemicals (Figure 11-33). OSHA mandates dental health care workers wear PPE when there is a potential for exposure to blood and OPIM to reduce risk of exposures to blood-borne pathogens. The recommended PPE includes:

● Gloves

● Protective clothing

● Masks

● Protective eyewear

Types of Gloves Used in Dentistry

Gloves are not a substitute for hand hygiene. Gloves are worn to help protect the DHCW from infectious pathogens, to prevent pathogenic microorganisms from being transmitted from the DHCW to the patient, and to reduce contamination of the DHCW's hands by organisms transmitted from one patient to another. Different types of gloves are used in the dental office, and the type chosen should be based on the procedure to be performed (Table 11-1).

Use of Examination Gloves in Dental Care Examination gloves must be worn during patient care activities that may involve exposure to blood or body fluids. Hands should be washed and dried before wearing (donning) gloves and immediately following the removal of the gloves (doffing). Refer to Procedure 11-4 for steps in donning and removing gloves. The DHCW must change gloves between tasks and remove gloves and wash hands immediately if a tear is suspected. Gloves should not be worn continuously. Table 11-1 provides information regarding glove use.

Despite wearing gloves, there is a potential for exposure to contaminated body fluids and potential for the patient to be exposed to the health care worker's skin flora and other contaminants. After two hours of wearing examination gloves, microscopic holes and wicking occurs. Approximately 30% of examination gloves fail to protect the wearer against contamination of their hands due to microscopic holes and wicking. Washing gloves while on hands is not recommended by the CDC, and hands must be washed immediately upon removal of gloves.

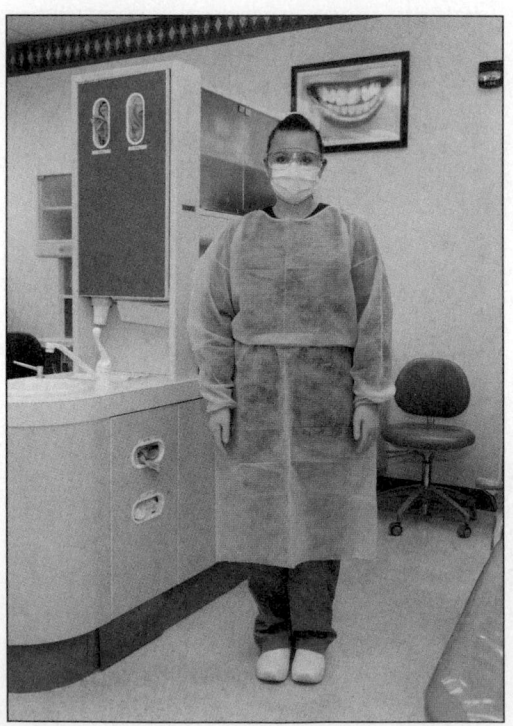

FIGURE 11-33
Dental assistant wearing personal protective equipment.

TABLE 11-1 Types of Gloves Used in a Dental Office

examination gloves	Dental personnel wear examination gloves during patient care procedures, when treatment may involve contact with blood, saliva, mucous membranes, and contaminated surfaces and instruments. These gloves can be worn on either hand and come in a variety of sizes ranging from extra-small to extra-large. It is important to note that these gloves are nonsterile, supplied by bulk in a box, and serve primarily as a protective barrier. Refer to the photos to the left to view examination gloves ([A] Vinyl exam gloves. [B] Latex exam gloves. [C] Lightly powdered nitrile exam gloves.) Examination gloves are single use; they should not be washed or reused and should be discarded after use. They are available in latex and latex free materials.
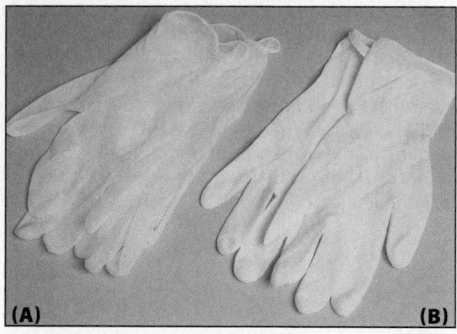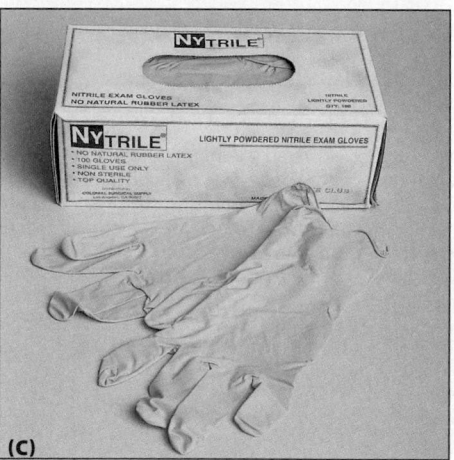	
sterile gloves	As the name suggests, these gloves are sterile and are prepackaged to ensure sterility until use. These gloves also are sized to specifically fit either the left or right hand. Surgical gloves are worn during any surgical procedure that exposes areas of the oral cavity. Sterile surgical gloves are worn for invasive surgical procedures involving the cutting of bone and significant amounts of blood. Surgical gloves should also be worn whenever handling sterile surgical instruments and items or coming in contact with an open wound.
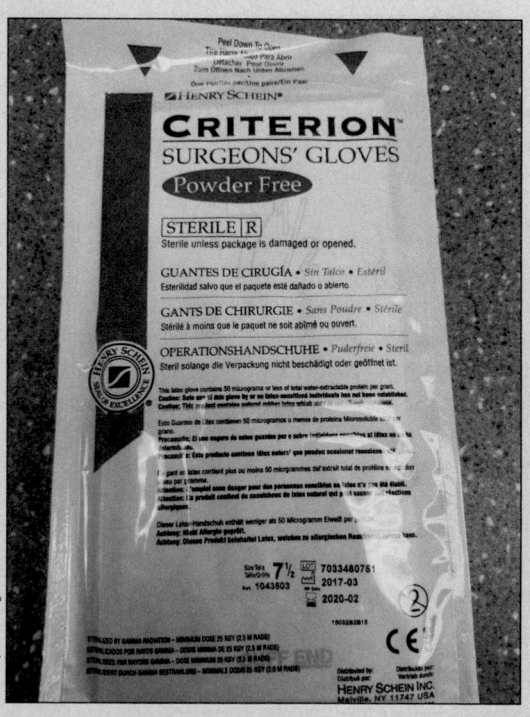	

(Continues)

TABLE 11-1 *(Continued)*

utility gloves	
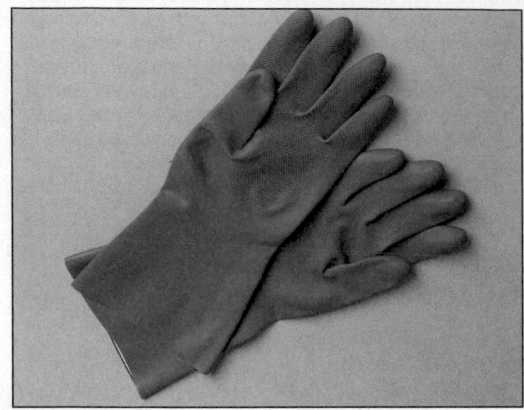	Utility gloves are thick rubber gloves that are resistant to chemicals and puncturing. Utility gloves resist the chance of **wicking** (microscopic punctures) that occurs in examination gloves when using plain soap, chlorhexidine, or alcohol. While sanitizing and disinfecting surfaces, instruments, and the treatment area, utility gloves are the gloves of choice. Utility gloves are not used for patient care. After each use, utility gloves are contaminated and must be disinfected appropriately. It is recommended that each staff member have their own utility gloves and assume responsibility for their disinfection to reduce the risk of **cross-contamination**. Utility gloves are replaced when they become cracked and lose the ability to function as a barrier.
overgloves	
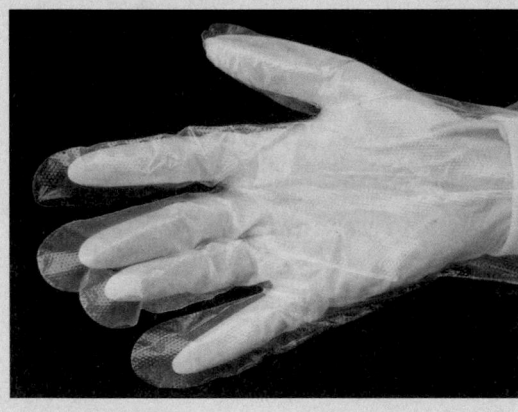	Overgloves are light, inexpensive, clear plastic gloves commonly referred to as "food handler" gloves. These are single-use, universal sized gloves typically worn over contaminated examination gloves to prevent cross-contamination. They are used to enter aseptic areas to prevent contaminating the area and materials and to prevent contaminating examination gloves. For example, overgloves can be put over examination gloves to enter data on a treatment room computer or to open a cabinet drawer.

Proper sizing of gloves is also important in reducing tears and wicking. Wearing gloves that are too small for long periods of time increases the risk of **carpal tunnel** syndrome.

Examination Glove Materials
Gloves are considered medical devices and are regulated by the FDA. All gloves used in the health care field must be FDA approved. The selection of the glove material is based on dentist and DHCW preference. The following should be considered in selecting glove material:

● Barrier protection with minimal leakage
● User comfort for flexibility in moving
● Cost effectiveness
● Availability of size ranges to minimize chance of carpal tunnel syndrome

Gloves are made of various materials:

● Natural rubber latex (NRL)
● Nitrile
● Polyvinyl chloride (synthetics)
● Polyethylene (plastic)

Latex has been used for over 100 years and is the best for all considerations; however, other materials are becoming preferred due to an increase in latex allergy.

Latex Allergy
Latex allergy ranges as high as 17% among health care workers. With the increase in the use of latex in dentistry (gloves, dental dam, prophy cups, orthodontic elastics), a detailed medical history is critical in identifying patients who may be allergic to latex. A DHCW with suspected latex allergy should obtain diagnosis from an appropriate health care provider. There are three major types of reactions that may occur related to the use of latex gloves (Figure 11-41). These include irritant dermatitis, delayed cutaneous hypersensitivity (Type IV allergic reaction), and Type I immediate allergic reaction. Types I and IV allergic reactions were covered in Chapters 14 and 15. Additional detail related specifically to latex is provided in Table 11-2.

Nonlatex Gloves
The use of nonlatex gloves has become increasingly important due to the increased incidence of latex allergy experienced by DHCWs and patients. The National Institute of Occupational Safety and Health (NIOSH) is the part of

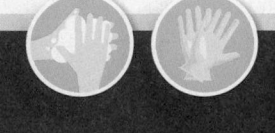

Procedure 11-4
Donning Gloves

Equipment and Supplies
- Sink
- Antimicrobial soap
- Disposable paper towels
- Gloves

Procedure Steps

1. Remove all jewelry from hands, perform handwashing technique, and select appropriately sized gloves.

2. Glove dominant hand first (in this image it is the right hand). Pick up one glove, holding the cuff of the glove with the left hand. Make certain to not contaminate the outside of the glove with bare hands. Manipulate the glove holding the cuff and inside of the glove (Figure 11-34).

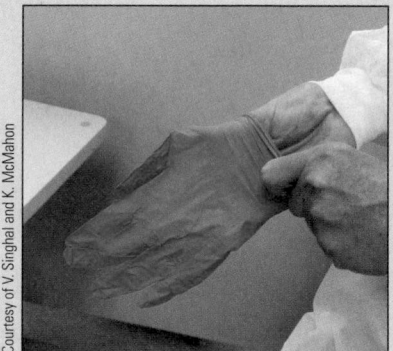

Courtesy of V. Singhal and K. McMahon

FIGURE 11-34

3. Line the thumb side of the glove up with the thumb side of the right hand while slipping the open end of the glove over the right hand.

4. Slip the open end of the glove over the right hand and thumb while positioning the fingers of the glove in line with the fingers of the right hand (Figure 11-35).

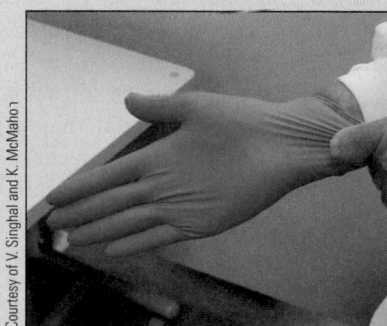

Courtesy of V. Singhal and K. McMahon

FIGURE 11-35

5. Stretch the palm side of the glove with the left hand and pull the glove on to the finger level (Figure 11-36).

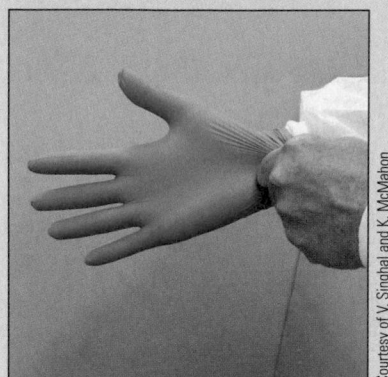

Courtesy of V. Singhal and K. McMahon

FIGURE 11-36

6. Pick up second glove with the gloved right hand. Line the thumb side of the glove up with the thumb side of the left hand (Figure 11-37).

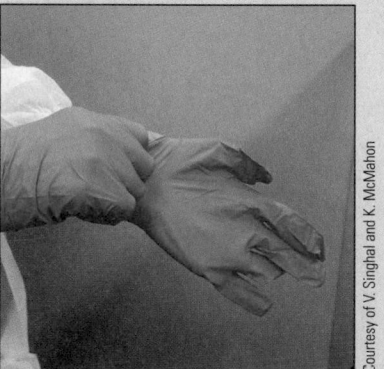

Courtesy of V. Singhal and K. McMahon

FIGURE 11-37

7. Slip the open end of the glove over the left hand and thumb. Stretch the palm side of the glove with the right hand, pull the glove on to the finger level, and position the fingers of the glove in line with the fingers of the left hand (Figure 11-38).

8. Once both hands are gloved, the remainder of the gloves can be pulled into position and adjusted for comfort (Figure 11-39).

9. Pull cuff of glove over the cuff of the gown (Figure 11-40).

(Continues)

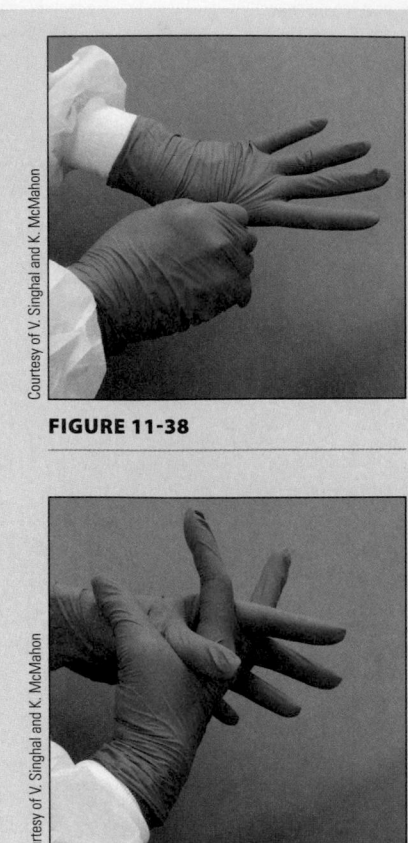

FIGURE 11-38

Courtesy of V. Singhal and K. McMahon

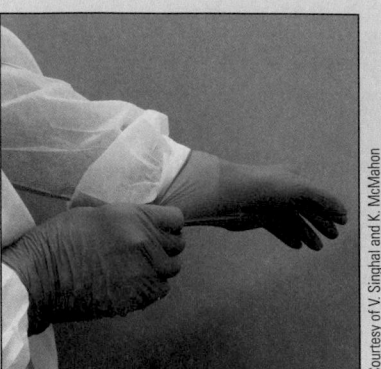

FIGURE 11-40

Courtesy of V. Singhal and K. McMahon

FIGURE 11-39

Courtesy of V. Singhal and K. McMahon

the CDC responsible for conducting research and making recommendations for the prevention of health-related illnesses. Based on the findings of NIOSH, the CDC has recommended that health histories specifically ask patients about a latex allergy, refer patients for a medical consultation if a latex allergy is suspected, provide a latex-safe environment in the dental office for

the health and safety of patients and DHCWs, and have an emergency kit with latex-free products available at all times.

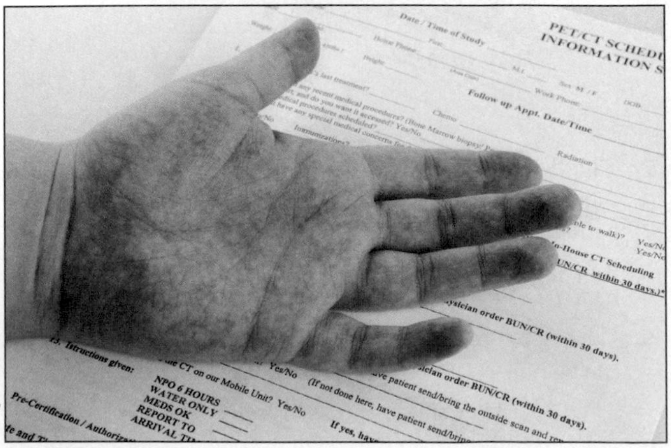

Protective Clothing

Various types of protective clothing (gowns and lab coats) are worn to prevent contamination of street clothing and to protect the skin of the DHCW from exposure to blood and body fluids. The type of protective clothing is dictated by the degree to which the employee will be exposed to blood and OPIM. Protective clothing includes reusable and washable or disposable clinic gowns, laboratory jackets, or uniforms and caps and shoe covers. The clothing material needs to prevent the penetration of blood or saliva through the material and onto personal clothing or skin. Fluid-resistant material is recommended during surgical procedures. For procedures that cause spatter, protective clothing with a high neckline and long sleeves with tapered cuffs to tuck into the gloves to protect the forearms are recommended. Ornamentation of protective clothing, such as buttons, zippers, ribbons, or other trims, should be kept to a minimum. Refer to Figure 11-33 for appropriate protective clothing for dental procedures.

Protective clothing should be changed daily or sooner if it becomes visibly soiled. Employers are required to provide disposable clothing or launder reusable protective clothing onsite or

© Angela Schmidt/Shutterstock.com

FIGURE 11-41
Latex allergy irritant dermatitis.

TABLE 11-2 Nonallergic and Allergic Reactions to Latex Gloves

irritant dermatitis	Skin irritation that does not involve the body's immune response is referred to as irritant **dermatitis**. It is not considered an allergic response. Frequent hand washing, scrubbing, and detergent break down skin and may result in irritant hand dermatitis. The skin becomes red, dry, irritated, and, in some cases, cracked. This allows for entry of sensitizing latex protein and glove chemicals that lead to latex allergy. This can be avoided by being careful to completely rinse soaps and antimicrobial agents from the hands after handwashing procedures, thoroughly drying the hands, and wearing nonpowdered gloves.
type IV hypersensitivity	Contact hand dermatitis is due to the chemicals (methacrylates, glutaraldehyde) used in latex glove production and not the latex itself. It is the most common reaction. Symptoms generally appear 24–48 hours after contact, but may be delayed up to 72 hours and do not involve the entire body (local reaction and not systemic). Type IV is not life threatening, but it does increase the risk to develop type I allergy.
type I hypersensitivity	This immediate reaction is not due to the chemicals used to process the gloves but to the actual latex proteins in the gloves. The immune system usually responds within two to three minutes of contact with the latex proteins, but response may occur hours later. Anaphylaxis is the primary cause of death associated with type I allergy. Type I allergy occurs from exposure to latex from cutaneous, mucosal, and aerosol contact. An allergic person cannot be in a room where latex is used.

with a commercial laundry. Protective clothing must be removed and placed in appropriate containers before leaving the work area. Contaminated clothing should never be worn outside the office to avoid the spread of contamination. Contaminated protective clothing should not be worn in the staff eating areas or when eating and consuming beverages. If an employee is going to leave the office during the course of the day, contaminated clothing should be changed for street clothing.

Masks

Masks protect patients against microorganisms generated by wearer and protect DHCW from large-particle droplet spatter that may contain bloodborne pathogens or OPIM from the patient. An examination mask needs to cover both nose and mouth and must be worn during procedures and patient care that likely generates splashes or sprays of blood or body fluids. Masks are supplied as flat or molded and have loops or ties (Figures 11-42A and 11-42B). In light of the COVID-19 pandemic, the CDC and OSHA currently require the use of N95 respirator masks (Figure 11-43) during aerosol producing procedures. Other infection control changes related to the pandemic will be discussed later in this chapter.

Masks are rated by the particle size filtering. A mask with 95% filtration efficiency for particles 3 to 5 micrometers in diameter is best. Visible spray from rotary instruments and equipment and air-water spray travel only a short distance and settle quickly on the floor, nearby equipment, operatory surfaces, personnel, or patients. Aerosols of 10 micrometers can remain airborne for extended periods and be inhaled. Masks must be changed between patients or during patient treatment if they become wet; moisture breaks down filtration. Masks should never be worn below the nose or on the chin. Remember that the outer surface of the mask is contaminated, so never lay it down on a clean surface.

Protective Eyewear

Eyewear should be worn to protect the mucous membranes of the eyes from contact with microorganisms. In addition to

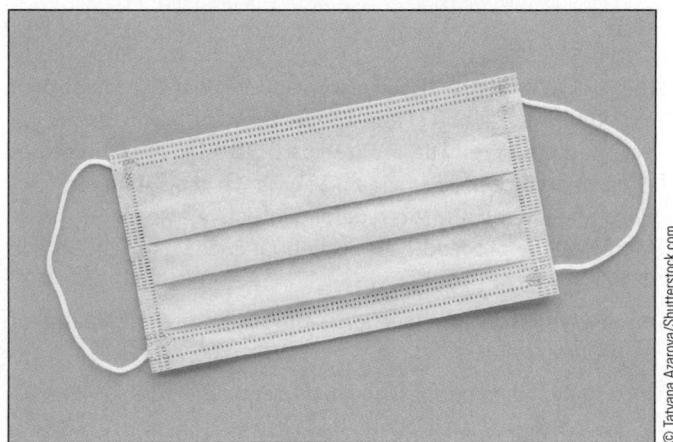

FIGURE 11-42A
Flat earloop face mask.

© Tatyana Azarova/Shutterstock.com

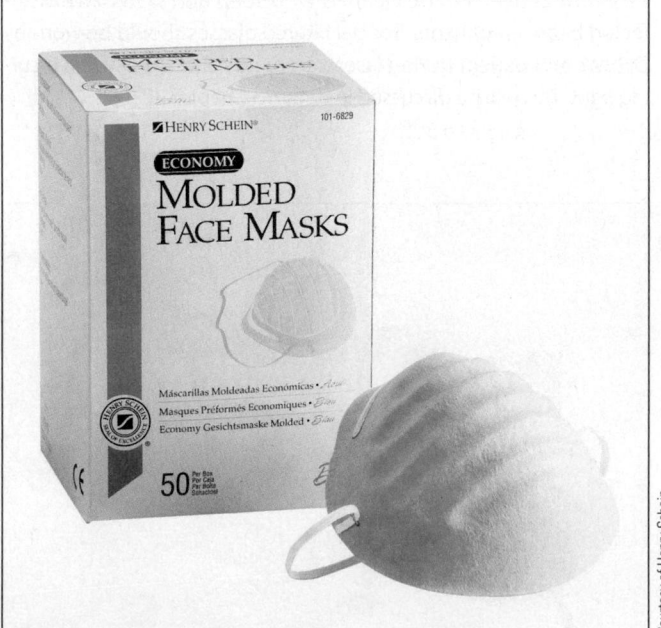

FIGURE 11-42B
Molded face mask.

Courtesy of Henry Schein

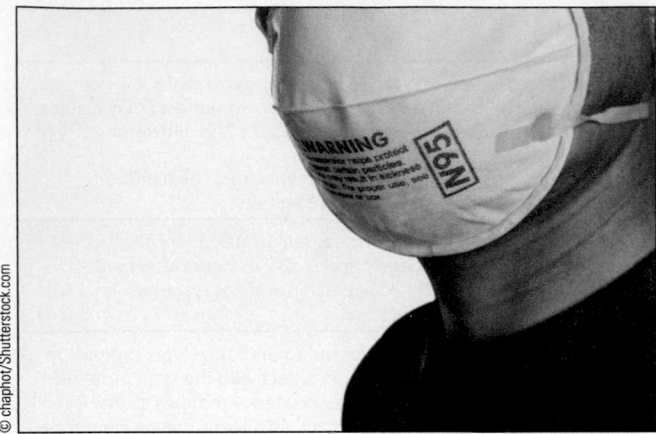

© chaphot/Shutterstock.com

FIGURE 11-43
N95 respirator mask.

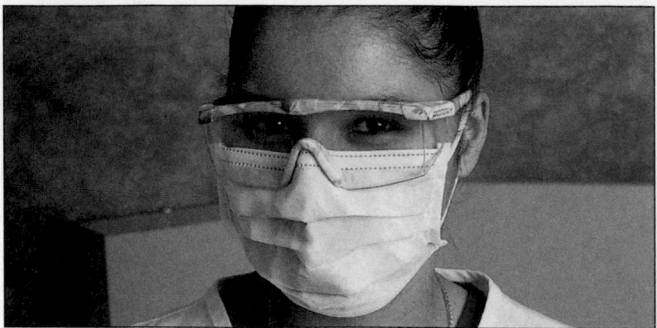

FIGURE 11-45
Assistant wearing goggles.

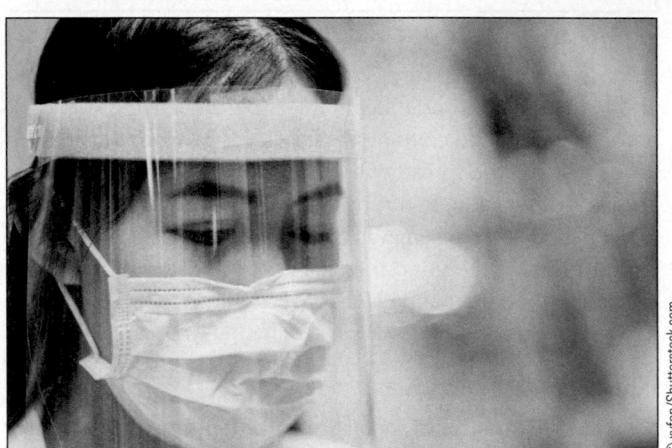

© xyfen/Shutterstock.com

FIGURE 11-46A
Dental assistant with face shield and mask.

the DHCW, patients should also wear eyewear to protect their eyes from spatter and self-infection. Eyewear protects the eyes against damage from aerosolized pathogens, such as the herpes virus; debris; tooth or amalgam fragments; and splattered solutions and chemicals. The type of protective eyewear is determined by the procedure and potential exposure to blood and OPIM:

- Safety glasses for chairside wear during patient treatment (Figure 11-44)
- Goggles when performing lab procedures (Figure 11-45)
- Face shields when there is a chance of high volume spatter and particles. Masks should be worn under shield (Figure 11-46A)

The DHCW wearing prescription glasses must wear side shield or safety glasses made to fit over prescription glasses (Figure 11-46B). All eyewear needs to be cleaned with soap and water and disinfected between patients. Special filtered glasses should be worn by DHCWs and patient during laser treatments and when using a curing light. This will be discussed in detail in Chapter 32.

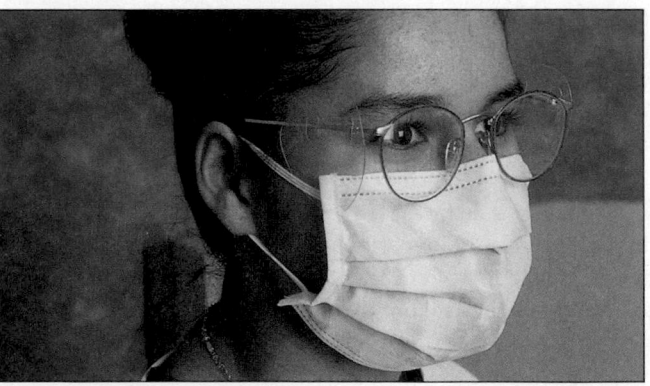

FIGURE 11-46B
Eyeglasses with side shield.

Changes in PPE related to COVID-19 pandemic

The COVID-19 pandemic has led to many changes related to infection control in dentistry. The guidelines for infection control were set by the CDC and OSHA and have evolved over time as more information regarding infection transmission became

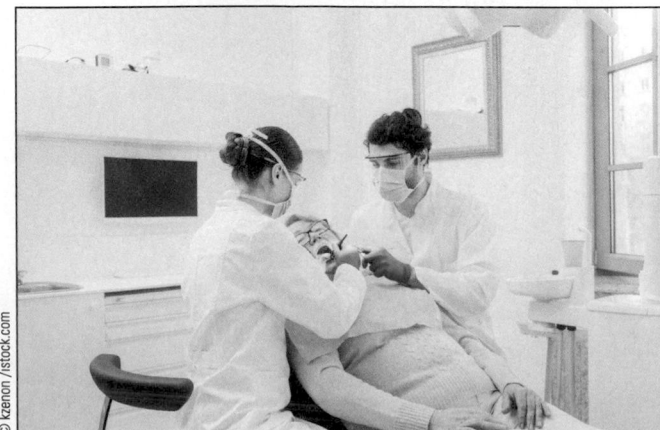

© Izenon /istock.com

FIGURE 11-44
Safety glasses during patient treatment.

available. The guidelines may change in different areas based on local transmission rate, reopening guidelines and risk to dental professionals and office staff.

During times of high transmission, OSHA recommends performing dental procedures only on an emergency basis. The guidelines recommend the postponement of elective and non-emergency procedures.

OSHA also recommends:

- The use of engineering controls such as dividers between operatories to be in place during patient treatment.

- Barriers to be placed between patients and the front desk staff (Figure 11-47).

- Not using aerosol producing equipment at this time (high-speed handpieces, air/water syringes, etc.). However, if such equipment must be used, OSHA recommends the use of high-speed evacuation and dental dams to minimize aerosols.

- Using local ventilation measures such as exhaust fans to move air from operatories to the external environment.

- Minimizing the number of people in the operatory during aerosol producing procedures and increasing the frequency of disinfection.

- Using administrative controls such as teledentistry when possible, limiting the number of people that accompany the patient to the dental office.

- Requiring that everyone wear cloth face coverings if not being actively treated.

- Extending office hours to minimize the number of patients in the office at the same time.

- All patients complete a health screening questionnaire to determine if they are a suspected COVID-19 or confirmed COVID-19 case. A patient who presents with symptoms and is determined to be an active COVID-19 case should be isolated and then sent home or to a medical facility for care.

- Training all dental personnel to avoid touching their faces and to complete as much as possible outside of the patient treatment area (e.g., entering information into the patient's record).

PPE requirements have also changed due to the COVID-19 pandemic. Box 11-2 provides OSHA guidelines related to PPE changes. All PPE must be provided by the dentist employer to the dental office employees.

Donning and Doffing PPE

The type of PPE used varies with the level of precautions required and types of exposure anticipated, splash or spray versus patient contact. CDC recommends a sequence for donning and removing full PPE to protect the DCHW from contamination. Refer to Procedure 11–5 for steps for donning and doffing PPE.

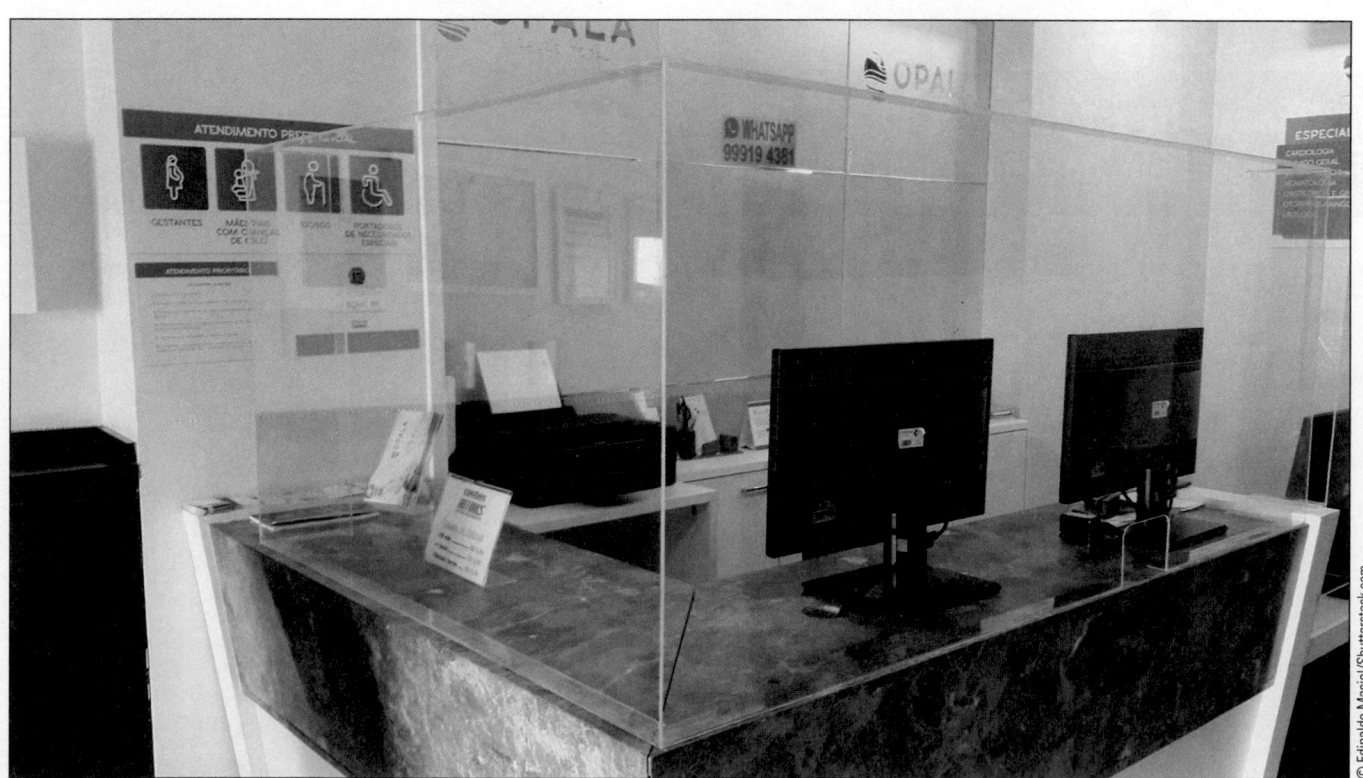

FIGURE 11-47
Barriers to be placed between patients and the front desk staff.

© Edinaldo Maciel/Shutterstock.com

BOX 11-2 OSHA Personal Protective Equipment Guidelines Related to the COVID-19 Pandemic

Providing patient care in an area where community transmission of COVID-19 has subsided.

- Non-aerosol producing procedures: use of PPE including a standard surgical mask.
- Aerosol producing procedures: use of PPE including surgical mask and faceshield or a NIOSH approved N95 respirator mask.

Providing patient care in an area where community transmission of COVID-19 continues in a local area.

- Non-aerosol producing procedures: use of PPE including surgical mask and faceshield or a NIOSH approved N95 respirator mask.
- Aerosol producing procedures: use of PPE including a NIOSH approved N95 respirator mask.

Providing patient care to a person with suspected or confirmed COVID-19 infection regardless of community transmission.

- Non-aerosol producing and aerosol producing procedures: use of PPE including a NIOSH approved N95 respirator mask.

Adapted from OSHA COVID-19 Control and Prevention/Dentistry Workers and Employers

Surface Sanitization

Sanitization refers to processes that reduce the number of microorganisms on inanimate objects to a safe level. It is generally referred to as a thorough cleaning process as it does not imply freedom from infectious microorganisms. The rationale for sanitization is to manage surface contamination.

The control of disease transmission depends on the cooperative efforts of all members of the dental team. The application of specific protective and preventive measures is required before, during, and after all patient appointments. The highest level of infection control possible will ensure a safe environment for both patients and the dental team. The CDC Guidelines for Infection Control in Dental Health-Care Settings 2003 have divided environmental surfaces into housekeeping surfaces and clinical contact surfaces.

Housekeeping Surfaces

Housekeeping surfaces include floors, walls, and sinks. These surfaces present a much lower risk for disease transmission than do clinical contact areas and patient treatment instruments. The CDC recommends that carpeting and cloth-upholstered furnishings in dental operatories, laboratories, and instrument processing areas should be avoided.

Housekeeping surfaces are cleaned with detergent and water or an EPA-registered hospital disinfectant or detergent. Mops and cloths need to be cleaned after use and allowed to dry thoroughly before storing and reuse, or use disposable, single-use mops and

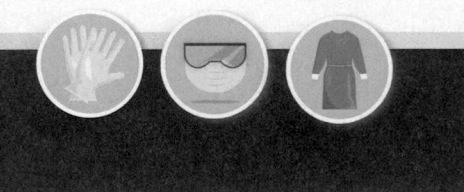

Procedure 11-5
Steps for Donning and Doffing PPE

Equipment and Supplies
- Gloves
- Protective clothing/gown
- Mask and protective eyewear

Sequence for Donning PPE

Procedure Steps

1. Select PPE by type of clinical interaction with patient.
   - ❏ Gloves—Use when touching blood, body fluids, secretions, excretions, contaminated items, mucus membranes, and nonintact skin.
   - ❏ Protective clothing/gown—Use during procedures when clothing or exposed skin may come in contact with blood, body fluids, secretions, and excretions.
   - ❏ Mask and protective eyewear—Use during procedures that may generate splashes or sprays of blood, body fluids, secretions, or excretions.

2. Don a gown without contaminating the outside of the gown (Figure 11-48).

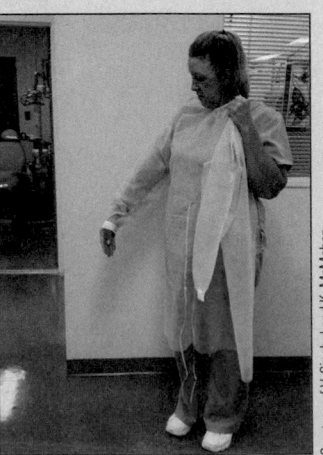

FIGURE 11-48

❑ Hold gown with left hand by the inside collar of the gown with opening of the gown toward the back.

❑ Slide right hand through the gown sleeve.

❑ Switch hands and hold the gown by the inside collar of the gown with the right hand.

❑ Slide the left hand through the gown sleeve (Figure 11-49).

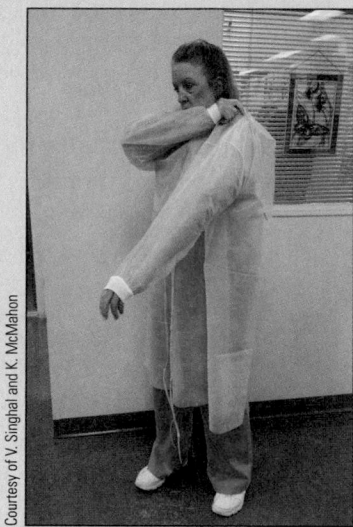

FIGURE 11-49

❑ Secure gown with neck and waist ties (Figure 11-50).

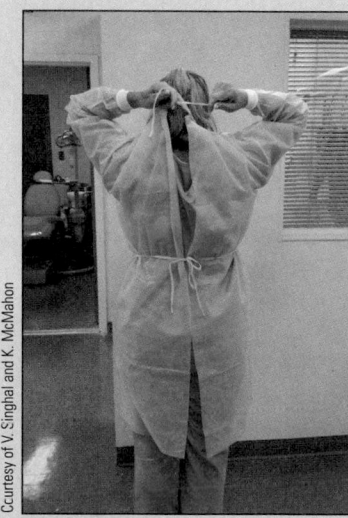

FIGURE 11-50

3. Don mask.

❑ Hold mask by the straps with the flexible nose piece facing upward (Figure 11-51).

❑ Pull mask to cover above the bridge of the nose and below the chin.

❑ Metal goes above the bridge of the nose and is pressed against nose for tight fit.

❑ Secure the mask on the head with ties or elastics.

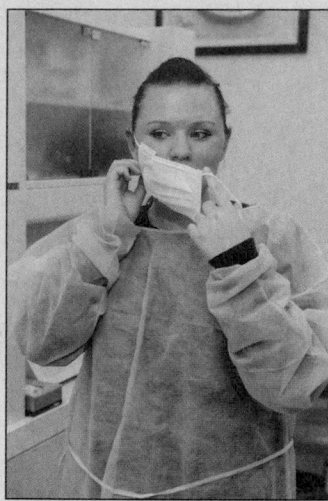

FIGURE 11-51
Wearing a mask

❑ When using ties, have one tie above the occipital bulge and the second below the ear.

❑ Pinch flexible nose piece against the bridge of the nose.

❑ Adjust the mask to completely cover the bridge of the nose, mouth, and chin.

4. Don protective eyewear (see Figure 11-45).

❑ Position eyewear over the eyes, resting on the bridge of the nose.

❑ Secure the eyewear to the head by adjusting the ear pieces.

5. Wash and dry hands as described in Procedure 11-1.

6. Don gloves, following steps as described in Procedure 11-4.

Sequence for Doffing PPE

Procedure Steps

1. Remove gloves—Gloves must be removed correctly in order to provide continued protection from contamination for the assistant. When removing gloves, it is critical that the outside of the glove does not come in contact with the assistant's skin. It is generally recommended to remove the glove with the dominant hand first because removing the first glove requires more dexterity.

❑ Grasp the left glove with the right hand (if right hand dominant) on the outside edge of cuff. Pull the glove away from the hand, turning the glove inside out while removing the glove from the left hand (Figure 11-52).

❑ Hold the removed glove in the right hand. Slide ungloved left index finger under the wrist of the right glove. Be careful not to touch the outside of the glove (Figure 11-53).

❑ Peel off the right glove from the inside. This creates a bag to hold both gloves by the inside of the glove to safely discard into the appropriate waste container.

(Continues)

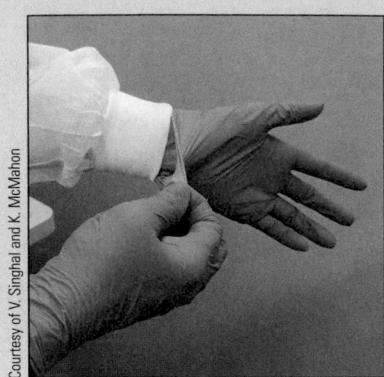

Courtesy of V. Singhal and K. McMahon

FIGURE 11-52

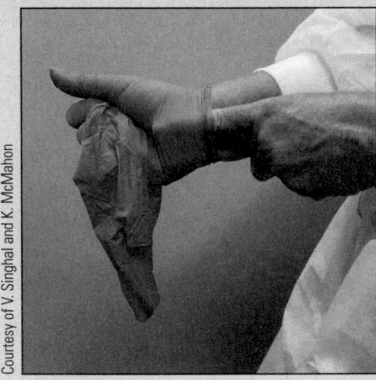

Courtesy of V. Singhal and K. McMahon

FIGURE 11-53

2. Remove protective eyewear.
   ❑ Grasp the ear piece with ungloved hands. Lift the eyewear from the face. Place eyewear in designated sanitizing area.

3. Remove gown.
   ❑ Unfasten ties.
   ❑ Hold gown by inside, neck area of the gown.
   ❑ Peel gown away from neck and shoulder (Figure 11-54).
   ❑ Turn contaminated outside of gown toward the inside.
   ❑ Fold gown into bundle taking caution to not touch contaminated outside of gown.
   ❑ Discard gown in designated area.

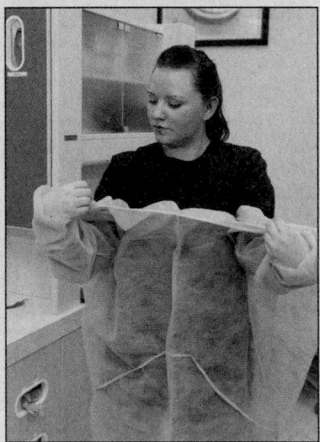

FIGURE 11-54
Doffing protective clothing.

cloths. Prepare fresh cleaning or EPA-registered disinfecting solutions daily and as instructed by the manufacturer. Clean walls and window coverings in the patient care areas whenever they are visibly dusty or soiled.

The dental office should be designed to present the least challenge to infection control measures. Treatment room features should maximize safe practice. Materials, shapes, and textures of floors, walls, sinks, countertops, dental units, dental chairs, clinician chairs, dental lights, and waste receptacles should facilitate easy cleaning and disinfecting and minimize the incidence of cross-contamination. Floors and walls and countertops should be as smooth and seamless as possible. Fabric drapery should be avoided. Surfaces should be nonabsorbent and easily cleaned (Figure 11-55).

Sinks should be smooth and have hands-free water faucets and soap and toweling dispensers. The sinks should be wide and deep enough for effective handwashing without splash and spatter. Paper toweling should be within easy reach of the sink. There should be a separate room or area with a sink for contaminated instrument care.

Clinical Contact Surfaces

Clinical contact surfaces are those surfaces directly contaminated with the DHCW's contaminated gloved hands and

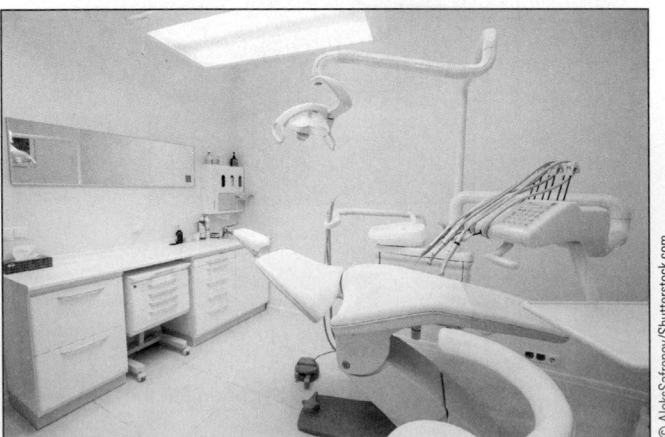

© AleksSafronov/Shutterstock.com

FIGURE 11-55
Dental office operatory.

contaminated instruments or by direct spray or spatter. Clinical contact surface must be precleaned and disinfected, protected with a surface barrier, or a combination of the two. The Office Safety and Asepsis Procedures (OSAP) Research Foundation recommends that clinical surfaces be classified and maintained under the following three categories: touch, transfer, and splash/spatter/droplet. Table 11-3 provides details regarding the various clinical contact surfaces.

TABLE 11-3 Clinical Contact Surfaces

Touch Surfaces

Touch surfaces are directly touched and contaminated during treatment procedures. These surfaces include dental light handles, dental unit controls, air-water syringe, mouthpieces for saliva ejector and high-speed evacuator, chair switches, chairside computers, pens, telephones, containers, and drawer handles.

The dental chair should have foot-operated controls to prevent contact with contaminated treatment gloves. The surface of the chair should be a smooth, seamless vinyl or plastic that can be easily cleaned and resist damage or discoloration from chemical disinfectants. Cloth upholstery should be avoided. Clinician chairs should also be smooth and seamless with a plastic seat cover that can be easily disinfected.

The dental light should be easy to clean or to apply a barrier to. Manufacturer's directions should be followed for cleaning and maintaining the integrity of the lens.

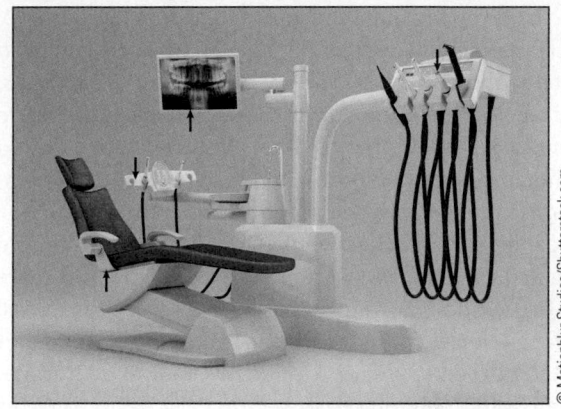
The dental chair.

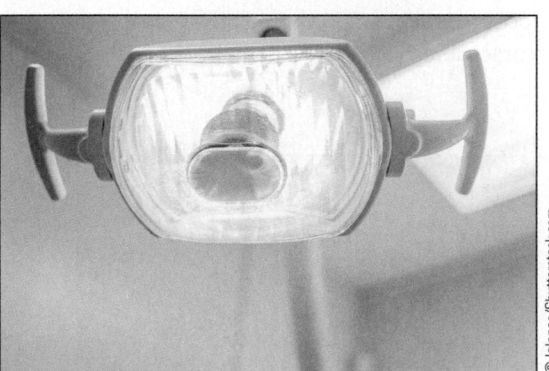
The dental light.

Transfer Surfaces

Transfer surfaces are not directly touched but may be subject to contaminated instruments. These surfaces include instrument trays, bracket trays (tables), and handpiece holders. The design of the dental unit should allow for easy cleaning and disinfection.

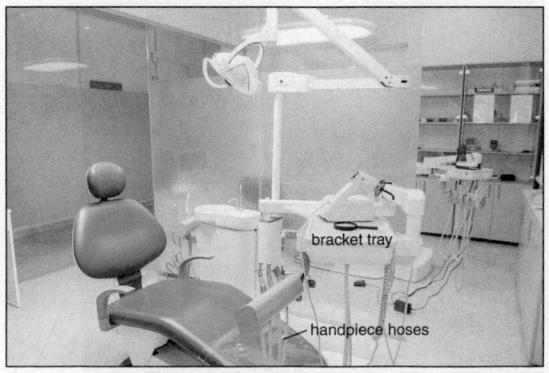

Splash, Spatter, and Droplet Surfaces

Splash, spatter, and droplet surfaces include countertops, walls, and floors within distance for air moisture. These surfaces are not touched by DHCW hands or contaminated instruments and supplies.

Precleaning Clinical Surfaces

There are two methods to handle surface contamination: preclean and disinfect surfaces between patients or prevent the surface from becoming contaminated with the use of a surface barrier. Precleaning is the process of reducing the number of microorganisms prior to disinfecting. It also removes blood and saliva, commonly referred to as **bioburden**. All contaminated surfaces must be precleaned before disinfecting, even if there is no visible blood on the surfaces (Figures 11-56A and B).

The clinician should use appropriate PPE when cleaning and disinfecting. Appropriate PPE includes gloves, eyewear, masks, and fluid repellant disposable gowns. Gloves should be puncture and chemical resistant (utility gloves). Protective eyewear and masks should be worn to protect the eyes and mucous membranes and to prohibit inhalation of airborne contaminants.

Precleaning is most effective on smooth, easily accessible surfaces. Regular soap and water may be used, but it is more efficient to use a disinfectant that has the ability to clean as well as disinfect. Clinical contact surfaces should be cleaned and disinfected between patients with an EPA-registered hospital disinfectant with an HIV, HBV claim, such as Cavicide or CaviWipes (Figure 11-57), unless they have been properly covered with an appropriate barrier (Figure 11-58).

The process of sanitization should always follow a standard operating procedure (SOP) that all dental personnel adhere to in order to ensure the chain of infection is not compromised. This maintains a safe environment for dental personnel, patients, and the community at large (Figure 11-59).

Use of Clinical Surface Barriers If a surface cannot be easily and thoroughly cleaned and disinfected, it should have barrier protection. A surface barrier is fluid-resistant and prevents microorganisms in saliva, blood, and other liquids from soaking through to contact the surface. Touch and transfer surfaces should be barrier protected and changed between patients to prevent cross contamination and reduce time and wear on surfaces. Hard-to-clean areas and all switches should also have barriers. This will prevent the entry of fluid into areas of electrical wiring.

There are several surface barriers available to keep microorganisms in water, saliva, blood or other liquids from making contact with the surface underneath. Barriers come in different types of materials, sizes, and shapes. Clear plastic is the most commonly used; plastic-backed paper, sticky tape, and aluminum foil can be used. Plastic bags are designed specifically to fit the shape of the dental chair, air-water syringes, intra-oral cameras, radiography tubeheads and sensors, hoses, and light handles (Figure 11-58). Plastic-barrier sticky tape may be used to protect smooth surfaces such as touch pads on equipment, electrical switches, and x-ray equipment.

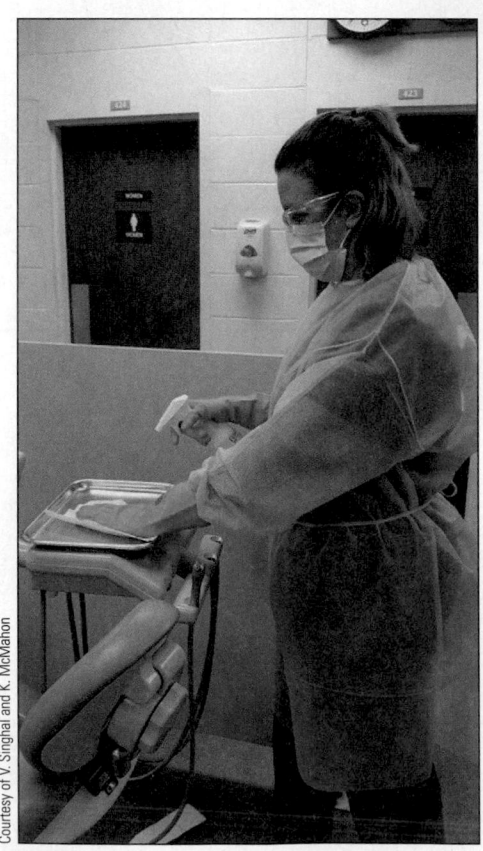

FIGURE 11-56A
Cleaning and disinfecting surfaces.

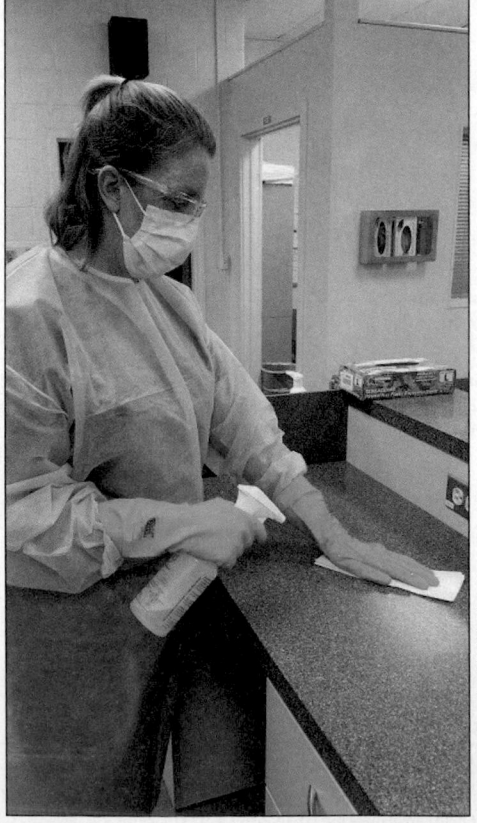

FIGURE 11-56B
Cleaning and disinfecting surfaces.

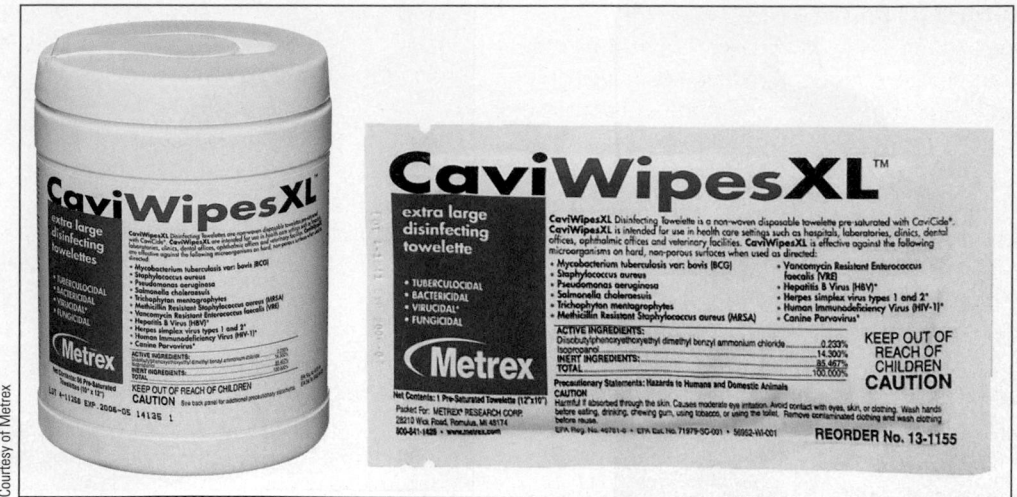

Courtesy of Metrex

FIGURE 11-57
CaviWipes for disinfection of surfaces.

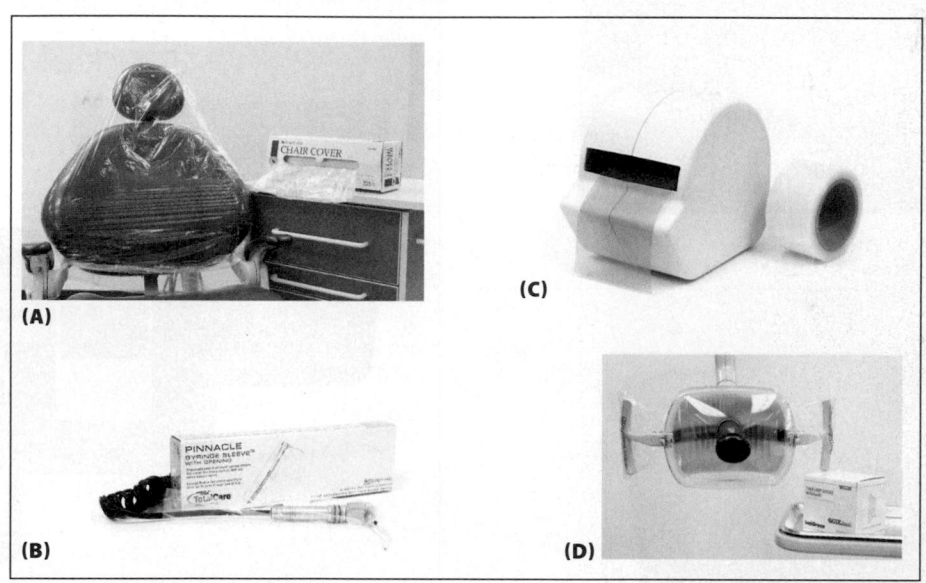

(A)

(B)

(C)

(D)

FIGURE 11-58
Various types of dental surface barriers.

Waste Disposal Federal, state, and local laws determine which categories of waste require special disposal, referred to as *regulated waste*. State and local public health authorities develop guidelines for medical waste handling and disposal methods. Although any item that has been in contact with blood or OPIM may be infectious, not all waste is regulated. Regulated medical waste found in the dental office includes soft waste such as cotton rolls and gauze that may be soaked with blood and/or saliva and contaminated sharps.

Regulated medical waste is capable of releasing blood or saliva during handling. Examples include waste soaked or saturated with blood or body fluids, extracted teeth, and surgically removed hard and soft tissues. Waste receptacles used for regulated soft medical waste need to be lined with heavy-duty plastic

bag liners that can be sealed tightly for disposal and bear a biohazard label (Figures 11-60 and 11-61). A separate, appropriately labeled biohazard receptacle should be placed in each treatment area for disposal of contaminated waste. Waste receptacles are color-coded red or yellow. States may also have guidelines for areas in the office to store medical waste, have storage times, and require special commercial waste pickup. Most states allow the discharge of fluid blood and OPIM into sanitary sewer lines. It is important that the DHCW contacts their state or county department of public health for specific guidelines.

Contaminated sharp items including needles, scalpel blades, burs, broken metal instruments, and orthodontic wire must be disposed of in sharps containers. Containers must be puncture resistant, leak-proof, tightly sealed, color-coded, and labeled with

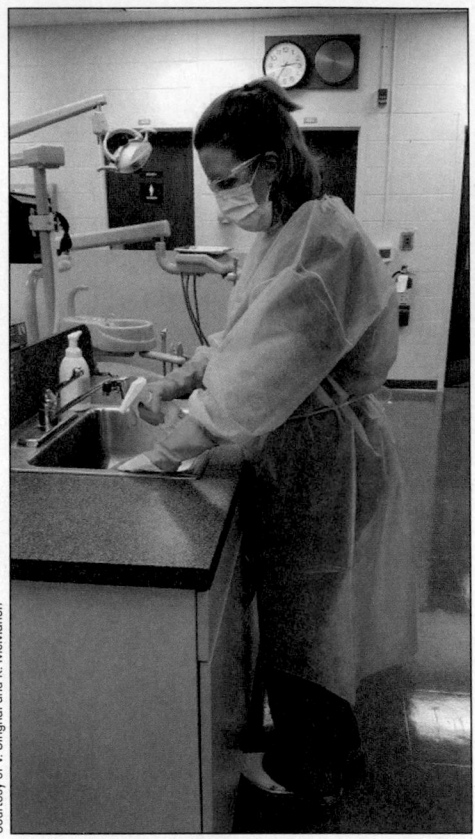

Courtesy of V. Singhal and K. McMahon

FIGURE 11-59
Disinfection of clinical surfaces.

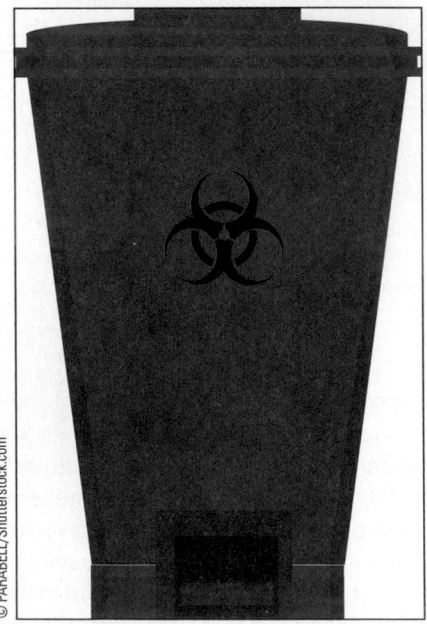

© PARABELL/Shutterstock.com

FIGURE 11-60
Biohazard container.

biohazard signage. A sharps container must be placed in each treatment area for disposal of contaminated sharps containers (Figure 11-62). Sharps containers should never be emptied and

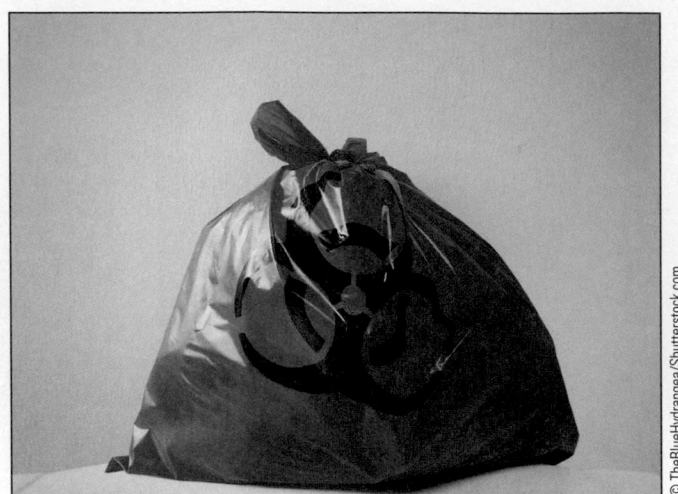

© TheBlueHydrangea/Shutterstock.com

FIGURE 11-61
Biohazard bag.

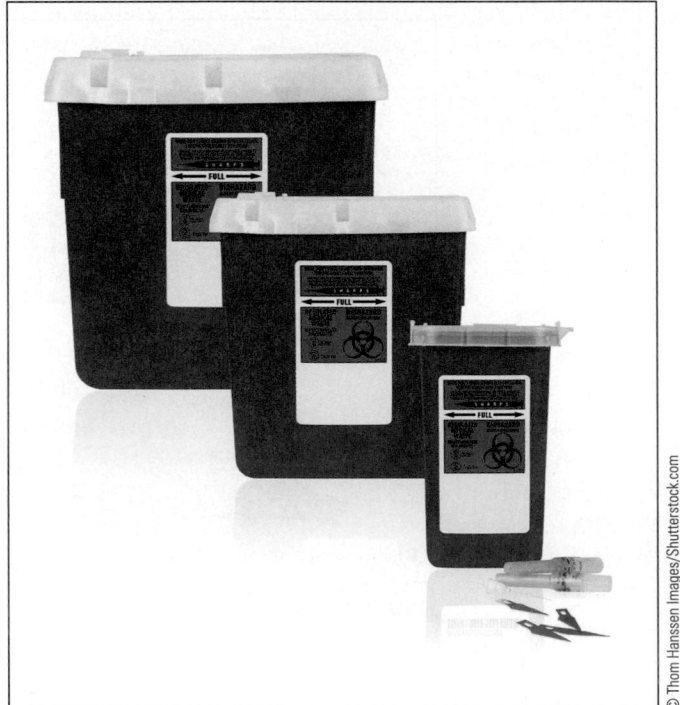

© Thom Hanssen Images/Shutterstock.com

FIGURE 11-62
Different sizes of sharps containers.

reused. There are companies that the office can contract with to collect the sharps containers when they become full. The companies will dispose of the sharps in a safe and appropriate manner. The sharps containers should be collected when the "fill-to" line has been reached.

Nonregulated medical waste is lightly contaminated articles including PPE, patient bib, surface barriers, tray covers, and paper toweling. This waste can be disposed of in lined regular trash containers with regular trash pickup.

In July 2017, the Environmental Protection Agency passed a law that requires amalgam, a silver colored filling material with trace amounts of mercury and other metals, to be disposed of via an amalgam separator. All dental offices will be required to have an amalgam separator installed by July 14, 2020. Amalgam separators prevent the material and the mercury from entering the waste water lines. Amalgam separators do fill up and need to be emptied and cleaned by a qualified and knowledgeable technician. The amalgam also must be recycled by a company that is qualified for this process. It is important to follow the regulations of your state regarding amalgam separators and amalgam recycling.

Although scope of practice regulations may vary significantly from state to state, some general rules remain a part of most waste disposal protocols:

- DHCW must wear PPE and carefully handle contaminated waste; never contact items with bare hands.
- Never compress waste by pressing down on top of trash.
- Remove waste bin liners and contents when emptying trash and dispose of the entire bag.
- Have biohazard waste removed from premises within state or county department of public health for specific guidelines and times.

Patient Treatment Instruments

Instruments and items used in the patient's mouth may be single-use items or processed and disinfected or sterilized to prevent cross-contamination.

Single Use Items

Many disposable items are used in dentistry to help reduce the chance of patient-to-patient contamination. These items are used only once and then discarded in the appropriate waste receptacle. They do not have to be cleaned, disinfected, or sterilized. Some items are manufactured to be either disposable or reusable. However, if an item presents a difficulty for cleaning, disinfecting, and sterilizing, it may be beneficial to switch to all disposable items.

Instrument Processing Area

Transporting and processing contaminated patient-care items requires attention to detail to minimize handling and avoid exposure to potentially infectious microorganisms through **percutaneous** cuts and contact with the mucous membranes.

A specific instrument processing area, or sterilization area, should be centrally located (Figure 11-63). This area should

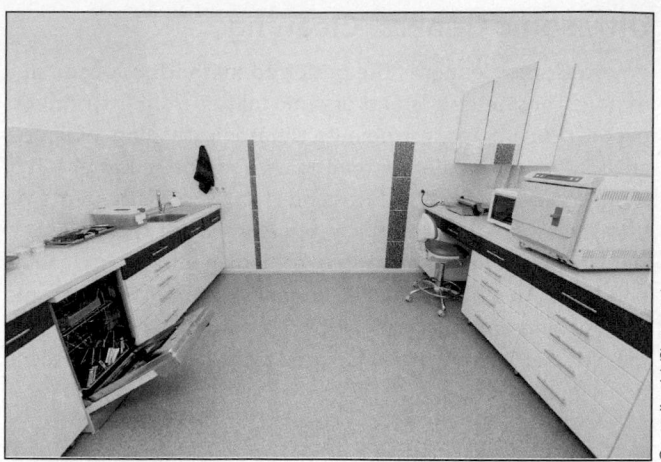

FIGURE 11-63
Dental office sterilization room.

not be a part of a common corridor that patients have to walk through. It should be separate from the treatment rooms and dental materials laboratory and should be reserved specifically for instrument processing. Good air circulation is essential for control of the heat generated by the sterilizers and any vapors that may be produced. A deep sink with hands-free controls, a hands-free trash receptacle, proper lighting, vacuum lines for flushing handpieces, and all other appropriate sterilization utilities and supplies are essential to ensure localized processing.

The processing area must be laid out in a way that prevents mixing of contaminated instruments with those that have been precleaned, packaged, and/or sterilized. Some offices employ a linear flow pattern; others employ a U-shaped flow pattern.

The contaminated instrument area is the initial receiving area. This is the area where initial cleaning is accomplished prior to disinfection and sterilization. All disposable items not already disposed of in the operatory are placed into the appropriate receptacle. If immediate cleaning is not possible, the contaminated instruments may be placed into a holding solution to prevent drying and caking of blood and debris on the instruments.

Processing of Contaminated Dental Instruments

There are eight steps involved in processing instruments. The process begins with the proper transportation of instruments. Table 11-4 provides the steps in processing instruments.

Infection Control

The CDC recommends using separate instrument processing area to limit the spread of contamination. The processing area should be divided physically into designated "dirty" and "clean" areas. In the dirty area, contaminated instruments are received and cleaned. It is important to always carry instruments in a covered container.

Ultrasonic General Cleaning

An ultrasonic cleaner is the preferred method to loosen and remove routine debris and organic matter from instruments over handscrubbing instruments. Ultrasonic cleaning minimizes cross infection, is safer for the DHCW, and does a better job of removing debris from surfaces and crevices of instruments. An ultrasonic general cleaning system consists of the ultrasonic cleaning unit, an instrument basket, and an ultrasonic cleaning unit cover. An ultrasonic general cleaning solution is placed into the cleaning unit main tank. A bur tray or mesh holder is used to hold small instruments and placed in the basket during operation (Figure 11-64).

Ultrasonic cleaners produce sound waves beyond human hearing that vibrate and create invisible bubbles in the ultrasonic cleaning solution. This formation of bubbles is called *cavitation*. Cleaning occurs by mechanical action when the bubbles burst and break inwardly (*implode*) causing a scrubbing action and by chemical action of the ultrasonic cleaning solution. The time for contaminated instruments to be exposed to this process varies from 5 to 15 minutes, depending on the efficiency of the unit and the amount and type of debris on the instruments. Follow manufacturer's directions and inspect instruments after processing to ensure instruments are visibly clean upon removal.

TABLE 11-4 Processing of Contaminated Instruments

Chairside sanitizing of instruments
The first step in processing instruments is sanitizing. Sanitizing is thoroughly cleaning an item with the complete removal of all debris and stain. It is best to sanitize instruments at the chair using utility gloves with a gauze soaked in hydrogen peroxide to make removing the debris easier. Instruments should be cleaned immediately after the procedure so the debris will not harden, making it more difficult to remove.

Transporting contaminated instruments	
After sanitizing, the tray is transported to the sterilization area. Proper transportation of instruments minimizes risk of exposure to self and environment when carrying items between the treatment and processing areas. The DHCW should wear appropriate PPE, place items on a rigid, leak-proof tray, and cover the tray before transporting.	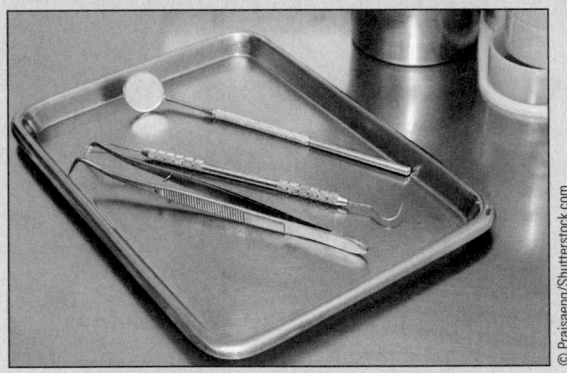 © Praisaeng/Shutterstock.com

Sterilization area sanitizing of instruments	
The CDC recommends the use of mechanical processes to sanitize instruments. An ultrasonic cleaner or instrument washer is generally used to sanitize instruments. Hand scrubbing is discouraged. Occasionally, if time does not allow for immediate cleaning, placing the instruments into a covered holding tank to allow them to presoak is the best alternative. This solution may be any noncorrosive liquid, a commercial enzymatic solution, or dishwasher detergent solution. The solution must be in a covered container and labeled with a biohazard label, indicating that it contains contaminated instruments and a chemical label indicating the type of cleaner. This solution should be changed whenever it becomes cloudy or, at least, daily.	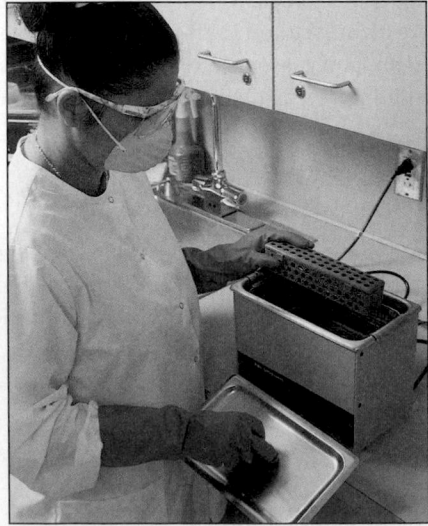

Disinfecting instruments

Once the instruments are free of debris, blood, and tissue fluids and thoroughly dried, the DHCW determines if the item requires disinfection or packaging for sterilization based on the CDC classification of instruments and procedures discussed earlier.

Sterilizing instruments

Items to be sterilized are packaged for sterilization. Instruments are run in the appropriate sterilizer for proper sterilization. Items that contact mucosa and cut tissues and are safe for sterilizers should be sterilized. Sterilization procedures are covered in later in this chapter.

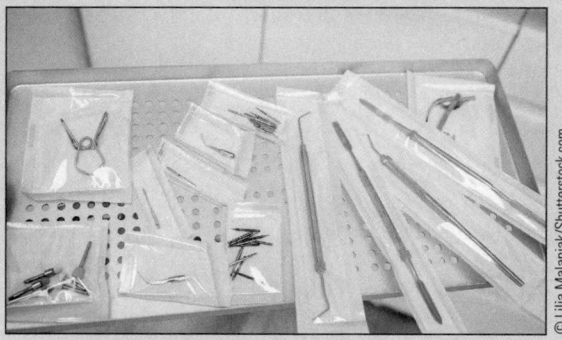

© Lilja Malanjak/Shutterstock.com

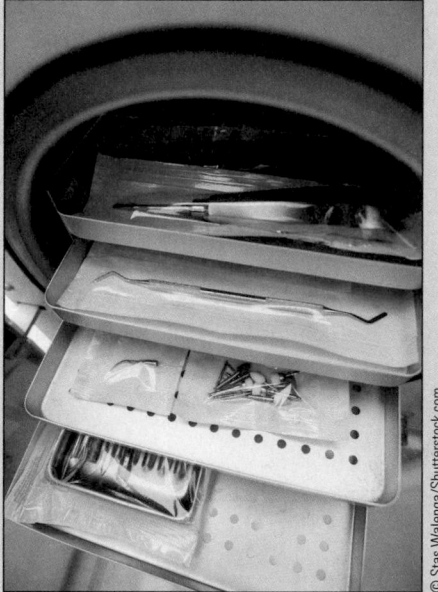

© Stas Walenga/Shutterstock.com

Storing disinfected and sterilized instruments

Disinfected and sterilized instruments must be stored in packages in a clean, dry environment to maintain the integrity of the package. Packages with tears requires that the instruments are re-cleaned, repackaged, and resterilized.

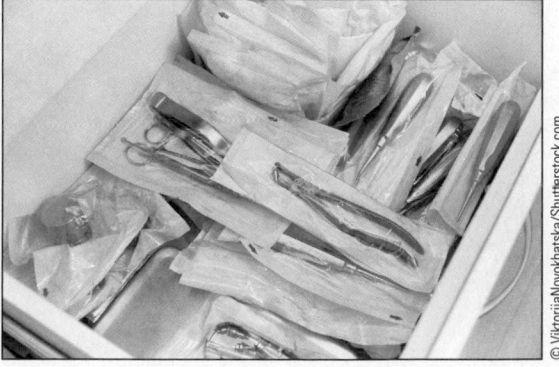

© ViktoriiaNovokhatska/Shutterstock.com

(Continues)

TABLE 11-4 *(Continued)*

Delivering processed instruments The DHCW inspects packages for damage, places packages on a tray, and covers them with bib/drape as processed instruments are carried to treatment area. Instrument packages are opened aseptically and covered with a bib/drape in the treatment area.	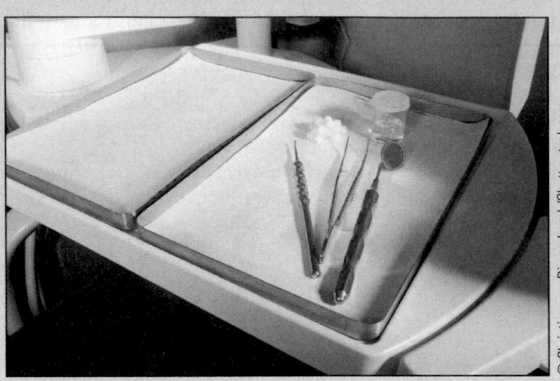 © Christine von Diepenbroek/Shutterstock.com

Ensuring processing quality

Dental offices are mandated to have a quality assurance infection control program. The program includes training, record keeping, maintenance, and testing for disinfection and sterilization of instruments. Quality assurance is discussed later in this chapter.

Some ultrasonic cleaning solutions have enzyme activity; others have antimicrobial activity. Neither type should be considered as a disinfectant. Their mechanism of action is to prohibit microorganisms from increasing in number. Only ultrasonic cleaning solutions recommended by the manufacturer's instructions should be placed in the main tank. The ultrasonic cleaning unit should be labeled with both a biohazard label and a chemical label indicating that it contains contaminated instruments and a chemical.

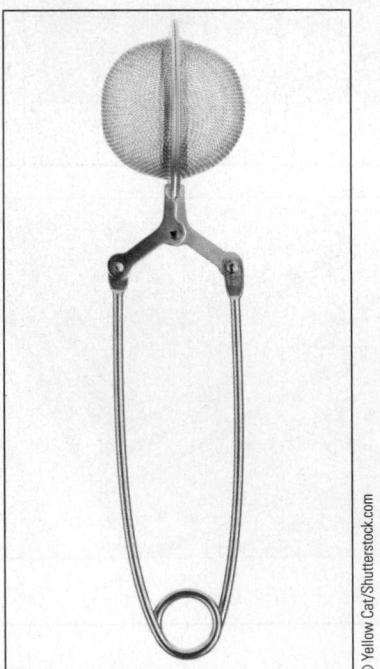

FIGURE 11-64
Bur basket for ultrasonic cleaner.

The ultrasonic cleaner solution must be inspected and discarded when it becomes cloudy or at least once a day. Wear protective clothing, mask, and eyewear for protection from exposure to chemical ultrasonic solution and contaminated aerosol.

When the solution is drained, the inside of the unit should be rinsed with water, disinfected, rinsed again, and dried. All appropriate PPE should be worn while changing solutions in the ultrasonic cleaner. Ensure the ultrasonic cleaning container contains the appropriate level of solution as recommended by the manufacturer. Instruments that are being cleaned must be completely submerged in the solution. Keep the ultrasonic cleaner covered while in use to reduce spatter and contamination of the processing area and to ensure operator safety. Wear utility gloves when placing instruments into the ultrasonic cleaner to avoid accidental injury. It is preferable to use instrument tongs to place loose instruments in the basket. If using instrument cassettes, place them into the basket. Keep lid on ultrasonic when not in use to prevent evaporation of the solution and minimize airborne contamination of the solution.

If instruments are not visibly clean after following manufacturer's directions, the ultrasonic cleaner may not be working properly. A simple test to check the effectiveness of the unit can be conducted using a piece of 5 x 5 inch aluminum foil. Hold the foil in a vertical position, half submerged in fresh, unused solution. Turn the unit on for 20 seconds. Remove the foil from the unit and hold it up to the light. The foil should be evenly marked with a tiny pebble-like appearance over the entire surface that was submerged in the solution. If there is not an evenly pebbled appearance, the unit should be serviced by the manufacturer.

Operating the Ultrasonic Cleaner Proper use of the ultrasonic cleaner is imperative to remove debris and organic matter from patient care instruments. Refer to Procedure 11-6 for steps in using the ultrasonic cleaner.

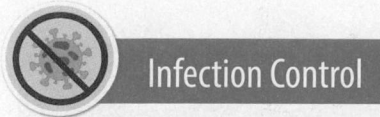

Infection Control

Follow all OSHA guidelines for exposure to chemical agents used for sanitization, disinfection, and sterilization. It is important to read and understand safety data sheets (SDSs) for all chemicals prior to using (Figure 11-65).

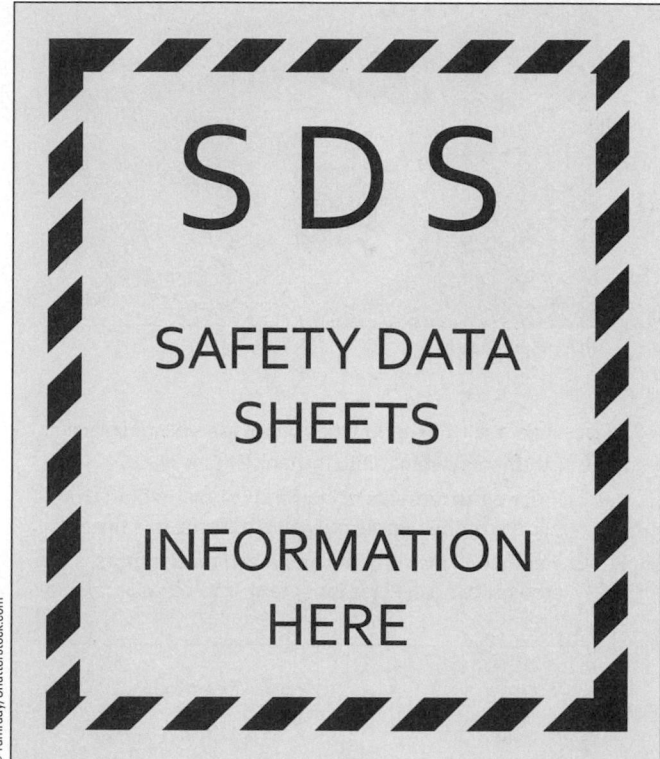

FIGURE 11-65
Safety Data Sheets.

Ultrasonic Cleaner: Special Solutions for Stubborn Stains There are different types of ultrasonic cleaning solution available. The general purpose cleaner is primarily used for routine debris (see Figure 11-73). It is available ready to use or as a superconcentrate (see Figure 11-74). There are stubborn stains that require the use of special ultrasonic solutions. Special stain removal solutions include tartar and stain remover for dentures; temporary cement remover for crowns; permanent cement remover for crowns; alginate, plaster, stone, and wax removers; and other hard-to-remove substances. Always follow manufacturer's directions for the product of choice. Improper use can permanently destroy instruments. For example, the finish of instruments can be damaged if an instrument is left in a permanent cement remover or if the instrument is not neutralized in the general cleaner or rinsed properly. When using special solutions, such as to clean a patient's removable dentures, a glass beaker is used to hold the solutions (see Figure 11-75). A beaker tray is placed over the tank to secure the beakers during operation. Follow the manufacturer's instructions for each type of solution.

Automated Washing/Disinfectors

Automated washing/disinfectors use hot water and detergents to remove organic material, similar to a household dishwasher. The FDA must approve these disinfectors for use with dental instruments. Instruments processed in automated washers/disinfectors are automatically dried and, upon removal, are wrapped and sterilized. The washers are the least hazardous for the assistant. The DHCW handles the instruments even less, thus reducing the risk of sticking themselves and getting infected (see Figure 11-76).

Handscrubbing Dental Instruments

Handscrubbing should be used as a last alternative after the instruments have been run through the ultrasonic cleaner solutions or washer if debris still remains on the instrument. In some states, OSHA actually prohibits handscrubbing. In these states, cleaning must be accomplished in an instrument washing machine or ultrasonic cleaner. Dental office personnel must be aware of state regulations. If handscrubbing cannot be avoided, a specific protocol must be followed. Wear all appropriate PPE, including protective clothing, goggle-type protective eyewear, and puncture-resistant gloves. Hold instrument in the middle of the handles and clean instruments one at a time using a long-handled brush, ensuring visibility of sharp instrument ends at all times. Scrub in a direction away from the body and into the sink bottom. Allow instruments to air-dry or pat them with thick toweling. *Never* roll or rub the instruments in a towel; this will increase the risk of accidental injury.

Procedures for More Difficult Stains

There are some debris and stains that require additional procedures to remove. Serrations and crevices in instruments also make the removal of debris challenging. Special instruments and chemical are needed to remove all this debris and stain. A bur brush is designed to remove hardened tooth debris from dental instruments such as burs used to drill decay or existing restorations (Figure 11-77).

Treatment of Contaminated Tray in Sterilization Area

After treating the patient, the DHCW transports the contaminated instruments to the processing area wearing utility gloves, protective clothing, protective eyewear, and mask. Instruments should be placed on the instrument tray and covered for safety during

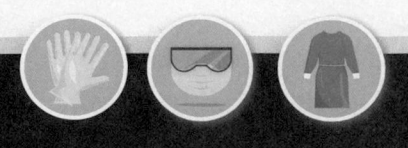

Procedure 11-6
Using an Ultrasonic Cleaner

Equipment and Supplies
- Personal protective equipment
- Ultrasonic cleaner
- General cleaner
- Dental instruments (to be cleaned)
- Towels

Procedure Steps

1. Check condition of the general cleaner and change as needed. Solution should contain minimal debris, be clear, and completely cover the instruments. Replenish tank of the ultrasonic above the instrument level with a general cleaner as needed between solution changes.

2. Change solution as needed.
   - ❏ Unplug unit and release latch to drain the tank (Figure 11-66).

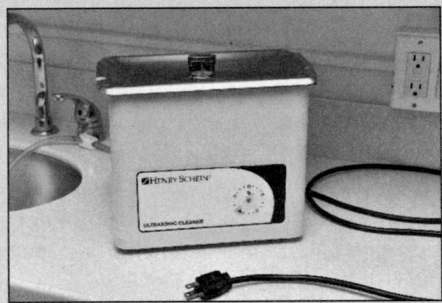

FIGURE 11-66
Ultrasonic unit unplugged.

   - ❏ Place inner tank in sink; rinse and thoroughly dry the tank (Figure 11-67).

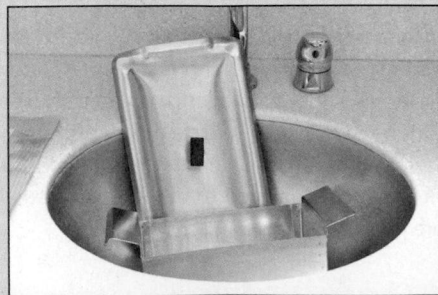

FIGURE 11-67

   - ❏ Place unit on counter, plug in unit, lock latch, and fill general cleaner to height that will cover the instruments (Figure 11-68).

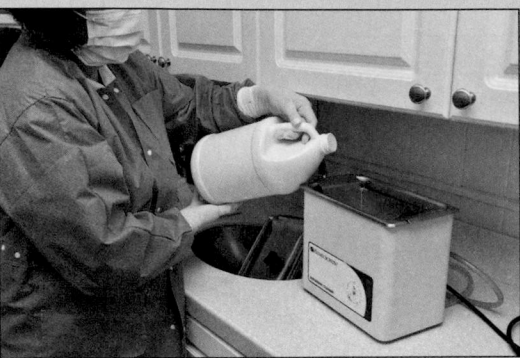

FIGURE 11-68

3. Place inner tank into upright position in the sink and place the instruments carefully into the tank (Figure 11-69).
   - ❏ Pick up instruments using tongs or by holding the middle of the handle only, two or three at a time.
   - ❏ Place small instruments into mesh holder (burs, crowns, bands). Place inner tank into ultrasonic unit.

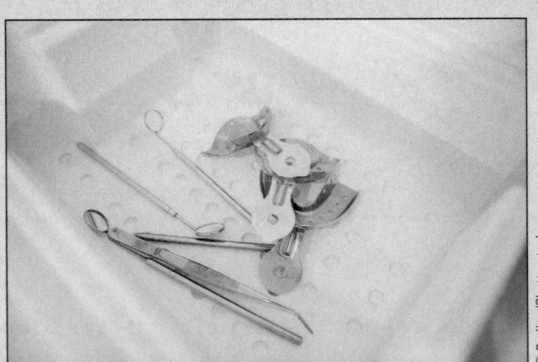

© Parilov/Shutterstock.com

FIGURE 11-69

4. Place cleaner lid on tank during operation.

5. Set the ultrasonic cleaner timer per the manufacturer's recommendation.

6. Lift the inner tank from the general cleaner after the recommended time (Figure 11-70). Allow excess solution to drain into the ultrasonic cleaner tank.
   - ❏ Place inner tank into sink and rinse instruments under water until all solution is rinsed free (Figure 11-71).

7. Place instruments onto towel and blot dry with a second towel. All excess water must be removed prior to disinfection or sterilization. Excess water will dilute the disinfectant and will cause rust or corrosion when sterilizing (Figure 11-72).

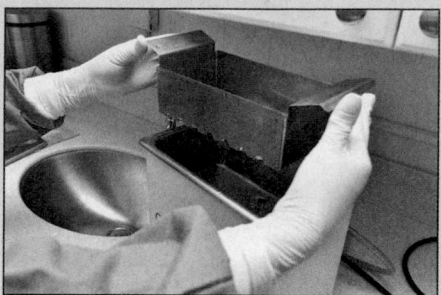

FIGURE 11-70

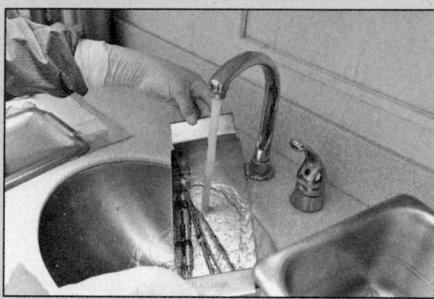

FIGURE 11-71

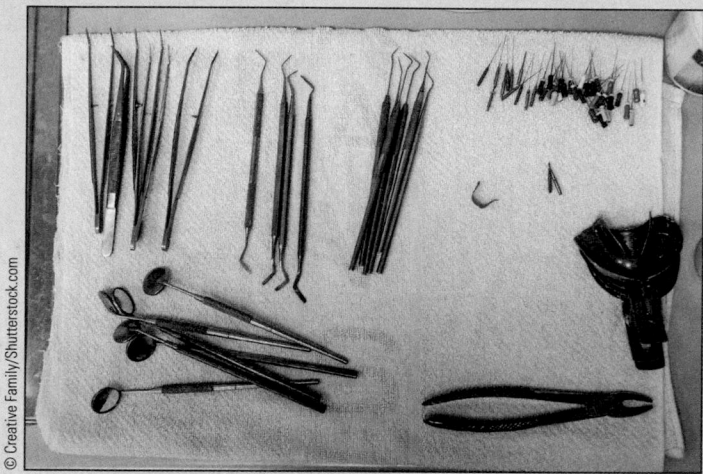

FIGURE 11-72

8. Inspect all instruments to ensure that they are debris free before bagging for sterilization.

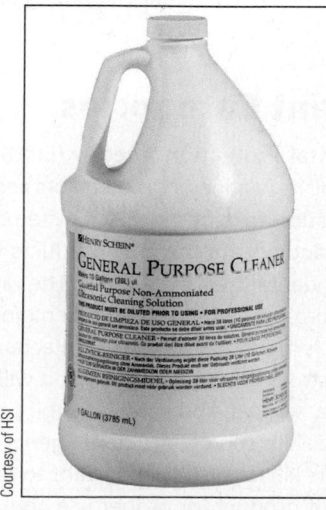

FIGURE 11-73
General ultrasonic solution.

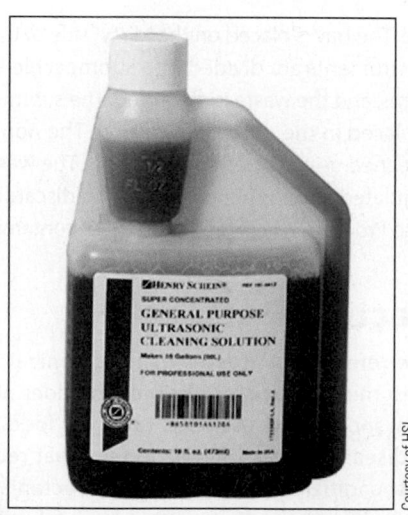

FIGURE 11-74
Superconcentrate of ultrasonic cleaning solution.

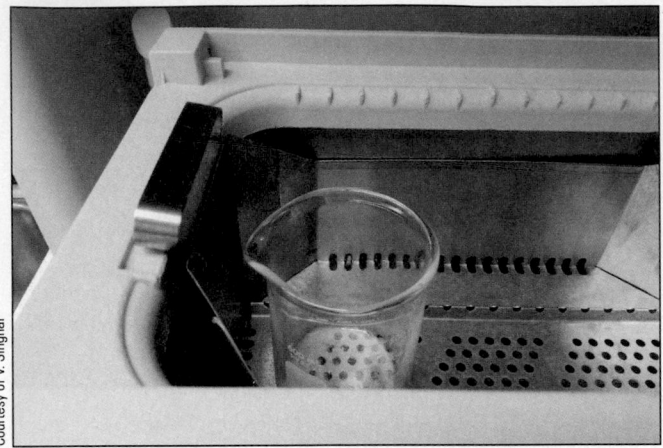

Courtesy of V. Singhal

FIGURE 11-75
Ultrasonic unit with beaker inside.

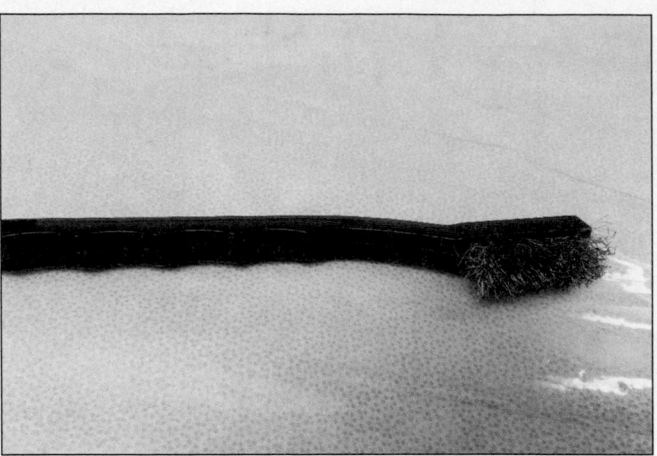

Courtesy of V. Singhal

FIGURE 11-77
Bur brush.

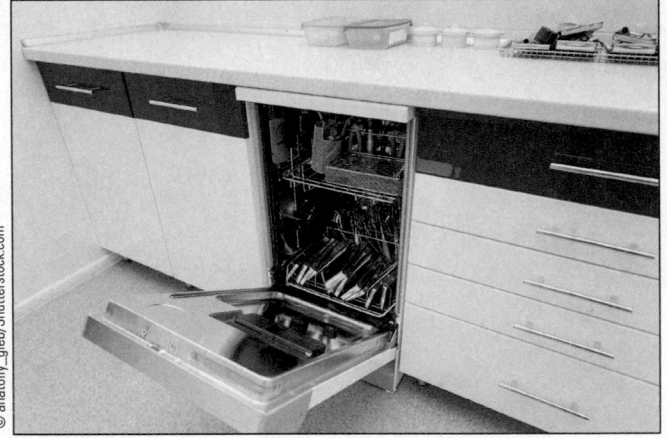

© anatoliy_gleb/Shutterstock.com

FIGURE 11-76
Automated dental dishwasher.

transporting. The tray is placed on the "dirty" side of the processing area. The instruments are divided into submersible and nonsubmersible items, and the waste is discarded. The submersible instruments are placed in the ultrasonic cleaner. The nonsubmersible items are cleaned using wipes and toweling. The waste is divided into nonregulated and regulated waste and discarded appropriately. Refer to Procedure 11-7 for treatment of contaminated tray.

Disinfection Protocols

Disinfection refers to processes using chemical agents that destroy most microorganisms. Disinfection does not kill resistant bacterial spores or viruses. The rationale for disinfection is to control disease-producing pathogens that remain on the surface after sanitizing procedures. Disinfectants should primarily be used for items that cannot be safely sterilized and general surfaces. In selecting the appropriate disinfectant, the dental assistant must be aware of the use of the area or item based on the CDC Classification of Instruments and the type of

contamination. Disinfection should not be confused with sterilization, which is the process of destroying all forms of life, including spores. Sterilization will be covered later in this chapter.

Classification of Instruments and Procedures

After items are free of debris and thoroughly dried, the dental assistant determines whether the item requires disinfection or sterilization based on the CDC Classification of Instruments and Procedures. Patient care items are categorized into three classifications based on the patient tissue the item or instrument comes in contact with and the function of the instrument. The degree of patient contact an item has suggests the risk of disease transmissions. The CDC recommends how items should be processed for reuse based on lowest to highest risk of disease transmission and categorized as noncritical, semicritical, and critical items. Table 11-5 provides details regarding each category of instruments.

Disinfectant Categories

The Environmental Protection Agency (EPA) is the agency responsible for the regulation of disinfectants according to their chemical classification. In dentistry, EPA registered products with **tuberculocidal** activity are the only products that should be used to disinfect dental treatment areas. The rationale for this is that the microorganism that causes tuberculosis, *Mycobacterium tuberculosis*, is highly resistant to disinfectants. Therefore, if a disinfectant destroys this microorganism, it will inactivate less resistant bacteria, viruses, and certain fungi. Chemical agents labeled **sporicidal** kills spores, **virucidal** agents kill viruses, and **fungicidal** agents kill fungi. It is important to read the label of every disinfectant product for proper use and handling, storage and disposal information, directions for use, shelf life, and safety warnings. The EPA has developed categories for chemical disinfectants as low, intermediate, and high level for ease in

Procedure 11-7
Treatment of a Contaminated Tray

Equipment and Supplies
- Personal protective equipment
- Contaminated tray, including high-speed handpiece
- Biohazard waste container
- Regular waste container
- Sharps container
- Ultrasonic cleaner
- Sink
- Dental high-speed handpiece
- Isopropyl alcohol
- Disposable paper towels

Procedure Steps

1. Divide items on tray into categories: waste, submersible, and nonsubmersible items. Select appropriate waste container.

2. Discard visibly contaminated disposable items in a biohazard container (Figure 11-78).

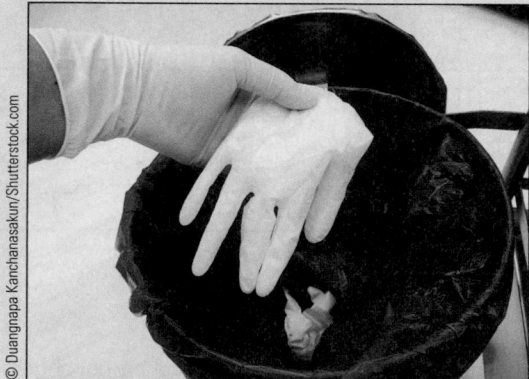

FIGURE 11-78
Dental assistant placing biohazard trash into biohazard container.

3. Discard lightly contaminated disposable items in the regular trash.

4. Dispose of contaminated sharps in the sharps container (Figure 11-79). Detach needle from anesthetic syringe using needle removal device on the lid of the sharps container. Allow the needles to drop into the sharps

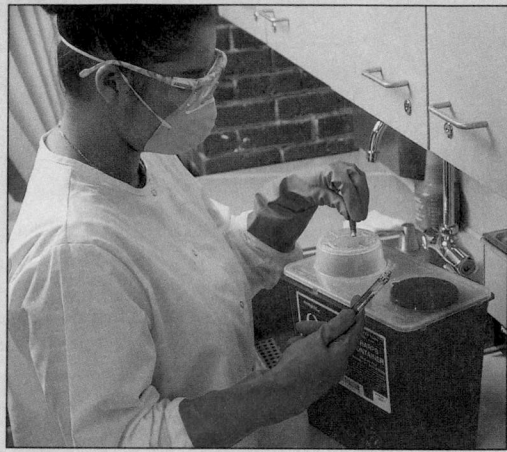

FIGURE 11-79
Dental assistant placing sharps in a sharps container.

container. Remove the anesthetic cartridge from the syringe and place into the sharps container.

5. Clean submersible instruments in the ultrasonic cleaner as outlined in Procedure 11-6.

6. Sanitize nonsubmersible items.
   - ❏ Rinse and dry safety glasses, instrument tray prepared for disinfection.
   - ❏ Prepare the dental high-speed handpiece per manufacturer's direction.
   - ❏ Run handpiece at unit after treatment or on air station in processing area (Figure 11-80).
   - ❏ Rinse and dry or wipe with isopropyl alcohol (Figure11-81).

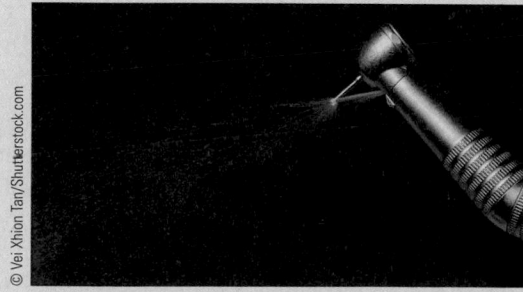

FIGURE 11-80
Dental handpiece being run at unit after treatment.

(Continues)

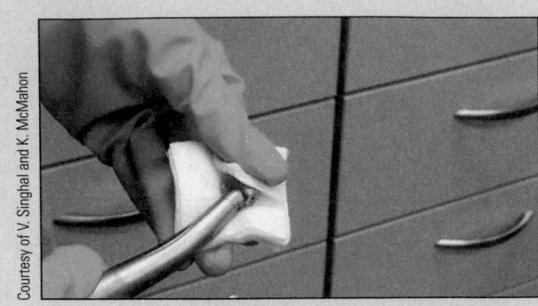

Courtesy of V. Singhal and K. McMahon

FIGURE 11-81
Disinfecting contaminated instruments.

7. Place all sanitized instruments into area designated for disinfection and sterilization.

8. Clean and disinfect the work area as outlined earlier in the discussion regarding clinical contact surfaces.

9. Clean utility gloves: Wash with soap and water under faucet, then remove and disinfect the utility gloves with surface disinfectant.

10. Remove PPE and discard in regular trash container.

11. Wash and dry hands.

TABLE 11-5 Three Categories of Risk of Transmitting Infection for Dental Instruments

Category	Procedure	Examples of Instruments	Infection Control
critical instruments	Penetrate soft tissue or bone; enter into or contact the bloodstream or other normally sterile tissue.	Surgical forceps, scalpels, bone chisels, and surgical burs	Sterilize after use. The items with the highest risk of disease transmission cut bone and hard structures or penetrate soft tissues. All critical items require sterilization. Sterilization techniques are discussed later in this chapter.
semicritical instruments	Do not penetrate soft tissues or bone; contact mucous membranes or nonintact skin.	Mirrors, reusable impression tray and amalgam condensers, radiographic image receptor holders, orthodontic pliers	Sterilize after use; when not feasible use high-level disinfection (registered with EPA as "sterilant/disinfectant")
noncritical instruments	Contact only intact skin.	Radiology machine heads, blood pressure cuffs and pulse oximeters, lead apron	Noncritical items can be barrier-protected or disinfected by using intermediate level disinfection (EPA registered hospital disinfectant with tuberculocidal claim). Low-level disinfectants that are nontuberculocidal can be used on surfaces and items that have not been contaminated with blood.

determining which disinfectant is most effective. Table 11-6 provides details about different levels of disinfectants.

Chemicals Not EPA Registered as Disinfectant

Although ethyl alcohol and isopropyl alcohol have bactericidal and tuberculocidal activity, they are not recommended to be used as a disinfectant. Due to their rapid evaporation, they are not effective in the presence of blood and saliva. Therefore, the American Dental Association (ADA), CDC, and OSAP do not recommend alcohol as a surface disinfectant. Dental equipment manufacturers do not recommend its use due to the damaging effects on plastics and vinyl. Alcohol is still used as a useful sanitizer to remove residue of disinfectants (iodophors) and shine metal surfaces.

Sodium hypochlorite (household bleach) is no longer recommended by the CDC as a disinfectant in the dental setting. It is still recommended as a sanitizer especially effective in removing blood from surfaces. Sodium hypochlorite is a rapid-acting, broad-spectrum disinfectant with bactericidal, sporicidal, and virucidal activities. It can degrade plastics, metals, and fabrics. Disadvantages of sodium hypochlorite include the need for daily preparation, strong odor, corrosiveness, and irritation to the skin and eyes.

Disinfecting Procedures

All health care team members must understand the importance of good infection control and follow all infection control procedures to maintain the highest level of safety for patients and the dental team. The two-step process of cleaning and disinfection of dental treatment rooms and instruments involves the use of chemicals and PPE.

TABLE 11-6 EPA Chemical Classification of Disinfectants

Chemical Category	Definition	Examples	Uses
high-level disinfectants	Destroys all microorganisms, save high numbers of bacterial endospores	glutaraldehyde, hydrogenperoxide, glutaraldehydephenate, hydrogen peroxide with peracetic acid, peracetic acid, orthophthalaldehyde	Heat-sensitive items; immersion only Not appropriate for environmental surface disinfection These disinfectants are used exclusively for semicritical items when the item cannot tolerate heat sterilization, such as plastic and rubber items used in the oral cavity. These items must be immersed in disinfectant. The only way to destroy microorganisms using the high level disinfectant is to submerge instruments in solutions to ensure all surfaces contact solution. Chemical agents with bacterial spore label claims containing glutaraldehyde are generally preferred. There are manufacturer claims for the high level disinfectants to be used as a disinfectant and as a sterilant. The recommended times for use as a disinfectant are less (90 minutes) whereas its use as a sterilant is longer (up to 10 hours) and may be active for up to 28 days. All sterilants and disinfectants are toxic to some degree. Glutaraldehyde is highly toxic, and manufacturer's instructions must be followed closely.
intermediate-level disinfectants	Destroys vegetative bacteria, most fungi, and viruses	EPA-registered hospital disinfectants with label claims of tuberculocidal activity. chlorine-based products, phenolics, iodophors, quaternary ammonium compounds with alcohol, bromides	Clinical contact surfaces and noncritical surfaces soiled with visible blood. Disinfectants in this category are recommended for disinfection of dental clinical areas where a noncritical item or surface and surfaces are visibly soiled with blood or saliva. Use only EPA registered hospital disinfectants with tuberculocidal label claims. The two most common intermediate disinfectants are *synthetic phenol* and *iodophor*. Synthetic phenol is recommended for flat, large areas that are not directly touched or used in the patient's oral cavity. Synthetic phenol compounds are broad-spectrum EPA-registered intermediate-level disinfectants. These products can be used on metal, glass, rubber, and plastic though they may leave a residual film on treated surfaces. Daily preparation is required. This disinfectant can be used as a spray-wipe-spray where the DHCW sprays the surface with the disinfectant, wipes the surface to sanitize, and sprays the surface the second time and spray is left for the time specified for disinfection. The DHCW can also use the saturate-wipe-saturate technique. Gauze squares are saturated in disinfectant or commercial wipes with disinfectant are used to wipe the item to sanitize, and a second saturated gauze remains wrapped around the item for the time specified for disinfection. Due to the increased aerosol produced by spraying the aerosol, the saturate-wipe-saturate method is preferred. Iodophor is a higher level of the intermediate disinfectants. It is recommended for items directly touched or used in patient's oral cavity. Only the saturate-wipe-saturate application should be used. Iodophors are rapid acting, broad-spectrum disinfectants with residual activity. These EPA-registered intermediate-level disinfectants have tuberculocidal action. They are recommended for disinfecting surfaces contaminated with potentially infectious microorganisms and are usually effective within 5–10 minutes. These products contain iodine, which may corrode or discolor metals, clothing, and vinyl surfaces. Another disadvantage is that iodophors must be mixed with distilled water because hard tap water will inactivate their activities.
low-level disinfectants	Can destroy vegetable bacteria, some fungi, and viruses Cannot inactivate *Mycobacterium bovis* (not tuberculocidal)	EPA-registered hospital disinfectants that lack label claims of tuberculocidal activity quaternary ammonium compounds	Housekeeping surfaces such as floors, walls, and noncritical surfaces without visible blood Clinical contact surfaces

Before starting the cleaning and disinfection process, don protective eyewear and clothing and heavy-duty utility gloves. Examination gloves used for patient care should not be used for cleaning and disinfecting because the chemicals will degrade them and allow both chemical and contaminants to penetrate to the skin. Ensure the products have been correctly prepared and are fresh. Read and follow manufacturer's directions and determine effectiveness of the disinfectant. Each disinfecting agent will have specified purposes, mixing directions, and expiration dates after which the disinfectant is no longer effective.

Disinfecting Clinical Contact Surfaces

Most dental offices use a combination of surface barriers and cleaning and disinfection procedures. The amount of direct patient contact and aerosol that contaminates the area must be considered in determining the appropriate disinfecting procedure. With minimal contamination, the spray-wipe-spray method is acceptable. When an area is highly contaminated, the cleaning and disinfecting products should be applied to a paper towel or gauze square to wipe the contaminated surfaces. Do not spray products directly onto contaminated surfaces. This can cause microorganisms to become aerosolized. After all surfaces have been cleaned, use a fresh paper towel or gauze square to apply the intermediate level disinfectant. Allow the surface to remain moist for the manufacturer's recommended time for tuberculocidal activity, usually ten (10) minutes. After the recommended time, the surfaces may be wiped dry. Water may be used to rinse residual disinfectant from surfaces that will come into contact with the patient's skin to avoid skin irritation and to avoid damage to the patient's clothing (see Figures 11-56A and B).

Disinfecting Transfer Surfaces

The higher intermediate level disinfectants (iodophors or quaternary ammonium) are used to disinfect surfaces touched by contaminated instruments and contaminated gloved hands during patient treatment such as handpiece holders, mouthpieces, and resin lights. Gauze squares are saturated in the disinfectant and surfaces are then disinfected using the saturate-wipe-saturate method. The disinfectant must remain in contact with the items surface for the manufacturer's recommended time (Figure 11-82).

Disinfecting Contaminated Instruments

The immersion method is used when disinfecting contaminated instruments that are heat sensitive and cannot be autoclaved. High level disinfectants are placed into an instrument tray and placed into a disinfecting dish. Care must be taken to make certain all the instruments are completely submerged and all hinged instruments are open to cover all areas with the disinfectant. The lid is closed and the instruments remain submerged for the time specified by the manufacturer's directions.

High level disinfectants are toxic and can irritate the eyes, mucous membranes, skin, and lungs. PPE should always be worn when using these chemicals. They should never be used for surface disinfection. The lid on the immersion container should always be closed to minimize fumes. The manufacturer's instructions should be followed when using high level disinfectants.

Factors Affecting Disinfectant Efficiency

Chemical disinfectants are balanced to give optimum disinfection. The effectiveness of the chemical agent depends on many variables. These variables are provided in Table 11-7.

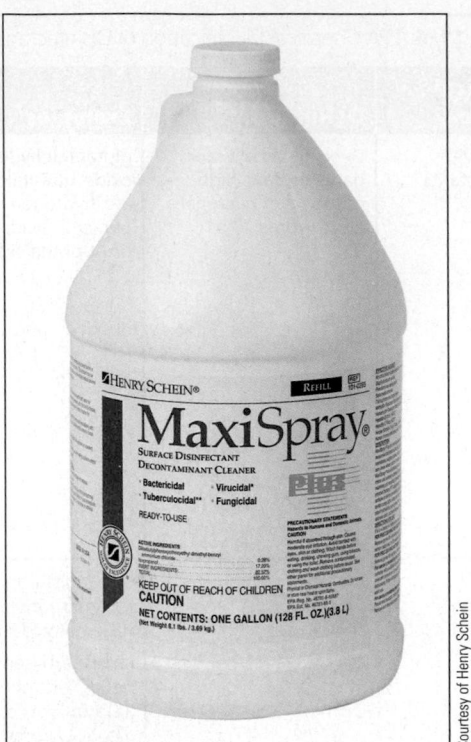

FIGURE 11-82
Surface disinfectant.

Disinfecting Waterlines

Untreated water used in dental units for patient treatment may contain high microbial counts and be potentially infectious. The water delivered by dental unit waterlines (DUWL) that connect the high-speed handpiece, air-water syringe, and ultrasonic scaler to the water supply must meet the EPA regulatory standards for safe drinking water of less than 500 bacterial colonies or colony forming units (CFU) of **heterotrophic** water bacteria per milliliter of water. Microbial counts greater than l,000,000 CFU/ml have been reported in dental unit waterlines. A case report published in 2012 by Dr. Maria Luisa Ricci addressed how an otherwise healthy 82-year-old woman contracted Legionnaire's disease after a dental visit. Previously, Legionnaire's sources of infection were primarily air-conditioning systems, hot-water systems, and spas. This case has proven that Legionnaire's can be acquired from dental unit waterlines. The aerosolized water from handpieces has been shown to be the most likely source of the infection in the dental office. Reports like this one demonstrate the importance of minimizing the contamination from dental unit waterlines and exposure of patients and staff.

Although there is a potential of high microbial counts through public waterlines, the dental unit waterline with its narrow-bore tubing, small volume of water, water in contact with the tubing inner surface, long times of stagnation, and "suck-back" that occurs during handpiece and air-water syringe use all contribute to increased bacterial growth and the development of biofilm. There are two types of microorganisms found in the DUWL.

TABLE 11-7 Variables Impacting Effectiveness of Chemical Agents

residual debris	Debris provides a barrier that hides microorganisms and prevents the disinfectant from reaching all the instrument surfaces. In order to disinfect or sterilize instruments, the instrument must be free of debris, blood, and tissue fluids and be thoroughly dry. Chemical disinfectants are used to kill microorganisms by coagulating proteins. Dirty instruments prevent chemicals from penetrating surface debris, thus preventing the instrument from being disinfected.
solution contaminator	Soap is the number one contaminator of disinfecting agents. It reacts with the disinfectant and weakens its effectiveness. Make certain the disinfecting dish is rinsed free of all soap residue and completely dry before adding new disinfectant. Care must be used when rinsing sanitized instruments that they are completely free of soap prior to placing into disinfectant.
disinfectant dilution	Make certain the accurate quantity of chemical is dissolved in distilled water per manufacturer's directions. Careful measurement of the disinfectant agent is absolutely essential to ensure effectiveness. The chemical can also be diluted by water carried over by improperly dried instruments. Added water will dilute and weaken the chemicals.
disinfectant temperature	Warm solutions are most effective in increasing the speed of the chemical reaction. Many manufacturers recommend using warm water in mixing the disinfectant.
disinfection time	The amount of time instruments need to remain in chemicals is stated in the manufacturer's directions. The time depends on the type of organisms and the instrument's use. If the instrument does not remain in the disinfectant the entire time recommended, the disinfection will be questionable.
disinfectant contact	The entire surface of the instrument must remain in contact with the disinfecting agent during the disinfection time. Do not overload the instrument tray in the disinfecting container and make certain instruments are completely immersed in disinfecting solution. Flat, smooth surfaces are easier to disinfect than those with crevices. Make certain to open all hinged items.
type of microorganism	Disinfectants are categorized and approved by the FDA by which microorganisms are killed, and the CDC classifies instruments and procedures for determining the method of disinfection. The DHCW needs to understand these recommendations in order to select which disinfectant and method is best practice for the type of microorganism that needs to be destroyed.
exhausted chemical	There are many ways the manufacturer uses to tell the condition and life of the disinfectant. Some manufacturer's directions specify how long the chemical is effective and provide expiration dates. Directions may describe the appearance of the chemical when the disinfectant is no longer effective. The most effective method is to use chemical strips and charts to examine the chemical activity.
storage and handling	After disinfection, all items need to be stored to protect against exposure to contamination. Instruments that have been disinfected must be wrapped or bagged to maintain their disinfection or prepackaged/wrapped in preparation for sterilization. Instruments may be stored in covered instrument trays and procedure tubs.

The first is **planktonic** (free-floating microbes found in natural water), and the second is microbes attached to the inside walls of the tubing, called biofilm. Biofilm is defined as any group of microorganisms (bacteria, protozoa, and fungi) that stick together on a hydrated surface and frequently form a matrix of **polysaccharide** slime layer that feeds and protects it. Biofilm will form on most nonshedding surfaces in nonsterile water or in a very humid environment. It can grow in showers, water and sewage pipes, and dental unit waterlines. The microorganisms multiply and can cause water line clogging and corrosion. If not immediately separated from the surface, microorganisms colonize and anchor themselves more permanently and cannot be removed by gentle rinsing. Biofilm in the dental waterline serves as a reservoir increasing the number of free-floating microorganisms in the water used for dental treatment. These microorganisms are released from the surface of the biofilm into the flowing water in the dental unit water line, and then the patients and clinical staff are exposed to microorganisms through aerosolized water from the high-speed handpiece, air-water syringe, and ultrasonic scaler.

Most microorganisms found in the dental unit biofilm are commonly found in water and are rarely a threat to patients with healthy immune systems. However, poor water quality is not acceptable in any health care facility and may affect the

health of immunocompromised patients. Water used through unit dental waterlines needs to be regularly treated and maintained to meet the drinking water standards. The best resource for proper treatment is the manufacturer of the dental unit. They will provide water quality control methods compatible with the unit. The dental assistant must carefully follow manufacturer's instructions, product directions, and maintenance protocol. Most manufacturers recommend chemical treatment, in-line microfilters, or a combination of these treatments to produce quality water. Manufacturers have been required since 1985 to have antiretraction valves in dental waterlines to eliminate suck-back. Periodic maintenance of antiretraction mechanisms must be a part of quality water control. The water quality monitoring is an important step in providing safe water. There are in-office testing kit and mail-in testing services offered in laboratories across the United States to estimate the number of free-floating heterotrophic bacteria that are present in the dental unit water.

Even with antiretraction, it is recommended that the waterlines and high-speed handpieces, air-water syringes, and ultrasonic scalers are flushed at the beginning of the clinic day and after each patient. Flushing does not affect the biofilm but is helpful to clear stagnant water and retracted contaminants during treatment.

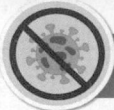 **Infection Control**

The CDC recommends that dental facilities take steps to improve dental unit water quality. Waters lines should be flushed at the beginning of the day for 30 seconds, which temporarily reduces the level of microbes in the water. Flush the air-water syringe and handpieces for 20 seconds after each patient to reduce patient-borne microbes that may have entered lines from suck-back.

Boil-Water Advisories Advisories are issued when the public water treatment equipment or processes have failed. Natural disasters such as floods, earthquakes, and tornados and water main breaks may damage the public water system. When the water tests above the safe drinking water standards or other standards are compromised, a public health announcement or "boil-water advisory" is sent to the public directing them to boil tap water before drinking.

The dental office water is also affected, and besides boiling water the CDC has many recommendations until the advisory is cancelled. No public water should be used when operating any equipment requiring water such as the air–water syringe, high-speed handpiece, and ultrasonic scaler. Public water should not be used for any dental treatment or added to materials including patient rinsing and staff handwashing. Self-contained water containers are still safe use, and bottled water can be used in mixing materials and patient rinsing as needed. Antimicrobial products that do not require water (alcohol-based hand rubs) or antiseptic towelettes should replace handwashing. If hands are visibly contaminated, use bottled water and soap.

Once the advisory is lifted, all the waterlines and equipment connected to the public water system and all faucets must be flushed for one to five minutes before using for patient or personal care. All flushed waterlines should be followed up with manufacturer's recommended disinfection.

Disinfecting Dental Vacuum Systems

All evacuator hoses must be flushed with water after each use and at the end of the day. High-volume evacuator and low-volume suction lines (saliva ejector) and solids collector traps should be flushed clean daily using an evacuation system cleaner according to dental system manufacturer instructions.

Evacuation cleaners dissolve dental debris including impression materials, organic tissue, blood, and saliva to provide optimal suction (Figure 11-83). It is critical to defer to manufacturer's directions in selecting evacuator cleaners and disinfectants. Solutions containing bleach or other chlorine disinfectants will interfere with amalgam collection, causing corrosion and failure of the evacuation system.

Changing or cleaning evacuator traps should be completed weekly. If the trap becomes clogged with debris sooner than a week, then it needs to be changed based on the amount of debris that it collects. It is recommended to use disposable traps. Amalgam contents should be disposed of appropriately. This will be discussed in detail in Chapter 12.

Disinfecting Dental Saliva Ejector Tubing Suck-back can occur from the very narrow and low-volume vacuum line of the saliva ejector tip into the patient's mouth. When the saliva ejector is used as a straw, there is more negative pressure in the patient's mouth than the evacuator tubing, which causes suck-back. The patient materials and biofilm can be aspirated into the mouth of the next patient. The saliva ejector tubing must be sanitized between patients and disinfected daily (Figure 11-84), and the patient must be instructed to not close their lips around the saliva ejector tip.

Studies have shown that gravity pulls fluid back toward the patient's mouth when the tubing is held above the patient's oral cavity. The tubing needs to be held below the patient's head when in use and after treatment. Suck-back also increases when there is a drop in pressure when the high volume evacuation is being used in an adjacent operatory. Although coordination of the use of the evacuators among different operatories within the office is not possible, it is important to realize the effect and use all precautions to avoid suck-back.

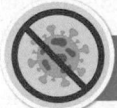 **Infection Control**

The ADA statement on dental unit waterlines since 1995 has been to improve water delivered to patients during nonsurgical dental procedures to contain no more than 200 CFU/mL The ADA further "urges the industry to continue to ensure that all dental units manufactured and marketed in the U.S.A. in the future have the capability to be equipped with a separate water reservoir independent of the public water supply." This allows for increased control of the source water quality and allows for uninterrupted dental care during "boil water" notices. Self-contained water systems greatly improve the quality of the treatment water. Self-contained water systems must be filled with distilled water and cleaned and disinfected according the manufacturer's instructions to avoid the containers from becoming highly contaminated.

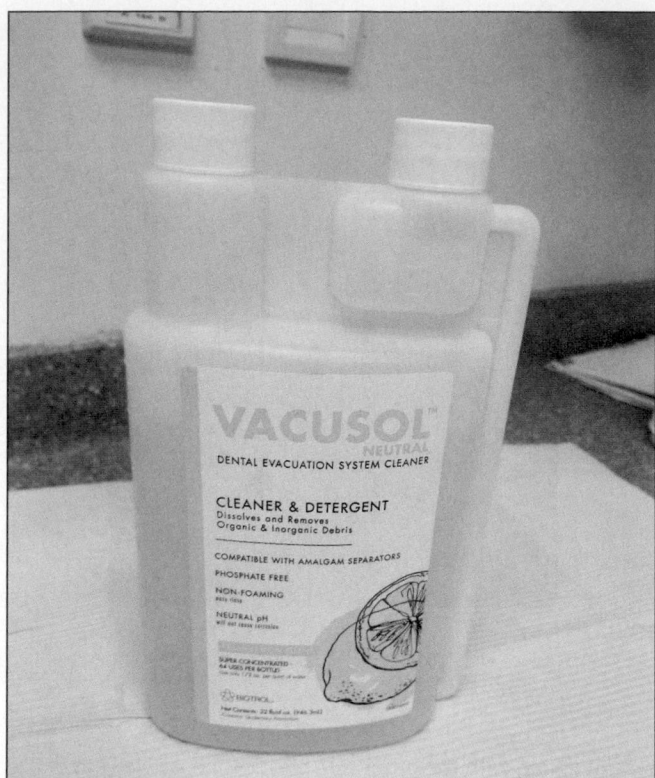

FIGURE 11-83
Evacuation system cleaner.

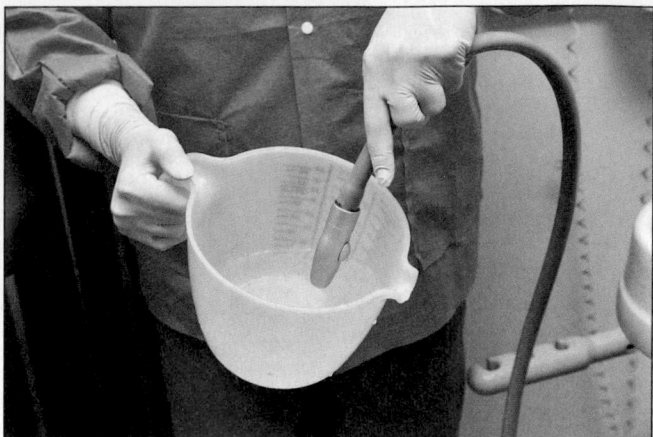

FIGURE 11-84
Dental assistant using saliva ejector cleaning solution at end of day to disinfect the tubing.

Sterilization

The highest level of infection control possible to ensure a safe environment for both patients and the dental team is sterilization. Sterilization is the process that inactivates all microbial life, including bacterial spores, viruses, bacteria, and fungi. The CDC recommends sterilizing critical and semicritical patient care items. The only exception would be items that would be damaged in the autoclave. These items should only be disinfected in a high level disinfectant as described earlier. Critical patient-care items are those that penetrate soft tissue or contact bone. Examples include surgical instruments, forceps, scalpels, bone chisels, scalers, and burs. The risk of disease transmission for these items is very high, and they must be **sterile**.

Preparation and Packaging for Sterilization

After the instruments have been thoroughly sanitized, rinsed, and dried, they are ready to be packaged for sterilization. Using an indelible ink pen, label the sterilizing package with the date sterilized, and identity of the sterilizer and the contents of closed packaging (Figure 11-85). This information is critical in the event a sterilizer fails sterilization testing. The assistant must wear utility gloves as the instruments are inspected for debris before packaging instruments for sterilization as these instruments are not sterile (Figure 11-86). Instruments are placed one at a time to prevent puncturing of the packaging material. Instruments need to fit loosely in a single layer in the package to allow for penetration of the **sterilant** during sterilization (Figure 11-87). Packaging of instruments allows them to remain sterile during storage until ready for use. Once instruments are exposed after sterilization, they are at risk of becoming contaminated. Wrapped packages of sterilized instruments must be examined for compromise of the package before opening in the treatment area. A package is compromised if the package is punctured, torn, wet, or open. Instruments of compromised packages need to recleaned, repacked, and resterilized. Sterile instruments must always be handled wearing gloves and using aseptic techniques.

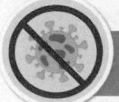 Infection Control

The CDC recommends the following when using saliva ejectors:
- Inform patient to not close lips around saliva ejector tip.
- Hold tubing below patient head when in use and after treatment.
- Rinse tubing between patients.
- Disinfect tubing daily.

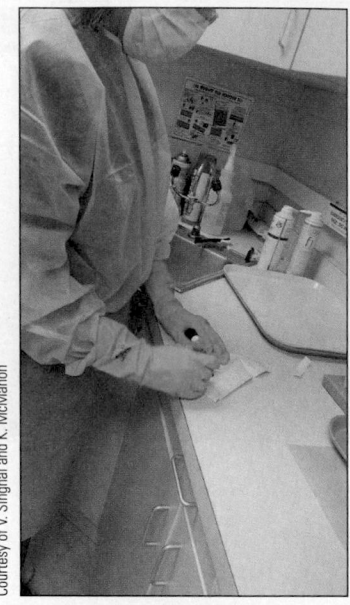

Courtesy of V. Singhal and K. McMahon

FIGURE 11-85
Assistant writing date on autoclave packaging.

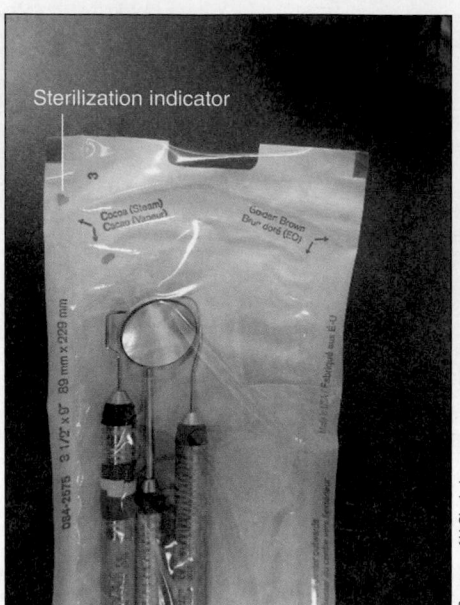

Courtesy of V. Singhal

FIGURE 11-87
Sterilization pouch with loosely packed instruments.

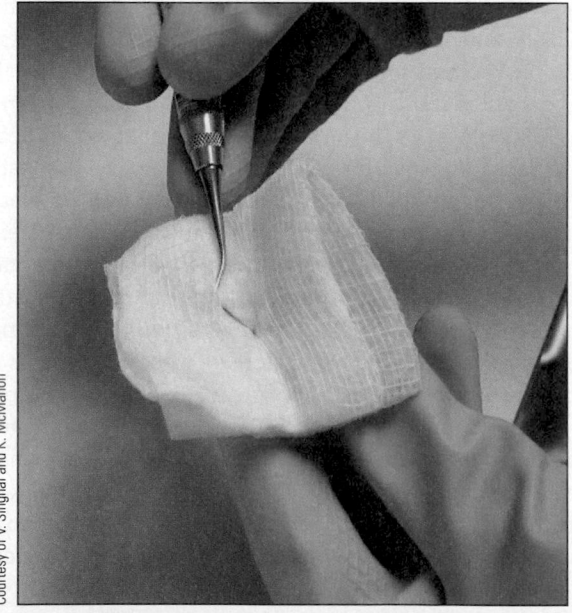

Courtesy of V. Singhal and K. McMahon

FIGURE 11-86
Assistant checking instrument to ensure that all debris has been removed.

Packaging Instruments There are many methods of packaging instruments for sterilization including pouches, wraps, and cassettes (refer to Figures 11-87 and 11-88). The assistant needs to select FDA approved packaging materials and cassettes used for sterilization processes, and the packaging materials must be compatible with the specific type of sterilization process. Types of packaging materials include paper wrap, paper/plastic pouches, cloth wraps, and wrapped perforated cassettes. Some pouches have one side paper to allow for

ease in drying with the other side plastic for easy viewing of the package content. Some pouches and paper wraps are self-sealing; others must be sealed with special *sterilization indicator tape* (Figure 11-89). The indicator tape has areas that turn dark to show that the package has been autoclaved. This, however, does not signify that the autoclave is working properly. Methods of testing the autoclave will be discussed later in this chapter.

Packaging materials are available in many sizes for packaging one instrument to an entire setup. Never substitute FDA-approved packaging and cassettes with plastic wraps, paper, or zipper-lock bags that are not approved; these may prevent the sterilization process from being effective and may melt. Never use safety pins, staples, paper clips, or other sharp objects that could penetrate the package.

Methods of Sterilization

All methods of instrument processing and sterilization require a consistent and disciplined protocol to prevent potentially infectious microorganisms from being transferred between patients, dental team members, and the community. You must *always* use PPE, including protective clothing, heavy-duty utility gloves, mask, and protective eyewear, when processing instruments.

Steam Sterilization A steam *autoclave* is used to sterilize patient-care items by means of steam and pressure of 15 pounds per square inch (psi). This process involves heating distilled water to produce steam and moist heat, both of which kill microorganisms. Autoclaves usually run through four cycles: heat-up, sterilizing, depressurizing, and drying. Some autoclave manufacturers have also added a presterilization cycle; others have added multiple steam cycles to purge air from the chamber before the

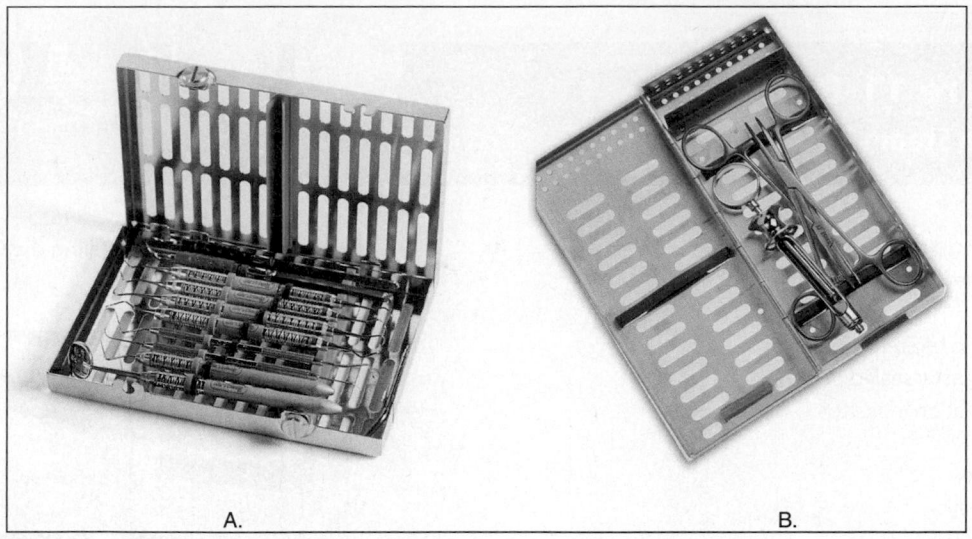

FIGURE 11-88
Instrument cassettes prior to wrapping.

sterilizing cycle. The temperature is maintained for specific times based on the temperature setting. Sterilization time ranges from 3 minutes at 273°F (134°C) to 30 minutes at 250°F (121°C) depending on the machine and the manufacturer (Figure 11-89).

Steam autoclaves are used for sterilizing heat-resistant plastics and glassware, dental handpieces, critical and semicritical patient care instruments, cotton rolls, gauze squares, and a variety of other dental accessories and instruments that are safe for autoclaving. The autoclave has some limitations; it can melt some plastics and rubbers, break nonautoclavable glassware, rust and corrode some metals, and dull sharp instruments. It is important to realize that loose items that are run through the steam autoclave are immediately contaminated upon removal from the autoclave simply by exposure to the environment. Therefore, it is imperative that all items be properly packaged prior to sterilization (Figures 11-87 and 11-90). A further advantage of packaging instruments is that they can be packaged in groups by their intended use and remain sterile while stored. Steam sterilization indicators should be included in every package prior to sealing and placing in the autoclave. These indicators monitor temperature, pressure, and the presence of steam during the autoclaving process. Steam sterilization indicators are an efficient way to monitor the functioning of the dental autoclaves. After instruments are pre-cleaned and packaged, they are ready for sterilization. The assistant must understand the operation of the autoclave for proper sterilization to occur. Refer to Procedure 11-8 for proper operation of a steam autoclave.

An autoclave is like a large pressure cooker that operates by using steam under pressure as the sterilizing agent (sterilant). Increasing the heat content increases the killing power. Steam has almost seven times the heat of boiling water and is considered the most dependable sterilizer. The autoclave has a reservoir

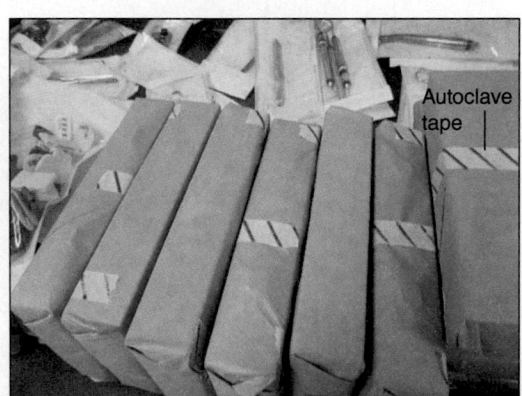

Autoclave tape

Courtesy of V. Singhal

FIGURE 11-89
Instrument cassettes with sterilization wrap and sterilization indicator tape.

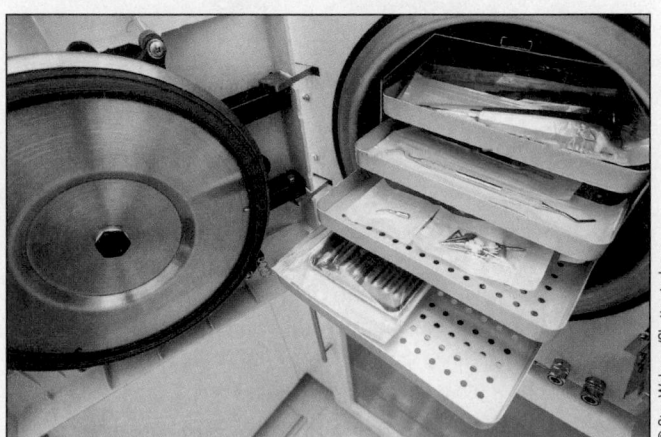

© Stas Walenga/Shutterstock.com

FIGURE 11-90
Dental autoclave with packaged instruments inside.

Procedure 11-8
Operating a Steam Autoclave

Equipment and Supplies
- Personal protective equipment
- Autoclave
- Instruments to be sterilized
- Disposable plastic sealed pouches
- Steam sterilization indicator
- Indelible pen
- Distilled water
- Procedural trays

Procedure Steps

1. Gather and don all PPE, following infection control guidelines.

2. Follow instructions in Procedures 11-6 and 11-7 for cleaning and disinfecting of instruments.

3. Ensure instruments are clean and examine each to ensure there is no damage, rust, corrosion, or other defect.

4. Place instruments loosely in bags, making certain not to puncture the bag. Insert steam sterilization indicator into package (Figure 11-91).

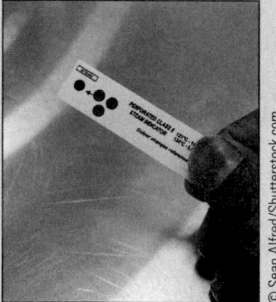

© Sean Alfred/Shutterstock.com

FIGURE 11-91
Steam sterilization indicator strips.

5. Package, seal, and label the instrument pack with date, sterilizer, and contents (see Figures 11-85 and 11-87).

6. Place bagged and sealed items onto an autoclave tray in a single layer to leave space between items to allow steam to circulate. Place larger packs on the bottom tray of the autoclave chamber to ensure the steam can flow properly. Never overload the autoclave. This will inhibit the flow of steam (see Figure 11-90).

7. Check reservoir and fill as needed. Most autoclaves require distilled water to avoid the buildup of deposits from tap water inside the chamber. Follow the

manufacturer's instructions for filling the water chamber (Figure 11-92).

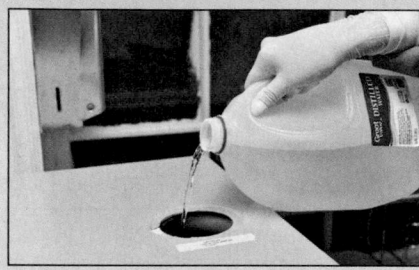

FIGURE 11-92
Dental assistant filling the autoclave water reservoir with distilled water.

8. Set autoclave controls for the appropriate time, temperature, and pressure, depending upon the autoclave and the size of the load. Lock the autoclave door (Figure 11-93). Follow the manufacturer's instructions.

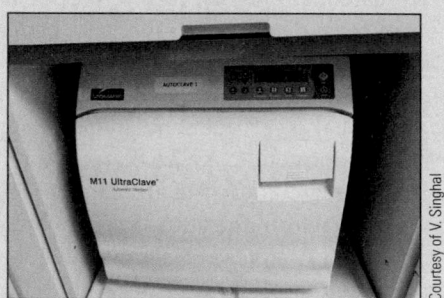

Courtesy of V. Singhal

FIGURE 11-93
Locked autoclave door.

9. After sterilization is complete, vent the steam from the chamber upon cycle completion if needed or sterilizer vents automatically. Open door when pressure gauge is at zero; most models self-vent. If manual venting is required, stand behind the door and open the door of the autoclave very carefully because the escape of steam can scald you. Leave door slightly cracked to allow the contents of the autoclave to dry and cool. The instruments should be allowed to dry and cool completely before being removed from the autoclave.

10. Remove the utility gloves, wash your hands, and put on clean patient examination gloves for handling sterile

packets and reassembling procedural trays. Remove the sealed packs from the autoclave using heat resistant gloves and place them in the area designated for sterile instruments in the instrument processing area (Figure 11-94).

11. Set up the appropriate procedural trays with the sealed packs and appropriate supplies. In some offices, instrument packs are stored in drawers or cabinets and procedural trays are set up as needed (Figure 11-95).

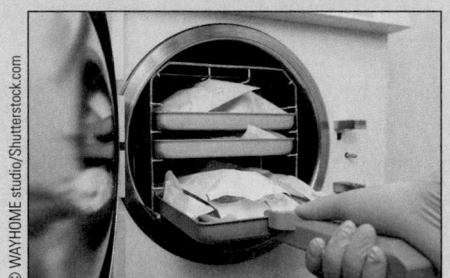

FIGURE 11-94
Dental assistant using holder to remove sterilized instruments from autoclave.

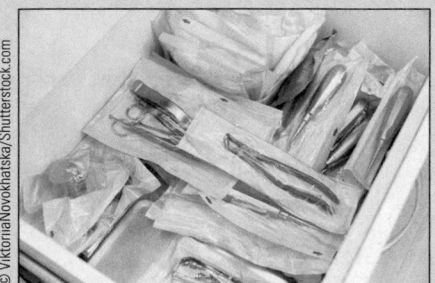

FIGURE 11-95
Sterile instruments in dental office drawer for storage.

that holds the sterilant (distilled water) to be used during the cycle. The chamber has stainless steel trays to hold the instruments during the sterilization cycle. The middle rows of trays are larger than the top and bottom trays, allowing for penetration of steam into sterilization packages. The autoclave door has a latch to securely close during operation.

The most commonly used method of instrument sterilization is steam sterilization. Other alternative methods that may be utilized in a dental office are dry heat sterilization and unsaturated chemical vapor sterilization.

Dry Heat Sterilization There are two types of dry heat sterilizers, which heat up air and transfer that heat directly to the instruments (Figure 11-96). Dry heat sterilization occurs at 320°F (160°C) to 357°F (190°C), higher temperatures than steam autoclaves and chemical vapor sterilizers. Follow manufacturer's directions for the appropriate length of time, based on temperature. All dry heat sterilizers need to be preheated for 15 to 30 minutes from a cold start, and the door should remain closed during the operation

The first type of dry heat sterilizer is the *static air sterilizer*, which is similar to an oven. Heating coils on the bottom of the chamber heat the air, which then rises, transferring the heated air to the instruments. This takes approximately 1–2 hours. This is referred to as static air because the air is not moving but rises from simple convection. The second type of dry heat sterilizer is forced air, which is also referred to as rapid heat transfer sterilizers. This type of sterilizer uses forced air at a high velocity to circulate the heated air (190°C/375°F) throughout the chamber, reducing the sterilization time to 6–12 minutes once the sterilizing temperature has been reached.

The dry heat sterilizer does not have the rusting and corroding problems presented by the steam autoclave. The higher temperatures do have limitations: nylon tubings and plastics can melt, and paper and cloth items can scorch. The dry heat does have a problem with air pockets that prevent an even exposure to heat, making it necessary to have items in a single row and never stacked. Refer to Procedure 11-9, sterilizing instruments using a dry heat sterilizer.

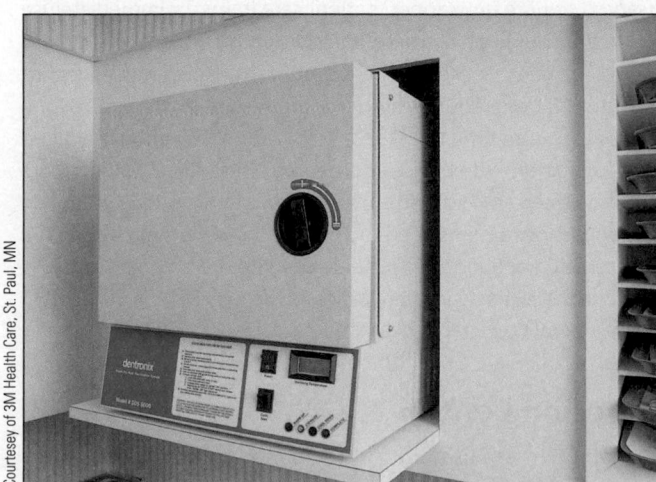

FIGURE 11-96
Dry heat sterilizer.

Unsaturated Chemical Vapor Sterilization *Unsaturated chemical vapor* sterilization is similar to steam autoclaving. Instead of using water to create a steam sterilant, chemical vapor sterilization uses a combination of alcohol, formaldehyde, ketone, acetone, and water to create vapor. The toxicity of these chemicals requires special consideration. OSHA mandates a Safety Data Sheet (SDS) for the chemical vapor solution. Adequate ventilation

Procedure 11-9
Using a Dry Heat Sterilizer

Equipment and Supplies
- Personal protective equipment
- Sanitized instruments safe for dry heat sterilizing
- Assortment of sterilization pouches specific for a dry heat sterilizer
- Indelible pen
- Dry heat sterilizer

Procedure Steps

1. Gather all items needed for sterilizing instruments. Always wear protective clothing, mask, eyewear, and utility gloves to avoid accidental injury. Read and follow the manufacturer's instructions for the dry heat sterilizer.

2. Ensure instruments are sanitized and examine each to ensure there is no damage, rust, corrosion, or any other defect (see Figure 11-86).

3. Prepare hinged instruments with their hinges opened to allow heat to reach all areas during the sterilization process.

4. Insert the process integrator into the instrument package.

5. Load the dry heat chamber with packages single file to permit adequate circulation of air around all packages.

6. Set the time and temperature according to the manufacturer's instructions for preheating. Do not add instruments to the load once the sterilization cycle has begun.

7. Set time for sterilization once the temperature has been achieved. Open the door when the timer rings to allow instruments to thoroughly cool and dry.

8. Set up the appropriate procedural trays with the sealed packs and appropriate supplies. In some offices, instruments packs are stored in drawers or cabinets and procedural trays are set up as needed (see Figure 11-95). Store the prepared trays in the designated area until it is needed in the treatment room.

---

is essential for control of the chemical vapors that escape when the unit is opened.

Standard packaging as used for steam autoclaving is used for unsaturated chemical vapor sterilization. Pressure within the unit should measure 29 psi, temperature should measure 270°F (131°C), and the time should be 20–40 minutes. Follow manufacturer's directions carefully.

Unlike the steam of the autoclave, the chemicals used prevents rusting, corroding, and dulling of metal objects. The chemical vapor sterilizer cannot be used with certain rubber and plastic objects and is not recommended for paper and cloth items. Refer to Procedure 11-10 for proper operation of the unsaturated chemical vapor sterilizer.

Liquid Chemical Sterilization
All dental health care workers should be trained on proper handling of liquid chemical sterilants, which must have an SDS. Liquid chemical sterilants are used for items that cannot withstand heat sterilization, such as plastic dental dam frames, shade guides, and radiographic film-holder devices. A liquid sterilant such as 2–3.4 percent glutaraldehyde must be used to sterilize these items. The sterilant must be tested with the chemical indicator strip to measure the level of active ingredients. Items being sterilized must remain immersed in the solution for 10 hours. Anything shorter than 10 hours is disinfection, not sterilization. The sterilant must be completely rinsed using sterile water to prevent harm to skin and tissue.

There are many limitations to the liquid chemical sterilant including that the FDA states that is does not convey the same sterility assurance as thermal and physical sterilization. The liquid does not adequately penetrate debris, and since items cannot be wrapped during the process, the sterility is lost following processing and during storage. This should not be the first choice for sterilization.

Immediate-Use Sterilization
Occasionally it may be necessary to sterilize unwrapped patient care items for immediate use due to a shortage of instruments or dropping an instrument with no replacement. Immediate-use sterilization, also referred to as flash sterilization, requires higher temperature and pressure for a shorter exposure time to achieve sterilization. This should only be used for instruments that are to be used immediately. Indicators must be placed among instruments during unwrapped cycles. The unwrapped instruments need to dry and cool while remaining in the sterilizer and transported in a sterile cover to the treatment area. To flash sterilize using steam sterilization is 134°C / 273° F at 206 kPa/30 psi for 3 minutes in a rapid heat autoclave (Figure 11-97).

Corrosion Control

Rust inhibitors are used to control for corrosion of carbon steel instruments and burs during steam sterilization. Sodium nitrate or other commercial products are available as a spray or dip solution to reduce rust and corrosion. An alternative to this is to use

Procedure 11-10
Using an Unsaturated Chemical Vapor Sterilizer

Equipment and Supplies
- Personal protective equipment
- Sanitized instruments safe for chemical vapor sterilizing
- Assortment of sterilization pouches specific for a chemical vapor sterilizer
- Indelible pen
- Chemical vapor sterilizer

Procedure Steps

1. Gather all items needed for sterilizing instruments. Read and follow the manufacturer's instructions for the untreated chemical vapor sterilizer. Always wear protective clothing, mask, eyewear, and utility gloves to avoid accidental injury. Follow infection control guidelines.

2. Ensure instruments are sanitized and examine each to ensure there is no damage, rust, corrosion, or other defect (see Figure 11-86). Insert the appropriate process integrator into the instrument package.

3. Place instruments loosely in bags, making certain to not puncture the bag and to ensure proper chemical vapor sterilization. Package, seal, and label the instrument pack with date, sterilizer, and contents.

4. Place bagged and sealed items onto an instrument tray in the chamber. Place larger packs on the bottom tray of the chamber to ensure the vapor can flow properly. Never overload the chamber. This will inhibit the flow of vapor.

5. Check reservoir and fill with chemical vapor solution as needed. Follow the manufacturer's instructions and precautions in the SDS for filling the reservoir. Set the controls for pressure, temperature, and time according to manufacturer's directions.

6. Vent the chamber upon cycle completion according to manufacturer's directions. Allow pressure gauge to reach zero, stand behind the door, and open the door of the sterilizer very carefully because the escape of steam can scald you. Leave door slightly cracked to allow the contents of the autoclave to dry and cool. Instruments should be allowed to dry and cool completely before being removed from the autoclave.

7. Remove the utility gloves, wash your hands, and put on clean patient examination gloves for handling sterile packets and reassembling procedural trays. Remove the sealed packs from the sterilizer and place them in the area designated for sterile instruments in the instrument processing area.

8. Set up the appropriate procedural trays with the sealed packs and appropriate supplies. In some offices, instrument packs are stored in drawers or cabinets and procedural trays are set up as needed. Store the prepared trays in the designated are until they are needed in the treatment room (see Figure 11-95).

unsaturated chemical vapor sterilization, which does not cause rusting and corrosion.

Some instruments, such as surgical scissors and forceps, are hinged and may need to be lubricated to maintain opening and closing. If lubrication is used, you must remove all excess lubrication before performing heat sterilization.

Handpiece Sterilization

Dental handpieces are exposed to blood, saliva, tooth fragments, and restorative materials. These may be retained within the handpiece and transferred between patients. Therefore, dental handpieces must be properly cleaned and heat sterilized, following specific protocols according to the handpiece manufacturer's directions.

The external surface of the handpiece should be wiped free of debris. Always follow manufacturer's directions for each handpiece. Some handpieces can be cleaned in the ultrasonic cleaner; others cannot be. Handpieces that cannot be submersed should be wiped with an alcohol gauze. Some handpieces require

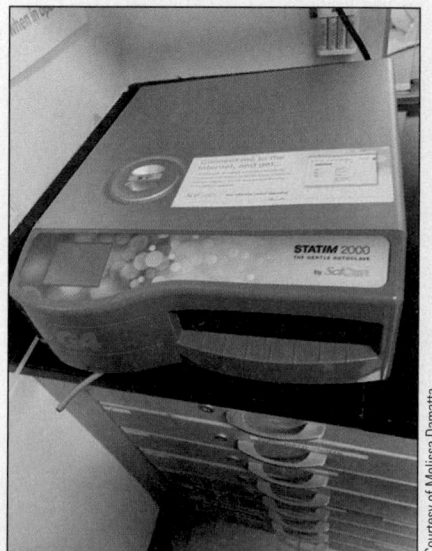

Courtesy of Melissa Damatta

FIGURE 11-97
Flash sterilizer.

lubrication prior to sterilization; others do not. There are also pressurized handpiece cleaners that can flush, clean, and lubricate the handpiece (Figure 11-98). The handpiece can now be packaged for sterilization. Only steam or chemical vapor sterilization is recommended for handpieces. Temperatures should not exceed 275°F (135°C).

Factors Affecting Sterilization

Dental instruments **must** be properly sterilized. It is difficult to determine whether sterilization has been achieved because pathogenic microorganisms are not visible to the eye. Sterilization failures occur when all surfaces are not in direct contact the sterilant for the required sterilization time. Improper instrument cleaning and packaging, improper loading of the sterilizer, and sterilizer malfunction can cause the sterilization process to fail. Therefore, sterilization monitoring is used to ensure sterility. Three forms of sterilization monitoring are currently used: physical, chemical, and biologic.

Monitoring Sterilization

Monitoring the sterilizers is an essential part of the dental office infection control program. Many factors can cause sterilization failure, including procedural errors like overloading or mechanical problems of the sterilizer. State and local regulations address the frequency and record keeping of monitoring sterilizers. The assistant should check with the state dental board for specific regulatory information. The CDC recommends monitoring the sterilization process using chemical indicators, mechanical techniques, and biological indicators. The chemical monitoring is the first indicator of operator failure to follow appropriate sterilization procedure or that the sterilizer may be malfunctioning.

Chemical Monitoring *Process indicators* and *process integrators* are chemical monitoring indicators. Process indicators are used externally; they are placed on the outside of instrument packages. Instrument bags and packages and indicator (autoclave) tape with color-change markers are process indicators. When exposed to a certain temperature, the color-change markers identify instrument packs that have reached that certain temperature. This does not indicate that the instruments packs have been exposed for the appropriate pressure or time. This type of monitoring system is referred to as single-parameter indicator as it only helps distinguish packages that have been processed from those that have not been. It does not indicate sterility.

Process integrators are used internally; they are placed inside instrument packages. These monitors are referred to as *multiparameter* indicators as they respond to pressure, temperature, and time. These, also, do not indicate sterility (see Figure 11-91). All packages must contain an internal chemical indicator to monitor the effectiveness of the sterilization procedure. If this indicator is not visible from the outside of the package, an external indicator must also be used. There are commercial pouches made with both the internal and external indicators. The operator must follow the sterilizer manufacturer directions as chemical indicators and integrators are sterilizer-specific.

Physical Monitoring Physical monitoring involves observing and recording the temperature, pressure, and exposure time displayed on the sterilizer gauges for each load of instruments. Incorrect readings indicate a problem. However, this type of monitoring is only an indication that the sterilization chamber has achieved the correct temperature, pressure, and time. If the chamber is overloaded or underloaded or instruments are improperly packaged, the instruments may not have reached the appropriate temperature to ensure sterility.

Biologic Monitoring *Biologic monitoring* is also referred to as spore testing. This is the preferred method of sterilization monitoring because it is the only way to determine whether sterilization has occurred, confirming that all bacteria and endospores have been killed. The CDC, the ADA, and OSAP recommend weekly biologic monitoring of sterilization equipment and a biological indicator with every load containing an implant device. Some states recommend cycle specific intervals. Dental office personnel must be aware of state regulations.

Biologic indicators (BIs) are bacterial spores that are highly resistant to sterilization. BIs are supplied in vials or strips of paper. Biological monitor can be performed using an in-office incubator and spore strips or a third-party mail-in spore monitoring program (Figure 11-99) The in-office testing will provide results in 24–48 hours, and the mail-in generally takes one week (Figure 11-100). The third-party program is considered more credible.

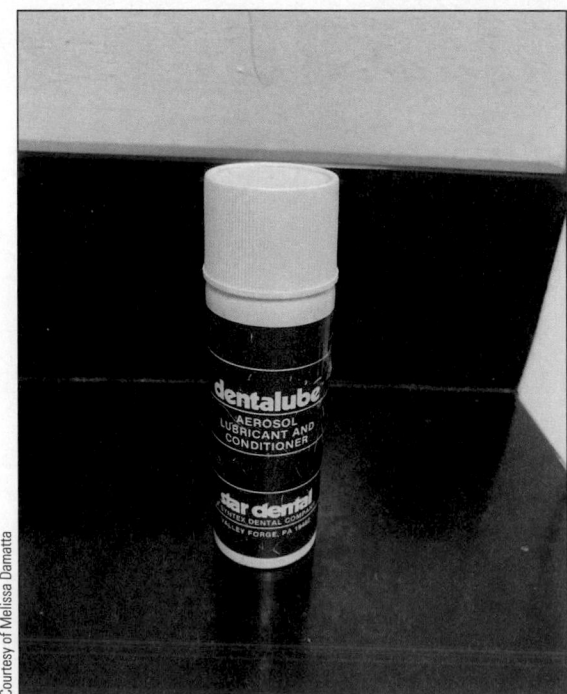

Courtesy of Melissa Damatta

FIGURE 11-98
Handpiece lubricant.

There are different types of BIs, dependent upon the method of sterilization. It is vital to follow manufacturer's directions to choose the appropriate BI to receive accurate results.

● Geobacillus *stearothermophilus* spore is used when testing a steam autoclave and chemical vapor.

● Bacillus atrophaeus spore is used to test dry heat sterilization.

Three spore strips are generally used to test the effectiveness of the sterilizing unit. Two strips are placed inside instrument packs and run through the sterilizer under normal conditions. The third BI is used as the control and is left in the packet. After sterilization, all three strips are **cultured**. A positive culture of a strip that has completed the sterilization cycle indicates that the spores survived the sterilization cycle and sterilization was not achieved. A negative culture of a strip that has completed the sterilization cycle indicates that the spores were killed and sterilization was achieved.

Monitoring Records All sterilization records must be maintained for chemical, mechanical, and biological monitoring in compliance with state and local regulations. If there is a positive spore test, the CDC recommends that the failing sterilizer not be used and all instruments sterilized in the sterilizer be resterilized in a sterilizer testing negative. The operator procedures should be reviewed to rule out operator failure, and the sterilizer needs to be retested using all three monitoring techniques. If the repeat monitoring is negative, the sterilizer can be put back in use. If the repeat test is positive, the sterilizer cannot be used until the cause is determined, the sterilizer is repaired, and the sterilizer is retested with biological indicator tests three consecutive empty-chamber negative sterilization cycles. All actions to re-establish proper sterilization should be recorded in the log for each sterilizer. All instruments that were processed since the last negative spore test must be resterilized.

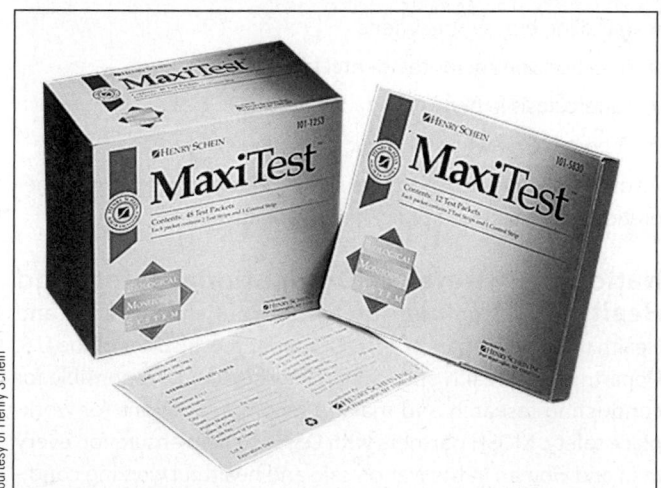

FIGURE 11-99
Mail in biological monitor for autoclave.

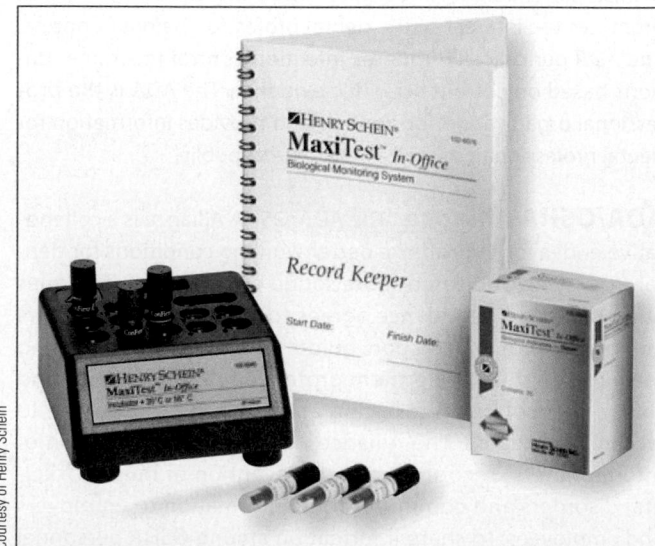

FIGURE 11-100
In-office biological monitor.

Sterilization Protocol

The CDC Guidelines for Sterilization of Patient Care Items have made general recommendations to ensure optimal infection control is achieved. Each recommendation is based on existing scientific data, theoretical rationale, and application to practice. They are as follows:

● Use only FDA-cleared medical devices for sterilization and follow manufacturer's instructions for correct use.

● Clean and heat-sterilize critical dental instruments before each use.

● Clean and heat sterilize semicritical items before each use.

● Allow packages to dry in the sterilizer before they are handled to avoid contamination.

● Process heat-sensitive critical and semicritical instruments by using FDA-cleared sterilants/high-level disinfectants or an FDA-cleared low temperature sterilization method. Follow manufacturers' instructions for use of chemical sterilants/high-level disinfectants.

● Single-use disposable instruments are acceptable alternatives, if they are used only once and are disposed of correctly.

● Do not use liquid chemical sterilants/high-level disinfectants for environmental surface disinfection or as holding solutions.

● Ensure that noncritical patient care items are barrier protected or cleaned or, if visibly soiled, are cleaned and disinfected after each use with an EPA-registered hospital disinfectant. If visibly contaminated with blood, use an EPA-registered hospital disinfectant with a tuberculocidal claim.

● Follow all OSHA guidelines for exposure to chemical agents used for disinfection and sterilization.

As a professional member of the dental health care team, dental assistants are legally and ethically responsible for performing sterilization procedures thoroughly and carefully. The CDC *Guidelines for Infection Control in Dental Healthcare Settings— 2003* protect patients, dental personnel, and the community at large from disease transmission. Additionally, the OSHA Bloodborne Pathogens Standard requires biologic monitoring of sterilizers and maintenance of records of the results. Many states have adopted specific infection control regulations that dental personnel need to be aware of and fastidiously abide by. The process of sterilization should always follow a standard operating procedure that all dental personnel adhere to in order to ensure the chain of infection is not compromised.

Guidelines for Infection Control in Dentistry

Differentiating recommendations from regulations and knowing where to turn for additional information is an important part of the infection control process. A guideline or recommendation is a representation of advisable action. Penalties are not imposed unless one of the enforcement agencies adopts the guidelines as part of their regulations. Examples of guidance organizations include the CDC, the ADA, and the ADA/OSHA Alliance and Office Safety and Asepsis Procedures Research Foundation (OSAP). While these organizations study and make recommendations and develop evidence-based guidelines concerning policies and procedures, they do not regulate action.

Nonregulatory Agencies and Infection Control

Many agencies function to educate and provide resources for health care workers and the public to adopt best management practices with regard to infection control. Nonregulatory agencies provide information to promote behavior change and to strengthen the work of regulatory agencies. Nonregulatory agencies were discussed previously in Chapter 3. This section will focus only on the role of nonregulatory agencies in infection control.

Centers for Disease Control and Prevention (CDC)

In 2003, the CDC published updated recommendations for dental infection control, which has been adopted as and considered to be the standard of care. This report, "Guidelines for Infection Control in Dental Health Care Settings—2003" was developed collaboratively by authorities on infection control in the CDC, the American Dental Association (ADA), and other private and professional organizations, as well as scholars in higher education and research.

Another significant CDC contribution was the 1985 development of the "universal precautions" concept to infection control procedures—"treat everyone as if known to be infectious for HIV and other bloodborne pathogens." This concept was changed in 1996 to "standard precautions" to expand the risk of health care associated infections to include all body fluids, secretions, and excretions, regardless of whether or not they contain blood.

The 2003 CDC guidelines address the following:

- educating and protecting dental health care personnel
- preventing transmission of bloodborne pathogens (including postexposure management)

- hand hygiene
- personal protective equipment
- contact dermatitis and latex hypersensitivity
- sterilization and disinfection of patient care items
- environmental infection control
- waste management
- dental unit waterlines and water quality
- biofilm
- dental handpieces and other devices that attach to dental unit airlines and waterlines
- radiology
- aseptic technique for parenteral medications
- disposable devices
- oral surgical procedures
- handling biopsy specimens
- infection control for the dental laboratory
- tuberculosis in dentistry
- program evaluation

All of the recommendations are based on scientific evidence, theoretical rationale, and applicability to dentistry.

National Institute for Occupational Safety and Health The National Institute for Occupational Safety and Health (NIOSH) is a part of the CDC under the auspices of the U.S. Department of Health and Human Services and is responsible for conducting research and making recommendations for workplace safety. NIOSH partners with OSHA to help ensure for "every man and woman in the Nation safe and healthful working conditions and to preserve our human resources."

American Dental Association (ADA) The ADA publishes frequent articles in the associations' publications to keep dentists current on the latest infection control developments and promotes the interest of the dental profession before Congress. The ADA periodically updates infection control recommendations based on current scientific evidence. The ADA is the professional organization for dentists and provides information for dental professionals as well as the general public.

ADA/OSHA Alliance The ADA/OSHA Alliance is a collaborative endeavor to promote better working conditions for dental employees and to promote sound ergonomic techniques and practices. The Alliance agrees to provide ADA members and others with information, guidance, and access to training resources that will help them protect employees' health and safety, particularly in reducing and preventing exposure to workplace hazards. The Alliance's goals include provision of information on recognition and prevention of musculoskeletal disorders and communicating information to employers and employees; to share information among OSHA personnel and health professionals regarding ADA's best practices; and to develop materials, training programs, workshops, seminars, and lectures.

Organization for Safety and Asepsis Procedures (OSAP)

The Organization for Safety and Asepsis Procedures (OSAP) is dentistry's nonprofit resource for infection control, safety information, occupational health issues, and education. It is composed of dentists, dental hygienists, dental assistants, government representatives, dental manufacturers, university professors, researchers, and dental consultants. OSAP is committed to providing and monitoring practical guidelines in infection control, promoting quality research relating to infection control, and interfacing with other regulatory agencies. OSAP has a bookstore containing multiple sources to help guide dental personnel to meet all CDC recommendations and OSHA regulations. Dental personnel can become a member of OSAP and receive practical guidance, updates, and trusted information. Members can earn continuing education for recertification by completing OSAP study packets.

Regulatory Agencies

Numerous agencies at local, state, and federal levels have responded to the concerns of health care consumers by establishing new or enhanced regulations that affect the practice of dentistry. Regulatory agencies were also discussed in Chapter 3. This section will focus on the role of regulatory agencies in dental infection control. In particular, three federal agencies have developed core standards with respect to infection control in health care settings: OSHA, the U.S. Food and Drug Administration (FDA), and the Environmental Protection Agency (EPA). The law requires regulations related to infection control practices in the dental setting to be followed. There are local authorities to enforce regulations, with fines or penalties, imprisonment, and loss of licensure for noncompliance. Examples of state regulatory agencies are the State Boards of Dental Examiners and State Boards of Health.

Occupational Safety and Health Administration

Enforcement authorities such as the Occupational Safety and Health Administration (OSHA) prescribe regulations or requirements regarding workplace safety, the Bloodborne Pathogen Standard, and the Hazard Communications Standard. OSHA is a federal agency created by Congress in 1970 and is the premier infection control education organization in dentistry. OSHA strives to ensure the safety and health of employees by establishing and enforcing standards providing training and education and to improve workplace safety. OSHA mandates that all dental offices have an infection control training manual available for training new employees as well as for implementing and maintaining OSHA standards. This manual must be updated on an annual basis. OSHA also requires that all dental offices offer annual infection control training for all employees to review and update them on current OSHA standards and regulations.

Occupational Exposure to Bloodborne Pathogens Standard

The Bloodborne Pathogen Standard is a comprehensive rule established by OSHA, which sets forth specific requirements intended to prevent the transmission of bloodborne diseases to employees. This standard applies to all employees who could "reasonably anticipate" to come in contact with blood and other infectious materials, including saliva. It imposes a number of requirements designed to protect employees, including the provision of PPE; establishing workplace controls; implementing specific housekeeping, laundering, and waste handling procedures; and maintaining employee medical and vaccination records.

Hazard Communications Standard

OSHA's Hazard Communications Standard (HCS) was first introduced in 1983. It resulted from a legal dispute between OSHA and employee unions. This standard is an extensive set of rules that requires employers to keep an inventory of hazardous chemicals in the workplace, maintain a file of Safety Data Sheets (SDS) for all products in the office, establish a labeling system for products used in the dental office to alert employees to potential dangers, and set up training programs for employees. The standard also sets forth significant recordkeeping responsibilities to document all the aforementioned regulations.

Food and Drug Administration

The Food and Drug Administration is an agency within the U.S. Department of Health and Human Services. Refer to Chapter 3 regarding the role of the FDA.

Environmental Protection Agency

The EPA is responsible for implementing federal laws designed to protect the environment by regulating the use and disposal of products that affect the environment. The EPA accomplishes its mission through efforts in research, monitoring, standard-setting, and enforcement activities.

The EPA affects the practice of dentistry in areas such as medical waste, amalgam, water fluoridation, sterilization agents, water quality, and sewage disposal. All chemical products used for disinfection, sterilization, or decontamination must be registered with the EPA. Products are tested either by the manufacturer or by independent laboratories using specific protocols for microbial efficacy, stability, and toxicity to humans. Data is then submitted to the EPA in an application for a registration number.

The EPA also provides explanations of chemical agent classification to aid in the selection of an approved product for a specific task, such as when to use high or intermediate level disinfection. It also provides assistance in evaluating the claims made by manufacturers on product labels. The EPA has varying jurisdiction with respect to hazardous waste and generator liability. In addition, many states and municipalities have laws regarding waste disposal; however, even in states with their own regulations, the EPA can take precedence if its regulations are more rigorous or if environmental contamination exists because of waste disposal.

State Board of Dental Examiners

Local dental societies and state dental boards can help with regulatory issues in your specific area. In addition, these boards respond to complaints from patients and from dental health care workers and employees. Please refer to Chapter 3 for detail regarding dental state boards.

Healthcare Environmental Resource Center The Healthcare Environmental Resource Center (HERC) provides pollution prevention and compliance guidelines for the health care sector. In dentistry, the focus of HERC is in regard to regulations on wastewater, identification of solid waste and its proper management and disposal, blood-soaked absorbents, sharps, chemicals related to processing of radiographs, sterilants, and disinfectants. Most state boards of health offices have enacted medical waste regulations to some extent and have regulations covering packaging, storage, and transportation of medical waste.

Chapter Summary

Infection control is a critical function of the dental assistant. The dental assistant and the staff must be trained for a safe workplace. Compliance with all regulations must be accomplished to ensure that the process of infection control will be adequate. Infection control training will occur at initial employment, when job tasks change, and annually thereafter.

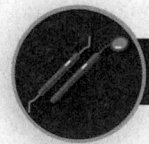

CASE STUDY

Victoria Scott, a dental assistant, received a personal telephone call during patient dental care. She left the dental treatment room, removed her latex gloves, and answered the telephone in the sterilization area. While in the area, she looked up another telephone number in the phone book, put instruments from the ultrasonic unit in water to rinse, placed them into the sterilizer, and then returned to the treatment room. Knowing that leaving the treatment area during patient care is not advocated, and focusing on asepsis, answer the following questions.

Case Study Review

1. What (if any) areas were contaminated?

2. What procedures should have been followed to prevent cross-contamination?

3. Identify the glove(s) that should have been used during each procedure.

Review Questions

Multiple Choice

1. It is important to perform hand hygiene after eating and before returning to patient treatment. It is not necessary to perform hand hygiene after treating patients and before eating.
   Select the correct response based on the statement above.
   a. Both statements are true.
   b. Both statements are false.
   c. The first statement is true; the second statement is false.
   d. The first statement is false; the second statement is true.

2. Which of the following is correct regarding clinical handwashing?
   a. It is acceptable to use bar soap in the dental office for clinical handwashing.
   b. If liquid soap containers are used, it is acceptable to top them off as needed.
   c. It is acceptable to wear jewelry while performing clinical handwashing.
   d. Attention should be given to areas such as under the fingernails and thumbs as these may be missed.

3. Which of the following statements is correct regarding examination gloves?
   a. Once the DHCW wears examination gloves, the potential to be exposed to contaminated body fluids is eliminated.
   b. It is acceptable to wash hands while wearing gloves.
   c. Wearing gloves that are too large may cause carpal tunnel syndrome.
   d. The DHCW must wash hands immediately upon removal of gloves.

4. Which of the following is correct regarding examination gloves?
   a. May be worn during sanitization of clinical surfaces
   b. Come in one size only
   c. May be washed and reused again
   d. Are available in latex, vinyl, and nitrile materials

5. Sanitization is a process that eliminates the number of microorganisms on inanimate objects. The rationale for sanitization is to manage surface contamination.
   Select the correct response based on these statements.
   a. Both statements are true.
   b. Both statements are false.
   c. The first statement is true; the second statement is false.
   d. The first statement is false; the second statement is true.

6. Which of the following is a clinical contact surface?
   a. treatment room walls
   b. treatment room floor
   c. treatment room sink
   d. dental chair light handle

7. Precleaning is the process of reducing the number of micro-organisms and bioburden prior to disinfecting. Clinical contact surfaces should be cleaned and disinfected between patients with an EPA-registered hospital disinfectant with an HIV, HBV claim unless they have been covered with a surface barrier.
   Select the correct response based on these statements.
   a. Both statements are true.
   b. Both statements are false.
   c. The first statement is true; the second statement is false.
   d. The first statement is false; the second statement is true.

8. Which of the following is not correct regarding clinical surface barriers?
   a. A surface barrier should be used when a surface cannot be cleaned and disinfected thoroughly.
   b. Touch and transfer surfaces should be barrier protected and changed between patients to prevent cross contamination.
   c. Placing barriers on switches will prevent fluid from entering into areas of electrical wiring.
   d. Clinical surface barriers are only available as a plastic material and are only available in one size.

9. Which of the following is correct regarding disposal of sharps in the dental office?
   a. It is optional to have a designated sharps container in the dental office.
   b. If the office has a sharps container, one container is sufficient for the entire office.
   c. Sharps containers may be emptied and reused.
   d. Sharps containers should be collected by a company that the office contracts with when the "fill to" line is reached.

10. Which of the following is correct regarding the instrument processing area layout?
    a. The instrument processing area should be located in an area of high patient traffic.
    b. The instrument processing area does not require ventilation.
    c. The initial receiving area should be where contaminated instruments are placed for cleaning.
    d. The processing area should be laid out so the contaminated instruments are in the same area as the instruments that have been sterilized.

11. What is the correct order of the steps of instrument processing?
    a. Chairside sanitizing of instruments, transporting of contaminated instruments, sterilization area sanitizing of instruments, disinfecting instruments, sterilizing instruments, storing disinfected/sterilized instruments.
    b. Chairside sanitizing of instruments, transporting of contaminated instruments, disinfecting instruments, sterilization area sanitizing of instruments, sterilizing instruments, storing disinfected/sterilized instruments.
    c. Chairside sanitizing of instruments, transporting of contaminated instruments, sterilization area sanitizing of instruments, disinfecting instruments, sterilizing instruments, storing disinfected/sterilized instruments.
    d. Chairside sanitizing of instruments, transporting of contaminated instruments, sterilizing instruments, sterilization area sanitizing of instruments, disinfecting instruments, storing disinfected/sterilized instruments.

12. The ultrasonic cleaner is the preferred method to loosen and remove routine debris and organic matter from instruments. Ultrasonic cleaners produce sound waves beyond human hearing that vibrates and creates invisible bubbles in the ultrasonic cleaning solution.
    Select the correct response based on these statements.
    a. Both statements are true.
    b. Both statements are false.
    c. The first statement is true; the second statement is false.
    d. The first statement is false; the second statement is true.

13. What is the correct order of the steps below in operating an ultrasonic cleaner?
    a. Place instrument bin in sink and place instruments into bin
    b. Check condition of ultrasonic cleaner and change as needed
    c. Place instrument bin into cleaner and place lid on cleaner
    d. Set ultrasonic cleaner time as per manufacturer's instructions
    e. Lift bin and allow excel cleaner to drain into ultrasonic unit
    f. Place instruments onto towel and allow to air dry
    g. Place bin into sink and rinse instruments in sink under water
    h. Inspect all instruments to ensure they are free of debris

14. Which of the following is correct regarding disinfection?
    a. Disinfection is the process of using steam and pressure to kill microorganisms.
    b. Disinfection kills resistant spores and viruses.
    c. Disinfection controls disease-producing pathogens that remain on the surface after sanitization.
    d. Disinfection and sterilization are synonymous.

15. Which of the following is correct regarding critical instruments?
    a. Critical instruments do not penetrate soft tissue or bone.
    b. Critical instruments include mouth mirrors and reusable impression trays.
    c. Critical instruments may be sterilized with a high level disinfectant when steam sterilization is not possible.
    d. Critical instruments enter into or contact the bloodstream or other normally sterile tissues.

16. Which of the following statements is correct regarding high level disinfectants?
    a. High level disinfectants may be used for surface disinfection.
    b. High level disinfectants may be used for sterilization of critical instruments that are sensitive to heat.
    c. High level disinfectants destroy all microorganisms save high numbers of bacterial endospores.
    d. High level disinfectants include chlorine based products.

17. The amount of direct patient contact and aerosol that contaminates the clinical contact surface must be considered in determining the appropriate disinfecting procedure When a clinical contact surface is highly contaminated, the spray-wipe-spray method is acceptable.

    Select the correct response based on these statements.
    a. Both statements are true.
    b. Both statements are false.
    c. The first statement is true; the second statement is false.
    d. The first statement is false; the second statement is true.

18. Which of the following is correct regarding dental unit water lines (DUWLs)?
    a. DUWLs need to meet the EPA regulatory standards of safe drinking water of less than 1,000 colony forming units of heterotrophic water bacteria per milliliter of water.
    b. There is one type of microbe found in DUWLs known as planktonic microbes.
    c. Biofilm is a group of microorganisms that stick together on a hydrated surface.
    d. Anti-retraction valves in DUWLs are optional.

19. Which of the following is correct regarding sterilizations?
    a. The CDC recommends sterilizing critical, semi-critical, and non-critical patient care items.

    b. Heat sensitive items that cannot be sterilized should be disinfected in an intermediate level disinfectant.
    c. The sterilizing package should be labeled with the date sterilized, identity of the sterilizer, and the contents of closed packaging.
    d. The dental health care worker should wear examination gloves while packaging the sanitized instruments for sterilization.

20. Match the agency with the correct contribution to infection control in dentistry.
    a. Centers for Disease Control
    b. Organization for Safety and Asepsis Procedures
    c. Occupational Safety and Health Administration
       1. Development of the "universal precautions" concept to infection control procedures.
       2. Mandates that all dental offices have an infection control training manual available for training new employees.
       3. Provides and monitors practical guidelines in infection control and promotes quality research relating to infection control.

Critical Thinking

1. What are the five steps to achieve asepsis in the dental office?

2. What is the sequence of steps in donning and doffing PPE?

3. What are the steps in managing a contaminated patient tray in the sterilization area?

Key Terms

Term and Pronunciation	Meaning of Root and Word Parts	Definition
asepsis (*uh*-**sep**-sis)	**a-** = without, not **sepsis** = presence of pathogenic microorganisms and their toxins	absence of the microorganisms that produce disease
bioburden (**bahy**-oh-**bur**-dn)	**bio** = life **burden** = to load oppressively, trouble, difficult to bear	the number of contaminating bacteria on a surface that has not been sterilized
bur (bur)	**bur** = a small surgical or dental drill	a rotary cutting tool made of steel used to remove dental decay and dental materials
carpal tunnel (**kahr**-p*uh* l) (**tuhn**-l)	**carpus** = wrist **-al** = pertaining to **tunnel** = passageway	passageway for nerve which runs from the forearm into the palm of the hand; syndrome involves the nerve becoming pressed and painful
cross-contamination (kraws) (*kuh* n-tam-*uh*-**ney**-sh*uh* n)	**cross** = to move from one side to the other **contaminate** = to make impure and unclean **-ation** = indicating a process	when disease-causing microorganisms are moved from one area, item, or person to another
culture (**kuhl**-cher)	**culture** = process of growing microorganisms in a controlled environment; nutritive substance (media)	a spore strip is placed into a culture media to determine if sterilizer is effective
dermatitis (dur-m*uh*-**tahy**-tis)	**dermat** = skin **-itis** = inflammation	inflammation of the skin
efficacy (**ef**-i-k*uh*-see)	**effect** = to bring about, produce a result **-acy** = quality or state	ability to produce a desired or intended result

Term and Pronunciation	Meaning of Root and Word Parts	Definition
ergonomics (ur-g*uh*-**nom**-iks	**ergo** = work **nomy** = management **ics** = relating to	an applied science concerned with design and arranging work areas for efficiency of people in the workforce
excretion (ik-**skree**-sh*uh*n)	**ex-** = out of **-cretion** = matter such as saliva and blood	to eliminate from the body
fungicidal (**fuhn**-j*uh*-sahyd-l)	**fungi** = fungus **cide** = act of killing **-al** = pertaining to	a chemical having the properties capable of destroying fungus
heterotrophic (het-er-*uh*-**trof**-ik)	**hetero** = different, other **trophy** = having nutritional habits or requirements **-ic** = relating to	organism that obtains food and energy from organic substances
planktonic (plangk-**ton**-ik)	**plankton** = passively floating organisms in water **-ic** = pertaining to	microscopic bacteria and protozoa floating in a body of water
percutaneous (pur-kyoo-**tey**-nee-*uh*s)	**per-** = through **cutaneous** = pertaining to the skin	passage of substances through the unbroken skin; passage by needle puncture
polysaccharide (pol-ee-**sak**-*uh*-rahyd)	**poly** = many, more than one **saccharide** = compound containing a sugar or sugars	a carbohydrate containing more than three simple sugars
post-exposure (pohst) (ik-**spoh**-zher)	**post** = after **expose** = to lay open to danger, harm **-ure** = action, result	occurring in the period of time after exposure to a disease
sanitizing (**san**-i-tahyz-ing)	**sanitary** = health or conditions affecting health; especially to cleanliness, precaution against disease **-ize** = to render, to make **-ing** = expressing action; or its result	to make free from dirt and germs, as by cleaning
secretion (si-**kree**-sh*uh*n)	**secrete** = discharge **-tion** = the action of	releasing a substance
sepsis (**sep**-sis)	**sepsis** = presence of pathogenic microorganisms and their toxins	the presence in tissues of pathogenic microorganisms or their toxins
serrations (se-**rey**-sh*uh*n)	**serrate** = notched on the edge like a saw **-tions** = a state, a condition	series of notches on an instrument used for cutting or gripping
sporicidal (**spawr**-*uh*-sahyd-l)	**spore** = a dormant, nonreproductive body formed by certain bacteria in response to adverse environmental conditions; highly resistant to dying **cide** = act of killing **-al** = pertaining to	a chemical having the properties capable of destroying spores
sterilant (**ster**-*uh*-l*uh* nt)	**sterile** = free from all living microorganisms **-ant** = causing or performing an action	a sterilizing agent
sterile (**ster**-il)	**ster-** = totally clean; free from living microorganisms **-ile** = expressing capability	free from all living microorganisms, especially pathogenic microorganisms
suck-back (suhk) (bak)	**suck** = to draw into the mouth by producing a vacuum by action of the lips and tongue **back** = to cause to move backward	microbes enter the tubing from dental patients during treatment; also called backflow
tuberculocidal (t*oo*-**bur**-ky*uh*-luh-sahyd-l)	**tuberculosis** = infectious disease that may affect almost any tissue of the body; especially the lungs characterized by tubercles (firm rounded nodule, swelling) **cide** = act of killing **-al** = pertaining to	a chemical having the properties capable of destroying mycobacterium tuberculosis organism, which is the causative organism for tuberculosis
virucidal (**vahy**-r*uh*-sahyd-l)	**virus** = an ultramicroscopic infectious agent **cide** = act of killing **-al** = pertaining to	a chemical having the properties capable of destroying viruses
wicking (**wik**-ing)	**wick** = a cord or strand of woven, twisted, or braided fibers that draws up fluid **-ing** = expressing the action or its result	penetration of liquids and small pathogens through minute holes in latex membranes

Management of Hazardous Materials

Specific Instructional Objectives

At the completion of this chapter, you will be able to meet these objectives:

1. Use terms presented in this chapter.
2. Identify the scope of the OSHA Bloodborne Pathogens Standard.
3. Describe the components of the OSHA Bloodborne Pathogens Standard.
4. Identify equipment to safeguard employees against injury.
5. Discuss requirements for work site safety.
6. Describe the employee training that is required to meet the OSHA standard for hazardous chemicals.
7. Explain the purpose of OSHA's Hazardous Communication Standard (HCS).
8. Identify the three major changes of the HCS to align with the *Globally Harmonized System of Classification and Labeling of Chemicals (GHS)*.
9. Describe the purpose of safety data sheet manuals.
10. Describe the required format of the new safety data sheets.
11. Identify the nine HCS pictograms.
12. Discuss the rationale for fire extinguishers.
13. Discuss the rationale for an evacuation plan.

Introduction

Infection control and the standards that relate to it are discussed in Chapter 11, "Infection Control." This chapter discusses the requirements of the Occupational Safety and Health Administration (OSHA) Bloodborne Pathogens Standard and Hazardous Communication Standard to manage biohazardous waste and hazardous materials, such as engineering controls, labeling, safety data sheets (SDSs), housekeeping, laundry, and the disposal of hazardous materials. Also included in this chapter is work site safety and the importance of fire extinguishers and an evacuation plan. Dental assistants must understand the entire Bloodborne Pathogens Standard as well as other OSHA requirements and how compliance is accomplished (Figure 12-1). The scope of the Bloodborne Pathogens Standards covers:

- Employee training, safety, and documentation requirements
- Exposure determination
- Infection control, standard precautions, and standard measures used to control possible exposures
- Postexposure follow-up
- Labeling/SDSs
- Housekeeping/laundry
- Disposal of biohazardous waste

Scope and Application

- The Standard applies to all occupational exposure to blood and other potentially infectious materials (OPIMs) and includes part-time employees, designated first aid providers, and mental health workers, as well as exposed medical personnel.
- OPIMs include saliva in dental procedures, cerebrospinal fluid, unfixed tissue, semen, vaginal secretions, and body fluids visibly contaminated with blood.

Methods of Compliance

- General—Standard precautions.
- Engineering and work practice controls.
- Personal protective equipment (PPE).
- Housekeeping.

Standard Precautions

- *All* human blood and OPIMs are considered infectious.
- The *same* precautions must be taken with all blood and OPIMs.

Engineering Controls

- Whenever feasible, engineering controls must be the primary method for controlling exposure.
- Examples include needleless IVs, disposable needle recapping devices, self-sheathing needles, sharps disposal containers, covered centrifuge buckets, aerosol-free tubes, and leak-proof containers.
- Engineering controls must be evaluated and documented regularly.

Sharps Containers

- Readily accessible and as close as practical to work area.
- Puncture resistant.
- Properly labeled or color coded.
- Leak proof.
- Closeable.
- *Routinely replaced* so there is no overflow.

Work Practice Controls

- Handwashing following glove removal.
- No breaking or bending of needles.
- When needle recapping is necessary use single-handed scoop method or use a needle guard.
- No eating, drinking, or smoking in work area.
- No storage of food or drink where blood or OPIMs are stored.
- Minimize splashing, splattering of blood, and splashing of OPIMs.
- No mouth pipetting.
- Specimens must be transported in leak-proof, labeled containers. They must be placed in a secondary container if outside contamination of primary container occurs.
- Equipment must be decontaminated before servicing or shipping. Areas that cannot be decontaminated must be labeled.

Personal Protective Equipment

- Includes eye protection, gloves, protective clothing, protective face masks, hair covering, and resuscitation equipment.
- Must be readily accessible and employers must require their use.
- Must be stored at work site.

Eye Protection

- Is required whenever there is potential for splashing, spraying, or splattering to the eyes or mucous membranes.
- If necessary, use eye protection with a mask, or use a chin-length face shield.
- Prescription glasses may be fitted with solid side shields.
- Decontamination procedures must be developed.

Courtesy of POL Consultants

FIGURE 12-1
Understanding OSHA's bloodborne pathogen and hazardous materials standard.

(Continues)

(*Continued*)

Gloves

- Must be worn whenever hand contact with blood, OPIMs, mucous membranes, non-intact skin, or contaminated surfaces/items or when performing vascular access procedures (phlebotomy).
- Must be changed if punctured or torn.
- Type required:
  — Vinyl or latex for general use.
  — Alternatives must be available if employee has allergic reactions (e.g., powderless, nitrile).
  — Puncture resistant utility gloves for surface disinfection and handling of contaminated materials and instruments.
  — Puncture resistant when handling sharps (e.g., Central Supply).

Protective Clothing

- Must be worn whenever splashing or splattering to skin or clothing may occur.
- Must be changed when clothing becomes soiled.
- Type required depends on exposure. Prevention of skin and clothes contamination is the key.
- Examples:
  — Low-level-exposure lab coats.
  — Moderate-level-exposure, fluid-resistant gown.
  — High-level-exposure, fluid-proof apron, head and foot covering.
- *Note*: If personal protective equipment (PPE) is considered protective clothing, then the *employer must launder it*.

Housekeeping

- There must be a written schedule for cleaning and disinfection.
- Contaminated equipment and surfaces must be cleaned as soon as feasible for obvious contamination or at end of work shift if no contamination has occurred.
- Protective coverings may be used over equipment.

Regulated Waste Containers (Non-Sharp)

- Closeable.
- Leak proof.
- Labeled or color coded.
- Placed in secondary container if outside of container is contaminated.

Laundry

- Handled as little as possible.
- Bagged at location of use.
- Labeled or color coded.
- Transported in bags that prevent soak-through or leakage.

Laundry Facility

- Two options:
  1. Standard precautions for all laundry (alternative color coding allowed if recognized).
  2. Precautions only for contaminated laundry (must be red bagged or biohazard labeled).
- Laundry personnel must use PPE and have a sharps container accessible.

Hepatitis B Vaccination

- Made available within 10 days to all employees with occupational exposure.
- Free to employees.
- May be required for student to be admitted to a college health program, as well as to an externship.
- Given according to U.S. Public Health Service guidelines.
- Employee must first be evaluated by a health care professional.
- Health care professional gives a written opinion.
- If the vaccine is refused, the employee signs a declination form.
- Vaccine must be available later if initially refused.

FIGURE 12-1
Understanding OSHA's bloodborne pathogen and hazardous materials standard.

Courtesy of POL Consultants

Postexposure Follow-Up

- Wash thoroughly with antimicrobial soap.
- Have a blood draw as soon as possible or within 2 hours.
- Document exposure incident.
- Identify source individual (if possible).
- Attempt to test source if consent is obtained.
- Provide results to the exposed employee.

Labels

- Biohazard symbol and word Biohazard must be visible.
- Fluorescent orange/orange-red with contrasting letters may also be used.
- Red bags/containers may be substituted for labels.
- Labels are required on:
  — Regulated waste.
  — Refrigerators/freezers with blood of OPIMs.
  — Transport/storage containers.
  — Contaminated equipment.

Information and Training

- Required for all employees with occupational exposure.
- Training required initially, annually, and if there are new procedures.
- Training material must be appropriate for the employees' literacy and education levels.
- Training must be interactive and allow for questions and answers.

Training Components

- Modes of HIV/HBV transmission.
- Explanation of exposure control plan.
- Explanation of engineering, work practice controls.
- Explanation of bloodborne standard.
- Epidemiology and symptoms of bloodborne disease.
- How to select the proper PPE.
- How to decontaminate equipment, surfaces, and so on.
- Information about hepatitis B vaccine.
- Postexposure follow-up procedures.
- Label/color code system.

Medical Records

Records must be kept for each employee with occupational exposure and include:

- A copy of employee's vaccination status and date.
- A copy of postexposure follow-up evaluation procedures.
- Health care professional's written opinions.
- Confidentiality must be maintained.
- Records must be maintained for 30 years, plus the duration of employment.

Training Records

Records are kept for 3 years from date of training and include:

- Date of training.
- Summary of contents of training program.
- Name and qualifications of trainer.
- Names and job titles of all persons attending.

Exposure Control Plan Components

- A written plan for each workplace with occupational exposure.
- Written policies/procedures for complying with the standard.
- A cohesive document or a guiding document referencing existing policies/procedures.

Courtesy of POL Consultants

FIGURE 12-1
Understanding OSHA's bloodborne pathogen and hazardous materials standard.

(Continues)

(*Continued*)

Exposure Control Plan
• A list of job classifications where occupational exposure control occurs (e.g., medical assistant, clinical laboratory scientist, and dental hygienist). • A list of tasks where exposure occurs (e.g., medical assistant who performs venipuncture). • Methods/policies/procedures for compliance. • Procedures for sharps disposal. • Disinfection policies/procedures. • Procedures for selection of PPE. • Regulated waste disposal procedures. • Laundry procedures. • Hepatitis B vaccination procedures. • Postexposure follow-up procedures. • Training procedures. • Plan must be accessible to employees and be updated annually.
Employee Responsibilities
• Go through training and cooperate. • Obey policies. • Use universal precaution techniques. • Use PPE. • Use safe work practices. • Use engineering controls.
Employee Responsibilities
• Report unsafe work conditions to employer. • Maintain clean work areas. Cooperation between employer and employees regarding the Standard will facilitate understanding of the law, thereby benefiting all persons who are exposed to HIV, HBV, and OPIMs by minimizing the risk of exposure to pathogens. Meeting the OSHA standard is not optional, and failure to comply can result in a fine that may total $10,000 for each employee.

Courtesy of POL Consultants

FIGURE 12-1
Understanding OSHA's bloodborne pathogen and hazardous materials standard.

OSHA's Bloodborne Pathogen Standard

In 1991, OSHA published the Occupational Exposure to Bloodborne Pathogens Standard. However, needlesticks and other sharps injuries continued to occur frequently, causing serious health effects. In 2001, according to OSHA, the CDC estimated that health care workers sustained nearly 600,000 percutaneous injuries annually involving contaminated sharps. Based on this information, the U.S. Congress passed the *Needlestick Safety and Prevention Act*, which directed OSHA to revise the bloodborne pathogens standard. The standard was revised and became effective in April 2001. Refer to Chapter 23 for details regarding this act.

Exposure Control Plan

A comprehensive infection control program should include a written Exposure Control Plan (ECP), which sets forth office policies and procedures that prevent or reduce the risk of disease transmission between dental office personnel, their families, patients, and the community. The plan should include the practices, procedures, products, and technologies that will help to prevent injury, illness, and disease transmission.

Goals and Objectives

The goals and objectives of the written ECP are clearly explained in the CDC's *Guidelines for Infection Control in Dental Health-Care Settings— 2003*. The evidence-based recommendations within this document apply to all settings in which dental health care is provided. The ultimate goal of the ECP is to reduce the acquisition and transmission of illness and infection. The main objectives are to prevent the transmission of infectious diseases within the dental office; maintain the safest possible environment for patients, employees, and the community; and eliminate or minimize occupational exposure to bloodborne pathogens in accordance with OSHA standard 29 CFR 1910.1030, "Occupational Exposure to Bloodborne Pathogens."

Two new requirements were added to the standard. First, the employer must solicit input from employees involved in direct patient care. These employees should be nonmanagerial, and the selection should be from a wide range of direct patient care interaction positions. Annually, the representative number of employees will give input after the employer has requested it.

The employer must document this input in the exposure control plan, as well as how, and from whom, they solicited said input. According to the *Revision to OSHA's Bloodborne Pathogens Standard, Technical Background and Summary*, the dentist can demonstrate that they are meeting the standard by:

- listing the employees involved and describing the process by which input was requested; or

- presenting other documentation, including references to the minutes of meetings, copies of documents used to request employee participation, or records of responses received from employees.

The employer must also:

- consider innovations in medical procedure and technological developments that reduce the risk of exposure; and

- document the use of appropriate, effective, and commercially available safer devices, and the considerations used to evaluate those devices.

The employer must select devices that are based on reasonable judgment:

- will not jeopardize patient or employee safety or be medically inadvisable; and

- will make an exposure incident involving a contaminated sharp less likely to occur.

The other addition to the standard is that, along with maintaining a log of occupational injuries and illnesses, the employer, under the new revision, must maintain a sharps injury log. As with all other employee records, this log must be kept in protection of the employee's privacy. The sharps injury log must contain the type and brand of the device involved in the incident, the location of the incident, and a description of the incident. The format of the log is set by the employer and may contain additional comments as long as the privacy of the employee is maintained.

Under engineering controls in the OSHA standard, the revision now specifies that "safer medical devices, such as sharps with engineered sharps injury protections and needle-less systems" constitute an effective engineering control and must be used where feasible.

"Sharps with engineered sharps injury protections" is a new term that includes nonneedle sharps or needle devices that contain built-in safety features, and are used for collecting fluids, administering medications or other fluids, or any other procedures involving the risk of sharps injury. This covers such devices as a syringe with a sliding sheath that shields the attached needle after use, and needles that retract into the syringe after use.

"Needleless systems" is a new term for devices that provide an alternative to needles for various procedures. This term is currently used more in medicine than in dentistry. It refers to such devices as jet injection systems or IV medication systems in which a port is used instead of a needle.

OSHA Compliance Directive

OSHA continues to revise and create compliance directives to further protect employees and clarify new standards for employers. These directives are a way to clarify the intent of the standard and the enforcement procedures for compliance. Employers and employees should continue to stay abreast of standards and requirements. The OSHA (http://www.OSHA.gov) and ADA (http://www.ADA.org) websites are good sources of information pertinent to dentistry.

Engineering/Work Practice Controls

The physical equipment and mechanical devices that employers provide to safeguard and protect employees at work are known as engineering and work practice controls. Examples of these are splash guards on model trimmers, puncture-resistant sharps containers, and ventilation hoods for hazardous fumes. The employer must provide this equipment to meet OSHA standards and provide a safe environment for employees. The employer must ensure that employees wash their hands immediately after gloves are removed and flush their eyes with water at an eye-wash station if contact with microorganisms or hazardous materials is suspected (Figure 11-4). The employer must ensure that employees flush any mucous membranes immediately if there has been possible contact with blood or other potentially infectious materials (OPIMs) in the office.

The employer sets up work practice controls to diminish harmful occupational exposure. OSHA defines occupational exposure as reasonably anticipated eye, skin, mucous membrane, or parenteral contact with blood or other OPIMs that may result from the performance of an employee's duties. It further defines parenteral as a means of piercing mucous membranes or the skin barrier through such events as needlesticks, cuts, and abrasions.

Sharps The Needlestick Safety and Prevention Act of 2000 requires dental offices to evaluate and select safer sharps devices as they become available. The dentist may purchase needle guards for dental needles to protect employees from unnecessary sticks. Several types are available (see Figure 23-12). Needles should never be recapped using the two-hand technique, because it is easy to stick the opposing hand or the other person's hand (refer to Chapter 23). Needles should also never be capped using the scoop method.

Upon completing a procedure, contaminated sharps and needles must be placed immediately in a labeled, leak-proof, puncture-resistant container (see Figure 11-68). Other sharps that are placed routinely in the sharps disposal containers are blades from knives used in surgery, broken glass, anesthetic capsules, and orthodontic wires. When the sharps disposal containers are full, they are sealed, sterilized using an autoclave if possible, and sent to an outside biohazard agency for safe disposal.

Occupational Exposure to Bloodborne Pathogens

The ECP should identify the level of exposure risk for each employee. For example, dentists, chairside dental assistants, and dental hygienists are all at risk for occupational exposure. The office manager and front desk assistant may not have any occupational exposure risk. However, if they at times may assist with hazardous waste management or sterilization procedures, this should be documented in the ECP as occasional occupational risk.

Any employee who has an occupational exposure incident must report it immediately (Figure 12-2). The employer must immediately make a confidential medical evaluation and follow-up available to the exposed employee. The medical evaluation and follow-up are made available to the employee at no cost. The dentist refers the exposed employee to a licensed health care professional to have the most current medical evaluation and procedures performed in accordance with the U.S. Public Health Service regulations. OSHA standards do not dictate the procedures to be performed but allow for the most current recommendations

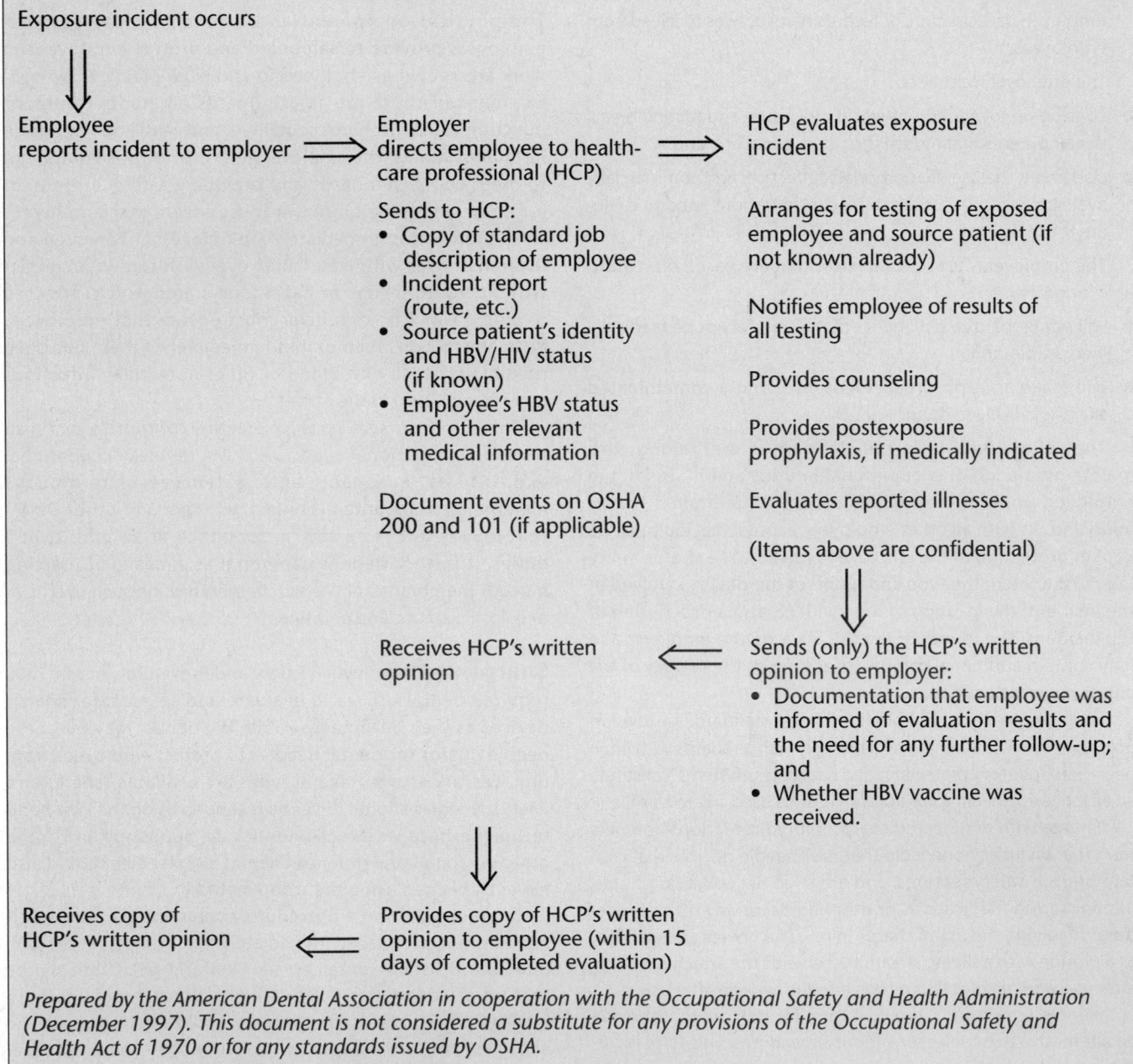

Exposure incident occurs

Employee reports incident to employer ⟹ Employer directs employee to health-care professional (HCP) ⟹ HCP evaluates exposure incident

Sends to HCP:
- Copy of standard job description of employee
- Incident report (route, etc.)
- Source patient's identity and HBV/HIV status (if known)
- Employee's HBV status and other relevant medical information

Document events on OSHA 200 and 101 (if applicable)

Arranges for testing of exposed employee and source patient (if not known already)

Notifies employee of results of all testing

Provides counseling

Provides postexposure prophylaxis, if medically indicated

Evaluates reported illnesses

(Items above are confidential)

Receives HCP's written opinion ⟸ Sends (only) the HCP's written opinion to employer:
- Documentation that employee was informed of evaluation results and the need for any further follow-up; and
- Whether HBV vaccine was received.

Receives copy of HCP's written opinion ⟸ Provides copy of HCP's written opinion to employee (within 15 days of completed evaluation)

Prepared by the American Dental Association in cooperation with the Occupational Safety and Health Administration (December 1997). This document is not considered a substitute for any provisions of the Occupational Safety and Health Act of 1970 or for any standards issued by OSHA.

Copyright © 1998 American Dental Association

Courtesy of the American Dental Association

FIGURE 12-2
Flowchart for occupational exposure to bloodborne pathogens.

to be applied. Reporting the incident immediately allows the dentist to carefully evaluate the circumstances surrounding the incident and to find ways to prevent the situation and exposure incident from happening again.

Documentation of Exposure Incident

The dentist documents the information from the exposure incident on a report. This report includes the route(s) of exposure, the circumstances that surrounded the exposure incident, and (if known) the identity of the source patient. The exposure incident report is placed in the employee's confidential medical record, and a copy of this report is provided to the health care professional who is providing the evaluation.

The employer is required to provide the licensed health care professional with a description of the employee's job duties and their relation to the incident; information about the route of the exposure; the circumstances surrounding the incident; relevant employee medical records, including vaccination status; a copy of the bloodborne pathogen standard; and the results of the source patient's blood testing (if available).

If the employer has over 10 employees, the employer may be required to complete OSHA Form 200 (Log and Summary of Occupational Injuries and Illnesses) and Form 101 (Supplemental Record of Occupational Injuries and Illnesses) to meet the recordable occupational injury requirement. Serious work related injuries must be logged and the records must be maintained for five calendar years.

In the case of a bloodborne pathogen exposure, the dentist must identify and document, in writing, the source patient, if known. Furthermore, the dentist must contact the source patient and request his or her consent to be tested for HBV and HIV, as well as to disclose the results of these tests to the exposed employee. If the source patient does not give consent for the testing, the dentist must document this on the report of the exposure incident. If the source patient agrees to be tested, the tests should be completed as soon as feasible. When the results are disclosed to the exposed employee, information regarding the source patient's rights to disclosure must be discussed (Figure 12-2).

Exposed Employee Blood (Collection and Testing)
The employee has the right to decline testing after an exposure incident or to delay the testing for up to 90 days. The employee may consent to have a baseline blood test that will determine the HBV and HIV serological status. The employee may choose to be tested only for HBV and not give consent for HIV testing at that time. The employee's blood sample must be saved for 90 days in case the employee elects to consent to the HIV testing. All tests must be performed by an accredited laboratory at no cost to the employee. The health care professional will notify the employee directly of all test results.

Postexposure Follow-Up Procedures
The procedure for evaluating the circumstances of an exposure incident should be clearly established and set forth in the ECP. The employee involved in the incident should first clean the wound with soap and water. If mucous membranes are involved, the affected area should immediately be flushed with cool water. Per OSHA, the dental office is required to have immediate access to eyewashes and showers in the event of a chemical exposure (refer to Figure 11-4). The employer or infection control coordinator should be immediately notified. The designated health care professional will be contacted for medical evaluation and follow-up. The employee involved in the exposure incident will then take a copy of the employee's standard job description, a copy of the exposure incident report, the source patient's identity and infectious status (if known and consent is obtained), the employee's HBV status, and all other relevant medical information and a copy of the OSHA Bloodborne Pathogens Standard to the designated health care provider. The designated health care provider will evaluate the exposure incident, employee, and source patient (with consent). Testing results and postexposure management will be provided as indicated. A written document will be sent to the employee and employer regarding all findings and diagnoses pertinent to the exposure.

A postexposure evaluation and follow-up procedure should be clearly established and written in the ECP. The employer must provide the exposed employee counseling, prophylaxis to prevent sexual transmission of any possible infection, and evaluation of reported illnesses. The provided counseling will aid the employee in interpretation of all tests, discussions about the potential risk of infection, and the need for further postexposure prophylaxis. The employee should also be counseled on the necessary use of protection during sexual contact.

Treatment may include, but is not limited to, an HBV vaccine if the employee has not had it, or chemoprophylaxis for high-risk cases of HIV transmission.

The health care professional also evaluates any reported illnesses that the exposed employee develops. The health care professional can evaluate the symptoms in relation to HBV and HIV infections. This allows the exposed employee to have immediate medical evaluation and referral for medical treatment, so that the treatment can be started as soon as possible. This does not mean that the employer is responsible for any costs associated with the treatment of the disease.

The health care professional sends the dental employer a written opinion about the evaluation, as well as notification that the employee was informed of the test results of the evaluation and of further follow-up. The dentist provides the employee with a copy of this written opinion and evaluation of the exposed employee within 15 days of the completion of the evaluation. The original document is placed in the employee's confidential record. The employer must maintain employee records in a confidential manner for the duration of employment plus 30 years, in accordance with OSHA's standard on Access to Employee Exposure and Medical Records, 29 CFR 1910.20.

Postexposure prophylaxis is provided according to the current recommendations of the U.S. Public Health Service. OSHA did not define this procedure in the bloodborne standard, due to ongoing changes that have developed in this area.

Employee Work Site Safety

The employer must provide a work site that is clean and sanitary. Each office must have a written schedule for infection control and decontaminating procedures for each area. Wastepaper baskets, floors, and all other surfaces that may have been contaminated with blood or OPIM must be included. The assistant must wear utility gloves while cleaning contaminated surfaces. All disposable items that are contaminated, including gloves, must be discarded in a biohazard container.

Broken Glass

Broken glass must be cleaned up with a broom (or brush) and dust pan (or cardboard). Dental assistants must never touch broken glass with bare hands or gloved hands, due to the risk of puncture. Broken glass must be placed in a leak-proof sharps container labeled "biohazard."

Laundry

Contaminated laundry must be handled as little as possible. Gloves must be used when placing it in a biohazard container or a red bag that is labeled with a biohazard symbol (Figure 12-3).

If the laundry is damp or wet, it must first be placed in a plastic bag to prevent blood or OPIM from seeping through it.

Laundry that is sent off site for cleaning is placed in a red biohazard bag for transportation. Dental assistants should take special care when removing protective clothing, especially items that are taken over the head. The chance for contamination of the face can take place if the outside surface of the clothing makes contact with it.

Hazardous Chemicals

The OSHA hazard communication standard is set up so that employees receive training about the risks of using hazardous chemicals and the safety precautions required when handling them. Employees must be trained in the identification of hazardous chemicals and the personal protective equipment to be utilized for each chemical. This training must occur within 30 days of employment or prior to the employee using any chemicals, and annually thereafter (Figure 12-4).

Employees must have a certificate available, or in their personnel files, that shows they have had the proper training. The certificate must identify that the employer has trained the employee in the proper handling of hazardous substances in the dental office (Figure 12-5).

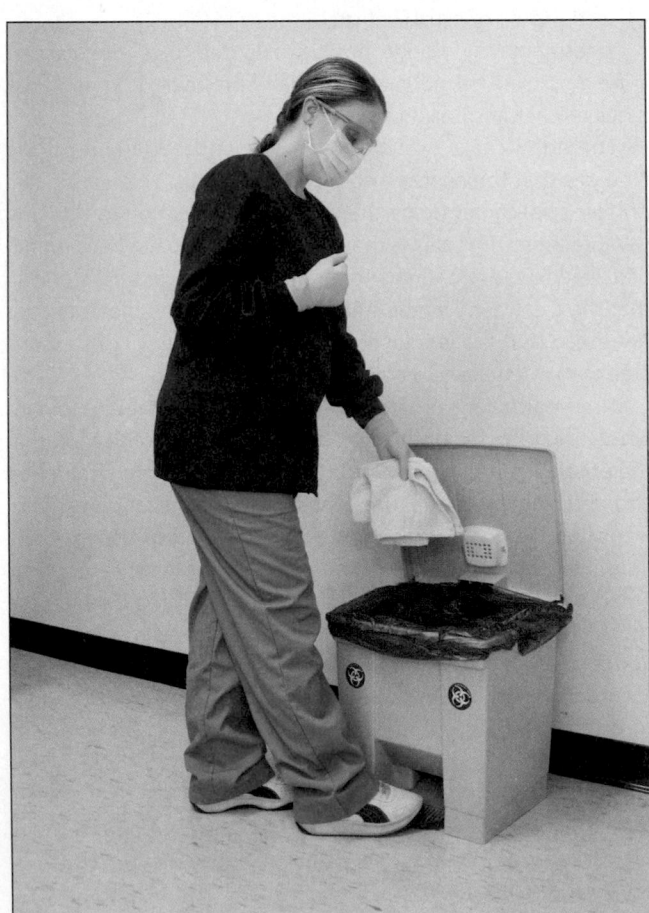

FIGURE 12-3
Proper disposal of contaminated laundry.

SAFETY TRAINING FORM

All employees receive safety training before those employees assume responsibilities that involve exposure to body fluids or chemicals or within 30 days of employment. Items that must be covered in the training session are as follows:

- Overall explanation of OSHA laws
- Explanation of the epidemiology and symptoms of HBV and HIV/AIDS
- Discussion about who is at risk in the dental office
- Transmission modes of microorganisms
- Methods of infection control in the workplace
- Universal/Standard Precautions
- Personal protective equipment
- Handwashing
- How spills are to be cleaned
- Postexposure incident procedure
- Coverage of the Hazardous Communication Standard
- Chemical labels and how to read them
- How to read SDSs, how to get SDSs, where SDSs are kept in the office, and interpretation of warning signs on SDSs
- How chemicals are to be stored and inventoried
- Hazardous waste laws and how to comply
- How to use sharps containers
- How to keep and who keeps records
- Medical consent forms
- HBV forms
- Engineering control records
- Safety training certification and when training is to take place

FIGURE 12-4
Safety training form.

OSHA HAZARD COMMUNICATION AND BLOODBORNE PATHOGEN STANDARD TRAINING CERTIFICATE

This certificate indicates your successful completion of the OSHA Hazard Communication and Bloodborne Pathogen Standard Training in the office of _____. The program instructed you of your rights as a worker, the responsibilities of your employer, and the proper knowledge and handling of hazardous substances and bloodborne pathogens in this dental office.

Date of employment _____

Date of training _____

Instructor's signature _____

Employee's signature _____

Employer's signature _____

FIGURE 12-5
Sample training form.

As with the Bloodborne Pathogen Standard, a written plan identifying employee training and detailing specific control measures used in the workplace must be compiled for the management of hazardous chemicals. If the office is not in compliance, penalties may be imposed on the employer.

All hazardous chemicals must be identified on a written form, such as a chemical inventory form (Figure 12-6). Other information required about the chemicals includes the quantity stored (each month or year), the physical state of the substance (liquid, solid, or gas), the hazardous class (health problem, fire hazard, and reactive), what PPE is required, and the manufacturer's name, address, and phone number.

OSHA's Hazardous Communication Standard (HCS)

The Hazardous Communication Standard, which is part of the Employee Right-to-Know Law, was revised in 2012. This revision included the adoption of the *Globally Harmonized System of Classification and Labeling of Chemicals (GHS)*. This means that chemicals and materials are classified and labeled the same way internationally, regardless of where the chemicals are manufactured, sold, or used.

Safety Data Sheets

One part of the 2012 revision to the HCS now requires manufacturers and employers to use specific criteria for classification of health and physical hazards; a label that includes a harmonized signal word, pictogram, and hazard statement for all categories; and a new 16-section format Safety Data Sheet (SDS, formerly Material Safety Data Sheet).

Every office must have a SDS manual that is alphabetized, indexed, and available to all employees. The SDSs are summaries that provide information about the potential hazards of a product as well as safety measures. The SDSs are usually written and provided by the product manufacturer or the product distributor. The SDS manuals can be in hard copy or on a computer. The manual contains the SDSs. These sheets come from the manufacturer. If SDSs are unavailable, the employer, or a designated employee (the safety assistant), must request it from the manufacturer, or it can be easily found on the manufacturer's website. The SDS form must include the following 16 sections, of which 12 are enforced by OSHA (Figure 12-7):

1. Description
2. Hazards
3. Composition
4. First aid
5. Fire fighting
6. Accidental release measures
7. Handling and storage
8. Exposure controls
9. Physical and chemical properties
10. Stability and reactivity
11. Toxicology
12. Ecology*
13. Disposal*
14. Transport*
15. Regulatory*
16. Other information

*These sections are enforced by agencies other than OSHA.

Harmonized Label

A second major change of the HCS requires that all labeling must now be done in the GHS format. The harmonized label includes a hazard statement that describes the hazard, a signal word that indicates the severity of the hazard, and an OSHA designated pictogram that indicates the type of hazard (Figure 12-8). There are nine pictograms that may be used, and OSHA enforces the use of eight of those. The pictograms communicate:

- health hazard (carcinogen and toxicity to organs or body systems);
- flame (flammable);
- exclamation mark (irritant or sensitivity);
- gas cylinder (gas under pressure);
- corrosion (skin, eye, or metal);
- exploding bomb (explosive or reactive);
- flame over circle (oxidizer);
- environment (nonmandatory); and
- skull and crossbones (acute toxicity or fatal).

Chemical Inventory Form

Date updated _____

Dental office _____

Chemical Name	Hazard Class				Physical State	Manufacturer	Comments
	(H)	(F)	(R)	(P)			

(H) Health
0—Minimal
1—Slightly
2—Moderate
3—Serious
4—Extreme

(F) Fire Hazard
0—Will not burn
1—Slight
2—Moderate
3—Serious
4—Extreme

(R) Reactivity
0—Stable
1—Slight
2—Moderate
3—Serious
4—Extreme

(P) Protection
A—Goggles
B—Goggles/gloves
C—Goggles/gloves/clothing
D—Goggles/gloves/clothing/mask
E—Goggles/gloves/mask
F—Gloves
G—Face shield/gloves

FIGURE 12-6
Sample chemical inventory form.

The *National Fire Protection Association's color and number method* is used to easily identify information about various hazardous ingredients on the SDS and product labels. While this labeling is not required, it may still be used along with the harmonized label (Figure 12-9).

Chemical Warning Label Determination

A third major change of the HCS requires that The National Fire Protection Association's color and number method is used to signify a warning to employees using chemicals (Figure 12-10). Four colors are used:

1. Blue identifies a health hazard.
2. Red identifies a fire hazard.
3. Yellow identifies the reactivity or stability of a chemical.
4. White indicates that PPE is needed when using the chemical.

The level of risk for each category is indicated by the use of numbers, zero to four—the higher the number, the greater the danger. Letters are used to identify the PPE needed.

A chemical warning label, a diamond-shaped symbol, displays the four colors with a place for the numbers to be written on each (Figure 12-10). The employee can quickly identify the hazard category, the risk for each, and the PPE equipment required. All hazardous chemicals must be labeled unless they are poured into separate containers for immediate use (Figure 12-11).

Quality Assurance/Updates

Maintaining the hazardous communication program requires a team effort. Efficiency and compliancy are dependent upon the everyday practices of the office staff and personnel. Each team member will need to do their part according to their job description to ensure proficiency. The hazardous communication program must be carefully planned. At least once every 12–18 months, evaluation of the program should occur. The designated officer may choose a specific month to schedule maintenance of the ventilation units in the office and may choose to stock up on disposable containers at that time as well. The business manager may review the budgeted costs for disposals around the same time and evaluate the expenses allocated to maintenance of the hazardous materials program.

Maintenance also includes replenishing any materials necessary, such as new labels or new postings. Have there been any

MERCURY
Safety Data Sheet
according to the federal final rule of hazard communication revised on 2012 (HazCom 2012)

Date of issue: 11/19/2013

SECTION 1: Identification of the substance/mixture and of the company/undertaking

1.1.   Product identifier

Trade name	: MERCURY
CAS No	: 7439-97-6
Other means of identification	: Colloidal Mercury, Quick Silver, Liquid Silver, NCI-C60399, Hydrargyrum

1.2.   Relevant identified uses of the substance or mixture and uses advised against

Use of the substance/mixture   : Variety of industrial, analytical and research applications.

1.3.   Details of the supplier of the safety data sheet

ABC Pharmaceuticals

1234 Chemcial Way
Amalgam Center, AL 31313

1.4.   Emergency telephone number

Emergency number   : 1-800-555-5656

SECTION 2: Hazards identification

2.1.   Classification of the substance or mixture

GHS-US classification

Acute Tox. 1 (Inhalation:dust,mist)	H330
Repr. 1B	H360
STOT RE 1	H372
Aquatic Acute 1	H400
Aquatic Chronic 1	H410

2.2.   Label elements

GHS-US labelling

Hazard pictograms (GHS-US)   :

          GHS06   GHS08   GHS09

Signal word (GHS-US)	: Danger
Hazard statements (GHS-US)	: H330 - Fatal if inhaled
	H360 - May damage fertility or the unborn child
	H372 - Causes damage to organs through prolonged or repeated exposure
	H400 - Very toxic to aquatic life
	H410 - Very toxic to aquatic life with long lasting effects
Precautionary statements (GHS-US)	: P201 - Obtain special instructions before use
	P202 - Do not handle until all safety precautions have been read and understood
	P260 - Do not breathe vapors, gas
	P264 - Wash skin, hands thoroughly after handling
	P270 - Do not eat, drink or smoke when using this product
	P271 - Use only outdoors or in a well-ventilated area
	P273 - Avoid release to the environment
	P280 - Wear eye protection, protective clothing, protective gloves, Face mask
	P284 - [In case of inadequate ventilation] wear respiratory protection
	P304+P340 - IF INHALED: Remove person to fresh air and keep comfortable for breathing
	P308+P313 - IF exposed or concerned: Get medical advice/attention
	P310 - Immediately call a POISON CENTER/doctor/...
	P314 - Get medical advice and attention if you feel unwell
	P320 - Specific treatment is urgent (see First aid measures on this label)
	P391 - Collect spillage
	P403+P233 - Store in a well-ventilated place. Keep container tightly closed
	P405 - Store locked up
	P501 - Dispose of contents/container to comply with applicable local, national and international regulation.

2.3.   Other hazards

other hazards which do not result in classification   : When inhaled, Mercury will be rapidly distributed throughout the body. During this time, Mercury will cross the blood-brain barrier, and become oxidized to the Hg (II) oxidation state. The oxidized species of Mercury cannot cross the blood-brain barrier and thus accumulates in the

FIGURE 12-7
Sample SDS.

(Continues)

(Continued)

MERCURY

Safety Data Sheet

according to the federal final rule of hazard communication revised on 2012 (HazCom 2012)

brain. Mercury in other organs is removed slowly from the body via the kidneys. The average half-time for clearance of Mercury for different parts of the human body is as follows: lung: 1.7 days; head: 21 days; kidney region: 64 days; chest: 43 days; whole body: 58 days. Mercury can be irritating to contaminated skin and eye. Prolonged contact may lead to ulceration of the skin. Allergic reactions (i.e. rashes, welts) may occur in sensitive individuals. Mercury can be irritating to contaminated skin and eyes. Short-term over-exposures to high concentrations of mercury vapors can lead to breathing difficulty, coughing, acute, and potentially fatal lung disorders. Depending on the concentration of inhalation over-exposure, heart problems, damage to the kidney, liver or nerves and effects on the brain may occur.

2.4.   Unknown acute toxicity (GHS-US)

No data available

SECTION 3: Composition/information on ingredients

3.1.   Substance

Not applicable

Full text of H-phrases: see section 16

3.2.   Mixture

Name	Product identifier	%	GHS-US classification
Mercury	(CAS No) 7439-97-6	100	Acute Tox. 2 (Inhalation), H330 Repr. 1B, H360 STOT RE 1, H372 Aquatic Acute 1, H400 Aquatic Chronic 1, H410

SECTION 4: First aid measures

4.1.   Description of first aid measures

First-aid measures general : Never give anything by mouth to an unconscious person. If exposed or concerned: Get medical advice/attention.

First-aid measures after inhalation : Remove to fresh air and keep at rest in a position comfortable for breathing. Assure fresh air breathing. Allow the victim to rest. Immediately call a POISON CENTER or doctor/physician. In case of irregular breathing or respiratory arrest provide artificial respiration.

First-aid measures after skin contact : Wash immediately with lots of water (15 minutes)/shower. Remove affected clothing and wash all exposed skin area with mild soap and water, followed by warm water rinse. Seek immediate medical advice.

First-aid measures after eye contact : Rinse immediately and thoroughly, pulling the eyelids well away from the eye (15 minutes minimum). Keep eye wide open while rinsing. Seek medical attention immediately.

First-aid measures after ingestion : Immediately call a POISON CENTER or doctor/physician. Rinse mouth. If conscious, give large amounts of water and induce vomiting. Give water or milk if the person is fully conscious. Obtain emergency medical attention.

4.2.   Most important symptoms and effects, both acute and delayed

Symptoms/injuries after inhalation : Short-term over-exposures to high concentrations of mercury vapors can lead to breathing difficulty, coughing, acute, chemical pneumonia, and pulmonary edema (a potentially fatal accumulation of fluid in the lungs) . Depending on the concentration of over-exposure, cardiac abnormalities, damage to the kidney, liver or nerves and effects on the brain may occur. Long-term inhalation over-exposures can lead to the development of a wide variety of symptoms, including the following: excessive salivation, gingivitis, anorexia, chills, fever, cardiac abnormalities, anemia, digestive problems, abdominal pains, frequent urination, an inability to urinate, diarrhea, peripheral neuropathy (numbness, weakness, or burning sensations in the hands or feet), tremors (especially in the hands, fingers, eyelids, lips, cheeks, tongue, or legs), alteration of tendon reflexes, slurred speech, visual disturbances, and deafness. Allergic reactions (i.e. breathing difficulty) may also occur in sensitive individuals.

Symptoms/injuries after skin contact : Symptoms of skin exposure can include redness, dry skin, and pain. Prolonged contact may lead to ulceration of the skin. Allergic reactions (i.e. rashes, welts) may occur in sensitive individuals. Dermatitis (redness and inflammation of the skin) may occur after repeated skin exposures.

Symptoms/injuries after eye contact : Symptoms of eye exposure can include redness, pain, and watery eyes. A symptom of Mercury exposure is discoloration of the lens of the eyes.

Symptoms/injuries after ingestion : If Mercury is swallowed, symptoms of such over-exposure can include metallic taste in mouth, nausea, vomiting, central nervous system effects, and damage to the kidneys. Metallic mercury is not usually absorbed sufficiently from the gastrointestinal tract to induce an acute, toxic response. Damage to the tissues of the mouth, throat, esophagus, and other tissues of the digestive system may occur. Ingestion may be fatal, due to effects on gastrointestinal system and kidneys.

Chronic symptoms : Long-term over-exposure can lead to a wide range of adverse health effects. Anyone using Mercury must pay attention to personality changes, weight loss, skin or gum discolorations, stomach pains, and other signs of Mercury over-exposure. Gradually developing syndromes ("Erethism" and "Acrodynia") are indicative of potentially severe health problems. Mercury can cause the development of allergic reactions (i.e. dermatitis, rashes, breathing difficulty) upon prolonged or repeated exposures. Refer to Section 11 (Toxicology Information) for additional data.

FIGURE 12-7

Sample SDS.

MERCURY

Safety Data Sheet

according to the federal final rule of hazard communication revised on 2012 (HazCom 2012)

4.3.	Indication of any immediate medical attention and special treatment needed

Treatment for Mercury over-exposure must be given. The following treatment protocol for ingestion of Mercury is from Clinical Toxicology of Commercial Products (5th Edition, 1984).

SECTION 5: Firefighting measures

5.1.	Extinguishing media

Suitable extinguishing media	: Foam. Dry powder. Carbon dioxide. Water spray. Sand.
Unsuitable extinguishing media	: Do not use a heavy water stream.

5.2.	Special hazards arising from the substance or mixture

Fire hazard	: Not flammable. Mercury vapors and oxides generated during fires involving this product are toxic.
Reactivity	: Stable. Reacts with (some) metals. Mercury can react with metals to form amalgams.

5.3.	Advice for firefighters

Firefighting instructions	: Use water spray or fog for cooling exposed containers. Exercise caution when fighting any chemical fire. Prevent fire-fighting water from entering environment. Do not allow run-off from fire fighting to enter drains or water courses.
Protective equipment for firefighters	: Do not enter fire area without proper protective equipment, including respiratory protection.
Other information	: Decontaminate all equipment thoroughly after the conclusion of fire-fighting activities.

SECTION 6: Accidental release measures

6.1.	Personal precautions, protective equipment and emergency procedures

General measures	: Uncontrolled release should be responded to by trained personnel using pre-planned procedures. Evacuate area. Evacuate personnel to a safe area.

6.1.1. For non-emergency personnel

Emergency procedures	: Evacuate unnecessary personnel.

6.1.2. For emergency responders

Protective equipment	: Equip cleanup crew with proper protection. In the event of a release under 1 pound: the minimum level "C" Personal Protective Equipment is needed. Triple-gloves (rubber gloves and nitril gloves over latex gloves), chemical resistant suit and boots, hard-hat, and Air-Purifying Respirator with Cartridge appropriate for Mercury. In the event of a release over 1 pound or when concentration of oxygen in atmosphere is less than 19.5% or unknown, the level "B" Personal Protective Equipments which includes Self-Contained Breathing Apparatus must be worn.
Emergency procedures	: Ventilate area.

6.2.	Environmental precautions

Prevent entry to sewers and public waters. Notify authorities if liquid enters sewers or public waters. Avoid release to the environment.

6.3.	Methods and material for containment and cleaning up

For containment	: For larger spills, dike area and pump into waste containers. Put into a labelled container and provide safe disposal.
Methods for cleaning up	: There are a variety of methods which can be used to clean-up Mercury spills. Use a commercially available Mercury Spill Kit for small spills. A suction pump with aspirator can also be used during clean-up operations. For larger release, a Mercury vacuum can be used. Calcium polysulfide or excess sulfur can be also used for clean-up. Mercury can migrate into cracks and other difficult-to-clean areas; calcium polysulfide and sulfur can be sprinkled effectively into these areas. Decontaminate the area thoroughly. The area should be inspected visually and with colorimetric tubes for Mercury to ensure all traces have been removed prior to re-occupation by non-emergency personnel. Decontaminate all equipment used in response thoroughly If such equipments cannot de adequately decontaminated, it must be discarded with other spill residue. Place all spill residues in an appropriate container, seal immediately, and label appropriately. Dispose of in accordance with federal, state, and local hazardous waste disposal requirements. (Refer to Section 13 of this SDS).

6.4.	Reference to other sections

See Heading 8. Exposure controls and personal protection.

SECTION 7: Handling and storage

7.1.	Precautions for safe handling

Additional hazards when processed	: Supervisors and responsible personnel must be aware of personality changes, weight loss, or other sign of Mercury over-exposure in employees using this product; These symptoms can develop gradually and are indicative of potentially severe health effects related to Mercury contamination.

FIGURE 12-7

Sample SDS.

(Continues)

(Continued)

MERCURY
Safety Data Sheet
according to the federal final rule of hazard communication revised on 2012 (HazCom 2012)

Precautions for safe handling	: As with all chemicals, avoid getting Mercury ON YOU or IN YOU. Do not handle until all safety precautions have been read and understood. Obtain special instructions before use. Wash hands and other exposed areas with mild soap and water before eating, drinking or smoking and when leaving work. Provide good ventilation in process area to prevent formation of vapor. Report all Mercury releases promptly. Open container slowly on a stable surface. Drums, flasks and bottles of this product must be properly labeled. Empty containers may contain residual amounts of Mercury and should be handled with care.
Hygiene measures	: Do not eat, drink or smoke when using this product. Always wash hands and face immediately after handling this product, and once again before leaving the workplace. Remove contaminated clothing immediately.

7.2. Conditions for safe storage, including any incompatibilities

Technical measures	: Follow practice indicated in Section 6. Make certain that application equipment is locked and tagged-out safely. Always use this product in areas where adequate ventilation is provided. Decontaminate equipment thoroughly before maintenance begins.
Storage conditions	: Keep container tightly closed. Store drums, flasks and bottles in a cool, dry location, away from direct sunlight, source of intense heat, or where freezing is possible. Store away from incompatible materials. Material should be stored in secondary container or in a diked area, as appropriate.
Incompatible materials	: Acetylene and acetylene derivatives, amines, ammonia, 3-bromopropyne, boron diiodophosphide, methyl azide, sodium carbide, heated sulfuric acid, methylsilane/oxygen mixtures, nitric acid/alcohol mixtures, tetracarbonylnickel/oxygen mixtures, alkyne/silver perchlorate mixtures, halogens and strong oxidizers. Mercury can attack copper alloys. Mercury can react with many metals (i.e. calcium, lithium, potassium, sodium, rubidium, aluminum) to form amalgams.
Prohibitions on mixed storage	: Mercury can attack copper alloys. Mercury can react with many metals (i.e. calcium, lithium, potassium, sodium, rubidium, aluminum) to form amalgams.
Storage area	: Storage area should be made of fire-resistant materials.
Special rules on packaging	: Inspect all incoming containers before storage to ensure containers are properly labeled and not damaged.

7.3. Specific end use(s)

No additional information available

SECTION 8: Exposure controls/personal protection

8.1. Control parameters

Mercury (7439-97-6)		
USA ACGIH	ACGIH TWA (mg/m³)	0,025 mg/m³
USA OSHA	OSHA PEL (Ceiling) (mg/m³)	0,1 mg/m³

8.2. Exposure controls

Appropriate engineering controls	: Ensure adequate ventilation. Ensure exposure is below occupational exposure limits (where available). Emergency eye wash fountains and safety showers should be available in the immediate vicinity of any potential exposure.
Personal protective equipment	: Avoid all unnecessary exposure. Gloves. Protective clothing. Safety glasses. Mist formation: aerosol mask.

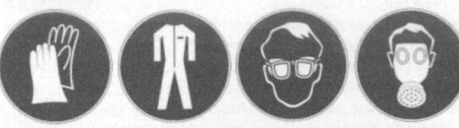

Hand protection	: Wear neoprene gloves for routine industrial use. Use triple gloves for spill response, as stated in Section 6 of this SDS.
Eye protection	: Splash goggles or safety glasses. For operation involving the use of more than 1 pound of Mercury, or if the operation may generate a spray of Mercury, the use of a faceshield is recommended.
Skin and body protection	: Wear suitable protective clothing.
Respiratory protection	: Maintain airborne contaminants concentration below provided exposure limits. If respiratory protection is needed, use only protection authorized in 29 CFR 1910.134 or applicable state regulations. Use supplied air respiration protection if oxygen levels are below 19.5% or are unknown.
Other information	: Do not eat, drink or smoke during use.

SECTION 9: Physical and chemical properties

9.1. Information on basic physical and chemical properties

Physical state	: Liquid
Colour	: Silver white.

FIGURE 12-7
Sample SDS.

MERCURY
Safety Data Sheet
according to the federal final rule of hazard communication revised on 2012 (HazCom 2012)

Odor	: Odorless.
Odor threshold	: Not applicable
pH	: Not applicable
Relative evaporation rate (butylacetate=1)	: No data available
Melting point	: No data available
Freezing point	: -38,87 °C (-37.97 F)
Boiling point	: No data available
Flash point	: Not applicable
Self ignition temperature	: Not applicable
Decomposition temperature	: No data available
Flammability (solid, gas)	: No data available
Vapour pressure	: 0,002 mm Hg at 25°C
Relative vapor density at 20 °C	: 6,9 (Air = 1)
Relative density	: No data available
Relative density of saturated gas/air mixture	: 13,6
Solubility	: No data available
Log Pow	: No data available
Log Kow	: No data available
Viscosity, kinematic	: No data available
Viscosity, dynamic	: No data available
Explosive properties	: No data available
Oxidizing properties	: No data available
Explosive limits	: Not applicable

9.2.   Other information

No additional information available

SECTION 10: Stability and reactivity

10.1.   Reactivity

Stable. Reacts with (some) metals. Mercury can react with metals to form amalgams.

10.2.   Chemical stability

Not established.

10.3.   Possibility of hazardous reactions

Not established. Hazardous polymerization will not occur.

10.4.   Conditions to avoid

Direct sunlight. Extremely high or low temperatures.

10.5.   Incompatible materials

Acetylene and acetylene derivatives, amines, ammonia, 3-bromopropyne, boron diiodophosphide, methyl azide, sodium carbide, heated sulfuric acid, methylsilane/oxygen mixtures, nitric acid/alcohol mixtures, tetracarbonylnickel/oxygen mixtures, alkyne/silver perchlorate mixtures, halogens and strong oxidizers. Mercury can attack copper alloys. Mercury can react with many metals (i.e. calcium, lithium, potassium, sodium, rubidium, aluminum) to form amalgams.

10.6.   Hazardous decomposition products

If this product is exposed to extremely high temperature in the presence of oxygen or air, toxic vapor of mercury and mercury oxides will be generated.

SECTION 11: Toxicological information

11.1.   Information on toxicological effects

Acute toxicity	: Fatal if inhaled.
Skin corrosion/irritation	: Not classified
	pH: Not applicable
Serious eye damage/irritation	: Not classified
	pH: Not applicable
Respiratory or skin sensitisation	: Not classified
Germ cell mutagenicity	: Not classified
	Based on available data, the classification criteria are not met
Carcinogenicity	: Not classified

FIGURE 12-7

Sample SDS.

(Continued)
MERCURY
Safety Data Sheet
according to the federal final rule of hazard communication revised on 2012 (HazCom 2012)

Mercury (7439-97-6)	
IARC group	3

Reproductive toxicity	: May damage fertility or the unborn child.
	Based on available data, the classification criteria are not met
Specific target organ toxicity (single exposure)	: Not classified
Specific target organ toxicity (repeated exposure)	: Causes damage to organs through prolonged or repeated exposure.
	Based on available data, the classification criteria are not met
	Causes damage to organs through prolonged or repeated exposure
Aspiration hazard	: Not classified
	Based on available data, the classification criteria are not met
Potential adverse human health effects and symptoms	: Based on available data, the classification criteria are not met. Fatal if inhaled.
Symptoms/injuries after inhalation	: Short-term over-exposures to high concentrations of mercury vapors can lead to breathing difficulty, coughing, acute,chemical pneumonia, and pulmonary edema (a potentially fatal accumulation of fluid in the lungs) . Depending on the concentration of over-exposure, cardiac abnormalities, damage to the kidney, liver or nerves and effects on the brain may occur. Long-term inhalation over-exposures can lead to the development of a wide variety of symptoms, including the following: excessive salivation, gingivitis, anorexia, chills, fever, cardiac abnormalities, anemia, digestive problems, abdominal pains, frequent urination, an inability to urinate, diarrhea, peripheral neuropathy (numbness, weakness, or burning sensations in the hands or feet), tremors (especially in the hands, fingers, eyelids, lips, cheeks, tongue, or legs), alteration of tendon reflexes, slurred speech, visual disturbances, and deafness. Allergic reactions (i.e. breathing difficulty) may also occur in sensitive individuals.
Symptoms/injuries after skin contact	: Symptoms of skin exposure can include redness, dry skin, and pain. Prolonged contact may lead to ulceration of the skin. Allergic reactions (i.e. rashes, welts) may occur in sensitive individuals. Dermatitis (redness and inflammation of the skin) may occur after repeated skin exposures.
Symptoms/injuries after eye contact	: Symptoms of eye exposure can include redness, pain, and watery eyes. A symptom of Mercury exposure is discoloration of the lens of the eyes.
Symptoms/injuries after ingestion	: If Mercury is swallowed, symptoms of such over-exposure can include metallic taste in mouth, nausea, vomiting, central nervous system effects, and damage to the kidneys. Metallic mercury is not usually absorbed sufficiently from the gastrointestinal tract to induce an acute, toxic response. Damage to the tissues of the mouth, throat, esophagus, and other tissues of the digestive system may occur. Ingestion may be fatal, due to effects on gastrointestinal system and kidneys.
Chronic symptoms	: Long-term over-exposure can lead to a wide range of adverse health effects. Anyone using Mercury must pay attention to personality changes, weight loss, skin or gum discolorations, stomach pains, and other signs of Mercury over-exposure. Gradually developing syndromes ("Erethism" and "Acrodynia") are indicative of potentially severe health problems. Mercury can cause the development of allergic reactions (i.e. dermatitis, rashes, breathing difficulty) upon prolonged or repeated exposures. Refer to Section 11 (Toxicology Information) for additional data.

SECTION 12: Ecological information

12.1.   Toxicity

Ecology - water	: Very toxic to aquatic life. Toxic to aquatic life with long lasting effects.

Mercury (7439-97-6)	
LC50 fishes 1	0,5 mg/l (Exposure time: 96 h - Species: Cyprinus carpio)
EC50 Daphnia 1	5,0 µg/l (Exposure time: 96 h - Species: water flea)
LC50 fish 2	0,16 mg/l (Exposure time: 96 h - Species: Cyprinus carpio [semi-static])

12.2.   Persistence and degradability

MERCURY (7439-97-6)	
Persistence and degradability	May cause long-term adverse effects in the environment.

12.3.   Bioaccumulative potential

MERCURY (7439-97-6)	
Bioaccumulative potential	Not established.

12.4.   Mobility in soil
No additional information available

12.5.   Other adverse effects

Other information	: Avoid release to the environment.

FIGURE 12-7
Sample SDS.

MERCURY
Safety Data Sheet
according to the federal final rule of hazard communication revised on 2012 (HazCom 2012)

SECTION 13: Disposal considerations

13.1.   Waste treatment methods

Waste disposal recommendations	: Dispose in a safe manner in accordance with local/national regulations. Waste disposal must be in accordance with appropriate federal, state, and local regulations. This product, if unaltered by use, should be recycled. If altered by use, recycling may be possible. Consult Bethlehem Apparatus Company for information. If Mercury must be disposed of as hazardous waste, it must be handled at a permitted facility or as advised by your local hazardous waste regulatory authority.
Ecology - waste materials	: Hazardous waste due to toxicity. Avoid release to the environment.

SECTION 14: Transport information

In accordance with DOT

14.1.   UN number

UN-No.(DOT)	: 2809
DOT NA no.	UN2809

14.2.   UN proper shipping name

DOT Proper Shipping Name	: Mercury
Department of Transportation (DOT) Hazard Classes	: 8 - Class 8 - Corrosive material 49 CFR 173.136
Hazard labels (DOT)	: 8 - Corrosive substances 6.1 - Toxic substances

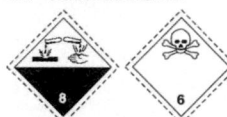

DOT Symbols	: A - Material is regulated as a hazardous material only when be transported by air, W - Material is regulated as a hazardous material only when be transported by water
Packing group (DOT)	: III - Minor Danger
DOT Packaging Exceptions (49 CFR 173.xxx)	: 164
DOT Packaging Non Bulk (49 CFR 173.xxx)	: 164
DOT Packaging Bulk (49 CFR 173.xxx)	: 240

14.3.   Additional information

Other information	: No supplementary information available.

Overland transport

No additional information available

Transport by sea

DOT Vessel Stowage Location	: B - (i) The material may be stowed "on deck" or "under deck" on a cargo vessel and on a passenger vessel carrying a number of passengers limited to not more than the larger of 25 passengers, or one passenger per each 3 m of overall vessel length; and (ii) "On deck only" on passenger vessels in which the number of passengers specified in paragraph (k)(2)(i) of this section is exceeded.
DOT Vessel Stowage Other	: 40 - Stow "clear of living quarters",97 - Stow "away from" azides

Air transport

DOT Quantity Limitations Passenger aircraft/rail (49 CFR 173.27)	: 35 kg
DOT Quantity Limitations Cargo aircraft only (49 CFR 175.75)	: 35 kg

SECTION 15: Regulatory information

15.1. US Federal regulations

Mercury (7439-97-6)	
Listed on the United States TSCA (Toxic Substances Control Act) inventory Listed on SARA Section 313 (Specific toxic chemical listings)	
EPA TSCA Regulatory Flag	S - S - indicates a substance that is identified in a proposed or final Significant New Uses Rule.
SARA Section 313 - Emission Reporting	1,0 %

15.2. International regulations

CANADA

FIGURE 12-7
Sample SDS.

(Continues)

(Continued)

MERCURY
Safety Data Sheet
according to the federal final rule of hazard communication revised on 2012 (HazCom 2012)

Mercury (7439-97-6)	
Listed on the Canadian DSL (Domestic Sustances List) inventory.	
WHMIS Classification	Class D Division 1 Subdivision A - Very toxic material causing immediate and serious toxic effects Class D Division 2 Subdivision A - Very toxic material causing other toxic effects Class E - Corrosive Material

EU-Regulations

Mercury (7439-97-6)
Listed on the EEC inventory EINECS (European Inventory of Existing Commercial Chemical Substances) substances.

Classification according to Regulation (EC) No. 1272/2008 [CLP]

Classification according to Directive 67/548/EEC or 1999/45/EC

Not classified

15.2.2.   National regulations

Mercury (7439-97-6)
Listed on the AICS (the Australian Inventory of Chemical Substances) Listed on Inventory of Existing Chemical Substances (IECSC) Listed on the Korean ECL (Existing Chemical List) inventory. Listed on New Zealand - Inventory of Chemicals (NZIoC) Listed on Inventory of Chemicals and Chemical Substances (PICCS) Poisonous and Deleterious Substances Control Law Pollutant Release and Transfer Register Law (PRTR Law) Listed on the Canadian Ingredient Disclosure List

15.3. US State regulations

Mercury (7439-97-6)				
U.S. - California - Proposition 65 - Carcinogens List	U.S. - California - Proposition 65 - Developmental Toxicity	U.S. - California - Proposition 65 - Reproductive Toxicity - Female	U.S. - California - Proposition 65 - Reproductive Toxicity - Male	No significance risk level (NSRL)
	Yes			

SECTION 16: Other information

Other information   : None.

Full text of H-phrases: see section 16:

Acute Tox. 1 (Inhalation:dust,mist)	Acute toxicity (inhalation:dust,mist) Category 1
Acute Tox. 2 (Inhalation)	Acute toxicity (inhalation) Category 2
Aquatic Acute 1	Hazardous to the aquatic environment — AcuteHazard, Category 1
Aquatic Chronic 1	Hazardous to the aquatic environment — Chronic Hazard, Category 1
Repr. 1B	Reproductive toxicity Category 1B
STOT RE 1	Specific target organ toxicity (repeated exposure) Category 1
H330	Fatal if inhaled
H360	May damage fertility or the unborn child
H372	Causes damage to organs through prolonged or repeated exposure
H400	Very toxic to aquatic life
H410	Very toxic to aquatic life with long lasting effects

NFPA health hazard   : 3 - Short exposure could cause serious temporary or
                               residual injury even though prompt medical attention was
                               given.

NFPA fire hazard   : 0 - Materials that will not burn.

NFPA reactivity   : 0 - Normally stable, even under fire exposure conditions,
                               and are not reactive with water.

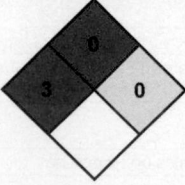

SDS US (GHS HazCom 2012)

This information is based on our current knowledge and is intended to describe the product for the purposes of health, safety and environmental requirements only. It should not therefore be construed as guaranteeing any specific property of the product

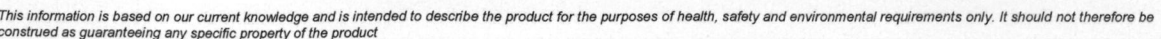

FIGURE 12-7
Sample SDS.

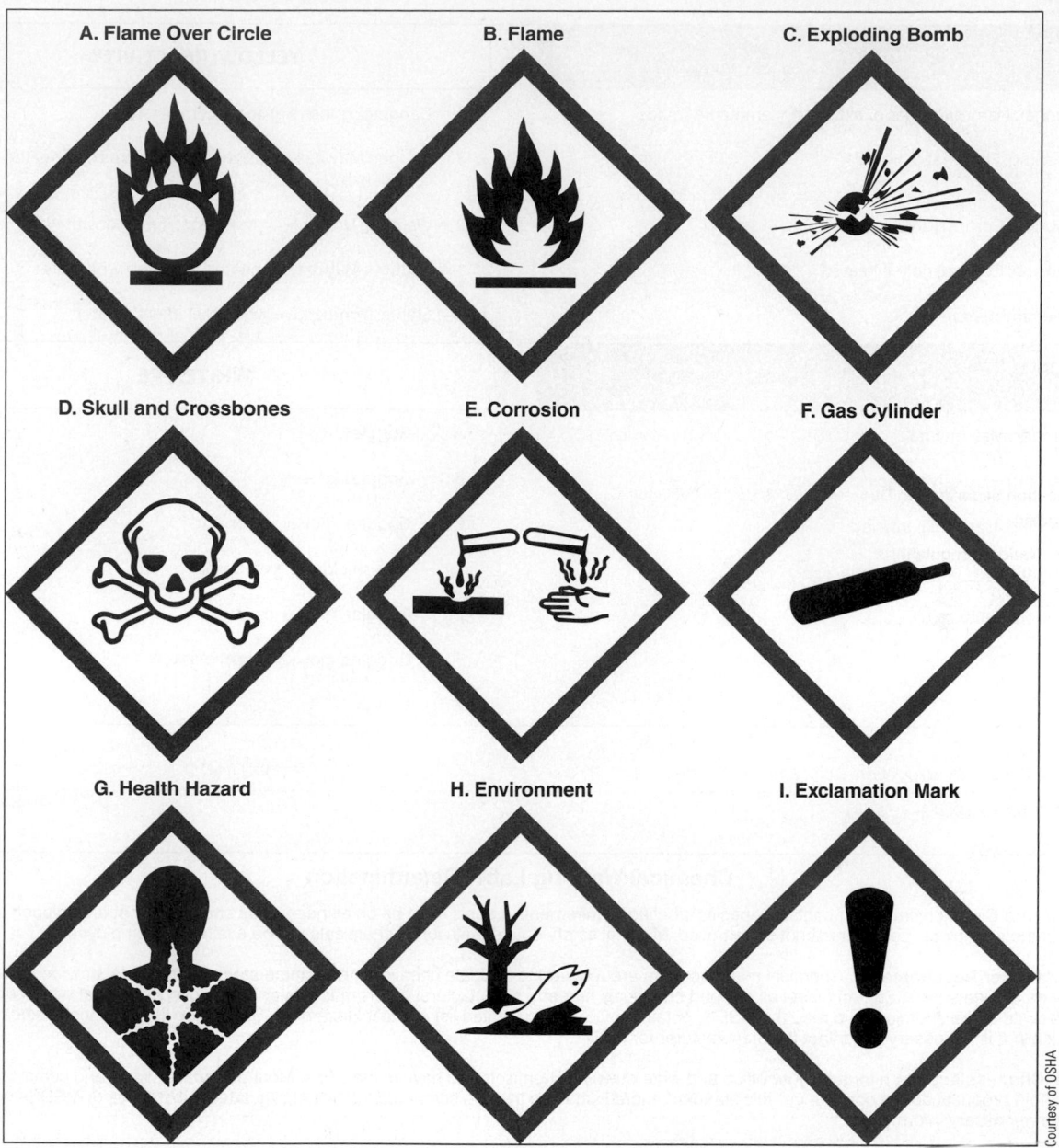

FIGURE 12-8
Hazard communication pictogram.

Courtesy of OSHA

incidences in the recent months that require new safety measures? Does the chemical spill kit or the emergency kit need new items? Keeping "on top" of the hazardous program will reduce potential health or accident risks. If appropriate, the facilitator may choose to conduct a mock chemical exposure scenario to make certain that all employees are aware of how to respond and treat hazardous situations. Regardless of how the maintenance program is organized, policies and relevant procedures must be included in the written program for reference and review. Taking the time to write, plan, implement, evaluate, and maintain the office hazardous communication program will ensure a safer environment for both the employees and the patients!

Evacuation Plans and Fire Extinguishers

All hazardous programs need to include evacuation plans that provide safe and accessible building exits in case of a fire or other emergency. The basic requirements include exit routes based on the number of employees in the office and a diagram of the evacuation routes posted in a visible location. The officer can obtain help in developing an evacuation plan through OSHA consultation services, office insurance company, or local fire or police service.

RED: FIRE HAZARD	YELLOW: REACTIVITY
4 = Danger: Flammable gas or extremely flammable liquids	4 = Danger: Explosive at room temperature
3 = Warning: Flammable liquid	3 = Danger: May be explosive if spark occurs or if heated under confinement
2 = Caution: Combustible liquid	2 = Warning: Unstable or may react if mixed with water
1 = Caution: Combustible if heated	1 = Caution: May react if heated or mixed with water
0 = Noncombustible	0 = Stable: Nonreactive when mixed with water

BLUE: HEALTH HAZARD	WHITE: PPE	
4 = Danger: May be fatal	A	Goggles
3 = Warning: Corrosive or toxic	B	Goggles, gloves
2 = Warning: Harmful if inhaled	C	Goggles, gloves, apron
1 = Caution: May cause irritation	D	Face shields, gloves, apron
0 = No unusual hazard	E	Goggles, gloves, mask
	F	Goggles, gloves, apron, mask
	X	Gloves

Courtesy of POL Consultants

FIGURE 12-9
National Fire Protection Association's color and number method.

Chemical Warning Label Determination

The Hazard Communication Act contains specific labeling requirements. Labels must be on all hazardous chemicals that are shipped to and used in the workplace. Labels must not be removed. Material safety data sheets for all chemicals will be available to employees.

Manufacturer Requirements: Chemical manufacturers are required to evaluate chemicals, determine status as hazards, provide material safety data sheets (MSDSs), and label all shipped chemicals properly. Manufacturer labels must never be removed. The best way to determine the hazards of the chemical is to read the MSDS, obtain an OSHA designated list or State Hazardous Substance list. For most mixed chemicals, it is necessary to contact the manufacturer for MSDS.

Office Chemicals: Search through your office and write down all chemicals you have in the office. Most pharmaceuticals and common household products do not come under this standard. Ingredients can then be compared to a list of regulated substances or MSDSs will provide necessary information.

Employer's Responsibility: Any hazardous chemical used in the workplace that is not in its original container **must** be labeled with the identity of the chemical and hazards. "Target Organ" chemical labels may be used. The label must include the chemical and common name, warnings about physical and health hazards, and the name and address of the manufacturer. The employer is to compile a chemical inventory list that is to be updated as needed. MSDS information should be located in a place where it is accessible to all employees. Label and MSDS information should be provided during the safety training program.

Identity: The term *identity* can refer to any chemical or common name designation for the individual chemical or mixture, as long as the term used is also used on the list of hazardous chemicals and the MSDS.

Note: If a chemical is poured into another container for immediate use, it does not need to be labeled.

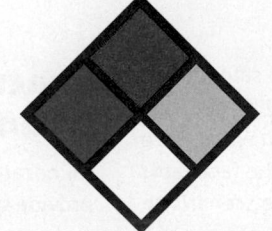

Chemical name

Common name

Manufacturer

Courtesy of POL Consultants

FIGURE 12-10
A chemical warning label.

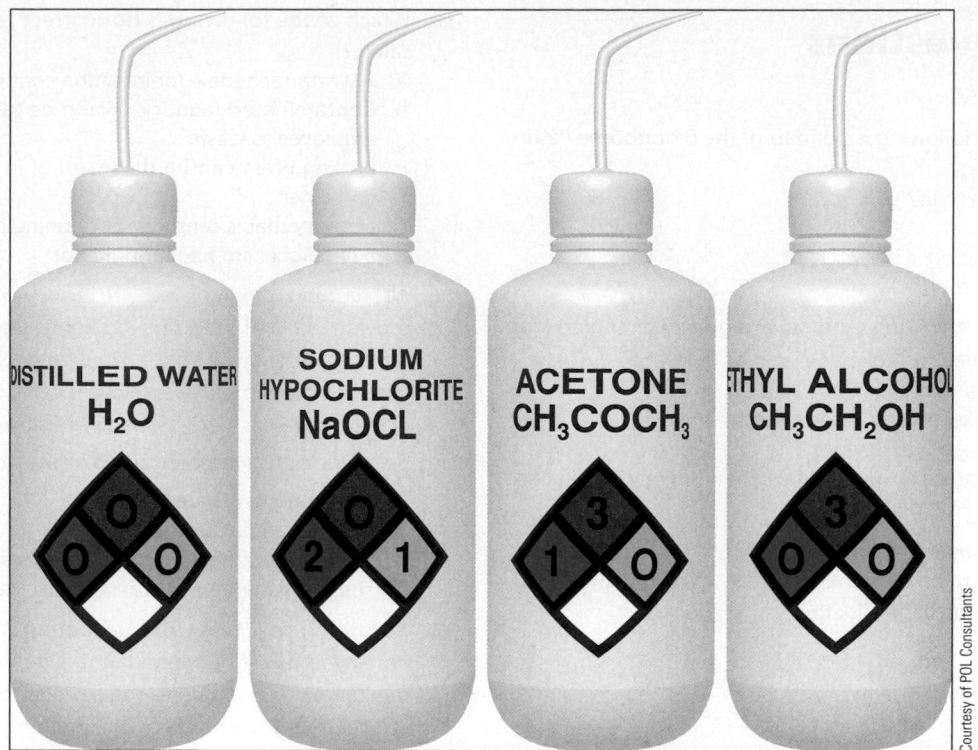

FIGURE 12-11
Containers with chemical warning labels.

The plan must also include mounted fire extinguishers rated not less than 2A that are readily accessible to employees without subjecting them to injury. The nearest fire extinguisher should not exceed 100 feet from treatment areas and should be included on the evacuation plan. A record must be kept of the inspection, maintenance, and testing for extinguishers.

Chapter Summary

OSHA regulations, including the hazard communication standard, are intended to require the employer to provide a safe work environment for all employees. The dental assistant must completely understand the entirety of the standard and how compliance is accomplished. Staff must be trained for a safe workplace. Compliance with all standards must be accomplished to ensure a safe workplace.

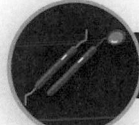 **CASE STUDY**

Rebecca Thomas, a 25-year-old, is a newly hired employee in the office of Dr. Charles. She is working as a chairside dental assistant. She will be completing her first month of employment. A fellow employee is discussing a case with Rebecca and accidentally knocks over a glass container. It breaks into several pieces. Rebecca received a cut on her finger from the broken glass and needed stitches.

Case Study Review

1. What training should Rebecca have completed?

2. What records of the incident must be kept by Rebecca's employer? For how long must they be kept?

3. What must be used to clean up the broken glass?

4. Where should the pieces of broken glass be disposed?

Review Questions

Multiple Choice

1. Which of the following is not part of the Bloodborne Pathogens Standard?
   a. employee training
   b. laundry
   c. housekeeping
   d. employment hours

2. Which of the following is not an example(s) of engineering or work practice controls?
   a. personal protective equipment
   b. splash guards on model trimmers
   c. needle recapping devices
   d. All of these are examples of engineering or work practice controls.

3. After an exposure incident, the employer provides a copy of the health care professional's written opinion within _____ days of a completed evaluation.
   a. 5
   b. 10
   c. 15
   d. 30

4. The color and number method often used to identify various chemicals was developed by the _____.
   a. Occupational Safety and Health Administration
   b. American Dental Association
   c. Environmental Protection Agency
   d. National Fire Protection Association

5. What does a skull and crossbone pictogram indicate?
   a. a health hazard
   b. acute toxicity or fatal
   c. corrosion
   d. PPE is needed

6. Where should pieces of broken glass be placed for disposal after clean up?
   a. a plastic bag
   b. a leak-proof sharps container
   c. a cardboard container
   d. a garbage container

7. Yellow on the chemical warning label determination identifies:
   a. a fire hazard.
   b. a health hazard.
   c. PPE is needed.
   d. the reactivity or stability of a chemical.

8. The OSHA hazard communication standard is set up so that the _____ receives training about the risks of using hazardous chemicals and the safety precautions.
   a. employee
   b. employer
   c. patient
   d. Both a and b

9. Which of the following is an accepted work practice control?
   a. two-handed recapping
   b. scoop method of recapping
   c. picking up large pieces of glass with gloved hands
   d. handwashing following glove removal

10. Which of the following is not correct regarding work site safety?
    a. A written schedule for infection control is not required.
    b. Contaminated laundry should be taken home by each employee to wash.
    c. Broken glass can be disposed of in the regular waste container.
    d. Laundry that is sent out for cleaning should be placed in a red biohazard bag for transport.

11. All hazardous programs need to include evacuation plans that provide safe and accessible building exits in case of a fire or other emergency. The basic requirements include exit routes based on the number of employees in the office and a diagram of the evacuation routes posted in a visible location.

    Select the correct response based on the statements above.

    a. Both statements are true.
    b. Both statements are false.
    c. The first statement is true; the first statement is false.
    d. The first statement is false; the first statement is true.

12. According to OSHA's Hazard Communication Standard, employees must be trained in the identification of hazardous chemicals and the personal protective equipment to be utilized for each chemical. This training must occur within 30 days of employment or prior to the employee using any chemicals, and every 2 years thereafter.

    Select the correct response based on the statements above.

    a. Both statements are true.
    b. Both statements are false.
    c. The first statement is true; the first statement is false.
    d. The first statement is false; the first statement is true.

13. Which of the following is not correct regarding the Safety Data Sheet (SDS) manual?
    a. The manual must be digital.
    b. The SDS in the manual must be from the manufacturer.
    c. The SDS forms in the must include all 16 sections.
    d. All of these are correct.

14. What does an exclamation mark pictogram indicate?
    a. a health hazard
    b. acute toxicity or fatal
    c. corrosion
    d. irritation

15. The 2012 revision of the Hazardous Communication Standard included the adoption of the *Globally Harmonized System of Classification and Labeling of Chemicals (GHS)*. This means that chemicals and materials are classified and labeled differently based on where the chemicals are manufactured, sold, or used.

    Select the correct response based on the statements above.

    a. Both statements are true.
    b. Both statements are false.
    c. The first statement is true; the first statement is false.
    d. The first statement is false; the first statement is true.

16. What does the skull and crossbone pictogram indicate?
    a. a health hazard
    b. acute toxicity or fatal
    c. corrosion
    d. irritation

17. What does the gas cylinder pictogram indicate?
    a. a health hazard
    b. acute toxicity or fatal
    c. corrosion
    d. gas under pressure

18. Which of the following is not correct regarding fire extinguishers?
    a. Fire extinguishers do not need to be mounted.
    b. The nearest fire extinguisher should be 150 feet away from the treatment area.
    c. It is not necessary to keep a record of fire inspection maintenance and testing.
    d. The fire extinguisher should not be rated less than 2A.

19. The Needlestick Safety and Prevention Act directed OSHA to revise the Bloodborne Pathogens Standard. This revision was based on the low number of percutaneous injuries that affected health care workers each year.

    Select the correct response based on the statements above.

    a. Both statements are true.
    b. Both statements are false.
    c. The first statement is true; the first statement is false.
    d. The first statement is false; the first statement is true.

20. You are working in a dental office and experience a sharps injury. Which of the following is correct?
    a. The exposure incident does not need to be documented by your employer.
    b. Your employer is not required to provide you with the source patient's blood test results if available.
    c. As an employee, you have the right to deny blood testing up to 90 days after exposure.
    d. If you do choose to get tested, you would be responsible for all test related expenses.

Critical Thinking

1. Would the scope of the OSHA Bloodborne and Hazardous Materials Standard cover the employee while traveling to the place of employment?

2. Employees have a lunchroom that becomes untidy and disorderly. The dentist never uses the lunchroom. If one of the employees has an accident in the room, who is responsible?

3. Standard precautions are issued by whom? To protect whom?

## CHAPTER 13

The Special Needs and Medically Compromised Patient

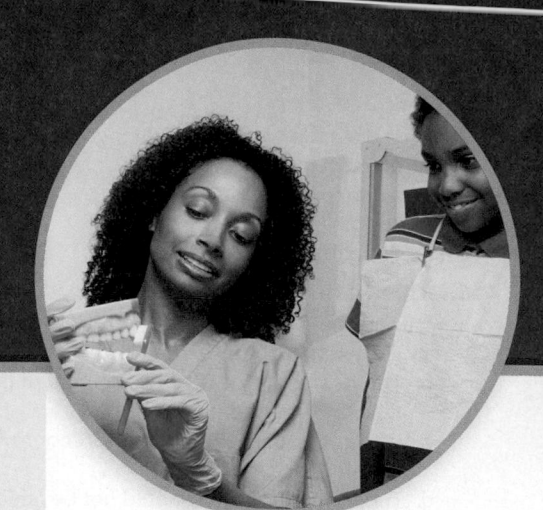

Specific Instructional Objectives

At the completion of this chapter, you will be able to meet these objectives:

1. Use terms presented in this chapter.
2. Differentiate between developmental and acquired disabilities.
3. Define special needs, the Americans with Disability Act (ADA) and a barrier free environment.
4. Summarize the special care for the patient with disabilities.
5. Describe one and two person wheelchair transfers.
6. Discuss dental management of the patient with a sensory disability.
7. Describe potential behavior of a patient with intellectual and developmental disabilities.
8. Describe oral findings of a patient with intellectual and developmental disabilities.
9. Discuss the effects of aging and dental management of the older patient.
10. Describe the cause, characteristics of disorders and diseases that define a patient who is medically compromised.
11. Describe the dental management of disorders and diseases that define a patient who is medically compromised.

Introduction

Many individuals with disabilities and who are medically compromised are living longer due to advances in medical treatment, and most reside in communities. This has increased the likelihood that they will be treated in a dental office setting. Patients with special needs and those who are medically compromised require special consideration when receiving dental treatment. Caring for these patients takes compassion, understanding, knowledge of their condition, recognition of the unique qualities of each patient, and knowing how to meet their needs. This chapter presents the more common types of patients with special needs and diseases that compromise the patient's health.

The Patient with Special Needs

Every patient is an individual with their own set of values and beliefs. Characteristics that make each patient special are gender, age, race, culture, language, economic status, and past dental experiences; all of these factors influence dental care. There are also patients who have a medical, physical, or mental disability that requires adaptations to dental care beyond routine. For some people special modifications are needed only at certain periods of life and not at others. Some individuals with severe medical or movement problems may need to be treated in a hospital, but those with a mild or moderate disability can be treated in a private practice.

Developmental disabilities occur during the period when most body systems of a child are developing before birth, at birth, or before the age of 22 years. Developmental disabilities usually last a lifetime. Those with this type of disability often have several **impairments** and may have limitations in learning, communicating, and living independently. Cerebral palsy and intellectual disability are examples of developmental disabilities. Acquired disabilities are the result of disease, trauma, or injury to the body and include spinal cord paralysis, limb amputation, and arthritis. Both categories of disabilities may require the aid of a caregiver. When providing dental care for individuals with disabilities we are treating "patients with special needs."

With greater numbers of people with disabilities residing in the community—54 million in the United States—the dental office will encounter such patients seeking care; the dental team must be knowledgeable and capable in order to handle treatment and dental management. The main objectives of care are to maintain oral health, prevent infection and tooth loss, and prevent the need for extensive treatment, which the patient may not be able to **tolerate** due to their physical or mental condition. By providing needed care the dental team can contribute to the oral health, overall wellness, and personal self-esteem of a patient with a disability.

The Americans with Disabilities Act

The Americans with Disabilities Act of 1992 prohibits discrimination against a person with a disability who is seeking access to services, including dental services. Some conditions that may allow one to qualify as disabled are orthopedic, visual, speech, and hearing impairments; cerebral palsy; muscular dystrophy; multiple sclerosis; intellectual disability; and specific learning disabilities. A person also may have a less obvious impairment such as epilepsy, cancer, heart disease, diabetes, emotional illness, drug addiction, or alcoholism.

A Barrier Free Environment The ADA sets standards and building codes for new construction to create "barrier free" environments that make the office space and services usable by everyone; the laws may vary by state, city, or county. The design code for most new buildings is usually "barrier free"

Barrier Free Facility

- Clearly marked designated wide parking spaces close to the building.
- Accessible front entrance with ramp and curb cut at appropriate grades and surfaces.
- Interior and exterior doors that are wide and easy to open.
- Wide corridors to allow a 360-degree turn in a wheelchair without bumping into the wall.
- Clear floor space with nonskid surfaces.
- Signs posted no higher than 5 foot from the floor.
- Elevators in buildings with 2 or more floors.
- Raised letters or Braille on elevator control buttons.

both inside and outside. According to Title 3 of the law, dental offices are required to make modifications to an existing building to allow access by persons with disabilities. Some simple changes to the office include a portable ramp at the entrance of the building, adding handrails to hallways and grab bars in restrooms, using lever type doorknobs, reception area with various chair heights and space for a wheelchair, magazine racks that are reachable, nonskid floor coverings, and eliminating hanging plants and area rugs.

General Treatment Considerations

A **holistic** view of oral health is required in order to provide a tailored care plan to meet the needs of each individual patient. For the special needs patient, communication with the entire health care team, family, caregiver, physician, social services, and dental team is essential.

Assessment, Planning, and Scheduling

Most patients with a disability or their caregivers will be prepared to discuss treatment issues when they first contact the office to schedule an appointment. An accurate and current health history is vital. Depending on the disability or medical condition, a consultation with the patient's physician, counselor, and other members of the **rehabilitation** team may be necessary to ensure treatment is safe and effective. Persons with disabilities may need more time to dress and prepare for the visit, so a mid-morning appointment may be best when the wait time is minimal and the patient and the staff is at their best. Pretreatment planning helps to determine what preparation is needed before the appointment, saves valuable time better spent caring for the patient, and makes the experience successful and positive for everyone. Table 13-1 outlines issues and questions that will help gather information for appointment scheduling, pretreatment planning and patient care.

Patient Care Modification

Dental care for the disabled patient usually requires additional staff members and treatment time and should be scheduled accordingly. Mobility and neuromuscular problems, mental capabilities, behavior problems, physical stamina, and sitting tolerance may require shorter chair time and minimal treatment per appointment.

Individuals with special needs may benefit from methods that help **desensitize** them to dental treatment. Strategies include:

- Practice oral manipulation with a daily tooth brushing routine at home; instruct caregivers in proper technique to avoid any injury (Figure 13-1).
- Reduce anxiety with strangers and unfamiliar environments— visit the dental office before care begins during times other than routine office hours.
- Observe a family member receiving care—the patient may mimic desirable behavior.

TABLE 13-1 Pretreatment Planning

Nature of the disability	Is physician consultation necessary? Assess mental ability, muscular coordination, dexterity, grip strength, sitting tolerance, involuntary movements. What do you need for the appointment (mouth prop, restraint, special oral hygiene aids, someone to help with the appointment)? Do you need to refresh your memory of special or modified radiographic techniques?
Degree of the patient's independence	Will someone accompany the patient to the appointment? Is the patient able to give consent to treatment? Is there a caregiver or guardian and if so are they legally appointed?
Dental history	Patient and/or caregiver attitude History of oral infection and oral habits Most recent care: procedures, fluoride therapy, success during treatment Current home care methods, degree of self-care
Social history	Patient attitude toward dentistry Cultural values and beliefs Can the patient shop for and prepare food?
Communication ability Hearing or vision loss	Does the patient speak English? Is there a need for an interpreter? Do you need writing materials to communicate? Is there a service guide dog?
Transportation	Does the patient come by themselves? Is the patient dependent on others for a ride? Does the patient rely on the schedule of public transportation?
Appointment time	When is the best time for the appointment? Dressing for the appointment Medicine and meal schedule Don't let the patient wait. Allow adequate time for the appointment.

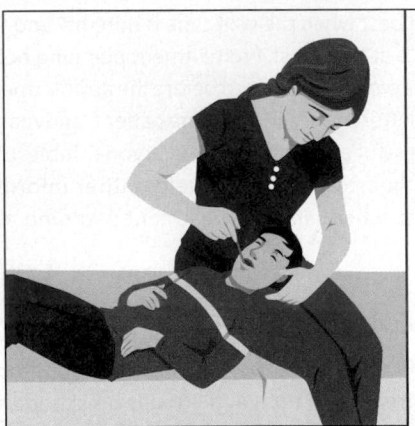
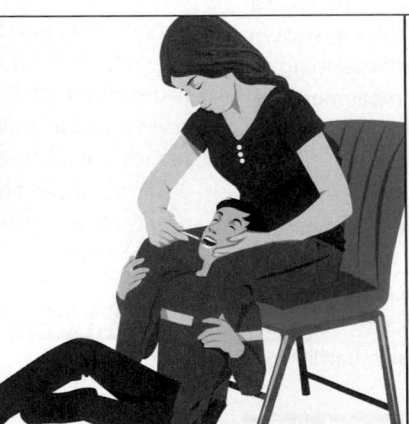
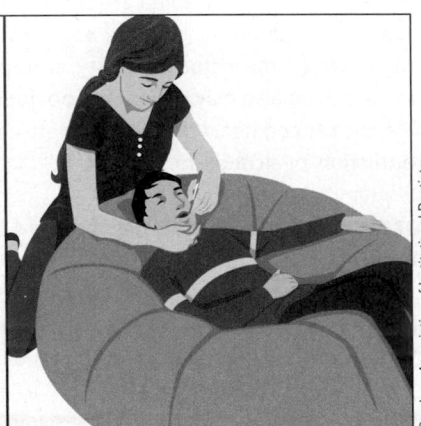

Patient's head in caregiver's lap   Patient sitting on the floor   Use of beanbag chair

Courtesy of Southern Association of Institutional Dentists

FIGURE 13-1
Head stabilizations.

- Treatment visits:

  First visit— the patient can sit quietly in the chair with a family member or caregiver nearby to offer reassurance; their teeth can be gently brushed.

  Second visit—follow the same routine, and if the patient remains relaxed, a minor dental procedure (cleaning, simple restoration) can be performed. If this process is successful, more complex treatment may be gradually added.

Monitor the patient's behavior during each visit.

- If the patient becomes uncooperative, the appointment should be terminated.
- If a restoration has been started and treatment must end, place a temporary filling.
- If these methods are not successful, dental procedures may have to be completed using sedation or protective stabilization.

Protective Body Stabilization

Disabled patients frequently have problems with support, balance, and even aggressive behavior. Sudden involuntary body movements such as muscle spasms can be a danger to the patient and the dental team during treatment. Severe cases could require sedation or general anesthesia, and hospitalization might then be appropriate. In the office, protective body stabilization may be used to make the patient feel comfortable and secure while allowing for safe and effective delivery of quality care. Methods for protective body stabilization include:

● Pillows, rolled blankets, or towels placed under the patient's knees and neck

● A bed sheet wrapped around a patient and secured with tape that can easily be cut if necessary

● A bean bag chair placed on the dental chair that will conform to the patient's body while filling the space between the patient and the dental chair

● Gently holding the patient's arms or legs in a comfortable position to minimize movement

● A child may lie on top of a caregiver in the dental chair, with the cargiver's arms around the child. Monitor this situation carefully because the caregiver can tire and easily lose control of the child during treatment.

● A commercially available full body wrap for patients who have extreme spasticity or severe behavioral problems; this method should not be considered for routine use (Figure 13-2).

Cautions for use of protective body stabilization are:

● Before treatment, obtain informed consent from the patient if they are mentally competent or a legal caregiver.

● Consider the regulations of your state's Dental Practice Act for additional education or a permit.

● Use of the least restrictive but safe and effective method.

● Use around extremities or the chest, must not actively restrict circulation or respiration.

● Procedure must be carefully monitored and terminated if the patient is severely stressed.

● Protective body stabilization should not be considered for those who cannot be immobilized safely due to associated physical or medical conditions such as asthma.

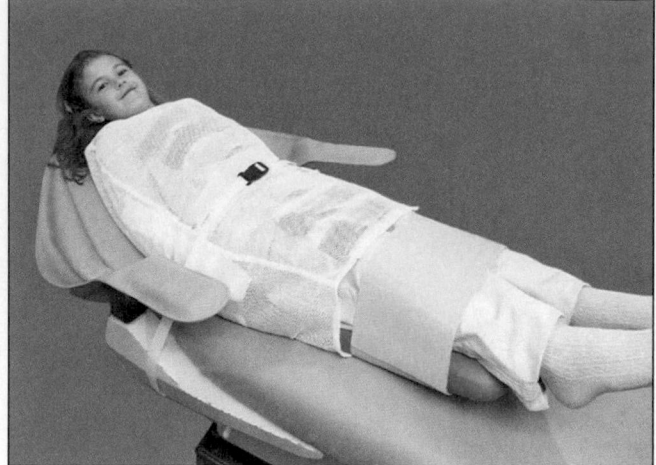

FIGURE 13-2
Protective body stabilization.

Courtesy of Specialized Care Co.

Use of a Mouth Prop

Mouth props may be necessary to provide care because a disabled person may lack ability, or may not want to keep their mouth open (Figure 13-3). Use of a mouth prop not only provides protection from the patient suddenly closing on fingers or instruments but also can improve access and visibility. Training on technique for safe use may be required. A long piece of dental floss should be tied through the hole in a commercially available prop and kept outside the mouth for easy removal in case of a breathing problem.

A custom mouth prop can be made using wooden tongue depressors, waterproof tape, and several pieces of gauze wrapped around one end (Figure 13-4). Use of a folded, moistened washcloth or several gauze squares folded together can also serve to keep the mouth open. Do not use plastic or stainless steel evacuator tips, and be aware of mobile teeth, which can be aspirated. Mouth props can cause fatigue of facial and masticatory muscles and the TMJ.

The Patient Who Uses a Wheelchair

Some patients with disabilities may be dependent on the use of a wheelchair in their everyday life; therefore, it is essential that the dental assistant be knowledgeable in patient transfer from

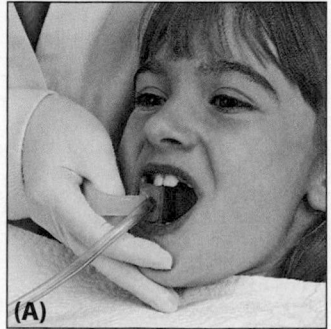 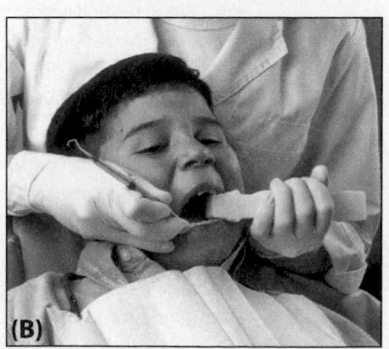

FIGURE 13-3
(A) Open Wide° Mouth Rest. (B) Open Wide° Re-Usable mouth prop.

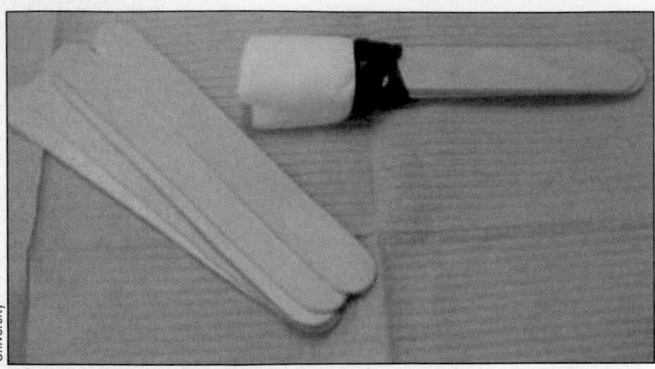

FIGURE 13-4
Custom mouth prop.

the wheelchair to the dental chair without causing injury to themselves or the patient. Some patients may use special padding or cushions to make the wheelchair more comfortable or to prevent their skin from breaking down. Persons who sit for long periods can develop pressure sores called **decubitus ulcers** that can become infected, causing a major health problem. Some persons with disabilities have no balance, coordination, strength, or body posture, and others cannot be safely moved at all. Bowel and bladder elimination schedules should be considered when planning for the appointment. Some patients may wear a gravity-drained device connected to tubing strapped to the inside of their leg, or a bag may be attached to the wheelchair. To avoid a medical emergency, care should be taken to ensure that any tubing remains intact (not bent or twisted) and in the original position required for draining. Ask the patient or caregiver if they are prone to spasms that can be stimulated by any movement or anxiety. Because spasms can be sudden and violent, you should

always be prepared to protect the patient and yourself from injury. Continuous spasms can be reduced by gently massaging the affected area.

Wheelchair Transfer

There are many factors to consider before, during, and after wheelchair transfer. It is important to remember that during the procedure the patient may be entirely dependent on you. Most wheelchair users have spent many hours in a rehabilitation program and physical therapy practicing skills that allow them as much independence as possible, but this may not be the case. Some patients need little or no assistance. Table 13-2 outlines preparation that is necessary before you start.

Ergonomics for Wheelchair Transfer

Remember to practice good **ergonomics** when attempting transfer:

- Position yourself as close to the patient as possible.
- Stand with your feet shoulder width apart to increase support and stability.
- Bend at the hips and knees keeping your back straight.
- Use momentum to lift by gently rocking the patient forward and back.
- Use leg and arm muscles to lift keeping the back straight.
- Avoid twisting your body at the waist; instead, take small steps as you turn or move.

One and two person transfer techniques are described and illustrated in Procedures 13–1 and 13–2.

TABLE 13-2 Assessment Before Wheelchair Transfer

• Plan and know each move before you start. • Explain each step to the patient as well as anyone who is providing help and what their responsibilities will be during the process. • No transfer should be attempted alone; another person should always be aware of a transfer and be available to provide help if needed.	
Assess the Patient	• Ask if they need help. • Does the patient understand what you say? • Patient size and weight • Mobility, balance, strength, endurance • Motivation • What method of transfer is safe and easiest? • Does the patient have a transfer preference? • Remember patients who use a wheelchair may have a greater chance of falling due of lack of coordination and may injure themselves and you.
Special Needs	• Is the patient stronger on their right or left side? • If they use chair padding or cushions, you need to transfer that to the dental chair first. • Elimination devices (bags or catheters) • Spastic movements
Prepare the Treatment Area	• Is the size of the treatment area large enough to accommodate a wheelchair, including the ability for it to turn? • Clear the area by moving the clinician stool, bracket tray, overhead light, hoses. • Check for any sharp or rough areas that could cause injury during transfer.

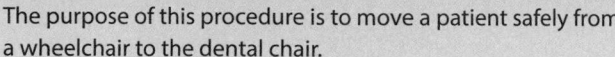

Procedure 13-1
One Person Wheelchair Transfer

The purpose of this procedure is to move a patient safely from a wheelchair to the dental chair.

Equipment and Supplies
- Dental chair
- Wheelchair
- Pillows or rolled blankets

Procedure Steps

1. Explain the procedure to the patient.

2. Clear the area by moving the clinician stool, bracket tray, headlight and hoses.

3. Check for any sharp or rough areas that could cause injury during transfer.

4. Place the front casters forward to prevent the chair from tipping.

5. Remove the foot rests or move them back.

6. Lock the wheels (Figure 13-5).

7. Lower the arm of the dental chair (Figure 13-6).

8. Position the wheelchair at a 30 degree angle to the dental chair with the seats aligned. Dental chair is slightly lower than wheelchair.

9. Transfer any padding the patient may use to the dental chair. Gently rock the patient forward while an assistant removes the padding from the wheelchair to the dental chair.

10. Position your hands under the patient's thighs and gently slide the patient forward to the front of the wheelchair seat (Figure 13-7).

11. Place the patient's feet together and hold them in place on either side by your feet. Come as close to the patient as possible, closing your knees on the patient's knees. This will reduce strain and help to support and stabilize the patient's legs as they rise from the chair. Place your feet shoulder width apart on either side of the patient's feet (Figure 13-8).

12. Place the patient's arms over your shoulders, and instruct the patient to rest their head on your shoulder. Do not allow the patient to grasp you around the neck (Figure 13-9).

13. Grasp the patient around the waist using wrist to wrist grasp (Figure 13-10).

14. Bend your knees, rock gently using your leg muscles to lift the patient off the seat (Figure 13-11).

15. Pivot on your foot closest to the dental chair to turn the patient toward the chair. Taking small steps maneuver the patient over the seat.

16. Lower the patient onto the dental chair (Figure 13-12).

17. Reposition the dental chair armrest. The patient can grasp the armrests to help you position them.

18. Lift the patient's legs into the dental chair (Figure 13-13).

19. Check to make sure any elimination devices are in place, arrange the patient's clothing so it is not wrinkled or binding against the skin.

20. If necessary stabilize the patient with pillows or rolled blankets.

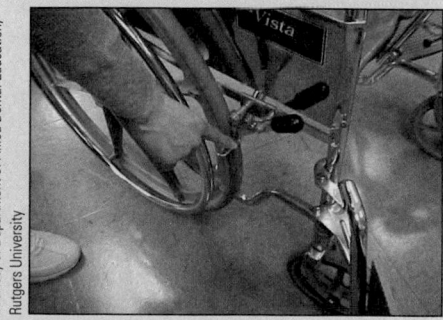

Courtesy of Department of Allied Dental Education, Rutgers University

FIGURE 13-5

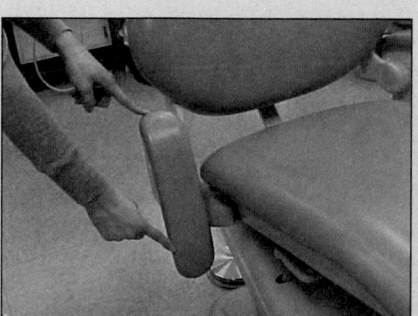

Courtesy of Department of Allied Dental Education, Rutgers University

FIGURE 13-6

(Continues)

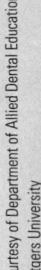

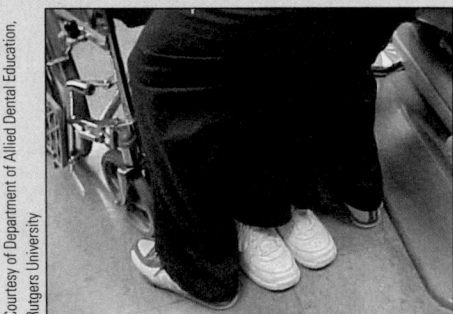

FIGURE 13-7

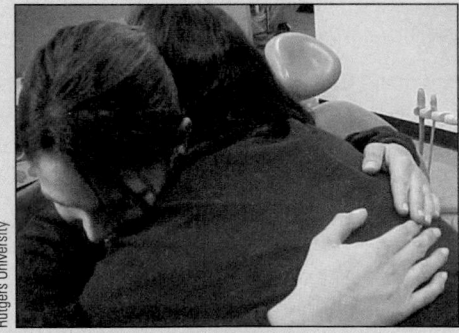

FIGURE 13-8

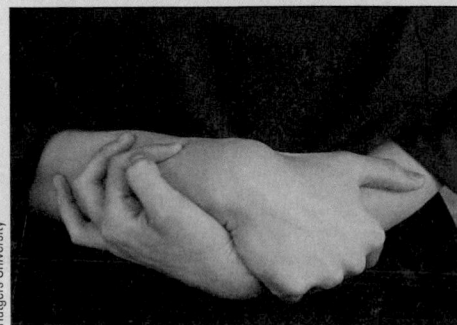

FIGURE 13-9

FIGURE 13-10

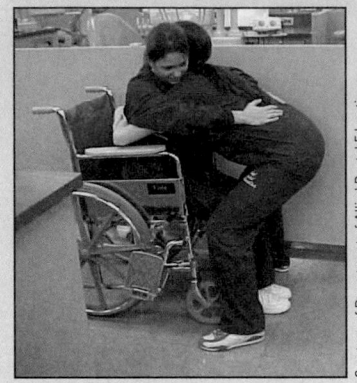

FIGURE 13-11

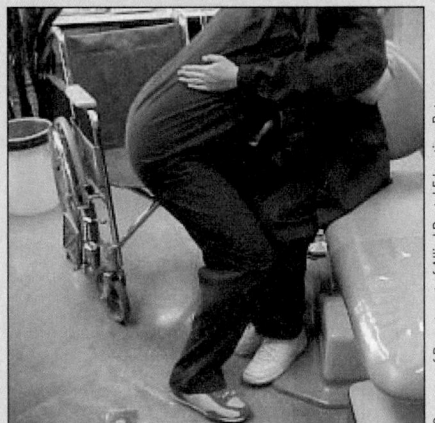

FIGURE 13-12

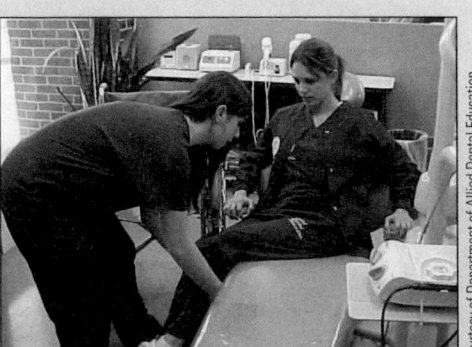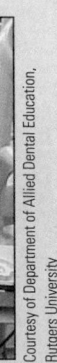

FIGURE 13-13

Procedure 13-2
Two Person Wheelchair Transfer

The purpose of this procedure is to move a patient safely from a wheelchair to the dental chair. Note that the dental chair is slightly higher then the wheelchair. Removing the headrest from the dental chair allows for easier lift over the chair (Figure 13-14).

Equipment and Supplies
- Dental chair
- Wheelchair
- Pillows or rolled blankets

Procedure Steps

1. Explain the procedure to the patient

2. Casters forward to prevent chair from tipping

3. Lock the wheels

4. Remove the footrests or move them back

5. Lower the dental chair arm

6. Wheelchair at a 30 degree angle to the dental chair

7. Make sure there are no sharp or rough areas that could cause injury

8. If necessary transfer any padding to the dental chair

9. The patient should cross their arms over their shoulders

10. First operator stands behind the patient and reaches around patient's torso slightly under ribcage and grasps wrist to wrist. (Figure 13-15). (*Note*: Stronger person should be placed behind the patient to support most of the patient's weight.)

11. Second operator slides hands under the patient's legs (Figure 13-16). One arm should be under the patient's thighs and one arm is placed under the patient's ankles to support the feet

12. Patient is lifted by both operators. The lift is done at a prearranged signal to the count of three.

13. The patient is lifted in one smooth motion and is placed into the dental chair (Figure 13-17).

14. The operator holding the patient's legs releases their grasp and repositions the patient.

15. The other operator does not release the patient until the patient is stabilized and the arm of the dental chair is replaced.

16. Follow steps 19 and 20 from Procedure 13-1.

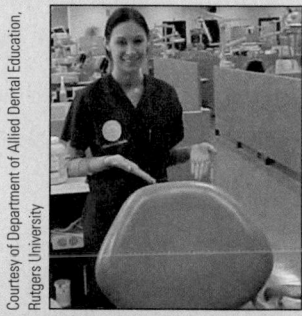

Courtesy of Department of Allied Dental Education, Rutgers University

FIGURE 13-14

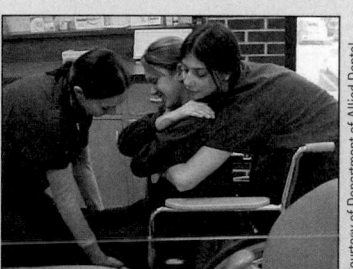

Courtesy of Department of Allied Dental Education, Rutgers University

FIGURE 13-16

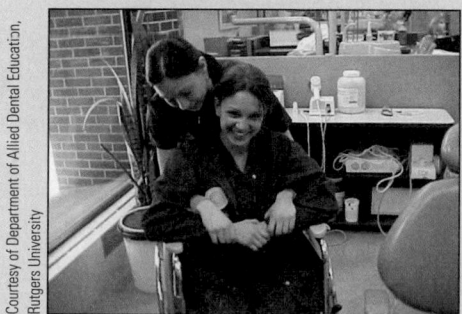

Courtesy of Department of Allied Dental Education, Rutgers University

FIGURE 13-15

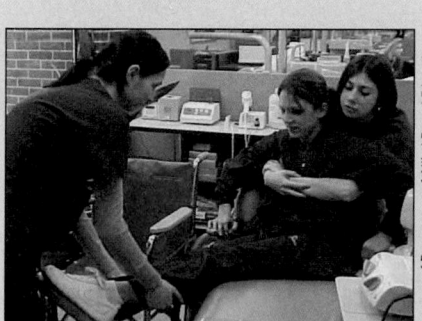

Courtesy of Department of Allied Dental Education, Rutgers University

FIGURE 13-17

Providing Treatment in the Wheelchair

Some patients who cannot be moved must remain in the wheelchair for treatment. These include patients using a device to help them breathe called a ventilator and persons who have varying degrees of **paralysis**. Dental treatment for these patients can be managed in the wheelchair with adequate head support and proper position (Figure 13-18). Treating the maxillary arch can be a challenge but is possible from a standing position. Remember to apply ergonomic principles when using the standing position. To avoid strain in your neck and back, keep procedures as short as possible. Include rest breaks for you and the patient to allow a recovery period for overworked muscles.

Sensory Disabilities

Sensory disabilities affect how a person sees and hears. More than 20 million Americans report having loss of vision including trouble seeing, even when wearing glasses or contact lenses; some persons are blind or unable to see at all. Hardness of hearing or deafness affects persons of all ages and is often referred to as the invisible disability because there may be no visual clues that there is any impairment. Hearing loss can be total or partial, affect one or both ears, and often impacts speech, language development, and motor activity; communication is often a major challenge. Vision and hearing impairments may require some modifications to treatment methods. It is important for you to recognize the mental and physical aspects of having a sensory disability in order to use your resources and imagination to help furnish care. Persons with sensory impairments, especially those with combined disabilities, present challenges for the dental team. Most can receive care in the private office with a few modifications to treatment. It is vital that you be informed and competent to provide treatment for the patient (see Table 13-3).

Vision Impairment

Not all visual impairments are the same. A legally blind person, even with optical correction, can see at 20 feet what a person with normal vision can see at 200 feet. Only 10% of people who are legally blind are totally without sight. Low vision is different from legal blindness and can interfere with a person's ability to perform everyday activities like reading, walking unassisted, and performing oral self-care. Vision impairment does not have any direct effect on oral health, but a person may not detect dental disease symptoms at an early stage that are typically recognized through vision. Other oral symptoms that could be present are lesions due to lip and cheek biting, occlusal wear due to bruxism, and trauma due to accidents.

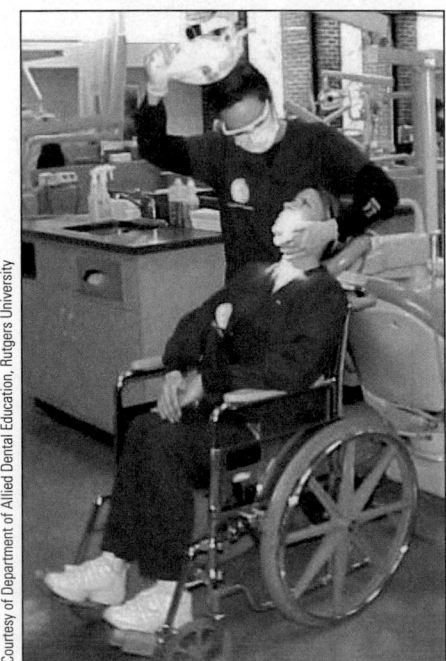

Courtesy of Department of Allied Dental Education, Rutgers University

FIGURE 13-18
Treatment for a patient in a wheelchair.

Guiding and Seating the Patient

- Have the operatory ready.
- Identify yourself and others who may be with you.
- Ask if the person needs help.
- Ask the person to take your arm.
  - Guide by walking as straight as possible half a step in front of the person.
  - Do not grab or pull the person by their arm; you may throw them off balance.
  - Do not hold onto or move a person's cane; it is part of their personal space.
  - Let the person you are guiding set the pace.
  - Avoid sudden, unexpected movements.
  - Point out obstacles.
  - Be specific.
- Guide dog or service animal
  - Walk on the side opposite the dog.
  - Do not touch or pet the dog, or offer food.
  - The dog may stay in the operatory with the person but out of the way.
- Patient seating
  - Put the person's hand on the back of the chair.
  - Position yourself near the chair as the person sits down; help if necessary.
  - Give a verbal description of where the chair is located in relation to the rest of the room.
  - If the person uses a cane, ask where they would like to keep it.
- Reverse seating procedures for patient dismissal; guide the patient if necessary.

TABLE 13-3 Dental Management of Sensory Disabilities

Vision Impairment
- Warn the patient before any change in chair position.
- If the person is sensitive to light, use dark glasses.
  - If you remove the person's own glasses, find out where is the best place to keep them.
  - Avoid shining the light in the patient's eyes.
- Explain every procedure slowly using descriptive words.
- Describe any smell and taste.
- Avoid surprise applications of suction, air, water, moving rubber prophy cup, and the vibration of motor driven instruments.
- With assistance, the patient may feel some of the instruments.
- Discuss rinsing options before it becomes necessary.

Deaf or Hard of Hearing
- If the patient uses a hearing aid, make sure it is turned on for conversation; ask the patient to remove or turn the hearing aid off when using power driven instruments; touching the hearing aid may create a whistle or buzz sound.
- Avoid the unpleasant sound created by shuffling the instruments against one another.
- When using local anesthesia, thoroughly explain the procedure and make sure anesthesia is complete before providing care.
- Watch the patient's facial expression to determine discomfort or other reactions.
- Create several common dental phrases written on index cards to use during the appointment.

Blindness in children may result from infection such as rubella or syphilis passed from mother to child during birth, neoplasm, and complications of premature birth. Causes of blindness in adults are due to accidents, eye disorders such as diabetic retinopathy, macular degeneration, glaucoma, and cataracts. When providing care for the person who is visually impaired, it is important to find out how much impairment they have, if they need your help, and how they prefer to communicate. Because a person with visual impairments may not pick up on nonverbal cues such as body posture, gestures, or facial expression communication, verbal communication must be descriptive.

Deaf or Hard of Hearing

The auditory system can be affected by injury, disease, or the aging process. Hearing loss can be the result of damage to one or several parts of the outer, middle, or inner ear, as well as the sensory pathways from the ear to the brain. *Deaf* is a term used to refer to people with degrees of hearing loss defined by the quietest sound a person can hear. *Hard of hearing* is a broad term that covers the full range of hearing loss from mild to profound.

Deafness can be caused before birth as the result of genetic defects; **prenatal** infections in the mother such as rubella, influenza, and **congenital** syphilis; **incompatible** mother/child blood type; and certain drugs. After birth infectious diseases, including mumps, measles, chicken pox, influenza, and even the common cold can cause deafness. Other causes are trauma to the head or any part of the ear, toxic effects of drugs such as antibiotics and aspirin, and loud noises. Age of onset of deafness can affect the development of speech and language. A problem with hearing, even a mild disability, has been shown to have an impact on a person's capacity to function socially.

Some deaf individuals are able to talk while others cannot or choose not to. People who wear a hearing aid may still have difficulty hearing. Offer the patient paper, pencil, and a hard surface to write on, such as a clipboard.

Intellectual and Physical Disabilities

Intellectual and developmental disabilities affect the mind as well as the body and last throughout a person's life. These disabilities are caused by problems before birth such as genetics, premature birth, or advanced maternal age; during the birth process by lack of oxygen to the baby or prolonged labor; and in infancy by trauma, brain tumors, infections, and toxins. It is important to be able to recognize signs of developmental delays and for the dentist to refer the patient to the appropriate expert. This is a dentist only task, not a decision for the dental assistant! The earlier the recognition and treatment of a developmental delay is started, the better the outcome for the child and their family. Mental capacity, mobility problems, uncontrolled body movements, and oral findings of increased caries and periodontal disease will present a challenge in providing care. Many persons with these disabilities may have additional medical issues such as cardiac and seizure disorders or vision and hearing impairments.

Intellectual Disabilities

Intellectual disability is often referred to as a **cognitive** disorder, mental challenge, or mental retardation. The level of intellectual function is made using standardized intelligence tests (IQ tests). Although a person with an intellectual disability appears to be an adult, dental care must be tailored to meet the needs of their mental age.

Classification of intellectual disabilities is as follows:

- Mild—IQ range of 50–69, adult mental age from 9–12 years, can be educated, can be employed and communicates well

- Moderate—IQ range 35–49, adult mental age from 6–9 years, can perform simple tasks, short attention span and memory, may need the support of a caregiver
- Severe—IQ range 20–34, adult mental age from 3–6 years, uses some speech, conforms to daily routine, needs continuous support of a caregiver
- Profound—IQ under 20, adult mental age below 3 years, delayed development, severe limitation, needs continuous support of a caregiver

Autism (ASD) Autism, also known as autistic spectrum disorder (ASD), is a complex, lifelong disability. Autistic disorders include different syndromes identified by their characteristics. Social interaction, language, behavior, and cognitive functions are all limited. While the cause of autism is unknown, genetics, neurological damage, chemical imbalance, and biochemical abnormalities are the most accepted causes. There is no medical test for autism; diagnosis is made by a team of specialists who observe behavior, perform educational and psychological testing, and document reports from cargivers.

Autism is found throughout the world in all racial, ethnic, and social backgrounds. While there is no cure, early diagnosis followed by intensive behavioral training may allow for better language and social skills. Other treatments include holistic and natural approaches such as vitamins, supplements, and special diets such as gluten-free and casein-free (wheat and milk are common allergens). Symptoms such as hyperactivity or self-injury may require medication. Characteristics, oral findings, and dental management of persons with intellectual and developmental disabilities are outlined in Table 13-4.

Down Syndrome (DS) Down syndrome is the most common chromosomal abnormality; it affects chromosome 21 during cell division. The abnormality causes a combination of physical characteristics that are constant throughout this population; individuals with DS tend to resemble one another. The disability can affect people of all races, cultures, and economic levels in every geographic region. Persons with Down syndrome may have

several medical conditions that are treatable, allowing for a life expectancy of 60 years.

Physical Disabilities

Physical disabilities are medical conditions that impair the patient's ability to perform daily tasks; to get around without crutches, wheelchairs, or other adaptive devices; and to live independently. The patient may have difficulty using, or cannot use, one or more limbs or may have problems with motor control. Some disabilities are congenital like cerebral palsy, and other are acquired later in life as with spinal damage and amputation.

Cerebral Palsy (CP) Cerebral palsy is a nonprogressive chronic neurologic condition caused by damage to the brain. While not curable, CP is not a progressive disease and does not get worse over time; however, affected individuals usually develop degenerative disorders such as osteoarthritis and respiratory problems. Symptoms of CP may vary from mild, needing no assistance, to severe, requiring use of a wheelchair and full time personal care. Use of adaptive devices such as a powered wheelchair and communication tools, speech and occupational therapy, medication to reduce or control movement, and possible surgery can maintain and even improve function (refer to Table 13-4 for more details).

The Medically Compromised Patient

According to former U.S. Surgeon General C. Everett Koop, M.D., "You are not healthy without good oral health." The relationship between dental health and systemic health is well documented; it has been shown that many systemic diseases and medical treatments have oral health **implications**. In fact, five of the six leading causes of death in the United States, heart disease, cancer, stroke, chronic lower respiratory disease, and diabetes, are believed to have a strong link to periodontal disease. To ensure the health of every patient, the dental team must be able to detect medical conditions that may

Communication Tips for Sensory Impaired

- Ask about the preferred method of communication
- Face the person and speak slowly and directly in a normal tone of voice; speak directly to the patient, not the person who accompanies them, but if necessary include a caregiver; avoid distractions such as people, noise from a radio, or open window.
- Give clear, concise instructions slowly, keep it simple, and stick to one topic or question at a time.
- The room should be well lit (note: standing in front of strong back lighting from a window or light can interfere with any residual vision and make it difficult for the person with limited vision or the person who reads lips to see you).

- Let the person know when you move from one place to another. Try not to startle them, and gain attention by speaking or lightly touching the person's arm before speaking.
- For visual impairment, use large print material, audio cassette, CD, Braille, or a designated reader.
- For deaf or hard of hearing, use lip or speech reading, American Sign Language, finger spelling, telecommunications devices, and hearing dogs.
- Interpreters translate spoken language to American Sign Language, and may be best for a difficult, complicated consultation. The Americans with Disabilities Act (ADA) requires the dental office to provide interpreter services if needed.

TABLE 13-4 Intellectual and Development Disabilities

	Characteristics	Oral Findings	Dental Management
Intellectual disabilities	Delayed growth and development, speech and language skills, malformations of the face, limitations in intellectual and social function	Lip thickness, delayed eruption, imperfect formation and missing teeth, increased periodontal infections and caries, clenching, bruxing, mouth breathing and tongue thrusting.	Evaluate for and adapt care modifications to the level of mental ability, function, and communication; "tell-show-do." Possible desensitization due to cooperation issues, possible protective body stabilization, short appointments, and frequent recare visits. Oral self-care instruction to the patient or if necessary the caregiver; fluoride varnish therapy.
Autism	Limited social interaction, eye contact, facial expression and gestures. Delay in language, repetitive use of language and body movements. Inflexible routines.	No specific oral findings except when other developmental disabilities are present. Damaging oral habits—bruxism, tongue thrusting, and self-injurious behavior. Increased dental disease, food pouching instead of swallowing. Side effects of medications—dry mouth and gingival overgrowth.	Possible desensitization due to cooperation issues. Evaluate ability to communicate; use verbal and nonverbal cues; "tell-show-do." Keep instruments out of sight and light out of the patient's eyes. Unusual sensitivity to sound, bright colors, and touch; minimize distractions. Same staff, dental operatory, and appointment time. Use praise to reinforce good behavior, and ignore inappropriate behavior. Provide comfort with soft music, stuffed animal or blanket, and a caregiver nearby. If necessary, use protective body stabilization. Short appointments, provide care when you can, and reschedule if necessary.
Down syndrome	Specific physical characteristics common to all persons with Down syndrome. Intellectual impairment in the mild to moderate range may be present. Increased risk for heart defects, respiratory and hearing problems, Alzheimer's disease, childhood leukemia, and thyroid conditions.	Higher incidence of periodontal disease due to decreased immune function rather than oral hygiene alone. Mouth breathing, fissured lips and tongue, obstructed airway issues due to macroglossia (enlarged tongue), increased secretions, obesity, enlarged tonsils, increased gag reflex, and adenoids. Reduced muscle tone can affect the mouth, contributing to an open bite and problems with chewing, swallowing, drooling, and speaking. Aphthous ulcers, oral Candida infection, and acute necrotizing ulcerative gingivitis are common. Delayed eruption, small or missing teeth, malocclusion, small maxilla, mandibular overjet, and posterior crossbite. Increased risk of caries due to poor food choices and effects of medications.	Possible physician consult and antibiotic premedication due to compromised immune system and possible heart problems. Determine level of mental function and ability to communicate. The patient can become aggressive and unmanageable if confused or disoriented; explain procedures and keep the atmosphere calm. Prevention is key, so provide oral hygiene instruction to the patient and if necessary their caregiver. Consider use of fluoride, treatments aimed at relieving dry mouth, and nutritional counseling; since the tongue may be fissured and can harbor bacteria, instruct the patient about cleaning the tongue every day with the toothbrush. Treat oral disease aggressively; topical and systemic antimicrobial agents and early periodontal therapy may be necessary. Provide a non-oil based lip balm during treatment. Ask if the patient needs help getting to the dental chair. Record successful strategies in the chart. Tendency for upper respiratory infections requires good fluid suction techniques. Provide pillows or a blanket to stabilize the patient and make them more comfortable. Early morning appointments when patient and operator are more rested may be best.
Cerebral palsy	Uncontrolled, involuntary body and mouth movements, seizure disorders, sensory impairment, speech and communication defects, some degree of intellectual disability may be present.	Increased dental disease, malocclusion, swallowing difficulty, enamel hypoplasia, mouth breathing, abnormal muscle and tongue movements (tongue thrusting), drooling, lack of lip closure, trauma from falls that can cause tooth fracture and avulsion, bruxism, and TMJ problems. Side effects of medications—dry mouth and gingival overgrowth.	Allow extra time. Anticipate uncontrolled body and mouth movements that create a danger to the patient and the dental team. Use stabilizing and protective devices. May need extra oral radiographs. Provide oral hygiene instruction, automatic modified toothbrush, flossing devices, antimicrobials, and fluoride rinse. If necessary, instruct caregiver.

have a negative impact on a patient's general health and oral health and may affect dental care. Timely referral to a physician for diagnosis and treatment can prevent problems. The goals for dental management of the medically compromised patient are to prevent a medical emergency from occurring in the dental office by obtaining a thorough medical history, maintain oral health, and prevent and control disease.

The Pregnant Patient

The oral health of a pregnant person affects the general health of her baby. For example, there is a relationship between gum disease and a baby born prematurely and/or with low birth weight. Therefore, it is extremely important for the health of the baby that the mother be free from oral disease before and during pregnancy.

A normal pregnancy is 40 weeks, while premature birth refers to a birth before 37 weeks. Pregnancy is divided into three stages or trimesters, each lasting three months. During the first trimester while all organ systems are forming, the **fetus** is at great risk for injury and malformation. **Teratogens** such as infections, use of drugs, smoking, or radiation can cause birth defects during the first trimester. Alcohol freely passes directly to the fetus, and no safe amount has been established for pregnant women. Pregnant women who drink alcohol are at risk for delivering a baby with fetal alcohol syndrome (FAS). FAS is characterized by damage to the central nervous system, which affects motor skills, behavior, and personality. Nutrition is especially important at this time. Spina bifida, a birth defect in which there is an opening in the spinal column, is preventable with the use of multivitamins containing folic acid.

It is worth noting that calcium is not taken from the mother's teeth during pregnancy. If there is not enough calcium in the diet, the baby will take what it needs from the mother's bones. Proper nutrition is essential so that enough calcium is available from the mother's diet for development of strong teeth and bones in the baby. During the second and third trimesters growth and development continue and the fetus gains weight.

Oral Problems during Pregnancy
Pregnancy causes hormonal changes that can lead to gingival inflammation (gingivitis), periodontitis, and caries. A *pyogenic granuloma*, more commonly called a "pregnancy tumor," can occur because of the greater amounts of bacteria that are present. The growth, usually located at the interdental gingival margin, is benign and may disappear after the pregnancy is completed. Surgical removal may also be necessary.

"Morning sickness," which causes nausea and vomiting, is common and can cause enamel erosion on the lingual of the maxillary anterior teeth; the weakened enamel is susceptible to demineralization from stomach acid. Brushing after vomiting is not recommended because the acid can be spread around the mouth and increase the chance of erosion. Rinsing with a teaspoon of baking soda dissolved in a cup of water can neutralize the acid. A soft toothbrush, low-abrasive toothpaste, and alcohol-free mouth rinses with fluoride are the best choices for oral self-care. If demineralization of the enamel has already occurred, a home use prescription fluoride is indicated.

Dental Management of the Pregnant Patient

Since dental care should be part of a healthy pregnancy, regular dental visits for exam and prophylaxis should continue. Care includes:

- Possible physician consultation
- Emergency care for infection or abscess any time
- First trimester— caution because the fetus is most susceptible to injury and malformation
- Second trimester— safest and most comfortable time to provide routine care
- Third trimester— the patient may be uncomfortable during treatment
  - To avoid compression of the **vena cava**, position the patient on left side using a pillow or rolled up blanket to elevate the right hip
  - Last half of the third trimester has greater risk of premature delivery
- Exposing radiographs—follow all methods for radiation safety and protection
  - Use a lead apron, a thyroid collar, and a second apron for the back to prevent secondary radiation from reaching the abdomen
- Ensure safety of patient and pregnant staff members— nitrous oxide (N2O) analgesia should not be used because it has been linked to a higher risk of miscarriage
- Know the U.S. Food and Drug Administration categories of prescription drugs for potential of risk to the fetus. Chapter 14 discusses this topic.

The Older Patient

The older population is one of the fastest growing segments in the United States. Experts estimate that by 2030 one in five Americans will be 65 years of age. As the baby boomer generation (those born between 1946 and 1964) ages, the numbers become even more significant. There will be many more people age 85 years and older seeking dental care. An average general dental practice will have about 260 or more patients age 65 years and older.

As the lifespan of a person increases, so does the occurrence of chronic diseases; however, good nutrition, exercise, and social interactions with others can maintain a healthier life. This diverse group of people has many complex needs that the dental professional must be prepared to meet.

As a healthy person ages, many changes take place inside and outside the body.

- Thin, wrinkled skin with increasing dark spots
- Loss of bone volume
- Curved spine
- Stiff joints
- Loss of muscle tone and strength

- Vision and hearing loss
- Reduced ability in organ system function
- Loss of elasticity in the blood vessels, with decreased cardiac output
- Slower mental ability, difficulty with complex tasks, short-term memory decline
- Immune system function weakens, chance of disease greater
- Decreased healing response, increase in the chance of secondary infection
- Chronic conditions—hypertension, arthritis, cardiovascular disease, and diabetes
- Multiple medications with potential side effects
- Psychological effects of aging—the patient may be happy to have time to enjoy their life or may experience the loss of their health and independence, loneliness, depression, or alcoholism

The Oral Effects of Aging The mouth undergoes changes with age; however, tooth loss does not occur because a person gets older. Americans turning 65 years old were the first to benefit from community water fluoridation and regular preventive dental care. In fact, many older adults have a full dentition and place a high value on maintaining and improving oral health. Oral effects of aging are:

Soft Tissues

- Oral mucosa is thin, less elastic, and less vascular
- Lingual varicosities
- Increased possibility of xerostomia, angular cheilitis, candidiasis, white patches from irritation, petechiae
- Burning tongue—smooth, shiny, atrophied papillae
- Decrease in taste **acuity**

Teeth

- Darker color
- Narrowing of pulp chambers, pulp calcification
- Attrition, abrasion, cracked enamel
- Root caries

Periodontium

- Bone changes—possible osteoporosis
- Cementum—increased thickness
- Gingiva—recession

Cardiovascular Diseases

Cardiovascular diseases are conditions that affect the heart and the blood vessels. Cardiovascular disease generally refers to a condition in which the blood vessels are narrowed due to **atherosclerosis**. Narrowing of the arteries may lead to

Older Adult Patient Recommendations

As with any patient, dental professionals must tailor care recommendations and treatment for the older adult patient based on their needs.

- Allow for extra time in the appointment, and schedule short late morning or early afternoon appointments (appointments should not last longer than 2 hours). Assessment of the patient and their individual needs starts with observation in the reception area (gait, balance, function, mental ability, etc.)
- Do not address the patient by their first name unless the patient suggests doing so; address the patient directly, and if necessary involve the caregiver.
- Ask if they need your help with walking to and from and with seating in the dental operatory.
- Screen with medical history for illness, possible physician consult, and antibiotic premedication.
- Be aware of side effects of medications.
- Evaluate oral conditions (xerostomia, root caries, etc.).
- Provide cushions and pillows for support, if needed, with possible upright or semi-supine chair position.
- Caution with **orthostatic hypotension**—change chair position slowly from supine to upright and allow the patient to sit for a minute before rising; if necessary provide support to help the patient out of the chair.
- Eliminate noise and distractions.
- Provide oral self-care instruction based on the patient's needs, in office and possible home fluoride therapy; assess nutrition related to dental needs.
- Schedule frequent recare appointments.

arrhythmias, heart attack, or a stroke. It is important the dental team is aware of the dental management needed in caring for a patient with cardiovascular disease (Figure 13-19).

Dental Management of the Patient with Cardiovascular Disease

- Know the patient's medical history.
- Take blood pressure at every visit.
- Plan for possible physician consultation and antibiotic premedication.
- Provide stress free environment.
- Reduce oral bacteria with preprocedural rinse and maintain high level of oral health.
- Change chair position slowly from supine to upright.
- Follow recommendations for use of vasoconstrictor in anesthesia and retraction cord.
- Recognize symptoms of heart disease that may affect dental treatment.

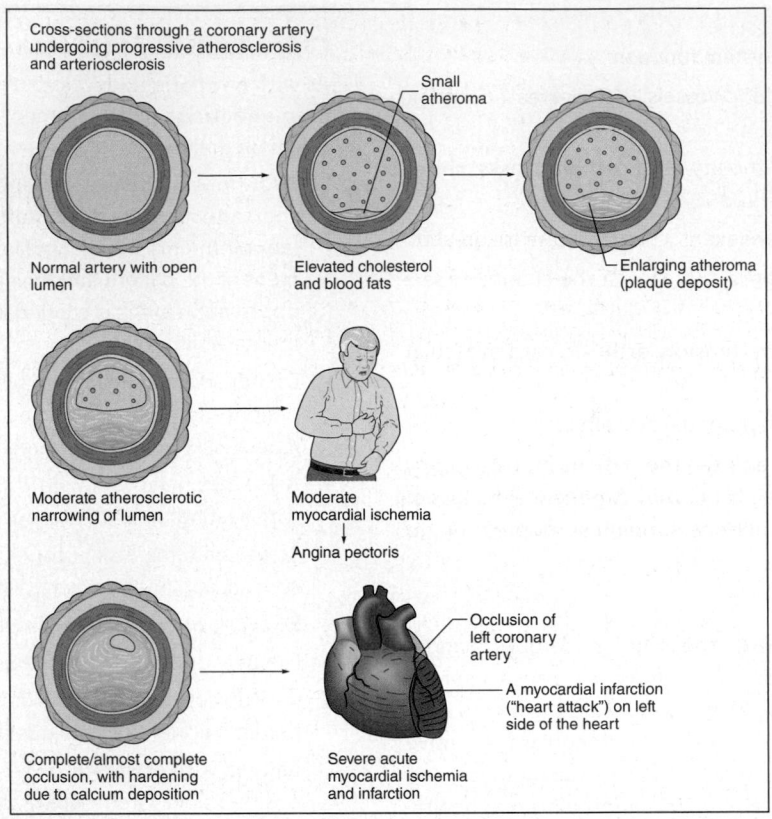

Cross-sections through a coronary artery undergoing progressive atherosclerosis and arteriosclerosis

Small atheroma

Normal artery with open lumen

Elevated cholesterol and blood fats

Enlarging atheroma (plaque deposit)

Moderate atherosclerotic narrowing of lumen

Moderate myocardial ischemia

Angina pectoris

Occlusion of left coronary artery

A myocardial infarction ("heart attack") on left side of the heart

Complete/almost complete occlusion, with hardening due to calcium deposition

Severe acute myocardial ischemia and infarction

FIGURE 13-19

Moderate atherosclerotic narrowing of lumen; moderate myocardial ischemia—angina pectoris.

Congenital Heart Disease Before birth, irregularities in the development of the heart can result in **anomalies** that affect its structure and function. There are several types of defects, but the most common involve the openings that allow exchange of blood and oxygen within the heart and between the heart and lungs (*ventricular sepal* defect, atrial septal defect, and *patent ductus arteriosus*).

The cause of congenital heart disease is often unknown. Genetics such as the chromosomal defects present in Down's syndrome may also result in congenital heart defects. Environmental factors such as a maternal viral infection of rubella may also result in congenital heart defects. Fatigue, fainting, **cyanosis** of the lips and nail beds, poor growth and development, chest deformity, heart murmurs, and congestive heart failure are symptoms that may occur with congenital heart disease. Although small defects often correct on their own, early diagnosis is essential because most cases require treatment before the age of 1 year such as heart medications and surgery.

Rheumatic Heart Disease Following **rheumatic** fever, the heart valves may become permanently damaged and may be susceptible to infective endocarditis. Rheumatic fever may appear 2–3 weeks after a strep throat infection (Streptococcal pharyngeal infection). The heart valves become scarred. The aortic and mitral valves are most commonly affected. Early

symptoms of rheumatic heart disease include **stenosis** of the valves, **murmurs**, and arrhythmias. Shortness of breath, **angina pectoris**, increased **diastolic** blood pressure, left ventricle enlargement, and congestive heart failure may appear.

Use of an antibiotic, such as penicillin, to cure a strep throat infection can prevent rheumatic fever and possible subsequent damage to the heart valves from developing. Antibiotic therapy, which may include long-term use of medication as prevention, is often given to avoid heart damage in those who have previously had rheumatic fever. To avoid the inflammation that can scar the heart, aspirin, steroids, or nonsteroidal medications are used. If damage does occur, surgery may be necessary to repair or replace a damaged valve. A heart murmur is a concern before any oral surgery because of potential infection of the heart valve and lining of the heart (endocarditis). Many dentists prescribe an antibiotic prior to any invasive procedure.

Infective Endocarditis (IE) Infective **endocarditis** is a microbial infection of the heart valves, endocardium, or cardiac **prosthesis** caused by a bacteremia. During invasive dental procedures that cause bleeding such as surgery, periodontal therapy, or endodontic procedures, microorganisms from the mouth can enter the bloodstream, infect, and damage normal heart valves. Damaged and prosthetic valves are more at risk for infection. IE is difficult to treat; therefore, prevention is important. Risk factors include previous history of IE, artificial heart valves, serious congenital heart conditions, and oral infections. IV drug abusers are at high risk because infected material from contaminated needles may be injected directly into the bloodstream.

Symptoms may appear two weeks after exposure and include fever, loss of appetite, weight loss, joint pain, and heart murmurs. In many cases IE is not diagnosed right away because the patient may feel as if they have the flu. Complications as a result of IE lead to susceptibility of reinfection, congestive heart failure, and stroke. Before the advent of antibiotics, IE was usually fatal. Medical management consists of antibiotic therapy and may include surgical intervention to repair significant damage.

Hypertension Hypertension or high blood pressure is the abnormal elevation of *arterial* blood pressure. The kidneys, heart, brain, and eyes are affected with sustained elevation of blood pressure. Hypertension is a risk factor for cerebral vascular accident (stroke), hypertensive renal disease, and ischemic heart disease. Risk factors include tobacco use, genetics, being overweight, diets high in salt, use of oral contraceptives, renal disease, medications, age (older people), race (African American males), and sex (male). Underlying medical conditions such as diabetes, kidney disease, endocrine disorders, obesity, and pregnancy are causes of secondary hypertension.

Hypertension is often called the "silent killer" because one third of the people who have it may have no symptoms. In fact, the dental office is often the first place hypertension is discovered. It is important to take and record each patient's blood pressure before every visit because many dental procedures and medications can cause an elevation in blood pressure. It is especially dangerous to provide treatment to the patient who is unaware they have sustained high blood pressure. If hypertension is discovered, routine dental care should be avoided until the patient seeks medical attention. Early symptoms may be occipital (back of the head) headaches, dizziness, visual disturbances, weakness, ringing in the ears, and tingling in the hands and feet. Later symptoms include chest pains, shortness of breath, mental confusion, convulsions, blurred vision leading to loss of sight, and nosebleeds.

The goal of treatment is to reduce blood pressure. Changes in diet, limiting alcohol, weight loss, smoking cessation, and daily physical activity control early hypertension. If lifestyle changes are inadequate to reduce blood pressure, then medication is prescribed by the physician. Depending on the medical condition of the patient, one (1) or more medications may be prescribed to manage the hypertension.

Angina and Myocardial Infarction Angina pectoris refers to a situation where a person feels an uncomfortable sensation or choking pain in their chest. This is due to either blocked arteries or disease in the coronary arteries, which results in lack of blood to the heart muscles. The lack of blood creates a deficiency in oxygen and other nutrients, making the heart work harder and at a faster rate. Angina usually lasts for a few minutes, is temporary, and ceases as soon as the blood supply to the heart returns to normal. There are many possible reasons for angina including physical exertion, emotional stress, heredity, or smoking. Person with angina are often prescribed nitroglycerin that can be self-administered during an attack. Dental treatment should be terminated early if the patient becomes overly anxious or complains of chest pains, and the patient should be encouraged to take their prescribed dose of nitroglycerin. There are two types of angina: stable and unstable. Unstable angina can lead to myocardial infarction. Angina pectoris is a syndrome that involves the heart, while myocardial infarction is a life threatening condition that can lead to an abrupt death.

Myocardial infarction (MI) is also referred to as a heart attack. This normally occurs when the coronary artery is blocked by unstable **plaque** surrounding arteries rupturing. The blocked arteries create a lack of blood supply and oxygen, which results in

Dental Management of the Patient with a Neurologic Disorder

- Preserve oral health and function and to prevent disease.
- Perform complex procedures before disease progresses.
- Office temperature should be comfortable and appointments scheduled in early daytime when the office is not busy.
- Use a caring and understanding approach to the patient.
- Possible wheelchair transfer or treatment in a wheelchair.
- Eliminate distractions and communicate using short words and sentences and direct eye contact; repeat instructions if necessary.
- Use cushions for stabilization, frequent position changes, and protective eyewear.
- Be aware of sudden, uncontrolled mouth movements.
- Use protective eyewear and practice good suction technique.
- Medication side effects include xerostomia, orthostatic hypotension, dizziness, nausea, and immunosuppression.
- Dental drug interactions may occur with epinephrine, erythromycin, narcotics, and general anesthetics.
- Self-care instruction— a power toothbrush may disturb some patients with AD; do not recommended mouth rinses for persons who cannot understand that swallowing the rinse may cause harm; consider the use of brush on fluoride gel; for patients who accumulate food on one side of the face because of numbness, suggest rinsing with water or oral irrigator after eating.
- Include the patient's family or caregiver in the appointment.

Remember, these discussions are confidential. By law, information in these conversations is considered "privileged information" and must not be shared outside of the office.

the death of heart muscle tissue. The common symptoms for MI include sudden and acute chest pain, shortness of breath, anxiety, **palpitations**, nausea, and sweating, and it can even cause death. A person suffering MI needs immediate medical attention, including oxygen supply and aspirin. The extent of heart tissue damage is permanent and evaluated using an electrocardiogram and echocardiography. When a patient reports that they have experienced a MI, their physician should be consulted before dental treatment. It is generally recommended that dental treatment is postponed a minimum of 6 months after the infarction to ensure the patient's safety.

Neurologic Disorders

The nervous system senses the external environment and controls the body. Any damage to any part of the system may cause functional loss. Although each neurologic disorder may have a different cause, many of the characteristics are the same. It is important for the dental team to be knowledgeable in the management of patients with a neurologic disorder.

Multiple Sclerosis Multiple sclerosis is a progressive disorder of the central nervous system (CNS) in which continuous destruction of the **myelin sheath** of nerves in the brain and spinal cord occurs. Sheath degeneration interferes with nerve impulse transmission. Although the cause is unknown, multiple sclerosis is thought to be autoimmune in nature. An infectious agent such as rabies, measles, or herpes may trigger the disease. Genetic and environmental factors may also play an important role.

Visual and motor disturbances make balance and walking difficult, and paralysis may affect use of the hands. Muscle weakness and spasticity are common and present a challenge during dental care. Oral symptoms include facial pain, TMJ dysfunction, and trigeminal neuralgia. Symptoms can be brought on by heat sources such as fever, physical exertion, bathing, sun exposure, and hot weather, and a local or systemic infection can stimulate a relapse. Other disturbances include loss of touch, pain, or speech and problems with concentration, temperature, and **proprioception**. Fatigue occurs in most of the patients and becomes worse later in the day.

About 85% of the patients who have multiple sclerosis present with stages of remission and relapse of the disease. Relapse attacks can last several days to weeks followed by a symptom free period, but with each attack, the condition becomes worse. Treatment includes the use of medications such as steroids and interferon and is aimed at relieving the symptoms. Exercise and rest may be helpful to manage fatigue.

Parkinson's Disease Parkinson's disease is a progressive, degenerative disorder of the CNS. Parkinson's disease affects the neurons that produce the chemical mediator dopamine, which is involved in nerve impulses related to muscle activity. The neurons that control posture, body support, and voluntary motion degenerate. The actual cause is unknown, but genetics and environmental factors are suspected. Other factors that can damage the cells include stroke, brain tumor, head injury, exposure to chemical toxins, and drug use.

People with Parkinson's have a loss of postural stability, making the body appear to be bent over; balance may be a problem as well. Generalized stiffness and shuffling contribute to a slow pace. A resting tremor in one or both hands, lips, tongue, and neck; a masklike facial appearance; diminished eye blinking; trouble swallowing with excessive salivation and drooling; and TMJ dysfunction present a challenge during dental treatment. Patients may need assistance with oral hygiene, and medications may cause xerostomia, leading to increased dental caries and periodontal disease. Treatment is aimed at controlling symptoms with the use of medications that replace dopamine. Deep brain stimulation (DBS) is a surgical procedure that uses an implanted device within the brain that is similar to a heart pacemaker. The battery-operated device delivers electrical stimulation to block nerve signals that cause some of the more **debilitating** symptoms of the disease such as tremors.

Amyotrophic Lateral Sclerosis (ALS) ALS is a progressive degeneration of the cells in the motor neurons of the spinal cord and cerebral cortex. Often diagnosed after the age of 55 years, the advance of **atrophy** continues with death in 3–5 years after diagnosis, usually from respiratory failure. The cause of ALS is unknown, but genetics, environmental factors, and viruses related to the **poliomyelitis** virus are suspected.

ALS affects more men than women. Symptoms include muscle cramping and weakness. Atrophy may begin in the hand and forearm, and weakness in the foot and ankle can be noticed early in the disease. The progressive deterioration of the muscles of respiration results in the inability to communicate or speak, and eventually to paralysis. Patients may need assistance in modifying oral care techniques or help from a caregiver. There is no cure for ALS. Medications such as corticosteroids and immunosuppressive drugs are used to improve symptoms. Exercise may help mobility, and custom devices can enhance function. As chewing and swallowing become difficult, a feeding tube may be required to provide adequate nutrition. Mechanical ventilation may be necessary, as weakness gets worse in the respiratory muscles.

Dementia and Alzheimer's Disease (AD) Dementia, which can affect any age group, is primarily a disease of aging. The slow, progressive, chronic decline in intellectual abilities affects thinking, memory, and judgment. Dementia is rarely reversible. Alzheimer's disease is a degenerative disorder of brain tissue and is the most common type of dementia. In rare cases early onset AD may strike as early as 30 or 40 years of age. Metabolic disorders such as anemia, **hypoxia, anoxia,** a brain tumor, trauma, infections, deficiency diseases, toxins, and medications may cause dementia. The cause of AD is unknown, but theories include genetics, environment, nutrition, and infectious agents.

Dementia differs from the normal decline that occurs with age. With age "mental processes become slowed, but the older healthy person still retains a firm grasp on reality, is oriented, can reason, has good judgment, and can continue to lead an active, self-supporting life" (Darby and Walsh). AD, which can extend up to 20 years, can be divided into stages where symptoms may overlap. In the early stages of AD the patient presents with memory loss of recent events, personality changes, and errors in judgment. Symptoms affect performance of everyday activities such as dealing with finances, following instructions, and driving. The middle stages present problems such as confusion and getting lost. In the early and middle stages of the disease, the patient may become combative, anxious, and depressed. The patient is unable to work and needs constant supervision. In advanced stages, seizures may occur, and the patient is often bedridden and unable to recognize family members; they may require care in a nursing facility.

Persons with AD have more dental disease than the normal elderly population. They may have forgotten how to perform oral self-care or be resistant to caregiver efforts with oral hygiene. Medications used to prevent seizures may cause gingival enlargement and salivary gland dysfunction. Oral injuries from falls and oral injury from using eating utensils are common. The edentulous patient may misplace or lose their dentures. There is no cure for dementia or AD; therefore, treatment is aimed at prevention. Once a patient is diagnosed, therapy is focused on slowing of symptoms and improvement of quality of life. Medications to manage the symptoms include antiseizure medication, antidepressants, antianxiety drugs, and antipsychotics. All these medications have oral effects, especially dry mouth.

Seizures
Symptoms of a seizure may include temporary confusion, staring spells, uncontrolled jerking movement of arms and legs, loss of consciousness or awareness, fear, and anxiety. Seizures can occur after a stroke, a closed head injury, an infectious illness, or high fevers, and many causes are unknown. Most seizures last from 30 seconds to 2 minutes. Most seizures can be controlled with medication; there are over 20 FDA-approved medications for epilepsy called antiepileptic drugs (AEDs). Seizures lasting more than 5 minutes are a medical emergency.

If there are two or more seizures or a tendency to have recurrent seizures, the patient is diagnosed as having epilepsy. An *epileptic seizure* is a sudden, uncontrolled electrical disturbance in the brain that disrupts the communication pathways of the neurons to create, send, and receive impulses to communicate. Anything that disrupts communication pathways can lead to a seizure. The dental assistant should question the patient with epilepsy if they have taken their prescribed levels of antiepileptic drugs prior to any treatment.

There are several types of seizures ranging in severity based on where and how they begin in the brain. The four main categories of seizures include the following:

- Nonepileptic seizures briefly change behavior and often look like epileptic seizures but are not caused by electrical disruptions in the brain.

- Absence seizure, previously known as petit mal seizures, are characterized by staring into space and subtle movements like eye blinking or lip smacking, and may cause a brief loss of awareness.

- Generalized tonic-clonic seizure, or grand mal seizure, can make the person cry out, lose consciousness, fall to the ground, and have muscle jerks or spasms. The person may feel tired after the seizure.

- *Status epilepticus seizures* are a continuous seizure, 30 minutes of uninterrupted seizure activity; any convulsions that last over 5 minutes require emergency attention.

Cerebrovascular Accident
Cerebrovascular accident (CVA) is the medical term for a stroke. A stroke occurs when blood flow to the brain is stopped by blockage (blood clot) or a blood vessel ruptures. This results in part of the brain being deprived of blood and oxygen that causes brain cells to die. A person who is suffering from a stroke should be treated immediately as a stroke left untreated too long may result in permanent brain damage. It is important to know the signs of a stroke using the acronym **FAST**:

- **F**ace: Does one side of the face droop? (Figure 13-20)

- **A**rm: If a person holds both arms out, does one drift downward?

- **S**peech: Is their speech abnormal or slurred?

- **T**ime: It's time to call 911 and get to the hospital if any of these symptoms are present

There is a recovery period after a stroke that may include rehabilitation, physical and occupational therapy, and neurology. The dental team should be particularly concerned about the risk of a

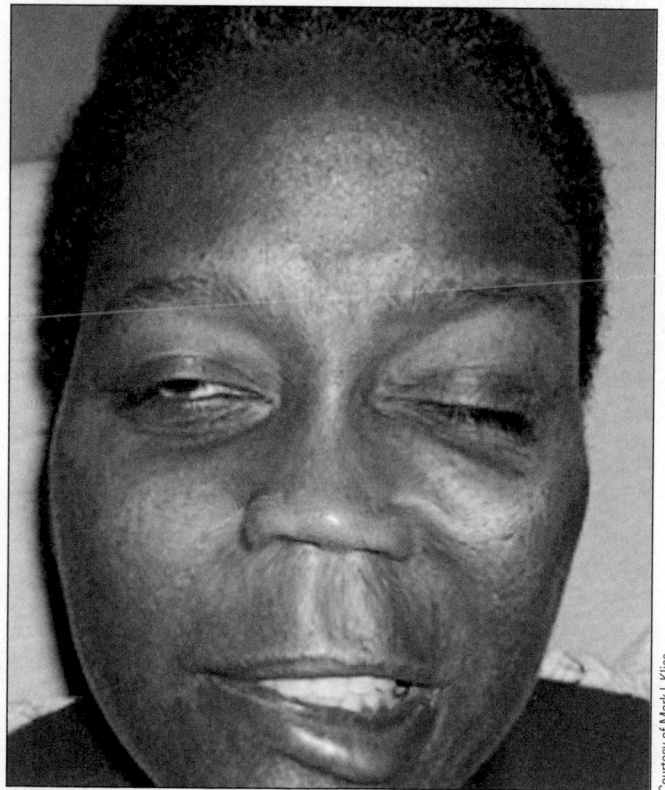

Courtesy of Mark L.Kliss

FIGURE 13-20
CVA: Facial features.

recurrence, assist patient in walking, be empathic to speech problems, and modify oral hygiene techniques due to loss of dexterity. Patients are often placed on anticoagulants, which may present a problem with excessive bleeding during dental treatment. The patient's physician should be consulted prior to treatment.

Blood Disorders

The dental team may be the first to notice a blood disorder through medical history and oral signs and symptoms. Increased bruising and bleeding from nose and mouth, shortness of breath, and recurrent infections and fevers are all signs that the patient may be suffering from a blood disorder. It is critical that the dental team follows up with the patient's physician and is aware of recommended dental management of patients with a blood disorder.

Dental Management of the Patient with a Blood Disorder

- A thorough medical history, possible physician consultation, and antibiotic premedication
- Knowledge of interactions with over-the-counter medications or herbs, as well as use of certain dental medications that can prevent excessive bleeding
- Provide a stress free environment
- Place radiographs, impression trays, and evacuation tips carefully to avoid injury
- Self-care instruction—extra soft toothbrush and careful flossing technique to prevent cutting the interproximal tissue will minimize the chance of infection
- Provide nutritional assessment and counseling

Red Blood Cell Disorders

Red blood cells, or erythrocytes, function to transport hemoglobin, carry oxygen to every cell, and also carry carbon dioxide from the cells. A large number of red blood cell disorders are anemias, which are a group of disorders of red blood cells in which there is an abnormally low level of hemoglobin or a decrease in the number of cells. Oxygen delivery to all cells is diminished as a result.

Each type of anemia has a different cause. Blood loss from trauma or slow internal bleeding can decrease red blood cells. The inherited disorders *thalassemia* and *sickle cell disease* cause abnormalities of hemoglobin. Certain chemicals such as benzene and arsenic, as well as radiation exposure, injure bone marrow and destroy red blood cells. Cancer, kidney, and liver disorders cause bone marrow suppression. Vitamin B_{12} and folate are essential for red blood cell production; therefore, a lack of these nutrients from inadequate intake or poor absorption causes anemias. Iron deficiency *anemia* is caused by excessive blood loss, poor intake, absorption, or increased demand, for example during pregnancy.

Muscle weakness and fatigue, palpations, shortness of breath, jaundice, pallor, and cracking and splitting of fingernails are all common findings. Oral signs include pallor of the mucosa and gingiva and angular cheilitis. The tongue may appear smooth and shiny with burning, painful sensations. The goal of treatment is to eliminate the underlying cause. It is helpful to suggest supplements and nutritional recommendations of foods high in iron, vitamin B_{12}, and folic acid. The dentist may recommend antimicrobial rinses along with an oral hygiene regiment to prevent periodontal disease and consult the physician to make certain the patient's condition is under control prior to dental treatment; usually there are no modification unless anemia is severe.

White Blood Cell Disorders White blood cells, or leukocytes, protect the body against pathogens and are an active part of the immune system. White blood cell disorders may occur because of a decrease (*leukopenia*) or increase in cell numbers (*leukocytosis*). Since white blood cells are involved in the immune response, dental patients with these disorders may experience delayed wound healing or infection that in some cases may be fatal.

Specific infections such as HIV/AIDS, influenza, measles, or bone marrow suppression or destruction can cause a decrease in white blood cells. Inflammation, infections, trauma, emotional stress, or exertion can cause an increase in cells. Leukemia is cancer of the white blood cells and is the most severe cause of an increase in cell numbers. Patients with leukemia exhibit the general symptoms of anemia. Tendencies to bleed easily and frequent infections are common. Oral signs include gingival enlargement, ulceration, and oral infection. Treatment is aimed at the cause. In most cases, treatment for increased white blood cell count is not necessary. Chemotherapy is used to treat leukemia. Treatment for leukopenia is aimed at reducing the risk of infection. Use of medications may stimulate white blood cell production.

Coagulation Disorders Platelets, or thrombocytes, are essential for blood clotting. A number of dental procedures may cause bleeding, and with a healthy patient, there is little or no risk. However, since bleeding disorders affect the ability of the blood to clot, it is essential that the dental team be aware of such problems to ensure the well-being of the patient. Bleeding disorders are due to problems with the structure and function of blood vessels, platelet dysfunction or deficiency, and coagulation factors. Infections, chemicals, collagen disorders, or certain types of allergy can damage blood vessels. The vessels become fragile and are unable to stop bleeding when injured. A platelet deficiency such as thrombocytopenia, or dysfunction of the platelets necessary to form a clot during bleeding, can be the result of bone marrow depression.

Hemophilia is a group of inherited blood disorders caused by low levels or absence of the protein essential for clotting. Liver disease and vitamin K deficiency may also cause coagulation disorders. Bleeding and bruising easily occur with minor trauma. Patients with coagulation disorders may bleed into joint spaces, creating severe disability. Severe or chronic bleeding can lead to anemia. Gingival bleeding is common. Oral signs seen in platelet disorders are **petechiae** and **ecchymosis**. After a consult with the physician, most patients with hemophilia can be treated in the dental office. Treatment depends on the type of disorder and can include coagulation factor replacement, plasma and platelet transfusion, immune therapies, and vitamin supplements.

Musculoskeletal Disorders

Musculoskeletal disorders affect the body's muscles, bones, joints, tendons, and ligaments, and range from mild discomfort and pain to serious disability. These patients require special dental management to make their dental office visits as comfortable as possible.

Dental Management of the Patient with a Musculoskeletal Disorder

- Assess mobility and need for assistance with walking.
- Question about joint replacement and possible antibiotic premedication.
- Provide cushions to help with patient positioning and change chair position slowly.
- Give frequent breaks to change body position and rest the TMJ.
- Self-care instruction—evaluate oral self-care ability and provide modifications, evaluate the patient's grip, strength, and ability to hold an automatic toothbrush.
- Use lifestyle and prevention strategies and nutritional counseling.
- Evaluate nutrition for adequate intake of vitamins and minerals.

Osteoarthritis (OA)
Osteoarthritis (OA), also known as degenerative joint disease, is a chronic and inflammatory ailment of the joints. In OA, degeneration occurs in the joint cartilage, causing pain and disability. OA affects older people because of the aging process or normal wear and tear. The disorder can be localized, affecting one joint, or generalized, where many joints are involved (Figure 13-21). Weight bearing joints such as the hips, knees, and spinal column are most involved. TMJ movement can also be compromised. Risk factors include obesity, repeated trauma, joint abnormalities, genetics, and metabolic factors.

There may be a cracking, grating sound in the joints with swelling and tenderness and limited range of motion in the TMJ. Pain, stiffness, and immobility are common and may be improved with mild activity. Over-the-counter pain medications such as aspirin, nonsteroidal anti-inflammatory drugs (NSAIDs), and acetaminophen are helpful to combat the pain and may allow movement. Skin cream and supplements such as glucosamine and chondroitin sulfate may provide relief of symptoms. Other treatments include corticosteroid injection and lifestyle changes such as diet, exercise, and weight loss. Since the condition may eventually require surgery and joint replacement, it is important

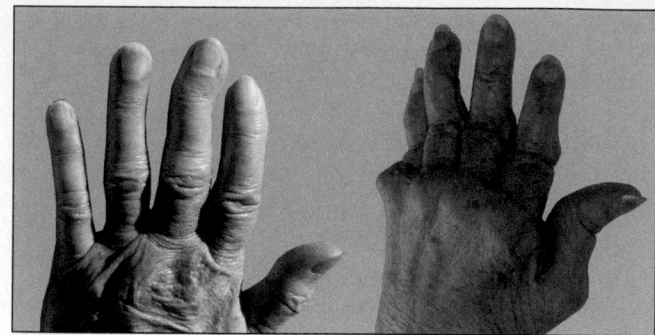

FIGURE 13-21
Comparison of (left) osteoarthritis and (right) rheumatoid arthritis; hands and joints.

to question the patient about any recent hospital stay because patients with joint replacement may need antibiotic premedication before dental visits.

Rheumatoid Arthritis
Rheumatoid arthritis (RA) is a chronic autoimmune disorder where the body's immune system mistakenly attacks the body's own tissue. Unlike the wear-and-tear damage of osteoarthritis, RA affects the lining of the joints, causing painful swelling that may result in bone erosion and joint deformity and physical disabilities. It attacks the lining of the membranes that surround the joints (*synovium*) resulting in a thickening of the synovium, which eventually destroys the cartilage and bone within the joint. The tendons and ligaments holding the joints together weaken and stretch, and the joint loses its shape and alignment and function. The dental care for RA needs to be modified to assist the patient in the loss of grasping a brush, and a pump up paste is easier for them. Studies show a strong connection between RA and periodontal disease; the bacterium that causes periodontal disease has been shown to increase the severity of rheumatoid arthritis.

RA is a chronic inflammatory disorder that can affect more than just the joints. It can damage many body systems, including the heart, lungs, blood vessels, skin, and eyes. Treatments can help manage RA, but there is no known cure. The patient is generally placed on an NSAID to reduce pain and inflammation, and they may also be taking a disease-modifying antirheumatic drug to help slow or stop RA from getting worse.

Osteoporosis
Osteoporosis is a disorder involving loss of mineral content and bone mass. More bone mass is being resorbed than reformed. Bone loss in osteoporosis is associated with increased age, the hormonal disturbances in menopause, calcium deficiency, and poor calcium absorption. Early stage bone loss, with levels below average, is a condition called osteopenia. Osteoporosis develops over many years. The condition, seen mostly in postmenopausal women, can also occur in men and in both men and women at an earlier age. Backaches are common, and with loss of support the person may exhibit a stooped posture. Loss of bone could affect the TMJ, presenting problems during dental care. Often the bones become fragile

and at risk for fracture. While osteoporosis itself does not cause periodontitis, it may affect the severity of the disease; evidence of bone changes can be seen in the mandible.

Treatment includes reducing risk factors such as high alcohol intake and using tobacco and caffeine. Protective factors can be maximized by increasing calcium and vitamin D intake and adding supplements to the diet. Exercise like weightlifting and walking can stimulate bone growth. Medications involve using hormone replacement therapy (HRT), parathyroid hormone (PTH) to stimulate bone formation, and bisphosphonates to inhibit bone resorption. Patients taking bisphosphonate drugs may be susceptible to **osteonecrosis** of the jaw. Before starting any drug therapy, the risks and benefits must be carefully considered for each individual patient.

Muscular Dystrophy (MD) MD is a progressive inherited disorder in which there is a degeneration of muscles causing severe weakness and loss of function. There are several types of the disorder, each progressing at a different rate and affecting specific muscle groups. Some cause little disability, such as fascioscapulohumeral MD (FSHD), while Duchenne MD is deadly. Duchenne MD, which occurs in childhood, accounts for about 50% of all muscular dystrophies. A defective gene causes MD. Because a woman may have no symptoms but still carry the gene, when there is a family history of muscular dystrophy genetic counseling is advised.

Symptoms vary with each type of the disorder, but progressive muscle weakness is the main indication. Specific groups of muscles may be affected. If the shoulder muscles are affected the patient may have difficulty raising their arms. Involvement of the facial muscles may make chewing and closing the eyes difficult. If the heart muscles are affected and become weak, there may be a disturbance in heart rhythm. Milder types of muscular dystrophy appear between the ages of 10 and 18 years. The more severe forms tend to occur in early childhood. Duchenne MD affects mostly boys and is detected when the child starts to walk. Signs include frequent falls, difficulty getting up from a lying or sitting position, waddling gait, and large calf muscles. The dental assistant should ask if the patient would like assistance and be prepared to help as needed. There may be learning disabilities present. Patients seen the dental office should be followed up with a physician consult particularly regarding anesthesia as there are adverse reactions, some of which are life-threatening.

There is no cure for muscular dystrophy, and current therapies are aimed at reducing deformities in the joints and spine and helping the patient stay mobile for as long as possible. Corticosteroids improve muscle strength and may delay the progression of certain types of the disease. Physical therapy exercises help preserve range of motion, and braces provide support and keep muscles and tendons stretched and flexible. Some people with severe muscular dystrophy may need a ventilator for breathing.

Endocrine Disorders

Endocrine disorders are grouped into two categories: hyposecretion, when the gland produces too little of an endocrine hormone, and hypersecretion of too much hormone production.

Hypothyroidism, hyperthyroidism, and diabetes are common endocrine disorders.

Hyperthyroidism Hyperthyroidism (overactive thyroid) is a common disorder and is caused by the thyroid gland producing too much of the hormone thyroxine. It can increase the body's metabolism, cause unintentional weight loss, a rapid or irregular heartbeat, palpitations, nervousness, anxiety, irritability, and increased appetite. If the patient is exhibiting symptoms, the dentist may defer elective treatment and consult their physician. The patient is generally prescribed an antithyroid medication. If left untreated it can result in heart problems and osteoporosis.

Hypothyroidism Hypothyroidism (underactive thyroid) is a common disorder in which the thyroid gland does not produce enough of certain crucial hormones to keep the body running normally. A number of symptoms such as intolerance to cold, feelings of tiredness, constipation, depression, and weight gain are presented. Occasionally a swelling of the front part of the neck due to goiter (enlarged thyroid gland) may appear. Patients with hypothyroidism are at an increased risk of heart disease and heart failure. Medicines that boost the levels of thyroid can help manage the condition, but there is no cure. The dental implications include xerostomia, which can cause accelerated tooth decay, greater risk of gum and oral infections, and burning mouth syndrome that causes a burning pain in the mouth.

Diabetes Mellitus Diabetes mellitus refers to a group of diseases that affect how the body uses blood sugar (glucose), which can lead to excess sugar in the blood. The pancreas releases insulin, which is the principal hormone that regulates blood glucose. Chronic diabetes conditions include type 1 diabetes and type 2 diabetes. In type 1 diabetes the immune system destroys the cells that produce insulin, and symptoms tend to come on quickly and are more severe. With type 2 diabetes the body's ability to respond to insulin is reduced and patients may not initially experience symptoms. Symptoms include increased thirst, frequent urination, extreme hunger with unexplained weight loss, fatigue, slow-healing sores, and frequent gum and skin infections. Treatment of diabetes concentrates on keeping glucose levels close to normal without causing low blood sugar, accomplished by dietary and exercise changes, minimizing stress, and if required insulin via injections or pumps. Diabetes is the most common endocrine disease, and the dental team is likely to encounter it frequently. Dental management should include scheduling short morning appointments, confirming the patient has eaten and taken all scheduled medications, and keeping stress to a minimum. Diabetes can turn into an emergency suddenly, making it crucial for the dental team to know the signs, symptoms, and emergency care (refer to Chapter 15).

Psychiatric Disorders

Psychiatric disorders may have both a psychological and biologic component where the patient experiences both mental and physical symptoms. See Chapter 17 for eating disorders.

Anxiety Disorder Most people experience some anxiety at times, and surprisingly, anxiety is often a strong source of motivation. Anxiety disorders include panic disorder, panic attacks, and post-traumatic stress disorder (PTSD). No single cause of anxiety disorder has been identified. The best explanation is thought to be a combination of psychosocial and biologic processes together. The condition, which often accompanies other psychiatric disorders such as mood disorder, personality disorder and schizophrenia, may be the result of emotional stress. Anxiety states are also associated with the use of certain drugs, hyperthyroidism, and mitral valve **prolapse**.

Anxiety is often felt mentally as a sense of danger, panic, tension, or dread that may or may not be real. The painful thoughts or impulses produced by these feelings are expressed physically as **tachycardia**, palpitations, chest pain, indigestion, headaches, shortness of breath, trembling or shaking, and sweating (clammy hands). Recurrent attacks characterize panic disorder. Panic attacks may occur unexpectedly and can be triggered by certain situations such as a **phobia**. PTSD is the result of a traumatic event associated with fear or threat to life such as war or disaster. Fear of going to the dentist is a common health care anxiety. Patients often have fear of the dental visit, particularly around claustrophobia, needles, sounds, or sensations. The dental team needs to use a number of calming techniques including showing empathy, taking time to listen to the patients voice their fears and concerns, and explaining procedures to help them relax.

Behavioral therapy includes relaxation, hypnosis, and biofeedback techniques as well as support from family and friends. It is essential to eliminate the use of caffeine, alcohol, and drugs

Dental Management of the Patient with a Psychiatric Disorder

- Avoid routine dental care until condition is stable.
- Review medical history, physician consultation may be necessary.
- Be alert for the signs of a psychiatric disorder.
- Do not rush; provide a comfortable, stress free environment, early appointments, and open communication; explain each step to the patient.
- Provide tinted protective eyewear, adjust dental light carefully, and change chair position slowly; patients with an anxiety disorder may need anti-anxiety premedication before dental treatment.
- Medication side effects— orthostatic hypotension, photosensitivity, xerostomia, taste changes, stomatitis, and glossitis.
- Self-care instruction—watch for signs of abrasion from vigorous tooth brushing, diet counseling, use of home fluoride, artificial saliva, and antimicrobial mouth rinses.
- Instruct caregiver.
- Consider use of local anesthesia.
- Determine if patient is legally able to make decisions.

of abuse because of the potential to intensify the disorder. Exercise often helps eliminate symptoms and gives the patient a sense of control. More severe cases require psychological treatment. Drugs used to manage the condition include antianxiety agents, antidepressants, and sedative hypnotics. The dental team needs to be aware of how to manage a patient with a psychiatric disorder.

Mood Disorders Sadness affects all people at some time in their life; however, people with mood disorders have symptoms that last most of the day. Mood disorders, which include major depression and bipolar disorder, have a complex set of symptoms, and both are characterized by periods of remission and recurrence. Reduced concentrations of the neurotransmitters norepinephrine and serotonin are suspected to cause depression, while increased concentrations of these chemicals may account for a manic episode. Bipolar disorder appears to have a strong genetic predisposition.

In general those experiencing major depression exhibit diminished interest in most activities, feel fatigue, have less ability to concentrate, have significant weight loss or gain, and may have recurrent thoughts of suicide. Depression can occur at any age and affects each age group differently. For example, children may be less motivated to learn and play while adolescents may exhibit antisocial behavior or turn to substance abuse. Depressed adults lack motivation and may have problems at work or in social interactions. The elderly may have feelings of isolation and worthlessness.

Persons with bipolar disorder experience a depressive phase as well as a **manic** phase. The depressive phase includes all the symptoms discussed for major depression. Extreme **euphoria**, hyperactivity, flight of thoughts, and excessive talking are characteristics of the manic phase. On the other hand, the mood may be irritable and angry. The dentist should refer patients found with signs and symptoms of mood disorder.

Depending on the disorder, mood stabilizing drugs and antidepressants are used for treatment. Depressed patients often have poor oral hygiene due to lack of disinterest in self-care and may develop xerostomia due to depression and drugs used for treatment. Individuals with mood disorder are often aware of the early signs of an episode and may be able to lessen its effects. Electroconvulsive therapy (ECT) may be considered for those patients who do not respond or are unable to take medication. Psychological and behavior therapy may benefit patients with lesser degrees of depression. In addition to medications, patients are encouraged to develop lifestyle changes that correct sleep disorders, diet modification, and exercise.

Schizophrenia Schizophrenia is a chronic, major **psychotic** disorder where the individual may be out of touch with reality. The cause of this disorder is unknown, but genetics and environment have been suspected. In susceptible individuals, certain events such as illness, drugs, and stressful psychological episodes appear to be the trigger. The cause has also been associated with an excess of dopamine at specific synapses in the brain. Onset of schizophrenia can be sudden or slow and can occur in late adolescence or early adulthood.

Disordered thinking, emotional changes, **delusions**, and **hallucinations** are hallmarks of the disorder. Function at work, social relations, and self-care decline. The patient may be confused, depressed, withdrawn, anxious, or without emotion. Some persons remain ill while others may experience periods of remission and recurrence. Antipsychotic medications reduce symptoms and improve the quality of life. Xerostomia is an oral side effect of medications and contributes to dental caries. Psychotherapy ensures compliance with medications, and vocational rehabilitation provides education and support that allow the patient to live a functional life.

Kidney Disease

The kidneys perform functions essential for life such as excreting waste, maintaining fluid balance, regulating acid–base balance of body fluids, regulating blood pressure, and producing red blood cells. Kidney disorders and disease can be acute or chronic. Acute conditions most frequently occur because of infection and inflammation; the disease runs its course and the kidney recovers. Chronic conditions can cause a slow, progressive loss of function.

The signs and symptoms of kidney disease may not be noticed, and many individuals are not diagnosed until there is irreversible damage. The continual destruction of the **nephrons** can lead to renal failure. Diabetes and hypertension are the main causes of end-stage renal disease.

Kidney disorders affect multiple body systems. With less kidney function, waste products are retained and **electrolyte** disturbance occurs. The patient may develop anemia, bleeding tendencies due to platelet dysfunction, and changes in bone production. Clinical signs and symptoms include edema, pallor, brown to yellow skin color, nausea, and vomiting. Oral findings are pale mucosa, increased gingival bleeding, increased calculus, petechiae, candidiasis, stomatitis, dry mouth, and ammonia taste. Radiographs may reveal bone changes, narrowing of the pulp chamber, abnormal calcifications in soft tissues, and a radiolucent **osseous** lesion. Laboratory and blood tests are used for diagnosis.

The goal of treatment is to slow the progress of disease and improve the quality of life. Conservative treatment includes diet modification to restrict protein and monitoring of fluid, sodium, and potassium intake. Control of associated conditions such as diabetes and hypertension is achieved with medication and lifestyle changes. As kidney function is reduced to a very low level, a medical procedure that artificially filters the kidney called dialysis may be necessary. The risks, benefits, type, frequency, and length of dialysis treatment are dependent on each individual patient. Because patients who are receiving dialysis may be using anticoagulation drugs, dental treatment should take place on any day other than the day of dialysis. End stage renal disease (ESRD) may require a kidney transplant. It is critical that the dental team follows dental management recommendations.

Respiratory Disorders

Respiratory disease—in particular, chronic obstructive pulmonary disease (COPD)—has been associated with poor oral health.

Dental Management of the Patient with Kidney Disease

- A physician consultation and antibiotic premedication may be necessary.
- Evaluate associated conditions and current medications.
- Dental treatment should take place on any day other than the day of dialysis.
- Monitor blood pressure at every visit but not in an arm with a dialysis access shunt.
- Watch dental chair position, do not place pressure on the arm with the shunt.
- Patients receiving dialysis are susceptible to blood borne disease transmission.
- Medication side effects— anticoagulant drugs may produce severe bleeding, immunosuppression, potential for toxic build-up of medications cleared by the kidneys—lidocaine/xylocaine, aspirin, nonsteroidal anti-inflammatory drugs, acetaminophen, penicillin, and clarithromycin
- Self-care instruction to eliminate any source of infection; the patient may be on a special diet that may affect oral health.

The most common forms of respiratory disorders encountered in the dental office are allergies and asthma. The dental management of patient with a respiratory disorder is important to avoid triggering an event in the dental office.

Dental Management of the Patient with a Respiratory Disorder

- Assess severity of disease; do not treat the patient if there is a respiratory infection present until the condition is stable with adequate breathing.
- To avoid respiratory discomfort, use upright or semi-supine chair position.
- If possible avoid use of dental dam.
- Avoid use of N2O sedation in severe cases.
- Avoid use of narcotics and barbiturates because they depress respiration.
- Use powdered materials such as alginate and gloves with caution.
- Avoid the use of power driven and air polishers and ultrasonic scaling devices.
- Self-care instructions—if necessary, initiate a smoking cessation program.

Allergies An allergy is initiated when the immune system mistakes a normally harmless substance for a dangerous invader. Allergies occur when the immune system reacts to a foreign protein (antigen) such as pollen, bee venom, pet dander, mold, and food that doesn't cause a reaction in most people. The immune system makes antibodies that identify a particular **allergen** as harmful. The immune system reaction with future allergen can inflame skin, sinuses, airways, or the digestive system. Allergic reactions can range from mild to severe. For example, hay fever can cause sneezing, itching of the eyes and nose, runny or stuffy nose, and watery, red, or swollen eyes (conjunctivitis). Allergies can trigger a life-threatening reaction known as **anaphylaxis**. Treatment includes avoiding known triggers, taking medications like antihistamines and corticosteroids to control symptoms, and using an **epi-pen** in case of an emergency. A patient may present with an allergy to a material used in the dental office such as a latex. A latex allergy may cause itchy skin, hives, or even anaphylaxis. Many offices have converted to all nonlatex materials.

Asthma

Asthma, also referred to as bronchial asthma, is a common condition in which there is an increased production of mucus and the airways of the lungs narrow and swell, causing a reversible obstruction. The symptoms include shortness of breath, chest tightness with pain, coughing, wheezing upon exhaling, and bronchospasms. Asthma can range from being a minor nuisance to a major problem that interferes with daily activities and may lead to a life-threatening asthma attack. Asthma worsens in the early morning, at night, and with exercise and cold. It is unknown why some people get asthma and others do not, but it is thought to be due to environmental and genetic factors. It cannot be cured, but its symptoms can be controlled through oral medication (corticosteroids) and delivery devices. There are several types of asthma inhalers; reliever inhalers that contain bronchodilators, preventer inhalers that usually contain a steroid, and long-acting bronchodilator inhalers (combination or nonsteroidal). The patient may also be prescribed a nebulizer that is a device that converts liquid medication into a fine spray of aerosols. Dental management includes requesting the patient to bring any prescribed inhalers with them to their dental appointment, and the inhaler should be placed next to the patient during treatment. If the patient has an asthma attack, dental treatment should be terminated, and the patient should be placed in upright position and assisted with the use of their inhaler.

Chronic Obstructive Pulmonary Disorder (COPD)

COPD is a general term used to describe pulmonary disorders that are characterized by obstruction of airflow to and from the lungs. In chronic bronchitis, inflammation causes a narrowing of the airway, and it becomes difficult to breathe in and out. In emphysema, there is a widening of the air spaces due to destruction of the alveolar walls. People with emphysema have difficulty exhaling.

Smoking is the main cause of COPD. The greater the number of cigarettes smoked, the greater the risk of developing disease. Other causes are underlying respiratory disease, genetics, long-term exposure to pollutants such as automobile emissions and household cleaning products, childhood problems such as underdeveloped lungs, and severe infection. People who have a deficiency in certain enzymes produced by the liver are also at risk.

COPD may take years to develop. Patients with bronchitis experience cough with large amounts of mucous, increased upper respiratory infection, and difficulty breathing. People with emphysema exhibit a dry cough and may have difficulty breathing with exertion; they may have to force the air from the lungs to exhale. Although bronchitis and emphysema are different, they often coexist, and patients may have symptoms of both diseases. There is no cure for COPD. Evidence of abnormalities for COPD may appear on a chest x-ray. People with the disease must reduce risk with smoking cessation and elimination of inhaled toxins. Use of vaccines to prevent infection such as pneumonia and flu is important. Medications include antibiotics, aerosol bronchodilators, and inhaled corticosteroids to reduce inflammation. Symptoms may be relieved with exercise, rehabilitation, and oxygen therapy. Surgical removal of part or all of one lung may be indicated for severe cases. A lung transplant may be an option for some individuals.

Cancer

Cancer is a group of diseases where abnormal cells spread by **metastasis** to other sites in the body, invading and destroying normal tissues. Although cancer is the second leading cause of death in the United States, early detection and effective treatment allow many more people to live longer. Cancer causing risk factors are smoking, alcohol abuse, obesity, poor nutrition, inactivity, overexposure to sunlight, and environmental or occupational exposure to chemicals such as asbestos.

Dental professionals play an important role in the detection of oral cancer and the management of complications related to therapy. In the United States, oral cancers, of which 9 out of 10 are **squamous cell carcinomas**, account for approximately 4% of all cancers with a 52% survival rate. Early detection of oral cancer is important for survival (Figure 13-22). The most common sites for squamous cell carcinomas are the ventral surface of the tongue, floor of the mouth, and oropharynx. If any of the signs

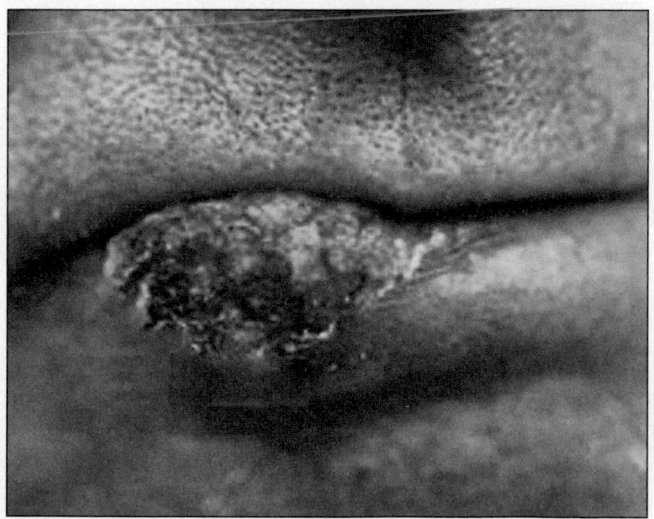

FIGURE 13-22
Cancer of the lip.

Courtesy of Mark L.Kliss

of oral cancer persist for longer than two weeks after removing irritants and therapy, then a biopsy must be considered to rule out oral cancer. Risk for oral cancer includes advancing age and any kind of tobacco use (cigarettes, cigars, pipes, and smokeless tobacco); the risk increases with amount and duration of tobacco use. There is added risk with the addition of heavy alcohol use. Other factors implicated but not proven are poor oral health, chronic trauma from ill-fitting dentures, and broken teeth.

Cancer causing agents alter the DNA of a cell. Mutated cells grow to form a tumor. **Malignant** cells can also penetrate the lymph and blood vessel walls and travel to other sites in the body. Most early cancers have no pain or other significant symptoms; however, it is important to recognize the early warning signs:

- A sore that does not respond to therapy
- Unusual bleeding or discharge
- Formation of a lump or mass
- Indigestion or difficulty swallowing
- Change in a wart or mole
- Chronic cough, hoarseness, sore throat
- Change in bowel or bladder habits
- Unexplained weight loss
- White patches inside the mouth or on the tongue

Surgery, radiation, and chemotherapy are the major ways to treat cancer and may be used alone or as a combination of all three. Therapy choice depends on the type of cancer and the size and location of the tumor. Immunotherapy shows promise and is being used to treat a growing number of malignancies. Other therapies include stem cell or bone marrow transplantation, use of hormones, vaccines, and biotherapy that is treatment to restore the ability of the body to fight disease. There are many complications that require the dental team to be knowledgeable of proper dental management of patients with cancer.

Dental Management of the Patient with Cancer

- Recognize signs and symptoms and educate the patient.
- Consult physician as to the best time to treat during therapy, and if antibiotic premedication is needed.
- Eliminate and prevent oral complications before cancer therapy.
- Examine dentures for pain, proper fit, irritation, and trauma.
- Treatment effects— chemotherapy may cause immunosuppression and bleeding problems, and if given before the age of 5–10 years may alter root development; radiation therapy to the body usually has no oral complications.
- Acute and chronic effects of head and neck radiation— may cause permanent dysfunction, mucositis, xerostomia, radiation caries, loss of taste, infections, **trismus**, or **osteoradionecrosis**.
- Oral self-care— oral hygiene instructions, tobacco and alcohol cessation, nutritional counseling, fluoride therapy.

HIV/AIDS

The human immunodeficiency virus (HIV) is a complex family of viruses that cause acquired immunodeficiency syndrome (AIDS). The virus causes impairment of the immune system allowing other health problems to occur. HIV/AIDS has become a worldwide public health problem.

The HIV virus can infect nearly all cells in the body, but the ones mainly affected are the CD4+ T-lymphocyte cells (T-helper cells) and macrophages, which are white blood cells that are an important part of the immune system. Once inside a cell, the virus multiplies and the cells are destroyed. HIV infection is confirmed with the use of blood tests. The number of T-helper cells is a marker used to evaluate the severity of disease. When a person is infected with the HIV virus, this count goes down, weakening the immune system. The lower the CD4 cell count is, the more likely it is that a person will get sick.

HIV virus is found in all body fluids, but only blood, semen, vaginal secretions, and breast milk contain enough viruses to transmit infection. Blood transfusion was once a source of HIV infection before testing and may still be in developing countries where tests are not available. While sexual contact is the main source of infection, intravenous (IV) drug users who share needles are at great risk. HIV+ mothers can transmit the virus to a fetus during pregnancy, during childbirth, or when breast feeding an infant.

Within 6–12 weeks after a person is first infected by the HIV virus, flu symptoms such as fever, lymph node enlargement, headache, rash, diarrhea, weight loss, and **pharyngitis** may appear. A

Dental Management of for the Patient with HIV/AIDS

- Dental professionals are ethically and legally obligated to treat persons who seek care who are HIV positive; they are protected by the Americans with Disabilities Act.
- Dental care for the HIV+ patient should be no different than any other patient; standard precautions must be followed for all patients.
- Careful intraoral and extraoral examination should detect signs and symptoms.
- Patients with a CD4+ cell count of more than 400 may receive all dental treatment; those with a cell count lower than 200 have increased susceptibility to infection and may need antibiotics before dental care.
- Physician consultation may be necessary.
- Effects of medications— xerostomia, nausea, and vomiting; evaluate for tooth erosion and caries
- Any source of oral infection should be controlled; use of chlorhexidine mouth rinse and fluoride varnish may be helpful.
- Oral self-care—immaculate oral hygiene and frequent recare visits to maintain oral health.

symptom free period of months to years may follow but the virus is still present and **replicating**. Signs of disease eventually reappear and opportunistic infections such as candidiasis begin to arise. Without treatment the disease progresses; CD4+ cell count falls below 200 and AIDS-defining diseases such as *pneumocystis carina pneumonia* (PCP) and Kaposi's sarcoma, a rare form of cancer can occur. Oral signs include oral **hairy leukoplakia** on the lateral borders of the tongue, **necrotizing ulcerative gingivitis** (NUG), oral warts, and recurrent herpes simplex virus.

There is no cure or prevention vaccine for HIV infection. Health education about risk, how the virus is passed from one person to another, and preventive measures to stop transmission is the first line of defense to stop the virus from spreading.

Current management to reduce the spread of the virus to healthy cells in the person infected with HIV includes the use of a combination of several antiviral drugs. A mix of drugs used in highly active antiretroviral therapy (HAAT) is commonly called an "HIV cocktail." The combination of drugs is more effective than the use of just one drug to control the spread of the infection. Using a cocktail of drugs also prevents the virus from mutating or becoming resistant and prolongs the life of HIV infected persons. The drugs are carefully monitored because of the serious side effects that range from headache and nausea to lipid abnormalities and organ failure. In order to give patients with HIV/AIDS the best care, the dental team needs to stay current with dental management recommendations.

Chapter Summary

Nearly one-fifth of all Americans have a physical, sensory, or intellectual disability according to the National Organization on Disability. The CDC reported that half of all Americans have a chronic disease. Many of these patients will seek help in the dental office. It is important for the dental assistant to be knowledgeable in how to manage patients with special needs and medically compromised patients who need special care. The dental assistant needs to be knowledgeable in how to modify routine procedures to accommodate these patients during dental office visits and to stay calm if something happens. The dental assistant needs to understand that disabled patients have the same needs as the nondisabled to be treated as equals and with respect.

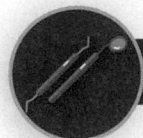 **CASE STUDY**

Aamira, a 52-year-old female patient, was just seated in the dental chair. The dental assistant began to explain the treatment for the day, which was to extract a severely fractured molar. At the end of the explanation, Aamira stated that she was having chest pain and began to show signs of shortness of breath, coughing, and wheezing upon exhalation.

Case Study Review

1. What condition exhibits all these signs?

2. What medication should the patient have been instructed to bring to the office and the assistant should have placed within easy access?

3. At what position should the dental chair be placed while the patient is taking their medicine?

Review Questions

Multiple Choice

1. All of these statements are true about developmental disabilities EXCEPT that they:
   a. are developed before birth.
   b. may develop at birth.
   c. are the result of disease, trauma, or injury.
   d. develop before age 22 years.

2. All of these disabilities are acquired EXCEPT:
   a. cerebral palsy.
   b. spinal cord paralysis.
   c. arthritis.
   d. limb amputation.

3. All of these accommodations are required by the Americans with Disability Act EXCEPT:
   a. designated wide parking spaces close to the building.
   b. special ordered dental chairs.
   c. hallways large enough for a wheelchair to turn around in.
   d. front entrance ramps.

4. Who is legally responsible to provide informed consent for the use of protective body stabilization?
   a. any patient over the age of 18
   b. any patient over the age of 21
   c. any mentally competent patient
   d. a legal caregiver

5. What causes a decubitus ulcer?
   a. caustic foods
   b. prolonged pressure on the skin
   c. strenuous exercise
   d. extreme heat

6. Which patient should not be moved from their wheelchair?
   a. patient who feels threatened
   b. patient who does not have a caregiver helping
   c. patient using a ventilator
   d. patients connected to any tubing

7. During the one person wheel chair transfer, where should the wheelchair be positioned to the dental chair?
   a. parallel
   b. 10 degrees
   c. 20 degrees
   d. 30 degrees

8. All of these are recommended in assisting a visual impaired patient EXCEPT:
   a. ask if they want help before giving it.
   b. let the patient set the pace.
   c. make service animals remain in the reception area.
   d. point out obstacles as they walk.

9. Which of these statements is true when communicating with a deaf or hard of hearing patient?
   a. All patients will be able to speak and read lips.
   b. Sign language can be used with all patients.
   c. Offer patient to write their preferred way to communicate.
   d. Speak slowly and loudly when addressing the patient.

10. Which oral findings may be present for a patient with cerebral palsy?
    a. imperfect formation and missing teeth, increased periodontal infections
    b. damaging oral habits, increased dental disease, food pouching
    c. abnormal muscle and tongue movement, swallowing difficulty
    d. increased disease due to decreased immune function, enlarged tongue and tonsils

11. With which disability would a patient exhibit trouble focusing, short attention span, and impulsive behavior?
    a. ADD/ADHD
    b. cerebral palsy
    c. autism
    d. Down syndrome

12. With which disability would a patient have limited social interaction and react negatively to sounds, bright colors, touching, and distractions?
    a. ADD/ADHD
    b. cerebral palsy
    c. autism
    d. Down syndrome

13. All of these are effects of aging EXCEPT:
    a. loss of elasticity in blood vessels.
    b. decreased cardiac output.
    c. slower mental ability.
    d. increase in tooth loss.

14. All of these are good dental management of the older patient EXCEPT:
    a. schedule appointments in late morning or early afternoon.
    b. schedule fewer recare appointments.
    c. address patient as Mr., Mrs., or Miss.
    d. ask if they need help walking and seating.

15. What disorder or disease would require that routine dental care be avoided until it is controlled?
    a. multiple sclerosis
    b. hypertension
    c. Parkinson's
    d. HIV

16. What disorder or disease's early detection in the dental office is important for the patient's survival?
    a. ALS
    b. COPD
    c. cancer
    d. coagulation disorder

17. Which disorder or disease requires the patient check their blood glucose level before dental treatment?
    a. muscular dystrophy
    b. diabetes mellitus
    c. HIV
    d. anemia

18. Which disorder or disease may result in life threatening bleeding during routine dental procedures?
    a. leukemia
    b. hemophilia
    c. endocarditis
    d. angina

19. Protective body stabilization may be needed for patient support, balance, and aggressive behavior. A full body wrap should be used for routine use with small children.
    a. Both statements are true.
    b. Both statements are false.
    c. The first statement is true; the second statement is false.
    d. The first statement is false; the second statement is true.

20. The ADA set standards to assist the dentist in creating a barrier free environment. Dental offices must follow state and city laws for persons with disabilities.
    a. Both statements are true.
    b. Both statements are false.
    c. The first statement is true; the second statement is false.
    d. The first statement is false; the second statement is true.

Critical Thinking

1. Defend the need for the Americans with Disabilities Act.
2. Describe when the term *special needs* would apply to a patient.
3. Why is a holistic view of oral health important when treating the special needs patient?
4. Why would it be difficult for the patient with a disability to tolerate dental care and the dental team to provide dental care?

Key Terms

Term and Pronunciation	Meaning of Root and Word Parts	Definition
acuity (*uh*-**kyoo**-i-tee)	**acus** = needle **-ity** = state or condition	sharpness, keenness
allergen (**al**-er-ju*hn*)	**allergy** = an abnormal reaction to a previously encountered substance **-gen** = that which produces	any substance, often protein, that induces a hypersensitivity that causes the body to react to contact; sneezing, itching, and skin rashes
anaphylaxis (an-*uh*-fu*h*-**lak**-sis)	**ana-** = up, upwards, again, against **prophylaxis** = protective treatment for disease	a severe, potentially life-threatening allergic reaction resulting from previous exposure to it; sudden drop in blood pressure, airway narrows, rash, nausea, vomiting
angina pectoris (**an**-ju*h*-nu*h*) (**pek**-tu*h*-ris)	**angina** = any attack of painful spasms; sensations of choking or suffocating **pectoris** = pectoral muscle; chest or breast	a syndrome characterized by constricting pain below the sternum; chest pain usually due to coronary artery disease
anomaly (*uh*-**nom**-*uh*-lee)	**anomalous** = irregular **-y** = inclined to	a deviation from the common rule, type, arrangement, or form.
anoxia (an-**ok**-see-*uh*)	**an-** = without **ox** = oxygen **-ia** = condition	an abnormally low amount of oxygen in the body tissues
anticoagulant (an-tee-koh-**ag**-yu*h*-lu*h*nt)	**anti-** = against, opposite of **coagulum** = clump, clot **-ant** = causing or performing an action	medicines that increase the time it takes for blood to clot; blood thinners
arrhythmia (*uh*-**rith**-mee-*uh*)	**a-** = without **rhythm** = uniform or patterned recurrence of a beat, accent **-ia** = denoting a condition	any disturbance in the rhythm of the heartbeat
atherosclerosis (ath-*uh*-roh-sklu*h*-**roh**-sis)	**athero-** = a mass of yellowish fatty and cellular substance forming in and below the lining of arterial walls; often causes obstruction of blood flow **scler-** = hard **-osis** = denotes condition	fat buildup in the arteries, hardening of the arteries; leading cause of stroke, heart attack, and peripheral vascular disease
atrophy (**a**-tru*h*-fee)	**a-** = not, without **tropho-** = nourishment **-y** = inclined to	a wasting away of the body or organ
cheilitis (kahy-**lahy**-tis)	**cheil** = lip **-itis** = inflammation	inflammation of the lips
cognitive (**kog**-ni-tiv)	**cognition** = something known **-ive** = function, connection	the mental processes of perception, memory, judgment, and reasoning
congenital (ku*h*n-**jen**-i-tl)	**con** = together **-gen** = that which produces **-al** = pertaining to	a condition present at birth
cyanosis (sahy-*uh*-**noh**-sis)	**cyan** = blue or dark blue **-osis** = denotes actions, conditions, or states, especially abnormal states	blueness of the skin, as from imperfectly oxygenated blood
debilitate (dih-**bil**-i-teyt)	**de-** = away from, out of **habilitate** = to make fit	to make weak or feeble

(Continues)

Term and Pronunciation	Meaning of Root and Word Parts	Definition
decubitus ulcer (dih-**kyoo**-bi-t*uh*) (**uhl**-ser)	**decubitus** = any position assumed by a patient when lying in bed **ulcer** = an open sore on the skin	open skin wound that forms where the pressure from body's weight pressing against the skin on a firm surface; referred to as bed sore
delusion (dih-**loo**-zh*uh* n)	**delude** = to mislead the mind; deceive **-sion** = the state of being	a fixed false belief that is resistant to reason or confrontation with facts
desensitize (dee-**sen**-si-tahyz)	**de** = indicates removal or separation **sense** = faculties as touch, sight, taste **-ize** = to make	to make indifferent or unaware in feeling
diastolic (dahy-*uh*-**stol**-ik)	**diastole** = normal rhythmical dilatation of the heart when chambers are filling with blood **-ic** = pertaining to	measurement of blood pressure; indicating arterial pressure during the interval between heartbeats
ecchymosis (ek-*uh*-**moh**-sis)	**ec** = out **chym** = juice **osis** = denotes action	a discoloration of the skin due to a bruise; passage of blood from ruptured blood vessel
electrolyte (ih-**lek**-tr*uh*-lahyt)	**electro** = electric; electricity **-lyte** = indicating a substance that can be decomposed or broken down	a solution or molten substance that conducts electricity
endocarditis (en-doh-kahr-**dahy**-tis)	**endo-** = within **card-** = heart **-itis** = inflammation	inflammation of the thin membranous lining (endocardium) of the heart's cavities.
epi-pen (**epee**-pen)	**epi-** = epinephrine; hormone secreted by central nervous system in response to stress **pen** = any of various instruments	auto-injector of epinephrine for emergency treatment of allergies
ergonomic (ur-g*uh*-**nom**-iks)	**ergo-** = work **-nomy** = distribution, management **-ics** = denotes principles	study of people in the work environment; design or modification of the work to make it most efficient and safe
euphoria (yoo-**fawr**-ee-*uh*)	**eu-** = good, well **phore** = person or thing that produces **-ia** = condition	state of intense happiness and self-confidence
fetus (**fee**-t*uh*s)	**fetus** = the young in the womb	a developing baby at the end of the second month of gestation
hallucination (h*uh*-loo-s*uh*-**ney**-sh*uh* n)	**hallucin** = wander in mind **-ate** = process **-tion** = indicating a state	a sensory experience of something that does not exist outside the mind
hemoglobin (**hee**-m*uh*-gloh-bin)	**hemo-** = blood **globulin** = any of several groups of blood plasma proteins	the oxygen-carrying pigment of red blood cells; gives cells their red color and conveys oxygen to tissues
holistic (hoh-**lis**-tik)	**holos** = whole **-ist** = hold certain principles, doctrines **-ic** = pertaining to; relating to	relating to the medical consideration of the complete person, physically and psychologically, in the treatment of a disease
hypoxia (hahy-pok-**see**-*uh*)	**hypo-** = decreased **oxy-** = oxygen **-ia** = condition, state	deficiency in the amount of oxygen delivered to the body tissues
impairment (im-**pair**-m*uh*nt)	**-impair** = to damage **-ment** = denoting action or state	the state to being physically or mentally diminished, weakened, or damaged
implication (im-pli-**key**-sh*uh* n)	**imply** = to indicate or suggest without being explicitly stated **-ate** = process **-tion** = indicating a state	something suggested as naturally to be inferred or understood
incompatible (in-k*uh*m-**pat**-*uh*-b*uh*l)	**in** = not **com** = exist together in harmony **-ible** = possessing power to do something	unable to exist together in harmony
jaundice (**jawn**-dis)	**jaundice** = yellowish discoloration of whites of eyes or skin caused by excess bile pigments in blood	a medical condition with yellowing the skin or whites of the eyes; typically caused by obstruction of the bile duct, liver disease, or breakdown of red blood cells
leukemia (loo-**kee**-mee-*uh*)	**leuk-** = white **-emia** = denotes condition of the blood	a malignant cancer of blood-forming tissues; increased number of immature or abnormal leukocytes that suppress the production of normal blood cells

Term and Pronunciation	Meaning of Root and Word Parts	Definition
malignant (m*uh*-**lig**-n*uh*nt)	**malign** = bad, injurious **-ant** = characterized by	tending to produce death; characterized by uncontrolled growth; cancerous, rapid spreading
manic (**man**-ik)	**mania** = excessive excitement or enthusiasm **-ic** = pertaining to	mental disorder characterized by excitement and delusion
metastasis (m*uh*-**tas**-t*uh*-sis)	**meta** = indicating change; alteration **stasis** = a state or condition in which there is not action or progress; static situation	transference of disease-producing organisms or malignant or cancerous cells to other parts of the body
murmur (**mur**-mer)	**murmur** = to continuously make a low or indistinct sound	an abnormal sound heard usually through a stethoscope.
myelin sheath (**mahy**-*uh*-lin) (sheeth)	**myel** = spinal cord; bone marrow **-in** = made of **sheath** = covering part or structure	wrapping around certain nerve axons; serving as an electrical insulator that speeds nerve impulse to muscles and other effectors
myocardial infarction (mahy-*uh*-**kahr**-dee-*uh*l) (in-**fahrk**-sh*uh*n)	**myo-** = muscle **cardium** = denotes tissue or organs associated with the heart **-al** = pertaining to **infarct** = a localized area of dead tissue resulting from obstruction of blood to that part **-ion** = denoting condition or action	death of heart muscle; another term for heart attack
necrotizing ulcerative gingivitis (**nek**-r*uh*-tahyz-ing) (**uhl**-s*uh*-rey-tiv) (jin-j*uh*-**vahy**-tis)	**necro-** = necrosis, death **-ize** = to convert into **ulcer** = open sore **-ive** = relating to **gingiv-** = gingiva; gums **-itis** = inflammation	progressive painful infection with ulceration, swelling, and sloughing off of dead tissue from the mouth and throat; trench mouth
nephron (**nef**-ron)	**nephron** = the functional unit of the kidney	the filtering and excretory unit of the kidney
oral hairy leukoplakia (**awr**-*uh*l) (**hair**-ee) (loo-k*uh*-**pley**-kee-*uh*)	**or-** = mouth **-al** = pertaining to **hairy** = consisting of or resembling hair **leuko-** = white **plaque** = flat, often raised patch **-ia** = denoting a disease or condition	condition common with weakened immune system; creamy white patches on tongue that can be wiped away
orthostatic hypotension (awr-th*uh*-**stat**-ik) (hahy-p*uh*-**ten**-shun)	**ortho-** = upright, correct **static** = pertaining to a stationary condition **hypo-** = decreased, lowered **tension** = pressure; blood pressure	abnormal decrease in blood pressure when a person stands upright
osseous (**os**-ee-uhs)	**oss-** = bone **-eous** = composed of	composed of bone; bony
osteonecrosis (osteo -n*uh*-**kroh**-sis)	**osteo** = bone **necr** = dead **-osis** = condition	death of bone tissue
osteoradionecrosis (os-tee-oh-rey-dee-oh-n*uh*-**kroh**-sis)	**osteo** = bone **radio** = radiation **necr** = dead tissue **-osis** = condition	bone tissue death induced by radiation
pallor (**pal**-er)	**pale** = light-colored or lacking in color **-or** = denoting a condition	an unhealthy deficiency of color of the face; as from fear, ill health, or death
palpitation (pal-pi-**tey**-shuhn)	**palpitate** = to pulsate, throb **-ion** = denoting action or condition	unpleasant sensation of irregular and/or forceful beating of the heart
paralysis (p*uh*-**ral**-*uh*-sis)	**para** = side by side **palsy** = paralysis; impairment or loss **-sis** = of action or condition	a loss or impairment of voluntary movement in a body part, caused by injury or disease
petechiae (pi-**tee**-kee-*uh*)	**petecchie** = rash, spot on skin	a minute, round, nonraised hemorrhage in the skin or a mucous membrane
pharyngitis (far-in-**jahy**-tis)	**pharynx** = throat; cavity that connects mouth and nasal passages with esophagus **-itis** = inflammation	inflammation of the mucous membrane of the pharynx; sore throat

(Continues)

Term and Pronunciation	Meaning of Root and Word Parts	Definition
phobia (**foh**-bee-*uh*)	**phobe** = fear **-ia** = denoting a condition	a persistent, irrational fear of a specific object
plaque (plak)	**plaque** = a flat patch on skin or organ	collection of fatty acids on the wall of the artery that bulges into the opening and potentially blocking passage
poliomyelitis (poh-lee-oh-mahy-*uh*-**lahy**-tis)	**polio** = gray matter in spinal cord **myel** = myelin sheath **-itis** = inflammation	an acute viral disease; inflammation of motor neurons of the brain stem and spinal cord resulting in paralysis; referred to as polio
prenatal (pree-**neyt**-l)	**pre** = before **natal** = pertaining to a person's birth	previous to birth or to giving birth
prolapse (**proh**-laps)	**pro** = forward, out **lapse** = to fall or deviate from a previous standard	medical condition where an organ or tissue falls out of place; generally slips down
proprioception (proh-pree-*uh*-**sep**-sh*uh* n)	**proprio** = one's own **perceive** = to become aware **-tion** = the act or faculty	the unconscious awareness of the position of one's body
prosthesis (pros-**thee**-sis)	**pros-** = in front of **thesis** = a setting down or placing	replacement of a missing body part with an artificial substitute
psychotic (sahy-**kot**-ik)	**psycho-** = indicating the mind or mental processes **-otic** = denoting relationship to an action; condition	a serious mental illness characterized by defective or lost contact with reality
rehabilitation (ree-h*uh*-**bil**-i-teyt)	**re** = again **habilitate** = to make fit **-ion** = denotes action	to restore to a condition of good health or ability to work.
replicate (**rep**-li-keyt)	**replica** = an exact copy or reproduction **-ate** = denoting action	to repeat, duplicate, or reproduce
rheumatic (roo-**mat**-ik)	**rheum** = watery discharge from mucous membrane **-ic** = having characteristics of	pertaining to rheumatism; inflammatory disorder of the extremities or back, characterized by pain and stiffness
squamous cell carcinoma (**skwey**-m*uh* s) (sel) (kahr-s*uh*-**noh**-m*uh*)	**squama** = a scale or scalelike structure **-ous** = possessing **cell** = the basic structural unit of all organisms **carcino** = cancer **-oma** = indicating a tumor	a malignant and invasive tumor covered with or formed by scales that spread by metastasis; cancer
stenosis (sti-**noh**-sis)	**steno** = narrow, close **-osis** = denotes actions, conditions	a narrowing or stricture of a passage or vessel
tachycardia (tak-i-**kahr**-dee-*uh*)	**tachy-** = swift, accelerated **card** = heart **-ia** = denotes an action	excessively rapid heartbeat
teratogen (t*uh*-**rat**-*uh*-j*uh*n)	**terato** = monster **-gen** = that which produces	a drug or other substance capable of interfering with the development of a fetus, causing birth defects
tolerate (**tol**-*uh*-reyt)	**tolerare** = to bear **-ate** = denotes function	to put up with
trismus (**triz**-m*uh* s)	**trismus** = a firm closing of the jaw due to tonic spasms of the muscles	a spasm of the jaw muscles that makes it difficult to open the mouth; lockjaw
vena cava (**vee**-n*uh* **key**-v*uh*)	**vena** = vein **cava** = hollow	either of two large veins discharging blood into the right atrium of the heart

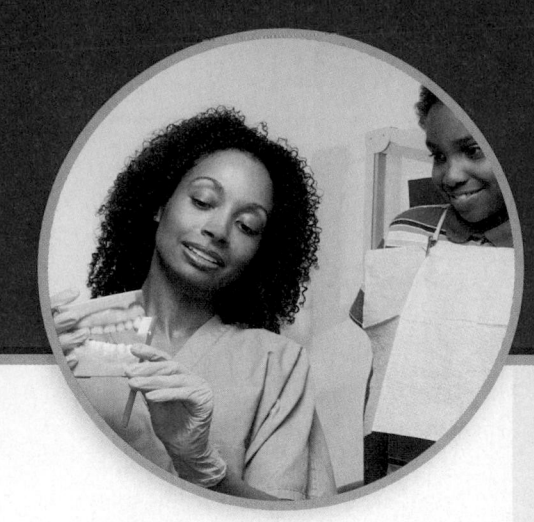

## CHAPTER 14

Pharmacology

Specific Instructional Objectives

At the completion of this chapter, you will be able to meet these objectives:

1. Use terms presented in this chapter.
2. State why it is important for the dental assistant to study pharmacology.
3. Discuss the significance of drug laws.
4. Explain the process of new drug development.
5. Recognize that a drug might be known by several names.
6. Identify the drug references available.
7. Discuss how drug dosages are calculated.
8. Compare and contrast the different routes of drug administration.
9. Outline the steps the body uses to process a drug.
10. Identify the information that belongs in each part of a prescription.
11. Provide the English meanings of the common Latin abbreviations used for prescriptions.
12. Discuss the regulations governing prescription drugs.
13. Recognize the signs of a substance use disorder in a dental patient.
14. Define what is meant by a therapeutic action of a drug.
15. Differentiate among the various types of adverse drug reactions.
16. Discuss the types of drugs commonly administered in a dental office.
17. Compare and contrast aspirin, ibuprofen and acetaminophen.
18. Discuss the dangers of inappropriate use of antibiotics.
19. Discuss the types of drugs commonly prescribed in a dental office.
20. Discuss the drugs that are specific to dental disease.
21. Recognize commonly used dental local anesthetics by name and concentration.
22. Discuss the reasons for selection of a local anesthetic with or without a vasoconstrictor.
23. Recognize medications on the medical history that may impact dental care.
24. Recognize common medications used for the following:
    a. cardiovascular disease
    b. endocrine disorders
    c. psychiatric disorders
    d. neurological disorders
    e. osteoporosis
    f. substance abuse

25. Explain the oral side effects of medications used for:

    a. cardiovascular disease

    b endocrine disorders

    c. psychiatric disorders

    d. neurological disorders

    e. osteoporosis

    f. cancer chemotherapy

26. Apply treatment modifications for patient management changes for patients taking:

    a. cardiovascular drugs

    b. endocrine drugs

    c. cancer chemotherapy

    d. osteoporosis medications

    e. Antabuse or methadone

Introduction

The terms *pharmacology* and *drugs* are normally associated with treating a disease, but they cover a much broader range of chemically induced changes in the body. The study of drugs, their properties, their reactions with each other, and their actions in the body is referred to as *pharmacology*. Pharmacology is constantly evolving due to emerging information and knowledge about drugs, new drugs being created, and existing drugs being altered. A *drug* is a substance that can change life processes within the body.

Drugs have never been as widely used and misused as they are today. The dental assistant needs to pay attention to patients' medical and dental histories, and carefully document the drugs used by each patient. The dental assistant must have knowledge about pharmacology, the side effects of drugs, and the interactions that take place when more than one drug is used.

Why Study Pharmacology?

A dental assistant may wonder, "Why should I learn about medications? Isn't that the dentist's job?" The dentist is ultimately responsible for making medication-related decisions, but the dental assistant needs to understand the drugs used or prescribed in the dental office and how these drugs may interact with other drugs the patient may be taking.

Knowledge of pharmacology will help you become a better consumer of prescription and over-the-counter (OTC) drugs. All health care professionals should have a working knowledge of basic pharmacology to be able to make wise decisions for their own medications and to help explain medications to patients. It is not reasonable to remember everything about every medication, but the dental assistant should know where to find the answers.

In most offices, it is a dental assistant who is responsible for maintaining inventory and ordering supplies. This includes drugs routinely used in the office and those needed in the emergency kit (Figure 14-1). In addition to ensuring an adequate supply of necessary medications, the assistant must check expiration dates of medications and store them according to manufacturer's requirements.

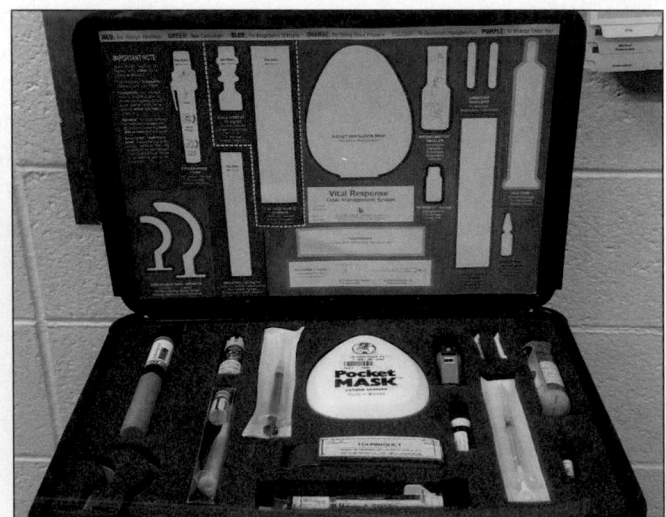

FIGURE 14-1
Emergency drug kit.

The dental assistant prepares the treatment room and has all necessary medications ready before the doctor and patient enter the room. By checking the scheduled treatment, the patient's medical history, and the doctor's preferences, the assistant anticipates the correct medication. If the dentist needs to write a prescription, the assistant will have the prescription pad ready and fill in some of the information on the prescription in advance. Some offices may provide electronic prescriptions directly to the patient's pharmacy. In that case a paper prescription is not provided and the patient would go to their pharmacy to pick up the prescription once it has been filled. Additionally, it is usually the dental assistant who discusses the medication with the patient. Patients often wait until the dentist has left the room to ask questions about their medication. Remember, these discussions are considered privileged information and are covered by HIPAA. The assistant should be prepared to answer questions intelligently and to refer to the dentist when necessary. This lesson will explain resources available to find information about medications. At the end of the appointment, it is usually the dental assistant who records the treatment notes in the patient's record. Documentation of medications administered or prescribed is part of the treatment record.

Scope of Dental Therapeutics

Most dental offices work with very few types of medication. There are three major groups of drugs the dental professional uses: anesthetics, **analgesics**, and **antibiotics**.

Local anesthetics and **topical anesthetics** are found in all offices, and most offices use a limited amount of antibiotics as well. Many offices also use **sedatives** and inhalation anesthetics or analgesics. Even the fluoride treatments administered in dental offices are considered drugs to be dispensed by prescription and under supervision of the dentist.

Laws require that the dentist prescribe medications only within the scope of practice. Additionally, a dentist may only prescribe medication for someone who is a patient of record in the dental practice and for conditions related to the dental treatment. The two most common dental conditions requiring medication are pain and infection, so analgesics and antibiotics are the drugs most often prescribed by dentists. In addition, some dentists prescribe medications for relaxation or relief of anxiety during treatment.

It is not difficult to become familiar with the medications a dentist administers or prescribes. A greater challenge is to have an understanding of all the medications a patient may be using, both prescription and over-the-counter (OTC), legal and illegal. It is important to know all of the medications and supplements a patient is using before administering or prescribing any medication in the dental office. All of these drug groups are explained further in later lessons.

Drug Laws

In 1906, the U.S. government passed *the Pure Food and Drug Act*. This law was enacted to control and regulate the composition, sale, and distribution of drugs. Prior to 1906, drugs were not regulated, and drugs of varying compositions and purity were sold. Many of these drugs were harmful for human consumption.

Other laws were passed to control the sale of **narcotic** drugs in the early twentieth century. *The Federal Food, Drug, and Cosmetic Act* was passed in 1938. This allowed only the United States Food and Drug Administration (FDA) to have control of all food, cosmetics, and drugs sold. The drugs and cosmetics must pass standards set by the FDA and obtain approval prior to sale. The FDA also controls advertising for all food, drugs, and cosmetics. This act was amended in 1951 and 1965 to add regulations to prevent tampering with foods, drugs, and cosmetics. It also required that certain preparations have warning labels, such as, "This product may cause drowsiness," or "Do not drive while taking this product." This act also includes a clause that states that any nonprescription or prescription drug must be shown to be effective as well as safe. Products may note on their packaging that they have met the rigid standards set by the FDA.

The *Comprehensive Drug Abuse Prevention and Control Act* of 1970 was established to identify drugs according to five schedules of abuse potential. Title II of this act deals with the control of drugs and enforcement of drug laws. The *Controlled Substances Act* gives the power of enforcement of this act to the DEA, which is part of the U.S. Department of Justice. Individuals who dispense drugs must have DEA-issued numbers to prescribe drugs. Dentists who dispense controlled substances improperly can have their offices closed and their licenses revoked. The dental assistants and the dentist must carefully check patients' medical and dental histories prior to writing any prescription.

Drug Development and Testing

FDA testing ensures that drugs are both safe and effective. In other words, a drug must be proven to achieve its effect, and it must cause no harm in doing so. Once the FDA determines that a drug is safe enough to be approved for sale to the public, it also determines whether the drug will be sold by prescription only or over the counter.

The FDA sets high standards for drug safety research, so drug development can take many years and cost millions of dollars. If a new drug performs well in testing, the drug company will apply for a **patent** on the formula. Once a patent is issued, no other company may produce this drug during the life of the patent, 17 years. Because of the cost and time involved in getting a new drug approved by the FDA, similar medications may be available in other countries sooner and at lower cost than they are in the United States. Some people travel to these countries to buy the medicine or purchase it over the Internet. Health care professionals should educate their patients that drugs purchased this way may not be as safe as drugs from the Unites States because they have not met the stringent testing that is required by the United States.

In addition to FDA testing, the American Dental Association (ADA) has a Seal of Acceptance Program for OTC dental health products. After evaluation and approval by the ADA Council on Scientific Affairs, companies may print the ADA Seal of Acceptance on their product packaging. This program is voluntary for companies who manufacture dental products, but it does involve time and cost to the company. Dental professionals and consumers should understand that FDA approval is mandatory and ensures that the product is safe and effective. The ADA seal shows that the manufacturer has gone beyond these requirements for a product. However, a product without the ADA seal is still a safe and effective product because it has passed the FDA standards.

Sources of Drugs

Many years ago, all drugs came from naturally occurring sources: plants, animals, or minerals that were accessible to the healers in a community. Remedies were passed down through generations and tested by trial and error. As medicine and pharmacology evolved, some of these natural remedies were discarded, but some were found to be effective. Today, some medicines are still made using these natural sources, and many of the drugs that we use today were originally derived from natural sources. Drugs derived from natural sources are known as nonsynthetic drugs. For example, penicillin was originally derived from a natural mold.

Other medicines are entirely manufactured in the laboratory. These drugs are called synthetic. Many medications are made using a combination of natural and synthetic ingredients. For example, the prescription pain reliever Tylenol #3 is a combination of acetaminophen, a synthetic, and codeine, a drug from plant sources.

Drug Names

Discussing drugs can be very confusing. A single drug may have a variety of names. It is important to recognize common drugs by their many names. Otherwise, a patient may take several medicines that have the same ingredients or take a medicine to which they have an allergy or other **adverse** reaction.

The first name a drug receives is a chemical name. This name is usually a long list of chemicals that make up the drug. Using this name in conversation would be like saying, "flour-yeast-sugar-water" when discussing bread. For example, acetylsalicylic acid (ASA) is aspirin. Except for chemists, drug company researchers, and pharmacology experts, the chemical name is used only in the early stages of research and drug development. When a drug has been tested and is ready to be sold to the public, the company owning the drug chooses a *proprietary*, or brand, name. This name is chosen to help sell the drug. It may provide some hint as to the drug's actions, or it may be chosen because it is easy to remember or pleasant-sounding. For example, Lopressor is a drug for hypertension. The name is made up of parts of the words "low" and "pressure." This name tells something about the drug. Inderal is also a drug for hypertension. This name gives no hint as to what type of drug Inderal is. Yaz is a common birth control medication. The name does not give any information about the drug's purpose, but it is short, simple, and easy to remember.

The brand (proprietary) name of the drug belongs to the company that developed the drug. Usually, this company has spent large amounts of time and money in the development process. The company profits only if the drug becomes successful. The company holds a patent on the formula for the drug and a trademark on the brand name. No other company may manufacture the drug or use the brand name for 17 years. This allows the company to regain the money spent on research and sometimes earn a profit. After the patent expires, other companies will be able to produce the drug under brand names chosen by each company. Thus, a popular drug that has been on the market for a long time may be sold under several brand names. Use of brand names can lead to confusion and misunderstanding by patients and dental professionals. When the patent expires on a brand name drug, any other manufacturer who wishes to sell the drug must meet FDA approval. The FDA checks each **generic** drug to ensure that it is equally as safe and **efficacious** as the original.

The third name a drug has is the generic name. The generic name for a drug never changes and is not capitalized, even if many companies sell the drug under different brand names. When reading about medications, an easy way to determine if the name used is the brand name or the generic name is to note whether the name is capitalized. Because the brand name is a proper noun, like your own name, it is always capitalized. The generic name is a common noun and is not capitalized. For example, *Kleenex* is a brand name. and *facial tissue* is a generic name. *Advil* and *Motrin* are brand names for ibuprofen.

It is advisable for the dental assistant to be familiar with the brand and generic names of all the drugs used or prescribed by the dentist. Also, when the assistant encounters an unfamiliar brand name in a patient's medical history, the assistant should look up the medication and fill in the generic name on the medical history.

Drug References

New drugs are being introduced to the market every day. The dentist and assistant must have a working knowledge of all the drugs administered or prescribed in the dental office. It is not possible to maintain this same level of knowledge for all the prescriptions, OTC drugs, and supplements that patients may be taking. Every dental office should have several drug references on hand. Drug references are now available in both print and electronic media. Printed drug references become outdated very quickly. An online drug reference that is updated regularly will have the most recent information on OTC and prescription medications.

The *Physician's Desk Reference* (PDR) is a comprehensive drug resource that is widely used and accepted. It is published yearly and is relatively inexpensive. The PDR is a very large book and so is not handy for use in the treatment area, but most dental offices will have at least one PDR in their library. The PDR can also be purchased as a CD-ROM, or dentists can join PDR.net, an online drug resource, at no cost. PDR.net can be accessed from a computer in the office or from a handheld electronic device such as a smartphone or a tablet. The print version of the PDR allows you to look up a drug by its generic name, brand name, classification, or manufacturer. There is even a section with photographs of many commonly used medications.

In addition to the standard PDR that covers prescription drugs, a second *PDR for Non-prescription Drugs, Dietary Supplements, and Herbs* is available. Dental professionals must remember that patients take a variety of agents in addition to their prescription medications. Nonprescription medications, supplements, and herbs can have interactions and side effects just as prescription medications do. A medication sold over the counter or claimed to be a "natural remedy" should never be assumed to be more safe or better than prescription medications.

The PDR provides highly technical information about drugs. Drug manufacturers pay the publisher to have their drugs listed in the PDR. This is both an advantage and a disadvantage for users of the PDR. Since the drug companies pay the publisher, this keeps the price of the book reasonable. However, the drug companies usually want to promote their newer drugs, which are still under patent. The company may choose not to purchase space in the book for a common medication, such as penicillin, that has been in use for many years. Therefore, all drugs do not receive equal space in the PDR.

Several drug handbooks are available as well for use as a drug reference. These handbooks are smaller and can be carried in a pocket or kept in a drawer in the treatment area. *Davis's Drug Guide for Nurses* is useful for any allied health worker. Information is divided into useful sections such as "Indications" and "Contraindications and Precautions." *Mosby's Dental Drug Reference* and *Lexi-Comp Drug Information for Dentistry* are drug handbooks written specifically for the dental office. All of these handbooks are available in print or electronic formats.

Dosages and Routes of Administration

For a drug to have an effect on the body, it must enter the body. The ways in which a drug is delivered are the routes of administration. Medications can be administered orally and swallowed, applied topically, sprayed, injected, or inhaled. Examples of oral forms are **tablets**, **capsules**, **suspensions**, **elixirs**, and **syrups**. Topical forms are creams and ointments. Medications inhaled through the respiratory system are mists, powders, and gases.

The route of administration can influence how effective a drug will be, how quickly the effects will begin, and the amount of medication needed. Some drugs can be delivered by several routes; others can be effective by only one. For example, aspirin is not an effective remedy for headache if applied topically to the head, but it works well when swallowed. Once the drug is administered, the body interacts with it through a series of processes.

Calculating Dosages

Standard prescription doses are based on an "average adult" weighing 150 pounds. While many adults weigh considerably more than 150 pounds, this is the weight at which most people have reached adult body functions in terms of ability to absorb, metabolize, and excrete drugs. Doses are not increased if the patient weighs more than 150 pounds. To avoid an overdose, a smaller dose may need to be calculated if the patient weighs less than 150 pounds. Patient medical histories should always include a patient's height and weight. This is especially important if the patient is a child. Many pediatric offices routinely weigh children at each dental checkup.

Most drug references will list children's dosages in terms of milligrams of drug per kilograms of body weight (mg/kg). In the United States, it is necessary to convert the child's weight from pounds to kilograms. Dividing the child's weight in pounds by 2.2 lbs/kg will do this. Most of the time, the dentist will do these calculations. The dental assistant can help by having the appropriate reference material ready.

Routes of Administration

In this section we will discuss routes of administration of medications.

Enteral Routes of Administration Many drugs are administered by means of the gastrointestinal tract, referred to as enteral. Oral and rectal administration must travel by way of the intestines.

Oral and Rectal Oral administration (swallowing) is one of the most common routes. Capsules, tablets, and liquids are all examples of oral dose forms. Oral administration is usually easy and generally well accepted by patients if the taste is not objectionable. Oral medications generally dissolve in the stomach and pass through to the intestines, where they are absorbed into the bloodstream in a manner that is similar to food.

Stomach acid can interfere with some medications, and so oral administration is not always the route of choice. Other medications may be too irritating to the stomach. The presence of food in the stomach may help with the absorption of some drugs and hinder absorption of others. Oral medications usually come with instructions as to whether they should be taken with food or on an empty stomach. Another disadvantage of oral administration is that it depends upon patient compliance. The oral route is convenient for medications that must be taken daily, but this requires the patient to self-administer the drug. There are a number of reasons, intentional and unintentional, why a patient may either fail to take their oral medicine or fail to take it correctly. The oral route of administration cannot be used if the patient is unconscious or vomiting.

A less common route that utilizes the GI tract is rectal administration. The dose form for rectal administration is called a *suppository*. This method is not as convenient as the oral route or well accepted by patients. It is a useful route if the patient is vomiting, and some medications for nausea are given in this manner.

Parenteral (Injections) Several types of injections may be used to deliver medications. Common injections are *intravenous* (IV), *intramuscular* (IM), and *subcutaneous* (SQ). The IV route places the medication directly into the bloodstream via the veins (Figure 14-2). This method gives very rapid and predictable results because there is no need to wait for the medication to be absorbed. In some offices, sedative (relaxing) drugs are delivered

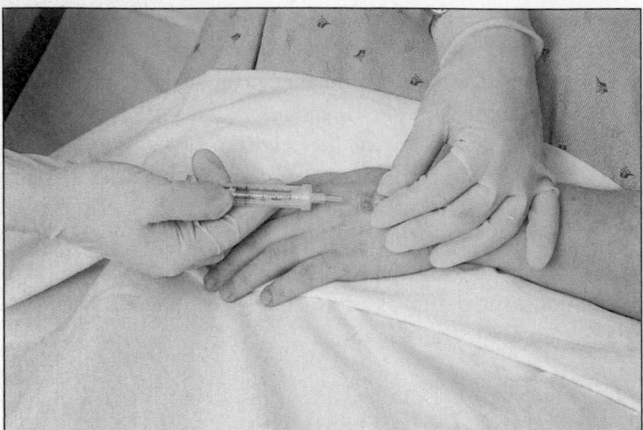

FIGURE 14-2
Administering a drug through an intravenous route.

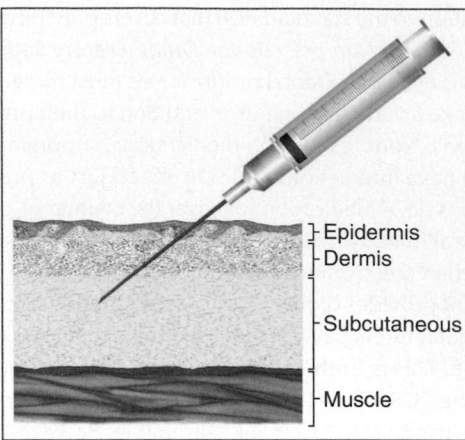

FIGURE 14-4
Administering a subcutaneous injection.

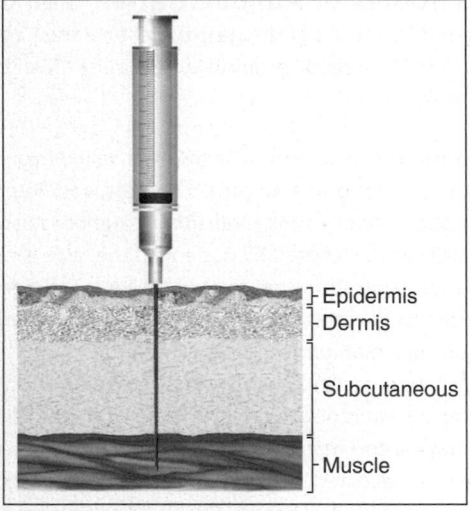

FIGURE 14-3
Administering an intramuscular injection.

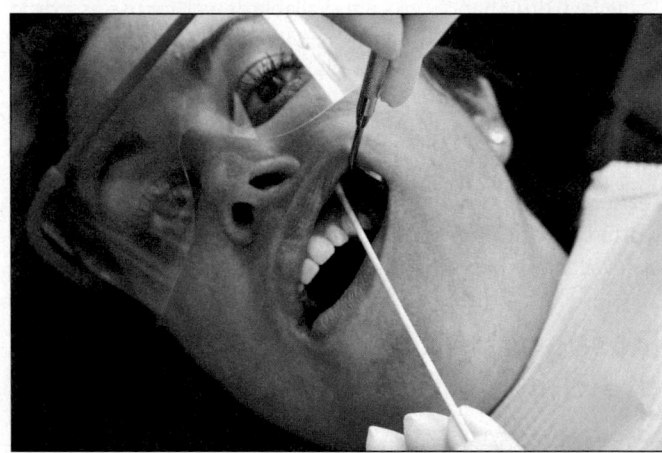

FIGURE 14-5
Topical anesthetic gel application.

by intravenous injection. However, the dentist requires special training before being allowed to administer sedatives to a patient intravenously. The IM route is used for medications that may be too irritating to be placed directly into a blood vessel (Figure 14-3).

The layer of skin directly below the epidermis is referred to as the dermis. Underneath the dermis is the subcutaneous layer. The subcutaneous injection is used to administer drugs into this layer (Figure 14-4). Injectable medications can be useful in an emergency situation because this technique provides a rapid response. However, only a trained operator can give an injection, so injections cannot be used in every situation.

Topical Administration Medication that is applied by rubbing on the skin or mucosa is called *topical*. Creams, salves, ointments, and lotions all fall into this category. In dentistry, a topical anesthetic is usually applied to the oral mucosa at the site where the dentist will inject the local anesthetic (Figure 14-5). The topical anesthetic numbs only the surface of the mucosa. It does not

take the place of the anesthetic injection, but allows the injection to be more comfortable for the patient. Two variations of the topical route of administration are sublingual application and the **transdermal patch.**

Sublingual Sublingual application takes advantage of the thin, **permeable** mucosa under the tongue. There are many blood vessels close to the surface here, and some medications can penetrate directly through the mucosa and into the blood vessels. Sublingual administration should not be confused with oral administration. The oral route involves swallowing and digesting the drug. Sublingual medicines enter the bloodstream without passing through the GI tract. Because of this, sublingual administration provides a rapid response to the drug and can be used for some emergency situations. Many pharmaceuticals are designed for sublingual administration, including cardiovascular drugs, steroids, enzymes, and some vitamins and minerals. Nitroglycerin sublingual pharmaceuticals are used in patients with coronary artery disease to relieve *angina pectoris* (chest pain) by relaxing

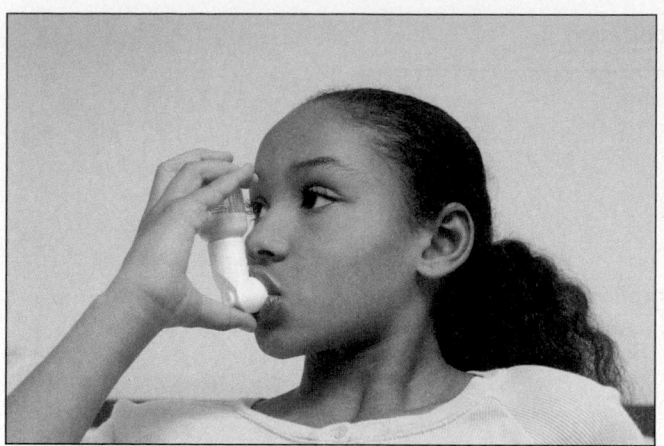

FIGURE 14-6
A bronchodilator is used to treat bronchial restriction in asthma.

blood vessels, widening the arteries, and increasing the supply of blood and oxygen to the heart.

Transdermal The transdermal patch holds medication against the skin in a way that allows small amounts of the medication to be absorbed over an extended period. A popular example of a transdermal patch is the nicotine patch used by many people who want to stop smoking. The patch is particularly useful for medicines that have unpleasant side effects. Because the patch delivers the medicine slowly and in tiny amounts, side effects may be less noticeable.

Inhalation Some drugs can be administered by inhaling them into the body. Sprays and mists used to treat respiratory problems such as asthma are administered in this manner (Figure 14-6). Inhalation is another route that gives rapid onset of effects, but only a small group of drugs can be administered in this manner. In dentistry, inhalation is used to administer nitrous oxide gas to relax or **sedate** a patient. Nitrous oxide sedation will be discussed in detail in Chapter 23. If a drug is to be inhaled, the dental assistant should verify that the patient is able to breathe freely through the nose. Something as simple as a stuffy nose can interfere with drug administration by inhalation.

Drug Processing by the Body

The route of administration is only the way the drug enters the body. Once administered, a drug goes through a series of processes and reactions as it moves around the body through the bloodstream, then it is broken down and removed from the body. These processes and reactions are called **absorption**, **distribution**, **metabolism** and **excretion**.

Absorption

Absorption is the movement of the drug from the site of administration into the bloodstream. In the oral route of administration, the site of absorption is the GI tract. Conditions in the GI tract may increase or decrease absorption. Some medicines are best absorbed if the stomach is empty, while others must be taken with food. The prescription label will provide instructions to the patient regarding whether to take the medication with food or on an empty stomach. Highly acidic conditions may increase the absorption of medicine so much that the patient receives more than the intended dose. With IM injections, the site of absorption is a large muscle, and the capillary vessels of the muscle slowly pick up the medicine. The IV method skips the absorption step by placing the medicine directly into the bloodstream (Figure 14-7).

Distribution

After a medication is absorbed into the bloodstream, it circulates in the body—wherever the blood vessels go. In order for the medicine to have its desired effect, it must reach its target tissues or organ. Along the way, the medicine reaches and affects many other tissues of the body. It is rare that a medicine is able to reach and affect *only* the target organ or tissue. The effects of the medicine on nontarget organs or tissues are called side effects and will be discussed later in this chapter. The delivery of the medication to various tissues and organs is called distribution. Some medications are better able to reach specific body tissues than others. In choosing a medication, the doctor must know if the medication is well distributed to the target tissues or organ (Figure 14-7).

A unique situation regarding distribution of medication is the case of a pregnant woman who needs to take a medication. Almost all drugs are distributed across the placenta and absorbed by the fetus. Dosage of a drug that may be perfectly safe for the mother may cause serious harm to her fetus. This situation will be discussed later in this chapter.

Metabolism

As the medication travels throughout the body, certain chemical reactions occur to break down the medicine into smaller components that can be more easily excreted (removed) from the body. This process is called metabolism. Specific chemicals, called enzymes, assist in breaking apart the large molecules. The resulting smaller molecules are called the *metabolites* or by-products of the drug. Some metabolites still have the ability to produce pharmacologic effects. These drugs may have to undergo several cycles of metabolism before being ready for the body to eliminate (Figure 14-7).

Enzymes produced and located in the liver metabolize most medications. Enzymes that circulate in the plasma of the blood metabolize a smaller number of drugs. Liver disease or damage, such as **cirrhosis** caused by alcoholism, can prevent a person from metabolizing drugs adequately, and the drug may become **toxic** in a patient with this health issue. For this reason, a dentist always reviews the health history for indication of liver disease before prescribing drugs or using local anesthetics.

In a healthy patient, the liver adapts to accommodate drugs that are given over a long period of time such as in the case of

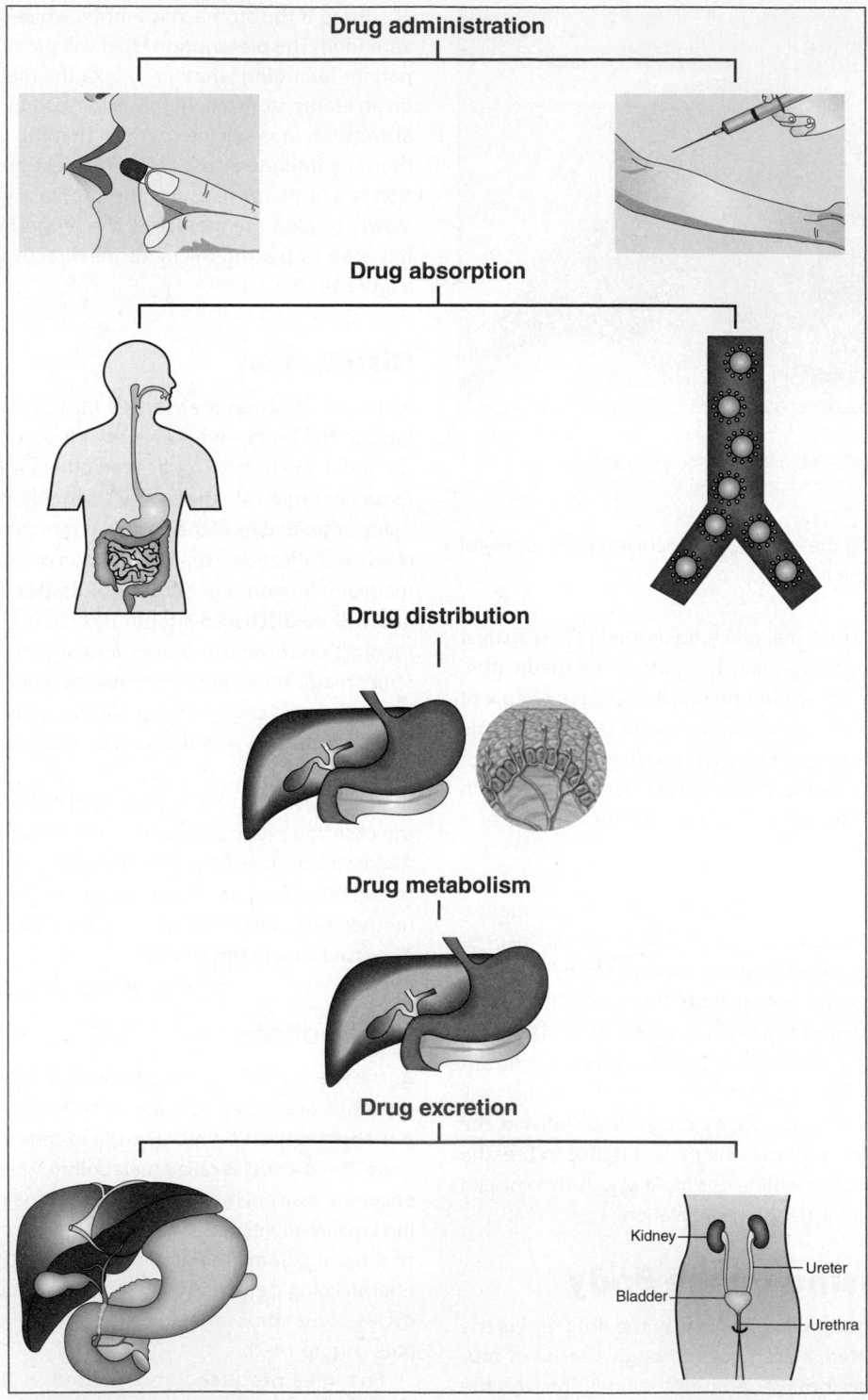

FIGURE 14-7
Pharmacokinetics: The stages of drug action in the body.

a chronic health problem that is being treated indefinitely. The liver begins to produce more of the enzymes needed to metabolize the drug. This accommodation is called *tolerance*. With tolerance, the effects of the drug do not last as long or are of lesser magnitude than when the drug was begun. Over time patients require more of the drug to achieve the desired effect.

Excretion

Excretion is the removal of toxic chemicals (such as drugs) and waste products from the body. The kidneys handle most of the burden for excretion of drugs and their by-products (Figure 14-7). Drug doses may have to be adjusted in patients with kidney

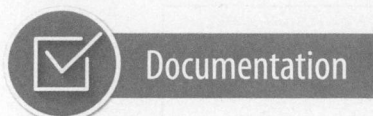 Documentation

10-13-2019 Reviewed medical history, no dental or drug allergies, no medications.
Nonsurgical extraction of #16, no complications. Anes: 2% lidocaine w/epi 1:100,000 X 1.5 carpules; Patient tolerated procedure well. Rx Tylox, disp #8, one tab q 4-6 h prn pain. M. Brown, DMD
10-20-2019 Arnold Green came to the office today requesting a copy of his treatment record for his employer. A workplace drug screening was performed yesterday and Arnold tested positive for opioids. Arnold threw away the prescription bottle and needs documentation of legitimate use of Tylox. A release of information form was signed and a copy of the 10-13-2011 treatment notes was given to Arnold. Katherine Evans, CDA.

disease. Some drugs are excreted intact and can be easily identified in the urine. Other times, drug by-products are present in urine It is important for dental professionals to record all drugs administered or prescribed in the patient's chart. This information may be needed at a later date.

While the kidneys are the most common organs of excretion, drugs are excreted to a lesser extent through virtually all body fluids including feces, perspiration, saliva, and breast milk. Some drugs are excreted by respiration as well; nitrous oxide, used in the dental office to relieve anxiety, is an example of a drug excreted through exhalation. One of the benefits of nitrous oxide is that it is absorbed quickly by inhalation and is excreted just as quickly through exhalation at the end of the procedure.

Writing a Prescription

Prescription drugs are those drugs available to the public only by order from a physician, dentist, or other licensed health care provider. A prescription is a specific set of written instructions, which includes directions to the pharmacist telling which drug and the amount of the drug to dispense as well as directions to the patient telling how and when to take the drug. By law, only the dentist can determine which drug is needed, how much is needed, and how it should be taken. The dental assistant may fill out the prescription for the dentist's approval and signature. Only the dentist can sign the prescription form. For this reason, dental assistants should understand the basics rules of prescription writing and the vocabulary used in a prescription.

Parts of the Prescription

Years ago, prescriptions were written in Latin and used words and symbols that were not easily understood by the general public. Today's prescriptions are much simpler and more straightforward. While some abbreviations of Latin terms can be used to save time, this is not required. It is perfectly acceptable to write a prescription using standard English. Likewise, it is preferable to use clear, legible handwriting to decrease the chance of prescription errors. Many drugs have similar sounding names but widely

different effects. Consider these popular prescription drugs: Zocor, used to treat high cholesterol levels; Zoloft, for depression; Zyrtec, for allergies. Therefore, spelling the drug name completely and correctly with good handwriting is necessary to ensure the correct drug is dispensed at the pharmacy.

A written prescription has three sections. These can be compared to the three sections of a formal business letter that has a heading, a body, and a closing (Figure 14-8).

Heading The heading of the prescription includes:
- name, address and telephone number of the prescriber (usually preprinted on the prescription pad)
- state license or Drug Enforcement Agency (DEA) number (if required)
- name, address, date of birth, and telephone number of the patient
- date of the prescription

Body The body of the prescription includes:
- the symbol Rx, which provides the instructions to the pharmacist regarding
- name of the drug and dosage form and size (e.g., 500 mg tablets)
- amount to be dispensed
- directions to the patient to be printed on the label of the drug package

Closing The closing of the prescription includes:
- the prescriber's signature and indication as to whether substitution of a generic drug is allowed
- refill instructions

Abbreviations and Units of Measure

Abbreviations of common instructions on the prescription can be used to save time and because space on the prescription form is limited. If abbreviations are to be used, the prescriber must be certain of the meaning intended and must print the abbreviation clearly. For example, the abbreviation *qid* means "four times

Dr. John Smith
123 ABC Way
Town, State, Zip

Phone: 000 000 0000   Date___April 6, 20XX___

NPI #___123456___

DEA#___8654321___   License #__123XYZ___

Name:__Joe Smith___   Patient's DOB:_April 2, 2000_

Address___123 Main Street Oakland, CA, 11111___

Rx

amoxicillin 500 mg tablets
Disp 21 (twenty-one)
Take 1 tab tid until complete

Substitute Yes or No

# of Refills_____one_____

Signature_____*Michael Jones*_____

FIGURE 14-8
Prescription format.

a day," but without the "i," *qd* means "per day." This would make a significant and potentially dangerous difference in the dosage (Figure 14-9).

The metric system should be used for all prescription writing. Pills, tablets, and capsules come in sizes measured in milligrams. Liquid medicines are usually measured in milliliters. While some prescription directions may be stated in terms of ounces, teaspoons, or tablespoons, it is wise to use medicine cups or syringes specifically made for measuring medications. Household utensils may not be the correct dose size (Figure 14-10).

Computer Generated Prescriptions

Most dental software programs have the option of using the computer to write the prescription. Using this feature can eliminate the problems of handwriting and spelling and can automatically provide documentation to the patient's chart. Prescriptions

```
gm = gram (1000 milligrams)
mg = milligram (0.001 grams)
ml = milliliter
cap = capsule
tab = tablet
q = every
d = day
h = hour
hs = at bedtime
prn = as needed
stat = immediately
PO = by mouth
q4h = every four hours
q6h = every six hours
qid = four times per day
tid = three times per day
bid = two times per day
disp = dispense
Rx = recipe, or "take thou"

Note: Some abbreviations should not be used because of high risk of error.
These include:
QD (write the word "daily" instead)
QOD (write "every other day")
U (write the word "units" instead)
```

FIGURE 14-9
Common abbreviations used in prescription writing.

```
1 kg = 2.2 pounds
30 gm = 1 ounce
30 ml = 1 fluid ounce
5 ml = 1 teaspoonful (tsp or t)
15 ml = 1 tablespoonful (tbsp or T)
```

FIGURE 14-10
Helpful conversions for prescriptions.

generated by the computer can be printed and given to the patient or transmitted electronically to the pharmacy.

Laws Governing Prescriptions

The prescribing of drugs is regulated by state and federal government laws. It is important for the dental assistant to be aware of these laws and follow all required procedures.

Who May Write a Prescription?

Prescriptions may be written only by a health care professional licensed to do so. Laws vary from state to state as to who may prescribe medications and which types of medications various providers may prescribe. Physicians, osteopaths, physician's assistants, nurse practitioners, dentists, optometrists, podiatrists, and veterinarians are among the professionals who may write prescriptions. Remember, these licensed professionals are limited to prescribing only the drugs necessary in their field of expertise.

Documentation

A dentist may write a prescription only for a patient of record in the practice. All medications dispensed, administered or prescribed in the dental office must be recorded in the patient's chart. For example, a dentist may dispense an antibiotic medication for the patient to take upon arrival at the office, then administer a local anesthetic for the procedure and write a prescription for the patient to take at home all in one appointment.

Patient Information

The dental assistant should be familiar with the medications routinely prescribed in the dental office and be prepared to give instructions to the patient about their use. The patient will also receive instructions from the pharmacy that fills the prescription. Federal law requires this for all patients who use Medicaid, but most state laws require that this benefit be extended to all patients. Most pharmacies provide this information by means of a computer generated information sheet. Despite this, many people do not take their prescription medication correctly. In the common situation of a dental patient being provided with two prescriptions, one for pain and an antibiotic for infection, it is important for the patient to know which is the antibiotic and which is the pain medication, the purpose of each drug, and how to take each medication.

HIPAA requires that all patient information is kept private and secure.

Controlled Substances

Over 74 million Americans currently admit to having used illegal drugs. In addition to this enormous number, misuse of prescription drugs and drug trafficking have affected countless additional family members, communities, and individuals. The Controlled Substances Act became law in 1970 to regulate the use of drugs that were commonly abused at that time. Over the next three decades, in response to public alarm about drug abuse, the law was continuously amended and strengthened. The DEA was created in 1973 to fight the growing use of illegal drugs in the United States. The DEA's Schedule of Controlled Substances provides a way of ranking the dangers and potential for abuse of various drugs, both legal and illegal.

Only drugs that have the potential to be misused or be addictive are listed in the schedule. The DEA regulates and enforces the manufacture, sale, and use of these drugs. The DEA is not involved with other prescriptions or OTC medications. There are five categories in the Schedule of Controlled Substances: Schedule I, Schedule II, Schedule III, Schedule IV, and Schedule V (Table 14-1).

Dentists who prescribe controlled substances must register with the DEA and with their state drug control agency. A DEA number is issued, and this number must appear on all prescriptions for controlled substances. Pharmacies are required to report all prescriptions for controlled substances to the DEA. The DEA monitors prescribers using the DEA number to see that use of controlled substances is appropriate for the type of practice.

TABLE 14-1 Five Schedules of Controlled Substances

	Regulations	Potential for Abuse	Examples
Schedule I	No legal prescription For approved research only	Very High	heroin, LSD, marijuana
Schedule II	Written prescription only No telephone Rx No refills	High	morphine, oxycodone, hydrocodone mixtures, amphetamines (e.g., Ritalin)
Schedule III	Written or telephoned Rx Limited refills	Moderate	codeine mixtures, **anabolic** steroids
Schedule IV	Written or telephoned Rx Limited refills	Low	diazepam (Valium), Halcion (triazolam), Ambien (zolpidem)
Schedule V	Formerly available OTC in the United States, and still available OTC in some countries	Very Low	cough remedies containing codeine or hydrocodone, Valium

Substance Use disorder

One of the growing problems in the United States is prescription drug misuse. Misuse occurs when a prescription drug is taken in a manner that it was not prescribed, for example, using another person's prescribed drugs or taking more than the prescribed amount. Taking a drug or medication for effects of **euphoria** is also misuse. Drug misuse will affect the patient's dental treatment, making it imperative that the dental team is aware of its potential danger. Illicit drugs such as marijuana, cocaine, and heroin also have a potential for abuse.

Recognizing Prescription Seeking Behaviors

In dentistry, there are times when it is necessary to prescribe a controlled substance for the relief of pain or anxiety. The dental patient typically needs these medications for a very short period of time, and so the chance of becoming addicted from a dental prescription is minimized. The dental assistant should be alert to two of the most common situations in which dental prescriptions could be abused. The first situation is when a patient may present to the dental office with existing addictions or drug misuse problems. The second situation is the "drug shopper" who is not a patient of record and who calls the office claiming a dental emergency.

The patient of record who has a history of drug misuse or who has an addictive personality will be discussed first. Drug misuse and addiction is a chronic problem in our society. Some patients of a dental practice have had experience with drug misuse. Some patients will indicate on the medical history that they have been through rehabilitation for alcohol of drug misuse. These patients are considered to be "in recovery" or "recovering abusers." Recovering patients will often ask that the dentist *not* administer or prescribe medications that could be addictive or misused. Even a short exposure to these substances could cause a **relapse** to the addictive behavior. Care must be taken to find alternative ways to control pain or anxiety. Other times, there will be no indication that the patient has an addiction problem until after a drug

has been prescribed. This patient may ask for refills of the prescription, claiming pain that continues long beyond normal for the dental procedure performed. This patient may also call the office asking for a different prescription, complaining that the medicine prescribed is not strong enough, or asking for specific medications, claiming "that is the only medication that works for me." These situations require both compassion and professional judgment. The response to pain is very personal and varies greatly from one individual to another. The patient of record who complains of excessive or lasting pain after a procedure should be asked to return to the office for evaluation.

The second scenario is related to individuals who are not patients of the office They may call or come to the office claiming dental pain and asking for a prescription. Dentists may legally prescribe medications only for patients of record. Therefore, a prescription should never be given to a stranger based only on a phone call. All persons who call the office in pain should be offered an examination appointment as soon as possible. After appropriate examination and diagnosis, the dentist will offer treatment options to solve the problem. Medications alone will never cure a dental problem. Prescriptions should be given only in combination with treatment. Many prescription-seeking individuals will ask for a prescription "to get me by until I can come in." This individual may even make an appointment and then fail to appear for the appointment once they have the prescription.

Currently, 49 states and the District of Columbia have implemented prescription monitoring programs (PMP). These programs require the practitioner to register for the program, providing access to the PMP site in their state. Prior to writing a prescription for a medication that has a misuse potential, the dentist must check the medication history of that patient. Since pharmacies are required to report all information regarding writing of prescriptions in Schedules II–V, the prescription history is available for all patients who have previously received a narcotic medication. The PMP sites have been set up in order to reduce prescription misuse and **diversion**.

The dental assistant should be alert to prescription seeking behavior. Many times the patient will say or do things in the presence of the assistant that are indictors of substance misuse. For

- Reports pain of excessive duration or severity for the procedure performed
- Claims allergies to common nonprescription pain relievers
- Asks for a specific drug by name or claims this is the only drug that works
- Calls late in the day or before a weekend or holiday and asks for medication to "get by" until Monday.
- Cancels appointments for treatment after receiving a prescription
- Asks for refills long before the prescription should have run out
- Visits numerous dental or other health care providers looking to obtain prescription medications

FIGURE 14-11
Warning signs of drug seeking behavior.

example, a patient may wear long sleeves and heavy clothing on a hot day in order to cover up needle marks from drug use. Another patient in the waiting room may be extremely impatient and want to see the dentist immediately. If an assistant has suspicions about a patient, the assistant should discuss them privately with the dentist (Figure 14-11).

Protecting the Office against Drug Diversion

People who are drug addicts or misuse substances are sometimes desperate to obtain what they want and can be very clever. All members of the staff should be trained to recognize addictive behavior. If a staff member suspects drug-seeking behavior, the dentist should be informed. Below are precautions that will protect the office from abusers.

Drug-seeking individuals may attempt to steal prescription pads and write their own prescription or alter a legitimate prescription. This behavior constitutes forgery and is illegal. Prescription pads should be stored in a secure place in the dental office. They should never be left in the open or left in the room with a patient. The doctor's DEA number should not be pre-printed on the prescription pad but should be written in by hand only when a controlled substance is prescribed. Some insurance companies are beginning to request the DEA number on all prescriptions, and some offices include the DEA number for this reason. This is not a secure practice, and other methods of providing information to the insurer are being developed. Some states require duplicate or triplicate forms for Schedule II prescriptions. In this case, the dentist keeps one copy in the office, the pharmacy keeps a copy, and one copy is sent to the state drug enforcement agency by the pharmacy.

Other precautions can be taken in the way a prescription is written. In the directions telling the pharmacist how many tablets or capsules to dispense, the number should be indicated in a secure manner. An abuser may attempt to alter the number, for example making 120 out of 12. If the prescriber uses Roman numerals (XII) or spells out the number (twelve), the prescription is more secure. Likewise, to indicate if the prescription may be refilled, the doctor should write "none" or "one" rather than "0" or "1."

A final precaution is to be well acquainted with the pharmacies in your practice area. Pharmacists and pharmacy workers are well trained in recognizing patients with prescription seeking behaviors. If a patient is acting in a suspicious manner or a written prescription has a suspicious appearance, the pharmacist may call the dental office for a consultation. Pharmacists become familiar with their regular prescribers' handwriting and with the prescriptions commonly prescribed by specific offices. If a patient with addictive behavior manages to obtain a prescription by dishonest means, the pharmacist may recognize it.

Therapeutic versus Adverse Drug Effects

The *therapeutic* effect of a drug is the desired effect, basically the reason a person would take the drug. All other effects are adverse effects. For example, a dental patient takes aspirin for a toothache. The desired effect is relief of pain. However, the patient may experience stomach irritation, reduced blood clotting, or an allergic reaction. Since these effects are unwelcome and have no positive effect on the toothache, they are considered adverse effects. If the same person takes a baby aspirin daily to prevent a heart attack, the reduced blood clotting is a therapeutic effect.

There are no "perfect" drugs that provide only therapeutic effects and no adverse effects. The effect of a drug cannot be limited to the specific body part needing treatment. Once a drug enters the body, it circulates and enters all body tissues, causing effects in many areas. In the best situations, the therapeutic effects can be maximized and the adverse effects reduced. Some adverse effects are serious enough to require selection of another drug for a patient.

Types of Adverse Reactions

There are a number of adverse effects possible. Some are predictable and expected and others cannot be predicted. Possible adverse effects are (1) toxicity; (2) allergic reaction; (3) side effects, including oral side effects; (4) teratogenic effects; and (5) interactions with other substances. As a dental assistant, you will be expected to discuss and explain these effects to patients.

Toxicity *Toxic* reactions are the simplest of all adverse reactions. A toxic reaction is simply "too much" of the therapeutic effect of the drug. For example, a drug taken to cause mild relaxation may cause loss of consciousness, or a drug that is used for treating high blood pressure (hypertension) causes the blood pressure to become too low (hypotension). Toxicity is usually associated with the dose of the drug. It is understandable that an excessive dose would produce excessive effects. Occasionally, a standard dose may produce excessive effects in a sensitive patient. Very young or older adult patients may be more sensitive to drug effects. Smaller than what is considered a standard dose may be needed for these individuals.

Allergic Reactions Allergic reactions are probably the most misunderstood of all adverse drug effects. Only a small percentage of adverse reactions are truly allergic. However, many people think that any unwanted drug effect is an allergic reaction. True allergic reactions fall into several easily identified categories ranging from mild and annoying to life threatening. A dental assistant must be able to distinguish an allergic reaction from other types of adverse reactions.

There are four types of allergic reactions. Types I and IV are the most common and easiest to recognize. Types II and III are more subtle, but the dental assistant must recognize them as well. Any other adverse reaction reported by a patient is *not* an allergy and will be handled differently by the dental team.

Type I: Immediate Hypersensitivity These are the most well known of the allergic reactions and include *erythema* or redness, *edema* or swelling (Figure 14-12), *urticaria* or hives (Figure 14-13), itching, runny nose, and difficulty in breathing. The difficulty in breathing is due to airway edema, which leads to narrowing of the airway. Immediate **hypersensitivity** reactions can quickly become life threatening because of the airway constriction and the severe drop in blood pressure (hypotension). A series of body chemicals, including histamine, cause these reactions. Thus, epinephrine administered intramuscularly (IM) in a concentration of 1:10,000 or intravenously (IV) in a concentration of 1:10,000 is the drug of choice for a severe immediate hypersensitivity reaction. Antihistamines alone are not powerful enough to reverse the airway edema and the hypotension. Epinephrine is the only drug with the capability of reducing these two severe components of immediate hypersensitivity reactions.

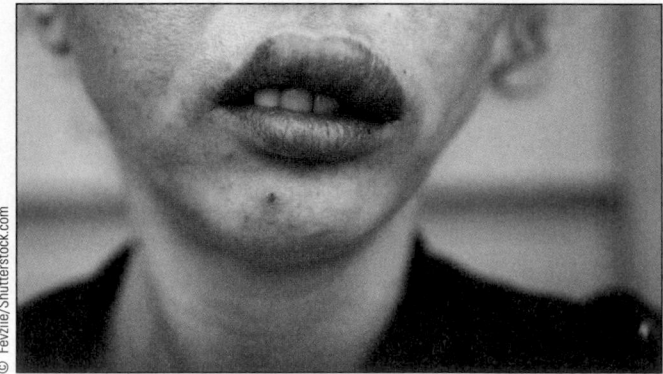

FIGURE 14-12
Edema of the lips.

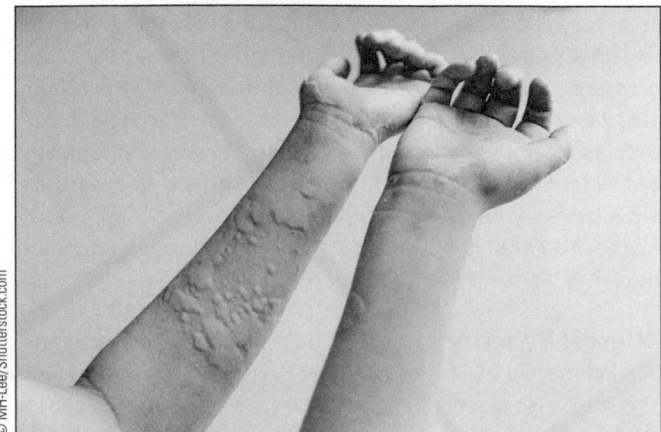

FIGURE 14-13
Urticaria.

Type II: Cytotoxic Hypersensitivity Reactions This type of allergic reaction is less common. It is often not recognized as an allergy. In this reaction, specific body tissues are damaged or destroyed. One example of this is hemolytic anemia, in which red blood cells are destroyed, causing severe anemia.

Type III: Immune Complex Hypersensitivity Reactions This reaction is similar to the Type II reaction in that specific body tissues are attacked. However, in this reaction tissues or cells are not destroyed immediately as with hemolytic anemia. Instead, certain body parts experience long-term inflammation with swelling and pain. This type of reaction is associated with autoimmune disease, such as rheumatoid arthritis and systemic lupus erythematosis.

Type IV: Delayed Hypersensitivity This allergic reaction lives up to its name by developing slowly. The first time a person is exposed to the drug or substance, there is no reaction. On further exposure, the reaction may take several days or weeks to occur. These reactions are generally mild, such as a skin rash (Figure 14-14). Repeated exposure to the allergen will bring on the reaction more rapidly with each exposure. Poison ivy is an example of delayed hypersensitivity. After an initial outbreak of poison ivy, each subsequent exposure causes a greater and speedier reaction. A dental assistant may experience this reaction to soaps or latex products such as gloves used in the dental office.

Side Effects The vast majority of all adverse drug reactions are side effects, *not* allergic reactions. Most side effects disappear if the offending drug is stopped. The severity of the side effect will increase or decrease with the amount of drug taken. Side effects are generally not life threatening, but they can be unpleasant enough to cause the patient to avoid using the medication as needed. The patient may not receive the beneficial effect of the drug if the side effect causes him or her to stop using it. Common side effects are gastrointestinal (GI) disturbances, drowsiness, **xerostomia**, **orthostatic hypotension**, effects on blood clotting, and suppression of the immune system.

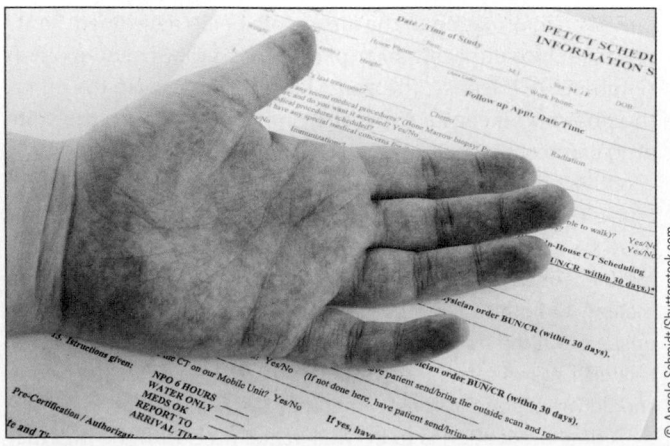

FIGURE 14-14
Allergic reaction caused by latex.

The dental assistant will discuss possible side effects with the patient to determine if the side effect may be a problem.

Gastrointestinal (GI) Side Effects Gastrointestinal (GI) side effects are common and can range from mild upset stomach to severe vomiting or diarrhea. The effects may be experienced with some of the pain relieving or anti-infection medications prescribed by dentists. In most cases, there is no long-term harm to the patient, but vomiting may interfere with optimal drug effects and/or healing. Additionally, the patient may stop taking the drug due to the unpleasant GI side effects; as a result, the patient is not receiving the beneficial effects of the medication. If a patient reports having these problems in the past, the dentist may select an alternate drug or suggest ways to minimize the effect.

Drowsiness Drowsiness occurs with certain pain medications or with drugs prescribed for anxiety (including dental anxiety). If these drugs are taken in combination, the effect is increased. The patient should be warned about this effect and the potential for it to be additive with other drugs that can also cause drowsiness, including alcohol. The dentist should be aware of all medications the patient uses and any alcohol use before prescribing drugs that cause drowsiness. Patients should be advised not to drink alcohol while taking these medications.

Xerostomia An adverse drug effect of special concern to dentistry is xerostomia or dry mouth. At least 150 commonly prescribed or OTC drugs are known to cause xerostomia. Without the cleansing and antmicrobial actions of saliva, dental plaque becomes stickier and food particles tend to cling to teeth and soft tissues. Patients with xerostomia have higher risk of dental caries and periodontal disease. Often, the xerostomia has developed over a long period of time and the patient is not aware of it. Dental professionals should recognize xerostomia in patients, educate the patient about the risks, and suggest solutions. It is usually not possible for the patient to stop taking the medication causing the problem.

The dental assistant must give advice to relieve the symptoms of xerostomia and prevent the related dental problems. A variety of OTC products are available to relieve symptoms of xerostomia, and the dental assistant should discuss these. The patient should be advised to avoid products containing harsh chemicals such as alcohol. While dental products containing alcohol do not actually cause dryness, these products can cause discomfort in a mouth that is already dry. Additional products to provide extra fluoride at home may be recommended. Changes in the patient's daily habits may minimize the impact of xerostomia. Sipping or rinsing with water throughout the day is helpful. Nutritional counseling about not consuming sugary foods and drinks is needed as well as these can increase the risk of decay in patients who experience xerostomia. The patient should avoid coffee and tea as these have a **diuretic** effect. The office should have informational materials for distribution to patients who have xerostomia.

Orthostatic Hypotension Orthostatic hypotension is dizziness or fainting that occurs when a person rises quickly from a sitting or reclining position. Dental assistants prevent this side effect from occurring after dental treatment by bringing the dental chair slowly to an upright position and asking the patient to remain seated for a few minutes. Certain medications, especially those for high blood pressure and psychiatric treatment, will increase this dizziness upon rising. The dental assistant should be aware of patients who use these medications and use extra care at the end of an appointment. Management of orthostatic hypotension will be discussed in detail in Chapter 15.

Effects on Blood Clotting Some medications change the blood's ability to clot. People who have survived a heart attack or stroke often take medications to decrease clotting. This can help prevent a second heart attack or stroke. In this situation, decreased clotting is the desired, therapeutic effect. However, on the day of dental surgery, failure to clot or taking much longer than normal to clot would be an adverse side effect. It is very important that the dental team be aware of any anticlotting medications the patient is taking. Some pain medications have a side effect of decreasing the ability to form a blood clot. If the patient is already taking an anticlotting medication and a pain medicine with this side effect, such as aspirin, is used by the patient to manage dental pain, there could be dangerous levels of bleeding.

Immune System Suppression Another side effect to consider is the effect of a medication on the patient's immune system. Medications that suppress the immune system put the patient at risk of infection. For example, patients who have had organ transplants must take immune suppressing medications to avoid rejection of the transplanted organ. Other situations are not so drastic. Patients may be taking a corticosteroid medication to manage allergies. Corticosteroids can suppress the immune system as well. Bacteria, viruses, or fungi easily infect the patient taking an immune suppressing medication. In a dental setting, this patient may appear with abscesses, periodontal disease, or an oral fungal infection known as *candidiasis*.

Teratogenic Effects The most heartbreaking of all adverse effects are *teratogenic* effects. A teratogen is a medication or substance that causes harm to a developing fetus. Until the 1960s, no relationship was recognized between medications used by a pregnant woman and any possible effect to her unborn child. Women were not counseled to avoid alcohol, smoking, or drugs during pregnancy.

Today, no medication is considered absolutely safe for pregnant women and their babies. New medications are not tested for potential fetal harm using human subjects. Animal testing is performed, and the FDA rates a medication's potential for fetal harm based on these results. The FDA has a rating system for

TABLE 14-2 Categories of Drugs Based on Potential Harm to the Fetus

Pregnancy Category	Evidence	Example Drugs in this Category
A	Adequate studies in pregnant humans have been done and show no danger to a fetus.	folic acid supplement Thyroid supplements if needed by the mother
B	Animal testing show no risk to the fetus. Some well-controlled human studies may have been done as well.	Tylenol Some antibiotics
C	Testing in pregnant animals showed harm to fetus, and/or there are no available studies in animals or humans.	Some antibiotics Some antidepressants
D	There is evidence that a human fetus could be harmed, but the drug may still be used in life-threatening situations for the pregnant woman.	Dilantin (phenytoin) lithium
X	Evidence of harm to the human fetus is proven and outweighs any benefit to the pregnant woman.	thalidomide Accutane

medications and pregnancy (Table 14-2). This rating system is not perfect. Since drugs cannot be tested on human pregnant females, few drugs are ever ranked in Category A. Category B is usually "as good as it gets" when searching for a medication that will be safe to prescribe to a pregnant woman. Category C basically means, "We don't know." Medications in this category may have caused harm in testing on animals and would never be tested in humans. Currently, the FDA is working to provide a more detailed and explanatory method of drug labeling for pregnancy.

There are other commonly used medications that have can cause birth defects. These include certain blood pressure medications, some medications used to treat psychiatric disorders, some prescription anticlotting medications, and some anticancer agents. Illegal drugs and alcohol are also known teratogens.

If the dentist will be prescribing a medication that has potential of harm to a fetus, the dental assistant should question all women of childbearing age as to the possibility of pregnancy. Further, the assistant should explain the reason for this question and explain the possible effects of the drug. What does "childbearing age" mean? It is best to err on the side of caution and ask most women. Pregnancies can occur as early as age 10 and as late as age 50-plus. This conversation should be clearly documented in the patient's chart, even if the woman states that she is not pregnant.

Interactions with Other Substances Some medications may have few adverse effects if taken alone. However, many individuals take a number of prescription and nonprescription medications as well as dietary supplements on a daily basis. Medications can interact with each other and even with food and drink. For example, the antibiotic tetracycline should not be taken with milk or other dairy products. The calcium in dairy products binds with the tetracycline and prevents its absorption by the body. It is important to know all of the medications a patient is taking, even those that the patient may not consider a medication, such as oral contraceptives or birth control pills, vitamins and other dietary supplements, or OTC medications such as aspirin. Some combinations will increase the effect of a medication, and some will block the medication's effectiveness. Other combinations will produce negative side effects that would not

occur with either medication alone. Many medications used in dentistry cause drowsiness or sedation. This effect is increased by the use of alcohol, even to the point of toxicity or harm to the patient. Cigarette smoking can alter the effects of some medication. It is the job of the health care worker to provide information about all possible interactions.

Commonly Used Medications in Dentistry

The dental office uses limited categories of medications. These medications will be discussed in this section.

Anesthetics

Anesthesia implies more than the absence of pain. Anesthetics can be general, local, or topical. A general anesthetic provides complete or partial loss of feeling, awareness, and consciousness and affects the entire body. A local anesthetic causes loss of feeling in a specific part of the body, and a topical anesthetic provides limited numbness only to the surface to which is applied.

General Anesthetics General anesthesia provides a reversible loss of consciousness and sensation. Patients under general anesthesia do not respond to words or touch. They cannot breathe on their own or protect their airway by coughing or gagging. Use of general anesthesia by a dentist requires additional extensive training or the services of an anesthesiologist or anesthetist. General anesthesia has several planes or levels that the patient goes through before reaching the surgical phase where procedures are completed. Stage I is analgesia, stage II is delirium, stage III is surgical, stage IV is respiratory arrest. Equipment to maintain respiratory function must be utilized when general anesthesia is being administered. Additionally, emergency life support equipment must be available. Because of the risks involved, this type of anesthesia is best used in a hospital operating room.

A variation of general anesthesia that is more often used in the dental office is *nitrous oxide* gas (laughing gas). Used correctly, nitrous oxide takes a patient only to stage I of general anesthesia or analgesia. Sensation of pain is reduced but not totally eliminated, and the patient is minimally sedated but not unconscious. The patient is able to respond to commands and answer questions and is able to maintain a patent airway. The gag reflex also remains functional in stage I analgesia. This natural protective reflex is important; in the event that a small object drops into the back of the throat, the patient is able to cough and prevent swallowing or inhalation of the object.

There are studies of increased rates of spontaneous abortion (miscarriage) among women who use or work with nitrous oxide, particularly during the first trimester. It is best to err on the side of caution in the dental office and not utilize nitrous oxide gas on a patient who is pregnant and in the first trimester or who is trying to become pregnant. It is not sufficient to ask, "Are you pregnant?" Instead, the patient should be asked, "Is there any possibility you *could be* pregnant?" Unfortunately, the risk includes not only patients but also dental and operating room workers exposed to nitrous oxide in the workplace. Pregnant female staff in the first trimester should also avoid being exposed to nitrous oxide. In the dental office, steps can be taken to minimize risk to team members. Nitrous oxide delivery systems should be equipped with a scavenger system to vent exhaled gases outside of the operatory. Additionally, equipment should be connected to the high-speed evacuation system to remove any trace gases from the operatory area. Monitoring equipment in the operatory can measure the concentration of nitrous oxide in the room. Some simple patient management techniques can significantly reduce the amount of nitrous oxide in the room. Instructing the patient to inhale and exhale through the nose allows exhaled gas to enter the scavenger system. Because nitrous oxide causes a state of deep relaxation, staff must continue to remind the patient to exhale through the nose in order for the gas to be beneficial to the patient.

Local Anesthetics

Safe, effective local anesthesia is one of the hallmarks of modern dentistry. Most dental services can be provided with only local anesthetic agents. While general anesthetics are inhaled in the form of a gas or injected into the bloodstream and affect the entire body, local anesthetics are injected near the site of the procedure to be performed. The goal is for the anesthetic liquid to bathe the nerve fibers. As long as the anesthetic remains in contact with the nerve fibers, the nerve is unable to send sensory messages to the brain. Depending on the amount of anesthetic used and the proximity to the nerve, sensations of temperature, pain, touch, and pressure will be blocked. Sometimes, the patient will lose motor function as in the patient who can only smile with one side of the mouth. Table 14-3 provides a summary of local anesthetics available for use in the United States.

Local anesthetics used by dentists today belong to a chemical group called *amides*. Allergic reactions to this group of anesthetics are extremely rare, and toxic reactions are uncommon when correct technique and dose are used. Novocaine (procaine), an earlier local anesthetic, is a member of a different chemical group, the *esters*. This group of anesthetics caused allergic and

TABLE 14-3 Local Anesthetics Available for Use in the United States

Brand Name	Generic Name	Percentage	Vasoconstrictor
Xylocaine	lidocaine	2%	epinephrine, 1:100,000
Octocaine	lidocaine	2%	epinephrine, 1:100,000
Carbocaine	mepivicaine	3%	none
Citanest	prilocaine	4%	none
Citanest Forte	prilocaine	4%	epinephrine 1:200,000
Marcaine	bupivicaine	0.5%	epinephrine 1:200,000
Septocaine, Septodont, Zorcaine	articaine	4%	epinephrine 1:100,000

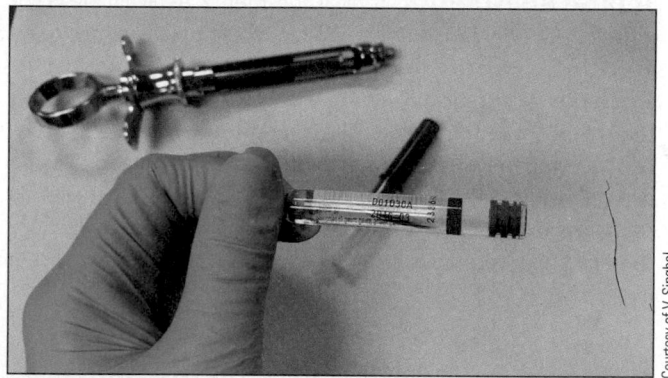

Courtesy of V. Singhal

FIGURE 14-15
Local anesthetic cartridge.

other adverse reactions. Novocaine and other esters are not used in dentistry today as a result. If a patient reports an allergy to local anesthetic, more information is needed. If the reaction occurred prior to 1960, it is possible that the patient was given Novocaine. The dental assistant must be aware that some people refer to all local anesthetics as "Novocaine." The patient may have had a reaction to other ingredients in the amide anesthetic solution, such as **bisulfites** that act as an **antioxidant**, or they may have had an adverse reaction that was not truly an allergy. Patients who are fearful of injections and faint upon receiving the local anesthetic may believe that they are having an allergic reaction to the local anesthetic. Use of the supine position in dentistry minimizes the risk of fainting or *syncope*. Asking the right questions will help the dentist choose an appropriate anesthetic.

A **vasoconstrictor** is added to many dental anesthetics to increase the duration of the anesthesia. Today, in the United States, epinephrine is the only vasoconstrictor used in dental local anesthetic cartridges (Figure 14-15). When the blood vessels are constricted, the blood flow is decreased, and the blood does not pick up the anesthetic and carry it away from the site of administration as quickly. Thus, the anesthetic lasts longer. The amount of vasoconstrictor used is minimal and is safe for most people. However, there are times when a vasoconstrictor should be avoided or administered in a limited dose.

The vasoconstrictor can increase heart rate and blood pressure. If the patient has existing heart disease that is not well managed, the vasoconstrictor can have a negative impact on the patient's heart condition. The vasoconstrictor may interact with other medications a patient is taking. Local anesthetics with vasoconstrictors include an antioxidant known as a *bisulfite*. It is contraindicated to use local anesthetics with vasoconstrictors in patients who have asthma or allergies to the bisulfites Some patients are allergic to bisulfites and as a result, a local anesthetic with vasoconstrictors should be avoided in patients who have allergies to bisulfites. Bisulfites can also trigger an asthmatic attack in patients who have a history of asthma. Local anesthetics with vasoconstrictors and bisulfites should not be used in a patient with a history of asthma. For all of these reasons, local anesthetics are available both with and without vasoconstrictor.

Topical Anesthetics Topical anesthetics are available in liquid, paste, or gel forms to be applied to the mucosa prior to an injection. The medication does not penetrate deep into the tissues, and the duration of action is only a few minutes to lessen the sharpness of the needle. These medications frequently contain an ester anesthetic, plus coloring and flavoring additives, so allergic reactions are possible although very rare. Most allergic reactions to topical anesthetics are limited to the area where the drug was applied, so topical anesthetics are relatively safe (Figure 14-16),

Anti-Anxiety and Sedative Medications

Anxiety about dental procedures prevents many individuals from seeking routine dental care. The best treatment for dental anxiety is a series of nonthreatening appointments that allow the patient

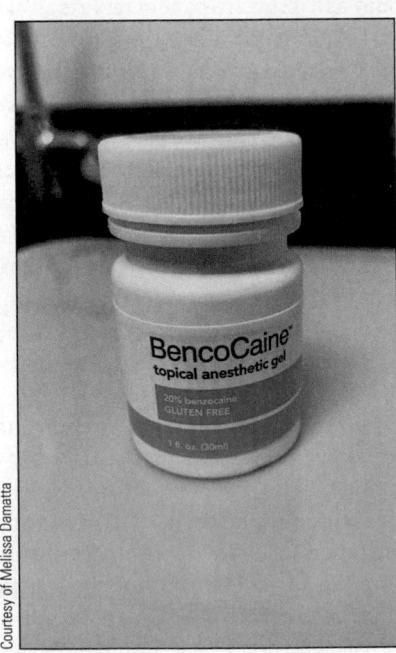

FIGURE 14-16
Topical anesthetic.

Courtesy of Melissa Damatta

Stress Reduction Protocol

- Establish rapport, be open to patient concerns
- Schedule short, morning appointments
- Avoid long waits in reception or treatment room
- Use topical anesthetic and gentle injection technique
- Ensure adequate anesthesia and post-procedure pain management
- Sedation with nitrous oxide may be beneficial

TABLE 14-4 Antianxiety/Sedative Medications Used in Dentistry

Brand Name	Generic Name	Drug Family	DEA Schedule	FDA Pregnancy Category
Valium	diazepam	benzodiazepines	IV	D
Ativan	lorazepam	benzodiazepines	IV	D
Versed	midazolam	benzodiazepines	IV	D
Noctec	chloral hydrate	hypnotic	IV	C
Pentothal	thiopental sodium	barbiturate	II	D
Seconal	secobarbital	barbiturate	II	D

to build trust in the dentist and staff. This process is known as *systematic desensitization therapy* and is appropriate for children and adults. The dental office can also utilize a stress reduction protocol for all patients (refer to feature box at top of page).

However, some patients may require the use of anti-anxiety medications to allow the patient to complete necessary treatment. The dentist may prescribe an oral medication to be taken before the appointment begins, use an intravenous (IV) medication during the appointment, or use a combination of the two. Examples of anti-anxiety or sedative medications are listed in Table 14-4.

The most common anti-anxiety medications used in dentistry belong to a family of medications called the **benzodiazepines**. Low doses of these drugs produce reduction in feelings of panic and anxiety. Higher doses produce drowsiness and sleep. Short-term use of benzodiazepines in the course of dental treatment is very safe. These drugs are Schedule IV controlled substances. While not highly addictive when used as directed, abuse of these drugs is possible if they are used excessively or combined with other substances, such as alcohol. The reversal agent for benzodiazepines is flumazenil. An office that uses benzodiazepines for sedation should also have flumazenil in the emergency kit in the event of an accidental overdose. Flumazenil is administered intravenously.

When a deeper sedation or unconsciousness is desired, a **barbiturate** drug may be used intravenously. Barbiturates are Schedule II controlled substances and are much more dangerous than benzodiazepines. Only an operator trained in advanced life-support and resuscitation techniques should administer barbiturates. Barbiturates cause both respiratory and cardiovascular depression, and equipment to maintain and monitor vital functions such as respiration must be utilized when barbiturates are administered. Barbiturates are never the drug of choice for relief of anxiety only, but may be used in a surgical setting for inducing short-term general anesthesia.

Chloral hydrate is a drug that is neither a benzodiazepine nor a barbiturate. For many years, chloral hydrate was used in dental offices for the sedation of children. It was administered as a liquid mixed with a flavored drink. Effects begin in about 30 minutes. Many dentists chose chloral hydrate because it was inexpensive and easy to use. Stomach upset is a common side effect of chloral hydrate, and effects of the drug vary from one child to another. Today, benzodiazepines are considered a safer and more reliable choice for children because there is a reversal agent for benzodiazepines in the event of overdose. There is no reversal agent for chloral hydrate.

If a sedative medication or nitrous oxide is to be used, the dentist and staff must take precautions to ensure the patient's safety and minimize liability for the office. Discussion of the treatment plan and informed consent must be obtained and documented prior to sedation. Recovery from nitrous oxide sedation is rapid and complete so that patients may drive themselves home after an appropriate amount of time. For all other forms of sedation, dental staff must ensure that the patient has safe transportation before the medication is administered. Some forms of sedation can cause fanciful thoughts or dreams of a sexual nature. It is advisable to have an assistant or observer of the same gender as the patient and to document this in the treatment notes. Many pediatric offices have observation windows so that parents may be assured that nothing inappropriate happens during treatment.

Both benzodiazepines and barbiturates are known to have teratogenic effects. Benzodiazepine use in the first trimester of pregnancy has been linked to cleft lip, cleft palate, and other conditions.

Women should always be questioned about potential pregnancy before administering or prescribing these medicines. In addition to questioning, the dentist or assistant should explain clearly the risks involved, and this conversation should be documented in the patient's chart with the patient's signature indicating understanding and consent.

Analgesics

It is important to understand that the response to pain varies greatly from one individual to another. Some people will tolerate a high level of pain, and others will demand relief for any hint of discomfort. While many factors are involved in the individual response to pain, fear and anxiety play a large role in the dental office. Anxious patients may report more pain involved with treatment. It is important to recognize all the issues involved in pain relief.

Analgesics are medications for relief of pain. Some analgesics also reduce inflammation. In dentistry, inflammation and pain

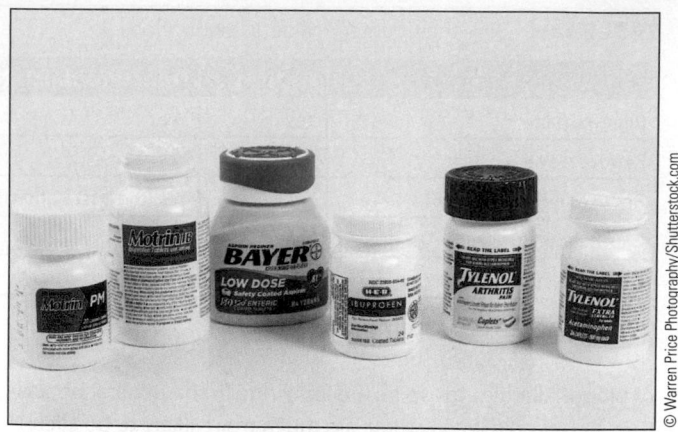

FIGURE 14-17
Over-the-counter pain medications.

© Warren Price Photography/Shutterstock.com

are closely linked, so medications that reduce both are especially helpful. Effective analgesics are available over the counter such as ibuprofen and aspirin. For severe pain, prescription medications may be needed. Many prescription pain medications are controlled substances because they contain opioid, or narcotic, substances. The nonopioid medications are discussed first in this section as most drugs with opioid ingredients also have nonopioid ingredients.

Over-the-Counter Analgesics Nonopioid analgesics are divided into three groups: the aspirin family, nonsteroidal anti-inflammatory drugs (NSAIDs), and acetaminophen (Figure 14-17). These medications are similar in many ways, but there are important differences. The assistant should understand when dentist recommends medications from each of these groups and, just as importantly, when medicines from each group should be avoided. Table 14-5 provides a summary of common OTC analgesics.

Aspirin (acetyl salicylic acid) is one of the oldest analgesics (Figure 14-17). Aspirin is sold as a stand-alone medication but is also an ingredient in many combination products, both OTC and prescription. Aspirin's primary therapeutic effects are relief of pain, reduction of inflammation, and reduction of fever. Onset of action is relatively fast, around 30 minutes. Adverse effects of aspirin are stomach irritation, increase in bleeding, and allergic reactions. Patients with any gastrointestinal problem, such as ulcers, gastroesophageal reflux disease (GERD), or colitis, should not take aspirin or any medication containing aspirin. Aspirin also reduces the clotting ability of blood. This can be an adverse effect if the patient takes aspirin prior to a surgical procedure. However, many people with cardiovascular disease take one baby aspirin every day to prevent blood clots based on recommendations made by their physicians. If a patient is taking a prescription medication such as Coumadin or Plavix to decrease blood clots, aspirin must be avoided. In some cases, the physician may advise the patient take aspirin along with the Coumadin or Plavix. However, the dentist should avoid recommending or prescribing aspirin to a patient who is taking a medication that reduces the clotting

TABLE 14-5 Over-the-Counter Analgesic Medications

	Aspirin	Nonsteroidal Anti-inflammatory Drugs (NSAIDs)	Acetaminophen
Relieves pain	Yes	Yes	Yes
Reduces fever	Yes	Yes	Yes
Reduces inflammation	Yes	Yes (the best option for dental pain barring any contraindications)	No
GI irritation	Yes	Yes	No
Decreases blood clotting	Yes	Minimally	No

of blood. Allergies to aspirin are fairly rare in the general population, but people with asthma are much more likely to be allergic to aspirin. Children who have a viral disease such as chicken pox or influenza and are treated with aspirin may develop a serious complication called Reye's syndrome. Reye's syndrome causes damage to the liver and kidneys and can be fatal. For this reason, aspirin is not used to treat fevers in children; a better option is acetaminophen. Aspirin also presents some risk for pregnancy, so it is not the drug of choice for pregnant women, infants, or children. Because the adverse effects of aspirin can be serious, it is important to know if a medication contains aspirin. Many OTC cold medications contain aspirin. It is important to read the box to determine what ingredients are contained in the medication.

The NSAIDs are a large group of drugs (Figure 14-17). NSAIDs such as ibuprofen and naproxen are similar to aspirin in both therapeutic and adverse effects. They are so similar that NSAIDs may be contraindicated in people who cannot use aspirin. For example, if a person is allergic to aspirin, they may be allergic to an NSAID as well. If a patient cannot take aspirin due to bleeding or gastrointestinal problems, an NSAID would also aggravate these problems. NSAIDs are more effective than aspirin in their effect on pain and fever and are better at reducing inflammation. Since dental pain is often associated with inflammation, the NSAIDs are the nonopioid drug of choice for dental pain *if* there are no medical contraindications to use.

The final choice for nonopioid pain relief is acetaminophen (Figure 14-17). Acetaminophen is considered an aspirin substitute. Acetaminophen is equal to aspirin in the relief of pain and fever. However, it is not anti-inflammatory and is not as effective as aspirin against dental pain. The advantage of acetaminophen is its lack of adverse effects in normal doses. It does not irritate the stomach and has no effect on bleeding. Large doses of acetaminophen are toxic to the liver. Acetaminophen combined with alcohol can cause liver damage in even small doses.

Prescription Analgesics Most prescription-strength analgesics are a combination an opioid drug and a nonopioid pain reliever. The weaker opioids given alone provide less pain relief than an NSAID. Stronger opioids, such as morphine, are not appropriate for dentistry. The combination drugs, with both opioid and nonopioid ingredients, make effective pain relievers. The success of combination drugs is explained by the way the two ingredients work together. Nonopioid drugs work by blocking pain-related chemicals at the site of the pain. Opioid drugs act within the

central nervous system to dull the response to pain ("I know that it hurts, but I really don't care."). Together, these drugs prevent pain messages from being sent to the brain and, for the messages that get through, they muddle the response to the message.

Common prescriptions for dental pain include drugs with codeine, hydrocodone, or oxycodone as ingredients, typically combined with aspirin or acetaminophen. It is important to know all of the ingredients of a drug. If a patient should avoid aspirin, the dentist should not prescribe a drug containing aspirin. Table 14-6 provides the ingredients of several prescription analgesics that may be used in dentistry.

These drugs are controlled substances in Schedules II or III. Meperidine (Demerol) is an opioid often requested by drug-seeking patients. Taken orally, it is no more, and perhaps less, effective for dental pain than the combination drugs, and it has significantly greater side effects. One of the most common side effects of all opioids is nausea and vomiting. It is best to discuss prior responses to opioid prescription medications before prescribing one. Even the best medication will not be effective if the patient cannot tolerate it.

Anti-Infective Drugs

There are three situations requiring anti-infective drugs in dentistry. Some patients arrive at the dental office with an existing

TABLE 14-6 Prescription Pain Medications Used in Dentistry

Brand	Ingredients (opioid, nonopioid)	DEA Schedule
Demerol	meperidine	II
Empirin #3	codeine, aspirin	III
Fiorinal #3	codeine, aspirin, butalbital, caffeine	III
Lorcet, Lortab, Norco, Vicodin	hydrocodone, acetaminophen	II
Percocet	oxycodone, acetaminophen	II
Percodan	oxycodone, aspirin	II
Tylenol #3	codeine, acetaminophen	III
Tylox	oxycodone, acetaminophen	II
Vicodin	hydrocodone, acetaminophen	II
Vicoprofen	hydrocodone, ibuprofen	II

dental or oral infection, others develop an infection after treatment, and occasionally a patient has a medical condition that requires the use of an antibiotic prior to treatment to prevent infection elsewhere in the body. This use of antibiotics is called *prophylactic* use because it prevents a potential medical problem. Most dental infections are bacterial in nature, but fungal and viral infections of the oral cavity are possible as well.

Antibiotics Drugs used to fight bacterial infections are antibiotics. Antibiotics can be either bactericidal or bacteriostatic. Bactericidal antibiotics destroy and kill the bacteria. Bacteriostatic antibiotics prevent the bacteria from replicating so the body's immune system can kill the bacteria. Antibiotics should not be prescribed routinely, but only when other means are not sufficient to remove the bacteria. Not every dental infection requires an antibiotic. For example, surgical drainage of an abscess or flushing of an area with saline or antimicrobial rinse may resolve a localized infection. Only when a dental infection threatens to spread to surrounding tissues is an antibiotic needed. Antibiotics have side effects, and overuse of antibiotics has serious consequences such as **resistance**.

Prophylactic Antibiotics The oral cavity is teeming with microbes. Any time the oral mucosa is penetrated, as in dental care, these oral microbes can enter the bloodstream. Immune cells in the bloodstream normally kill off the bacteria within a couple of hours. Some individuals have medical conditions that increase the risk that these transient bacteria may set up a colony within the body. Taking a large dose of antibiotic just prior to a dental procedure can provide protection for these at-risk individuals. The feature box below lists dental procedures that generally require antibiotic prophylaxis for at-risk patients.

The feature box above lists conditions requiring antibiotic prophylaxis and conditions that do *not* generally require it.

2007 Guidelines from the American Heart Association for Use of Prophylactic Antibiotics Based on Procedure to Be Performed

Prophylaxis Recommended
Prophylaxis is recommended for *all dental procedures* that involve manipulation of gingival tissue or the periapical region of the teeth, or perforation of the oral mucosa.

Prophylaxis Not Necessary
- oral radiographs
- routine anesthetic injections through noninfected tissues
- delivery of removable prosthetic appliances
- placement or adjustment of orthodontic brackets and appliances
- occlusal sealants or supra-gingival restorations
- fluoride treatments

2007 Guidelines from the American Heart Association for Use of Prophylactic Antibiotics Based on Medical Condition

Prophylaxis Recommended
- prosthetic heart valve or prosthetic material used for defective cardiac valve repair
- previous infective endocarditis
- congenital heart disease (CHD)
- unrepaired cyanotic CHD
- CHD that has been completely repaired with prosthetic materials (first 6 months after procedure)
- Repaired CHD with residual defects still present
- Cardiac transplant patients who develop valvulopathy

Prophylaxis Generally NOT Necessary
- heart murmur
- mitral valve prolapse
- history of cardiac bypass surgery

Prophylaxis MAY Be Necessary (consult physician)
- renal dialysis
- systemic lupus erythematosis
- severe sickle cell disease

Prosthetic Joints
In 2014 a panel was formed by the American Dental Association. This panel conducted a study and concluded that prophylactic antibiotics given prior to dental procedures are *not recommended* for patients with prosthetic joint implants.

Other conditions that may require prophylactic antibiotics are systemic lupus erythematosis, sickle cell anemia, and kidney dialysis. The antibiotic of choice is amoxicillin, which is in the penicillin family. If the patient is allergic to penicillins, the drug of choice is clindamycin. Table 14-7 provides the most recent American Heart Association (AHA) guidelines for antibiotic dosage for patients presenting for specific dental procedures and with a medical condition that requires antibiotic premedication.

Today, joint replacements for knees and hips are becoming more common. Until 2014, the AHA required that patients with prosthetic joints be premedicated with antibiotics in order to prevent prosthetic joint infections (PJI).

A physician's consultation may be needed to determine if the prophylaxis is needed. Remember, a patient is not required to give consent for their physician and dentist to share information *if* the information impacts the safety of the patient. If the patient refuses to give consent, the dental office can refuse treatment as treatment without complete information may result in harm to the patient.

 As soon as the patient arrives at the office, the dental assistant should confirm that the patient has taken the necessary premedication, and this should be recorded in the patient's chart.

TABLE 14-7 Antibiotic Prophylaxis Regimen for Patients with a Medical Condition

Condition	Medication	Regimen: Single dose 30-60 minutes before procedure for adults
Able to take oral medications	amoxicillin	2 grams
Unable to take oral medications	ampicillin **OR** cefazolin or ceftriaxone	2 g IM or IV 1 g IM or IV
Allergic to penicillins or ampicillins and able to take oral medications	cephalexin **OR** clindamycin **OR** azithromycin or clarithromycin	2 gm 600 mg 500 mg
Allergic to penicillins or ampicillins and unable to take oral medications	cefazolin or ceftriaxone **OR** clindamycin	1g IM or IV 600mg IM or IV

Adapted from the American Heart Association

Precautions for Antibiotic Use Antibiotics should only be used for infections caused by bacteria; antibiotics are ineffective against viral or fungal infections. In addition, antibiotics should not be used if the infection can be resolved by other means, such as debridement of the infected area. Overuse of antibiotics leads to formation of resistant strains of bacteria. In addition, antibiotics have significant side effects including diarrhea, reduction in blood clotting, failure of oral contraceptives, and secondary infections by organisms such as yeast. Most side effects are due to the fact that antibiotics kill not only the harmful bacteria causing the infection but also the "good" bacteria that help the body with such things as digestion and formation of vitamin K (necessary for blood clotting).

Common Antibiotics The antibiotics most often used in dentistry are the penicillins, cephalosporins, macrolides, tetracyclines, and clindamycin. Penicillins are **bacteriocidal,** have been used for many years, and are a good choice for dental infections. Penicillins are rapidly absorbed and distributed and they are effective against a wide range of bacteria. For this reason, amoxicillin, a member of the penicillin family, is the first drug of choice for prophylactic antibiotic premedication. Unfortunately, some people have allergies to penicillin, and the allergic reaction can, in rare cases, be life threatening. Patients should always be questioned about prior experience with penicillin. Names of commonly used penicillins are Pen VK, Amoxil (amoxicillin), and Augmentin (amoxicillin and potassium clauvulanate).

Cephalosporins are similar to penicillins and may be used for bacteria resistant to penicillin. Because the two antibiotics are so similar, about 10% of people who are allergic to penicillin are also allergic to cephalosporins. Names of common cephalosporins are Keflex (cephalexin), Ceclor (cefaclor), Suprax (cefixime), and Omnicef (cefdinir).

The macrolides are a group of **bacteriostatic** drugs that includes erythromycin, clarithromycin, and azithromycin. These drugs are effective against the same bacteria as penicillin and are the drugs of choice if the patient is allergic to penicillin. Because macrolides are "-static" instead of "-cidal," penicillin is always the better choice if the patient is not allergic. Names of common macrolides are E-mycin (erythromycin), Zithromax (azithromycin), and clarithromycin (Biaxin).

The tetracyclines are antibiotics with unique interest to dentistry, both positive and negative. Tetracyclines are of little use for infections of the teeth or bone, such as a periapical abscess, but they are especially useful against periodontal disease. This is because the tetracyclines aggregate in the fluid in the gingival sulcus. This makes them effective against periodontal disease. Tetracyclines are used in both topical and systemic forms to fight advanced periodontal conditions. The topical form of tetracycline is injected into the gingival sulcus. One brand name is Arestin, and another is Oraqix. There is also a low-dose tetracycline tablet, Periostat, taken orally by patients with aggressive periodontal disease. Other commonly used periodontal products contain the antimicrobial chlorhexidine; the common brand name is Periostat. Chlorhexidine rinses are available by prescription only.

Until the more recent discovery of periodontal benefits, tetracyclines were widely known for the permanent staining they cause in teeth. The tetracycline molecule attaches to any calcifying tissue. If tetracycline is given during tooth or bone development, the drug becomes part of that structure. The structure is just as strong and healthy as normal, but the tetracycline creates a grey or brown discoloration. If tetracycline is given during pregnancy, the child's deciduous teeth will be affected. If tetracycline is given between birth and age six, the permanent teeth will be permanently stained. Names of common tetracyclines are Sumycin (tetracycline), Vibramycin (doxyclycline), and Minocin (minocylcine).

Cleocin (clindamycin) is not related to any other group of antibiotics, even though the name looks similar. Adverse reactions to clindamycin are more serious than to other antibiotics, so it is never the first drug of choice for dental infections. Clindamycin is sometimes used for endocarditis prophylaxis in patients who are allergic to penicillin.

The assistant should be aware that different antibiotics may have similar sounding names. This is a situation in which the type of drug cannot be deduced by the name alone. If in doubt, consult a drug reference.

Antiviral and Antifungal Drugs In addition to bacterial infections, the viral infection herpes simplex and the fungal infection candidiasis (yeast) are often seen in dental practice. Antibiotics are not effective against either of these.

While it is not always possible to "cure" a viral infection, medication can lessen the severity and duration of the lesion. If the individual is otherwise healthy and has only occasional episodes of herpes labialis, the infection can be allowed to run its course. Patients troubled by frequent outbreaks or patients with compromised immune systems, such as people living with AIDS or cancer, can benefit from antiviral medication. These medications

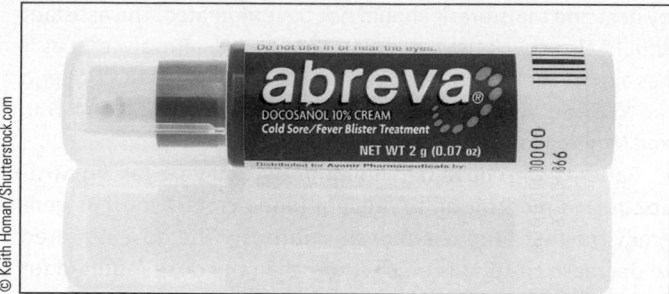

FIGURE 14-18
Abreva.

are also useful for the healthy patient who develops a herpes lesion just prior to an important event such as a wedding. Abreva (doclosanol) is available without a prescription (Figure 14-18) and Zovirax (acyclovir) and Denavir (penciclovir), a more potent drug, are both available by prescription for treatment of herpes simplex labialis. All of these medicines are applied directly to the affected area and work best if applied at the first sign that an outbreak is about to occur.

Oral yeast infections are common in infants and in the frail elderly. They also occur in patients of any age who wear complete dentures. Yeast grows well in a warm, moist environment. Dentures that are not removed and cleaned daily create a perfect environment for yeast to flourish. If the patient is not an infant, elderly, or a denture-wearer, an oral yeast infection may be a sign of a compromised immune system. Oral yeast infections occur in HIV positive patients and can be an indicator that HIV infection is progressing to full-blown AIDS. Other conditions that may contribute to yeast infections are leukemia, cancer chemotherapy, and long-term antibiotic use. Nystatin is the drug of choice for yeast infection. It is available as a liquid to be swished and spit out or swallowed. Other drugs for yeast are clotrimazole (Mycelex) and ketoconazole (Nizoral). Clotrimazole is available as a lozenge that can be held in the mouth. Unfortunately, these oral preparations are high in sugar content.

Patient Risk Assessment

Before any drug is administered or prescribed in the dental office, the risks and benefits to the patient must be weighed. The medical history is the starting place for risk assessment. In many offices, the dental assistant Is the first person to review the medical history. The dental assistant should ensure that the written or computerized medical history in the patient's record is current and up to date, even if the patient was just treated recently. Simply asking, "have there been any changes since your last visit?" is not adequate. Significant facts and changes should be noted for the dentist's review.

Allergies to any substance should be documented in the medical history. Then, questions about a specific drug should be asked prior to administering or prescribing the drug. New allergic reactions can occur at any time. Every time a drug is used, these questions should be asked. Patients should also be asked if they

are currently taking any medications, prescription or OTC. This, too, can change from one dental visit to the next. This question has three purposes. The dental staff needs to be aware of any potential drug interactions that may occur with dental drugs. We also need to look for oral side effects of the patient's medication and be prepared to discuss them with the patient. Finally, there may be patient management considerations related to the patient's medication. For example, many medications cause orthostatic hypotension. This side effect of many medications, such as blood pressure lowering medications, causes a sudden drop in blood pressure when the patient rises from a supine position. The patient can suddenly become unconscious as a result. For patients taking medications that can cause orthostatic hypotension, the dental assistant should take care that the patient does not stand up quickly from a supine position. The patient should be brought from supine to upright slowly in stages, and the dental assistant should stand near the patient in case of loss of consciousness.

For all female patients of childbearing age, the dental assistant should inquire about possible pregnancy before any medications are administered or prescribed. Most expectant mothers will joyfully announce this without questioning, but some may not be aware of the relevance to dental care. Other women may suspect that they are pregnant but have not yet confirmed it. A question from the dentist or assistant will prompt information that may not otherwise be offered.

ASA Classification System

The American Society of Anesthesiologists (ASA) physical status classification system is covered in detail in Chapter 15. This system was created in order to establish the patient's physical status prior to selecting an anesthetic or prior to performing surgery. This classification should be considered whenever anesthesia is administered, including local anesthesia or nitrous oxide in the dental office. Obviously, some medications and some procedures carry more risk than others. Recognizing medical issues and addressing stress and anxiety can lower the risk of an adverse event with a fearful patient. Likewise, recognizing medications the patient is taking for systemic disease will help in understanding the severity of the disease and the appropriate ASA category.

Dental Implications of Medications for Systemic Disease

While it would be impossible to remember every oral and systemic adverse effect for every drug, some effects are common to many groups of drugs. When in doubt, do not hesitate to consult a drug reference.

Cardiovascular Medications

All practices that treat adult patients will see a large number of patients who take cardiovascular medications. Cardiovascular disease is a leading cause of death and disability in the United States. With early diagnosis and advances in treatment, many affected individuals will not die from their cardiovascular disease but will live in treatment for many years. The diseases include hypertension, hyperlipidemia or elevated cholesterol, angina pectoris or chest pain due to blockages in the vessels that supply the heart, coronary artery disease, and congestive heart failure. Congestive heart failure is a condition in which the heart is not efficiently working as a pump. The practice will also see many individuals who have survived a heart attack (myocardial infarction, MI) or stroke (cerebrovascular accident, CVA). Patients with all of these conditions take medications, often multiple medications. The number of medications a patient takes to control their condition can be an indicator of the severity of the condition.

Digitalis was one of the first medications used to treat heart disease, beginning in the 1700s as a remedy made from the foxglove plant. Today, the most common form of digitalis is *digoxin* (Lanoxin). Digitalis can be used to treat congestive heart failure and *arrhythmias* or abnormal heart rhythms, but is usually limited to use for patients who have both conditions. Digitalis drugs have serious side effects and can result in toxicity if the patient is not monitored closely by their physician. For this reason, other, safer medications are tried first. Digitalis is used only if other medications are not effective. When the medical history shows the use of digitalis, the assistant should surmise that the patient's heart condition is serious. A drug interaction with local anesthetics containing vasoconstrictors is possible. Vasoconstrictors should be used in limited amounts or not at all. The patient's physician should be consulted prior to treatment to determine whether or not the patient can receive a local anesthetic with epinephrine and whether or not the patient can be treated safely in the dental office. The medical consult should be received in a written format and saved in the patient's record. While many cardiovascular medications cause xerostomia, digitalis is one of the few drugs that cause an increase in salivation, especially at toxic levels of the drug. Other patient management considerations are that patients with congestive heart failure may not be comfortable in a supine position, and the dental assistant should monitor the patient's pulse to check for arrhythmia.

Nitroglycerin is another cardiac medication that has been used for many years. Its primary use is in the treatment and prevention of angina pectoris. Nitroglycerin is a powerful *vasodilator*. By dilating coronary vessels, nitroglycerin allows more oxygen to reach the heart muscle. Unfortunately, vasodilation is not limited to the vessels of the heart but occurs all over the body. After a dose of nitroglycerin, patients may experience headaches from dilation of cranial blood vessels as a side effect. This is another situation where vasoconstrictors should be used with caution. If too much vasoconstrictor enters the bloodstream, the patient may have an attack of angina due to the narrowing of the blood vessels. However, pain due to inadequate anesthesia may also trigger an attack of angina. At each appointment the dental assistant should ask the patient if they have their medicine with them. It is best to use the patient's own medication in case of an attack as it is the correct prescribed dose for the patient. However, the office should keep nitroglycerin in the emergency kit as well. The assistant should ask the patient to put the nitroglycerin in a location that can be easily reached if needed. Nitroglycerin is inactivated

by heat and moisture. It should not be refrigerated. The assistant should also check the expiration date on the nitroglycerin as it has a short shelf life Commonly prescribed forms of nitroglycerin are NTG and Nitrostat for acute attacks, and Nitro-Bid, Nitro-Dur, and Minitran for daily preventive use.

Patients who have had an MI or CVA may be taking **anticoagulant** medication to prevent blood clots. Aspirin is generally the first drug used for this purpose. The dose required to decrease clotting is much lower than the dose required for pain relief. Still, some patients cannot tolerate aspirin due to the side effects such as gastrointestinal irritation. The prescription drug Plavix (clopidogrel) may be used for these patients instead. Both aspirin and Plavix affect the platelets. The drug Coumadin (warfarin) works in a different way. Of the three drugs, warfarin has the greatest number of drug interactions and precautions.

Care must be taken with patients taking any drug that decreases blood clotting. This patient is in danger of excessive post-operative bleeding during and after surgical procedures. Simple restorative and preventive procedures can usually be performed with no adverse consequences. A consultation with the patient's physician is recommended when surgical procedures are needed. Pain medication containing aspirin must be avoided.

Cardiovascular disease is treated with many medications from a number of drug groups. Some drugs are effective for more than one type of cardiovascular disease. For example, a *diuretic* may be used to treat congestive heart failure by causing excess fluid to leave the body. This allows the heart to pump more efficiently. A diuretic may also be used to manage hypertension. Common diuretics include HCTZ (hydrochlorothiazide) and Lasix (furosemide). Diuretics can cause a potassium deficiency known as *hypokalemia* that leads to muscle cramps or cardiac arrhythmias.

Another popular cardiovascular drug group is the ACE (angiotensin converting enzyme) inhibitors. ACE inhibitors can be used to treat congestive heart failure and hypertension. They are considered a safer choice than the digitalis drugs for heart failure. Long-term use of NSAID pain relievers may decrease the effectiveness of both diuretics and ACE inhibitors. Common ACE inhibitors are Capoten (captoppril), Vasotec (enalopril), and Prinovil or Zestril (lisinopril). The letters "-pril" at the end of the generic name can help the dental assistant recognize drugs in this group. Likewise, the drug family known as beta blockers can be recognized by the letters "-olol" at the end of the generic name. Beta blockers reduce the effects of epinephrine and norepinephrine normally produced by the patient's body. So, use of epinephrine should be limited to the cardiac dose of epinephrine or two cartridges of lidocaine 1:100,000 epinephrine concentration. Epinephrine should be avoided in the *retraction cord* that may be used to take impressions for a fixed prosthesis. Common beta blockers are Inderal (propranolol), Tenormin (atenolol), and Lopressor (metoprolol).

Yet another cardiovascular drug group is the calcium channel blockers. This group has an oral side effect of gingival enlargement. No other cardiovascular drug group has this effect. The gingival overgrowth is triggered by irritation from plaque and calculus. The dental assistant can help the patient control this effect by encouraging excellent oral hygiene and teaching plaque control techniques.

Some calcium channel blockers can be recognized by the ending "-ipine" on the generic names. Some calcium channel blocking drugs are Procardia (nifedipine), Norvasc (amlodipine), Cardizem (diltiazem), and Calan (verapamil). Calcium channel blockers and beta blockers are effective for both hypertension and the prevention of angina pectoris. Calcium channel blockers and ACE inhibitors share the adverse effect of *dysgeusia*, or altered taste. Other adverse effects of several cardiovascular drugs are xerostomia and orthostatic hypotension. The dental assistant should be aware of these.

HIPAA requires that all patient information is kept private and secure.

Patients who have high cholesterol or hyperlipidemia may be on cholesterol lowering medications. High cholesterol can lead to fat buildup in blood vessels. If not controlled through diet and medications, the buildup may cause narrowing of the blood vessels, which can lead to a myocardial infarction or a stroke. Lipitor is an example of one drug in this group.

Endocrine Medications

Drugs that act on the endocrine system are many and varied. Most of them are replacements for a particular hormone that is deficient in a patient's body. A few endocrine drugs act to block the action or production of a hormone.

Diabetes is a disease that is increasing in prevalence, and the dental office will treat many patients taking medication for diabetes. If the medical history shows that a patient is taking insulin, this indicates that the patient has Type I (insulin-dependent) diabetes or a more severe case of Type II diabetes. This patient is much more likely to have a diabetic emergency during dental treatment than a Type II diabetic who controls their diabetes with diet and exercise only. The dental assistant should be watchful for signs of a diabetic emergency and be prepared to respond as described in Chapter 15. Patients with Type II diabetes may also be taking an oral medication to help regulate their blood sugar. These medicines include Diabinese (chlorpropomide), Glucotrol (glipizide), Glucophage (metformin), and many others. Both Type I and Type II diabetics should be questioned as to when they last had a meal, and whether they have taken their medicine and checked their blood sugar.

Patients with thyroid disorders can have either too much thyroid hormone (hyperthyroid) or too little (hypothyroid). Sometimes the thyroid gland is removed from a patient who is hyperthyroid, making the patient hypothyroid. So, the most common thyroid drug is a thyroid hormone replacement. A few of these are Synthroid (levothyroxine), Cytomel (liothyronine), and Euthyroid or Thyrolar (liotrix). Thyroid disorders and the impact on dental treatment is further discussed in the Medical Emergencies chapter of this textbook.

A number of female patients will be taking drugs to alter the levels of various female sex hormones. This includes drugs used to prevent pregnancy (contraceptives) as well as drugs taken to increase fertility. There is some indication that women taking contraceptive drugs may be more likely to develop a dry socket after tooth extraction. A woman taking drugs to increase fertility, such as Clomid (clomiphene), should be treated as if she is already pregnant as this is a powerful fertility drug. If dental treatment is necessary and requires the use of any drugs, treatment should be scheduled during the first days of the menstrual cycle when it is unlikely the patient is pregnant. Postmenopausal women may be taking estrogen replacement drugs such as Premarin (conjugated estrogen). Any female hormonal medications can influence the gingiva. Redness, bleeding and swelling as associated with pregnancy-related gingivitis may be seen in women taking any of these drugs.

Androgens, the male sex hormones, and the anabolic steroids have some limited therapeutic uses. Androgens may be used to treat certain types of breast cancer in females. Anabolic steroids are synthetic versions of the male hormone testosterone and may be used to replace the hormone when the body does not produce enough. However, these medications are more often used in illegal ways. Athletes may abuse the androgens to rapidly increase muscle mass while reducing fat. Used in this manner, doses up to 100 times the therapeutic dose may be used. The adverse effects of high cholesterol, liver disease and aggressive behavior, increase with increased doses. Anabolic steroids have similar effects and abuse potential. These drugs alter the normal balance of tissue buildup and breakdown. These too, have very serious adverse effects. For this reason, anabolic steroids are controlled substances in Schedule III.

The *corticosteroids*, such as prednisone, are used for management of inflammatory and allergic conditions. With short-term use, these drugs give excellent relief of symptoms. Patients with chronic conditions, such as arthritis, who use these drugs indefinitely have serious adverse effects and may require special management in the dental office. Because corticosteroids suppress the immune response, patients who take them for long periods are at increased risk of infection and have poor wound healing. This is a consideration if dental surgery is needed. Long-term use of corticosteroids can also lead to *osteoporosis*, or a reduced density of bone. Susceptibility to infection plus osteoporosis puts the patient at risk for periodontal disease. If periodontal disease is present, it will have a more rapid course and will not respond as well to treatment. Some dental patients with asthma use an inhaler that contains a bronchodilator and may also contain a corticosteroid (see Chapter 15). These patients may develop a localized oral fungal infection at the spot the inhaled medicine contacts the oral tissues due to the corticosteroids. The dental assistant should advise patients to rinse their mouth with water after each use of the inhaler. Flovent (fluticasone) and Advair (fluticasone/ salmeterol) are just two of the many inhalers containing corticosteroids. Dentists sometimes prescribe topical steroids, such as Kenalog (triamcinolone), to treat **aphthous** ulcers. Not all patients need an inhaler with a corticosteroid. The steroid helps to reduce inflammation in the airways, reducing the symptoms of the asthmatic attack. Some patients may be using an inhaler that contains only the bronchodilator. One example of a bronchodilator is a beta-2 agonist. These medications work on the beta-2 receptors in the lungs to relax the muscles and open the airways. The patient in the dental office should always be asked to bring their asthma pump with them in the event the patient experiences an asthmatic attack while in the office. This will be discussed in further detail in Chapter 15.

Psychiatric Medications

As with many other medical conditions, psychiatric disorders are often treated on an outpatient basis. Many of the psychiatric drugs have side effects and drug interactions that affect dental health and dental treatment. The three types of psychiatric disorders most often encountered in the dental office are psychosis, depression, and bipolar disorder.

Medicines for psychosis and bipolar disorder have the most serious adverse effects, including xerostomia, orthostatic hypotension, sedation, and neuromuscular problems called *extrapyramidal effects*. Extrapyramidal effects can cause uncontrollable movements that affect the face, lips, and tongue with tremors and muscle spasms. These can make dental treatment difficult and can cause TMJ problems. Additionally, oral hygiene home care is difficult for those who suffer from extrapyramidal effects. Antipsychotic medications also lower the seizure threshold and produce sedation. Any additional medication that causes sedation, such as opioids, should be avoided. Common antipsychotic drugs are Haldol (haloperidol), Thorazine (chlorpromazine), Abilify (aripiprazole), and Risperdal (risperidone).

A wide variety of drugs are available for treatment of depression. The older drugs, tricyclic antidepressants and monoamine oxidase inhibitors (MAOIs), have many side effects and are used only for depression that does not respond to other treatment. The newer class of antidepressants is the selective serotonin reuptake inhibitors (SSRIs). Examples of SSRIs are Prozac (fluoxetine), Zoloft (sertraline), and Celexa (citalopram). Xerostomia is a side effect of these drugs, but not as severe as seen with the older antidepressants. Welllbutrin (buproprion) is an antidepressant with a secondary use; it can help people stop smoking. This medicine is also used for smoking cessation under the brand name Zyban.

Medications for Neurological Disorders

Medications for neurological disorders such as Parkinson's disease, muscular sclerosis, and seizure disorders have many of the same side effects as the psychiatric drugs, especially xerostomia and sedation. One antiseizure medication, Dilantin (phenytoin), is of particular interest to dentistry because it causes gingival overgrowth. Like gingival overgrowth associated with calcium channel blockers, excellent oral hygiene can prevent much of this oral effect. However, the gingival overgrowth associated with phenytoin is more likely to occur and is more generalized

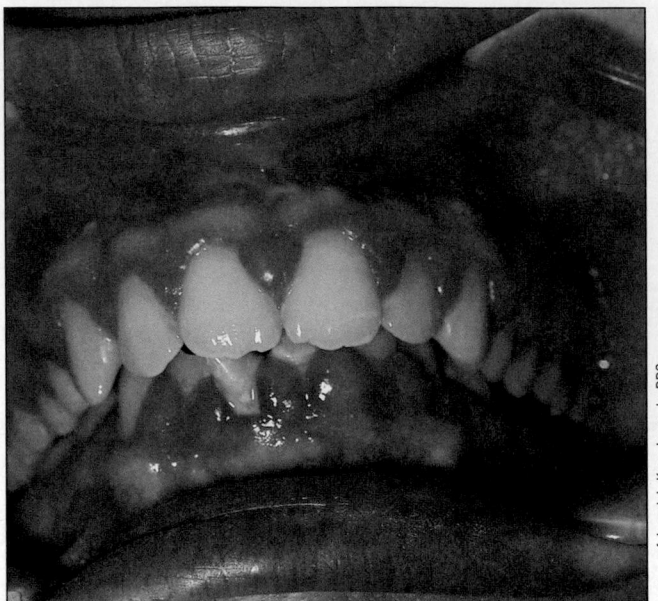

FIGURE 14-19
Gingival hyperplasia.

Courtesy of Joseph L. Konzelman, Jr., DDS

and severe than that associated with calcium channel blockers. This condition is sometimes referred to as Dilantin induced gingival hyperplasia, and the tissues tend to be thick and fibrotic (Figure 14-19).

In some cases, surgery is needed to remove the excess tissues (gingivectomy). The tissue will eventually grow back if oral hygiene is not improved. Many medications for seizure disorders also have teratogenic effects.

Cancer Chemotherapy

As cancer treatments become more successful, more patients will survive cancer or live longer with cancer. The dental office will see patients who have had cancer chemotherapy, are currently in chemotherapy, or are about to begin chemotherapy. The word *chemotherapy* in this case means the use of drugs to kill or slow the growth of cancer cells. Since cancer cells reproduce themselves at a rapid rate, chemotherapy drugs tend to target all cells that are reproducing themselves. Tissues that are constantly growing or repairing themselves, such as bone marrow, hair, skin, and nails, will be adversely affected by cancer chemotherapy. Likewise, mucosa of the oral cavity and GI tract can become very fragile. This adverse effect is called *mucositis*. Xerostomia is also common with chemotherapy. Various types of anemia may occur during chemotherapy because, in health, blood cells are continually produced in the bone marrow. The patient may be low on red blood cells, white cells, platelets, or all three. Low white cell counts put the patient at risk of infection. Because the immune system is depressed, patients may develop oral yeast infections. Low platelets increase the risk of bleeding. Low red cell counts deprive all of the tissues of oxygenation and cause fatigue.

Ideally, the patient should have a dental evaluation prior to the start of chemotherapy. The dentist treats any potential sources of infection and performs other necessary treatment. This ideal situation rarely occurs. After a diagnosis of cancer, there is further testing, possible surgery, and consultations with various medical specialists. Patients generally feel overwhelmed. There is often little time between the diagnosis and the beginning of chemotherapy. When a patient calls the dental office for an appointment prior to chemotherapy, it is important to offer an appointment that allows for evaluation and treatment before chemotherapy begins. Dental staff can talk to the patient about potential oral side effects of chemotherapy and offer ideas for managing them.

Dental treatment during chemotherapy involves more risk. Because of the bone marrow suppression that often occurs, the patient is at increased risk for infection, bleeding, and/or delayed healing. If treatment is necessary, consultation with the oncologist and blood counts should be obtained prior to treatment. The oncologist may prescribe medications to stimulate blood cell production to bring red cells, white cells, or platelets into the acceptable range for dental care. The patient's blood counts will be highest on the day before the next dose of chemotherapy.

After chemotherapy, most adverse effects will subside. Hair, skin, and mucosa will heal and regrow. This process of returning to normal can take many months. However, blood counts will improve in several weeks. Dental care can resume as soon as the patient's blood counts are normal. Some patients report that the xerostomia and oral sensitivity never completely go away. Dental workers can be extremely helpful in recommending appropriate oral care products.

Osteoporosis

Osteoporosis is a serious health hazard in the aging population. The incidence of osteoporosis increases with age. Women tend to develop osteoporosis earlier in life. After age 70, osteoporosis occurs equally in both men and women. A group of medications called the bisphosphonates strengthen bones weakened by osteoporosis. Some bisphosphonates are taken orally, and some are given as an IV. *Osteonecrosis* or localized death of the bone, especially in the mandible (ONJ, osteonecrosis of the jaw), is a rare but serious complication of bisphosphonate use and most commonly occurs with the IV form of bisphosphonates.

Fosamax (alendronate) and Boniva (ibandronate) are oral bisphosphonates, while Reclast (zoledronic acid) is an IV form. Osteonecrosis of the jaw is usually related to trauma. Normally uneventful dental situations such as oral or periodontal surgery or irritation from a dental appliance can trigger this effect. As bisphosphonate use increases with the increase in the aging population, dental professionals will see more of osteonecrosis.

Medications Used to Treat Substance Use Disorders

Recovering substance abusers present a special challenge to dental care providers. These patients must avoid all medications that can trigger relapse, such as opioids and anti-anxiety medications. Also, some recovering addicts take medications that can impact dental care.

Recovering alcoholics may be taking Antabuse (disulfiram). While taking this medication, any contact with alcohol will produce a severe, unpleasant reaction characterized by nausea and vomiting, headache, chest pain, racing heartbeat, and hyperventilation. Care must be taken that the patient is not exposed to alcohol in the course of dental treatment. Even alcohol-containing mouth rinses or disinfectant wipes may trigger this reaction.

Individuals recovering from narcotic use disorders should not be prescribed any scheduled substances. Any mood-altering drugs can trigger a relapse. In addition, the patient may have developed tolerance to these substances so that the usual therapeutic dose is not effective. Some recovering addicts take an opioid drug called Dolophine (methadone). Methadone prevents the addicted patient from experiencing withdrawal symptoms. However, opioid pain medication will be ineffective and could cause an overdose. NSAIDs are the best choice for dental pain relief in this case.

Chapter Summary

At no other time have drugs been as widely used and misused as they are today. The dental assistant will need to pay attention to the patient's medical and dental history and carefully document the drugs used by the patient. The dental assistant will have to become knowledgeable about pharmacology, the side effects of drugs, and drug interactions. Dental assistants are concerned with prescribed drugs, but they must also have knowledge about the illegal drugs that patients may be using and what will happen if the two types of drugs interact. It is also important to know the signs and symptoms that individuals may experience if under the influence of drugs. Background knowledge about drugs and their effects aids the dental assistant in providing better patient care.

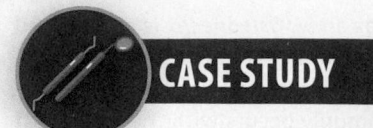

CASE STUDY

Jordan Taylor, a 20-year-old male, comes in because an upper anterior tooth has decay. This is his first visit to the office and he is from out of town. He states that he has pain and that the over-the-counter pain medications do not work for him. He also states that when he returns home he will go to his regular dentist for treatment and for now he just needs something to help alleviate his pain. He claims that the only medication that has helped to alleviate his pain in the past is Percocet. He seems nervous and anxious.

Case Study Review

1. What should the patient be told regarding treatment?

2. What database should be checked before writing a prescription for a narcotic pain medication?

3. Should the patient be given a prescription for Percocet?

Review Questions

Multiple Choice

1. Dental assistants should study pharmacology so that they can write prescriptions properly and so they can make better choices for themselves regarding OTC medications. *Select the correct answer based on this statement.*
   a. Both statements are true.
   b. Both statements are false.
   c. The first statement is true; the second statement is false.
   d. The first statement is false, the second statement is true.

2. Which of the following is correct regarding synthetic versus nonsynthetic drugs?
   a. Synthetic drugs are derived from natural sources.
   b. Nonsynthetic drugs are made in a laboratory.
   c. Some medications are a combination of synthetic and nonsynthetic sources.
   d. None of these choices are correct.

3. Which of the following is correct regarding drug names?
   a. The first name given to a drug is a brand name.
   a. The chemical name given is how the drug is marketed.
   b. Once the patent expires after 15 years, other companies may manufacture generic drugs.
   c. The FDA requires that the generic drug must be as efficacious as the original drug.

4. Which of the following is correct regarding the Physician's Drug Reference (PDR)?
   a. The PDR is available in print format only.
   b. The PDR allows the dental professional to look up drugs by brand name only.
   c. Manufacturers pay for space in the PDR.
   d. The PDR is published every 2 years.

5. Enterally administered drugs are administered by means of the gastrointestinal tract. Oral and rectal methods of administration are considered enteral.
   Select the correct response based on these statements.
   a. Both statements are true.
   b. Both statements are false.
   c. The first statement is true; the second statement is false.
   d. The first statement is false; the second statement is true.

6. The intravenous method of administration avoids absorption *because* the drug is placed directly into the bloodstream. Select the correct response based on this statement.
   a. Both statements are true.
   b. Both statements are false.
   c. The first statement is true; the second statement is false.
   d. The first statement is false; the second statement is true.

7. Which of the following Latin abbreviation used on a prescription means two times per day?
   a. qid
   b. prn
   c. bid
   d. tid

8. Tylenol with codeine is under which schedule number of controlled substances?
   a. Schedule I
   b. Schedule II
   c. Schedule III
   d. Schedule IV

9. Which of the following is not correct regarding patients with prescription seeking behaviors?
   a. The patient may have a history of past drug abuse.
   b. The patient may not be a patient of record but may call the office claiming a dental emergency.
   c. The patient may request refills claiming pain that is lasting longer than anticipated.
   d. Patients with drug seeking behaviors do not steal prescription pads, and as a result, it is not necessary to secure the pads.

10. The therapeutic action of a drug is the desired effect resulting from the action of the drug on nontarget organs or tissues. The adverse reactions are those that occur due to the action of the drug on target organs or tissues.
    Select the correct response based on these statements.
    a. Both statements are true.
    b. Both statements are false.
    c. The first statement is true; the second statement is false.
    d. The first statement is false; the second statement is true.

11. The group of local anesthetics used today are amides. The ester local anesthetics are no longer used due to the risk of allergic reactions.
    Select the correct response based on these statements.
    a. Both statements are true.
    b. Both statements are false.
    c. The first statement is true; the second statement is false.
    d. The first statement is false; the second statement is true.

12. A patient presents with stomach ulcers and needs a nonprescription pain medication to help minimize discomfort from the treatment completed. Which medication would be the best option for the patient?
    a. acetaminophen
    b. aspirin
    c. ibuprofen
    d. acetaminophen with codeine

13. Which of the following is not a reason for a patient to take an antibiotic?
    a. an existing dental infection
    b. a dental infection that develops after treatment
    c. the presence of an oral fungal infection
    d. prophylactically to prevent a potential medical infection

14. Which of the following are not commonly used or prescribed drugs in a standard dental office setting?
    a. local anesthetics
    b. general anesthetics
    c. antibiotics
    d. pain medications

15. Which of the following is a prescription based home use antimicrobial rinse used to manage periodontal disease?
    a. fluoride
    b. Periostat
    c. Oraqix
    d. antibiotics

16. Which of the following is a contraindication for a local anesthetic with epinephrine?
    a. controlled hypertension
    b. controlled Type II diabetes
    c. allergy to pollen
    d. allergy to bisulfites

17. Nitroglycerine is used for the management of _____.
    a. hypertension
    b. congestive heart failure
    c. angina pectoris
    d. blood clots

18. Osteonecrosis of the alveolar bone is a rare but serious side effect of bisphosphonates. Osteonecrosis is more likely to occur in the maxilla.
    Select the correct response based on these statements.
    a. Both statements are true.
    b. Both statements are false.
    c. The first statement is true; the second statement is false.
    d. The first statement is false; the second statement is true.

19. Medications used to treat psychiatric disorders may lead to extrapyramidal side effects. These uncontrollable movements of the jaws and face can make dental care more difficult.
    Select the correct response based on these statements.
    a. Both statements are true.
    b. Both statements are false.
    c. The first statement is true; the second statement is false.
    d. The first statement is false; the second statement is true.

20. Which of the following is correct regarding treatment for cancer?
    a. Patients do not need to have an oral evaluation prior to the start of cancer chemotherapy.
    b. It is not important to correct all sources of potential infection from the oral cavity.
    c. The patient can safely have dental treatment at any time during cancer chemotherapy.
    d. Xerostomia is a common side effect of cancer chemotherapy.

Critical Thinking

1. Calculate how many milligrams of amoxicillin should be given to a child that weighs 70 pounds. Dosing is 30 mg/kg/day. 3 divided doses for a child under 88 pounds.

2. What are the parts of the prescription and the information that belongs in each part?

3. What are the signs and symptoms of the four types of allergic reactions?

Key Terms

Term and Pronunciation	Meaning of Root and Word Parts	Definition
adverse (ad-**vurs**)	**adverse** = contrary, opposite	opposing one's interests or desire; occurrence of effect that is not desired
anabolic (an-*uh*-**bol**-ik)	**ana** = up, building up **-ism** = indicating an action, process	constructive metabolism; building up of body tissues
analgesic (an-l-**jee**-zik)	**-an** = without **-algia** = pain **-ic** = relating to	a drug that relieves pain
antibiotic (an-ti-bahy-**ot**-ik)	**-anti** =against **bios** =life **-ic** = relating to	a drug that destroys microorganisms or stops their growth and reproduction
antioxidant (an-tee-**ok**-si-d*uh* nt)	**anti-** = against, opposite **oxide** = any compound of oxygen with another element **-ize** = to make **-ant** = serving the capacity of	a substance, such as vitamin C, vitamin E, or beta carotene, that counteracts the damaging effects of oxidation in a living organism
aphthous ulcers (ăf'th*ə*s) (**uhl**-ser)	Aphtha = eruption Ulcus = sore	mucosal ulcer
bisulfite (bahy-**suhl**-fahyt)	**bi-** = two **sulphur** = a yellow nonmetallic element occurring widely in nature; used in the manufacture of pharmaceuticals and many sulfur compounds, especially sulfuric acid **-ite** = used to name salt or ester	a salt of sulfurous (containing sulfur) acid
capsule (**kap**-s*uh* l)	**caps** = covering, or top to **-ule** = indicating smallness	a gelatinous case enclosing a dose of medicine
cirrhosis (si-**roh**-sis)	**cirrh-** = liver **-osis** = condition	a chronic disease of the liver
diuretic (dahy-*uh*-**ret**-ik)	**diuretic** = tending to increase the discharge of urine	drug that increases urine output
diversion (dih-**vur**-*zhuh* n)	**divertere** = turn	to turn away or redirect from proper course
efficacious (ef-i-**key**-*shuh* s)	**efficient** = performing or functioning in the best possible manner with the least waste of time and effort **-acious** = given to, inclined to	capable of having the desired result or effect; effective as a means, measure, remedy

Term and Pronunciation	Meaning of Root and Word Parts	Definition
elixir (ih-**lik**-ser)	**elixir** = cure all, a remedy for all diseases	a sweetened, aromatic solution of alcohol and water containing, or used as a vehicle for, medicinal substances
euphoria (yoo-**fawr**-ee-*uh*)	**eu** = well **pherein** = to bear	state of intense happiness
generic (j*uh*-**ner**-ik)	**genus** = stock	referring to all members of a group; general
local anesthetic (**loh**-k*uh* l) (an-*uh* s-**thet**-ik)	**locus** = a places, specific location **-al** = pertaining to **an** = without **aesthesia** = sensation, feeling **-ic** = relating to	anesthetic drug that produces loss of feeling in a body part without affecting feeling or consciousness in other parts of the body, usually by injection
narcotic (nahr-**kot**-ik)	**narcosis** = a state of stupor or drowsiness produced by a chemical agent **-tic** = relating to	a class of substances that produce stupor or sleep
opioid (**oh**-pee-oid)	**opium** =dried juice of the opium poppy **–oid** = form, shape	drug containing or derived from opium or a synthetic derivative of opium; used in medicine as an analgesic
orthostatic hypotension (awr-th*uh*-**stat**-ik)	**ortho** = upright; straight **stat** = immediately **-ic** = pertaining to	a decrease in the blood pressure to below normal that occurs when a person assumes a standing position after rising from a bed or chair
patent (pat-nt)	**patent** = an invention or process protected by law	the exclusive right granted by a government to an inventor to manufacture, use, or sell an invention for a certain number of years
permeable **pur**-mee-*uh*-b*uh*l	**permeare** = pass through	capable of being passed through
relapse (**ree**-laps)	**re** = back **labi** = to slip	recurrence of symptoms of a disease after a period of recovery
resistance (ri-**zis**-t*uh* ns)	**resist** = to withstand the action or effect of **-ance** = indicating an action	the capacity to withstand something, especially the body's natural capacity to withstand disease
sedate (si-**deyt**)	**sedate** = to calm or quiet	to calm or to soothe fear or nervousness by means of a sedative drug
suspension (s*uh*-**spen**-sh*uh* n)	**suspend** = hold up **-ion** = denoting action or condition	a system consisting of small particles kept dispersed by agitation (mechanical suspension) or by the molecular motion in the surrounding medium (colloidal suspension)
syrup (**sir** *uh* p)	**syrup** = any of various thick sweet liquids	a concentrated sugar solution that contains medication or flavoring
tablet (**tab**-lit)	**tablet** = a flattish cake of some substance	a medicinal formulation made of a compressed powdered substance containing an active drug
topical anesthetic (**top**-i-k*uh* l) (an-*uh* s-**thet**-ik)	**-topo** = place of external surface **-al** = pertaining to **an** = without **aesthesia** = sensation, feeling **-ic** = relating to	local anesthetic drug that is applied directly to skin or mucosa

(Continues)

Term and Pronunciation	Meaning of Root and Word Parts	Definition
transdermal patch (trans-**dur**-m*uh* l) (pach)	**trans** = across **derm** = skin **-al** = pertaining to **patch** = a small piece of adhesive material	a method of delivering medicine by placing it in a special, adhesive patch that is applied to the skin
toxic (**tok**-sik)	**toxin** = any poison **-ic** = pertaining to	poisonous
vasoconstrictor (vas-oh-k*uh* n-**strik**-ter)	**vaso** = vessel **constrict** = to draw of press in; to contract **-or** = a person or thing	drug causing constriction or narrowing of the blood vessels
xerostomia (zeer-*uh*-**stoh**-mee-*uh*)	**xero** = dry **stom** = a mouth or mouthlike **-ia** = abnormal condition	dry mouth

## CHAPTER 15

Medical Emergencies

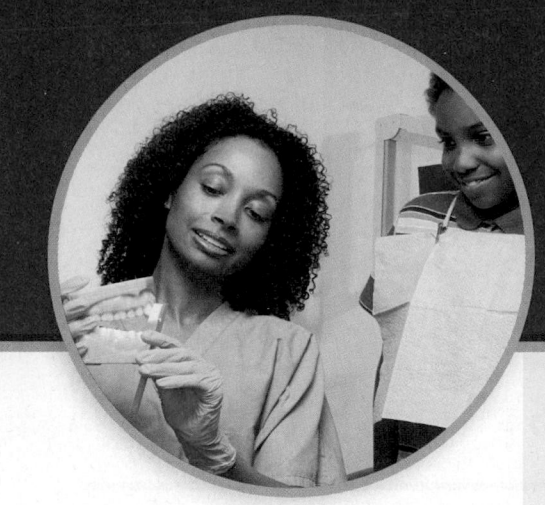

Specific Instructional Objectives

At the completion of this chapter, you will be able to meet these objectives:

1. Use terms provided in this chapter.
2. Discuss prevention of a medical emergency through collection of an accurate patient history.
3. Recognize signs of an anxious or fearful patient.
4. Discuss ASA classifications of medical risk.
5. Explain prevention of a medical emergency through staff preparation.
6. Explain prevention of a medical emergency through office preparation.
7. Compare and contrast the management of postural hypotension and vasovagal syncope.
8. Compare and contrast the signs and symptoms of postural hypotension and vasovagal syncope.
9. Identify the predisposing factors to postural hypotension.
10. Compare and contrast the signs and symptoms of asthma and hyperventilation.
11. Compare and contrast the management of asthma and hyperventilation.
12. Discuss the management of chronic obstructive pulmonary disease.
13. Define adrenal disorders.
14. Discuss the management of an acute adrenal crisis in the dental office.
15. Describe the anatomical structure of the thyroid gland.
16. Compare and contrast hypothyroidism and hyperthyroidism.
17. Describe the protocol in managing a thyroid related medical emergency in the dental office.
18. Differentiate between type I, type II, prediabetes, and gestational diabetes.
19. Discuss the complications of diabetes.
20. List the steps in managing a diabetic emergency in the dental office.
21. Compare and contrast angina and myocardial infarction.
22. Discuss the management of an angina attack in the dental office.
23. Discuss the management of a myocardial infarction in the dental office.
24. Define cardiac arrest.
25. Define congestive heart failure.
26. Discuss the protocol for managing acute pulmonary edema in the dental office.
27. Differentiate between epilepsy and seizures.
28. Discuss generalized seizures.
29. Outline the steps in the management of a seizure in the dental office.
30. Differentiate between an ischemic cerebrovascular accident and a hemorrhagic cerebrovascular accident.

31. Outline the steps in the management of a cerebrovascular accident in the dental office.
32. Identify common dental allergens.
33. Outline the steps in the management of an allergic reaction in the dental office.
34. State the protocol for managing an airway obstruction in the conscious patient.
35. State the role of the dental assistant in managing a medical emergency.

Introduction

Though medical emergencies do not occur frequently in a dental office setting, they can occur at any time. It is important the office staff prepares to handle an emergency should it arise. Preparation is accomplished through prevention of a medical emergency as well as through maintaining basic life support and CPR skills. Office practice drills on managing medical emergencies are also important in preparation should an emergency take place.

Prevention

Collection of an accurate medical history for every patient is a critical step in the prevention of a medical emergency. The front desk receptionist of the dental office is usually responsible for requesting the patient to complete the health history form. The dental assistant should update the medical history form at each visit, even if only a few days have passed between visits. This is because the patient may have visited the physician in between dental visits and the health status may have changed.

Medical History

Once the patient is seated in the dental operatory by the dental assistant, it is important the assistant reviews the medical history verbally with the patient. This will ensure that nothing has been inadvertently omitted (Figure 15-1). The medical history form reviews any possible past and present conditions of the various body systems. Some patients may have difficulty understanding the terminology and as a result may need assistance in completing the form. The physician's information should be listed on the form in case a consultation is required. The form may contain questions regarding the patient's dental history. Questions regarding past dental experiences may provide clues as to how the patient feels about dental treatment. A highly anxious patient is more likely to suffer from a medical emergency than one who is not apprehensive. Apprehensive patients may benefit from sedation and additional methods to reduce anxiety regarding their dental visits.

It is important to ask the patient to list all medications they may be taking including over-the-counter medications and natural medications such as vitamins and herbal supplements. If the patient is unsure of the names of the medications, request that they bring them to the office in their original containers so that all necessary information can be recorded on the health history form. Since some medications treat more than one disorder, it may be necessary to ask the patient for what condition the medication is prescribed. If the patient is unsure, the physician may need to be consulted. The drug references discussed in Chapter 14 may be used to review the patient's medications.

Any areas on the medical history form to which the patient provided a *positive response* or "yes" must be questioned thoroughly by the clinician. For example, if a patient states that they have a history of high blood pressure or hypertension, the clinician must question further. Some important questions that may need to be asked are: Is the patient currently under treatment by a physician? Is the patient taking medications to control the elevated blood pressure? If so, what are the side effects the patient is experiencing from the medications? How well controlled is the blood pressure? If the patient has hypertension, does it require any modifications to dental treatment?

Vital Signs

Vital signs are important as they provide information regarding the patient's level of functioning. Once you have reviewed the medical history, the patient's vital signs should be recorded. The vital signs that should be observed are pulse rate, blood pressure, temperature, and respiration rate. The vital signs vary depending on the age, gender, weight, and physical health of the patient. Since the patient is usually less apprehensive at the initial consultation visit, it is important to record vital signs at this time. These vitals will provide a baseline or reading that the operator can use for reference in case an emergency were to occur.

Time 12:21 PM

Rutgers-SHRP

Date 9/13/2015

Eaglesoft Medical History 2(Copy)(Copy)(Copy)(Copy)

Patient Name: (1265) Vaishali Singhal   Birth Date: 3/11/1967   Date Created: 9/13/2015

Although dental personnel primarily treat the area in and around your mouth, your mouth is a part of your entire body. Health problems that you may have, or medication that you may be taking, could have an important interrelationship with the dentistry you will receive. Thank you for answering the following questions.

Are you under a physician's care now?	○ Yes ○ No	If yes
Have you ever been hospitalized or had a major operation?	○ Yes ○ No	If yes
Are you taking any medications, pills, or drugs?	○ Yes ○ No	If yes
Do you take, or have you taken, Phen-Fen or Redux?	○ Yes ○ No	If yes
Have you ever taken Bisphosphonates such as Fosamax, Boniva, Actonel ?	○ Yes ○ No	If yes
Are you on a special diet?	○ Yes ○ No	If yes
Do you use tobacco?	○ Yes ○ No	If yes
How much alcohol do you drink?	○ Yes ○ No	If yes
Any diseases run in your family?	○ Yes ○ No	If yes
Do you use controlled substances?	○ Yes ○ No	If yes
Have you had radiation therapy?When? For what? Where?How long?	○ Yes ○ No	If yes

Women: Are you...

☐ Pregnant/Trying to get pregnant?   ☐ Nursing?   ☐ Taking oral contraceptives?

Are you allergic to any of the following?

☐ Aspirin   ☐ Penicillin   ☐ Codeine   ☐ Acrylic
☐ Metal   ☐ Latex   ☐ Sulfa Drugs   ☐ Local Anesthetics

Other allergies?   ☐   If yes

Do you have, or have you had, any of the following?

AIDS/HIV Positive	○ Yes ○ No	Cortisone Medicine	○ Yes ○ No	Hemophilia	○ Yes ○ No	GERD/Acid Reflux	○ Yes ○ No
Alzheimer's Disease	○ Yes ○ No	Diabetes	○ Yes ○ No	Hepatitis A	○ Yes ○ No	Recent Weight Loss/Gain	○ Yes ○ No
Anaphylaxis	○ Yes ○ No	Drug/Alcohol Addiction	○ Yes ○ No	Hepatitis B or C	○ Yes ○ No	Renal Dialysis	○ Yes ○ No
Anemia	○ Yes ○ No	Easily Winded	○ Yes ○ No	Herpes	○ Yes ○ No	Rheumatic Fever	○ Yes ○ No
Angina	○ Yes ○ No	Emphysema/COPD	○ Yes ○ No	High Blood Pressure	○ Yes ○ No	Rheumatism	○ Yes ○ No
Arthritis/Gout	○ Yes ○ No	Epilepsy or Seizures	○ Yes ○ No	High Cholesterol	○ Yes ○ No	Scarlet Fever	○ Yes ○ No
Artificial Heart Valve	○ Yes ○ No	Excessive Bleeding/Nosebleeds	○ Yes ○ No	Skin Disorders/Hives or Rash	○ Yes ○ No	Shingles	○ Yes ○ No
Artificial Joint/Prosthesis	○ Yes ○ No	Excessive Thirst	○ Yes ○ No	Hypoglycemia	○ Yes ○ No	Sickle Cell Disease	○ Yes ○ No
Asthma	○ Yes ○ No	Fainting Spells/Dizziness	○ Yes ○ No	Irregular Heartbeat	○ Yes ○ No	Sinus Trouble	○ Yes ○ No
Blood Disease	○ Yes ○ No	Frequent Cough	○ Yes ○ No	Kidney Problems	○ Yes ○ No	Spina Bifida	○ Yes ○ No
Mumps/ Measles/Rubella	○ Yes ○ No	Frequent Diarrhea	○ Yes ○ No	Leukemia	○ Yes ○ No	Stomach/Intestinal Disease	○ Yes ○ No
Breathing/Respiratory Problems	○ Yes ○ No	Frequent Headaches	○ Yes ○ No	Liver Disease	○ Yes ○ No	Stroke	○ Yes ○ No
Bruise Easily	○ Yes ○ No	Genital Herpes	○ Yes ○ No	Low Blood Pressure	○ Yes ○ No	Swelling of Limbs/Joints	○ Yes ○ No
Cancer	○ Yes ○ No	Glaucoma	○ Yes ○ No	Lung Disease	○ Yes ○ No	Thyroid Disease	○ Yes ○ No
Chemotherapy	○ Yes ○ No	Hay Fever/SeasonalAllergies	○ Yes ○ No	Mitral Valve Prolapse	○ Yes ○ No	Tonsillitis	○ Yes ○ No
Chest Pains	○ Yes ○ No	Heart Attack/Failure	○ Yes ○ No	Osteoporosis	○ Yes ○ No	Tuberculosis	○ Yes ○ No
Cold Sores/Fever Blisters	○ Yes ○ No	Heart Murmur	○ Yes ○ No	Pain in Jaw Joints	○ Yes ○ No	Tumors or Growths	○ Yes ○ No
Congenital Heart Disorder	○ Yes ○ No	Heart Pacemaker	○ Yes ○ No	Parathyroid Disease	○ Yes ○ No	Ulcers	○ Yes ○ No
Convulsions	○ Yes ○ No	Heart Trouble/Disease	○ Yes ○ No	Psychiatric/Mental Disorders	○ Yes ○ No	Venereal Disease	○ Yes ○ No
Yellow Jaundice	○ Yes ○ No	Difficulty Swallowing	○ Yes ○ No	Dry Skin	○ Yes ○ No	Weakness/Sleepiness	○ Yes ○ No
Urinary problems	○ Yes ○ No	Frequent Infections	○ Yes ○ No	Sjogren's Syndrome/Dry Mouth_Eyes	○ Yes ○ No	Halitosis/Bad Breath	○ Yes ○ No
Transfusions	○ Yes ○ No	Tattos	○ Yes ○ No	Serious Head/Neck Injuries	○ Yes ○ No		

To the best of my knowledge, the questions on this form have been accurately answered. I understand that providing incorrect information can be dangerous to my (or patient's) health. It is my responsibility to inform the dental office of any changes in medical status.

Signature of Patient, Parent or Guardian:

X _____   Date:_____

Courtesy of Eaglesoft

FIGURE 15-1
Medical history form.

Blood Pressure

Blood pressure is recorded using a blood pressure cuff or *sphygmomanometer* and a *stethoscope* (Figures 15–2A and B). It is essential that the patient be relaxed and that an appropriately sized blood pressure cuff be used. Large cuffs may be used for blood pressure measurements on larger patients, and pediatric sized cuffs are available for use on children and small adults. An inappropriately sized cuff will produce erroneous readings.

Blood pressure is recorded in units of millimeters of mercury, or mm Hg, and expressed as two numbers, for example, 120/80. The upper number (in this case, 120) is the **systolic** blood pressure. This is the pressure required for the left ventricle to pump the blood to the remaining vessels in the body. The lower number (in the example above, 80) is the **diastolic** blood pressure. This number is the pressure is of the heart muscle at rest while it is refilling with blood.

HIPAA requires that all patient information is kept private and secure.

While listening for blood pressure using a sphygmomanometer and a stethoscope, various heart sounds such as thuds and swishes will be audible to the operator. These sounds are known as Korotkoff sounds and are a result of the blood re-entering the vessels as the pressure of the cuff is being released. Either the right or the left arm may be used to record the blood pressure; however, blood pressure in the right arm will usually be approximately 10 mm Hg lower than in the left arm.

Based on American Dental Association (ADA) recommendations, blood pressure should be obtained at the initial visit for each new patient as a screening tool for undiagnosed hypertension. If an elevated blood pressure is obtained, notify the patient, wait 5 minutes, and take a second reading. Record both readings in the chart. At the next appointment, a third reading should be obtained. If all three readings are elevated, it is possible that the patient may be suffering from undiagnosed hypertension and should be referred to his or her physician for further evaluation. Box 15-1 provides the blood pressure classifications for adults.

Clinical management of a patient with hypertension may require some modification in treatment. It is important to ensure good pain management techniques and implement stress reduction protocol. Short appointments will be less stressful for patients with hypertension. Nitrous oxide sedation for relaxation will be beneficial. Use of epinephrine in the local anesthetic should be limited to 0.4 mg or two cartridges of lidocaine with 1:100,000 epinephrine concentration.

Pulse Another important vital sign is the pulse as it can provide information about the rhythm of the heart. The pulse

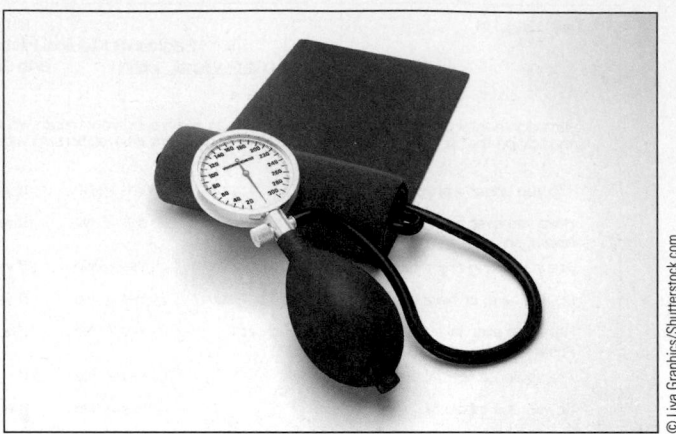

FIGURE 15-2A
Sphygmomanometer.

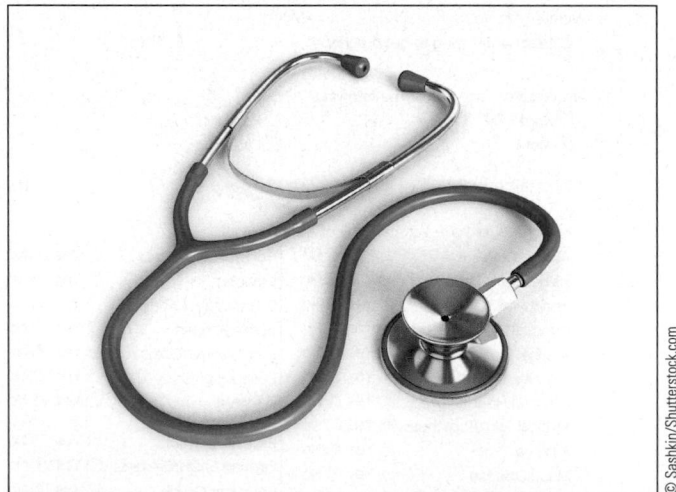

FIGURE 15-2B
Stethoscope.

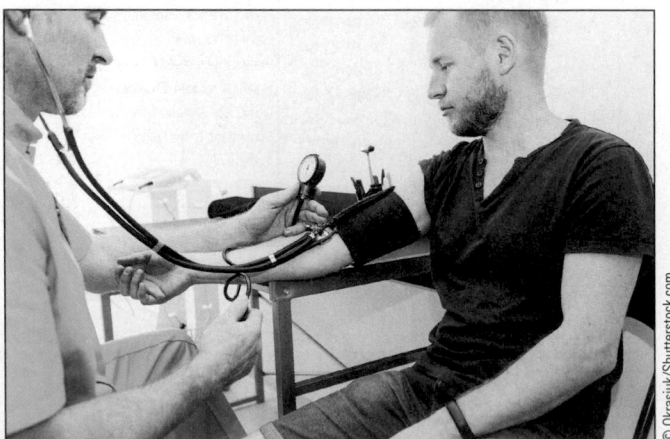

FIGURE 15-2C
Cuff of the sphygmomanometer placed snugly around the patient's upper arm, approximately one inch above the antecubital fossa with gauge visible to the operator.

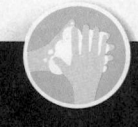

Procedure 15-1
Taking Blood Pressure

Equipment and Supplies
- Sphygmomanometer
- Stethoscope
- Medical and dental history forms

Procedure Steps
1. Assemble equipment and supplies.
2. Wash and dry hands.
3. Greet patient and introduce self.
4. Explain procedure and purpose to patient.
5. Review medical history of patient.
6. The patient should be seated with the arm at heart level.
7. Support elbow on a solid surface.
8. Remove all air from the sphygmomanometer by squeezing the cuff.
9. Expose the patient's arm and place the cuff of the sphygmomanometer snugly around the upper arm, approximately one inch above the antecubital fossa with gauge visible to the operator (see Figure 15-2C).
10. Turn small knob near the inflating bulb clockwise to close it (see Figure 15-2A).
11. Place eartips of the stethoscope in your ears; be sure that they are facing toward the front. This will allow a more comfortable placement into the ears as well as a better fit.
12. Place the bell (chest piece portion) of the stethoscope over the brachial artery in the antecubital fossa (see Figure 15-2C).
13. Inflate the cuff to a reading of 180 mm Hg.
14. Slowly release the valve to begin deflation of the cuff, and listen for sounds through the stethoscope.
15. The first sound heard is the systolic blood pressure or the upper number.
16. The final sound heard through the stethoscope is the diastolic reading or the lower number of the blood pressure.
17. Record blood pressure on medical history form.

is felt when the arteries expand and contract based on the beating of the heart. The most common artery to use to record pulse in a dental office setting is the radial artery in the wrist. The carotid artery, located in the neck, may also be used and is the preferred artery during a medical emergency because it supplies blood to the brain and the head.

The first and second fingers of the hand may be used to record the pulse by placing them over the radial artery (Figure 15-3). The thumb should not be used to for taking this recording, because the thumb has its own pulse.

A normal adult pulse rate ranges from 60 to 100 beats per minute. A pulse that is fast may be a sign of **tachycardia** (rapid heart rate); whereas a slow pulse rate may be a sign of **bradycardia** (slow heart rate). A well trained athlete may have a pulse rate of 40 beats per minute. A pulse with an abnormal rhythm may signify an arrhythmia (abnormal heart rhythm). Medications may also cause a change in the pulse rate. The cause of an abnormal pulse rate should be investigated to determine the cause. Patients with a high pulse rate should not be scheduled for elective dental care until the cause of the elevated pulse rate is determined and brought to a safe level.

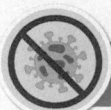 **Infection Control**

Disinfection of Stethoscopes

Studies have found that the majority of stethoscopes are contaminated and as a result may transmit nosocomial infections. *Isopropyl alcohol* or rubbing alcohol may be used to disinfect stethoscopes regularly and is less corrosive to the metal and rubber components of this instrument than other germicides.

Beginning with the earpieces, wipe the stethoscope, including the bell and diaphragm. To thoroughly wipe the diaphragm, take it apart to remove any particles by wiping with an alcohol gauze and then reassemble.

BOX 15-1 Blood Pressure Classifications and Dental Management Protocol

Classification	Systolic Blood Pressure in mm Hg	Diastolic Blood Pressure in mm Hg	Dental Management	ASA
normal blood pressure	Less than 120	Less than 80	• Routine dental treatment • Recheck in 6 months	I
elevated	120-129	Less than 80		
stage I hypertension	130-139	80-89	• Monitor for three consecutive appointments and refer to physician if consistently elevated • Stress reduction protocol • Routine dental treatment	II
stage II hypertension	Greater than or equal to 140	Greater than or equal to 90	• Recheck blood pressure after 5 minutes • Refer for medical consult if elevated • Palliative dental management only in office • Required dental treatment must be performed in a hospital setting	III or IV

Respiration Respiration is the third vital sign that should be recorded in the patient's chart. Respiration is the process of exhalation and inhalation. Normal respiration ranges for an adult is 12–18 breaths per minute. A faster than normal respiration rate is known as *tachypnea*, and a lower than normal respiration rate is known as *bradypnea*. Tachypnea and bradypnea may be caused by disease processes. Tachypnea or bradypnea should be evaluated for causes prior to the start of dental treatment.

Respiration should be recorded by the assistant while the patient is seated in the dental chair. Respiration should be observed for a minimum of 30 seconds and then may be doubled for the 1-minute respiration rate. This observation should be conducted without the patient being aware the respiration is being observed to prevent a subconscious change in the respiration by the patient.

Temperature Temperature, which is not taken frequently in the dental office setting, is the fourth vital sign. It may be recorded prior to a surgical procedure or in case of patient illness. Body temperature may be recorded with the use of a digital, oral, or ear thermometer (Figure 15-4A). Disposable

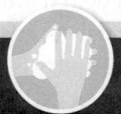

Procedure 15-2
Measuring Radial Pulse

Equipment and Supplies
- Watch with a second hand
- Medical and dental history forms

Procedure Steps
1. Assemble equipment and supplies.
2. Wash and dry hands.
3. Greet patient and introduce self.
4. Explain procedure and purpose to patient.
5. Review medical history of patient.
6. Rest patient's arm and hand on a support like the armrest of the dental chair.

7. Face patient's palm upward.
8. Place fingers properly on thumb side of wrist (see Figure 15-3).
9. Count pulse for at least 30 seconds time and multiply number of pulses counted by 2. Count for at least 1 minute if irregular pulse is detected.
10. Counts pulse accurately within plus or minus 2 of instructor's count.
11. Describe if pulse is normal, fast, or slow.
12. Record pulse on medical history form.

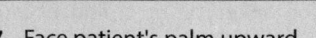

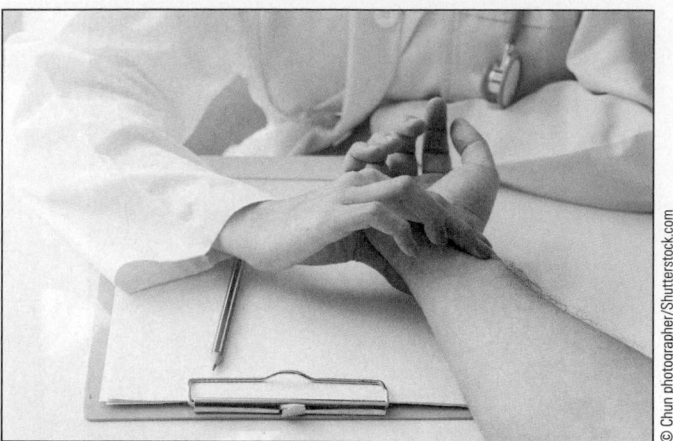

FIGURE 15-3
Operator places fingers properly on thumb side of wrist.

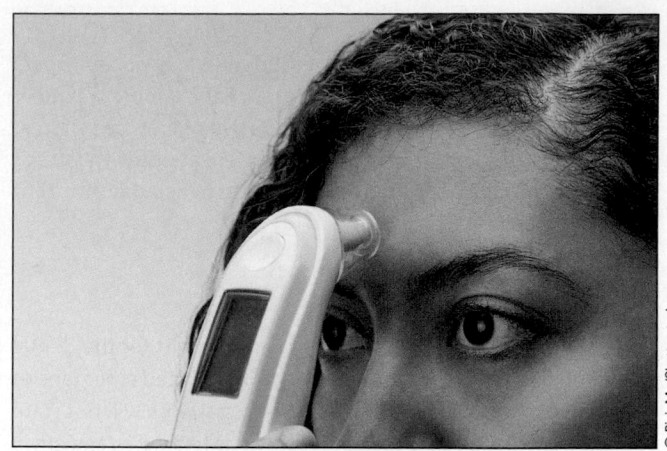

FIGURE 15-4A
Digital thermometer.

paper thermometers are also available (Figure 15-4B). Body temperatures vary throughout the day for each person, and the average is 98.6°F (37°C) and ranges from 97°F to 99°F (36.11 to 37.22°C) for an adult. Body temperature for a child of school age may range from 98°F to 99°F (36.67 to 37.22°C). To prevent the transmission of bacteria from an ear or an oral thermometer, single use, disposable probe covers are recommended. The office may also choose to use a disposable thermometer. It is important to record all vital signs in the patient's record.

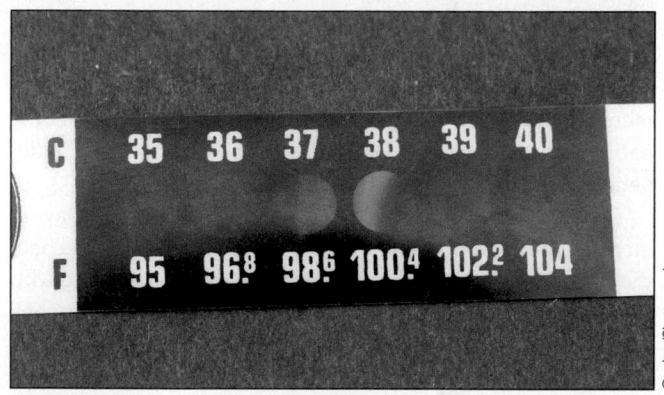

FIGURE 15-4B
Disposable forehead thermometer.

 Documentation

Documentation of Vital Signs

Date	Blood Pressure	Pulse	Respiration
2/1/XX	124/82 in right arm	65/minute	14/minute

Procedure 15-3
Observing and Recording Respiration

Equipment and Supplies
- Medical and dental history forms

Procedure Steps
1. Assemble equipment and supplies.
2. Wash and dry hands.
3. Greet patient and introduce self.
4. Review medical history of patient.
5. While patient is seated in the dental chair, count respirations while patient is unaware of this.
6. Count regular respirations for 30 seconds and multiply by 2. If an irregular respiration is noted, count respirations for one full minute.
7. Describe respirations by depth and rhythm.
8. Record respirations on patient's medical history form.

Physical Exam

In addition to the vital signs discussed above, a visual inspection of the patient should be completed. For example, a patient with cold, clammy skin may be apprehensive or may be suffering from hypoglycemia or **hypothyroidism**. A patient with speech difficulties may have suffered from a **cerebrovascular accident** (CVA) in the past.

Anxious Patients

Identification of the anxious patient is important for the dental practitioner in order to minimize any anxiety related emergencies that may occur in the dental office. Many patients will not state that they are anxious. Inclusion of questions related to anxiety in the medical history is important in helping to determine possible dental fears. A follow-up conversation helps to identifying the anxious patient (Table 15-1).

Observation of the patient will also aid in recognition of the anxious patient. A patient who is severely *phobic* or fearful will let the dental office staff know and in many cases will avoid appointments except in cases of severe discomfort. Severely phobic patients are best treated with intravenous (IV) sedation or under general anesthesia.

Patients who have a more moderate fear may display an increase in blood pressure and pulse rate. In the dental chair, the patient may display signs of fear and anxiety by sitting with a stiff posture and being *diaphoretic* (excessive sweating). They may also exhibit "white knuckle syndrome" in which they grip the arms of the dental chair so tightly that the knuckles of the hands are white (Figure 15-5). These patients may not admit to their fears, and it is important for the practitioner to discuss the cause of the anxiety and offer management options that will allow for more comfortable dental treatment.

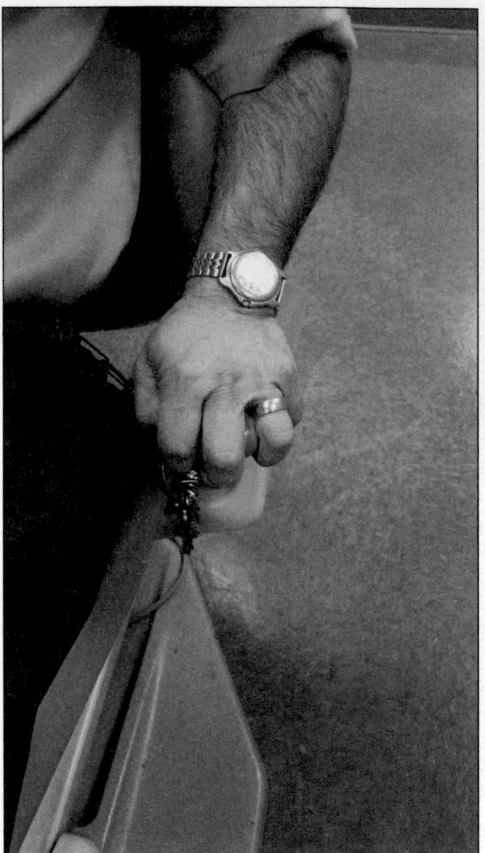

FIGURE 15-5
Patient gripping arm of chair.

American Society of Anesthesiologist (ASA) Classification

Based on the medical history, dental history, physical exam, and anxiety questionnaire, the clinician must determine the patient's ASA classification to estimate the medical risks associated with anesthesia during a surgical procedure. Table 15-2 provides details regarding the ASA classifications. Stress reduction protocol may be necessary for patient who are at a risk for a medical emergency in a dental office. Table 15-3 provides guidelines for stress reduction protocol in the dental office.

Medical Consult

Once the medical history and dental history are obtained and a physical and oral exam have been completed, a treatment plan should be formulated. If a medical consult is warranted, the patient's physician can then be contacted to discuss the patient's health status. The dental practitioner should discuss his or her assessment of the patient's physical status and ask the physician for further information regarding the patient. The dental treatment plan should be presented to the physician along with an explanation of medications that may be used and the level of stress the patient may experience. A written record of the conversation should be maintained in the patient's chart (Table 15-4).

TABLE 15-1 Medical History Questions to Help Identify an Apprehensive Patient

1. How do you feel about an upcoming dental appointment?
   a. I enjoy the appointment.
   b. I am neutral about the appointment.
   c. I am somewhat anxious about the appointment.
   d. I am afraid of going to the dental office.
   e. I am extremely fearful of going to the dental office.
2. How do you feel when you are in the waiting room of the dental office?
   a. Calm and relaxed
   b. Slightly anxious
   c. Very anxious
   d. Frightened
3. How do you feel when you are in the dental chair?
   a. Calm and relaxed
   b. Slightly anxious
   c. Very anxious
   d. Frightened
4. How do you feel about the sound of the drill and other instruments?
   a. Calm and relaxed
   b. Slightly anxious
   c. Very anxious
   d. Frightened

TABLE 15-2 American Society of Anesthesiologists (ASA) Classifications for Medical Risk

ASA Classification	Examples	Treatment Modifications
ASA I	Healthy patient with no systemic diseases	None
ASA II	Mild systemic disease such as controlled hypertension or controlled **diabetes mellitus**.	Stress reduction protocol
ASA III	Significant systemic disease such as **stable angina**.	Stress reduction protocol
ASA IV	Severe systemic disease which is a constant threat to life; such as someone who has **unstable angina**.	Treatment should be conservative, in the form of palliative care until the patient's physical status improves.
ASA V	End stage form of a disease such as cancer or an infectious disease and is not expected to live for more than 24 hours.	Elective dental treatment is a contraindication. Palliative treatment for pain management may be necessary for these patients.

TABLE 15-3 Stress Reduction Protocol in the Dental Office

- Premedicate for anxiety if needed.
- Morning appointments with minimal wait times are best.
- Appointment length is determined by anxiety level and/or physical ability to tolerate longer appointments.
- Administer nitrous oxide sedation as needed.
- Use good pain control methods during and after procedure as needed.
- Make follow-up phone call to patient later in the same day.

TABLE 15-4 Medical Consult Form

Request for Medical Consultation and Response

Patiient's DOB   Patient's Full Name
Patient's Chart ID
Patient's Address   phone #

To Dr: _____
Pertinent Medical History and Pertinent Physical Findings:

Reason for Request:
The patient above is a registered patient of _____, who will be receiving dental treatment. Treatment may include extractions, endodontics, or minor surgeries.
Additional procedures:

Please Advise Before the Next Scheduled Visit:
Please include Patient Medical Status and contra-indications/recommendations. Include also the need for prophylactic antibiotic coverage, with initial dose requirements. Indicate if patient is cleared for dental treatment.

From: Dentist Name
Dentist Signature:
Patient Signature for Authorization for Medical Consult:

Staff and Office Preparation

Staff and office preparation is a critical component of managing a medical emergency should it arise. This includes maintenance of current credentials in basic life support (BLS), also known as cardiopulmonary resuscitation (CPR). Updating of credentials may require that the dental assistant participate in a refresher course offered at local organizations and hospitals. Additionally, each member of the team should be assigned to a specific role in the event of a medical emergency. For example, it may be the role of the dental assistant to obtain the emergency kit and bring it to the location of the emergency in the office. Emergency phone numbers should be maintained at the front desk in an easily accessible location so that help can be called for immediately in the event of a medical emergency. Office preparation also includes the availability of certain medications to either maintain the patient until emergency medical services (EMS) arrives or reverse an emergency condition. Medications that should be maintained in the dental office emergency kit will also be discussed in this chapter.

Basic Emergency Kit

Many emergencies that occur in the dental office may need the use of medications for management. Every dental office should maintain a basic emergency kit that is easily accessible in case of a patient emergency. Figure 14–1 provides an image of the emergency kit. Keep in mind that BLS is always implemented prior to the use of medications if warranted. At a minimum, the medications discussed in Table 15-5 should be available in the dental office emergency kit.

Optional Emergency Kit Items

Dental offices may also opt to have some *adjunct* or accessory drugs available in the office for use. These additional adjunct drugs and equipment are identified in Table 15-6 and should be available only if the dentist is comfortable with their use and administration.

Team Effort in Emergency Management

The dental team should practice office emergency management drills in order to be prepared should an actual emergency occur. An emergency can occur not only to a patient but also a staff member. During a medical emergency in the dental office, it is critical each member have a specific role in aiding emergency management. The staff member with the patient at the time of the emergency is the one to initiate BLS and signal the remainder of the staff that the office emergency system needs

TABLE 15-5 Components of a Basic Dental Office Emergency Kit

Component	Description	Example
ammonia vaporole	Aromatic ammonia is available in a *vaporole* or capsule form and should be crushed and held under the patient's nose to stimulate respiration in vasodepressor **syncope**.	
epinephrine	1:1000 concentration of epinephrine in the emergency kit for intramuscular (IM) administration in case of an anaphylactic allergic reaction.	
histamine blocker	An injectable histamine blocker such as *chlorpheniramine (Chlortrimetron)* or diphenhydramine *(Benadryl)* should be readily available in the dental emergency kit to reverse a mild to moderate allergic reaction.	
nitroglycerine	Nitroglycerine is a vasodilator utilized to manage the chest pain associated with angina or an acute myocardial infarction, also known as a heart attack.	

Component	Description	Example
bronchodilator	Bronchodilators are used to alleviate asthma symptoms and allergic reactions with symptoms of respiratory difficulty.	© New Africa/Shutterstock.com
sugar source	Cake icing or non-diet soda or orange juice or chocolate used in the event of a hypoglycemic episode.	© Stephanie Frey/Shutterstock.com
aspirin	Used in the event of a suspected myocardial infarction or as an anticoagulant in patients with a history of a myocardial infarction or a cerebrovascular accident.	© Hurst Photo/Shutterstock.com
oxygen	An E size portable oxygen tank should be available in the dental office for use. In addition to the oxygen tank, pediatric and adult sized masks that allows oxygen administration must also be available as part of the dental office's emergency kit.	

(Continues)

TABLE 15-5 Components of a Basic Dental Office Emergency Kit (*Continued*)

Component	Description	Example
automatic external defibrillator (AED)	Used in the event of cardiac arrest.	© Quaity Stock Arts/Shutterstock.com

TABLE 15-6 Adjunct Drugs for Dental Office Emergency Kit

naloxone	Reversal agent for narcotic analgesic agents such as morphine, meperidine, codeine, and oxycodone that may be used in emergency for pain management. Narcotic analgesics can result in central nervous system depression.
hydrocortisone	Hydrocortisone sodium succinate is used to manage an acute allergic reaction and acute **adrenal insufficiency**.
phenylephrine	**Phenylephrine** effectively aids in relieving mild to moderate hypotension but must be used with caution in patients who have hyperthyroidism or an underlying heart condition.
injectable antihypoglycemics	50% dextrose intravenous solution or glucagon intramuscularly may be administered to a patient who is unconscious due to hypoglycemia.
diazepam (Valium)	Emergency drug to treat prolonged seizures that are not self-limiting.
flumazenil	Reversal agent for overdose and CNS depression due to administration of benzodiazepines.
tourniquets, syringes and needles	**Syringes** and needles are adjunct equipment and should be available in the emergency kit in order to be able to administer drugs requiring IV or IM administration. **Tourniquets** are used to aid in the administration of IV medications.
cricothyrotomy equipment	In the case of an airway obstruction, a **cricothyrotomy** is a last resort option which is performed in the trachea below the obstructed area. (**Scalpels** designed to perform this procedure can utilized by the dentist trained in advanced life-saving procedures.
airway equipment	In an unconscious patient, the use of **oropharyngeal** or **nasopharyngeal** airway equipment may be warranted if traditional methods of maintaining an open airway are not successful. Both are available in adult and pediatric sizes.

to be activated. The signal may be a code word used by the staff members as an internal alert to prevent other patients from being aware the emergency is occurring.

The staff members not with the patient at the time of the emergency should be assigned duties such as retrieving the emergency kit and the oxygen tank. Also assign a staff member to the role of preparing the necessary emergency drugs. Remember, however, to cross train each staff member in all of the necessary duties in case one member of the team is unavailable.

In case of an emergency, the receptionist should notify EMS. Keep phone numbers for hospitals, nearby physicians, and dentists trained in ACLS current and near office telephones. Upon contact with EMS, the receptionist should explain the type of emergency that is occurring as well as the location of and phone number of the office, and also provide his or her name as well as the name and age of the patient. In the case of a life threatening and serious emergency, it may be necessary to reschedule any patients in the waiting room and any remaining patients for that day.

Syncope

Fainting or syncope is one of the most common medical emergencies that occurs in the dental office today, although this condition has decreased over the past several years due to the implementation of the **supine** position during patient treatment (Figure 15-6). Syncope may be the result of a psychological reaction (*vasovagal syncope*) or a physiological reaction (*postural hypotension*). In this section, both the psychological causes and the physiological causes of syncope will be discussed as well as prevention and management.

Vasovagal Syncope

Also known as *vasodepressor syncope* or simple faint, vasovagal syncope most commonly arises in an anxious patient. Recognition of such anxiety in a patient is important in the prevention of a syncopal episode. Anxiety recognition can be accomplished partially through the use of the anxiety questionnaire discussed

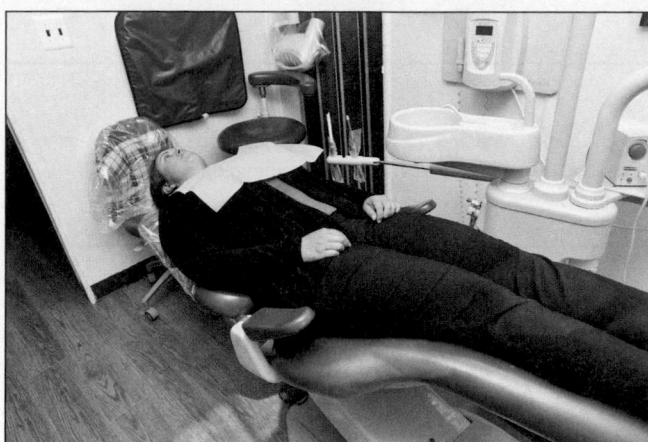

FIGURE 15-6
Supine position.

TABLE 15-7 Presyncopal Signs and Symptoms

- Pale appearance
- Sweat
- Nausea
- Dizziness
- Tachycardia
- Hypotension
- Bradycardia
- Syncope

previously. Monitoring of vital signs also aids in identification. Vital signs not within normal limits should encourage the dental assistant to investigate their cause. An anxious patient may exhibit tachycardia and an elevated blood pressure as well as sweating. Once the anxiety is determined, methods for stress reduction can be implemented to prevent vasovagal syncope. The stress reduction protocol is outlined in Table 15-3.

Physiology of Vasovagal Syncope
An anxious patient in the dental office experiences a "flight or fight" reaction while in the dental chair, caused by activation of the sympathetic autonomic nervous system (SANS), and resulting in a release of epinephrine from the adrenal glands. The physiological effects of epinephrine are widespread due to its action on receptors in the skin, skeletal muscle, heart, and beta 2 receptors in the lungs. Epinephrine leads to vascular *constriction* or narrowing and an increase in blood pressure. This action of peripheral vasoconstriction sends the blood to the center of the body and to the skeletal muscles to be used in the flight-or-fight situation. Additionally, epinephrine acts on the ventricular heart muscle to increase the *chronotropic* (rate) and *inotropic* (force of contraction) of the heart. As a result, the heart is more efficiently pumping blood to the skeletal muscle in order to enable the body to respond to the crisis. Epinephrine also causes bronchodilation, allowing the body to receive more oxygen.

The body's response to epinephrine is critical for rapid response. However, in the dental office, such a response may lead to vasodepressor syncope because the peripheral vasodilation effect leads to pooling of the blood in the skeletal muscles of the extremities, resulting in **hypotension** This in turn results in a deficiency of oxygenated blood being supplied to the brain and finally syncope.

Syncope usually occurs while the patient is upright, not while supine, because the supine position allows gravity to ensure a sufficient oxygen supply of blood flow to the brain (Figure 15-6). Vasodepressor syncope occurs with a progression of signs and symptoms. Table 15-7 provides the presyncopal signs and symptoms the patient will experience as they progress from early presyncope to syncope. If the dental assistant identifies the **prodromal** signs of presyncope in a patient, repositioning of the patient in the supine position can reverse the symptoms and prevent vasodepressor syncope from occurring.

Management of Vasodepressor Syncope
If vasodepressor syncope does occur, the CPR/BLS algorithm must be implemented. Table 15-8 outlines the protocol for management of vasodepressor syncope.

After an episode of vasodepressor syncope, a patient who rises too soon may lose consciousness again. It is important to keep the patient in the supine position. Reschedule treatment for another day as recovery from vasovagal syncope may take several hours. Determine what led to the syncopal episode. Question the patient as to whether or not the syncope may have been caused by fear or anxiety during the procedure. Also ask the patient about when their last meal was eaten. Once the cause is determined, treatment modifications may be made for the next appointment.

Release the patient with a family member or friend once it has been determined that the syncopal episode was not caused by an underlying medical condition. If the dentist believes that the episode was caused by a medical problem, EMS should be called and the patient taken to the hospital for further evaluation. EMS should also be called if the patient does not regain consciousness rapidly once they are positioned. Once released, advise the patient to refrain from driving since the possibility of a second syncopal episode is higher during the several hours that follow the first.

Postural Hypotension

Another condition that may lead to a loss of consciousness is postural or orthostatic hypotension. The cause of this is significantly different than for loss of consciousness in vasodepressor syncope. Whereas vasovagal syncope has a psychogenic cause, postural hypotension results from an underlying physiological problem.

Physiology of Postural Hypotension
Loss of consciousness due to postural hypotension occurs in patients undergoing a positional change from a prolonged supine or sitting position to upright. In some cases, a patient's body may not be able to adjust to the change in position and the patient will

TABLE 15-8 Protocol for Management of Vasodepressor Syncope

- Assess the situation and activate the office emergency system.
- Assess circulation by palpation of the carotid artery.
- Place patient supine to ensure brain receives adequate circulation and ensure patent airway via the head tilt, chin lift method. (Patient should breathe spontaneously now—if not, another serious emergency should be considered and BLS implemented).
- Crush and place ammonia vaporole under patient's nasal cavity to initiate movement.
- Administer oxygen via nasal cannula (Figure 15-7).

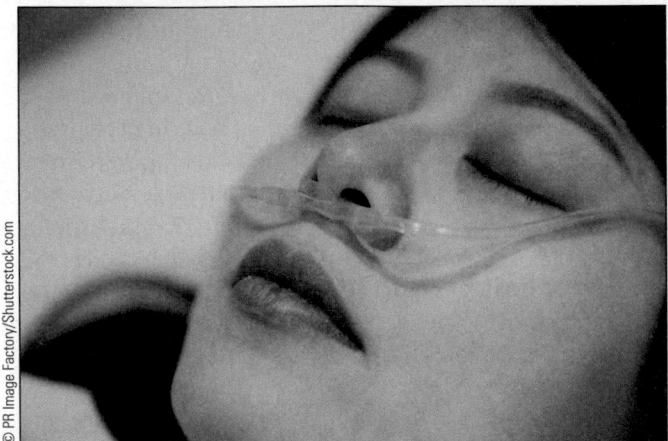

FIGURE 15-7
Oxygen delivery via nasal cannula.

suddenly lose consciousness. This occurs because gravity allows the blood to flow to the brain more readily when the patient is in the supine position. When the patient is placed upright, the blood vessels are unable to instantaneously constrict, and blood pressure drops, eliciting unconsciousness.

One key difference between vasovagal syncope and postural hypotension is that there are no prodromal signs or symptoms in postural hypotension as there are in vasodepressor syncope. Additionally, orthostatic hypotension occurs very rapidly.

Predisposing Factors of Postural Hypotension Predisposing factors in orthostatic hypotension are varied. Table 15-9 identifies predisposing factors. A thorough medical history will reveal to the dental practitioner any conditions the patient that could result in orthostatic hypotension. It is also important to question whether or not the patient has lost consciousness in the past.

Prevention of Postural Hypotension Table 15-10 provides the steps the practitioner should implement in order to prevent an episode of postural hypotension.

If the cause of the loss of consciousness was postural hypotension and the patient has experienced loss of consciousness in the past, the appointment may proceed if both the practitioner and the patient see fit. At the end of the session, the patient may be dismissed without an escort because once the body has adjusted to the positional changes, a second syncopal episode is not likely to occur. However, if this syncopal episode has occurred for the first time, the patient should be dismissed with a family member. A physician should determine the cause of the syncope, and the dental appointment should be rescheduled.

Respiratory Disorders

Two medical emergencies that may be classified under the umbrella of respiratory disorders are asthma and hyperventilation. However, each significantly differs from the other with relation to cause and physiological occurrences. This section also discusses

TABLE 15-9 Predisposing Factors to Postural Hypotension

elderly patients	Varicose veins may be one cause.
pregnacy first or second trimester	Due to circulatory system expansion and a decrease in blood pressure.
pregnancy third trimester	Caused by female lying supine for several minutes. Turning the patient to her left side will reduce the pressure on the vena cava and prevent loss of consciousness.
heart conditions	Myocardial infarction, heart valve defects or congestive heart failure can result in decreased blood pressure caused by poor circulation.
medical conditions	Hypoglycemia in a patient with diabetes, hypothyroidism, adrenal insufficiency (Addison's disease) can result in a drop in blood pressure.
many commonly used medications	Blood pressure medications, tricyclic antidepressants, antipsychotic medications, PDE5 inhibitors used for **erectile dysfunction**, sedative agents used in the dental office.
Being in a **recumbent** position for a long period of time such as long appointments	Move dental chair into upright position slowly to allow patient to adjust to change in position.

TABLE 15-10 Protocol for Prevention of Postural Hypotension

Return dental chair slowly to an upright position.
• From supine raise chair to a semi-supine position and allow patient to sit for 2 or 3 minutes.
• Raise chair to fully upright position and allow patient to sit for 2 or minutes while the body adjusts.
• Allow patient to rise from chair slowly to a standing position. The practitioner should stand near the patient in case of loss of consciousness.

the different ways each of these emergencies is managed by the dental auxiliary.

Asthma

Asthma is a chronic lung disorder characterized by constriction of the bronchioles. This causes wheezing on exhaling and coughing due to limited airflow. The patient may also feel short of breath and experience tightness in the chest due to constriction of the airways.

Patients suffering from asthma may be sensitive to certain *allergens* or triggers. Exposure to these allergens results in sensitization of the airways, which in turn causes inflammation and narrowing of the air passages and at times great difficulty in breathing. Inflamed airways produce more mucus than noninflamed airways, and this can cause further airway constriction. Patients with mild asthma may suffer from one or two attacks per week, whereas those with severe asthma can suffer from daily continual symptoms. Asthma may be intrinsic or extrinsic. Table 15-11 provides details of both types of asthma.

Medications to Treat Asthma Asthmatic patients manage acute symptoms with bronchodilators. Although epinephrine is an effective bronchodilator, its action on the beta 1 and alpha 1 receptors results in unwanted side effects such as tremors and palpitations. This has led to a preference for other more selective bronchodilators, such as albuterol, for management of acute asthmatic attacks, which have fewer undesirable side effects. Table 15-12 provides details on the types of medications that are used by an asthmatic patient.

Dental Management of an Asthmatic Patient A thorough medical history review aids in the identification of the asthmatic patient. Table 15-13 provides the medical history questions that are related to asthma. Stress reduction as identified in Table 15-3 is important in prevention of an asthmatic attack. A patient with mild asthma that may be managed with inhalers is an ASA II. A patient with moderate to severe asthma may be an ASA III. Patients who have been hospitalized previously for asthma are also an ASA III.

Management of an Asthmatic Attack In the dental office, stress is a trigger for an asthma attack. The patient's inhaler should be placed in the operatory for accessibility should it be required. Table 15-14 provides the protocol for management of an asthmatic attack.

TABLE 15-11 Types of Asthma

Intrinsic Asthma or Nonallergic Asthma	*Extrinsic* Asthma or Allergic Asthma	Status Asthmaticus
Most common in adults.	Most common in younger adults and children.	Serious, life threatening asthmatic attack.
Trigger for intrinsic asthma is exercise or stress or pollution.	Usually triggered by an allergen such as food, pollen, medications.	Does not respond to the patient's normal medications.
Symptoms are present even between attacks and daily medications are needed to control the asthma.	Determine the trigger to ensure the patient is not exposed to that particular allergen in the dental office.	Attack continues and may go on for hours or days if left untreated.
Poor prognosis as the patient will not outgrow it and symptoms may worsen with time.	Patient usually outgrows this form of asthma.	Patient needs to be hospitalized for aggressive treatment.

TABLE 15-12 Medications to Manage Asthma

Beta-2 (B2) Agonists	Corticosteroids
For management of acute symptoms	For management of severe asthma
Bind to the beta 2 receptors in the lungs, resulting in a relaxation of the bronchial smooth muscle and dilation of the airways	Used in combination with B2 agonists to prevent an asthmatic attack or minimize the severity of an asthmatic attack
Examples include albuterol delivered through a metered dose inhaler	Inhaled corticosteroid reduce bronchiole inflammation; examples include *beclomethosone* (Qvar), *fluticasone* (Flovent)
	Patients with severe asthma may be taking oral corticosteroids such as *prednisone*
	Inhaled corticosteroids use may result in oral candidiasis.

TABLE 15-13 Medical History Questions Related to Asthma

Do you have difficulty breathing?
If the patient has a diagnosis of asthma, it is important to find out the following:
• What triggers an asthma attack?
• How often do they occur?
• How are the asthma attacks managed?
• Have you ever been hospitalized for an asthma attack?
• What medications are you taking?

TABLE 15-14 Protocol for Management of an Asthmatic Attack in the Dental Office Setting

• Assess the situation.
• Check circulation by palpating the carotid artery.
• Check airway and breathing.
• Position patient upright for comfort.
• Provide the patient with their own inhaler, preferably. If the patient did not bring their inhaler, provide the one from the emergency kit.
• If needed administer oxygen via a nasal cannula, full face mask or nasal hood.
• If asthma is not relieved by the inhaler, administer 0.3 ml of epinephrine 1:1,000 concentration intramuscularly.
• If asthma persists, call EMS to transport patient to hospital as this may be a case of status asthmaticus.

Hyperventilation

Hyperventilation is breathing in excess of what the body requires and is usually caused by a state of anxiety or panic.

Prevention of Hyperventilation One of the more common medical emergencies in the dental office is hyperventilation. In this setting, such an emergency is usually caused by stress and anxiety. The patient who suffers from anxiety usually tries to hide it. The fear and anxiety builds up until it emerges as a hyperventilation episode. Identification of the anxious patient is important in the prevention of an episode. The anxiety questionnaire in Table 15-1 may aid in identifying the anxious patient. The patient may also be asked about previous unpleasant experiences in the dental office.

Use vital signs as well for aid in identification. The apprehensive patient may have an elevated blood pressure and pulse rate. It is critical to obtain baseline vitals when the patient is not anxious, preferably at the initial visit.

Those who suffer from hyperventilation are usually adults in the age group of 15 years to 45 years, an age common for hiding emotions such as fear and anxiety.

Physiology of Hyperventilation Hyperventilation is characterized by *tachypnea* or rapid breathing and deeper than normal breathing. As a result, carbon dioxide (CO_2) in the body is blown off and there is an excess of oxygen (O_2) in relation to the CO_2. The result is hypocarbia and respiratory alkalosis, which must be reversed in order to restore a normal oxygen and carbon dioxide balance.

Signs and Symptoms of Hyperventilation If the rapid respiration goes unnoticed by the clinician, the patient may begin to suffer symptoms of hyperventilation. The hypocarbia leads to vasoconstriction of the cerebral blood vessels. As a result, the patient complains of dizziness and confusion. The patient may also feel as if they are suffocating and experiencing chest pain. Other symptoms may be numbness and tingling of the extremities and perioral areas. Syncope may occur if the problem is not recognized and managed appropriately.

Management of Hyperventilation in the Dental Office The dental assistant must remain in control of the situation when managing a medical emergency. Table 15-15 provides the protocol for management of an episode of hyperventilation in the dental office.

Oxygen should *not* be administered to the hyperventilating patient since oxygen levels are already higher than normal. Hyperventilation is the one medical emergency in which oxygen is contraindicated.

Chronic Obstructive Pulmonary Disease (COPD)

COPD is a chronic progressive lung disorder which also results in difficulty in breathing. However, the underlying cause of COPD is different from the underlying cause of asthma and hyperventilation.

COPD includes chronic bronchitis and emphysema. Most patients diagnosed with COPD suffer from both. The condition usually progresses and worsens over time. Most people who have been diagnosed with COPD have a history of smoking. COPD may also be caused by air pollution and exposure to chemical fumes.

In a healthy person the alveolar sacs expand and contract when air is inhaled and exhaled. In a patient with COPD, the alveolar sacs lose their elasticity and some sacs are also destroyed, resulting in less surface area for air exchange between the lungs and the blood (Figure 15-9). Mucus also builds up and increases the difficulty in breathing.

TABLE 15-15 Protocol for Management of Hyperventilation in the Dental Office Setting

- The dental professional must remain in control of the situation.
- Calm the patient down by speaking to the patient in a quiet and reassuring manner.
- Patient should cup their hands and cover their nose and mouth (Figure 15-8).
- Encourage the patient to breathe the exhaled, carbon dioxide rich air slowly as this will reverse the hypocarbia.
- If this is not successful, valium may need to be administered to the patient; in this case the patient will need to be driven home by a family member.

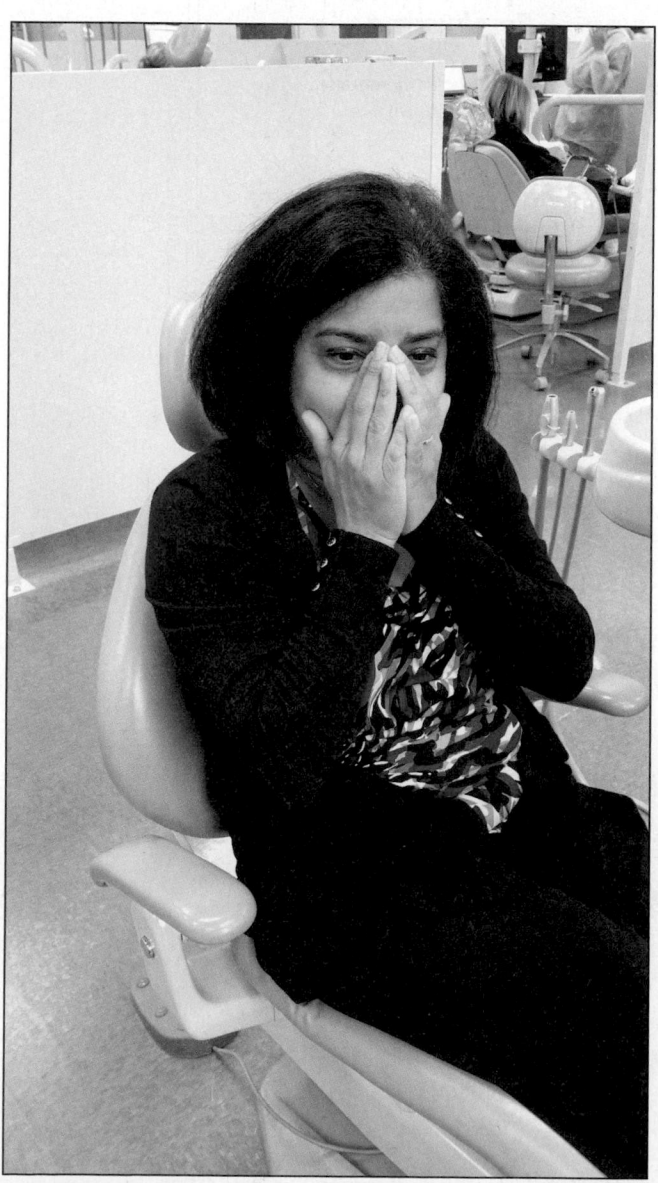

FIGURE 15-8
Hyperventilating patient cupping their hands and covering their nose and mouth.

The COPD patient needs to be managed with the use of the stress reduction protocol as outlined in Table 15-3. However, oxygen administration for routine stress management is contraindicated with the COPD patient because they depend on blood oxygen levels for the drive to breathe. Additional oxygen administered to the COPD patient may result in cessation of respiration. However, oxygen can be administered to the COPD patient for the management of a medical emergency.

The COPD patient may be taking medications to manage the disorder. These could include theophylline and steroid medications. Avoid administering narcotic pain medications for pain management as these medications suppress the respiratory centers in the brain. Valium is also contraindicated for administration to a COPD patient as is nitrous oxide and oxygen. A medical consult from the physician should be obtained prior to treating the COPD patient.

Adrenal Disorders

The *adrenal glands* are small glands located on top of both of the kidneys. These glands produce many hormones, most of which do not have essential functions in the body. Each gland is composed of two parts: the cortex, which is the outer portion of the gland, and the medulla, which is the inner portion of the gland. Each part has a separate and distinct function (Figure 15-10). Table 15-16 provides detail regarding important hormones produced by the adrenal cortex.

Some patients suffer from adrenal dysfunction, which may lead to either excess secretion (*hypersecretion*) of cortisol or insufficient secretion (*hyposecretion*) of cortisol. Table 15-17 provides detail regarding adrenal disorders.

Acute Adrenal Insufficiency

In nonstressful situations, the daily output of cortisol by the adrenal glands is approximately 20 milligrams. The body often requires higher levels of cortisol to adapt to a stressful situation. In the patient who has adrenal insufficiency, the adrenal cortex is unable to produce the necessary levels. During acute adrenal insufficiency, the patient suffers from sudden lower back pain, dehydration, vomiting, diarrhea, hypotension, and loss of consciousness. An acute crisis of adrenal insufficiency, if not immediately and appropriately managed, will lead to death. The main cause of death due to an acute adrenal crisis is hypotension or hypoglycemia.

Medical History and Prevention and of Acute Adrenal Insufficiency

A thorough and complete medical history that includes medications taken in the past two years helps to identify the patient who may have adrenal insufficiency and is at risk for an acute adrenal crisis. Table 15-18A provides

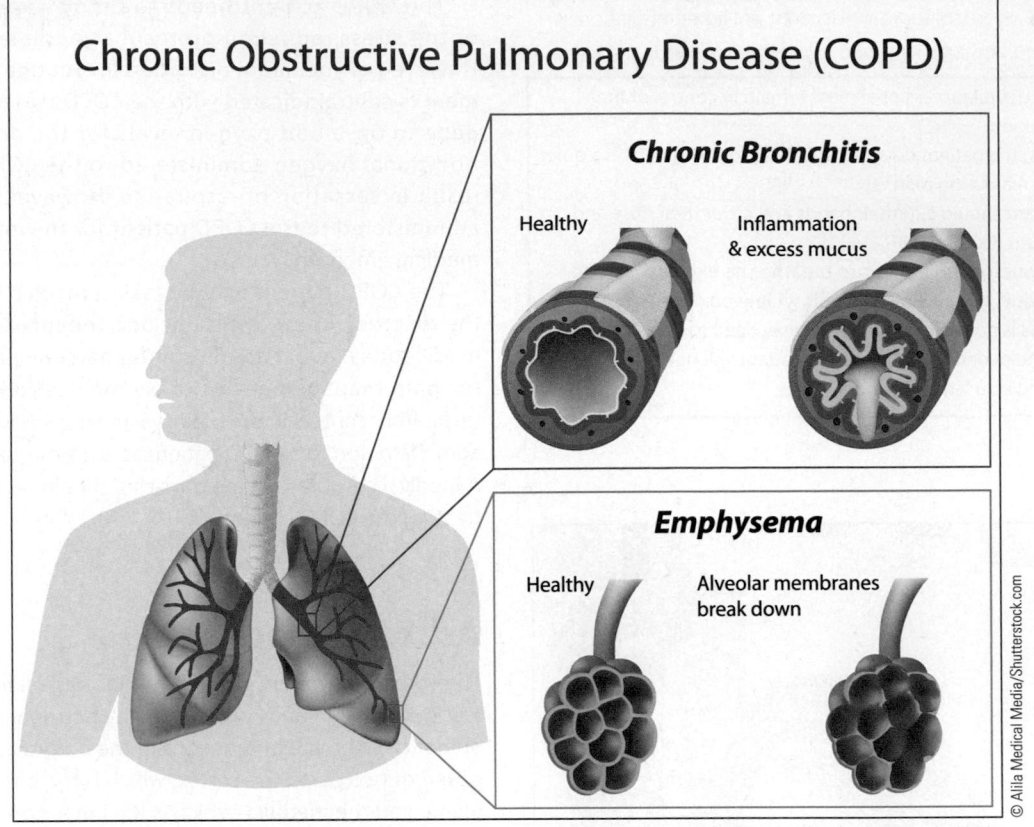

FIGURE 15-9
Chronic obstructive pulmonary disease.

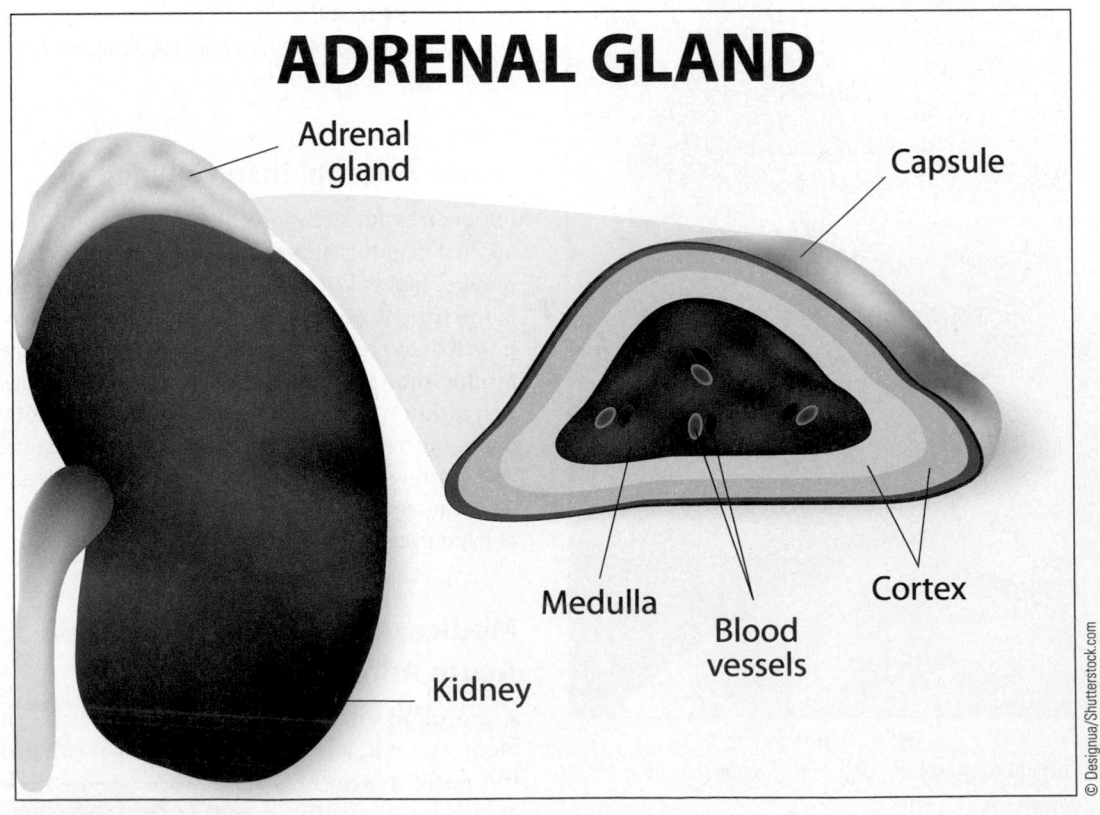

FIGURE 15-10
Adrenal glands.

TABLE 15-16 Hormones Produced by the Adrenal Cortex

Hormone	Function
glucocorticoids	Regulate glucose and its metabolism
mineralocorticoids	Regulate minerals and water in the body
cortisol (hydrocortisone)	Helps body adapt to stressful situations

the medical history questions that pertain to adrenal insufficiency. The Rule of Twos aids in identification of a patient who may have adrenal insufficiency based on prescription steroid use. The Rule of Twos is provided in Table 15-18B

TABLE 15-17 Adrenal Disorders

Disorder	Clinical Manifestations	Causes/Treatment
hypersecretion—Cushing's syndrome		Can be caused by medications or a tumor. Removal of part of the adrenal gland to allow the remainder to function or removal of the entire gland, which can lead to insufficiency. If the entire adrenal gland is removed, the patient is then placed on daily corticosteroids for life.
hyposecretion—Addison's disease (primary insufficiency)		A slowly progressing disorder usually caused by an autoimmune destruction of the adrenal cortex. Symptoms of adrenal insufficiency become noticeable when approximately 20% of the cortex is functioning. Once diagnosed, the patient is placed on cortisol therapy.
hyposecretion—secondary insufficiency		Caused by insufficient release of adrenocorticotropic hormone (ACTH) by the pituitary to stimulate adrenal glands. This leads to cortisol not being released by adrenal glands. Most commonly occurs because patient is taking corticosteroids to manage another medical condition such as asthma. Leads to disuse atrophy of the adrenal cortex. If the patient stops taking the prescribed corticosteroids, the atrophied adrenal cortex may not be able to produce enough to handle stress, sending the patient into an acute crisis of adrenal insufficiency.

TABLE 15-18A Medical History Questions Related to Adrenal Insufficiency

Do you have asthma, arthritis, or inflammatory skin disease?
If the patient responds yes to the above question, ask the following:
• How are the conditions managed?
• Are you being treated by a physician?
• What medications have been prescribed?
If the patient is taking corticosteroids, ask the following questions:
• Is the medication topical, oral, or administered by an injection?
• What is the dose of the medication?
• Are you still taking the medication? If not, when was it stopped?

TABLE 15-18B Rule of Twos

Rule of Twos
• Patient has taken 20 mg or more of hydrocortisone or its equivalent
• Orally or via an injection for at least two weeks
• Within the past two years

If adrenal suppression is suspected, contact the patient's physician. If the physician's records indicate that the patient suffers from adrenal insufficiency and is at risk for an acute adrenal crisis, supplemental steroids at two to four times the normal daily output can be prescribed by the doctor to alleviate any stress of a dental procedure.

Management of an Acute Adrenal Crisis in the Dental Office

The dental office must be equipped to manage such a crisis, should it occur. If the signs and symptoms of an acute adrenal crisis begin to develop, immediate intervention by the clinician is necessary.

In the event of acute adrenal insufficiency, provide basic life support as required for the conscious or unconscious patient. Provide oxygen and monitor and record vital signs. Summon EMS and administer 100 mg of hydrocortisone via an IV or IM from the emergency kit. EMS will transport the patient to the hospital, where additional corticosteroids will be administered along with **electrolytes**.

Thyroid Disorders

As one of the largest endocrine glands in the body, the thyroid gland has many important functions, such as regulating the body's metabolism and balancing calcium.

Thyroid Anatomy

The thyroid gland is located at the front portion of the neck, consists of two lobes, and sits below the larynx. The lobes rest on each side of the trachea and are connected together by a thin band of tissue called an *isthmus* (Figure 15-11).

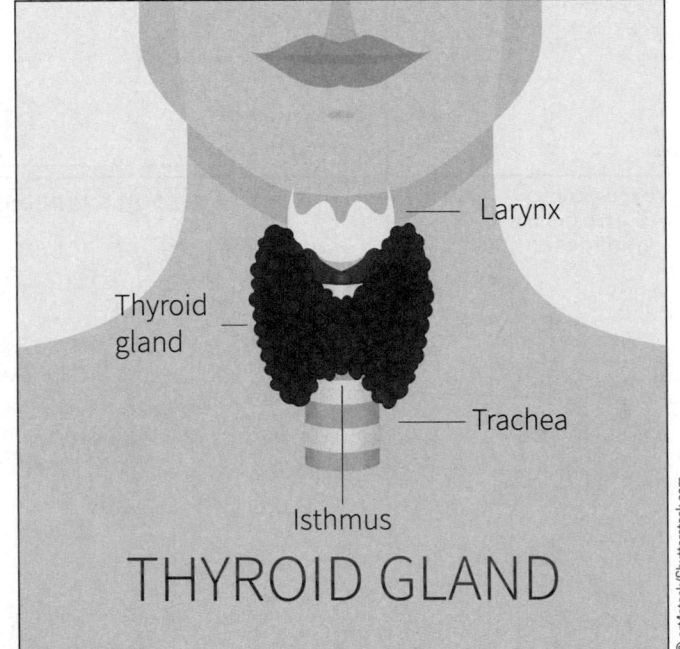

FIGURE 15-11
Thyroid gland.

Hormones Produced by the Thyroid Gland

The thyroid gland produces several hormones; the main ones are T4 (*thryoxine*) and T3 (*triiodothyronine*). The cells of the thyroid gland require iodine to produce these hormones. Iodine is not produced by the body and must be ingested in foods. Natural sources of iodine include sea vegetables such as seaweed and marine life such as fish and shellfish. Without iodine, T3 and T4 are not produced so the thyroid cannot produce its hormones. The thyroid then begins to *atrophy* or slowly diminish in function due to underuse. This is known as a simple goiter. The availability of salt containing iodine has significantly reduced the number of cases of simple goiter in the world.

Tyrosine, an amino acid, is also used to manufacture T3 and T4. These two important hormones are responsible for controlling body metabolism, growth, and development. In addition, the thyroid gland produces *calcitonin*, which regulates calcium levels in the body.

Hyperthyroidism and Hypothyroidism

Patients suffering from thyroid disorders may experience either hypothyroidism or hyperthyroidism. These two disorders present clinically different signs and symptoms and may result in life threatening emergencies if undiagnosed or untreated. Table 15-19 provides details about hypothyroid and hyperthyroid disorders.

Medical History and Prevention of Thyroid Disorder Related Medical Emergencies

A thorough medical history obtained by the clinician will aid in the identification of the hypothyroid patient. In the case of a positive response to a thyroid disorder, it is important to determine whether or not the patient has a history of hypothyroidism or hyperthyroidism.

TABLE 15-19 Thyroid Disorders

Disorder	Clinical Manifestations	Causes/Treatment
hypothyroidism-low levels of thyroid hormone	Hypothyroidism usually occurs over a long period of time and progresses slowly. Patient may feel tired and fatigued and become more sensitive to cold. A hoarse voice may become evident. The hypothyroid patient may also gain weight despite efforts to diet and exercise, and may also feel more depressed. 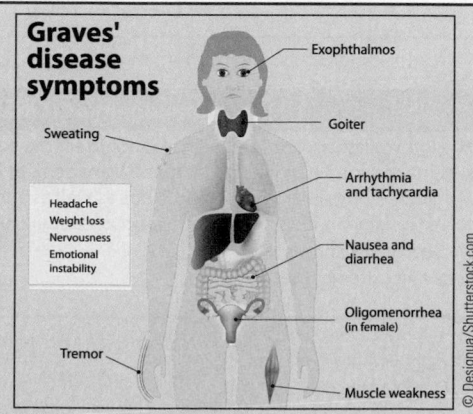	**Hashimoto's thyroiditis** is the most common cause of primary failure of the thyroid gland in the United States. The thyroid gland is regulated by a feedback mechanism, and failure of the pituitary (secondary failure) or failure of the hypothalamus (tertiary failure) may also occur. An overactive thyroid gland may be removed or destroyed, resulting in hypothyroidism. Hypothyroid patients are treated with synthetic thyroid hormone and are considered to be *euthyroid*. Untreated hypothyroidism may lead to myxedema **coma**.
hyperthyroidism (thyrotoxicosis)		Most common cause is an autoimmune disorder called Grave's disease. The undiagnosed and/or untreated hyperthyroid patient usually appears anxious or apprehensive in the dental office and may also exhibit **exophthalmos**. Sedation options may not be beneficial as it is a hormonal imbalance causing the anxiety. These patients are extremely sensitive to epinephrine, and administration of a local anesthetic with epinephrine may result in tachycardia. Untreated hyperthyroidism may lead to thyroid storm.

TABLE 15-20 Medical History Questions Related to Thyroid Disorders for Patients with a Confirmed Thyroid Disorder

- Do you have hypothyroidism or hyperthyroidism
- Are you seeing a physician?
- How well is your thyroid disorder managed?
- What medications are you taking to manage your thyroid disorder?

Physical observation of the patient may aid in identifying a patient with a thyroid disorder. Table 15-19 provides signs and symptoms that may be presented by a patient who has an undiagnosed thyroid disorder. Table 15-20 provides medical history questions that are related to thyroid disorders.

Untreated hyperthyroidism can lead to thyroid storm. Elective dental care should be postponed for the severely uncontrolled hyperthyroid patient until the medical condition has been brought under control. Long term, undiagnosed hypothyroidism can lead to myxedema coma if the patient is put into a stressful situation. In the case of a thyroid disorder, the physician should be consulted to determine the patient's condition and risk level. The disorder should be brought under control by the physician before the patient is treated in the dental office.

The uncontrolled hyperthyroid or hypothyroid patient is considered to be an ASA III risk. The alert clinician can utilize the medical history to identify the patient with a thyroid disorder. Adequate identification of the patient aids in the prevention of a thyroid related crisis.

Management of Thyroid Disorders in the Dental Office

In the event of a thyroid related emergency, dental treatment should be immediately terminated. Table 15-21 provides the protocol for management of thyroid storm or myxedema coma in the dental office.

Diabetes

Diabetes mellitus is an endocrine disorder that effects the regulation and balance of blood glucose levels. Patients with diabetes have elevated levels of glucose because of an insulin deficiency. The deficiency may be partial or complete. **Insulin** deficiency is due to

a dysfunction of the beta cells located in the *islets of Langerhans* areas in the pancreas (Figure 15-12). The pancreas also produces another hormone called glucagon. Both insulin and glucagon are responsible for maintaining adequate physiological levels of glucose. The functions of these two hormones is provided in Table 15-22. Diabetes may result in a variety of acute and chronic problems (discussed later in this section).

In a nondiabetic patient, blood glucose levels are maintained between 70 mg/dl and 150 mg/dl by the body. Blood glucose levels are lowest in the morning upon waking and rise after a meal is eaten. If the blood glucose level drops to 60 mg/dl or below, the patient may suffer from the signs and symptoms of *hypoglycemia*. Glucose greater than 150 mg/dl may be an indication of *hyperglycemia* or elevated blood sugar. When glucose levels rise to 160 mg/dl or more, the glucose is excreted out with the urine. Urine tests for diabetes will detect the glucose.

Types of Diabetes

Recognizing the type of diabetes is crucial in determining the proper treatment at the time of a crisis.

Type I Diabetes Type I diabetes was previously referred to as insulin dependent or juvenile onset diabetes. Though it usually occurs in younger adults and children, it can develop at any age. Table 15-23 provides detail about Type I diabetes

Type II Diabetes Type II diabetes is the most common form of diabetes and was known in the past as non-insulin-dependent diabetes mellitus or adult onset diabetes. This form of diabetes has a genetic component, though there is a link between obesity and the development of Type II diabetes. Additionally, the incidence of type II diabetes is rising in children, due to the increase in childhood obesity related to the consumption of

TABLE 15-21 Medical Emergencies Related to Thyroid Disorders and their Management

Medical Emergency	Clinical Manifestations	Management/Treatment
myxedema coma	True coma in this extreme state of hypothyroidism is rare. The main clinical manifestation of myxedema coma is deterioration of the mental state of the patient. Additionally, myxedema coma results in hypotension, depressed respiration, electrolyte imbalance, **hypovolemia**, and **hypothermia** and is normally precipitated by stress. In rare and extreme cases, coma and death may result.	Once diagnosed, the patient must be admitted to the hospital. Management includes replacement of electrolytes and fluids as well as administration of large doses of intravenously administered T3 and T4.
thyroid storm	The extreme end result of untreated hyperthyroidism. The main differentiating factor between hyperthyroidism and thyroid storm is the resulting **hyperpyrexia**. Thyroid storm is a result of massive doses of thyroid hormone circulating in the blood of the patient. In the event of thyroid storm, the patient must be immediately admitted to the hospital.	Management includes administration of medications that will stop the production and release of thyroid hormones. Beta blockers will also be administered intravenously to counteract the effect on the cardiovascular system. Cold packs may be utilized to counteract the hyperpyrexia.

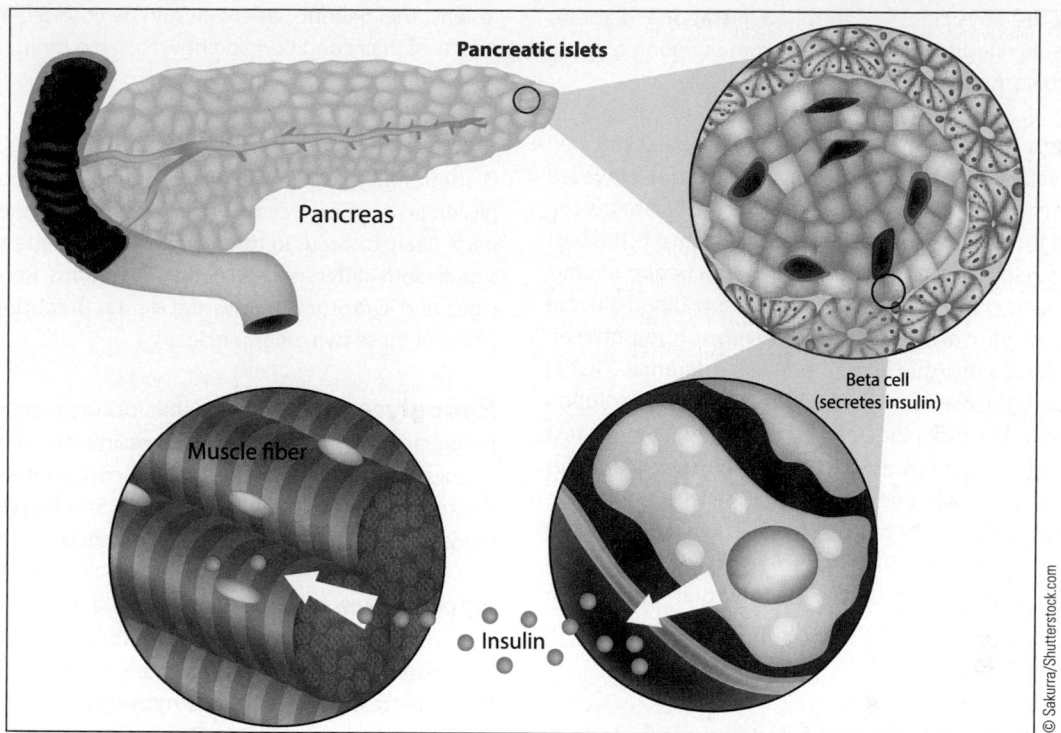

FIGURE 15-12
Pancreatic beta cells.

TABLE 15-22 Functions of Insulin and Glucagon

insulin	Lowers blood sugar levels in the body by taking glucose from the bloodstream and allowing the body to store the glucose in the cells as glycogen through a process called *glycogenesis*.
glucagon	If blood glucose levels decrease, *glucagon* slowly breaks down the glycogen through a process known as *glycogenolysis* and releases it back into the blood as glucose.

TABLE 15-23 Types I Diabetes

- Has a genetic component that results in the destruction of the beta cells of the pancreas that produce insulin. With the beta cells no longer able to produce insulin, blood glucose levels rise. In the untreated patient, glucose in the body is not taken into the cells and stored.

- When the cells in the body do not have glucose available for use, the body starts to break down stored fats for energy. The breakdown of fats releases *ketone bodies* into the blood stream to be used for energy. When the ketone bodies are broken down for energy, acetone (an aromatic chemical) is released. This acute condition is known as *ketoacidosis*. Ketone bodies are excreted in the urine, which would be used in diagnosing Type I diabetes. If the patient is not treated and ketoacidosis continues, the body breaks down muscle for energy, resulting in weight loss and muscle wasting.

- Prior to diagnosis. the patient may exhibit signs and symptoms such as **polydipsia**, **polyuria**, and **polyphagia** and weight loss that is unexplained.

- Patient will have a hot dry flushed appearance due to fluid loss

- Untreated ketoacidosis can lead to a coma

- Management of the type I diabetic includes daily insulin injections as well as balancing carbohydrate intake.

processed foods and a sedentary lifestyle. Table 15-24 provides additional details about Type II diabetes.

Gestational Diabetes *Gestational* diabetes occurs in pregnant females. Elevated blood glucose levels may occur in the pregnant female because pregnancy hormones interfere with the function of insulin. Predisposing factors to gestational diabetes are a family history of diabetes and a previous delivery of a baby weighing greater than 9 pounds. In most cases of gestational diabetes, the elevation of glucose is mild and does not pose a threat to the baby. However, a healthier diet will be recommended by the physician. If this alone does not lower blood glucose to healthy levels, oral medications or insulin injections may be implemented. The patient will be closely

TABLE 15-24 Types II Diabetes

- Blood glucose elevation occurs because either the beta cells of the pancreas do not produce enough insulin to allow glucose to be taken up by the cells of the body or the cells of the body are resistant to the insulin produced by the beta cells.
- The type II diabetic usually produces sufficient levels of insulin to prevent ketoacidosis.
- Initially, for prediabetes or a slightly elevated glucose level in the type II diabetic, the physician recommends a healthy diet, implementation of daily exercise, and weight loss. In the compliant patient, glucose levels may decrease, and the patient may not need medications.
- If the type II diabetic is not compliant with the physician's recommendations or if the lifestyle modifications alone do not reduce blood glucose levels, oral antidiabetic medications may be prescribed for the patient.

monitored by the physician. Uncontrolled gestational diabetes may harm the developing baby. In most women, blood glucose levels return to normal postpartum.

Prediabetes The prediabetic patient is one who has elevated blood glucose levels. However, the levels are not elevated enough for the diagnosis of diabetes. Diagnosis of diabetes can be conducted through a variety of tests. The A1C test is the best measure of a person's blood glucose levels over a period of time. The fasting plasma glucose (FPG) test will measure blood glucose levels after fasting overnight. The FPG levels range between 100 mg/dl and 125 mg/dl. The oral glucose tolerance (OGTT) measures blood glucose levels two hours after an oral solution containing sugar has been ingested by the patient. Such a test is conducted in the laboratory of the physician's office under supervision. In the prediabetic patient, glucose levels will range between 140 mg/dl and 199 mg/dl. Prediabetic patients do not exhibit signs and symptoms of diabetes. Obesity may be a factor in many cases. Implementation of a healthy diet and regular exercise can aid in significantly reducing blood glucose levels in the prediabetic patient.

Acute and Chronic Complications of Diabetes

It is usually the Type I diabetic patients who face many acute and chronic complications. Table 15-25 provides details on the types of complications experienced by Type I diabetics.

Because the periodontal tissues are highly vascular, the diabetic patient is at risk for periodontal disease. A well-controlled diabetic is not at significantly higher risk than a nondiabetic patient, but uncontrolled diabetics are not able to respond appropriately to the bacteria found in plaque. Periodontal diseases in the diabetic patient progresses at a faster rate and has a poorer prognosis than in nondiabetics. Also, diabetics are prone to xerostomia (dry mouth), which increases the risk of carious

lesions. The diabetic patient should be counseled about the oral effects of their condition and how to avoid them.

Management of Diabetes

Diabetics may suffer from either of two acute condition, hypoglycemia or hyperglycemia. The extremes of these conditions are more likely to occur in the Type I diabetic patient. Both present significantly different clinical manifestations. Recognition of the signs and symptoms allows the dental practitioner to manage either of these two emergencies.

Hypoglycemia Hypoglycemia occurs more commonly and progresses quickly, leading to unconsciousness if not immediately managed. The patient will become confused and behave in a bizarre manner, and may be sweating. Some bystanders mistake this behavior for a person who is intoxicated.

Hyperglycemia Hyperglycemia and ketoacidosis are not something that can be managed in the dental office. The patient must be referred to a physician for treatment of the diabetes. The conscious hyperglycemic patient should be referred to a physician. The unconscious hyperglycemic patient should be managed until EMS arrives to transport the patient to the hospital.

Medical History and Prevention of Diabetic Complications in the Dental Office

A detailed medical history will aid in the identification of the diabetic patient and in prevention of a medical emergency in the dental office. Medical history questions related to diabetes are outlined in Table 15-26.

TABLE 15-25 Acute and Chronic Complications of Type I Diabetes

Acute complications	• The most common acute complication, the one of most concern for the dental practitioner, is hypoglycemia. If the patient takes the normal insulin dose and does not eat the usual quantity of food, the blood glucose levels may drop below the minimum 60 mg/dl, resulting in hypoglycemia. Vigorous exercise or stress may also result in hypoglycemia. • The signs and symptoms of hypoglycemia are confusion, mood swings, and anxiety. If left untreated, the patient may lose consciousness and suffer from seizures.
Chronic complications	• Damage to both the small and large blood vessels leads to issues in many organs in the body as they become progressively starved of blood supply. **Microangiopathy** leads to diabetic retinopathy, which may lead to blindness. Other eye problems that are more common in the diabetic are **cataracts** and **glaucoma**. • Incidence of cardiovascular disease, such as angina or a myocardial infarction, is higher in Type I diabetics. • Blood vessel damage also leads to a greater incidence of stroke. • Higher incidence of **nephropathy** may result in the need for dialysis or a kidney transplant. • Microangiopathic changes also lead to poor blood flow and circulation, particularly in the extremities. This may lead to gangrene in the feet, resulting in amputations. • **Neuropathy** can result in a loss of sensation in the feet. In the well-controlled diabetic, the incidence of chronic problems is less than in the patient who is unable to manage the disease.

TABLE 15-26 Medical History Questions Related to Diabetes

Have there been any recent changes to your overall health?
Have there been any recent hospitalizations?
Has there been any recent weight loss?
Are you frequently thirsty?
Are you taking any prescription or non-prescription medications?
 	
If the patient has a history of diabetes it is important to find out whether it is Type I or Type II. For the Type I diabetic, ask about:
    ● Frequency of insulin injections
    ● Episodes of ketoacidosis or hypoglycemia

Management of the Diabetic Patient in the Dental Office

An uncontrolled diabetic patient should also be evaluated by their physician for organ damage, particularly the renal system and the cardiovascular system. Table 15-27 outlines the protocol for management of a diabetic patient in the dental office.

The most common medical emergency related to diabetes is an episode of hypoglycemia. Table 15-28 outlines the protocol for management of hypoglycemia in the dental office.

Angina and Myocardial Infarction

Angina is not a disease; rather it is symptom of an underlying disease, specifically *atherosclerosis* or narrowing of the blood vessels (Figure 15-13). Though the heart supplies blood to all parts of the body, it too needs a supply of oxygenated blood in order to function efficiently. Chapter 4 discusses the anatomy of the heart in detail. The student should refer to that chapter as needed for this section. An *occlusion* or blockage of a coronary blood vessel significantly reduces blood flow and oxygen supply

to the heart and results in angina. Angina chest pain is difficult to differentiate from pain related to an **infarct** of the myocardium; however, there are some differences between the two. The difference will be discussed later in this section. Though angina pain is not a myocardial infarction, if it remains uncorrected, the patient may eventually suffer from an infarction.

Angina

Angina pain is usually located in the substernal area. The pain may radiate to the left jaw, back, left shoulder, or the left arm (Figure 15-13). Though the underlying cause of the angina pain is similar in both stable and unstable angina, there are differences between the two forms. Table 15-29 provides additional details regarding signs and symptoms of stable and unstable angina. Table 15-30 provides factors that predispose a patient to angina.

Nitroglycerine

Nitroglycerine alleviates the pain of an acute angina attack by creating a temporary dilation of blood vessels, including the coronary blood vessels, thus allowing oxygen rich blood to

TABLE 15-27 Management of the Diabetic Patient in the Dental Office

● Schedule morning appointments at a time that allows the patient to eat and take medicine and check glucose levels prior to appointment. ● Do not schedule appointments at meal times. ● Follow stress reduction protocol outlined in Table 15-3. ● Extensive treatment should be broken up into multiple appointments. ● Prior to treatment, ask about the last meal eaten and when glucose levels were last checked.

TABLE 15-28 Management of Hypoglycemia

conscious patient	● In the conscious patient, a sugar source such as glucose tablets, chocolate, orange juice, apple juice, or a non-diet soda may be administered. ● Upon ingestion of the sugar source, the signs of hypoglycemia reverse very rapidly. In many cases, the patient will have a sugar source with them. ● If a sugar source is not administered, the patient may lose consciousness.
unconscious patient	● An IV glucose solution may be administered. In case an IV is not practical, cake icing may be placed in the mucobuccal fold of the patient. The sugar from the icing will be absorbed slowly through the oral mucosa and recovery may take up to 30 minutes. The patient should be monitored at all times and a patent airway should be maintained. ● DO NOT ADMINISTER JUICE OR SODA TO THE UNCONSCIOUS DIABETIC PATIENT.

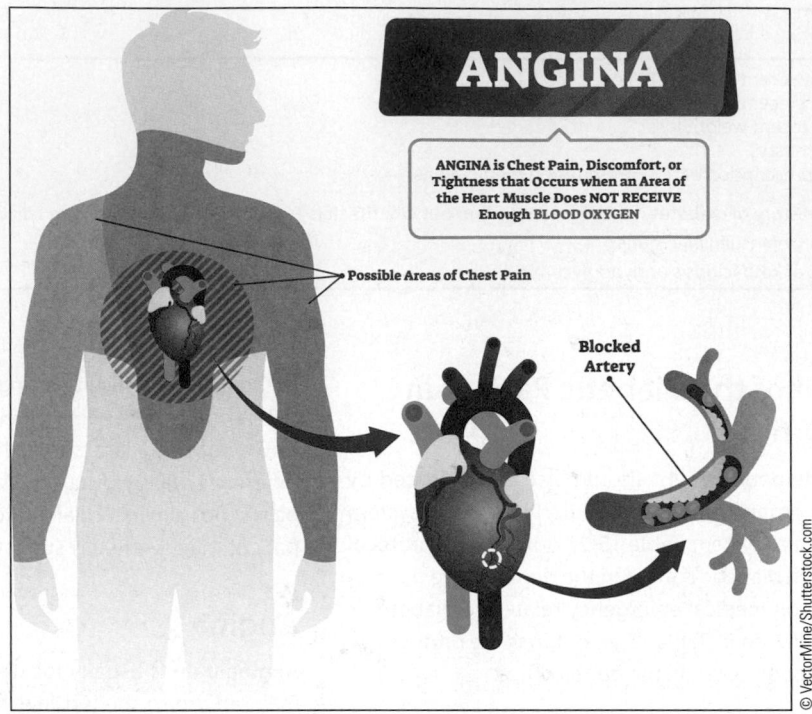

FIGURE 15-13
Angina.

© VectorMine/Shutterstock.com

TABLE 15-29 Signs and Symptoms of Stable and Unstable Angina

stable angina	<ul><li>The intensity of the pain and how long it lasts, what triggers the attack, and its responsiveness to medications are predictable.</li><li>Angina attacks usually last up to 5 minutes and are relieved by rest and nitroglycerine, a vasodilator.</li><li>Patients may state the pain is a squeezing discomfort.</li><li>Patients may display a cold sweat, look pale, and feel lightheaded and nauseous.</li><li>An arrhythmia may be present during an attack.</li><li>Angina attack is usually brought on physical exertion, stress, hot or cold weather, or ingestion of a heavy meal.</li></ul>
unstable angina	<ul><li>Acute unpredictable attacks that may occur even at rest. They vary in length of duration and can last for 15–20 minutes.</li><li>Nitroglycerine may or may not relieve the angina pain.</li><li>**Atherosclerotic plaque** buildup is more significant than in the patient with stable angina, thereby creating a greater risk for suffering from a myocardial infarction.</li></ul>

flow more readily to the heart muscle satisfying the demand of the heart for oxygen and relieving the pain of the attack. The vasodilating activity of nitroglycerine results in several transient side effects such as facial flushing, headache, and hypotension.

Nitroglycerine is available as sublingual tablets or a sublingual spray. The tablets have a short shelf life, approximately 3–6 months from the time the bottle is opened, depending on how well sealed the container is. Nitroglycerine tablets should be stored in the original container away from light, moisture, and heat. Patients often keep several bottles in various locations such as work, home, purse, and car. Sometimes these tablets remain unused and expire. In the case of an acute angina attack, it is better to use the patient's own tablets, which have been dosed appropriately. An active nitroglycerine tablet, when placed sublingually, produces a tingling sensation and will have a bitter taste. If a patient states that there are no such sensations, the tablet is most likely expired

and the nitroglycerine will not relieve the angina pain. In that case, retrieve the nitroglycerine sublingual spray from the emergency kit and administer to the patient. Due to the highly vascular nature of the sublingual tissues, administration of nitroglycerine in this area allows a rapid absorption of the medication and a rapid pain relieving effect. Patients may also be taking beta blockers or calcium channel blockers to manage angina.

Medical History and Prevention of an Acute Angina Attack in the Dental Office

The dental practitioner can take several measures to prevent an angina related emergency. A thorough medical history is vital in identifying the patient with a history of angina, including questions about previous occurrences and medications. Table 15-31 provides information regarding the importance of the medical history information to prevent an angina attack in the dental office.

TABLE 15-30 Predisposing Factors to Angina

- Diabetics are more prone to developing cardiovascular problems and as a result angina.
- High blood pressure, if left untreated, leads to cardiovascular damage and angina.
- Hypertension can cause angina.
- Obesity—in most cases, obesity is due to poor diet and a sedentary lifestyle.
- Family history of cardiovascular disease increases the risk of angina.
- Elevated cholesterol levels are linked to angina.
- Males over the age of 45 are prone to cardiovascular disease.
- Smokers are more likely to develop cardiovascular disease, leading to angina.

TABLE 15-31 Medical History and Prevention of an Acute Angina Attack

- Patients who had a myocardial infarction or a cerebrovascular accident in the past could also be on aspirin therapy and may also be taking potent **anticoagulants** such as **warfarin** to prevent a recurring incident.
- Question the patient about previous heart disease or a family history heart disease.
- Diabetics and those with adrenal and thyroid disorders are at a significantly higher risk for cardiovascular disease than those without these disorders.
- Those with a positive history of angina should be questioned regarding the frequency and duration of episodes as well as the factors that trigger an angina attack. Record details about the radiation of the pain during an attack and how well nitroglycerine alleviates an attack must be explored.
- For those with a history of angina, request that the patient bring their nitroglycerine to each appointment; be sure to check the expiration date of the medication. At each appointment, the patient's nitroglycerine should be kept within reach in the event of an angina episode during dental treatment.

Management of a Patient with a History of Angina

The dental practitioner must be able to manage the patient with a history of angina in the dental office. A patient with stable angina is an ASA II patient and may be treated in the dental office following a medical consult with the patient's physician. The patient with unstable angina should not be considered for elective dental care since they are at a significant risk for a myocardial infarction. Table 15-32 provides the management protocol for the patient with a history of stable angina.

The unstable angina patient experiencing dental pain must be managed palliatively with pain medication and antibiotics. Consult the physician and delay treatment until the patient's cardiac condition improves. If treatment is a must, the unstable angina patient should be treated in a hospital operating room with full resuscitation equipment available in the case of a cardiac event.

Management of an Acute Angina Attack in the Dental Office An angina episode may occur in the dental office. In this case, all dental procedures must be stopped and the situation assessed. In most cases of angina, the patient will be able to maintain circulation, airway, and breathing, and will prefer the upright position. Table 15-33 provides the steps the dental assistant should take in the event a patient experiences an attack of angina.

Myocardial Infarction

A myocardial infarction may also occur while the patient is in the dental office. Stress may trigger an attack in those at risk. The dental assistant should be able to identify patients based on medical history. Appropriate patient management aids and minimizes the risk of such an occurrence.

TABLE 15-32 Management of the Dental Patient with a History of Stable Angina

- Stress reduction protocol is important in preventing an angina episode: Schedule patients in the morning after a full night's rest; keep appointments short since patients with a history of angina may not be able to tolerate the stress of long appointments; provide good pain control.
- Use of 100% oxygen provided through a nasal hood may be beneficial to the patient with stable angina.
- Nitrous oxide and oxygen sedation would be beneficial as it will cause anxiolysis and provide additional oxygen.
- Utilize good pain control through the use of local anesthesia. Limit the amount of epinephrine to 2 carpules of 1:100,000 epinephrine concentration, which is equivalent to the cardiac dose of 0.04 milligrams of epinephrine.
- As a preventive measure, the angina patient may also take their nitroglycerine prior to the start of the dental procedure.

TABLE 15-33 Management of an Acute Angina Attack in the Dental Office

- Place the patient upright. One dose of the patient's nitroglycerine should be administered by placing under the patient's tongue.
- Supplemental 100% oxygen can be beneficial by providing the additional oxygen the heart is demanding.
- Pain should be alleviated in approximately 1 to 2 minutes, but a second dose of nitroglycerine may be necessary.
- If the angina pain is not relieved, it may be because the nitroglycerine has expired and is no longer effective. In that case, the nitroglycerine sublingual spray may be retrieved from the emergency kit and one or two sprays administered.
- Up to 3 doses of nitroglycerine may be administered within 15 minutes. If the angina pain is still not relieved, the patient may be suffering from a myocardial infarction and EMS should be summoned immediately.
- The patient with no history of angina suffering from chest pain should be treated as a possible myocardial infarction. Summon EMS immediately in these cases.

Causes of a Myocardial Infarction

Despite advances in medicine, one of the leading causes of death throughout the world is an acute myocardial infarction, caused by coronary artery blockage. The predisposing factors to an acute myocardial infarction are similar to those for angina listed in Table 15-30. The blockage significantly reduces blood and oxygen to the myocardium, resulting in an infarct. This blockage may result in angina and can progressively increase and result in a myocardial infarction. A myocardial infarction may also occur without warning in a patient with no history of angina pain. In many cases, this condition results in damage to a portion of the heart muscle and leads to other cardiovascular issues, such as congestive heart failure. It is important for the dental practitioner to be aware of these complications. Survivors of an infarct may appear healthy but may have significant heart problems.

Signs and Symptoms of a Myocardial Infarction

The signs and symptoms of an acute myocardial infarction are similar to those of an acute angina attack but may be more painful (Table 15-29). The signs vary from patient to patient.

Medical History and Prevention of a Myocardial Infarction

A complete and thorough medical history aids in identification of a previous acute myocardial infarction or undiagnosed heart disease. Identifying the patient through questioning about their medical history will aid in the prevention of a myocardial infarct in the dental office. Table 15-34 provides questions that should be asked to aid in the identification of a patient with a history of diagnosed or undiagnosed cardiovascular disease.

The post myocardial infarction patient may be an ASA II, III, or IV depending on the number of past incidents and residual complications. A thorough medical history and consult with the physician, if necessary, will aid in the determination of the ASA classification of the patient who has suffered from a myocardial infarction. Table 15-35 provides examples of ASA classifications of post myocardial infarction patients. Table 15-36 provides the common medications that a post myocardial infarction patient may be taking.

The post myocardial infarction patient should be managed in the same manner that the patient with a history of angina is managed. Refer to Table 15-33 for management protocol of a post myocardial infarction patient.

Management of a Myocardial Infarction in the Dental Office

In the event of a myocardial infarction in the dental office, it is critical to implement the emergency care protocol including activation of EMS as rapidly as possible. In the angina patient, initial management is for angina. In the event that the pain is more severe than what the patient usually experiences or if the three doses of nitroglycerine do not alleviate the pain, myocardial infarction management should be implemented. In the patient without a history of angina and suffering from chest pain for the first time, the steps should be implemented for myocardial infarction management. The signs and symptoms of a myocardial infarction are provided in Table 15-37. Table 15-38 outlines the steps to implement in the event of a suspected myocardial infarction in the dental office.

TABLE 15-34 Medical History Questions to Determine if Patient Has a History of a Previous Myocardial Infarction or Undiagnosed Heart Disease

- Previous episodes of chest pain
- History of heart disease, diabetes, or thyroid and adrenal disorders
- Diagnosis of diabetes or thyroid and adrenal disorders
- Previous hospitalizations
- Note all surgeries and medications in the chart and ask reason for hospitalization.
- Evaluate for hypertension and blood pressure.
- If the patient has a history of a previous myocardial infarction, ask when it occurred and if there has been more than one occurrence.

TABLE 15-35 ASA Classifications of Post Myocardial Infarction Patients

ASA II	More than 6 months post myocardial infarct and has no residual complications
ASA III/IV	Myocardial infarction more than 6 months ago and demonstrates complications such as arrhythmias or congestive heart failure; considered to be an ASA III or IV depending on the severity of the complications
ASA IV	Less than 6 months post myocardial infarct—no elective care

TABLE 15-36 Medications that a Post Myocardial Infarct Patient May Be Taking

- Anticoagulant medication to prevent clotting and reduce the risk of future myocardial infarctions (these may result in excess bleeding during dental treatment)
- Daily aspirin regimen to prevent clotting
- Beta blockers, calcium channel blockers, ACE inhibitors to reduce pressure and allow the heart to function more efficiently
- Diuretics to help the body get rid of excel fluid so heart can pump with less resistance
- nitroglycerine
- Anticholesterol medications to reduce plaque buildup in the blood vessels

TABLE 15-37 Signs and Symptoms of a Myocardial Infarction

Patients may experience:
- A silent infarct, which is more likely to occur in females and diabetics
- Intense pressure or squeezing in the chest
- Pain that may or may not radiate to the jaw, teeth, shoulder, back and arm
- Dyspnea along with **diaphoresis**
- Syncope
- Stomach pain, which may be thought to be acid reflux. Medical care may be delayed, resulting in death.
- Restlessness in an attempt to alleviate the pain
- Hypertension

TABLE 15-38 Management of a Suspected Myocardial Infarction in the Dental Office

- Assess the situation, check circulation by palpation of the carotid artery, monitor breathing, and maintain an open airway.
- Keep the person calm in order to minimize strain on the heart.
- Morphine or nitrous oxide may be administered to the patient for pain.
- Oxygen may be administered to the patient.
- Administer 325 milligrams of aspirin to chew and swallow.
- Vital signs should be monitored and recorded every 5 minutes.
- EMS will transport the patient to the hospital for further treatment.

Cardiac Arrest

Sudden cardiac arrest is a condition in which the heart suddenly stops beating, resulting in lack of blood flow to the brain and other vital organs. If this is not reversed quickly, death will result.

Basic Life Support

The American Dental Association (ADA) Council on Scientific Affairs recommends that all staff members, including those who do not have constant patient contact, be trained in basic life support (BLS) at the health care provider level. Training of all staff members allows rapid recognition of a medical emergency should it occur, resulting in more efficient management. After initial training in BLS, refresher courses may be required to maintain certification. The American Heart Association (AHA) offers courses throughout the year in BLS. Implementation of BLS is always the primary step in the management of a medical emergency; use of medications is secondary. BLS courses should also include instruction on the use of an automatic external defibrillator (AED).

Congestive Heart Failure

Nearly 5 million people in the United States currently suffer from *congestive heart failure* (CHF), a condition in which the heart is unable to adequately provide oxygenated blood to the organs in the body, significantly impacting the quality of life for those it affects. When the heart starts to fail as a pump, the heart tries to compensate by enlarging and thickening, leading to heart failure. The incidence of CHF has increased. Today, many people suffering from CHF are living longer due to modern medical advances. Congestive heart failure, which is irreversible and in most cases becomes progressively worse over time. Many times, one side of the heart fails first, followed by the second. It is important for the clinician to identify patients who suffer from congestive heart failure in order to appropriately manage dental treatment.

Causes of Congestive Heart Failure

Several underlying causes can lead to the development of congestive heart failure. Table 15-39 provides a summary of the predisposing factors to congestive heart failure.

Left and Right Ventricular Failure The left ventricle of the heart is more prone to failure before the right. Right ventricular failure usually follows the left, though either can occur alone. Table 15-40 provides the signs and symptoms of left and right ventricular failure.

Medical History and Prevention of an Emergency Related to Congestive Heart Failure

The medical history plays an important role in identifying the patient with congestive heart failure. Questions that should be asked related to congestive heart failure are outlined in Table 15-41.

ASA Classifications

The ASA classifications of a patient with a diagnosis of congestive heart failure varies based on the extent and the progression of the disease. Table 15-42 provides some examples of ASA classifications of patients with congestive heart failure.

Dental Management of the Patient with Congestive Heart Failure

The dental clinician should obtain a medical consult from the patient's physician for the ASA III or IV patient prior to treatment. The ASA IV patient may be best treated in a hospital setting.

TABLE 15-39 Predisposing Factor to Congestive Heart Failure

- Previous myocardial infarction with residual damage to the heart muscle
- *Congenital* heart defects which are present from birth and significantly alter the function of the heart
- Abnormal heart valves resulting in blood not flowing in the correct direction and instead backing up into the previous chamber
- History of uncontrolled hypertension, which causes the heart to continuously pump against very high pressure
- Uncontrolled hypothyroidism, hyperthyroidism, and diabetes

TABLE 15-40 Signs and Symptoms of Left Ventricular and Right Ventricular Failure

left ventricular failure	<ul><li>Lung congestion leading to dyspnea</li><li>Pink tinted **sputum** upon coughing, due to the red blood cells in the lungs</li><li>*Orthopnea* or difficulty breathing while lying down; may sleep with multiple pillows</li><li>*Paroxysmal nocturnal dyspnea*, or shortness of breath at night which is relieved by sitting up for some time</li></ul>
right ventricular failure	<ul><li>fatigue</li><li>dyspnea</li><li>**peripheral pitting edema** (Figure 15-14)</li><li>**nocturia**</li><li>**distended jugular veins**</li></ul>

In order to prevent an acute pulmonary edema, implementation of stress reduction protocol is important in the management of a patient with congestive heart failure. This life threatening medical emergency is discussed below. Additionally, orthopnea may prevent placement of the patient in the supine position. The patient with more advanced congestive heart failure patient may be more comfortable in the semisupine or upright position. Oxygen supplementation may be administered to the patient during dental treatment.

Management of Acute Pulmonary Edema in the Dental Office

Acute pulmonary edema is a truly life threatening emergency caused by an acute exacerbation of congestive heart failure. Acute pulmonary edema takes place when fluid leaves the pulmonary vasculature and enters the alveoli of the lungs. The fluid build-up causes extreme dyspnea, which may be slow in onset or rapid in onset. The

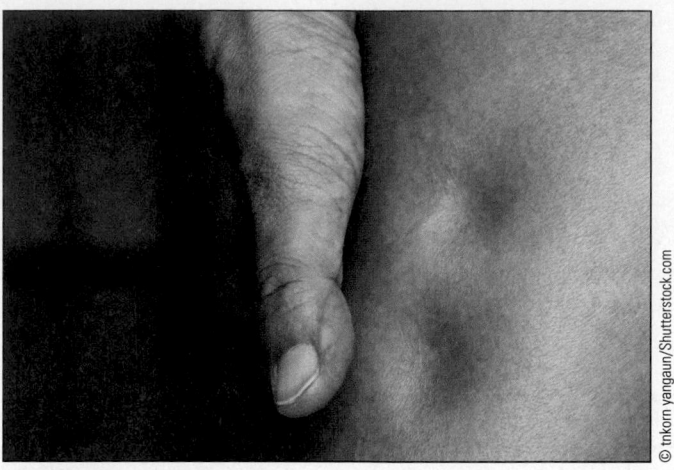

FIGURE 15-14
Peripheral pitting edema.

patient may also become anxious and show signs of cyanosis. A cough with pink-tinted sputum may be present.

Stress in the dental office can trigger acute pulmonary edema in the CHF patient. These events may be more common in patients who may not be compliant with diuretics and other prescribed medications to manage the condition. Summon EMS in the event of acute pulmonary edema in the dental office, as treatment for this event must be aggressive and more definitive than what the dental professional can provide. Until the arrival of EMS, the dental professional must manage the situation. Table 15-43 describes the protocol for management of an episode of acute pulmonary edema.

Epilepsy and Seizures

Seizures, also known as fits or *convulsions*, are a group of disorders which occur due to an abnormally large discharge of electrical activity. Nearly 3 million Americans, of all ages, suffer from

---

TABLE 15-41 Medical History Questions Related to Congestive Heart Failure

- Past myocardial infarction, angina, hypertension
- Valvular defects or congenital heart defects
- Medications such as diuretics, calcium channel blockers, ACE inhibitors, and beta adrenergic agonists
- Past hospitalizations
- If the patient has a confirmed diagnosis of CHF, ask about:
  - The extent of the disease
  - Ability to perform daily activities, such as walking up a flight of steps without having to stop and rest
  - Sleeping with multiple pillows
  - Waking at night because of difficulty in breathing
  - Swelling of ankles; also view the ankles for edema
  - Examine the jugular vein for distention when the patient is upright
  - Recent significant weight gain

TABLE 15-42 ASA Classifications of Patients with Congestive Heart Failure

ASA II	Patient is able to perform normal daily activities with only slight fatigue and slight dyspnea
ASA III	Moderate fatigue and dyspnea during routine activities Needs multiple pillows to sleep at night May stop several times during normal activities to rest
ASA IV	Dyspnea and fatigue even at rest

TABLE 15-43 Management of an Episode of Acute Pulmonary Edema in the Dental Office

- Keep the patient calm and comfortable.
- Terminate all dental treatment.
- Position patient upright as this will be more comfortable.
- Administer oxygen to the patient via a nasal cannula or a nasal hood.
- Record vital signs every 5 minutes until the arrival of EMS.
- EMS will transport the patient to the hospital, where intravenous diuretics will be administered to aggressively reduce fluid via urine excretion.
- The dental practitioner must investigate the reason for the acute pulmonary edema and modify future treatment to prevent a subsequent episode.

epilepsy and seizures. The incidence of epilepsy is highest in those under the age of 2 and over the age of 65.

Temporary problems such as drug use, high fever, or abnormal glucose levels may be the cause of some seizures, which usually doesn't occur again once the cause has been corrected. Since these seizures occur only once, the patient does not have epilepsy. Patients may suffer from partial seizures, which affect one side of the brain and generally do not result in a loss of consciousness, or generalized seizures, which affect both sides of the brain and may result in a loss of consciousness. The classical type of seizure most people recognize is the *grand mal* or *generalized tonic clonic seizure* (GTCS).

Generalized Seizures

This section will focus on two types of generalized seizures and their management, the absence seizure and the GTCS. *Status epilecticus*, a life threatening emergency related to the GTCS, will also be discussed in this section. Table 15-44 provides signs of each type.

TABLE 15-44 Signs and Symptoms of Absence Seizures, Generalized Tonic Clonic Seizures, and Status Epilepticus

absence seizures (Figure 15-15)	No loss of consciousness Patient may be in a "trance-like" state Lasts for 10–20 seconds and may go undiagnosed for a long time No **prodromal** or **postictal** phase Usually begin in childhood
generalized tonic clonic seizures (Figure 15-16)	Tonic phase of muscle contraction and rigidity followed by a clonic phase of rhythmic muscle contraction and relaxation Prodromal phase during which patient experiences an aura such as a smell or sound only they experience. Patient falls to the floor and releases an epileptic cry, followed by the ictal phase which is the seizure and lasts for about 5 minutes During the grand mal seizure, the patient may clench their teeth or bite their cheek or tongue, resulting in visible blood in and around the oral cavity. Frothing at the mouth, due to saliva mixing with air, can also occur as well as loss of bladder or bowel control. The patient may have difficulty breathing, causing cyanosis. Blood pressure may become extremely elevated. Postictal phase—upon termination of the seizure, the patient goes into a deep sleep and may be confused upon awakening. The patient will also be tired due to the physiological impact on the muscles of the body.
status epilepticus	Any grand mal seizure that lasts for more than 5 minutes is considered to be a grand mal status seizure or *status epilepticus*. This form of GTCS is a life threatening emergency due to the stress on the body. The cardiovascular system is severely overworked, and blood pressure rises to extreme highs. Additionally, brain damage occurs due to hypoxia. If the seizure is not terminated through medical intervention, death results from cardiac arrest.

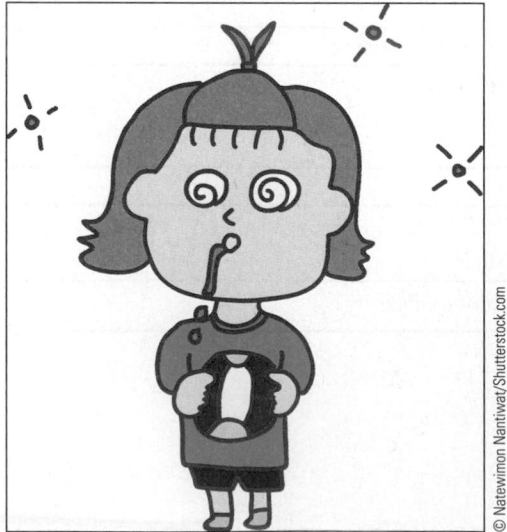

FIGURE 15-15
An absence seizure.

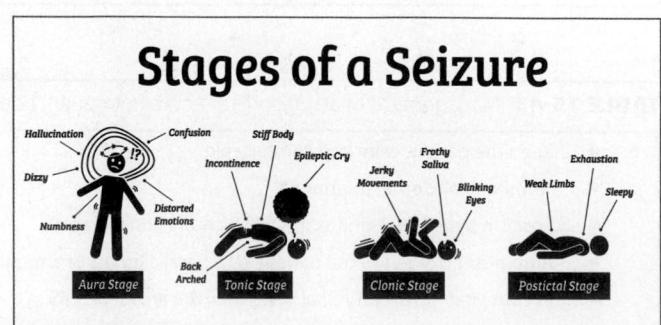

FIGURE 15-16
Stages of a seizure.

Status Epilepticus

Medical management includes administration of intravenous anticonvulsive agents such as diazepam (Valium) or midazolam. Status epilepticus usually happens to patients who are noncompliant with medications to control seizures or who have other underlying medical disorders such as brain tumors. Illicit drug use can also cause grand mal status seizures.

Causes of Epilepsy and Seizures

Approximately 70% of cases of epilepsy are idiopathic in nature. Despite the fact that most cases have an unknown cause, certain triggers, such as flashing lights, will cause a seizure in those with the disorder. For the remaining 30% of the cases, the cause is usually identifiable. Table 15-45 provides details regarding identifiable causes of seizures.

Medical History and Prevention of Seizures in the Dental Office

A thorough medical will aid the dental professional in the identification of the patient with a history of seizures. Table 15-46 provides medical history questions related to seizures or epilepsy that the dental professional should ask a patient.

The medications used to manage epilepsy are central nervous system depressants. As a result, patients may experience drowsiness. Some of the medications cause stomach upset, and xerostomia is a side effect of many of the medications. As a result of reduced salivary flow, the patient may be more prone to decay and therefore should be educated regarding management of xerostomia. Many patients will suck on candy or drink sugar-containing beverages to relieve the dry mouth symptoms, increasing the risk of caries. Patients should be advised to use sugar-free gum or candy and drink water. Saliva substitutes such as Moi-Stir® or Xero-Lube® may also be recommended.

Management of Epilepsy and Seizures in the Dental Office

Implementation of stress reduction protocol as outlined in Table 15-3 reduces the risk of a seizure in the dental office setting. However, the dental professional should be aware of how to manage an epileptic seizure should it occur. Table 15-47 provides the protocol for management of an epileptic seizure in the dental office setting.

Cerebrovascular Accident

A *cerebrovascular accident* (CVA) is also known as a stroke or brain attack. The underlying cause of a stroke is arteriosclerosis of a blood vessel that supplies the brain. The occlusion caused by the plaque buildup leads to decreased blood and oxygen to that area of the brain. If the occlusion is significant enough, the result is a stroke. Patients who suffer from a CVA may recover completely, or

TABLE 15-45 Predisposing Factors to Epilepsy

- Trauma to the brain
- Genetics
- Diagnosis of Down's syndrome
- Brain tumors
- **Electrolyte** and metabolic imbalances can lead to seizures, but may be reversed by treating the condition
- Certain medications
- In newborns, a lack of oxygen during childbirth or maternal drug use
- Alzheimer's disease is the most common cause in the elderly
- Stroke and head trauma
- **Febrile** seizures
- Hypoglycemia
- Local anesthetic overdose in the dental office

TABLE 15-46 Medical History Questions Related to Seizures and Epilepsy

- Returning patients should be questioned about recent hospitalization and any changes in medical history.
- Those with a history of seizures should be asked about the type of seizures experienced and what triggers a seizure. Some patients are well controlled due to the medications and others may continue to experience seizures despite medications. A medical consult should be obtained from the treating physician prior to dental treatment of a patient who continues to experience seizures despite treatment.
- Patients with a history of seizures should be questioned about their aura so the practitioner is aware a seizure may be forthcoming.
- Ask about how long the seizures last and any hospitalizations related to the condition.
- Also note how often the patient sees the physician for management as well as the physician's phone number in the patient chart.
- Question the patient about medications used to control the seizures. Dilantin, valproic acid, carbamezapine, ethosuximide, and phenobarbital are some common medications a patient may be taking to manage epilepsy.

TABLE 15-47 Management of the Absence and Generalized Tonic Clinic Seizure

absence seizures	<ul><li>Minimal intervention required.</li><li>Prevent injury to the patient by terminating dental treatment and removing all objects from the patient's mouth and out of their way.</li><li>Offer reassurance and remain with the patient until the seizure terminates.</li><li>Usually last for less than 30 seconds and seizure may be unnoticed at times.</li><li>Treatment may continue if the patient and practitioner believe that it is appropriate to do so.</li><li>Determine what may have triggered the seizure so modifications may be implemented for future treatment.</li><li>If the seizure does not terminate within 5 minutes, EMS should be summoned and BLS implemented as necessary.</li></ul>
generalized tonic clonic seizures	<ul><li>If the practitioner is made aware of the aura and if time allows, remove all objects from the patient's mouth, move all objects from the treatment area to prevent harm to the patient, and move the patient to the floor.</li><li>If the seizure begins without prior warning, it may not be possible to move the patient to the floor. Instead, lower the chair and place the patient supine.</li><li>Summon EMS.</li><li>Maintain a patent airway with the head-tilt, chin lift method.</li><li>Use soft suction tips to suction the airway of blood and saliva. Do not place anything between the patient's jaws.</li><li>Gently restrain the patient only to prevent injury. Protect head by placing a soft blanket underneath</li><li>Monitor and record vital signs.</li><li>Upon termination of the seizure, prepare to manage the postictal phase. During this phase, the patient will sleep and should be placed in a supine position. Respiratory, cardiovascular and central nervous system depression also occur during the postictal phase.</li><li>Oxygen may be administered to the patient and the airway should be maintained with the head tilt chin lift method. Monitor and record vital signs. The patient may take up to 2 hours to recover. A determination must be made to discharge the patient to a hospital or send the patient home with a friend or family member. Only release the patient to go home upon return of vitals to normal and confirmation of no confusion or disorientation. If in doubt, EMS will transport the patient to a hospital.</li><li>In the event that the GTCS does not terminate within 5 minutes, it should be considered a grand mal status epilepticus seizure and managed aggressively.</li></ul>
status epilepticus	<ul><li>For the practitioner unfamiliar with administering IV anticonvulsants, the patient should be maintained until EMS arrives. Upon administration of IV anticonvulsant medications, the seizure will terminate. In all cases of grand mal status, the patient must be transported by EMS to a hospital for further management and evaluation.</li></ul>

the CVA may be severe enough to cause permanently disability or death. The end result depends on the type of stroke, the extent of damage to the brain, and how quickly the patient receives medical care.

Types of Cerebrovascular Accidents

Eighty-seven percent of strokes are *ischemic* strokes. Hemorrhagic strokes make up approximately 13% of all cases of strokes (Figure 15-17). Table 15-48 provides details on both the ischemic and hemorrhagic stroke.

Transient Ischemic Attack (TIA)

A transient ischemic attack (TIA) is not a true stoke but is a mini stroke or a warning stroke, similar to angina in the heart. Table 15-48 provides additional details about a TIA.

Predisposing Factors to a Cerebrovascular Accident

There are several predisposing factors that may lead to a CVA; some are modifiable and some are not. Table 15-49 outlines the modifiable and nonmodifiable risk factors for a CVA.

Medical History and Prevention of a Cerebrovascular Accident

A thorough medical history will aid the dental professional in identifying the patient who may have suffered from a stroke in the past or is at higher risk for a CVA. Medical history questions that are related to cerebrovascular accident are outlined in Table 15-50.

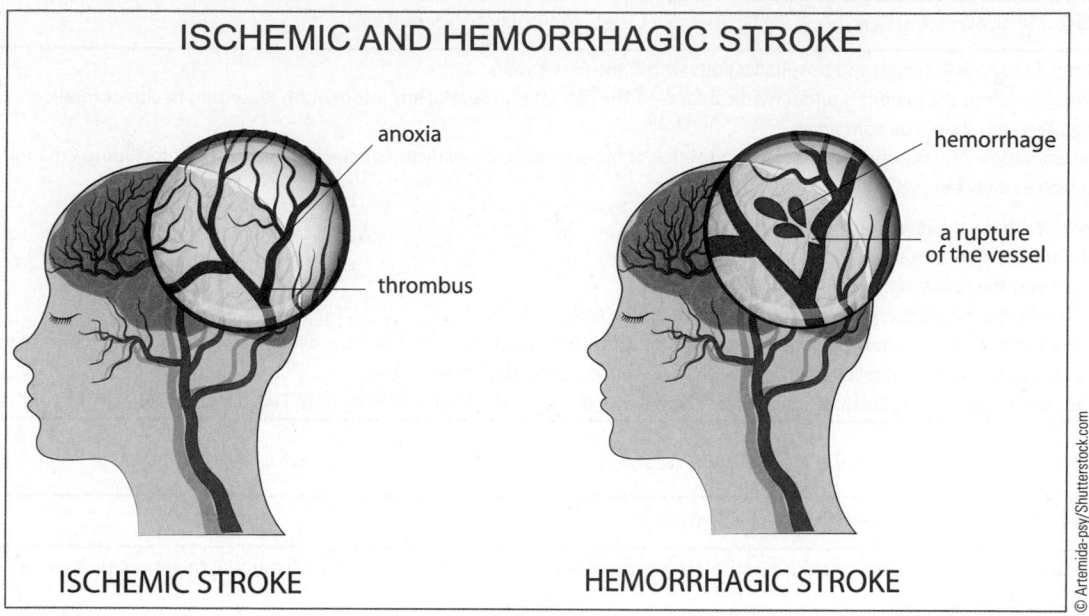

FIGURE 15-17
Ischemic and hemorrhagic stroke.

TABLE 15-48 Comparison of Ischemic Stroke, Hemorrhagic Stroke, and Transient Ischemic Attack

ischemic stroke	Occurs when a blockage due to atherosclerotic plaque buildup or a **thrombus** or **embolus** in a blood vessel supplying an area of the brain is present.
hemorrhagic stroke	Occurs when an **aneurysm** ruptures. Hypertension may lead to a rupture. In the dental office, stress can elevate blood pressure and cause an undiagnosed aneurysm to burst, resulting in a hemorrhagic CVA.
transient ischemic attack	Caused by an occluded blood vessel.
	Referred to as a warning stroke or a mini stroke and is similar to an angina attack to the heart.
	Not a true stroke but the signs and symptoms of a TIA are very similar to that of a stroke
	Usually lasts less than a minute.
	When the TIA subsides, there are no residual effects and no permanent damage to the brain.

TABLE 15-49 Risk Factors for a Cerebrovascular Accident (CVA)

Modifiable Risk Factors for a CVA	**Nonmodifiable Risk Factors for a CVA**
• Hypertension-reducing blood pressure through diet, exercise, and medications can reduce the risk of a stroke • Smoking cessation • Diabetes leads to elevated cholesterol and hypertension, thus increasing the risk of a CVA • Arteriosclerotic plaque buildup • Physical inactivity • History of TIA	• After the age of 55, the risk of suffering from a stroke doubles for each decade of life • Race— African Americans are at a higher risk for obesity, hypertension, and metabolic syndrome resulting in a higher risk for a CVA as compared to Caucasians • Family history of CVA • Those with a previous history of stroke are at a greater risk of a second CVA

Dental Management of the Patient with a History of a Cerebrovascular Accident

Patients who have suffered from a CVA in the past six months are not candidates for elective dental care. The risk of a second stroke occurring is considered to be much higher during the six-month period following an incident than it is once the six-month time period has passed. Patients may receive palliative care until the six months has passed. If treatment is necessary, it should be performed in a hospital setting in case of the event of an emergency. Table 15-51 provides management protocol for a patient with a history of a CVA. Table 15-52 provides the ASA classifications of a patient who has a history of a CVA.

TABLE 15-50 Medical History Questions Pertaining to a Cerebrovascular Accident (CVA)

- Overall changes in health and hospitalizations within the past 3 years
- Whether or not the patient is under medical care—if the patient is unsure of any information regarding health or medical events, the treating physician should be contacted
- Patients should be questioned regarding presence of hypertension, visual disturbances, and medications including OTC and prescription as well as daily baby aspirin

For the patient who has a positive history of a stroke:
- When the CVA occurred
- What was the cause of the CVA
- What was the blood pressure reading at the time of the CVA?
- Is the patient now on antihypertensive medications and is the blood pressure now controlled? How long was the patient hospitalized?
- Question the patient on recovery from the damage that occurred due to the stroke.
- The patient should also be questioned about whether or not he or she is still suffering from TIAs despite medical intervention.

TABLE 15-51 Dental Management of a CVA Patient

- Implementation of stress reduction protocol which includes short morning appointments. Extensive treatment plans should be broken up into multiple visits.
- Good pain control with local anesthesia–epinephrine should be limited to the cardiac dose.
- Nitrous oxide and oxygen sedation.
- Patient taking anticoagulant medications may experience prolonged bleeding. Dentist can request blood test result which included bleeding time. Consult with physician to determine best course of action for treatment. Physician may opt to reduce dose of anticoagulant thus reducing bleeding time or may request that the dentist use local measures such as sutures and cellulose sponges to enhance clotting and healing. Dentist may opt to alter treatment plan to minimize bleeding.

TABLE 15-52 ASA Classification of Patients with a History of a CVA

The patient with no or very minor residual neurological effects due to the CVA is an ASA II classification. The patient with significantly impaired speech or impaired mobility that requires assistance is an ASA III classification. The ASA IV post CVA patient will have significant residual mental effects and may be immobile due to the severity of the CVA. This patient may also suffer from significant **dysphagia** or **aphasia**.

Management of a Cerebrovascular Accident in the Dental Office

A CVA is a life threatening emergency and must be managed quickly and with accuracy. Rapid recognition of the signs and symptoms will allow appropriate management. Table 15-53 provides details regarding the signs and symptoms of an ischemic stroke and a hemorrhagic stroke. Table 15-54 provides the protocol for the management of a suspected CVA in the dental office setting.

TABLE 15-53 Signs and Symptoms of a Stroke

ischemic stroke	- Slow onset - **Hemiparalysis** or paralysis on one side of the body. Paralysis will occur on the contralateral side of the cerebral infarct. - aphasia and dysphagia - Loss of vision or double vision - **ataxia** - Headache and dizziness
hemorrhagic stroke	In addition to the signs and symptoms of an ischemic stroke, the patient experiencing a hemorrhagic stroke may exhibit the following: - Sudden onset - Headache - Vomiting - Loss of consciousness results in a poor prognosis

TABLE 15-54 Protocol for Management of a Suspected CVA in the Dental Office

- Terminate dental treatment and remove all objects from the patient's mouth.
- Palpate carotid artery to assess circulation.
- Ensure that the patient has a patent airway and is breathing. In most cases, the patient will be able to maintain an airway without assistance.
- Position the patient in Fowler's position or semi-upright to reduce pressure on the brain and aid in minimizing damage.
- Monitor vital signs and record every 5 minutes. This information can then be provided to EMS. Keeping the patient calm is important. Summon EMS so patient can be transported to a hospital.
- Oxygen may be administered to the patient.
- It is important to not administer any sedative agents or other central nervous system depressants. These will mask symptoms and make diagnosis more difficult for EMS and the hospital staff.
- If the patient loses consciousness, the CVA may be extensive and time becomes critical for the patient. In the event of loss of consciousness, place the patient supine and perform BLS as needed. Once the patient has been transported to the hospital, more definitive care will be administered.
- In the event that the patient is suffering from a TIA, the symptoms should subside. It is best not to continue treatment at this time. The patient should be sent to a physician for evaluation. Treatment should resume once patient has received medical care and after consult with the patient's treating physician.

Allergic Reactions

Certain people experience allergic reactions when they come in contact with a particular allergen. The allergen may be a food, bee sting, or medication. Some people may be sensitive to certain allergens whereas others are not. Exposure may occur through contact with the skin, inhalation, or ingestion of the allergen. The reaction may range from mild, such as a skin irritation, to life threatening such as anaphylaxis and anaphylactic shock. Allergies are more common in those who have a family history. In most cases, the first exposure to the antigen is the sensitizing dose. An allergic reaction will normally not occur on initial exposure. The second exposure to the antigen, now known as an allergen, will result in an allergic reaction in a sensitized patient. The second dose is also known as the challenge dose

Most adverse reactions, such as an overdose to an agent, need a minimum dose. However, for an allergic reaction to occur no minimum dosage is required; exposure to the tiniest amount of the allergen may trigger a reaction in those who have been sensitized. This section will discuss the physiological aspect of an allergic reaction, types of allergic reactions that may occur, and management of allergic reaction.

Physiology of an Allergic Reaction

The immune system is highly complex and designed to protect us from the millions of microorganisms and other invaders we face every day. However, that protective mechanism can become life threatening if the body's immune system responds to an invader through a heightened allergic response.

Regardless of the severity of the allergic reaction, the underlying chemical and physiological aspects are very similar. The body has a variety of defense mechanisms that prevent the entry of an antigen. Table 15-55 summarizes the different mechanisms the body uses to defend itself against a potential antigen or allergen.

The antibodies are constantly circulating in the blood and lymph fluid. This system is critical in protecting the body against invaders that have managed to bypass the initial defenses. However, the activation of this system also causes the allergic reaction, which, at times, can be life threatening. As a result, allergic reactions do not occur on the exposure to the sensitizing dose; they occur on exposure to the challenge dose.

When a person is initially exposed to the sensitizing dose of the antigen, an antibody, specifically *Immunoglobulin E* (IgE), is produced. Each IgE is specific to a particular allergen. These antibody

TABLE 15-55 The Body's Defense Mechanisms Against a Potential Allergen/Antigen

First Line of Defense—Physical Barriers

- Skin is the largest barrier and prevents entry of a potential allergen and antigen.
- The tiny hairs that line the nasal passages that trap particles and prevent antigen entry into the airways.

Second Line of Defense—Cells and Chemical Barriers

- Interferons and other chemicals
- Phagocytes which activate to engulf and destroy the allergen/antigen

Third Line of Defense—Immune System Cells with Memory Which Are Formed by the Bone Marrow, Spleen, and Thymus

- B lymphocytes produce antibodies specific to the antigen/allergen
- T lymphocyte destroy the antigen once it has been identified by the antibody
- Macrophages which will "clean up" the remains of the antigen destroyed due to the specific immune response

molecules then travel to mast cells, which are found mostly in the nose, the gastrointestinal (GI) tract, eyes, lungs, and blood vessels. Once they arrive at the mast cell, they attach. Upon second exposure to the allergen, IgE becomes active. This results in degranulation of the mast cells, which then release their contents, causing other chemical mediators to arrive at the site of the mast cells. This cascade of events leads to an allergic reaction.

The main chemical released by the mast cell degranulation is histamine. The release of histamine results in several physiological effects that can range from mild to severe and life threatening. Table 15-56 summarizes the progressing physiological effects of an allergic reaction from mild to moderate to severe.

Mild allergic reactions are usually self-limiting or may be managed with histamine blockers. Severe allergic reactions require aggressive intervention to reverse the laryngeal edema and hypotension.

Common Dental Allergens

Though we are exposed to many potential allergens every day, the dental practitioner utilizes certain substances that have significant potential to be allergenic. Some patients, who may be hypersensitive to these substances, may suffer from an allergic reaction in the dental office that can range from mild to severe. Table 15-57 summarizes common dental allergens.

Medical History and Prevention of an Allergic Reaction

A thorough medical history will aid the dental professional in identification of the patient with allergies, thus avoiding a potential emergency. It is also important to remember that just because a patient never had a reaction to a potential allergen in the past does not mean that an allergic reaction may not develop in the future. Evidence demonstrates that repeated exposure to an antigen can result in an allergic reaction even with no previous history of a reaction. Additionally, those with allergies to multiple substances are more likely to have a reaction to a substance utilized or administered in the dental office. Table 15-58 provides the medical history questions that should be asked regarding previous allergic reactions.

Management of an Allergic Reaction in the Dental Office

Allergic reactions are managed based on clinical manifestations. If a patient exhibits signs of an allergic reaction while in the dental office, treatment should be terminated and the potential cause of

TABLE 15-56 Progression of Severity of Physiological Effects of an Allergic Reaction

mild	Localized skin reactions such as erythema, urticaria, **pruritus**, and edema
moderate	**Rhinitis** and **conjunctivitis** with possibly generalized erythema, urticaria, pruritus, and edema
severe	Dyspnea and abdominal cramping as well as rhinitis and conjunctivitis with generalized erythema, urticaria, pruritus, and edema
anaphylaxis	All of the above plus laryngeal edema and hypotension which may lead to death if not reversed

TABLE 15-57 Common Dental Allergens

local anesthetics	The most common reactions to local anesthetic administration are that psychogenic-fearful patients may undergo syncope due to the sight of the needle. Some patients may be allergic to bisulfites, which are antioxidants found in local anesthetic carpules containing epinephrine to prevent the oxidation of epinephrine and preserve the shelf life of the carpule. Bisulfites are also found in many commonly used products such as cosmetics and many foods. Patients who are allergic to bisulfites should not be administered a local anesthetic with epinephrine. One cannot be allergic to epinephrine as it is an **endogenous** substance. If a patient to claims to have a true allergy to all local anesthetics, it is important to investigate further prior to treating the patient. Question the patient regarding the experience. Some patients have palpitations from sensitivity to the epinephrine and believe this is an allergic reaction. If, upon questioning the patient, it is determined that a possible allergy to local anesthetics may exist, refer the patient to an allergy specialist for further testing and evaluation. The patient may be treated palliatively until a final determination is made.
antibiotics	Though any antibiotic has the potential to cause an allergic reaction, some are more allergenic than others. Penicillin antibiotics are well known for causing reactions in patients who have been sensitized. Patients who claim to have an allergy to penicillin should not be administered this particular antibiotic; a different appropriate antibiotic should be selected. All patients should be questioned carefully regarding allergy to penicillin and other antibiotics. Any positive responses should be noted in the chart. Patients with a history of allergy to penicillin may be prescribed erythromycin as an alternative.
analgesics	Analgesics, narcotic and non-narcotic, are another group of drugs commonly prescribed in the dental office for pain management. Patients with nasal **polyps** and asthma are more likely to suffer from sensitivity to aspirin than are those without. Those who are allergic to aspirin may also be allergic to nonsteroidal anti-inflammatory agents (NSAIDs) such as ibuprofen and naproxen. These patients should not be administered any aspirin or NSAID containing pain medications. The drug of choice for pain management for these patients should include acetaminophen. Codeine is a commonly prescribed narcotic agent for pain management in the dental office. Though allergy to codeine is uncommon, some patients may be sensitive to this medication. Codeine does have other adverse drug reactions such as constipation, nausea, and vomiting. Some patients confuse these with an allergy. In this case an alternative such as an NSAID may be prescribed.

(Continues)

TABLE 15-57 (Continued)

sedatives	Sedative agents may be utilized for patients who are anxious or who are unable to cooperate due to a disability, either mental or physical. Though sedative agents do not commonly cause allergic reactions, some patients may have sensitivity to a particular sedative agent. If it is necessary to use a sedative agent, one from a different group that the patient is not sensitive to may be selected for use.
latex	Prior to 1987, latex allergy had not been heard of. However, since then, the incidence of allergic reactions to natural rubber latex (NRL) has been on the rise. Latex is a material commonly found in the dental office. Nitrile, vinyl, and *neoprene* gloves are available as an alternative. Nasal hoods for sedation dentistry and dental dams are also available as a nonlatex alternative. Dental tubing can be purchased in a nonlatex form. and prophy cups are available also as a plastic rather than latex. The decrease in latex use has reduced the incidence of an allergic reaction for both the professional and the patient.

TABLE 15-58 Medical History Questions Pertaining to Allergic Reactions

Ask about known food and drug allergies. Asthmatics are more sensitive to aspirin and NSAIDs than are nonasthmatics. A history of asthma may be a relative contraindication to the use of aspirin and NSAIDs. Patients with multiple allergies to foods and medications are more likely to be sensitive to a substance administered in the dental office.

In the event a patient has a positive response regarding allergies, further questioning should take place regarding the type of reaction and its cause. Many patients are not aware that side effects such as stomach upset from pain medications or heart palpitations caused by epinephrine administration in a local anesthetic cartridge are not true allergic reactions. Some patients also may claim that they suffered from syncope during administration of a local anesthetic. This is a *psychogenic* reaction and not an allergic reaction. Such an event can be prevented by placing the patient supine during treatment. If the patient is unsure of the cause of the reaction and the events surrounding the possible allergic reaction, the clinician should contact the treating physician. Was the patient hospitalized for the reaction? Was the reaction localized. or was it systemic? Until a final determination can be made regarding the existence of an allergy, the patient should be treated as if they are allergic to the substance in question.

the reaction removed from the area if possible. If latex is the likely cause, the latex item should be removed. The patient should be able to maintain circulation, airway, and breathing during a mild allergic reaction. Most patients will be more comfortable in the upright position. Table 15-59 provides the protocol for management of an allergic reaction.

Airway Obstruction

In the dental office, the potential for a foreign body airway obstruction exists. For example, if a tooth is being extracted and slips from the instrument, it may lodge in the airway. Other items commonly used in dentistry such as restorative materials, cotton ro;ls, or gauze may also be lodged in the airway. In this case, the patient will usually give the universal sign of choking (Figure 15-18).

In the case of an obstructed airway, the Heimlich maneuver may be performed on the conscious patient. If the object does

not dislodge and the patient becomes unconscious, CPR and BLS should be initiated.

The Role of the Dental Assistant in Managing a Medical Emergency

Prevention of a medical emergency is key. The medical history plays a vital role in prevention. The dental assistant should review the medical history with every returning patient at each visit to ensure that there are no changes. The dental assistant should thoroughly review the medical history with every new patient. The dental assistant and all dental office staff should be up to date with basic life support at a minimum. The office should conduct regularly scheduled practice drills in managing an emergency should it occur. The well-prepared dental assistant should be ready and able to help in the event of a medical emergency.

TABLE 15-59 Management of an Allergic Reaction

- Delayed reactions that do not progress usually manifest initially as skin reactions, and diphenhydramine or chlorpheniramine may be administered. The patient should then be monitored for progression of signs and symptoms. Diphenhydramine may cause drowsiness, and the patient should not be allowed to drive home.
- In the event the symptoms are spreading but the airway is not involved, IM administration of diphenhydramine is recommended. The patient should also be provided with an oral antihistamine to be taken for 3 days to prevent recurrence of the allergic reaction. Patients should not be released until all symptoms have resolved. In the event that a patient calls the office after leaving, stating that an allergic reaction is occurring, request that the patient return to the dental office for management or to the nearest hospital.
- Allergic reactions that result in bronchospasm may also occur. In such a reaction, the clinical manifestations are limited to the bronchioles, and the reaction may not progress to an anaphylactic reaction. The clinical signs and symptoms are that of a nonallergic asthmatic reaction, and the reaction should be managed as such with the use of an inhaler.
- If the allergic reaction initiates as a skin reaction and progresses rapidly, and the airway becomes compromised due to laryngeal edema, the management must be aggressive to prevent an anaphylactic reaction. Circulation, airway, and breathing must be assessed and maintained by the clinician as necessary. Oxygen should be administered to the patient, and 0.3 ml of epinephrine 1:1000 should be administered IM. Epinephrine will counteract the effects of histamine, reversing the vasodilation and hypotension as well as the airway edema and bronchoconstriction. In this instance, EMS must be summoned. The patient will be transported to the hospital for further evaluation.

Heimlich Maneuver

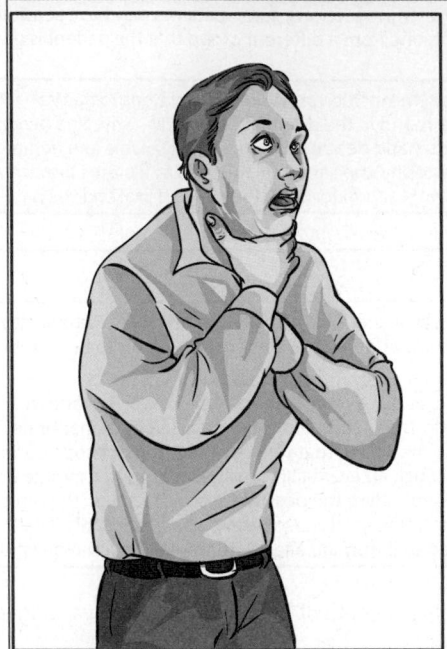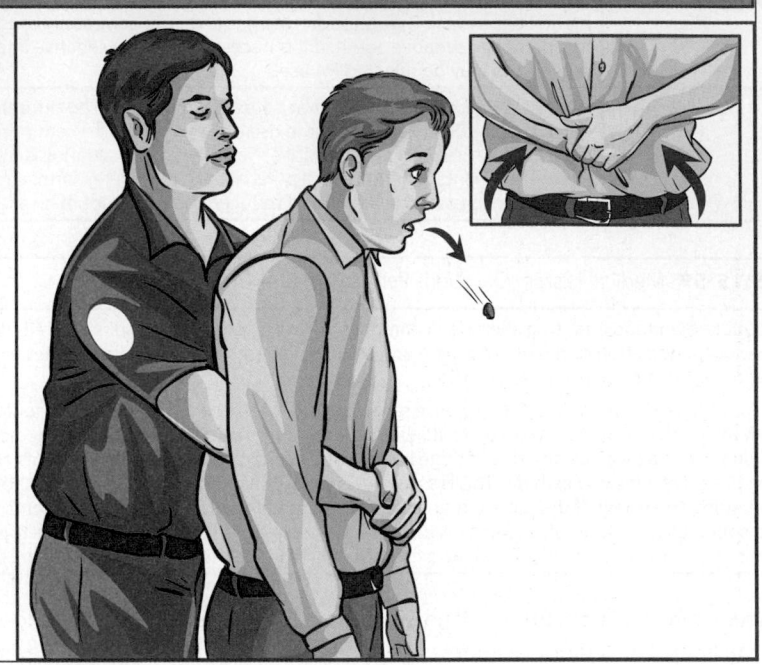

© Drp8/Shutterstock.com

FIGURE 15-18
Universal choking sign and Heimlich maneuver.

Chapter Summary

Even though the number of emergencies is not high in a dental office, the dental assistant must always observe the patient and be prepared to prevent and respond to emergencies. Emergencies may also happen to the dentist and to other dental auxiliaries. When an emergency arises, the dental team must react automatically. Any hesitation at such a time may cost a life. It is best if a routine is established so that everyone can ensure that everything is addressed. The assistant has a vital role in the prevention of emergencies and in emergency care. Maintaining a thorough medical history and patient observation at all times assists in the evaluation for prevention.

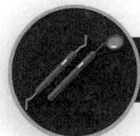 **CASE STUDY**

A 56 year-old female patient presents to the office for treatment. She has a history of Type I diabetes. She was rushing to her 9 AM appointment and did not have time to eat her usual breakfast. She did take her usual insulin medication. She is now in the dental chair, and you notice that the patient is conscious but becoming confused and is behaving strangely.

Case Study Review

1. What is this patient experiencing?
   a. Hyperglycemia
   b. Hypoglycemia
   c. Ketoacidosis
   d. None of these

2. How would you manage the patient to reverse the signs and symptoms the patient is experiencing?
 a. Provide orange juice.
 b. Provide diet cola.
 c. Provide water.
 d. Place the patient in supine position.

3. The patient now becomes unconscious. You place the dental chair in the supine position. What is your next course of action?
 a. Provide orange juice.
 b. Provide diet cola.
 c. Provide water.
 d. Place cake icing in the mucobuccal fold.

Review Questions

Multiple Choice

1. Which of the following is correct regarding the medical history that should be obtained from the patient?
 a. It is not necessary to include the medications the patient is taking in the medical history.
 b. Once the patient completes the medical history form, it is not necessary to verbally review it with the patient.
 c. Since the treatment in a dental office is only related to the teeth, it is not important to obtain an accurate medical history.
 d. The medical history form may include questions about past dental experiences to determine how the patient feels about dental treatment.

2. Normal respiration ranges from 60 to 100 breaths per minute.
 a. True
 b. False

3. Which of the following statements is correct regarding a fearful or anxious patient?
 a. A fearful or anxious patient will usually keep their scheduled appointments.
 b. A fearful or anxious patient will usually voice their anxiety to the dental practitioner.
 c. Fearful or anxious patients will have normal blood pressure and heart rate.
 d. Anxious patients may demonstrate "white knuckle syndrome."

4. Which of the following is not considered to be part of the stress reduction protocol?
 a. Premedication for anxiety if needed
 b. Late appointments so the patient can relax in the reception room
 c. Nitrous oxide sedation as needed
 d. Good pain control during and after the procedure

5. All dental office should have an updated CPR/BLS certification. It is not necessary for each dental office staff member to be assigned to a role in the event of a medical emergency.

Select the correct response below based on the statements above.
 a. Both statements are true.
 b. Both statements are false.
 c. The first statement is true; the second statement is false.
 d. The first statement is false; the second statement is true.

6. Which of the following is not considered to be part of the protocol for management of an episode of vasovagal syncope in the dental office?
 a. Assess circulation by palpating the radial artery.
 b. Place patient supine to ensure brain receives adequate circulation.
 c. Ensure a patent airway by using the head tilt, chin lift method.
 d. Crush an ammonia vaporole under the patient's nose.

7. Postural hypotension has prodromal signs and symptoms such as pale appearance and a feeling of nausea. Vasovagal syncope has a sudden onset, and there are no prodromal signs and symptoms.

Select the correct response below based on the statements above.
 a. Both statements are true.
 b. Both statements are false.
 c. The first statement is true; the second statement is false.
 d. The first statement is false; the second statement is true.

8. A patient who is recumbent for a long period of time such as during a long dental appointment may suffer from postural hypotension upon rising from the dental chair. The dental assistant should rapidly put the chair upright and allow the patient to rise quickly to avoid an episode of postural hypotension.

Select the correct response below based on the statements above.
 a. Both statements are true.
 b. Both statements are false.
 c. The first statement is true; the second statement is false.
 d. The first statement is false; the second statement is true.

9. Asthma is characterized by constriction of the bronchioles. Patients who suffer from asthma exhibit a wheezing sound on exhalation.

Select the correct response below based on the statements above.
 a. Both statements are true.
 b. Both statements are false.
 c. The first statement is true; the second statement is false.
 d. The first statement is false; the second statement is true.

10. Which of the following is part of the management protocol for hyperventilation?
    a. Request patient to place cupped hands over the nose and mouth and breathe.
    b. Administer a bronchodilator.
    c. Administer oxygen.
    d. Place the patient in the supine position.

11. What is the main cause of death in an acute adrenal crisis?
    a. hypotension
    b. vomiting
    c. diarrhea
    d. lower back pain

12. The thyroid gland sits in the posterior portion of the neck *and* is composed of two lobes separate by a band of tissues known as an isthmus.

    Select the correct response below based on the statements above.
    a. Both statements are true.
    b. Both statements are false.
    c. The first statement is true; the second statement is false.
    d. The first statement is false; the second statement is true.

13. Which of the following statements is correct regarding hyperthyroidism?
    a. Undiagnosed hyperthyroid patients are sensitive to cold.
    b. Undiagnosed hyperthyroid patients may experience weight gain.
    c. In hyperthyroidism the thyroid gland produces insufficient thyroid hormones.
    d. Grave's disorder is the most common cause of hyperthyroidism.

14. Thyroid storm is the acute emergency related to hypothyroidism. Thyroid storm is managed in the hospital by administration of medications that will stop the production and release of thyroid hormones.

    Select the correct response below based on the statements above.
    a. Both statements are true.
    b. Both statements are false.
    c. The first statement is true; the second statement is false.
    d. The first statement is false; the second statement is true.

15. Type II diabetics do not produce any insulin, which leads to a rise in blood glucose levels. The breakdown of fats for fuel results in ketoacidosis in Type II diabetics.

    Select the correct response below based on the statements above.
    a. Both statements are true.
    b. Both statements are false.
    c. The first statement is true; the second statement is false.
    d. The first statement is false; the second statement is true.

16. Which of the following is the most common acute complication of diabetes?
    a. hyperglycemia
    b. ketoacidosis
    c. hypoglycemia
    d. nephropathy

17. Which of the following is not correct regarding angina?
    a. Patient who have had a myocardial infarction in the past may suffer from angina.
    b. The patient with angina should be questioned about the intensity and duration of the angina attack.
    c. Since nitroglycerine is in the dental office emergency kit, the patient does not need to bring their own nitroglycerine with them to the dental office.
    d. Implementation of stress reduction protocol is important for the patient with a history of angina.

18. The 11 AM patient is a 55-year-old overweight male with a history of angina. The patient brings his nitroglycerine with him, and you place it on the work area in the treatment room for easy access in case it is necessary. During treatment, the patient starts to experience a squeezing pain in his chest. You and the dentist stop treatment and position the chair upright. The patient states that what he is feeling is his usual angina pain. The best way to manage this patient would be to:
    a. Leave him alone and let the angina pain subside.
    b. Call EMS immediately.
    c. Provide him with a sugar source.
    d. Provide him with his nitroglycerine.

19. Which of the following is not a step in the management of a myocardial infarction in the dental office?
    a. Keep the patient calm to minimize strain on heart.
    b. Administer nitrous oxide for pain management.
    c. Administer oxygen.
    d. Administer 325 milligrams acetaminophen to chew and swallow.

20. Sudden cardiac arrest is when the heart begins to fail as a pump, resulting in lack of blood flow to the brain and other vital organs. If this is not reversed quickly, death will result.

    Select the correct response below based on the statements above.
    a. Both statements are true.
    b. Both statements are false.
    c. The first statement is true; the second statement is false.
    d. The first statement is false; the second statement is true.

Critical Thinking

1. A 62-year-old female patient with a history of chronic obstructive pulmonary disease (COPD) presents to the office for routine preventive care. As the dental assistant, identify what your role is in the management of this patient and the patient's COPD.

2. What is the difference between Cushing's syndrome and Addison's disease?

3. How can the Rule of Twos help identify a patient with an adrenal disorder?

Key Terms

Term and Pronunciation	Meaning of Root and Word Parts	Definition
adrenal insufficiency (Addison's disease) (*uh*-**dreen**-l) (in-*suh*-**fish**-*uh* n-see)	**adren** = endocrine gland that produces steroidal hormones, epinephrine and norepinephrine **-al** = pertaining to **in-** = without **sufficient** = enough **-cy** = indicating quality	diminished activity of the adrenal glands; also known as Addison's disease
alkalosis (al-*kuh*-**loh**-sis)	**alkali** = various bases, neutralize acids **-osis** = condition	an abnormal condition of increased alkalinity of the blood and tissues compared to normal health
anaphylactic (an-*uh-fuh*-**lak**-sis)	**ana** = against **prohylaxis** = prevention of or protective treatment for disease **-ic** = characterized by	a life threatening severe allergic reaction and state of shock
anaphylactic shock (an-*uh-fuh*-**lak**-tik)	**anaphylaxis** = hypersensitivity induced by preliminary exposure to a substance **-ic** = relating to **shock** = a state of profound depression of the vital processes of the body	a severe and sometimes fatal allergic reaction to second exposure; rapid swelling, acute respiratory distress, and collapse of circulation, fainting, itching, and hives
anaphylaxis (an-*uh-fuh*-**lak**-sis)	**anaphylaxis** = hypersensitivity induced by preliminary exposure to a substance	hypersensitivity (as to foreign proteins or drugs) resulting from sensitization following prior contact with the causative agent
aneurysm (**an**-yuh-riz-*uh* m)	**aneurysm** = a sac formed by abnormal dilation of the weakened wall of a blood vessel	weakening of the wall of an artery leading to a bulging and possible rupture
antecubital fossa (**an**-tee **kyoo**-bi-tl **fos**-*uh*)	**ante** = before, in front of **cubutus** = elbow **fossa** = depression	depression in front of the elbow
anticoagulant (an-tee-koh-**ag**-*yuh*-*luh*nt)	**anti-** = against **coagulate** = change from the liquid state to a solid or gel; clot **-ant** = agent	agent that prevents blood clotting
antigen (**an**-ti-j*uh*n)	**anti-** = against **body** = physical structure **gen** = that which produces	substances(toxins, bacteria, viruses, and other foreign substances and the cells of transplanted organs) that stimulate the production of antibodies
aphasia (*uh*-**fey**-zh*uh*)	**a-** = loss of **-phasia** = speech disorder	loss of speech
ataxia (*uh*-**tak**-see-*uh*)	**ataxia** = an inability to coordinate voluntary muscular movements	uncoordinated walk
atherosclerotic plaque (ath-*uh*-roh-skl*uh*-**roh**-sis) (plak)	**atheroma** = yellowish fatty and cellular material; in and beneath inner lining of the arterial walls **sclerosis** = a hardening of a tissue or cell wall by thickening **plaque** = abnormal patch, film	deposition on the arterial walls of fat and lipid, resulting in a narrowing of the blood vessels
bradycardia (brad-i-**kahr**-dee-*uh*)	**brady** = slow **card** = heart **-ia** = condition	slow heart rate, usually less than 60 beats per minute.
cataracts (**kat**-*uh*-rakts)	**cataract** = an abnormality of the eye, opacity of the lens, causing impairment of vision or blindness	cloudiness in the lens of the eye
cerebrovascular accident (se-ree-broh-**vas**-ky*uh*-ler) (**ak**-si-d*uh* nt)	**cerebro** = affecting the cerebrum; anterior and largest position of the brain; controls voluntary movements and coordinates mental activity **vascular** = pertaining to vessels **accident** = unexpected bodily event	a sudden, nonconvulsive loss of neurologic function caused by ischemia or a hemorrhagic vascular event in the brain; also known a stroke
chronic (**kron**-ik)	**chronic** = marked by long duration, frequent recurrence over a long time, often by slowly progressing seriousness	long term as in a disease
coma (**koh**-m*uh*)	**coma** = profound unconsciousness caused by disease, injury, or poison	deep sleep with unresponsiveness

(Continues)

Term and Pronunciation	Meaning of Root and Word Parts	Definition
conjunctivitis (ku*h*n-juhngk-t*uh*-**vahy**-tis)	**conjunctiva** = mucous membrane lining inner eyelid and exposed surface of eyeball **-itis** = inflammation	inflammation of lining of inner eyelid, may be caused by infection or allergy
cricothyrotomy (**krahy**-koid- **thahy**-roid-**ot**-t*uh*-mee)	**cricoid** = cartilage at lower part of larynx **thyroid** = largest cartilage of the larynx, Adams's apple **-tomy** = cutting, incision	an emergency procedure in which an incision is made between the cricoid cartilage and the thyroid cartilage to maintain a patent airway
diabetes mellitus (dahy-*uh*-**bee**-tis) (**mel**-i-t*uh* s)	**diabetes** = any of several disorders characterized by increased urine production **mellitus** = a disorder of carbohydrate metabolism, characterized by inadequate production or utilization of insulin	metabolic disorder of elevated blood glucose, signs and symptoms include excess urination, thirst, and hunger
diaphoresis (dahy-*uh*-fuh-**re-sis**)	**diaphoresis** = technical term for sweating **-tic** = having characteristics of	producing perspiration; increasing perspiration
diastolic (dahy-*uh*-**stol**-ik)	**diastole** = the passive rhythmical expansion or dilation of the cavities of the heart as they fill with blood **-ic** = pertaining to	post-systolic relaxation of the heart, particularly referring to the ventricles.
distended jugular veins (dih-**sten**-did) (**juhg**-y*uh*-ler) (veyns)	**distended** = enlarged or stretched out **jugular** = relating to the throat or neck **veins** = vessels that carry blood from the capillaries toward the heart	enlarged jugular veins
dysphagia (dis-**fey**-j*uh*)	**dys** = bad, difficulty **-phagia** = swallowing	difficulty swallowing
electrolytes (ih-**lek**-tr*uh*-lahyt)	**electro** = conducting electrical currents; major force in controlling fluid balance within the body **lyte** = used in forming compound words; denotes something subjected to a certain process	ions such as sodium, potassium, or calcium which are necessary for body functions
embolus (**em**-b*uh*-l*uh* s)	**embolus** = a mass (an air bubble, a detached blood clot, or a foreign body) circulating in the blood	blood clot that detaches and travels from a larger vessel to a smaller one, resulting in occlusion of the smaller vessel
engulf (en-**guhlf**)	**engulf** = to swallow up	special cells that infold around foreign particle and swallow it up; important bodily defense against infection
erectile dysfunction (ih-**rek**-tl) (dis-**fuhngk**-sh*uh* n)	**erectile** = tissue capable of filling with blood and becoming rigid **dys-** = bad, abnormal, faulty **function** = to perform a specified action	unable to maintain a penile erection, impotence
exophthalmos (ek-sof-**thal**-m*uh* s)	**ex-** = beyond, from **ophthalm** = eye	bulging of eyes from the socket; most common cause is Grave's disease
febrile (**fee**-br*uh* l)	**febr-** = fever **-ile** = marked or caused by	related to fever
glaucoma (glaw-**koh**-m*uh*)	**glaucoma** =a disease of eye; increased pressure within the eyeball, can result in damage to the optic disk and gradual loss of vision	disease of the eye related to high pressure of intraocular fluid
Hashimoto's thyroiditis (hahsh-ee-**moe**-toe) (thahy-roi-**dahy**-tis)	**Hashimoto** = physician **thyroid** = thyroid gland **-itis** = inflammation	autoimmune disorder which results in destruction of the thyroid gland
hemiparalysis (hem-ee-p*uh*-**ral**-*uh*-sis)	**hemi-** = half **paralysis** = a loss or impairment of voluntary movement in a body part	paralysis on one side of the body; can occur due to a stroke
hyperpyrexia (hahy-per-pahy-**rek**-see-*uh*)	**hyper** = excessive **pyrex** = fever **-ia** = condition	elevated body temperature
hypocarbia (**hahy**-poh-**kahr**-bee*uh*)	**hypo** = reduced **carb** = carbon dioxide **-ia** = condition	**state of reduced** carbon dioxide **in the** blood **resulting from deep or rapid breathing, known as** hyperventilation
hypotension (hahy-p*uh*-**ten**-sh*uh* n)	**hypo** = less than normal **tension** = pressure, being stretched	low blood pressure

Term and Pronunciation	Meaning of Root and Word Parts	Definition
hypothermia (hahy-p*uh*-**thur**-mee-*uh*)	**hypo** = subnormal **therm** = temperature **-ia** = condition	low body temperature
hypothyroidism (hahy-p*uh*-**thahy**-roi-diz-*uh* m)	**hypo** = less than normal **thyroid** = endocrine gland that regulates growth and metabolism **-ism** = describing condition	a disorder in which there is a decreased secretion of hormones from the thyroid gland; causing a slowing of metabolism causing myxedema; in infants and young children, the result is cretinism; the leading to developmental abnormalities
hypovolemia (hahy-p*uh*-**vol**-**nee**-mee-*uh*)	**hypo** = abnormally low **vol** = volume **-emia** = condition of the blood	low volume of circulating blood in the body
infarct (**in**-fahrkt)	**infarct** = a localized area of dead tissue; from obstruction of the blood supply to that part	tissues that undergo necrosis due to lack of blood supply
insulin (**in**-*suh*-lin)	**insulin** = hormone, secreted in the pancreas by the islets of Langerhans, controls glucose in the blood	hormone secreted by the islets of Langerhans in the pancreas to regulates carbohydrate metabolism
interferons (in-ter-**feer**-ons)	**interferon** = protein produced by cells after they have been exposed to a virus	proteins produced by cells in response to a virus to block viral replication
microangiopathy (mahy-kroh-an-jee-**op**-*uh*-thee)	**micro** = small **angio** = blood vessels **pathy** = disease	disease which affects the small blood vessels of the body; may occur in a diabetic patient
nasopharyngeal (ney-zoh-f*uh*-**rin**-jee-*uh* l)	**naso** = nose **pharynx** = throat, cavity connecting mouth and nasal passages to esophagus **-al** = pertaining to	referring to the nasal cavity and the portion of pharynx posterior to the nasal cavity
nephropathy (nuh-**frop**-*uh*-thee)	**nephro** = kidney **-pathy** = disease	kidney damage, may occur in a diabetic
neuropathy (noo-**rop**-*uh*-thee)	**neuro** =nerve **-pathy** = disease	damage to the peripheral nerves, may occur in a diabetic
nocturia (**nok**t- **yoo r**-ee*uh*)	**nocturn** = during the night **urine** = waste matter excreted by the kidneys **-ia** = abnormal condition	frequent urination at night
oropharyngeal (awr-oh-f*uh*-**rin**-jee-*uh* l)	**or** = mouth **pharynx** = throat, cavity connecting below soft palate to epiglottis **-al** = pertaining to	related to the mouth and the pharyngeal area
palliative (**pal**-ee-ey-tiv)	**palliate** = to relieve or lesson without curing **-ive** = pertaining to	relieving symptoms of a disease or disorder without offering a cure
perioral (pe-**Ree**- **ohr**-*uh* l)	**peri-** = around, surrounding **or** = mouth **-al** = relating to or involving	area around the oral cavity
peripheral pitting edema (p*uh*-**rif**-er-*uh* l) (**pit**-ing) (ih-**dee**-m*uh*)	**periphery** = outermost part or region within a precise boundary **-al** = pertaining to **pitting** = making hollows or indentations especially in a surface of an organism **edema** = swelling from accumulation of excessive amount of watery fluid in cells, tissues, or serous cavities	abnormal accumulation of fluid in the intercellular spaces resulting in fluid build-up in the periphery; results in an indentation on the skin when pressed
phagocytes (**fag**-*uh*-sahyts)	**phago** = eating, destroying **cyte** = cell	cell that engulfs and destroys invaders such as bacteria and viruses
phenylephrine (fen-l-**ef**-reen)	**phenyl** = derived from benzene; used in manufacturing of pharmaceuticals **ephrine** = epinephrine, vasoconstrictor	adrenergic vasoconstrictor
polydipsia (pol-ee-**dip**-see-*uh*)	**poly** = excessive **dips** = thirst **-ia** = disease, abnormal condition	excess thirst, one of the symptoms of a diabetic
polyp (**pol**-ips)	**polyp** = projecting mass of swollen mucous membrane; hypertrophied or tumorous	growth protruding from a mucous membrane

(Continues)

Term and Pronunciation	Meaning of Root and Word Parts	Definition
polyphagia (pol-ee-**fey**-jee-*uh*)	**poly** = excessive **phag** = eating, feeding on **-ia** = disease, abnormal condition	excess hunger, one of the symptoms of a diabetic
polyuria (pol-ee-**yoo r**-ee-*uh*)	**poly** = excessive **urine** = waste matter excreted by kidneys **-ia** = disease, abnormal condition	excess urination, one of the symptoms of a diabetic
postictal (pohst-**ik**-t*uh*l)	**post** = following, after; a seizure **ictus** = sudden stroke or seizure **-al** = pertaining to	time period following a seizure
prodromal (**proh**-drohm-*uh*l)	**prodrome** = any symptom that signals the impending onset of a disease **-al** = pertaining to	signs or symptoms that mark the onset of a disease
pruritus (proo-**rahy**-t*uh* s)	**pruritus** = intense sensation of itching	itching of the skin
recumbent (ri-**kuhm**-b*uh* nt)	**recumbent** = lying down	reclining or supine position
retinopathy (ret-n-**op**-*uh*-thee)	**retina** = membrane lining inner eye; contains the rods and cones **-pathy** = disease	disease of the retina of the eye that may lead to blindness
rhinitis (rahy-**nahy**-tis)	**rhin-** = nose **-itis** = inflammation	inflammation of the mucous membrane of the nose
scalpel (**skal**-p*uh* l)	**scalpel** = small, light knife used in surgery	knife or surgical instrument
sputum (**spyoo**-t*uh* m)	**sputum** = matter, as saliva mixed with mucus or pus, expectorated from the lungs and respiratory passages	substance coughed up from the airway via the oral cavity
stable angina (**stey**-b*uh* l)(an-**jahy**-n*uh*)	**stable** = able or likely to continue or last **angina** = any attack of painful spasms characterized by sensations of choking or suffocating	a sudden intense chest pain caused by a temporary decrease in oxygenated blood to the heart muscle; patient is usually aware of causes, intensity, and duration of attack
supine (soo-**pahyn**)	**supine** = lying on back face upward	reclined position with knees and nose in the same plane
syncope (**sing**-k*uh*-pee)	**syncope** = faint, loss of consciousness resulting from insufficient blood flow to the brain	loss of consciousness
syringe (s*uh*-**rinj**)	**syringe** = an instrument for injection of medicine or withdrawal of bodily fluids; consists of a hollow barrel fitted with a plunger and a hollow needle	instrument used to withdraw liquid from the body or inject a liquid into it
systolic (si-**stol**-ik)	**systole** = of blood pressure; the maximum arterial pressure occurring during contraction of the left ventricle of the heart **-ic** = pertaining to	contraction of the heart, particularly the ventricles
tachycardia (tak-i-**kahr**-dee-*uh*)	**tachy** = rapid, accelerated **card** = heart **-ia** = condition	rapid heart rate, usually greater than 100 beats per minute
thrombus (**throm**-b*uh* s)	**thrombus** = a clot of blood formed within a blood vessel and remaining attached to its place of origin	blood clot in a vessel that leads to occlusion
tourniquet (**tur**-ni-kit)	**tourniquet** = any device for arresting bleeding by forcibly compressing a blood vessel	a tight band used to control bleeding from a large artery
unstable angina (uhn-**stey**-b*uh* l) (an-**jahy**-n*uh*)	**un** = not **stable** = able or likely to continue or last **angina** = any attack of painful spasms characterized by sensations of choking or suffocating	a sudden intense chest pain caused by a temporary decrease in oxygenated blood to the heart muscle; patient is usually aware of causes, intensity, and duration of attack
warfarin (**wawr**-f*uh*-rin)	**warfarin** = a crystalline anticoagulant, preparation used in management of potential or existing clotting disorders	drug which reduces the risk of a blood clot
wheezing (**weez**-ng)	**wheeze** = a wheezing breath or sound **-ing** = expressing action	high pitched sound that occurs usually on exhaling; occurs due to constricted airways such as in asthma

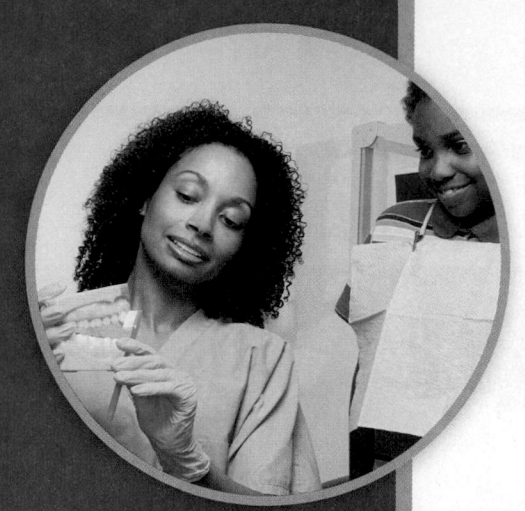

## CHAPTER 16

Oral Health and Preventive Techniques

SECTION IV
Prevention and Nutrition

Specific Instructional Objectives

At the completion of this chapter, you will be able to meet these objectives:

1. Use terms presented in this chapter.
2. Explain how biofilm affects the tooth, gingiva, and periodontium.
3. Describe strategies that are part of a good prevention plan.
4. Identify oral hygiene tips that will aid each age group.
5. Order activities for good oral self-care practice.
6. Provide guidance in selection of the ideal toothbrush.
7. Explain special considerations for the use of a toothbrush.
8. Demonstrate tooth brushing techniques.
9. Describe the purpose of the ingredients contained within most dentifrices.
10. Recommend different types of dental floss based on oral findings.
11. Demonstrate proper dental flossing.
12. Evaluate oral self-care using disclosing agents and biofilm indices.
13. Compare oral hygiene aids and their uses.
14. Describe fluoride and its use in good self-care.
15. Discuss benefits and mechanism of systemic and topical fluoride.
16. Select oral hygiene aids for patients with prosthetic appliances.
17. Compare the design of products to assist patients with disabilities to perform oral self-care effectively.
18. Describe the mission of dental public health.

Introduction

Dentistry is more than filling teeth; it is about preventing dental disease. Dental assistants have an important role in preventive dentistry by educating the public on how to prevent disease and achieve optimal oral health. They must be knowledgeable about the many products available that aid patients in maintaining their teeth and gums, be a good listener, and evaluate the needs of patients. Dental assistants must be able to motivate patients of all ages and oral conditions. To be effective in preventive dentistry, the dental assistant needs to be a model of good oral hygiene. The first step is for the assistant to care for their own teeth properly, practice good nutrition, and have a fresh, clean smile.

Dental Disease

There are two types of dental disease, dental caries and periodontal disease, that are directly affected by oral hygiene. Periodontal disease affects the gingiva and the periodontium. Dental disease is the result of many factors, including the bacteria that live in the mouth, the diet, and the patient's susceptibility to disease. Lifestyle choices such as smoking and the patient's ability to perform oral self-care are also important. When a person has dental disease, they may be unable to chew and speak.

Soft and Hard Deposits

There are soft and hard deposits that build up in the mouth. The acquired pellicle, biofilm (Figure 16-1), supra (above) and sub (below) gingival calculus (Figure 16-2), and materia alba all cause or contribute to dental disease. The acquired pellicle, or dental pellicle, is a clear protein film that forms from saliva and attaches on all surfaces of teeth within seconds after brushing. This is the first step in biofilm formation. These deposits are summarized in Table 16-1.

Biofilm hides between teeth and under the gum line and is one of the major causes of dental caries and periodontal disease. It is a mass of bacteria that grows on surfaces of pellicle within the mouth. Initial biofilm formation takes as long as 2 hours. It is an invisible, sticky, and colorless deposit at first and becomes a pale yellow color as it grows into colonies. The bacteria in the biofilm when fed by the sugar in food produce acids that attack the teeth and gingiva. The acids cause a demineralization, in which minerals, calcium, and phosphate are lost from the enamel surface. Demineralization appears as a whitish area on the tooth (Figure 16-3). The dentist may decide to watch this area and hope that, with special care, remineralization may occur in the patient's tooth or may

Dental Decay (Caries) Equation
Sugar + biofilm = acid + tooth = dental caries

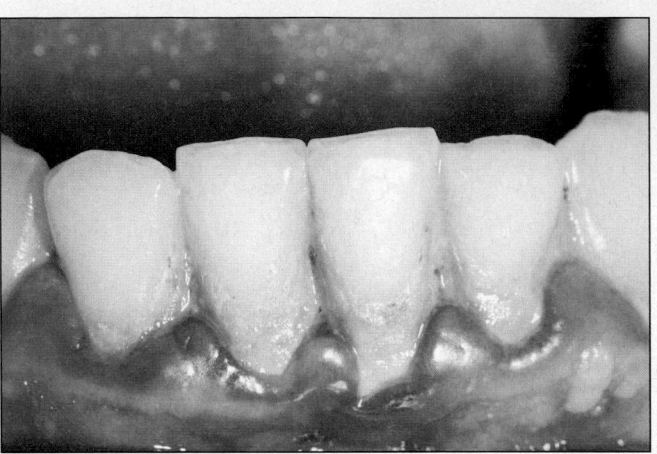

FIGURE 16-1
Biofilm.

consider the area as incipient decay and elect to restore the tooth before it becomes carious.

If biofilm is not removed within 24 to 72 hours, minerals are deposited into the biofilm and it hardens into calculus. Calculus is strongly bonded to the teeth and can only be removed by a dental professional. Approximately 68% of adults have calculus. When calculus is not removed it may cause receding gum and bone loss, which are symptoms of periodontal disease. Materia alba is a white cheese-like accumulation of biofilm, food debris, tissue cells, and blood cells deposited around the teeth at the gum line.

TABLE 16-1 Soft and Hard Deposits

Era	Events
acquired pellicle	Clear, sticky substance that adheres to teeth, restorations and calculus. It is made from mucus and proteins from saliva and its purpose to provide protection against acids. Immediately after cleaning, the pellicle begins to reform.
biofilm	Within 1-hour colonies of bacteria attach to the pellicle above and below the gumline. Biofilm is only visible with the use of staining or disclosing agents. As the biofilm ages, (7-14 days) the bacteria increase and become more harmful causing caries and periodontal disease. Specific bacteria in biofilm quickly metabolizes acid from the fermentable carbohydrates (sugar) eaten by an individual. The acid formed by the biofilm dissolves the calcium and phosphate minerals in tooth enamel and dentin causing caries. The frequency of intake of sugary foods has a strong effect on how much acid is produced. Other bacteria in biofilm cause gingival inflammation, infection and eventually lead to destruction of the periodontal supporting tissues. Biofilm can only be mechanically removed with brushing and flossing.
calculus	Calculus (tartar) is biofilm that has been mineralized (become hard) by calcium and phosphate from the saliva. Mineralization occurs within 24 to 72 hours. Calculus has a rough surface that allows biofilm to easily attach. Each layer of biofilm then becomes hard and can only be removed with instruments by a dental professional. The bacteria in calculus above the gumline (supra gingival) and below the gumline (subgingival) contributes to periodontal inflammation and disease.
materia alba	Loose deposit of bacteria, cellular debris, salivary products and broken down food debris. Materia alba sticks to the teeth, appears white to yellow in color and is easily visible (has a cottage cheese appearance). The bacteria within material alba contribute to gingival inflammation and demineralization of tooth structure. Materia alba is easily removed with water spray or irrigation.

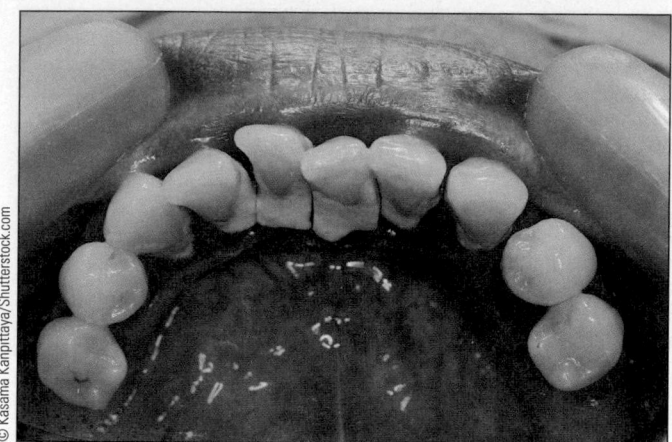

FIGURE 16-2
Super and subgingival calculus.

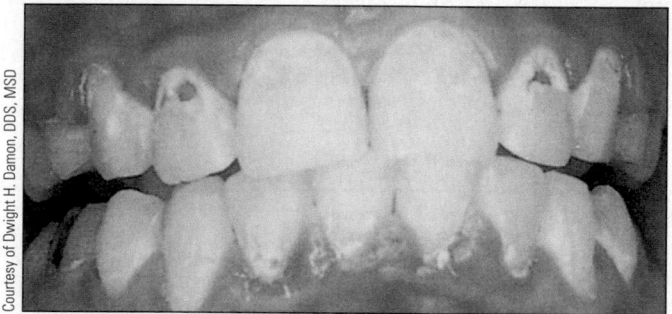

FIGURE 16-3
Demineralization of the tooth enamel appears as a white chalky area.

Preventive Dentistry

The goal of any dental prevention care plan is to maintain a healthy mouth, preserve oral function, and avoid pain and possible expensive dental treatment. It is important to first access the needs and ability of each patient, and design a prevention plan including education and monitoring.

Regular dental visits with examination, radiographs, **oral prophylaxis**, and oral self-care instruction are critical parts of a good prevention plan. Other strategies include fluoride, **dental sealants**, diet counseling to reduce the use of fermentable carbohydrates, and antimicrobial mouth rinses to reduce or eliminate harmful bacteria. Habits such as tobacco use (smoking and chewing) are harmful to the oral environment. If a patient uses tobacco, **cessation** should be part of the prevention plan.

Patient Motivation

Preventing dental disease is ultimately the responsibility of the patient, but dental auxiliaries spend a great deal of time educating and motivating patients to care for their teeth and oral cavities. The first aspect of patient motivation is for the dental assistant to assess oral hygiene and to listen to the patient. Listening to the patient gives insight into the patient's attitude toward oral hygiene and allows the assistant to get a better idea

how to communicate with, and motivate, the patient. It is best to work with patients to help them recognize their dental problems and develop solutions, and then provide motivation and help them set oral hygiene goals.

Age Characteristics

Each patient should be treated as an individual, taking into consideration the patient's age, oral hygiene knowledge, skills, attitude, and any special considerations (Figure 16-4). Different age groups have characteristics that are normally identifiable; however, these characteristics are not absolute. A few general characteristics pertaining to each age group are discussed in Table 16-2.

Home Care

Patients are ultimately responsible for caring for their oral health at home. The dental assistant can suggest ideas that will make this task simpler while still having every section of every tooth cleaned every day. The dental assistant's goals should closely resemble the ideas that stimulated the patient's desire to meet these goals. These ideas, of course, will differ for each patient. If what patients have been doing is working, and they are not developing periodontal disease or dental decay, then acknowledge that they are doing a good job and encourage them to keep it up.

If a patient is missing areas, the dental assistant should help them modify their technique. Patients should be made aware that the gingival tissue may be sore and may bleed when they first start a vigorous oral hygiene program. This means that the tissues are not healthy, but they will improve over time. It is much like the rest of the body. For instance, if a body is out of shape and an exercise program including sit-ups is started, the abdominal area will be sore for a week or so until the area is in shape. The same is true for gingival tissue. In about a week, the tissue will firm up and become healthier if the patient maintains the program. Patients should be

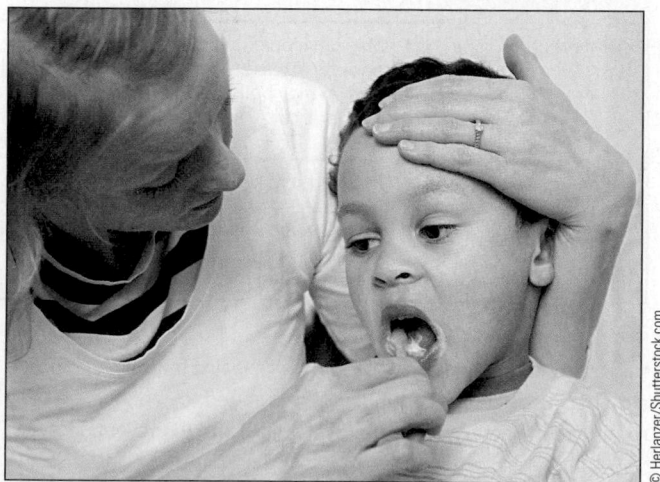

FIGURE 16-4
Parent brushing her child's teeth. Instruct mother to sit behind her child to be in the same position as when brushing their own teeth. Have mother support their child's head with their non-dominant hand.

TABLE 16-2 Tailoring Preventive Care to Age

Age Range	Characteristics	Needs	Teaching
Infants (birth to one year)	• Unable to care for teeth on their own	• Must be accomplished by parent or guardian • Needs to be a positive experience • Make it fun	• Positioning child in arms or sitting in chair • How to hold hand and use washcloths or infant tooth brushes (see Figure 16-4)
Preschool (one year to four years)	• Lacks highly developed motor skills • Attention span of about 5 minutes • Unable to read • Loves to imitate parents	• Use visual aids (fun toothbrush or puppet) • First appointment with dentist around the age of one • Should be positive and pleasant • Still need parental assistance	• Use "Mr. Air" to blow "wind" on the tooth • Use "Mr. Water" to give the child a drink • Count the "upstairs" and "downstairs" teeth • Demonstrate use of the toothbrush to "tickle" the teeth • At home, sit and watch TV or listen to a story while brushing teeth • Have parents role play • Must get a thorough monitored brushing at least once a day (at bedtime) but twice a day is best • Try to floss between molars once per day
Five through eight years	• Attention span increases to 10 to 15 minutes • Learning to read • Expanding vocabulary • Likes to please adults and enjoys learning • Loves facts • Requires constant guidance • Dexterity is improving	• Use positive reinforcement • Make it fun and entertaining	• Teach better brushing techniques • Teach how to floss • Use cartoon videos for demonstration and teaching • Coloring sheets, matching, and finding items in pictures make learning fun • ADA has videos for use in teaching
Nine through twelve years	• Wants to fit in with peers • Very curious • Are able to brush and floss proficiently • Attention span around 30 minutes	• Mixed dentition may need special care	• Use realistic visual aids • Give rewards for good hygiene • Take pictures for an honor wall in the office or online with parental permission • ADA has videos for use in teaching
Thirteen through Fifteen years	• Motivated by peer pressure and personal appearance • May be uncoordinated	• Improved nutrition • More diligence with hygiene • Provide positive reinforcement	• May need practice flossing • Teach good nutrition
Sixteen through nineteen years	• Peer pressure continues to be a factor • Questioning of authority • Wants to avoid bad breath • Improved coordination	• Improve nutrition habits • Improve techniques	• Teach good nutrition • Allow them to take responsibility • Teach about the role of sugar in tooth health, biofilm formation, and decay • Demonstrate improved brushing and flossing techniques
Twenty through sixty years	• May develop gingivitis or periodontal disease • Biofilm may build up with lack of dental care	• Have more specialized needs and concerns that are individualized • Must be involved and motivated	• Teach how to unlearn bad habits • Assistance with identifying problems • Teach that bleeding indicates care or attention is required
Sixty plus years	• Motivated to keep teeth for lifetime • May develop physical impairments • May be taking medications	• Repair or replacement of restorations and appliances	• Teach value of routine appointments • Discuss age-related changes that impact oral health • Techniques to adapt to arthritis • Discuss impact of medications on oral health

told to expect soreness and bleeding for the first few days and not to stop because of it. They should be encouraged to continue the daily routine to maintain healthy gingival tissues and to prevent decay.

Fluoride

Fluoride has been shown to reduce the chance of caries by 60%. Fluoride can be taken **systemically** in dietary supplements and community water sources while the teeth are forming. **Topical** fluoride can be obtained in toothpaste, mouth rinses, and in-office professionally applied topical fluoride treatments. This chapter discusses these various ways of adding fluoride to a patient's preventive plan.

Dental Sealants

A dental sealant is a plastic covering applied to tooth surfaces that are most susceptible to biofilm accumulation and caries.

The sealant is a smooth surface that is easy to clean and acts as a barrier to protect the enamel from biofilm and acids. Sealants reduce the risk of dental caries by 80%. The related sealant procedures are covered in more depth in Chapter 26, "Dental Sealants."

Biofilm Control and Oral Self-Care

Oral self-care practices such as brushing the teeth, using dental floss, and cleaning the tongue reduce harmful bacteria (biofilm) that cause dental disease. Biofilm must be mechanically removed; it cannot be rinsed or blown off the teeth. The objective of oral self-care is to clean biofilm and stains from all tooth surfaces, massage soft tissue, and replace fluoride lost from the tooth. Since biofilm forms quickly, oral self-care should be performed at least twice daily, especially before bedtime. Perform oral self-care in the following order:

- Use dental floss first—Dental floss cleans the two **interproximal** tooth surfaces, mesial and distal. Thoroughly cleaning these spaces before you brush effectively allow the fluoride in toothpaste to reach all tooth surfaces. If tooth brushing is performed first, the teeth may feel clean and flossing may be neglected.

- Tooth brushing—A toothbrush cleans three tooth surfaces: facial, lingual, and occlusal/incisal. Toothpaste (**dentifrice**) is used for some stain removal, for topical fluoride, and for a clean mouth feeling.

- Tongue cleaning—Because the tongue also contains bacteria that cause dental disease, it must be cleaned daily.

Manual Tooth Brushing

A manual toothbrush is the most common method used to clean the teeth. There are many different styles and types. Most toothbrush bristles are made of nylon and have rounded ends to prevent injury to the teeth and gums (Figure 16-5). Soft bristles are recommended over medium and hard because they do not abrade the tooth or the gingiva. The type of toothbrush that is recommend should be based on the patient's individual needs and preferences. Factors that influence selection include manual **dexterity**, position and health of the teeth, and gingiva and patient preference. The ideal toothbrush should be the correct size and shape for the patient's mouth and effectively remove biofilm without harming the teeth or surrounding tissue.

Brushing Tips for Best Results

The main objective of tooth brushing is to remove biofilm from all surfaces, to control **inflammation** and prevent disease. The patient should use a systematic sequence starting and ending in the same place so that no areas are missed. When placing the brush, overlap the previous stroke to ensure coverage of every surface. The health and anatomy of the gingiva and position of the teeth require variations in brush placement and selection of toothbrush method.

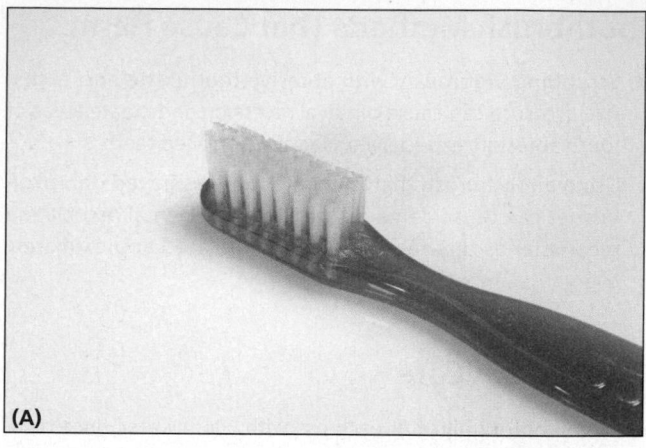

(A)

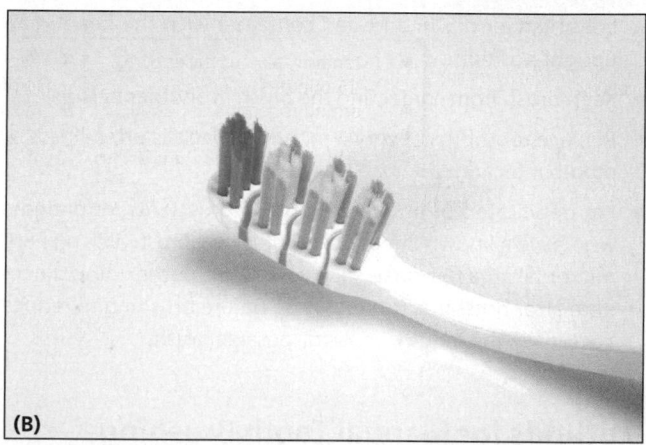

(B)

FIGURE 16-5
Types of manual toothbrushes.

Time

- 2 minutes is ideal.
- Patient counts brush strokes before moving to the next section (5-10 strokes based on patient need).
- Use a clock or egg timer.
- Power toothbrushes may have a timer.
- Timers can be helpful for patient motivation.

Frequency

- Brush two times a day because not all areas of the mouth are reached each brushing time. Brushing twice daily will ensure complete removal of bacteria.
- Brush before bedtime and after sleeping.

Pressure

- The pressure a patient exerts on the brush is difficult to measure. Too little and biofilm will not be removed; too much will cause harm to the tooth and gingiva.
- Careful observation of existing conditions such as abrasion and gingival **recession** may indicate excessive force used during brushing.

Toothbrush Methods That Cause Harm

- Scrubbing vigorously with abrasive toothpaste and excessive pressure can cause gingival recession and create areas of tooth abrasion, especially on facially displaced teeth.

- Using a toothbrush that is worn out or has frayed or broken bristles can cause damage. The American Dental Association recommends that toothbrushes be replaced approximately every three months. (Figure 16-6)

Toothbrush Care

- Clean thoroughly after each use with warm water, rinse completely, and tap out excess water.

- Let brush air dry in an open container with the head in an upright position.

- Keep brush from contacting the brush of another person.

- Replace toothbrush every 3 months especially after illness or mouth infection.

- For debilitated or immunosuppressed patients, or patients who have a known infection, disinfect the brush with an antimicrobial spray or rinse such as 0.12% chlorhexidine gluconate after brushing, use oral rinse before brushing to reduce bacteria in the mouth, or use disposable brush.

Methods for Manual Tooth Brushing

Each toothbrush method is designed for different cleaning problems and patient skill levels; therefore, more than one toothbrush method at a time may be necessary. For all methods, clean only two or three teeth at a time, and overlap strokes as you move to the next area. For occlusal surfaces, position the brush parallel to the chewing surface and gently press the bristles into the pits and fissures using a back-and-forth horizontal stroke. Using too much force will bend the bristles and not reach into the pits and fissures. Make sure to overlap strokes until the entire chewing surface is clean. The following methods are illustrated in Procedure 16–1: Bass (sulcular), Stillman, Charter, Roll Stroke, Fones, and Horizontal Scrub. The Bass, Stillman, and Charter methods can be modified by adding a roll stroke toward the occlusal surface in a vertical motion after the prescribed method is completed. Modification ensures cleaning all tooth surfaces.

Tongue Brushing

It is important to clean the surface of the tongue. Bacteria can collect in the irregular dorsal (top) surface of the tongue. A conventional toothbrush is most often used to ensure cleaning of the tongue surface. The size of the toothbrush head may limit access to the posterior area of the tongue because it may initiate gagging. To clean the tongue, the toothbrush should be placed as far back as is comfortable and then be drawn forward to the tip of the tongue, allowing the bristles to clean the debris that has accumulated. Repeat this process until the entire tongue has been cleaned. The toothbrush should be rinsed in water and not contain toothpaste as the chemicals may irritate the tongue.

There are several tongue cleaners on the market that are also used to scrape moderate to heavy debris and biofilm that is difficult to remove with the toothbrush alone. (Figure 16-13). The head of the cleaner is placed at the most posterior area of the tongue. Using light pressure, drag the cleaner to the tip of the tongue; too much pressure will damage the **papillae** of the tongue. After each pass, rinse the cleaner with water and repeat the process until the device is clean. After the tongue cleaning is complete, wash and dry the cleaner and store in a clean, dry place.

Dentifrices

A dentifrice or toothpaste is used with a toothbrush to clean the teeth. It is not needed for actual biofilm removal but helps in removing stains, polishes the teeth, and provides fluoride. As with any other recommendation made for patients, the selection of a dentifrice should be based on individual patient needs and preferences.

Types of Dentifrice

Dentifrices come in powders, gels, and paste. The active ingredient in a dentifrice provides a therapeutic and/or cosmetic benefit. Therapeutic agents include fluoride for caries prevention, antibacterial agents such as Triclosan (Colgate® Total®) that can help prevent periodontal disease, or agents that work in various ways to improve hypersensitive teeth. A small pea-sized amount of dentifrice is placed onto the toothbrush for use. It should not be ingested as some contents may upset the stomach. Calculus

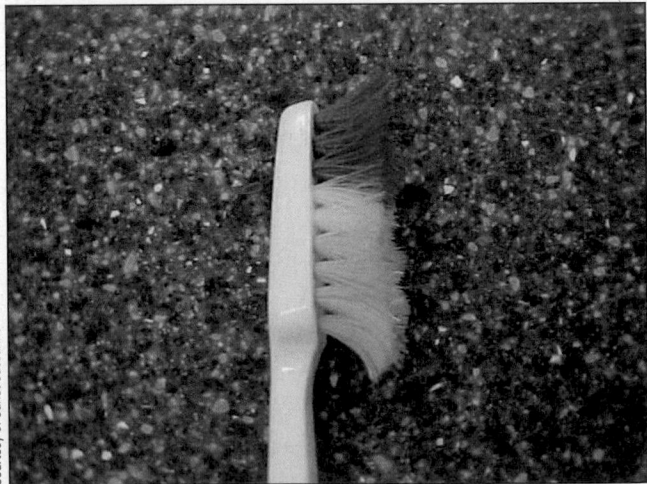

Courtesy of Janet Jaccarino

FIGURE 16-6
Worn out toothbrush is less effective and may damage soft tissue.

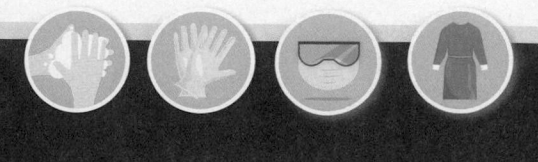

Procedure 16-1
Toothbrushing Methods

The dental assistant or dental hygienist determines which tooth brushing method is best for the patient based on the patient's skill level and oral hygiene needs. The assistant or hygienist demonstrates and instructs the patient on the selected brushing method. More than one method may be selected to adequately meet all the patient's needs.

Equipment and Supplies

- Manual toothbrush selected for patient's mouth size
- Dentoform or patient
- PPE: protective clothing, mask, glasses, and examination gloves on during patient demonstration
- Patient mirror if demonstration is intraoral

Bass (Sulcular) Brushing Method

Method Indication

- Periodontal health and maintenance
- Clean gingival margin and sulcus
- Presence of periodontal disease (gingivitis and pocketing)

Procedure Steps

1. Grasp the brush and place the tips of the bristles angled apically into the sulcus at 45° (Figure 16-7).

2. Use gentle, short vibratory strokes without removing the bristles from the sulcus.

3. Lift the brush and continue into the next group of teeth until all teeth have been cleaned.

4. For the lingual side of anterior teeth, hold the brush vertically with the bristle tips in the sulcus.

Stillman Brushing Method

Method Indication

- Gingival message and stimulation
- Clean cervical and interproximal areas

Procedure Steps

1. Place the toothbrush with the bristles directed apically and placed partly on the gingiva and partly on the cervical area of the tooth (Figure 16-8).

2. Use light pressure on the bristles until there is slight gingival blanching.

3. Use short back-and-forth vibratory strokes.

4. Move the brush head toward the occlusal.

5. For the lingual side of anterior teeth, hold the brush vertically with the bristle tips placed on the gingiva, rotating and sweeping toward the incisal edges.

Charters Brushing Method

Method Indication

- Clean interproximal surfaces
- Clean around surgical sites
- Orthodontic and fixed prosthetic appliances

Procedure Steps

1. Grasp the toothbrush and direct the bristles toward the occlusal at a 45° angle to the tooth (Figure 16-9).

2. Gently press the bristles into the interproximal area.

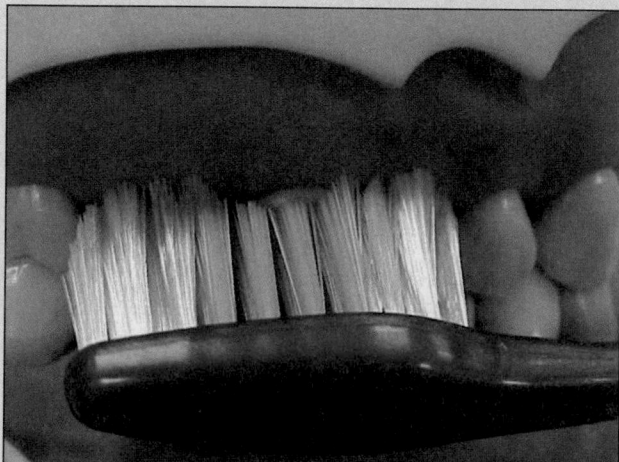

FIGURE 16-7

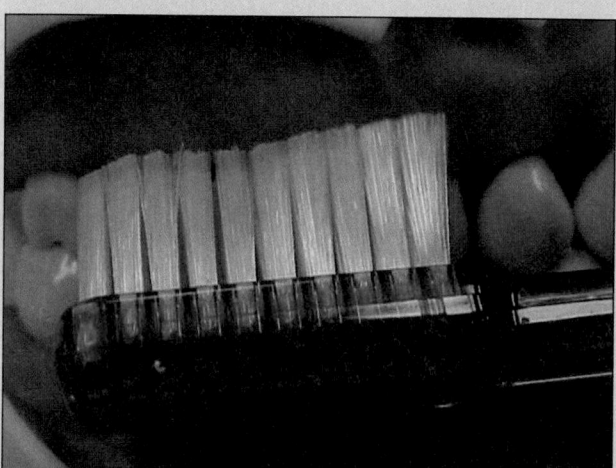

FIGURE 16-8

(Continues)

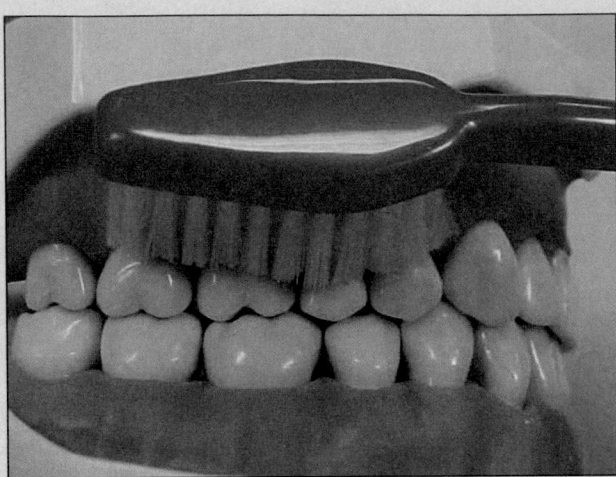

FIGURE 16-9

3. Move brush in a circular motion over the maxillary and mandibular teeth.

4. Anterior teeth are edge to edge. Hold the brush horizontally with the bristle tips placed on the maxillary and mandibular teeth.

5. Continue circular motion.

Horizontal Scrub Brushing Method

Method Indication
- Clean facial and lingual surfaces
- Can cause toothbrush abrasion

Procedure Steps

1. With the teeth closed, place the brush inside the cheek.

2. Position bristles at 90° angle against the posterior maxillary and mandibular teeth (Figure 16-11).

3. Move brush in a horizontal back-and-forth scrub motion over the maxillary and mandibular teeth.

4. Avoid excessive pressure.

Roll Stroke Brushing Method

Method Indication
- Clean gingival margin and clinical crown
- Children with healthy gingiva
- Used to modify Bass, Stillman, and Charter methods

Procedure Steps

1. Grasp the toothbrush with the bristles positioned apically against the attached gingiva at a 45° angle (Figure 16-12).

3. Move toothbrush in back-and-forth pattern using vibratory strokes.

Fones Brushing Method

Method Indication
- Clean facial and lingual surfaces
- Young children with primary teeth
- Can easily damage teeth if done too vigorously

Procedure Steps

1. With the teeth closed, place the brush against the inside of the cheek.

2. Position bristles at 90° angle against the posterior maxillary and mandibular teeth (Figure 16-10).

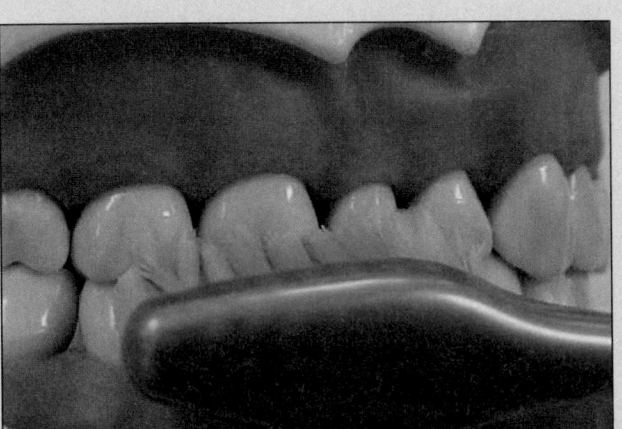

FIGURE 16-10

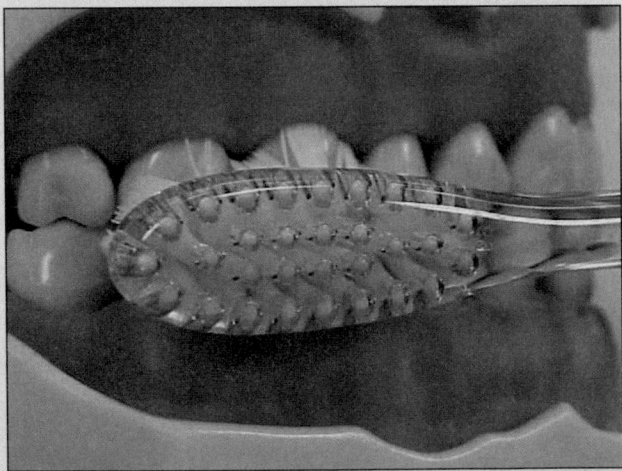

FIGURE 16-11

2. Roll the brush slowly over the teeth toward the occlusal in a vertical motion.

Modified Bass, Stillman, and Charter

Method Indication

After the prescribed method is completed, add a roll stroke toward the occlusal surface in a vertical motion to ensure cleaning all tooth surfaces.

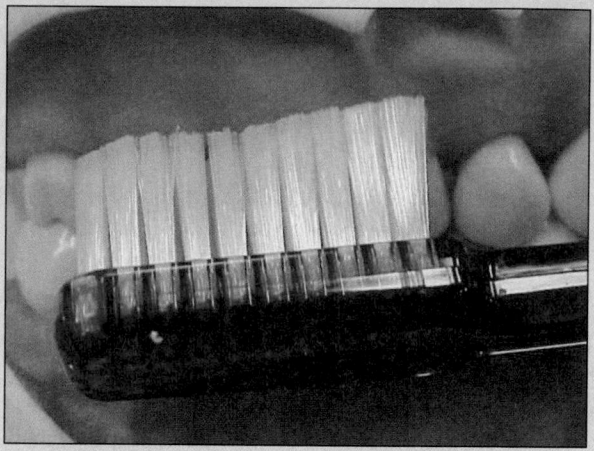

FIGURE 16-12

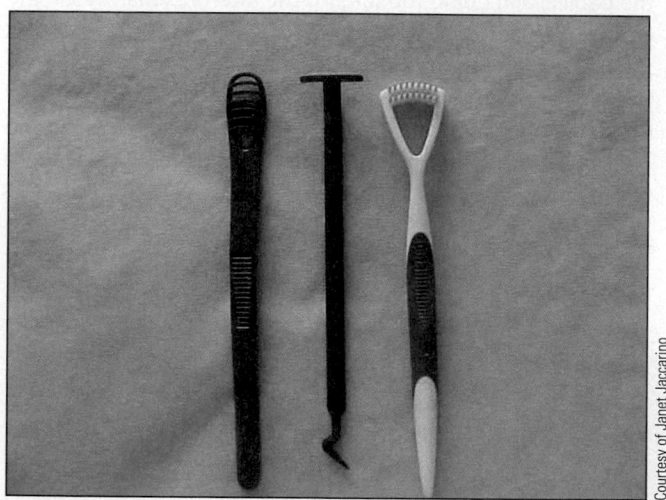

Courtesy of Janet Jaccarino

FIGURE 16-13
Manual tongue cleaners.

control, stain removal and whitening agents provide cosmetic benefits. Ingredients contained in most dentifrices are:

- Detergent— cleans and foams
- Abrasive—cleans and polishes
- Moisture stabilizer (humectant)—prevents water loss and hardening
- Preservative—inhibits microorganism growth
- Flavoring—sweetener
- Binder—thickener
- Water—hydrates binders, stabilizes ingredients
- Coloring—enhances appearance
- Active ingredient—provides therapeutic or cosmetic benefit

Be aware that some dentifrices contain strong abrasives, which can wear away tooth structure. In addition, there are wide varieties of natural dentifrices that contain herbal and organic

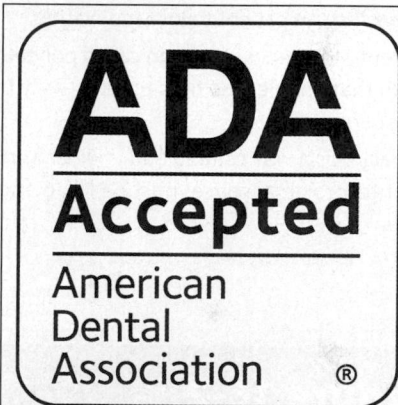

Reproduced with permission of the American Dental Association

FIGURE 16-14
American Dental Association Seal of Acceptance.

ingredients. Before recommending any product for your patient, make sure it has the American Dental Association Seal of Acceptance. The seal means that a product has met the criteria for safety and effectiveness established by the ADA's Council on Scientific Affairs and that all claims for effectiveness have been verified (Figure 16-14).

Dental Floss

Dental floss is used to remove biofilm from between the teeth where the toothbrush cannot reach. Daily flossing has been shown to reduce the risk of gingivitis and caries. When recommending dental floss to your patient, take into consideration the type of contact between the teeth, contour of the gingiva, roughness of interproximal surfaces, and the patient's dexterity and preference.

Types of Dental Floss

Most dental floss is made of nylon. Colors, flavorings, and therapeutic agents such as whiteners or fluoride may be added

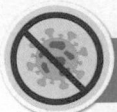

Infection Control

Infection Control: Toothpaste Tube Contamination

Bacteria and viruses that cause disease can be transmitted from one user to another when a contaminated toothbrush comes in contact with the opening of a toothpaste tube. Family members should have their own tube of toothpaste to prevent cross-contamination and to meet each person's individual needs.

to dental floss to enhance its effectiveness. Types of dental floss include the following:

- Waxed—a wax covering provides strength and may enable the floss to slide more easily between the teeth, especially where there are tight contacts or rough tooth surfaces.
- Unwaxed—unwaxed floss is thinner and may be helpful for tight contact areas. Be aware that unwaxed dental floss may fray when rubbed over a rough tooth surface, calculus, or restoration, causing the patient to lose motivation.
- Monofilament—coated with a resin called polytetrafluoroethylene (PTFE) that enables the floss to slide easily between the teeth without fraying.
- Tape—usually has a wax coating and is wider and flatter than floss. The interproximal space must be large enough to use dental tape.

Dental Flossing Technique

Proper dental flossing takes practice and may not be easy for the patient to master. Provide careful instruction and observe the patient's technique to be sure that no gingival trauma is caused. Trauma may be caused by snapping the floss into the contact area, too much interproximal pressure, failing to wrap the floss around the tooth in a "C" shape when inserting the floss under the papilla, and going too far into the interproximal area. If the gingiva is inflamed, bleeding may occur when the patient starts flossing. Be sure to explain that bleeding is not a sign to stop flossing but a sign of infection or poor flossing technique. In most cases, the bleeding will stop when biofilm is removed and the gingiva returns to health. Procedure 16–2 illustrates proper dental flossing.

Procedure 16-2
Dental Flossing Technique

The dental assistant or dental hygienist determines, demonstrates, and instructs the patient on how to floss.

Equipment and Supplies
- Floss container
- Dentoform or patient
- PPE: protective clothing, mask, glasses, and examination gloves for patient demonstration
- Patient mirror if demonstration is intraoral

Procedure Steps
1. Remove approximately 18 inches of floss from the container.
2. Wind floss around middle fingers of each hand.
3. Pinch floss between thumbs and index fingers, leaving a 1 to 2 inch length in between (Figure 16-15).

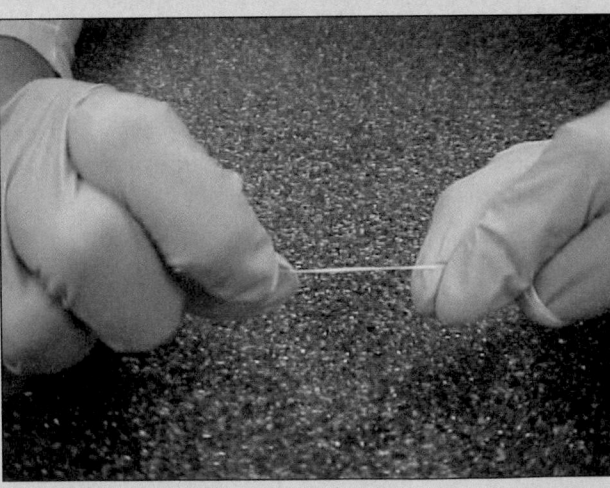

FIGURE 16-15

4. Keeping the floss tight between fingers, use index fingers or a combination of index finger and thumb and place the floss between two teeth (Figure 16-16).

5. Guide the floss gently between the teeth by using a see-saw motion until the floss is below the contact. To avoid injury to the gingiva do not snap the floss between the teeth.

6. Curve the floss in a "C" shape tight against the tooth (Figure 16-17).

7. Slide the floss gently under the gumline (Figure 16-18).

8. Remove biofilm and debris by scraping up and down several times. To avoid injury to the gingiva, do not use too much force to push the floss and do not go too far under the gumline (Figure 16-19).

9. Lift the floss over the interproximal papillae just below the contact area without removing the floss from between the teeth.

10. Move the floss to the adjacent tooth and repeat the procedure.

11. Remove the floss gently from between the teeth. If the floss tears when sliding past the contact area, gently place the floss below the contact area and pull between the teeth.

12. Wind the floss on the fingers to allow for a fresh section to be used.

13. Using a clean piece of floss, move between the next two teeth and repeat the procedure.

14. Floss each tooth thoroughly until the entire mouth is clean.

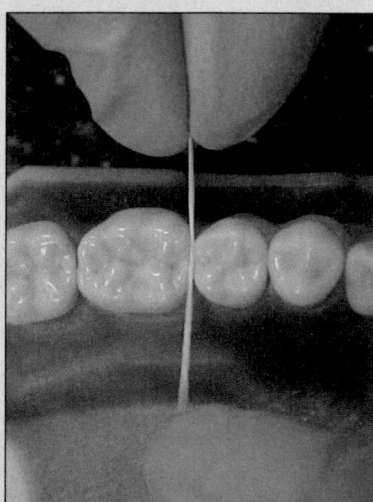

FIGURE 16-16

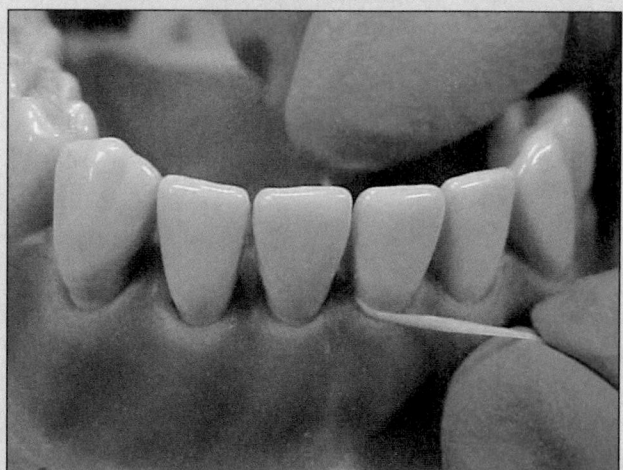

FIGURE 16-17

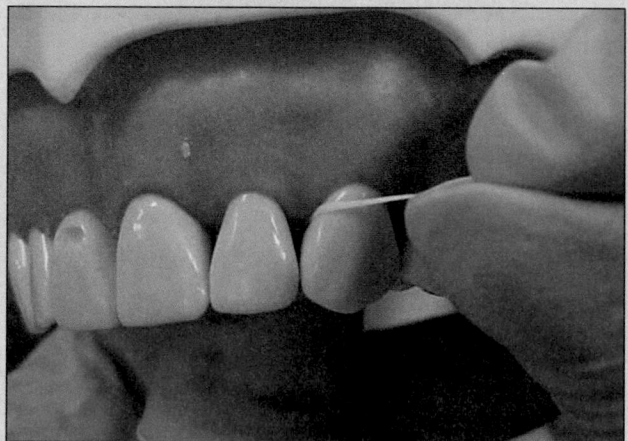

FIGURE 16-18

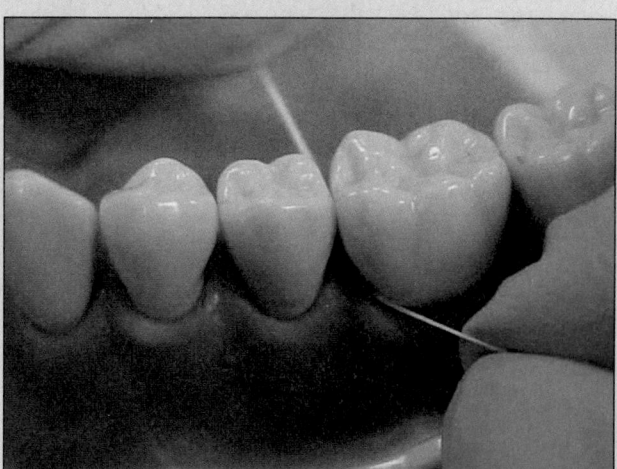

FIGURE 16-19

Oral Self-Care Assessments

There are many ways the patient can assess their new hygiene technique. They will often share that it doesn't hurt to brush and floss any more. Patients may also notice a decrease or no bleeding after brushing and flossing. An astute patient may find the gingival tissue is no longer swollen and red and has a healthier pink color. However, biofilm is invisible or at least hard to see. The dental team may instruct the patient in the use of a disclosing agent.

Disclosing Agents

Soft deposits and biofilm, which is otherwise invisible, pick up the color and become easily identified using disclosing agents (Figure 16-20). Disclosing agents are a helpful tool used for evaluation and assessment, providing motivation for patients during instruction for oral self-care and research.

A disclosing agent is supplied as a liquid or tablet that contains a dye or coloring agent. The agent is a temporary coloration that is usually red, blue, or purple that lasts for 30 minutes. Some agents will highlight older biofilm blue and newer biofilm as red (Figures 16–21and 16–22). Before use, it is advisable to place petroleum jelly on the lips to prevent the color from sticking to the tissue. There are also fluorescent disclosing agents which glow under a blue light and do not leave a stain after disclosing.

Precautions When Applying Disclosing Agents

In general, the use of a disclosing agent is not harmful to patients; however, a few precautions before starting the procedure will avoid any problems. A careful medical history is essential to ensure that the patient is not allergic to any of the ingredients contained in the disclosing agent. Tooth colored and crown and bridge restorations may become stained by the coloring agent, and removal may not be possible. Applying a

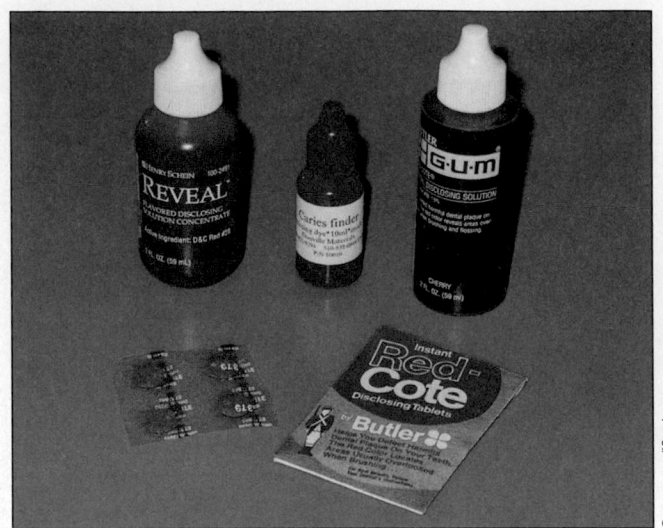

FIGURE 16-21
Examples of disclosing agents (liquids and tablets).

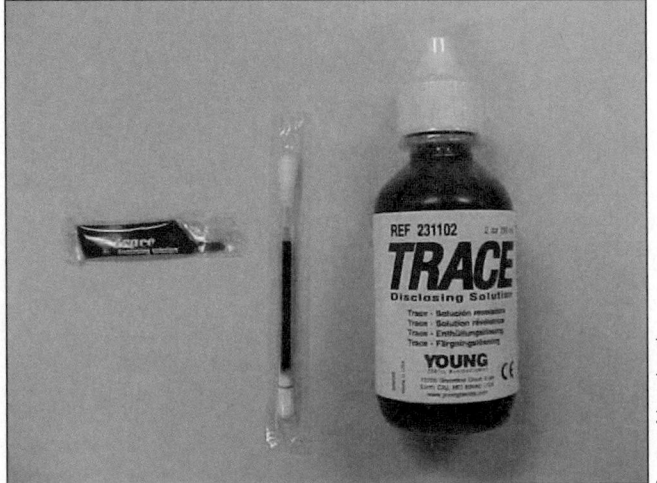

FIGURE 16-22
Example of one use disclosing solution packet, one time use disclosing solution swab and a bottle of disclosing solution.

water-based lubricant to the restoration may avoid staining. Disclosing agents should not be applied before sealant placement because the color may become incorporated into the sealant. Refer to Procedure 16–3 for the disclosing procedure.

Measure Patient's Oral Hygiene

Indices are used to measure a patient's oral hygiene status, to educate and motivate individual patients during oral self-care instruction, to recommend proper treatment, and to collect data to determine the oral health of community populations. The most common index used to evaluate biofilm in the clinical setting is the biofilm control record.

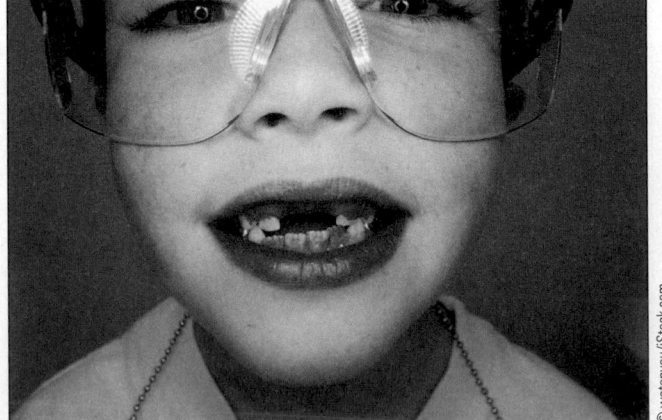

FIGURE 16-20
Disclosing solution on the patient's teeth indicating where improved oral hygiene is needed.

Procedure 16-3
Applying Disclosing Agent for Biofilm Identification

The dental assistant or dental hygienist performs this procedure. During the hygiene appointment, disclosing would be done to identify biofilm and its location for the patient and operator. Means of removing the biofilm are then discussed and demonstrated.

Equipment and Supplies
- PPE: protective clothing, mask, glasses, and examination gloves
- Dental mouth mirror and hand mirror
- Saliva ejector and air/water syringe tip
- Cotton-tip applicators (2)
- Petroleum jelly (lubricant)
- Disclosing agent (liquid, tablet, or swab) and disposable cup

Procedure Steps

1. While seating the patient, review the medical and dental history with the patient.

2. After washing hands and donning PPE, examine the oral cavity.

3. Place lubricant onto a cotton-tip applicator and apply it to the patient's lips. Some dentists may want lubricant applied on any tooth-colored restorations to prevent staining.

4. Place a couple drops of the liquid disclosing agent into a disposable cup. Use a cotton-tip applicator to absorb the agent and apply it to the patient's teeth. All accessible surfaces of the teeth should be covered with the disclosing solution. If using the tablet method, instruct the patient to chew for 15 seconds.

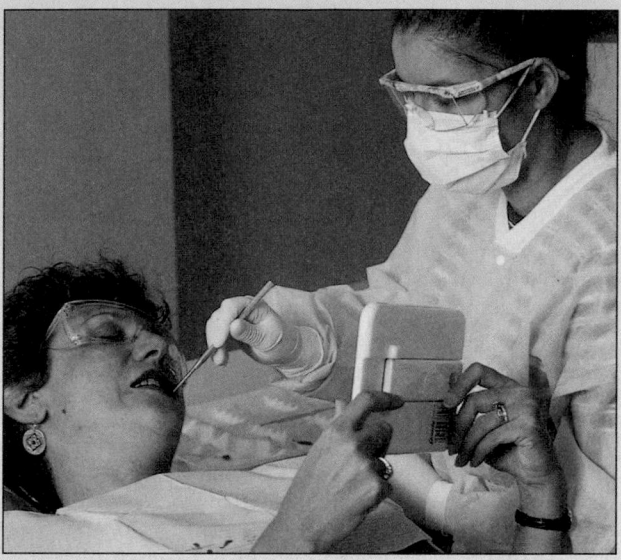

FIGURE 16-23
Dental assistant working with a patient to identify biofilm after disclosing the patient's teeth.

5. Rinse the agent from the teeth using a gentle spray of water from the air/water syringe and suction the mouth using the saliva ejector tip.

6. Hand the patient a hand mirror to see the biofilm, and use a mouth mirror to help the patient identify the areas with biofilm (Figure 16-23).

7. Demonstrate for the patient the methods of brushing and flossing for biofilm removal.

Biofilm Control Record

The biofilm control record is a rapid assessment tool used to record the presence of biofilm on individual tooth surfaces. (Refer to Figure 16-24.) Four surfaces are recorded on the mesial, distal, facial, and lingual surfaces. Six surfaces may also be used. Refer to Procedure 16–4 for how to take a biofilm score.

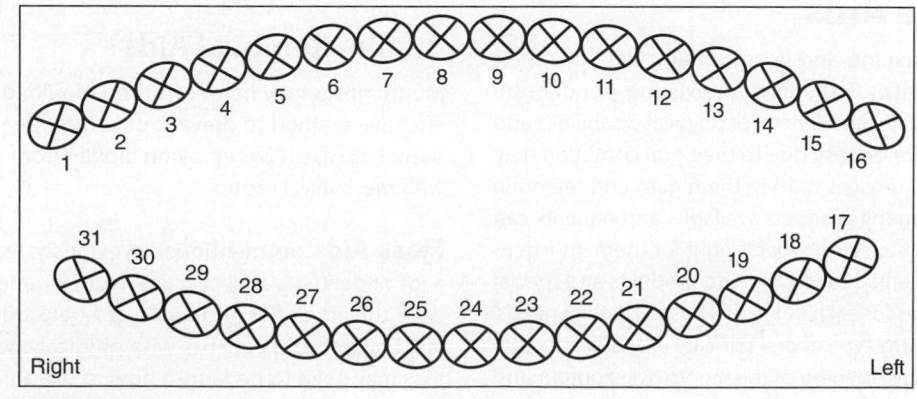

FIGURE 16-24
Biofilm control record.

Procedure 16-4
Completing the Biofilm Control Record

After the dental assistant has applied a disclosing agent for biofilm identification, the biofilm control record is completed as a visual of the patient's oral hygiene.

Equipment and Supplies
- PPE: protective clothing, mask, glasses, examination gloves, and overgloves
- Dental mouth mirror
- Biofilm chart and red pencil, or software program

Procedure Steps

1. Place overgloves over examination gloves after disclosing the patient's mouth to record biofilm on the biofilm chart or on the computer. (It should be noted that some states do not allow overgloves to be used for any type of treatment, even in the case of placing them over examination gloves to write on a chart. The dental assistant would then have someone else chart for them, or place a barrier on the computer or writing utensil to allow for charting to occur.)

2. Mark a red horizontal line through all missing teeth.

3. Examine each surface for biofilm at the gingival margin using the dental mouth mirror.

4. Record by coloring with the red pencil on the appropriate space on the record form.

5. Calculate the biofilm score.
   - ❏ Determine the number of total surfaces for the teeth present. Multiply the number of teeth present by 4 (or 6) depending on which form is being used.
   - ❏ Determine the number of biofilm stained surfaces by counting all the surfaces recorded in step 4.
   - ❏ Determine the percentage of biofilm present in the mouth by multiplying the number of biofilm stained surfaces by 100 and dividing by the total number of available surfaces.

Calculation Example for Biofilm Control Record

1. Multiply the number of teeth present by 4 or 6.

   Example has 26 teeth present ($26 \times 4 = 104$ surfaces)

2. Percent of biofilm

   Number of surfaces with biofilm (example has 8 surfaces with biofilm) $\times 100 = 800$
   Divide by number of total surfaces (104)
   800 divided by 104 = 7.6%

Interpretation: 0% is the ideal score; however, less than 10% is considered good.

Patient Biofilm Score and Oral Hygiene Instructions

In some offices, a record of biofilm location and the patient's biofilm score are referred to during future appointments to evaluate the patient's progress. The assistant should also document what oral hygiene instructions were provided for reference.

Oral Hygiene Aids

For most patients brushing and flossing daily will keep their mouth clean and healthy. Patients with existing periodontal problems, restorations and appliances, or physical disabilities and those who are at risk for disease due to their oral condition may need special oral care devices to help them gain and maintain oral health. There are many products available, and patients can be overwhelmed trying to select what is right for them. As a dental professional it is essential to recommend products and special oral hygiene techniques for each individual based on their needs. When recommending any type of oral self-care aid, take into consideration the size of the opening of the mouth, the contour and position of the teeth, size of the interdental spaces, anatomy of

the gingiva, **periodontal pocket** depths, types of **prostheses**, orthodontic appliances, and the patient's dexterity and preference. Remember if a patient's self-care routine is effective in keeping their mouth healthy, there may be no need to recommend additional products. Often reinforcement and encouragement of their behavior is all that is necessary. It is important to keep in mind that the simpler the task, the greater the chance of getting it accomplished. Adding a large number of steps will make it more difficult for the patient to accomplish the task daily.

Biofilm Removal Aids

Mouth rinses may help to control biofilm growth, but the most effective method to prevent or control dental caries and periodontal disease is by removing biofilm from all areas of the tooth with mechanical action.

Floss Aids As mentioned previously, learning to floss takes a lot of dexterity and practice. Not all patients are able to conquer the art of flossing and need help from a caregiver or an aid. Children and patients' with physical and intellectual disabilities may need to be taught how to use a floss aid to be able to independently complete their oral hygiene. There are many floss aids including floss holders, floss threaders, tufted floss and the adapted use of gauze squares

Floss Holder A floss holder is recommended for patients with a strong gag reflex, those who lack manual dexterity, caregivers, and the physically and mentally challenged. The holder has a handle with a yolk-like device, or two prongs in a Y shape. The prongs are 1 to 2 inches apart. Floss is secured between the prongs, and the handle is grasped to guide the floss between the teeth (Figure 16-25). Refer to Procedure 16–5. It may be difficult to load the floss and maintain tension of the floss between the prongs. When the patient is away from home there are on-the-go flossers they can use. Flossers are C shaped, prethreaded, one-time use devices that may be easier for most patients to use. Orthodontic flossers are similar with the exception that the flosser collapses, allowing it to get beneath the orthodontic appliances (Figure 16-26). Floss holders such as Gum Chucks® make it easy for even the youngest patient to clean between their teeth (Figure 16-27).

Floss Threader A floss threader is used to reach into closed contacts where traditional flossing techniques cannot reach the interproximal areas. It allows the patient to clean between bridge spaces, under pontics, around orthodontic wires and retainers, through teeth that are splinted together or severely overlapped, and under bars between **implants** (Procedure 16–5). A floss threader is similar in function to a sewing needle threader. It is a thin straight piece of plastic with a loop at one end (Figure 16-28). A length of dental floss is threaded through the loop.

Tufted Floss Tufted floss is used to clean between bridge spaces, under pontics, around orthodontic wires and retainers, and under bars between implants (Procedure 16–5). Tufted floss may be more effective than regular floss in removing biofilm from interproximal root concavities, sites where recession

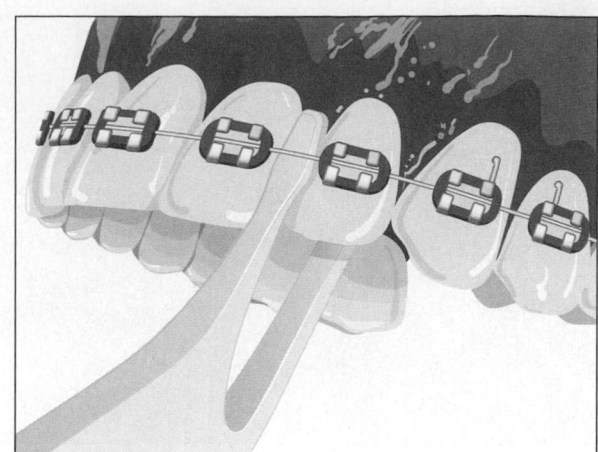

FIGURE 16-26
Orthodontic flossers.

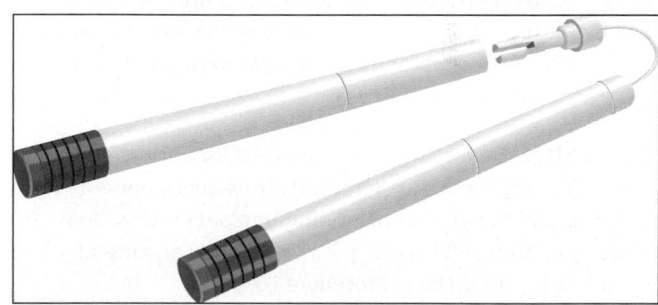

FIGURE 16-27
Gum Chucks®.

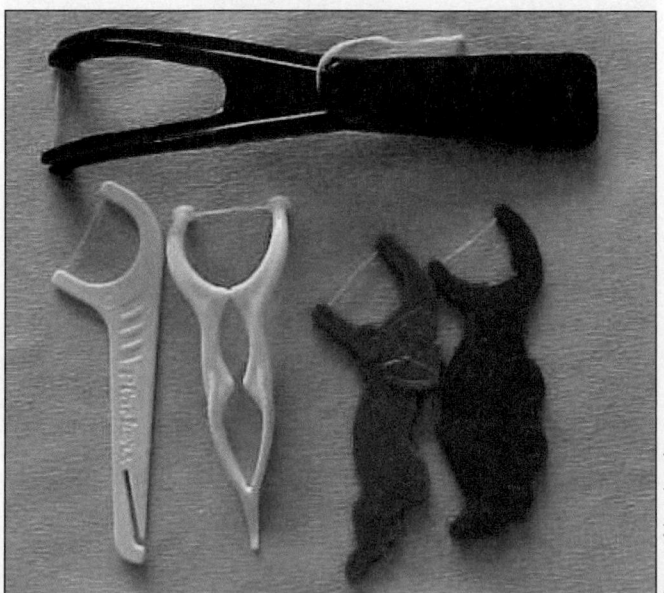

FIGURE 16-25
At top is a Y shaped floss holder and the bottom row shows flossers.

Courtesy of Janet Jaccarino

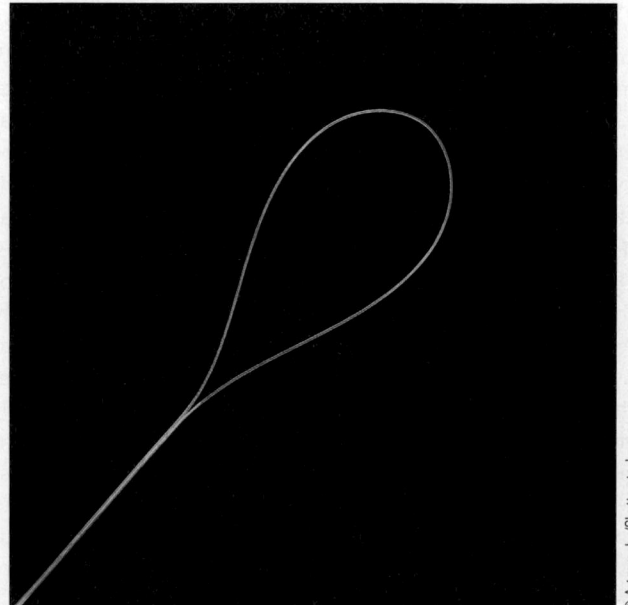

FIGURE 16-28
Eez-Thru Floss Patterson Dental Supply.

© Artography/Shutterstock.com

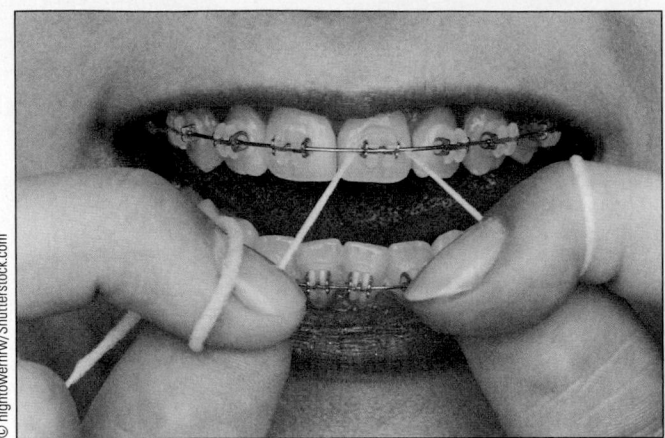

FIGURE 16-29
Tufted floss.

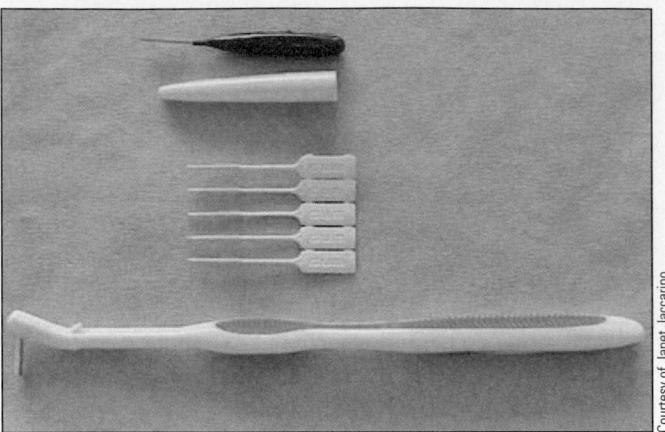

FIGURE 16-30
Interdental brushes; travel brush and insert brush with handle.

and bone loss expose **furcations**, areas with open contacts, and wide spaces between the teeth. One end of dental floss may be plastic or stiff floss and is attached to a thicker piece of tufted or fluffy floss. A length of regular dental floss may also be attached (Figure 16-29).

Gauze Strip Gauze strips may be used for very wide spaces between teeth, teeth next to **edentulous** areas, under pontics and bars, and between implants and implant crowns. Strips are made by cutting or folding 2 × 2 inch or larger squares of gauze into a 1 inch strip. (Refer to Procedure 16–5).

Interdental Brush An interdental brush (also called a proxy brush) is used in larger interproximal spaces to clean biofilm from under and around orthodontic and fixed appliances, interproximal root concavities, furcations, areas with open contacts, teeth next to edentulous areas, and areas that are difficult to reach with other methods for interproximal cleaning. The interproximal brush is used without cleaning agents. The brush can also be used to deliver antimicrobial agents into interproximal spaces and periodontal pockets.

The interdental brush is made of soft nylon filaments that are twisted into stainless steel or plastic wire. The brushes are available in different sizes and shapes (small and large cylindrical and tapered) to accommodate individual interproximal areas (Figures 16-30 and 16-31). There are two types of brush heads. One type is the insert type brush head used with a plastic or metal handle that is angled for easy access to areas in the mouth. A travel size is also available with the brush head that is attached to a small handle. When selecting a brush, it should be slightly larger than the interproximal space to ensure that the bristles thoroughly clean the teeth. (Refer to Procedure 16–5.) After the teeth have been cleaned, rinse the bristles thoroughly using warm water, tap out excess water, and let the brush air dry in an open container. It is important to monitor the bristle integrity so that no trauma is caused to the tooth surface or soft tissue from exposed wire or plastic during movement of the brush. Dispose of and replace the brush when it is worn out.

End Tuft Brush The end tuft brush is used for areas with open contacts, teeth next to edentulous areas, and areas that are difficult to reach with other methods for interproximal cleaning.

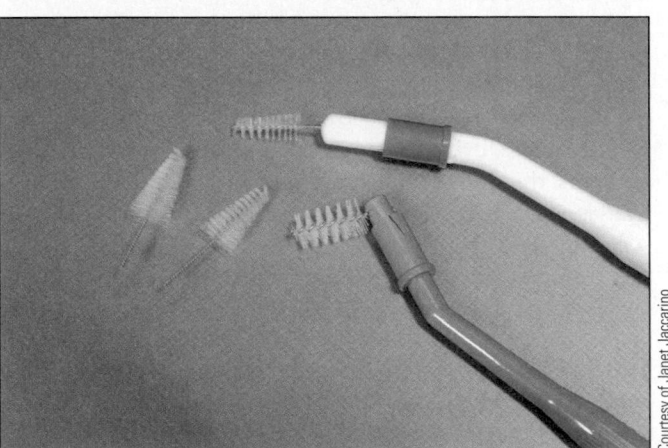

FIGURE 16-31
Assortment of sizes and shapes interdental brushes and handles.

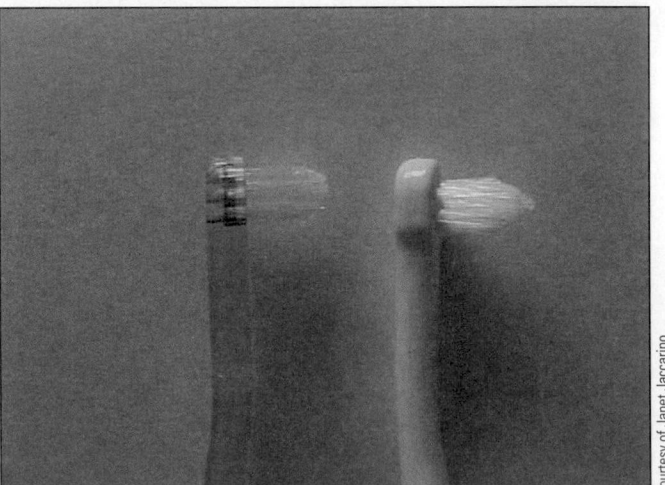

FIGURE 16-32
End tuft brushes.

(Refer to Procedure 16–5.) It has a small brush head attached at a right angle to a plastic handle (Figure 16-32). After the teeth have been cleaned, rinse the bristles thoroughly using warm water, tap out excess water, and let the brush air dry in an open container.

Toothpick The toothpick is used to remove biofilm from just under the gingival margin especially in areas with orthodontic appliances, periodontal disease with exposed furcation areas, posterior lingual areas, and in concave proximal spaces. (Refer to Procedure 16–5.) A toothpick is also useful to deliver antimicrobial agents or to burnish fluoride into areas of sensitivity. Only round tapered wooden toothpicks should be used. The toothpick can be handheld or placed in a perio-aid handle designed to hold the toothpick, which offers better extension to for hard-to-reach areas (Figure 16-33). After use, dispose of the toothpick; wash and dry the handle and store in a clean dry place.

Stimulators

Stimulators are designed to promote healthy and firm gingiva by massaging the gingival tissues and stimulating blood flow. They also help to dislodge food particles and biofilm, but they are not a replacement for mechanical biofilm removal techniques. There are many stimulators available: rubber tip stimulators, wooden wedge stimulators, and oral irrigators, which are covered in this chapter under the "Automated Oral Hygiene Devices" heading.

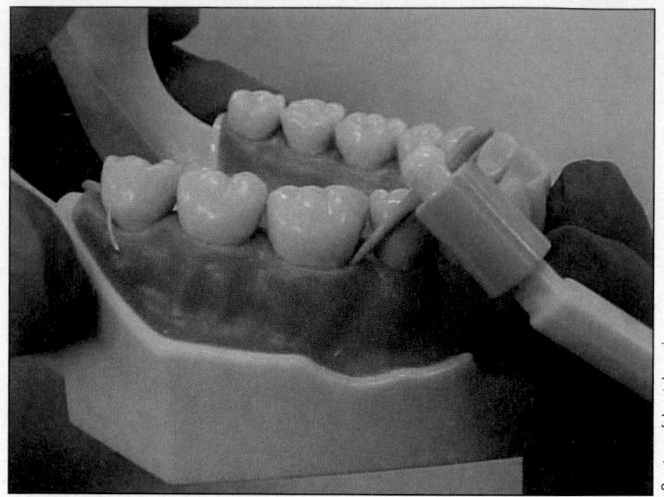

FIGURE 16-33
Toothpick inserted into perio-aid handle.

Procedure 16-5
Demonstrate Biofilm Removal Aids

Equipment and Supplies
- Dentoform
- Floss holder
- Dental floss
- Floss threader
- Tufted floss
- 2 × 2 gauze square
- Interdental brush
- End tuft brush
- Round tapered wooden toothpick and adjustable handle

Procedure Steps: Y Shape Floss Holder

1. Grasp the handle of the floss holder (Figure 16-34).

2. Slide the floss gently between the teeth using a back-and-forth motion until the floss is below the contact area.

3. Slide the floss gently under the gumline and scrape up and down several times.

4. Lift the floss over the interproximal papillae, floss the adjacent tooth, and scrape up and down several times.

5. Remove the floss gently from between the teeth. Move between the next two teeth and repeat the procedure. Floss each tooth thoroughly until the entire mouth is clean.

6. Clean the floss holder once flossing is complete. Remove and dispose of the floss, wash and dry the handle, and store in a clean, dry space.

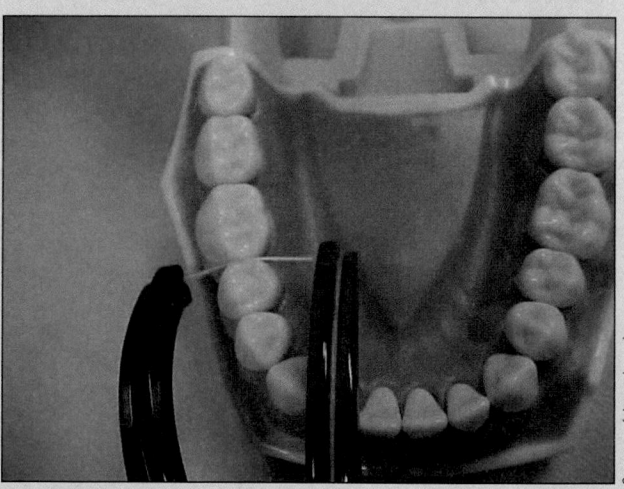

FIGURE 16-34
Y shaped floss aid.

Procedure Steps: Floss Threader

1. Insert the straight piece of plastic into the interproximal space from the facial. Care should be taken not to injure the gingiva when inserting the straight piece of plastic through the interproximal space (Figure 16-35).

2. Remove the floss from the loop and follow the same technique as for finger flossing. (Refer to Procedure 16–2.)

(Continues)

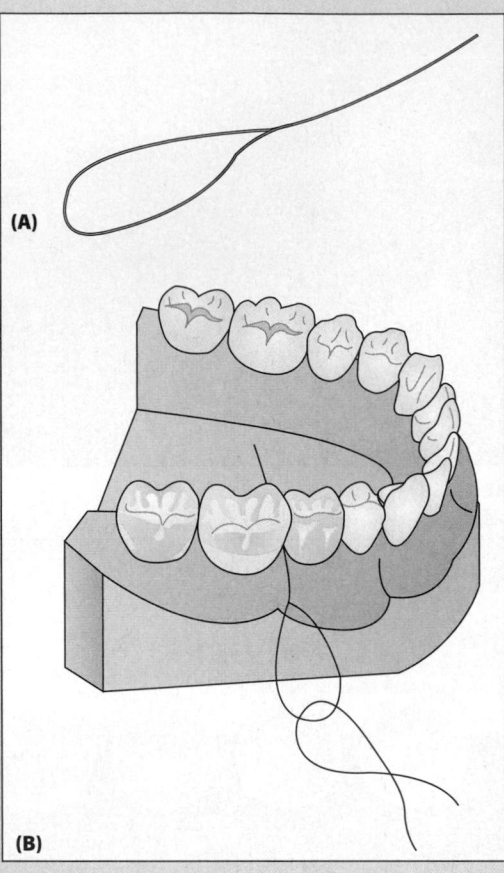

FIGURE 16-35
(A) Floss threader. (B) Floss threader threaded under the pontic area of a bridge.

3. Remove the floss by pulling through the interproximal space and dispose of the used floss.

Procedure Steps: Tufted Floss

1. Thread the stiff end of floss into the interproximal space.

2. Follow the same technique as for finger flossing. (Refer to Procedure 16–2).

3. Remove the floss by pulling through the interproximal space and dispose of the used floss.

Procedure Steps: Gauze Squares

1. Cut or fold gauze square into a 1 inch strip.

2. Hold the gauze strip on both ends.

3. Position the gauze on the tooth surface near the cervical area.

4. Move the gauze strip in a back-and-forth shoe-shine motion several times (Figure 16-36).

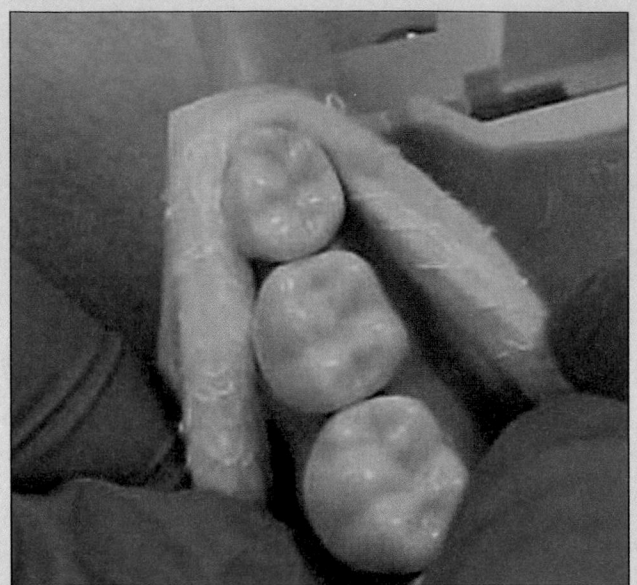

FIGURE 16-36

Procedure Steps: Interdental Brush

1. Select the size and shape of bristles that are slightly larger than the interproximal space.

2. Insert the brush head into the adjustable end of the handle and secure into place.

3. Moisten the bristles and place into the interproximal space near the cervical area and move the handle and brush in an in-and-out motion. Care should be taken not to injure the gingiva during insertion (Figure 16-37).

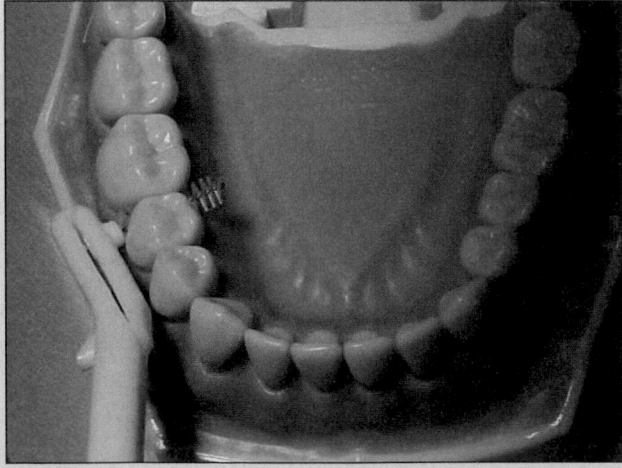

FIGURE 16-37

Courtesy of Janet Jaccarino

4. Bend the brush head to access periodontal pocket. Remove biofilm using an in-and-out and an up-and-down motion.

Procedure Steps: End Tuft Brush

1. Direct the tip of the tuft into the desired area to be cleaned.

2. Use a rotating vibratory motion similar to the Bass toothbrush method.

Procedure Steps: Toothpick

1. Insert the toothpick into the adjustable end of the handle, twist the toothpick to make sure it is held tight and secure into place. Break off the excess end of the toothpick

2. Moisten the end with saliva to soften the wood.

3. Place the tip at the gingival margin slightly into the sulcus at a 45° angle.

4. Remove biofilm by tracing the gingival margin around the tooth with the tip maintaining contact with the tooth (see Figure 16-33).

5. Clean furcation areas with an in-and-out motion and concave proximal spaces with an up-and-down motion. Care should be taken not to force the teeth apart in interproximal areas or injure the gingival tissue upon insertion.

Rubber Tip Stimulator The rubber tip stimulator is used to stimulate or massage the gingiva to improve circulation and increase keratinization. Rubber tips can be used to remove biofilm from just above and slightly below the gingival margin, in large spaces between teeth, and in exposed furcation areas. Stimulators do not adequately remove biofilm from tooth surfaces. The dentist may also recommend a rubber tip stimulator to re-contour the gingiva after periodontal surgery.

This stimulator has a cone-shaped flexible rubber tip attached to the end of a plastic or metal handle or the end of a toothbrush (Figure 16-38). The tip is placed on a 90° angle to the tooth above and just below the gingival margin. Move the tip, tracing along the contour of the tooth. Insert interproximally and move the tip in an in-and-out motion. Aggressive use of stimulators and increased pressure can wear away the tissue and papilla. After use, wash and dry the tip and handle and store in a clean, dry place. Replace the rubber tip when it is worn or cracked.

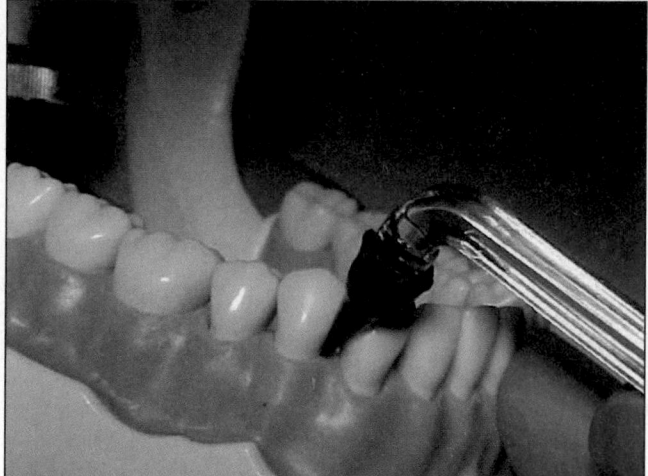

FIGURE 16-38
Rubber tip stimulator.

Wooden Wedge Stimulator This stimulator is used for larger spaces between teeth where the papilla does not completely fill the space and between exposed furcations. The wooden wedge stimulator is made of soft wood such as balsa or birch. The wedge is approximately 2 inches long and triangular in shape (Figure 16-39). The wedge tip must be moistened with saliva before use. The wedge is inserted between the teeth from the buccal aspect with the base or flat surface of the triangle near the gingiva. If the wedge meets resistance, stop and reposition the stick. Once between the teeth, use moderate pressure to move the tip in an in-and-out motion. Clean the side on one tooth and then the adjacent tooth. If debris builds up on the wedge, rinse under running water. Once cleaning is complete, dispose of the wedge. Wooden dental stimulators are not recommended as often as they used to be as improper use can cause a flattening of the interdental papilla and the sharp pointed end can cause injury to the gingiva.

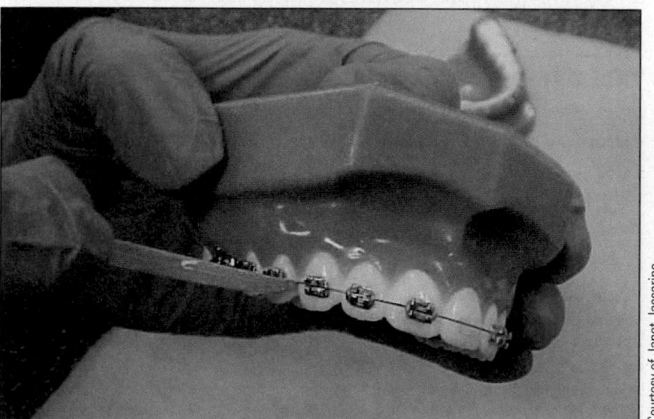

FIGURE 16-39
Wooden wedge stimulator.

On-the-Go Aids

A number of oral hygiene aids are available to supplement the hygiene techniques and to assist with biofilm removal when brushing is not possible. The dental assistant should stay abreast of the dental aids on the market and know how they can help specific patients.

Mouth Rinses Mouth rinses have been used for many years for preventive, therapeutic, and cosmetic purposes (Figure 16-40). Remember that recommendations for oral self-care must be based on individual needs. While some mouth rinses can be purchased over the counter, others may need a prescription. Mouth rinses contain an active ingredient that provides therapeutic benefits such as **antiseptics** and **antimicrobials** that are **bactericidal** or **bacteriostatic**. Products also contain inactive ingredients such as dyes, preservatives, water, alcohol, sweeteners, and flavoring (Table 16-3). Preventive and therapeutic uses include control of oral malodor, caries, and periodontal disease reduction and relief of **xerostomia**. Mouth rinses are also recommended to improve postsurgical healing, management of oral **mucositis**, and maintenance of the health of peri-implant tissues. Cosmetic mouth rinses contain agents that reduce stain and whiten teeth.

Mouth rinses containing alcohol are contraindicated for the recovering alcoholic, as well as children under the age of six and those with mental and physical disabilities, because these patients may not understand or have the ability to spit the mouth rinse out after use. Since xerostomia can be made worse by the addition of alcohol, some mouth rinses are available without this ingredient.

The assistant should instruct the patient to always follow directions for frequency of use, amount of rinse, and length of time in the mouth. The patient should take the recommended amount of rinse into their mouth and close their lips and teeth. The rinse should be forced through the interdental spaces as well as to the front and back and the right and left sides of the mouth. When rinsing is complete, the patient should spit into the sink.

When brushing, flossing, or mouth rinsing is not possible, just using water to swish around and between the teeth helps loosen debris, dilute bacteria, and reduce bacterial activity. If a sink is not available to spit the water out, simply swallow. This technique is referred to as the "swish and swallow."

Chewing Gum If nothing else is available, a good alternative for biofilm and loose debris removal as well as reduction of oral

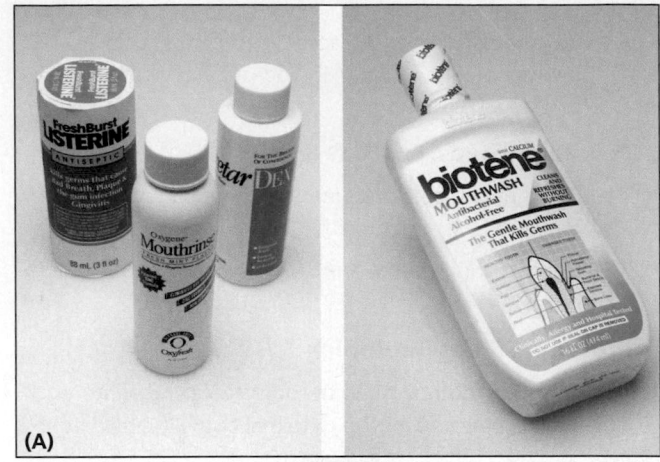

(A)

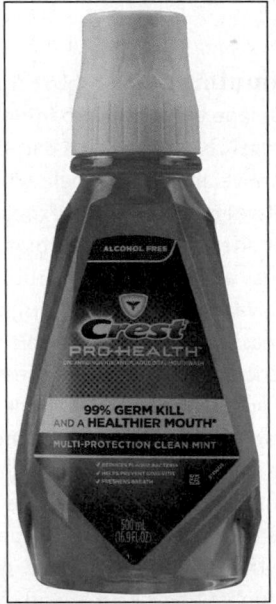

(B)

FIGURE 16-40
(A) Antimicrobial mouth rinses. (B) Multi Protection Oral Rinse.

TABLE 16-3 Active Ingredients in Mouth Rinses

Ingredient	Function
Essential Oils (thymol, eucalyptol and menthol)	Alters bacterial cell walls and inhibits the cell's enzymatic activity Adverse effects – burning associated with alcohol in the formula and light staining of the teeth
Quanternary Ammonium Compounds (cetylpyridinium chloride (CPC)	Bacterial cell wall lysis, decreased cell metabolism, decreased ability for bacteria to attach to tooth surfaces Adverse effects – staining of teeth, burning sensation and increased supragingival calculus formation
Oxygenating Agents (hydrogen peroxide)	May offer beneficial effects by creating an **aerobic** environment destroying some bacteria Adverse effects - use of mouth rinses containing hydrogen peroxide with concentrations greater than 3% for longer than 30 days may cause damage to the oral tissues
Chlorhexidine (by prescription 0.12% concentration)	Reduction in pellicle formation, alteration of bacterial adsorption and/or attachment to teeth, bacterial cell wall lysis. Also available without alcohol Adverse effect – staining of teeth, restorations and tissues, increased supragingival calculus, altered taste, irritation of soft tissue
Triclosan (at this time FDA approved and only available in US in dentifrice, outside US in mouth rinses)	Broad spectrum antibacterial agent acts on bacterial cell wall causing lysis Adverse effects – may contribute to the development of antibiotic-resistant germs
Herbal Extracts (echinacea, goldenseal, alovera)	Antimicrobial and anti-inflammatory properties Adverse effects- sanguinarine-containing products may cause mild burning sensations

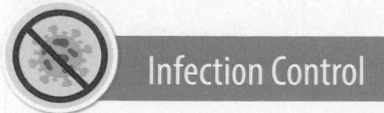

Infection Control

Use Mouth Rinse to Reduce Microorganisms

Before dental care is provided, the patient should use a mouth rinse to reduce the number of microorganisms in the mouth and prevent contamination by the aerosols produced by handpieces and ultrasonic devices.

malodor is to chew gum. Chewing gum increases saliva production that buffers and washes away the biofilm acids that have the potential to cause tooth decay after eating. The chewing action also helps dislodge particles from the teeth. To date the American Dental Association seal of acceptance is given to chewing gum that contains sugars that do not produce caries (Figure 16-41). **Xylitol** is a sweetener that tastes like sucrose but has the benefit of inhibiting the attachment and transmission of bacteria. The use of xylitol-containing gum may enhance remineralization of the teeth and inhibit future recolonization of biofilm bacteria. Xylitol is proven safe for people of all ages. In addition to gum, xylitol is available in oral rinses, toothpaste and gels, sprays, wipes, lozenges, and lollipops for children and adults. Xylitol can be used as part of a patient's caries prevention program.

Tooth Wipes and Swabs Tooth wipes and swabs can be used to clean biofilm from the teeth when brushing is not possible. They are made of soft material and treated with mouthwash or flavoring. The wipe is made to fit over the index finger, and the swab has a piece of absorbent material on a stick (Figure 16-42). The entire tooth surface should be cleaned from the gingival margin to the biting and chewing edges, from both the cheek and tongue side areas. Tooth wipes are not intended to replace the use of a toothbrush and floss.

Automated Oral Hygiene Devices

Automated devices may increase patient compliance with oral self-care and are useful for patients who have difficulty reaching specific areas of the mouth. The large diameter of the handle of

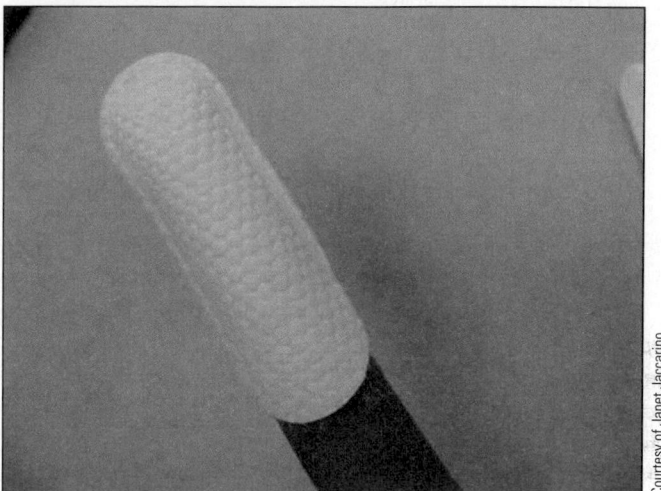

FIGURE 16-42
Tooth swab.

the automated toothbrush may be easier to hold for those with disabilities and more convenient for caregivers. Vigorous rinsing of the mouth with water will aid in removing loose debris and may help return the oral environment to a normal pH after acid production. While rinsing may flush the entire mouth, the use of an oral irrigator will target specific areas and, based on individual needs, should be part of a regular oral self-care regimen.

Automated Toothbrushes Automated toothbrushes come in many designs and are activated by electricity (Figure 16-43). They have larger handles and chargers (the handles have to be larger to hold the rechargeable battery and circuit board). The heads of the mechanical toothbrush can move in several different directions and are available in different sizes and shapes for all oral health needs. Dental assistants must be familiar with each motion to be able to recommend the appropriate tooth brushing method for each motion. The motions can be reciprocating, orbital, vibratory, arched, elliptical, or a combination of two or more of these motions (Figure 16-44). Newer models also incorporate sonic action that seems to be particularly effective in removing biofilm and **extrinsic** stains. Some of the automatic units have built-in timing devices that allow 30 seconds for each of the four quadrants and stop when 2 minutes have elapsed. Studies suggest that when using an automated toothbrush with a 2-minute timer, subjects tended to brush for a longer period of time than those who brush with a manual toothbrush. An automatic toothbrush can be used in place of a manual toothbrush. Care should be taken to apply light pressure and to let the action

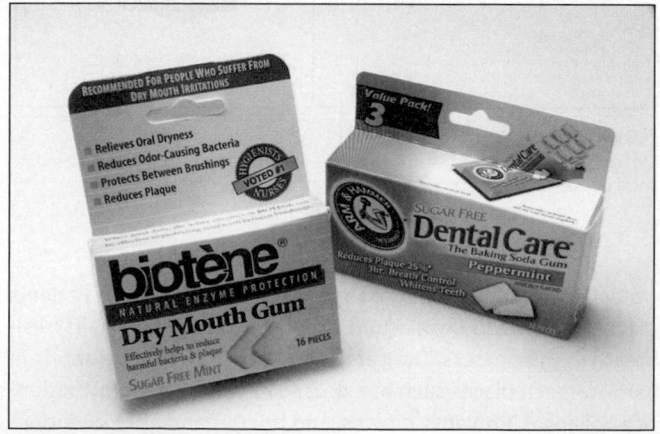

FIGURE 16-41
Xylitol-containing chewing gum used to prevent tooth decay.

of the bristles clean the teeth and gums. When used properly these devices are safe and effective; however, to achieve optimal use of automated devices requires instruction and should be monitored by a professional. Some automated toothbrushes come with flossing and tongue cleaning attachments.

Advanced mechanical toothbrushes incorporate the latest oral technology (Figures 16–45A and 16–46B). These toothbrushes connect with a smartphone through Bluetooth. This allows for personalized guidance, tracks performance over time with graphs and charts, and stores up to 6 months of brushing data. It senses when the patient is brushing too hard, has unique adjustable settings based on dental professional input, and motivates the patient to brush with news, reminders, recommendations, and rewards.

Oral Irrigator An oral irrigator or water jet uses a specially designed supra- and subgingival tips to deliver a steady or pulsating stream of water. These devices have been shown to reduce gingivitis. (Figure 16-47) An oral irrigator does not remove biofilm and should not replace brushing and flossing. The pulsating

Motion	Illustration
Reciprocating motion— moves back and forth in a line	
Orbital motion— moves in a circle	
Vibratory motion— vibrates quickly back and forth	
Semicircular motion— moves in an arc	
Elliptical motion— moves in an oval	

FIGURE 16-44
Motions of mechanical toothbrushes.

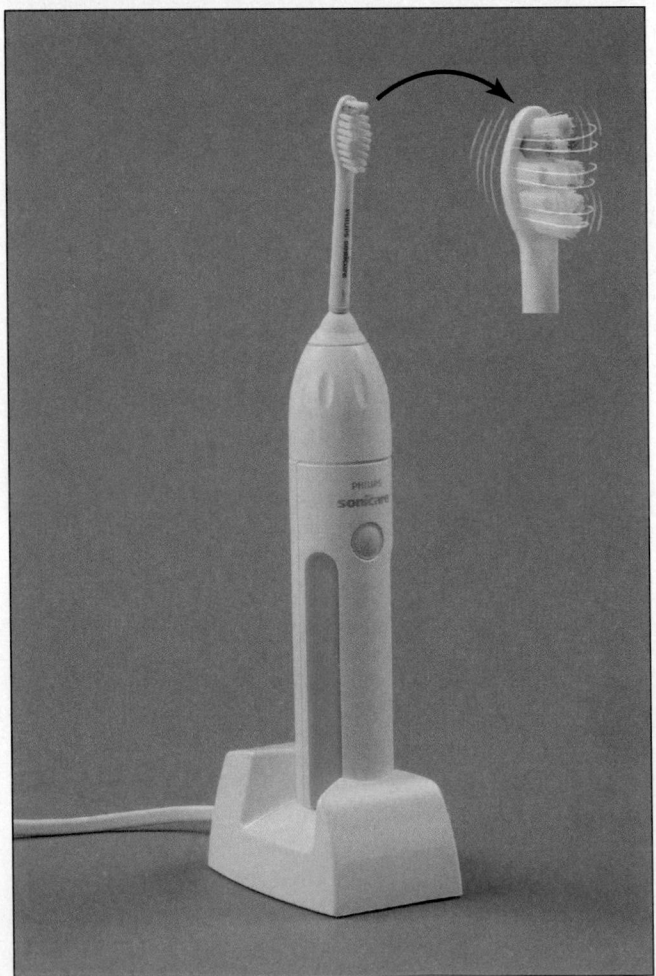

FIGURE 16-43
Phillips Sonicare dynamic action gently and effectively reaches deep between teeth and along gumlines.

water flow allows food debris to be removed easily. Some patients place mouthwash in the fluid-holding container to gain fresh breath in the process. They are useful to remove loose debris in hard-to-reach places such as exposed furcation areas, orthodontic appliances, implants, crowns, and bridges and after periodontal and oral surgery. A subgingival irrigation tip has been shown to be a better mechanism to deliver antimicrobial agents such as

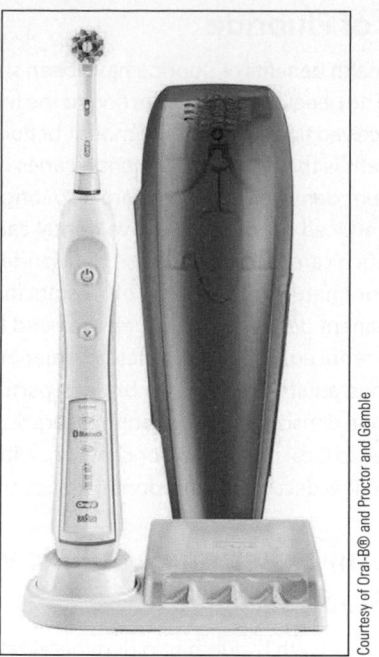

Courtesy of Oral-B® and Proctor and Gamble

FIGURE 16-45
Oral B pro 5000 automatic toothbrush with Bluetooth communication.

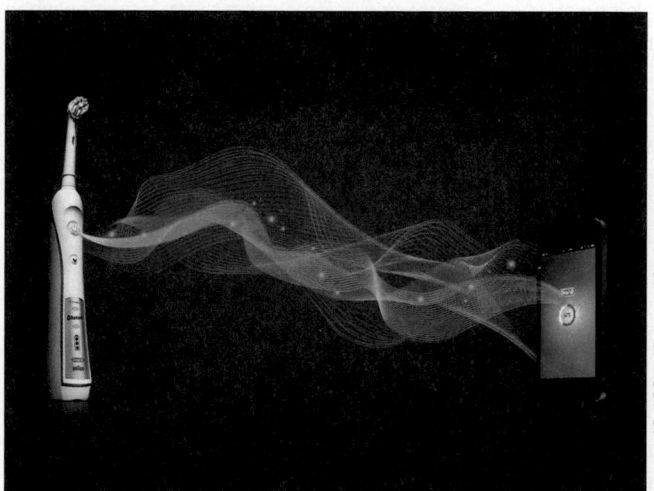

Courtesy of Oral-B® and Proctor and Gamble

FIGURE 16-46
Action with Bluetooth communication.

0.12% chlorhexidine into deeper pockets more effectively than using a toothbrush, interdental aid, or rinsing. A specialized tip to clean the tongue can also be used with this device.

The patient should be instructed on the importance of carefully using the oral irrigator. Improper use can cause tissue damage when turned on high and directed toward the gingival sulcus. The device could force debris into the tissue and damage the periodontium. The irrigator should be used at a low speed and in a direction that forces debris to be pushed away from the gingival area. The patient should first fill the fluid-holding container with fresh water, an antimicrobial agent, or mouthwash to gain fresh breath in the process (Figure 16-48). The water pressure is set to the lowest setting to prevent injury to the gingiva.

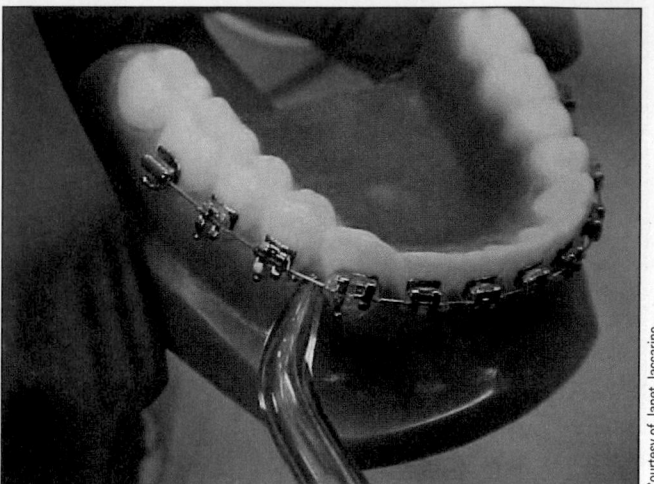

Courtesy of Janet Jaccarino

FIGURE 16-47
Oral irrigation tip placement.

The pressure can be increased over time as directed by the dentist. The desired tip is selected and attached to the unit. The patient is instructed to lean over a sink to allow the water to flow from the mouth. Place the tip in the mouth and turn the unit on. To clean supragingivally, direct the tip at a 90° angle to the tooth. Activate the flow of water and trace the gingival margin of the entire tooth buccal, lingual and interproximal. Stop the flow of water and move to the next area to repeat the process. For subgingival irrigation use the specialized thin plastic or rubber tip designed for this purpose and direct slightly below the gingival margin.

Fluoride

Fluoride is a natural mineral nutrient (fluorine) which has been found to be safe and effective by the Centers for Disease Control (CDC) and the World Health Organization (WHO) when used following established guidelines. For some patients self-applied fluoride may be a valuable addition to their home oral self-care program. Fluoride is essential to the formation of healthy bones and teeth, just as calcium and phosphorus are. When the fluoride content of the teeth is increased to the optimum level, there is a significant reduction in dental caries. Fluoride for home use is available over the counter or by prescription as dentifrices, mouth rinses, dietary supplements, and prescription gels.

Fluoride Content in the Bones and Teeth

- Normal bone contains 0.01 to 0.3 percent fluoride.
- Dental enamel contains 0.01 to 0.02 percent fluoride.
- Carious teeth contain as little as 0.0069 percent fluoride.

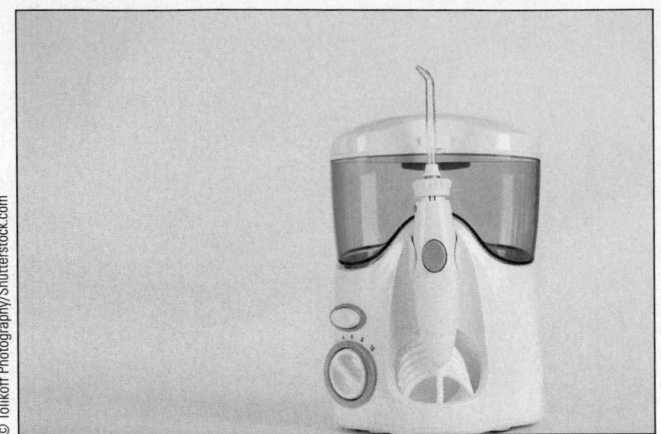

FIGURE 16-48
Oral irrigation device.

History of Fluoride in Dentistry

Early in the 1900s, Dr. G.V. Black and Dr. F. McKay of Colorado first revealed that people with **mottled enamel** (discolorations) did not have as much dental decay. In the 1930s, a chemist found a definite relationship between fluoride and mottled enamel. Eventually, an optimum level of fluoride was found. This level prevented dental caries without mottling the teeth. The optimum level was found to be 1 part per million (1 ppm). *Note: This level has since changed to 0.7 ppm. In some climates, this level may be adjusted slightly.* For example, in hot climates where people are likely to drink more water, the level may be reduced.

How much fluoride is in water?

At 1 ppm, one part of fluoride is diluted in a million parts of water. 1 ppm can be represented as:

1 inch in 16 miles
1 minute in 2 years
1 cent in $10,000

Source: American Dental Association. Water Fluoridation

Benefits of Fluoride

The dental health benefits of fluoride have been shown in numerous studies. The benefits are in proportion to the length of time an individual received fluoride and the amount of fluoride given. The primary benefit is the reduction of dental caries in both primary and permanent dentition, but there are also long-term benefits, such as the reduced need for extensive dental care and the time and cost of such care. Through the use of fluoride, primary teeth are not lost prematurely to decay. This results in less malocclusion in permanent dentition; therefore, the need for orthodontic treatment is reduced. There is also less permanent tooth loss at early ages. Thus, adults require fewer bridges, partials, or dentures. Improved bone density can affect bone resorption, loss of bone, and resistance to local mastication or chewing. With stronger alveolar bone and less decay, the periodontal tissues stay healthier.

Mechanism of Action: Systemic versus Topical Fluoride

Fluoride protects teeth by inhibiting demineralization, enhancing remineralization, and inhibiting bacterial activity. Fluoride works systemically when it is incorporated into a tooth while it is developing before it **erupts** into the mouth. Teeth are composed of minerals, one of which is **hydroxyapatite**. During tooth formation when fluoride is taken into a tooth, a fluoride **ion** replaces a hydroxyl ion and makes an improved mineral called **fluorapatite**. Fluorapatite is stronger, less **soluble**, and more resistant to the acids that cause tooth decay. Systemic fluoride comes from drinking water and ingesting supplements and food. After eruption, fluoride can be applied to the teeth topically. Topical uptake means the fluoride **diffuses** into the surface of the enamel of an erupted tooth. Topical fluoride is applied to the teeth by using toothpaste containing fluoride, mouth rinses, and professional application. It has been found that the most benefit from fluoride is through topical uptake.

Patient Assessment

Fluoride does have harmful effects such as nausea and vomiting associated with **ingestion** and dental **fluorosis**. When

TABLE 16-4 Self Applied Fluoride Therapies

Therapy	Fluoride Content	Indication for Use
Dentifrice (OTC)	1000-1100 parts per million (ppm). Sodium fluoride (Neutral pH) 0.24%, sodium monofluorophosphate 0.76%, and stannous fluoride 0.45%	Caries prevention
Prescription gel (Rx)	5000 parts per million (ppm). Sodium fluoride (Neutral pH, NaF) 1.1%, Acidulated sodium fluoride (3.5 pH, APF) 1.1%	High caries risk, control demineralization, orthodontic appliances, protect against post radiation caries
Mouth rinse (OTC and Rx)	OTC – NaF 0.05% and 0.022% OTC and Rx - NaF and APF 0.044% Rx - 0.2% NaF	Moderate – high caries risk, exposed root surfaces, hypersensitivity, control demineralization, orthodontic appliances,
Dietary supplements (Rx)	Rx – 0.25mg, 0.50mg and 1.0 dosage of NaF	For children ages 6 mos. -16years who do not have access to community water fluoridation, or a water supply containing less than 0.6 ppm. High risk of developing caries.

recommending home fluoride use, the benefits must be weighed against the potential harm (Table 16-5). During patient assessment, factors to consider include the patient's age, frequency of dental care, diet and nutrition, oral self-care practices, and the amount of fluoride the patient is receiving from other sources such as community water, school programs, and other home and professional therapy. Some well water contains natural fluoride and should be tested during the patient assessment before adding fluoride.

Fluoridation

Fluoridation is the process of adding fluoride to the community water supply. Adding fluoride to community water supplies is a controversial issue in many areas. Although it has been proven that adjusting the amount of fluoride to the optimum level does reduce dental caries, some people oppose fluoridation. Much has been written about the fluoride controversy, and dental assistants need to be current on what is going on in their dental communities. Knowing whether the water is fluoridated, the benefits of fluoridation, and the effects of too much fluoride will better prepare the assistant to answer patients' questions.

Fluoride Toxicity

Fluoride, like many other substances, can be **toxic** when absorbed in excessive amounts. Today, fluorides are regulated carefully by occupational health legislation and governmental agencies. Over the years, it has been found that the toxicity of fluoride depends on the duration and dosage of ingestion. Fluoride used in dentistry presents little or no risk for acute toxicity. However, the dental assistant should be aware of the possibilities of fluoride poisoning, and when and where it has occurred, because patients may have questions.

Fluoride Ingestion When large amounts of fluoride are ingested, inhaled, or absorbed into the body at one time, **acute** fluoride poisoning occurs; it is extremely rare. The lethal dose varies from 2.5 to 10 grams in adults to as low as 0.25 grams in infants. A medical doctor should be contacted whenever excessive amounts of fluoride are ingested at one time. When there is suspected toxicity, the patient should drink milk and then seek medical treatment immediately. Milk acts as a demulcent, a medicine that soothes irritated mucous membranes. It also helps with the mild nausea the patient may have.

Ingestion of high fluoride levels in water, or combinations of several fluoride sources over a period of time, results in **chronic** fluoride poisoning. Two effects of chronic fluoride overdose are crippling fluorosis (skeletal hypermineralization of ligaments) and mottled enamel. (Figures 16–49 and 16–50) With today's health and safety controls in industry, crippling fluorosis can be avoided. Mottled enamel is caused by excess exposure to fluoride during the time of tooth development. When the fluoride level is from 1.8 to 2.0 ppm, the enamel shows varying degrees of white areas or brown lines, a condition called enamel hypoplasia (Table 16-5). Because high levels of fluoride occur naturally in some areas, mottled enamel would be more common in those areas unless the amount of fluoride in the water supply were adjusted to the optimum level.

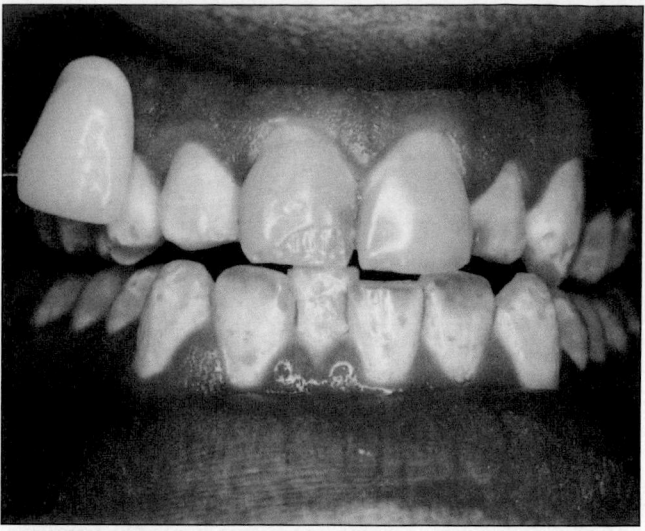

FIGURE 16-49
Dental fluorosis on a new patient who was seeking cosmetic dentistry. Notice the shade guide to the side.

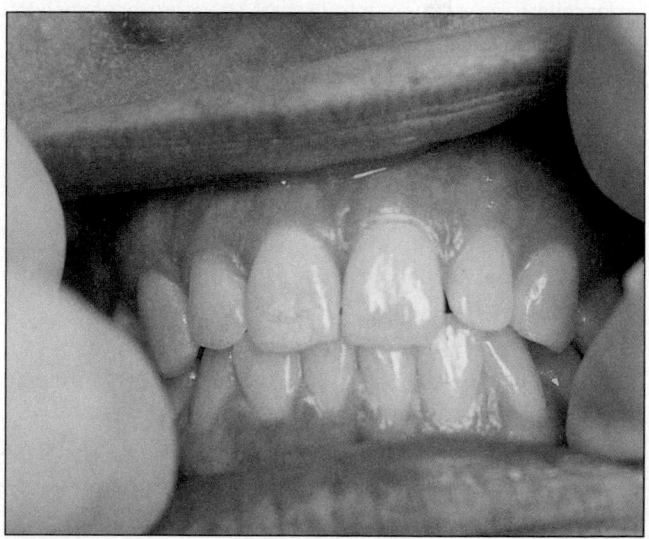

FIGURE 16-50
Mild dental fluorosis.

Mottled enamel is pitted because of a deficiency in the number of ameloblasts (enamel-forming cells) and chalky because of a lack of mineral deposits.

Systemic Fluoride

Systemic fluoride is ingested and then circulated through the body to the developing teeth. Sources of systemic fluoride include fluoridated water, food containing fluoride, and fluoride dietary supplements.

- Fluoride may be added to the community or school water supply. The level of natural fluoride is evaluated to adjust water supplies to the optimum level prescribed for dental health. Sodium fluoride is used in the community water supply. Foods such as meat, vegetables, cereals, and citrus fruits

TABLE 16-5 Appearance of Teeth with Exposure to Different Levels of Fluoride

Amount of Fluoride Exposure	Appearance of the Teeth
Exposure between 0.7 and 1.2 ppm (the optimum level depending on average temperature of the area)	Teeth are white, opaque, and shiny without blemishes.
Exposure up to 1.8 ppm	The structure of the enamel is not affected, but chalky bands or flecks can be seen on the surface.
Exposure over 1.8 ppm	Chalky bands or flecks appear on the surface and the enamel structure is affected; this is known as **enamel hypocalcification**. The chalky bands and flecks discolor with time. With increased exposure to fluoride, the enamel may become cracked and pitted.

naturally contain small amounts of fluoride. Tea and fish have slightly higher amounts of fluoride.

- Fluoride dietary supplements supplied as tablets, drops, and lozenges require a prescription from a dentist or physician. Vitamins with fluoride are also available. According to the ADA Council on Scientific Affairs, no fluoride supplements should be prescribed before the age of 6 months. Recommendations are for children ages 6 months to 16 years. Drops are recommended for children under 2 years of age and should be swallowed, tablets for children from 2 to16 years old should be chewed, and lozenges for children 2 to 16 years old should be retained in the mouth until dissolved. When using fluoride supplements avoid taking with any calcium-containing product such as milk to ensure complete **bioavailability** of the fluoride.

- The ADA's Council on Dental Therapeutics recommends that specific amounts of fluoride be prescribed according to the child's age and weight.

- Studies have shown a 50 to 65% reduction in caries for patients who have received the optimum prescribed amount of fluoride during tooth development.

- Not all bottled water contains fluoride. Be sure to check the label if fluoride benefits are desired and bottled water is the water supply.

The amount of natural fluoride in a water supply can be determined by tests done by private laboratories, as well as by state and county agencies. In rural areas and cities without fluoridated water, children should receive fluoride supplements. The dentist should assist the parents in determining the methods and amount of fluoride the child should receive for maximum benefit. It is important that the fluoride supplement be taken continuously during tooth development to be most effective.

Topical Fluoride

Topical fluoride is another method that makes the tooth more resistant to demineralization, and also assists in the remineralization of decalcified areas. Because topical fluoride only penetrates the outer layer of the enamel, it is most effective if the tooth is cleaned before application. Cleaning can be accomplished by tooth brushing or a professional rubber-cup polish. Topical fluoride application in the Dental Office is discussed in Chapter Dental Prophylaxis and Recare Appointment.

Dual Benefit of Chewing Fluoride Tablets

If fluoride tablets are chewed before being swallowed, the teeth benefit from both the topical and systemic fluoride applications.

Types of Self-Applied Topical Fluoride Therapy Self-applied fluoride for home use is available over the counter or by prescription as dentifrices, prescription gels, and dietary supplements. Fluoride in biofilm binds within bacteria and causes an antibacterial effect that inhibits the production of acids responsible for dental decay.

- Brushing with a fluoride dentifrice approved by the ADA is readily available and cost effective. It is one of the best ways to incorporate caries prevention as part of a thorough oral self-care strategy.

- Fluoride at greater strengths is available through prescription and is used as a supplement in office professional applications. The gel can be used with a brush-on technique or applied with the use of a custom tray.

- Mouth rinses containing fluoride are available over the counter and at greater strengths through prescription. Some mouth rinses contain alcohol and should be used with caution in certain patient populations.

Hygiene Care of Prosthetic Appliances

A patient may have prosthetic appliances that require special oral hygiene care for obtaining the desired biofilm-free result each day. Professional knowledge and guidance will aid patients in the care of their prosthetic appliances, such as full or partial dentures, fixed bridges, implants, and orthodontic brackets.

Full and Partial Dentures

Since biofilm, debris, and calculus can accumulate on a partial or full denture, it is important for the patient to know how to thoroughly clean these appliances and the surrounding tissues daily. The dentures should be removed following a meal and overnight. Failure to remove the denture can result in a bacterial or fungal

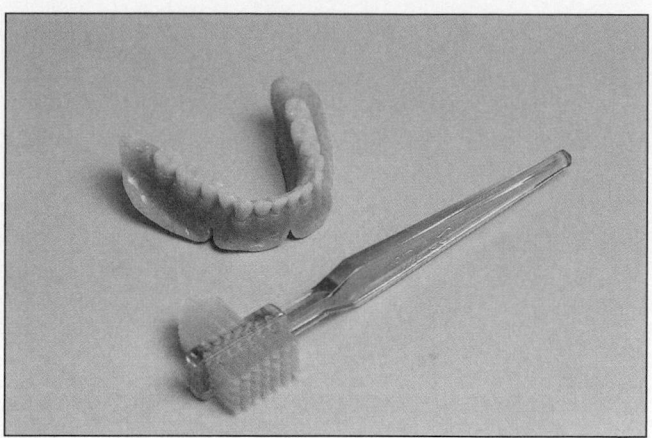

FIGURE 16-51
Denture and denture toothbrush.

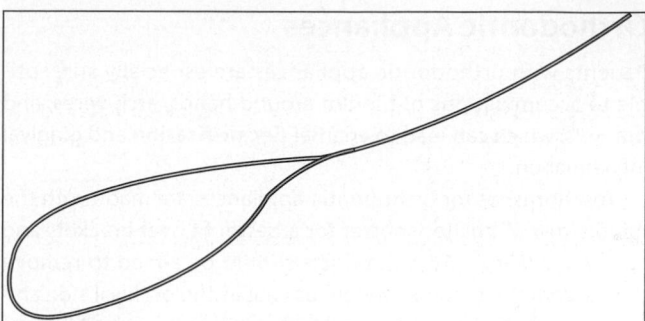

FIGURE 16-52
A Floss threader.

infection, irritation of the soft tissue, increased resorption of the alveolar bone, and oral **malodor**. Whenever a denture is out of the mouth, it should be stored in water to prevent shrinkage and distortion of the acrylic. Clean dentures using commercial cleaning agents and a brush designed for this purpose. Using a specially formulated chemical soak has the advantage of reaching all parts of the denture whereas just brushing alone may miss some areas. A combination of soaking and brushing may more thoroughly clean the denture (Figure 16-51). Abrasive powder or paste and mouthwashes containing essential oils or alcohol are not recommended for denture cleaning because they can cause damage to the plastic.

Before cleaning the denture, fill a basin with water and line with a towel to prevent damage. Remove the denture and rinse away any saliva, debris, and denture adhesive. Hold the denture over the basin and use the brush to clean all areas including any clasps. Rinse the denture under running water, being sure to remove any cleaner, and store in a container with water.

After a patient receives a denture they may feel their dental care is over. They think that if they do not have teeth then they do not have to see a dentist. Patients need to be instructed on oral hygiene and encouraged to have routine dental office visits. Every night the patient needs to rub and massage their gums and palate with a coarse, cheap, wet washcloth. The patient should be scheduled for a yearly dental visit for oral cancer exams and evaluation of the jawbone and gingiva regarding the fit of the denture and dental health.

Fixed Bridges

A fixed bridge that is anchored on both sides with a **pontic** in the middle will not allow for normal flossing. The patient will need special instructions on how to use a floss threader (see Procedure 16-5 and refer to Figures 16–52 and 16–53) to remove biofilm and debris from under the bridge. The patient may also need special brushing instructions to clean the gingival area more carefully.

Implants

Patients with implants must be diligent about oral self-care because biofilm can easily accumulate, causing dental disease. Peri-implant inflammation can occur around an implant with

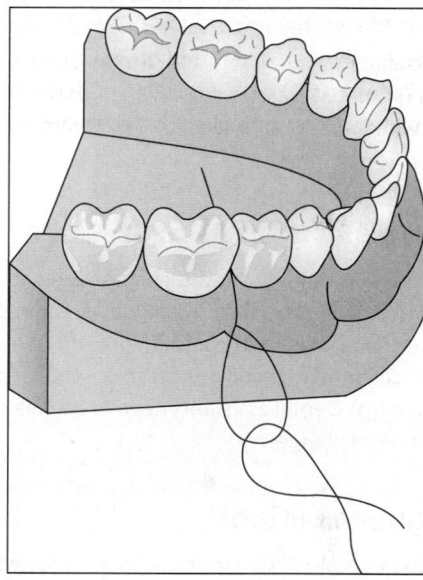

FIGURE 16-53
Floss threader threaded under the pontic (false tooth) area of a bridge.

subsequent bleeding, **suppuration**, and eventual bone loss. It is critical to use a soft toothbrush and low-abrasive toothpaste to avoid damage to the implant and surrounding tissues. The Bass position of 45° angle toward the gingiva is recommended. A power brush can be as useful for implants as it is for natural teeth. In addition, the toothbrush or any of the aids mentioned here can be dipped in an antimicrobial mouth rinse such as 0.12% chlorhexidine gluconate to reduce bacteria around the implant.

An interdental brush can reach between implants from the buccal and lingual areas. It is best to choose a brush with nylon-coated wires rather than metal wires to avoid damage to the implant. A rubber tip can clean around the implant and be used to message and stimulate the soft tissue. If the space is tight dental floss or dental tape can be placed around the implant; crisscross the floss and use it in a shoe-shine motion on the buccal and lingual areas. An end tuft brush can be used to clean around individual implants. Oral irrigation is also useful to remove loose debris and deliver an antimicrobial mouth rinse.

Orthodontic Appliances

Patients with orthodontic appliances are especially suscepti-ble to accumulations of biofilm around bands, arch wires, and brackets, which can lead to enamel **decalcification** and gingival inflammation.

Toothbrushes for orthodontic appliances are made with the middle row of bristles shorter for a better fit over brackets and arch wires (Figure 16-54). Efforts should be aimed to remove debris from the gingival margin as well as the occlusal side and gingival side of the bracket and arch wires using a combination of the Bass, Stillman, and Charters brushing positions.

Interdental cleaning can be challenging, but there are many products designed for this purpose such as an Orthodontic Flosser shown in Figures 16–55A and 16–55B. Flossing can also be accomplished with the use of a floss threader (Figure 16-56). An interdental brush or an end tufted brush can be used to clean around and between the arch wires. A wooden wedge or rub-ber tip stimulator is useful to clean brackets and message the papillae.

Challenges to Oral Self-Care

As you have learned throughout this chapter dental care for each patient should be based on their individual needs including oral self-care. There are however those patients whose oral environ-ment or physical or mental abilities present a challenge to effec-tive biofilm control. Dental assistants need to be creative to meet the oral hygiene challenges.

The Pregnant Patient

Pregnant patients may require special dental hygiene techniques because of the nausea that often accompanies pregnancy. Regur-gitation will repeatedly bring acid from the stomach over the

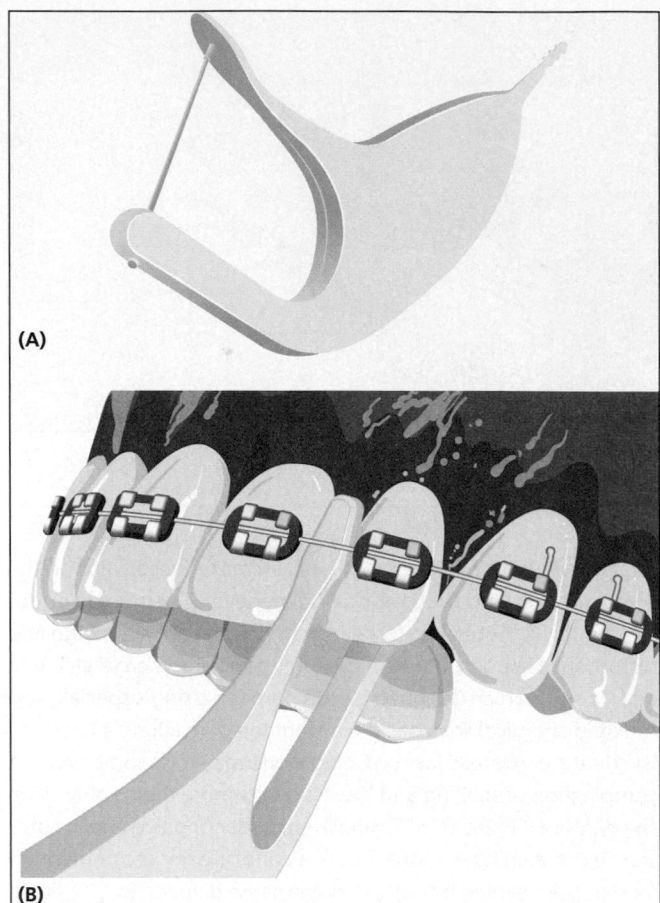

(A)

(B)

FIGURE 16-55
Orthodontic Flosser.

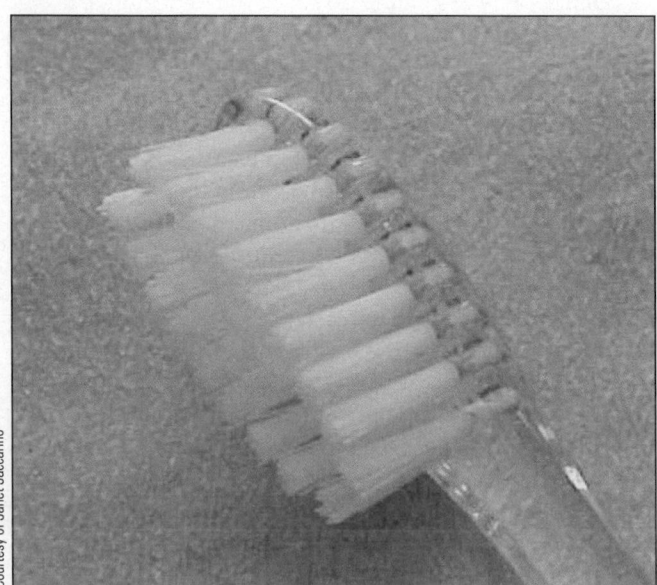

Courtesy of Janet Jaccarino

FIGURE 16-54
Orthodontic toothbrush.

surface of the teeth (this will also be a concern for patients with bulimia). Patients should be educated on the possible destruc-tion of the teeth from this acid repeatedly contacting the teeth. In addition, placing a toothbrush into the mouth may cause the patient to gag. Problem solve with the patient, and find a way to meet the goal of proper oral hygiene. Normally, eliminating toothpaste, and identifying specific times of the day when the pregnant patient is less nauseated, allows tooth brushing and flossing to be made more comfortable during pregnancy. The dental assistant should tell the pregnant patient that increased gingival bleeding is normal and that routine prophylaxis (clean-ing) is recommended during pregnancy. The patient's physician should approve any dental treatment.

The Infant Patient

Baby teeth start to form before birth; therefore, it is important for the mother to have a healthy pregnancy. The mother's diet defi-ciencies may result in abnormal tooth formation and calcification, so it is important for pregnant women to eat a well-balanced diet and take daily vitamin and mineral supplements. Pregnant women should have a complete dental exam, and any dental disease should be treated. The American Academy of Pediatric Dentistry

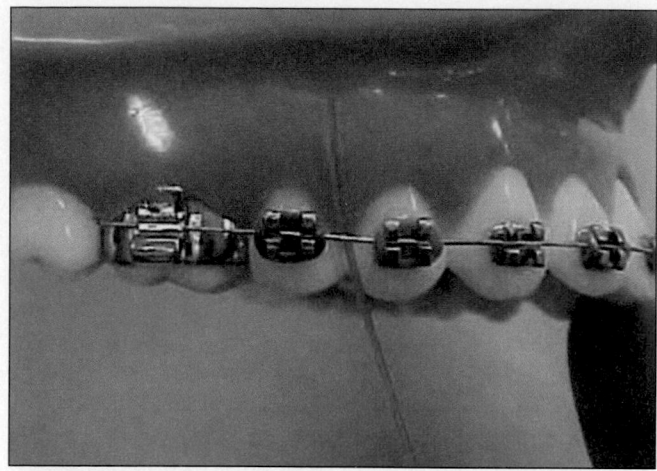

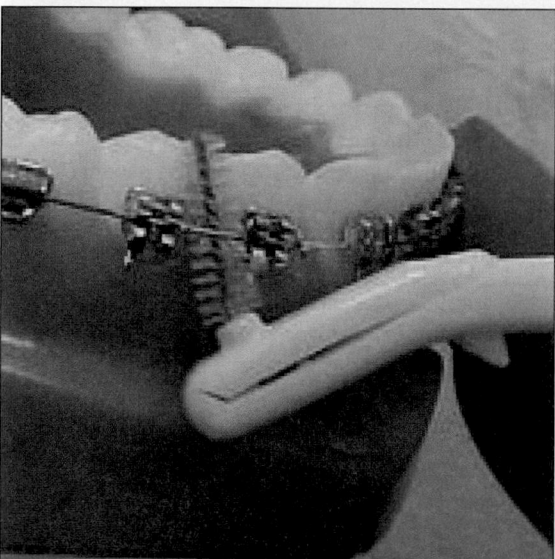

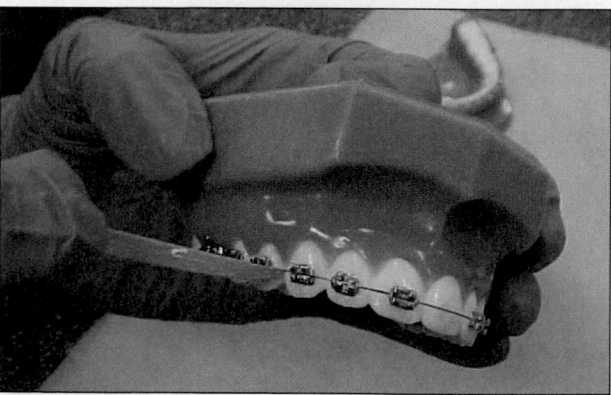

Images courtesy of the Department of Allied Dental Education, Rutgers University

FIGURE 16-56
Interdental cleaning for orthodontic appliances.

recommends that a child should see a dentist as soon as the first tooth comes in between 6 months and 1 year of age. Dental problems and pain can lead to trouble chewing, speaking, and learning. An early examination and prevention program will establish good oral self-care and eating habits for a lifelong healthy mouth.

Even though an infant does not have teeth, it is still important to clean their mouth daily especially after feeding and at bedtime.

Cleaning the baby's gums will prevent bacteria from adhering to the area and damaging the teeth as they come into the mouth. Gently wipe the baby's gums with a soft, moistened washcloth or a piece of gauze. A finger cot which fits over the finger can also be used and is especially made for this purpose. After the teeth erupt, continue to use a cloth or switch to a soft-bristled, infant-sized toothbrush. Clean between the teeth using a floss holder designed for children. By the time the molars first appear around age 1, it is best to use a toothbrush all the time.

The Older Patient

For many older patients with arthritis, holding floss and a toothbrush is difficult. There are toothbrushes with large, soft handles that help these patients. A floss holder can be used to secure the floss tightly as it is placed between the teeth. Listen to these patients and keep in mind that they want to save their teeth to be able to eat properly. Many are afraid of having dentures. The wonderful thing about older patients is that they often have time to listen carefully to oral hygiene directions, and to ask questions to clarify what is required to meet their oral hygiene goals.

The Patient with Cancer

Patients with cancer may have a number of oral manifestations due to the cancer and the therapy. Loss of muscle function, gingival bleeding, rampant caries, and xerostomia may compromise the skills of good oral hygiene. Xerostomia is abnormal dryness of the mouth and may be due to radiation or chemotherapy treatments. The patient may have a number of problems to overcome, such as root caries. Home topical fluoride treatments are often suggested to help eliminate these problems. Listen and problem solve with the patient. It will be important that infection does not perpetuate in the oral cavity and compound the patient's condition. The dental assistant may suggest that an extra-soft toothbrush, or a moistened foam toothbrush, be used on the tender tissues along with a nonabrasive fluoride toothpaste. Maintaining the teeth and tissues will allow the patient to eat properly and regain a healthier state. Use empathy, encouragement, and sincerity to motivate the patient.

The Patient with Heart Disease

Patients with heart disease may express a number of the same problems that cancer patients have due to medication usage. Many have xerostomia, gingival bleeding, and rampant caries. Patients with congestive heart disease will be uncomfortable in the chair if the chair is reclined (this brings increased fluid around the heart, and patients feel as if they are suffocating). Be aware of the patient's health status, address the problems that are identified, aid the patient through education, and be understanding when seeking a method to accomplish good oral hygiene.

The Patient with Disabilities

Poor oral hygiene and dental disease may be more prevalent in persons with disabilities due to the effects of their condition and medication on the oral environment. For example, some patients, especially those with arthritis, cannot grasp a toothbrush or even bend their elbow to reach their mouth. Persons with developmental disabilities may have **malocclusion** or teeth with developmental defects. Persons with a mental disability may have oral habits such as pouching of food. Some patients may have poor physical coordination. These issues may inhibit the ability for self-care, contributing to poor oral hygiene. Many medications that a patient with disabilities may be taking have side effects such as xerostomia, which may contribute to the development of dental disease. These issues may contribute to poor oral condition that may have serious health implications. For these reasons it is essential for the dental assistant to assess each patient's needs and provide oral self-care education to help them or their caregiver develop the skills to prevent oral disease and maintain health. A daily preventive program should be effective, simple to use, and low cost.

Assessment and skill evaluation can help determine if the patient can do what you want them to do. Can the patient brush and floss on their own, or are they partially or totally dependent on a caregiver? Is the patient able to understand and follow directions? How does the patient's disability affect self-care, and what modifications will be necessary to enable the patient to be as independent as possible? Watching the patient's current technique will help to determine their skill level. Be sure to ask them to reach the most difficult areas of the mouth such as the lingual of the lower molars. Ask the patient questions to determine if they will understand and follow directions.

The dental assistant may need to design a custom device for self-care. It is important to judge the patient's physical and mental limitations that will affect its use. For example, before recommending an automatic toothbrush, make sure the patient is strong enough to lift it and hold it for at least 2 minutes. Oral care products can be modified so that the patient will be able to perform daily oral hygiene. A tennis ball or bicycle handle grip can be attached to the end of a toothbrush to make the handle bigger, providing

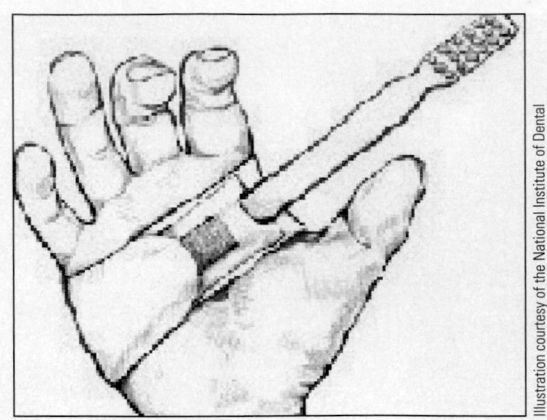

FIGURE 16-58
Velcro® strap.

Illustration courtesy of the National Institute of Dental and Craniofacial Research, National Institutes of Health

a better grip for the patient with arthritis. Foam tubing, available from health care catalogues, may also be helpful (Figure 16-57).

For the patient who cannot close their hand around a toothbrush, a Velcro® strap used to hold food utensils can be modified to hold a toothbrush (Figure 16-58). The patient can also purchase a commercially available modified product such as the Surround® Toothbrush available from the Specialized Care Company. This toothbrush is designed to clean the buccal and lingual tooth surfaces at the same time using only one motion (Figure 16-59).

Any custom oral self-care device should be easy to use, inexpensive, light-weight, and have parts that are easy to replace (Figure 16-60). In addition it should not cause damage to the teeth or gingiva. Remember the size of the toothbrush brush head selected for the patient is determined by the size of their mouth and their ability to open. A soft bristle, rounded, nylon toothbrush is the best choice.

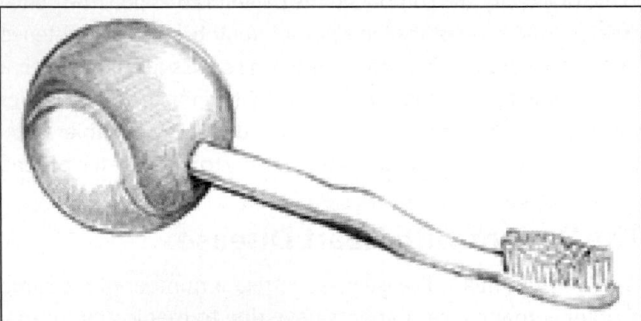

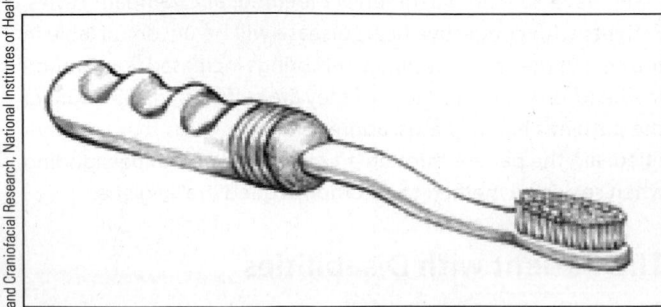

Illustrations courtesy of the National Institute of Dental and Craniofacial Research, National Institutes of Health

FIGURE 16-57
Make the toothbrush handle bigger.

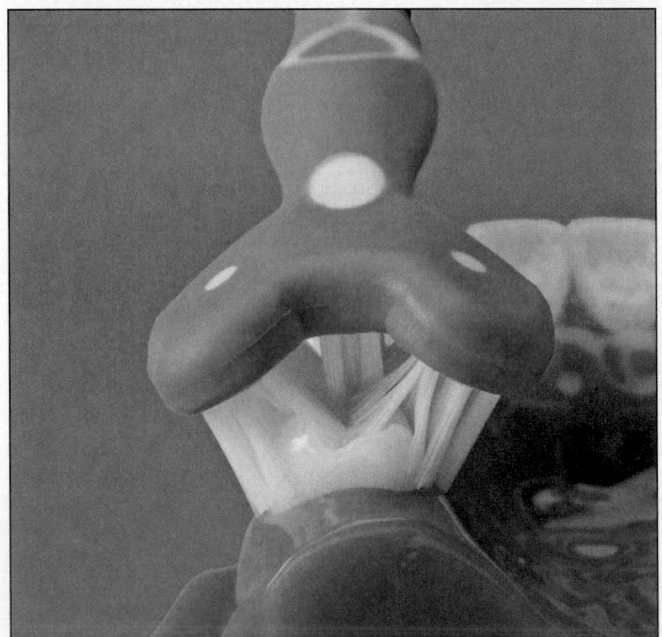

Image courtesy of the Specialized Care Company, Hampton, NH

FIGURE 16-59
Surround® Toothbrush.

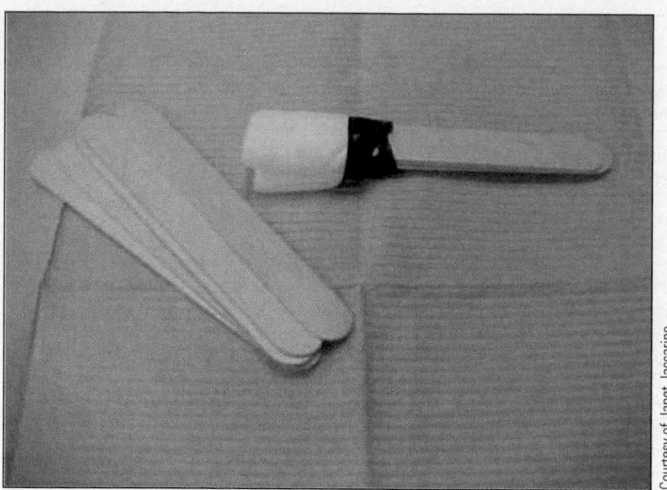

FIGURE 16-60
Custom handle for patients unable to grasp regular sized handles.

Dental Public Health

Dental public health, part of the much larger public health infrastructure (Table 16-6), is recognized by the American Dental Association as one of the dental specialties and focuses on oral health issues in communities and populations. Examples of dental public health include fewer caries because of school and water fluoride programs, less periodontal disease because of education and access to quality care, and less oral cancer because

of tobacco cessation and screening programs, research, and evidence-based practice.

Healthy People 2020

"Healthy People is a set of goals and objectives with 10-year targets designed to guide national health promotion and disease prevention efforts to improve the health of all people in the United States." Healthy People recognizes the impact of oral disease and overall health and has set 17 goals to help improve oral health. The goals include the reduction of dental disease through increased access to care and programs aimed at prevention of disease. The various public health organizations track the progress of these objectives.

Surgeon General's Report on Oral Health

In 2000 the Office of the Surgeon General released the first-ever report that highlights the importance of oral health to general health and well-being. While the report states that great progress has been made to reduce the extent and severity of oral diseases, it also notes the fact that not all Americans are experiencing the same degree of improvement. There are certain populations that are at greater risk for oral disease. Children, the elderly, members of racial and ethnic groups, low socioeconomic status populations, and those with disabilities often face challenges in obtaining oral care. The report calls for practitioners, communities, and lawmakers to form partnerships that will improve the oral health of all individuals.

TABLE 16-6 Public Health Organizations

World Health Organization (WHO) - the directing and coordinating authority for health within the United Nations system. It is responsible for providing leadership on global health matters, shaping the health research agenda, setting norms and standards, articulating evidence-based policy options, providing technical support to countries and monitoring and assessing health trends
Pan American Health Organization (PAHO) - an international public health agency working to improve health and living standards of the people of the Americas
U.S. Department of Health and Human Services (USDHHS) - government's principal agency for protecting the health of all Americans and providing essential human services, especially for those who are least able to help themselves
Centers for Disease Control (CDC) - a federal agency under the Department of Health and Human Services. Its main goal is to protect public health and safety through the control and prevention of disease, injury, and disability. The CDC focuses national attention on developing and applying disease control and prevention
Food and Drug Administration (FDA) - responsible for protecting the public health by assuring the safety, efficacy and security of human and veterinary drugs, biological products, medical devices, our nation's food supply, cosmetics, and products that emit radiation. Also has responsibility for regulating the manufacturing, marketing and distribution of tobacco products to protect the public health and to reduce tobacco use by minors
National Institutes of Health (NIH) - mission is to seek fundamental knowledge about the nature and behavior of living systems and the application of that knowledge to enhance health, lengthen life, and reduce illness and disability
Office of the Surgeon General - The Surgeon General of the United States is the nation's leading spokesman on matters of public health.
National Institute of Dental and Craniofacial Research (NIDCR) - is a branch of the U.S. National Institutes of Health. The institute aims to improve the oral, dental, and craniofacial health through research and the distribution of important health information to the American people.
Indian Health Service (IHS) - within the U.S. Department of Health and Human Services (HHS). IHS is responsible for providing medical and public health services to members of federally recognized Tribes and Alaska Natives. IHS is the principal federal health care provider and health advocate for Indian people, and its goal is to raise their health status to the highest possible level
Health Resources and Services Administration (HRSA) - an agency of the U.S. Department of Health and Human Services, is the primary Federal agency for improving access to health care by strengthening the health care workforce, building healthy communities and achieving health equity. HRSA's programs provide health care to people who are geographically isolated, economically or medically vulnerable

TABLE 16-7 Dental Care Programs Supported by the Government

Medicaid - is the largest government program that finances dental care for eligible low income populations in the United States. Each state is required to provide dental benefits to eligible children; however states may choose whether or not to provide dental benefits for adults. (Medicaid.gov)
Children's Health Insurance Program (CHIP) - provides oral health care for children in families with incomes too high to qualify for Medicaid, but can't afford private coverage. CHIP provides federal matching funds to states to provide this coverage. (Medicaid.gov)
Maternal and Child Health Bureau (MCHB) - the goal of the bureau is to promote comprehensive, community-based oral health care for women, infants and children through government program grants. (MCHB - HERSA.gov)
Federally Qualified Health Centers (FQHC) - are also known as "safety net" dental clinics. They provide care to the uninsured, underinsured, patients with Medicaid, Medicare and private insurance. Fees are based on your ability to pay and no one is ever turned away for lack of funds. (HERSA.gov)
State-based Oral Disease Prevention Programs - started by the CDC this program provides financial support to state oral health programs to enable them to provide oral health promotion and disease prevention programs. (CDC.gov)
Access to Care - There are solutions to the problem of access to care for those living in underserved areas. These include mobile dental services that use vans and trailers set up to provide care and teledentistry which uses communication technology for long distance diagnosis and consultation with specialists in other parts of the country. Finally, dental professionals can volunteer their services in many ways through community and their organization efforts.

While progress has been made in reducing dental disease, there remain many people in the United States who do not receive regular dental care. Barriers that prevent use of regular oral health care include cost, family structure and limited family income, lack of dental insurance, lack of education and health literacy, lack of perceived need for regular dental care, inability to take time off from work, and place of residence and geographic location which affect the available providers and transportation. In addition, those who depend on others, those with disabilities, and those who are institutionalized often face the problem of access to regular care.

Government Financing of Dental Care

Without private dental insurance the expense of treatment can be a great burden for vulnerable populations. Treatment in private dental offices is impossible for some; however, there are government and state programs that provide services to those who qualify (Table 16-7).

Community Oral Health Prevention Programs

Health care professionals realize that it is much more cost effective to prevent a disease or condition than it is to actually provide treatment. For populations at risk most oral diseases are preventable through programs that provide oral health education and intervention. Community and school-based programs provide dental sealants, oral cancer screening, and tobacco cessation. Many of these programs involve partnerships that charitable organizations, universities, community health agencies, and federal, state, and local governments as well as volunteers from the dental profession. Dental public health departments have been instrumental in implementing community fluoridated water. The addition of small amounts of fluoride to community water supplies provides cost effective protection against caries for the greatest number of people living in that community. Studies show that community water fluoridation reduces dental decay by 20 to 40% even with the use of other products containing fluoride. The United States now has over 60 years of practical experience with community water fluoridation. Its remarkable longevity is testimony to fluoridation's significance as a public health measure. In recognition of the impact that water fluoridation has had on the oral and general health of the public, in 1999, the Centers for Disease Control and Prevention named fluoridation of drinking water as one of 10 great public health achievements of the twentieth century.

Chapter Summary

In order to be effective in preventive dentistry, dental assistants must first care for their own teeth properly. Becoming knowledgeable about the oral disease process will aid the dental assistant in educating patients on its prevention. The dental assistant must have the knowledge to solve oral hygiene concerns, know what preventive aids are available, and then aid patients in maintaining their teeth and gums. The dental assistant should encourage the patient to follow a good preventive program consisting of these practices:

- Brush and floss daily to remove biofilm and bacteria.
- Periodically disclose to evaluate the effectiveness of brushing and flossing.
- Follow a fluoride program while the teeth are developing to allow them to be strong and decay resistant. The fluoride program includes office applications and home treatments.

- See a dentist for routine care and, especially, when teeth newly erupt in order to have the dentist evaluate if dental sealants need to be placed in areas where there are faulty unions in the enamel. (See Chapter 26, "Dental Sealants.")
- Follow a good nutrition and exercise program to maintain overall health. Good nutrition over a lifetime allows strong teeth and bones to develop and be maintained (See Chapter 17, "Nutrition").
- Schedule regular dental visits for a thorough examination, cleaning, and any necessary dental treatment.

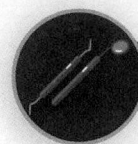 **CASE STUDY**

Heidi Ann Jones, a 17-year-old, came into the dental office concerned with the discoloration of her teeth. After a thorough examination by the dentist, the findings showed that she had no caries, one restoration, and marginal gingivitis.

Case Study Review

1. What further questions would be important to ask Heidi?
2. What preventive techniques would benefit Heidi?

Review Questions

Multiple Choice

1. A sticky mass that contains bacteria and grows in colonies on the teeth is called what?
   a. caries
   b. demineralization
   c. biofilm
   d. acid

2. How soon after brushing their teeth may a patient expect biofilm to begin forming?
   a. within seconds
   b. 2 hours
   c. 4 to 6 hours
   d. 12 hours

3. If biofilm is left undisturbed on the tooth and sugar is introduced, what may happen?
   a. caries
   b. fluorosis
   c. xerostomia
   d. poisoning

4. What is the primary cause of gingivitis?
   a. poor nutrition
   b. biofilm
   c. xerostomia
   d. demineralization

5. What can be applied to developing teeth to allow them to be strong and decay resistant?
   a. disclosing solution
   b. fluoride
   c. fermentable carbohydrates
   d. mouth rinses

6. At what age can motivating the patient that oral hygiene will help them fit in with peers and brushing and flossing proficiently can be taught?
   a. 5–8 years
   b. 9–12 years
   c. 13–15 years
   d. 16–19 years

7. Which of the following is the recommended order to complete oral self-care?
   a. tooth brushing, tongue cleaning, and flossing
   b. flossing, tooth brushing, and tongue cleaning
   c. tongue cleaning, flossing, and tooth brushing
   d. tooth brushing, flossing, and tongue cleaning

8. Why is it recommended to have a nylon bristled toothbrush?
   a. for ease of cleaning
   b. to prevent teeth and gum injury
   c. to reduce the cost of the brush
   d. to last longer

9. Which brushing technique has the bristles pointed at a 45° angle into the sulcus while using a gentle, short vibrating motion?
   a. Bass
   b. Fones
   c. Stillman
   d. Charters
   e. Roll

10. Which toothpaste ingredient and brushing technique used together is more likely to injure the teeth?
   a. fluoride and Charters
   b. detergents and Fones
   c. abrasives and scrub
   d. whiteners and Bass

11. What motion should be used when guiding the floss between the teeth?
   a. snapping
   b. see-saw
   c. straight pressure
   d. depends on how tight the contacts are

12. Since patients may have difficulty in identifying biofilm, what can be used to help them see it more easily?
   a. a flashlight
   b. a mouth mirror
   c. disclosing agent
   d. fluoride

13. A patient has all teeth except the third molars are missing. After disclosing you indicate that there are 20 areas of biofilm. Using the biofilm control record assessment, what would be the patient's biofilm score?
   a. 10
   b. 15
   c. 18
   d. 20

14. A patient has open contact areas and large amount of periodontal bone loss. What aid would remove biofilm from this area?
   a. flosser
   b. floss threader

   c. interproximal brush
   d. interdental stimulator

15. When fluoride is incorporated into a tooth during development it makes an improved mineral called what?
   a. hydroxyapatite
   b. hydroxyl ion
   c. fluorapatite
   d. xylitol

16. How can the patient obtain systemic fluoride?
   a. drinking fluoridated water
   b. fluoride containing food
   c. fluoride supplements
   d. all of these

17. Which toothbrush is advocated for orthodontic tooth brushing?
   a. All bristle rows are even in height.
   b. The outer row of bristles is shorter.
   c. The middle row of bristles is shorter.
   d. There are five rows of bristles.

18. Why may a person with disabilities be at a higher risk of poor oral hygiene and dental disease?
   a. They have higher incidence of oral developmental defects.
   b. They may have poor physical coordination.
   c. Many medications have oral side effects.
   d. All of these may exist.

19. What is the largest government program that finance dental care for low income populations?
   a. CHIP
   b. CDC
   c. Medicaid
   d. Access to Care

20. What is the optimal level of water fluoridation?
   a. 0.7 ppm
   b. 1 ppm
   c. 10 ppm
   d. 25 ppm

Critical Thinking

1. Why would it be advantageous for the patient to brush using a wet toothbrush and floss before applying fluoride to the toothbrush and brushing?

2. How can disclosing agents and biofilm indices be used to educate and motivate a patient during oral self-care instruction?

3. What should the dental assistant consider before adding more oral hygiene aids to a patient's oral hygiene plan?

Key Terms

Term and Pronunciation	Meaning of Root and Word Parts	Definition
acquired pellicle (*uh*-**kwahy***uh* rd) (**pel**-i-*kuh* l)	**acquire** = to obtain or begin to have something **pellicle** = very, thin layer of protein; acts as a protective layer	thin, clear film of insoluble proteins, fats, and other materials from saliva that forms within minutes of removal; provide breeding ground for biofilm and calculus
acute (*uh*-**kyoot**)	**acute** = sharp or severe; intense	brief and severe symptoms of a disease
antimicrobial (an-tee-mahy-**kroh**-bee-*uh* l)	**anti-** = against **microbe** = microorganism **-al** = pertaining to	destructive to or inhibiting the growth of microorganisms
antiseptic (an-t*uh*-**sep**-tik)	**anti-** = against **sepsis** = invasion by pathogenic microorganisms or their toxins **-ics** = having characteristics	free from or cleaned of germs and other microorganisms
bactericidal (bak-**teer**-*uh*-sahyd l)	**bacteria** = bacterium; one-celled organisms; may be involved in infectious diseases **cide** = act of killing **-al** = pertaining to	capable of killing bacteria
bacteriostatic (bak-teer-ee-*uh*- **stat**-ik)	**bacteria** = bacterium; one-celled organisms; may be involved in infectious diseases **stasis** = stoppage; cause to stand still **-ic** = having characteristics	preventing the further growth of bacteria
bioavailability (bahy-oh-*uh*-vey-l*uh*-**bil**-i-tee)	**bio-** = life, living organisms **available** = ready for use **-able** = having necessary power **-ity** = expressing state	the extent to which a nutrient or medication can be used by the body
biofilm (**bahy**-oh)	**bio-** = life **film** = a thin layer or coating	a sticky mass that contains mucus and bacteria and grows in colonies on the teeth; also referred to as dental plaque
calculus (**kal**-ky*uh*-l*uh*s)	**calc** = stone **-ule** = indicating smallness	hard, calcified deposit of mineralized biofilm that forms on teeth, restorations, and dental appliances; also known as tartar
cessation (*se*-**sey**-*shuh* n)	**cease** = to stop, delay, inactivity **-tion** = indicating action or process	a temporary or complete stopping
chronic (**kron**-ik)	**chron** = time **-ic** = relating to	continuing for a long time; constantly recurring
decalcification (dee-kal-suh-fi-**key**-shuh n)	**de-** = removal of or from something **calc** = calcium **-fication** = action or state	the act or process of loss of calcium from bone and tooth
demineralization (dee-**min**-er-*uh*-lahyz-shuhn)	**de-** = removal of or from something specified **mineral** = any of a class of substances occurring in nature, usually comprising inorganic substances, usually of definite crystal structure, but sometimes **-ize** = to convert into **-ate** = denotes function **-ion** = denotes action or condition	to remove minerals from; deprive of mineral content
dental caries (**den**-tl) (**kair**-eez)	**dent** = tooth **-al** = relating to **caries** = death	dental cavities; tooth decay

(Continues)

Term and Pronunciation	Meaning of Root and Word Parts	Definition
dental sealant (**den**-tl) (**see**-l*uh* nt)	**dent** = tooth **-al** = relating to **seal** = to close or block **-ant** = serving in the capacity of	a resin material used to seal pits and fissures on the enamel surface to prevent future decay
dentifrice (**den**-t*uh*-fris)	**denti** = tooth **fric** = to rub **-ice** = indicating state	a paste, powder, liquid, or other preparation for cleaning the teeth
dexterity (dek-**ster**-i-tee)	**dexter** = skillful **-ity** = denoting state or condition	skill in using the hands or body; agility
diffuse (dih-**fyooz**)	**dif** = differ **fuse** = to become united or blended	to spread over an area, to pass through a tissue or substance
edentulous (ee-**den**-ch*uh*-l*uh* s)	**e-** = without **dent** = teeth **-ulous** = inclined to do	lacking teeth; toothless
erupt (ih-**ruhpt**)	**erupt** = to burst through	when developing teeth break through the gums
extrinsic (ik-**strin**-sik, -zik)	**exterior** = outer; being on the outside **-ic** = having characteristics	being outside; outward or external; coming from without
fluorapatite (floo r-**ap**-*uh*-tahyt)	**fluor** = fluorine, fluoride **apatite** = mineral composed of calcium fluorophosphates or chlorophosphate	a crystalline mineral, $Ca_5(PO_4)_3F$, formed from hydroxyapatite in the presence of fluoride, that has a hardening effect on bones and teeth
fluoridation (floor-i-**dey**-sh*uh*n)	**fluor** = fluorine, fluoride **-ide** = used to name chemical compounds **-ation** = indicating process, action, result	the process of adding fluoride to the water supply
fluoride (**floor**-ahyd)	**fluor** = fluorine, fluoride **-ide** = used to name chemical compounds	a natural mineral nutrient derived from fluorine; essential to the formation of healthy bones and teeth
fluorosis (fl*oo*-**roh**-sis)	**fluor** = fluorine, fluoride **-osis** = denotes actions, conditions or states	an abnormal condition caused by excessive intake of fluorides; also called mottled enamel
furcation (**fur**-key-sh*uh*n)	**furcate** = forked, branching **-ation** = indicating process, action, result	a dividing point of a multirooted tooth; division of the roots
hydroxyapatite (hahy-drok-see-**ap**-*uh*-tahyt)	**hydroxyl** = chemical compound; principal storage form of calcium and phosphorous in bone **apatite** = mineral composed of calcium fluorophosphates or chlorophosphate	a mineral, $Ca_{10}(PO_4)_6OH_2$, that is the principal storage form of calcium and phosphorus in bone
implant (im-**plant**)	**im-** = in **plant** = to put or set in	an artificial tooth placed permanently within the bone of the jaw
indices (**in**-d*uh*-seez)	**index** = number indicating the relation of one part or thing to another **-ces** = plural form	the plural of index, which is a listing or an indicator
inflammation (in-fl*uh*-**mey**-sh*uh*n)	**inflame** = to cause redness and heat **-ation** = the state of being	body's defense against infection or trauma; symptoms of redness, heat, pain, and swelling may occur
ingestion (in-**jest**-ch*uh* n)	**ingest** = to take (food or liquid) into the body **-tion** = indicating process	consuming something orally, whether it be food, drink, medicine, or other substance; it is usually referred to as the first step of digestion
ion (**ahy**-*uh* n)	**ion** = a charged subatomic particle	an atom or molecule with a net electric charge due to the loss or gain of one or more electrons

Term and Pronunciation	Meaning of Root and Word Parts	Definition
interproximal (in-tur-**prok**-suh-muh l)	**inter** = between **proximity** = adjoining; nearest next **-al** = pertaining to	also called interdental area; is the gap that exists between teeth and that is occupied by the gums; spaces facilitate the appearance and accumulation of oral biofilm (bacterial plaque), as they are hard to clean even when teeth are in a normal position
keratinization (ker-uh-tn-ahy-**zey**-shuh n)	**keratin** = a fibrous protein that occurs in the outer layer of the skin and in hair, nails, feathers, hooves **-ize** = to convert into **-ation** = indicating a process	the development of or conversion into keratin
malocclusion (mal-uh-**kloo**-zhuh n)	**mal-** = bad **occlude** = to close, shut **-ion** = denoting condition	faulty occlusion; irregular contact of opposing teeth in the upper and lower jaws
malodor (mal-**oh**-der)	**mal-** = bad **odor** = a sensation perceived by the sense of smell; scent	an unpleasant or offensive odor; stench
materia alba (muh-**teer**-ee-uh) (**ahl**-buh)	**matter** = a kind of substance **alba** = white matter	a white cheese like accumulation of food debris, microorganisms, tissue cell, and blood cells deposited around the teeth at the gumline
mottled enamel (**mot**-ld) (ih-**nam**-uh l)	**mottle** = spotted or blotched in coloring **-ed** = indicating a condition **enamel** = the hard, glossy, calcareous covering of the crown of a tooth, containing only a slight amount of organic substance	also referred to as hypomineralization; a condition caused by excessive amount fluoride during tooth formation resulting in a white chalky appearance to the enamel
mucositis (myoo-**koh**-sahy-tis)	**mucosa** = a lubricating membrane lining an internal surface of an organ, as the alimentary, respiratory, and oral cavity. **-itis** = inflammation	painful inflammation and ulceration of the mucous membranes of the mouth and lining the digestive tract
oral prophylaxis (**ohr**-uhl) (proh-fuh-**lak**-sis)	**or-** = mouth **-al** = relating to **pro-** = for or in favor of **phylaxis** = process of guarding	removal of hard deposits and polishing of the teeth with a rubber cup
papilla (puh-**pil**-uh) **papillae** (plural form)	**pap** = something resembling teat or nipple **-illa** = small, tiny	small raised projection covering the top of the tongue; or interdental papilla small raised projection of gingiva between two adjacent teeth
periodontal disease (per-ee-uh-**don**-tl) (dih-**zeez**)	**peri-** = surrounding **-odont** = tooth **-al** = relating to **dis-** = away, negative **ease** = freedom from pain or physical annoyance	common infection that damages the soft tissue and bone supporting the tooth; bone is slowly and progressively lost
periodontal pocket (per-ee-uh-**don**-tl) (**pok**-it)	**peri-** = surrounding **-odont** = tooth **-al** = relating to **pocket** = a small enclosed or isolated area	a diseased space between the inflamed gum and the surface of a tooth
periodontium (per-ee-uh-**don**-shuh m)	**peri-** = surrounding **-odont** = tooth **-ium** = indicating groups	the bone, connective tissue, and gum surrounding and supporting a tooth
pontic (**pon**-tik)	**pont** = replaces natural teeth **-ic** = pertaining to	a portion of a bridge that replaces the missing tooth; false tooth
prosthesis (pros-**thee**-sis)	**prosth(o)-** = substitute for a missing or defective part of the body **-eses** = plural suffix	a device, either external or implanted, that substitutes for or supplements a missing or defective part of the body

(Continues)

Term and Pronunciation	Meaning of Root and Word Parts	Definition
recession (ri-**sesh**-uhn)	**recess** = withdrawal **-ion** = the act of	movement of gingival tissue away from the tooth
remineralization (ree-**min**-er-uh-lahz-shuhn)	**re-** = back again **mineral** = natural substances such as calcium, phosphorus **-ize** = to convert, transform **-ation** = denoting action	the minerals are replaced in the tooth
soluble (**sol**-yuh-buh l)	**sol-** = solution; liquid **-uble** = capable of being	capable of being dissolved or liquified
suppuration (suhp-yuh-**rey**-shuhn)	**suppurate** = produce or discharge pus **-tion** = the process of	process of pus forming; matter from a sore
systemic (si-**stem**-ik)	**system** = an organism or body considered as a whole, especially with regard to its vital processes or functions **-ic** = having characteristics	pertaining to or affecting the body as a whole
topical (**top**-i-kuh l)	**topo** = place, local **-ic** = having characteristics **-al** = relating to	applied to the surface of the body; applied externally
toxic (**tok**-sik)	**toxin** = poison **-ic** = affected with, pertaining to	containing or being poisonous material; causing death or serious debilitation
xerostomia (zeer-uh-**stoh**-mee-uh)	**xero-** = dry **stom** = mouth or mouthlike **-ia** = denoting condition	dryness of the mouth caused by diminished function of the salivary glands due to aging, disease, drug reaction
xylitol (**zahy**-li-tawl)	**xylose** = a colorless, crystalline pentose sugar; derived from xylan, straw, corncobs **-itol** = indicating that certain chemical compounds are polyhydric alcohols	a naturally occurring pentose sugar alcohol, $C_5H_{12}O_5$, used as a sugar substitute

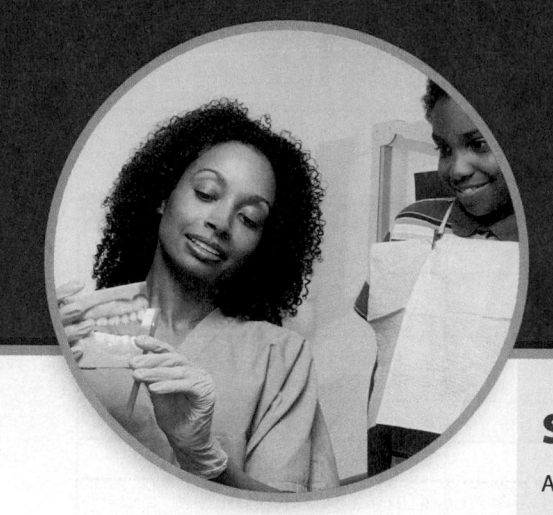

Specific Instructional Objectives

At the completion of this chapter, you will be able to meet these objectives:

1. Use terms presented in this chapter.
2. Describe the role of nutrition in the health of the human body and oral development.
3. Discuss the six classes of nutrients and their functions and sources.
4. Identify the food groups and their nutrients.
5. Discuss calories, metabolic rate, and BMR.
6. Interpret food labels.
7. Summarize food safety issues.
8. Compare governmental dietary recommendations.
9. Explain the feature of MyPlate in selecting food groups.
10. Explain the role of nutrition upon dental caries, gingivitis and periodontal disease.
11. Describe the role of carbohydrates in the diet and its effect on the teeth.
12. Discuss the relationship between nutrition and systemic disease.
13. Explain the special dietary needs of patients in specific dental situations.
14. Describe religious and cultural considerations regarding diet.
15. Discuss the implications of eating disorders
16. Discuss the dental assistant's role in nutrition.

Introduction

Nutrition is closely linked to the health of the entire body. It directly impacts how an individual feels and functions throughout the day. The dental assistant needs to be knowledgeable of how poor nutrition affects the oral cavity in order to educate and counsel their patients. It is critical that a dental assistant is a model for the patient and maintains good health through good nutrition. This chapter covers nutrients, food groups, interpretation of food labels, dental and systemic diseases associated with poor nutrition, and the oral implications of eating disorders. Knowledge of nutrition allows the individual to make sound decisions. The old saying, "You are what you eat" is true.

Health and Nutrition

The most valuable possession we have is our health, yet many people do not realize it until it is lost. Health is not simply the absence of disease, but the state of genuine well-being. At a minimum, health means freedom from physical disease, mental disturbances, and emotional stress. At a maximum, health means complete wellness of mind and body. **Nutrition** is the process of providing or obtaining the food necessary for health and growth. A well-balanced **diet** consists of a variety of all foods such as fruits, vegetables, whole grains, dairy products, meats, and beans. Good nutrition plays a key role in maintaining good health.

The body can never be better than the food it is provided. Often, painful degenerative conditions develop due to poor lifestyles and diets that are deficient in nutrients.

Healthy eating begins with learning the correct way to eat. One important aspect is limiting food intake that contains a lot of fat, salt, and refined sugar. Healthier eating includes understanding about balance, variety, and moderation. Foods can be balanced by selecting foods from each of the food groups (food groups are covered later in this chapter). Variety is the spice of life, so choose foods that might normally be avoided. For example, do not choose an orange every time when reaching for a piece of fruit; add variety by choosing kiwi or melon. Healthy eating also includes moderation; try not to have too much or too little of any one type of food. All foods, even some sweets, can be a part of healthy eating when they are used in moderation.

Many patients may have the meaning of the word *diet* confused with weight loss. Everything taken into the mouth is the diet. People can eat large amounts of food and still be undernourished or lacking the correct nutrients for the body. A disorder resulting from being undernourished is **malnutrition**. More than 60% of Americans are overnourished, leading to obesity and diseases related to obesity. Americans are eating an abundance of fast foods that are high in fat content. That, along with the lack of exercise, contributes to the overall population gaining a minimum of a half a pound a year.

Nutrition and Oral Health

Good nutrition to maintain health and prevent disease is important not only during times of development and growth but throughout a person's life.

Nutrition and Oral Structures before Birth

Primary teeth begin to mineralize during the third or fourth month of pregnancy. At birth the crowns of primary teeth are just about formed and by the age of 1 year the crowns of permanent teeth are almost completely calcified. Lack of certain nutrients at this time is related to decreased tooth size, less mineralization, and delayed eruption and may even affect the growth and development of the maxillary (upper) and mandibular (lower) bone. Teeth that are well formed and calcified are more resistant to dental **caries**. If salivary development, composition, and flow are affected because of poor nutrition, the protective effects for the mouth are diminished. Healthy periodontal tissues that resist disease are also forming at this time. It is especially important that pregnant women maintain a healthy diet so that the developing baby will have healthy oral structures throughout their lifetime.

Nutrition during Growth and Development of the Mouth

Poor nutrition during periods of growth and development can have consequences throughout a person's life. Some deficiencies that occur during this time may or may not be reversible depending on when the problem occurs. For example, if a nutritional

TABLE 17-1 Impact of Nutritional Deficiency on Tooth Development

Nutritional Deficiency	Effect on Tooth Development
vitamin C	• Disturbance of dental formation
vitamin A	• Disturbance of enamel formation • Delayed eruption
vitamin D	• Poor mineralization • Pitted enamel
calcium	• Poor mineralization
phosphorus	• Poor mineralization
magnesium	• Underdeveloped enamel
iron	• Increased caries susceptibility
zinc	• Increased caries susceptibility
fluoride	• Increased caries susceptibility

deficiency or **toxicity** occurs at the time when enamel is forming, the results are usually permanent. Teeth that are malformed are more susceptible to caries and may not be able to chew food adequately, which could affect the development of the jaws. Salivary glands that function well to produce high quality saliva depend on enough water intake to avoid dehydration-induced **xerostomia** (Table 17-1).

Nutrition for a Lifetime of Oral Health

Nutritional concerns for our patients do not end with growth and development. Intake of appropriate foods in adequate amounts is essential to maintain a healthy mouth throughout a person's life. Critical times for nutrition awareness exist across the life span:

- Infancy—a time of growth and development; proper nutrients are needed
- Young childhood—caregivers have an opportunity to set a good example for healthy eating habits
- School-aged children—a lifelong relationship with food is forming, and children are making their own snack choices; vegetables may be a last choice and children are hungry after school, so caregivers should keep the refrigerator stocked with healthy, ready-to-eat snacks and drinks; be aware of caries development
- Teenagers—a time of rapid physical growth and hormonal changes; bone structure is developing, nutrient and energy needs are greater, and diets are influenced by peer pressure; acne control, weight control, and muscle building may be of concern; a busy lifestyle can lead to poor food choices, and caregivers should be aware of the development of eating disorders, caries development because of food choices, and development of gingivitis because of poor oral hygiene
- Adults—nutrient needs are still important but may be reduced due to busy lifestyle; choosing a vegetarian diet may require additional nutrients not obtained in food; inadequate nourishment can cause oral epithelium to become more

TABLE 17-2 Impact of Nutritional Deficiencies on the Oral Mucosa

Nutritional Deficiency	Effect on Oral Mucosa
vitamin A	• White patches caused by irregular keratinization of epithelium • Generalized gingivitis
vitamin C	• Dark red, inflamed gingiva • Gingival edema • Bleeding gingiva • Ulceration of the gingiva
vitamin B₁ (thiamin)	• Hypersensitivity and burning sensation
vitamin B₂ (riboflavin)	• Bluish to purple mucosa
vitamin B₃ (niacin)	• Thin and fragile epithelium • Stomatitis (inflammation of mucosa) • Reddened marginal and attached gingiva • Burning sensation
vitamin B₆ (pyridoxine)	• Stomatitis
vitamin B₉ (folic acid)	• Inflamed gingiva with erosions and ulcerations • Pale mucosa if anemia is present
vitamin B₁₂ (cyanocobalomine)	• Stomatitis • Pale or yellowish mucosa
iron	• Painful sore mouth with ulcerations • Pale or ashen gray mucosa
zinc	• Thickening of the epithelium

susceptible to infection; be aware of oral changes such as cracked lips and lesions at the corners of the mouth as well as the onset of more advanced periodontal disease

• Elderly—good nutrition keeps the body free from disease and loss of teeth; the side effects of some medications (including xerostomia) result in the loss of the protective effects of saliva, which can make eating difficult; be aware of the special problems of this population such as taste changes, swallowing problems, altered GI motility, economic and psychological issues, root caries, and the development of periodontitis (Table 17-2)

Dental professionals need to be aware of populations that are especially at risk for nutrient deficiencies leading to certain diseases and conditions, nutritional needs of vegetarians, and the effects of alcohol and drug abuse.

Nutrients

The health benefits of nutritious food choices are abundant. Good nutrition can prevent a number of diseases including heart disease, stroke, high blood pressure, Type II diabetes, **osteoporosis**, and even some types of cancers. Healthy eating provides nutrients, vitamins, and minerals needed for body functions and tissue repair. When a body is receiving all necessary nutrients in the amounts that it requires, the outcome is a longer life, a healthy weight, and the avoidance of future health problems.

A nutrient is a substance that is necessary for the functioning of a living organism. Nutrients serve three functions:

1. Provide body with fuel which, when **oxidized**, releases energy for activities
2. Supply materials for upkeep and building of body tissues
3. Regulate body processes

There are six classes of nutrients:

• carbohydrates
• proteins
• fats
• vitamins
• minerals
• water

Carbohydrates

Carbohydrates are compounds that consist of carbon plus hydrogen and oxygen in the same proportion as they are found in water. Carbohydrates provide the body with 4 **Calories** per gram and are considered the body's main source of fuel. They are the cheapest, most easily obtainable nutrient, and the most rapidly digested form of fuel for the body.

Sources of Carbohydrates Carbohydrates primarily come from plants and are found in grain, fruits, and vegetables. The only animal products that contain carbohydrates are milk and milk products (**lactose**).

Functions of Carbohydrates The functions of carbohydrates are as follows:

• Provide energy and act as fuel for the body
• Maintain blood **glucose** levels
• Provide fuel for central nervous system and nerves.
• Spare proteins for the body so it does not burn protein for energy
• Assist in burning fat for fuel
• Provide bulk in the diet (**fiber**)
• Function as a protective and detoxifying agent in the liver.

Recommended Dietary Allowance (RDA) Since the exact number of carbohydrates needed per day varies from person to person, it is given as a percentage of total daily caloric intake. It is recommended that 55% to 65% of the total Calorie intake should be from carbohydrates. In addition, 25 to 35 g of the percentage should be from fiber. Based on a 2,000-Calorie diet, this would equate to between 225 and 325 g of carbohydrates daily. It is also suggested that refined sugar in the diet be limited to less than 20% of total Calorie intake.

Classification of Carbohydrates Carbohydrates are classified as follows:

• *Simple sugars* (monosaccharides and disaccharides)—monosaccharides are absorbed without further digestion.

Foods that contain simple sugars are usually sweet to the taste such as ripe fruits, candy, cookies, cake, and soda. Milk, ice cream, cheese, and yogurt are disaccharides. Disaccharides are formed by linking two monosaccharides together. All of the monosaccharides and disaccharides can be used by **biofilm** as a food source and are therefore considered **cariogenic**. Sucrose (simple sugar) is considered the most cariogenic of sugars.

- *Complex carbohydrates* (polysaccharides)—made up of many monosaccharides linked together. Foods high in complex carbohydrates include cereal grains, potatoes, legumes, and whole grains contain vitamins, minerals, fiber, and water. In an effort to lose weight, some people eliminate complex carbohydrates from the diet, which can result in an insufficient intake of B vitamins, iron, and fiber. (Refer to the box "Classification of Carbohydrates.")

Proteins

The word *protein* means "of prime importance." Proteins are composed of the elements carbon, hydrogen, oxygen, and nitrogen. Protein is a nutrient that is necessary for the growth and repair of all of the body's tissues. Proteins provide the body with 4 Calories

TABLE 17-3 Essential and Nonessential Amino Acids

Essential Amino Acids	Nonessential Amino Acids
arginine	alanine
histidine	asparagine
isoleucine	aspartate
leucine	cysteine
lysine	glutamate
methionine	glutamine
phenylalanine	glycine
threonine	proline
tryptophan	serine
valine	tyrosine

per gram. A molecule of protein is made up of 24 different **amino acids**. Think of amino acids as the letters in the alphabet and the protein as the word made up from the letters. The human body can produce some amino acids. The others, called essential amino acids, must be consumed daily (Table 17-3).

Sources of Protein   Meat and milk products provide most dietary protein. Other sources of protein include soy, pinto beans, fish, eggs, peanut butter, lentils, cooked macaroni, oatmeal, rice, nuts and seeds, and some vegetables and fruits.

Functions of Protein   The functions of proteins are as follows:

- Responsible for growth and maintenance of all cells and tissue
- Help to build and repair tissues
- Form antibodies, hormones, enzymes, transport proteins, and chemical messengers

Recommended Dietary Allowance (RDA)   Protein requirements vary with age, and during periods of growth and development the requirements are greater. At least 10% of daily calories should be from protein.

Classification of Proteins   Proteins are classified as complete and incomplete proteins.

- Complete proteins are those foods that contain all the essential amino acids in amounts necessary to maintain life and support growth. Sources of complete proteins are usually foods that come from animals: meat, dairy products, eggs, and fish.
- Incomplete proteins contain some but not all of the essential amino acids. These foods alone will not support life and growth and must be eaten with complimentary foods that supply the missing essential amino acids. Foods that can be combined to supply all of the essential amino acids include rice and beans, soy milk or tofu, and whole grains and nuts.

Classification of Carbohydrates

Monosaccharides: simple sugars

- *Glucose*—also known as dextrose is the principle product of the digestion of disaccharides and polysaccharides. Found in fruit, sweet corn, corn syrup, and honey.
- *Fructose*—also called laevulose; found in fruits, vegetables, and honey. Can also be manufactured.
- *Galactose*—one of the end products of digestion. Produced from lactose milk sugar.

Disaccharides: composed of two simple sugars or monosaccharides

- *Sucrose* yields glucose and fructose. Known as table sugar.
- *Lactose* yields glucose and galactose. Known as milk sugar
- *Maltose* yields two molecules of glucose. Maltose is the result of the breakdown of starch.

Polysaccharides: complex carbohydrates made up of multiple monosaccharides

- *Starch* is found in cereals, grains, and bulbs; once ripened, the starch turns to glucose. Salivary **amylase** in the mouth breaks starch down.
- *Glycogen*, also known as animal starch; the form in which humans and animal store carbohydrates in the liver and muscles to provide energy.
- *Fiber* provides roughage for gastrointestinal health and gives a sense of fullness. Hemicellulose, also known as bran, is an indigestible grain fiber.

Fats

Fats, also referred to as lipids, are composed of the same three elements that are found in carbohydrates: carbon, hydrogen, and oxygen. Fat provides the body with 9 Calories per gram in a more concentrated form of fuel, yielding 2.25 times as much energy per gram as carbohydrates. Triglycerides make up 95% of fats found in foods and are stored in body tissues. Dietary fats are essential for oral health because they are incorporated into tooth structure.

Sources of Fat Fats are obtained from animal foods such as meat, dairy products, and fish. Fat is also found in plants, nuts, seeds, and oils. Some foods are processed with fat such as chips, crackers, granola bars, and french fries. Obvious sources of fat include margarine, butter, mayonnaise, salad dressing, and meats with marbling or visible fat.

Functions of Fat The functions of fats are as follows:

- Build healthy cell membrane, without which the cell cannot function
- Cushion organs against injury
- Maintain body insulation and temperature
- Provide a good source of energy
- Give a sense of fullness and slow digestion
- Improve the texture and taste of food
- Carry the fat-soluble vitamins A, D, E, and K
- Provide the body with essential **fatty acids**

Recommended Dietary Allowance (RDA) Fat is essential in the diet. Total fat includes all types of dietary fat. Limit total fat intake to 20 to 35% of daily Calories. Based on a 2,000-Calorie-a-day diet, this amounts to about 44 to 78 grams of total fat a day. Eating foods rich in the "good fats," monounsaturated and polyunsaturated fats, helps maintain heart-healthy habits while staying within the total fat allowance.

Classification of Fats Fats are classified as saturated and unsaturated fats.

- *Saturated fats* are fatty acid molecules that have hydrogen atoms bonded at all possible locations. Saturated fats have a significant health impact such as increased risk of cardiovascular disease, hypertension, and cancer. Examples of saturated fats are butter, shortening, coconut oil, beef fat, and bacon grease. Saturated fats are usually solid at room temperature.
- *Unsaturated fats* are known as "good fats" because they may decrease the risk of heart disease. These fats have at least one unfilled hydrogen bond. **Monounsaturated** fats, found mostly in plants, have only one hydrogen bond. **Polyunsaturated** fats are also called essential fatty acids because they cannot be made by the body and must be obtained from food sources. Unsaturated fats are usually liquid at room temperature. Examples of unsaturated fats include olive oil and canola oil.

Types of Essential Fatty Acids

- Linoleic acid is an omega-6 fatty acid found in corn, soybean, and safflower oils.
- Linolenic acid is the omega-3 fatty acid found in cold water fish and flax seeds.
- Arachidonic acid is found in animal fat.

Vita comes from the Latin word meaning "life." The first vitamins were discovered by a group of scientists in 1913. They named the first vitamin "A," the second vitamin "B," the third "C," and so on. Later, they found that Vitamin B was not a single vitamin but several, so they added numbers to the letter B (e.g., Vitamin B_1, B_2, and B_3). Some of the other vitamins were given names rather than letters or numbers. In the 1940s, a committee of scientists named the vitamins A, B, C, D, E, and K with number subscripts where applicable.

Vitamins

Vitamins are a group of Calorie-free micronutrients needed in small amounts by the body. Vitamins do not provide energy; rather they function to regulate **metabolic** processes. By acting as **catalysts** and **coenzymes**, vitamins release the energy in foods.

Sources of Vitamins Some vitamins can be manufactured by the body, such as vitamin D from sun exposure and vitamin K from bacteria in the gut. However, food needs to be eaten to get most of the vitamins; therefore it is essential that a variety of foods are eaten to provide the body with all the nutrients it needs.

Recommended Dietary Allowance (RDA) The RDA for vitamins is different for each vitamin based on the average daily level of intake sufficient to meet the nutrient requirements of nearly all (97%–98%) healthy people. At certain times vitamins may be needed in greater amounts, for example in disease states, pregnancy, periods of growth and development, or due to increased energy use. In addition, lifestyle factors can affect vitamin absorption. These including smoking, and abuse of alcohol or other drugs. There are many oral implications of vitamin deficiencies. However, too much of certain vitamins can cause harm, such as a buildup of excess fat-soluble vitamins resulting in nausea, diarrhea, cramps, bleeding, interference with certain drugs, and even birth defects. Therefore tolerable upper intake levels (UL) have been set. UL is the maximum daily intake of a vitamin that is unlikely to cause adverse health effects.

Classification of Vitamins Vitamins are either fat-soluble or water-soluble.

- Fat-soluble vitamins are absorbed more slowly and stored in the liver and fat cells. Fat-soluble vitamins are vitamins A, D, E, and K. Absorption of these vitamins can be reduced by the use of mineral oils and other laxatives. Fat-soluble vitamins tend to be stable in food and losses in cooking a minimal (Table 17-4, "Fat-Soluble Vitamins").

TABLE 17-4 Fat-Soluble Vitamins

Fat-Soluble Vitamins	Function	Sources	Deficiency	Toxicity
vitamin A (RDA 5,000–50,000 IU)	Acts as an antioxidant, supports tissue healing and immune response, promotes healthy eyes, helps maintain healthy skin	Carotene plant form Retinol animal form Carrots (raw or juices), pumpkins, yams, tuna, cantaloupe, mangos, turnip, beets, greens, spinach, fish, eggs	Poor night vision; macular degeneration; increased risk of cataracts dry skin; hearing, taste, smell, and nerve damage	Nausea, vomiting, headaches, dry skin, joint pain and constipation
vitamin D (RDA 400–800 IU)	Promotes bone development, helps absorb and metabolize calcium, aids the immune system	Sun exposure, sardines, salmon, mushrooms, eggs, fortified cereals, herring, liver, tuna, cod liver oil, margarine	Rickets, delayed tooth development, weak muscles, softened skull in infant, irreversible bone deformities; in adults, osteoporosis, osteomalacia, hypoglycemia	Nausea, vomiting, headaches, diarrhea, constipation, fatigue, loss of appetite, and excessive thirst
vitamin E (RDA 30–1,200 IU)	Acts as a powerful antioxidant, helps repair tissues, increases circulation, reduces blood pressure	Vegetable and nut oils, including soybean, corn, and safflower; whole grains, wheat germ, and sunflower seeds; spinach	Anemia (rare) Edema (rare)	Generally nontoxic, but stomach upset, dizziness, and diarrhea may occur.
vitamin K (RDA 80 mcg)	Aids in blood clotting, maintains bone health	Green leafy vegetables, including spinach, kale, collards, and broccoli	Rare except for newborns when bleeding tendencies are possible; can interfere with the effects of anticoagulant medications	Generally nontoxic, but a type of jaundice may occur in premature infants

- *Water-soluble vitamins* are easily absorbed, cannot be stored, can be destroyed by cooking, and are excreted within hours. Water-soluble vitamins include B complex and C vitamins. The body maintains the balance of water-soluble vitamins through the kidney; any excess is excreted through urine. Vitamin B_6 or niacin can become toxic when intake is excessive because the kidneys cannot easily eliminate the surplus (Table 17-5).

- *Antioxidants* are molecule that inhibits the oxidation of other molecules. Oxidation can cause a chain reaction that produces free radicals that can damage DNA and may be harmful to the body. Some cells can heal, while others are permanently damaged. Scientists believe free radicals may contribute to the aging process, as well as diseases like cancer, diabetes, and heart disease. Vitamin A, C, E, and beta carotene are antioxidants.

Minerals

As with vitamins, minerals are also essential in a healthy diet plan. Minerals are needed to regulate many of the body's functions. Minerals are found in hormones and enzymes and form the greater portion of all the hard tissues of the body: bone, teeth, and nails. Some of the minerals that are positive or negatively charged are called **electrolytes**. When a person is healthy, the electrolytes are in balance.

Recommended Dietary Allowance (RDA) As with vitamins, minerals are needed by the body only in small amounts.

Each mineral has it's own RDA. There are times when the body needs more of certain minerals such as diets that restrict or eliminate foods, anorexia nervosa, severe alcoholism, and in women monthly blood loss. As with vitamins, there are UL recommendations for minerals. For example, overconsumption of processed foods that contain large amounts of sodium and chloride (table salt) is a risk factor for hypertension.

Classification of Minerals

- *Major minerals*—Humans need some minerals in relatively large amounts (more than 100 mg) each day.
- *Trace elements*—These are required in very small amounts. Even though the RDA of these minerals is very small, these elements are still just as necessary for health as the major minerals (Table 17-6).

Water

Water is the principle constituent of all living organisms and the most abundant component of the human body. It is essential to all body biochemical processes; a person can live about 28 days without food but only 3 days without water. A turnover of 5% of total water each day is experienced by the average human adult. In excessive heat, the body requires additional intake of water to prevent **dehydration**. Water contains no calories. The human body is roughly 70% water.

Sources of Water One-third of the water our body needs comes from foods and two-thirds comes from beverages. Good

TABLE 17-5 Water-Soluble Vitamins

Water-Soluble Vitamins	Function	Sources	Deficiency	Toxicity
The Vitamin B Complex				
vitamin B_1 (thiamine) (RDA 25–300mg)	Promotes proper heart function Aids with digestion Promotes nerve function	Rice bran, breads, wheat germ, enriched pastas and cereal, pork, beef, ham, oranges, fresh peas, beans	Mild: appetite and weight loss, nausea, vomiting, severe **beriberi**, and muscle weakness Severe: beriberi and muscle weakness	Generally nontoxic
vitamin B_2 (riboflavin) (RDA 25–300 mg)	Promotes red blood cell formation Prevents **cataracts**	Poultry, fish, yogurt, milk, cheese, broccoli, turnip greens, asparagus, spinach, fortified grains and cereals	Cracks and sores in the corners of the mouth and on the tongue, dizziness, hair loss, inability to sleep, sensitive to light, red eyes	Generally nontoxic
vitamin B_3 (niacin) (RDA 25–300 mg)	Promotes adrenal gland function Assists in expelling toxins Helps to maintain muscle tone	Chicken, tuna, veal, beef liver, fish, pork, eggs, milk, peanuts, fortified breads and cereals, brewer's yeast, broccoli, carrots, turnip greens, dates, tomatoes, potatoes	Dizziness, fatigue, headaches, inability to sleep, loss of appetite, indigestion, diarrhea, **halitosis**, **dermatitis**, mouth ulcers	Nausea, vomiting, cramps, diarrhea, liver damage, **gout**, **arthritis**, severe rash to large portions of the body
vitamin B_5 (pantothenic acid) (RDA 5 mg)	Promotes red blood cell production Aids in the breakdown of fats and carbohydrates for energy Helps maintain healthy digestive tract	Brewer's yeast, corn, whole grains, egg yolk, beef, duck, lobster, tomatoes, sweet potatoes	Fatigue, **insomnia**, stomach pains, upper respiratory tract infections	Generally nontoxic
vitamin B_6 (pyridoxine) (RDA 1.3 mg)	Promotes healthy nerve and brain function Helps with absorption of vitamin B_{12}	Brown rice, whole grain flour, bran, shrimp, fish, lentils, nuts	Muscle weakness, depression, nervousness, short-term memory loss	**Peripheral neuropathy** of hands and feet with numbness, tingling, pricking, and burning
vitamin B_7 (biotin) (RDA 30 mg)	Aids in the metabolism of carbohydrates, fats, and amino acids	Brewer's yeast, nut butters, soy beans, legumes, organ meats, cooked eggs	(Rare) hair loss, dry scaly skin, cracking in the corners of the mouth, swollen tongue	Generally nontoxic
vitamin B_9 (folic acid) (RDA 400 mg, 600 during pregnancy)	Aids in the production of DNA and RNA Required for proper brain development and function	Whole grains, wheat germ, salmon, milk, spinach, asparagus, avocado, root vegetables (carrots and potatoes), orange juice	Birth defects including **spina bifida**, **cleft palate**, and brain damage to the infant if a pregnant woman does not have adequate folic acid intake	Generally nontoxic
vitamin B_{12} (cyanocobalamin) (RDA 25–500 mg)	Promotes proper iron function, regulates red blood cell formation	Clams, ham, cooked oysters, king crab, herring, salmon, tuna, lean beef, liver, bleu cheese, gorgonzola cheese	Unsteady gait, **depression**, dizziness, drowsiness, headaches, inflammation of the tongue, constipation and digestive upset, anemia, chronic fatigue	Generally nontoxic
vitamin C (ascorbic acid) (RDA 60–5,000 mg)	Acts as an antioxidant Helps the body resist infection Promotes adrenal gland function Aids in collagen production Can reduce high blood pressure and cholesterol	Cantaloupe, kiwi fruits, oranges, pineapple, peppers, pink grapefruit, strawberries, avocados, lemons, mangos, broccoli, asparagus, collards, kale, watercress, onions, radishes	Poor wound healing, bleeding gums, bruises easily, nosebleeds, joint pain, lack of energy, susceptibility to infection; severe deficiency called scurvy	Generally nontoxic

TABLE 17-6 Essential Minerals

Major Minerals	Function	Sources	Deficiency	Toxicity
calcium (RDA 1,000–1,500 mg)	Supports development and maintenance of strong bones and teeth Promotes heart, nerve and muscle function	Milk, cheese, yogurt, dark green vegetables, prunes, canned salmon, tofu	Muscle spasms, osteomalacia, osteoporosis; severe deficiency is called rickets	Generally nontoxic
magnesium (RDA 500–750 mg)	Necessary for contraction and relaxation of muscles Transports energy in cells Aids in production of proteins	Brown rice, oatmeal, dried beans, broccoli, bananas, avocados, spinach, fish	Sleep disturbances, irritability, confusion, rapid heartbeat, muscle spasms, stomach upset	Generally nontoxic
phosphorus (RDA 1,200 mg)	Required for maintaining strong bones and teeth	Fish (especially halibut and salmon), lean beef, milk, oatmeal, dried beans, dried fruits	Fatigue, irritability, loss of appetite, weakness, bone pain, skin sensitivity	Generally nontoxic
potassium (RDA 3,500 - 4,700 mg)	Essential for kidney, heart, digestive and nerve function	Bananas, dried apricots, baked potatoes	Dry skin, acne, edema, thirst, diarrhea, chills, muscle spasms, increased cholesterol and blood pressure	Generally nontoxic
sodium (RDA 1,500 mg but no more than 2,300 mg)	Maintains balance of body fluids Necessary for nerve function Necessary for muscle contraction/relaxation	Largest source is commercially processed foods	Hyponatremia (rare), tiredness, disorientation, headache, muscle cramps, nausea; severe hyponatremia can lead to seizures, coma, and death	Hypernatremia, swelling in the extremities, and hypertension

Trace Minerals	Function	Sources	Deficiency	Toxicity
chromium (RDV 200–600 mcg)	Aids in metabolism of fats and carbohydrates Aids in insulin metabolism	Brewer's yeast, wine and beer, grape juice, whole grains, brown rice, dried beans, corn, potatoes, mushrooms, dairy products, eggs, ham, chicken	Alteration in metabolism of fats, carbohydrates, amino acids	Generally nontoxic
iron (RDA 18 mg)* *more for pregnant, nursing or menstruating women	Works with hemoglobin in red blood cells to deliver oxygen to the body The most abundant trace mineral in the body	Beef, liver, eggs, soybeans, green leafy vegetables, dried beans, pumpkin seeds, dried fruits	Anemia, fatigue, mental confusion, nervousness, pallor, dizziness, dry coarse hair, hair loss, dysphagia, cracked lips and tongue	Rare from food sources, but poisoning and death can occur from overdose of supplements
manganese (RDA 15–30 mg)	Aids in bone formation Metabolism of fat and proteins	Wheat bran, wheat germ, nuts, shellfish, dairy products, cocoa, tea, pineapple juice, apples, apricots, peaches	Rare	Rare
zinc (RDA 25–50 mg)	Acts as an antioxidant Promotes immune system function Helps to regulate appetite, taste and smell	Cooked oysters, beef, lamb, fish, poultry, whole grains, nuts, lima beans, yogurt	Changes in taste and smell, impaired night vision, thin and fragile nails, hair loss, delayed sexual maturation	Nausea, vomiting, abdominal pain, fatigue
iodine (RDA 150 mcg)	Regulates thyroid hormone Aids in metabolism	Iodized salt, saltwater fish, shellfish, seaweed products, soy milk, soy sauce	Enlarged thyroid gland (goiter), fatigue, depression, weight gain	Goiter, nausea, vomiting, abdominal pain

foods sources of water are soup, salads, fruits, and vegetables. Even dry foods such as crackers and nuts contain some water. Caffeinated beverages such as coffee, tea, and colas act as a **diuretic** and cause the body to lose water.

Functions of Water Water is used by the body in several ways, but the primary function is as a solvent for biochemical reactions. For instance, a large part of the blood is composed of water, and this allows for transport and necessary reactions to occur. This solvent action also serves to remove toxic waste from the body. Water acts as a lubricant, especially in the digestive system and the joints. It also helps control body temperature, releasing excessive heat through perspiration, and dispersing heat evenly throughout the body.

The functions of water are as follows:

- Provide an **aqueous medium** for bodily fluids
- Act as a transporter
- Dilute and remove wastes
- Build and cushion tissue
- Aid in digestion
- Regulate body temperature
- Moisten mucous membranes

Recommended Dietary Allowance (RDA) Every day the body loses water through breath, perspiration, urine, and bowel movements. For the body to function properly, it must replenish its water supply by consuming beverages and foods that contain water. The Institute of Medicine determined that an adequate intake (AI) for men is roughly about 13 cups (3 liters) of total beverages a day. The AI for women is about 9 cups (2.2 liters) of total beverages a day. Too much or too little water in the body can cause harm.

- *Water* intoxication is very rare and may happen if the kidneys are not functioning properly. Too much water in the body can put pressure on the brain, causing seizures or death and may cause the blood volume of water to drop causing circulatory shock.
- *Water deficiency* the first sign of dehydration is thirst followed by headache, heartburn, stomach cramps, low-back pain, or fatigue. Severe dehydration is very dangerous and can cause weakness, exhaustion, **delirium**, and even death.

Food Groups and Healthy Eating

It is often difficult for people to choose foods that offer the most health benefit. Which foods, and how much, should be consumed each day? The USDA has developed nutritional guidelines dividing foods into food groups and recommended daily servings of each group for a healthy diet called MyPlate. A food group is a collection of foods that share similar nutritional properties. MyPlate uses food groups and the familiar place setting to remind consumers to build a healthy meal (Figure 17-1). An 1,800 to 2,000 Calorie diet with choices from all of the food groups based on MyPlate is adequate for most healthy adult females, and 2,200 to 2,400 is adequate for most adult males. Adjustments can be made based on the individual's age, health-related issues such as cardiovascular disease or diabetes, activity level, and personal preference. Calories can be added or subtracted if the goal is weight gain or loss. MyPlate will also help with portion control, which is often difficult to determine. A portion is the specific amount of food a person eats in one setting. The USDA website, *ChooseMyPlate.gov*, offers tips and interactive tools to help educate consumers to smarter, healthier nutrition choices.

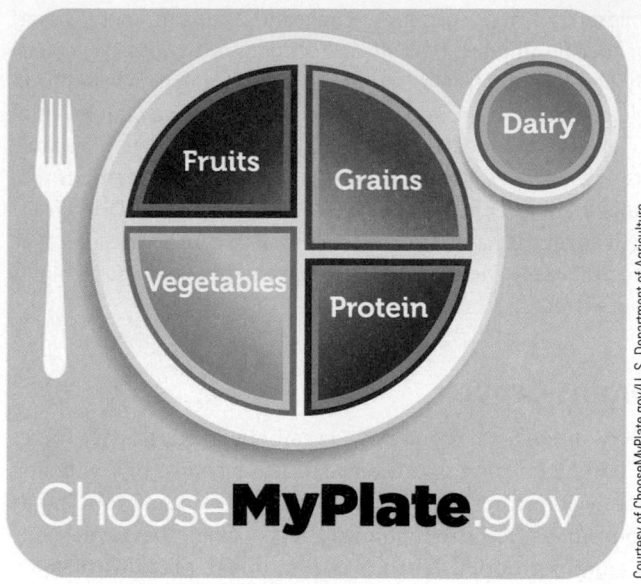

Courtesy of ChooseMyPlate.gov/U. S. Department of Agriculture

FIGURE 17-1

MyPlate new generation food icon. When making up a plate, the USDA recommends to make half your plate fruits and vegetable, make at least half of your grains whole grains, and switch to fat free or low fat (1%) milk.

The five food groups are vegetables, fruits, grains, dairy, and protein foods.

Vegetables Group

Vegetables provide many nutrients, especially vitamins A, C, E, and folic acid. In addition they are a good source of potassium and dietary fiber. A diet rich in vegetables and fruits can lower the risk of cardiovascular disease, diabetes, and certain types of cancer. In general, 1 cup of raw or cooked vegetables or vegetable juice, or 2 cups of raw leafy greens are considered as 1 cup from the vegetable group. For a healthy diet include at least 1 cup for children, 2 ½ cups for women, and 3 cups for men. The guidelines recommend eating a variety of different vegetables throughout the week. Dark green vegetables like broccoli and spinach; red and orange vegetables such as carrots, sweet potatoes, and tomatoes; starchy vegetables for example corn and potatoes as well as other types of vegetables like cauliflower, green beans, and mushrooms will help provide all the nutrients needed. Listed in the vegetable group are beans and peas, which are unique foods because they can be counted as both vegetables and proteins.

Fruits Group

Like vegetables, fruits are a good source of vitamins, potassium, and dietary fiber and provide many of the same benefits. The USDA recommends that half the plate be fruits and vegetables. In general, 1 cup of fruit or 100% fruit juice, or ½ cup of dried fruit can be considered as 1 cup from the fruit group. Fruits may be fresh, canned, frozen, or dried, and may be whole, cut up, or pureed. A healthy diet should include at least 1 cup for children, 1 ½ to 2 cups for women, and 2 cups for men. A chart for specific amounts of fruits that count as one cup is available at MyPlate.gov. It should be noted that beverages labeled "fruit juice drink" contain very little fruit juice and have high levels of sugar. Commonly eaten fruits include apples, bananas, grapefruit, grapes, oranges, peaches, plums, and raisins. Remember that fruits are higher in sugar content than vegetables. Dried fruits such as raisins have a greater potential to cause caries because the fruit easily sticks to the tooth surface and the sugar is highly concentrated.

Grains Group

Foods in the grain group provide carbohydrates, an easy source of energy for the body. Grains are also a source of B vitamins, which help turn carbohydrates into energy. Any food made from wheat, rice, oats, cornmeal, barley, or another cereal grain is a grain product. Bread, pasta, oatmeal, breakfast cereals, tortillas, and grits are examples of grain products. A healthy diet should include at least 1 ½ ounce for children, 3 ounces for women and 4 ounces for men. In general, 1 slice of bread, 1 cup of ready-to-eat cereal, or ½ cup of cooked rice, cooked pasta, or cooked cereal can be considered as 1 ounce equivalent from the grains group. A chart for specific amounts of grains that count as one ounce equivalent of grains is available at MyPlate.gov. Grains are divided in two subgroups, whole grains and refined grains.

● Whole grains contain the entire grain kernel and all of its nutrients and fiber. Whole grain foods include whole-wheat flour, cracked wheat, oatmeal, cornmeal, and brown rice.

● Refined grains have been milled, a process that removes the bran and germ. This is done to give grains a finer texture and improve their shelf life, but it also removes dietary fiber, iron, and many B vitamins. Some examples of refined grain products are white flour, degermed cornmeal, white bread, and white rice. Most refined grains are *enriched*. This means certain B vitamins (thiamin, riboflavin, niacin, folic acid) and iron are added back after processing. Fiber, which provides many health benefits, is not added back to enriched grains.

Dairy Group

Dairy products provide calcium, which is necessary for strong bones and teeth; many dairy products are fortified with vitamin D, which promotes absorption of calcium. All fluid milk products and many foods made from milk are considered part of the milk group. Common dairy products are skim milk or low fat milk, buttermilk, cheeses, and yogurt. Calcium-fortified soymilk (soy beverage) is also part of the dairy group. Foods made from milk that have little to no calcium, such as cream cheese, cream, and butter, are not part of the dairy group. In general, 1 cup of milk, yogurt, or soymilk (soy beverage), 1 ½ ounces of natural cheese, or 2 ounces of processed cheese can be considered as 1 cup from the Dairy Group. A healthy diet should include at least 2 cups for children, and 3 cups for women and men. Serving amounts should be increased for pregnant women. Dairy products can

contain high levels of milk fat; therefore fat-free or low-fat products should be chosen whenever possible.

Many individuals have difficulty digesting products made from cow's milk due to a condition known as lactose intolerance. Lactose-free products are available, or enzyme supplements may be suggested to help these individuals consume dairy products. As an alternative, soy, almond, coconut, rice, and cashew milk or products made from goat milk may be consumed. These products are a good source of calcium but may not contain the essential nutrients found in cow's milk. Select alternatives that contain at least 120 mg of calcium per 3.4 ounces (100 ml).

Protein Group

Proteins are needed for building bones, muscles, cartilage, skin, and blood. Proteins are also required to produce some enzymes and hormones. All foods made from meat, poultry, seafood, beans and peas, eggs, soy products, nuts, and seeds are a part of the protein group. The USDA recommends choosing lean or low-fat meat and poultry. Select a variety of protein foods to improve nutrient intake and health benefits, including at least 8 ounces of cooked seafood per week. Young children need less, depending on their age and Calorie needs. In general, 1 ounce of meat, poultry, or fish; ¼ cup cooked beans; 1 egg, 1 tablespoon of peanut butter, or ½ ounce of nuts or seeds can be considered as 1 ounce equivalents from the protein foods group. A healthy diet should include at least 2 ounces for children, 5 ½ ounces for women, and 6 ½ ounces for men from the protein group. Lean meats prepared by roasting, broiling, or poaching are recommended to avoid the consumption of unnecessary fats. People who do not eat animal products have options in the protein foods group that include beans and peas, processed soy products, nuts, and seeds. This group of people include vegetarians, lacto-ovo vegetarians, and vegans.

● *Vegetarian*—a large number of people practice some type of vegetarian lifestyle. Some individuals eat some animal products, but not all. Many people avoid beef or pork for religious reasons. These individuals can obtain their protein from poultry or fish.

● *Lacto-ovo vegetarian*—these people do not eat meat but will consume eggs and milk products. There are complete proteins in these foods.

● Vegan—the strictest vegetarians are known as vegans. These individuals avoid all products made from animals. A vegan must consume plant products containing complimentary amino acids in order to provide the protein needed by the body. This is possible with careful planning. Nonmeat sources of amino acids include dried beans and peas (kidney, pinto, and lima beans, black eyed peas, lentils), seeds, and nuts.

Oils

Oils are fats that are liquid at room temperature. Oils come from many different plants and from fish. They are not considered a food group, but because they provide essential nutrients such as fatty acids, the USDA includes them in the recommendations for what to eat. A healthy diet should include at least 3 teaspoons of recommended oils for children, 5–6 teaspoons for women, and 6–7 teaspoons for men.

Some common oils include canola oil, corn oil, cottonseed oil, olive oil, safflower oil, soybean oil, and sunflower oil. Foods that are naturally high in oils are nuts, olives, some fish, and avocados. Other foods that are mainly oil include mayonnaise, salad dressings, and soft (tub or squeeze) margarine with no trans fats.

Solid fats are fats that are solid at room temperature and come from many animal foods and can be made from vegetable oils through hydrogenation. Solid fats include butter, milk fat, meat and poultry fat, shortening, and hydrogenated oil.

The USDA recommends that most of the fats eaten should be polyunsaturated or monosaturated fats. Good sources of beneficial oils are olive oil, canola oil, fish, and nuts.

Balancing Energy

Ideally, people should take in enough nutrition to equal the amount of energy used daily. The amount of energy a substance can supply is measured in the form of Calories. One Calorie of food energy is understood to mean one kilocalorie. A kilocalorie is equivalent to one thousand nondietary calories, with a lower-case "c". When referring to a Calorie, always capitalize it or abbreviate it by using a capital C or Cal. Carbohydrate and protein grams yield 4 Calories per gram; in contrast, 1 gram of fat yields 9 Calories. For example:

- 5 grams of carbohydrates $\times$ 4 Calories = 20 Calories of carbohydrates
- 5 grams of proteins $\times$ 4 Calories = 20 Calories of protein
- 5 grams of fat $\times$ 9 Calories = 45 Calories of fat

The total of all three categories would be 85 Calories. Fats are more energy rich than carbohydrates or proteins.

Calories are taken into the body to use as energy for everything from running to breathing. The body uses what it needs and stores the rest as fat. The physical and chemical changes that take place in relationship to the usage of energy are called the metabolic rate. If the rate of metabolism is less than the consumed Calories, then the person will store fat; if the rate of metabolism is greater, the stored fat will be used.

The energy that is used when a person is at rest is called the basal metabolic rate (BMR). The BMR will be higher for pregnant women, children, and leaner individuals because it takes more energy to fuel muscle than it does to store fat in the body. Optimum energy balance would include the same amount of Calories taken into the body as are used. Ideally, most Calories would come from carbohydrates. Fats and protein should make up less than half the Calories taken in.

Nutrition Labels

For dental assistants to make good choices and be able to advise patients to do the same, they must be knowledgeable about nutrition labels on food products. Information is provided on the label according to government standards. Manufacturers of food products know that people are attracted to descriptive words on the product packages such as "lite" or "healthy." These terms may or may not describe the product, so it is important to read the details on the nutrition label. Consumers should pay more attention to the Calories and fat content when they compare two similar items. Information about preservatives (the chemicals added to food to keep it fresh for a longer period) and artificial flavors and colors is also found on the food label.

Standard information is listed on nutrition labels. The government requires that the labels be easy for the consumer to read, so nutritional information is most often listed in a standard format. The Nutritional Labeling and Education Act requires manufacturers to list all ingredients in the product. Individuals who have special dietary needs can readily identify ingredients, and all consumers can make comparisons from one product to another. The labels provide the serving size, percent of daily nutritional value, Calories, fat and cholesterol, sodium, carbohydrate, and other pertinent information. In 2016 the nutrition label received an update making it more consumer-friendly (Figure 17-2). On the new label serving sizes have been updated, and the serving size and calories are now in bold and larger print. Daily values have been updated. There are new requirements to include added sugars. The label includes nutrients required and the actual amounts present in the product. It also contains a new footnote relating daily values to a 2,000 Calorie diet.

If the product packaging indicates that it is organic or organically grown, it must have been grown without the use of herbicides, chemical pesticides, or fertilizers. In addition, to qualify as organically grown, plant seeds must not have been prepared with the use of hormones or any other enhancement.

The *serving size* is listed on the label in a measurement or number of the product (for instance, ½ cup, or 2 cookies on a cookie package). It also gives the total number of servings per package. The rest of the information pertains to a single serving size.

The *ingredients* and *percent of daily value* are also listed. The daily value percent is based on a diet of 2,000 Calories per day for one adult. So, if the amount listed for total carbohydrate is 15 grams, this indicates that it is 5% of the daily value required according to calculations for the carbohydrate group.

Total *Calories* per serving are noted along with specific Calories derived from fat. The Calories from fat should total less than 30% of total Calories. Remember that this is the Calories in one serving and not the entire package.

Fat and *cholesterol* notations are valuable to the consumer because of various health concerns, including heart disease and weight control. The listing on the sample label in Figure 17-2 breaks out total fat as well as saturated fat. Saturated fat primarily comes from animal sources, while unsaturated fat primarily comes from vegetable sources. The total cholesterol content for one serving is also noted on the label.

Patients with heart disease or other diseases on sodium-restricted diets will want to watch the levels of *sodium* in foods. The total amount of sodium for one serving is listed on the nutritional label.

SIDE-BY-SIDE COMPARISON

Original Label

Nutrition Facts
Serving Size 2/3 cup (55g)
Servings Per Container About 8

Amount Per Serving

Calories 230   Calories from Fat 72

	% Daily Value*
Total Fat 8g	12%
Saturated Fat 1g	5%
Trans Fat 0g	
Cholesterol 0mg	0%
Sodium 160mg	7%
Total Carbohydrate 37g	12%
Dietary Fiber 4g	16%
Sugars 1g	
Protein 3g	
Vitamin A	10%
Vitamin C	8%
Calcium	20%
Iron	45%

*Percent Daily Values are based on a 2,000 calorie diet. Your daily value may be higher or lower depending on your calorie needs.

	Calories:	2,000	2,500
Total Fat	Less than	65g	80g
Sat Fat	Less than	20g	25g
Cholesterol	Less than	300mg	300mg
Sodium	Less than	2,400mg	2,400mg
Total Carbohydrate		300g	375g
Dietary Fiber		25g	30g

New Label

Nutrition Facts
8 servings per container
Serving size   **2/3 cup (55g)**

Amount per serving

Calories   230

	% Daily Value*
Total Fat 8g	10%
Saturated Fat 1g	5%
Trans Fat 0g	
Cholesterol 0mg	0%
Sodium 160mg	7%
Total Carbohydrate 37g	13%
Dietary Fiber 4g	14%
Total Sugars 12g	
Includes 10g Added Sugars	20%
Protein 3g	
Vitamin D 2mcg	10%
Calcium 260mg	20%
Iron 8mg	45%
Potassium 235mg	6%

*The % Daily Value (DV) tells you how much a nutrient in a serving of food contributes to a daily diet. 2,000 calories a day is used for general nutrition advice.

Courtesy of the FDA

FIGURE 17-2
Food label.

The total amount of *carbohydrate* is also listed, which may be broken down into dietary fiber (complex carbohydrates) or sugar (simple carbohydrates).

The nutritional labels show other information, such as the protein, vitamins, and minerals in the product.

Disease Prevention and Health Promotion

The U.S. Department of Health and Human Services (HHS) estimates that unhealthy eating and lack of physical inactivity contribute to as many as 580,000 deaths each year in this country. Six of the leading causes of death in the United States, heart disease, diabetes, obesity, hypertension, stroke, and many cancers, are directly related to diet. Americans consume too much saturated fat, sodium, and sugar and not enough fruits, vegetables, whole grains, calcium, and fiber. Most experts agree that preventing diet-related diseases through education could prevent

at least $71 billion per year in medical costs, lost productivity, and lost lives. Fortunately there are resources available that help promote healthy eating habits. ChooseMyPlate (as discussed previously) and the Dietary Guidelines for Americans are the cornerstone of federal food, nutrition education, and information policies. These two federal initiatives offer practical advice to help individuals make food and activity choices for a healthy, active life.

Dietary Guidelines for Americans

The Dietary Guidelines for Americans emphasizes three major goals for Americans:

- Balance Calories with physical activity to manage weight.
- Consume more of certain foods and nutrients such as fruits, vegetables, whole grains, fat-free and low fat dairy products, and seafood.

- Consume fewer foods with sodium (salt), saturated fats, *trans* fats, cholesterol, added sugars, and refined grains.

The guidelines also contain key recommendations for the general population and specific groups such as pregnant women. In addition the guidelines recommend balancing healthy eating with daily exercise.

Reliable Sources of Nutritional Information

With so much attention on diet and health via commercials, magazines, newspapers, television, and the Internet, it is very difficult and confusing to decide whether or not nutritional information is accurate. Reliable sources of information include professional health organizations, government health agencies, volunteer health agencies, and certain consumer groups.

Consumers should be wary about any claims that state a product is natural or nontoxic because this does not mean that the product is safe. Also, be aware of claims that state the product is a scientific breakthrough or that there is a secret ingredient included that will cure disease. And last, if there is a money back guarantee for the product, one should be cautious of its claim.

Health Monitoring Devices

Today's health conscious individual has numerous devices to aid them in maintaining health and wellness. Most of the devices track food choices and exercise on tablets and smartphones. A popular health monitoring device is the Fitbit. It can track the steps taken, distance covered, Calories burned, floors climbed, active minutes, and sleep habits. It also has a WiFi Smart Scale that measures weight, BMI, lean mass, and body fat percentage. The **body mass index** (BMI) is a value derived from the mass and height of an individual.

Numerous apps are available online that can be downloaded to aid in weight management, provide diet information and recipe suggestions, improve health, and track your fitness stats. One example is *Fooducate,* which serves as a dietary partner and health eating educator, and encourages those who have health concerns. It has a barcode scanner that can be used for the foods eaten or to give healthy alternatives to consider before choosing foods. Another example, *Lose It*, helps set goals and track progress to success. Its barcode scanning is used to track eating habits only. There are options to appeal to everyone's lifestyle and needs, including *Weight Watchers, Cronometer, SparkPeople, Calorie King*, and *Techlife* just to name a few. Individuals should research the apps to identify the one that meets their needs. Almost all of them work with the iPhone or Android, and many have a built-in message center. Getting healthy is getting easier with the help of technology.

Energy Drinks and Shots

Energy drinks and shots have become popular. People take these drinks to give them a boost, making them more alert. Most of them contain large amounts of caffeine, with added sugar, vitamins (B vitamins), legal stimulants, amino acids (found in meat and fish), and substances that helps metabolize fat. A clinical dietitian at the Mayo Clinic states, "The concern is that these ingredients are at much higher concentrations than naturally found in food and plants and the effects when combined especially with caffeine may be enhanced."

Unlike drugs and supplements, energy drinks do not get tested for safety by the FDA. Experts are increasingly concerned that their ingredients could have unintended health risks. It is recommended that an individual does not have more than two drinks each day to stay within a safe level. The Journal of the American Heart Association found that caffeinated energy drinks altered the heart's electrical activity and raised blood pressure. The World Health Organization warns they may pose a danger to the public health, and the American Academy of Pediatrics states that children should not consume them. However, the European Food Safety Authority research confirms energy drinks are safe for consumption.

As the consumption of energy drinks remains controversial, the consumer should be cautious and ask the advice of their physician. Health studies have found that these drinks may cause dehydration, seizures, insomnia, and heart problems and that people who take certain prescribed or OTC medications or have a heart condition could be at an increased risk of a fatal arrhythmia (irregular heartbeat). The dental concerns come from repeated sugar over the teeth, which may cause decay.

Nutrition and Dental Disease

Nutrition (or lack of) affects the body locally and systemically. Locally, the effects result from the interaction of food and the oral bacteria that lead to biofilm formation. Good oral hygiene with biofilm control as well as regular dental visits are vital to help prevent or control dental disease. It is important for the dental assistant to understand the relationship between nutritional deficiencies and dental disease (Figure 17-3).

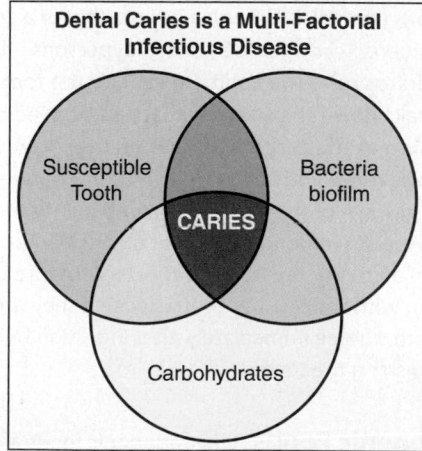

FIGURE 17-3
Chain of dental caries.

Dental Caries

In the caries process (tooth decay), tooth enamel is **demineralized** first. Demineralized enamel allows bacteria to reach the dentin, and a carious lesion (dental cavity) is the result. Remember caries is a dynamic process of demineralization and remineralization (refer to Chapter 16). Other factors that affect caries production are the presence of specific bacteria (*Streptococcus mutans* and *Lactobacillus*) and **fermentable** carbohydrates at the same time as well as saliva, fluoride exposure, and oral hygiene. See Chapter 9 on Oral Pathology for a complete discussion of the caries process.

There are six factors involved with the beginning of the caries process and its continued destruction of the tooth; they are:

- a caries-susceptible tooth
- specific biofilm bacteria
- readily fermentable carbohydrates (sugar) in contact with biofilm on the tooth surfaces
- saliva
- lack of fluoride
- poor oral hygiene

The chain of dental caries includes susceptible tooth + fermentable carbohydrate + bacterial biofilm → acid → breakdown/demineralization of tissue = dental disease.

If this chain is broken at any point, dental caries will not occur.

Cariogenic Foods

Carbohydrates are foods that contain both sugar and starch, both of which can support bacterial growth. However, the impact of these carbohydrates on caries depends on the type (consistency) and frequency (number of exposures) of consumption. The most cariogenic foods are simple sugars that are highly fermentable carbohydrates, have a sticky consistency, break into small particles in the mouth, cause an acid environment in the mouth, and are highly processed. Examples include mints, cookies, candy, soft drinks, presweetened cereals, cakes, dried fruits, crackers, bread, muffins, and potato chips. Although fermentable carbohydrates are considered the major cause of caries, all carbohydrates have the ability to demineralize tooth enamel. Although a potato chip or a cracker may not be considered cariogenic by most laypersons, these types of carbohydrates have the ability to stick to the tooth. Salivary amylase breaks down the starches that can be used by the biofilm for as long as the carbohydrate is on the tooth. Now think of a cracker covered with sweet jelly sticking between and on the occlusal surface of the teeth. This combination of starch and sugar in the mouth for long periods of time is perhaps the most damaging of all to the teeth. It is important to note that sugars can be eaten without causing tooth decay if they are removed from the tooth surface immediately after ingestion by rinsing the mouth or brushing the teeth.

Low Cariogenic Foods

Low cariogenic foods are relatively high in protein and fiber, have moderate amounts of fat, minimal amounts of carbohydrates, and a high concentration of calcium and phosphorus; are nonacidic; and stimulate saliva secretion. Examples include cheese, peanuts, meat, milk, eggs, raw vegetables, fresh fruit, cocoa products, and sugarless gum.

Importance of Saliva Any foods that stimulate the saliva will assist in protecting against caries formation. Saliva dilutes acid-producing bacteria, exerts antibacterial action, and provides protective minerals such as calcium and phosphorus, which promote **remineralization** of the tooth enamel. The process of remineralization is the replacement of lost minerals in hard dental tissues. It can halt, slow down, and, in some cases, reverse the caries process. Saliva has the ability to neutralize acids and remineralize tooth enamel; the amount and quality of saliva is important. Saliva has a natural cleansing ability, as does rinsing with water immediately after consuming sugar. When the saliva flow is poor, there is less natural cleansing in the mouth and the caries rate may increase.

Soda and Caries Many patients drink soft drinks all day long. Regular sodas are very acidic; each can of soda equals 10 teaspoons (tsp) of sugar (Figure 17-4). Even diet sodas are very acidic, and the effects of artificial sweeteners are not yet known. Noncola drinks and iced teas are also harmful because of additives that contribute to demineralization of the enamel.

Caries Risk Assessment It is important to assess the risk for caries from high to low based on the amount, type and the time foods are consumed. Research shows that sugar causes acid production in the mouth for 20 minutes after exposure as it returns to a neutral state. Acid can be cleared by **dilution**, neutralization, and **buffering**. The following equation will help patients understand the damage that their diet may be causing to their teeth.

Number of exposures × 20 minutes = time of sugar-acid production

For example, 32 single exposures × 20 minutes = 640 minutes or 10.6 hours of possible decay from sugar. The demineralizing effect may last 40 to 60 minutes after the cariogenic food has been introduced.

The higher cariogenic type of sugar that sticks to the teeth remains on the tooth until it is physically removed (caramels and gummy candies) has a spike in acid production. Some of the worst culprits are ones that remain in the mouth until they are dissolved, like mints, hard candy, and suckers. During this time the sugar-acid production clock remains ticking.

Another caries risk factor is when the sugar-containing food is eaten (see box below).

Cariogenic Sugar Risk Factors (Highest to Lowest)

Type of Sugar	Time/Frequency of Consumption
Sticky sucrose	Between meals or before bed
Liquid sucrose	Between meals or before bed
Sticky sucrose	Eaten during meals
Liquid Sucrose	Eaten during meals

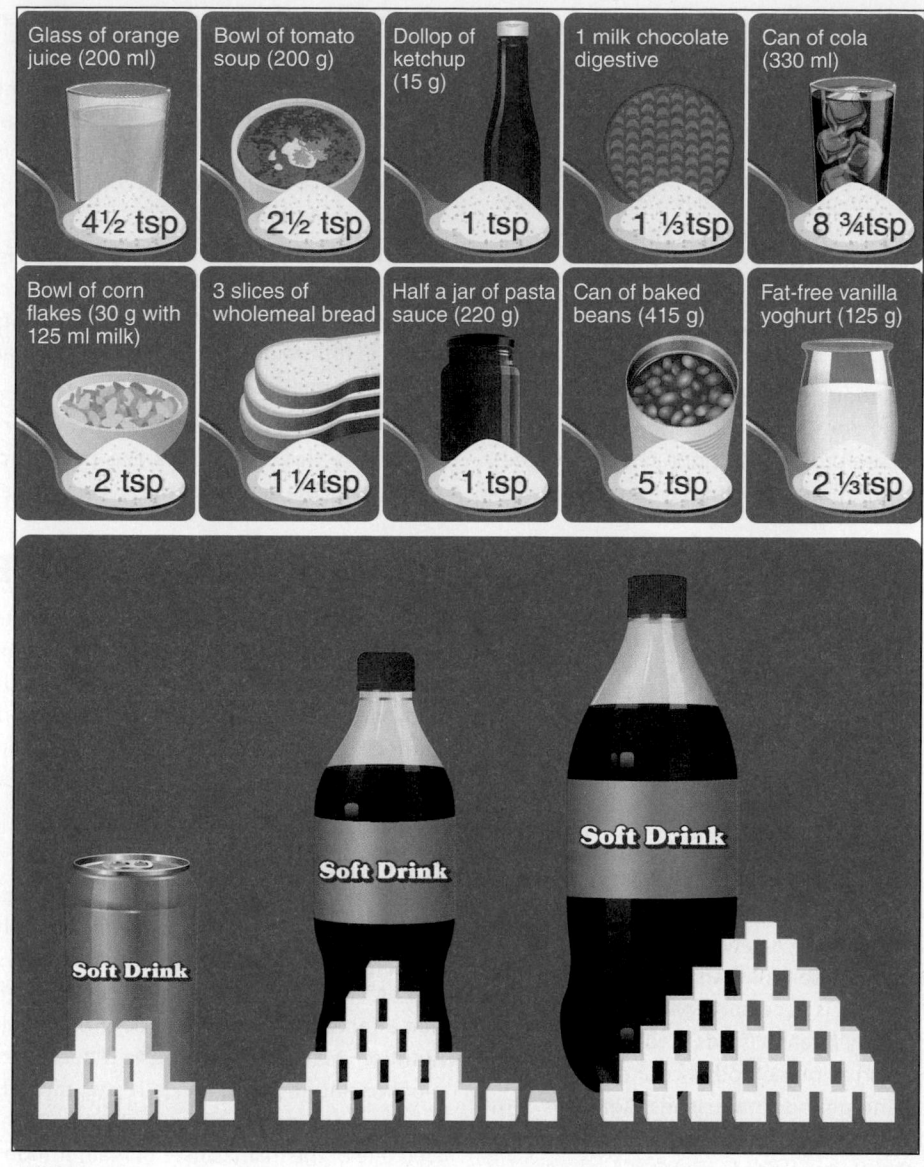

FIGURE 17-4
Amount of sugar in foods.

Diet Counseling for Caries Through diet counseling, the patient becomes aware of the sucrose-containing foods they consume. The cariogenic potential of foods depends on these variables:

- ability to form acid
- ability to dissolve enamel
- ability of food to stick to teeth
- solid and sticky sugar foods are more cariogenic than sugar in solution (liquid)

Recommendations for reducing caries potential are as follows:

- Restrict and, if possible, eliminate snacking between meals with sugar containing foods.
- Avoid snacking at bedtime, which is the worst time to consume sugar-containing foods, especially if teeth are not brushed before bed. Salivary flow is decreased during sleep, causing the mouth to act as an incubator for bacteria.
- Use fluoridated water.
- Use sugar sparingly.
- Brush and floss between meals.
- Visit the dentist regularly.
- Eat a balanced diet and include low cariogenic foods

Periodontal Disease

Periodontal disease affects the tissues of the periodontium (tissues that surround, support, and nourish the tooth). The factors involved in periodontal disease development are as follows:

- susceptible periodontium
- presence of local irritants, dental biofilm, and calculus
- nutritional deficiencies

Impact of Nutritional Deficiencies on the Periodontal Tissue The periodontium is more susceptible to breaking down when the nutrients needed during development are missing from the diet. Adequate nutrition is needed throughout life for the periodontal tissues to maintain and repair themselves and resist disease. The alveolar bone requires the presence of calcium, phosphorus, vitamin D, and fluoride. The soft tissues need a continuous supply of vitamin C. Although the imbalance of nutrition does not cause periodontal disease, it can accelerate the disease process. Nutritional factors to prevent or control periodontal disease can be addressed with patient counseling.

Gingivitis Gingivitis is the inflammation of gingiva surrounding the tooth. There are three primary factors involved in the development of gingivitis:

1. susceptible gingiva due to systemic factors
2. presence of local irritants like biofilm
3. fermentable carbohydrates that come in contact with the gingiva

Gingiva is more susceptible to gingivitis when there is a vitamin deficiency. A deficiency of vitamin C can lower the gingiva's resistance to the accumulation of biofilm. The lack of vitamin C does not cause gingivitis; however, a deficiency allows the tissue to become more inflamed and painful than if the deficiency did not exist. Adequate vitamin C is necessary for tissues to be able to repair themselves properly. Vitamin C aids in the production of collagen, which is found in all of the body's connective tissues, including the gingival and periodontal tissues. Again, as with caries, the lack of protective foods along with an abundance of carbohydrates, affects the progression of gingivitis.

Periodontitis Periodontitis is a continuation of inflammation from the gingival tissue to the supporting tissue around the tooth, alveolar bone and periodontal ligament. The primary factors which cause gingivitis are the same for periodontitis. A diet rich in omega-3, calcium, and vitamin D helps to make the tissues more resistant to disease. A reduction in fermentable carbohydrates will help in the reduction of biofilm and consequently calculus formation. Research shows that smoking, poor diet, and high body weight have a direct and strong association with periodontal disease.

Diet Counseling for Periodontal Disease The relationship between periodontal disease and nutrition is not very clear. However, we know that good nutrition is especially important during times of growth and development of the oral tissues and certainly poor nutrition can make an existing periodontal condition worse. Certain nutrients help build, maintain and repair periodontal tissue and enhance the immune system to fight infection. Specific issues to discuss with the patient include the following:

- Gingival sulcus—because of the fast turnover of these tissues (3 days), the body needs an adequate supply of nutrients to build and maintain healthy soft tissue and bone. Recommend foods rich in vitamins C, A, B complex, and D as well as calcium and magnesium.
- Periodontal infection—the body needs nutrients that will help repair diseased tissue. Inadequate nutrition may impair the repair process. Recommend nutrients that repair and aid in the formation of collagen such as vitamin C, protein, iron, zinc, copper, and selenium.
- Food consistency—eating crunchy, fibrous foods increases salivary flow, exercises the periodontal ligament, and increases the density of the alveolar bone.

Nutrition and Systemic Effects

Research shows that adopting eating habits that are consistent with the nutritional guidelines will promote optimum overall health as well as oral health. Nutrition (or lack of it) affects the body locally and systemically. A systemic effect depends on the nutrients in one's food choices. This influences general health, growth, development, and resistance to disease.

Malnutrition

Malnutrition simply defined is bad nutrition. It may be caused by not having enough to eat, not eating enough nourishing foods or being unable to use the food that has been eaten. Malnutrition and oral health have an interdependent relationship; malnutrition affects oral health, and poor oral health may lead to malnutrition. Malnutrition causes a reduced resistance to microbial biofilms and reduced tissue repair capacity, which affects the development of the oral cavity disease. Poor oral health is considered one of the main causes of malnutrition in the United States; teeth dictate what you are and are not able to eat. Research has found that malnutrition caused by poor oral health leads to functional decline, decreased quality of life, and higher risk of death. Improving the oral health of senior citizens can help improve their overall health. Malnutrition can lead to serious health issues including stunted growth, diabetes, eye problems, and heart disease. The WHO say malnutrition is the gravest single threat to global public health.

Marasmus is an example of a disorder due to malnutrition. Marasmus has a higher incidence in babies and young children. It leads to dehydration and weight loss. This disorder is a form of starvation. The symptoms include weight loss, dehydration, chronic diarrhea, and stomach shrinkage. There is an increased risk among those living in a rural area where it is difficult to get food.

Diabetes

Diabetes mellitus is a chronic disorder of carbohydrate (glucose) metabolism and is characterized by abnormally high blood glucose levels (hyperglycemia). This results from problems with the hormone insulin, which include defective insulin that does not work effectively to lower blood glucose levels, or increased insulin resistance due to obesity. Oral manifestations include the presence of candida albicans, xerostomia (dry mouth), increased progression and severity of periodontal disease with hyperplastic and red gingiva, periodontal bone loss, tooth mobility, and early tooth loss. These conditions are more common in diabetics whose disease is not well controlled. Well-controlled diabetics are far less likely to experience these adverse effects.

Nutritional management of the diabetic patient:

- Instruct patient to read labels carefully for sources of carbohydrates.
- Eat foods that have a low glycemic index (low in sugar).
- Consume foods that have protective factors against periodontal infection.
- Balance diet and medications. The patient must eat so that their insulin levels remain balanced with the medications.

Phenylketonuria

Phenylketonuria (PKU) is a genetic disorder characterized by the inability of the body to utilize the essential amino acid phenylalanine. Oral manifestations include prominent cheek and upper jaw bones, widely spaced teeth, poor development of tooth enamel, and decreased body growth.

Protein Energy Malnutrition

Protein energy malnutrition, also referred to as protein calorie malnutrition, is a form of malnutrition caused by an inadequate amount of protein intake. Mostly affecting older children, an acute form is known as kwashiorkor, which is characterized by edema, bulging of the abdomen, an inability to grow or gain weight, irritability, anorexia, ulcerating skin lesions, and fatty liver infiltrates. Other populations that may be susceptible to protein energy malnutrition are those on kidney dialysis and chemotherapy treatment. Oral manifestations include delayed eruption of teeth, caries-prone teeth, poor cementum deposition, degenerative change in gingiva and periodontium, irregular predentin layer, poor calcification, and reddening of the tongue with loss of papilla.

Cancer

All types of cancer as well as its treatment and complications from surgery, chemotherapy, radiation, and stem cell transplant create many challenges to adequate nutrition. Treatment may impair a patient's appetite and ability to taste food, chew, and swallow. Radiation treatments and/or chemotherapy can cause xerostomia, nausea, loss of appetite, radiation caries, stomatitis, and glossitis. Dietary modifications for the cancer patient must be individualized to address the specific needs.

Nutritional management of the patient with cancer:

- Smooth, bland foods that are nutrient-rich are good for many situations.
- Choose high protein, high Calorie foods to help wounds heal.
- Avoid foods and drinks that can cause gas.
- If constipation is a problem, choose foods high in fiber.
- For glossitis or stomatitis, the texture of the food is particularly important. Hard or crunchy foods could injure the mucosa. In addition, acidic foods, such as tomatoes or citrus fruit, may cause pain.
- For xerostomia choose foods with a high liquid content. Cariogenic foods should be avoided for both generalized xerostomia and radiation-induced xerostomia. Chewing sugarless gum, holding ice chips in the mouth, or using saliva substitutes, such as Biotene or Salivart, can help with severe xerostomia.

Immune System Disorders

A healthy immune system is the body's defense against disease. The immunocompromised patient does not have the ability to fight infection. Causes of immune deficiency are malnutrition, human immunodeficiency virus (HIV), cancer, organ transplant, and autoimmune diseases. The drugs used to treat these conditions can also cause immune depression. Because the oral tissues have a high rate of turnover, dental professionals may be the first to recognize symptoms of immune deficiency such as xerostomia, mucositis, esophagitis, stomatitis, and candidiasis. Nutritional requirements must be specific to meet each person's individual needs.

Nutritional management of the patient with an immune system disorder:

- Screen for nutritional risk.
- Screen for smoking cessation and alcohol dependence.
- Provide appropriate recommendations such as a diet high in Calories, protein, and all other nutrient rich foods.
- Suggest nutritional supplements for added Calories and other nutrients.
- Refer to a registered dietitian.

Osteoporosis

Osteoporosis is a condition in which there is a decrease in the total amount of bone in the body but bone composition remains normal. Some loss of bone is associated with the normal aging process. With osteoporosis bone mass decreases and the bone becomes more fragile; the skeleton may be unable to withstand ordinary stresses, and fractures become more common. Oral bone loss may increase the risk of tooth loss. Risk factors include race, female gender, advancing age, slight body build, low estrogen status, family history, history of poor calcium and vitamin D intake, lack of physical activity, certain medical conditions and medications, and excessive intake of caffeine, alcohol, and tobacco.

Nutritional management of the patient with osteoporosis:

- Prevention throughout life is important with adequate intake of calcium and vitamin D; moderate amounts of sodium, protein, and phosphorus (soda); regular weight-bearing exercise (walking, jogging, cycling, and weight lifting); and avoiding tobacco.

- Consume three to four servings of foods rich in calcium and vitamin D.
- For those who cannot tolerate milk products, advise calcium rich soy products such as tofu and calcium fortified orange juice.
- Advise calcium and vitamin D supplements.
- For postmenopausal women, advise regular bone health screening.

Physical and Mental Conditions

There are many nutritional problems suffered by patients with special needs. The inability to properly brush and floss their teeth causes significant dental problems leading to nutritional deficiencies and disease. These patients may exhibit food texture aversions; drug and food interactions; exaggerated gag, cough, bite, and swallow reflexes; absence of or weak sucking response due to a cleft lip or palate; poor arm and head control; and inadequate jaw, lip, and tongue control.

For patients with special needs, the diet may need to be modified. Work with the family and caregiver when recommending any changes.

Nutritional management for the patient with special needs:

- Educate the family and/or caregiver on dietary problems that may be caused from poor oral health as well as dental disease that is related to diet.
- Ensure that the diet is nutritionally stable.

Refer to a professional dietitian if the nutritional needs require ongoing management.

Diet Management for Patients with Special Dental Needs

There are times when the dental team will need to modify a patient's diet to meet the special requirements for specific dental treatments such as oral surgery, orthodontic treatment or learning to eat with a new denture.

Oral Surgery

After dental surgery (extractions, implants, periodontal surgery), patients face the challenge of maintaining good nutrition while the mouth is healing. Good nutrition will speed the healing process, but this can be difficult if the oral tissues are tender and chewing or swallowing is difficult. Furthermore, care must be taken not to disturb the surgical area. Side effects of anesthesia and pain medications may include loss of appetite and nausea.

Nutritional management for the patient after oral surgery:

- Drink plenty of fluids.
- A liquid diet should be followed for the first few days. The liquid diet may include high-protein liquid products fortified

with vitamins and minerals such as Boost, Ensure, Sustacal, or Instant Breakfast.

- After the first few days, a soft diet can be introduced, gradually adding more solids until the patient can return to a normal diet.
- Patients should avoid smoking, alcohol, spicy and crunchy foods, alcoholic beverages, and hot liquids that may cause injury to the surgical site or induce bleeding.

Oral Trauma

Patients who have suffered injury to the mouth or jaws have significant difficulty maintaining an ordinary diet. Caution is required to avoid further damage to the injured area. Again, pain medication may play a role in reducing the appetite.

Nutritional management for the patient with oral trauma:

- As with oral surgery, the trauma patient may require a liquid diet at first, progressing to a soft diet, and then solid food that has been cut into small pieces.
- Patients should not eat foods that require a biting or tearing action by the affected teeth. It is important that no chewing pressure be placed on the injured area.
- Patients who have suffered a fractured jaw may have their maxillary and mandibular jaws fixated (wired together) for a number of weeks.
- Great creativity is needed to design a liquid diet that can provide optimal nutrition for a lengthy period.

Orthodontic Treatment

Orthodontic patients require a special diet for several reasons. After initial placement of brackets or bands and each subsequent orthodontic adjustment appointment, there is a period of tenderness and possible tooth mobility. The patient will require a soft diet for a few days. In addition, some foods may damage the orthodontic appliances, and these foods should be avoided for the duration of treatment.

Nutritional management for the patient with orthodontic appliances:

- Foods to be avoided by orthodontic patients include any sticky or retentive food or candy, gum, nuts, cookies, popcorn, pretzels, raw celery and carrots, soda, hard bagels, and pizza crust.
- Crunchy foods such as apples and carrots may be eaten if they are sliced.
- The patient should be informed that chewing on ice should be especially avoided.

New Dentures

Eating with dentures is a challenge for new denture wearers. Dentures do not function like natural teeth. With the acrylic material covering the palate and alveolar ridges, sensations caused by food in the mouth are reduced. The denture wearer is less aware of temperature and texture of food or the location of the food in the mouth. There will be an adjustment period of days or weeks as the patient learns to use the dentures.

Nutritional management for the patient with new dentures:

- Initially, a liquid diet is advised.
- When the patient is comfortable swallowing liquid, while wearing the dentures, soft foods can be added. Avoid sticky or hard foods.
- Later, the patient can try solid foods cut into small pieces.
- Chew foods slowly, on both sides, with the back teeth to prevent tipping of the denture.
- Use caution with food and drinks of hot temperature. Since the denture covers the palate, the heat may not be felt until the food is on the way down.
- Eventually, most patients will be able to eat a full range of foods.
- If the patient reports difficulty eating particular foods, such as fruits and vegetables, the dental staff may be able to suggest alternatives that provide the same nutrition.

Temporomandibular Joint Disorders

The patient with **temporomandibular joint** disorders may have difficulty eating a full diet. The patient may have joint or muscle pain upon opening the mouth, restricted opening, or pain when chewing pressure is applied.

Nutritional management for the patient with temporomandibular joint disorders:

- A soft diet with eating events divided into several small meals a day to limit the amount of chewing at one sitting.
- Recommend liquid supplements such as Boost, Ensure, Sustacal, or Instant Breakfast.
- Foods that require opening wide such as whole, raw apples or large sandwiches can be cut into small pieces.
- Chewing gum should be omitted from the diet.

Stomatitis

Stomatitis is inflammation of the mucosal lining of any of the structures in the mouth. It can involve the cheek, lips, tongue, gums, throat, and/or roof or floor of the mouth. Stomatitis can result from poor oral hygiene, dietary protein deficiency, poorly fitting dentures, thermal burns from hot foods or drinks, allergic reactions, and cancer chemotherapy.

Similarly, nutritional deficiencies have specific effects on the oral mucosa. Because the oral mucosa continues to repair and replace itself through life, adequate nutrition is necessary at all stages of life. A lack of specific nutrients will result in oral disease.

A healthy salivary flow also helps to protect the mucosa and teeth from the many insults that occur on a daily basis. It is important to assess patients for xerostomia because this dryness predisposes the mouth to stomatitis.

Nutritional management for the patient with stomatitis:

- Recommend products that help relieve dry mouth such as Biotene.
- Drink plenty of fluids.
- Recommend foods such as fruits, vegetables, grains, nuts, and seeds.
- Special emphasis should be placed on whole grains, cereals, fruits, and vegetables that are either raw or cooked lightly to stimulate saliva flow. Sprouted seeds like green gram beans and alfalfa are also healthy foods to eat.
- Avoid candies, processed food, pickles, soft drinks, refined foods, tough or fibrous meats, coffee, tea, white flour, sugar, and condiments.

Religious and Cultural Diet Considerations

In many cultures, food is an important part of social rituals or religious observance. Religious rules can affect food choices. For example, Hindus do not eat meat, fish, poultry and eggs; Jewish people do not eat non-kosher meat and fish or birds of prey; Islamic countries exclude pork or alcohol in any form; and Thai farmers give blessings at every stage of a rice crop's growth.

It is necessary to understand that the role of food in cultural practices and religious beliefs is complex and varies among individuals and communities. This understanding is vital in helping to develop a dietary plan that will work for your patient. **Compliance** is the key. So where do we find information on cultural diversity? There are associations, administrations, universities, resource centers, web links, continuing education courses, and articles published in dental journals that provide professionals with up-to-date information. To become a culturally **competent** dental professional, it is important to be well informed about the populations we serve in the area we practice. Always remember to respect the sensitivity of different religious and cultural backgrounds. Dental assistants will come into contact with patients who come from a variety of cultural backgrounds. As stated in Chapter 1, each patient must be treated as an individual, and stereotyping must be avoided. Patients may eat foods that are unfamiliar to the dental assistant. Some examples include cultures that may drink specific teas that stain the teeth, or they may come into the United States and go from eating fruits and vegetables to a high-carbohydrate diet. Dental assistants should be informed of patients' diet choices so they can make suggestions that will aid them in achieving and maintaining good oral habits.

Eating Disorders

In today's society, it seems as if everyone is either overeating or doing everything possible to stay thin. The media and the fashion industry have brought forth the idea that all individuals should aspire to be thin. Advertisers repeatedly assert that taking this or that pill will allow for significant weight loss within a short time.

Eating disorders such as chronic dieting syndrome, compulsive overeating, bulimia, and anorexia nervosa are widespread and can be serious and even life-threatening. They can have psychological, physical, and medical implications. The population most affected is females (at a ratio of 10 females to 1 male), aged 12 to 30, and often from white, affluent families.

Chronic dieting syndrome causes the individual to experience continuous weight loss and gain, and compulsive overeating can cause a number of psychological, physical, and medical implications that increase risk factors for diabetes and other diseases. Bulimia and anorexia can become life-threatening.

Chronic Dieting Syndrome

Chronic dieting syndrome is commonplace. A large percentage of people are ingesting pharmaceuticals or diet supplements to control their weight. This is important to dental assistants because the drugs may cause problems in dental treatment. The dieting may cause the heart to race or chemical imbalances. Adding the anxiety of dental treatment may be enough to cause problems for the patient. Paying special attention to patients' medical and dental histories will be extremely beneficial.

Bulimia

Bulimia is classified as an eating disorder characterized by restricting food intake for a period of time, followed by an over-intake or binging period that results in feelings of guilt or low self-esteem. Self-induced vomiting or purging, laxative abuse, excessive exercise, or overuse of diuretics usually follows the binge period.

Bulimia may occur when other weight loss attempts do not work. Once tried, it quickly becomes obsessive, resulting in an out-of-control cycle of overeating and purging. An estimated 3 to 5% of women in the United States have been affected by bulimia at some time in their lives. Far fewer men are affected with this disorder. Bulimia and anorexia nervosa behaviors are very secretive and therefore difficult to diagnose. Individuals with bulimia may experience weight gains and losses but normally do not show extreme weight loss such as in anorexia nervosa. The overeating (binging) is not caused by the desire for food but is a response to stress or depression. Eating brings about overwhelming happiness or a euphoric feeling that is quickly followed by the feeling of self-hatred and depression because of the binging. The individual experiences loss of control and then begins the purging or other behaviors that allow them to feel that they have regained control. Individuals may take laxatives, participate in excessive exercise, take diuretics, or use other weight loss methods to rid the body of the weight gained during the overeating.

There are a number of oral and systemic complications that can result from bulimia (Figure 17-5). Oral manifestations include severe dental **erosion** from exposure to stomach acids due to vomiting, especially seen on the lingual (facing the tongue) surfaces of the upper anterior (front) teeth. When the enamel has thinned or completely eroded, the teeth are more susceptible to decay and are more sensitive to heat or cold. The recurring regurgitation (vomiting) can cause the parotid glands and the saliva

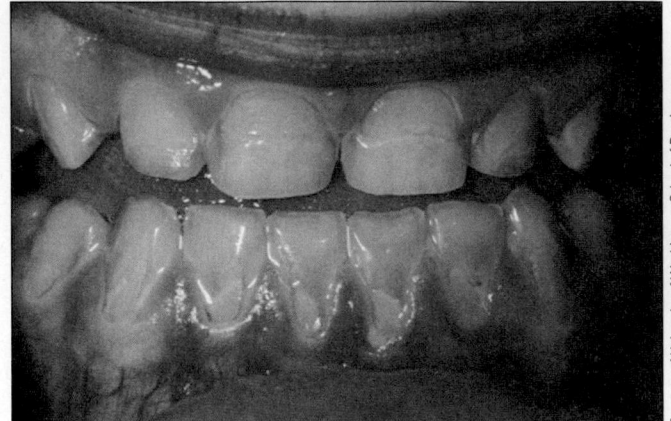
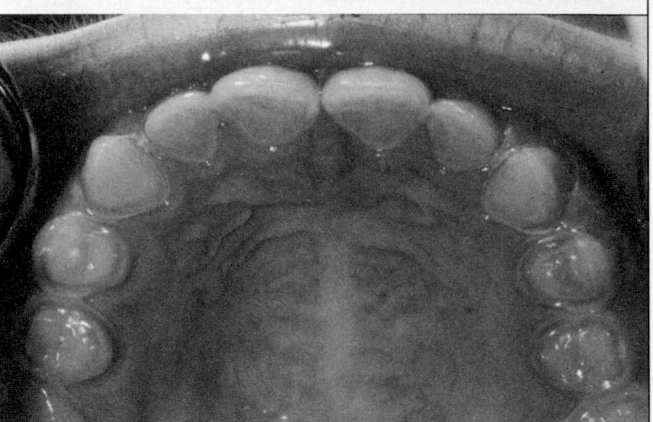
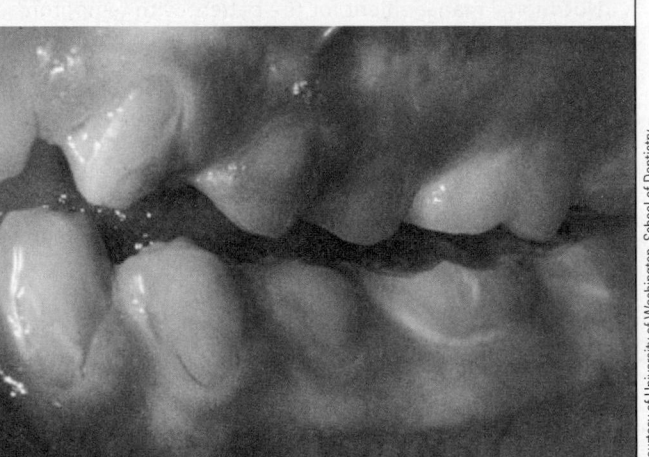

Courtesy of University of Washington, School of Dentistry

FIGURE 17-5
Eroded tooth structure shown of the facial, lingual, and buccal surfaces of the teeth due to bulimia.

glands to become tender and swell, which can be very uncomfortable. Oral trauma to the lining of the mouth or throat may be evident due to fingers or objects used to induce vomiting.

Anorexia Nervosa

Anorexia nervosa is classified as both an eating and emotional disorder, resulting in a prolonged avoidance of eating. This disorder is characterized by severe weight loss, emaciation, an extreme aversion to food, decreased sleep, an extreme fear of being fat, and psychological disturbance. Individuals with this disorder have a distorted body image and see themselves as fat even though they may be overly thin. This psychological disorder centers on control, and behavioral symptoms focus on the fear of putting on weight or eating foods that contain fat or carbohydrates. Individuals with anorexia nervosa may have psychological, physical, and behavioral symptoms such as flaky skin, brittle nails, thinning of hair on the head, amenorrhea (absence of monthly menstrual periods), heart complications, kidney function issues, gastrointestinal complications, impaired organ function, lanugo (baby-like hair) on the body, food obsession, extreme use of laxatives, depression, social withdrawal, and obsessive exercising. The individual often feels intensely hungry but will deny fulfillment of this need. Individuals with anorexia nervosa are obsessed with food and thinking of food. They may find it difficult to go out to eat with others. They usually have eating rituals and may cut their food into small pieces and arrange and rearrange it on their plate; typically anorexics know every Calorie in each bite consumed. Individuals suffering from this disorder may prepare Calorie-laden foods for others but would feel extreme distress if they had to eat it themselves. The disorder is not focused on the weight loss or food intake but on control and other fears relating to the body.

Treating this disease is difficult. It is much easier to diagnose in the later stages because of emaciation, or extreme thinness. It is more complicated to diagnose in the early stages due to secrecy and attempts to hide the disorder from others. There are numerous types of therapies that can be helpful to people with anorexia nervosa, including psychological therapy, group therapy, family therapy, cognitive behavior therapy, and drug therapy, along with numerous hospital treatments that focus on correcting the malnutrition. Intravenous feeding may be recommended to treat the malnutrition. Working with a nutritionist during any of these therapies may enhance the outcome. The individual may require day treatment or longer inpatient care. Even if the treatment is successful, relapses can easily occur because the slightest stress triggers the disorder again. Of the individuals who have been hospitalized for anorexia nervosa, an estimated 8 to 10% later die from suicide or starvation. This condition is on the rise in the United States; an estimated 1 in every 100 adolescent females has anorexic symptoms.

The individuals that come to the dental office with this disorder have numerous physical problems, so special attention to the medical and dental history is crucial. They may also be very uncomfortable lying back in the dental chair if the dental treatment continues for any length of time. The oral cavity may show signs of the disorder, such as sore tissues resulting from poor periodontal health. The binging and purging may be reflected in the state of the teeth, as noted in the section on bulimia. Calcium intake may be limited; therefore, the teeth may not be as strong as normal, and decay may progress more rapidly. Oral manifestations include tooth enamel and dentin erosion, occlusal changes, thermal sensitivity and abnormal swallowing, susceptibility to gingivitis and periodontitis, and poor healing. Since the anorexic patient avoids all foods, the oral mucosa could show any of the signs of deficiency described previously.

Female Athlete Triad Syndrome

Female athlete triad is a medical condition that affects physically active females, especially those who engage in sports in which a low body weight and lean physique are desired (like dancers, gymnasts, and runners). It involves three basic symptoms (a triad): low energy with or without an eating disorder, menstrual dysfunction, and low bone density. This syndrome may not be completely reversible, making early diagnosis and intervention critical. Since the original discovery of the syndrome there have been many more components that have been identified. The International Olympic Committee has proposed changing the name to relative energy deficiency in sports (RED-S) because there are many more components that may be involved including endocrine (hypothalamic dysfunction), metabolic, hematologic, growth and development, cardiovascular, gastrointestinal, and immunologic effects of energy deficiencies. If the athlete is diagnosed with an eating disorder, they will have the same oral effects as mentioned previously.

Role of the Dental Assistant in Nutrition

It is important for dental professionals to treat each patient as a whole individual and not just consider their dental condition. Part of that responsibility is to recognize the signs and symptoms of patients suffering from nutritional deficiencies, and to provide the proper care or a referral needed. While it is not possible to provide in-depth nutritional counseling to every dental patient, certainly there are those who would benefit the most from nutritional advice. The high-risk patients include pregnant women, adolescents, older adults, individuals with rampant caries or severe periodontal disease, patients with special dental needs, edentulous (all teeth missing) patients, and patients undergoing cancer treatment. Other factors to consider are knowledge of dental staff, scheduling issues, availability of space to counsel the patient, and individual patient needs.

As discussed before, a person's diet has a great impact on their oral health, and oral problems affect what a person eats and their nutritional status. For these reasons it is important that the dental team be able to identify dietary concerns and be able to provide advice and/or referral. A diet assessment should be completed including a comprehensive evaluation of a person's food intake (food habits) and lifestyle (buying practices, cooking methods, likes and dislikes, and whether the patient is able to shop for themselves). In addition, a thorough medical history is essential. Once the information is collected, the dental assistant can assess the nutritional status of the patient and then work with the patient to design a nutritional plan to maintain health or stop or heal dental disease.

Diet Assessment Tools

There are several tools that will help the dental assistant and the patient record the diet history, including eating patterns, what determines food selection, how the food is prepared, and even snacking patterns.

- *24 hour recall*—the patient records all food consumed during a single day. This tool provides a good analysis of basic nutritional adequacy, variety of nutrients, and the cariogenic potential of foods eaten in one day. In addition, snacking patterns are easily revealed. However, the day the patient chooses may not be a typical day, and the recall of the diet may be inaccurate.

- *Food frequency questionnaire*—the patients write down how often they consume a specific type of food in a day or week. With this tool the dental assistant can see how much of a food group a patients eats, including carbohydrates. The food frequency questionnaire is not specific and does not provide enough data to evaluate the patient's total nutrition. The best use of the questionnaire is to use it in conjunction with 24 hour recall to give a total picture.

- *Food diary*—this tool is the most effective method of recording food intake. The patient records food and drink consumption for 3 to 7 days. A great advantage is that the patient is involved in the process; however, patient cooperation for 7 days may be difficult.

The guidelines for these procedures are outlined in the "Guidelines for Recording Food Intake" box.

After the selected food list is completed, put each food listed into the appropriate food group using MyPlate as a guide. Compare the amounts eaten with what is recommended or needed. Evaluate foods for nutritional adequacy, evaluate nonessential foods or foods that can cause harm, and finally look for excesses in any one food, especially foods that have the potential to cause caries. The dental assistant can develop a list of foods that provide

Guidelines for Recording Food Intake

- Be as accurate as possible.
- Record soon after eating.
- Record all meals and snacks for each day, including one weekend day.
- Record portion size and how the food was prepared.
- Include added sugar.
- For combination dishes (soups, casseroles, chili) record each ingredient separately.
- Use brand names.
- Enter the time eaten.
- Record miscellaneous food such as mints, gum, and cough drops.

the necessary nutrients, but it is important that the patient choose foods they are likely to eat. It does no good to advise specific foods if the foods are unpalatable or offensive to the patient. Utilizing a nutritional assessment will allow to meet the needs of everyone.

Diet Counseling

Once the data is complete, the dental assistant can determine the nutritional status of the patient, assess the potential for dental disease and then help the patient establish realistic goals for a healthy mouth and body. Remember the goal of any education program should be to modify the patient's behavior to result in better habits. If possible, a quiet, private room other than the dental operatory is the ideal place to counsel patients.

There are two approaches to counseling patients:

- *Direct approach*—the counselor assumes an authoritative role. The patient provides information about their diet and then acts as a passive listener. The counselor analyzes and evaluates the diet and makes any necessary recommendations for improvement. Although easier for the counselor because it requires less time, it is not ideal because the patient is not involved in making the diet and lifestyle choices.

- *Indirect or behavior modification approach*—the patient is encouraged to become involved in the decision-making process regarding the dietary recommendations for a healthier lifestyle. The counselor provides the information about the etiology of dental disease, the importance of a healthy diet, and the tools needed to make that change in lifestyle. The patient then chooses from among the recommended strategies to achieve the goal. Although more time and effort is required from both parties, there is a greater probability that the plan will be accepted by the patient.

It is necessary to put a time limit on any patient education effort. If a particular strategy is not working then the dental assistant and the patient need to come up with an alternative plan that actually works. A follow-up appointment at a predetermined time is necessary to evaluate for success.

Cariogenic Foods Counseling

Evaluating cariogenic foods in patients' diets can be accomplished by the dental assistant reviewing the patient's food diary and identifying cariogenic foods with the patient. Evaluation of each food in the patient's diet provides a better understanding of which types of foods are cariogenic. Dental assistants will need to advise patients on carbohydrates because they are potentially cariogenic. Explain how cariogenic foods break down into simple

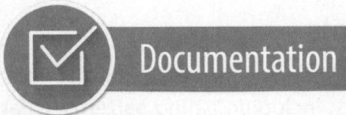 **Documentation**

As with any treatment, documentation in the patient's record is required. Make sure to include all information: what tools were used, the plan or strategy, whether the plan was successful, and any modifications needed.

sugars in the mouth that can be used by bacteria to cause dental caries. Most patients will be aware that carbohydrates already broken down into simple sugars, such as candies, soft drinks, and sweet desserts, cause decay. It will be the other carbohydrates that patients are unaware of that may cause decay, such as raisins, crackers, fruits, and a few vegetables. The intake of fruits and vegetables normally is not a problem because fruits and vegetables do not stick to the teeth and are not converted to simple sugars until they reach the stomach.

The assistant can discuss the following:

- The texture of the foods and whether they are retentive sugars, such as caramels, that stick in a concentrated sugar form on the tooth. Suggest to patients that they choose carbohydrates that will not remain on the teeth for long periods.

- The number of times cariogenic foods are being eaten.

- What time of day cariogenic foods are eaten. Eating cariogenic foods at bedtime, when the flow of saliva decreases, increases the chance of decay. Saliva is a buffer to the acid, and if the flow rate of the saliva is inadequate, the cariogenic substances may not be washed away.

- The more often the teeth are exposed to cariogenic food, the greater the probability of decay; for instance, the person who drinks a soft drink very slowly and allows the sugar to soak on the teeth over and over will have a greater chance of decay.

- Eating cariogenic foods with other foods may offer some neutralization of the acid that feeds the bacteria.

- When medicines and mouth fresheners containing sugars dissolve in the mouth, bathing the teeth with sugar for a long period may cause a large number of caries over time.

- Infants who have erupted teeth and are given bottles of milk, fruit juice, or sweet substances for long periods may develop nursing bottle syndrome (NBS) or baby bottle tooth decay (BBTD). This extensive decay of newly formed teeth is due to the sweetened liquid frequently bathing the teeth, often at bedtime. Parents should be informed and advised of the possibility of NBS so they can take preventive measures.

It is important for the dental professional to recognize nutritional deficiencies and their relationship to oral and total body health. However, before thinking about any nutrition counseling for a patient, it is important to remember that the dental professional should only counsel patients in relation to their oral health. If it is discovered that a patient needs diet recommendations for a medical problem, it is beyond the scope of the dental practice and the patient must be referred to a registered dietitian or a physician.

Chapter Summary

Dental assistants need to have a background in nutrition to maintain good overall health as well as aid patients in diet modification to increase foods with nutritional value and decrease cariogenic foods. Everyone can benefit from knowledge of how to read nutrition labels and select food wisely. One of the responsibilities of the dental assistant is to instruct patient on postoperative instructions after dental treatment requiring changes in the patient's diet. Having an understanding of eating disorders may prove beneficial in the work environment with other coworkers and patients.

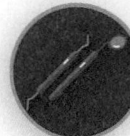 **CASE STUDY**

Maci Smith is a 17-year-old who had been involved in chronic dieting to keep her weight down. Recently when Maci came into the dental office, staff members noticed that she had lost an extreme amount of weight. Signs of erosion on the lingual surface of her teeth were also noted. Maci told the dentist that her teeth were sensitive to heat and cold.

Case Study Review

1. What should the dental assistant do if they observe this condition?

2. What diagnosis may be indicated with these symptoms?

3. Should the dentist discuss with Maci the possibility that she has been purging?

4. What other areas in the oral cavity could be examined?

Review Questions

Multiple Choice

1. Which foods should be limited to maintain good health?
   a. protein, milk, and sugar
   b. whole grains, meats, and salt
   c. fat, salt, and refined sugar
   d. beans, fats, and grains

2. What are the consequences of nutritional deficiency or toxicity that occurs at the time when enamel is forming?
   a. Malformations of teeth are usually permanent.
   b. Malformed teeth are more susceptible to caries.
   c. Inadequate chewing may occur.
   d. All of these are likely.

3. Which of these nutrients is considered the body's *main* source of fuel?
   a. fats
   b. vitamins
   c. minerals
   d. carbohydrate

4. Which of these nutrients are responsible for growth and maintenance of all cells and tissues of the body?
   a. fats
   b. vitamins
   c. minerals
   d. proteins

5. Water-soluble vitamins include:
   a. B_1, B_2, D, and niacin.
   b. D, E, K, and C.
   c. D, E, B, and K.
   d. B_1, B_2, C, and niacin.

6. Which nutrient is potentially cariogenic and must be evaluated in a patient's diet?
   a. fats
   b. proteins
   c. carbohydrates
   d. minerals

7. Which food group is a good source of carbohydrates?
   a. fruits
   b. vegetables
   c. proteins
   d. grains

8. The _____ food group is necessary for strong bones and teeth.
   a. protein
   b. grains
   c. dairy
   d. fruits

9. Which is a measurement of energy a substance supplies?
   a. RDA
   b. DRI
   c. DV
   d. calorie

10. Food labels daily values are based on a _____ calorie diet.
    a. 1,200
    b. 1,500
    c. 2,000
    d. 2,400

11. At what temperature should the refrigerator be set to minimize the chance of bacterial growth and food poisoning?
    a. 70°F
    b. 60°F
    c. 40°F
    d. 0°F

12. Which federal government guideline emphasizes food portions for better eating?
    a. Dietary Guidelines for Americans
    b. MyPlate
    c. food labels
    d. Food and Drug Administration

13. Which focuses on the amount of particular nutrients needed to prevent deficiencies?
    a. DRIs
    b. RDAs
    c. MyPlate
    d. Healthy People 2020 Report

14. A continuous supply of _____ is needed for healthy soft tissues.
    a. vitamin C
    b. vitamin D
    c. calcium
    d. phosphorus

15. Which tissue needs calcium, phosphorus, vitamin D, and fluoride present for healthy development?
    a. soft tissue
    b. muscle
    c. bone
    d. nerves

16. Which is the most cariogenic?
    a. fats
    b. proteins
    c. fermentable carbohydrates
    d. vegetables

17. Which may be a result of poor calcium and vitamin D intake?
    a. phenylketonuria (PKU)
    b. diabetes
    c. kwashiorkor
    d. osteoporosis

18. A patient has just had their orthodontic appliances placed. Which foods should the dental assistant direct the patient to avoid?
    a. soda
    b. popcorn
    c. gum
    d. all of these should be avoided.

19. The eating disorder characterized by bouts of gross overeating followed by purging resulting in tooth erosion is called:
    a. anorexia nervosa.
    b. bulimia.
    c. pica.
    d. chronic dieting syndrome.

20. What is the dental assistant's primary nutritional task?
    a. Monitor weight changes.
    b. Monitor food and drug interactions.
    c. Counsel patients with compromised oral integrity.
    d. Record reactions to foods.

Critical Thinking

1. How can knowledge of nutrition benefit the dental assistant?

2. How should food labels be used in selecting food and planning a healthy diet?

3. How can using MyPlate help the patient get the nutrients that they need?

4. Using MyPlate, do you have any areas that you need to improve?

5. If the dental assistant learns that a patient is bulimic, what should the dental assistant do? Should this information be disclosed to the dentist? What information should be offered to the patient about the effects on the oral cavity?

6. Explain why it is better to eat more of a candy at once than throughout the whole day.

7. Complete your personal food diary. Make a list of the foods and beverages that you have consumed in a 7-day period. Look at each item on the list. Consider why you chose that particular food or beverage. Was it out of habit, convenience, or because it was a better choice nutritionally? In reviewing your list, you may learn a great deal about yourself from your food choices. This will also enable you to educate your patients so that they will be able to make better food choices for optimal health and wellness.

8. Using your completed food diary and MyPlate as a guide, assess your diet by comparing the amounts eaten with what is needed for nutritional adequacy. Identify foods that are cariogenic.

Key Terms

Term and Pronunciation	Meaning of Root and Word Parts	Definition
amino acids (*uh*-**mee**-noh) (**as**-idz)	**amine** = class of compound derived by replacement of one or more hydrogen atoms with organic groups **-o-** = combining vowel to connect elements in a compound word **acid** = any class of compounds that form hydrogen ions when dissolved in water	compounds that link together to form proteins
amylase (**am**-*uh*-leys)	**amylo** = indicating starch **-ase** = indicating an enzyme	an enzyme primarily found in saliva and pancreatic fluid that converts starch and glycogen into simple sugars
arthritis (ahr-**thray**-tis)	**arthro-** = joint **-itis** = inflammation	acute or chronic inflammation of a joint
aqueous medium (**ey**-kwee-*uhs*) (**mee**-dee-*uh*m)	**aqua** = water **-eous** = composed of **medium** = a means of effecting or conveying something	a solution in which the solvent (has ability to dissolve molecules) is water; nearly all biochemical reactions take place in this medium
beriberi (**Ber**-ee-**ber**-ee)	**beri** = weakness	a disease of the nervous system due to thiamine (vitamin B_1); symptoms of pain, difficulty walking, paralysis of extremities, emaciation and swelling
biofilm (plak) (**bahy**-oh-film)	**bio-** = involving life or living organisms **film** = a thin layer or coating	well-organized community of bacteria that adheres to tooth surfaces, primary cause of most periodontal disease and caries
body mass index (**bod**-ee) (mas) (**in**-deks)	**body** = refers to the entire physical structure of an individual **mass** = physical volume or bulk of a solid body **index** = a number indicating the relation of one part or thing to another in respect to size, capacity, or function	a measurement of the relative percentages of fat and muscle mass in the body
buffer (**buhf**-er)	**buff** = to reduce or deaden the force of **-er** = designating person or object	a substance that prevents change in the acidity of a solution
Calorie (**kal**-*uh*-ree)	**Calorie** = an amount of food having an energy-producing value of one Calorie (kcal)	heat required to raise 1 kilogram of water 1 degree Celsius

(Continues)

Term and Pronunciation	Meaning of Root and Word Parts	Definition
candida albicans (**kan**-di-d*uh*) (**ahl**-b*uh*-kanz)	**candida** = yeast-like fungi that may cause athlete's foot, vaginitis, or thrush **alba** = white **-an** = belonging to or relating to	a yeast species that is the principle cause of candidiasis; parasitic fungus that can infect the mouth, skin, intestines, or vagina
caries (**kair**-eez)	**caries** = decay, decompose	progressive decay of bone or tooth
cariogenic (kair-ee-*uh*-**jen**-ik)	**cari(es)** = dental caries; tooth decay **gen** = that which produces **-ic** = pertaining to	contributes to the production of dental caries
carotene (**kar**-uh-teen)	**carrot** = orange or yellow root of this plant can be eaten raw or cooked **-ene** = denotes origin or source	any of three yellow or orange fat-soluble pigments found in plants (especially carrots) and transformed to vitamin A in liver
catalyst (**kat**-l-ist)	**cata-** = something that causes activity; chemical reaction **-lysis** = breaking down, loosening	substance that starts or speeds up a chemical reaction; enzyme in saliva is a catalyst in digestion
cataracts (**kat**-uh-rakt)	**cataract** = degeneration; opaque area (cloud-like)	a loss of transparency of the lens of the eye; reducing vision or blindness
chemotherapy (kee-moh-**ther**-uh-pee)	**chemical** = a drug that interacts with atoms or molecules **therapy** = treatment of diseases or disorders	treatment of disease using chemicals that have a toxic effect on the disease-producing microorganisms to selectively destroy cancerous tissue
cleft palate (kleft) (**pal**-it)	**cleft** = split **palate** = roof of the mouth	a congenital defect of the palate; crack in the middle of the hard palate
coenzyme (koh-**en**-zahym)	**co** = molecule providing the transfer site for biochemical reactions **enzyme** = group of complex proteins produced by living cells; act as catalysts in biochemical reactions	a chemical compound that is bound to a protein; required for protein's biological activity
collagen (**kol**-uh-juhn)	**colla** = glue-like **-gen** = that which produces	tough fibrous proteins found in bone, cartilage, skin and connective tissue; most plentiful protein in the body
competent (**kom**-pi-tuh nt)	**compete** = to strive to outdo another for acknowledgement **-ent** = causing or performing an action	having suitable skill, knowledge and experience for a specific purpose; properly qualified
compliance (k*uh* m-**plahy**-*uh* ns)	**comply** = to act or be in accordance with requirements **-ance** = indicating an action	the act of confirming, cooperation or obedience
dehydration (dee-hahy-**drey**-sh*uh* n)	**de-** = removal, separation **hydro** = water **-ate** = denoting a function **-ion** = denoting action or condition	an abnormal loss of water from the body, especially from illness or physical exertion
delirium (dih-**leer**-ee-*uh* m)	**delirare** = to be crazy **-ium** = denoting associated status	a more or less temporary disorder characterized by restlessness, excitement, delusions, and hallucinations
demineralization (dee-**min**-er-*uhl*-ahy-zey- sh*uh*n)	**de** = removal of **mineral** = any of a class of naturally occurring solid inorganic substances **ize** = to convert **tion** = indicating action	loss of mineral salts, especially from the teeth or bones
depression (dih-**presh**-*uh*n)	**depress** = to make sad or gloomy **-sion** = act of or state of	a condition of emotional withdrawal and sadness greater and more prolonged than reasonably warranted
dermatitis (dur-muh-**tahy**-tis)	**derm-** = indicating skin **-itis** = inflammation	inflammation of the skin
dialysis (dahy-**al**-uh-sis)	**dia-** = passing through **-lysis** = breaking down, loosening	the process which removes uric acid and urea from the blood using a machine (dialyzer), which is a substitute for the normal function of the kidney
diet (**dahy**-it)	**diet** = food and drink a person regularly consumes	a specific allowance or selection of food

Term and Pronunciation	Meaning of Root and Word Parts	Definition
dilution (dih-**loo**-sh*uh* n)	**dilute** = to make a liquid thinner or weaker by the addition of water or the like **-ion** = denoting action or condition	the act of reducing the concentration of a mixture or solution
diuretic (dahy-*uh*-**ret**-ik)	**diuret** = increase the flow of urine **-ic** = of, relating to	a medical substance that increases the volume of urine excreted; used to reduce swelling and high blood pressure
electrolyte (ih-**lek**-truh-lahyt)	**electro-** = electric or electricity **-lyte** = pertaining to a process	any of various ions, such as sodium or chloride, required by cells to regulate the electric charge and flow of water molecules across the cell membrane
erosion (ih-**roh**-zh*uh*n)	**erode** = eat into or away **-ion** = denoting action or condition	the wearing away of a tooth by chemical or abrasive action
esophagitis (ih-**sof**-*uh*-jahy-tis)	**esophagus** = a muscular passage connecting the mouth or pharynx with the stomach **-itis** = inflammation of an organ	inflammation of the esophagus
fatty acids (**fat**-ee) (**as**-idz)	**fat** = large number of oily compounds found in plant and animal tissues; serve as source of energy **-y** = characterized by **acid** = any class of compounds that form hydrogen ions when dissolved in water	are the building blocks of fat in the body and in food; body breaks down fats into fatty acids during digestion
fermentable (**fur**-ment-t*uh*-b*uh* l)	**ferment** = any of a group of living organisms such as yeasts, molds, and certain bacteria that cause a chemical reaction to change complex compounds to simple substances **-able** = capable of	any of a group of chemical reactions that split complex organic compounds into simple substances; sugar to alcohol by yeast
fiber (**fahy**-ber)	**fiber** = thread-like matter from tissue or parts of plants	dietary material containing substances which are resistant to the actin of digestive enzymes; indigestible carbohydrate that is important for digestive health
glossitis (glaw-**sahy**-tis)	**gloss/o** = tongue **-itis** = inflammation	inflammation of the tongue
glucose (**gloo**-kohs)	**gluc** = sugar **-ose** = full of; forms the names of sugars	sugar that serves as a major source of energy to the body; found in most plant and animal tissue
gout (gout)	**gout** = defective metabolism of uric acid causing acute pain	acute, recurrent disease of painful inflammation of the joints; mainly in the feet and hands; elevated levels of uric acid
halitosis (hal-i-**toh**-sis)	**halitus** = breath, exhale **-osis** = denotes condition or state	a condition of having offensive-smelling breath; bad breath
hyperplastic gingiva (hahy-per-**plas**-tik) (jin-**jahy**-v*uh*)	**hyper** = above, over, or in excess **plast** = grow, develop, or change **-ic** = having characteristics **gingiv(a)** = the gums	overgrowth of gum tissue around the teeth; symptom of poor oral hygiene or certain medications
immunocompromised (im-y*uh*-noh-**kom**-pr*uh*-mahyzd)	**immune(o)** = protected from disease **compromise** = to expose or make vulnerable to danger **-ed** = indicating a condition	having an impaired immune system and incapable of an effective immune response
inflammation (in-fl*uh*-**mey**-sh*uh*n)	**inflame** = to cause redness and heat **-ation** = the state of being	body's defense against infection or trauma; symptoms of redness, heat, pain, and swelling may occur
insomnia (in-**som**-nee-*uh*)	**in-** = negative force, not **somni-** = sleep **-ia** = denoting disease or pathological disorder	sleeplessness; inability to obtain sufficient sleep
intoxication (in-tok-si-**key**-sh*uh* n)	**in-** = in, into, within **toxic** = poison **-ate** = denotes function **-ion** = denoting action or condition	drunkenness caused from excess of a potentially poisonous substance
lactose (**lak**-tohs)	**lact** = milk **-ose** = full of; forms the names of sugars	a sugar present in milk

(Continues)

Term and Pronunciation	Meaning of Root and Word Parts	Definition
malnutrition (mal-noo-**trish**-*uh* n)	**mal-** = bad **nutri** = to nourish **-tion** = act or process	insufficient food, unbalanced diet, or faulty digestion or utilization of food
metabolic (met-*uh*-**bol**-ik)	**metabolic** = chemical processes by which cells produce the substances and energy needed to sustain life	chemical reactions that occur within the body to sustain life.
monounsaturated (mon-oh-uhn-**sach**-*uh*-rey-tid)	**mono-** = one, single **saturate** = to unite with the greatest possible amount of another substance **-ed** = indicating a condition or quality	relating to fats that are liquid at room temperature; mostly from foods such as olives, avocados, and nuts
mucositis (myoo-koh-**sahy-tis**)	**muco-** = mucous membrane, lubricating membrane lining of an internal surface **-itis** = inflammation	painful inflammation and ulceration of the mucous membranes lining the mouth and digestive tract
nutrition (noo-**trish**-*uh* n)	**nutri** = to nourish **-tion** = act or process	the process of nourishing or being nourished, especially the process by which a living organism assimilates food and uses it for growth and replacement of tissues
osteomalacia (os-tee-oh-m*uh*-**ley**-sh*uh*)	**oste** = bone **malaco** = soft **ia** = condition	abnormal softening of the bones
osteoporosis (os-tee-oh-p*uh*-**roh**-sis)	**oste** = bone **pore** = small opening, space **osis** = condition	loss of bone tissue resulting in porous bones from lack of calcium
oxidize (**ok**-si-dahyz)	**oxide** = compound of oxygen with another element **-ize** = to make	combine an element with oxygen and take away hydrogen
peripheral neuropathy (p*uh*-**rif**-er-*uh*l) (noo-**rop**-*uh*-thee)	**periphery** = near the surface or outside **-al** = pertaining to **neuro-** = nerve; nervous system **-pathy** = disease; suffering	a result of damage to the nerves outside the brain and spinal cord (peripheral); causes weakness, pain, and numbness generally in hands and feet
polyunsaturated (pol-ee-uhn-**sach**-*uh*-rey-tid)	**poly** = many **un** = not **saturate** = to unite with the greatest possible amount of another substance **-ed** = indicating a condition or quality	organic compound, fat, or oil, containing several bonds usually of plant origin; regarded as healthier in the diet than saturated fats
remineralize (ree-**min**-er-uh-lahz)	**re-** = back again **mineral** = natural substances such as calcium, phosphorus **-ize** = to convert, transform	the minerals are replaced in the tooth
resistance (ri-**zis**-t*uh* ns)	**resist** = to make a stand or make efforts in opposition **-ance** = indicating an action	the act or power of opposing or withstanding
retinol (**ret**-n-awl)	**retinol** = another name for vitamin A$_1$	known as vitamin A$_1$, found in food and used as a dietary supplement; animal form of vitamin A; responsible for transmitting light sensation to the retina of the eye
spina bifida (**spahy**-n*uh*) (**bif**-i-d*uh*)	**spina** = spine or spine-like projection **bifida** = split into two	a congenital defect that involves an imperfectly closed spinal column; causes neurological abnormalities including paralysis
stomatitis (stoh-m*uh*-**tahy**-tis)	**stoma** = mouth **itis** = inflammation	inflammation of the oral tissues
temporomandibular joint (tem-p*uh*-roh-man-**dib**-y*uh*-ler) (joint)	**tempor/o** = temporalis area **mandibul** = mandible; lower jaw **-ar** = pertaining to **joint** = encapsulated area between two bones	the hinge joint between the temporal bone and the lower jaw
toxicity (tok-**sis**-i-tee)	**toxin** = any poison produced by an organism **-ic** = having the **-ity** = expressing state or condition	the quality or degree of being poisonous
xerostomia (zeer-*uh*-**stoh**-mee-*uh*)	**xero** = dry **stome** = mouth; opening resembling mouth **-ia** = disease, pathological or abnormal condition	dryness of the mouth by diminished function of the salivary glands due to aging, disease and drug reaction

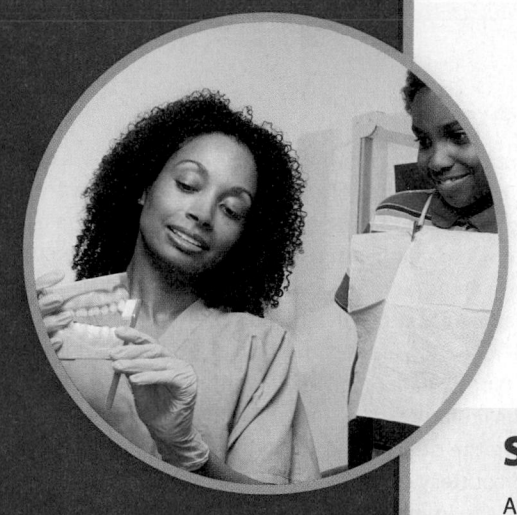

The Dental Office

Specific Instructional Objectives

At the completion of this chapter, you will be able to meet these objectives:

1. Use terms presented in this chapter.
2. Describe the design of a dental office, explaining the purpose of each area.
3. Follow safety rules in operating dental equipment.
4. Describe appearance and function of the equipment in the treatment room.
5. Select the best method to sanitize and disinfect equipment.
6. Describe the daily routine to open and close the dental office.
7. Prepare the treatment room for patient seating.
8. Greet and escort the patient to the treatment room.
9. Seat the patient.
10. Dismiss the patient.
11. Assist patients requiring seating accommodations.

Introduction

Dental offices have a variety of designs, including a single building, a medical/dental complex of individual units, a remodeled home, a suite in an office building, or space in a mall. Dental professionals go to great lengths to ensure that their offices are clean, convenient, and offer pleasant settings for patients. The dentist's vision and expectations are reflected in the office design, which should always consider the patients the dentist serves. The practice may serve families, primarily children, or primarily adults and may be in a rural or an urban setting. The most successful practices encompass all facets into a welcoming atmosphere where dental treatment can be provided.

The appearance of the dental office makes a statement about the dentist, the dental staff, and the quality of the dental care. This chapter describes the rooms in the dental office, the specific equipment used by dental professionals, and preparation for and seating a patient.

Dental Office Design

The dental office has several basic components designed to meet the dentist's individual preferences and needs. Innovations in dental offices include more open designs with partial walls and greater access to the patient treatment rooms and sterilization area. Higher ceilings, open doorways, and more windows also create the feeling of openness for the patient and the dental team. The office should have a climate control system that remains at a comfortable temperature throughout the year, regardless of the weather conditions. Architects and decorators often work with dental professionals to achieve the look the dentist desires.

The office may be small with two or three patient treatment rooms, or it may have a clinic setting with any number of treatment rooms (Figure 18-1). The sizes and numbers of these rooms vary (Figure 18-2).

The primary goal of the office design is to attract patients and make a warm, welcoming atmosphere to make the patient comfortable and to be efficient in delivering patient care. A dental practice which treats children needs to be child-friendly, consider special safety needs, and have bright, playful decorations. A prosthodontist or cosmetic dentist serving primarily adult patients will reflect a classic design more appealing for adults.

Architects and decorators often work with professionals in dental supply houses to achieve the look the dentist desires. Dental professionals have spent a lot of time and money researching what helps make a patient comfortable, decreases patient anxiety, and increases dental efficiency. Research has found the following to be desirable: room temperature at 68–72°F, good airflow to minimize dental smells, soothing color tones (light blue and white), relaxing designs, sound control between rooms, soft instrumental background music, patient privacy, open design with partial walls for easier access to multiple chairs, and staff with smiles and caring attitudes.

Dental offices, no matter how different they are in their layout and appearance, are all similar with basic rooms, areas, and equipment. Most offices have a reception area, business office, treatment area, sterilization area, film processing room, dental **laboratory**, restroom, storage area, and private office. Offices may also include a radiography room, storage, patient education area, **consultation** room, staff lounge, and laundry room.

Reception Area

The reception area is the first room the patient enters. This is the first impression the patient has of the office. The reception area needs to be clean, adapted to the type of patient, and have an area for the patient's coat and umbrella. There are many different types of reception areas ranging from very playful child themes to beautiful, classic areas with relaxing aquariums and plant life (Figure 18-3). All reception areas should have current magazines suitable for the type of patient, an activity area for children, and patient education literature.

Patients judge the quality of care by the office appearance, cleanliness, and courtesy of the staff. The office staff should face the reception area to immediately greet all patients. Dental staff should refrain from the use of the term *waiting room*. The office should be organized and on schedule so that a patient should not have a long wait before being seen. Upon arrival, the patient should be greeted promptly, with a smile and by name.

Business Office

The business office is the center of the dental office communication. Business office staff coordinates all the activities of the office. They need to be centrally located to be aware of all office activities and for effective communication with the patient and the dental team. Generally there is a counter or window between the reception area and the business office so the office personnel are able to see the patient enter (Figure 18-4). The business office must also provide a private area to discuss patient treatment and finances and a secure area to file all private information.

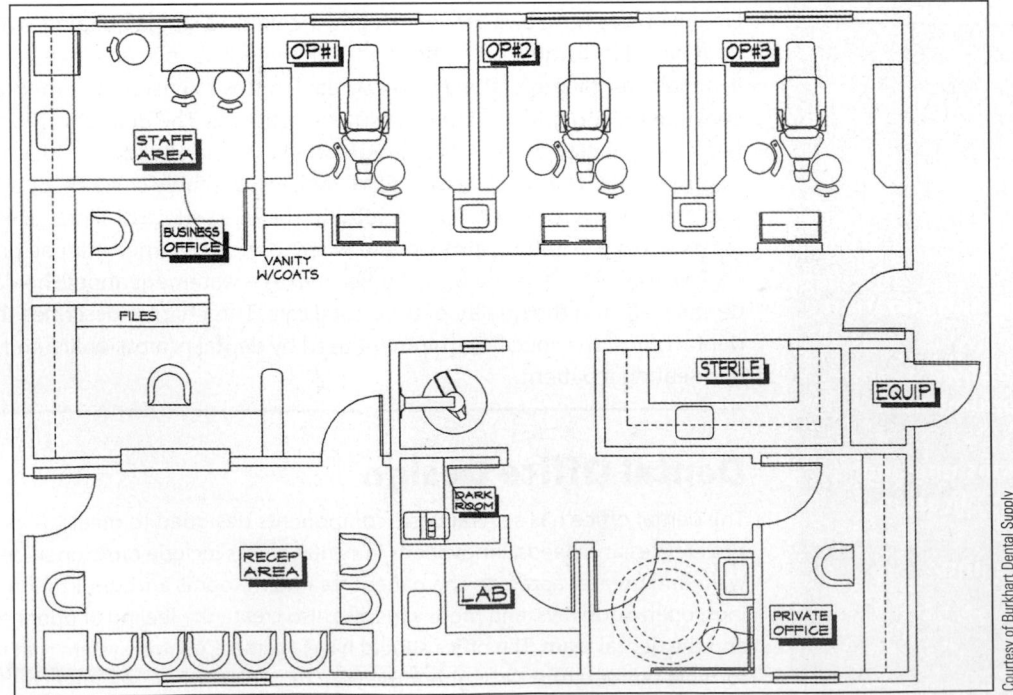

FIGURE 18-1
Small dental office blueprint.

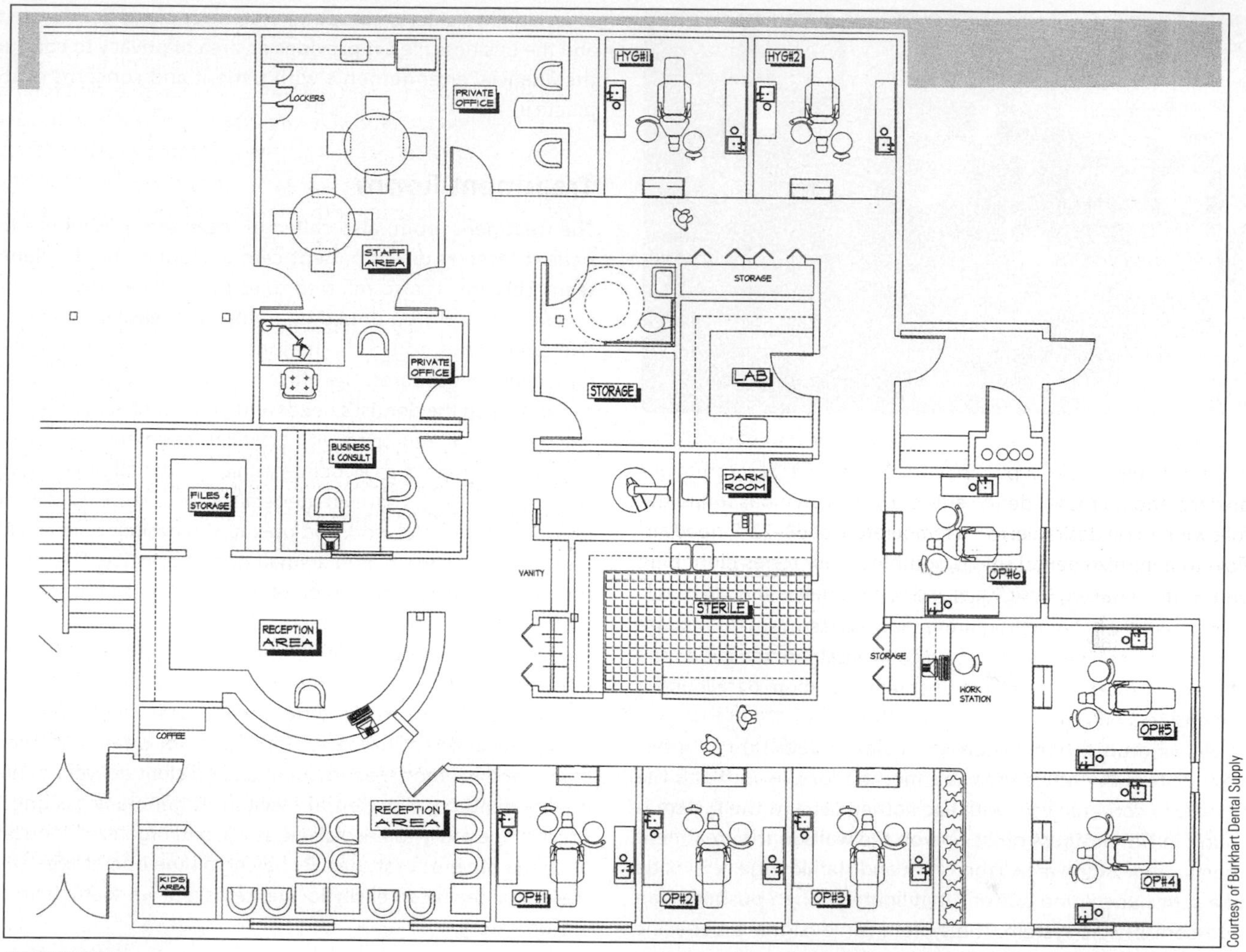

FIGURE 18-2
Large dental office blueprint.

Courtesy of Burkhart Dental Supply

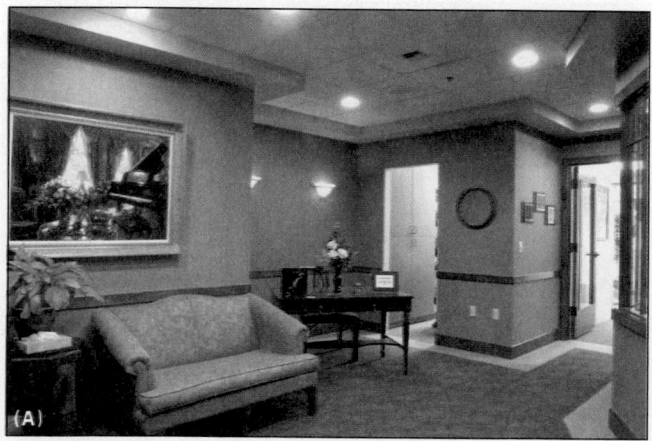
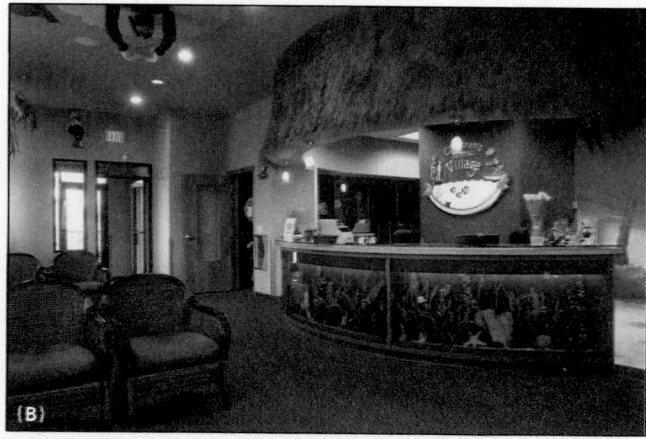

FIGURE 18-3
Reception areas can be designed to appeal to the patient population. (A) The reception area in a cosmetic dentistry office of Dr. Charles Regalado. (B) The pediatric dental practice of Dr. Jay Enzler.

HIPAA requires that all patient information be kept private and secure.

The primary responsibility of staff working in the business office is communication and handling phone calls, making appointments, keeping patient records, and managing the patient flow. Equipment located in this area includes a

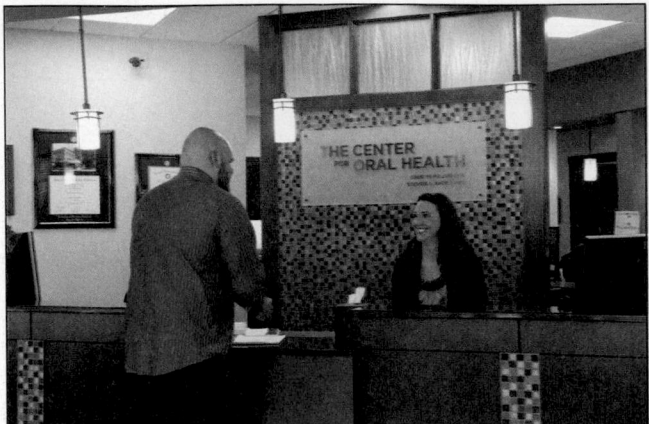

FIGURE 18-4
The reception desk and business office of Dr. Charles Regalado.

business desk and chair, phone system, communication system, computer system, copier, calculator, fax machine, and filing cabinets. Dental offices are requiring more space to accommodate high-technology equipment and to facilitate increased dental insurance processing. (Refer to Chapter 44 for more details about the business office.)

A communication system is a color-coded light or intercom system the office uses as a method for the staff and the dentist to communicate with each other. Usually, the system is found in the business office and on the walls in the treatment rooms, sterilization area, laboratory, and staff lounge. It is made of a series of colored buttons that light up when pushed or an intercom/phone system. The system can designate a specific message or call a member of the dental team. For example, the hygienist lets the dentist know the patient is ready for examination, or the receptionist tells everyone that the next patient has arrived. These systems can be customized for the individual needs of an office.

Hands-free communication systems are rapidly gaining popularity. With these systems a hands-free ear piece is used by the dental team. There are many types of systems with features that work in smaller dental offices with a few staff members as well as features that work in large dental clinics. These systems allow the office staff to directly contact and communicate with one another using headsets that are linked over a wireless local area network. Some of the characteristics of these systems are that they are lightweight and can be easily worn by the user. Systems allow users to make outgoing calls, pick up incoming calls, and communicate with other staff members. They are also great for maintaining privacy and prevent cross-contamination since there is no need to push buttons on the colored light systems. Offices have found that with the hands-free communication system there is immediate communication among the whole dental team, so they can provide superior service to the patients.

Many offices have a designated administrative area where the office manager or business assistant manages the business part of the dental practice. This area is close to the front of the

office and has a desk, computer system, copier, phone system, and the business files. It provides an area of privacy to conduct the financial arrangements with patient and concerns of the practice.

Treatment Room

The treatment room, also called an **operatory**, is where the patient receives direct patient care performed by the dental team. This area is also referred to as the **clinical** area and has several identically equipped operatories for ease of operation. The operatories house the major equipment needed to perform dental procedures. The office may have several operatories depending on the dentist's needs and number of active patients. The operatory is equipped with a patient treatment chair, operator's chair, assistant's chair, delivery unit, and dental cabinets with sinks (Figure 18-5). There are generally two or more operatories for **operative** dental work and operatories designed specifically for the dental hygienist in a small dental practice. The operatory design is dictated by type of practice, types of procedures performed, and dentist's preference.

Dentists design the dental office and operatories to more efficiently coordinate the steps in the dental procedures. This enables the dentist to move from one operatory to another as the dental assistant prepares the patient for treatment, allowing for optimal time management and efficient delivery of high quality dentistry. The dental assistant is generally assigned a specific operatory to keep clean, stock, and organize identically to all the other operatories. By having all the operatories alike, the dental team can easily locate items and work efficiently in any operatory.

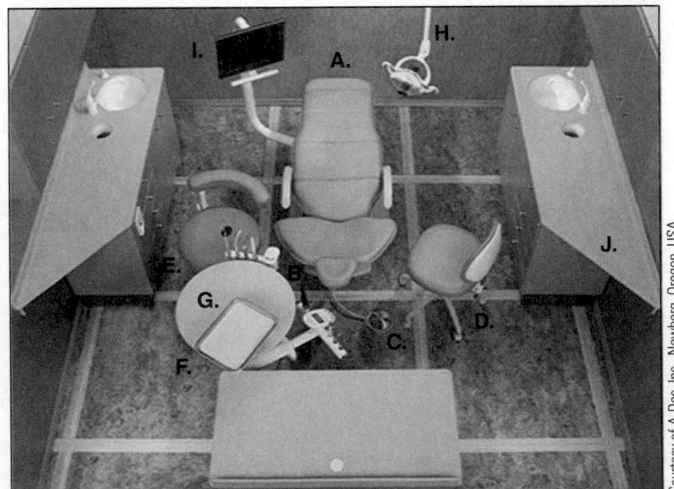

FIGURE 18-5
Operatory equipped with rear delivery system for delivering patient dental care. (A) Patient dental chair. (B) Patient dental chair adjustments (not pictured). (C) Rheostat to control handpieces. (D) Operator chair with lumbar support. (E) Assistant chair with extended arm. (F) Dental unit. (G) Bracket table. (H) Dental light. (I) Computer screen for digital radiographs and patient information. (J) Dental cabinets with sinks and countertops.

Sterilization Area

The sterilization area should be centrally located near the treatment area. All dental instruments are thoroughly cleaned, *sterilized*, and prepared for the next patient. The area has a sink, counter space, storage space, and equipment and chemicals for sanitization, disinfection, and sterilization of dental instruments and items (Figure 18-6). The counter space has three areas: contaminated area (where all instruments from the operatory are returned), clean area (where instruments are free of debris and ready to be sterilized or disinfected), and sterile area (where instruments are placed once they have been removed from the sterilizer). The sterilization area must always be organized, neat, and clean. This area is also used for local storage of dental supplies for immediate use.

Sterilizing equipment, a sharps container, a hazardous waste container, ultrasonic equipment, and a *handpiece* cleaner/lubricating machine are all housed in the sterilization area. It is important to have good air circulation to protect everyone from the chemical fumes and exhaust from the sterilizing equipment. (The sterilizing equipment is discussed in Chapter 11, "Infection Control.")

Dental Office Laboratory

This area is where the basic dental laboratory procedures are performed: pouring impressions, trimming and finishing models, fabricating custom trays, adjusting and polishing appliances, and preparing cases to be sent to a commercial laboratory. The amount of lab work in the dental office depends on the type of procedures performed in the office and the dentist's preference. General dentists who do a lot of prosthodontic work, prosthodontists, and orthodontists require the most laboratory work and equipment in the dental office.

The laboratory area will have a work bench, stools, heat and air source, sink, exhaust fan, and cabinets (Figure 18-7). The basic laboratory equipment includes a dental vibrator, model trimmer, lab handpieces, vacuum former, and dental lathe. Cabinets provide storage for instruments such as lab knives, spatulas, and rubber bowls. As materials may have been in the patient's mouth before being brought to the lab, all aseptic precautions must be followed. The staff should wear protective glasses and masks to prevent dust and debris from causing injuries when working with the equipment. (Refer to Chapter 33 for more details about dental laboratory procedures.)

Film Processing Area

The film processing room is a small room near the treatment area. Most offices that use standard radiographic film process the film using an automatic processor with a daylight loader. The daylight loader has a cover that screens out the white light so that the film can be processed with the white light on. This eliminates the need for a darkroom. The area needs a sink and counter space to maintain the processor and to mount the film (Figure 18-8). A darkroom may still be necessary for practices that use panoramic or cephalometric films.

It is still a good practice to have a backup manual processing tank. The manual technique requires a darkroom. This room receives its name because all white light has to be sealed out to develop the x-rays using the manual tanks. A safelight is used to develop the x-rays when light-tight facilities are needed. When manual processing is used, a sink and counter space for processing and mounting are needed. (Refer to Chapter 27 for more details about radiographs.)

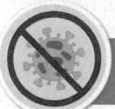 **Infection Control**

OSHA has specific requirements for the sterilization area so that instruments, trays, and all items used on patient flow from dirty areas to clean areas to minimize the chance of cross contamination.

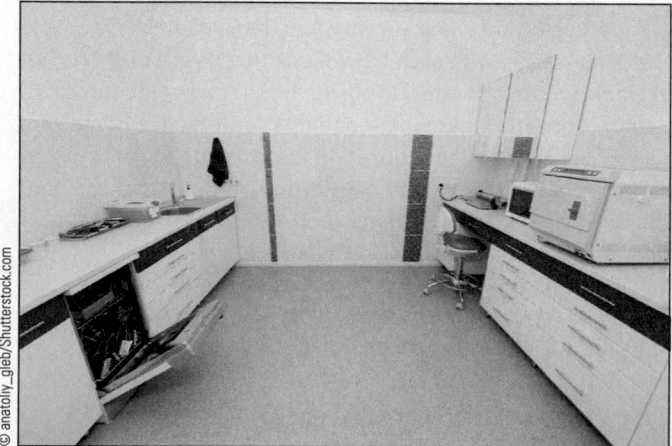

© anatoliy_gleb/Shutterstock.com

FIGURE 18-6
Sterilization area with (from left to right) contaminated/sanitization area; clean/sterilization area, and storage area for sterilized items.

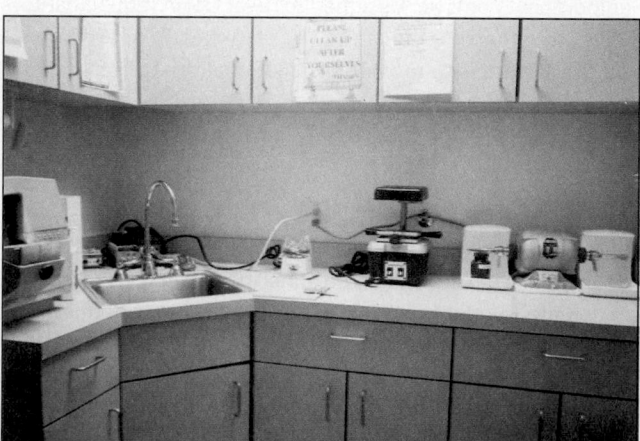

FIGURE 18-7
Laboratory work bench area with dental laboratory equipment. See Chapter 33 for details of equipment in the photo.

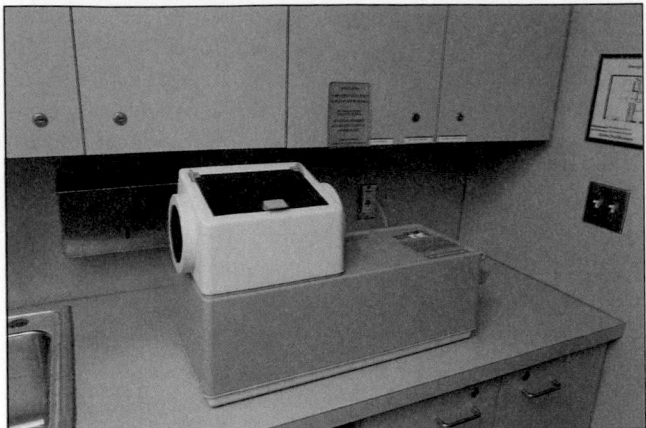

FIGURE 18-8
Film processing area with sink, counter space, storage, and automatic processing unit with daylight loader.

An office that has switched to **digital radiography** no longer needs a darkroom to process the films. The image of the tooth is taken using a **sensor** and is transmitted onto a computer. The images are stored and viewed on the computer.

Radiography Room

Most dental offices have an intraoral radiography unit in each treatment room to expose intraoral radiographs. Sometimes the **x-ray tubehead** is housed between two rooms to slide out into either room. The controls are found outside the room so that the dental assistant is not exposed to radiation. (Further information about the x-ray unit can be found in Chapter 27). The extraoral radiography equipment (**panoramic** and **cephalometric x-ray machine**) is housed in a separate radiography room. This room is generally out of the traffic area of the dental office where radiographs can be safely exposed without the worry of radiating persons other than the patient (Figure 18-9). Guidelines come from the state health department, and periodic inspections may be required by state agencies.

Radiography rooms are designed to meet OSHA requirements when using ionizing radiation. The state health department sets specifications to provide occupational safety from radiation when exposing radiographs.

Dentist's Private Office

The private office is the dentist's personal area. This area is where they maintain personal and personnel information in locked files, participate in telephone conferences with other dentists and physicians, and evaluate patient cases. The dentist may show the patient their recommendation for treatment on radiographs, models, and patient educational programs. The private office has the dentist's desk, chair, computer, locked file cabinets, and professional library. The private office is generally located in the back part of the dental office. This is the dentist's private area, and dental staff should not enter without permission.

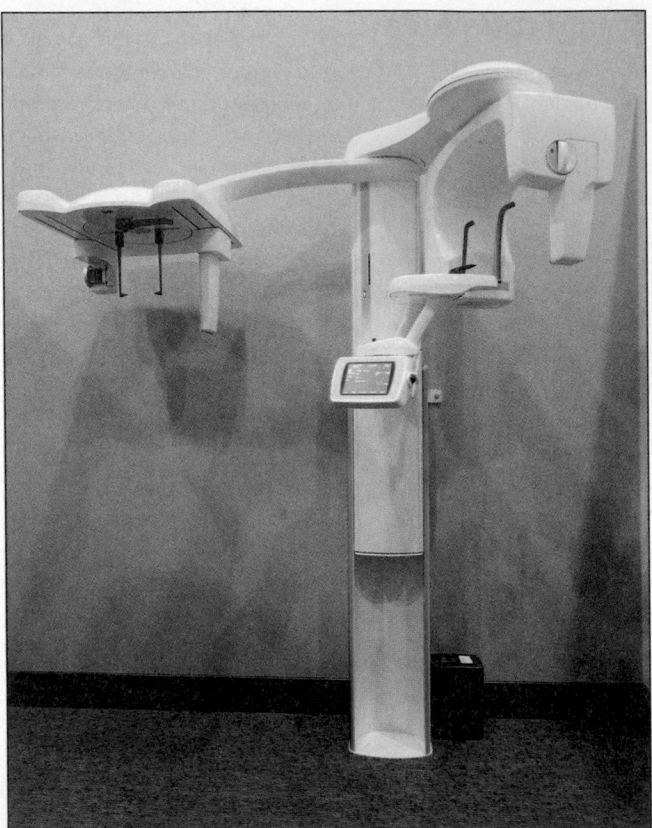

FIGURE 18-9
Panoramic x-ray machine area in radiography room.

Staff Lounge

The lounge is a designated area for staff breaks, lunch, relaxation, and sometimes staff meetings. The lounge is generally supplied with a refrigerator, microwave, table, chairs, coffee maker, and lockers. If the area is used for meetings, there will be audiovisual equipment. A washer and dryer may also be in this area.

Patient Education Area

A patient education area is a very functional and diverse area in the dental office. With each type of practice, its use may vary; for example, in the orthodontic office, the space may be furnished with mirrors and sinks where patients can practice home care techniques. The patient education area may be an information center containing a variety of information on dental care and treatments available to patients, such as bleaching treatments or dental implants.

Often this room has a sink, a counter or table with chairs, and multimedia equipment including a television and DVD equipment. This area may also be used for consultations with the patient.

Consultation Room/Area

Some offices have a designated consulting area with a table and chairs. The dentist discusses diagnosis and treatment with the patient in privacy. There is generally audiovisual equipment, pamphlets, an x-ray viewbox, or a computer to see digital radiographs and models to assist the dentist in the case presentation (Figure 18-10). If there is not a separate consultation room, the dentist may use the private office or patient education area for consultation.

Storage Area

This is generally a large closet area designed to store bulk **expendables** and dental materials. Many storage areas also house the dental support equipment that run the dental unit; water supply, central vacuum system, and air compressor. Keeping the utilities in a room away from the operatories helps to muffle the noise. The area should be maintained at an even 70° F, and care must be taken to follow manufacturer's guidelines when storing chemicals.

The support equipment includes:

● main switch provides electricity to turn on the dental unit; always check the electrical plug when the unit and utilities do not turn on.

● master water valve runs the water of the air/water syringe and handpiece (Figure 18-11).

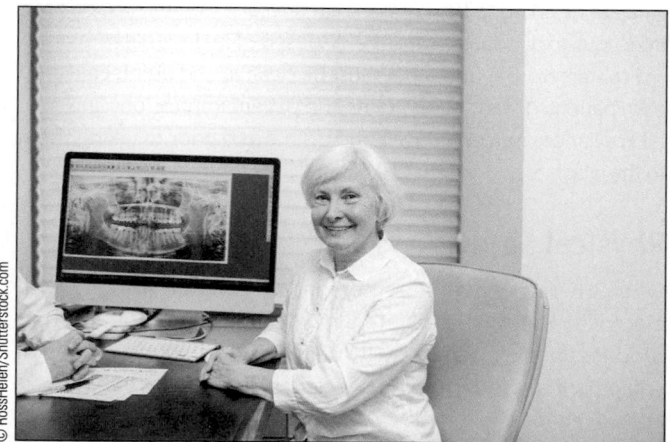

FIGURE 18-10
Consultation room.

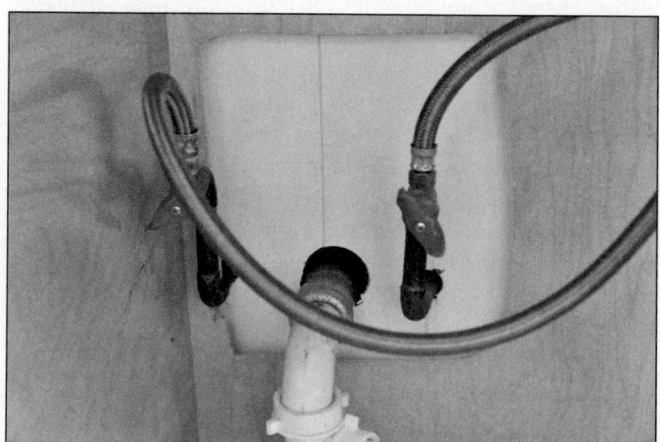

FIGURE 18-11
Master water valve.

● air compressor runs the air of the air/water syringe and handpieces (Figure 18-12).

● central evacuation system provides the suction for the saliva ejector hose and high velocity evacuation hose (Figure 18-13).

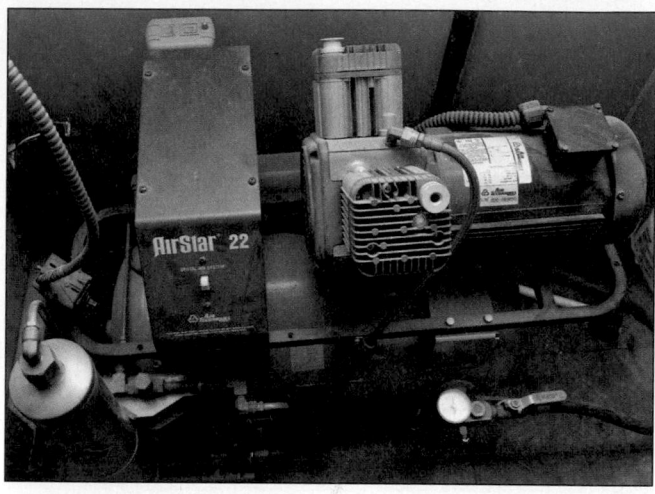

FIGURE 18-12
Air compressor generates ultradry dental air, which runs and protects valuable handpieces from premature failure due to the effects of moist air and the build-up of oil residue. A dental compressor prevents the introduction of an oily film to a prepared surface, which could compromise resin retention and restorations, wasting chair time. Most importantly, the patients' health is protected with ultradry air that provides an environment that is not conducive to bacterial growth.

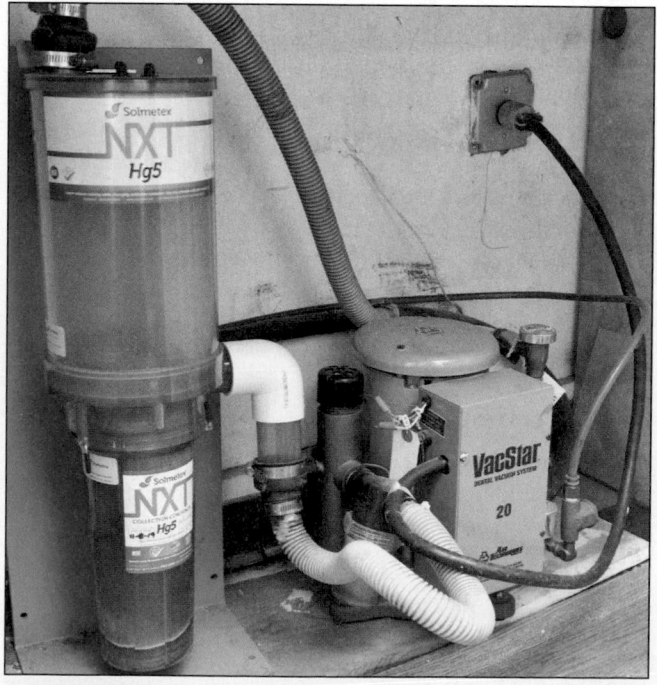

FIGURE 18-13
Central evacuation system.

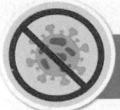

Infection Control

Care and Maintenance of Support Equipment

Each piece of equipment has specific care and maintenance needs that are described in detail by the manufacturer. A maintenance log needs to made and followed to keep the most important equipment in the office working smoothly. Ongoing maintenance for the air compressor is critical. It is important that the filters be changed routinely and the compressor be checked for condensation in the lines. A quick check for condensation is blowing air from the air/water syringe onto a mirror. If the mirror remains clear, there is not condensation. If moisture appears on the mirror, there is condensation occurring; the line may have particles, moisture, and algae. These contaminants may work their way into the dental handpieces and the oral cavity. If condensation is apparent, call for dental service to correct the problem. The central evacuation system filters or traps must be cleaned regularly to keep this system working to capacity.

Laundry Room

The laundry room has a washer, dryer, folding area, closet, and sometimes a changing area. OSHA regulations state that the employer is responsible for laundering staff uniforms or providing a laundering service.

Staff cannot wear or launder uniforms outside of work. The employer is responsible to clean, launder, repair, and replace uniforms if infection control gowns are not provided by the dentist.

Safety Rules in Operating Clinical Dental Equipment

When operating equipment or handling materials, safety comes first. The dental team must follow infection control procedures and safety precautions recommended in the manufacturer's directions and Safety Data Sheet (SDS). The dental office must have written policies and safety rules to protect all employees, patients, and visitors. It is important for the staff to know how to use and maintain equipment to prevent accidents.

There are three areas of safety the dental team must be aware of when working with dental equipment and materials: biohazard safety, physical safety, and chemical safety.

Biohazard Safety

All items in the clinical areas, as well as items brought into the business office and dental laboratory from the treatment room, are potentially contaminated. Exposure control procedures must be followed when using every item in the clinical area. All patient records must be kept in protective covers or handled using clean hands, uncontaminated gloves, or overgloves. When records are not in use, they should be placed in an area away from potential exposure. All items that are used with the patient that cannot be sterilized must be cleaned and disinfected before returning them to operatory storage. Those items to be sterilized need to be placed on a tray to be taken to the contaminated area in the sterilization area. Infectious expendables must be disposed of in designated biohazard containers. The operatory must be cleaned and disinfected after each patient. All laboratory items and patient impressions and dental appliances must be rinsed and disinfected prior to taking them to the laboratory. (Refer to Chapter 11, "Infection Control.")

Physical Safety

When operating dental equipment, you will be working with electricity, items that rotate at high speeds, equipment that produces heat, and items with sharp cutting edges. All dental equipment is safe if you start by reading the manufacturer's operation directions, follow all safety rules, and keep all equipment in good working condition.

When working with electricity, make certain the plug is secure, that the wiring is intact, and that you never operate the equipment with wet hands or around water. You must always wear safety eyewear, keep hair pulled back, make certain jewelry and loose clothing like scarves and large sleeves will not enter the work area, and keep on task when operating rotary equipment. Hold any piece of equipment that cuts or produces heat firmly by the handle, secure a finger rest to prevent slippage of the equipment, and securely hold the item being cut. Do not overrun the equipment at a high speed for a long time as this causes unnecessary heat and undue wear on the equipment. You not only need to know how to run the equipment safely, you need to know how to handle an emergency.

Documentation

It is important not only to keep all equipment in good working condition but also to document routine maintenance and to keep all original manufacturer's directions. This will ensure that all warranties are accepted and that all equipment will run safely and efficiently.

Know the location of the fire extinguisher and how to use it. You should also know the fire escape routes.

Chemical Safety

Many dental materials used throughout the office contain chemicals that are potentially dangerous and hazardous if the manufacturer's directions are not followed. They may be caustic, toxic, carcinogenic, or combustible. Caustic chemicals may have strong acids or bases, which can cause irritation and severe burns. Chemicals may be hazardous and potentially dangerous if the manufacturer's directions are not followed. Toxic chemicals are poisonous, and carcinogenic chemicals may contribute to the development of cancer. Chemicals can enter the body by direct contact with skin or mucous membranes and by ingestion or inhalation. The dental staff must read the manufacturer's directions, follow SDS guidelines for safe usage, and be aware of emergency steps if needed. The SDS explains how to handle materials as well as what PPE is recommended to avoid inhaling the chemical (mask), absorbing it by direct contact (gloves, eyewear, and protective clothing), and ingesting it (mask). The SDS also explains how to handle a chemical emergency including immediate eyewash, first aid procedures, and information necessary for the physician if injury requires EMS.

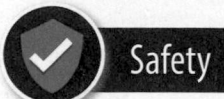

OSHA requires that manufacturers must have a label on all products that are potentially hazardous. Labels identify chemicals and any hazard warning. (Refer to Chapter 12 for more information about OSHA regulations.)

Some chemicals are combustible and may burst into flame or explode. Those chemicals labeled reactive may have a dangerous reaction when combined with another chemical. The reaction may be toxic fumes released, or the mixture may explode. A corrosive label indicates that the chemical may eat away other substances if in direct contact. Following is an important safety rules checklist the dental assistant needs to strictly adhere to:

SAFETY RULES CHECKLIST

- Follow manufacturer's instructions before operating equipment.
  Note: As a student, never use equipment prior to training, demonstration, and/or detailed reading of the manufacturer's operation directions. When in the dental office, ask staff to demonstrate any equipment that you have not learned in class.
- Read SDSs, follow precautions, and be aware of emergency procedures.
- Make certain the equipment is well maintained to ensure its safe operation.
  - Check the operation of the equipment prior to its use.
  - Use equipment shield when running lab instruments.
  - Use machine or central evacuation when available.

- Report all faulty equipment, accidents, and incidents to dentist immediately.
- Keep focused on the work at hand.
  - Most reported accidents are due to being distracted while working.
  - Use good lighting while working.
- Never leave equipment running.
  - Turn off all equipment when done with work, especially rotary equipment, hot equipment, and running water.
  - Always unplug equipment before cleaning or performing maintenance.
- Wear PPE recommended by manufacturer.
  - Always wear eye protection when running rotary instruments.
  - Wear mask when running equipment that creates dust or when working with powder (polishing powder).
- Wear recommended PPE when working with potential infectious items, dental spray, rotary instruments, and chemicals.
- Keep hair pulled back.
- Avoid wearing dangling jewelry or clothing.
- Wear gloves whenever exposure to blood or OPIM is possible.
- Never leave an area contaminated.
- Make certain contaminated items are placed in the contaminated area in the sterilization area when immediate decontamination is not possible.
- Decontaminate all items prior to returning to storage or moving item to an uncontaminated area. For example, patient mirrors and equipment used on patient must be sanitized and disinfected before returning to dental cabinet. Dental impressions must be rinsed and disinfected prior to taking it to the lab.
- No eating, drinking, cosmetics, or smoking are permitted in any area.

Clinical Dental Equipment

Dental equipment is continually being developed to accommodate new dental techniques, advanced procedures, changing dental concepts, and specialty areas. Plus, each dental equipment manufacturer creates their product just a little differently from the other manufacturers. The dental team must become acquainted with a large assortment of equipment and learn the care and maintenance for each. Dental equipment is expensive and, with careful maintenance, is meant to last for years. Someone in the office often is assigned to perform the routine maintenance of the equipment. A dental equipment technician is called when more substantial problems occur.

Patient Dental Chair

The dental chair is for seating the patient for clinical examination and dental treatment. It is designed to provide patient comfort and to assist the operator and/or assistant in providing treatment comfortably and efficiently. There is a wide variety of dental chairs due to modernization, accommodation for dental procedures, and dentist's preference. There are chairs for general dentistry and specialties including surgical and orthodontic treatment. The most common is the contour dental chair. It is a lounge type chair that is cushioned for the patient's comfort and supports the patient's entire body. The dental chair is available in different sizes for children and adults.

The dental chair (also called the treatment chair) is easily manipulated to various positions to view and access all areas of the mouth, to perform different dental procedures, and for operator ease in performing dentistry. The dental chair has several parts that can be adjusted independently for specific patient positioning desired by the operator: headrest, backrest, seat, footrest, armrest, and base.

The headrest securely holds the patient's head and neck. It can be adjusted to patient height and for comfortable positioning for treatment. The backrest and seat supports the patient's upper and lower back, lumbar area, bottom and knees. The backrest can be moved to an **upright** position or recline to a lying down position. The seat of the chair can be raised and lowered for the height of the operator and to a comfortable position to perform treatment. The footrest generally moves up as the backrest reclines. The armrest supports the arms, elbows, and hands. The armrest may raise or move aside for patient seating and dismissal. Not all armrests are movable. The base is the part of chair that rests on the floor and is the main support of the chair.

The parts of the chair can be manipulated by hand controls located on each side of the chair and on the back of the backrest, by digital control on the dental unit, or by foot using a **rheostat** (foot controller is preferred for infection control; Figure 18-14). With the controls, the dental team can make independent movement of the chair. The team can raise and lower the entire chair, recline the backrest and raise the footrest, or place the backrest in upright position and lower the footrest. Most chairs have a control that automatically makes a combination of moves from sitting up to reclining and from reclining to sitting up. There is a swivel lever attached to the base that allows the chair to be rotated side to side (left to right). This lever should be in the locked position when seating the patient.

There are three positions used when treating patients depending on the area of the mouth being treated, the type of procedure being performed, and operator's preference: upright position, **supine** position, and **subsupine** position. The dental assistant should be able to place chair into these positions with ease.

Upright Position: The back of the treatment chair is at a 90 degree angle to the floor, and the seat is at its lowest possible point. The upright position allows ease for the patient to be seated and dismissed. This position is used when taking some radiographs and taking impressions. The entire chair can be raised or lowered in the upright position to accommodate patients or operators of different sizes (Figure 18-15).

Supine Position: The patient is reclined into a lying down position with their knees and head at approximately the same level; or nose and toes are even. This is the best position for sit-down dentistry. It allows for easy delivery of four-handed dentistry (the two hands of the dentist and two hands of the chairside assistant) while performing dental procedures. The patient's head is positioned in the headrest over the operator's

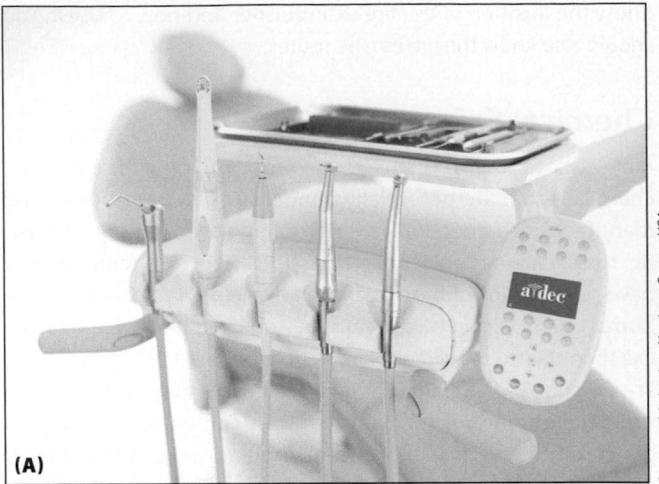

Courtesy of A-dec, Inc., Newberg, Oregon, USA

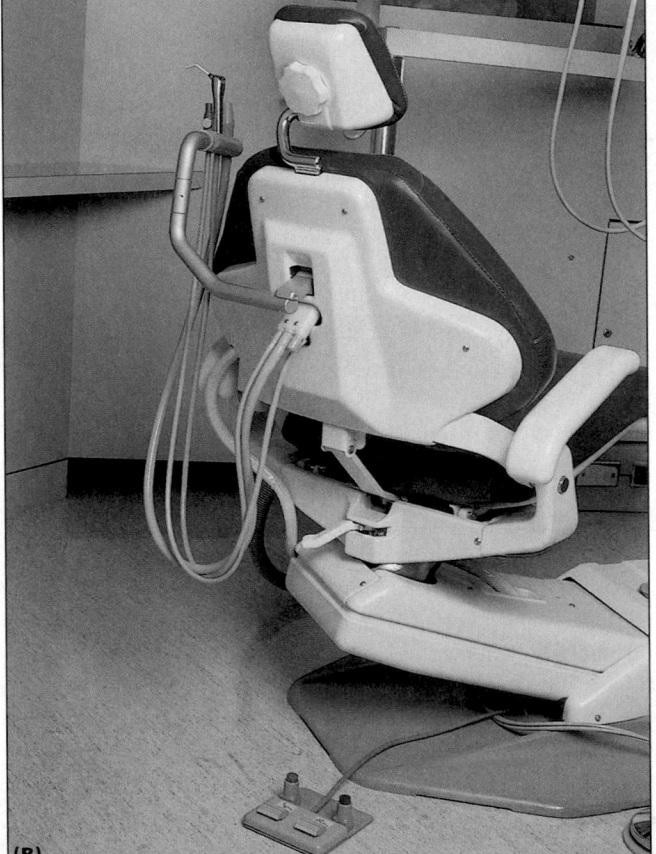

© bikeriderlondon/Shutterstock.com

FIGURE 18-14
(A) Digital controls for adjusting the dental chair position. (B) Dental chair with foot controls for adjusting the chair.

lap, allowing for ease and efficiency for the operator. The supine position is utilized for most dental procedures (Figure 18-16). This positions the patient's feet above their chest, which is also desirable for improved blood circulation during procedures.

Subsupine Position: The patient is reclined with their head lower than their feet. This position is used for emergency treatment and for treating unconscious patients; it is also referred to as the **Trendelenburg position**. This position is uncomfortable for routine treatment (Figure 18-17).

Procedure 18-1
Positioning Patient Dental Chair

Place chair in upright, supine, and subsupine positions.

1. Become familiar with the operation of the dental chair.
   - ❏ Use the chair controls to raise and lower the chair.
   - ❏ Use the chair controls to recline and raise the backrest of the chair.
   - ❏ Unlock chair lever to swivel the chair and lock lever in place.

2. Place the dental chair in the upright position (Figure 18-15) by using the chair controls to:
   - ❏ Place the chair in its lowest position.
   - ❏ Place the back of the chair to a 90 degree angle to the floor.
   - ❏ Raise the chair to a height accessible for the operator.

3. Place the dental chair in the supine position (Figure 18-16) by using the chair controls to:
   - ❏ Raise the chair 6 inches.
   - ❏ Recline the backrest to a 45 degree angle to the floor.
   - ❏ Raise the chair another 6 inches.
   - ❏ Recline the backrest until the head and knees are even.

4. Place the dental chair in the subsupine position (Figure 18-17) by using the chair controls to:
   - ❏ Place chair into supine position as described above.
   - ❏ Recline the backrest approximately 4 inches until the head is lower than the knees.

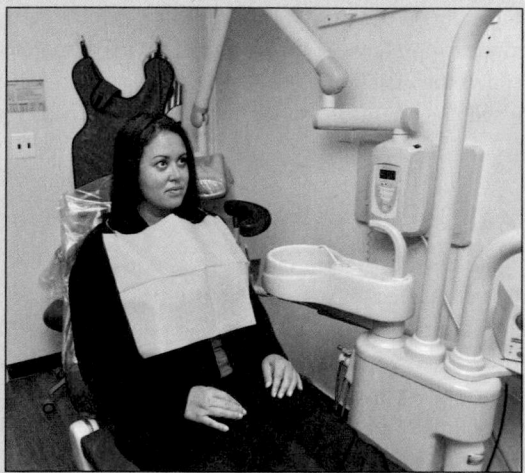

FIGURE 18-15
Upright position.

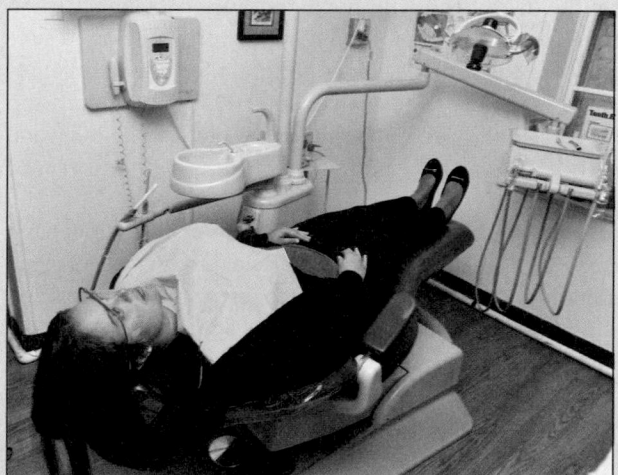

FIGURE 18-16
Supine position.

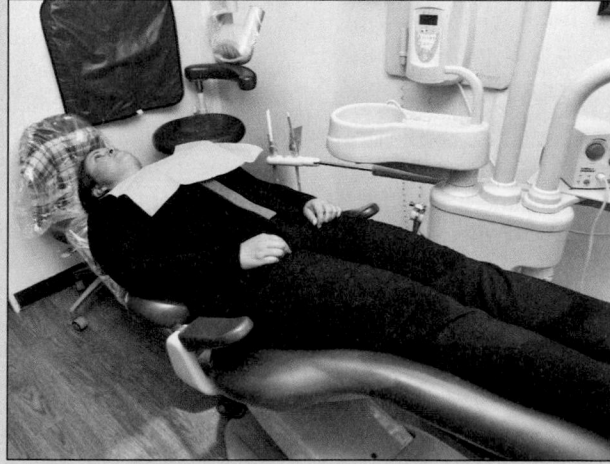

FIGURE 18-17
Subsupine position.

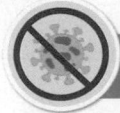

Infection Control

Infection Control for Patient Dental Chair

The dental chair is made of material that provides patient comfort and is easy to clean and disinfect between patients. The staff should wipe away bits of debris, sanitize and disinfect the dental chair following manufacturer's directions between patients, or use a chair barrier which is changed between patients. The dental chair is classified as a noncritical item requiring an EPA intermediate level disinfectant. The dental staff should use the saturate–wipe–saturate technique on the chair controls or cover the controls with barriers. At the end of the day, the chair should be placed in the upright position and lifted to the highest level for easy cleaning. Per manufacturer's directions, most chairs should be washed with soap and water, and crèmes should be applied weekly to keep the material's moisture to prevent drying and cracking from the use of disinfectants.

Dental Stools

Dental stools are needed by the operator and the assistant during most procedures. **Ergonomic** studies have resulted in the improved design of dental stools to provide comfort and prevent fatigue during dental procedures. When selecting stools, the dentist and staff should try a variety of stools to find the one that meets their requirements, provides good support, and is comfortable. There is more information on ergonomics and the dental team in Chapter 20. The operator's and assistant's stools have some similarities but also have several differences.

Operator Chair/Stool The operator's chair or stool has a cushioned flat or saddle seat that is adjustable to the height of the operator to allow the operator's feet to rest firmly on the ground (Figure 18-18). Most have a back with an adjustable support for the operator's lumbar area. The wheels of the stool are small and sturdy to withstand movement around the dental chair to obtain the best view and access to the patient's mouth for efficiency and ease in performing dental procedures. A proper ergonomic operator's stool will help reduce fatigue and back pain.

Assistant Chair/Stool The assistant stool has an adjustable foot ring for the assistant to set their feet, which provides

stability for the assistant regardless of their height. The stool has an attached side support bar (abdominal arm) that fits around the assistant's rib cage (Figure 18-19). The arm is easily adjusted to add comfort for the assistant while assisting with procedures. It supports weight as the assistant leans toward the patient. This allows the assistant to lean in and view the oral cavity without placing strain on their back. The assistant's stool should be positioned approximately 4–6 inches higher than the operator's stool. This allows the assistant to have a clear view of the patient's oral cavity over the operator's hands and head and provides for better access.

Dental Delivery Unit

The dental **unit** is the primary piece of equipment in the treatment area. It provides the basic utilities needed to run the attached dental equipment to perform dental procedures. The unit provides electricity, water, compressed air, and vacuum. There are different types of delivery units depending primarily on the type of practice, procedures performed, and dentist's preference.

There are three distinct types of instrument delivery systems that have evolved to accommodate the various ways in which dentists position and use their instruments. These are front delivery, rear delivery, and side delivery (Figure 18-20).

Front Delivery Unit: The unit is mounted on the treatment chair and is placed over the patient; it is also referred to as transthorax (over-the-patient) system. The unit is easily reached by the operator (Figure 18-21). Over-the-patient delivery places the dental instruments on a moveable tray attached to a post on the dental chair. Over-the-patient systems are best for smaller treatment rooms and operators working alone (dental hygienists) because

Safety

OSHA requires that the base of both the operator's and assistant's chairs should have five spokes with wheels to avoid tipping.

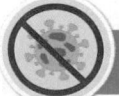

Infection Control

Infection Control for Dental Stools

The chairs are classified as noncritical items and should be sanitized and disinfected between patients using an EPA intermediate level disinfectant. The dental staff can use the saturate–wipe–saturate technique. The stool adjustment levers should be covered with a barrier. In order to prevent the chairs from drying, manufacturer recommended crèmes should be applied weekly.

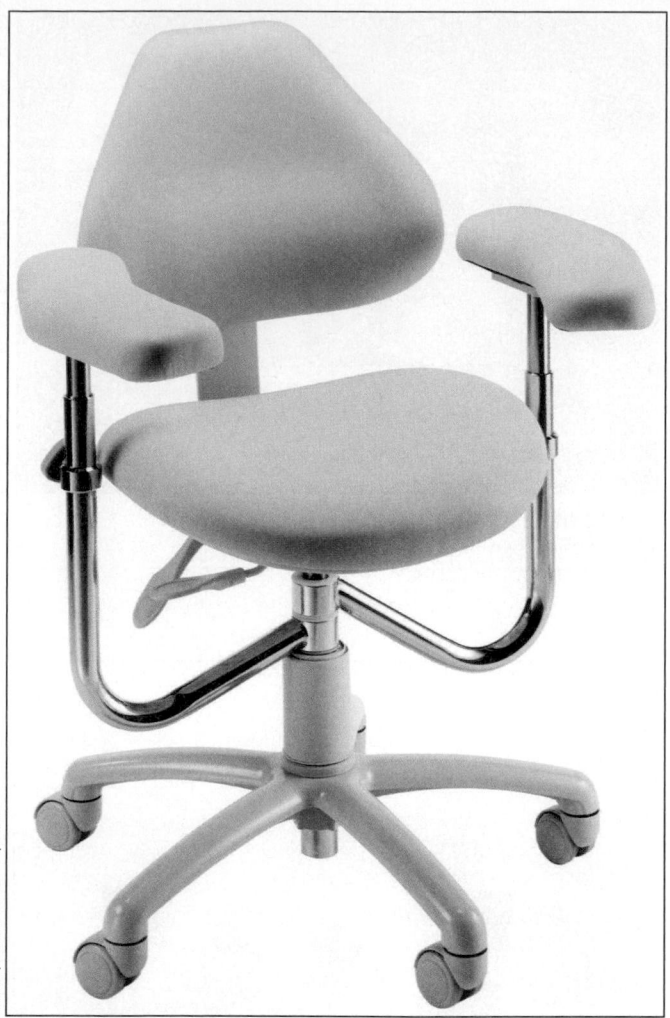

Courtesy of KaVo Dental Corporation

FIGURE 18-18
Operator's stool with back support, broad base, comfortable seat, and casters.

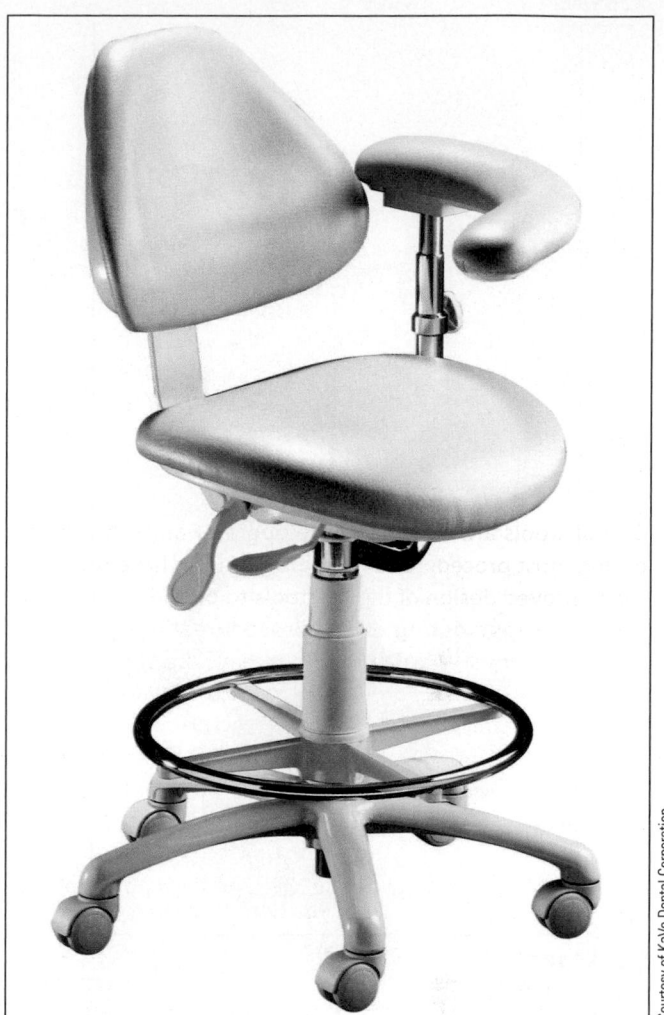

Courtesy of KaVo Dental Corporation

FIGURE 18-19
Assistant's stool with front arm support, comfortable seat, broad base, foot rest, and casters.

of their simple, integrated design. However, over-the-patient delivery presents a cluttered appearance, the close proximity of the instruments may make the patients anxious, and it is not conducive to four-handed dentistry.

There are two styles of over-the-patient units: standard and left/right style. With a standard over-the-patient unit, the arms for the dental instruments and light originate from a fixed position on the side of the chair. The placement of this unit is dependent on whether the doctor is right or left handed. With a left/right style unit these arms mount below the chair, allowing them to be rotated around the chair to either a right or left-handed delivery position.

Rear Delivery Unit: The rear delivery unit is behind the patient treatment chair and accommodates both the assistant and the operator (Figure 18-22). Rear delivery places all of the instrumentation out of the patient's view and facilitates the smooth transfer of instruments between assistant and doctor. It also provides for easy left hand/right hand conversion. Rear delivery may require deeper or wider treatment rooms depending on the size of the rear cabinet. The rear cabinet is the most common type of rear delivery system, but wall-mounted units and carts can also be used.

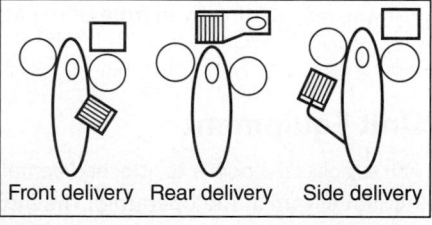

Front delivery   Rear delivery   Side delivery

FIGURE 18-20
Front delivery (transthorax), rear delivery, and side delivery units.

Side Delivery Unit: The side delivery unit is situated on either side of the patient treatment chair. There is an operator's and an assistant's unit. Each has their own dental equipment needed to perform dental procedures. The operator unit generally has handpieces, a curing light, and an air/water syringe. The assistant's unit has an air/water syringe, oral evacuator mouthpiece, and saliva ejector mouthpiece (Figure 18-23). Side delivery gives the treatment room a clean appearance because it places the instrumentation on a pull-out arm that is mounted inside a side

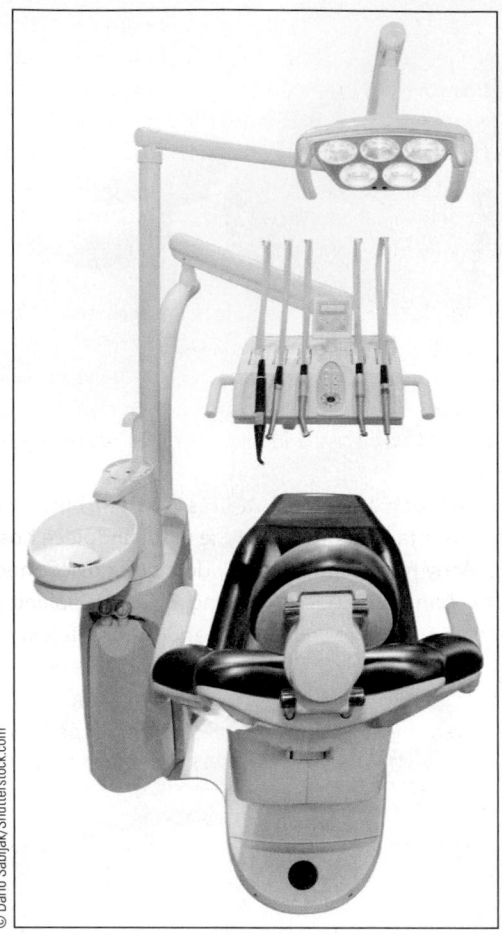

FIGURE 18-21
Front delivery system.

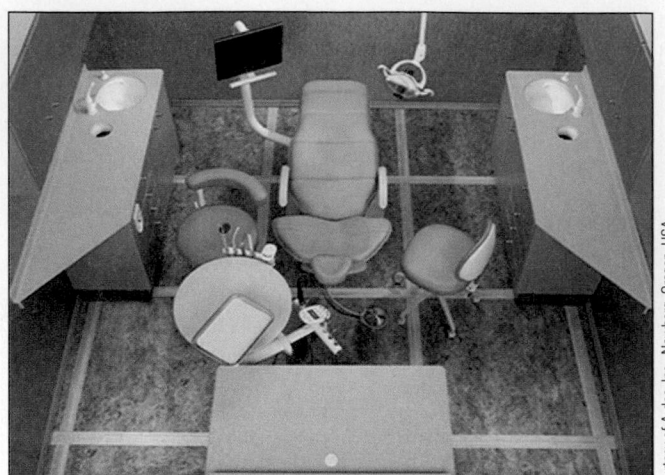

FIGURE 18-22
Rear delivery system.

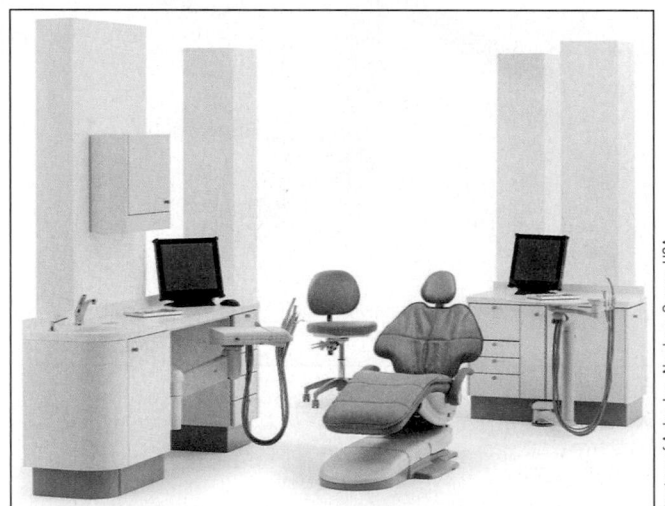

FIGURE 18-23
Side delivery system.

cabinet, leaving the chair uncluttered. When the dentist uses side delivery, the assistant's instrumentation can be located on the chair, in the rear, or directly in front of the assistant on a mobile cart.

Dental Unit Equipment

The dental unit supplies the power to attached dental equipment for delivering dental care in the operatory. The most common equipment generally includes dental handpiece connectors, saliva ejector hose, oral evacuator hose, air/water syringe, and a bracket table (Figures 18-24 and 18-25). The electricity to the unit is turned on by the main switch. The main switch must be turned on to run the dental unit equipment. Some units have an accessory switch to turn on all other utilities.

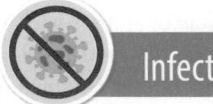 **Infection Control**

Infection Control for Dental Units

The staff should wipe away bits of debris, sanitize and disinfect the dental unit following manufacturer's directions between patients, or use a barrier that is changed between patients. The dental unit is classified as a noncritical item requiring an EPA intermediate level disinfectant. The dental staff should use the saturate–wipe–saturate technique on the unit controls or cover controls with barriers.

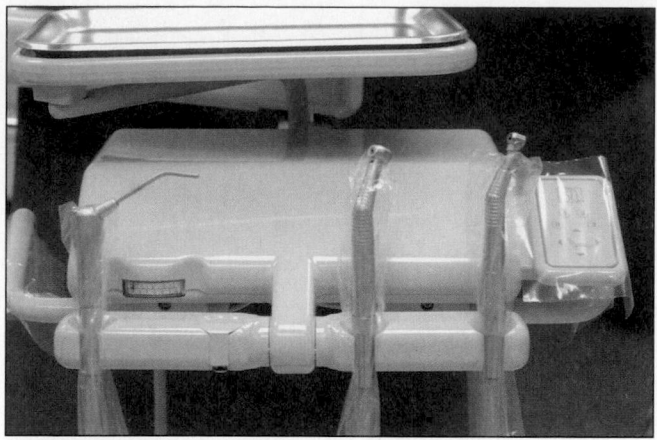

FIGURE 18-24
Operator's dental unit with (shown from left to right) air/water syringe, high-speed handpiece, and low speed dental handpiece.

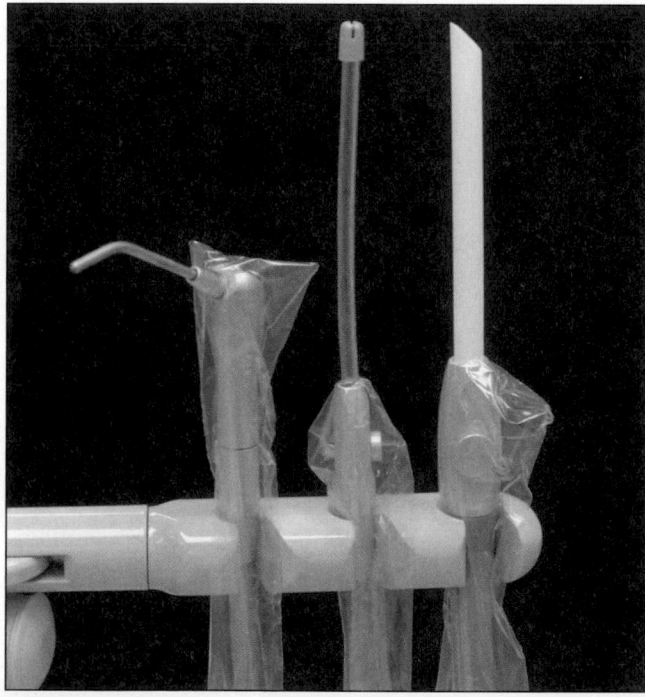

FIGURE 18-25
Assistant's dental unit with (shown from left to right) air/water syringe with disposable air/water syringe tip, saliva ejector with disposable saliva ejector tip, and oral evacuator hose with disposable HVE tip and bracket table.

Dental Handpieces The *dental handpiece* is the single most crucial piece of equipment needed to perform dental procedures. Handpieces are used to cut, finish, and polish tooth structures, restorations, and dental appliances. Handpieces are used to cut tooth structure, to remove caries, and prepare the cavity (shape the remaining tooth structure) to place a restoration (filling); the handpiece is referred to as the drill by laypersons, but professional language is preferred for dental personnel.

Burs (small cutting bits) are placed into the handpiece and are rotated to do the cutting (Figure 18-26). There are two types of handpieces used to cut structures: the high-speed and low-speed handpieces. The handpieces at the higher rpms are classed as high-speed handpieces, and lower rpms are called low-speed handpieces.

The high-speed handpiece utilizes an air turbine to rotate the bur and is attached directly to the unit handpiece hose by a coupling. Many manufacturers provide a quick disconnect that attaches the handpiece to the coupling. By gently pulling on the handpiece, the handpiece can be changed very quickly. Some couplings must be pressed before the handpiece is released. Each handpiece has a holder and selector (safety switch) attached to the unit. When the handpiece is removed from the handpiece holder, it automatically selects the handpiece to be used. This

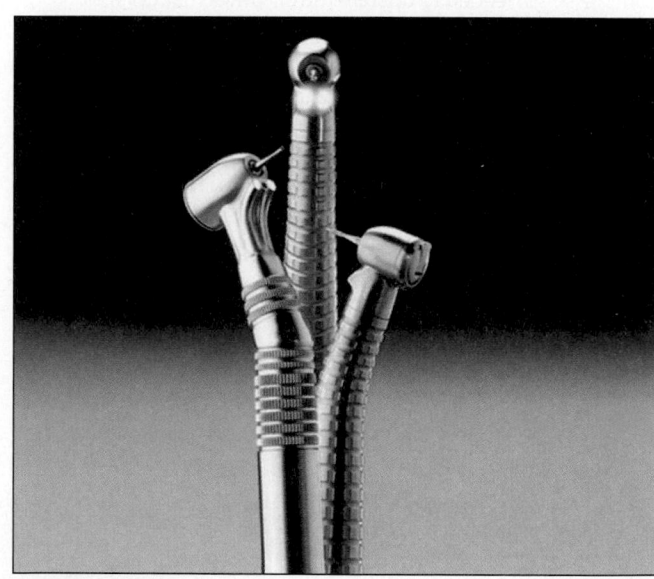

FIGURE 18-26
Burs placed into a variety of high-speed handpieces.

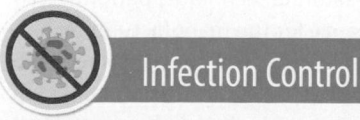

Infection Control

Infection Control for Dental Unit Equipment

All unit equipment must be disinfected by manufacturer's directions or have barriers placed. Hoses and switches should be disinfected by an EPA intermediate disinfectant after each patient using the saturate–wipe–saturate technique.

system allows only the selected handpiece to run when the rheostat is depressed.

Some handpieces have fiber optic systems that provide light directly onto the tooth surface being cut. The fiber optic handpieces are attached to a fiber optic adaptor that is attached to the unit handpiece hose. When attaching high-speed handpieces to the unit, it is important to connect the handpiece to the correct coupling. Care must be taken when connecting or removing the low speed attachments to the corresponding motor. Failure to do so may break the handpiece or motor. Most handpieces can be sterilized, but always follow the manufacturer's guidelines for disinfection or sterilization. The high-speed handpiece should never be submersed in liquids or be placed in the ultrasonic cleaner. Burs should be cleaned and sterilized after use; some burs are one-time use and disposed of in the appropriate biohazard container.

Dental unit handpieces are air-driven. Compressed air enters the handpiece and turns the **turbine** of the high-speed handpiece and the motor of the low-speed handpiece. A rheostat is used to run the handpieces (Figure 18-27). The *rheostat* is a foot controller that works similarly to a car accelerator. The more pressure placed on the rheostat, the more air pressure is released through the handpiece, causing the rotary instrument to rotate faster. The handpiece is removed from the automatic handpiece holder and the rheostat is pressed to run the handpiece; a rotary instrument must always be placed in the handpiece before running. The air compressor is needed to operate the air-driven handpieces.

The handpieces also have water lines that run to the handpieces to provide water to help cool the tooth (coolant) when it is being prepared (shaped for the placement of a restoration). There is a switch on the rheostat to select the use of air alone or air and water together. The air and water pressure are controlled by dials on the dental unit for each handpiece.

Air/Water Syringe The air/water syringe (a/w syringe) is a piece of equipment that delivers a stream of water, or air, or a spray of water and air combined. The controls for the syringe are on the handle and should be easy to operate with the thumb of one hand (Figure 18-28). When the button marked A is pressed;

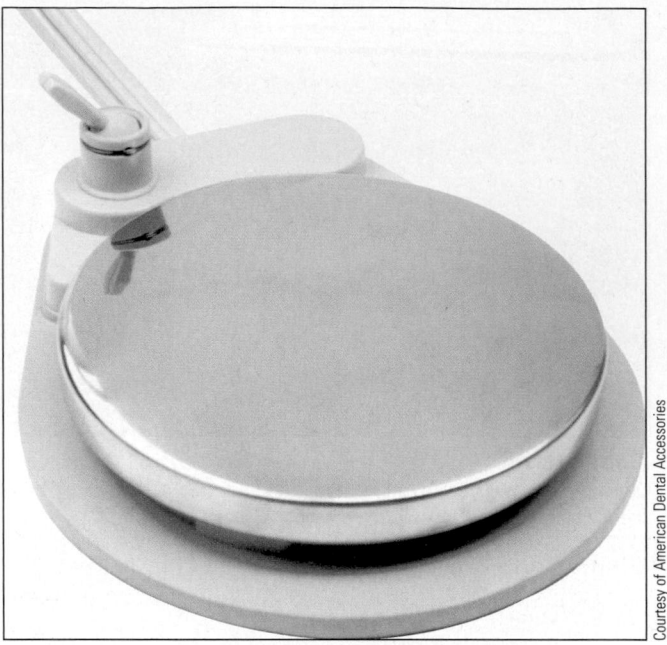

Courtesy of American Dental Accessories

FIGURE 18-27
Handpiece rheostat with water control switch.

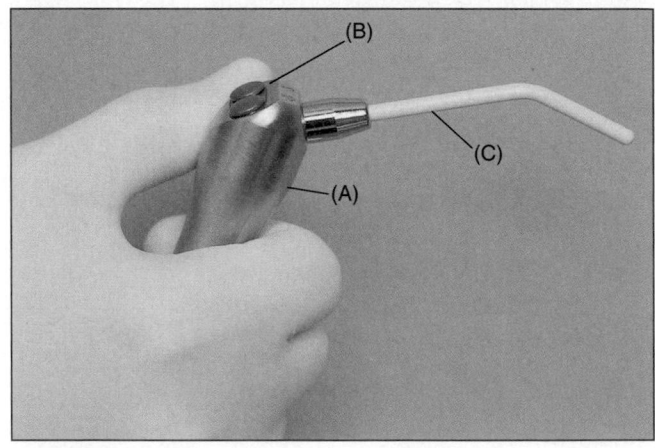

FIGURE 18-28
Air/water syringe. (A) handle, (B) air/water controls, and (C) removable and disposable air/water tip.

Infection Control

Infection Control for Dental Handpieces

The handpieces are classified as critical items. They must be removed from the unit, covered on the tray, and taken to the sterilization area to be sterilized. Handpiece holders, switches, adaptors, and motors are classified as semicritical items and should be sanitized and disinfected using an intermediate level disinfectant. High level disinfectants are not used for surface disinfection because of fumes and their caustic nature on the skin. Most directions require using the saturate–wipe–saturate technique, performed by first wiping with gauze saturated in disinfectant to remove debris and then leaving a second gauze for the manufacturer recommended time. Many offices use presoaked gauze to minimize fumes. Some units require that the handpiece hoses be flushed with water after each patient due to potential biofilm buildup on the inside of the waterlines. The handpiece hose is flushed by switching the toggle control and pressing the rheostat to flush the handpiece and handpiece hoses for 20–30 seconds after each patient. Most units now have antiretraction hoses, making flushing hoses unnecessary. The handpieces should be flushed for 20–30 seconds by a unit rheostat or placed in a handpiece air station prior to sterilization procedures. A barrier is recommended to cover handpiece hoses where the handpiece and hose coupling joins.

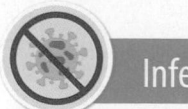
Infection Control

Infection Control for Air/Water Syringe

The air/water syringe tips should be disposed of and waterline hose should be flushed for 30 seconds after each patient. The syringe is a semicritical item, which needs to have a barrier or be disinfected with an intermediate level disinfectant using the saturate–wipe–saturate technique. The disinfectant needs to remain in contact for the time recommended by the manufacturer. New barriers are placed on the syringe handle and the tubing for each patient (Figure 18-29).

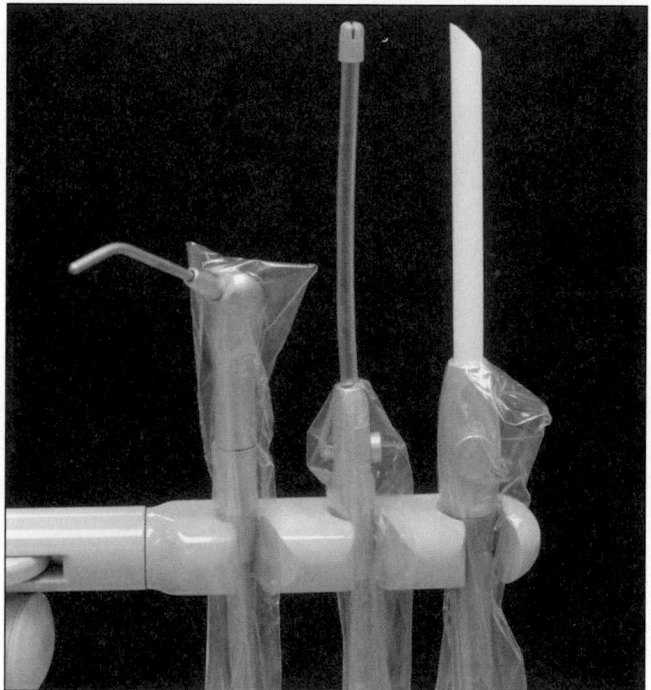

FIGURE 18-29
Air/water syringe, saliva ejector, and oral evacuator with barriers in place.

only air is released. The W button releases water only. When both buttons are pressed, a spray of air and water is released. An a/w syringe tip is placed into the syringe and is used to rinse and dry the patient's mouth during dental procedures. The air compressor and water supply are needed to operate the a/w syringe.

Saliva Ejector
The saliva ejector provides a gentle suction. The small saliva ejector hose and mouthpiece are connected to the dental unit (Figure 18-29). A saliva ejector tip is placed into the mouthpiece of the saliva ejector hose (Figure 18-30). The saliva ejector tip is placed into the patient's mouth and is used to suction saliva during procedures. The saliva ejector should be used to suction only fluid matter; solid material will block the small ejector hose. The ejector tip may be used to hold the tongue away from the work site and help keep the area dry for the placement of dental materials. The central vacuum system

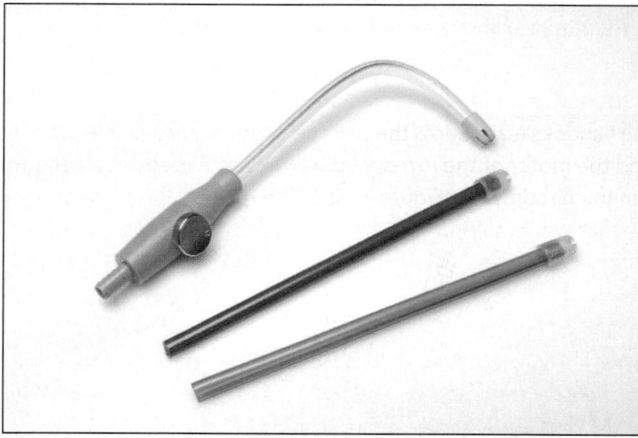

FIGURE 18-30
Saliva ejector tip is placed into the saliva ejector mouthpiece. The tips are available in assorted colors and can be bent into desired shape for better placement into the mouth.

provides the suction for the saliva ejector. The suction is turned on by turning a knob or level on the mouthpiece.

Oral Evacuator
The oral evacuator is used to aspirate solid debris and large volumes of fluid from the oral cavity. The oral evacuating hose is a larger hose than the saliva ejector and has a much greater suctioning ability (Figure 18-29). The evacuator is also referred to as the high velocity evacuator (HVE). An aspirating tip is placed into the oral evacuator mouthpiece. The central vacuum system provides the suction for the oral evacuator (Figure 18-31). The suction is turned on by turning a knob or level on the mouthpiece.

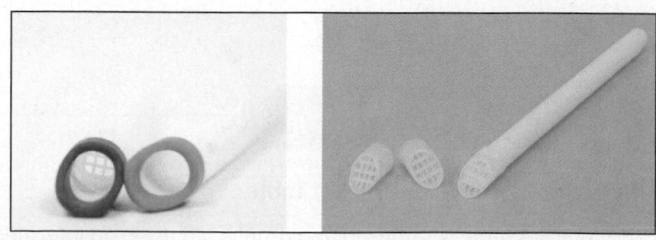

FIGURE 18-31
Oral evacuator (HVE) disposable tips.

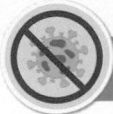

Infection Control

Infection Control for Saliva Ejector and Oral Evacuator

The saliva ejector and oral evacuator tips should be disposed of after use, and the hoses need to be flushed after every patient using a cup of water. The dental staff needs to flush a quart of water at the end of each day and clean the hoses once a week using a commercial vacuum cleaner and disinfectant. The dental unit has a trap that collects solids suctioned through the hoses (Figure 18-32). This trap must be cleaned weekly. Some manufacturers recommend daily trap inspection and cleaning. The saliva ejector and oral evacuator mouthpieces and control knobs are semicritical items that need to be disinfected with an intermediate level disinfectants using the saturate–wipe–saturate technique. The disinfectant needs to remain in contact with the equipment for the period of time recommended by the manufacturer. Each unit supplies directions for maintenance procedures. Barriers may be placed over the mouthpiece and hose during patient treatment.

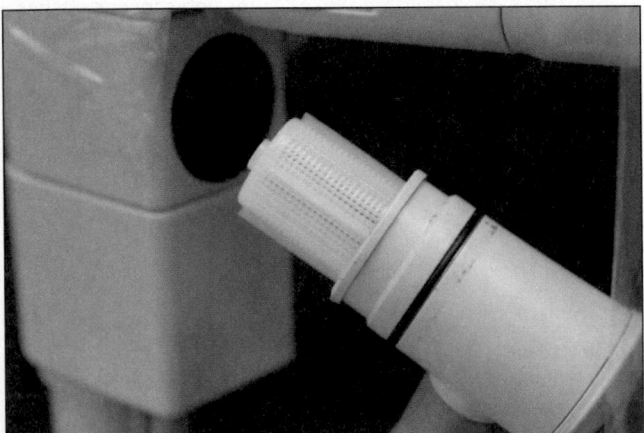

FIGURE 18-32
High-volume evacuator disposable trap.

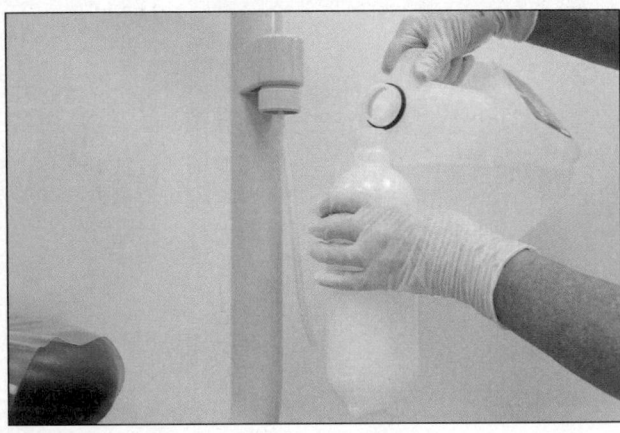

FIGURE 18-33
Self-contained water reservoir plastic bottle is attached to the dental unit. The bottle is filled with distilled water.

Bracket Table The bracket table is the working surface of the dental unit. The bracket table is used to hold instrument trays and dental materials needed for the dental procedure. Some bracket tables have an area to also hold procedure tubs and containers for expendables (see Figure 18-5).

Self-Contained Water Reservoir Most dental units have a self-contained water reservoir (bottle). Many of the systems have a removable water bottle that is refilled using distilled or sterile water (Figure 18-33). Air pressure is supplied to the water bottle, which forces water through the unit and on to the handpieces and air/water syringe.

Dental Operating Light The oral cavity is a small, dark opening that needs to be illuminated while performing procedures. The dental light (lamp) is attached to an arm and can be mounted off the side of the dental chair or from the ceiling (Figure 18-34). The dental light is very bright, using mostly halogen bulbs to provide the needed light for clear vision. Both the operator and the assistant should be able to adjust the position of the light. The light's arm allows the dental staff to direct the light to all areas of the mouth. A switch is generally located at the junction of the light and the arm. Most lights have dimmer switches to change the intensity of the light.

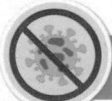

Infection Control

Infection Control for Bracket Table

The bracket table is sanitized and disinfected using an intermediate disinfectant. The flat working surface is disinfected using the spray–wipe–spray technique, and the holders and switches are disinfected using the saturate–wipe–saturate technique. The table and switches may be covered by a tray barrier during patient treatment.

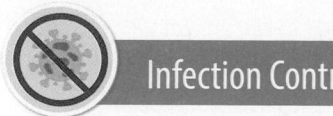

Infection Control for Water Reservoir

To help clean the water lines and to bring in fresh water, the handpieces and air/water syringe should be flushed for 20–30 seconds after each patient. Each system has directions to be followed for periodic sanitizing and disinfection of the reservoir.

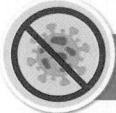

Infection Control for the Dental Light

The light switches and handles should be disinfected with an intermediate disinfectant using the saturate–wipe–saturate technique. Barriers may be used to cover the light handles and switch (Figure 18-35). Newer lights may have motion sensor switches to aid in infection control. The light covers are easily scratched. The manufacturer provides specific directions in caring for the light cover, disinfection, and changing the lightbulb.

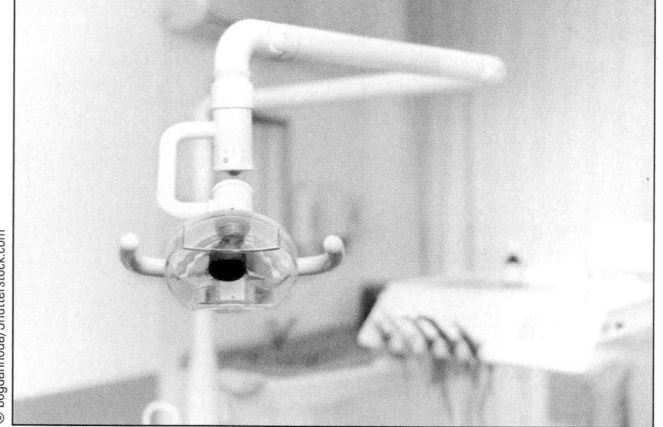

FIGURE 18-34
Dental operating light attached to the dental chair.

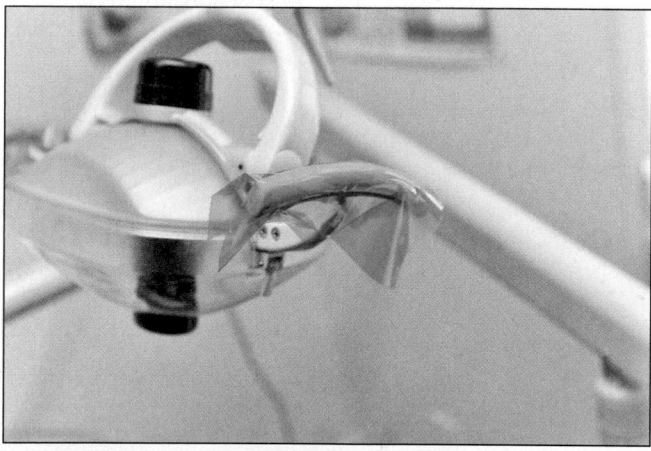

FIGURE 18-35
Light handles covered with plastic sleeves.

Computerized Equipment

Many offices are computerized with terminals in the treatment rooms as well as the business office. Computer systems allow the office to be paperless and to be more efficient at completing specific tasks, such as billing. Some systems allow the dentist and staff to enter treatment plans, chart the condition of the patient's mouth, make the patient's next appointment, bill the insurance company, and give information and instructions. The number of computers and the programs or systems used in the office are determined by the dentist. To use the computers efficiently and effectively, additional training and cooperation of all staff members are required.

Computer digital radiography equipment is also part of the technology found in the dental office (Figure 18-36). A computer is displayed in every treatment room. (Digital radiography equipment is discussed in Chapter 29, "Extraoral and Digital Radiography.")

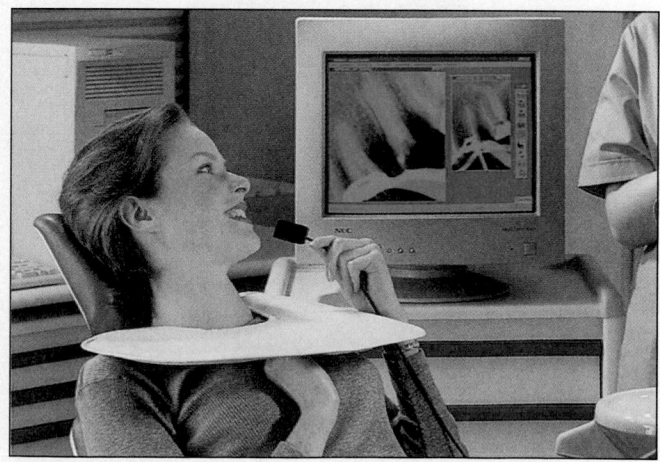

FIGURE 18-36
Computer digital radiography equipment.

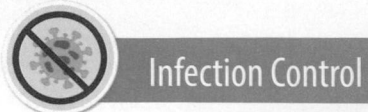

Infection Control

Infection Control for Computerized Equipment

A barrier should be placed over the keyboard and mouse or touch-screen computer monitors. Clean and disinfect surfaces using a germicidal wipe containing a hospital disinfectant by wiping the surface with friction for five seconds once a day and when soiled. The intraoral camera barrier should be changed for each patient.

Computerized equipment includes an intraoral camera and a computer terminal. An intraoral wand contains a small camera that transmits to the computer monitor (Figure 18-37). The wand is placed in the patient's mouth, and the image is displayed on the monitor. The computer freezes a picture on the screen or prints it out. The intraoral camera allows the patient to see areas and conditions in their mouth while the dentist is discussing them.

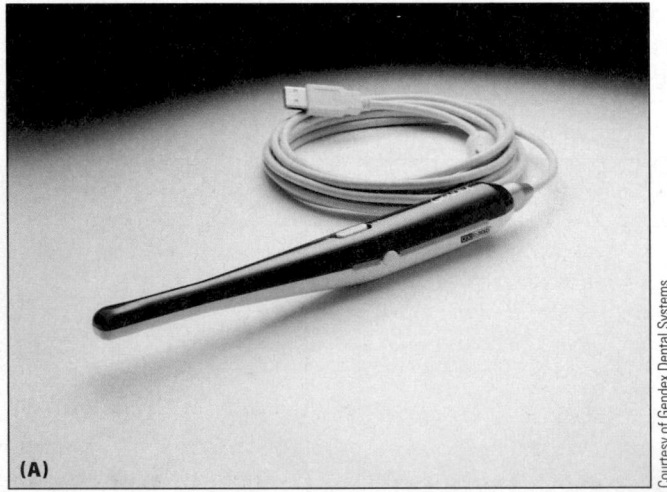

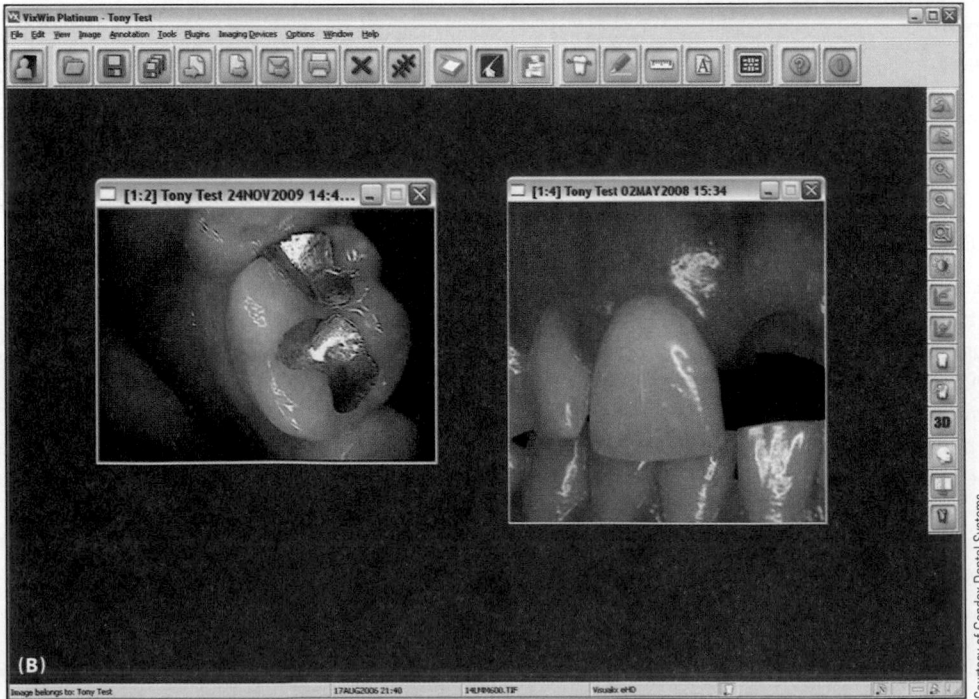

FIGURE 18-37
(A) Intraoral camera. (B) Images of the patient's mouth using the intraoral camera.

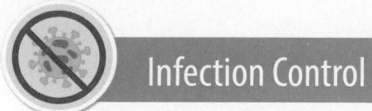

Infection Control

Infection Control for Dental Viewbox

The viewbox is disinfected with an intermediate disinfectant using the saturate–wipe–saturate technique. A barrier can be placed over the viewbox switch.

Dental Viewbox

The dental viewbox is used to illuminate the standard dental radiographs for better viewing. The viewbox is usually placed on the counter near the dentist or mounted on the wall. It is turned on using a switch generally found on the top of the box (Figure 18-38).

Dental Cabinets

Cabinets are located in the operatory for easy access to dental materials. Dental cabinets have instrument drawers, compartments for dental supplies, storage for dental equipment, and pull-out drawers to be used as a working area (Figure 18-39). There is generally an operator's sink and an assistant's sink. Operatory sinks have foot controls or light and motion sensor devices which allow for hands free operation. The staff can use the sink quickly without contaminating sink faucets or their hands. The sinks should be easy to clean and have an area nearby for soap and towel dispensers.

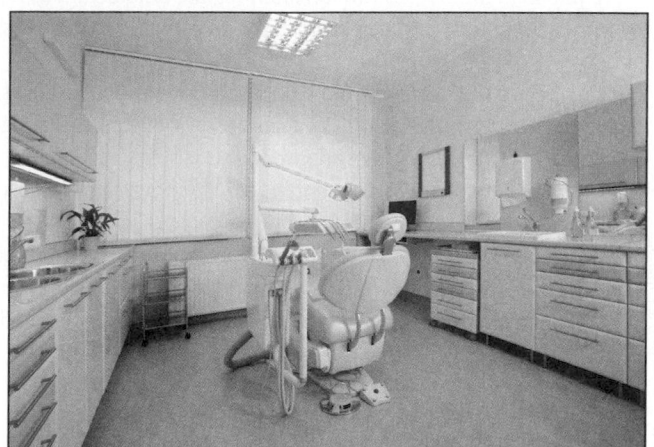

FIGURE 18-39
Dental treatment with ample counter space and storage.

Some dental cabinets have built-in areas for the viewbox or computer to view digital radiographs, communication/intercom system, TV/stereo, and storage for instruments setups and procedure tubs.

Routine Office Care

With the amount of equipment being operated in the dental office, a routine schedule needs to be in place to ensure proper maintenance control, and items should be checked off when accomplished. Often this responsibility is given to the dental assistants. Usually, the office is cleaned professionally, but the assistant should periodically check the overall appearance of the office.

Daily, weekly, or monthly maintenance tasks might include changing x-ray processing solutions, cleaning the inside of the sterilizers, changing ultrasonic solutions, performing monitoring activities to check the effectiveness of the sterilizers, and making miscellaneous equipment repairs. It is necessary to keep

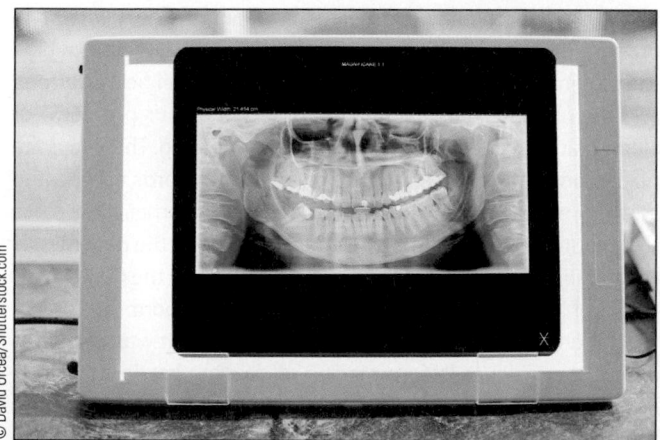

FIGURE 18-38
Dental viewbox.

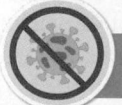

Infection Control

Infection Control for Dental Cabinets

The flat working surfaces, drawer handles, sink, and faucet handles need to be sanitized and disinfected with an intermediate disinfectant using the spray–wipe–spray or saturate–wipe–saturate technique after each patient. The inside of the drawers and cabinets need to be disinfected weekly. Special barriers are available for electronic equipment such as computer keyboards.

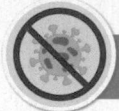

Infection Control

Summary of Clinical Equipment Disinfection Guidelines

Equipment disinfected with an intermediate disinfectant using the spray–wipe–spray or saturate–wipe–saturate technique: dental chair, operator and assistant stools, bracket table, cabinet flat working surfaces, drawer handles, inside drawers and cabinets, sink, and faucet handles

Equipment disinfected with an intermediate disinfectant using the saturate–wipe–saturate technique: all unit hoses, unit switches, handpiece holders and selectors, light switches, light handles, and all equipment used during patient care prior to returning to storage

Equipment disinfected with a high level disinfectant using the saturate–wipe–saturate technique. Disinfectant must remain on equipment surface per manufacturer's directions: all mouthpieces attached to unit hoses (saliva ejector mouthpiece and HVE mouthpiece), air/water syringe, handpiece adaptors, and motors

Equipment varies with different manufacturers. Need to follow manufacturer's directions: light cover, self-contained water system, and dental unit trap

Equipment requiring flushing of waterlines: air/water syringe and handpieces with coolant and hoses

Equipment requiring flushing with recommended vacuum cleanser: saliva ejector and HVE hoses

Equipment that is sanitized and sterilized in sterilization area: HVE funnels and all handpieces

replacement parts on hand for equipment that needs routine care (e.g., the O-rings in the air/water syringe, which must be changed when air or water leaks).

Opening and Closing the Dental Office

The daily routine of opening and closing the dental office usually falls to the dental assistants. These tasks are sometimes divided, with one assistant opening the office and the other closing the office. If there are numerous staff members, these responsibilities are often divided by the week or month.

Whoever is responsible to open the office in the morning usually arrives 30–45 minutes early and completes the routine (Procedure 18-2) before the other staff members arrive.

To close the office, the responsible person stays after the last patient and makes sure that everything is turned off and the office is ready for patients the next day (Procedure 18-3).

Receiving and Dismissing Patients

Specific procedures are necessary to prepare the treatment area for receiving patients. Often you have less than five minutes between patients to clean the area used by a previous patient and have it ready to receive the next patient. You must have a standardized method to receive patients to be organized and time efficient. Items not prepared or forgotten will cause a delay in treatment and frustration for the patient and dental team.

It is vital to patient care that the dental team follows a standardized routine in preparing for receiving patients. Most routines include these steps:

- Prepare the treatment area.
- Prepare tray setup.

- Prepare for patient seating.
- Greet and seat the patient.

Prepare the Treatment Area

Once all items used on the previous patient have been removed from the treatment area and the area is completely disinfected, the dental assistant is ready to prepare for seating the next patient. In order to prepare for the patient, the assistant must first examine the patient chart to discover what procedures will be performed and the patient's medical history for any previous problems or alerts that may affect treatment or patient seating. The x-rays are placed on the viewbox, and the charts and records are located away from the treatment area or covered with a barrier. If the office is computerized, the dental assistant should open the patient's file to have the information, chart, and x-rays ready for the dentist. Any model or lab work is brought into the treatment room.

Using the office protocol, the dental assistant washes hands and puts on gloves before placing all routine barriers to cover equipment in preparation for receiving the next patient. Once all the barriers have been placed, the assistant retrieves and places the setup on the bracket table. The tips (aspirating, saliva ejector, and air/water tips) are retrieved from the setup tray and placed into their respective mouthpieces or syringe. A biohazard bag should be placed near the working area to dispose of expendables throughout the procedure. Many offices have a routine patient seating setup that is placed on the counter or bracket table space. The patient seating setup may include the following items.

A patient napkin is placed over the patient's chest to protect the patient's clothing from dental spray and soiling. It is generally made of impervious backed paper that prevents soaking through to patient clothing. The backing should be placed against the patient (Figure 18-40).

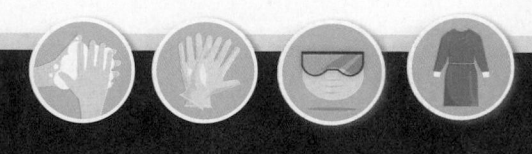

Procedure 18-2
Daily Routine to Open the Office

These tasks are done by the assistant each morning. The assistant arrives at the office early to open the office and prepare for the day's schedule. The dentist should be immediately alerted about any equipment that is not running smoothly.

Procedure Steps

1. Turn on all the lights in the office.

2. Turn on the master water valve, the central vacuum system, the air compressor, and the master and accessory switches to each dental unit.

3. Wash hands, don gloves and protective eyewear.

4. Fill self-contained water reservoir.
   - ❏ Turn switch to change water reservoir.
   - ❏ Remove water reservoir.
   - ❏ Empty reservoir in sink and fill with distilled water.
   - ❏ Reattach reservoir and turn switch back to original position.

5. Check the air/water syringe.
   - ❏ Press air button to check air flow for 20–30 seconds.
   - ❏ Hold syringe over sink and press water button to check water flow for 20–30 seconds.
   - ❏ Hold syringe over sink and press air and water buttons to check spray for 20–30 seconds.

6. Check oral evacuator.
   - ❏ Turn knob or lever to "on" position.
   - ❏ Place mouthpiece into cup of water and check suction strength.

7. Check saliva ejector.
   - ❏ Turn knob or lever to "on" position.
   - ❏ Place mouthpiece into cup of water and check suction strength.

8. Check low-speed handpiece.
   - ❏ Place low-speed handpiece into low speed motor.
   - ❏ Insert rotary instrument into handpiece.
   - ❏ Select air only on rheostat.
   - ❏ Press rheostat to check air pressure and rotation of rotary instrument.

9. Check high-speed handpiece.
   - ❏ Place high-speed handpiece onto high speed coupling.
   - ❏ Insert rotary instrument into handpiece.
   - ❏ Select air only on rheostat.
   - ❏ Press rheostat to check air pressure and rotation of rotary instrument.
   - ❏ Switch to water on rheostat.
   - ❏ Hold handpiece over sink and press rheostat to check flow of water.

10. Check dental light.
    - ❏ Hold dental light facing the dental chair.
    - ❏ Turn on the dental light switch.
    - ❏ Test dimmer switch.

11. Check the reception room, straighten the magazines and the children's area, and unlock the patients' door to the office.

12. Turn on the communication system, check the answering machine or the answering system, start the computers, unlock the files, and organize the business area.

13. Post copies of patient schedules in designated areas throughout the office according to HIPAA regulations.

14. Turn on all equipment in the film processing area.
    - ❏ Change the water in the processing tanks and replenish solutions, if necessary.

15. Remove PPE and wash hands.

16. Change into appropriate clinical clothing, following OSHA guidelines.

17. Review the daily patient schedule.

18. Prepare treatment rooms for the first patients.
    - ❏ Check supplies, place barriers, and review patient records.
    - ❏ Prepare the appropriate trays and lab work for the first patients.

19. Turn on any sterilizing equipment and check solution levels.
    - ❏ Prepare new ultrasonic and disinfection solutions.
    - ❏ Complete overnight sterilization procedures.

20. Replenish supplies needed for the day.

Napkin clips, also referred to as alligator clamps, are used to hold the patient napkin in place. They are placed around the patient's neck and attached to both sides of the napkin. Many napkins come with adhesive on both sides of the neck area or with a disposable napkin holder to eliminate the need for a clip, leaving one less item to be disinfected (Figure 18-41).

Protective eyewear is worn by the patient and dental team during use of rotary instruments (handpieces) to protect the eyes from dental materials, debris, and bacteria.

A handheld mirror is available to allow the patient to remove and apply cosmetics before and after procedures. The mirror is also a helpful educational tool to allow patients

Procedure 18-3
Daily Routine to Close the Office

These tasks are done by the assistant at the end of the day. The office evening routine includes closing the office for the evening and preparing for the next day. As with the opening routine, the assistants usually share the responsibility of closing the office. Each office has specific details, but the following are general tasks.

Procedure Steps

1. Wash hands, don gloves and protective eyewear.

2. Clean the treatment rooms. This may include an in-depth cleaning of the dental chair and dental unit.
   - ❏ Flush the handpieces and air–water syringes, run solutions through the evacuation hoses, clean traps and filters, and maintain water reservoirs.

3. Position the dental chair for evening housekeeping.

4. Turn off all master switches, air compressor, and central vacuum system.

5. Process, mount, and file x-rays. Follow the manufacturer's instructions to shut down automatic processors.
   - ❏ Turn off water supply to manual processing tanks.
   - ❏ Wipe counters and turn off the safe light.

6. Sterilize all instruments and set up trays for the next day.
   - ❏ Empty ultrasonic solutions and turn off all equipment.
   - ❏ Restock supplies.

7. Make sure all laboratory cases have been sent to the lab and early-morning cases have been received from the lab.

8. Remove PPE and wash hands.

9. Confirm and complete appointment schedule for the next day, insurance forms, and daily bookkeeping responsibilities.
   - ❏ Pull charts for the next day or review patient information on computer.

10. Turn off business office equipment and turn on the answering machine or service.
    - ❏ Lock patient and business office files.

11. Straighten the reception room.
    - ❏ For the security of the office, all doors and windows should be locked.

12. Change from uniform to street clothes, following OSHA guidelines.

13. Turn off machines in the staff lounge and clean tables and counters.

14. Turn off all the lights in the office and lock the door as you leave.

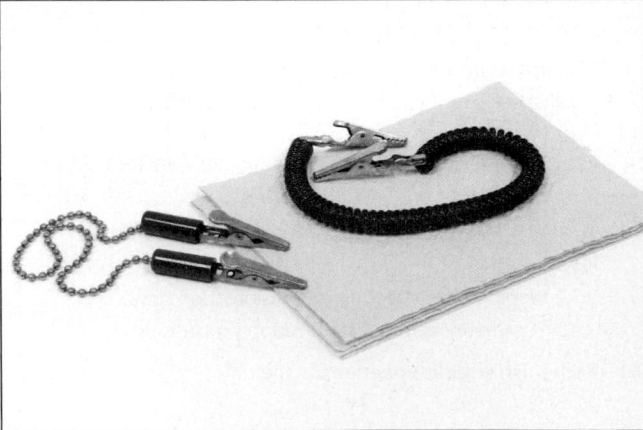

FIGURE 18-40
Patient disposable napkin with napkin clips.

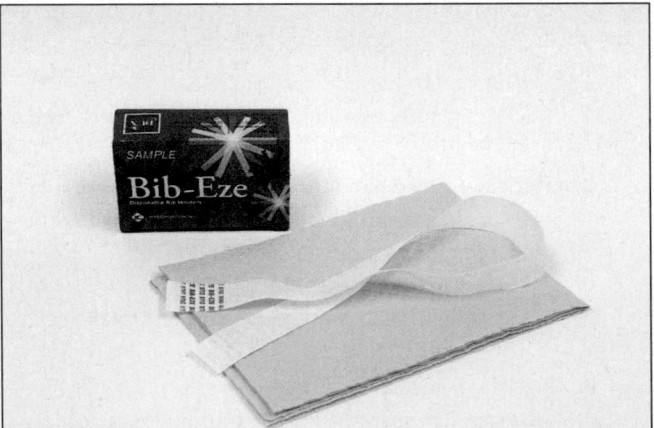

FIGURE 18-41
Patient disposable napkin and disposable napkin holder.

to see specific areas in their mouth and to view some dental procedures.

Facial tissues are provided to the patient to remove cosmetics and clean areas of the face after dental procedures. For some, it adds comfort to be able to blot any saliva or moisture they may feel on their face during procedures.

Antimicrobial mouth wash and disposable cups are provided for a preprocedural mouth rinse. This reduces the number of

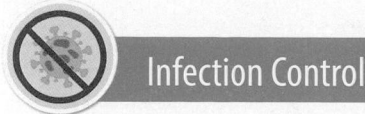

Infection Control

All expendables used in patient seating should be disposed of in contaminated waste. The napkin clips should be disinfected using immersion disinfectant. Protective eyewear and the hand mirror can be disinfected using the spray–wipe–spray technique and intermediate disinfectant.

microorganisms released in the form of aerosols and splatter that can contaminate the dental team and the patient.

Prepare Tray Setup

The appropriate setup is assembled, placed on the bracket table, and covered with the patient napkin until the patient is seated. Setups should remain covered until use to protect items and materials from being contaminated and to prevent the patient from seeing the instrument while being seated. Details about dental instruments and setups are covered in Chapter 19.

Prepare for Patient Seating

The patient chair is placed in an upright position at a height for the individual patient's seating with the armrest positioned to receive the patient. The chair height is then adjusted so the seat of the chair is directly behind the back of the patient's knee. A pathway to the chair needs to be cleared for safe seating. The dental light, dental units, rheostats, and stools should be moved into positions that will not interfere with the patient path to the chair during seating.

Once the treatment area is disinfected and prepared for patient seating, the dental assistant should stand back and take one last look and see the area as a patient will. It is important that the treatment area look clean, organized, and welcoming.

Greet and Seat the Patient

Once the treatment area is prepared to receive the next patient, the dental assistant is responsible for greeting, escorting, seating, and preparing the patient for the scheduled appointment. The dental assistant should review the chart to know what type of patient is to be escorted. The greeting and manner of escort depends on the patient's age; physical, mental and emotional needs; and language. For example, a 2-year-old and an 80-year-old have very different needs and require different escort techniques. Ambulatory patients and those in a wheelchair or using a walker require different accommodations that the assistant needs to be aware of prior to entering the reception area to greet the patient. Special accommodations are discussed later in this chapter. (Also refer to Chapter 13.) Following is the greeting and escort procedure for older children and adult patients.

The dental assistant should always be pleasant and courteous, maintain eye contact, and address the patient in a proper and professional manner. One of the important roles the dental assistant plays is to put the patient at ease and to begin to establish a rapport with the patient. This begins when the dental assistant greets and escorts the patient to the treatment area. They

should enter the reception area and call the patient by their first name, followed by their title and last name: for example, "Jane, Mrs. Smith." Wait until the patient answers, make eye contact, smile, and say, "Mrs. Smith, the doctor will see you now." Avoid a greeting that may be intimidating or cause confusion. Never say, "The doctor is ready for you" as this may sound threatening. Also avoid asking, "Do you want to come in?" The patient might say "no," causing an awkward moment.

Allow the patient time to gather their belongings, and offer to help if the patient has a lot of personal items with them. Offer to hang up the patient's coat if needed. Extend your arm as you ask the patient to please follow you to the chair you have reserved especially for them. Introduce yourself as you lead the patient into the operatory. Explain how glad you are to see the patient today and make them feel welcome.

After the patient has been greeted and escorted toward the treatment area, the assistant should direct the patient to the treatment chair. If the patient is holding personal items, offer to place the items into a cabinet within the patient's view for safe keeping. It is important that the patient can keep an eye on the area that is storing their personal items to avoid accusations of items missing later. The assistant should ask the patient to take a seat in the chair reserved for them. While the patient is being seated, the assistant should stand next to the chair backrest and offer a hand to help the patient to be seated. The patient should be instructed to sit on the edge of the dental treatment chair and to swing legs into position (Figure 18-42). The patient should

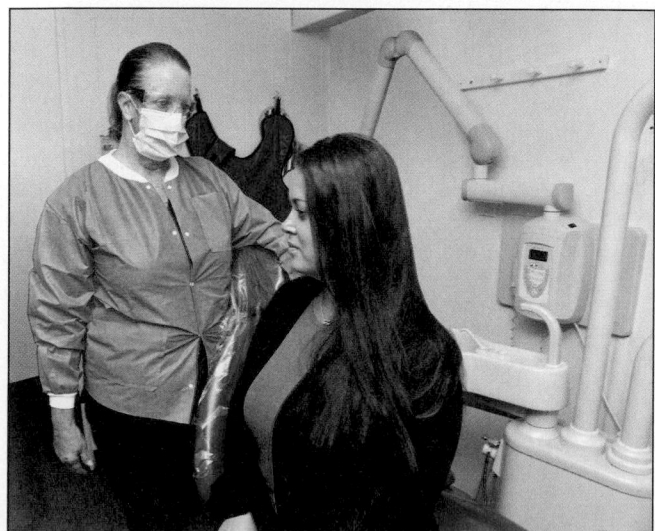

FIGURE 18-42
Assistant stands next to chair back rest while patient is instructed to sit on edge of dental chair.

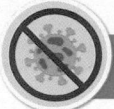

Infection Control

A preprocedural antimicrobial mouth rinse reduces bacteria in the mouth and keeps the patient and dental team safer. The CDC recommends it to be a standard of care.

be seated so that the buttocks and shoulder blades are flush against the back of the treatment chair.

Once the patient has been seated, the armrest is returned to the closed position. Ask the patient to sit with their back against the backrest and position the headrest to support the patient's head beneath the occipital area. It is extremely important always to inform the patient what you are doing so that they are not surprised by any sudden or unexpected movement of the chair during the seating process. The assistant should also ask patients to silence their cell phones so as not to startle the dental team or other patients.

Inform the patient that you are going to raise the chair slightly and recline the back of the chair. Raise the chair a few inches and recline the chair to a 45 degree angle. This is a good position to drape the patient with the protective patient napkin as the patient's head will lean forward slightly. The napkin clip should be clipped on the opposite side the assistant is standing prior to placement. This allows the assistant to clip the side closest to them once it is placed around the patient's neck to prevent leaning over the patient (Figure 18-43). This allows for ease in placing the napkin over the patient's chest with the chain of the clip around the neck.

As the assistant is draping the patient with the napkin, this is a good time to explain what procedures are scheduled for this appointment and to ask if the patient has any concerns or questions for the dental team. As the primary dental assistant, you spend a great deal of time with your patients. They often feel as if they can express concerns to you since they feel comfortable

with you. Any questions that you can have ready for the dentist prior to their arrival into the treatment area will increase productivity and expedite the patient's visit.

After the napkin is placed, explain the office protocol for infection control practices and how the dental team takes patient health and safety seriously. Present the protective eyewear for the patient's use while the dentist performs procedures that may result in dental spray. The patient is asked to rinse their mouth using a mouth rinse before treatment. Offer the hand mirror and tissue to patients who are wearing lipstick. Explain how the lipstick may be smeared during procedures and ask them to remove it. Review and update the patient's medical and dental history.

Explain to the patient that the dentist will need the patient lying down in a position where their head and knees are level. Inform the patient that you will need to raise and lower the chair until this position is obtained. Then raise the chair slightly and recline the chair halfway to the supine position. Ask if the patient is comfortable. Positioning movement increases some patients' apprehension. Remember, you work in this environment every day; the sights, sounds, and smells are not that familiar to the outside world. The assistant can ease this anxiety by taking a seat in the operator stool behind the treatment chair while positioning the chair into the supine position. From this position, you can also tell when the patient's head and knees are parallel (Figure 18-44).

Continue to lower the backrest until the patient is in a supine position. Many dentists prefer to have the patient still in the upright position when they enter the room in order to greet them for the first visit. The height of the backrest should be 2 inches above the dentist's thighs. The dentist should need to only make

FIGURE 18-43
Patient placed in 45 degree position. Assistant places patient napkin on the side they are standing.

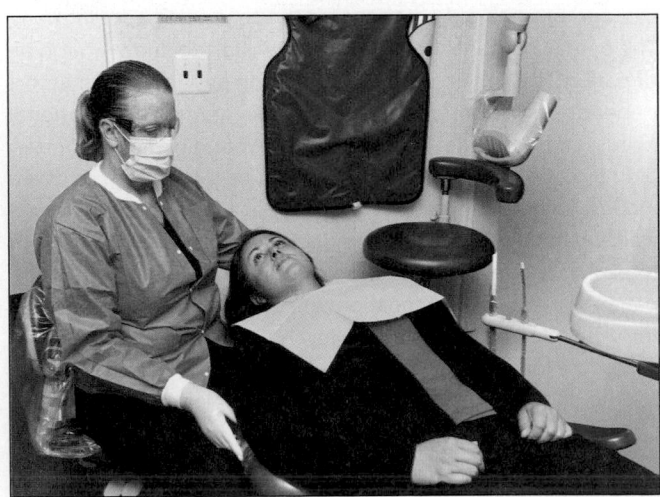

FIGURE 18-44
Assistant in operator stool while placing patient in supine position.

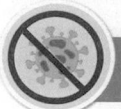 **Infection Control**

Having the dental team wash their hands and open sterilized instrument packages in front of the patient gives the patient confidence that the office staff is following infection control standards.

a slight adjustment of this height to be ready to begin the procedure. Ask the patient once again if they are comfortable and make certain the patient's head is near the end of the headrest.

Once the patient is lying in the supine position, make certain that their head is comfortably supported by the headrest at the end of the chair. The dental light should be positioned over the patient's chest and preadjusted for the operator's use. The face of the light should be directed toward the patient's chest approximately 36 inches above the patient. The assistant should turn on the light and direct the light to touch the tip of the patient's nose. Turn off the light until the dentist is ready to start the procedure. With the light in this position, the dentist will be provided with the best illumination of the patient's mouth and light will not be shining in the patient's eyes.

The operator's stool and rheostat can be moved to the operator's preference, and the assistant's stool can be positioned for the procedure to begin. The assistant communicates to the dentist that the treatment area is ready for them. The assistant should wash their hands in front of the patient, don the PPE necessary for the procedure, be seated on the assistant's stool, and open sterilized instrument packages in front of patient.

It is important to establish rapport with the patients and make them feel welcome and at ease. Remember to talk to the patients and show an interest in what they have to say. Ask them about subjects they are involved with and are comfortable discussing. People like to talk about themselves, their families, work, vacations, and hobbies. Note points of interest on the treatment chart so continued reference can be made. Often, patients will ask questions about dental concerns. General information can be given by the dental assistant. The dentist can answer specifically when they come into the treatment room. Communication with patients begins when they walk into the office and should continue until they leave.

When the dentist enters the room, they will wash hands, don fresh PPE, and welcome the patient. The dental assistant should introduce the patient to the dentist if this is the patient's first visit to the office or the first time being treated by this dentist. Again, this cannot be done appropriately if the patient is already in the supine position. The elder person should be introduced first. An appropriate introduction would be to say, "Mrs. Smith, this is Doctor Jones. Doctor Jones, this is Mrs. Smith." The dentist will greet the patient, make some comforting remarks, and then take their position at the chair.

After the dentist's greeting, the dental assistant will turn on the dental light and adjust the light for maximum illumination of the area where the dental treatment is being performed. For the mandibular teeth, the light is raised and the beam is directed downward (Figure 18-45). For the maxillary teeth, the light is lowered and the beam is directed upward (Figure 18-46).

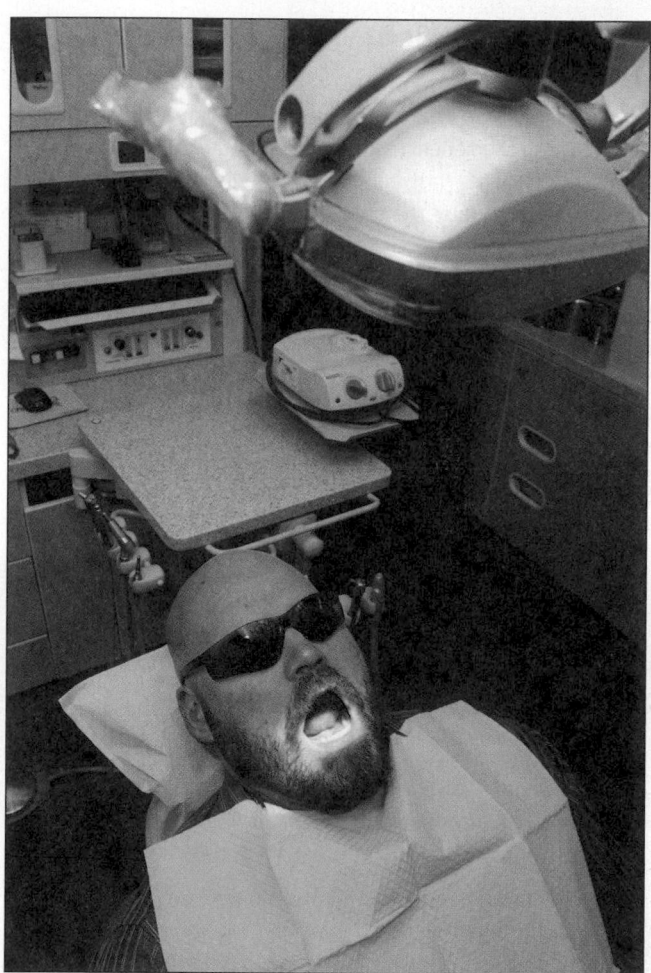

FIGURE 18-45
Patient seated and light adjusted for the mandibular arch.

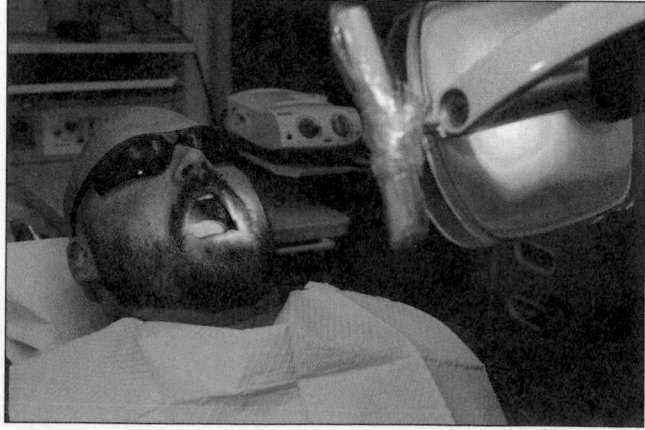

FIGURE 18-46
Patient seated and light adjusted for the maxillary arch.

The dentist will signal that they are ready to begin the procedure by placing their hands on either side of the patient's head; the assistant will pass dental instruments for the dentist to examine the area, and the procedure will begin. During the procedure, the light may need to be adjusted periodically. The assistant must be observant to keep the field of operation well lit.

Dismiss the Patient

At the completion of the procedure, the assistant should take precautions to remove from the patient's vision any soiled items that might disturb the patient (such as bloody materials) and dispose of them in appropriate trash containers. When dismissing the patient, it is important to raise the backrest slowly and in stages. Rapidly returning to an upright position after lying in the supine position for some time may cause the patient to feel lightheadedness, which is referred to as **postural hypotension**. The assistant should raise the backrest to the 45 degree angle, remove the patient napkin, ask the patient how they feel, and examine how they look. Tell the patient you are returning them to the upright position.

The assistant should also examine the patient's face for any debris. Anything that might disturb the patient (such as blood) should be

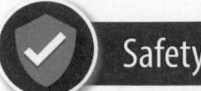

Safety

If you notice that the patient's pupils are dilated, their breathing is strained, or their skin feels clammy, the patient is at risk of syncope (fainting). The patient should be asked to rest a while until they are feeling better. If it takes the patient more than a few minutes, the dentist should be informed.

removed by the assistant using a gauze moistened in water. The assistant should also offer the patient the hand mirror and facial tissue and allow the patient to wipe their own face before being dismissed. During this time, the assistant should deglove, wash hands, and complete the necessary patient records. The patient's personal items should be returned to the patient, and the assistant should escort the patient to the business office and provide the office business personnel with the patient's completed records. The dental assistant should provide the patient with pleasant parting words. For example, tell the patient good bye and what a pleasure it was to have them as a patient. Once the patient is dismissed, the assistant returns to the treatment area to prepare the next patient.

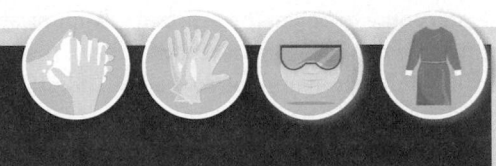

Procedure 18-4
Seating the Dental Patient

This procedure is performed by the dental assistant to prepare the patient for the dental treatment. The dental assistant has already decontaminated the dental treatment area and equipment. The following procedure follows non-pandemic guidelines.

Note: Follow interim guidelines for patient seating during COVID-19 pandemic (refer to Chapter 11 for more details). Instruct patient to wear facemask upon entering the patient check-in area and to sanitize hands with alcohol-based sanitizer.

Screen patients for fever (100.4 degrees F). Question patient if they know if they have been exposed to COVID-19 in the last few days and if they have had these symptom in the last 14 days: cough, shortness of breath and new loss of taste or smell.

Greet screened patients in the reception area wearing recommended PPE (examination mask and gloves)

Equipment and Supplies

PPE and barriers (placed on counter) (Figure 18-47)
- Patient's medical and dental records
- Infection control barriers for dental chair, hoses, counter light switches, and controls:
    - ❑ barrier sleeves (A)
    - ❑ barrier tape (B)
- Operator and assistant PPE
    - ❑ protective clothing (C)
    - ❑ protective eyewear (D)

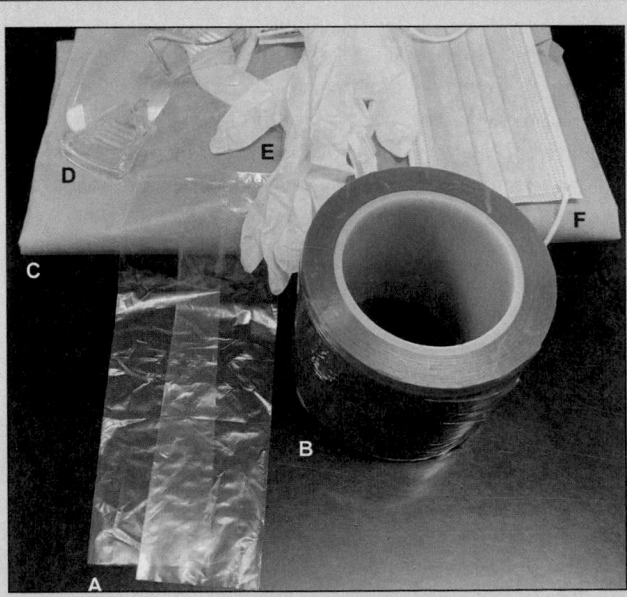

FIGURE 18-47
PPE and barriers.

    ❑ examination gloves (E)
    ❑ mask (F)

Patient PPE (Figure 18-48):
- hand mirror (A)
- patient napkin (B)

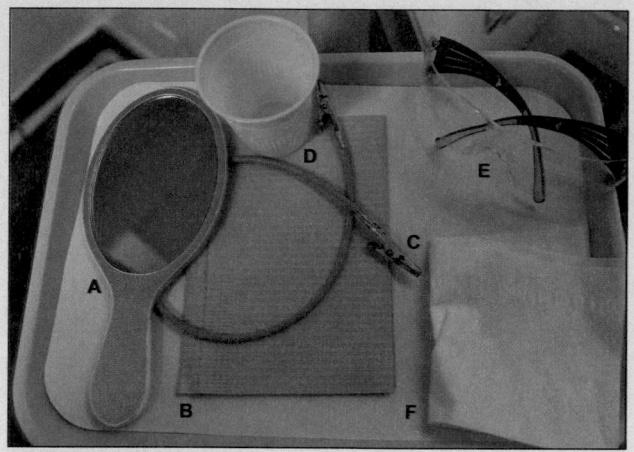

FIGURE 18-48
Patient PPE.

- napkin clip (C)
- antimicrobial mouth rinse and disposable cup (D)
- patient protective eyewear (E)
- facial tissue (F)
- instrument tray with packaged sterile setup for scheduled procedure (A) (Figure 18-49)
- saliva ejector (B)
- evacuator (HVE) (C)
- air/water syringe tips (D)
- 2 × 2 gauze squares (E)
- trash and biohazard containers

Procedure Steps

1. Wash hands and don gloves.

2. Open patient file on treatment area computer.
   - ❏ Review patient chart for name, age, special considerations, and scheduled procedure.
   - ❏ Pull up patient's radiographs.
   - ❏ Place barriers on keyboard, mouse, and touch screen.

3. Place barriers on the dental chair, light handles and switch, all dental unit hoses and switches, stool adjustment levers, counters, and unit mouthpieces and hoses (Figure 18-50).

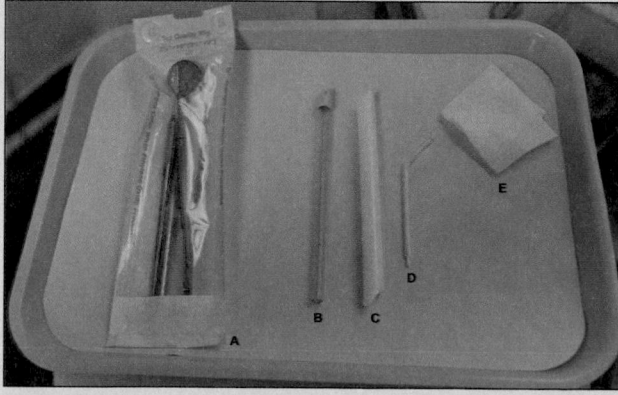

FIGURE 18-49
Instrument tray.

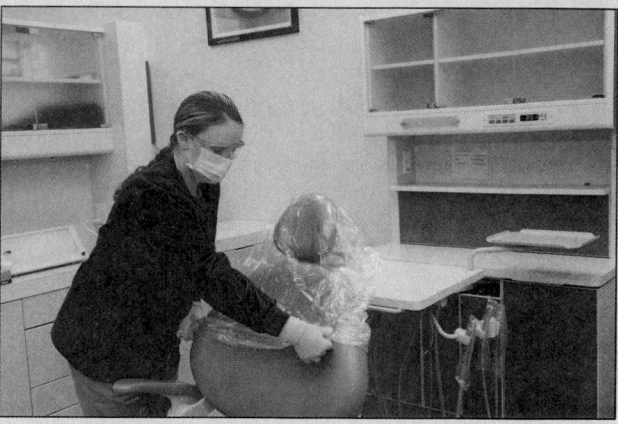

FIGURE 18-50
Dental assistant placing barriers.

4. Place patient seating setup and dental team PPE on countertop.

5. Bring instrument tray with packaged sterile instruments into treatment area and place on bracket table.

6. Ensure that handpieces, air/water syringe, and suction of saliva ejector and oral evacuator are working properly.

7. Place dental chair in upright position at comfortable height for patient with the armrest to receive the patient.

8. Prepare pathway for patient safe seating.

9. Greet and escort the patient to the treatment room.
   - ❏ Remove PPE.
   - ❏ Enter reception area and call the patient by first name, followed by title and last name.
   - ❏ Make eye contact with patient and say, "the doctor will see you now."
   - ❏ Ask patient to follow you to chair reserved for them.
   - ❏ Place patient's belonging in cabinet within their view.
   - ❏ Some offices offer mouthwash to the patient at this time.

10. Seat the patient in the dental chair while standing next to the dental chair back rest to be able to help the patient to be seated.
    - ❏ Instruct patient to sit on the edge of the chair and swing legs onto footrest.
    - ❏ Have the patient sit all the way back in the chair with buttock and shoulder against the backrest.
    - ❏ Place armrest in closed position and place headrest supporting the patient's head beneath the occipital area.

11. Position the chair for dental treatment.
    - ❏ Inform patient before each movement of the chair.
    - ❏ Raise chair a few inches while reclining backrest to 45 degree angle.
    - ❏ Clip napkin on the opposite side you are standing, place napkin over patient's chest, and clip napkin on side closest to you.
    - ❏ Offer hand mirror and tissue to remove lipstick.

(Continues)

❏ Review and update patient's medical and dental history and provide a brief explanation of scheduled treatment for the day.

❏ Explain office protocol for infection control and present protective eyewear for patient to wear.

❏ Continue to recline chair backrest to supine position 2 inches above the dentist's thighs.

❏ Adjust the head rest until the patient's head is well supported.

12. Position the dental light 36 inches above and toward the patient's chest.

❏ Turn on the light and slowly move the light to the tip of the patient's nose.

❏ Turn off light until the start of the procedure.

13. Position the operator's stool and the rheostat.

14. Position the assistant's stool.

15. Put on mask and protective clothing and eyewear.

16. Wash hands and don gloves before being seated chairside.

17. Open sterile instrument packaging and position the tray setup.

18. Place dental handpieces, saliva ejector, evacuator, and air/water syringe tips into their respective couplings or mouthpieces.

19. Inform dentist the patient has been seated.

20. Carry on a conversation with patient, establish rapport, and make them feel welcome.

21. Introduce the patient to the dentist if this is the patient's first time being treated by this dentist.

22. Turn on the light and adjust for maximum illumination of the dental treatment area.

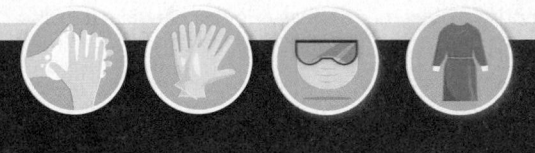

Procedure 18-5
Dismissing the Dental Patient

This procedure is performed by the dental assistant after the dental procedure has been completed.

Equipment and Supplies
The following items were set up for the procedure and now must be handled as the assistant dismisses the patient.

- contaminated treatment area from previous patient
- patient's medical and dental history (on computer or in patient file)
- utility gloves
- disinfectants for both spray–wipe–spray and saturate–wipe–saturate methods
- paper towels
- gauze squares
- contaminated and biohazard waste containers

Procedure Steps

1. Rinse and evacuate the patient's mouth thoroughly at the completion of the procedure.

2. Turn off dental light and position out of the patient's way.

3. Remove from patient's vision any items that might disturb the patient.

4. Remove assistant mask and protective eyewear.

5. Inform patient that you are returning them to upright position.

❏ Raise the backrest to 45 degree angle, remove the patient napkin, place it over the tray setup, and ask patient to remove protective eyewear.

❏ Remove debris from patient's face with moistened gauze square.

❏ Ask patient how they feel and examine their eyes and breathing.

❏ Offer hand mirror and tissue.

❏ Raise backrest to upright position if patient is stable.

6. Deglove, wash hands, and complete patient records or wear overgloves (Figure 18-51).

❏ Provide any postoperative instructions.

7. Clear path to escort patient and position the armrest to release the patient.

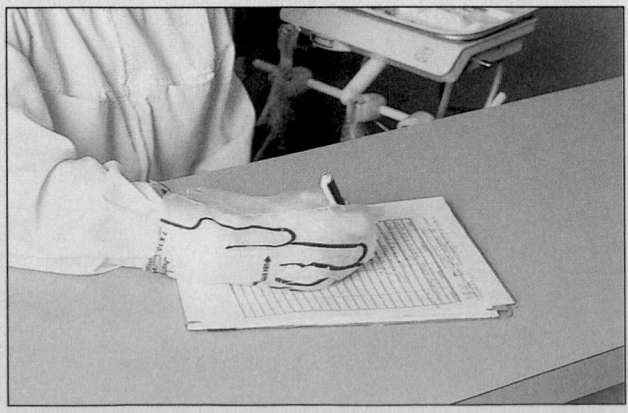

FIGURE 18-51
Dental assistant wearing overgloves while writing on a patient's chart.

8. Return patient's personal items, escort them to the business office, and provide pleasant parting words.

9. Return to the treatment area and prepare for the next patient.

   ❏ Don utility gloves and appropriate PPE.

   ❏ Remove all items used on the patient. Place all contaminated tips, handpieces, and instruments onto patient tray, cover tray with patient napkin, and transport to sterilization area.

   ❏ Remove all barriers with soiled outer side toward the inside of the barrier and dispose of immediately using office protocol. Do not shake a barrier free of debris. If area under barrier becomes contaminated, disinfect using method required for that particular item.

   ❏ Remove the chair cover from the dental chair, inverting it so that any splatter or debris remains on the inside of the bag (Figure 18-52).

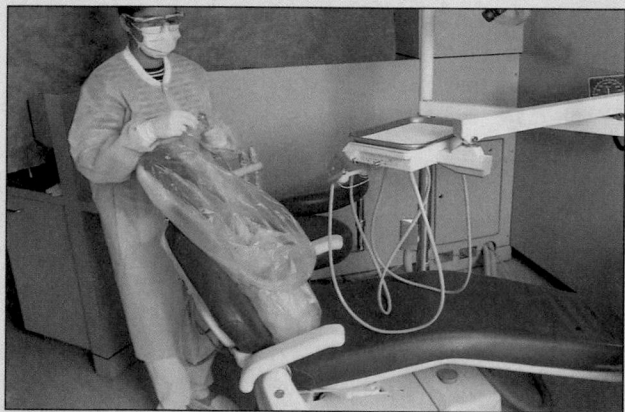

FIGURE 18-52
Invert chair cover so any splatter or debris remains on the inside.

   ❏ Remove all barriers and place them in the inverted bag.

   ❏ Disinfect air/water syringe, HVE and saliva ejector mouthpieces, and handpiece motors and adaptors using the saturate–wipe–saturate method. Use two gauze squares saturated in high level disinfectant for each item. Use the first to wipe all debris from the item. Use the second gauze to wrap the item to disinfect for the time recommended by manufacturer. Many manufacturers recommend that gauze soaked in alcohol be used to remove any disinfectant residue.

   ❏ Saturate–wipe–saturate using intermediate level disinfectant to disinfect all operatory equipment not covered by barriers (patient mirror, viewbox, material dispensers) or area exposed beneath torn barriers and return to storage.

   ❏ Disinfect flat surfaces with intermediate level disinfectant using saturate–wipe–saturate or spray–wipe–spray dictated by office protocol; sinks, countertops, bracket table, dental cabinets, operator, and assistant stools (Figure 18-53).

   ❏ Clean and disinfect face of dental light per manufacturer's directions.

   ❏ Clear water lines for 30 seconds each: air/water syringe and handpieces.

   ❏ Suction a cup of water through evacuation lines for 30 seconds each: oral evacuator and saliva ejector.

10. Remove all PPE when treatment area is decontaminated or disinfected and wash hands thoroughly.

11. Return operatory seating to closing position specified by office protocol.

12. Stand back and examine area for cleanliness and orderliness.

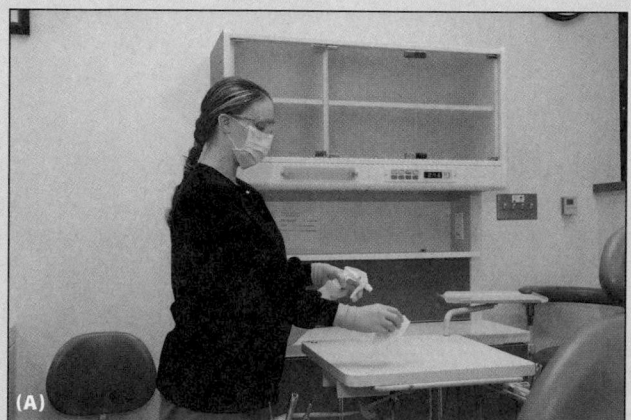
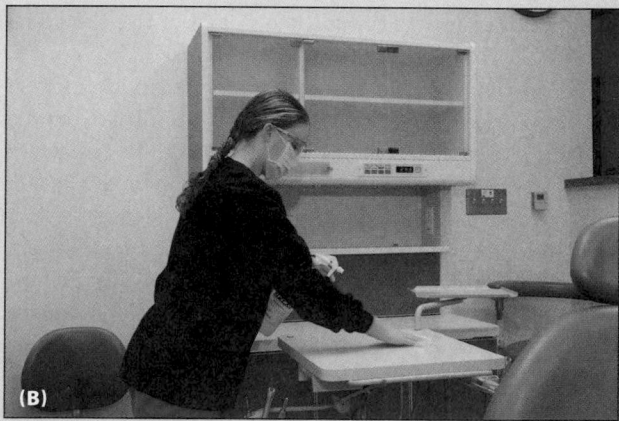

FIGURE 18-53
(A) Spraying the area with disinfectant to sanitize. (B) Wiping and spraying the area again for time recommended by manufacturer for disinfection.

Patients Who May Need Seating Accommodations

Although most patients can be seated in a routine manner, some patients need special considerations. With most of these patients, planning and preparing before their appointment eliminates problems. This chapter covers seating for small children, older patients, pregnant patients, patients with sensory disabilities, patients with wheelchairs or walkers, and non-English-speaking patient. Patients with intellectual and physical disabilities are discussed in Chapter 13.

Small Children

Many of the steps in seating a child patient are the same as when seating an adult. However, some changes are needed to adapt to the child's size, maturity, and age. Preparing the patient's records is the same, except the child's caregiver (parent or guardian) should be consulted when reviewing the medical history. Children five years of age and under may present challenges. Most doctors prefer that the mothers of young patients remain in the reception area, so the dental assistant must know the office protocol. The caregiver must be told about this protocol prior to attempting to escort the child patient. One reason for this protocol is the fact that the caregiver may not be able to handle seeing their child receive **intrusive** dental procedures (e.g., an injection) or the sight of their child's blood. Children can read a caregiver's fear, which will cause the child to be more fearful. The caregiver may also interfere with the doctor obtaining the child patient's attention, for example, by speaking to the child during the procedure. The dentist needs the child's undivided attention for patient cooperation and safety. In addition, there is not enough room in a small treatment area for an extra person, and more people in the room raises the issue of being able to perform proper infection control procedures. Occasionally there is a need for the caregiver to be in the operatory to comfort the child, but this should be determined by the dentist on an individual basis.

When the dental assistant steps into the reception room, it is important to greet both the caregiver and the child, but the focus should be on the child. Do not call the child caregiver's name at the reception door. If the child is playing on the floor in front of the caregiver, the dental assistant should leave the door between the reception area and treatment area open. The assistant bends down just to the side between the caregiver and the child. The assistant should try to build confidence and rapport by showing an interest in what the child is doing and take time to start up a light conversation. Once you make contact, tell the child and caregiver that the doctor will see them. Hold the child under the armpit and walk to their side. This allows you to lift the child up if they decide to drop to the floor. This also places you to the side if the child throws a kicking tantrum. After the child is seated, have another assistant stay with the child for a moment and return to the caregiver to tell them that the child is doing fine and reemphasize the rationale for the separation.

If the child is sitting on the caregiver's lap, the assistant should try to complete the escort as described previously. If

The patient's privacy is of utmost importance. The child's situation should be discussed in privacy; perhaps the caregiver could be invited to step inside the reception door to explain how their child is doing.

the child latches onto the caregiver's neck, the assistant may need to help the caregiver release the child's grip. The assistant can use a technique very similar to the water safety lifesaving release technique.

The dental chair is lowered to accommodate the child. A booster chair, pillow, or cushion may be used to elevate the child in the chair. If the child is too small to reach the headrest, some operators just remove or reposition it so that it does not interfere with treatment or the patient's comfort, and the patient napkin can be folded to accommodate the size of the child. To prevent the child from sliding down in the dental chair, have them sit with legs crossed (Figure 18-54). Answer any questions the child has using language appropriate to their level of understanding. More information on dealing with the child patient appears in Chapter 34, "Pediatric Dentistry." Once the procedure is

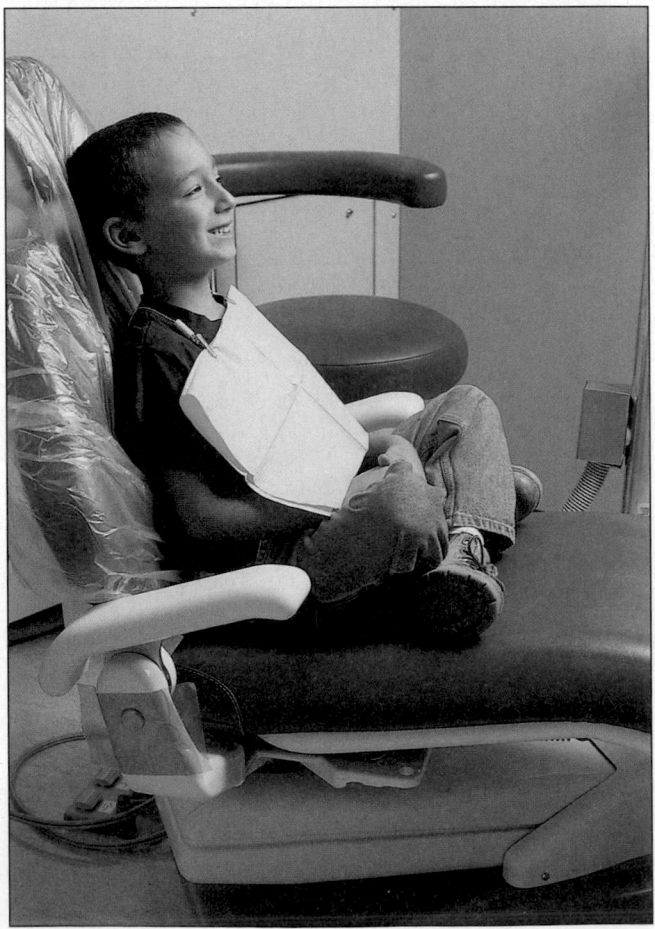

FIGURE 18-54
Child patient seated with legs crossed to prevent them from sliding down in the chair. The patient napkin is folded to fit the size of the patient.

completed and the child is dismissed, escort them to the reception area and inform the caregiver about the treatment performed. Postoperative instructions for the child should be repeated to the caregiver.

Older Patients

This escort is similar to that for the ambulatory adult. The main difference is to consider the patient's physical needs, including their ability to hear you. Speak to the older patients directly so they can see you speak. Speak when you are in close proximity and preferably in a quieter area. With senior patients, assistance may be needed. The dental assistant should be careful not to offend these patients by challenging their ability to take care of themselves. Usually, the older patient will ask for help if it is needed. Review the medical history for any changes in health and medication. Treatment can be broken into shorter segments to accommodate restroom and stretching breaks. The senior patient may not be comfortable in the reclined position for long periods, so the dental assistant should position the patient upright whenever possible.

Pregnant Patients

When a pregnant woman is sitting in a reclined position, it may be difficult for her to breathe. The dental assistant can allow her to sit upright until the dentist is ready to begin the procedure. During the first trimester of pregnancy, women may find dental treatment uncomfortable because of nausea. The safest and most comfortable time to schedule dental appointments is during the second trimester of pregnancy. Restroom breaks may become more necessary for women in the third trimester of pregnancy.

Patients with Sensory Disabilities

When a patient has hearing difficulties, the dental assistant must be in a position where the patient can observe lip movement and facial expression. Remove the mask and speak normally but slowly; make eye contact and ask questions to be sure the patient understands. To make the patient feel comfortable and show that the assistant really cares about them, the assistant may consider learning a few words in sign language.

The patient who is blind may be escorted by someone, but they are often very independent. Good communication requires information about their abilities and concerns. The dental assistant should talk to the blind patient throughout the procedure and explain what is happening or what is about to be done. (Refer to Chapter 13 for more details.)

Patients with Wheelchairs or Walkers

If a patient comes into the office in a wheelchair or using a walker, they may need some assistance getting into the dental chair. The pathway to the treatment room should be cleared as much as possible. If the patient is using a walker, give assistance when needed. Usually, the patient has a routine and will tell you if help is needed. The wheelchair patient often needs someone to lift or move them from the wheelchair to the dental chair. (Refer to Chapter 13 for more details.)

Patients with special needs know their abilities. Communicate with them to understand their needs and treat them the same as all other patients.

Non-English-Speaking Patients

Some dental practices have patients who neither speak English nor understand the procedures. The dental staff needs to assist these patients in any way they can. Sometimes an interpreter, a relative, a friend, or someone from a church or social agency comes with the patient. This is very helpful, especially during the first several visits. The staff may try to learn key words in the patient's language to assist in communication as well as to show that the office cares and is making an effort to understand the patient. The dental staff may research and find information about the patient's country or culture to identify something in common with the patient. Pictures help when trying to make the patient understand what is involved in a procedure and what to expect.

Finding means of communicating with patients from other cultures who speak languages other than English is important. Placing yourself in that situation should help you imagine how you would feel if you have a dental problem when traveling or living abroad. Think of ways to work with these patients. There are many apps that can turn your phone into an interpreter. Some apps can translate 103 different languages. You can translate both ways. You can enter what you wish to say in English and have it translated into the patient's language or vice versa. These apps are worth a try as many more non-English-speaking patients are being seen in the dental office.

Chapter Summary

It is important for the dental assistant to understand the various dental office designs and how each area relates to patient care. Each dentist lays out their office to meet the needs of the practice. The assistant learns the function of each area in the dental office and the equipment that is used in this area. Responsibilities and the job description of the dental assistant are discussed in relation to preparing for the patient and seating and then dismissing the patient. The dental team goes to great lengths to provide an infection free environment and to ensure patient and employee safety.

Examining the needs of the various needs of patients gives the dental assistant the information to plan and prepare for these patients to eliminate problems and make their experience a positive one.

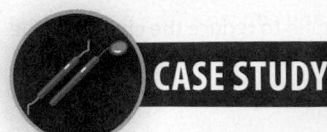

CASE STUDY

Maxine Rodrigez, age 77, had several restorations completed during her hour-long appointment. She is in good health but was in the supine position for most of her appointment.

Case Study Review

1. What can the dental assistant expect will happen once the procedure is complete and the patient is again seated upright?

2. How can the assistant aid Maxine before escorting her to the reception area?

3. Is there anything the dental assistant can do to prevent patients from experiencing discomfort resulting from positioning during treatment?

Review Questions

Multiple Choice

1. A patient would be escorted to what room for the dentist to perform operative procedures?
   a. dental office laboratory
   b. consultation room
   c. treatment room
   d. business area

2. The ultrasonic equipment is located in which of the following areas or rooms?
   a. treatment room
   b. sterilizing area
   c. x-ray processing area
   d. storage area

3. Where can the dental personnel locate safety rules in operating clinical equipment?
   a. equipment manufacturer directions
   b. Safety Data Sheets
   c. office written policies
   d. all of these are correct.

4. Where can an assistant find the best explanation of how to handle materials and handle a chemical emergency?
   a. Safety Data Sheet
   b. office safety manual
   c. asking another assistant
   d. material's directions

5. If the saliva ejectors and oral evacuators at each dental unit fail to suction, what piece of equipment needs to be turned on?
   a. rheostat
   b. dental unit
   c. air compressor
   d. central vacuum system

6. What chair position has the patient's nose and knees on the same plane?
   a. upright
   b. supine
   c. subsupine
   d. ergonomic

7. The assistant should aspirate a cup of water into the saliva ejector and oral evacuator hoses:
   a. before each patient.
   b. after each patient.
   c. at the end of the day.
   d. once a week.

8. How long should handpiece hoses and air/water syringes be flushed after each patient?
   a. 5 seconds
   b. 10 seconds
   c. 30 seconds
   d. 60 seconds

9. All of these procedures are performed during closing routines EXCEPT:
   a. change from uniform to street clothes.
   b. start the sterilizer.
   c. in-depth cleaning of dental chair and dental unit.
   d. turn off all master switches.

10. All of these procedures are performed during opening routines EXCEPT:
    a. review daily patient schedule.
    b. prepare treatment rooms for first patients.
    c. prepare new ultrasonic solution.
    d. flush all hoses.

11. By what means are items in the treatment area contaminated?
    a. direct spatter
    b. indirect spatter
    c. assistant's gloved hands
    d. All of these are capable of contaminating the area.

12. When must the area or equipment be disinfected after treatment?
    a. barrier torn
    b. barrier improperly removed
    c. barrier not used
    d. All of these are correct.

13. The professional greeting in addressing a patient in the reception area is:
   a. title and last name.
   b. last name and title.
   c. last name only.
   d. first name only.

14. After obtaining the patient's attention, the assistant should tell them:
   a. The doctor is ready for you.
   b. Do you want to come in?
   c. The doctor will see you now.
   d. It is time for your appointment.

15. After the patient is seated, what should be positioned first to prevent the patient from falling?
   a. headrest
   b. backrest
   c. armrest
   d. footrest

16. Where should the sterile bags or trays of instruments be opened?
   a. in the sterilization room
   b. in the treatment room before the patient is seated
   c. in the treatment room after the patient is seated
   d. there is no preference

17. What can the dental assistant do to reduce the chance of the patient experiencing postural hypotension symptoms after being in the supine position?
   a. Slowly return patient to upright position.
   b. Have patient remain in upright position for a few minutes.
   c. Ask patient how they are feeling and examine their pupils.
   d. All of these steps should be followed.

18. Which dental chair position may be uncomfortable for a senior patient for long periods of time?
   a. upright
   b. supine
   c. 45 degree angle
   d. 30 degree angle

19. Which dental chair position may make it difficult for a pregnant patient to breathe?
   a. upright
   b. supine
   c. 45 degree angle
   d. 30 degree angle

20. When treating a _____ patient, the mask may need to be removed occasionally.
   a. senior
   b. child
   c. hearing-impaired
   d. blind

Critical Thinking

1. A three-year-old child is scheduled for a new patient examination. The receptionist explains to the parent that the office protocol is that caregivers do not accompany their child into the treatment area. As the dental assistant enters the reception area to escort the child for treatment, the child screams and says they will not go. The parent insists that they have to be with the child during treatment. What should the assistant do if the parent becomes angry?

2. During opening routines, neither the air/water syringe nor any of the handpieces will work. What should the assistant do next?

3. An emergency appointment has run over the scheduled time. The next patient is in the reception area. What should the assistant do? What steps in preparing the operatory for the next patient can be omitted to save time?

Key Terms

Term and Pronunciation	Meaning of Root and Word Parts	Definition
cephalometric x-ray machine (sef-*uh*-**loh**-me-trik) (**eks**-rey) (*muh*-**sheen**)	**cephalo-** = head **meter** = measure **-ic** = relating to **x-ray** = electromagnetic radiation used in taking radiographs **machine** = apparatus that performs some kind of work	a machine that takes an x-ray of the head capturing an image of the side of the face; used for diagnostic and treatment planning
clinical (**klin**-i-k*uh*l)	**clinic** = place where outpatients are treated **-al** = pertaining to	conducted in or as if in a clinic; based on actual observation of signs
condensation (kon-den-**sey**-sh*uh*n)	**con-** = with **dense** = closely compacted together **-ate** = possessing	water collecting as droplets when contacted with humid air
consultation (kon-s*uh*l-**tey**-sh*uh*n)	**consult** = to give professional advice **-tion** = action, process	a conference between doctor and patient to discuss condition and treatment

(Continues)

Term and Pronunciation	Meaning of Root and Word Parts	Definition
digital radiography (**dij**-i-tl) (rey-dee-**og**-ruh-fee)	**digit** = symbols of number system, as 0 or 1 in binary **-al** = pertaining to	uses a digital image capture device instead of x-ray film; transfers data to computer system
ergonomic (ur-guh-**nom**-iks)	**ergo** = therefore, in consequence of **nomic** = science of	modification of work necessary to prevent repetitive strain injuries
expendable (ik-**spen**-duh-buh l)	**expend** = to put out or away **-able** = fit for	designed for a single use; not reusable
handpiece (**hand**-pees)	**hand** = part of body at the end of the forearm **piece** = portion of something	dental drill; used to perform a variety of dental procedures
intrusive (in-**troo**-siv)	**intrude** = to thrust oneself without permission or welcome **-ive** = expressing tendency	when a situation becomes worrisome, troublesome, irritating, disturbing
laboratory (**lab**-ruh-tawr-ee)	**labor** = work **-tory** = a place equipped to work	a workplace to make dental appliances
operative (**op**-er-uh-tiv)	**operate** = to perform surgical procedure **-ive** = expressing tendency	relating to treatment requiring dental procedures
operatory (**op**-er-uh-tawr-ee)	**operate** = to perform surgical procedure **-tory** = a place equipped to work	a room in which a dentist (or assistant) performs tasks for the patient
panoramic x-ray machine (pan-uh-**ram**-ik) (**eks**-rey) (muh-**sheen**)	**pan-** = unobstructed wide view **-orama** = display or spectacle **-ic** = relating to **x-ray** = electromagnetic radiation used in taking radiographs **machine** = apparatus that performs some kind of work	x-ray head evolves around the patient's head capturing and image of the upper and lower jaw on one radiograph
postural hypotension (**pos**-cher-uhl) (hahy-puh-**ten**-shuhn)	**posture** = assume a bodily position **-al** = pertaining to **hypo-** under **tense** = taut or strain **-ion** = denoting action or condition	a sudden drop in blood pressure due to a change in body position; person moves from lying down to sitting/lying down position
rheostat (**ree**-uh-stat)	**rheos** = a flowing, stream **stat** = regulating device	a device that uses resistance to regulate electrical current to run equipment
sensor (**sen**-sawr)	**sense** = to detect, perception **-or** = denoting property	a device that responds to a physical stimulus and transmits a resulting impulse
sterilize (**ster**-uh-lahyz)	**steril** = render free of microorganisms **-ize** = function of	procedure to make free from bacteria
subsupine (sub-soo-**pahyn**)	**sub-** = from below **supine** = turned or thrown backward	lying with head lower than body; used mostly in emergencies
supine (soo-**pahyn**)	**supine** = turned or thrown backwards	lying face upward
Trendelenburg position (trend-**el**-uhn-burg) (puh-**zish**-uhn)	**Trendelenburg** = Friedrich Trendelenburg, German surgeon; used to increase blood flow to the heart **position** = reference to place; location; situation	a supine position with head inclined at a 45 degree angle; pelvis is higher than head
turbine (**tur**-bahyn)	**turbid** = something that spins **-ine** = of the nature of	a part within a handpiece for producing continuous power when rotors revolve by a fast-moving flow of air
unit (**yoo**-nit)	**unit** = single thing regarded as a member of a group	structure or other equipment regarded as a structural or functional constituent of a whole
upright (**uhp**-rahyt)	**up** = elevated position right = something standing erect; right angle	position at right angles to the horizon
x-ray tubehead (**eks**-rey) (toob-hed)	**x-ray** = electromagnetic radiation used in taking radiographs **tube** = hollow, cylindrical part **head** = resembling a head in function	part of x-ray machine housing the x-ray tube that has the specific function of producing radiation

Dental Instruments and Tray Systems

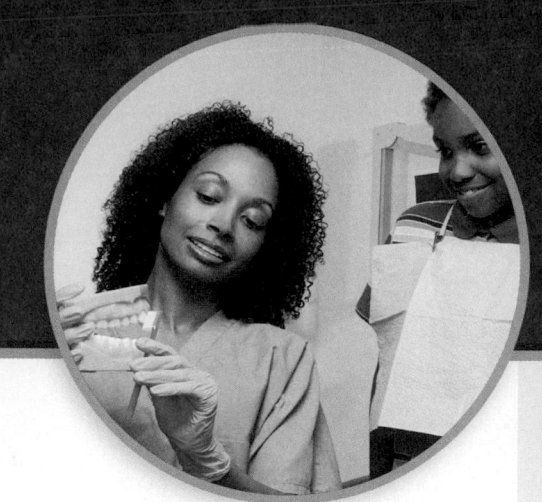

Specific Instructional Objectives

At the completion of this chapter, you will be able to meet these objectives:

1. Use terms presented in this chapter.
2. Recall the names, functions, and parts of hand instruments.
3. Describe expendable materials and their uses.
4. Describe types of handpiece power sources.
5. Identify handpiece types, parts, and their use.
6. Compare and contrast the emerging handpieces.
7. Identify the classification of cavities.
8. Name parts of a rotary instrument.
9. Select a rotary instrument appropriate for each type of handpiece.
10. Identify cutting burs by name and number series.
11. Compare and contrast cutting, surgical, vulcanite, and finishing burs.
12. Discuss types of abrasive rotary instruments and mandrels.
13. Compare and contrast care of burs, abrasive rotary instruments, and polishing instruments.
14. Defend need for standardized procedures and tray setups.
15. Describe preparation of tray setups.

Introduction

Dental instruments are continually developing as technology changes and dental materials require instruments of specific designs or materials. Most instruments are made of stainless steel, and a few consist of a high-tech plastic or resin or anodized aluminum. Dentists select the instruments that they feel the most confident and comfortable using. Each procedure requires special instruments to accomplish the task. For example, when examining the pits and grooves of the teeth, the dentist uses an explorer. The ends of all explorers are pointed and sharp but designed with different angles to reach all surfaces of the tooth.

The dental assistant is responsible for keeping the instruments sterilized and in working condition. The dental assistant orders new instruments as needed, prepares setups, and keeps the instruments in sequence while assisting during the procedure.

Instruments are generally categorized into handpieces, rotary instruments, and hand instruments. In this chapter, the basic instruments used in general dental procedures, various tray systems, and how to prepare an instrument tray are discussed Instruments used in dental specialty procedures will be covered in the specialty chapter; for example, the root canal instruments are found in Chapter 37, "Endodontics." Those instruments used in professionally cleaning teeth are discussed in Chapter 24.

Hand Instruments

In order to prepare tray setups, the assistant must know what instruments are needed for the procedures and be able to identify the instruments. Hand instrument is the name given to the instruments included in the tray setups that are held in the operator's or assistant's hands to perform dental procedures. At first glance, the instruments may look similar to one another. Throughout the assisting chapters, you will discover features that will help you tell them apart. Each instrument's design is determined by how the dentist will use it in performing a specific procedure, for the particular area of the mouth, and to accommodate the personal preference of the dentist.

Parts of Hand Instruments

Hand instruments are rodlike instruments that typically are made of stainless steel, carbide steel, or plain steel. Stainless steel is preferred in making surgical instruments for its ability to resist corrosion that can occur as a result of sterilization procedures. However, it is a weaker form of steel and not a good choice for instruments requiring strength. Carbide steel is the strongest and can be sharpened to the keenest edge. It is preferred when strength is required; for example, in cutting hard tooth structures. Plain steel is weak and is the least expensive. It is preferred for disposable items that are to be used once and then thrown away. Both carbide and plain steel corrode when sterilized. Some instruments may be made of plastic and special rubber materials.

The hand instrument consists of three parts: the handle, working end, and shank (Figure 19-1).

● The handle is designed to be gripped in the operator's hand. It is usually hexagonal (six sided), which provides for a better grip, and may be smooth or serrated. Depending on how the instrument is to be used, the handles may be small or large. The larger, lighter handle is preferred for ergonomic designs, which are larger with finger rests and grooves (Figure 19-2). Other handles are covered with a soft, rubberlike material that makes the instruments easier to hold and grip. A few instruments are designed with a cone socket handle, which allows the working ends to be replaced.

● The working end is the functional part of the instrument. The design is based on the instrument's use. Some common working ends used in dentistry include tines (sharp points), beaks (tweezer-like tips), blades (cutting surfaces), and nibs (blunted ends to condense materials).

● The shank is the tapered portion of the instrument that connects the handle to the working end. The angle of the shank to the handle is designed for best access to hard-to-reach areas of the mouth. Some common shanks used in dentistry include straight angle (working end is in line with handle), curved, monangle (working end is set at an angle to the handle), binangle (two angles in the shank), and triple angled (three angles in the shank provide access to posterior areas in the mouth) (Figure 19-3). Usually, instruments that are used in the posterior areas of the oral cavity have more angles, while instruments with fewer angles are used in anterior areas.

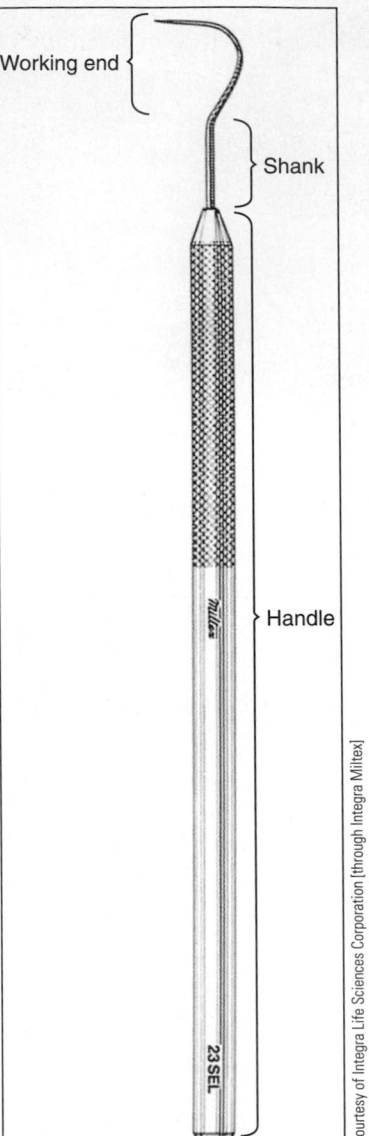

Courtesy of Integra Life Sciences Corporation [through Integra Miltex]

FIGURE 19-1
Parts of the single-ended dental instrument.

Identifying Hand Instruments

The dental team generally refers to hand instruments by instrument names, instrument numbers, or a combination of the two. The instrument's name may describe the use of the instrument's working end (explorer), or it may have the name of the designer. When the name of the designer is used, the person's proper name is used. For example, two common restorative instruments are the Wall and Hollenbeck carvers. The dental manufacturer assigns a number that **universally** represents the instrument. This number is also used as the stock number. The **stock** number is used when ordering the instrument. For example, a contouring plier is called the Howe 110 pliers, also referred to as the straight contouring pliers. The stock number is written on the end on the instrument handle (Figure 19-4).

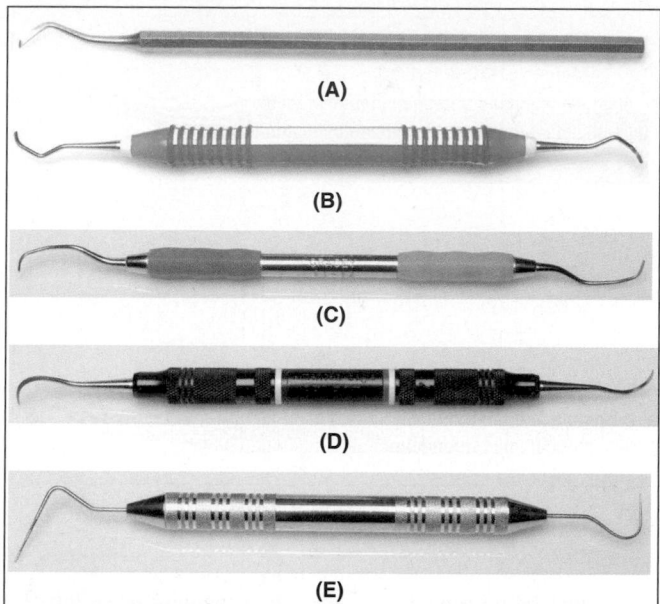

FIGURE 19-2
Variety of instrument handle styles. (A) Standard handle. (B-E) Ergonomic handles.

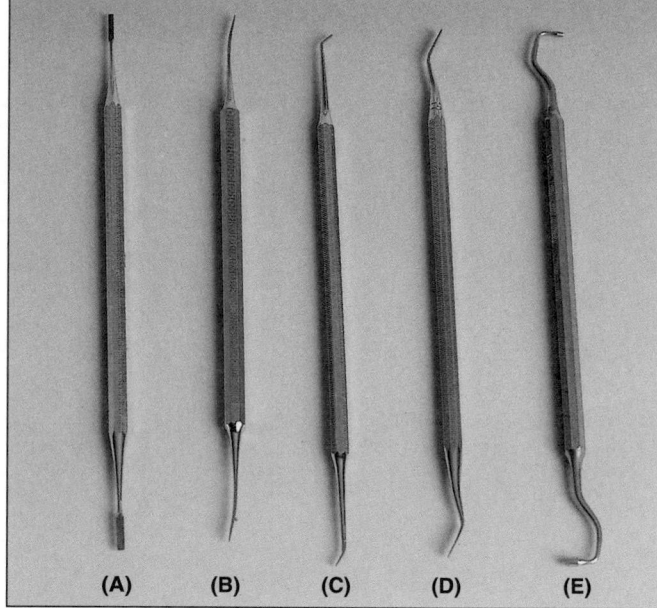

FIGURE 19-3
Instrument shanks. (A) Straight. (B) Curved. (C) Monangle. (D) Binangle. (E) Triple angle.

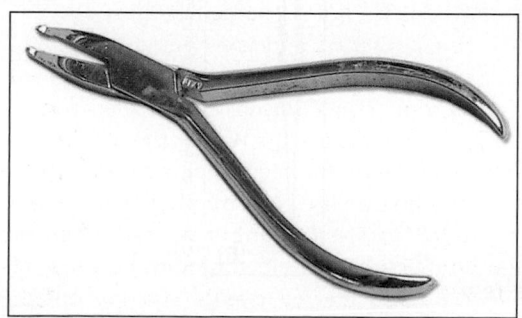

FIGURE 19-4
Howe pliers with stock number 110 written on the end on the instrument handle.

Instruments may also be identified by the instrument's formula to standardize the exact size and angulation of the instrument. G. V. Black's instrument formula describes the dimensions of the working end and angulations of the shank. A common restorative instrument has three numbers identifying the details of the instrument. The first number is the instrument's working end width; the second number is the working end's length; the third number is the angulation of the shank (Figure 19-5). There is also the four-number formula used to further describe the angle of the cutting side to the blade (Figure 19-6). Some instruments, such as chisels, hatchets, and hoes, have a series of three numbers, and some, such as angle formers and gingival margin trimmers, have four numbers. Formulas minimize discrepancies in the production of instruments from one manufacturer to another and simplify ordering instruments.

Instruments supplied with one working end are referred to as single-ended (SE). Double-ended (DE) instruments have working ends at each end of the handle. The DE instruments are designed with working ends at opposite angles to provide better access to different areas in the mouth. In some DE instruments each working end has the same angle, but they

Black's Three-Number Formula

1. The first number is the width of the blade in tenths of a millimeter. In the formula 20 9 14, the first number (20) indicates that the blade is 2.0 mm wide.

2. The second number is the length of the blade in millimeters. In the formula 20 9 14, the second number (9) indicates that the blade is 9 mm long.

3. The third number gives the angle of the blade to the long axis of the handle, in degrees centigrade. In the formula 20 9 14, the third number (14) indicates that the instrument has a blade at an angle of 14/100 of a circle.

Black's Four-Number Formula

1. The first number is the same as that in the three-number formula, representing the width of the blade in tenths of a millimeter. In the formula 15 85 8 12, the first number (15) indicates that the blade is 1.5 mm long.

2. The second number, differing from that in the three-number formula, represents the degree of the angle of the cutting edge of the blade to the handle of the instrument. In the formula 15 85 8 12, the second number (85) indicates that the cutting edge forms an 85° C angle with the handle.

3. The third number is the same as the second number in the three-number formula. Using the formula 15 85 8 12, the third number (8) indicates that the blade is 8 mm long.

4. The fourth number is the same as the third number in the three-number formula. Using the formula 15 85 8 12, the fourth number (12) indicates that the blade forms a 12° C angle with the handle of the instrument.

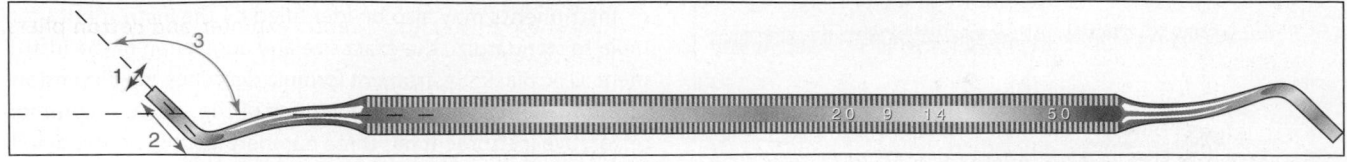

FIGURE 19-5
Hatchet with Black's three-number formula.

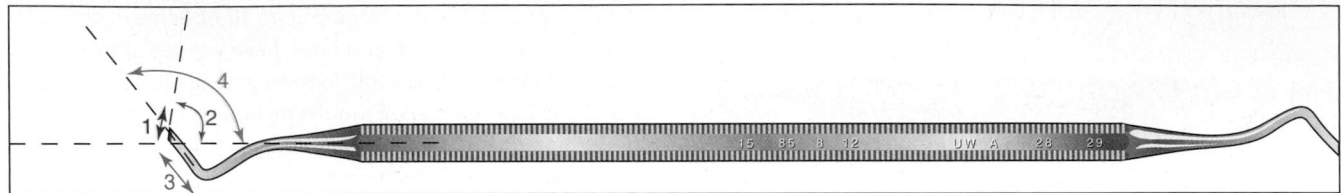

FIGURE 19-6
Angle former with Black's four-number formula.

are curved in opposite directions so that they can be used on either side of the arch or **cavity preparation** (e.g., a gingival margin trimmer) (Figure 19-7). The two ends may have similar function with one end larger than the other (e.g., an amalgam condenser) (Figure 19-8). The DE design is also time efficient for sequential procedures requiring one type of working end followed immediately by a different working end. For example, the flat end of the plastic filling instrument (also call Woodson) is used to place the material, and the nib is used to condense the material into the cavity preparation (Figure 19-9).

Some working ends are designed to work specifically on the right or left side. The instrument may have a capital R written next to the instrument number. R represents working end designed for the maxillary right and the mandibular left (these opposite sides of the mouth require the same angle). The opposite side

would be L (although not imprinted) for use on maxillary left and mandibular right. Some instruments are universal, have no markings, and can be used on right or left on the same arch.

Categories of Hand Instruments

There are four categories of instruments used in operative procedures: examination, hand cutting, restorative, and accessory.

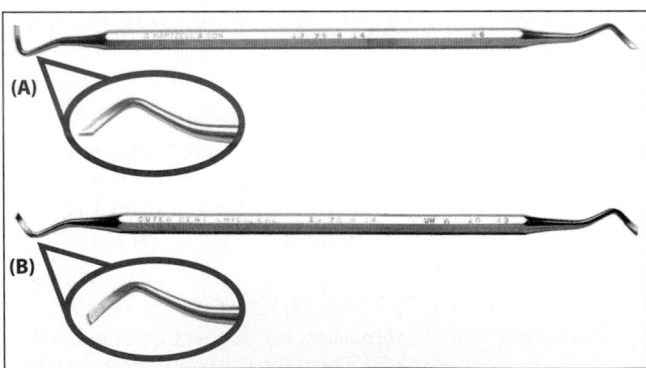

FIGURE 19-7
Gingival margin trimmer. (A) Distal gingival margin trimmer. (B) Mesial gingival margin trimmer.

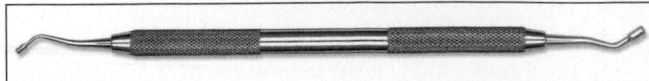

FIGURE 19-8
Amalgam condenser.

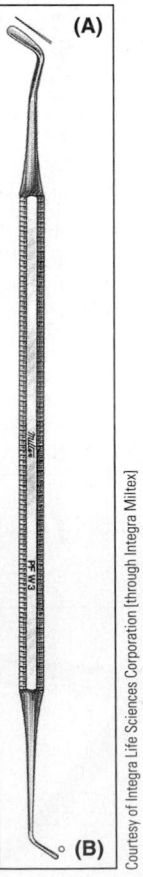

FIGURE 19-9
Plastic filling instrument. Working end (A) is flat to insert the dental material and (B) has nib for condensing the material.

- *Examination instruments*—used by the operator to examine the oral cavity and restorations.
- *Hand cutting instruments*—held in operator's hand to cut tooth structure and dental materials. Used to remove decay from carious lesion and to smooth the remaining tooth structure for placement of a restoration; also referred to as cavity preparation instruments.
- *Restorative instruments*—hand held by operator to place and finish restorative materials.
- *Accessory instruments*—variety of instruments used to assist in completing dental procedures. Instruments are not necessarily included on the tray but are kept in cabinets and tubs, for example, expendables, scissors, and forceps.

Examination Instruments

No matter what procedure is to be completed, the patient's tray will always have three basic hand instruments for use by the operator, known as the basic tray setup. These instruments include the mouth mirror, dental explorer, and cotton pliers. Some offices include the articulating forceps and periodontal probe in the basic setup and expendable materials. These instruments are included in the examination category of operative dentistry.

Mouth Mirror Mouth mirrors are small magnifying mirrors available in different sizes that are used for indirect vision of the oral cavity, retraction of soft tissue (cheek and tongue) for better vision, tissue protection (to block the tongue in case the handpiece slips), and reflection of light when viewing the mouth (Figure 19-10). It may be made of metal or plastic, have a handle with a cone socket for easy replacement of the mirror head, or come in one piece (Figure 19-11). The mouth mirror may be sterilized or disposable. The types of mirror heads are the plane surface (gives a ghost image), front surface (eliminates ghost images), and concave (magnifies the image) surface. The mirror head sizes are identified by number; the most commonly used are numbers 4 and 5.

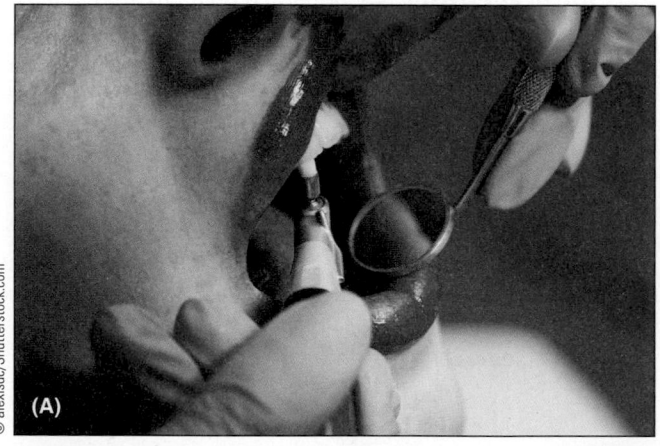
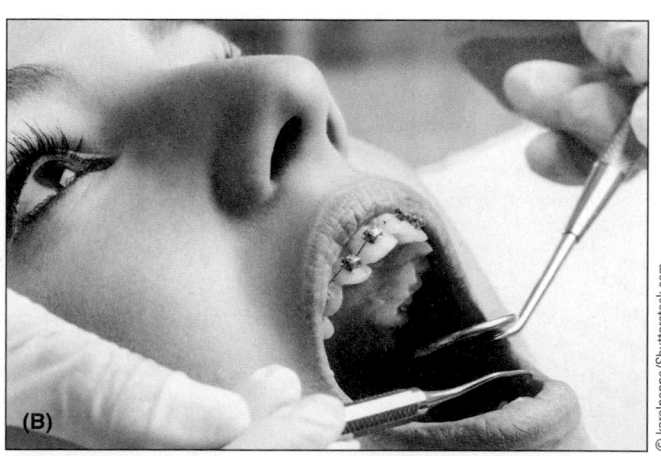
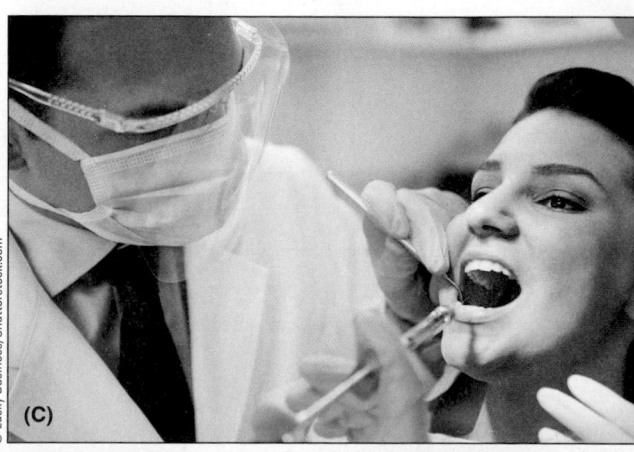
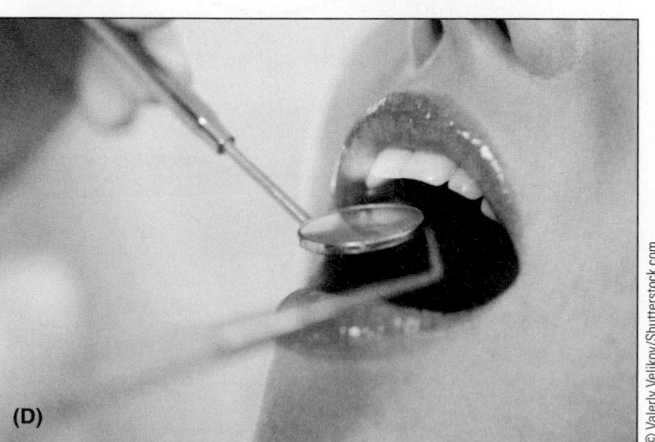

FIGURE 19-10
Use of the mouth mirror. (A) Using the mouth mirror to indirect vision gives the operator a view of areas of the oral cavity not seen with direct vision. (B) Reflecting the light from the overhead dental light to illuminated areas in the oral cavity. (C) Retracting with the mouth mirror to hold the tongue and/or cheeks away from the working area during a procedure. (D) Transillumination, shown here with the mirror reflecting the light through a tooth surface as well as using reflection, retraction, and indirect vision.

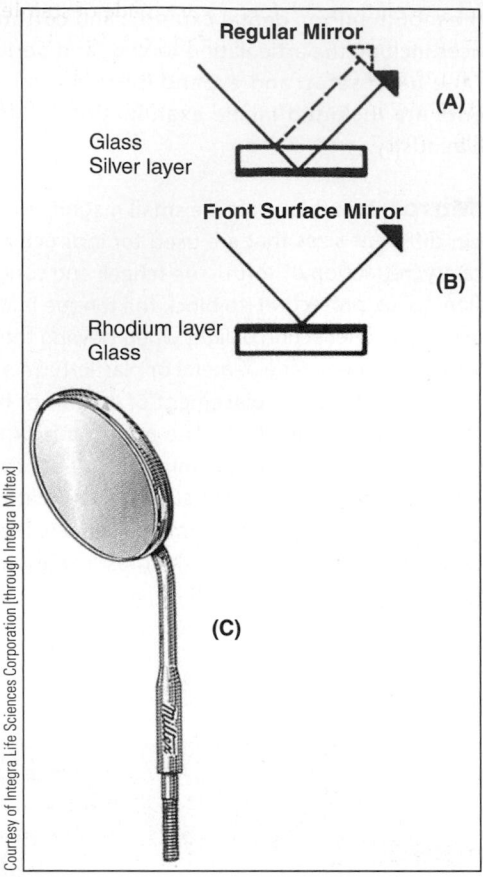

Courtesy of Integra Life Sciences Corporation [through Integra Miltex]

Regular Mirror

(A)

Glass
Silver layer

Front Surface Mirror

(B)

Rhodium layer
Glass

(C)

FIGURE 19-11
(A) Plane (regular) surface mirror. (B) Front surface mirror. (C) Cone socket mirror.

Dental Explorer Explorers are fine, sharp **tines** made of flexible steel used to examine indentations of the teeth (pits and fissures), check for presence and depth of carious lesions, and check cavity preparations and dental restorations. They are available as either single-ended or double-ended instruments. Double-ended explorers may have a sickle probe (Shepherd's hook) on one end and a pigtail, right angle, or Orban (also called #17) on the other end (Figure 19-12). Some may have a periodontal probe on one end of the instrument that has markings at millimeter intervals; these are called expros (Figure 19-13). This is very functional and reduces the number of instruments on the tray. The mirror and explorer are used together at the beginning of most procedures to inspect the area being examined or treated.

Cotton Pliers Cotton pliers, also called cotton forceps, are used to transfer items to and from the oral cavity or to retrieve materials from drawers and containers to avoid contamination. The pliers resemble tweezers and may be nonlocking or locking. The tips (beaks) of the cotton pliers can be plain or **serrated** (Figure 19-14).

Periodontal Probes Periodontal probes are used to measure the depth of the gingival sulcus utilizing the millimeter measurement. They may be single- or double-ended instruments. The working end of the probe is a blade that is rounded or blunted and is marked in millimeters (mm). There are variations in the indication of calibrations, including color coding (Figure 19-15).

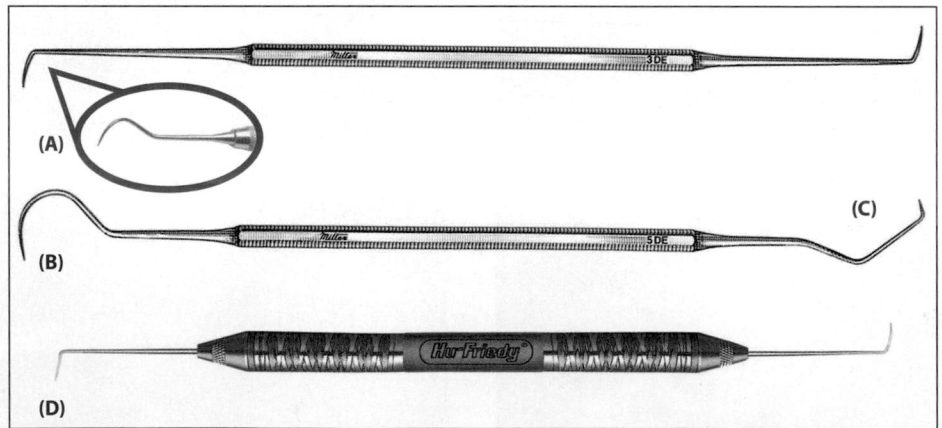

FIGURE 19-12
Working ends of an explorer. (A) Pigtail. (B) Shephard's hook. (C) Orban. (D) Right angle.

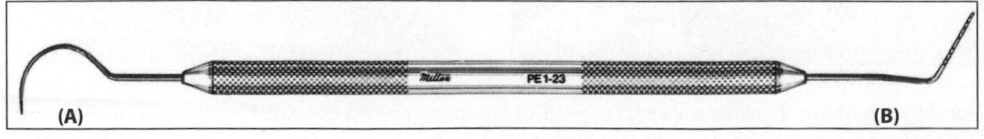

FIGURE 19-13
Expro. (A) Shephard's hook explorer end. (B) Periodontal probe end.

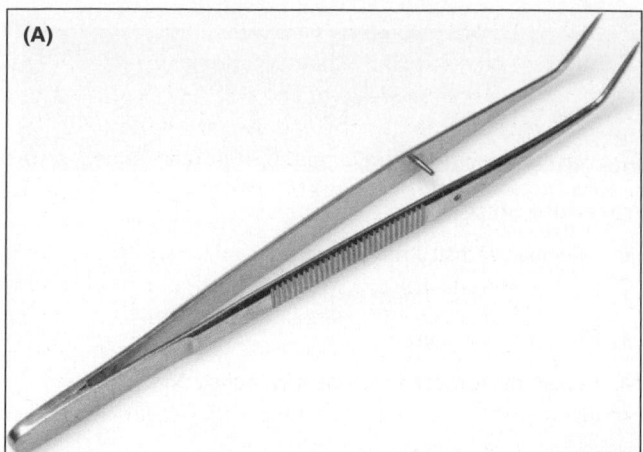

(A)

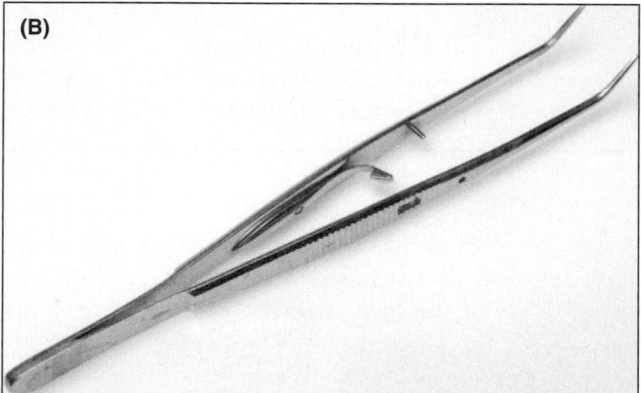

(B)

FIGURE 19-14
Cotton pliers. (A) Nonlocking and (B) locking cotton pliers.

the natural articulation. The forceps are made of stainless steel or disposable plastic and are opened and closed by placing pressure on the handle (Figure 19-16). Sometimes cotton pliers, especially locking cotton pliers, are used in place of articulating forceps.

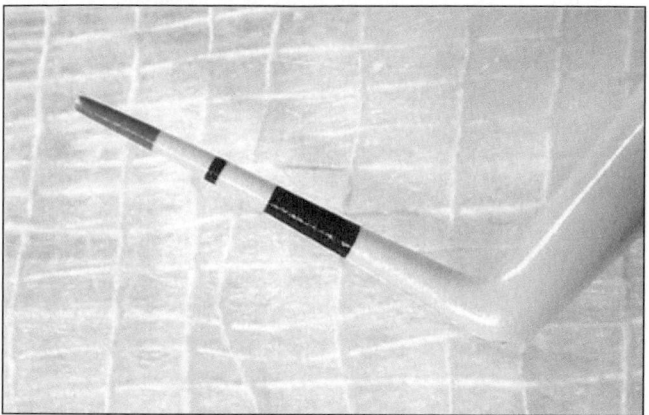

Courtesy of Hu-Friedy Mfg., Co., Inc.

FIGURE 19-15
Periodontal probe with color-coded markings of millimeters.

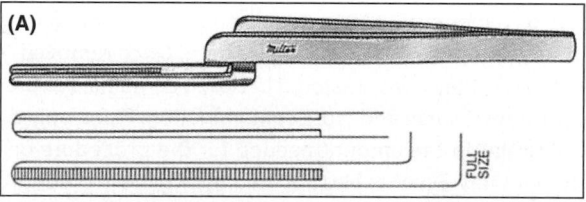

(A)

FULL SIZE

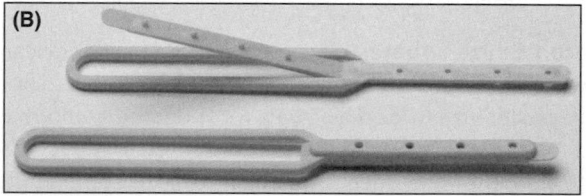

(B)

FIGURE 19-16
(A) Articulating forceps. (B) Disposable articulating forceps.

Articulating Forceps Articulating forceps are used to hold articulating paper when checking the patient's **articulation** and occlusion. Articulating paper (a piece of carbon paper) that leaves a blue marking on the teeth and is used to see how the teeth meet (articulate) when the patient bites to make certain the occlusion is healthy. It can also be used to make certain that any restoration that is placed duplicates

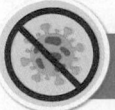

Infection Control

All hand instruments should be sanitized and sterilized in the sterilization area prior to reuse or storage. All dental instruments must be properly cared for, maintained, and sterilized to ensure that the instruments will last a long time, function as designed, and be used safely. Instruments should be cleaned as soon as possible after use. When this cannot be done, the instruments should be placed in a presoak solution to prevent blood and debris from drying on the instruments.

To properly clean the instruments, place them in an ultrasonic cleaner or other instrument washer for the designated amount of time. The instruments should be covered with the ultrasonic solution and spread out as much as possible. Instrument **cassettes** enhance handling of the instrument by reducing the possibility of damage to the instrument and providing more organization and efficiency. The cassettes also reduce the risk of injury to the dental assistant during the cleaning and sterilization of the instruments.

Procedure 19-1
Identify Examination Instruments

This procedure is performed by the dental assistant to identify the examination instruments and explain their use.

Equipment and Supplies
- mouth mirror
- dental explorer
- expro
- cotton pliers
- periodontal probes
- articulating forceps

Procedure Steps
1. Examine the instrument closely.
2. Identify the instrument by name.
3. Explain how it is used.
4. Explain the numbering system identified on the instrument.
5. List the procedure(s) where the instrument may be used.

Expendable Materials Along with the hand instruments, there are several expendable materials needed for performing dental procedures. Expendables are items that are used once and thrown away, referred to as one use items. They consist of cotton or paper products and are supplied in bulk in packages or in smaller amounts in sterile packaging. Once removed from the package, they must be stored in closed containers to protect against dental spray and cross contamination. Place only those expendables in the amount needed for the procedure on the instrument tray. Expendables not used during the procedure cannot be returned to the expendable container and must be properly disposed.

Cotton Gauze Squares Gauze squares are used for cleaning and disinfecting, for moisture absorption, for patients to bite on after procedures to stop bleeding, for sponging hemorrhages, and for applying materials. They are also used to retract tissues such as the tongue, cheeks, and lips; keep instruments clean; and receive debris during chairside procedures. Gauze material is shaped into 2 × 2 or 4 × 4 inch squares that are also referred to as sponges. They may be supplied filled or unfilled with cotton layers; filled is much thicker and more absorbent. Gauze squares are supplied as sterile and nonsterile in bulk packages and individual presterilized packets of two cotton-filled gauze squares (Figure 19-17).

Cotton Pellets Cotton pellets are used to dry the tooth cavity and small areas in the oral cavity and to place medications. Pellets are made of small, round balls of cotton. They are sized from 1 to 4 with 1 being the smallest (11/32 inches in diameter). Pellets are often kept in a metal dispenser with a tilt top lid for easy dispensing, which is referred to as a tilt top dispenser (Figure 19-18).

Cotton Rolls Cotton rolls are used for isolation, to help control saliva (placed in mucobuccal fold and floor of mouth to absorb moisture), and to retract tissues. They are also used to apply

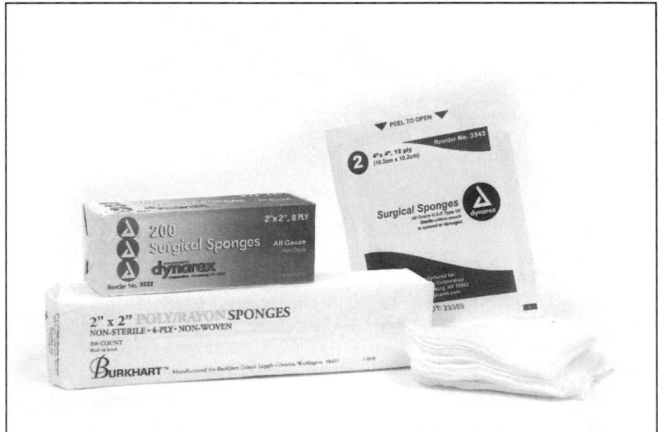

FIGURE 19-17
Gauze squares are available in various sizes and packaging.

topical anesthetic and medications. They are made of rolled up cotton and supplied in 2 and 6 inch rolls. Cotton rolls are smooth or braided and sterile or nonsterile (Figure 19-19).

Cotton Tip Applicator Cotton tip applicators are used to apply topical anesthetic and medications to mucous membranes. They are one-ended wood sticks with tightly wrapped cotton tips that resemble a Q-tip. Applicators may be supplied in 3 inch and 6 inch lengths in bulk packaging or individually in sterile packaging (Figure 19-20).

Articulating Paper Articulating paper is used to test the articulation of teeth and restorations. It is made of blue, red, green, and black carbon paper. The patient bites on the paper and it leaves marks where the teeth meet (Figure 19-21).

Dental Floss
Floss is used to remove debris or clean between the proximal surfaces of adjacent teeth. It can also be used to check

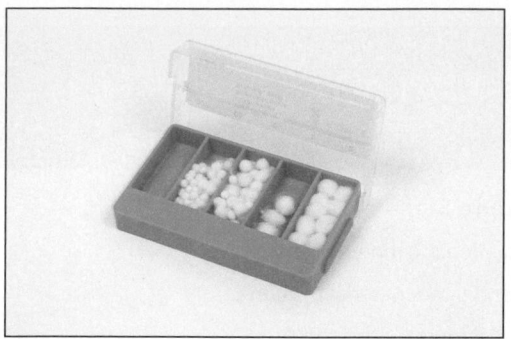

FIGURE 19-18
Cotton pellets come in different sizes and containers designed for easy dispensing.

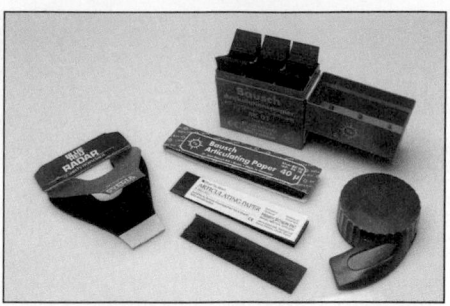

FIGURE 19-21
Articulating paper is available on rolls, as individual strips, and in horseshoe shapes. It can be stored in easy-access dispensers.

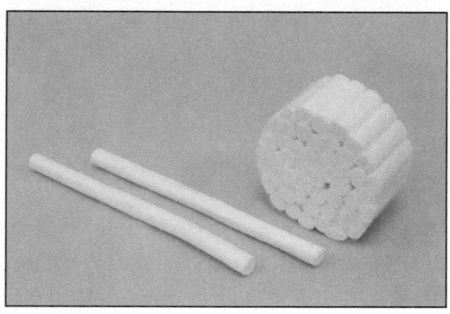

FIGURE 19-19
Cotton rolls supplied as 6 inch and 2 inch rolls of superabsorbent cotton.

patient's mouth. Floss looks like a string and is supplied waxed and unwaxed and **bonded** and unbonded. Floss may be supplied within its own dispenser or as replacement spools to be placed into floss dispensers.

Hand Cutting Instruments

Hand cutting instruments are used to assist in the design of the cavity preparation. Most cutting during the cavity preparation is performed with burs in low and high-speed handpieces. Hand cutting instruments may also be needed for refining details of the cavity preparation after using cutting burs or before using the burs to remove soft decay. There are two primary groups of hand cutting instruments used during the cavity preparation procedure: hatchets and chisels. Hand cutting instruments are often designed double ended with one end used on the mesial surface and the other end the distal.

the tightness or lack of contacts between teeth and restorations. Floss may be used as a **utility** expendable for many dental procedures and to secure dental dam clamps and bite blocks to prevent items from falling into the back of the

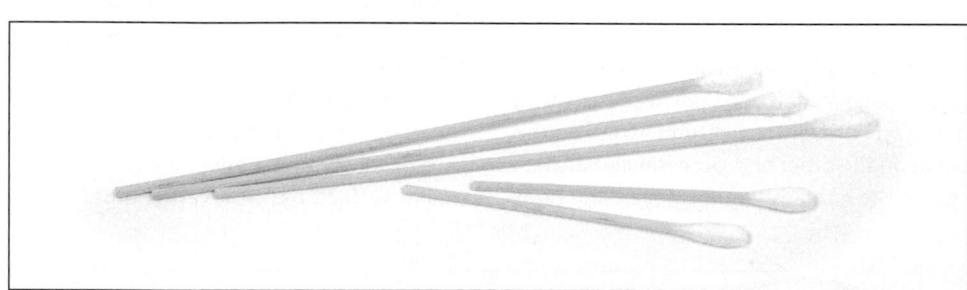

FIGURE 19-20
Cotton tip applicators supplied in 3 and 6 inch lengths.

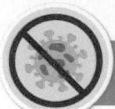 **Infection Control**

Most expendables come supplied in sealed packages, sterile and nonsterile. Once a package is opened, it is exposed to contaminants. It is important to place expendables directly into an aseptic container with a lid. Expendables should only be removed from containers with sterile forceps (sterile cotton pliers). Hands (bare hands and/or gloved hands) should not enter an aseptic expendable container.

Blood soaked or saturated in OPIM expendables must be disposed of in biohazard containers.

Procedure 19-2
Identify Expendable Materials

This procedure is performed by the dental assistant to identify the expendable materials and explain their use.

Equipment and Supplies
- cotton gauze squares
- cotton pellets
- cotton rolls
- cotton tip applicator
- articulating paper
- dental floss waxed
- dental floss unwaxed

Procedure Steps
1. Examine the material closely.
2. Identify the material by name.
3. Explain how each is used.
4. Explain the available sizes.
5. List the procedure(s) where the material may be used.

Hatchets Hatchets are designed with the cutting edge parallel to the plane of the instrument (cutting blade is in line with the handle of the instrument). The more common hatchets are the excavators, enamel hatchet, and gingival margin trimmer.

Excavators Excavators are used to remove soft carious dentin from the cavity preparation. The blades are curved and rounded with cutting edges to be able to scoop matter from the cavity. The spoon excavator, also called the discoid spoon, is round, and the blade excavator, also called the banana spoon, is a long blade with a rounded end (Figure 19-22).

Enamel Hatchet The hatchet, also called enamel hatchet, has a straight blade and is basically the same shape as a woodsman's axe (Figure 19-23). There is an angle in the shank of a hatchet, and the blade is flat. Hatchets are paired left and right, with a bevel on one side of the blade on one end of the instrument and on the reverse side of the blade on the other end. Sometimes, hatchets are marked with rings on the handles to indicate left and right

ends. They are used in a downward motion for removing hard carious tissue, **cleaving**, and **planing** (removal of unsupported, undermined enamel) of the remaining tooth structure. Hatchets are used to refine lines and angles within the cavity preparation to obtain retention for the restorative material.

Gingival Margin Trimmer The gingival margin trimmer resembles the hatchet. Instead of a straight blade there is a curved blade with an angled cutting edge (Figure 19-24). It is used to reach and bevel the mesial and distal boxes of the gingival margin walls of cavity preparations involving the mesial and distal surfaces. With the double ends of the instrument, one end curves toward the left and the other end curves toward the right.

Chisels
Chisels have the cutting edge at a 90° angle (perpendicular) to the plane of the instrument. They are designed to refine and smooth cavity preparation. A chisel is used to shape and plane (make surface flat or level) enamel and dentin walls of the

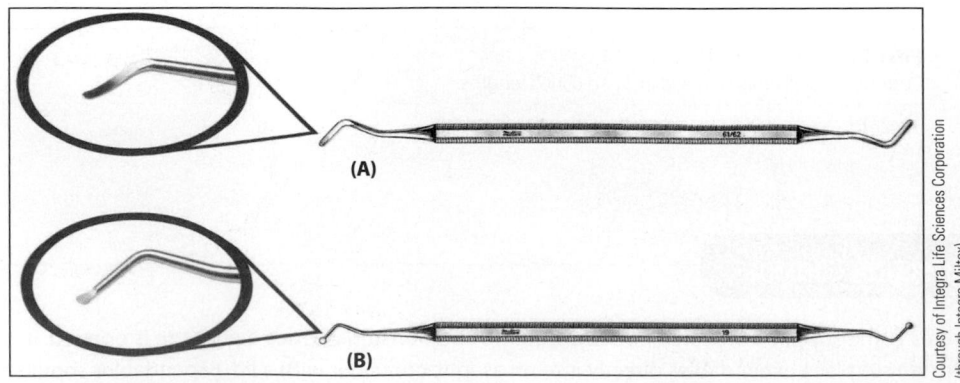

(A)

(B)

FIGURE 19-22
Excavators. (A) Blade excavator. Close-up view of working end of blade excavator. (B) Spoon excavator. Close-up view of the working end of the spoon excavator.

Courtesy of Integra Life Sciences Corporation (through Integra Miltex)

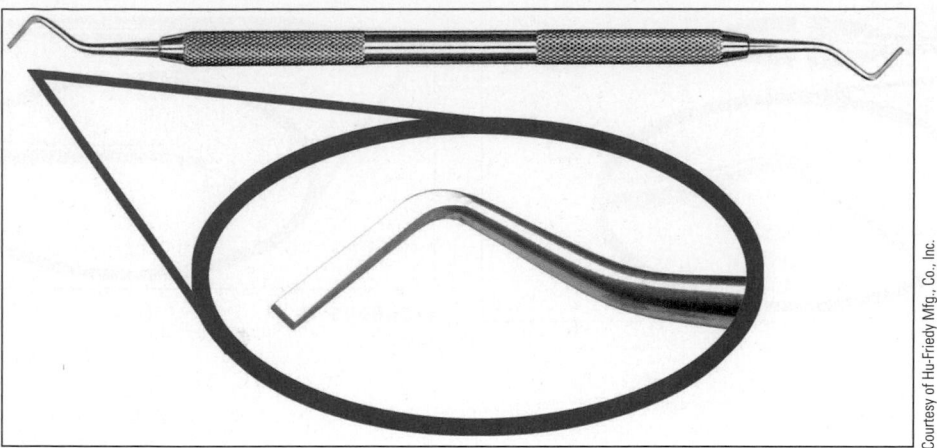

FIGURE 19-23
Paired left and right hatchet.

Courtesy of Hu-Friedy Mfg., Co., Inc.

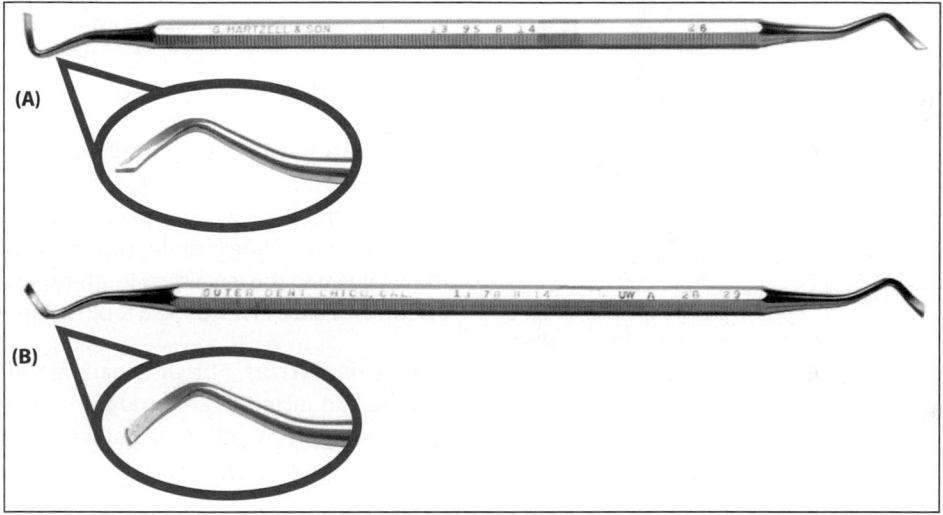

FIGURE 19-24
Gingival margin trimmers (GMT). (A) Distal GMT. Close-up of the working end of the distal GMT. (B) Mesial GMT.
Close-up of the working end of the mesial GMT.

cavity preparation. The more common are chisels, hoes, and angle formers.

Chisels come in several designs depending on the shape of the shank.

- *Straight chisel*—the blade is straight with the handle and shank (Figure 19-25).
- *Binangle chisel*—the shank has two bends (Figure 19-26).
- *Wedelstaedt chisel*—curved shank (Figure 19-27).

Hoes Hoes are designed to shape and smooth the floor of the preparation. They are shaped like a garden hoe, with the working end at a right angle to the shank (Figure 19-28).

Angle Formers Angle formers are similar to the chisel except the cutting edge of the blade is angled. They are used to help in

forming the proximal boxes, line, and point angles of the cavity preparation (Figure 19-29).

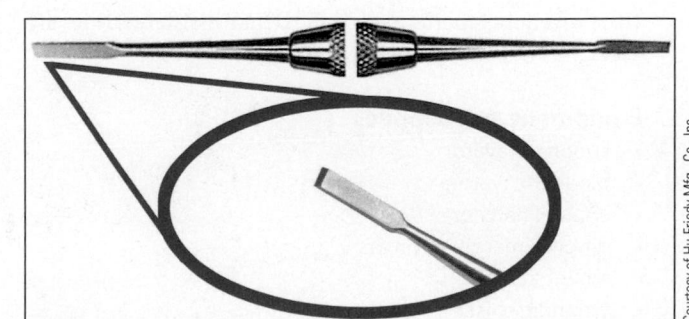

FIGURE 19-25
Straight chisel.

Courtesy of Hu-Friedy Mfg., Co., Inc.

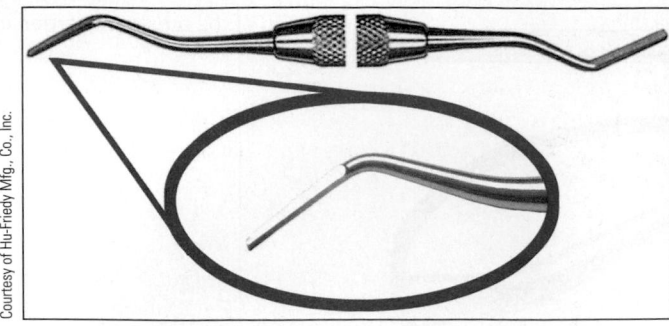

Courtesy of Hu-Friedy Mfg., Co., Inc.

FIGURE 19-26
Binangle chisel.

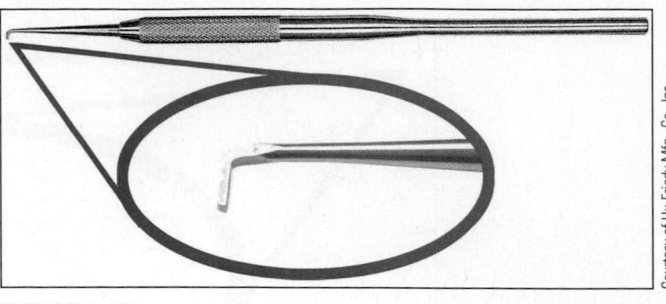

FIGURE 19-28
Hoes.

Courtesy of Hu-Friedy Mfg., Co., Inc.

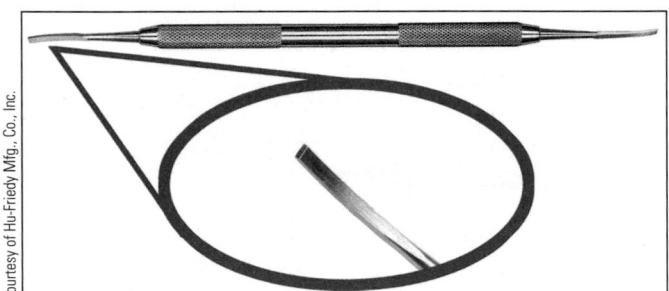

Courtesy of Hu-Friedy Mfg., Co., Inc.

FIGURE 19-27
Wedelstaedt chisel.

Restorative Instruments

The most common **direct restorations** used in operative dentistry are **dental amalgam** and **resin composites**. Dental amalgam, referred to as a silver filling, has been used in dentistry for more than 150 years and is still commonly used because it is a strong, long-lasting restoration and is less likely to break under the pressure and wear from chewing. It is often recommended in large cavity preparations and **bruxism**. Amalgam also requires less time in the dentist's chair, is less costly than other materials, and has better dental insurance coverage. (Read Chapter 31 to learn more about dental amalgam.)

Amalgam Restorative Instruments Restorative instruments are used to restore a tooth to its original contour and anatomy after the cavity preparation procedure. The amalgam restoration procedure includes placing, condensing, and carving the amalgam to the remaining tooth structure. Following are the instruments used in restoring a tooth using dental amalgam.

Amalgam Carrier The amalgam material is supplied in a capsule and mixed in an **amalgamator** to a soft putty consistency (Figure 19-29). An amalgam carrier, a thick-handled,

Procedure 19-3
Identify Hand Cutting Instruments

This procedure is performed by the dental assistant to identify the hand cutting instruments and explain their use.

Equipment and Supplies
- spoon excavator
- blade excavator
- enamel hatchet
- gingival margin trimmers
- straight chisel
- binangle chisel
- Wedelstaedt chisel
- hoe
- angle former

Procedure Steps
1. Examine the instrument closely.
2. Identify the instrument by name.
3. Explain how it is used.
4. Explain the numbering system identified on the instrument.
5. List the procedure(s) where the instrument may be used.

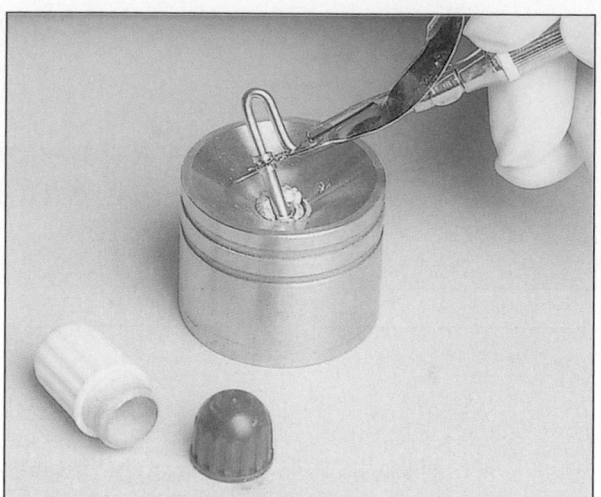

FIGURE 19-29
Placing the amalgam material into the amalgam carrier.

double-ended instrument with a small hollow barrel on one end and a large hollow barrel on the other end, is loaded and used to carry the amalgam to the cavity preparation. Most carriers are made of stainless steel, and some have Teflon or coated barrels to prevent clogging. Each end has a lever that dispenses the amalgam out of the hollow barrel and into the tooth preparation when depressed (Figure 19-30).

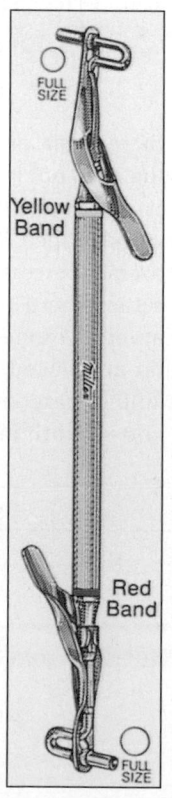

FIGURE 19-30
Double-ended amalgam carrier.

Amalgam Condensers Once each end of the amalgam carrier has been emptied into the preparation, an amalgam condenser (plugger) pushes and **condenses** the amalgam material into the tooth preparation. There are hand condensers and mechanical condensers. The condensers have nibs sized 0 to 4 to allow the operator to reach all areas of the preparation; the smaller the number, the smaller the nib. The amalgam carrier and condenser are interchanged until the tooth preparation is slightly overfilled with amalgam. The hand condensers are usually double-ended and are available in a wide variety of working ends. The locations and designs of cavity preparations have required that condensers be diverse in design. The working ends may be plain (smooth) or serrated. They may be round, ovoid, rectangular, diamond, or cone shaped (Figure 19-31). The shanks of condensers may be monangled, binangled, or triple angled.

Mechanical condensers, also called **pneumatic** condensers, are used to pack and condense amalgam through vibrations into the cavity preparation. These condensers are attached to the dental unit and operated with compressed air. Packing points come in a variety of shapes and sizes. The action of the condenser is like a woodpecker, with short, quick movements.

Burnishers The operator may choose to **burnish** the condensed amalgam. Burnishers are blunt, rounded instruments that come in a variety of shapes (Figure 19-32). Burnishing is controversial as some research is concerned that burnishing may possibly weaken the amalgam and increase tarnish and corrosion. Other research shows that it smooths the amalgam, increases the marginal seal, and brings excess mercury to the top of the amalgam overfill to be removed through carving.

Carvers The operator **carves** the amalgam to restore the anatomy and function of the tooth by gently scraping and shaping the amalgam with carvers. There is a large assortment of carvers to duplicate the numerous anatomical landmarks, sizes of teeth, and preparation locations.

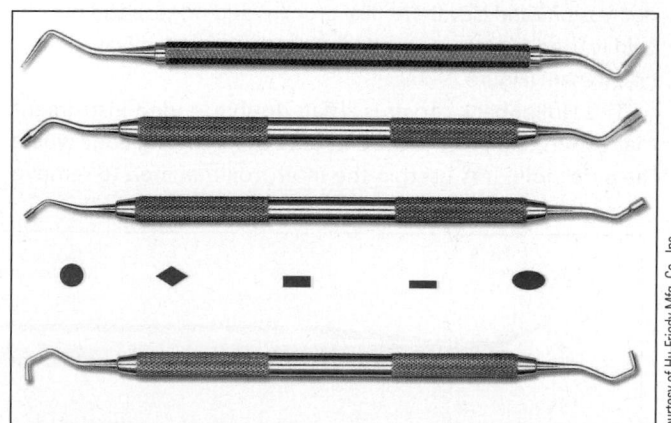

FIGURE 19-31
Various designs of amalgam condensers. Shown in red are the various shapes of the working ends. The last condenser is called a back-action condenser and gets in difficult-to-reach areas.

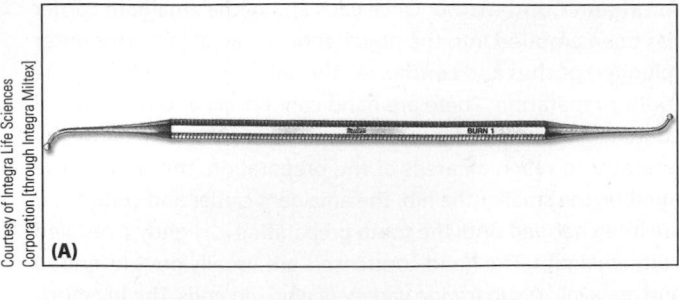

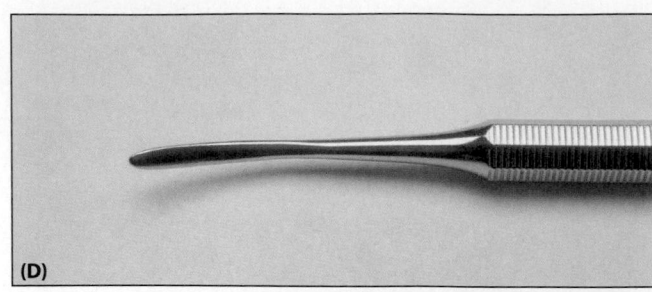

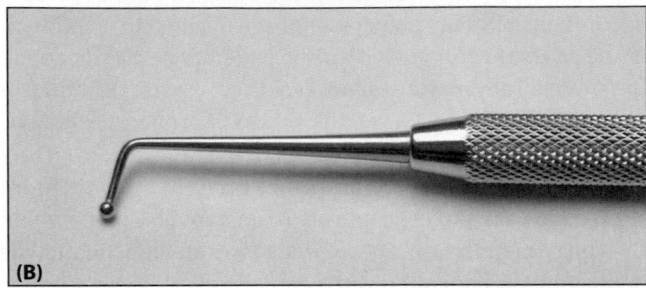

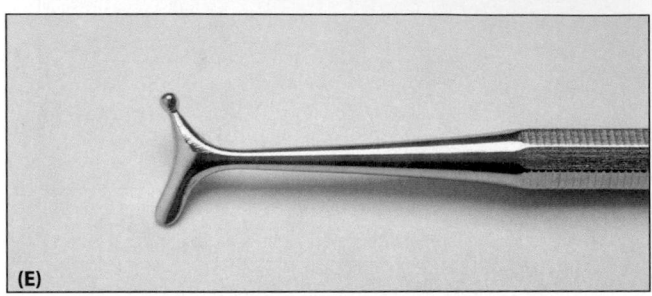

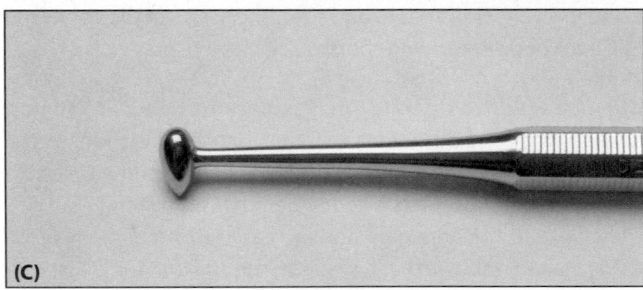

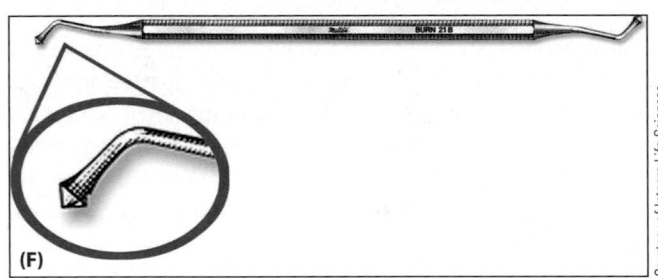

FIGURE 19-32
(A) Double-ended ball burnisher. Close-ups: (B) Ball burnisher. (C) Football (or egg) burnisher. (D) Beaver tail burnisher. (E) T-ball burnisher. (F) Acorn burnisher.

Wall's carver is a double-ended instrument referred to as the shovel and hoe end. This carver is used to establish the primary anatomy of a larger restoration (Figure 19-33).

The cleoid-discoid carver is a double-ended instrument containing a disc and spade shaped end. The cleoid establishes linear depressions and elevations (like grooves and ridges), and the discoid is used to restore rounded, dished out anatomical features (like fossae) (Figure 19-34).

The Hollenback carver is a flat, double-ended instrument that comes to a point at the end but has its cutting edge where the sides join. It is used in the interproximal area to remove and smooth amalgam where mesial and/or distal surfaces are involved. If the restoration does not include an interproximal area, the Hollenback is not used (Figure 19-35).

The T-3 carver has one end shaped like a disc, and the other end is a blade. It is used to remove excess restorative material and to carve and shape occlusal anatomy (Figure 19-36).

The interproximal carver instrument (IPC) has long, thin blades on each end that are placed at different angles. It is used to trim excess filling material in the interproximal surface and to carve and smooth interproximal surfaces (Figure 19-37).

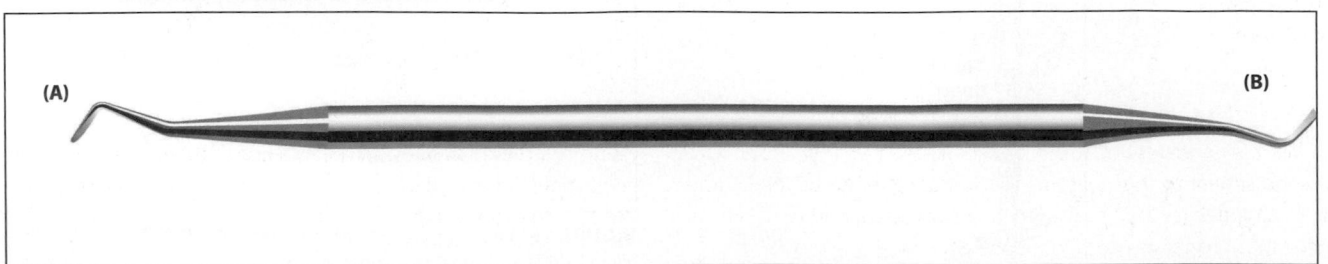

FIGURE 19-33
(A) Wall's carver shovel end and (B) carver hoe end.

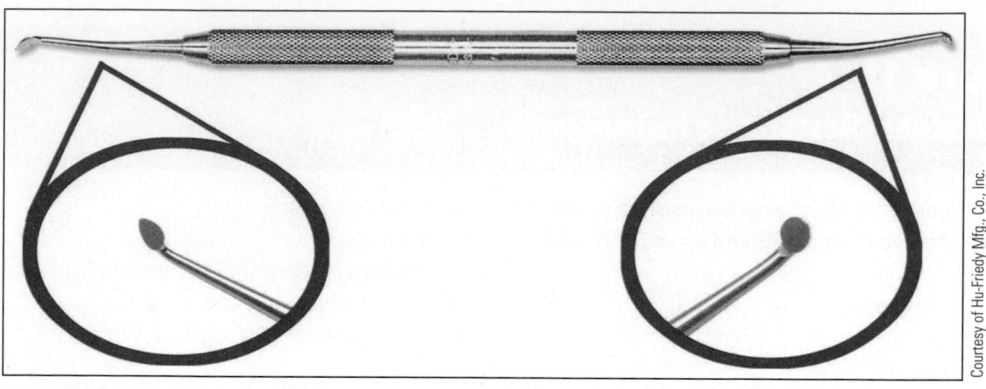

FIGURE 19-34
Double-ended instrument with two different ends. Cleoid end looks like a claw or spade and is pointed. Discoid end is round and looks like a disc.

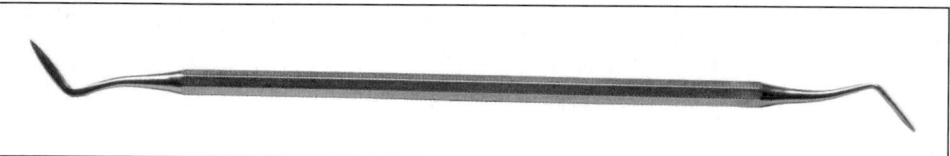

FIGURE 19-35
Hollenback carver double-ended with working ends positioned at different angles.

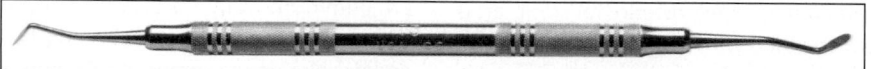

FIGURE 19-36
T-3 Carver.

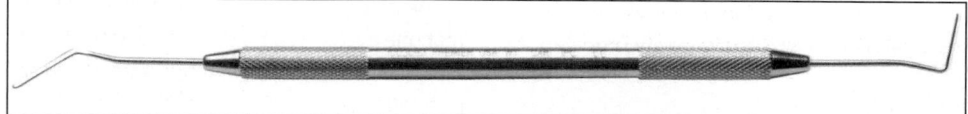

FIGURE 19-37
Interproximal Carver Instrument (IPC).

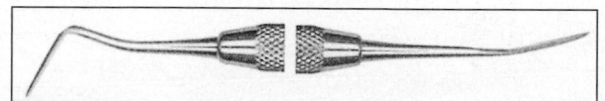

FIGURE 19-38
Ward's carver.

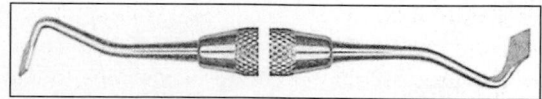

FIGURE 19-39
Frahm carver.

Ward's carver is a double-ended instrument with one end shaped similar to the Hollenback and the other end curved similar to a Wedelstaedt. It is used to carve amalgam and also as a lab instrument to carve wax (Figure 19-38).

Frahm's carver is shaped similar to a kite with two angled cutting sides meeting at a point. It is used to carve triangular ridges and the central groove (Figure 19-39).

Procedure 19-4
Identify Amalgam Restorative Instruments

This procedure is performed by the dental assistant to identify the amalgam restorative instruments and explain their use.

Equipment and Supplies
- amalgam carrier
- amalgam condensers
- ball burnisher
- football burnisher
- beaver tail burnisher
- T-ball burnisher
- acorn burnisher
- Walls' carver
- cleoid-discoid carver
- Hollenback carver
- T-3 carver
- interproximal carver instrument (IPC)
- Ward's carver
- Frahm's carver

Procedure Steps

1. Examine the instrument closely.

2. Identify the instrument by name.

3. Explain how it is used.

4. List the procedure(s) in which the instrument may be used.

Composite Restorative Instruments Composite, tooth-colored materials are being used more often than amalgam probably due to their cosmetic value. They cannot be used in every situation. Composites are not as strong as amalgam, wear faster, and are not recommended in the posterior for some large restorations or patients diagnosed with bruxism. Read Chapter 32 to learn more about composites. Composite resin material is made from a mixture of acrylic resin, powdered particles similar to glass, and are supplied in shades that can match the patient's natural tooth color. The composite material is packaged as a one-paste composite system with a syringe for several applications or as a single-dose cartridge that is used in a composite syringe (Figure 19-40). The material is injected into the cavity preparation from the syringe or placed on a paper pad for delivery with a composite placement instrument.

Metal instruments will scratch and discolor composite materials. Composite instruments are made of stainless steel with an aluminum-titanium coating (XTS) (Figure 19-41) or Teflon (Figure 19-42), which are nonadhering, hard, and prevent scratching and discoloring the composite. Composite instruments come in a wide variety of shapes that are designed for the different functions required when doing a composite filling. These include placement, condensing, carving, contouring, and burnishing the composite or other tooth-colored materials. The instruments may have the same shape on each end but different sizes, or they may be designed so that one end is used on the right and the other on the left. Some are designed to be used on anterior restorations and others for posterior restorations.

Once the composite is placed, it is **cured** using a curing light and contoured, refined, and polished using handpieces and composite **burs**.

FIGURE 19-40
(A) Composite one-paste syringe. (B) Composite syringe. (C) Single-dosage cartridges used with the composite syringe.

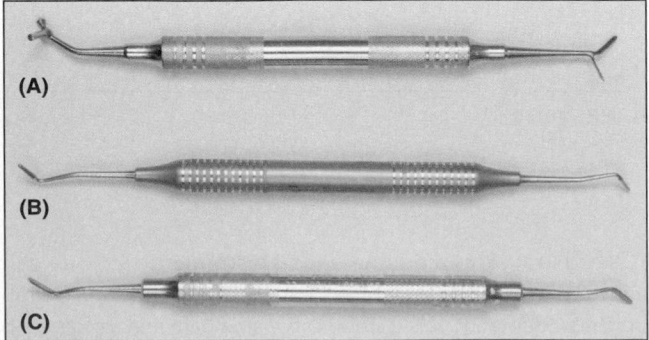

FIGURE 19-41
XTS composite instruments. (A) IPC. (B) Tindilly. (C) Garrisons's.

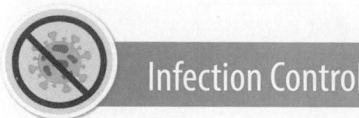
Infection Control

The XTS composite instruments cannot be placed in the ultrasonic sterilizer but are instead cleaned separately with mild detergent. Check the manufacturer's information.

Procedure 19-5
Identify Composite Restorative Instruments

This procedure is performed by the dental assistant to identify the composite restorative instruments and explain their use.

Equipment and Supplies
- composite syringe
- IPC composite instrument
- Tindilly composite instrument
- Garrison's composite instrument
- plastic filling composite instrument
- teflon filling composite instrument

Procedure Steps
1. Examine the instrument closely.
2. Identify the instrument by name.
3. Explain how it is used.
4. List the procedure(s) in which the instrument may be used.

Accessory Instruments

Accessory instruments are instruments that are needed for a procedure and not necessarily included in a tray setup. These instruments are typically kept in the dental treatment area unit carts with drawers, in dental cabinet drawers, or in tub systems.

A plastic filling instrument, also referred to as a Woodson instrument, is a double-ended instrument that has a paddle on one end and a small condenser on the other end. The paddle end is used to place materials such as **dental cements** into the cavity preparation, and the condenser end packs the material (Figure 19-43).

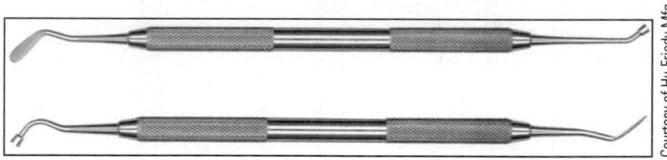

Courtesy of Hu-Friedy Mfg., Co., Inc.

FIGURE 19-43
Woodson plastic filling instrument.

The liner applicator is smaller instrument with a small-balled tip. It is used to place **liners** into the cavity preparation (Figure 19-44).

There is a variety of spatulas used in the dental office. A cement spatula is used to mix cements, **bases**, and liners (Figure 19-45). A plastic spatula is used to mix composite resin

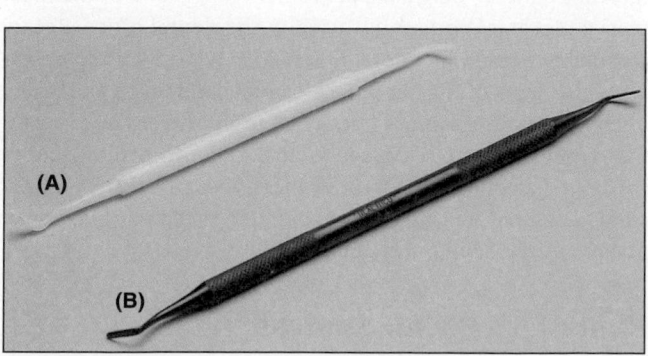

(A)

(B)

FIGURE 19-42
(A) Plastic and (B) Teflon composite instruments.

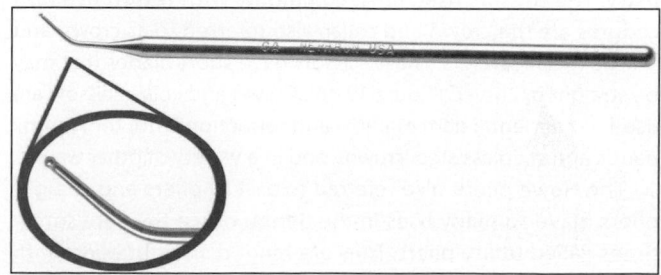

FIGURE 19-44
Liner applicator.

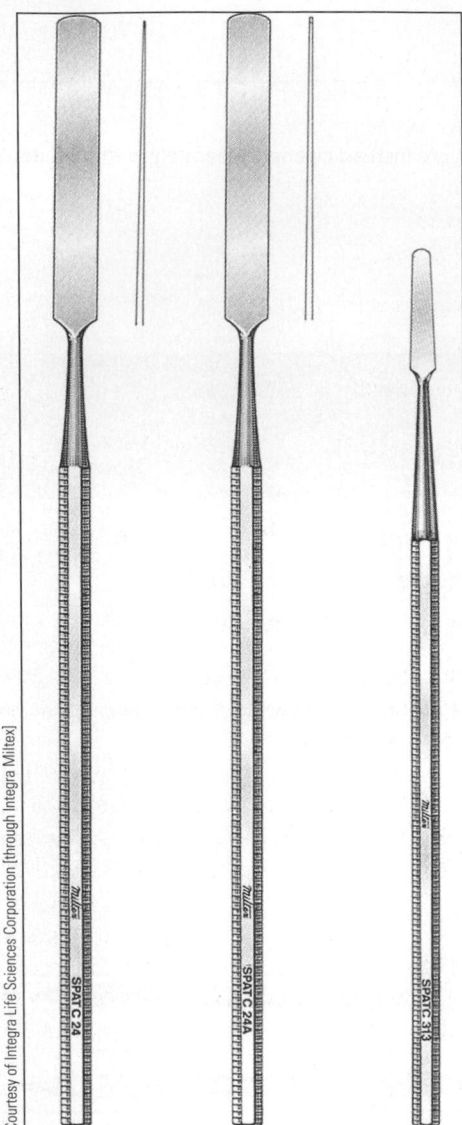

FIGURE 19-45
Cement spatulas.

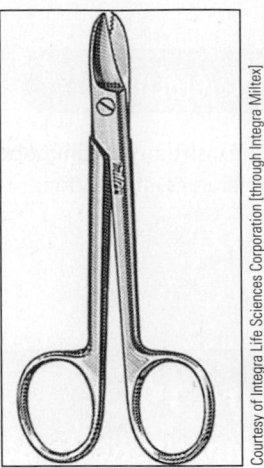

FIGURE 19-46
Straight crown and collar (bridge) scissors.

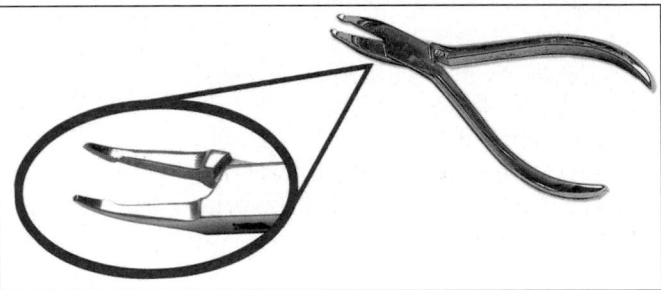

FIGURE 19-47
Howe pliers.

materials. These spatulas are usually double ended and may be disposable. Laboratory spatulas are used to mix a variety of laboratory materials. These spatulas are larger and have longer, wider blades. Laboratory spatulas are made entirely of plastic or with metal blades and wooden handles.

There are many different types of scissors used in dentistry. The scissors used most commonly with restorative procedures are the crown and collar, also referred to as crown and bridge (C&B), scissors. These scissors have short blades that may be straight or curved (Figure 19-46). Crown and collar scissors are used to cut dental dam material and retraction cord, trim matrix bands and stainless steel crowns, and in a variety of other ways.

The Howe pliers, also referred to as 110 pliers and straight pliers, have so many uses in the dental office they are sometimes called utility pliers. They are hinged straight pliers with straight or curved beaks that have a flat, rounded, serrated end (Figure 19-47). Howe pliers are handy when you need to grasp something tightly and to carry items to and from the oral cavity, place matrix bands, place and remove wooden wedges, and in a variety of ways in orthodontic procedures.

Dental Handpieces

The work of a dentist is most often associated with a drill. The drill is the layperson's term for the **dental handpiece**. A wide variety of dental handpieces are available to meet the needs of dental procedures, both in the oral cavity and in the laboratory. It is a metal, pencillike instrument and is one of the most crucial pieces of equipment used in the dental office. Rotary instruments, resembling drill bits, held in handpieces complete the actual work of the handpiece. Dental handpieces and rotary instruments are the most frequently used instruments in dentistry. They are used to remove tooth structure and bone and to cut, polish, and finish dental appliances. There are many types of handpieces that are categorized according to the combination of **power source**, speed, and design.

Handpiece Power Sources

There are **gears** within the head of the handpiece that spin around when the operator presses the rheostat to turn rotary

Procedure 19-6
Identify Accessory Restorative Instruments

This procedure is performed by the dental assistant to identify accessory instruments and explain their use.

Equipment and Supplies
- Woodson plastic filling instrument
- liner applicator
- cement spatulas
- crown and collar (bridge) scissors (straight and curved)
- Howe pliers (110)
- Teflon filling composite instrument

Procedure Steps

1. Examine the instrument closely.

2. Identify the instrument by name.

3. Explain how it is used.

4. List the procedure(s) in which the instrument may be used.

---

instruments held tightly in its **chuck** (Figure 19-54). There are a variety of power sources used to run the handpiece, depending on the particular use needed by the operator.

Belt-driven Since the 1800s handpieces have been used in dentistry. The belt-driven handpiece was the first type developed to rotate instruments used to cut oral structures. The gears within the handpiece are powered by a **belt and pulley**. The original handpieces were operated by the dental assistant, who pumped a foot-treadle dental engine to run the belt, turn the gears, and spin the rotary instruments. As this type was improved, a motor powered by electricity was added to power the belt-driven handpiece

Motor-driven Improvements of the dental handpiece have evolved rapidly over the years. The next type used was a small motor attached to the end of the handpiece, and electricity powered the gears inside the handpiece rotating the rotary instrument (Figure 19-48). This type is used in the dental laboratory.

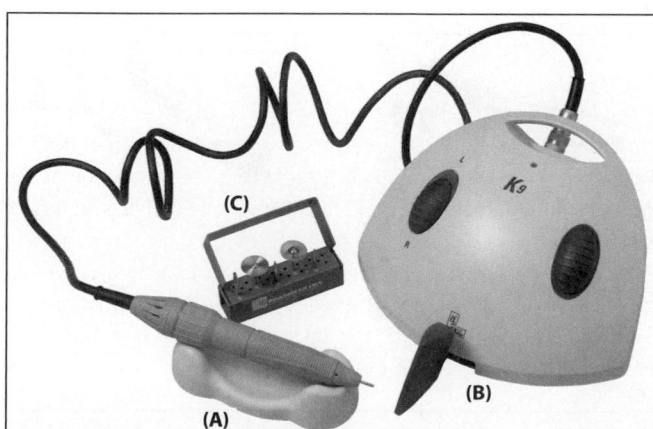

FIGURE 19-48
Laboratory motor-driven handpiece. (A) Handpiece with holder. (B) Foot control. (C) Selection of laboratory rotary instruments.

Some types are modified to be used in **portable dental units** where an air compressor is not available. In more recent years, manufacturers have improved this handpiece for chairside use, discussed later in this chapter.

Air-driven Handpieces used in patient care today generally use air under pressure to produce the energy to run the handpiece. The main function of air is to rotate the air **turbine** that has replaced the gears at specific **revolutions per minute** (rpms). An air compressor supplies air under pressure. The air-driven handpieces can turn the turbine much faster, rotating the instruments at a higher speed; these handpieces are also referred to as **airotors**. Modern commercial laboratories are also using air-driven handpieces.

Handpiece Speed

Rotary instruments need to be used at different speeds to perform specific functions. Dental handpieces are designed to rotate instruments at low speeds, high speeds, and ultraspeeds. The speed at which the handpiece turns rotary instruments is measured in revolutions per minute (rpm). Compressed air drives the turbines in the handpiece. To activate and control the speed of the handpiece, a rheostat (foot control) is operated, much like the accelerator on a car. Handpieces can rotate the rotary instruments forward and backward. The assistant should always check the setting for the rotation before passing the handpiece to the operator.

Low-Speed Handpieces Low-speed handpieces, also referred to as slow speed, have speeds ranging from 6,000 to 30,000 rpm. These handpieces have many uses in dentistry including polishing teeth, removing soft decay, defining cavity preparations, and finishing and smoothing restorations. Low-speed handpieces may be driven with belt, motor, or air power sources. There are many handpiece designs and attachments to accommodate the varying uses of low-speed handpieces, including **straight**, **right angle**, and **contra-angle handpieces**.

Safety

Protective Eyewear when Operating Handpieces

When the dentist prepares a patient's tooth using a handpiece, a dental spray is produced containing tooth debris, infectious microorganisms, water, saliva, and particles of restorations. It is vital that the dental team and patient are protected from the potential harm this spray may cause. The patient and dental team should wear protective eyewear to protect their eyes from particles being sprayed. This dental spray can contain matter that can cut the eye and potentially cause an eye infection. The dental team should also wear masks when using any rotary instruments to prevent inhalation of infectious microorganisms. General safety guidelines for the dental team are to wear protective eyewear and a mask whenever operating a rotary device.

High-Speed Handpieces   Speeds for high-speed handpieces range from 100,000 to 400,000 rpm. The handpieces that rotate at higher speeds are often referred to as **ultraspeed handpieces**. Air-driven is the only power source that can drive the high-speed handpieces at these rotations. The high-speed handpieces are used by the dentist to remove old restorations and decay, cut tooth structure to develop a cavity outline, and finish restorations.

Rotary instruments turning at these higher speeds create heat and friction that can potentially harm the pulp and cause discomfort for the patient. Most high-speed handpieces are manufactured with **coolants**. The dentist can select on the rheostat to deliver a spray of air or an air/water spray to be delivered from the handpiece coolant to minimize the heat and friction produced. Low-speed handpieces do not have coolants because they do not rotate at the speeds that heat up the tooth or tissue. Special handpieces are made to cut oral structures during oral surgery. (Refer to Chapter 36 for more details.)

Handpiece Designs

Over the years, the design of handpieces has changed to provide varying speeds, to hold different types of rotary instruments, to offer better access to areas in the oral cavity, to complete lab work, and to meet ergonomic needs. The dental assistant needs to be able to recognize all types of handpiece designs and identify them by name.

Straight Handpiece   The straight handpiece was one of the first designs used in dentistry (Figure 19-49). It gets its name from its straight shape. One end of the handpiece is attached to a low-speed motor. The low-speed motor is connected to the unit's handpiece hose designated for low-speed handpieces. The other end houses the chuck that secures rotary instruments and handpiece attachments. The chuck is opened and released by pressing a button or twisting the handpiece. The straight handpiece is primarily used outside the mouth for lab work. It receives a laboratory rotary instrument to cut and polish dental appliances. The

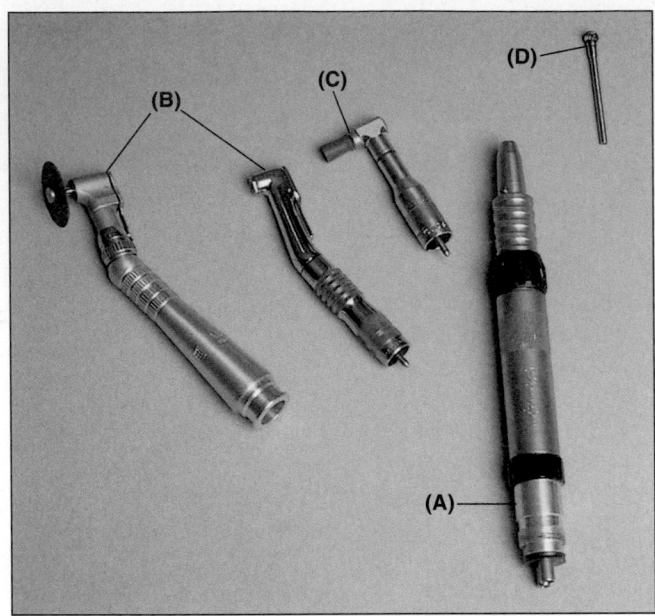

FIGURE 19-49
(A) Low-speed straight handpiece with nose cone for insertion of long-shank rotary instruments or handpiece attachments and motor.
(B) Contra-angle attachment shown with and without a disc. (C) Right-angle attachment with rubber cup inserted. (D) Long-shank rotary instrument.

straight handpiece has attachments to be used in the mouth. A right angle and contra-angle can be attached for better access in the patient's mouth.

Right-Angle Attachment   The right-angle attachment is designed with its working end at a 90° angle (right angle) (Figure 19-49C). This design allows for better access into the patient's mouth and is primarily used during **prophylaxis** to clean and polish the patient's teeth, also referred to as a prophy angle. Most offices use plastic right angles that are made for one time use and are disposed of after each patient (Figure 19-50). The rotary instruments for the right angle either screw into the chuck or snap into place (snap-on).

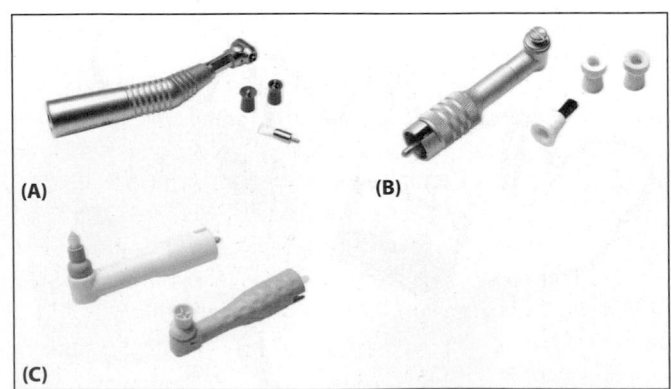

FIGURE 19-50
(A) Low-speed handpiece with screw type right-angle attachment. (B) Snap-on right-angle attachment. (C) Disposable right angle attachments with a cup and brush.

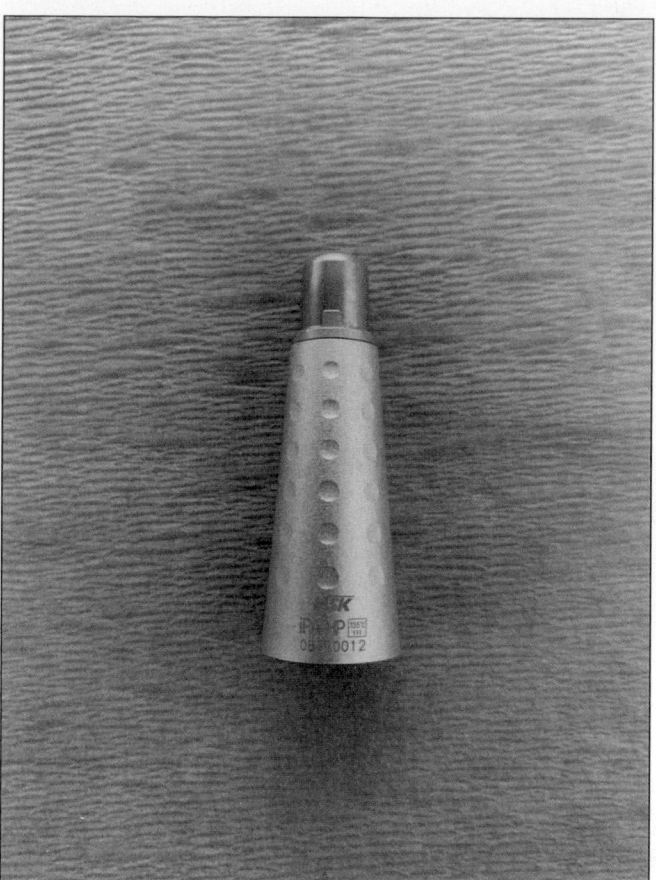

FIGURE 19-51
U-style adaptor for attachment for right angle attachment.

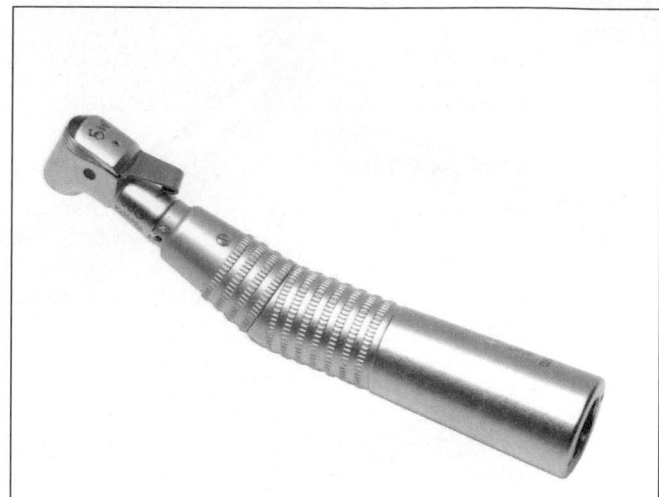

FIGURE 19-52
Low-speed handpiece with latch type contra-angle attachment.

The right angle attachment can be attached directly to a low-speed motor, a straight handpiece, or a U-style adaptor. The U-style adaptor, also called a prophy adaptor, is smaller and lighter than using a straight handpiece (Figure 19-51).

Contra-Angle Attachment The contra-angle attachment is designed with contrasting angles that provides better access to all areas of the mouth (Figure 19-49B). It is used to remove decay, define cavity preparations, and finish and smooth restorations. The low-speed handpiece does not have or need a water supply, but in some procedures the dental assistant periodically applies air or water to the tooth or restoration to prevent any heating of the tooth. The contra-angle can be attached directly to a low-speed motor or to a straight handpiece. There are two types of chucks to hold the rotary instrument: the latch type and autochuck. The latch is opened for the insertion of the rotary instrument and closed to secure the instrument (Figure 19-52). The autochuck has a release that is pressed to open and close the chuck to hold the rotary instrument.

High-Speed Handpiece Design The high-speed handpiece is also designed with contrasting angles that provides access to all areas of the mouth. The earlier handpieces were heavy and bulky, producing poor ergonomics for the operator. The modern head sizes are smaller, allowing for better visibility and access to the operative site, and the patient does not have to open their mouth as wide for greater comfort. High-speed handpieces are being designed with ergonomics in mind that are more comfortable, lighter weight, have less vibration, and are less tiring for the dentist. These handpieces are used to cut cavity preparations and to finish restorations. The high-speed is connected directly to the unit high-speed hose. High-speed handpieces are made to insert rotary instruments using a bur tool or with autochucks (Figure 19-53).

Parts and Features of Dental Handpieces

The dental assistant must be able to recognize handpiece parts and rotary instruments that fit into the handpiece and be able to care for them properly. Following is a description of the parts and features of handpieces.

Head The head or working end of the handpiece is where the rotary instruments are inserted (Figure 19-54). Options for the head include a standard size and a smaller size for pediatrics and smaller mouths.

Chuck The chuck is the part of head that holds the rotary instruments. The rotary instrument is inserted into a small hole in the chuck (Figure 19-55). Models of handpieces have a variety of methods to open and close the chuck. There are bur tools, latches, and autochuck releases on the handpiece head. The bur tool is used to insert and remove the rotary instruments, the latch is opened and closed, and the autochuck built-in button is pressed, eliminating need for a tool or latches.

Coolant High-speed handpieces generate heat and friction, which can damage the pulp and cause patient discomfort.

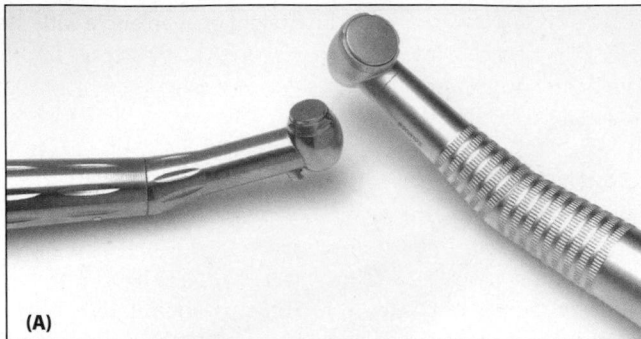

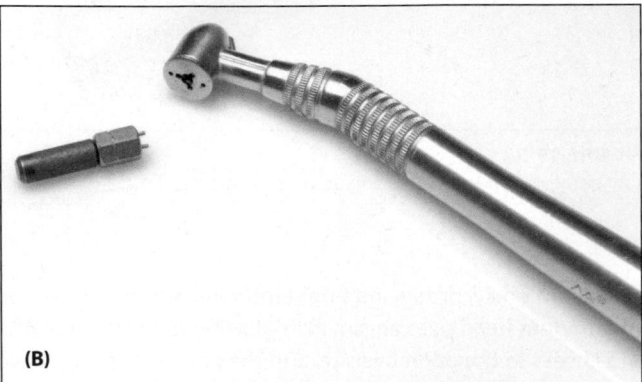

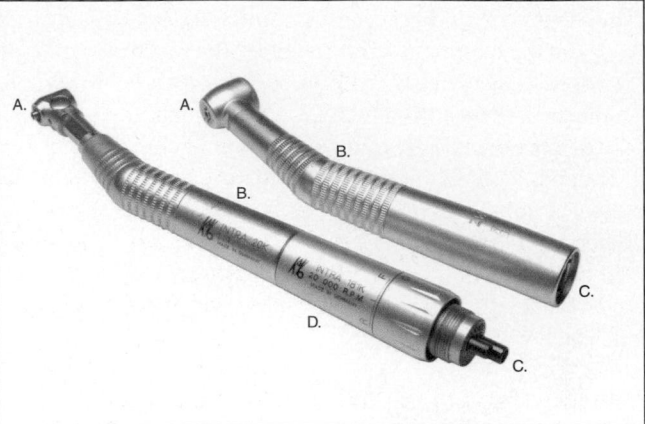

FIGURE 19-54
Shown on the left is the low-speed handpiece and motor with right angle attachment. On the right is a high-speed handpiece. Parts of the handpieces. (A) Head. (B) Shank-handle portion. (C) Connection end attaches to dental unit hose couplings.

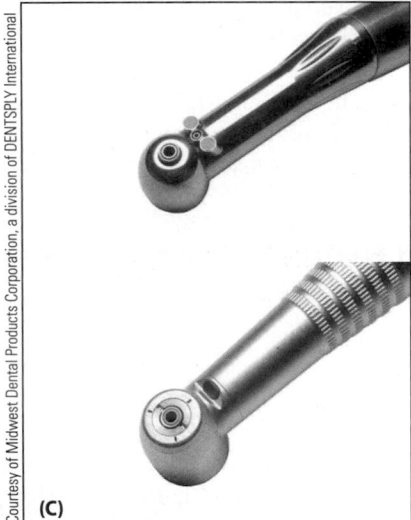

Courtesy of Midwest Dental Products Corporation, a division of DENTSPLY International

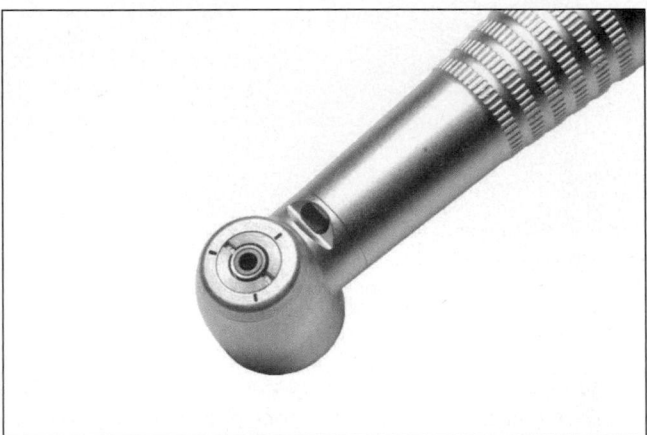

FIGURE 19-55
The rotary instrument is inserted in the chuck (small hole) in the center of the head.

FIGURE 19-53
(A) High-speed handpieces with autochucks; push-button back to place and remove the bur. (B) High-speed handpiece with a bur tool to place and remove the bur. (C) Hole in center of handpiece head is the chuck.

A coolant is housed in the handpiece head, which has a water or air-water spray that helps to keep the tooth cool (Figure 19-56). The selector to control the desired coolant is generally located on the handpiece rheostat. One of the responsibilities of the dental assistant during the cavity preparation is to efficiently use the HVE to suction this spray to keep the patient comfortable and maintain a clear field of vision for the dentist.

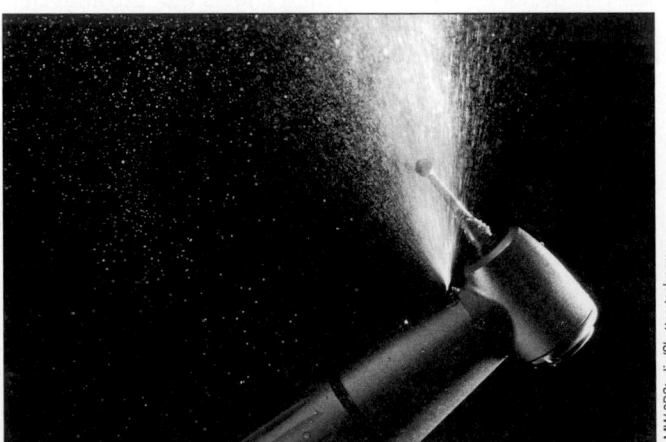

© MW 3DStudio/Shutterstock.com

FIGURE 19-56
Handpieces with coolants help cool the tooth with water or air/water spray.

Fiber-Optic Light Because the mouth is a deep dark place to work and the operator's hand can block the overhead light, the high-speed handpieces often have a **fiber-optic** light source to illuminate the operative site (Figure 19-57). A fiber-optic system is added to the dental unit with an electronic control module, with fiber optics running through the handpiece tubing to the handpiece. The light source is channeled through the handpiece by a fiber-optic bundle. There are two focused lights that emit white light toward the bur, making visibility inside the oral cavity much easier. Halogen bulbs are used on either side of the chuck opening (Figure 19-58).

Handle and Shank The handle, also referred to as the shaft, is the part of the handpiece held in the operator's hand, located between the head and connection end of the handpiece. The shank is the part located between the head and the handle

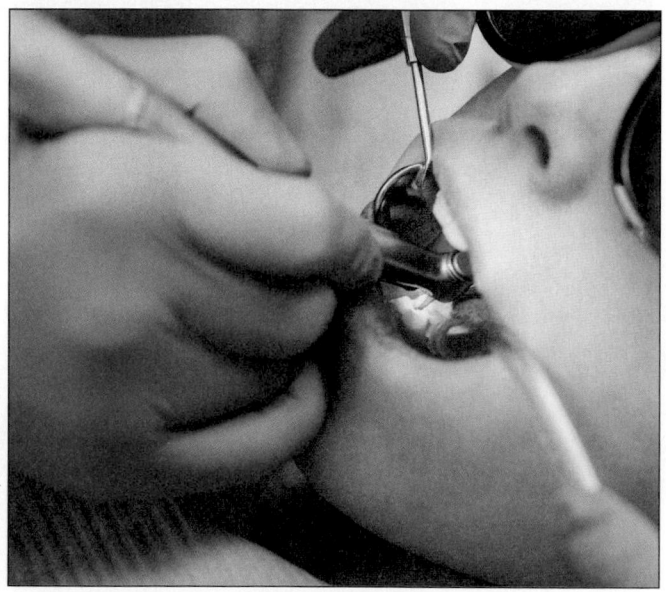

FIGURE 19-57
Fiber optics provide a light while in use, providing direct illumination of the operative site.

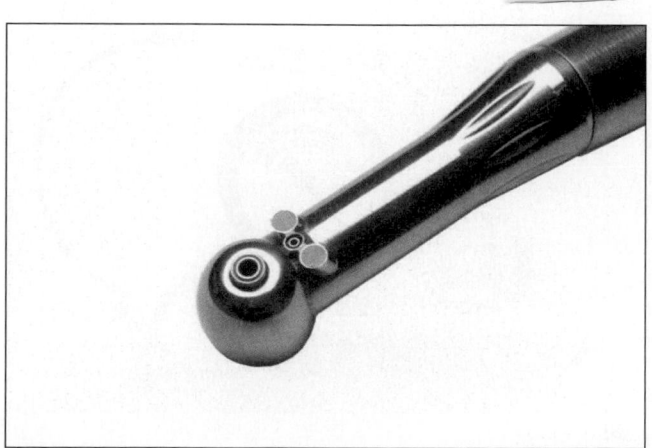

FIGURE 19-58
Fiber-optic light on either side of the chuck.

(Figure 19-54B). The shank can be straight or at an angle with the head. The right-angle has the head at a 90° angle to the handle. The contra-angle has two contrasting angles to improve access and visibility of the operative site.

Connection End The connection end attaches the handpiece to the power source. The connection end of the low-speed handpiece is attached to the low-speed motor, and the motor is attached to the unit handpiece hose coupling. High-speed handpieces are attached directly to the coupling of the handpiece hose (Figure 19-54C). The handpiece hose encloses wires from the power source, transports air and water, and contains the fiber-optic cord for the light source. The dental assistant needs to prevent entanglement of these hoses to prevent any interference in the efficiency of the handpiece. Forward and reverse controls for the low-speed handpiece are also located on the connection end.

Handpiece Holder When the handpiece is not in use, the handpiece needs to be secured on the handpiece holder. The holder is attached to the dental unit. Many of these units have automatic switches built into the holder. When the handpiece is placed in the holder, the handpiece selector is pressed by the handpiece, turning off the power to the handpiece. Again, once the handpiece is removed from the holder, the selector is released, turning on the power to the handpiece. For safety, the handpiece should be placed in the holder with the rotary instrument facing toward the unit.

Emerging Handpiece Technologies

The handpieces covered previously in this chapter are the standard equipment used in most dental offices. Handpieces are continually evolving with the practice of dentistry and dental technology. Following are the highlights of the latest technologies and developments in handpieces.

Standard Handpiece Advancements There are many improvements and advancements being made for the standard dental handpieces. Some of the most recent are sensors and LEDs being used to improve the handpieces.

Sensors There have been many breakthroughs in handpiece technology. New on the market is a sensor called the speed-sensing intelligence. It monitors the bur speed by detecting vibrations from the rotating bur and signals the increase of air pressure and speed. This feature provides exceptionally fast cutting action and minimized wear on the turbine.

Illumination LEDs (light-emitting diodes) are an improvement over the halogen bulbs used in current fiber optics. The LEDs provide better illumination using a neutral daylight color, last 10 times longer, and do not get as hot as the halogen bulb.

Electric Handpieces An electric handpiece is an alternative to the air-driven handpieces mainly used by dentists today. They have greatly improved and are becoming more popular countertop units (Figures 19-60A and B). They consist of the base unit, control panel, foot switch, air pressure gradient (varies the pressure in small increments), handpiece, abrasive flow control, and external suction device. Each unit requires an air pressure source (most can use air lines to the dental unit) and the abrasive. The air abrasion handpiece releases a powerful air stream of small, fine aluminum oxides particles that blasts away decay and

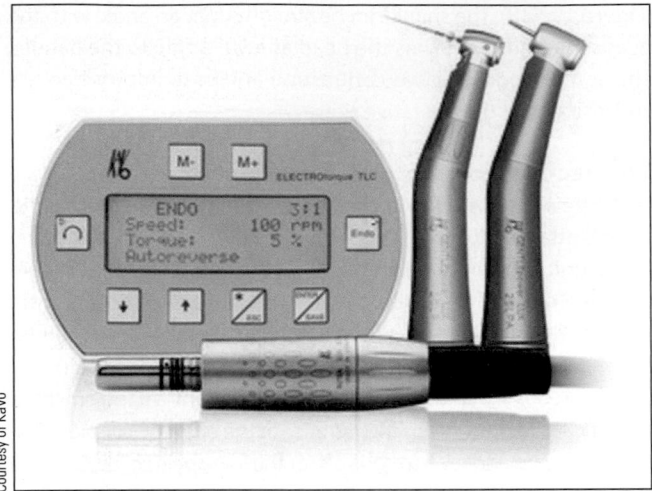

Courtesy of KaVo

FIGURE 19-59
Electric handpiece control unit with motor and hose, high-speed attachments with fiber optics, slow-speed, endodontic, and straight attachment.

in the dental office. The electric handpieces are quiet, vibration free, efficient, and sterilizable. They allow for smoother cuts and refined margins with higher torque and precision. Electric handpieces use a control unit to supply electrical power to operate the handpiece at speeds from 20 to 200,000 rpm and have lightweight cellular optic rods that deliver illumination (Figure 19-59). With these speed variations, one electric handpiece can be used for both high-speed and low-speed procedures. A coolant system must be used to minimize heat and friction. The units can be calibrated to be used with existing air pressure and rheostats.

Air Abrasion Air abrasion, also called microabrasion, is an effective alternative to the standard dental handpiece. It is used much like sandblasting is used to remove graffiti from walls. Air abrasion base units come in movable floor models or small

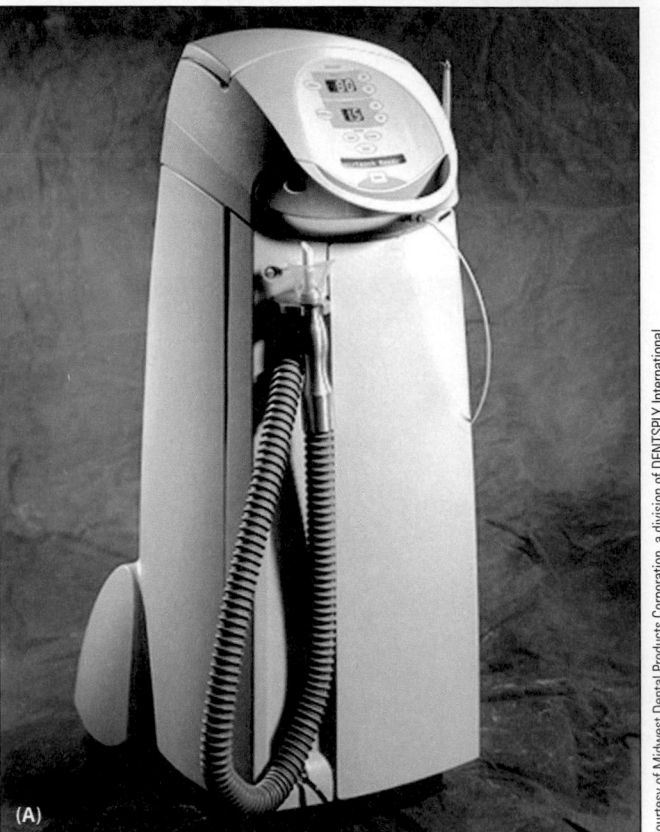

(A)

Courtesy of Midwest Dental Products Corporation, a division of DENTSPLY International

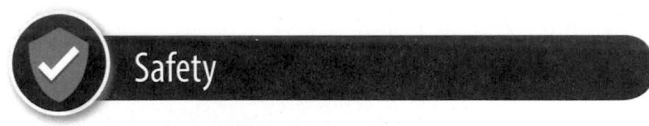

Safety

Overheating of Electric Head

The electric handpiece tends to overheat. Cases have been reported of patient burns, including third-degree burns, linked to overheating of the handpiece head. The FDA is alerting dental professionals about possible patient burns from overheating electric dental handpieces. Burns can occur when the electric handpiece is worn or clogged. The increased power is sent to the handpiece head to maintain performance generating heat at the head or the attachment. This can burn the patient very quickly without warning because the patient is anesthetized and may not be able to feel the heat. The operator is not aware of the overheating because they are protected from the heat by the handpiece housing. The FDA recommends steps to prevent burns from electric handpieces.

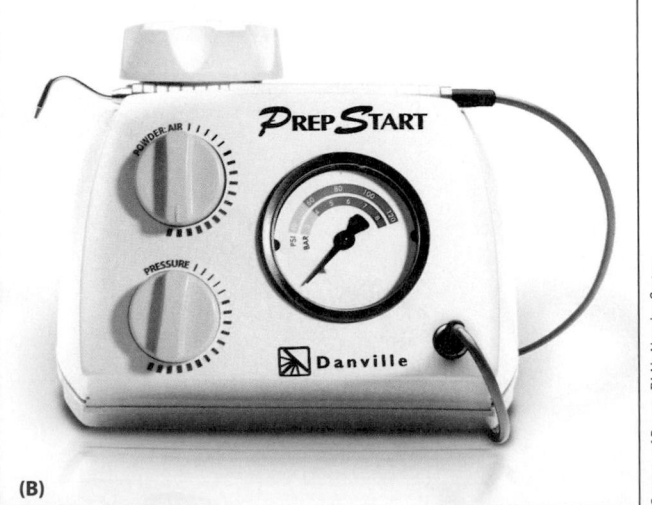

(B)

Courtesy of Prepstar™ Air Abrasion System

FIGURE 19-60
(A) Air abrasion floor model. (B) Air abrasion countertop unit.

tooth structure. Its most common use is to prepare cavities for the placement of composite restorations, veneers, and sealants, all requiring an etched surface for the materials to adhere. It is also used to repair tooth structure cracks and discolorations and to prepare tooth surfaces for bonding procedures.

Air abrasion is less painful, more precise, and removes less tooth structure than using the standard handpiece and rotary instruments. There is no vibration and no heat from the handpiece. In most cases, a coolant and an anesthetic injection are not necessary when using air abrasion. Air abrasion technology does not harm soft tissue, operates very quietly, and usually has shorter treatment time. This procedure produces a large spray of dusty particle debris. The dental team must follow safety recommendations; see box "Safety with Air Abrasion." The air abrasion cannot be used as an alternative to the standard dental handpiece in every procedure like crown and bridge preparation and surgery.

The **microetcher** is a smaller version of the air abrasion unit. It is about the size of a pen and has an abrasive reservoir with an interchangeable jar. The reservoir is attached to the microetcher and holds the abrasive. The microetcher comes with several different tips called nozzles (Figure 19-61). It can be hooked up in an operatory or a lab where there is an air line for compressed air of 40 to 100 psi. Microetchers are used for many procedures including etching for sealants and composite restorations and to roughen surfaces for bonding orthodontic bands and brackets.

Lasers Laser use in dentistry has increased over the past few years. Instead of rotary instruments to cut structures, a **laser** beam is used to **cauterize** soft tissue and **vaporize** decayed tooth structures (Figure 19-62). The appearance of the laser handpiece resembles the standard handpiece and has the laser conducted through a fiber-optic cable. With the use of a laser, the patient generally does not need anesthesia, and the laser beam completes the procedure in less time. The laser still uses an air and water coolant to minimize heat and discomfort for the patient.

Safety

Safety with Air Abrasion

Air abrasion is safe when using the recommended precautions. The dental team and patient need to wear protective eye wear to prevent eye irritation from the spray. The dental assistant needs to suction particles to help reduce the dental spray, and the dental team needs to wear masks to prevent breathing the dust particles into the lungs.

A **dental dam** should be placed to protect the areas of the mouth that are not being treated and to prevent abrasion debris from building up in the back of the patient's throat.

Lasers have many applications in dentistry. They are effective in small cavity preparations, removal of caries and composite restorations, etching and treatment of dentinal sensitivity, caries prevention and bleaching, controlling bleeding, removal of biopsy tissue, endodontic therapy, and treatment of lesions. There are some special considerations when using a laser; amalgam restorations should not be removed using a laser due to potential release of mercury; the laser etching is inferior to standard etching techniques. All uses are not yet fully documented or explored; however, it is thought that lasers may revolutionize cavity design and preparation with the continued development of adhesive dentistry. It is thought that in the future using the laser may result in adhesion without acid etching. The dental laser is a medical device that must be used following safety recommendations.

Ultrasonic Handpiece The **ultrasonic handpiece** is not only used for scaling procedures and root canal therapy but also may be used to remove bonding materials after cementing

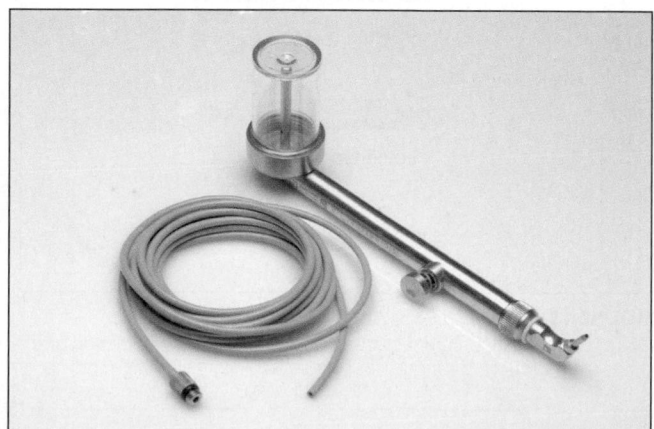

FIGURE 19-61
Microetcher with hose and abrasive reservoir.

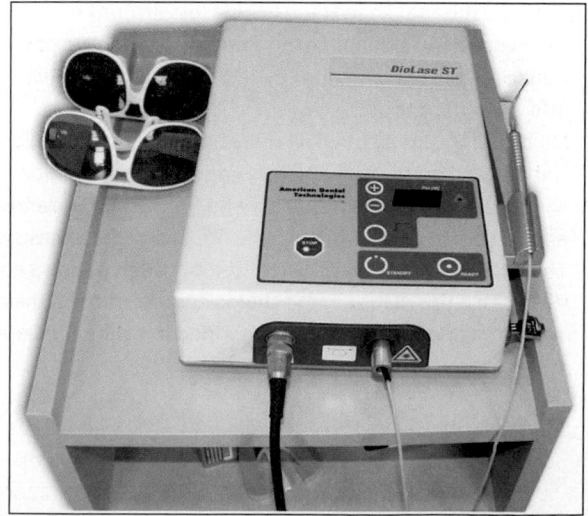

FIGURE 19-62
Dental laser unit with handpiece attachment and safety glasses.

Safety

Safety with Lasers

When a laser handpiece is being used, it is critical to establish laser safety protocols for the dental office and adequate training of all staff involved. The laser beam is extremely hot and can cause damage to the eye and skin. Due to its extreme heat, it is a fire potential. There are several potential dangers in using the laser handpiece that can be controlled with the proper training and precautions:

- Laser safety goggles recommended by the laser manufacturer's directions must be worn by the dental staff and patient at all times. Special loupe inserts must be used to protect the operator's eyes.
- Laser energy can be reflected. It is imperative that the operator reduce or avoid the number of reflective surfaces in the operating field. A distance of within 10 feet of the laser is potentially dangerous for unprotected dental team members. Signs of potential danger must be posted.
- The level of radiation exposure must be closely monitored to remain below the level to which an unprotected person may be exposed without experiencing adverse biological changes to the eye or skin.
- As the laser interacts with tissue, a smoke plume results that not only hinders vision but also contains debris. The debris includes not only infectious microorganisms but also toxic gases. This debris is referred to as laser-generated air contaminants. High velocity evacuation is critical in reducing the amount of air contaminants. It is recommended to place the HVE within 4 cm of the target site and that the dental team wear masks capable of filtering to 0.1 mm.
- Due to the thermal component of the laser, there is a risk of fire if it contacts combustible materials or gases. Care must be taken in the use of lasers around nitrous, oxygen, or any alcohol based materials (alcohol-soaked gauze squares and alcohol-based topical anesthetics) and aerosol products.
- Oil-based lip products, which may be flammable, should not be used on the patients. A syringe of saline solution should be kept on the dental tray for immediate use and easy access to a working portable fire extinguisher ensured.
- The fiber-optic tip must be sterilized between patients and disposable tips placed in the sharps container. The remainder of the laser unit should be wrapped in a barrier recommended by the laser manufacturer.

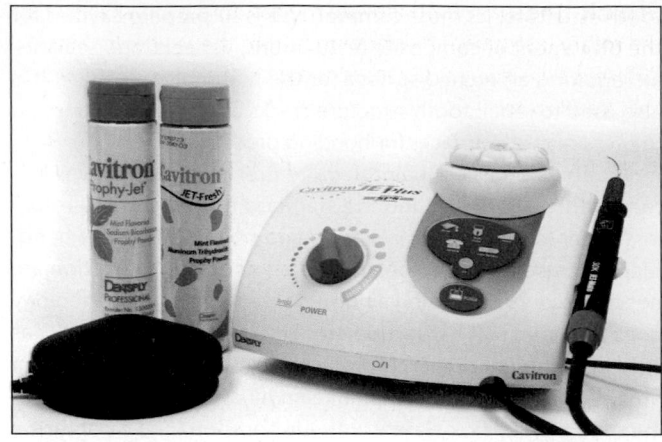

FIGURE 19-63
Ultrasonic handpiece.

crowns and orthodontic appliances. The handpiece is attached to the ultrasonic scaler unit. The unit converts electrical energy into ultrasonic vibrations that are transmitted to the handpiece. There are specific connections on the dental unit for the electrical and water needed for the ultrasonic unit. Ultrasonic handpieces are controlled by a foot pedal (Figure 19-63).

Dental Rotary Instruments

Rotary instruments are used in dental handpieces at chairside and in the dental laboratory. There are hundreds of different rotary instruments, each with their own specific use. They are named by their composition, use, shape, and type of shank. The main types of instruments are burs, abrasives, and polishing rotary instruments.

Parts of Rotary Instruments

A rotary instrument has three parts: shank, head, and neck (Figure 19-64).

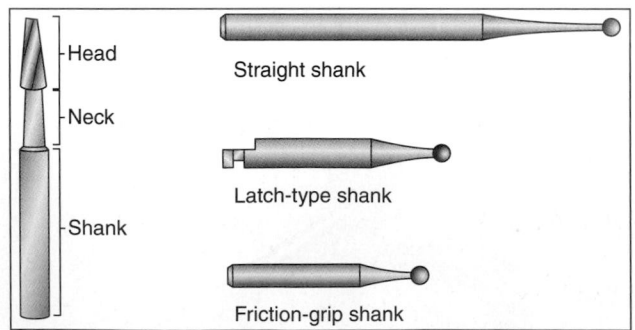

FIGURE 19-64
(A) Parts of a bur. (B) Different shanks: straight, latch type, and friction grip.

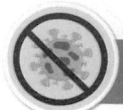

Infection Control

The manufacturer's directions for maintaining and sterilizing the handpiece should be followed carefully. Handpieces that are used for patient treatment must be sterilizable; disinfecting handpieces is not acceptable. Refer to Chapter 11 for details.

Shank The shank is placed into the handpiece chuck and holds the rotary instrument by gripping it from the inside. It comes in different sizes and shapes depending on the type of handpiece chuck it fits into.

Sizes of Shanks There are three different lengths of rotary instrument:

- *Long shank* (LS) is placed into straight handpieces. It is primarily used in the laboratory outside the patient's mouth to adjust and polish dental appliances.
- *Short shank* (SS) is placed in the low-speed contra-angle and high-speed handpieces. The smaller size shank fits inside the patient's mouth and is used for cutting tooth structures.
- *Pedodontic shank* (PS) is placed in the low-speed contra-angle and high-speed handpieces. The smaller size shank fits inside a small child's mouth and is used for cutting tooth structures.

Shapes of Shanks The end of the shank that fits into the handpiece chuck is designed to fit the different types of handpieces:

- *Latch type shank* (LA) has a short shank. It has a notched area at the end of the shank that is placed into a latched low-speed contra-angle handpiece. The lever of the handpiece is closed holding the rotary instrument secure. It is primarily used in the patient's mouth on low speed only.
- *Friction grip type shank* (FG) is designed with both the long shank and short shank. It is straight and is held in the handpiece grip by friction. The long shank FG fits into the low-speed straight handpiece. The short FG shank fits into the high-speed handpiece. The short FG shank also fits into FG low-speed contra-angle handpieces. The low-speed contra-angle can be designed to hold either LA or FG shank rotary instruments.
- *Screw and snap-on shanks* are the designs used for prophy cups and prophy brushes used in the low-speed right angle handpieces (prophy angles).

Head The head is the working end of the instruments. The use of the rotary instrument determines what type of head is needed. The working end (head) comes in different shape and sizes for different purposes. Some of the different types of heads include burs, stones, diamonds, discs, and wheels. Naming the various heads is covered later in this chapter.

Neck The neck is tapered and connects the shank to the head.

Burs

Burs are used for removing decay, removing old restorations, cavity preparations, occlusal adjustments, dental appliance adjustments, finishing and polishing restorations, and surgical procedures. They are made of steel. There are a variety of steels used in the manufacturing of rotary instruments depending on

the purpose. Stainless steel rotary instruments are primarily used during surgery. Stainless steel sterilizes well without rusting. But it is not the strongest choice to easily cut enamel and restorative materials. Tungsten carbide steel is reinforced steel made tougher and stronger and can be made sharper than stainless steel. It is primarily used in cutting tooth tissue and dental materials. With proper sterilization procedures, carbide rotary instruments can be used more than once. Plain steel is weaker and the least expensive of the three. It dulls and rusts easily and is generally used once and thrown away.

Cutting Burs When the dentist removes caries and shapes the tooth for a restoration using a handpiece and hand cutting instruments, it is called a cavity preparation. Teeth have many different shapes, and there are many types of restorative materials. The dentist decides the appropriate restorative material and what cavity preparation is required.

Cavity Classifications In the early 1900s, G. V. Black developed a classification of cavities based on the tooth type and the cavity location (tooth surfaces involved) and method to restore teeth that is still used widely today. The original classification system placed cavities into five groups indicated by a Roman numeral and the word *Class*. Class I, Class II, Class III, Class IV, and Class V were used to describe the carious lesions. Later Class VI was added to Black's classifications of caries lesions to describe further cavities that involve the incisal or occlusal surface that has been worn away due to attrition (Box 19-1).

Types of Cutting Burs A cutting bur contains flutes (6 to 8 blades) and is the most frequently used rotary instrument to cut hard tissue (tooth/bone). The bur is mainly used to remove caries, cut tooth structure, and define the preparation for the placement of a restoration. The bur is named by shape and size of the head. Some shapes include round, inverted cone, straight, tapered, and pear (Table 19-1). The bur is also given a number representing the shape and size; the smaller the number, the smaller the bur head. The dental assistant needs to recognize the burs by shape and recall the bur's number series (Figure 19-73).

Surgical Burs Surgical burs are made of stainless steel. They are not as strong as the cutting burs, but as mentioned earlier, they can be sterilized without rusting. They are supplied in similar shapes and sizes as the cutting burs (Figure 19-88). Surgical burs are manufactured in extra-long shanks to enable the dentist to reach an area deep within patient tissue that needs cutting. Surgical burs are used in a low-speed handpiece to reduce and contour the alveolar bone and tooth structure.

Laboratory Burs Laboratory burs are referred to as a vulcanite or acrylic bur. These burs are also cutting burs that are used outside the mouth for laboratory work. Laboratory burs are used to make adjustments and in the fabrication of dental appliances, used on denture bases, custom trays, mouth guards,

BOX 19-1   Cavity Classifications

Class I

Class I caries include the following three types of developmental cavities in the pit and fissures of teeth:

- Occlusal surfaces of the posterior teeth (premolars and molars) (Figure 19-65).

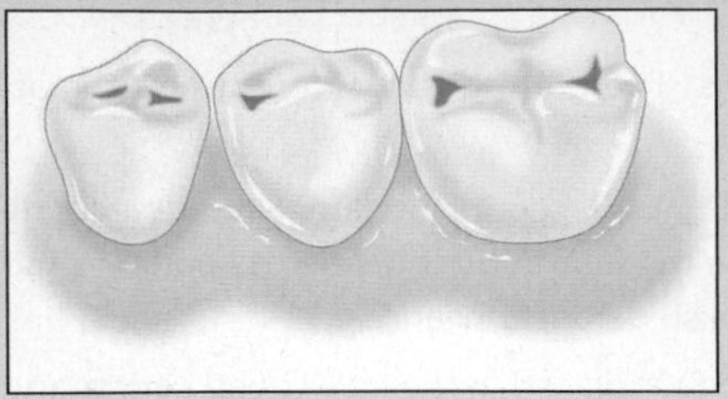

FIGURE 19-65
Class I posterior occlusal surface.

- Buccal or lingual pits on the molars (Figure 19-66).

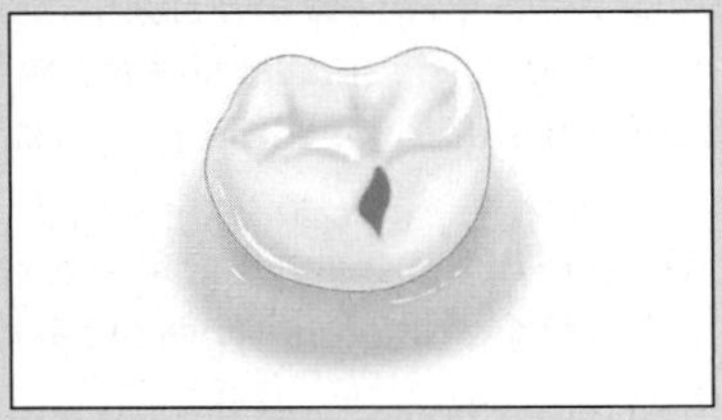

FIGURE 19-66
Class I buccal or lingual pit.

- Lingual pit near the cingulum of the maxillary incisors (Figure 19-67).

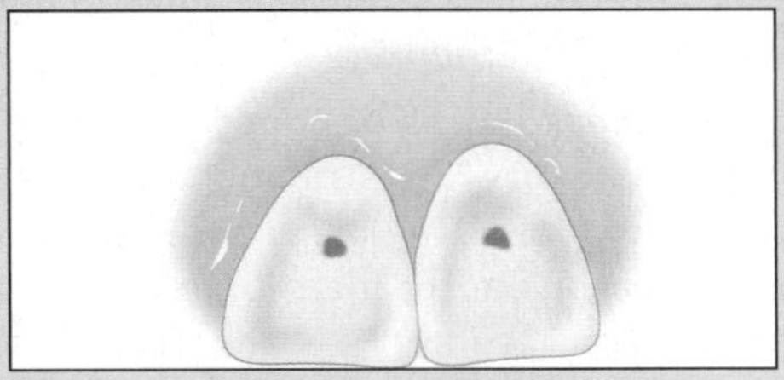

FIGURE 19-67
Class I anterior pit.

Class II

Class II caries are on the proximal (mesial or distal) surfaces on the posterior teeth (premolars and molars) (Figure 19-68).

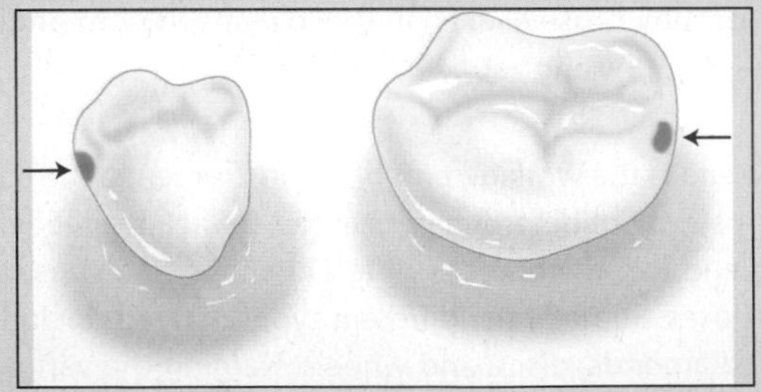

FIGURE 19-68
Class II posterior proximals.

Class III

Class III caries are on the interproximal surface (mesial or distal) of anterior teeth (canines, lateral incisors, and central incisors) (Figure 19-69).

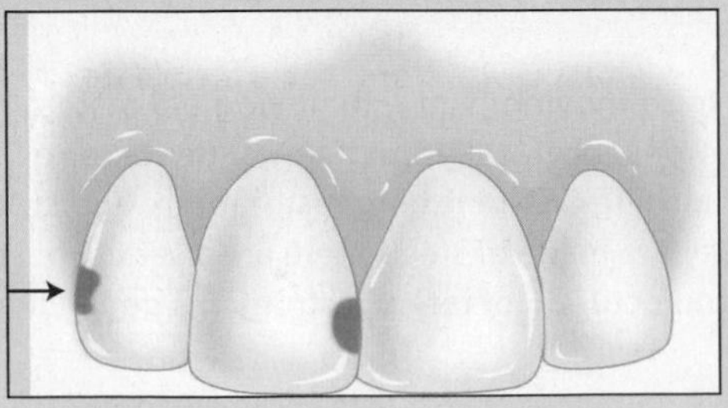

FIGURE 19-69
Class III anterior proximals.

BOX 19-1 Cavity Classifications

Class IV

Class IV caries are on the interproximal surface (mesial or distal) of anterior teeth and include the incisal edge (Figure 19-70).

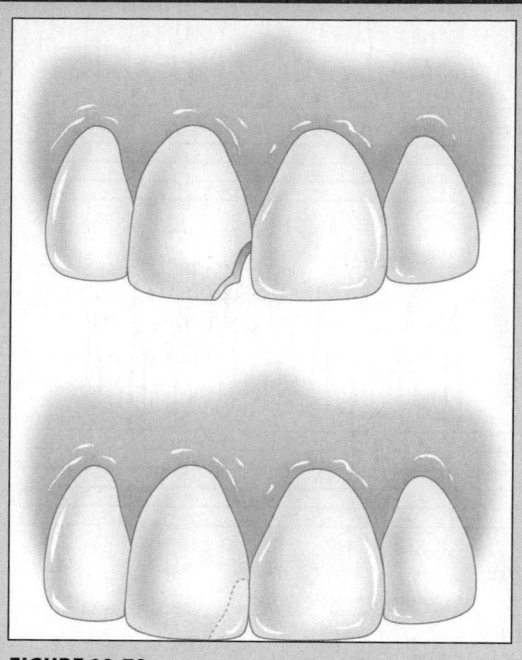

FIGURE 19-70
Class IV anterior involving proximals and incisal edge.

Class V

Class V caries occur on the cervical third of the facial or lingual surface of the tooth (Figure 19-71). Often, Class V caries occur because the patient regularly sucks on sweets. Additionally, the dental assistant may see several Class V caries in one quadrant because the patient takes medications, chews gum, or drinks sodas over long periods of time.

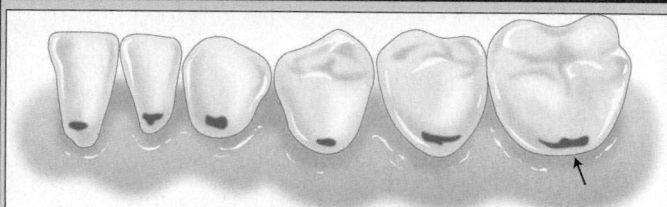

FIGURE 19-71
Class V cervical third.

Class VI

Class VI caries involve the incisal or occlusal surface that has been worn away due to abrasion (Figure 19-72).

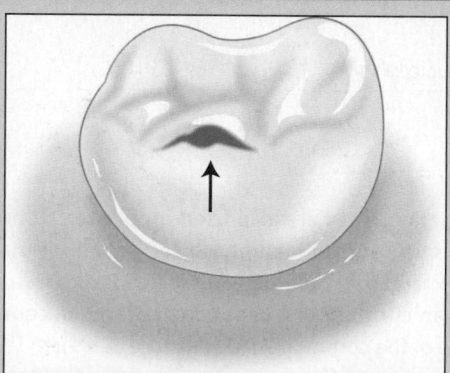

FIGURE 19-72
Class VI incisal/occlusal abrasion.

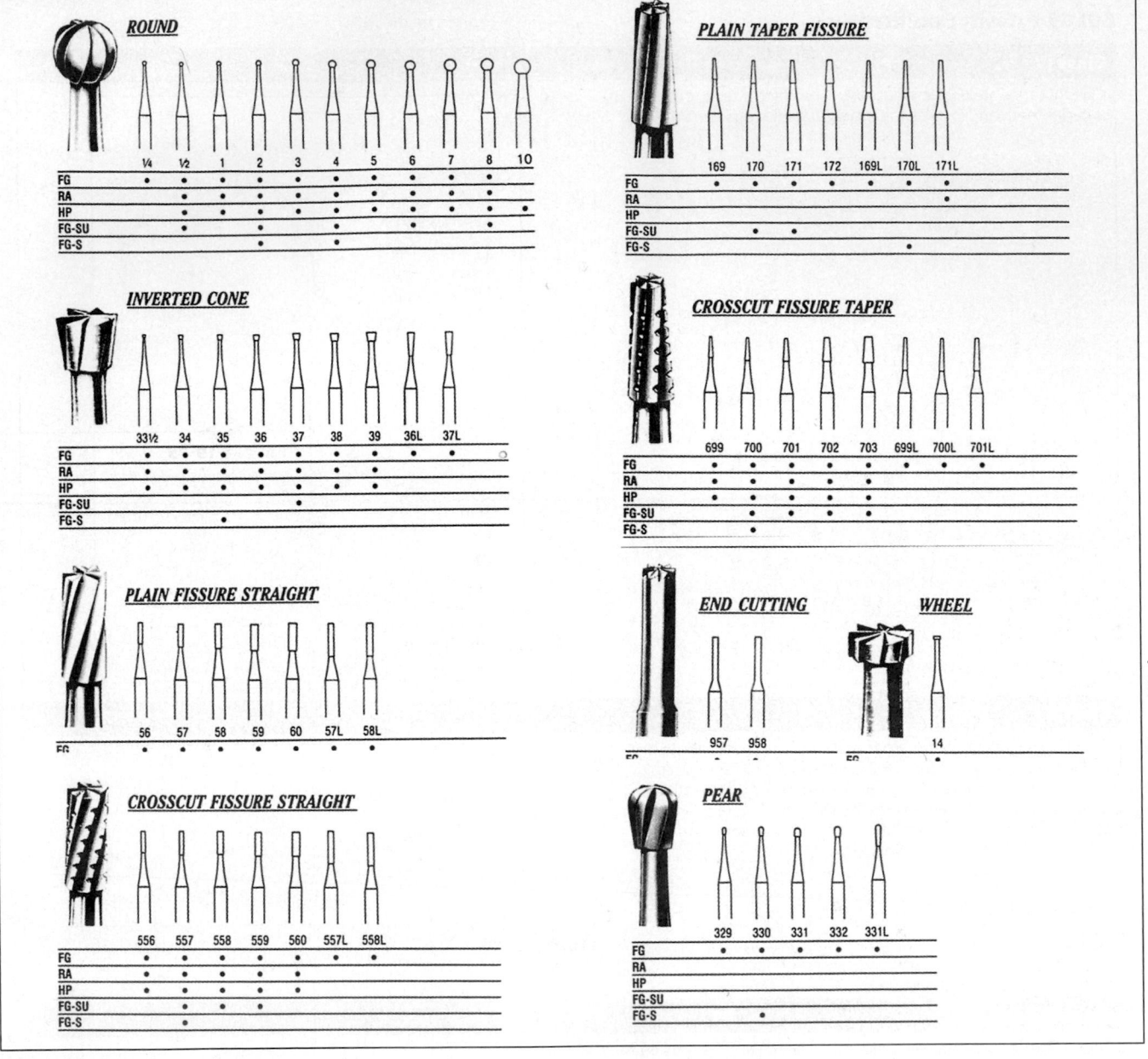

FIGURE 19-73
Bur shapes and number ranges.

and bleaching trays. They are also used on plaster, stone, and metal materials. The vulcanite bur has a long shank, is made of carbide steel, is named by the shape of the head, and has a much larger head than cutting burs. Pear, tapered, round, cone, and barrel are some of the common shapes (Figure 19-89).

Finishing Burs The **finishing** burs contain a greater number and finer flutes (30 blades) than the cutting burs. Finishing burs smooth, trim, and finish metal restorations and natural

tooth–colored materials. These burs are used to final finish restorations and to polish older restorations. The finishing burs smooth surfaces and removes scratches, pits, and **flash** from restorations. When used on older restorations, they help in removing tarnishing and corrosion. Finishing burs are supplied in shapes and sizes similar to cutting burs. They have many additional shapes including flame, cone, and barrel (Figure 19-90). They are identified by the manufacturer's number. Some are color coded for easy identification. A red band indicates 8 and 12 blades on the finishing

TABLE 19-1 Cutting Burs and Their Functions

Cutting Bur Name and Function	Image and Number Series	Example of Uses
Round Burs Ball shaped head used first to open the cavity and remove carious tooth structure (Figure 19-74). Larger round burs in low-speed handpieces used to remove carious tissue from larger cavities. Since the bur turns slowly, the dentist can feel the bur hitting solid healthy tooth and stop to prevent pulpal exposure. Small round burs prepare decayed pits and fissures and make retentive points in the preparation to help retain restorations (Figure 19-75).	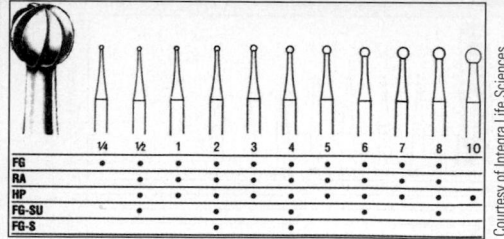 Number series is ¼, ½, 2, 4, 6, 8, and 10. **FIGURE 19-74** Round bur series.	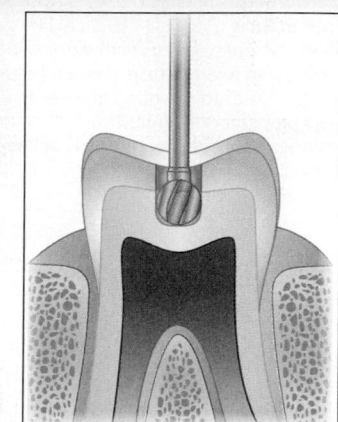 **FIGURE 19-75** Round bur use.
Inverted Burs A cone (triangular shape) turned upside down (inverted) onto the neck of the bur (Figure 19-76). Removes caries and the points of the inverted cone make retentive points and undercuts in the cavity preparation to help hold the restoration in the cavity while cutting a flat floor of the cavity preparation (Figure 19-77).	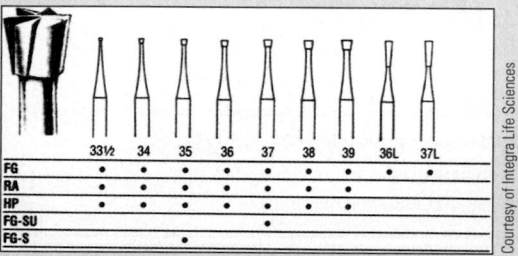 Number series is the 30s (33-1/3 to 39). **FIGURE 19-76** Inverted bur series.	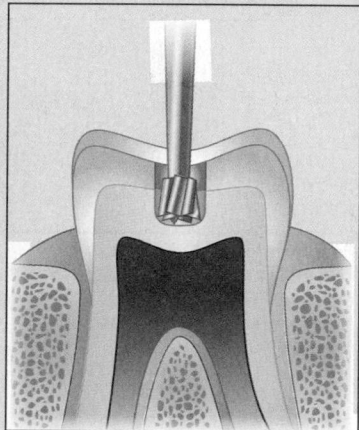 **FIGURE 19-77** Inverted bur use.
Straight Burs Cylindrical in shape and have vertical grooves called fissures; also referred to as straight fissure burs (Figure 19-78). Used to open a tooth and make walls of the preparation straight and perpendicular to the pulpal floor (Figure 19-80). For a smooth slow cut, a *plain cut straight fissure bur* is used to prepare the tooth. For a faster, rough cut a *cross-cut fissure straight bur* may be preferred. They have horizontal grooves along the fissures called cross cuts (Figure 19-79). Normally, the fissure burs are flat on the end, but some fissure burs have rounded or dome-shaped working ends. The number range for these burs differs from that for the regular fissure burs.	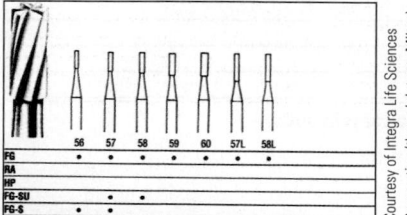 Number series is in 50s. **FIGURE 19-78** Plain straight bur series. 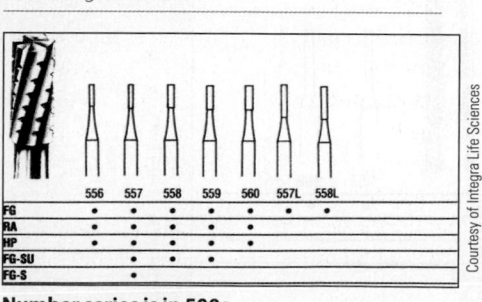 Number series is in 500s. **FIGURE 19-79** Cross-cut straight bur series.	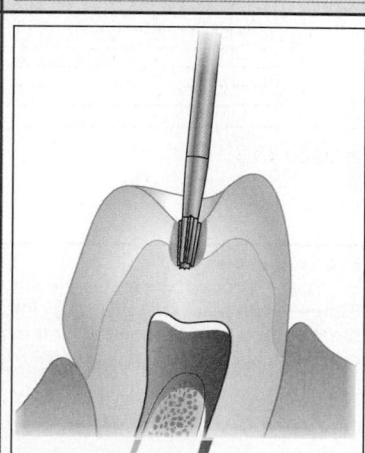 **FIGURE 19-80** Straight bur use.

(Continues)

TABLE 19-1 *(Continued)*

Cutting Bur Name and Function	Image and Number Series	Example of Uses

Tapered Burs
Cylindrical, pointed burs with vertical grooves also referred to as tapered fissure burs. Cut detailed retention grooves in the cavity preparation (Figure 19-83). Fissures are either *plain cut* (Figure 19-81) or have *cross cuts* (Figure 19-82).

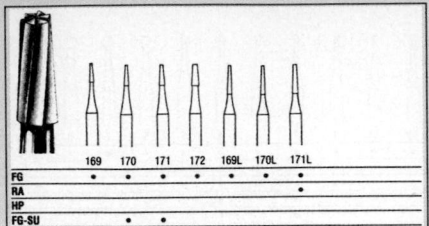

	169	170	171	172	169L	170L	171L
FG	•	•	•	•	•	•	•
RA							•
HP							
FG-SU		•	•				
FG-S				•			

Courtesy of Integra Life Sciences Corporation (through Integra Miltex)

Number series is in 160s and 170s.

FIGURE 19-81
Plain tapered bur series.

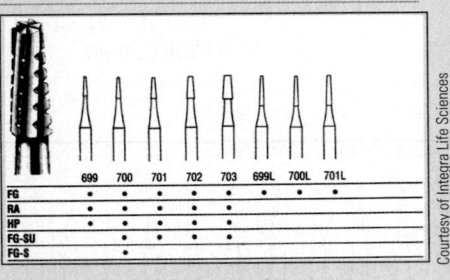

	699	700	701	702	703	699L	700L	701L
FG	•	•	•	•	•	•	•	•
RA	•	•	•	•	•	•		
HP	•	•	•	•	•			
FG-SU		•	•	•	•			
FG-S		•						

Courtesy of Integra Life Sciences Corporation (through Integra Miltex)

Number series is in 160s and 170s.

FIGURE 19-82
Cross-cut tapered bur series.

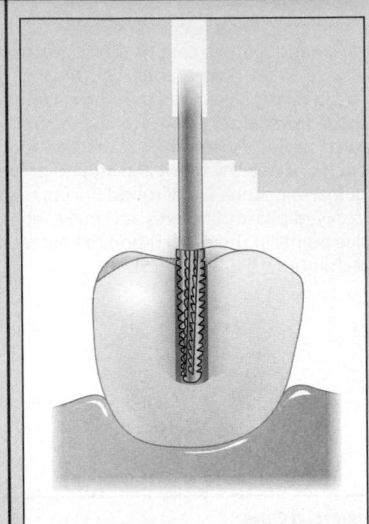

FIGURE 19-83
Tapered bur use.

Pear Burs
Resemble a pear inverted onto the neck of the shank (Figure 19-84). Designed to open and shape small cavity preparations (Figure 19-85).

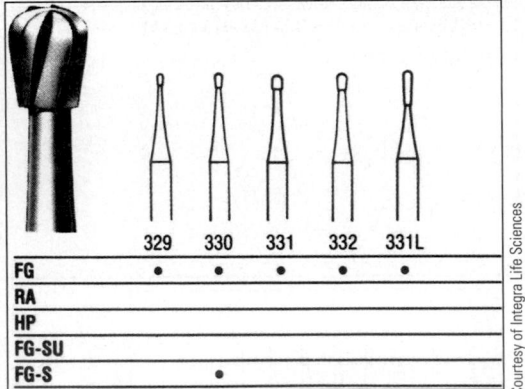

	329	330	331	332	331L
FG	•	•	•	•	•
RA					
HP					
FG-SU					
FG-S		•			

Courtesy of Integra Life Sciences Corporation (through Integra Miltex)

Number series is in 300s.

FIGURE 19-84
Pear bur series.

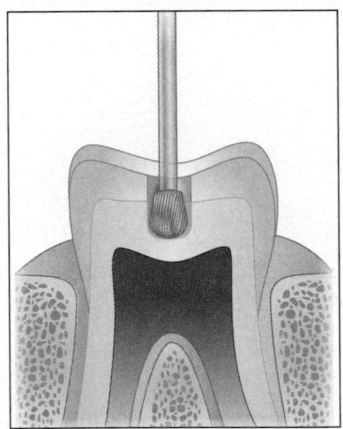

FIGURE 19-85
Tapered bur use.

End Cutting Burs
Have cutting edge at the end of the bur (Figure 19-86). Make the initial entry into the tooth and create a shoulder for the margin of a crown preparation (Figure 19-87).

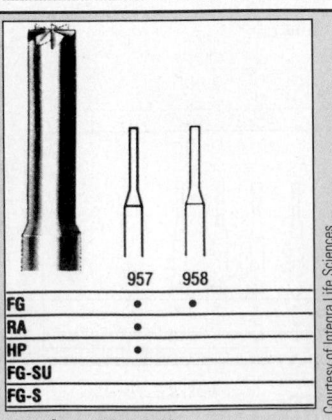

	957	958
FG	•	•
RA	•	
HP	•	
FG-SU		
FG-S		

Courtesy of Integra Life Sciences Corporation (through Integra Miltex)

Numbers 957, 958

FIGURE 19-86
End cutting bur series.

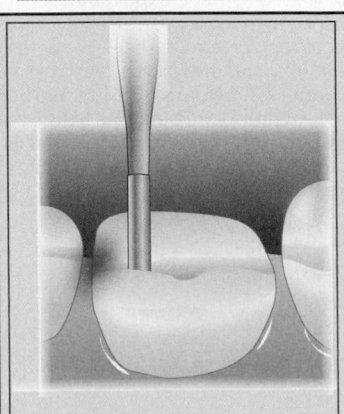

FIGURE 19-87
End cutting bur use.

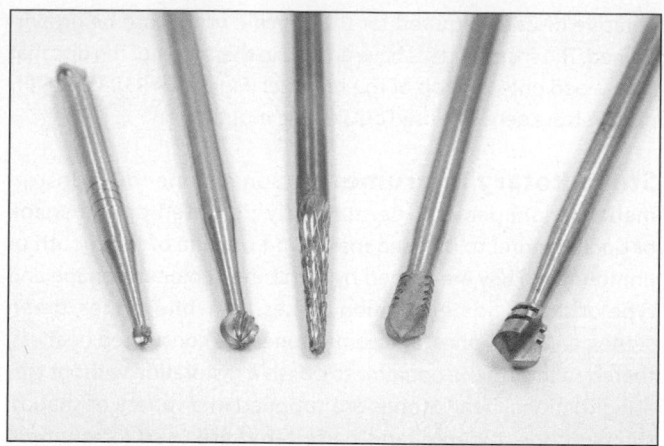

FIGURE 19-88
Surgical burs.

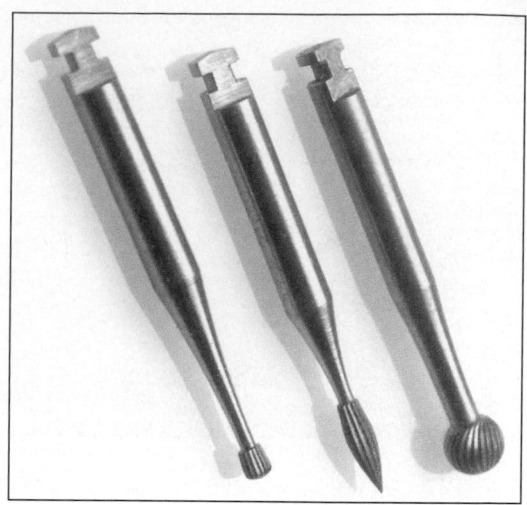

FIGURE 19-90
Finishing burs in various shapes.

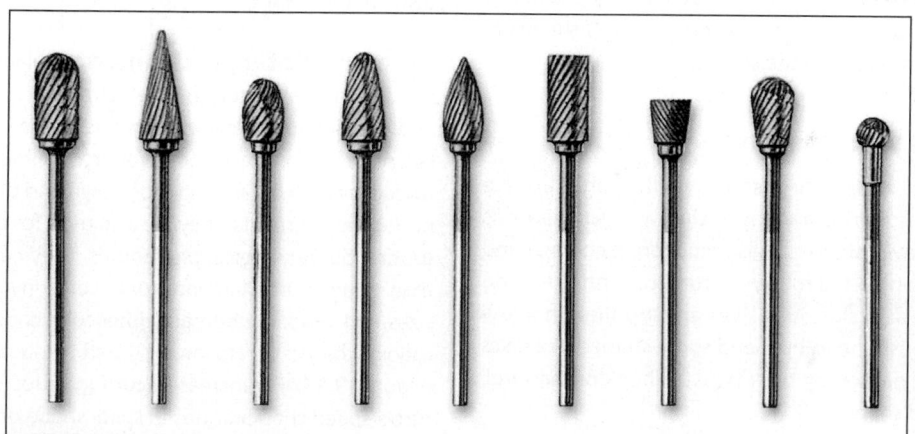

FIGURE 19-89
Laboratory burs.

Courtesy of Integra Life Sciences Corporation [through Integra Miltex]

bur. A yellow band indicates 16 and 20 blades, and a white band indicates a 30-blade finishing bur.

Fissurotomy Burs

Fissurotomy burs are extremely small (0.33 mm). Made of carbide, they are used to explore the occlusal surface and to allow for effective diagnoses and treatment while preserving healthy tooth structure. These burs cut quickly, leaving a smooth, minimally invasive groove in suspicious pits and fissures. Fissurotomy burs are designed as depth gauges, giving the burs minimal access to the fissures and permitting virtually pain-free fissure cavity preparation (Figure 19-91).

Bur Blocks

Rotary instruments are stored in a bur block. There are many variations and designs, such as round or rectangular shapes. Bur blocks come with covers and may be magnetic. Both friction-grip and latch-type burs can be stored in bur blocks. They are made of metal or plastic (Figure 19-92).

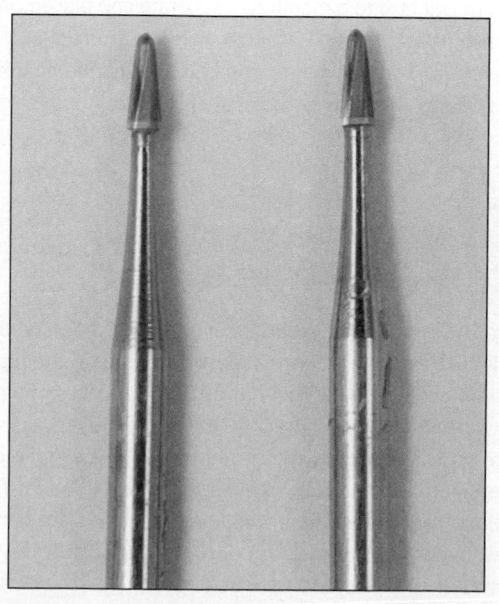

FIGURE 19-91
Fissurotomy burs.

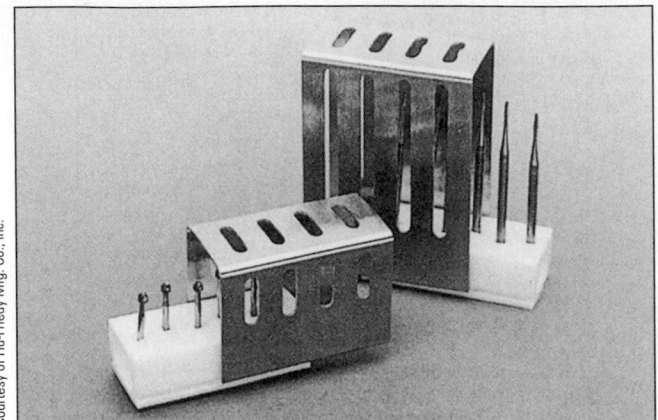

FIGURE 19-92
Bur block with covers, magnetized and made of metal.

Some bur blocks can be sterilized with the burs they hold. If the bur blocks cannot be sterilized, the burs are placed in a mesh holder that looks like a tea strainer and run through the ultrasonic cleaner, and then placed in the sterilizer.

Abrasive Rotary Instruments

Abrasive materials are held onto metals by adhesion. Abrasive rotary instruments can perform many of the same functions as the cutting burs; however, some can also function to cut finer and smoother. They are nonbladed rotary instruments and are made of a variety of stone particles. Abrasives are supplied in many forms, some similar in shape to burs and some shaped like discs and wheels. They are named by their type of shank or mandrel, abrasive material, and shape.

Mandrels
A **mandrel** is a rod used in low-speed handpieces with various abrasives. The abrasives are either permanently attached (mounted) to a mandrel or separate and placed on a mandrel (unmounted). Mandrels are available in short-shank latched (SS LA) and short-shank friction grip (SS FG) and long-shank friction grip (LS FG) and with a screw-on or snap-on mounting to exchange

abrasive discs as required for the specific procedure being performed. The snap-on discs have an area in the center of the disc that is snapped onto the top of the mandrel (Figure 19-93). The LS FG mandrels are generally used outside the mouth.

Stone Rotary Instruments
Some stone rotary instruments are shaped and permanently mounted onto a shank or on a mandrel to be used inside and outside of the mouth or unmounted. They are named by the stone's color and shape and type of shank. Some common stones are white stones, green stones, and red stones, and some stones are considered heatless, thereby allowing the operator to polish a restoration without creating frictional heat. Stones are supplied in a variety of shapes, such as cone, tapered, and barrel, that are used for multiple purposes in dentistry including cutting, polishing, and finishing restorations and appliances (Figure 19-94). White stones, also miscalled resin burs, are used to finish resin materials. It is important when working on resin materials to use materials that will not discolor the resin.

Diamond Rotary Instruments
Diamond chips are imbedded in materials through an electroplating or a bonding process and are used to make precision cuts of harder structures. Diamond rotary instruments are often preferred to finish composite resin restorations and the refinement of crown and bridge preparations and occlusal adjustments. They are also used for bone and gingival contouring during surgical procedures. They cut faster and smoother than cutting burs. Diamond stones come in a wide variety of shapes, sizes, and **grits**. The burs are either color coded for easy grit identification or have letters following the stone numbers to indicate the grit (Figure 19-95). For increased cutting reduction of tooth structure, turbo/speed cut diamonds in spiral shape or dual cross cut may be used. These instruments, however, are more costly, maintained differently, and often stored separate from the cutting burs. They are often inaccurately referred to as diamond burs; remember burs have flutes.

Abrasive Discs
The abrasive discs are round and flat or concave. An abrasive stone can be shaped as a disc and permanently mounted onto a shank or mandrel. The discs are also designed

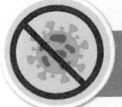 Infection Control

Due to the structures that burs cut and their shape, debris collects in the grooves between the flutes. Burs need to be cleaned thoroughly by being placed into a mesh container in the ultrasonic general cleaner. The assistant needs to inspect each bur and remove any remaining debris with a bur brush prior to disinfection or sterilization. The assistant should hold the bur by its shank and brush downward into the sink until all debris is removed. Burs can be disinfected with laboratory use only provided the bur did not come in contact with biohazard contamination. When in direct contact with a patient, the bur is a convenient carrier of disease and must be sterilized. The assistant should read directions for specific rotary instruments. Some manufacturers recommend the use of an autoclave, and others prefer dry heat oven. Burs are generally stored in bur blocks placed in specified positions in the block for easy retrieval. Many bur blocks are designed to be autoclaved with the burs in position for use. Although this process saves money, it dulls the bur. To help decrease dulling the burs, the burs need to be dried prior to being placed in the sterilizer. Some dentists prefer using a bur once and disposing of it in the sharps container.

Procedure 19-7
Identification of Dental Burs

This procedure is performed by the dental assistant to identify the parts of a bur, types of shanks, names of burs, and number series for cutting burs.

Equipment and Supplies
- round burs (¼, ½, 2, 4, 6, 8, and 10)
- inverted burs (33-1/3 to 39)
- straight fissure plain cut bur (50s)
- straight fissure cross-cut bur (500s)
- tapered fissure plain cut bur (160s and 171s)
- tapered fissure cross-cut bur (600s and 700s)
- pear burs (300s)
- end cutting burs (957 and 958)

- diamond burs
- finishing burs
- surgical burs
- vulcanite laboratory burs
- fissurotomy burs

Procedure Steps
1. Examine the instrument closely.
2. Identify the instrument by name.
3. Identify the type of shank (SS LA, SS FG, LS LA, LS FG).
4. Recall the instrument's number series and/or shapes.
5. List the procedure(s) where the instrument may be used.

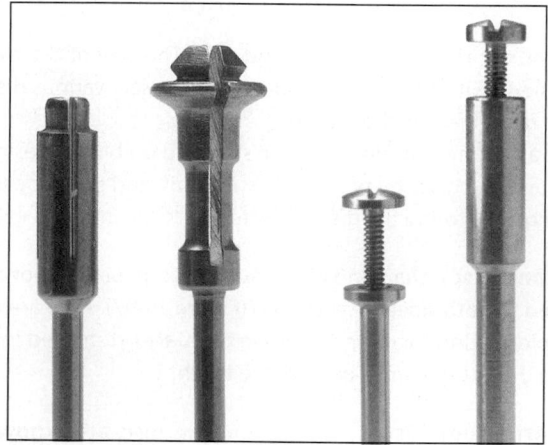

FIGURE 19-93
Mandrels with different heads. Two mandrels shown on the left are snap-on and the two on the right are screw-type mandrels.

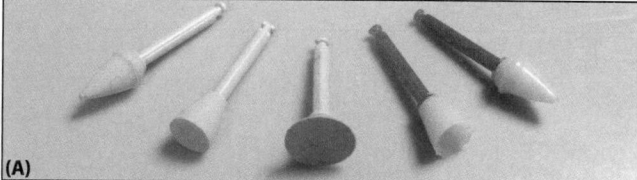
(A)

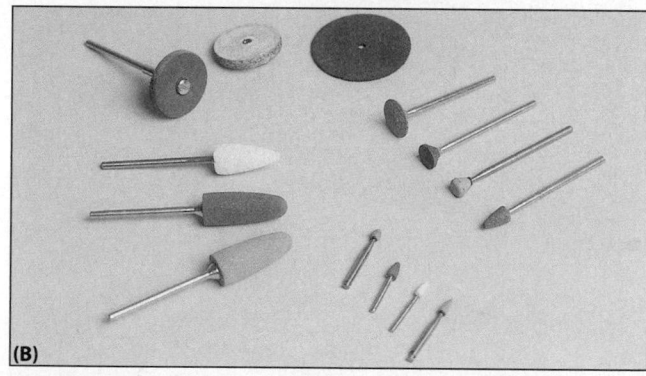
(B)

FIGURE 19-94
(A) Various points, cups, and wheels to define, polish, and finish composite restoration. (B) Various types and grits of stones, wheels, and points.

with a hole in the center of the disc to be mounted onto a screw-on mandrel or with a metal reinforced hole to be placed onto a snap-on mandrel.

Abrasive materials are also supplied as discs of metal, plastic, or paper with abrasive material on one or both sides. With abrasives on both sides, they can cut with both sides of the disc. When cutting between the teeth, the disc with abrasives on one side is often preferred to cut only the tooth being prepared. These discs are often referred to as separating discs and also known as safe-sided discs since they will not harm the adjacent tooth. The discs may be rigid or flexible and are available in a variety of sizes and **grits**. The abrasive material may be made of several different materials, such as **garnet**, diamond, quartz, sand, and **carborundum**. When ordering abrasives, the size, grit, abrasiveness, and mandrel type must be specified.

Sandpaper Discs Some discs have sandy particles from stones attached to the disc. These are referred to as sandpaper discs; this name is given even when attached to plastic discs. Sandpaper discs are described by the type of abrasive, its grit, and the size of the disc. The more common types of abrasive used are **cuttle**, sand, garnet, and **emery** (Figure 19-96).

The grit of the disc is determined by the size of the abrasive particle. The larger the particle size, the faster and rougher the cut. The grit is described as extra-coarse, coarse, medium, fine, and extra-fine. This is named very similar to sandpaper used to

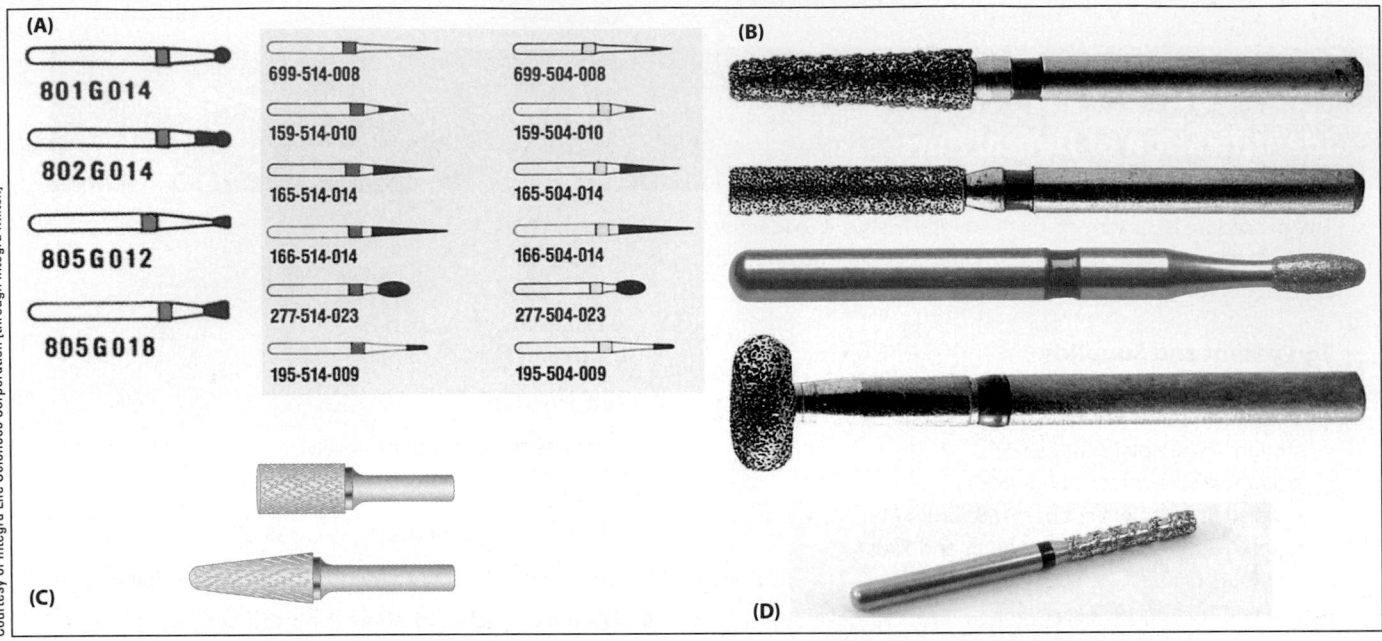

FIGURE 19-95
(A) Various shaped diamond rotary instruments in: coarse, fine, and extra-fine. (B) Variety of diamond stones. (C) Turbo spiral shaped. (D) Dual-crosscut.

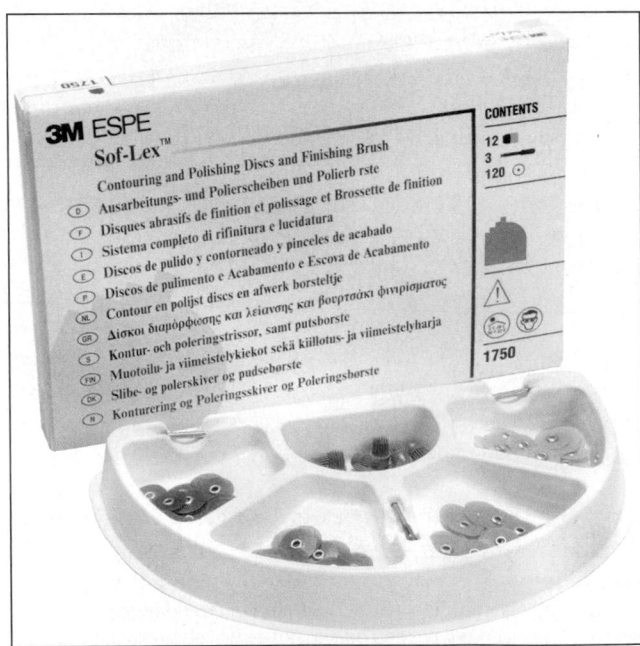

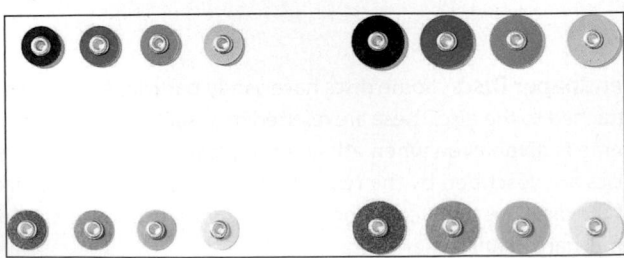

FIGURE 19-96
Sandpaper discs in various shapes, sizes, types, and grits. The cuttle discs are white, sand is sand color, garnet is a redder brown, and emery is black.

finish surfaces of wood, walls, and cars. The size of the disc is measured by its diameter. The operator will select various diameters to reach areas in the mouth.

An assortment of discs may be supplied on blocks designed to display the discs by type of abrasive, grit, and size for ease in locating and storing the discs. They may also be arranged in kits.

Diamond Discs Diamond discs have diamond particles or chips bonded to both sides of steel discs (Figure 19-97). They are used for rapid cutting. Diamond concave discs are often used in preparing the interproximal areas of the tooth.

Carborundum Discs A **carborundum** disc, also known as a Jo-dandy disc and separating disc, is a thin, brittle disc that breaks easily. They are double-sided and are used primarily in the dental laboratory to cut and finish gold restorations, but they can be used intraorally as well (Figure 19-98).

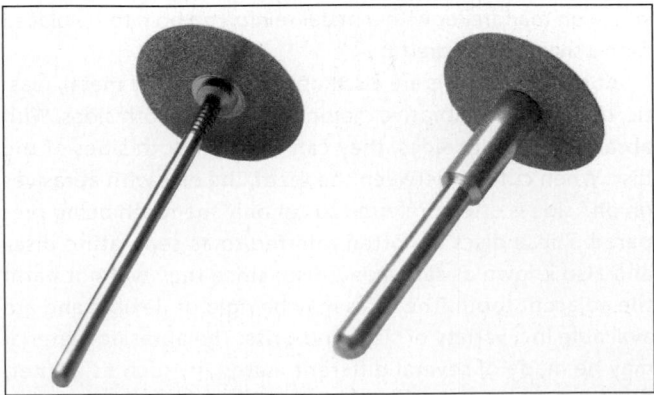

FIGURE 19-97
Diamond discs for rapid cutting.

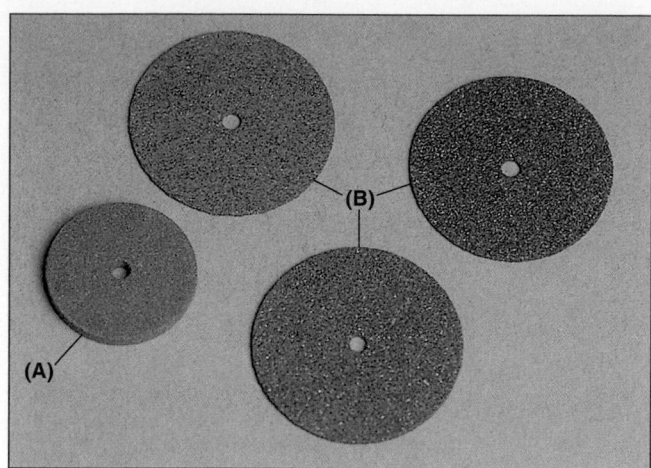

FIGURE 19-98
(A) Rubber wheel. (B) Carborundum discs.

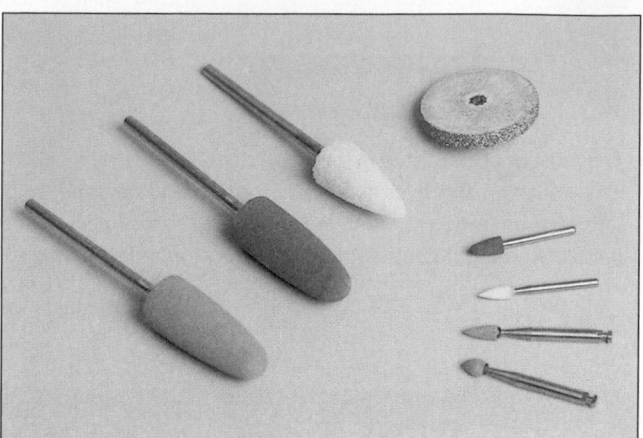

FIGURE 19-99
Wheels and points.

Abrasive Wheels Abrasive wheels are thicker than discs (Figure 19-98). Wheels can be used outside the mouth for laboratory work and intraorally to adjust the height of appliances and for **equilibration**. One of the more common wheels is the heatless stone. This stone can cut while producing minimal heat.

Rotary Polishing Instruments There are many polishing instruments designed to apply abrasive agents in the oral cavity. Rubber cups (prophy cups) are used to remove stain and biofilm and to clean and polish teeth and restorations. Powder, paste, and gel agents are applied to the tooth surfaces using the rubber cup attached to a right angle (prophy angle). Prophy brushes remove stain and clean and polish the pits and fissures of teeth and restorations. The brushes are also attached to right angles. Most prophy cup and brushes are made for one time use. In situations where these are reused, they must be cleaned in the ultrasonic cleaner and placed in a sterilant per manufacturer's directions.

There are polishing instruments to apply abrasives to polish dental appliances in the laboratory area. Some of the more common instruments are burlew rotary instruments, bristle brushes, and ragwheels.

Rubber (Burlew) Rotary Instruments The rubber **burlew** rotary instruments are made from soft to hard rubber to remove scratches from appliances and restorations. They are supplied as discs, wheels, and tips (Figures 19-98A and 19-99). The mandrels utilized with these instruments may be LS or SS permanently mounted or screw on. Wheels are made of rubber material impregnated with an abrasive agent. They come mounted and unmounted and are available in various grits. They are used for finishing and polishing. Rubber points come in a variety of sizes and grits. They are made of rubber material impregnated with abrasive agents. Points are used to polish and are especially adaptable when defining anatomy in the restoration.

Bristle Brush The bristle brush resembles a chimney brush and initially polishes appliances in the laboratory outside the mouth. Since the brush itself is not abrasive, the operator needs to add abrasives to the brush. The operator uses various abrasive compounds in cake form or gritty pumice in a water/pumice slurry.

Rag/Feltwheel A ragwheel resembles small rags held together. The operator applies coarse to fine pumice to polish appliances to a high luster outside of the mouth. A rouge compound that is a very fine abrasive is used with the ragwheel to polish metal structures. A felt wheel, made of felt material, is another option. Ragwheels must be sterilized after each use or be used for one time only.

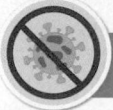 Infection Control

Most abrasive rotary instruments used intraorally are made for one time use. All other abrasive rotary instruments should be cleaned using the ultrasonic cleaner, disinfected, rinsed, and dried well. Employing a bur brush to remove debris will remove the abrasive particles and should never be done. Brushing one abrasive instrument against another will help with hard-to-remove debris without damaging the surface. High heat may melt the adhesion holding the abrasive; therefore, it is important to check the manufacturer directions before sterilization. Most directions will state that diamonds made for direct patient care are safe to be sterilized using heat sterilizers.

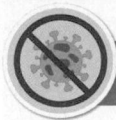

Infection Control

The most important step in handling dental appliances is adequately cleaning and disinfecting before beginning work in the laboratory. Polishing abrasives in powder form should be disposed of after use, and abrasive compound should be sprayed with disinfectant recommended in manufacturer's directions. Polishing rotary instruments can be brushed against each other to remove loose debris, then should be cleaned in the ultrasonic cleaner and submerged in high-level disinfectant.

Procedure 19-8
Identification of Abrasive and Polishing Rotary Instruments

This procedure is performed by the dental assistant to identify types of mandrels and mountings, and abrasive and polishing rotary instruments.

Equipment and Supplies
- assortment of mandrels
- stone rotary instruments (white, green, red, and heatless)
- diamond rotary instruments
- sandpaper discs (cuttle, sand, garnet, and emery and extra-fine, fine, medium, coarse, and extra-coarse)
- diamond disc
- carborundum (Jo-dandy) disc
- abrasive wheel
- rubber (burlew) wheel
- rubber (burlew) points
- bristle brush
- rag/feltwheel

Procedure Steps

1. Examine the instrument closely.
2. Identify the instrument by name.
3. Identify the type of mandrel (SS LA, SS FG, LS LA, LS FG).
4. Identify the type of mounting (permanently, screw-on, snap-on).
5. Explain how it is used.
6. List the procedure(s) where the instrument may be used.

Procedure 19-9

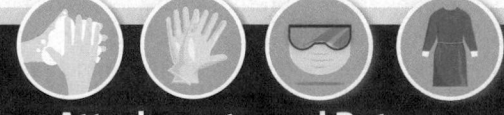

Identify and Attach Dental Handpieces, Handpiece Attachments, and Rotary Instruments

This procedure is performed by the dental assistant to identify various dental handpieces and handpiece attachments, demonstrate how to assemble and attach to the dental unit, and place a rotary instrument.

Equipment and Supplies
- high-speed handpiece
- low-speed straight handpiece
- contra-angle/latch attachment
- prophy/right-angle attachment
- variety of dental rotary instruments shanks (SS LA; SS FG; LS FG)

Procedure Steps

1. Identify the high-speed handpiece.
   - ❏ Attach it to the high-speed dental unit coupling/hose (Figure 19-100).
   - ❏ Align the receptors properly so the handpiece fits securely.
2. Place the rotary instrument into the high-speed handpiece.
   - ❏ Select SS FG bur.
   - ❏ Open the chuck by pressing on the autochuck or with a bur tool.

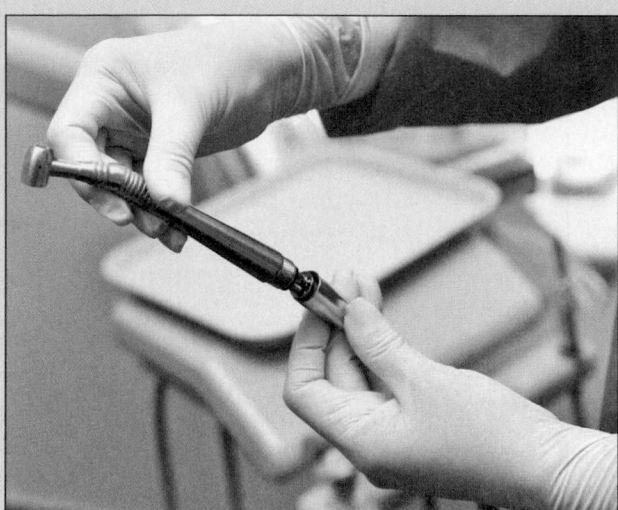

FIGURE 19-100
Attach high-speed handpiece to dental unit coupling/hose.

❏ Insert into the high-speed handpiece (Figure 19-101).
❏ Release the autochuck or tighten using the bur tool for the chuck to grasp the bur.

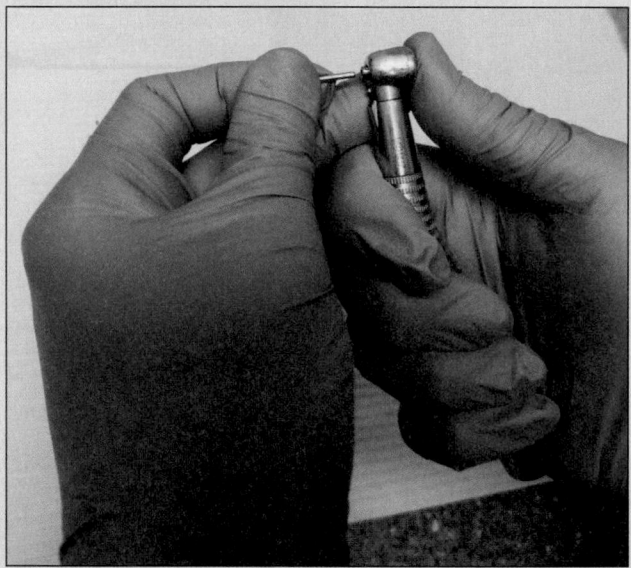

FIGURE 19-101
Insert SS FG into high-speed handpiece using autochuck.

❏ Check to be sure that the bur is secure by tugging on the bur between fingers.

3. Identify the low-speed handpiece.
   ❏ Attach it to the low-speed dental unit coupling/hose (Figure 19-102).
   ❏ Align the handpiece with the receptors so the handpiece fits securely.

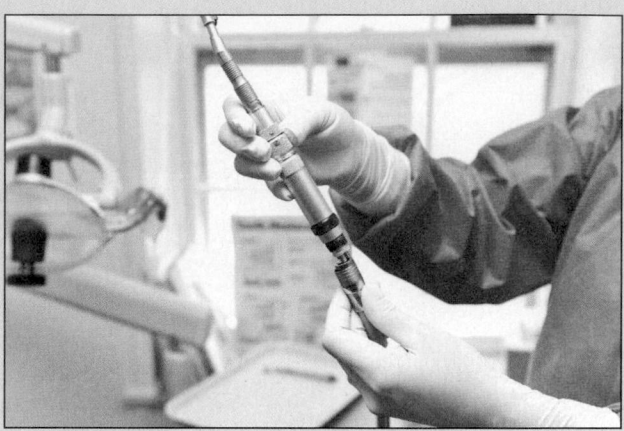

FIGURE 19-102
Attach the low-speed handpiece into dental unit coupling/hose.

4. Place the rotary instrument into the low-speed straight handpiece.
   ❏ Select an LS FG bur.
   ❏ Insert it into the chuck of the low-speed handpiece (Figure 19-103). Depending on the handpiece, twist or press the control to open the chuck to receive the bur.

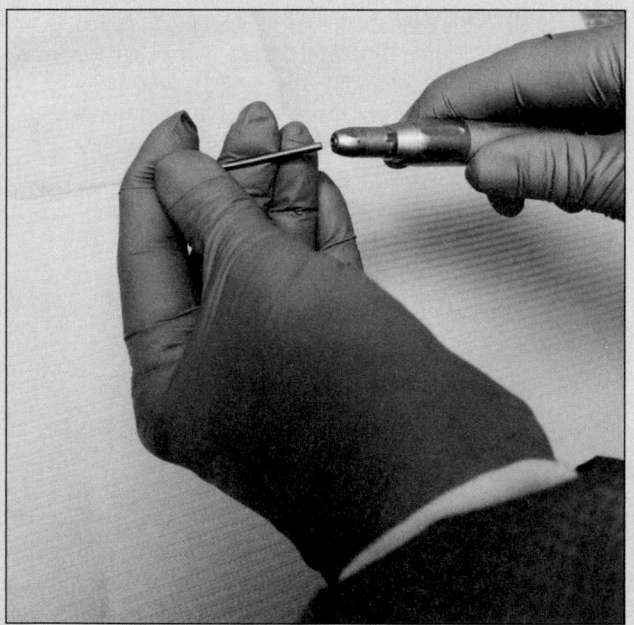

FIGURE 19-103
Insert LS FG into low-speed handpiece.

❏ Twist the control on the handpiece to lock it in place.
❏ Check to be sure that the bur is secure by tugging on the bur between fingers.

5. Identify the contra-angle attachment.
   ❏ Attach to the low-speed handpiece by slipping it over the working end of the straight handpiece (Figure 19-104).

(Continues)

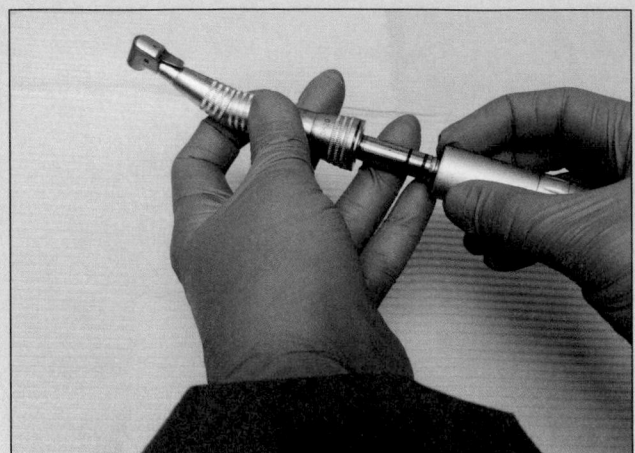

FIGURE 19-104
Attach contra-angle to straight low-speed.

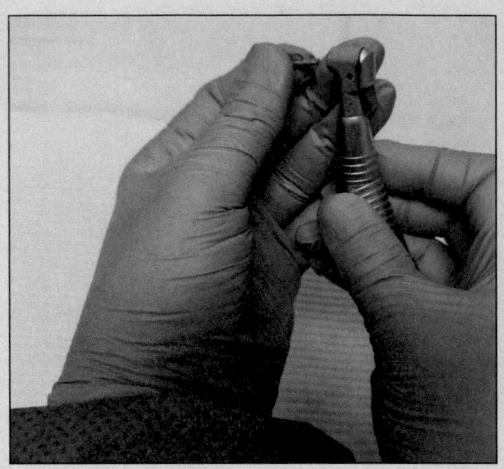

FIGURE 19-105
Insert bur into latched contra.

6. Place the rotary instrument into the low-speed handpiece.
   - ❏ Select an SS LA (some low-speed handpieces have an autochuck like the high-speed and will use an SS FG bur).
   - ❏ Open the contra-angle latch, insert the bur into the chuck (Figure 19-105), and check that it went to end of the chuck.
   - ❏ Close the lever and check to be sure the bur is secure.
7. Identify the prophy/right-angle attachment.
   - ❏ Attach it to the low-speed handpiece by slipping it over the working end of the straight handpiece or U-style adaptor (Figure 19-106).
   - ❏ Twist the control on the handpiece to lock it in place.
   - ❏ Select a prophy cup or brush and place on prophy angle.

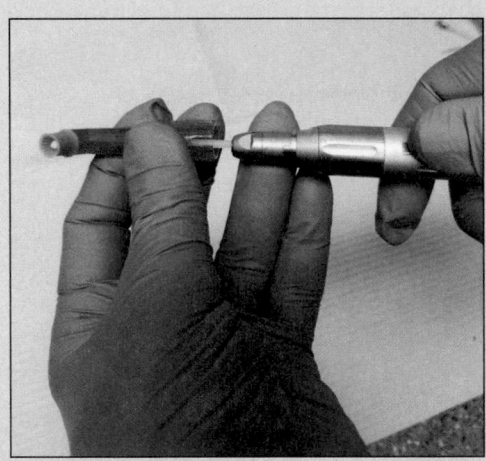

FIGURE 19-106
Right angle onto U-style.

Tray Systems

A preset tray system is most commonly used in dental offices. It provides an efficient means of transporting instruments to the treatment room, which saves time for the dental assistant. There are many systems available, including plastic or metal trays, tubs, or the cassette system.

Trays and Tubs

Trays, tubs, and accessories can be color coded for efficient handling and storage (Figure 19-107). Plastic or paper barriers are used before placing instruments on the tray, especially for ribbed trays. These barriers help with tray disinfection. The tubs hold the materials needed to complete a particular procedure (Figure 19-108).

Cassette System for Instruments

Cassette systems are designed to carry instruments for use in treatment rooms, through the cleaning and sterilizing processes,

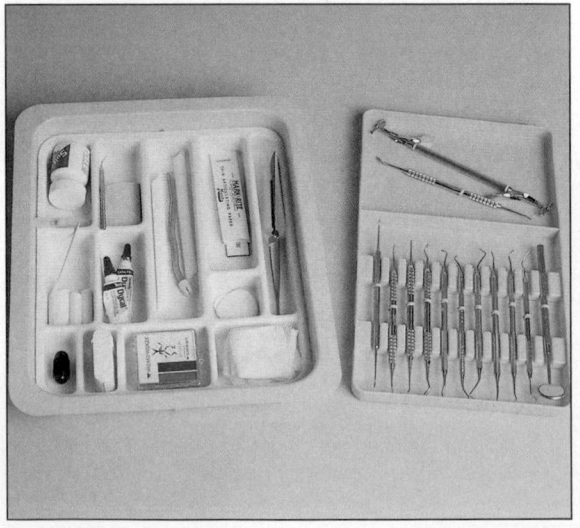

FIGURE 19-107
Tub, tray, and instruments all color coded. Shown are the instruments on the tray and the materials needed for an amalgam procedure in the tub.

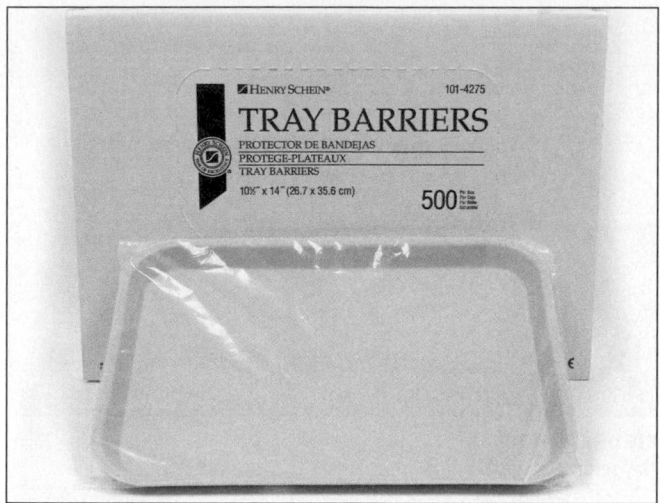

FIGURE 19-108
Tray barriers are used to cover the tray. They protect the tray from moisture and liquid that may occur during a procedure.

and then into storage (Figure 19-109). Instruments for a certain procedure are color coded and then placed in a cassette. The cassette provides an efficient and safe means for handling instruments. Also, when the cassette is open, it provides its own tray. After being used for a procedure, the cassette is carried to the sterilization area. Here the instruments are reorganized and placed in the cassette. When the cassette is closed, the instruments remain securely in place. The cassette is then placed in the ultrasonic or instrument washer. When this process is complete, the cassette is rinsed thoroughly and then wrapped or packaged and labeled, sterilized, and stored until needed. In the treatment room, the cassette is unwrapped on the counter top or cart, ready for use. The wrap acts as a barrier between the tray and the counter.

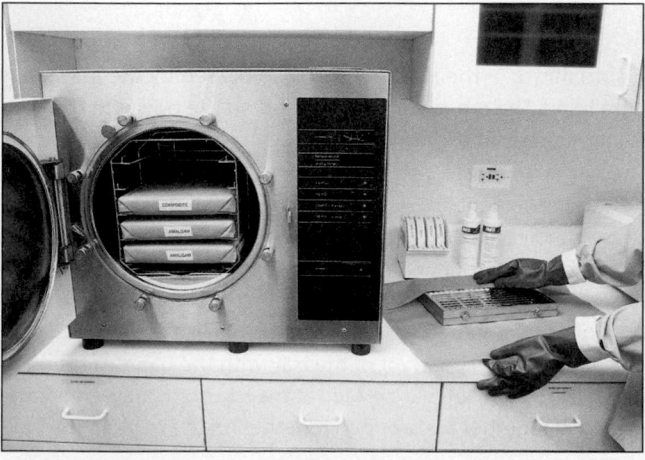

FIGURE 19-109
Cassette system. Cassettes are wrapped in paper and taped with label tape and then placed in sterilizer.

The cassette system efficiently keeps instruments together at all times. It increases safety by reducing the possibility of puncture injuries during cleaning and sterilizing. The cassettes come in different sizes and can be stored vertically or horizontally because the instruments are held into position. The wrapped cassettes are labeled with tape that is premarked for all procedures performed in the office. This makes it easy to identify the tray set that is needed in the treatment rooms. For more information, refer to Chapter 11, "Infection Control."

Prepare for Tray Setup

Anticipation and preparation for the scheduled appointments throughout the day allow for time efficiency, productivity, high-quality patient care, and a smooth running day. Many offices have a brief staff meeting to review the day and post daily schedules before patients arrive. If meetings are not a part of the office routine, the dental assistant needs to review the procedures for the day to be knowledgeable of the upcoming procedures. The assistant should also check the posted schedule for updates. This will help the assistant to be ready with preset tray setups and with any needed supplies, equipment, and laboratory work.

The first step in preparing the tray setup for the next patient is to review the patient's records for medical alerts, that day's treatment, and anticipated procedures. There are as many different tray setups as there are dentists and procedures. As an assistant, you need to know the setup for each given procedure—all instruments and materials. Prior to the patient being seated, the assistant needs to be sure that they are prepared for the next scheduled appointment, have acquired the correct patient chart, and know the setup for the proper procedure. Not equipping the tray setup with the appropriate materials, instruments, and expendables will waste valuable time, productivity, and money.

Set Up Patient Tray Having standard procedures and tray setups enhances the quality of service. Tray setups consist of specific instruments that are needed for various procedures. Dental assistants complete the setup in an orderly fashion and place instruments on the tray by **sequence** of use during the procedure. This enhances productivity and eliminates confusion during procedures. The dentist will need particular instruments and materials to complete the procedure. The efficient dental assistant learns to anticipate what instruments the dentist needs. To assist in this, the dental assisting staff prepares standard setups. Specific instruments included in each setup will vary in different offices based on the dentist's preference.

The dental assistant selects which setups are needed for the next procedure, places sterile hand instruments onto an instrument tray, transports them to the patient treatment area, and places the tray on the bracket table. The setup may remain in the sterile cassette, be kept in sterile instrument bags on an instrument tray, or be placed onto a bracket table covered with a barrier. Items to be used on a patient should never be placed directly onto a working surface. All areas need to be covered to protect the patient from cross infection and protect the surface from infection and staining. Commercial tray barriers are made to cover the instruments trays, and bracket table covers are made to cover flat surface working areas.

No matter what procedure is to be completed, the patient's tray will always have three basic hand instruments, known as the basic tray setup. These instruments include the mouth mirror, dental explorer, and cotton pliers. Some offices include the articulating forceps in the basic setup. These instruments are included in the examination category of operative dentistry.

Every operator has preferences on the instrumentation for a procedure. However, there are some basic considerations:

- Clear plastic tray barriers may be placed.
- Instruments are placed in order of use.
- The basic tray setup (mouth mirror, explorer, and cotton pliers) is placed first.
- Instruments should be grouped according to functions; for example, all the carvers are placed together.
- Cotton supplies are usually arranged across the top of the tray.
- Scissors or other hinged instruments are placed on the far right of the tray for easy access.
- Return instruments to their original positions after receiving them from the operator. This ensures that an instrument can be found easily if the operator needs to use it again.
- Keep instruments clean and free of debris before returning them to the tray. Gauze sponges on the tray aid with the immediate removal of cement, blood, or debris, which will harden on the instrument after use.

Positioning Instruments
The instrument is placed onto the bracket table in with the tray lengthwise (tray's greatest length placed vertically) or widthwise (tray's greatest length placed horizontally) in front of the dental assistant depending on type of dental unit, available work space, and personal preference. When setting up a lengthwise tray, begin placing hand instruments from the bottom of the tray (end closest to you) to the end of the tray; the mirror is the instrument closest to the assistant (Figure 19-110). With the widthwise tray, begin placing instruments from the left of the tray to the right; the mirror is furthest towards the assistant's left hand (Figure 19-111).

The instruments are also positioned for ease in picking up, passing, and returning instruments to the tray. Dental assistants use the left hand to pass instruments to the dentist's right hand and use the right hand to pass instruments to the dentist's left hand. Note: Setting up for a right-handed operator and left handed-operator is different. This text will refer to setups and procedures for a right-handed operator.) The instruments are placed differently for the two tray positions to accommodate the ease in transferring instruments.

Setting Up for Lengthwise Tray
The general rule in placing hand instruments onto the lengthwise tray is that the instrument handles face the direction of the hand that the dental assistant will use to pass the instrument. For example, the dentist uses the

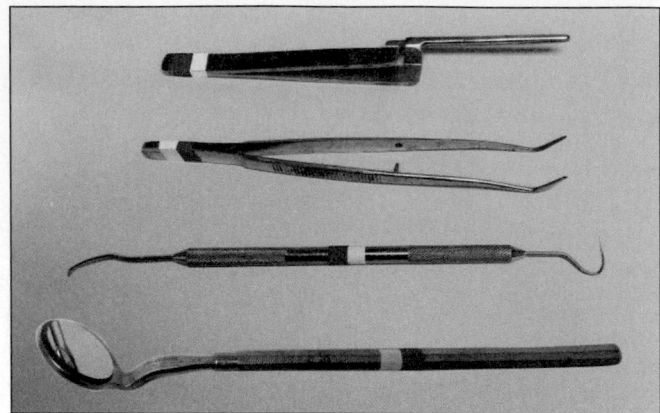

FIGURE 19-110
Tray setup prepared lengthwise.

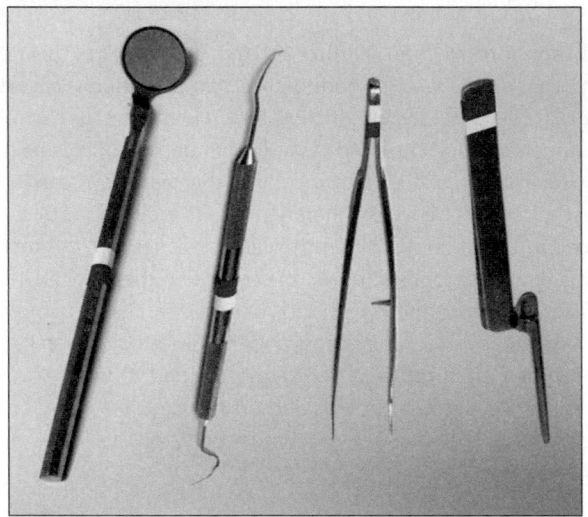

FIGURE 19-111
Tray setup prepared widthwise.

mouth mirror in their left hand, so it is passed by the assistant's right hand. The mouth mirror is placed on the tray with the handle facing toward the right side of the tray for the assistant's ease. The dental explorer, cotton pliers, and articulating forceps are passed to the dentist's right hand from the assistant's left hand. These handles are placed on the instrument tray with the handles facing toward the left. When placing a double-ended instrument, the end used most frequently or used first is placed facing toward the right of the tray. Accessory instruments like forceps and scissors are placed to the right of the tray with the handles facing to the right. Expendables are placed at the top of the tray, and materials used together are grouped together on the tray.

Setting Up for Widthwise Tray
The rule in placing instruments onto the widthwise tray is that the instruments passed with the

assistant's right hand have the handles toward the assistant (facing down). Instruments passed with the assistant's left hand have the handles toward the top of the tray (facing up).

Color-Coding Systems

Color coding is a method for easily identifying instruments and trays (Figure 19-112).

The color coding may be set up to indicate the following:

- Procedures, such as amalgam or composite.
- Treatment rooms, where the instruments are stored or used.
- Additional sets of instruments (there may be four composite setups, each marked for the procedure and then a second color for the set).

- Individual operators. The dentist may have two tray setups for prophylaxis and the hygienist may have four additional prophylaxis tray setups. Color coding keeps the dentist and the hygienist tray setups separate.
- Sequence. Instruments can be color coded diagonally to indicate the sequence of use.
- Any combination of these.

There are several types of materials used to color-code dental instruments, including plastic rings and colored coding tape. Color-coding tape may also be used to color-code tubs and trays, bur blocks, and tray mats. Also available are color-coded systems where the tubs, trays, tray mats, bur blocks, and mouth mirrors are all one color. Color-coding materials must be autoclavable and durable (Figures 19-104A to C).

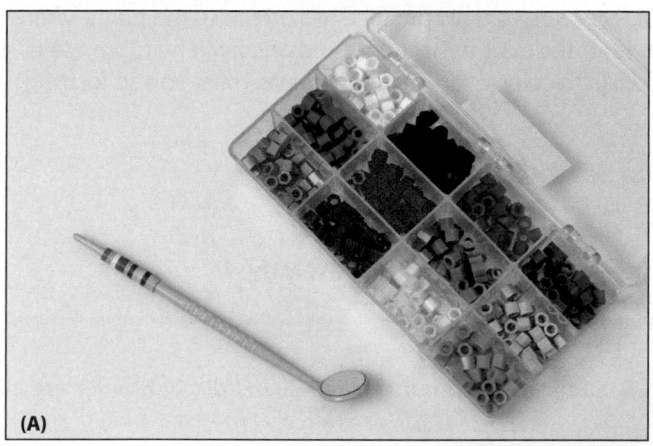

(A)

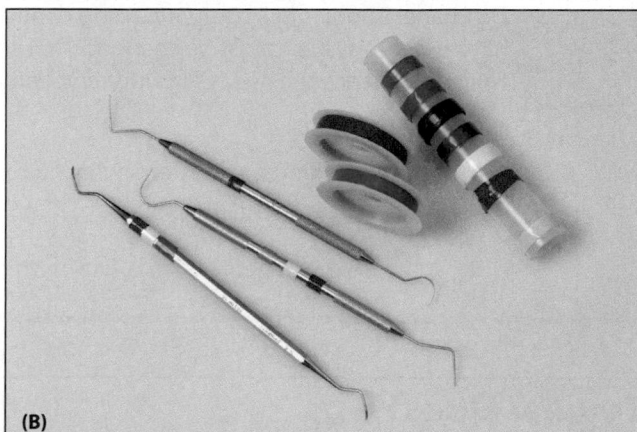

(B)

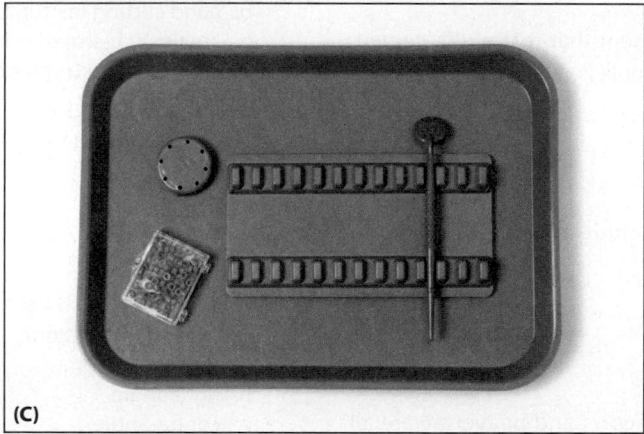

(C)

FIGURE 19-112
Color-coding materials. (A) Plastic rings. (B) Tape. (C) Tray, instrument mat, mouth mirror, bur block, and colored rings all color coordinated.

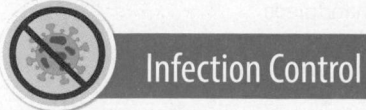 Infection Control

Chairside Infection Control

Once the instruments are placed on the bracket table, they should be covered to protect the instruments and materials from being contaminated and to prevent the patient from seeing the instruments while being seated. A biohazard bag should be placed near the working area to dispose of expendables throughout the procedure. The sign of an efficient assistant is when the tray is as organized and clean at the end of the procedure as it was at the beginning. Instruments should be returned to sequence for orderliness, and when time allows, the instrument should be wiped with a wet gauze prior to being replaced on the tray.

Chapter Summary

In this chapter you have studied that one of the very important responsibilities of the dental assistant is to be able to recognize, name, and maintain dental instruments and handpieces used in general dental procedures. The assistant is also responsible for keeping the instruments sterilized, organized, and in working condition. As each procedure and operator requires specific instruments, the efficient assistant learns to anticipate what instruments and materials are needed to complete the procedure in order to prepare and set up the patient tray. The assistant needs very good organizational skills to develop standard procedures and utilize various tray systems.

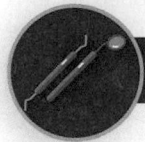

CASE STUDY

Dr. Charles Thomas has been practicing dentistry for five years, and his practice has grown to the point where his tray setup system must be changed. Dr. Thomas has three treatment rooms and one hygiene room. He is willing to finance the necessary updating and would like to color-code his instruments, trays, and so forth.

Case Study Review

1. Before deciding on a system, what factors must be considered?

2. Suggest some color-code combinations.

3. What are the benefits of an office in which a color-coding system is effectively used?

Review Questions

Multiple Choice

1. The part of the dental instrument that is straight, curved, monangle, binangle, or triple angle is called the _____.
   a. handle
   b. shank
   c. working end
   d. shaft

2. The mouth mirror's uses include all of the following EXCEPT:
   a. indirect vision.
   b. light reflection.
   c. retraction.
   d. direct vision.

3. Egg shaped, T-ball, football, acorn, and beavertail are all shapes of _____.
   a. finishing knives
   b. burnishers
   c. plastic filling instruments
   d. gingival margin trimmers

4. There is moisture in the tooth cavity, and it is ill-advised to use the air syringe. What expendable could the assistant pass the dentist?
   a. cotton gauze
   b. cotton pellet
   c. cotton roll
   d. cotton tip applicator

5. Burnisher, condensers, and cleoid-discoid carver are all _____.
   a. examinations instruments
   b. hand cutting instruments
   c. amalgam restorative instruments
   d. composite instruments

6. Which power source is most commonly used in today's restorative procedures?
   a. belt-pulley
   b. motor-driven
   c. air-driven
   d. electric-driven

7. Which handpiece is used to remove decay and develop the cavity for a restoration?
   a. straight
   b. right angle
   c. contra-angle
   d. high-speed

8. The part of the handpiece where rotary instruments and attachments are held is called the _____.
   a. working end of the handpiece
   b. shank of the handpiece
   c. connecting end of the handpiece
   d. holder

9. Which handpiece with its many applications is revolutionizing dentistry, especially in the continued development of adhesive dentistry?
   a. electric handpiece
   b. air abrasion
   c. laser
   d. fiber-optic

10. Which cavity classification involves the proximal surfaces on the posterior teeth?
    a. Class I
    b. Class II
    c. Class III
    d. Class IV

11. What part of the rotary instrument is inserted into the handpiece chuck?
    a. head
    b. shank
    c. neck
    d. handle

12. What handpiece rotates long shank burs?
    a. high-speed handpiece
    b. right angle
    c. straight handpiece
    d. contra-angle

13. Which of the following handpiece types would accept a notched bur?
    a. high-speed handpiece
    b. right angle
    c. straight handpiece
    d. contra-angle

14. What is the number series for a straight fissure cross-cut bur?
    a. 30s
    b. 50s
    c. 160s and 170s
    d. 500s

15. The _____ bur is used for rapid reduction of tooth structure, and _____ burs are used to reduce and contour the alveolar bone and tooth structure.
    a. diamond; surgical
    b. diamond; laboratory
    c. cutting; finishing
    d. fissurotomy; cutting

16. The rotary instrument also known as a Jo-dandy is the _____.
    a. diamond bur
    b. sandpaper disc
    c. carborundum disc
    d. rubber wheel

17. Which mandrel is generally used outside the mouth?
    a. SS LA
    b. SS FG
    c. LS FG
    d. LS LA

18. Abrasive rotary instruments should be cleaned using _____.
    a. a bur brush
    b. gauze square and disinfectant
    c. alcohol solvent
    d. ultrasonic cleaner

19. Color-coding systems are set up to indicate all of the following EXCEPT:
    a. procedures.
    b. which dental arch/tooth the instrument is used on.
    c. treatment rooms.
    d. individual operators.

20. The assistant is positioning the hand instruments lengthwise on the tray for a right handed dentist. What direction should the handle of the mirror face?
    a. left side of the tray
    b. right side of the tray
    c. top of the tray
    d. bottom of the tray

Critical Thinking

1. Which handpiece would the dental assistant select if the procedure included polishing the patient's teeth? Would an attachment be required?

2. What is the recommended procedure for setting up tray? Explain why.

3. What should the assistant review prior to setting up the patient's tray?

Key Terms

Term and Pronunciation	Meaning of Root and Word Parts	Definition
abrasion (*uh-**brey**-zhuhn*)	**abrade** = to scrape off **-ion** = indicating an action	the process of scraping or wearing down by friction
amalgamator (*uh-**mal**-guh-meyt-or*)	**amalgam** = an alloy of mercury with other metals **-ate** = denotes function **-or** = denotes machine	device that mixes by shaking amalgam capsules containing mercury and alloy particles
airotor (*air-**oh**-ter*)	**air** = mixture of gases that surround earth	another name for air driven high-speed handpiece

(Continues)

Term and Pronunciation	Meaning of Root and Word Parts	Definition
articulation (ahr-tik-*yuh*-**ley**-sh*uh*n)	**articulate** = to be united or connected by or as if by a joint **-tion** = indicating an action	teeth meet when the temporomandibular joint closes
base (beys)	**base** = bottom layer or coating	material placed on the floor of the preparation to protect the pulp
belt and pulley (belt) (**pool**-ee)	**belt** = an endless flexible band passing about two or more pulleys **pulley** = a wheel with a grooved rim mounted on a shaft; driven by or driving a belt passing around it	consists of two fixed pulleys connected by a belt; one pulley powered by an electrical motor and energy transferred to second pulley the belt to turn rotary instrument
bonded (**bon**-did)	**bond** = something that holds together **-ed** = indicating a result	one material attached to another by a chemical process or adhesive
bruxism (**bruhk**-siz-*uh*m)	**brux** = to clench teeth **-ism** = denoting action	habit of teeth grinding
bur (bur)	**bur** = a rotary cutting instrument	rotary instrument used in dentistry to remove decay, shape and reduce tooth structure
burlew (**bur**-loo)	**burlew** = rubber infused or permeated with abrasive substances	an abrasive infused rubber wheel used in dentistry for polishing
burnish (**bur**-nish)	**burnish** = to make smooth	the process of adapting and polishing a restoration
carborundum (kahr-b*uh*-**ruhn**-d*uh*m)	**carborundum** = various abrasive materials; esp. consisting of silicone carbide	silicon carbide instrument used to cut metal or gold; known as separating disc or a Joe Dandy
carve (kahrv)	**carve** = to form something by cutting	act of anatomically shaping dental restorations
cassette (k*uh*-**set**)	**case** = container, box **-ette** = denoting small	container used to store instruments during cleaning and sterilization procedures; keeps instruments in an orderly fashion during treatment
cauterize (**kaw**-t*uh*-rahyz)	**cautery** = an agent or instrument used to burn, sear, or destroy tissue **-ize** = to cause to become	to destroy tissue, as in surgery, by burning, searing, or cutting; including caustic agents, electric currents, and lasers
cavity preparation (**kav**-i-tee) (prep-*uh*-**rey**-sh*uh*n)	**cavity** = a hollow place in the tooth produced by caries **prepare** = to make ready for something **-tion** = expressing action	used as a verb; the process of dental instruments to mechanically remove caries and diseased and unsupported tooth structures
chuck (chuhk)	**chuck** = a device for holding a drill bit	a device in the head of the dental handpiece that holds the rotary instrument
cleave (kleev)	**cleave** = to split or divide by cutting along a natural line division	unsupported and undermined tooth structures are cut and removed at the line of healthy and unhealthy structures
condense (k*uh*n-**dens**)	**condense** = to make more compact	to pack filling material into the prepared cavity of a tooth
contra-angle handpiece (**kon**-tr*uh*) (**ang**-g*uh*l) (hand- **pees**)	**contra** = in contrast to **angle** = a figure formed from two lines that meet at a common place; sides of a triangle form three angles **handpiece** = handheld dental device that holds revolving instruments	handpiece with two contrasting angles; permits access to difficult or impossible areas to reach with a straight handpiece
coolant (**koo**-l*uh*nt)	**cool** = comfortably free from heat; neither warm nor cold **-ant** = agent that performs an action	air or water used to reduce the temperature of tissue and cool the working end of the handpiece during operation
cure (kyoor)	**cure** = to harden or accelerate	a method to promote and accelerate the hardening process of composites
cuttle (**kuht**-l)	**cuttle** = white internal shell of cuttlefish (squid); cuttlebone used as a mineral supplement for cage birds and as a polishing agent	white abrasive particle made from cuttlebone of cuttlefish; used to cut, polish, and finish structures

Term and Pronunciation	Meaning of Root and Word Parts	Definition
dental amalgam (**dent**-tl) (*uh*-**mal**-g*uh*m)	**dent** = teeth **-al** = relating to **amalgam** = an alloy of mercury with other metals	an alloy of mercury with other materials to fill cavities in teeth
dental cement (**den**-tl) (si-**ment**)	**dent** = teeth **-al** = pertaining to **cement** = material that hardens for mending or adhering objects	dental material used as a base, temporary restoration, or for adhering appliances to the tooth
dental dam (**den**-tl) (dam)	**dent** = teeth **-al** = pertaining to **dam** = barrier to obstruct the flow of water	rubber material used to isolate and keep the operative site dry
dental handpiece (**den**-tl) (hand- **pees**)	**dent** = teeth **-al** = pertaining to **handpiece** = handheld dental device electrically or air powered that holds revolving instruments	dental drill, used to remove decayed tooth structure, prepare remaining structure for insertion of a dental filling, finish restorative materials, and perform oral surgery procedures
direct restoration (dih-**rekt**) (res-t*uh*-**rey**-sh*uh*n)	**direct** = straightforward **restore** = bring back to use **-ate** = denote function **-ion** = denoting condition	all of the work to fabricate and complete the restoration is completed within the mouth
emery (**em**-*uh*-ree)	**emery** = hard grayish-black mineral; used as an abrasive and polishing agent	a grayish-black particle of aluminum oxide rock; used to cut, polish, and finish structures
equilibration (ih-**kwil**-*uh*-brey-sh*un*)	**equilibrium** = a state of balance due to the equal action of forces **-ate** = product of a process **-tion** = indicating an action or process	the tooth structure and restorations are reshaped to alleviate pressure on individual teeth and balance the biting force; state of bodily balance
excavate (**eks**-k*uh*-veyt)	**excavate** = to remove by digging or scooping out	hand cutting instruments are used to remove decayed dental tissue
expendable (ik-**spen**-d*uh*-b*uh*l)	**expend** = to use up **-able** = capable	consumed in use and thrown away
flash (flash)	**flash** = a ridge of thin metal or plastic formed by extrusion of excess material	when there is excess restorative material over the margins of the preparation
fiber-optic (fahy-ber-**op**-tik)	**fiber** = a fine, threadlike piece **optic** = of or relating to eye, vision	thin transparent fibers of glass or plastic that are enclosed in a cable; transmits light throughout the length of cable to the head of the dental handpiece
finishing (**fin**-ish-ing)	**finish** = to bring to completion **-ing** = expressing action	process of creating a smooth and glossy surface
garnet (**gahr**-nit)	**garnet** = group of hard glassy minerals; used as a gem and as an abrasive	deep-red transparent abrasive particle used to cut, polish, and finish structures
gears (geerz)	**gear** = wheel with teeth around its rim that mesh with the teeth of another wheel to transmit motion	a part of the handpiece, having cut teeth that mesh teeth in another part to rotate chuck and rotary instrument
grit (grit)	**grit** = the texture or grain of an abrasive	the size of abrasive particles resulting in rough to smooth surfaces; extra-fine (smooth) to extra-coarse (rough)
laser (**ley**-zer)	**laser** = acronym for **l**ight **a**mplification by **s**timulated **e**mission of **r**adiation	laser handpiece; converts electromagnetic radiation of mixed frequencies to highly amplified radiation used to cut and dissolve tissue
liner (**lahy**-ner)	**line** = to cover the inner side or surface **-er** = designate person or thing	a thin layer of material placed over exposed dentin within cavity preparation; protects the pulp
mandrel (**man**-dr*uh*l)	**mandrel** = a shaft on which a working tool is mounted (disc, wheel) on one end and the other end is held in a workpiece	one end of the mandrel shank is held in the handpiece and the other end holds various rotary instruments

(Continues)

Term and Pronunciation	Meaning of Root and Word Parts	Definition
microabrasions (mahy-kroh-uh-**brey**-zhuhn)	**micro** = too small to be seen by unaided eye **abrade** = to scrape off **-ion** = indicating an action	extremely small scratches making uniform rough surface
microetcher (**mahy**-kroh-ech-uhr)	**micro-** = small **etch** = to cut or wear away **-er** = designate person or thing	handheld dental sandblasting unit for intraoral and lab applications; increases surface bonding
planing (**pleyn**-ing)	**plane** = flat or level surface **-ing** = expressing action	hand cutting instruments are used to make tooth surfaces flat and level
pneumatic (noo-**mat**-ik)	**pneuma** = blow, wind **-ic** = having characteristics	operated by air or by the pressure of air
portable dental unit (**pohr**-tuh-buhl) (**den**-tl) (**yoo**-nit)	**port** = area for passage **-able** = capable dent = teeth **-al** = pertaining to	equipment used to complete dental procedures that is easily carried or transported
power source (**pou**-er) (sohrs)	**power** = force of engine to operate **source** = to furnish or supply	hardware component that supplies power to an electrical device that causes the dental handpiece to rotate
prophylaxis (proh-fuh-**lak**-sis)	**prophylaxis** = the prevention of disease or control of its possible spread	professional cleaning of the teeth by a dentist or dental hygienist
resin composite (**rez**-in) (kuhm-**poz**-it)	**resin** = synthetic material used as a filler; plastic **composite** = to put together; made up of separate parts or elements	fillers (glass and glass ceramics) and different types of synthetic resins (plastics) are put together to make the resin composite; used in dentistry as restorative material or adhesives
revolutions per minute (rpm) (rev-uh-**loo**-shuhns) (pur) (**min**-it)	**revolve** = to cause to turn around, to rotate **-tion** = indicating action **per** = for each **minute** = a period of time equal to 60 seconds	rate of revolutions of a motor within a minute
right angle handpiece (rahyt) (**ang**-guh l) (hand-**pees**)	**right angle** = an angle measuring ninety degrees, formed by the intersection of two perpendicular lines **handpiece** = handheld dental device electrically powered that holds revolving instruments	head operates at a 90° angle to the handpiece handle to gain better access to working area and to reduce strain of operator's hand
serrated (**ser**-ey-tid)	**serrate** = notched or having grooves **-ed** = indicating a result	having a jagged or notched surface; help prevent instruments from slipping
sequence (**see**-kwuhns)	**sequel** = an event or circumstance following something **-ence** = indicating a quality	an action or event that follows another
stock (stok)	**stock** = supply of goods kept on hand	stock number is written on instruments for ease in naming and ordering
straight handpiece (streyt) (hand-**pees**)	**straight** = without a bend or angle **handpiece** = handheld dental device electrically powered that holds revolving instruments	a handpiece where the handpiece handle is in line with the rotary instrument
tine (tahyn)	**tine** = a sharp, projecting point or prong, as of a fork	a sharp, point used as the working end of an instrument
topical anesthetic (**top**-i-kuhl) (an-uhs-**thet**-ik)	**topo-** = place, local **-ic** = having characteristics **-al** = pertaining to **an-** = without **esthesia** = sensation or feeling **-ic** = relating to	agent applied to soft tissue to numb the area
turbine (**tur**-bahyn)	**turbine** = any of various machines having a rotor (blades) driven by pressure converted to rotary motion	part of dental handpiece that converts air pressure to rotary motion causing the chuck to rotate
ultrasonic handpiece (uhl-truh-**son**-ik) (hand-**pees**)	**ultra** = beyond, extreme **sonic** = having speed about equal to sound in air **handpiece** = handheld dental device that holds revolving instruments	handpiece with a tip supplying high-frequency vibrations; removes deposits on teeth such as bacteria, calculus, and other substances

Term and Pronunciation	Meaning of Root and Word Parts	Definition
ultraspeed handpiece (**uhl**-tr*uh*-speed) (hand- **pees**)	**ultra** = beyond, extreme **speed** = full rate of motion **handpiece** = handheld dental device that holds revolving instruments	handpiece that rotates at the maximum speed; holds rotary instruments
universally (yoo-n*uh*-**vur**-s*uh*-lee)	**uni-** = one **verse** = to turn **-ally** = every	everywhere or in every case
utility (yoo-**til**-i-tee)	**utile** = useful **-ity** = quality of	having or made for a number of useful or practical purposes rather than a single, specialized one
vaporize (**vey**-p*uh*-rahyz)	**vapor** = a substance that is in a gaseous state at extreme heat **-ize** = to cause to become	to destroy by being turned into gas as a result of extreme heat; to evaporate or cause to evaporate
vulcanite bur (**vuhl**-k*uh*-nahyt) (bur)	**vulcanite** = hard rubber produced by vulcanizing (treat with heat and sulfur) natural rubber **bur** = a small cutting tool	a rotary instrument used to cut hard rubber and plastic materials; mouth guards and denture bases

CHAPTER 20
Ergonomics and Instrument Transfer

Specific Instructional Objectives

At the completion of this chapter, you will be able to meet these objectives:

1. Use terms presented in this chapter.
2. Recognize the risk factors that may cause work-related injuries.
3. Describe recommended ergonomics in dentistry.
4. Demonstrate proper positioning for operator, assistant, and patient during four-handed dentistry.
5. Employ motion economy while assisting chairside.
6. Describe team positions, postures, and use of fulcrum in achieving good transfer techniques.
7. Utilize recommended instrument transfer zones.
8. Demonstrate the types of instrument grasps and transfer of instruments for a procedure.
9. Defend the importance of teamwork in four-handed dentistry.

Introduction

As the profession of dentistry seeks to improve the working environment and reduce stress, dental ergonomics has become an important issue. The term ergonomics refers to the study and analysis of human work, including the anatomical and psychological aspects of people and their work environments. Ergonomics must be learned and then applied to benefit individuals. All members of the dental team should be aware of work-related injuries and be involved in applying ergonomic concepts in the dental office. This chapter presents recommended ergonomic practices and instrument transfers for the operator and assistant to save time and prevent muscle strain and fatigue.

Work-Related Injuries in the Dental Office

Without the knowledge of potential work-related injuries and their prevention, the assistant may be at risk for musculoskeletal disorders (MSD). A dental team without a proper work environment, equipment, and training in ergonomics may inadvertently contribute to their own work-related injuries. The greatest risk factors for the chairside assistant are twisting and turning of the back, extended reaching to access instruments and materials, and long periods of time sitting in one position. The most frequent

MSD occurs in the lower back, upper back, and shoulders. Injuries can be aggravated by not obtaining the proper body position and posture while working chairside and not seeking early medical attention (Figure 20-1).

With the increased intraoral functions performed in expanded functions, the expanded function dental assistant (EFDA) may experience repetitive contraction of muscles in the wrist, hand, and fingers during fine motor control motions. Like dentists, they are placing restorations and handling dental handpieces. The EFDA also experiences the traditional neck and shoulder strain from sitting with the neck in a head-down position that

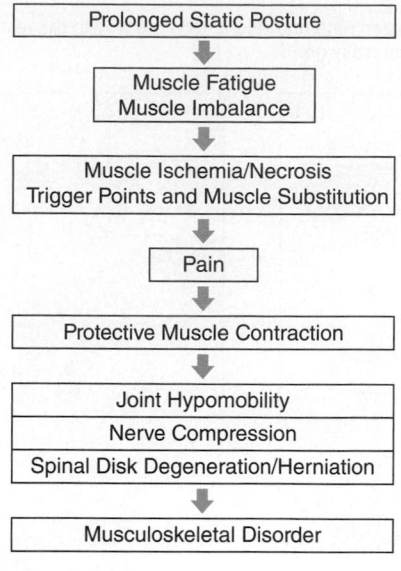

FIGURE 20-1
Progression of MSD.

has been attributed to procedures previously performed only by the dentist. When motions are repeated frequently for long periods of time, muscle–tendon **strain** and fatigue occurs. Tendons and muscles can recover by stretching. Stretching and relaxation techniques can help reduce stress as well as preventing long term injury (Figure 20-2 and Table 20-1).

Lower Back Pain

Lower back pain is at epidemic levels in the United States, second to the common cold for patients seeking medical attention. The **lumbosacral** spine has tissue (muscles, ligaments, nerves) and structures (joints, discs, bones) that all have the potential for generating pain. Physical causes for such pain include continuous **lumbar flexion** and rotation that increases the risk of injury to the **lumbar discs**. The chance of injury is increased by inflexibility of hips and pelvis and weak abdominal and **gluteal** muscles. Thus, we find a greater incidence of lower back pain in a population with inadequate conditioning.

The risk for lower back pain is increased in dentistry primarily due to prolonged periods of time in a seated position. In a sitting position, the upper and lower **erector spinae** muscles are generally strained in an unsupported sitting posture. In addition, this position creates a low back compressive load in the lumbar spine region. This causes an increased load on the soft tissues of the lumbar spine and discs, resulting in back discomfort. Poor body position, poor posture, and twisting while sitting chairside increase the risk of lower back pain. More stress is placed on the discs and muscles with the back bent or twisted compared to when the back is straight (Figure 20-3).

Upper Back and Shoulders

Repeated and continuous bending or twisting impose increased stresses on the upper back and shoulders. Again, body position and posture play an important role in preventing these injuries. Having the assistant stool and work area at the proper height when reaching will reduce upper back and shoulder strain. The assistant sitting at a height usually a few inches (4–6) higher than the dentist provides better access to the patient's mouth for instrument transfer and oral evacuation.

Neck and Shoulders

Pain in the neck and shoulders is related to indirect viewing of the patient's mouth, poor lighting, providing a comfortable position for the patient at the operator's expense of comfort, and extended time spent in the same position. This causes contraction of the upper **trapezium** to maintain this position without armrests, leading to fatigue and discomfort of the neck and shoulder area. This injury can be reduced by adjusting patient position, proper posture, and body position including using a lower arm position to compensate for the lack of an armrest.

Wrist and Hands

Hand and wrist problems have been associated with the dental operator's repetitive and forceful exertion using instruments. Two of the more common are **carpal** tunnel syndrome and **trigger** finger.

Carpal tunnel syndrome (CTS) is a diagnosis that is all too common to dental professionals. The carpal tunnel is the area of the wrist through which pass the flexor tendons and the median nerve (Figure 20-4). Repeated forceful motions of the hand and wrist cause swelling and place pressure on this nerve, which can lead to CTS. Proper body, hand, and finger position; holding the instrument correctly; and stabilization of the fingers in the mouth can reduce the chance of injury. Frequently resting your wrist and hands is the most important measure in helping to prevent CTS. Slowly opening and closing the hands will also help warm the muscles and joints of your hand. If your discomfort continues or worsens, you should seek professional assistance to prevent further damage to your muscles and nerves.

Trigger finger (**tenosynovitis**) is generally caused by a sustained, forceful power grip with a repetitive motion. The **tendon** becomes inflamed and narrow, which prevents the smooth movement of the finger. A **nodule** forms on the tendon, causing a "clicking" or "triggering" movement. The assistant will feel pain with the movement of the tendon, warmth, swelling, and pain upon palpation.

Hand, wrist, and forearm stretches are used to prevent sprain. Practice these exercises between patients, at lunch, on the way to the restroom, at home—whenever you can to keep your hands, wrists, and forearms stretched. They also feel really good.

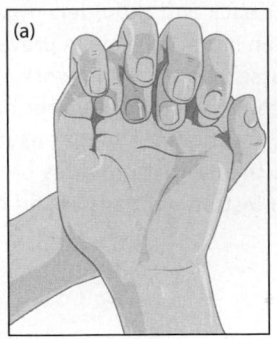
(a)

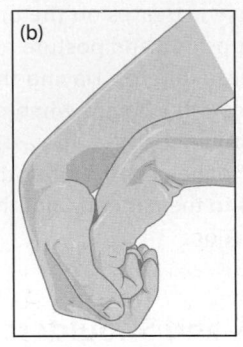
(b)

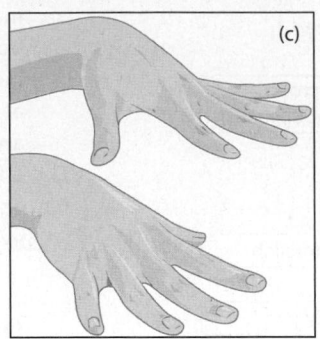
(c)

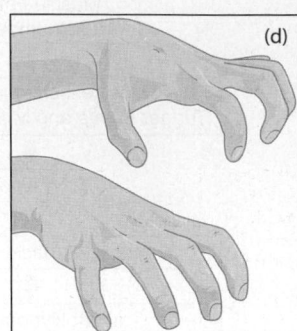
(d)

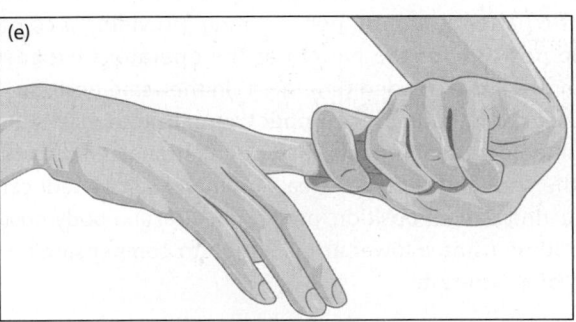
(e)

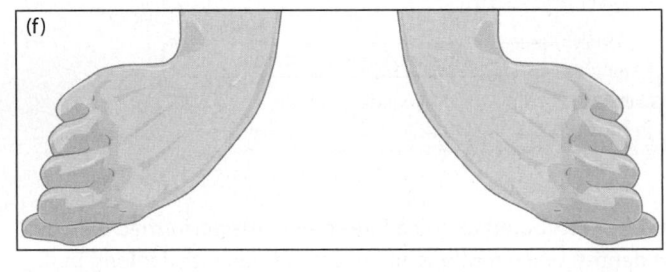
(f)

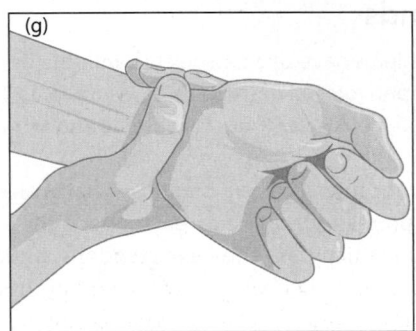
(g)

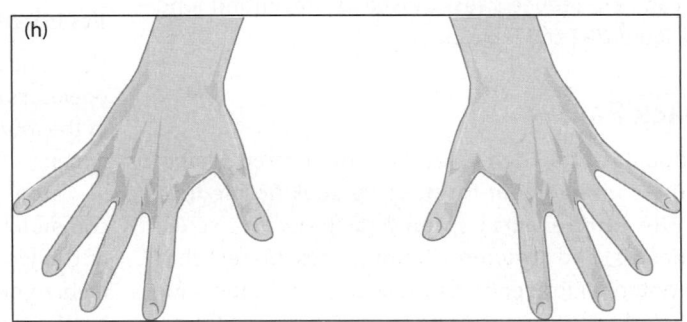
(h)

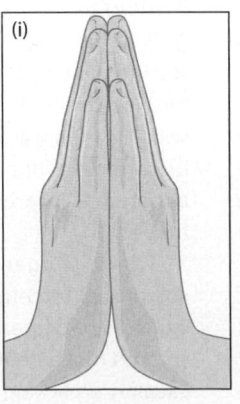
(i)

FIGURE 20-2
Stretching and relaxation techniques.

TABLE 20-1 Routine Stretching Exercises

These exercises have been adapted from Cooper and Brian's published routine stretching exercises that can help prevent work related injury and relax the body. They recommend that stretching be performed every hour while exhaling into the stretches slowly. Each exercise only needs to be repeated 3–5 times. The dental assistant will have to be creative and find time to do these stretches while performing routine duties (exercise fingers while washing hands) and during lunch breaks.

Neck Rotation Exercises	Lower Back Exercises
Head Rotation Drop head forward. Rotate head to right shoulder. Rotate head to left shoulder. Return head to front.	*Backward Lean* Place hands on buttocks and lean backward. Hold for 5 seconds. *Spine Rotation* Sit in chair and place left hand on right knee. Look over right shoulder and feel spine rotation. Repeat on other side. *Forward Bend* Bend forward at waist. Try to touch toes. Hold for 5 seconds.
Shoulder and Upper Back Exercises	
Shoulder Rotation Rotate right shoulder. Rotate left shoulder. *Shoulder Shrug* Shrug shoulders by raising them. Hold this position for 5 seconds. *Overhead Reach* Place hands and arms straight over head and stretch. Hold for 5 seconds. *Elbow Spread* Interlock fingers behind head. Move elbows backward. Hold for 5 seconds. *Arm Straightening* Interlock fingers behind back and straighten arms. Hold for 5 seconds.	**Wrist and Finger Exercises**
	Finger Curl Stretch fingers out. Curl fingers toward palm of hand. *Finger Pull* Pull fingertips of one hand back with the other. Repeat with other hand.

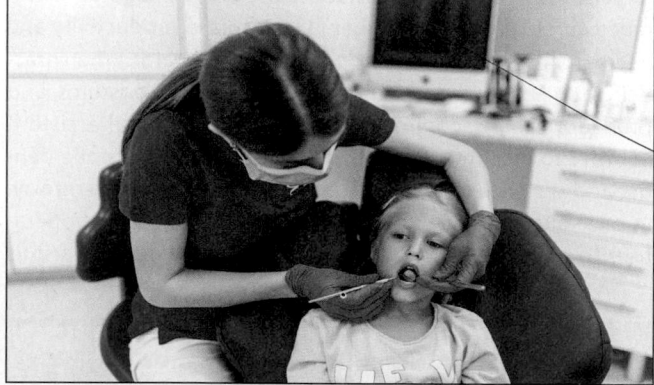

© F8 studio/Shutterstock.com

FIGURE 20-3
This position not only looks awkward, but also it will potentially result in muscles being strained from an unsupported sitting posture. MSDs may occur from chronic low back compressive pressure on the lumbar spine region.

Stress

It is important to consider the psychological as well as the physical demands of a job. Musculoskeletal and psychological stress seem to be interrelated. Various studies have identified the main **stressors** in dentistry as the demands of doing meticulous surgical procedures of long duration, time and management pressures, and fatigue from MSD. Many of these stressors are shared by the assistant as they are the dentist's right hand at the chair (Table 20-2).

TABLE 20-2 Factors in Work-Related MSD Injuries

Awkward positions
Poor posture
Remaining in one position for extended periods of time
Stress
Infrequent breaks
Inappropriate use of dental stools
Poor postural muscle strength
Poor flexibility
Risk factors are only part of the story. Plan nonwork activities that include rest and conditioning to strengthen muscles for posture and to reduce stress.

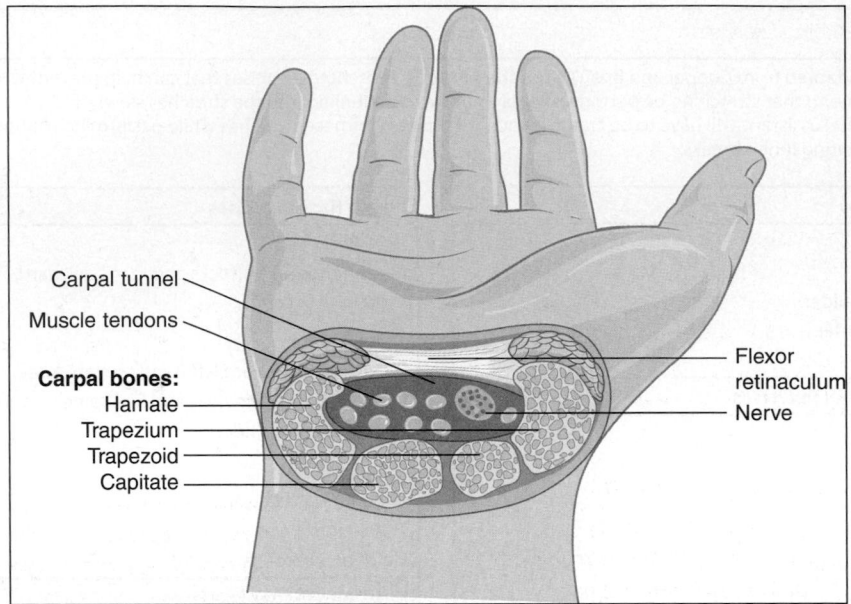

FIGURE 20-4
Anatomical view of carpal flexor tendons and median nerve in tunnel.

Safety

"Fit of Gloves"

The fit of examination gloves is important not only in infection control but also in the musculoskeletal health of the worker's hands. The NIH has found a correlation between increased tears and compression **neuropathies** and examination gloves that are too small and tight fitting. When the gloves are too tight, the hands are chronically compressed, held in uncomfortable positions, and don't rest for long periods of time. If these ill-fitting gloves or ambidextrous gloves are worn continuously, it can cause pain and numbness in the hand, particularly at the base of the thumb.

If the assistant notices these symptoms, changing to a larger glove size or switching to a hand-specific glove may help. In selecting gloves, the assistant should make sure the glove is not too tight across the palm or constricting at the wrist, and the finger length should be adequate to allow for comfortable finger movement. Wearing gloves that are too large can also be injurious. A glove too large results in less dexterity for the wearer, causes a problem in grasping instruments, and results in a higher incidence of puncture injuries.

A properly fitting glove should feel almost like not wearing any glove at all. There are some ergonomic gloves that are designed to the natural shape of the hand. These gloves do not interfere with the freedom of movement and provide a greater tactile sense. Gloves that are microtextured allow the assistant to get a better grasp of an instrument with more ease. Wearing examination gloves that meet these recommendations helps prevent slippage and reduces the chance of acquiring a hand related MSD. These gloves may cost more, but what price is put on preventing MSD?

Ergonomics in Dentistry

Dental ergonomics is the science of designing equipment to maximize productivity by reducing operator fatigue and discomfort. Successful use of ergonomics increases productivity and worker satisfaction and decreases illnesses and injuries. Ergonomics plays a significant role in the practice of modern dentistry.

Modern dentistry is based on the concept of four-handed dentistry, in which the assistant provides chairside assistance in transferring instruments to increase productivity and decrease physical stress on the dentist or operator. When practicing four-handed dentistry, specific positions, postures, and procedures are recommended for the dentist and assistant in order to most effectively utilize the two hands of the dentist and the two hands of the assistant working in **harmony**. In previous chapters we discussed how to set up the operatory to maximize efficiency and how the design of various

What Do OSHA Guidelines Recommend?

Employers must discuss ergonomic issues with their employees. Employees need to be aware of work related MDSs, their signs and symptoms, and the importance of reporting them early. This means that all current and new employees should be trained in these areas.

Why Should These Guidelines Be Followed?

According to OSHA information, a total of 626,000 work days were lost due to MSD, and 34% of all work related injuries were due to MSD.

instruments facilitates ergonomics. These are both aspects of applied ergonomics in the dental profession. The dental assistant can help prevent MSD by following the ergonomic recommendations.

Body Mechanics

Ergonomics begins with good body mechanics. Body mechanics is the application of **kinesiology** to the use of proper body movement in everyday activities and to preventing and correcting problems related to posture as well as to enhancing coordination and endurance. As dental personnel, we need to make certain that we move our bodies correctly and utilize each muscle and bone **efficiently** as we go about our daily routines.

The assistant has many duties that require moving and lifting equipment and supplies. Using proper body mechanics reduces stress and strain, which lessens fatigue and helps us to remain healthy and injury free. To ensure you are using proper body mechanics, follow the guidelines listed in Table 20-3.

Dental Team Positioning

When delivering treatment, the dental team consists of the patient, operator, and assistant. The positioning of the entire team affects not only the efficiency of delivering care but can help in preventing MSD.

Patient Seating As discussed in Chapter 18, the patient should be positioned in a supine or subsupine (depending on the procedure) position. These positions allow the operator and assistant to have maximum and easy access to the oral cavity while maintaining patient comfort. The height of the patient chair should be adjusted so that the operator and assistant can utilize proper body mechanics while seated in their respective chairs. Simple requests to have the patient raise or lower their chin or turn toward the right or left can improve view and access to the operative site. Often, music is offered to help the patient relax and withstand sitting for longer periods of time.

Operator Seating The operator's position is key to the arrangement of the patient, assistant, and equipment. The operator must be seated in a comfortable position to perform the dental procedure efficiently, with easy access to the oral cavity and a clear view of the operating field. For maximum comfort and to reduce stress and strain, the operator stool should be positioned in such a manner that the feet are flat on the floor, thighs parallel to the floor, with knees pointed down at a slight angle, and the lower portion of the back up against the backrest of the stool. The back and neck are in an upright position with the top of the shoulders parallel to the floor.

The operator's arms should be bent at the elbows, and forearms should be parallel to the floor and close to the body. It is

TABLE 20-3 Body Mechanics

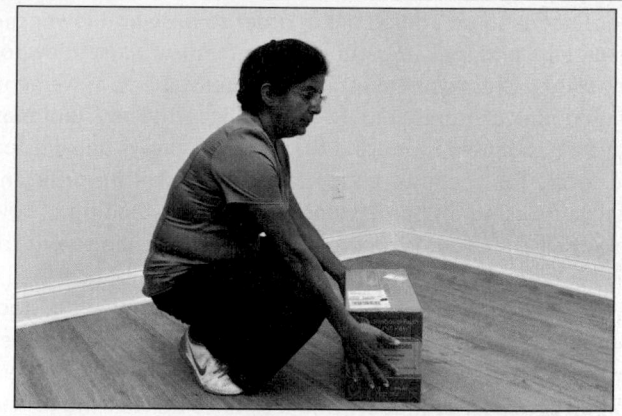

- Always establish a broad base of support when lifting a heavy object. Keep your feet approximately shoulder width apart, one foot slightly in front of the other, with your weight distributed evenly on both feet.
- Get as close as possible to an object before attempting to lift it, and carry it as close to your torso as possible.
- Always bend from your hips and knees, keeping your back straight.
- Lift with your legs, since they contain your strongest muscles.
- Use the weight of your body to help push or pull heavy objects on the floor.
- Try not to twist your body when working; instead turn with feet or the entire body.
- Try not to bend for long periods of time.
- Always ask for help if a job is too big for one person.

recommended to have the forearms resting on stool armrests (Figure 20-5). The operator should position their legs under the headrest with the chair approximately 2 inches above the thighs. The distance between the operator's face and the patient's oral cavity is approximately 14–18 inches. Operators may also use dental loupes to improve the stress from indirect viewing of the patient's mouth and poor lighting (refer to the box below). The rheostat and handpieces should be positioned within easy reach of the operator.

Dental loupes (telescopes) are the most frequently used tools for magnification in dentistry. Research has shown that using loupes reduces the risk of work-related injuries by lessening eye strain and enhancing the posture and positioning of the operator (the operator's head must be held farther forward when not using a loupe). In addition, the use of loupes equipped with lights eliminates the need to reach for and adjust the dental light. There are many designs of loupes available.

Assistant Seating The assistant is positioned across from the operator on the opposite side of the patient. The assistant's stool needs to be adjustable in order to raise and lower the chair, arm, and foot ring. All of these features must allow for any stature of assistant to establish proper stability, movement, and comfort (Figure 20-6). In some offices, the assistant may have a designated room, and the stool will always be adjusted perfectly for them. In other cases there will be different assistants using the same stool, so the understanding of how to adjust the stool is of the upmost importance to ensure proper ergonomics.

It is recommended that the assistant sit straight in the stool 4–6 inches higher than the operator. This position provides an unobstructed view of the operative site, improves access to oral cavity for aspiration, and facilitates transferring instruments to the operator. The foot ring and arm (abdominal bar) are designed to reduce fatigue and stress and eliminate back pain. The assistant should place their feet on the foot ring with thighs parallel to the floor and knees pointed down at a slight angle. The assistant stool should be positioned so the thigh closest to the patient is parallel to and touching the backrest of the dental chair with the front edge of the stool even with the patient's mouth. Resting your side against the arm eases the strain on the lower back. The assistant's arms should be bent at the elbows, and forearms should be parallel to the floor. It is recommended to have the forearms resting on the arm of the stool. The instrument tray, aspirating hoses, and equipment to be used during the procedure should be positioned within easy reach of the assistant.

Ergonomic Dental Equipment As you have learned, there are different types of dental units and delivery systems, but they should all have one thing in common: easy access. The operator and assistant should have easy access to each type of unit, allowing for minimum movement and twisting to obtain necessary instruments and equipment. Utilizing the proper type of dental unit, operator's stools, and assistant's chairs will make for a well-oiled procedure. If the treatment area uses a cart, it should be positioned so there is easy access and entry to the entire cart, usually at the 2:00 position.

Safety

Although the stool is ergonomically designed, if you do not take the proper position you will not receive the benefits of its design. In fact, improper positioning may lead to MSD. The stool is on wheels and the side arm moves, making it a little difficult to mount, so you should practice sitting in and exiting the chair. You should also know how to adjust the chair to the proper position to suit your individual comfort.

Activity Zones The clock concept envisions the work area and positioning of the operator and assistant at the patient chair as a circle and divides it into activity zones that correspond to the position of numbers on an analog clock (one that has hands that move around a dial). For example, in this system the top of the patient's head corresponds to the top of the clock dial, so it is referred to as the 12:00 position. The chin corresponds to the bottom of the clock dial, so it is said to be in the 6 o'clock position. Table 20-4 outlines the various parts of the work area as viewed from above the patient and their assigned clock positions for a right-handed operator, and Table 20-5 does so for the left-handed operator.

Motion Economy

In the dental field, the part of the body that becomes most fatigued is the lower back. Delivering patient care involves a great deal of reaching, twisting, and turning from the seated position. Motion economy deals with understanding the types of movements used in the practice of dentistry and identifying the ones that are effective and the ones that are not. Motions that place the team in an awkward, stressed, or strained position for prolonged periods of time are not necessary; they are harmful and should be eliminated.

A motion is classified according to the identity and number of body parts used in making it. Table 20-6 lists the five classifications of motions routinely used by the dental assistant. The more muscles involved in a movement, the less precise the movement becomes. Therefore, the operator should rely on using mostly Class I, II, and III motions, which allow the most efficient and effective movements. Class IV and Class V should be eliminated or at least reduced to maintain proper body mechanics and reduce stress, strain, and fatigue.

Principles of work simplification can be used selectively in dentistry to decrease stress, tension, and the occurrence of MSD. The principles of work simplification in dentistry are Rearrange, Eliminate, Combine, and Simplify (Table 20-7). The dental assistant should consider work simplification principles as they perform duties. These steps will be discussed in more detail in the sections on instrument transfer.

Assistant as Operator

With the increase of intraoral procedures performed by the dental assistant, you will find yourself in the operator's stool. It is important to use good posture and position at the chair to minimize MSD. The dental assistant should sit with the back resting against the back rest with their arms parallel to floor and elbows bent. When working from the back of the patient, the view and access is best with the assistant sitting at the 11:00 position (Figure 20-7). In situations where working from the front of the patient is better, the assistant sits at the 7:00 position (Figure 20-8).

DENTAL ERGONOMIC POSTURE

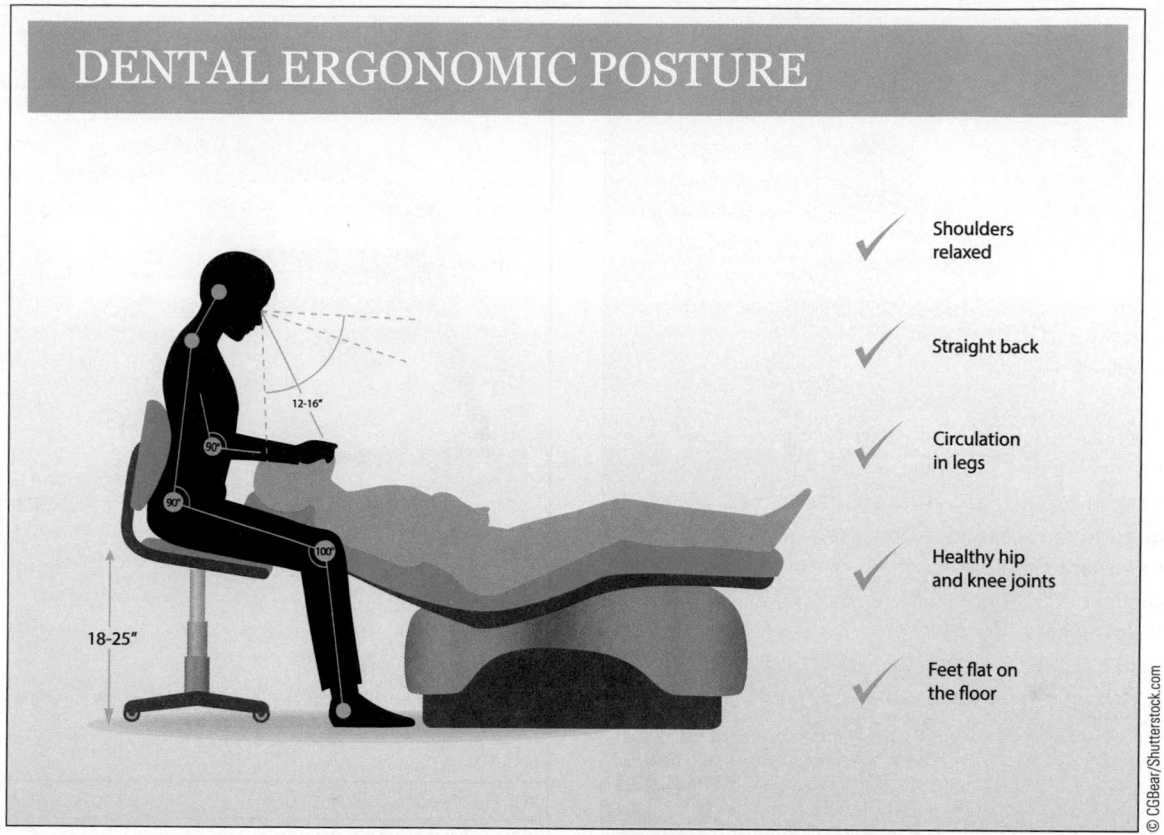

Shoulders relaxed

Straight back

Circulation in legs

Healthy hip and knee joints

Feet flat on the floor

© CGBear/Shutterstock.com

FIGURE 20-5A

Optimal working posture that should be maintained to reduces stress on muscles, ligaments, tendons, spinal discs, and surrounding tissue. The operator is modeling good position and posture. The operator is sitting back in the stool with his back straight and supported by the back rest. The dental chair is adjusted to 2 inches above the operator's thighs, and the operator is seated below the dental chair headrest. Their feet are flat on the floor, thighs are parallel to the floor, and knees are pointed at a slight angle.

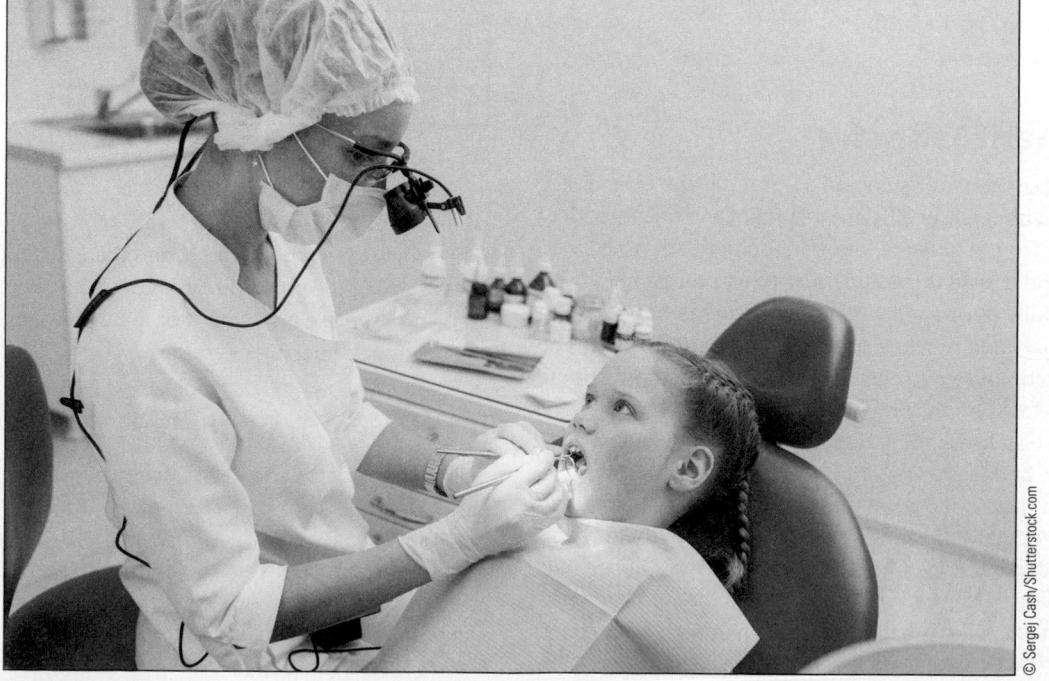

© Sergej Cash/Shutterstock.com

FIGURE 20-5B

The operator is wearing dental loupes to prevent bending over to view the patient's mouth, and their arms are parallel to the floor.

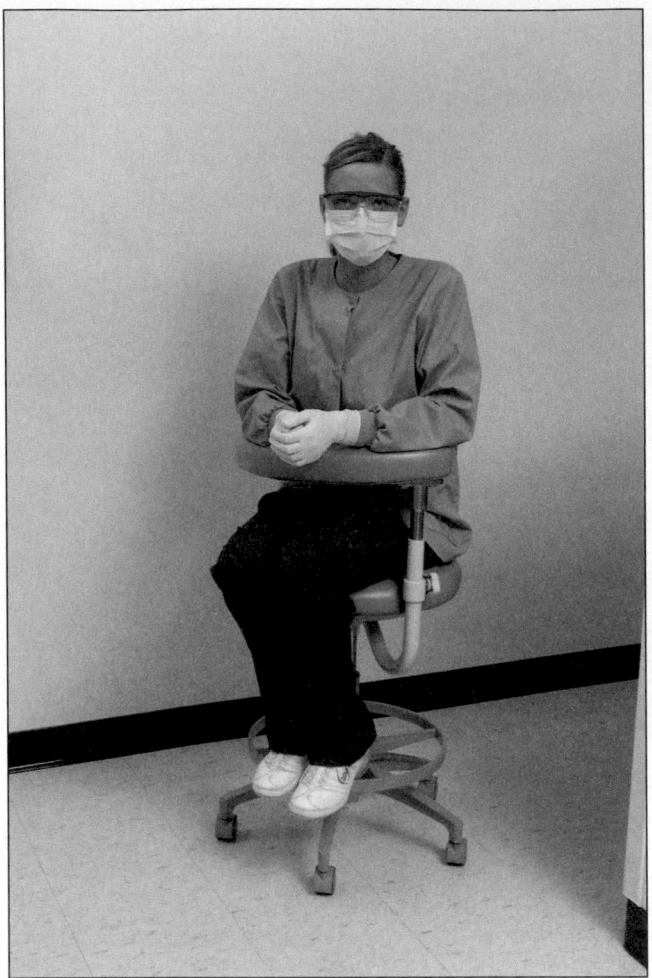

FIGURE 20-6
Dental assistant properly positioned on assistant stool with feet resting on foot rest, thighs parallel to the floor, and back upright.

TABLE 20-4 Activity Zones for a Right-Handed Operator, with Assistant on the Left

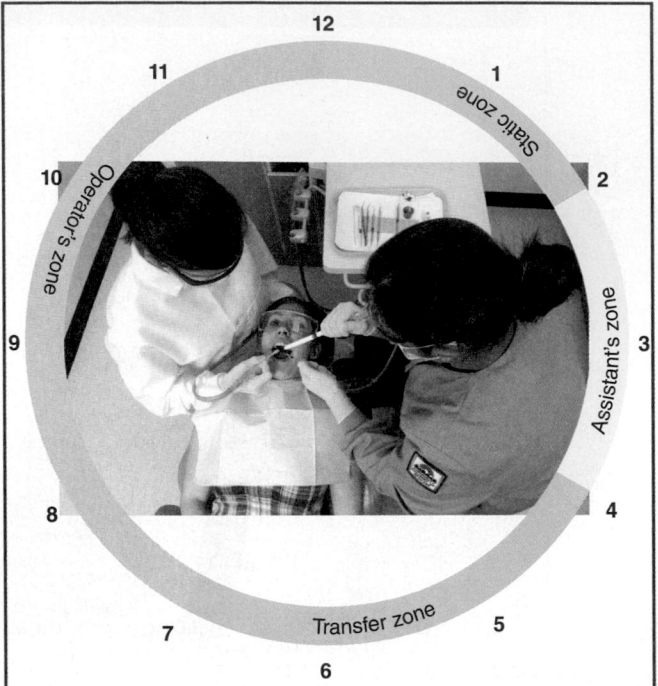

●	*Top of patient's head:* 12:00
●	*Static zone:* 12:00–2:00
This zone is reserved for the mobile cart, nitrous oxide, and any item that might not be suitable to deliver over the patient.	
●	*Assistant's zone:* 2:00–4:00
●	*Patient's chin:* 6:00
The assistant does not move as much as the operator, but this zone should still be kept clear to provide movement and access equipment.	
●	*Transfer zone:* 4:00–7:00
●	This area is used to transfer instruments, medications, and supplies.
●	*Operator zone:* 7:00–12:00

Instrument Transfer

The primary purpose for having an assistant at the chair assisting the dentist is to deliver efficient treatment and quality patient care. In order for the goals of four-handed dentistry to be met, the dentist and assistant must learn to function as a team. This teamwork is fully developed when both team members coordinate procedures and practice specific instrument **transfer** and **exchange** techniques. Ideally the dentist and assistant should work in such close harmony that verbal exchange is unnecessary.

Transfer procedures should be coordinated to the point where the sequence and exchange of instruments is continuous. The first step is to have good communication between the dentist/operator and dental assistant. The dental assistant should have a thorough understanding of how the dentist/operator wants the procedure to be performed so they can have the work area prepared with the necessary instruments and materials beforehand and be able to anticipate the sequence of procedural steps. Failure to have the complete **armamentarium** for a procedure will result in inefficient use of time locating missing items and lengthening the patient chair time. When the assistant has a thorough knowledge of the procedure, they are able to anticipate the next step and have the instrument or material ready to be passed to the operator before it is needed.

Instrument Transfer Positions

The four-handed dentistry concept begins with specific positions, postures, and procedures to enhance the dentist's and assistant's ability to work as a team. With the assistant seated across from the dentist in the assistant's zone (2–4 o'clock) and the dentist in the operator's zone (7–12 o'clock), the dental team can best utilize the two hands of the dentist and the two hands of the assistant working in harmony to save time and reduce stress and fatigue.

TABLE 20-5 Activity Zones for a Left-Handed Operator, with Assistant on the Right

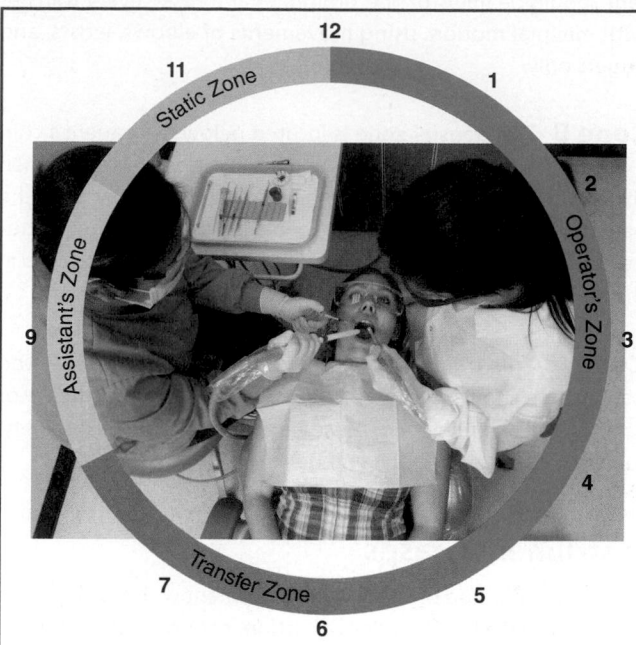

- *Top of patient's head*: 12:00
- *Operator zone*: 12:00–5:00
- *Transfer zone*: 5:00–8:00

This area is used to transfer instrument, medications, and supplies.

- *Assistant's zone*: 8:00–10:00

The assistant does not move as much as the operator, but this zone should still be kept clear to provide movement and access equipment.

- *Static zone*: 10:00–12:00

This zone is reserved for the mobile cart, nitrous oxide, and any item that might not be suitable to deliver over the patient.

TABLE 20-6 Classification of Motion

Class I:	Movement of the fingers only (picking up instruments from the patient tray)
Class II:	Movement of fingers and wrist (mixing materials on the tray, typing on computer)
Class III:	Movement of fingers, wrist, and elbow (transferring instruments to operator, using computer mouse)
Class IV:	Use of entire arm and shoulder (repositioning dental light, sending a fax)
Class V:	Use of entire arm and upper torso (rotating and reaching for items on the counter)

TABLE 20-7 Work Simplification Steps

Rearrange: Place equipment into position that will eliminate unnecessary movement.
Eliminate: Remove unnecessary equipment, movements, or steps to procedures.
Combine: Use double ended instruments, instead of single ended instruments.
Simplify: Eliminate as many variables as possible.

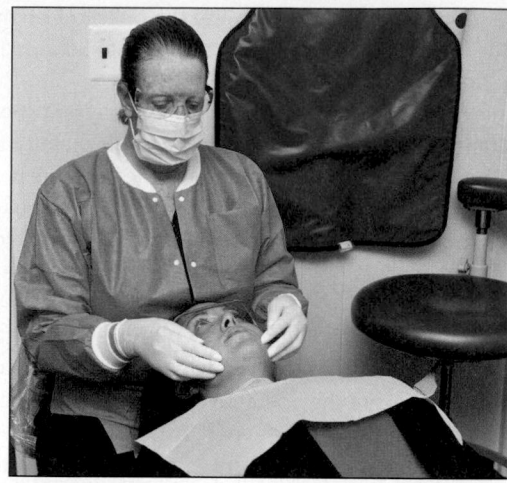

FIGURE 20-7
Back position. The assistant is sitting at the right-handed position at 11–12 o'clock. Her back and neck are straight with her forearm parallel to the floor.

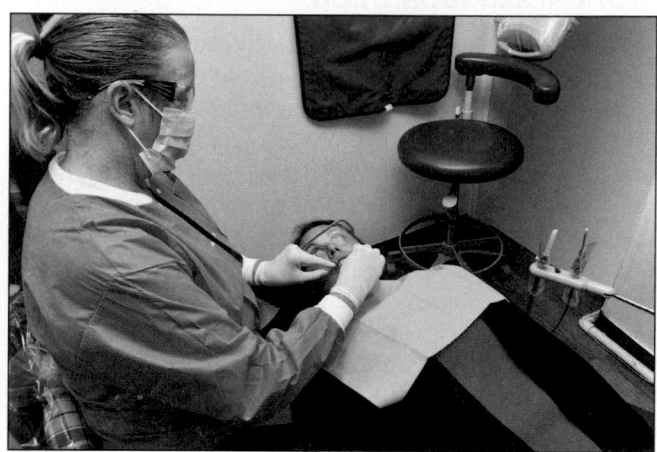

FIGURE 20-8
Front/side position. The assistant is sitting at the right-handed position toward the front of the patient at 7 o'clock. Her back and neck are straight with her forearm parallel to the floor.

Once the dental team has taken their positions at the chair, it is important that they assume the recommended posture to maximize efficiency and minimize strain. The dentist/operator should be seated at the chair and obtain the best position for easy access to the area in the patient's mouth where they will be working. The operator signals they are ready for an instrument transfer by placing their hands on either side of the patient's face and establishing a finger rest (Figure 20-9). The operator will receive and hold the instrument using the thumb, index finger, and middle finger. With the fourth and fifth fingers, the operator obtains a finger rest by resting their fingers against hard structures of the patient's mouth near the area where the work is being performed. Generally, the operator will rest the ring finger against tooth surfaces in the immediate vicinity of the operative site or opposite arch and stabilize the position by resting the little finger against another tooth or patient tissue. The finger rest works as a **fulcrum** for stabilization and working pivotal movement of the instruments. It is also used to stabilize the operator's hand and reduce the likelihood of slippage and uncontrolled movements that may cause injury.

In achieving good transfer technique, the assistant should be able to transfer instruments while the operator maintains their eyes on the operative site and maintains the finger rest during the transfer of instruments. When an effective transfer occurs, the operator should be able to receive an instrument without looking away from the operative site and without moving from the established finger rest.

The dental assistant should be in the position at the chair that provides the best view of the operative site and easy access to transfer instruments to the operator, maintain moisture control, and retract patient tissues as needed. This position is generally 4–6 inches higher than the operator to obtain an unobstructed view with the bracket table at the 1–2 o'clock position within easy reach.

Work Area Preparation

The transfer techniques begin with the placement of instruments and materials in order of use with the handles directed for ease of transfer. As you recall, hand instruments passed to the operator's right hand are passed with the assistant's left hand. For ease in picking up the instrument, the handles should be placed with the handles toward the assistant's left. Hand instruments passed to operator's left hand are passed with the assistant's right hand. Instruments should be placed with the handles facing the assistant's right. Larger instruments, forceps, and scissors are placed to the right of the tray with the handles facing toward the right. Expendables are placed at the top of the tray with those items used together placed together.

Correct technique in passing and receiving instruments and materials to the operator is a skill that must be practiced to mastery level to achieve the most out of four-handed dentistry. In order for the assistant to be **proficient** in this skill, they need to not only understand the sequence of each individual procedure and be able to anticipate when and what the next instrument needed will be, but also know the instrument transfer zones, what grasp the dentist/operator desires to hold the instrument, and what transfer technique works best for each instrument and material.

Instrument Transfer Zones

There are three instrument transfer zones (A, B, and C) designated for transfer for specific types of instruments and materials. These zones are used for ease and safety of instrument transfer (Figure 20-9).

Zone A The Zone A transfer area is located below the patient's eyes to the chin. Most hand instruments are transferred in this area. The operator is able to maintain their finger rest when instruments are passed in this area. In order to transfer instruments to the operator, the assistant must bring the instruments over the patient's chest and into Zone A. This is to make certain instruments are not seen by the patient and are not accidentally dropped on the patient's face. The assistant should be mindful of ergonomics and make every transfer with minimal motion, using movements of elbows, wrists, and fingers only.

Zone B This transfer zone is located below the patient's chin extending in a 12-inch square over the chest. Zone B is used when the instruments or items need to be transferred away from the patient's face for safety. This would include passing larger instruments (forceps, scissors), medicaments, and instruments not used in the mouth.

Zone C This transfer zone is located behind and over the patient's left shoulder. Zone C is used when the object is heavy or **caustic** and when the item passed may enhance patient anxiety, for example, the anesthetic syringe.

Instrument Grasps

A grasp is a method of holding an instrument with the fingers in a manner that allows freedom of action, control, tactile sensitivity, and **maneuverability**. In the dental field, there are different types of grasps for different types of procedures and instruments used by both the dentist/operator and dental assistant. The dental assistant must be skilled in securely grasping instruments for use and be able to transfer instruments for the dentist's/operator's preferred grasp.

Pen Grasp The pen grasp is most frequently used with hand instruments passed in transfer Zone A. The instrument is held in the position shown in Figure 20-10, just as one would hold a pen or pencil. The instrument is supported between the index finger, middle finger, and thumb.

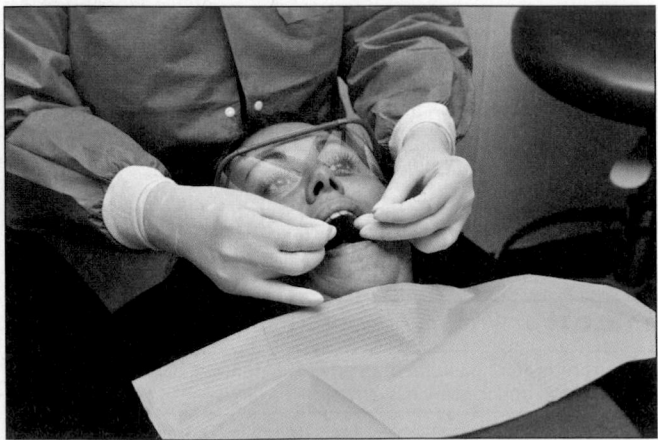

FIGURE 20-9
Instrument transfer zones: proper finger rest of operator to receive an instrument.

Modified Pen Grasp This is similar to the pen grasp, except the pad of the middle finger is placed on the handle of the instrument. This grasp allows for more strength and stability. This grasp may be used in holding the HVE and when mixing and condensing materials (Figure 20-11).

Palm Grasp The instrument or equipment is held securely in the palm of the hand. This grasp is used mostly for instruments with hinges and bulky instruments, such as forceps and the air/water syringe (Figure 20-12).

Palm–Thumb Grasp The instrument is held in the palm of the hand, and the thumb is used to stabilize and guide the instrument. The operator may use this grasp with instruments that require a more vertical movement, such as when using a chisel or an oral evacuator for retraction purposes. With the

operator's thumb toward the working end, they can perform a scraping motion such as when using a chisel (Figure 20-13). The thumb away from the working end allows movement for a digging, pulling action as needed when using an oral evacuator for retraction purposes. This is also known as the thumb-to-nose grasp and reverse palm–thumb grasp (Figure 20-14).

Types of Instrument Transfers

Efficient instrument transfer is one of the basic skills the dental assistant must learn in order to be productive and successful assisting in procedures. In the dental field, there are three common instrument transfers: single-handed, two-handed, and hidden. All procedures discussed pertain to a right-handed operator, unless otherwise stated. When working with a left-handed operator the positions are reversed.

Single-Handed Transfer

Single-handed dental instrument transfer is the most common transfer technique and is used for efficiency. The assistant transfers the instrument with the left hand, which frees the assistant's right hand to hold the oral evacuator or air/water syringe.

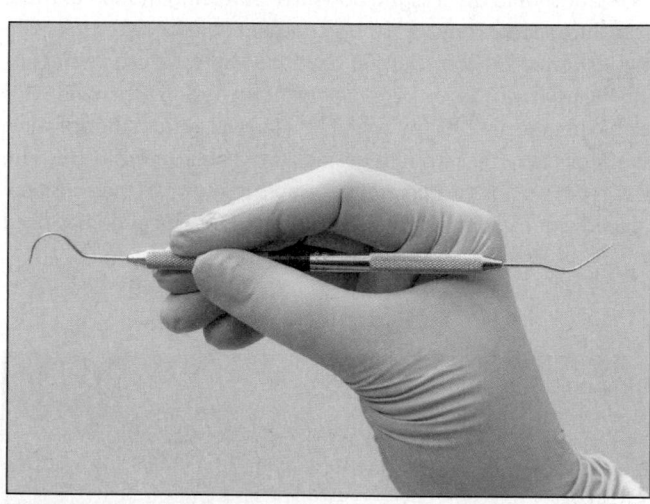

FIGURE 20-10
Pen grasp.

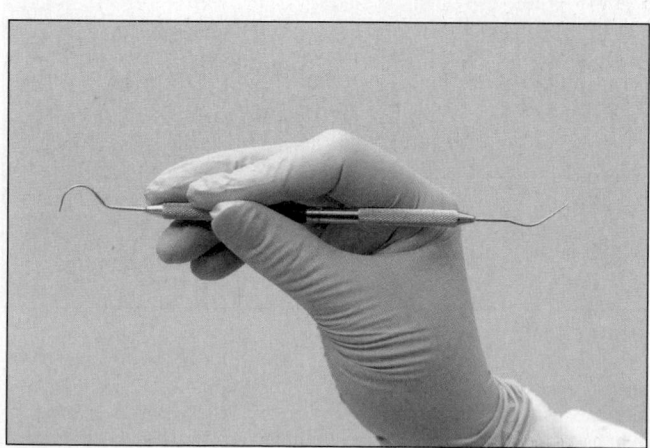

FIGURE 20-11
Modified pen grasp.

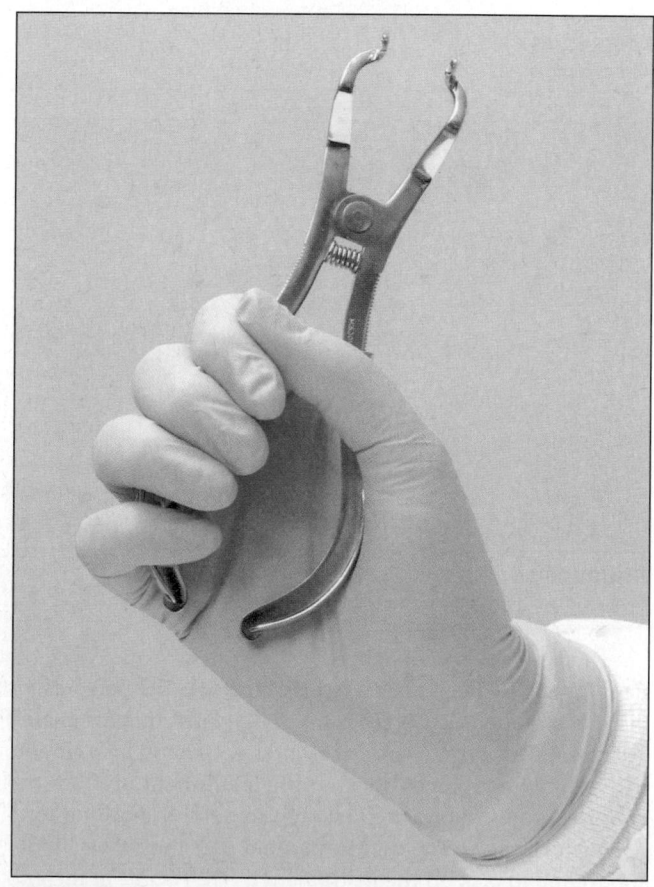

FIGURE 20-12
Palm grasp.

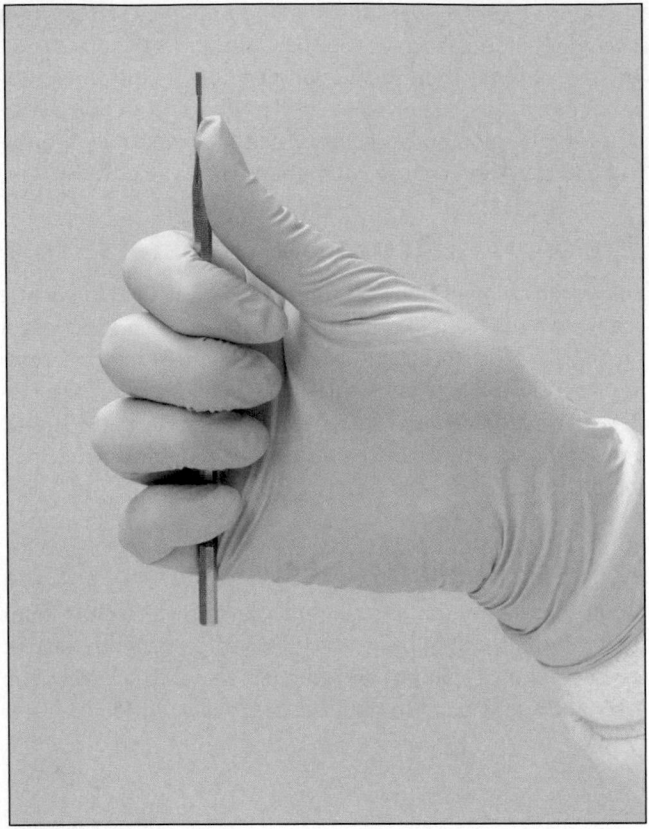

FIGURE 20-13
Palm–thumb grasp.

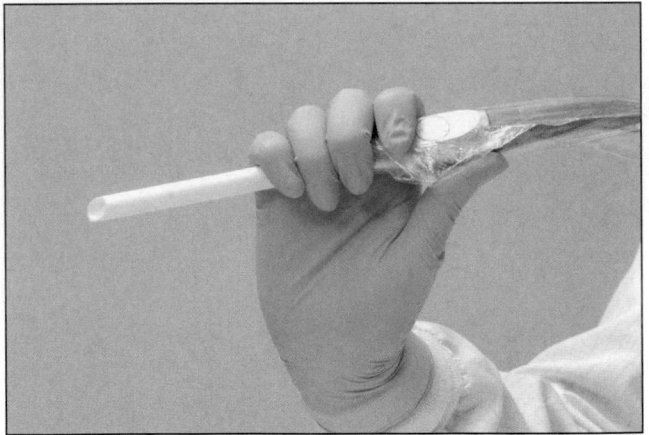

FIGURE 20-14
Reverse palm–thumb grasp.

Pen Grasp—Transfer and Retrieval

The pen grasp is the most frequently used to transfer hand instruments passed in Zone A. This type of transfer works with hand instruments and dental handpieces. Picking the instrument up from the prepared tray setup is the first step to get into position for a successful transfer. The dental assistant uses their index finger and thumb to pick up the instrument by the handle at the end opposite the one used by the operator. The assistant allows the instrument to stabilize on the instrument tray as the instrument slips between the opening of their index finger and thumb (Figure 20-15). The assistant rotates the instrument into a pen grasp by holding the instrument between the index finger, middle finger, and thumb. The middle finger is placed below the instrument to stabilize the instrument. The instrument is in ready position to be transferred to the dentist/operator and into the recommended transfer zone to be used in pen grasp. The assistant brings the instrument below the patient's chin into Zone A, ready to be passed. The assistant must never pass instruments near the patient's eyes as this may cause patient anxiety and is a safety risk.

The operator signals they are ready for instruments by placing hands on either side of the patient's face and establishing a finger rest (Figure 20-16). The assistant directs the working end in the position of use. The assistant places the working end of the instrument into the patient's mouth in the area the operator is working. The instrument should be placed firmly between the operator's index finger and thumb at the junction of the handle and the shank. The assistant should use a slight, downward pressing motion to make sure the operator is aware of the instrument transfer before releasing the instrument. A good transfer can occur without the operator taking their eyes off the work area and without moving their hands. This eliminates the need for the operator to look away from the operative site, move from their fulcrum position, or fumble for the instrument. It is important for the operator to be able to maintain their position; movement may disrupt the procedure, and the operator may need

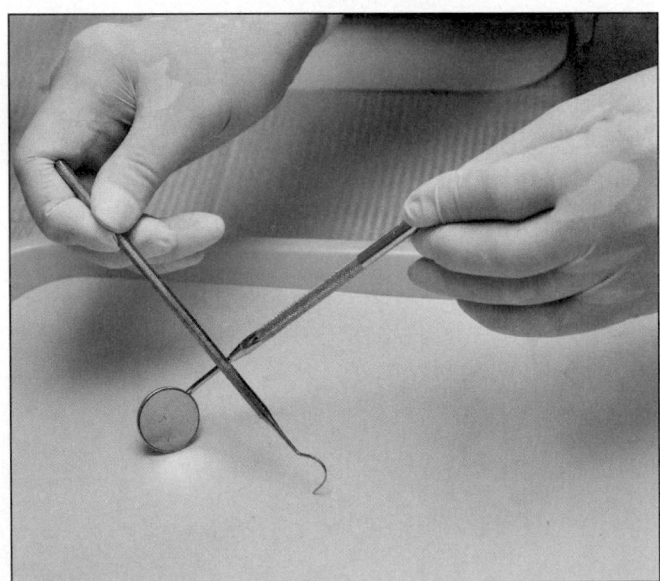

FIGURE 20-15
Pen grasp transfer. Remove instrument from instrument tray. Assistant picks up instrument between index finger and thumb while resting instrument on tray on the opposite side of the working end. Assistant picks up mirror in right hand and explorer in left. Rest instrument on tray while the instrument is allowed to move between opening of index finger and thumb.

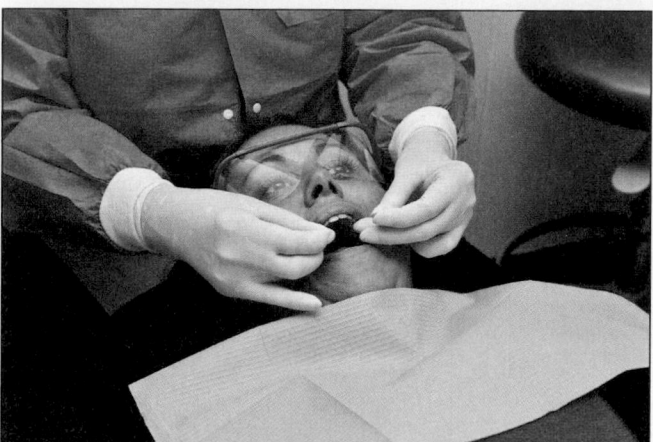

FIGURE 20-16
Dentist signals for receiving mirror and explorer at beginning of procedure by establishing finger rest.

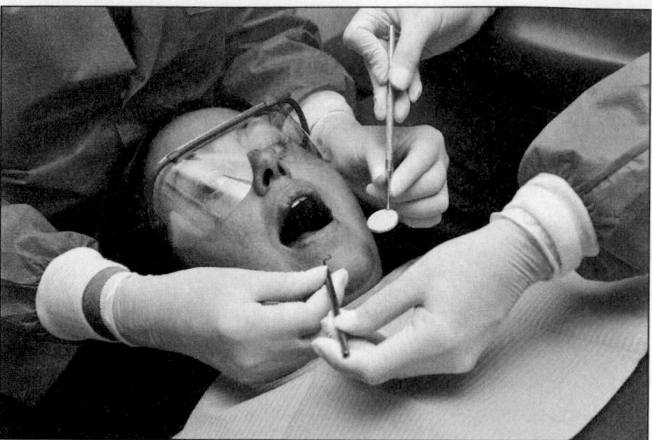

FIGURE 20-17
Pen grasp transfer. Assistant picks up the mirror and explorer and rests middle finger under instruments to secure the instruments. Mirror and explorer are faced toward the maxillary arch and passed at the same time to examine the maxillary anterior teeth.

In dentistry, instruments, handpieces, and equipment are transferred in the "position of use." Position of use refers to when the assistant positions the instrument so it is ready to be used by the operator without adjustments. For example, the working end of the instrument is positioned for the proper dental arch; the working end should be positioned upward for the maxilla and downward for the mandible. When the assistant retrieves the instrument from the tray, they should pick up the instruments from the opposite end of use.

to keep the area isolated or may be retracting tissue and keeping an area dry. Movement will cost the operator needless time and loss of focus or concentration.

The dentist/operator lifts the end of the handle to signal that they are finished with the instrument and ready for it to be retrieved. The operator should make certain there is enough of the handle to be grasped by the assistant. The assistant retrieves the instrument by grasping the end of the handle with their index and middle finger and thumb to remove the instrument from the operator's hands. Once an instrument has been retrieved, debris from the used instrument should be wiped clean with a gauze square using the right hand before replacing the instrument on the tray in its original order of use. The assistant returns the instrument to the instrument tray and places it into sequence by resting it on the tray and allowing the instrument to slide through the opening between the thumb and index finger.

It is unusual that the assistant will need to pass two instruments — one in each hand. The mirror and explorer are exceptions. These two instruments are transferred simultaneously by the assistant at the beginning of most procedures (Figure 20-17). This is a good place for assistants to begin practice in transferring instruments. Pick up the dental mirror by the handle using the right hand while picking up the explorer with the left hand. Hold

both instruments in the pen grasp. When the operator places hands on either side of the patient's head, the assistant passes both of the instruments to the operator while pressing down simultaneously.

Pen Grasp— Baton Technique Sometimes when passing a double-ended instrument, the operator requests the opposite end than the assistant has ready to pass. To get the desired end into position to be passed, the assistant needs to use the baton technique. The baton technique resembles the maneuver made by drum majors as they rotate and spin the baton as they lead the band.

While holding the instrument in the pen grasp the assistant brings their index finger to the same side of the handle as the thumb. With the instrument now being held between the index and middle finger, the assistant moves the thumb on the same side as the middle finger. By pulling the thumb toward the assistant, the ends of the instrument are rotated. The assistant can return to holding the instrument in pen grasp and move up to the opposite end of the handle. Once the pen grasp is secure, they are ready to transfer the opposite working end to the operator.

Safety

In order to maximize efficiency and safety during instrument transfer, it is important to continuously observe the patient's movement, especially during transfer of an anesthetic syringe and sharp objects. To be safe during the transfer procedures, the team should maintain firm control of the instruments at all times, using only the transfer zone over the patient's chest. Instruments or materials should never be laid on the patient's napkin.

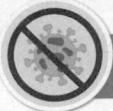

Infection Control

During the instrument transfer techniques, the working end should never be contaminated by touching it with your hands or any nonsterile item. While performing the baton technique, move to the middle of the instruments before rotating the instrument.

Palm Grasp—Transfer and Retrieval This transfer is used when the procedure requires that the operator hold the instrument firmly in the palm of their hand. This grasp is used for pliers, scissors, forceps, and instruments not to be used in the mouth. The operator signals the palm grasp transfer by bringing their hand in Zone B with palm up or down depending on the area and operator preference. The assistant picks up the instrument above the junction of the working end (flat portion between working end and handle of the instrument) between thumb and index and middle finger (Figure 20-18). The assistant should curve the palm of their hand away from the working end of the instrument to ensure that the working end is not touched or contaminated, the glove is not torn, and the assistant is not injured. The assistant holds the instrument using a modified pen grasp and slightly opens the hinge. The assistant places the instrument into the palm of the operator's hand with a slight pressing motion (Figure 20-19). The operator grasps the instrument with all fingers and thumb supporting it.

The operator signals that they are finished with the instrument by returning the instrument into Zone B. The assistant retrieves the instrument by holding the instrument above the junction of the working end using a modified pen grasp. The instrument is returned to its position on the tray with the handles facing toward the right.

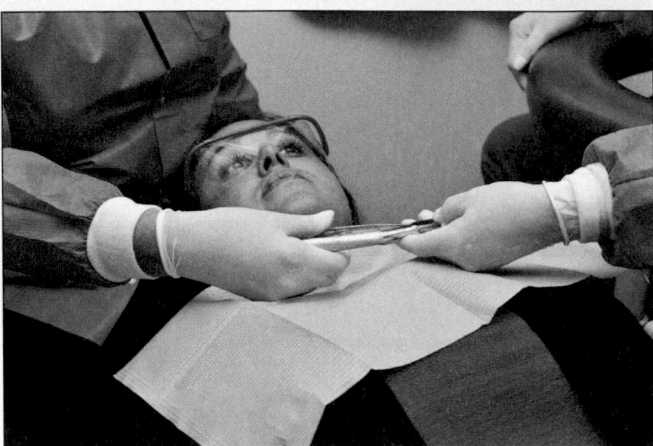

FIGURE 20-19
Palm grasp transfer. The assistant holds the forceps above the junction of the instrument handles with left hand, and the operator grasps the instrument's handles.

There is a slight modification when transferring and retrieving scissors. The assistant slightly opens the scissors and holds them until the operator is able to insert their fingers into the scissors rings before releasing the instrument (Figure 20-19). When retrieving scissors, the assistant holds the instrument above the junction of the blades until the operator removes their fingers from the scissor rings.

Palm–Thumb Grasp—Transfer and Retrieval The operator uses this grasp when they are using a scraping or digging motion. Instruments that are to be transferred using the palm–thumb grasp need to be placed on the instrument tray with the working end facing the assistant's left. The assistant picks up the instrument above the junction of the handle and the shank and turns the instrument with the handle facing the operator (Figure 20-21). The operator signals transfer by bringing their hand into Zone B with palm up or down. The assistant places the instrument firmly in the operator's palm using a slight pressing motion to make the operator aware of the pass (Figures 20–22A and B). When the operator is finished with the instrument, they should rotate the instrument into pen grasp and lift the handle of the instrument to signal ready for retrieval. The instrument is retrieved by the assistant using the pen grasp retrieval technique and returned to the instrument tray.

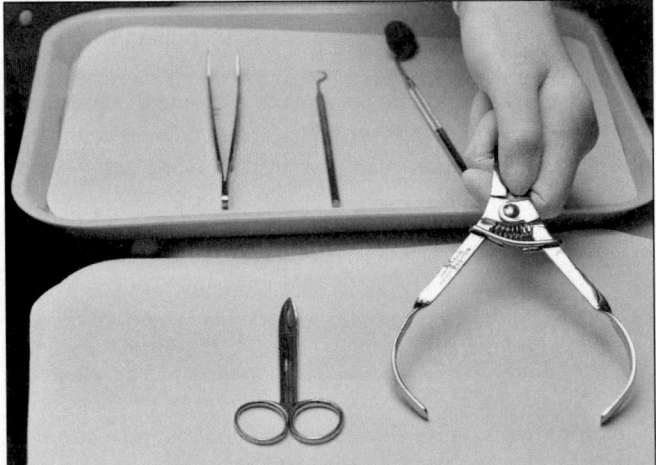

FIGURE 20-18
Palm grasp. Assistant picks up forceps using modified pen grasp above the junction of the working end between the thumb and index and middle finger. The palm of hand is curved away from working end to make certain the end is not contaminated.

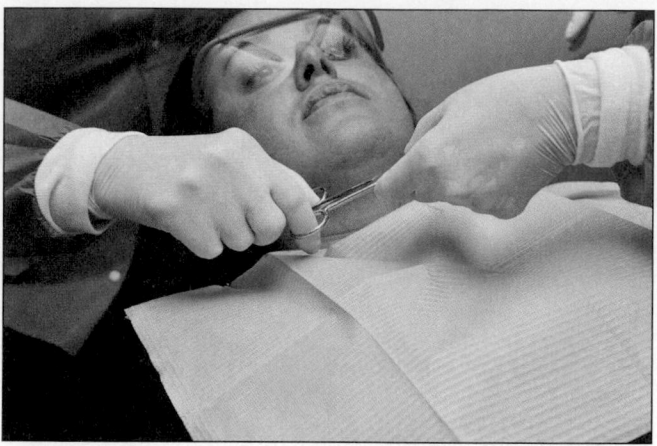

FIGURE 20-20
Scissors transfer. Assistant holds scissors in left hand above the junction of working end while slightly opening the hinge with right hand. Dentist signals by bringing their hands into Zone B. Assistant holds scissors below the dentist's hand with left hand. The scissors are held until the dentist inserts fingers into the rings.

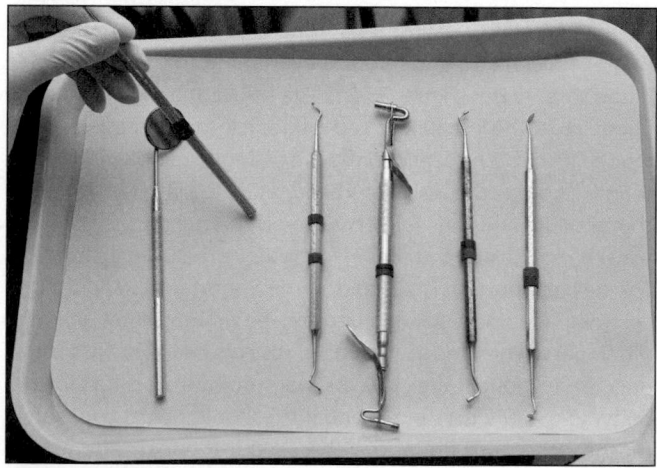

FIGURE 20-21
Palm–thumb grasp transfer. The assistant picks up the instrument on the working end side.

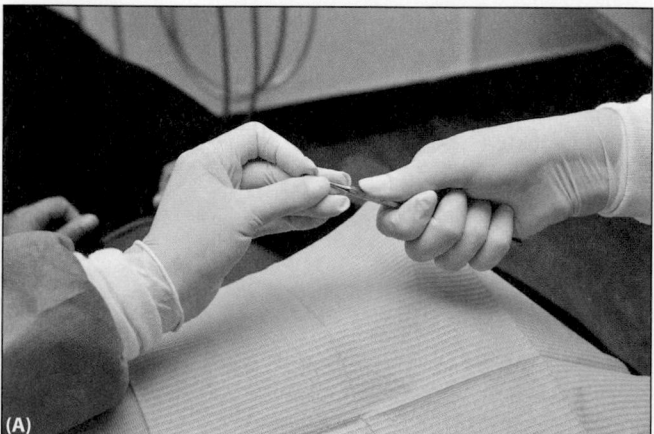

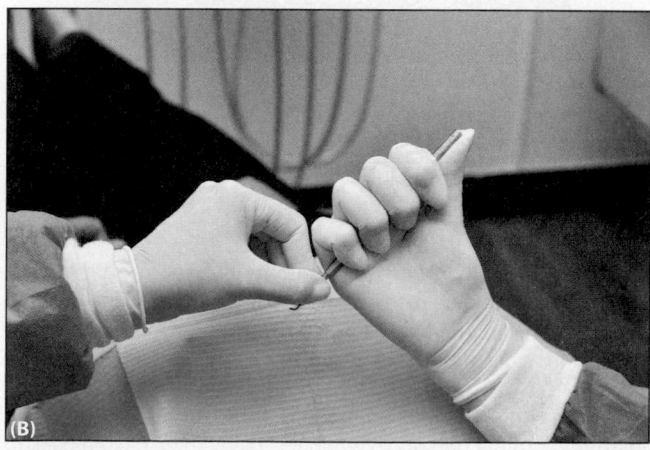

FIGURE 20-22
There are two versions of the palm–thumb grasp for scraping or digging. (A) The operator holds the scaler with thumb toward the working end to scrape calculus from the patient's teeth. (B) The chisel is held with the thumb away from the working end to dig and pull tissue from the cavity preparation.

Double Instrument Exchange

When assisting the dentist during procedures, the dental assistant will not always pass just one instrument at a time. As the operator finishes with one instrument, they generally need another immediately. The assistant needs to anticipate the next instrument and have it ready to be passed. There is a double instrument exchange for all three of the instrument transfers.

Pen Grasp—Double Instrument Exchange When using the pen grasp double instrument exchange, the assistant uses five steps: working step, signal, pretransfer step, mid-transfer, and roll technique.

Working Step The alert assistant already has the next instrument in their left hand ready for transfer. The assistant picks up the instrument from the tray using the left hand. The dental assistant uses the index finger and thumb to pick up the instrument by the handle at the end opposite the one used by the operator. The assistant brings the new instrument toward the instrument in the operator's hand (Figure 20-23). When ready for the exchange, the assistant needs to make certain to hold the instrument parallel to and just above the one held in the operator's hand.

Signal The operator signals they are done with the first instrument. They raise the handle of the instrument slightly from the operative site while maintaining a finger rest (Figure 20-24). The operator should hold the instrument in the middle of the handle (allow enough room for the assistant to grasp the handle) and keep the handle parallel to the patient's pupils.

Pretransfer The assistant extends their ring and small finger of the left hand to grasp the used instrument near the end of the handle. The assistant retrieves the used instrument by curling the extended fingers around the instrument and pulling the instrument back and parallel with their forearm. The assistant is now in position to retrieve the first instrument. Make certain to not rotate the instrument above Zone A, never beyond the nose and around the eyes. This technique makes the pass easier and safer.

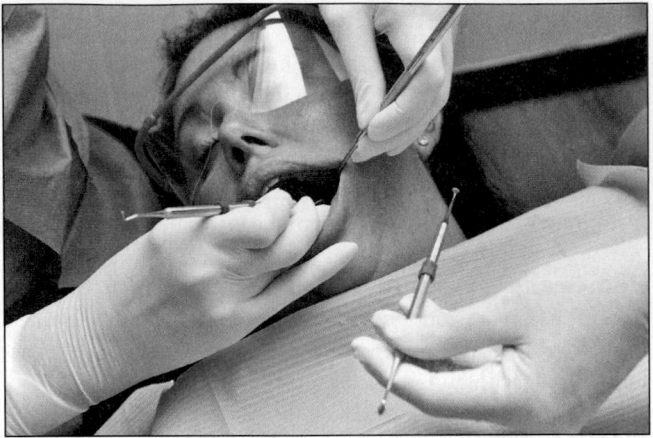

FIGURE 20-23
Working step. Assistant holds instrument in Zone B in ready position to transfer.

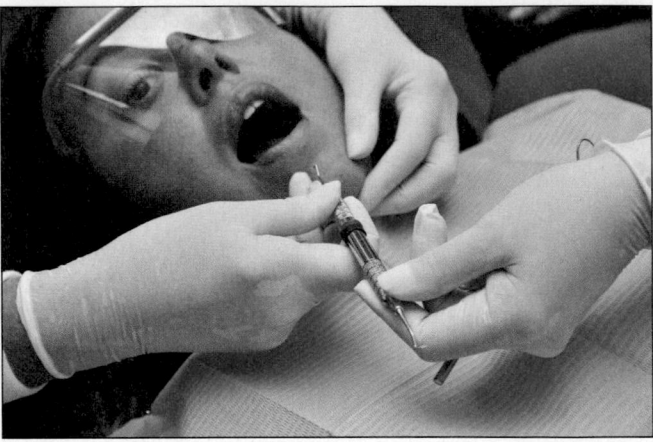

FIGURE 20-25
Pretransfer. Assistant extends last two fingers, retrieves instrument from dentist, and draws the instrument toward the forearm. Mid-transfer. The new instrument is transferred to the dentist.

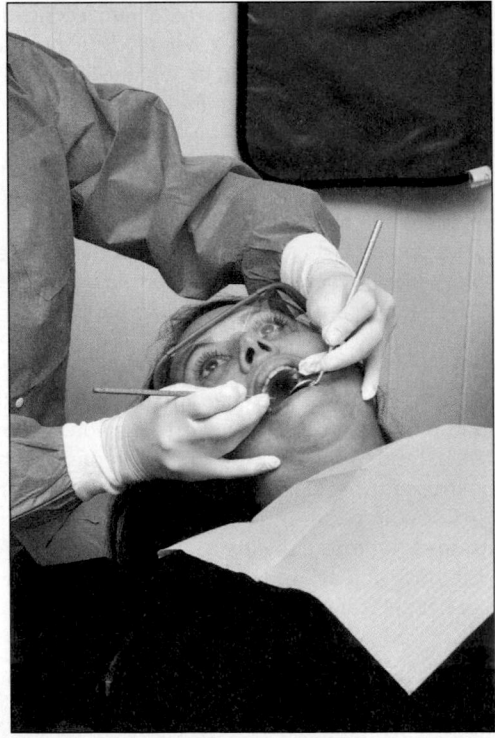

FIGURE 20-24
Signal. Dentist maintains finger rest and lifts handle of the used instrument to signal for instrument exchange.

The assistant presses the instrument between the thumb and ring or small finger and rolls the instrument to the top knuckle of the small finger (Figure 20-26). The assistant brings the middle finger under the instrument and rotates it into pen grasp by holding the instrument between the index finger, middle finger, and thumb. Imagine the assistant's hand is divided into two portions, the "pick up" and the "delivery." The pickup portion of the hand uses the fourth and fifth fingers to retrieve the used instrument. The delivery portion is the part of the fingers and hand used to complete the single-handed transfer, the thumb, index, and middle fingers. When receiving a used instrument, some assistants may use just one finger, but this does not always allow for stability, so two fingers (fourth and fifth) should be used for safety reasons; the third finger may be used if the instrument feels unstable.

Mid-transfer With the first instrument out of the way, the assistant delivers the new instrument to the operator using the pen grasp technique (Figure 20-25). A Class II motion (fingers and wrist) is the only motion necessary to deliver the new instrument.

Roll Technique The roll technique is used to return the retrieved instrument to the pen grasp when it is ready to be passed back to the operator or to return it to its place on the instrument tray. This technique gets its name because the instrument is actually rolled up the ring and little finger.

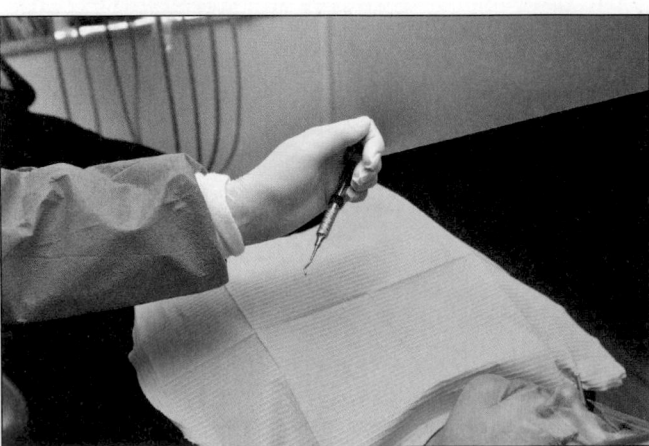

FIGURE 20-26
Roll technique. Assistant brings retrieved instrument into Zone B and rolls it into pen grasp before returning it to the patient tray in sequence.

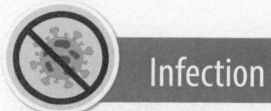

Infection Control

If a member of the dental team is cut by the working end of an instrument or gets a tear in the glove, the procedure should be stopped and the worker must immediately remove the glove and perform clinical handwashing using an antimicrobial soap. They should don a new pair of gloves, return to the treatment area, and replace the contaminated instrument with a sterile instrument to complete the procedure. The second worker remaining with the patient should explain to the patient what has just occurred. This is an OSHA guideline. An incident form must completed before the end of the day.

OSHA requires that employers provide gloves for infection control. There is no specification for the type and sizing of the glove; however, ill-fitting gloves may increase the chance of slippage, poor instrument transfer, and increased possibility of tearing and puncturing the glove and of acquiring MSD.

Whenever the integrity of the examination glove is in question, the assistant should go immediately to the sterilization area to remove the glove and inspect their hands. If there is a tear in the glove but the skin is intact, the hands should be washed with antimicrobial soap. There is no need for an incident report to be completed. If the skin is open, the assistant should take immediate emergency care and complete the incident report (Figure 20-27).

Palm–Thumb Grasp—Double Instrument Exchange

When the operator is holding an instrument at the time the dental assistant is passing an instrument using the palm–thumb grasp, the dental assistant needs to retrieve the first instrument with the left hand using the pen grasp. The second instrument is held in the assistant's right hand at the junction of the hand and shank with the blade facing the operator. The operator grasps the instrument around the handle with their thumb toward or away from the working end. When the operator is finished with the instrument, they rotate the instrument to the pen grasp before signaling exchange. The instrument exchange is completed with the pen grasp retrieval in assistant's left hand.

Two-Handed Transfer

Generally the assistant retrieves instruments with the same hand used to transfer; however, if two large instruments are being exchanged, both hands may need to be used.

OFFICE INCIDENT REPORT	
Subject of Incident (last name, first name, middle initial):	Date of Incident:
Employee or Patient (Circle One)	
Permanent address:	
Description of Incident (to be state clearly in subject's own words):	
_Office dental assistant Anna Graves tears glove while working with Dr. Casey on patient Mrs. Davis. Patient presented for restorative. During transfer of instruments, a spoon excavator caught Anna's gloves and caused a tear. The tear was initially not noticed and the work progressed. Anna noticed the tear a few minutes later into the treatment visit.	
Subject's Signature	
Witness 1 Name and Address and Phone Number	
Witness 2 Name and Address and Phone Number	
Witness 3 Name and Address and Phone Number	
Was the subject examined by a physician in hospital? Yes or No (circle one)	
Physican's Name (please print)	
Signature and title of person preparing report	

Courtesy of Dr. V. Singhal

FIGURE 20-27
Office incident report.

Procedure 20-1
Single-Handed Pen Grasp Double Instrument Transfer

The double instrument transfer is performed at the dental unit by the dental assistant and the operator. The dental assistant uses their left hand to transfer instruments for a right-handed dentist. This is reversed for a left-handed operator. The dental assistant's free hand may hold the evacuator or retract oral tissues.

Equipment and Supplies
- Basic setup: mouth mirror, explorer, and cotton pliers
- Assortment of hand instruments

Procedure Steps
1. Prepare instruments for procedure.
   - ❏ Place instrument tray lengthwise, close to patient in 2 o'clock position.
   - ❏ Place instruments on tray in order of use.
   - ❏ Face handles passed with the right hand toward the right.
   - ❏ Face handles passed with the left hand toward the left.

2. Prepare for instrument transfer.
   - ❏ When beginning the procedure, the dentist will always utilize the mouth mirror and explorer to inspect the areas to be treated.

3. Simultaneously pick up mirror and explorer.
   - ❏ Pick up explorer with left hand and mirror with right hand with first finger and thumb at opposite ends of the working end.
   - ❏ Move the instrument into position to pass by resting the instrument on the middle finger.
   - ❏ Position instrument for use: working end up for maxillary and down for mandibular.

4. Watch for dentist's signal (places hands and establishes finger rest) to transfer first instrument.
   - ❏ Move instrument into the transfer zone over patient's chest.
   - ❏ Place instruments into dentist's hands between the thumb and first finger.

   - ❏ Provide a slight pressing down motion as releasing the instrument.

5. Pick up next instrument needed in procedure sequence.
   - ❏ Hold instrument to be transferred in transfer zone over patient's chest.

6. Watch for dentist's signal for an instrument exchange. (maintains finger rest, and with pivotal action rotates working end away from patient's oral cavity and lifts handle of instrument)

7. Hold transfer instrument parallel to the instrument in use and out of operator's way.
   - ❏ Retrieve the used instrument.
   - ❏ Extend last two fingers and grasp used instrument.
   - ❏ Tuck the used instrument and brace it securely against the palm. Bring used instrument parallel to forearm with the pickup portion of the hand.

8. Simultaneously, extend the new instrument with working end pointed in the position of use.
   - ❏ Place instruments into dentist's hands between the thumb and first finger.
   - ❏ Provide a slight pressing down motion as releasing the instrument.

9. Roll used instrument and return to holding position.
   - ❏ Hold instrument between last two fingers and thumb.
   - ❏ Press against the instrument and roll the instrument until above first knuckle of the ring finger.
   - ❏ Fold index and middle fingers under the handle and return instrument to holding position.
   - ❏ Bring fingers around the end of the instrument and obtain pen grasp.

10. Hold instrument parallel to the instrument in use and out of operator's way if the instrument is to be used again or return used instrument to its original position on the tray and pick up the next instrument to be passed.

Palm Grasp The two-handed transfer is used when transferring bulky items or instruments such as forceps or scissors. This type of double instrument exchange requires that the assistant pick up the used instrument with one hand and deliver the new instrument with the other hand. The dental assistant holds the next instrument to be passed in their left hand. The operator signals by bringing their hand into Zone B. When ready to pass, the assistant retrieves the first instrument with the right hand and places the second instrument above the operator's right hand (Figure 20-28). The assistant brings the second instrument down into the operator's hand and transfers the new instrument with the left hand while taking the used instrument with the right hand. The assistant returns the used instrument to sequence with the right hand. This exchange involves more movement (Class III) and does not allow the assistant to use the air/water syringe or HVE while transferring.

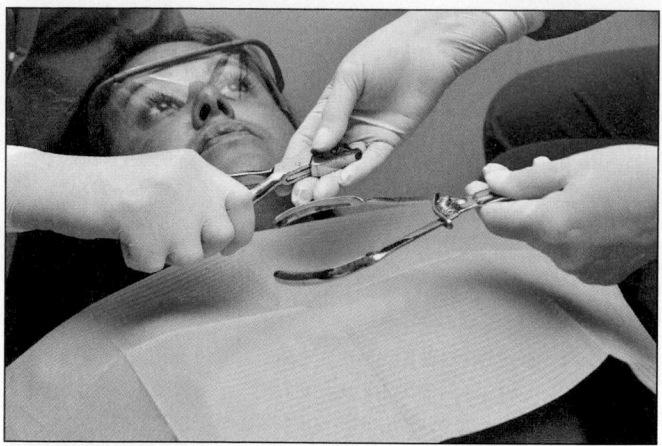

FIGURE 20-28
Dentist signals for transfer of forceps by placing hand palm up into Zone B for a mandibular position of use. The assistant faces the beaks toward the mandibular anterior (downward), takes the instrument being retrieved, and places handles of new instrument into dentist's palm with slight pressing motion.

Instrument Transfer Modifications

There are times when the transfer must be modified. The operator may have to move away from the patient's mouth to receive some instruments, or the size or weight of some instruments may require the transfer to be modified.

Transferring Heavy and Large Instruments Dental handpieces are bulky, but they can be transferred with the one-handed transfer. The assistant picks up the handpiece near the hose attachment, away from the working end. Handpieces are heavier and, with the hose attachment, are difficult to transfer, but with time and practice the transfer will be smooth and manageable. If both hands are free, use the two-handed pass to transfer the handpieces.

To pass the air/water syringe, the assistant holds the end of the syringe covering the nozzle and tip with the palm of the hand. The handle of the syringe is projected toward the operator for easier grasping. The operator receives the syringe at the

Procedure 20-2
Two-Handed Palm Grasp Double Instrument Transfer

The two-handed transfer is performed when two hinged instruments need to be exchanged at the dental unit by the dental assistant and the operator. The assistant passes the new instrument with their left hand and retrieves with their right hand.

Equipment and Supplies
- Assortment of forceps and pliers
- Scissors

Procedure Steps

1. Assemble instruments for procedure.
   - ❏ Place instrument tray lengthwise, close to patient in 2 o'clock position.
   - ❏ Place instruments on tray in sequence of use.
   - ❏ Face handles passed with the right hand toward the right.
   - ❏ Face handles passed with the left hand toward the left.
   - ❏ Place forceps and scissors to right of tray with handles facing right.
   - ❏ Place expendables at the top of the tray.

2. Prepare for instrument transfer.
   - ❏ Pick up the forceps with left hand using a modified pen grasp.
   - ❏ Hold instrument above the junction of the working end (flat portion between working end and handle of the instrument) between thumb and index and middle finger.
   - ❏ Curve palm of hand away from working end of the instrument to prevent touching or contaminating working end.

   - ❏ Slightly open the hinge with right hand.
   - ❏ Position instrument for use: working end up for maxillary and down for mandibular.

3. Watch for dentist's signal.
   (signals palm grasp transfer by bringing hand in Zone B with palm up or down depending on the area and operator preference)

4. Pass forceps to dentist.
   - ❏ Move forceps into the transfer zone over patient's chest.
   - ❏ Place the instrument into the palm of the operator's hand with a slight pressing motion.

5. Pick up next instrument needed in procedure sequence.
   - ❏ Pick up the scissors with left hand using a modified pen grasp.
   - ❏ Hold instrument above the junction of the working end (flat portion between working end and handle of the instrument) between thumb and index and middle finger.
   - ❏ Curve palm of hand away from working end of the instrument to prevent touching and contaminating working end.
   - ❏ Slightly open the hinge with right hand.
   - ❏ Position instrument for use: working end up for maxillary and down for mandibular.

6. Hold instrument in left hand to be transferred in Zone B over patient's chest.

7. Watch for dentist's signal for an instrument exchange.
   - ❏ Return forceps into Zone B.

(Continues)

8. Prepare for instrument exchange.
   - ❏ Place scissors below the operator's right hand.
   - ❏ Retrieve used forceps with right hand holding above the junction of the working end in modified pen grasp.
   - ❏ Hold scissors until operator is able to insert fingers into rings before releasing the instrument.
   - ❏ Return forceps to its position on the tray.

9. Watch for dentist's signal for an instrument retrieval.
   - ❏ Return scissors into Zone B.

10. Hold the scissors above the junction of the blades until the operator removes their fingers from the scissor rings.

11. Retrieve scissors.

12. Return scissors to its position on the tray.

handle. For the return transfer, the assistant receives the syringe in the same manner it was passed, by covering the nozzle and tip with the palm of the hand. This process can be accomplished by either the one- or two-handed exchange (Figure 20-29).

Hidden Transfer This transfer is so named because it takes place out of the view of the patient, under their chin in Zone C. It is used when transferring dental materials, caustic materials, and anxiety-producing items (anesthetic syringe). It allows the operator to receive the material out of the patient's line of vision, thus lessening the anxiety of the patient. This transfer

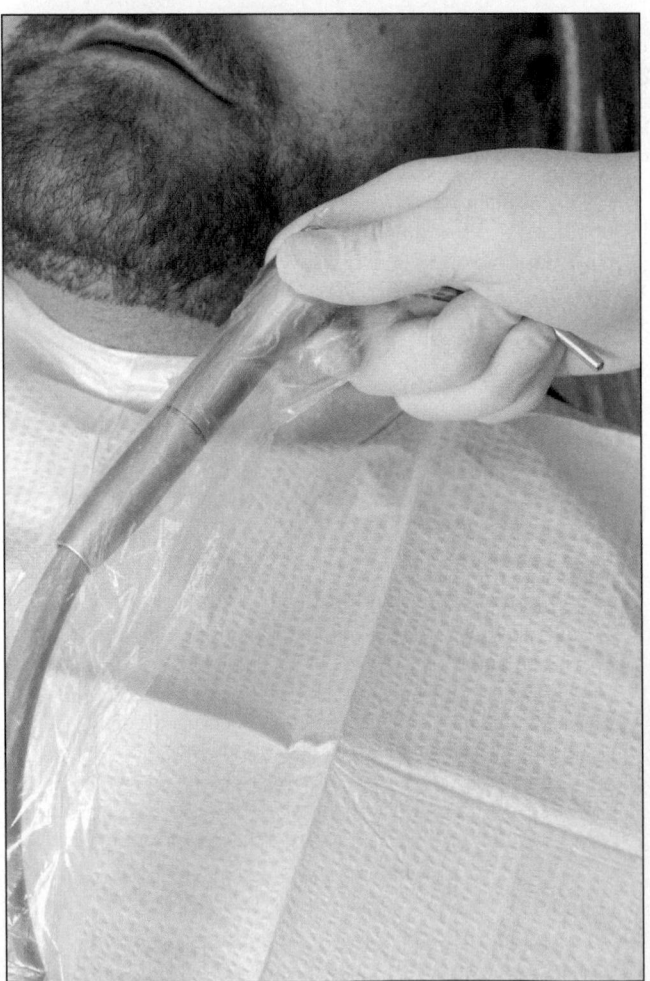

FIGURE 20-29
Air/water syringe transfer. The assistant holds the air/water syringe near the handle in transfer position.

can also be performed behind the patient's head (in the **static** zone) to avoid possible needlesticks or spillage of caustic materials (Class V movement) (Figure 20-30).

Transferring Dental Materials and Medicaments Small amounts of dental materials and medicaments are generally passed on a glass slab, paper pad, or dappen dish. The materials are held under the patient's chin and over the patient's chest in the A transfer zone in the right hand near the treatment site. The assistant passes the application instrument in the left hand and then holds a gauze square in the left hand to wipe excess material from the application instrument (Figure 20-31). The paper pad is held in a tripod-type grasp (thumb, forefinger, and middle finger) to stabilize if the dentist presses down with applicator.

Transferring Expendables When transferring expendables, cotton tip applicators, cotton rolls, and gauze squares, the assistant can pass the item with their hands using the pen grasp. In passing small expendables like cotton pellets, the assistant should use cotton pliers.

It is easier to pass materials using locked cotton pliers. If the assistant needs to pass materials using nonlocking pliers or if the material is too large for the pliers to lock, they must maintain a tight grasp on the pliers until the transfer is completed and the operator has established a grip to hold the material. When the pliers are retrieved, the working end should be grasped in the palm of the assistant's hand to prevent dropping the material held in

✓ Safety

Both dentist and assistant need to not only pay attention to what they are doing but also be aware of what the team member is doing. A signal between the team to make the other (and not the patient) aware of a situation is critical for the safety of the patient and team.

The use of a nonverbal signal is important not only to prevent patient anxiety when there is a potential anxiety provoking situation but also because repetitious verbal communication throughout every workday can become tedious.

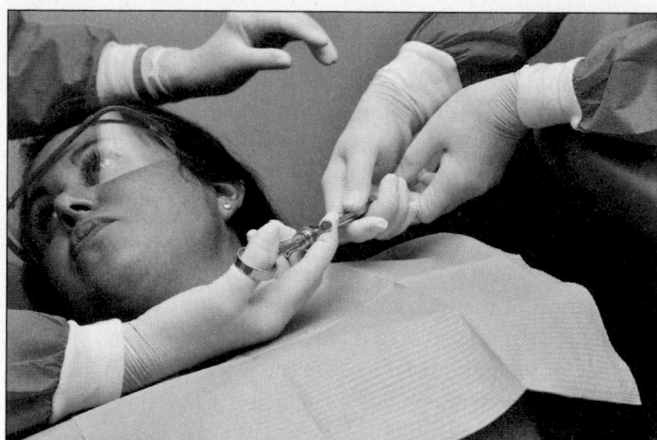

FIGURE 20-30
Hidden transfer—syringe pass. Assistant holds the barrel of the syringe in palm of right hand and moves syringe behind the patient's head. Operator reaches over to receive syringe.

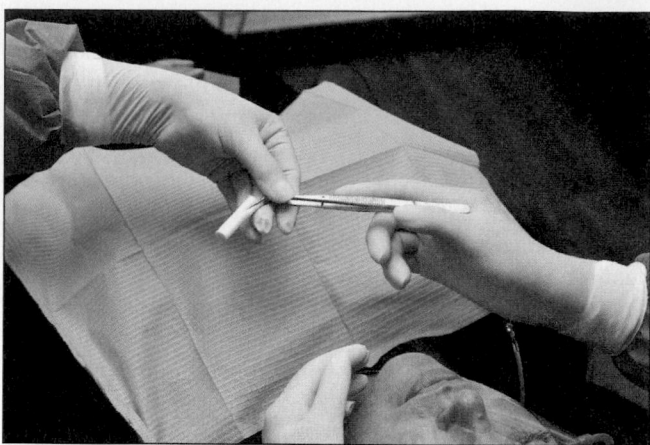

FIGURE 20-32
Transfer expendables. When retrieving expendables, the assistant retrieves the pliers near the beaks using the left hand or grasps the item from the pliers holding a gauze square in the right hand.

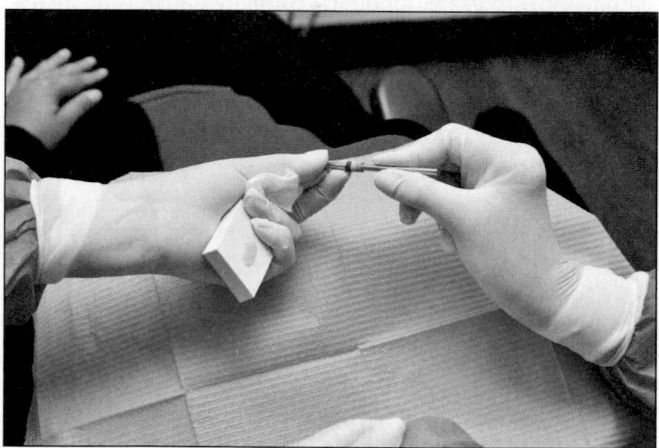

FIGURE 20-31
Transfer dental materials. The assistant mixes the material on the mixing pad while placed on the bracket table and then holds mixing pads with mixed material under the patient's chin. Assistant passes placement instrument with left hand.

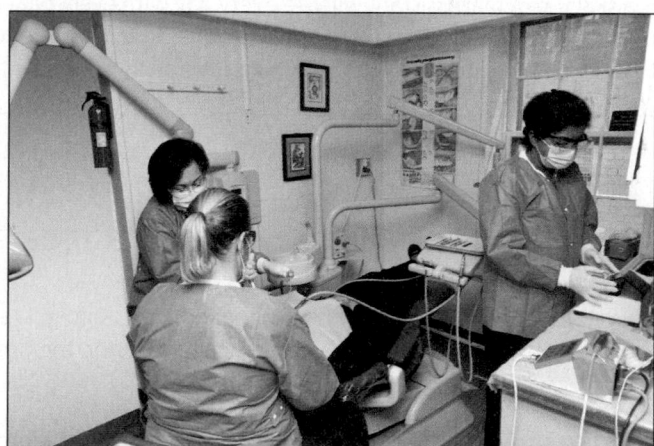

FIGURE 20-33
Six-handed transfer. The operator is finishing up the preparation of the tooth to receive an amalgam restoration. The assistant holds the air/water syringe in the left hand and the HVE in the right. The third team member is mixing the amalgam in the amalgamator.

the pliers (Figure 20-32). The beaks of the working end should be in the palm when transferring, not just when retrieving.

Six-Handed Transfer

In some special circumstances, a third set of hands may be valuable and necessary. When performing tasks such as charting, manipulating multiple materials, or working in a surgery setting, the assistant and operator may be so involved in the procedures at hand that a third set of hands may be requested. The third person may need to chart, prepare materials, or retract soft tissue, as well as anticipate the needs of not only the operator but also the assistant (Figure 20-33).

Developing Teamwork

It is important when the dentist and assistant are working closely together as a team that they develop and learn to communicate verbally and nonverbally. Thoroughly knowing each procedure will enhance the team's four-handed transfer skills. Practice of these procedures will increase their **psychomotor** skills and proficiency of the task at hand. Both the dentist and assistant have equally important roles in making successful instrument transfers and making it a smooth, continuous procedure.

Teamwork is defined in *Webster's New World Dictionary* as "a joint action by a group of people, in which each person subordinates his or her individual interests and opinions to the unity and efficiency of the group." Each member of the team is still important; however, working as a team means that effective and efficient teamwork goes beyond the individual's accomplishments. The most effective teamwork is produced when all individuals involved harmonize their contributions and work toward a common goal.

The dentist needs to be comfortable telling the assistant exactly how they want the instrument transferred. If the assistant isn't using enough pressure when placing the instrument into the dentist's hand or not hitting the exact spot, the dentist should not only tell but demonstrate what they want. Team communication should be open enough that the assistant can tell the dentist what they can do to help make transferring instruments easier. If the dentist is holding the instrument in a position that is difficult

for the assistant to reach in picking up the instrument, the assistant should not only be able to tell but demonstrate what they want. When each member of the team understands the procedure, communicates throughout the workday, and anticipates each other's needs, the dental team (dentist and assistant) can develop an efficient standardized routine for the performance of dental procedures.

Safety for the patient and dental team should always be of utmost importance. The assistant should always be aware of the location of the instrument's working end. Many ends are designed to cut tissue. Just a moment of inattentiveness or slight slippage of the hand may result in the working end accidently cutting the patient or one of the dental team.

Chapter Summary

Four-handed, sit-down dentistry has changed the role of the dental assistant. Working right at the chair with the dentist or dental hygienist, the assistant has become an important aspect of performing dental procedures on patients. Transferring instruments is a skill the dental assistant will use every day with every patient. Learning how to use ergonomics, correctly transferring instruments, understanding what needs to be done during a procedure, and anticipating the next step will enable the dental assistant to be a great asset to the operator and a comfort to the patient.

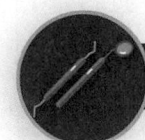 **CASE STUDY**

Dr. Danton and the dental assistant, Kaitlin, are placing a composite filling on Chance Garrett. Kaitlin wants to prove her skills and efficiency during the procedure by having instruments ready.

Case Study Review

1. What can Kaitlin do to prepare for the procedure so that everything will keep moving smoothly during the procedure?

2. What instrument(s) should she be prepared to pass first?

3. When the dentist is done with the composite filling instrument, what should Kaitlin do?

Review Questions

Multiple Choice

1. What area(s) of the body is at epidemic levels of MSD in the United States and has increased in dentistry, which needs improved strength and flexibility to reduce the pain?
   a. upper back and shoulders
   b. neck and shoulders
   c. wrist and hands
   d. lower back pain

2. When assisting a right-handed operator, what zone is from 2–4 o'clock?
   a. static zone
   b. assistant's zone
   c. transfer zone
   d. operator zone

3. At what position is it recommended for an EFDA to sit when working from the back of the patient for best view and access?
   a. 12
   b. 11
   c. 10
   d. 1

4. Which classifications of motion are most effective and should be incorporated to minimize MSD?
   a. Classes I, II, and III
   b. Classes II, III, and IV
   c. Classes III, IV, and V
   d. Classes IV and V

5. Which classifications of motion should be reduced or eliminated to reduce stress and fatigue?
   a. Classes I, II, and III
   b. Classes II, III, and IV
   c. Classes III, IV, and V
   d. Classes IV and V

6. What class of motion is reaching for and rotating items while chairside assisting?
   a. I and II
   b. III
   c. IV
   d. V

7. How does the operator let the assistant know that they are ready to begin the procedure and instrument transfer?
   a. Use a predetermined verbal request.
   b. Adjust the dental light.
   c. Establish a finger rest.
   d. Move their stool into position.

8. A _____ is a point on which the fingers are stabilized and can pivot or move.
   a. finger rest
   b. fulcrum
   c. grasp
   d. zone

9. At what position is the operator seated to begin four-handed transfer of instruments?
   a. 12–2 o'clock
   b. 2–4 o'clock
   c. 4–7 o'clock
   d. 7–12 o'clock

10. What zone is located below the patient's chin to a 12-inch square over the patient's chest?
    a. A
    b. B
    c. C
    d. D

11. In what zone are most hand instruments transferred?
    a. A
    b. B
    c. C
    d. D

12. How does the operator let the assistant know that they are ready to receive the next hand instrument?
    a. Lower the handle.
    b. Lift the handle.
    c. Place the instrument over the patient's chest.
    d. Use a predetermined verbal request.

13. All of the following are instrument grasps EXCEPT:
    a. palm–index finger grasp.
    b. modified pen grasp.
    c. palm grasp.
    d. pen grasp.

14. Which grasp is generally used with instruments that have plier-like (hinged) handles?
    a. pen grasp
    b. modified pen grasp
    c. palm–thumb grasp
    d. palm grasp

15. How does the assistant retrieve the used instrument when performing the pen grasp double instrument exchange?
    a. extends middle and ring finger
    b. extends ring finger and small finger
    c. uses the baton technique
    d. waits for operator to bring it into Zone B

16. Where is the new instrument placed in relation to the used instrument when exchanging forceps?
    a. below
    b. above
    c. next to
    d. behind

17. Which of the following instruments require the transfer to be modified?
    a. cotton pliers
    b. scissors
    c. air/water syringe
    d. All of these

18. How does the operator let the assistant know that they are ready to receive the next forceps?
    a. Lower the handle.
    b. Lift the handle.
    c. Place the instrument over the patient's chest.
    d. Use a predetermined verbal request.

19. When is the hidden transfer used?
    a. to keep out of the view of the patient
    b. when transferring dental material
    c. when holding caustic materials
    d. All of these

20. When may a six-handed transfer be needed?
    a. during charting
    b. preparing materials
    c. retracting soft tissue
    d. All of these

Critical Thinking

1. What is CTS? What can the dental team do to reduce the risk of CTS?

2. How can the lack of good ergonomics affect the future and longevity of your career as a dental assistant?

3. How can the fit of the examination glove affect the health of the dental assistant's hands? Too small? Too large?

4. How does harmonizing affect teamwork? What do you plan to do to harmonize with the dentist you choose to work with?

5. What can you do as a student to become an effective part of the dental team?

Key Terms

Term and Pronunciation	Meaning of Root and Word Parts	Definition
armamentarium (ahr-m*uh*-m*uh*n-**tair**-ee-uhm)	**armament** = process of equipping **-arium** = indicating a place for something	the assembling of equipment, methods, and techniques to carry out a procedure
carpal (**kahr**-p*uh*l)	**carpus** = wrist **-al** = pertaining to	any bone of the wrist
caustic (**kaw**-stik)	**caust** = burning **-ic** = having characteristics	capable of burning, corroding, or destroying living tissue by chemical action
efficient (ih-**fish**-*uh*nt)	**efficient** = functioning in best possible manner	ability to complete a job with minimum expenditure of time and effort
erector spinae (ih-**rek**-ter **spahy**-nee)	**erectus** = upright **spina** = thorn like; backbone **erector** = a muscle that raises or keeps a part erect	a deep muscle along the length of the back; attached to sacrum (backbone at level of pelvis) to small of back; functions to straighten back and rotate to one side or other
ergonomics (ur-g*uh*-**nom**-iks)	**ergo-** = work **-nomy** = management **-ics** = relating to	an applied science concerned with design and arranging work area for efficiency of people in workforce
exchange (iks-**cheynj**)	**exchange** = trade, to give up something for something else	to retrieve one instrument while transfer a second instrument
fulcrum (**fool**-kr*uh*m)	**fulcrum** = a prop, a support	point of rest to support hand for balanced movement
gluteal (**gloo**-tee-*uh* l)	**glute** = rump, buttock **-al** = pertaining to	any one of the three large muscles that form the human buttock and move the thigh
harmony (**hahr**-m*uh*-nee)	**harmony** = agreement in action	simultaneous action without need of verbalization
kinesiology (ki-nee-see-**ol**-*uh*-jee)	**kinesis** = motion **-ology** = study of	study of muscles and body movement
lumbar disc (**luhm**-bahr) (disk)	**lumbus** = loins **-ar** = belonging to **discus** = a flat circular plate	a broad disc of cartilage separates vertebra of spine situated in the part of back and sides between the lowest ribs and pelvis; acts as a shock absorber
lumbar flexion (**luhm**-bahr) (**flek**-shuhn)	**lumbus** = loins **-ar** = belonging to **flex** = to bend **-ion** = denoting action	a bending movement in the part of the back and sides between the lowest ribs and pelvis
lumbosacral (luhm-boh-**sey**-kruhl)	**lumbus** = loins **sacrum** = a bone from fusion of vertebrae between lumbar and coccygeal (tail/end of spine)	relating to the lumbar vertebrae and the sacrum
maneuverability (m*uh*-**noo**-ver-*uh*-bil-i-tee)	**maneuver** = a planned and regulated movement **able** = having skill **-ty** = denoting state	a movement or action requiring dexterity and skill
neuropathy (noo-**rop**-*uh*-thee)	**neuro-** = nerve, nervous system **-pathy** = disease	disease resulting from damaged or malfunctioning nerves causing weakness, numbness, and pain
nodule (**noj**-ool)	**node** = small round knot **-ule** = small, little	a small, abnormal, knobby bodily protuberance; calcification or tumor near an arthritic joint
proficient (pr*uh*-**fish**-*uh*nt)	**proficient** = competent, well-advanced	expert, skilled, experienced, skillful
psychomotor (sahy-koh-**moh**-ter)	**psych** = mind **motor** = muscles that induce movement	characterizing movements of the body associated with mental activity
static (**stat**-ik)	**static** = having no change	lack of movement or change
strain (streyn)	**strain** = to draw tight or taut	to impair, injure, or weaken (a muscle, tendon, ligament) by stretching or overextension

Term and Pronunciation	Meaning of Root and Word Parts	Definition
stressor (**stres**-er)	**stress** = burden, pressure **-or** = denoting a thing or person	force exerted when body part presses on, pulls on, pushes against, compresses, or twists another body part that causes stress
tendon (**ten**-d*uh*n)	**teno/tendo** = to stretch **-on** = name a part	a band of tough, fibrous, inelastic connective tissue that joins a muscle to a bone
tenosynovitis (ten-oh-sin-uh-**vahy**-tis)	**teno** = tendon **synovia** =clear, lubricating fluid secreted by membranes in joint cavities, tendon, sheaths, and bursae **-itis** = inflammation	inflammation of a tendon sheath from trauma, repeated strain, or systemic disease
transfer (trans-**fur**)	**transfer** = to convey or remove from one place or person to another	to pass from one person to another
trapezium (tr*uh*-**pee**-zee-*uh*m)	**trapezia** =bone in the wrist **-ia** = denoting condition	a bone in the wrist at the base of the thumb
trigger (**trig**-er)	**trigger** = to become active, activate	anything, as an act or event; that serves as a stimulus and initiates a reaction or series of reactions

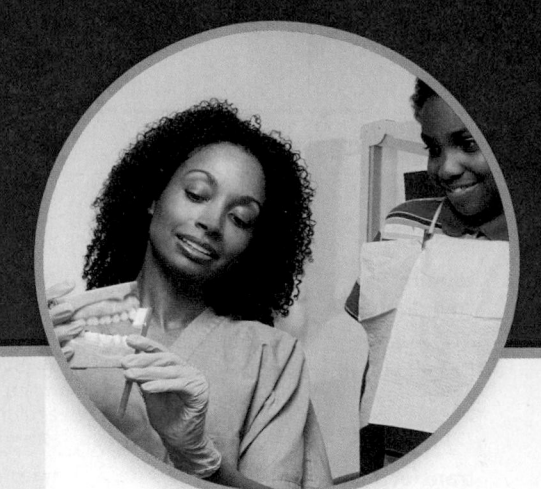

CHAPTER 21

Moisture Control

Specific Instructional Objectives

At the completion of this chapter, you will be able to meet these objectives:

1. Use terms presented in this chapter.
2. Defend the importance of effective moisture control in clinical practice.
3. Select appropriate aspiration technique given a clinical situation.
4. Demonstrate proper positioning and placement of saliva ejector, HVE, and air/water syringe.
5. Select appropriate isolation technique given a clinical situation.
6. Prepare tray setup and the dental dam material for placement.
7. Demonstrate placement of absorbent materials and dental dam.
8. Recall when pharmacological methods are recommended for moisture control.

Introduction

The oral cavity is a difficult environment in which to work. One of the greatest challenges is the presence of saliva. Excess saliva can obstruct the dentist's view of the operative site, make it difficult to use dental instruments, and cause **restoration** failure. An assistant skilled in moisture control techniques can keep saliva out of the **operative site**, allowing for greater visibility, and prevent saliva from contacting the teeth during treatment. A dry tooth surface is important for the dentist to clearly view, access, and check the cavity preparation for any remaining caries. Caries has a leathery texture that can be easily observed in a dry tooth. It is much more difficult to detect remaining caries if the tooth surface is moist, increasing the likelihood of not removing all the caries.

Most dental **resin** composite restorative materials require that the tooth surface be **etched** in order to achieve a **bond** with the tooth. Saliva contacting the tooth can create **mucinous** deposits that block the **micropores** in the enamel surface and prevent the bonding material from adhering to the tooth surface. Any amount of saliva on an etched surface will produce mucinous deposits.

Saliva, blood, and other sources of moisture will interfere with the properties of many different dental materials. Moisture can affect the set and hardness of dental material(s) and may cause biological damage to the patient. For example, if saliva mixes with **amalgam** before the amalgam is able to set, the saliva may cause the release of hydrogen gas within the restoration. The resulting increase in internal pressure causes excessive expansion of the amalgam, weakening it and leading to corrosion, fracturing, voids at the cavity margins, and eventually **secondary caries**. The patient will also feel pain from pressure on the pulp, pain when biting down due to high points in **occlusion**, and eventual pain from fracturing of the remaining tooth structure. A dry operative site is critical to achieving optimal results during many dental procedures.

Moisture control is not only important for the success of the procedure but for patient comfort and safety. The build-up of saliva, blood, tooth debris, and dental materials in the back of the patient's throat is discomforting for the patient and is potentially dangerous. The build-up makes the patient feel as if they are choking or need to swallow. A more serious danger is the potential for the patient to aspirate foreign bodies. Inhaled objects may obstruct the patient's breathing or become lodged in the patient's lungs.

Moisture Control Techniques

A primary responsibility of the dental assistant is to maintain a clean and dry field of operation while the dentist or operator is performing oral procedures. Two primary techniques are employed in the dental office to control moisture: aspiration and isolation.

Aspiration Techniques

The dental assistant needs to become proficient in using the aspirating equipment to suction saliva and debris and to rinse and dry the operative site. The equipment used for aspirating techniques include the saliva ejector, oral evacuator, and air/water syringe. An efficient assistant selects the appropriate equipment for each situation and maintains an operative field that is free of excess saliva, water, blood, excess materials, and tooth particles. Some procedures require that the assistant follow the dentist's work with either the saliva ejector or oral evacuator. There are procedures where the assistant will be evacuating with the right hand and rinsing the operative site with the air/water syringe in the left hand, all while not interrupting the dentist's treatment.

The assistant must also be able to assist the dentist in retracting patient tissue, not only to maintain the field of vision, but also to protect the patient's soft tissue. The patient may choke on saliva as it builds up in the back of the throat. With good aspiration techniques the assistant controls saliva buildup and prevents items from falling into the patient's throat. It takes a lot of practice to master the skills of aspiration and develop the dexterity needed to evacuate, rinse, dry, retract tissue, and transfer instruments simultaneously.

OSHA requires that whenever there is a chance of producing dental spray the assistant must wear full PPE whenever aspirating, rinsing, and drying the patient's mouth. The PPE includes mask, protective glasses, protective clothing and examination gloves. The patient should also be provided glasses to protect their eyes from dental spray and foreign objects.

Saliva Ejector

The saliva ejector is used to aspirate saliva and other liquid substances. It is not meant to suction debris or blood. The ejector has low suction, and the saliva tip has a small diameter, which makes it easy to maneuver and avoid trauma to the oral mucosa. The suction is low enough that the tip can be placed under the tongue to help control saliva during procedures. The standard saliva ejector tips are made of a flexible plastic. They have a flexible wire that runs the length of the tip. The tips are supplied preshaped (like a question mark), or they can be straight to be shaped to suit the patient's anatomy and the procedure.

Placement of Saliva Ejector Tip When the tip is shaped like a question mark, the top of the question mark should rest against the mandibular teeth and gently lie in the sublingual area opposite the side on which the operator is working. In this position, it is stationary and stays out of the operator's way. The tip efficiently removes fluid while not interfering with the operator's work space. The saliva ejector is often placed in the stationary position while performing a prophylaxis or cementing a crown, and beneath the dental dam while the dentist is preparing the tooth (Figure 21-1).

The ejector tip may be used to aspirate excess saliva buildup in the mouth. Held in the assistant's right hand, it can be used to follow the air/water syringe, but only when the rinse produces a completely liquid rinse free of larger debris. The assistant can use the tip in its straight position or modify the shape for better aspiration access. Never allow a patient to close their mouth around a saliva ejector tip. This causes a back vacuum as well as an unpleasant—and unhealthy—contamination in the patient's mouth from the dental line.

Patients' lips should never be placed over the end of the standard ejector tip during aspiration. This may cause retraction of infectious materials into the patient's mouth.

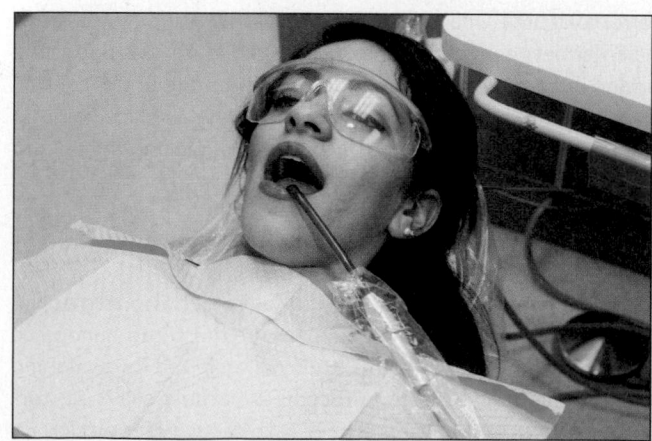

FIGURE 21-1
Saliva ejector in the patient's mouth. Notice the handle control on the hose and the flexibility of the saliva ejector, which is bent to stay in the patient's mouth.

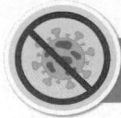

Infection Control

Saliva ejector tips and HVE tips are made for one use and should be disposed of in a biohazard waste container. Metal tips need to be sterilized. Aspirating hoses should be rinsed between patients, allowing each hose to suction 6–8 ounces of water through the hose. The aspirating mouthpieces should be wrapped using intermediate disinfecting solution for the time recommended by the manufacturer between patients. As a closing routine, the hose should be suctioned with 6–8 ounces of evacuator disinfecting solution.

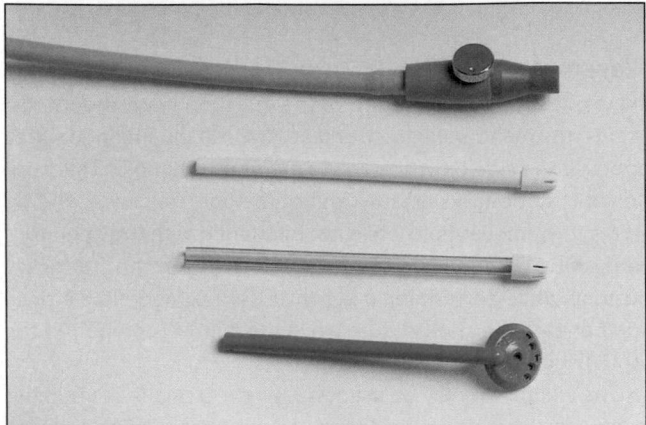

FIGURE 21-2
Saliva ejector hose with controls and attachment with several different types of saliva ejectors.

Types of Ejector Tips There are many types of saliva ejector tips available. Some tips have a sponge attached to the end of the ejector because patients often feel that the hard end of the standard tip is uncomfortable when placed in the stationary position for long periods of time. The cushioned tip not only increases patient comfort but also improves the aerosol capturing abilities of the tip and serves as a cheek retractor. Another tip is designed as a flat coil with a series of small holes. It can be bent to fit in the floor of the mouth, in the vestibule, and behind the retromolar area. One tip contains a small, flat restraint that forms a barrier between the patient's tongue and teeth. This tip has the added advantage of keeping the wiggly tongue under control. Some suction tips have a soft funnel end that is placed around the patient's lips to remove saliva instead of placing the tip into the patient's mouth (Figure 21-2).

Oral Evacuator (HVE)

Moisture control refers not only to saliva but also to gingival bleeding from the operative field, tissue fluid, and handpiece spray. High volume evacuators (HVE) are preferred for suctioning the mouth during operative procedures because saliva ejectors remove water too slowly and have little capacity for picking up solids. The HVE hose and tip have larger diameters and are more suitable for removing large particles, blood, and water from a high-speed handpiece and the air/water syringe. The HVE can be used as a valuable tool in retracting the tongue and cheek away from the field of operation.

The HVE may be made of disposable plastic or sterilizable stainless steel and is either straight or designed with a slight angle in the middle. The working end is beveled with one side (open) to allow for better suctioning, and the other side is straight and has a nonbeveled side (closed) to be used for retraction; some HVE tips are beveled on both ends, one for anterior and one for posterior. Surgical suction tips are much smaller in circumference than normal to provide more concentrated suction in a smaller space. For sterile purposes, the surgical tips are only made of stainless steel.

HVE Grasps

The HVE is held in the assistant's right hand using the palm–thumb or pen grasp. The "palm grasp" without the thumb extended is also very effective, especially if the HVE tubing is not very cumbersome. The dental assistant should try both grasps to see which feels the most comfortable, is the easiest to direct, and is the most proficient. The best grasp is what feels and works best for the assistant.

Palm–Thumb Grasp In the palm–thumb grasp the assistant holds the tip with fingers curled around the tip and mouthpiece; the thumb rests against the mouthpiece facing away from the patient's mouth. The thumb can be used to change direction and/or exert a little pressure for tissue retraction. This grasp is more secure for suctioning and retraction (Figure 21-3).

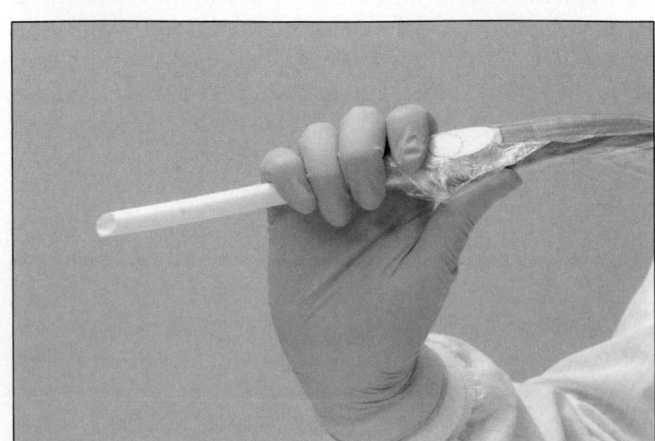

FIGURE 21-3
Using palm-thumb grasp with HVE.

Pen Grasp In the pen grasp the assistant holds the tip between the thumb and index and middle finger like holding the hand instrument in pen grasp. The pen grasp is better for directing the tip in a specific area.

HVE Suctioning Guidelines

Proper positioning and placement of the HVE will allow for better access, retraction, and suctioning. Following the guidelines below will help the novice dental assistant develop good suctioning skills.

Position of HVE

While obtaining the chosen grasp, the assistant should always position the bevel to face the tooth and the closed side toward the soft tissue. By making certain the bevel is adjusted properly, the assistant will not have to make adjustments in the patient's posture and position to obtain the best access to the mouth.

The HVE tip should be placed first to retract the cheek and tongue as needed to provide space for the operator. The assistant should position the tip posterior (when possible) and close to the work area. It should not be so close as to direct the water spray away from the rotary instrument. This position will be out of the field of vision and draw the dust and spray away from the work area, dentist, patient, and assistant. Keep the bevel parallel to the buccal or lingual surface of the work area (opposite the operator's position when possible) and even with the occlusal/incisal edge. In some cases, you can place the tip slightly above the occlusal or incisal to get getter suction. When preparing teeth, this position helps suction debris immediately and cuts down the spray.

Once the operator places the instrument, the assistant should make certain the HVE bevel is directed toward the operative site and place the length of the tip against a hard structure (tooth) to maintain a secure position. This will also act as a rest to take the stress off the assistant's hand and stabilize the tip. The HVE should not be moved once the operator is in position. Movement may bump the operator causing the instrument to slip or block the operator's view.

Placement of HVE

The placement of the HVE depends on the quadrant, specific work area, and type of suctioning desired. There are eight recommended placements of the HVE; a placement for each of the posterior quadrant work areas and four anterior placements. The tip is placed where it is not only out of the operator's vision and work area, but also where the assistant can access it easily while providing no harm to the patient.

Safety

Remember, the assistant's poor posture and position may increase the risk of developing MSD. It is important to make certain the bevel is positioned and secure before the operator's instrument is placed in the patient's mouth. Strained, unbalanced position may also result in uncontrolled movement that may **impinge** on the patient's tissue or bump the operator's instruments, resulting in injury to the patient's tissue.

Maxillary Right Quadrant When working in the maxillary right quadrant, the tip is placed on the lingual surface of the teeth (work area) between the work area and the tongue. With the bevel toward the work area and the closed end of the tip toward the tongue, it prevents the tongue from touching the work area. The assistant should obtain a rest on the maxillary left quadrant hard tissue to secure the tip and take stress off their hand. This is the easiest quadrant to gain access and suction. This would be a good place for the novice assistant to start. (Refer to Procedure 21-1, Figure 21-4.)

Mandibular Right Quadrant When working in the mandibular right quadrant, the tip is placed on the lingual surface of the teeth, between the work area and the tongue, as was done with the maxillary placement. This time, however, the tongue will be in the way. The assistant needs to make certain the closed end of the tip is toward the tongue, place the end of the bevel close to the hard tissue of the arch, and depress and retract the tongue and sublingual mucosa in one motion. Make certain the bevel is parallel to and open just above the occlusal surface and posterior to the work area. Obtain a rest on the mandibular left quadrant hard tissue to secure this placement. This placement is much trickier than the maxillary placement. Do not become alarmed if you suck the patient's tongue into the tip as you are learning this skill. (See Procedure 21-1, Figure 21-5.)

Safety

Occasionally, the patient's soft tissue will be sucked into the HVE. This may occur if the patient has a very small mouth, tight lips, a large tongue, or a very curious tongue that is always seeking the HVE and/or work area. This cannot always be avoided. Remain calm. It makes an awful sound but should not harm the patient. The tissue generally can be released by gently turning the bevel to release the suction. If this does not work, turn off the HVE suction and the tissue will be immediately released. Do not pull the patient's tissue with the HVE.

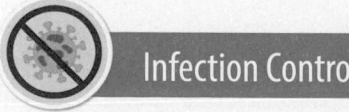

Infection Control

With the use of good suctioning, bacterial aerosol production is minimized. This reduces the dental spray in the treatment area for the dental team, dental equipment, and patient.

Maxillary Left Quadrant When working in the maxillary left quadrant, the tip is placed on the buccal surface of the teeth. The closed end of the tip is used to help retract the cheek and lip. This is best accomplished by holding the tip in the center of the mouth first. Then insert the tip gently inside the commissure while retracting the cheek. Be careful not to stretch the tissue. If the assistant places the tip at the commissure first, the tissue will be impinged from pulling back to get the tip into position. The bevel should be placed parallel to and open just below the occlusal surface and posterior to the work area. (See Procedure 21-1, Figure 21-6.)

Mandibular Left Quadrant When working in the mandibular left quadrant, the tip is placed on the buccal surface of the teeth. The closed end of the tip is used to help retract the cheek and lip as was accomplished in the maxillary left quadrant. The tip should be placed in the center of the mouth first, inserting the tip gently inside the commissure while retracting the cheek. The bevel should be placed parallel to and open just above the occlusal surface and posterior to the work area. (See Procedure 21-1, Figure 21-7)

Maxillary Anterior—Lingual Work Area The position of the HVE tip is on the facial surface when the dentist is working on the lingual. The assistant will need to use the closed side of the tip to retract the lip. Place the bevel just below the lip line, position the tip between the lip and the teeth, and gently retract the lip. A gentle rolling of the tip to get it under the lip is more comfortable for the patient. The bevel should be placed toward the teeth and parallel to the incisal edge. There is not a structure for a rest in this position. The assistant can reduce the stress of this position by holding the upper arm against the body. (See Procedure 21-1, Figure 21-8.)

Maxillary Anterior—Labial Work Area The position of the HVE tip is on the lingual surface when the dentist is working on the labial. The assistant places the bevel toward the teeth and parallel to the incisal edge. The closed side of the tip is toward the tongue to prevent the tongue from entering the work area. The assistant can use the occlusal surface of the maxillary left posterior teeth to rest the tip. (See Procedure 21-1, Figure 21-9.)

Mandibular Anterior—Lingual Work Area The position of the HVE is on the labial surface when the dentist is working on the lingual. The assistant will need to use the closed side of the tip to retract the lip. Place the bevel just above the lip line, position the tip between the lip and the teeth, and gently retract the lip. The assistant should place the bevel toward the teeth, parallel to and just above the incisal plane. There is not a structure for a rest in this position. The assistant can reduce the stress of this position by holding the upper arm against the body. This is one of the harder placements to hold. The assistant may need to change seating position or the dentist may need to assist in providing access by moving the patient's head. (See Procedure 21-1, Figure 21-10.)

Mandibular Anterior—Labial Work Area The position of the HVE tip is on the lingual when the dentist is working on the labial. The assistant will need to use the closed side of the tip to depress and retract the tongue to prevent the tongue from entering the work area. The bevel is placed toward the teeth, parallel to and just above the incisal plane. The assistant can use the occlusal surface of the mandibular right posterior teeth to rest the tip. (See Procedure 21-1, Figure 21-11.)

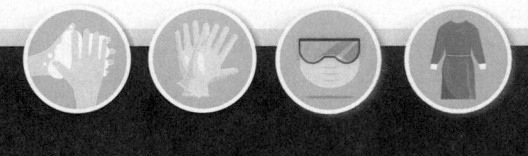

Procedure 21-1
Positioning and Placement of HVE

This procedure is performed by the dental assistant during dental treatment. The oral cavity is maintained to keep the area clear and clean for the operator and for the comfort of the patient. Each area of the mouth requires different evacuator tip positioning. The following illustrates how to position the HVE tip for posterior and anterior placements when assisting a right-handed operator.

Equipment and Supplies
- Basic setup: mouth mirror, explorer, and cotton pliers
- HVE tip and air/water syringe tip
- cotton rolls
- dental handpiece

Procedure Steps *(Follow aseptic procedures)*
1. Select preference of grasps.
   - ❏ Hold HVE using palm–thumb grasp or pen grasp given clinical situation.

2. Position HVE close to operative site.
   - ❏ Place tip before and out of operator's field of vision.
   - ❏ Place bevel facing the tooth with closed side toward soft tissue.
   - ❏ Position tip posterior to the work area.
   - ❏ Keep bevel parallel to buccal/lingual surface of work area.
   - ❏ Keep bevel even with occlusal/incisal edge.
   - ❏ Rest length of tip against hard structure to secure placement.
   - ❏ Take caution to not impinge patient's tissue.

HVE PLACEMENT FOR MAXILLARY RIGHT QUADRANT (FIGURE 21-4)

3. Place HVE to evacuate maxillary right quadrant.
   - ❏ Place bevel of tip toward the lingual surface of the work area.

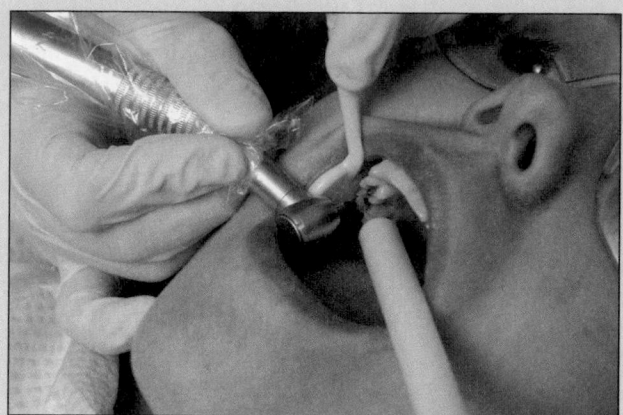

FIGURE 21-4
Maxillary right posterior tip placement.

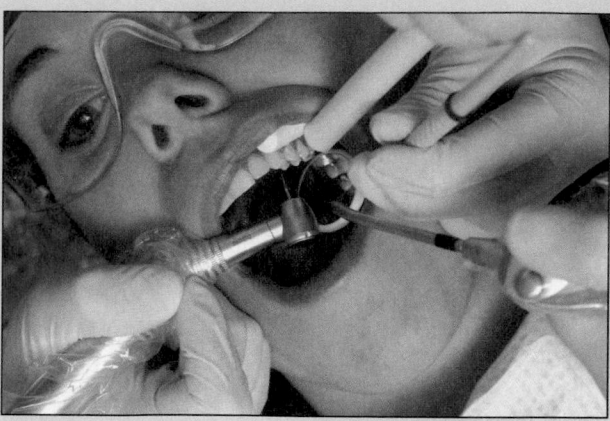

FIGURE 21-6
Maxillary left posterior tip placement.

❏ Place closed end of tip between work area and tongue to prevent tongue from entering work area.
❏ Obtain a rest on the maxillary left quadrant hard tissue to secure this placement.

HVE PLACEMENT FOR MANDIBULAR RIGHT QUADRANT (FIGURE 21-5)

4. Place HVE to evacuate maxillary right quadrant.
   ❏ Place bevel of tip toward the lingual surface of the work area.
   ❏ Place closed end of tip between work area and tongue.
   ❏ Depress and retract the tongue and sublingual tissue.
   ❏ Obtain a rest on the mandibular left quadrant hard tissue to secure this placement.

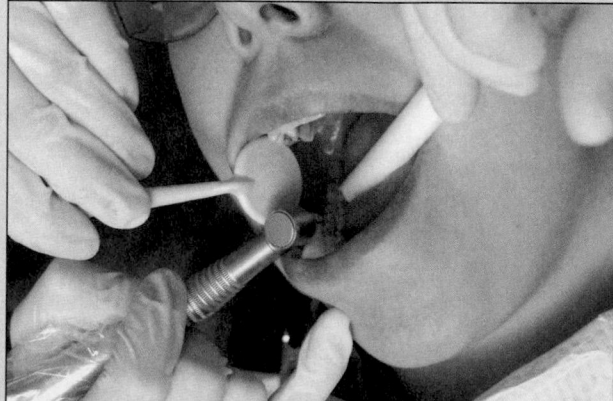

FIGURE 21-5
Mandibular right posterior tip placement.

HVE PLACEMENT FOR MAXILLARY LEFT QUADRANT (FIGURE 21-6)

5. Place HVE to evacuate maxillary left quadrant.
   ❏ Place closed end of tip toward the cheek.

❏ Retract cheek without impinging or stretching patient's soft tissue.
❏ Place bevel of tip toward the buccal surface of the work area.
❏ Obtain a rest by gently steadying tip against cheek muscles.

HVE PLACEMENT FOR MANDIBULAR LEFT QUADRANT (FIGURE 21-7)

6. Place HVE to evacuate mandibular left quadrant.
   ❏ Place closed end of tip toward the cheek.
   ❏ Retract cheek without impinging or stretching patient's soft tissue.
   ❏ Place bevel of tip toward the buccal surface of the work area.
   ❏ Obtain a rest by gently steadying tip against cheek muscles.

HVE PLACEMENT FOR MAXILLARY ANTERIOR WITH LINGUAL WORK AREA (FIGURE 21-8)

7. Place HVE to evacuate maxillary anterior with lingual work area.
   ❏ Place closed end of tip toward the lip.
   ❏ Retract lip without impinging or stretching patient's soft tissue.
   ❏ Place bevel of tip toward the labial surface of the work area.
   ❏ Obtain a rest by holding upper arm against the body.

HVE PLACEMENT FOR MAXILLARY ANTERIOR WITH LABIAL WORK AREA (FIGURE 21-9)

8. Place HVE to evacuate maxillary anterior with labial work area.
   ❏ Place closed end of tip toward the tongue.
   ❏ Prevent tongue from entering work area.
   ❏ Place bevel of tip toward the lingual surface of the work area.
   ❏ Obtain a rest by holding tip against occlusal surface of maxillary right teeth.

(Continues)

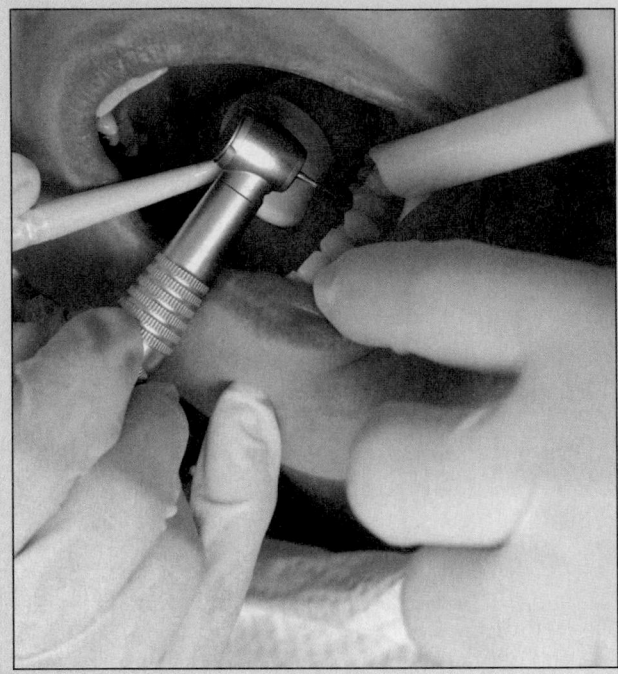

FIGURE 21-7
Mandibular left posterior tip placement.

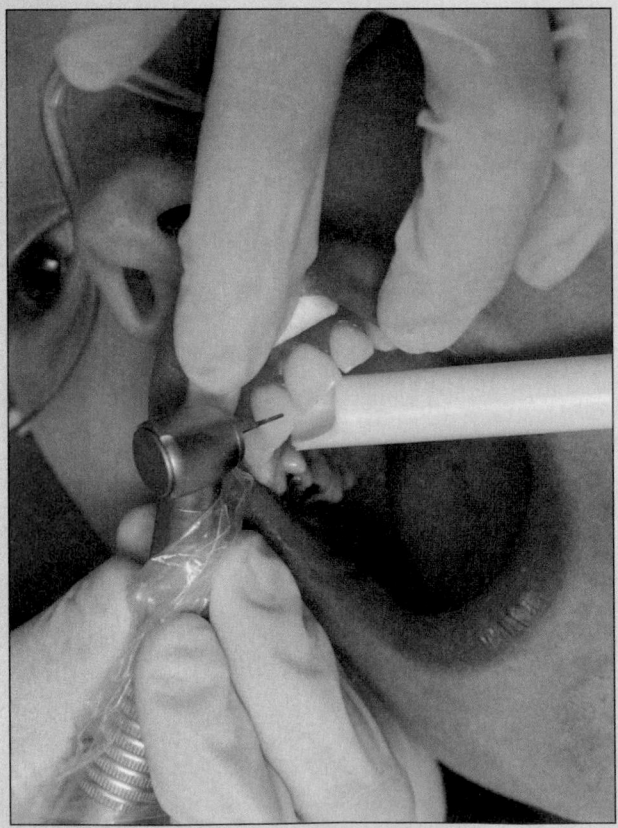

FIGURE 21-8
Maxillary anterior lingual tip placement.

HVE PLACEMENT FOR MANDIBULAR ANTERIOR WITH LINGUAL WORK AREA (FIGURE 21-10)

9. Place HVE to evacuate mandibular anterior with lingual work area.
   - ❑ Place closed end of tip toward the lip.
   - ❑ Retract lip without impinging or stretching patient's soft tissue.
   - ❑ Place bevel of tip toward the labial surface of the work area.
   - ❑ Obtain a rest by holding upper arm against the body.

HVE PLACEMENT FOR MANDIBULAR ANTERIOR WITH LABIAL WORK AREA (FIGURE 21-11)

10. Place HVE to evacuate mandibular anterior with labial work area.
    - ❑ Place closed end of tip toward the tongue.
    - ❑ Depress and retract the tongue and sublingual tissue.

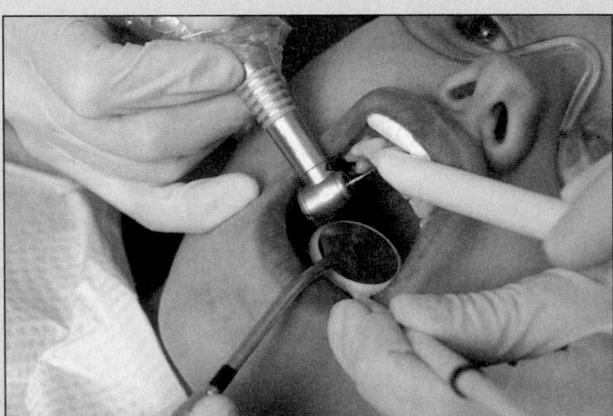

FIGURE 21-9
Maxillary anterior facial tip placement.

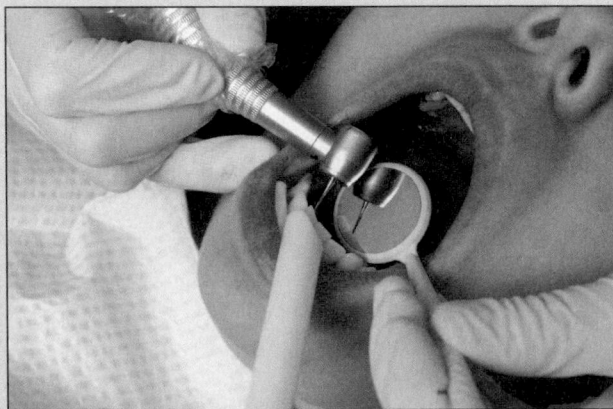

FIGURE 21-10
Mandibular anterior lingual tip placement.

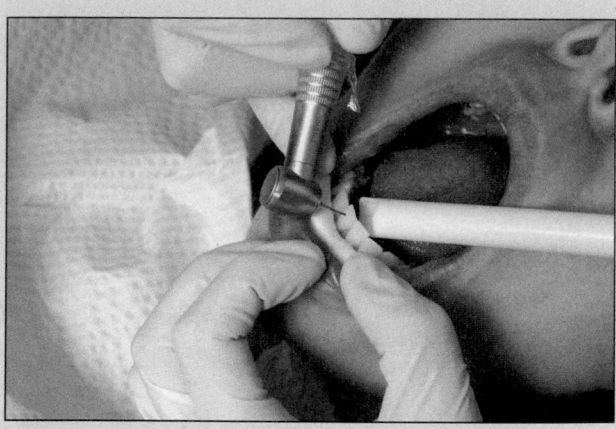

FIGURE 21-11
Mandibular anterior facial placement.

❑ Place bevel of tip toward the lingual surface of the work area.
❑ Obtain a rest by holding tip against occlusal surface of mandibular left teeth.

Rinse and Dry Mouth

At various times the work area needs to be rinsed and dried before completing the next step. The assistant completes the rinse by holding the air/water (A/W) syringe in the left hand to rinse and then dry the area. The HVE is held in the right hand to suction. There are times during a procedure that the operator will need to exchange instruments. When this occurs, the assistant holds the A/W syringe and HVE in the right hand while exchanging instruments for the operator with the left. Once the instrument has been replaced on the tray, the assistant moves the A/W syringe back to the left hand.

There are two types of rinses needed before, during, and after procedures. When the assistant needs to clean just the preparation area, they use a *limited area rinse*. For example, if the dentist has just completed preparing a tooth for a restoration, the preparation needs to be rinsed and dried before placing the restoration. In this case, the assistant would use a limited area. If the entire mouth needs to be rinsed, the assistant would use the *full mouth rinse* technique. For instance, if a patient has a lot of soft debris covering the teeth but there is no time to brush and floss the patient's teeth before the exam, a full mouth rinse would be used to clean away the soft debris. Also, after the operator has polished the patient's teeth during a **prophylaxis**, a full mouth rinse is needed to remove all the polishing paste before releasing the patient.

Limited Area Rinse The dental assistant uses the limited area rinse to maintain a clear work area for the operator and for the patient's comfort and safety. The limited rinse is performed frequently throughout the procedure. An alert assistant will know to rinse and dry when the handpiece stops. The assistant positions the HVE in the right hand as instructed previously. The A/W syringe is held in the left hand with the syringe tip directed toward the tooth or operative site on the opposite side of the HVE.

The assistant should keep the syringe tip close to the tooth to direct the spray and air to the desired location. Press the water button only if a gentle rinse is desired. If the debris is **tenacious**, use a dental spray by pressing both the air and water buttons at the same time and directing the tip at approximately a 45 degree angle toward the tooth or teeth. Make certain not to direct the water at a direct right angle to the tooth; this will cause the water to splatter. If the area needs to be dried, press the air button only and keep the HVE in position to hasten the drying process and to keep the tongue out of the work area. The assistant can help the operator maintain clear vision by using the air on the mirror to remove loose debris.

When rinsing, water tends to pool in the mandibular retromolar area. The assistant should check and evacuate this area after every rinse. It is most efficient to have the patient lean toward the assistant. The water will then pool in the retromolar area closest to the assistant, providing better access. Following are the guidelines for rinsing and drying each area of the mouth.

Maxillary Right Posterior Have the patient face forward. Hold the syringe on the facial surface and gently retract the cheek with the A/W syringe tip. Position the HVE on the lingual surface between the tooth and tongue just below and parallel to the occlusal surface. Adjust the bevel to just below and parallel to the occlusal surface. Determine if the procedure requires a gentle rinse or if a dental spray is needed. Rinse and dry as needed.

Mandibular Right Posterior Have the patient face forward. Hold the syringe on the facial surface and gently retract the cheek with the A/W syringe tip. Position the HVE on the lingual surface between the tooth and tongue to depress and retract the tongue. Adjust the bevel to just above and parallel to the occlusal surface (Figure 21-12).

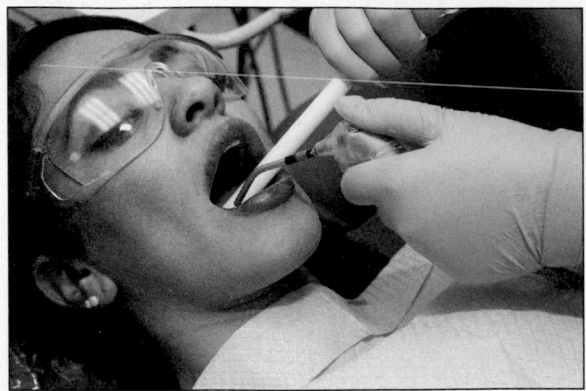

FIGURE 21-12
Assistant using the HVE and the air/water syringe positioning for the mandibular right posterior.

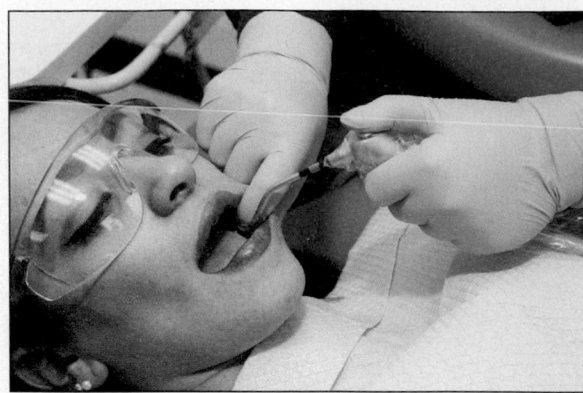

FIGURE 21-13
Assistant using index finger for retraction while spraying with air/water syringe.

Maxillary Left Posterior The assistant should instruct the patient to turn toward them to provide the assistant with a better view and afford access to the maxillary left posterior. Hold the syringe on the lingual surface between the teeth and the tongue. The assistant may need to use the syringe to keep the tongue out of the work area as well to as rinse. The closed end of the HVE tip is used to help retract the cheek or lip as well as to evacuate. Adjust the bevel to just below and parallel to the occlusal surface. Rinse and dry as needed.

Mandibular Left Posterior The assistant should instruct the patient to turn toward them. Hold the syringe on the lingual between the teeth and tongue. The assistant will need to use the syringe to depress and retract the patient's tongue to keep it out of the work area as well as to rinse. The closed end of the HVE tip is used to help retract the cheek or lip as well as to evacuate. Adjust the bevel to just above and parallel to the occlusal surface. Rinse and dry as needed. This position may require a little more practice due the location of the tongue (Figure 21-13).

Maxillary Anterior The assistant should instruct the patient to turn slightly toward them. Hold the syringe on the facial surface. The assistant will need to use the syringe to retract the patient's lip to keep it out of the work area as well as to rinse. The closed end of the HVE tip is placed between the maxillary teeth and the tongue to keep the tongue out of the work area. The open end of the HVE is just below and parallel to the incisal edge.

Mandibular Anterior The assistant should instruct the patient to turn slightly toward them. Hold the syringe on the facial surface. The assistant will need to use the syringe to retract the patient's lip to keep it out of the work area as well as to rinse. The closed end of the HVE tip is placed between the teeth and the tongue. The assistant will need to depress and retract the tongue as well as to evacuate.

Full Mouth Rinse In completing a full mouth rinse, the assistant incorporates all the A/W syringe and HVE positions and placements as for a limited area rinse. The difference is that the entire mouth is rinsed. It is easier if you start the full mouth rinse in the area farthest from you and bring the water toward you to provide better access and visibility. It is also better to rinse the maxillary before the mandibular. The most efficient way to conduct a full mouth rinse is as follows: Rinse the maxillary right with the patient facing forward, then have the patient move toward you slightly as you rinse the maxillary anterior. With the patient leaning toward you, rinse the maxillary left area. Check the retromolar area toward you and evacuate as needed. Instruct the patient to face forward again and rinse the mandibular right, then have the patient move toward you slightly as you rinse the mandibular anterior. With the patient leaning toward you, rinse the mandibular left area. Make a final check of the retromolar area toward you and evacuate as needed.

After completing the full mouth rinse, ask the patient how the mouth feels and if there is any area they would like to have you rinse more. Remember the ergonomic principles you learned previously: if the patient position or your position makes it difficult to perform a task, the patient is generally easier to reposition than you or the equipment. Protect yourself from MSD.

Isolation Techniques

There are many materials and techniques that help to isolate the operative site and control moisture. Absorbent materials can be placed to control salivary flow while retracting soft tissue. Absorbent materials used in moisture control include cotton rolls, dry guards, gauze squares, and cotton pellets. These absorbent materials provide only short term moisture control and are not effective against high volumes of moisture and active tongues. These materials may need to be replaced with fresh absorbents as they become saturated during a procedure.

The placement of a dental dam also isolates selected teeth from being exposed to saliva, acts as a barrier between the teeth and the soft tissues, and provides better moisture control, access, and visibility for the operator. No single device works well in every situation, and some situations require the use of more than one product. This means that the assistant needs to be versatile in their thinking and abilities when performing isolation techniques.

Cotton Rolls

Cotton rolls control small amounts of moisture and also retract soft tissue. They absorb saliva and other fluids for short periods of time for procedures like examinations, sealants, and fluoride application. The assistant may use additional moisture control techniques like the saliva ejector tip to help control the excess saliva and the A/W syringe for keeping the tooth dry.

Cotton rolls generally are placed in the facial (mucobuccal fold) and/or in the lingual (resting against the floor of the mouth and tongue) with the muscles keeping the cotton rolls in position. The cotton roll can also be placed over the parotid duct (Stenson's duct) to control flow of saliva from the parotid gland. Plastic cotton roll holders or stainless steel Garmer clamps can be used to assist in holding the cotton securely in place. The holders come as a pair: one that fits the right side and one for the left. The cotton rolls are placed into both sides of the holder, which is placed in the mouth with the bend of the holder resting on the mandibular incisors and the clamp securing its placement under the chin. When removing the cotton rolls, it is important to moisten them with a spray of water from the A/W syringe. As the saliva is absorbed the epithelium becomes dry and sticks to the cotton roll. Sudden removal of a dry cotton roll can remove epithelial tissue and cause pain for the patient (Figure 21-14).

Dry Angles

Also referred to as dry guards and cellulose wafers, dry angles are used primarily to control small amounts of moisture from the parotid gland duct opening. The dry guard is a flat, triangular absorbent pad that resembles a wafer. One side is made of absorbent cotton, and the other side consists of moisture-proof backing. Some are foil-covered to reflect more light in the oral cavity, thus improving visibility. The dry guard is placed against the buccal mucosa and is held between the cheek muscles and the teeth. Dry guard holders may be used to secure positioning of the guards. Like a cotton roll, the dry guard must be moistened with the A/W syringe to prevent injuring the epithelium when being removed (Figure 21-15).

Gauze Squares Gauze squares are mainly used to absorb blood during surgical procedures; they are also referred to as sponges. Only sterile gauze should be used during surgical

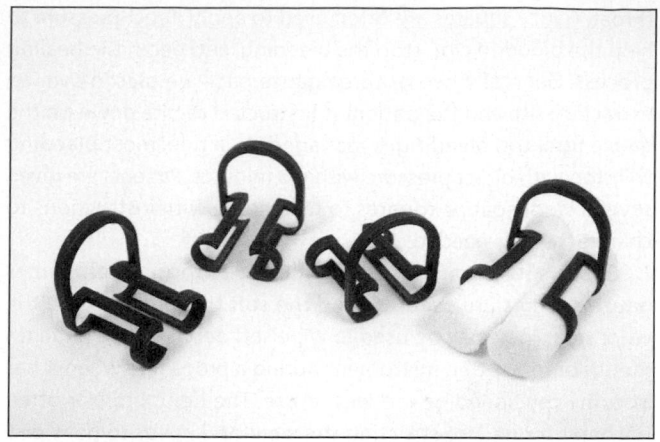

FIGURE 21-14
A cotton roll holder is a one-piece plastic device with two clamps sized to hold a cotton on each side connected with a flexible bow.

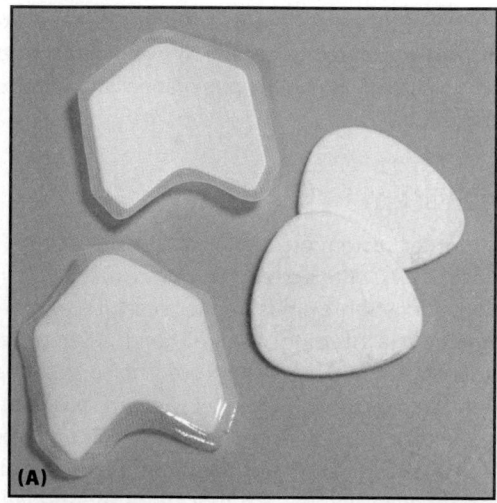

(A)

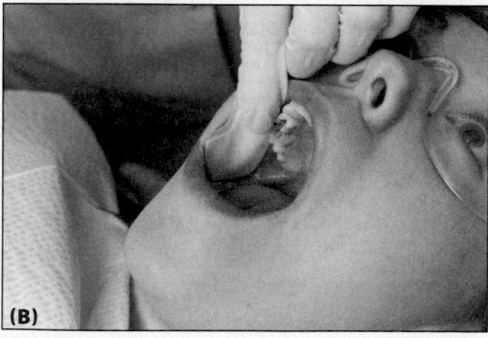

(B)

FIGURE 21-15
(A) Assortment of dry angles. (B) Assistant placing dry guard into patient's mouth.

procedures. The gauze square is made of interwoven threads with a filling usually made of cotton. When there is a lot of bleeding, a sterile gauze may be placed posterior of both retromolar areas to absorb the blood and keep it from draining into the patient's throat. Gauze squares are often used to apply direct pressure to help the blood to clot, stop the bleeding, and begin the healing process. Generally two or three gauze pads are placed over an extraction site and the patient is instructed to bite down on the gauze until the bleeding is managed. As a rule, most bleeding will stop with direct pressure within 5 minutes. Patients are given several sterile gauze squares to take home with instructions to change them as needed.

Gauze squares are used for multiple purposes. Sometimes gauze squares are used to keep the soft tissue away from the work area. They may be used to wipe soft debris from a patient's mouth or to wipe an instrument during a procedure when it has become too soiled or too wet to use. The dental mirror often becomes fogged, obstructing the view, and needs to be wiped with a gauze square.

Cotton Pellet

When it is hard to access the cavity preparation and drying, a cotton pellet often is the best option. When there are very deep preparations with less tooth structure over the pulp, there is a greater chance of damaging the pulp by overdrying it with the air syringe. In such cases, drying the preparation with a cotton pellet is often preferred.

Isolite System

There is another system used to maintain a clear, dry field for the operator. The Isolite system provides isolation, retraction, evacuation, and a light source in one piece of equipment. The system includes a titanium control head, a power/vacuum hose, and a one-time-use mouthpiece. The control head contains a light emitter, a dual-channel vacuum, and controls for both. This system is connected to the dental unit's vacuum system and an electrical source. The mouthpieces are attached to the control head before each procedure and then placed in the patient's mouth.

The mouthpiece is made of a soft flexible material and comes in a variety of sizes. The mouthpiece includes a tongue and cheek protector, throat barrier, vacuum channels, and an integrated bite block (Figure 21-16). Once the mouthpiece is placed, the operator can work on either the upper or lower quadrants. The patient is comfortable with the bite block in place, and the tongue, cheeks, and throat are protected. The dental assistant is free to perform other functions during the procedure. The mouthpiece is disposed of after each use to prevent cross-contamination.

The Isolite system is used with many different procedures, including crowns and bridges, fillings, implants, sealants, veneers, CERAC dentistry, and laser dentistry, as well as some oral surgery and orthodontic and periodontic procedures. Procedure times have been reduced by over 20% with use of this system. It is becoming increasingly popular with dentists, dental assistants, and dental hygienists. The main disadvantage is the cost of the mouthpieces, and the learning curve.

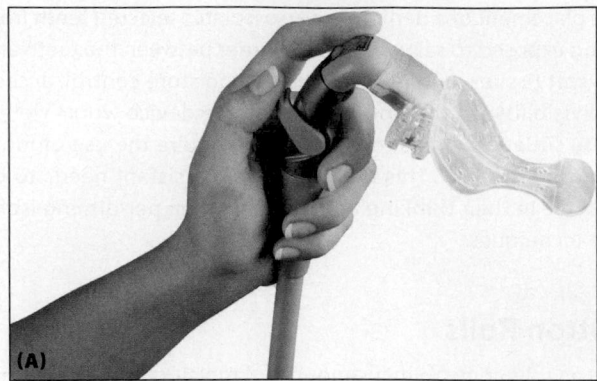

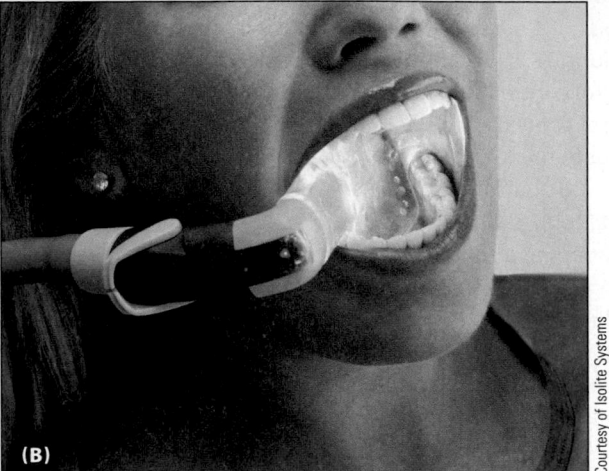

Courtesy of Isolite Systems

FIGURE 21-16
Isolite system. (A) Provides evacuation, isolation, retraction, and light source. (B) It also serves as a mouth prop for the patient to help keep their mouth open.

Dental Dam

Working in the patient's mouth to restore teeth requires that the dentist work in a small, dark, and wet environment. Only the dental dam completely isolates the operative field from saliva, moisture, bleeding, and tissue fluids. This is especially important when working with materials that are affected by moisture contamination. Although not all patients are familiar with the dental dam, it has been used in dentistry since 1864. The dental dam remains the most effective and easiest way to keep the mouth dry during a dental procedure. The American Dental Association Council on Dental Materials and Equipment acknowledged the need for using the dental dam when stating, "The use of **rubber dam** to maintain a dry field is essential." Moisture control is the most cited advantage in using the dental dam. Use of the dental dam also helps the dentist overcome many environmental problems found in the oral cavity, improves visibility and access, and aids in patient management.

The dental assistant helps prepare for and assist in the placement of the dental dam. In some states the dental assistant places the dental dam; this is considered an expanded function (Figure 21-17). While it is possible for a lone operator

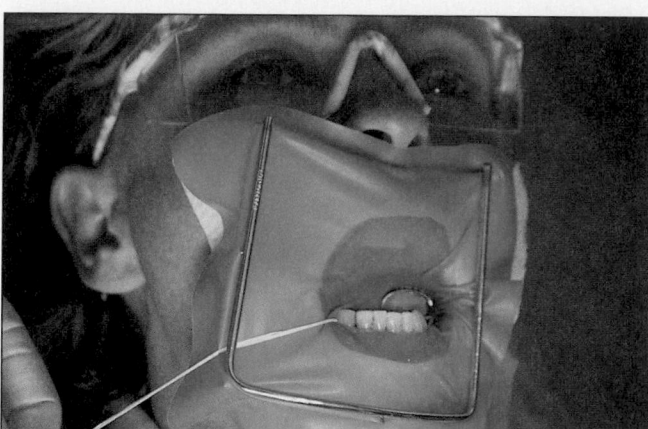

FIGURE 21-17
Dental dam placed in the mouth.

to place the dental dam, it is much more efficient if an operator and assistant work together, using a four-handed technique. A skilled dental operator can place the dental dam within 3 to 5 minutes, which is usually the time needed for the anesthetic to take full effect.

Advantages of Using a Dental Dam
The dental dam was used originally for isolation purposes when performing **endodontic** procedures to maintain asepsis. Once the pulp is removed and the cavity is cleaned, the dental dam isolates the area from further contamination. The dental dam is the standard of care for endodontic procedures and is generally placed during operative procedures when the dentist needs to cut tooth structure and replace a restoration.

Placement of the dental dam may be new and frightening to the patient. Teaching the patient about the benefits and explaining the steps in placement may reduce fears caused by something unfamiliar. When demonstrating the need to the patient, it is helpful to show how the dental dam helps both the dentist and patient. It is important for the dental assistant to be prepared to tell the patient the advantages of using the dental dam. The assistant can explain that the dental dam saves time, ensures that the dental restoration will not be contaminated, and is safer for the patient.

Timesaving: The dental dam provides maximum access and visibility. It acts as a physical barrier to moisture and retracts the soft tissues. Once the dental dam is in place, there is no need for the patient to rinse or spit. The dental dam maintains a dry, clean operating field. It keeps saliva out of the work area and also helps in **retracting** soft tissue. The dental assistant will not have to retract tissue during the procedure and will have minimal need to rinse and evacuate. The dentist can work faster because the field of vision remains clear. The dental dam material provides a dark, nonreflective background that contrasts to the operating site, enhancing the visibility. The dental dam provides the ideal conditions for the operator to perform restorative procedures.

Ensured Properties of Dental Materials: As you recall, dental materials deteriorate when contaminated by moisture. Many materials lose potential strength, resulting in adverse effects for the patient, and other materials won't even set. The dental dam prevents contamination and ensures that the patient receives the best possible results. Teeth that are prepared and restored using dental dam isolation are less prone to postoperative complications and pain or sensitivity related to contamination from oral fluids.

Safety: The dental dam protects both patient and operator. It protects the patient from aspirating or swallowing debris or small instruments associated with operative procedures. The patient does not need to worry about debris falling into their throat or tasting the various materials. The dental dam keeps the lips, cheeks, gingiva, and tongue out of the way of the work area. This prevents injury to structures and allows the dentist to maintain a more stable fulcrum. The dental dam also acts like a physical barrier between the patient's oral fluids and the operator, thus protecting the dental team by reducing contact with harmful bacteria from the patient's mouth and minimizing aerosol production.

Increased Productivity: The dental dam enhances efficiency and increases the productivity of four-handed dentistry, allowing the assistant the freedom to perform functions other than simply rinsing and evacuating. Use of the dental dam is essential when the operator is working alone. Expanded function dental assistants (EFDA) who use dental dams have found that the dental dam does some of the patient management for them. It keeps saliva and blood out of the operational field, minimizes the need to rinse the area of debris, retracts soft tissue, and improves access to the operating site. The dental dam also reminds the patient to hold their mouth open and minimizes talking, which can contaminate the working area.

Disadvantages in Using a Dental Dam
Although the dental dam has many advantages, placement is not necessary for all procedures. The most frequently cited disadvantages of using the dental dam are time consumption of placing the dental dam and patient objection. Placing the dental dam does require dexterity and practice to master the skill. Sometimes the operator is not able to use the dental dam because the teeth may be **malpositioned**, partially erupted, severely broken down, or missing, which makes the placement more challenging. If the cavity is below the gingival margin, a clamp may not be able to fit beneath the cavity. This causes the operator to modify the placement technique.

Occasionally a patient is too nervous to use the dental dam. With the dental dam in place, the patient may feel **claustrophobic**, which is exaggerated by the patient's decreased ability to communicate with the dental team. The operator can help reduce these feelings by explaining the use and steps in placing the dental dam, by making certain that the dental dam material does not cover the patient's nose, and by arranging alternative ways of communicating with the patient. Sometimes simply telling the patient to raise their hand if something is needed will help alleviate any feelings of lack of control. Patients suffering from obstructed nasal passages and respiratory diseases that

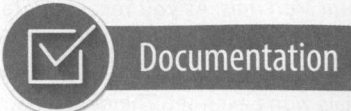
Documentation

Patient's Refusal to Use a Dental Dam

Some dentists document the patient's refusal to use a dental dam. Following is an example of how the conversation with Mrs. Engle can be documented.

Mrs. Engle expressed concern about having a dental dam placed in her mouth. The necessity of the dental dam was explained to her by the assistant (Chris) and Dr. Tyler. Mrs. Engle insisted that she did not want the dental dam. Dr. Tyler requested that Mrs. Engle sign a statement that Dr. Tyler had explained the need for a dental dam and was refusing to use the dental dam. Dr. Tyler used isolation by cotton holder and cotton rolls. Although Dr. Tyler is meticulous in his procedure, he is concerned that some moisture may have contaminated the restoration.

make breathing through the nose difficult may not tolerate the dental dam. A patient may feel sensitivity to the material, and for those patients, dental dams are available in a nonlatex material. There are dental dam napkins that can be placed between the dental dam and the patient's face. In these cases, the operator may need to use one of the alternative isolation techniques discussed previously.

Dental Dam Setup
Most offices have a standard setup consisting of materials and instruments that the dental assistant prepares for the placement of the dental dam.

Dental Dam Material
The dental dam material is a stretchy piece of rubber available in both natural latex rubber and a non-latex rubber (Figure 21-18). Holes are punched in the material, and the teeth are placed through the material for isolation. Dams come in many different sizes, colors, and **gauges**. The dental dam material is supplied as a continuous roll (125 mm or 150 mm) or in precut square sheets (5 × 5 or 6 × 6 inch). The 5 × 5 dental dam is used for primary dentition and the 6 × 6 for permanent dentition. The traditional color is gray, and a light or dark gray can be ordered. Dark gray is preferred as it reduces glare and offers the greatest contrast of the tooth against the dental dam. Now dental dam material can be ordered in just about any color the dentist prefers, including pastel blue, green, or lavender. The gauge is the thickness of the material. The dental dam material is available in thin gauge (0.00 g), medium, heavy, extra heavy, and special heavy (0.014 g). The medium and heavy gauges are usually preferred because the material doesn't tear as easily and retracts gingiva better. Dental dams have a shelf life of 9 months at 21 degrees C. Warmer temperature will reduce the shelf life and the flexibility of the material, causing rips and tears during placement.

Dental Dam Punch
The dental dam punch is a precision instrument with a rotating punch plate of progressive hole sizes. The plate is rotated to select the desired hole size, and the operator squeezes the handles together to press the floating stylus (cutting tip) through the hole (Figure 21-19). This procedure is used to punch perfect, tear-resistant holes in the dental dam material, providing the correct opening through which teeth may slide. Selecting the corresponding hole size for the tooth being isolated is important (Figure 21-20).

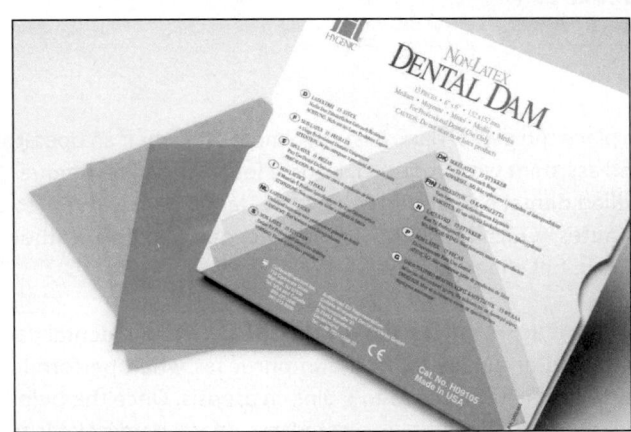

FIGURE 21-18
Various sizes, colors, and gauges of dental dam material.

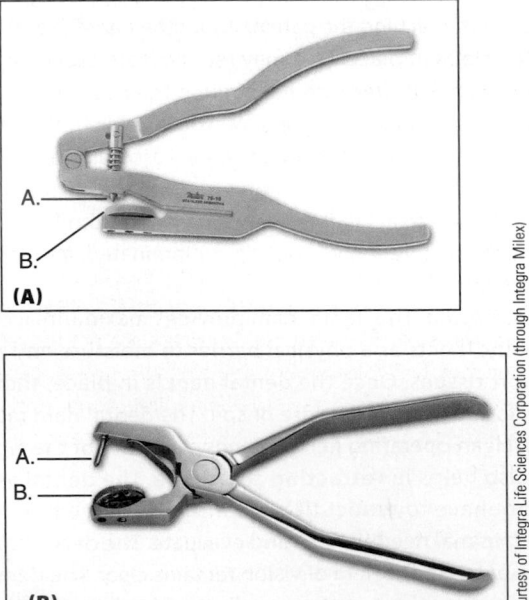

FIGURE 21-19
Dental dam punch. (A) Stylus, which is a sharp projection to punch through the dental dam. (B) Punch plate or table, which is a rotating disc containing several hole sizes.

Courtesy of Integra Life Sciences Corporation (through Integra Milex)

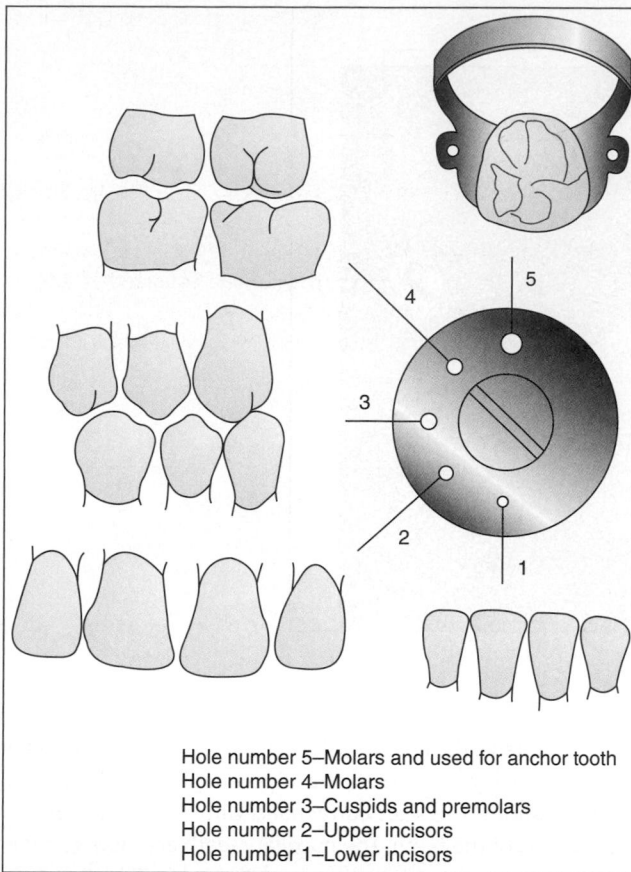

Hole number 5–Molars and used for anchor tooth
Hole number 4–Molars
Hole number 3–Cuspids and premolars
Hole number 2–Upper incisors
Hole number 1–Lower incisors

FIGURE 21-20
Dental dam punch table with corresponding teeth.

The size of hole punched for each tooth depends on several factors:

● whether the hole being punched is for a tooth that is going to be a clamp bearing tooth (anchor tooth) or if the tooth is just going to be isolated

● the cervical diameter of the tooth

● the elasticity of the dental dam material being used

A hole that is too small may tear as the dental dam material is being placed over the tooth. A hole that is too large may permit saliva to leak around the tooth during the procedure. Each hole is given a numerical value representing the size of the hole; the larger the number, the larger the hole. There are many types of dental dam punches available from single-hole to six-hole punches.

Dental dam punches need to be handled properly and should be regularly checked for wear and tear. The three main areas of concern are:

1. The punch should produce clean cut holes in the rubber sheet. When the hole starts to become ragged around the edges, it is due to the blunting of the sharp cutting edges of the stylus. This usually occurs due to prolonged use of the punch. The dental dam is more likely to tear during placement when the holes are not clean cut.

2. The punch floating stylus gets jammed going through the rubber sheet and does not punch without tearing. This may be due to damage to the punch stylus and/or hole as a result

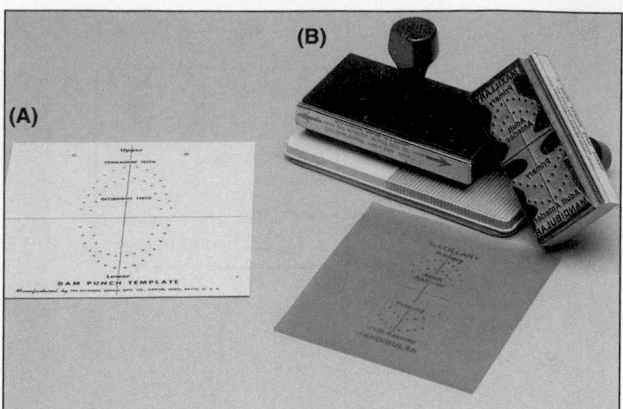

FIGURE 21-21
Dental dam punch guides: (A) Template. (B) Stamp with inkpad.

of incorrect alignment. When the disc is turned, a click can be heard as the disc falls into position, aligning the hole to be punched by the stylus. If the plate is not properly aligned, the assistant will feel resistance in the movement of the plate and the stylus as it is brought into the hole. This dulls the cutting edges of the stylus and the hole.

3. The plate will not turn or is hard to turn. Dental dam material can build up in the plate. This can be removed easily with an explorer. The workings of the punch can corrode with improper care. Make certain to care for the punch according to the manufacturer's directions.

Dental Dam Punching Guides There are many punching guides available to help position the placement of the holes in the dental dam material (Figure 21-21). There is a plastic **template** approximately the same size and shape of the unstretched dental dam with holes representing the placement of the teeth in dental arches. The template is laid over the dental dam, and the holes are marked onto the rubber sheet. A dental dam stamp that has a diagram of hole placement can be placed into an ink pad and placed onto the rubber sheet marking the hole positions.

The dental dam guides are perfect adult and pediatric dental arches, so they will not fit every patient. Instead, the markings act as guides. The operator should examine the oral cavity before punching the dental dam to adjust positioning for the specific patient's dentition. As the dental assistant becomes proficient in punching the dental dam, there should no longer be a need for using a template.

Dental Dam Clamp A dental dam clamp acts like a retainer to anchor and stabilize the dental dam in the mouth. The dental dam can be used to isolate only the tooth being prepared (single isolation), or it can be used to isolate several teeth. When multiple teeth are being isolated, the clamp is usually placed on the tooth most posterior to be isolated with the dam; it is referred to as the clamp bearing tooth or anchor tooth.

The standard clamp is designed for fully erupted teeth. The clamp has five parts: forceps holes, jaws, prongs, bow, and wings (Figure 21-22).

● Forceps holes are holes on either side of the clamp where the clamp forceps are inserted.

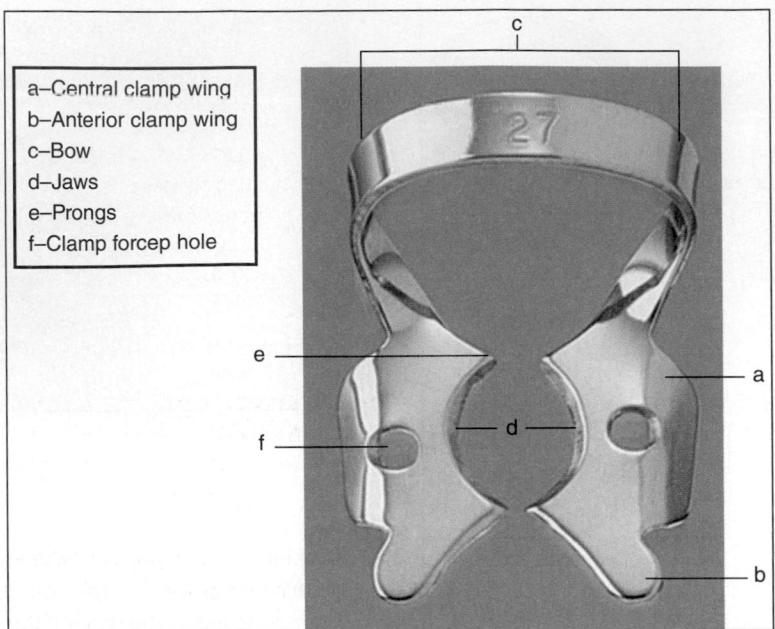

a–Central clamp wing
b–Anterior clamp wing
c–Bow
d–Jaws
e–Prongs
f–Clamp forcep hole

FIGURE 21-22
Parts of the dental dam clamp.

- Jaws are the part of the clamp that the clamp forceps spread open to go over the contour of the tooth and then spring back to fit snugly around the cervix of the tooth being clamped (Figure 21-23).

- Prongs are flat, sharp, and have a four-point bearing clasp to fit snugly around the cervix of the tooth so as not to impinge on tissue.

- Bow is placed toward the posterior of the mouth and used to extend the dental dam to the distal.

- Wings are small flanges on either side of the clamp that allow the clamp to be retained in the dam during placement and hold the dental dam on the facial and lingual once placed.

Standard clamps are recognized by the flat jaws and the prongs that point directly toward each other. The clamp is designed to grasp the tooth at or above the gingival margin, causing minimal gingival damage. Clamp jaws are available in a variety of sizes and shapes to fit all types of teeth and to accommodate different cavity preparations. The sizes correspond with the **circumference** of the cervix of the teeth. The maxillary teeth are more rounded and the mandibular are more squared in shape. The clamps are designed to adapt to the shape differences; maxillary clamps are more rounded than the mandibular clamps. Several companies manufacturer clamps; however, most companies use **universal** numbers to identify the clamps (Table 21-1).

There are specialty clamps designed with jaws directed more gingivally with longer prongs to grasp partially erupted teeth well below the gingival margin. These clamps are designated with a capital A following the clamp number. Serrated clamps have serrated jaws that give a tiger-like grip on broken teeth. These clamps are identified by a capital T after the clamp number. To be able to access distal caries, clamps are designed with distally extended bows and are marked by a capital D after the clamp number. Specialty clamps are also designed without wings to fit into smaller areas in the most posterior areas of the mouth. These clamps are designated with a capital W in front of the clamp number. Clamps are also designed to help retract the gingiva to access cervical caries.

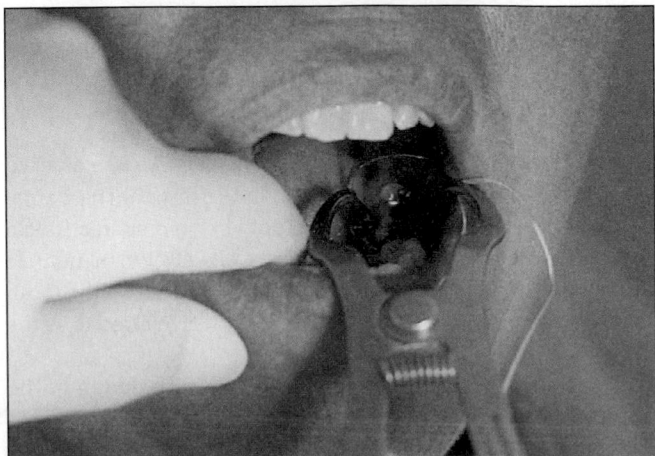

FIGURE 21-23
The clamp forceps open the jaws with a spring motion.

Safety

Safety Ligature Tie

Clamps can break in two, snap, or spring off during placement. A piece of floss is tied around the bow of the dental clamp to avoid swallowing or aspirating the clamp and is wrapped around the operator's finger while placing the clamp. This allows the clamp to be easily withdrawn. This is a critical safety step and must never be omitted.

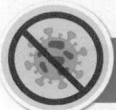

Infection Control

Dental dam clamps come in contact with saliva, blood, and tissue fluids. All clamps need to be thoroughly cleaned to make certain all debris is removed and then need to be sterilized. Clamps should also be checked to make certain they are not sprung; the prongs should be parallel and close together. Keeping clamps open locked in clamp forceps for extended time will result in a stretched out (sprung) clamp.

TABLE 21-1 Dental Dam Clamps

Universal Dental Dam Clamps		
Mandibular molar clamps	#7 winged clamp	#W7 wingless clamp
Maxillary molar clamps	#8 winged clamp	#W8 wingless clamp
Smaller molar clamps (will also fit most D. 2nd molars)	#3 smaller lower molars	#4 smaller upper molars
Premolar clamps (will also fit most D. 1st molars)	#2 winged clamp	#W2 wingless clamp

Courtesy of Henry Schein

(*Continues*)

TABLE 21-1 *(Continued)*

Universal Dental Dam Clamps		
Premolar clamps (will also fit smaller D. 1st molars)	#00 winged clamp	#W00 wingless clamp
Anterior clamps	#6	#9

Specialty Dental Dam Clamps		
Partially erupted molars	#14	#W14A
Tiger clamp	Tiger clamp #14T molar	Tiger clamp/distal access #14DT molar

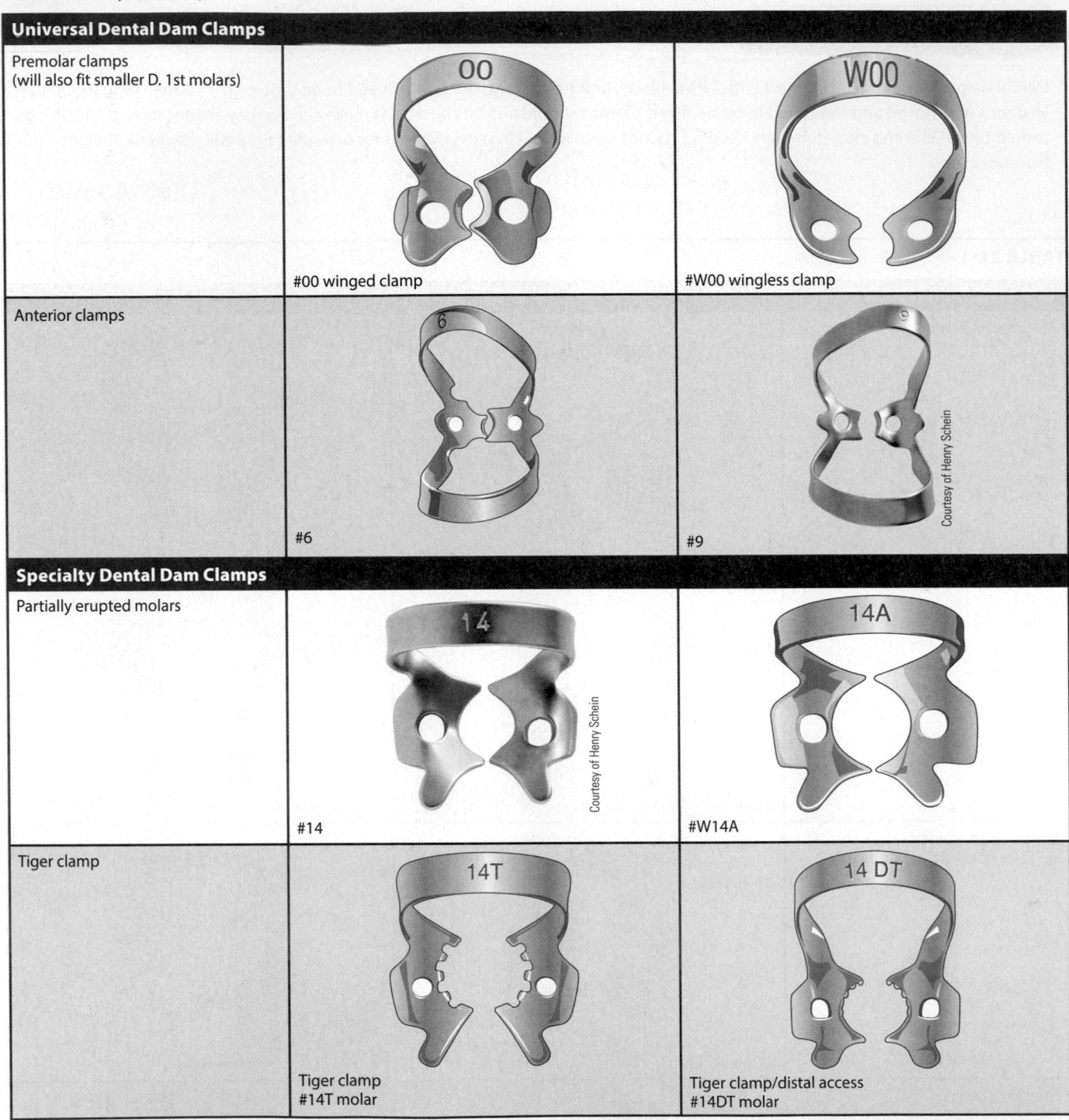

The assistant is often expected to select the appropriate clamp for the procedure and always have it ligated. (Refer to Procedure 21-2, Figure 21-28). A dental assistant is expected to become familiar with clamps by shapes or numbers and be able to select the appropriate clamp for the individual tooth or special situation.

Dental Dam Clamp Forceps The forceps are used to place and remove the clamp from the anchor tooth (Figure 21-24). The beaks of the forceps are placed into the clamp forceps holes, entering on the side away from the bow. The clamp is opened by squeezing the forceps to spread the jaws enough to slip over the crown of the tooth. The clamp forceps open wider when the handle is squeezed closed. There is a sliding ring between the hinge and the forceps handles that can hold the forceps and the jaws open. By holding the handles downward and gently squeezing the handles together, the sliding ring will slide down and keep the forceps in the locked position, holding the clamp in an open position. Leaving the forceps in a locked position after the clamp has been placed in the mouth will wear out the forceps spring and shorten the life of the forceps. The clamps will also be **sprung**

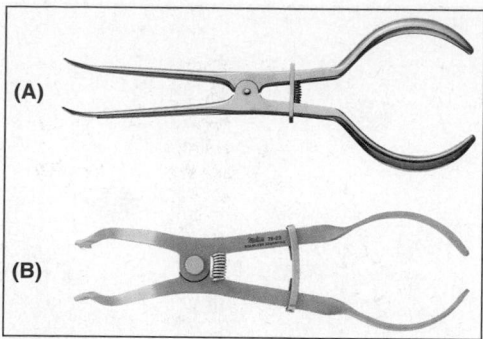

FIGURE 21-24
Dental dam clamp forceps.

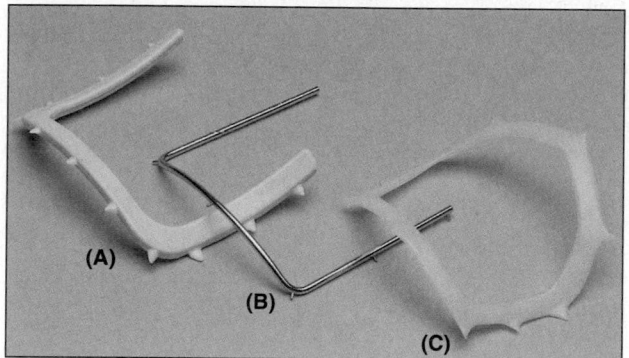

FIGURE 21-25
Dental dam frames. (A) U-frame. (B) Metal Young frame. (C) Ostby frame.

if they are left in the locked position. Make certain to sterilize and care for the forceps according to the manufacturer's directions.

Dental Dam Frame The dental dam frame is used to support the edges of the dental dam, hold the dental dam in place, and keep the material out of the field of operation. There are several types of frames. A popular one is the Young's frame, a metal U-shaped dental dam frame with a series of pegs on the frame (Figure 21-25). The open end of the U allows the upper edge of the dental dam material to fall slightly forward and below the tip of the patient's nose. The material is stretched over the pegs to secure the dental dam material to the frame. These pegs can be broken if the frame is dropped; care needs to be taken in handling the metal frames. The U-shaped frame is also available in plastic.

Another type of dental dam frame is a complete circle with broad blunt pegs that supports the upper edge of the dental dam material. These are primarily made of radiolucent plastic allowing for radiographic exposures with the dental dam in place during endodontic treatment. The more popular is the Otsby frame. Assistants need to follow manufacturer's directions for recommended infection control procedures

Lubricant Once a tooth has been slipped through the punched hole in the dental dam material, the material between the holes needs to be placed between the teeth. The material between the holes is referred to as the dam **septum**. When there are tight

contacts or crowded or rotated teeth, it is often difficult to get the dam **septae** between the teeth. A lubricant can be placed on the underside of the dam to help pass the dental dam material between the teeth. To prevent damage to the rubber, a water-soluble lubricant must be used. Dental dam lubricant is commercially available. Avoid oil-based lubricants like baby oil, petroleum jelly, or cooking oil lubricants because they weaken the dental dam material, resulting in leakage. Lubricant should be placed on a gauze square from the lubricant container and applied to the dental dam using a cotton tip applicator to prevent cross-contamination.

A lubricant can also be used to prevent drying and irritation of the patient's lips and corners of the mouth. The dental assistant can apply cocoa butter or non-petroleum jelly with a cotton tip applicator or even permit the patient to apply a personal lip balm.

Waxed Dental Floss Waxed dental floss has many uses in placing the dental dam. It is used to tie around the bow of the clamp as a safety ligature, to check the tightness of contacts prior to placing the dental dam, to help ease dam septae between the contacts, and to ligate the most anterior tooth to anchor the anterior portion of the dental dam. It can also be used to help remove any dental dam scraps of material that may remain after the dental dam has been removed. Waxed floss is used so much during this procedure, that is difficult to have enough precut pieces of floss or to take the time to cut a piece from the floss dispenser. Making butterfly ties helps to solve this problem (Procedure 21-2, Figure 21-29).

The assistant makes butterfly ties by cutting a 12-inch piece of waxed floss. The assistant holds one end of the floss between their thumb and index finger of one hand and gently wraps all but an inch of the floss around the index and middle finger. The assistant removes their fingers, making a loop of floss. The center of the floss is twisted, which holds the butterfly tie together until ready for use. The assistant holds each end of the floss and pulls, providing an already cut piece of floss ready for use.

Plastic Instrument (Woodson) The plastic instrument is used in many steps during the application of the dental dam. The paddle end is used to remove the dental dam from the wings of the clamp during placement, to hold floss at the cervix of the tooth when placing a ligature tie around a tooth, and to help **invert** (tuck) the dam around the teeth to prevent leakage.

Safety

Review the patient's medical history prior to using the dental dam. When there is a notation of an allergy to latex, the dam napkin should be used or avoid the use of a latex dental dam material. There is also a connection between food allergies and latex allergies known as a latex-food syndrome. There is an increased risk of being allergic to latex if the patient is allergic to banana, avocado, passion fruit, kiwi, papaya, mango, peach, fig, melon, and pineapple. Caution should also be taken in using the dental dam with these patients.

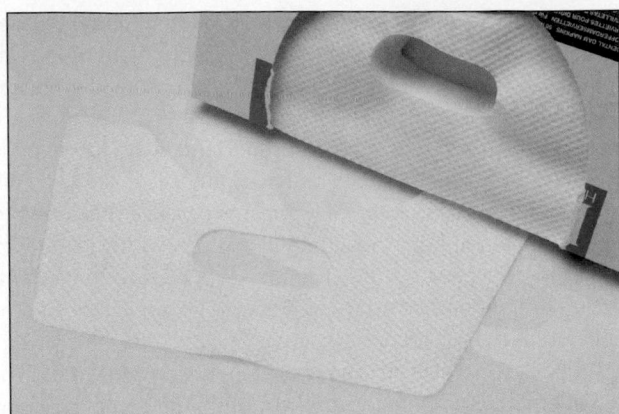

FIGURE 21-26
Dental dam napkin.

Crown and Bridge Scissors The crown and bridge scissors have many uses in the dental dam procedure. When directed away from anatomic structures, the curved scissors make it easier to cut materials without cutting tissue. When using the dental dam material, they can be used to adjust the length of floss ties, cut a hole in the dental dam for placement of a saliva ejector, and cut dam septae for removal of the dental dam.

Dental Dam Napkin A disposable dental dam napkin is primarily used for patient comfort (Figure 21-26). It can be placed between the dental dam and the patient's skin to prevent skin contact with the dental dam material for patients sensitive to latex. The napkin reduces the possibility of an allergic reaction, absorbs saliva that may seep at the corners of the patient's mouth, and acts as a cushion between the frame and the patient's face.

Stabilizing Cord The stabilizing cord is an elastic cord that comes in different sizes and colors (Figure 21-27). It is stretched and then placed interproximally to secure the dental dam material. The cord is used to stabilize the dental dam placement at the opposite end of the clamp or for individual teeth. For example, instead of using a dental dam clamp, use the stabilizing cord for an anterior dental dam placement (Figure 21-34).

Prepare Tray Setup for Dental Dam Placement In preparing to assist in placing the dental dam, the dental assistant will need to include the basic setup, expendables, and dental dam instruments on the instrument tray. For the dental dam procedure in this chapter, the tray is placed lengthwise on the bracket table (Procedure 21-2). The hand instruments should be placed on the instrument tray in the order of use with handles passed to operator's left hand facing the right of the tray. The mirror is placed in this manner. Those passed to the operator's right hand and facing the left of the tray are the explorer, cotton pliers, and plastic instrument. The dental dam instruments are placed to the right of the tray with the handles facing the right in order of use, and expendables are placed at the top of the instrument tray.

Once the patient is seated, an experienced assistant can select the clamp by viewing the patient's chart and mouth. The safety

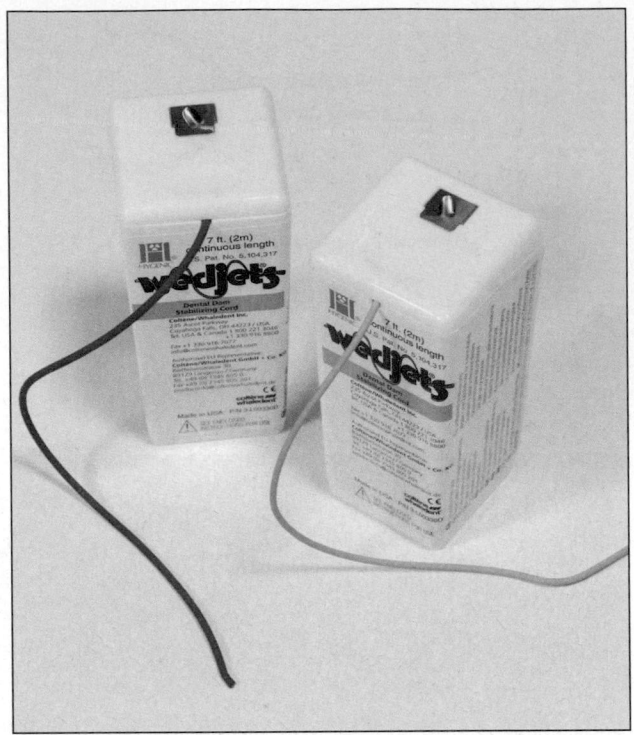

FIGURE 21-27
Stabilizing cord.

ligature should be tied around the clamp before the dentist **anesthetizes** the patient. The area is now ready for the placement of the dental dam.

Prepare the Dental Dam Material for Placement
The assistant reviews the patient's chart and examines the tooth that is to be **prepared**, the location of the preparation, the position of the teeth in that quadrant, and what tooth will be the anchor tooth before punching the dental dam material. The first step in preparing the dental dam material is to determine the number of holes that need to be punched.

Determine the Number of Holes to Punch The location of the **preparation** will determine which tooth needs to be clamped and how many teeth need to be isolated. G. V. Black's system of classification of cavities is used in determining the number of holes to be punched. The classification, what teeth are present and their position, what teeth need to be isolated, and which tooth needs to be clamped determines the number of holes to be punched. The dentist or skilled assistant will determine what holes need to be punched and perform the actual punching of the dental dam material. Following are guidelines; however, ultimately the number of holes is the operator's preference.

Class I Placement As you recall, a Class I cavity includes lingual pits of anterior teeth and occlusal surfaces of posterior teeth. When the cavity involves one surface a single isolation is generally used. The tooth being prepared is the only tooth

Procedure 21-2
Preparing the Dental Dam Setup

The dental assistant prepares all the instruments and materials needed to assist the operator in placing the dental dam.

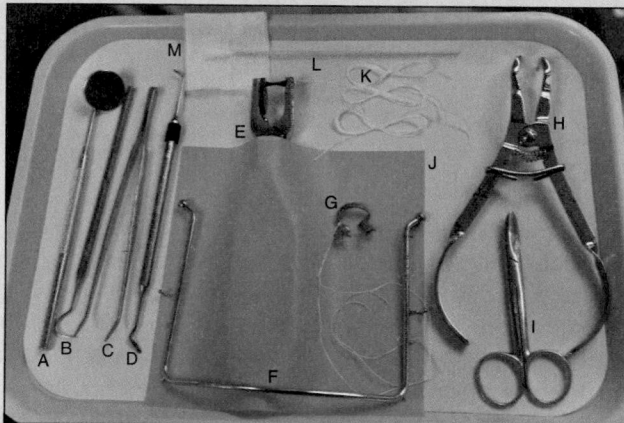

FIGURE 21-28
Completed dental dam tray setup.

Equipment and Supplies
- Basic setup
  - ❏ mouth mirror (A)
  - ❏ explorer (B)
  - ❏ cotton pliers (C)
- Plastic instrument (D)
- Dental dam instruments
  - ❏ dental dam punch (E)
  - ❏ dental dam frame (F)
  - ❏ selected dental dam clamp with safety ligature (G)
  - ❏ dental dam clamp forceps (H)
- Crown and bridge scissors (curved) (I)
- Dental dam expendables
  - ❏ dental dam material (6 × 6) (J)
  - ❏ prepared "butterfly" dental floss (K)
  - ❏ lubricant on cotton-tip applicator (L)
  - ❏ gauze squares (M)

Procedure Steps *(Follow aseptic procedures)*
1. Place the materials and instruments on instrument tray.

2. Carry tray to the treatment area and place on the bracket table lengthwise.

3. Place basic setup on tray in order of use with handles facing the passing hand:
   - ❏ *Face handles passed by assistant's right hand toward right.*
     - ❏ mirror

   - ❏ *Face handles passed by assistant's left hand toward left.*
     - ❏ dental explorer
     - ❏ cotton pliers

4. Place plastic instrument next with handles facing left.

5. Place dental dam instruments to right of tray in order of use with handles facing right:
   - ❏ dental dam punch
   - ❏ dental dam clamp forceps
   - ❏ Young's dental dam frame
   - ❏ crown and bridge scissors

6. Place dental dam material over dental dam frame.

7. Select dental dam clamp based on patient's chart and observation of patient's mouth.
   - ❏ Tie safety ligature around the bow of the clamp (Figure 21-29).
   - ❏ Tear off a 12–18 inch piece of floss.
   - ❏ Hold the ends of the floss making a loop in the middle.
   - ❏ Insert the loop through the bow of the clamp.
   - ❏ Pull the ends of the floss through the loop and tighten the floss against the bow.

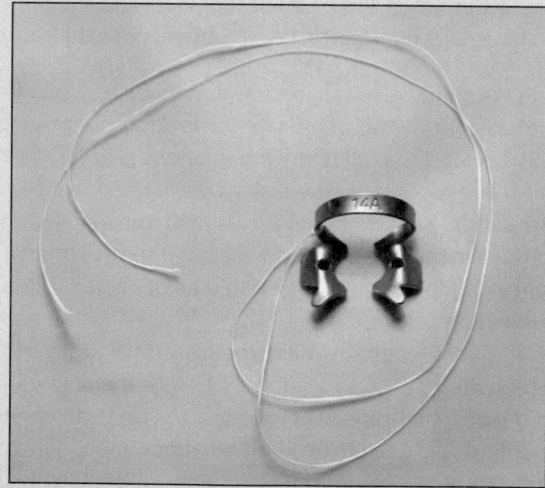

FIGURE 21-29
Safety tie around bow of the clamp.

8. Place expendables at top of tray:
   - ❏ Place lubricant on gauze square using cotton tip applicator.
   - ❏ Place applicator on gauze square.

(Continues)

❑ Prepare and place number of waxed floss (butterfly ties) to be used (Figure 21-30).
  ❑ Cut a 12-inch piece of waxed floss.
  ❑ Hold one end of the floss between thumb and index finger of one hand.
  ❑ Gently wrap all but an inch of the floss around the index and middle finger.
  ❑ Remove fingers making a loop of floss.
  ❑ Twist the center of the floss loop to hold the waxed floss together until ready for use (when ready to use the floss, hold each floss end and pull to provide an already cut piece of floss ready for use).

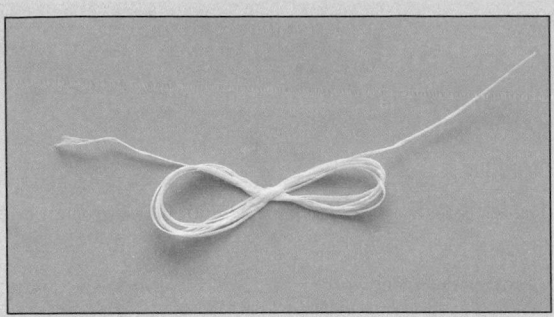

FIGURE 21-30
Prepared butterfly tie.

isolated and is also used for the placement of the clamp; it is the **clamp-bearing** (or anchor) tooth.

Only one hole needs to be punched. For example:

- Tooth #10 is being prepared and has lingual pit caries (#10 Lingual caries); one hole for #10 would be punched.

- Tooth #30 has occlusal caries (#30 occlusal caries); one hole for #30 would be punched.

If a posterior cavity includes the buccal or lingual pits, three holes may need to be punched for better access. A hole is punched on either side of the tooth being prepared, the most posterior tooth is clamped, and the most anterior tooth and tooth being prepared are isolated. For example:

- Tooth #30 has occlusobuccal caries (#30 OB caries); #31 would have a hole punched and be the anchor tooth and #30 and #29 would have holes punched for each tooth and would be isolated.

Class II Placement A carious lesion that involves a proximal surface (mesial or distal) of a posterior tooth is considered a Class II lesion. Most Class II cavity preparations also involve the occlusal surface to allow the dentist access to the proximal surfaces. The dentist prefers to gain access to the proximal surface through the occlusal surface of the diseased tooth. Otherwise, the neighboring (proximal) tooth would be damaged trying to remove the decay.

Class II cavities would be mesio-occlusal (MO), disto-occlusal (DO), and mesio-occlusodistal (MOD). Since the preparation involves the proximal surface at least one to two teeth anterior and posterior would need to be punched. For example:

- Tooth #19 DO; #17 would be the anchor tooth, and #18, #19, #20, and #21 would have holes punched for each tooth and would be isolated.

Most Class II cavities need to have a **matrix band** for proper placement of the restoration. For room for the matrix and better interproximal access for the bur, most operators prefer two teeth anterior and two teeth posterior if possible.

Class III Placement A carious lesion that involves a proximal surface (mesial or distal) of an anterior tooth is considered a Class III lesion. The mesial and distal can be accessed with anterior teeth

through the lingual or the facial, so the incisal surface would not need to be involved. Class III cavities would be M or D. As with the Class II, there needs to be room for a matrix and bur access interproximally. It is better to place the clamp on a posterior tooth because it is easier to clamp and there is less patient trauma and better access for preparation. Generally the first premolar on the same side of the mouth as the tooth to be prepared is the anchor tooth that holds the clamp. Holes are punched for all teeth from the anchor tooth to two teeth beyond the tooth to be prepared. Class III usually requires punching a minimum of five holes. For example:

- Tooth #7 D; #5 is the first premolar and would be the anchor tooth and #6, #7, #8 and #9 would have holes punched for each tooth, and would be isolated.

Class IV Placement A carious lesion that involves the incisal surface of an anterior tooth is considered a Class IV lesion. Most times this classification will also involve the proximal surfaces. Class IV cavities would be I, MI, DI, and MID. As with the Class III, there needs to be room for the matrix and bur access interproximally. The punching for the Class IV is the same as for the Class III and usually requires punching a minimum of five holes. For example:

- Tooth #8 MI; #5 is the first premolar and will be the anchor tooth, and #6, #7, #8, #9 and #10 would have holes punched for each tooth and would be isolated.

Notice that this example requires six holes to include the two teeth needed to be mesial to the tooth being prepared (#8) and punching to a premolar for clamp placement.

Class V Placement A carious lesion that involves the gingival one third on the facial or lingual surface of either an anterior or posterior tooth is considered a Class V lesion. The type of isolation needed is determined by how close to the gingiva the cavity is located. Class V cavities at the level of and below the gingiva (subgingival) may require single isolation and placement of a gingival retraction clamp. If the cavity is coronal to the gingiva (supragingival), clamping one tooth posterior and isolating one tooth anterior will allow for better access.

For example: If the maxillary right canine (#6) has a Class V labial gingival 1/3 cavity preparation, the assistant punches for a single isolation and with a gingival retraction clamp such as clamp #6.

Safety

There is a potential concern for safety when trying on the clamp. If the clamp is not securely placed around the cervix of the tooth, it can pop off. The operator should secure and hold the clamp with their index finger on the clamp while placing the clamp. For additional safety, the operator can wind the end of the safety tie about one of their fingers (Figure 21-31). The clamp can be quickly retrieved from the mouth if it should pop off.

Try On Clamp After determining what tooth needs to be clamped, the dental dam clamp should be tried on the tooth to be prepared. The dental dam clamp should be selected as described previously. The assistant should tie the safety ligature of dental floss to the bow of the clamp with the loop placed on the facial side of the clamp. The beaks of the dental dam clamp forceps are inserted into the dental dam clamp holes with the bow facing away from the forceps. The assistant locks the forceps and passes it to the operator with the beaks facing down for the mandibular arch and up for the maxillary.

The operator opens the jaws of the clamp and places the clamp below the **height of contour** of the tooth, first on the lingual surface and then the facial surface. The operator then gently allows the clamp jaws to close around the tooth, secures the lingual of the clamp with index finger, and releases the forceps from the clamp. Using both fingers the clamp is pressed into position around the cervix of the tooth. All four prongs should contact the lingual and facial surfaces at the cervix. The clamp should be stable and should not rock or impinge or **blanch** the gingival tissue. After the clamp is tried on it is removed and returned to the assistant. To remove the clamp, the forceps are inserted into the clamp holes and the jaws are opened to pass the height of contour of the tooth.

Check Contacts of Teeth to Be Isolated After the operator determines that the clamp can be placed securely, the contacts of the teeth to be isolated should be checked. The assistant should pass a 12-inch piece of floss to the operator, holding the ends of the floss while the operator winds the floss around their middle fingers. The operator flosses between the teeth checking that the floss can freely enter each interproximal space. Anything that obstructs the floss will also obstruct the septum of the dental dam material, making placement difficult if not impossible. Obstructions like calculus may need to be removed and rough edges of existing restorations may need to be smoothed prior to dental dam placement.

Determine Hole Placement Once the operator has checked the clamp and the teeth to be isolated, the dental dam is ready to be punched. The dentist or skilled assistant punches the dental dam using the teeth as a guide. Adjustments may need to be made for missing teeth, misaligned teeth, or fixed prosthetics. The dental assistant passes to the operator the dental dam punch with the dental dam wrapped around the punch. Some operators like to punch the dental dam while it is secured on the dental dam frame. The frame helps keep the dental dam **taut**, making the punching easier.

An assistant who is able to punch the dental dam for the dentist is a great asset. This is a skill the novice assistant should aspire to acquiring. Novice assistants can use one of the templates to help guide them in the placement of the holes. In learning how to place the holes without the use of a template, operators can use the following guidelines in dividing the dental dam to determine the placement of the holes.

The dental dam is first divided into sixths (Figure 21-32). One way to mark the divisions is to fold and then crease the dental

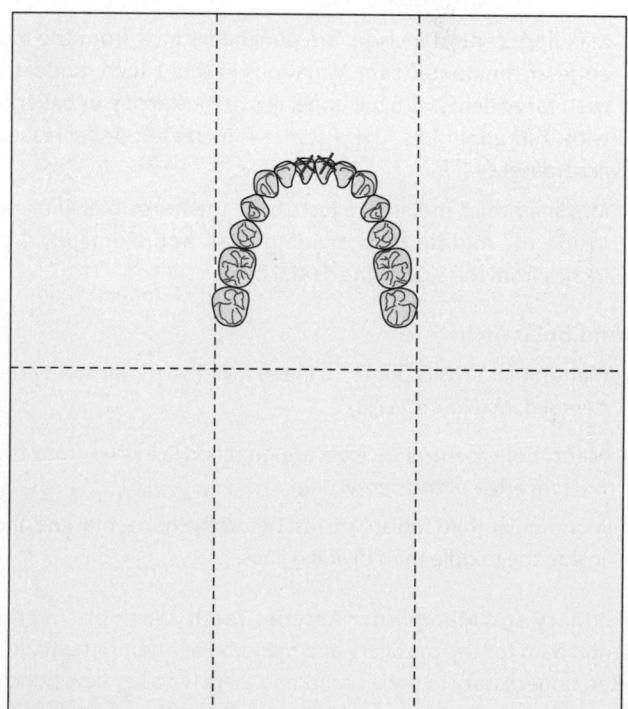

FIGURE 21-32
Dental dam divided into sixths with a maxillary arch punched for work on the maxillary central incisors.

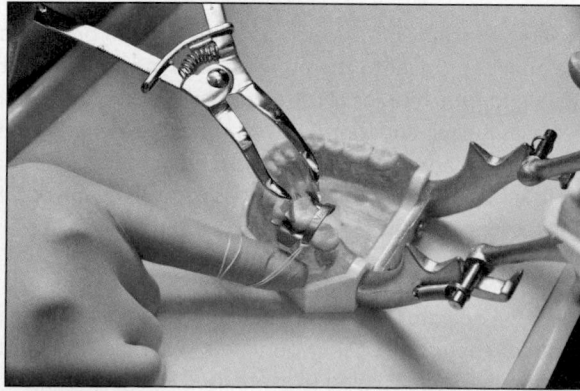

FIGURE 21-31
Use of safety ligature.

dam. This leaves a faint mark on the dam for the operator to use when punching the dam.

To begin, fold the dam in half and then crease the fold. This horizontal line is the division between the maxillary and mandibular arches. With the dam folded in half, fold the dam vertically into equal thirds and crease along each fold. The center third is where the dam will be punched. This represents the width of the arches of most patients. Some operators prefer to divide the dam into thirds only, and some divide the dam into quarters and mark the center point as a reference point before punching.

Punch the Dental Dam After the dental dam is divided, it is ready to be punched for placement. Often, the key hole punch is punched first. The key hole punch is the largest hole punched in the dental dam and is the hole for the clamp-bearing tooth (anchor tooth). The next holes are punched about 3 to 3.5 mm apart (distance between the holes on the punch plate). This distance is needed to allow the septal dental dam to slide between the teeth. It is important for the operator to visualize the patient's arch on the dental dam and follow the natural curvature of the patient's arch. Notice the natural curvature of normally positioned teeth in the occlusal view of the dental arch. The molars are fairly straight, premolars begin to curve, the canine is at the peak of the curve, and the centrals are straight across from each other. Following are guidelines for various hole placement needs.

Maxillary Arch

- Maxillary arch is punched in the upper middle sixth portion of the dental dam (Figure 21-32).

- Maxillary central incisors are punched 1 inch from the top edge of the dental dam. Variations in this 1-inch guide are used for patients with full upper lips or mustaches, or patients with thin upper lips. The distance is increased or decreased accordingly.

- Maxillary third molars are just above the horizontal line and inside the middle third dividing lines, approximately 1 ½ inches from the side of the dental dam.

Mandibular Arch

- Mandibular arch is punched in the lower sixth portion of the dental dam (Figure 21-33).

- Mandibular central incisors are punched 2 inches from the bottom edge of the dental dam.

- Mandibular third molars are just below the horizontal line and inside the middle third dividing lines.

Maxillary and Mandibular Anterior Teeth When placing the dental dam for the maxillary and mandibular anterior teeth, it is often unnecessary to use a clamp, and there is no key hole punch. Dental floss is doubled, and a piece of dental dam or stabilizing cord is placed in the distal interproximals of each canine. This is usually enough to hold the dam in place without the placement of a clamp (Figure 21-34).

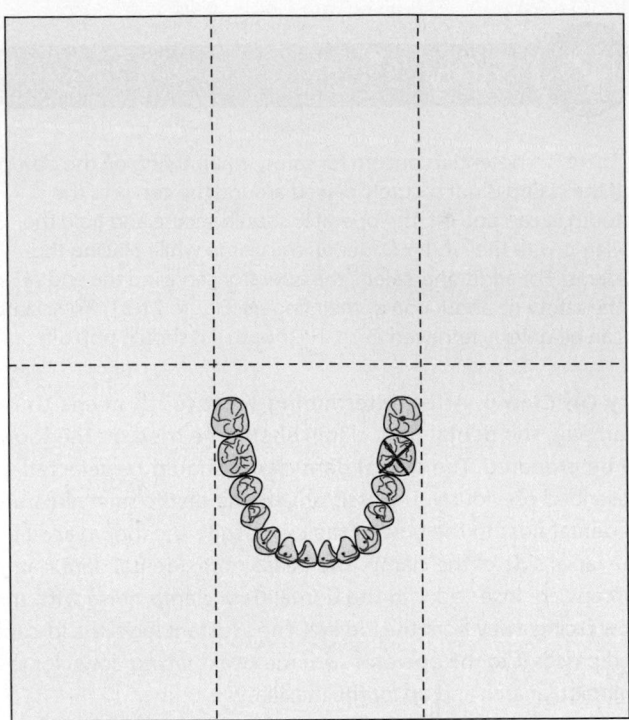

FIGURE 21-33
Mandibular arch punched for work on the mandibular.

Missing or Malpositioned Teeth Punching for patients who have missing or malpositioned teeth is accomplished by the operator following the pattern of the teeth in the patient's mouth as the dental dam is being punched.

- When teeth are malpositioned (out of normal alignment or position), they often are positioned either buccal or lingual of the normal curve of the arch, so the corresponding holes must be positioned either toward the buccal or the lingual to match the arch.

- Missing teeth or edentulous areas are accommodated by leaving a space on the dam between holes punched for teeth present in the mouth. So, if tooth #5 is missing, then tooth #4 would be punched, a space would be left, and then teeth #6, #7, and so on would be punched.

Bridgework Placement Patterns for patients with bridgework require punches similar to the punches with missing teeth. It is impossible to punch holes for the pontics (portion of a bridge that replaces the missing tooth), so the punches are made for the abutment teeth, and spaces are left for the number of pontics. Slits are cut between the holes with scissors to allow the pontics to be exposed.

Determine Hole Size While determining the placement of the holes, the operator rotates the punch disc to the appropriate hole size for each tooth being punched. When using an adult five-hole punch, the following sizes are used as a guide:

- The first hole is the smallest hole and is designed for mandibular incisors.

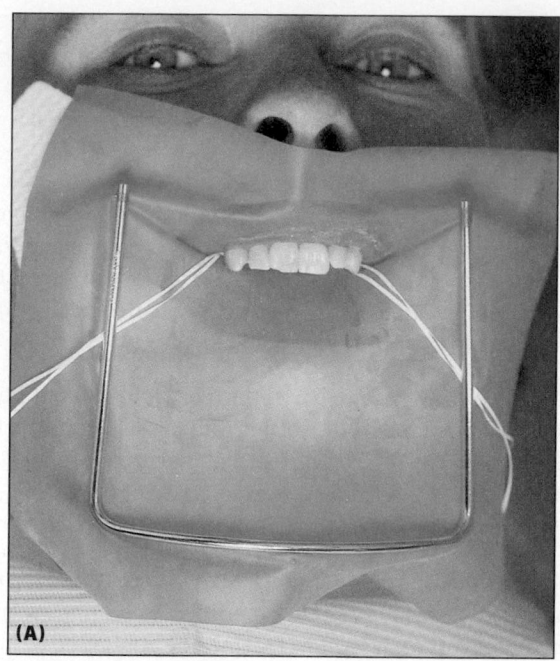
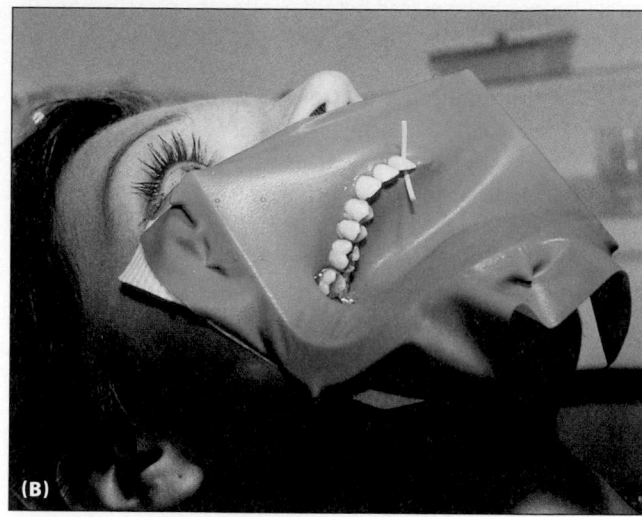

FIGURE 21-34
(A) Maxillary anterior placement with floss used as ligatures. (B) Patient with stabilizing cord securing dental dam in place.

- The second hole is designed for maxillary incisors and canines.
- The third hole is designed for premolars.
- The fourth hole is designed for molars.
- The fifth hole is designed for clamp-bearing molars.
- When clamping for all other teeth, the general rule is to use the next larger hole size.

The same guidelines are followed when using the five-hole pediatric dental dam punch:

- The first hole is the smallest hole and is designed for primary mandibular incisors.
- The second hole is designed for primary maxillary incisors and canines.
- The third hole is designed for primary first molars.
- The fourth hole is designed for primary second molars.
- The fifth hole is designed for clamp-bearing molars.
- When clamping for all other teeth, the general rule is to use the next larger hole size.

There is a six-hole dental dam punch that is used for mixed dentition. Holes 1 through 5 are used as the five holes of the pediatric dental dam punch. Holes 2 through 6 are used as the five holes of the adult dental dam punch.

Common Errors When Punching a Dental Dam

- Punching the arch too flat or wide results in folds or bunching and stretching on the lingual; punching the arch too curved or narrow results in folds and stretching on the facial. These errors make tucking the dental dam into the gingival sulcus difficult. The curve of the arch should match the arch curve of the patient.

- Tearing or leaving a tag of dental dam material around the hole, which may be caused by a dull stylus or improperly lining up the punch hole with the stylus. This error will cause the dental dam to tear more easily when being stretched for placement, and the dental dam may leak once in place.

- If the holes are too close together, there will not be enough material to seal around each tooth, but the dam will be stretched and gingival tissue will be exposed. If the holes are too far apart, there will be excess material between the teeth. It may be difficult to get all the dam material interproximal when placing the dental dam, and the bunched dental dam material may get in the operator's way during the procedure. The hole spacing should match the space between the patient's teeth.

- Upper lips are not covered by the dental dam. The dental dam was punched with less than 1 inch for the maxillary centrals from the upper dental dam edge. The nose is covered by the dental dam. There is more than 1 inch space from the maxillary centrals to the upper dental dam edge. This can remedied by cutting out an area for the nose using crown and bridge scissors.

Placement of the Dental Dam Dental assistants help the dentist with the dental dam in states where it is not legal for them to place the dental dam, but in states where dental assistants can place the dental dam, the assistants punch the dam, select the clamp, and place and remove the dental dam without the chairside presence of the dentist. Once the dental dam has been punched, the underside of the dental dam material can be lubricated as needed and the patient can be offered a water soluble lubricant to be applied to their lips and corners of the mouth.

The operator is ready to place the dental dam. There are many methods used in placing the dental dam. The method selected depends on the position and eruption of the tooth, the location of the cavity preparation, and the dentist's or operator's preference. Clamps can be placed before or after the placement of the dam or along with the dental dam material as one unit.

Placement of Clamp before Dental Dam Placing the clamp before the dental dam (Procedure 21-3) is the best option when the anchor tooth is partially erupted (specialty A clamp) or the anchor tooth is the last tooth in the arch and there is not enough room for the placement of a winged clamp (specialty W clamp). Both the A clamp with extended prongs and the W clamp that is wingless cannot be held in the dental dam during placement. The extended prongs tear the dental dam material and the wingless clamp cannot be secured in the punched hole as with the winged clamp.

Placement of Clamp First After the dental dam is punched, the clamp needs to be placed around the anchor tooth with the safety ligature attached. With this technique the clamp is tried on the tooth to confirm selection of the dental clamp, and then the dental dam is punched. The A clamps are used to clamp hard-to-clamp teeth, and the placement has a much higher level of difficulty. The operator has to place the clamp just below the height of contour and then very carefully press the clamp into position. The prongs, although designed to grip below the gingiva, can impinge, abrade, lacerate, or irritate the gingival tissue. This often causes gingival bleeding especially when the patient has gingivitis and the tissue is swollen. It is common that these areas have gingivitis because these areas are hard to reach with a toothbrush, and partially erupted teeth are more difficult to keep clean.

Safety

The jaws of the clamp have **prongs** that help to secure the clamp around the cervix of the tooth. These prongs are somewhat sharp and can damage tissues and restorations. Minor damage to marginal gingiva and cervical cementum may occur if the operator is not careful in the release of the clamp around the tooth. Damage to restorations and crowns can occur if the prongs are allowed to grip or scrape across the margins during placement and removal of the clamp.

Placement of the Dental Dam The operator stretches and places the dental dam over the bow of the clamp with the index fingers. The anchor hole is stretched over the bow first and then under the jaws. A medium to heavy gauge material is preferred as this stretching may cause thinner material to tear. If the napkin is used, the operator gathers the dental dam in one hand and inserts the other hand through the napkin opening to grasp the material and pull it through. The napkin and frame are adjusted and the dental dam is attached to the dental dam frame. The safety ligature is passed under the dental dam frame and attached to the dental dam frame.

Isolate Teeth The operator places the most anterior hole around the most anterior tooth to be isolated. This tooth is ligated to help the dental dam stay secure. The remaining teeth are isolated, and the dental dam is inverted around the cervix of each tooth. The area is rinsed and evacuated before the dentist begins treatment.

Removal of the Dental Dam The assistant rinses and evacuates the area and passes the operator the crown and bridge scissors. The operator cuts each septum, making one continuous cut, and the dental dam is pulled through the lingual side until all of the material is free from the contacts. The assistant passes the clamp forceps. The operator releases the clamp and removes the dental dam and frame as a unit. The assistant rinses and evacuates the patient's mouth. The operator checks the dental dam to see if it is complete, and any remaining material is removed using a piece of waxed dental floss. The operator may gently massage the gingiva to help the blood return to the area to reduce postoperative pain.

Placement of Clamp after the Dental Dam The steps in preparing the dental dam material for placement of the clamp after the dental dam are the same as the previous method. The primary difference is that the clamp is placed after the dental dam. Placing the clamp after the dental dam is the best option when the cavity to be prepared is a Class V. The dentist needs to retract the gingiva for better access to the cavity. In this case, the tooth to be prepared is also the anchor tooth. This requires a single isolation with only one hole punched.

A gingival retraction clamp is the best choice to isolate the Class V cavity. The dam cannot be stretched over the gingival retraction clamp with the large bows (butterfly clamp). The method used in placing the gingival retraction clamp is to place the dental dam over the anchor tooth first and then place the clamp. The dental dam is stretched away from the gumline of

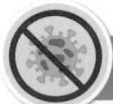

Infection Control

Patients with cardiac conditions are at risk for infective **endocarditis** with dental procedures. Placement of the dental dam has been ranked as a medium risk of causing **bacteremia** due to the possibility of damaging gingiva and causing bleeding. Infectious disease specialists such as the AHA produce guidelines that state when **antibiotic prophylaxis** is indicated. The risk is increased with use of the extended prong clamps if the gingiva is pierced or in the presence of gingivitis and bleeding.

Procedure 21-3
Assist Operator in Placing Clamp before Dental Dam

This procedure is performed by the dentist or dental assistant. The patient has been anesthetized before placement of the dental dam and before the cavity preparation begins. The dental assistant has prepared all equipment and supplies needed for the entire procedure. With this procedure the assistant is assisting the dentist or operator. Black font represents the assistant's functions, and **blue** font represents dentist/operator functions. *Note*: The student assistant can complete this procedure as either the operator or assistant depending on state regulations.

Equipment and Supplies
- Basic setup
  - ❏ mouth mirror
  - ❏ explorer
  - ❏ cotton pliers
- Plastic instrument
- Dental dam instruments
  - ❏ dental dam punch
  - ❏ dental dam clamp forceps
  - ❏ dental dam frame
  - ❏ assortment of dental dam clamps
- Crown and bridge scissors (curved)
- Dental dam expendables
  - ❏ dental dam material (6 × 6)
  - ❏ dental dam napkin
  - ❏ lubricant
  - ❏ cotton-tip applicator
  - ❏ gauze squares
  - ❏ dental floss
  - ❏ stabilizing cord (optional)

Procedure Steps *(Follow aseptic procedures)*

1. Prepare dental dam setup as described in Procedure 21-2.

2. Demonstrate exemplary skills in assisting placement of dental dam.
   - ❏ Anticipate each step of the procedure.
   - ❏ Perform instrument exchange.
   - ❏ Maintain proper team position.
   - ❏ Maintain clean work area and return materials to storage.

   Dentist anesthetizes area prior to placing dental dam (details in Chapter 23).

3. Explain dental dam procedure to patient.
   - ❏ Lubricate lips and corners of patient's mouth using cotton tip applicator.

   Operator examines patient's mouth to determine the anchor tooth, shape of the arch, tooth alignment, missing teeth, the presence of crowns and bridges, and dental clamp.

4. Pass mirror and explorer.

   Operator checks tightness and ease of floss passing through interproximals (Figure 21-35).

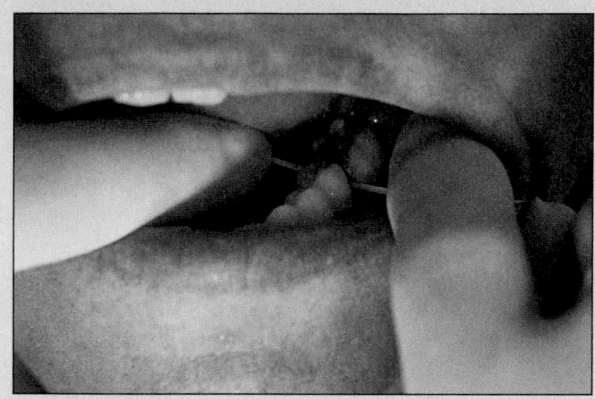

FIGURE 21-35
Dental operator checking patient's contacts with floss.

5. Pass floss to operator, holding ends of floss as they wrap their fingers around the floss.

6. Prepare for removal of calculus or smoothing of roughness as needed.
   - ❏ If calculus is present, pass the operator's favorite scaler.
   - ❏ If there is interproximal roughness due to restoration, pass the operator's preferred instruments: sandpaper strip, **lightening strip**, etc.

   Operator places the selected dental dam clamp for try-on.

7. Assist in try-on of clamp.
   - ❏ Tie safety ligature around bow of selected clamp.
   - ❏ Engage forceps into clamp forceps holes with clamp bow facing toward the lingual of the cavity and lock forceps.
   - ❏ Pass forceps to operator with beaks facing toward the operative site (up for maxillary and down for mandibular).

   Operator passes clamp over contour of crown.
   - ❏ *Places the clamp on lingual surface and then buccal.*
   - ❏ *Releases lock to ease clamp around just below contour of crown and above the gingiva.*
   - ❏ *Holds lingual of clamp with index finger as forceps are removed.*

8. Retrieve clamp forceps and hold ready to return to operator.

   Operator secures clamp with index fingers on lingual and facial surfaces (Figure 21-36).
   - ❏ *Checks for proper fit of clamp.*

(Continues)

❏ Clamp is stable with no rocking.
❏ All four prongs are against facial and lingual surfaces.
❏ Clamp does not pinch gingiva and gingival tissue is not blanched.

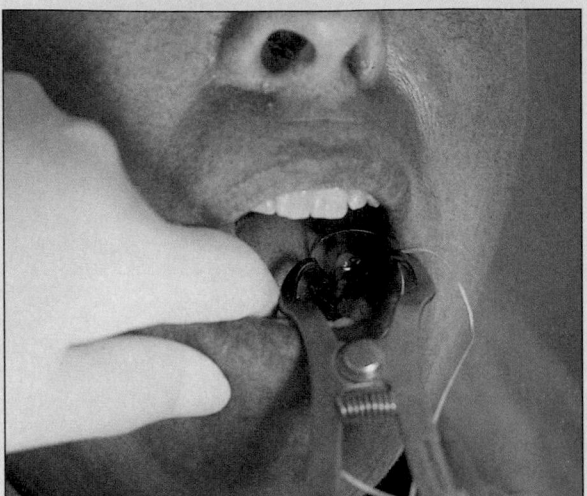

FIGURE 21-36
Dental dam clamp placed on anchor tooth.

9. Pass clamp forceps to remove clamp. Retrieve clamp forceps and clamp after try-on and return forceps to position on tray.

10. Anticipate assisting in punching the dental dam.
    ❏ Pass the dental dam punch and dental dam material while retrieving the clamp forceps.

    Operator punches the dental dam material (Figure 21-37).

    ❏ Follows the guidelines for hole placement.
    ❏ Divides the dental dam material into sixths.

❏ Punches the dental dam, aligning the stylus and the holes carefully.
❏ Centers the punch in the upper middle third of the dental dam for maxillary placement or lower middle third for mandibular.
❏ Punches holes according to the size of the tooth, with the key hole punch being the largest to accommodate the anchor tooth and the clamp.
❏ Punches following the pattern of the patient's arch.
❏ Lubricates the dental dam on the tissue side of the dam with a water-soluble lubricant.

11. Pass dental dam lubricant on cotton tip applicator (at operator request).

12. Anticipate operator's placement of the clamp.
    ❏ Engage forceps into clamp forceps holes with clamp bow facing toward the lingual of the cavity.
    ❏ Pass forceps to operator with beaks facing toward the operative site in locked position (up for maxillary and down for mandibular).

    Operator places the selected dental dam clamp.

    ❏ Squeezes forceps handle slightly to release locking bar.
    ❏ Passes clamp over contour of crown.
    ❏ Places the clamp on lingual surface and then buccal.
    ❏ Releases lock to ease clamp around just below contour of crown and above the gingiva to evaluate the clamp position.
    ❏ Holds lingual of clamp with index finger as forceps are removed.

13. Retrieve clamp forceps.

    Operator secures clamp with index fingers on lingual and facial surface.

    ❏ Checks for proper fit of clamp (Figure 21-38).
    ❏ Clamp is stable with no rocking.

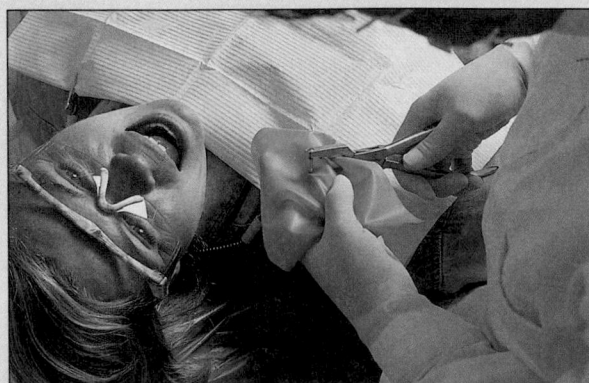

FIGURE 21-37
Dental operator punching dental dam material.

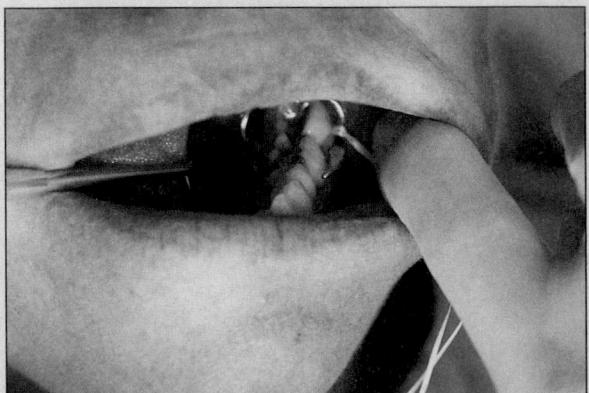

FIGURE 21-38
Evaluate clamp placement and patient comfort.

❏ All four prongs are against facial and lingual surface.

❏ Clamp does not pinch gingiva and gingival tissue is not blanched.

❏ Confirms with patient that the clamp position is comfortable.

14. Anticipate assisting in placement of dental dam.

    ❏ Retrieve clamp forceps and pass punched dental dam material.

    ❏ Return forceps to position on tray.

Operator places the dental dam over the clamp bow.

    ❏ **Places index fingers on each side of the key hole punch.**

    ❏ **Spreads hole wide enough to slip over the clamp.**

    ❏ **Stretches hole over the anchor and one side of the clamp.**

    ❏ **Exposes the other clamp jaw making entire clamp and anchor tooth exposed.**

    ❏ **Pulls the safety tie through the dental dam and drapes to side of patient's mouth.**

15. Anticipate need and pass operator's preference floss or stabilizing cord.

    Operator isolates the most anterior tooth punched (Figure 21-39).

    ❏ **Secures material with floss or stabilizing cord.**

16. Pass dental dam napkin as needed.

    Operator places napkin around patient's mouth, pulls dental dam material through napkin hole and adjusts evenly around the mouth (Figure 21-40).

17. Anticipate need and pass dental dam frame.

    Operator places the frame either under or over the dental dam material, depending on the type of frame and operator preference.

    ❏ **Stretches dental dam and attaches to pegs on frame.**

18. Anticipate need and pass floss to isolate remaining teeth.

    Operator isolates remaining teeth using dental floss through each contact area (Figure 21-41).

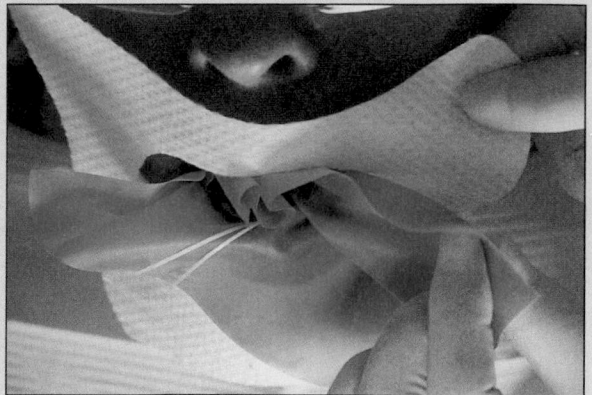

FIGURE 21-40
Dental napkin being placed around patient's mouth.

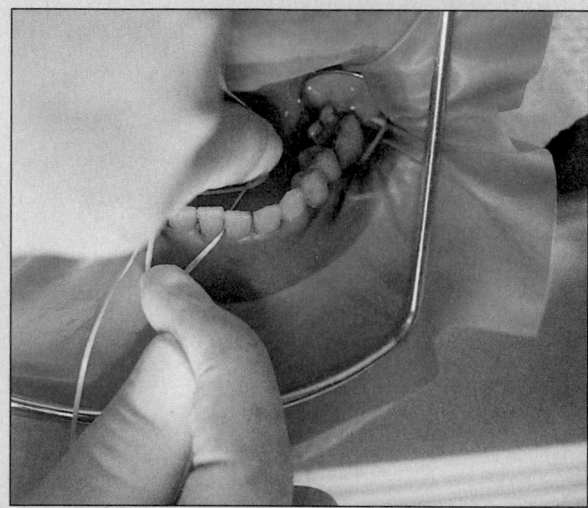

FIGURE 21-41
Dental operator placing dam between contacts with floss.

19. Dry teeth with air/water syringe to facilitate the placement of the dental dam material.

20. Anticipate need and pass plastic instrument to invert dental dam material.

    Operator inverts/tucks the dental dam material (Figure 21-42).

    ❏ **Uses plastic instrument to tuck edge of the dental dam material that surrounds the tooth into the gingival sulcus to seal tooth and prevent leakage.**

21. Use air from air/water syringe to dry the surface as the operator tucks the material.

22. Retrieve plastic instrument and pass saliva ejector as needed.

23. Rinse and evacuate.

    Operator checks with patient to be sure dam is comfortable after the dental dam is placed (Figure 21-43).

    ❏ **Places saliva ejector on opposite of operative site as needed.**

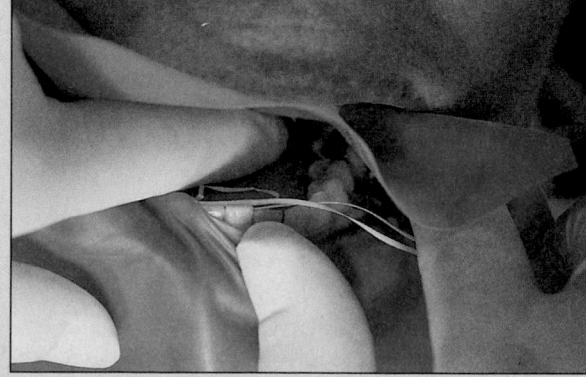

FIGURE 21-39
Clamp with dental dam material on tooth and most anterior tooth ligated with floss.

(Continues)

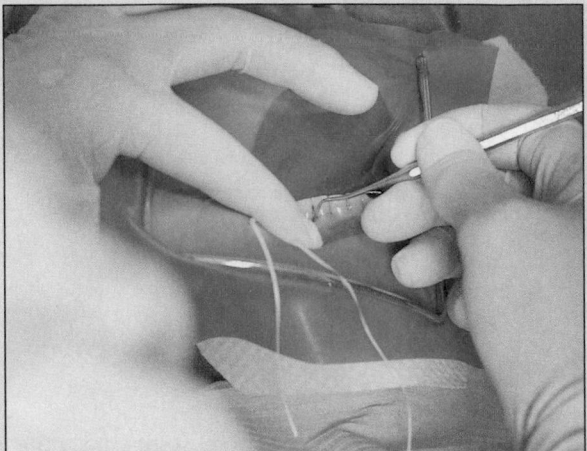

FIGURE 21-42
Dental dam is in place and the dental operator is tucking the dental dam material with a plastic instrument.

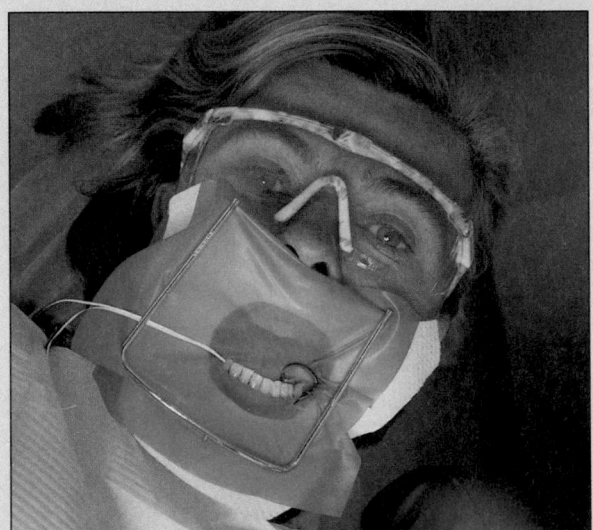

FIGURE 21-43
Patient with dental dam on and ready for dentist.

24. Assist during restorative procedures.

Operator completes scheduled treatment.

25. Assist in removal of dental dam at the completion of the restorative procedure.
   ❏ Rinse and evacuate before removal of dental dam.

Operator removes saliva ejector and clamp.

26. Retrieve saliva ejector and pass clamp forceps to operator.

27. Retrieve clamp forceps and clamp.

Operator removes dental dam material (Figure 21-44).

   ❏ Stretches dental dam away from restored tooth and cuts the septal dam.
   ❏ Slips index or middle finger underneath dental dam material.
   ❏ Stretches and pulls material facially and away from the tooth.

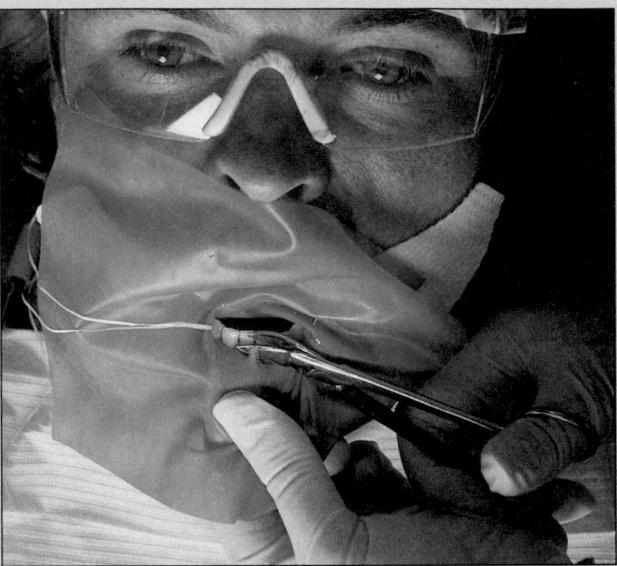

FIGURE 21-44
Pulling dental dam material toward facial, the operator cuts the interseptal material.

   ❏ Slants scissors toward occlusal surface and cuts the interseptal dam.

28. Pass curved crown and bridge scissors.

29. Retrieve scissors at operator's signal.

30. Anticipate need and pass dental dam clamp forceps.

Operator removes dental dam clamp.

   ❏ Places the forceps in clamp holes and squeezes the handles to open clamp jaws.
   ❏ Gently lifts clamp straight off the tooth.

31. Retrieve clamp forceps.

Operator releases the dental dam material from the pegs on dental dam frame.

   ❏ Removes frame from the material.

32. Retrieve dental dam frame.

Operator removes the dental dam material.

   ❏ Pulls the interseptal dam from between the teeth and removes entire material as one piece.

33. Retrieve dental dam material.

Operator removes the dental napkin and wipes area around the mouth.

34. Retrieve dental napkin.

35. Rinse and evacuate patient's mouth and pass floss as needed.

Operator examines the dental dam material for any tears and to make certain all interseptal material is present.

   ❏ Checks interproximals for dental dam material.
   ❏ Flosses to remove any remaining dental dam material as needed.
   ❏ Massages gingiva around anchor tooth to increase circulation of the area.

the anchor tooth, and the jaws of the clamp are opened placing the lingual side first and then the facial to retract the gingiva.

To remove the dental dam, the clamp is removed first and then the single hole will slide off the tooth. The assistant rinses and evacuates the patient's mouth and massages the gingiva. After having the clamp in place for a long period of time, a patient may experience postoperative discomfort when the anesthetic wears off. To alleviate the discomfort, the operator may gently massage the gingiva to stimulate blood flow to the area.

Placement of Dental Dam as a Single Unit The method of placing the clamp along with the dental dam material can be used when the anchor tooth is fully erupted and a clamp with wings can be placed. Placing the dental dam as a unit is especially helpful when the operator is working alone. Generally the operator punches the dental dam while it is on the frame, and then the wings of the clamp are inserted from the top of the anchor hole. A safety ligature is placed on the bow of the clamp. The dental dam material is loosened on the frame by moving the pegs to the outer edge of the material. The clamp forceps are inserted into the clamp forceps holes (Figure 21-45). The operator positions the dental dam and frame over the patient's mouth, spreads the jaws of the clamp open, locks the forceps with the sliding ring, and looks through the opening in the jaws of the clamp to see the tooth to be clamped. The jaws of the clamp are placed beneath the tooth's height of contour; the jaws are placed against the lingual side of the tooth to help stabilize the placement on the buccal side and then gently released just above the gingiva. The operator places their index finger on the lingual side to secure the clamp while the forceps are being removed. The assistant retrieves the clamp forceps.

The operator places their other index finger on the buccal side of the clamp and gently slides the clamp apically on the tooth to obtain a four-point contact centered on the tooth. The clamp should be stable without any rocking. The assistant passes the plastic instrument to the operator to remove the dental dam material from the wings of the clamp. The operator slides the paddle end between the dental dam and the wings to gently slide the material off the wings.

The operator extends the dental dam until the most anterior hole covers the most anterior tooth to be isolated. The operator places two fingers on either side of the dental dam and stretches the material around the tooth and between the contacts. If the dental dam does not slide through easily, a piece of floss can be used to help slide the dental dam between the teeth. The floss is placed through the contact and left in place, and then it is flossed through a second time using another part of the floss. The floss should be pulled from beneath the contact by sliding the floss out sideways rather than snapping it back out the contact point. If it is pulled back through the contact, the dental dam will come back out with the floss. The most anterior tooth can be ligated to keep the dental dam in place while isolating the remaining teeth. Floss is entered through the mesial contact, wrapped around the lingual of the tooth, and entered through the distal contact. The floss is pushed down at the cervical of the tooth with the paddle end of the plastic instrument, and the floss is tied once while continually pulling the floss toward the gingiva. The floss is tied two more times to secure it at the cervical of the tooth.

The operator continues to slide each tooth to be isolated through the punched holes and floss dental dam septa as needed. Once all the teeth have been isolated, the operator inverts the dental dam at the cervix of each tooth. The dental dam is adjusted on the frame to make the material smooth. The safety ligature is attached to the dental dam frame. The dental assistant should rinse and evacuate before the dentist begins the preparation procedure.

Alternative Methods in Placing the Dental Dam

There are many alternative methods and materials in placing dental dams available. Some place the dental dam with anchors other than standard metal clamps, and some methods are clampless. There are times when the placement of the standard clamp is not possible. The operator may try using ligature ties around the neck of the anchor tooth to stabilize the dental dam. Interdental wedges or rubber strips can be placed into the embrasure beneath the contacts for retention. When teeth are so tightly contacted together that floss cannot pass through, wedges can be placed between teeth to provide slight spacing. This allows the floss to pass through the contact area.

An alternative to the full dental dam placement is the quick-dam. This is an oval piece of dental dam that has a border of flexible plastic. This dental dam comes with its own template to mark each tooth and is punched using a regular punch and the same size holes as the standard dental dam method. After the holes have been punched, the dam frame is folded and inserted into the patient's mouth, lying in the vestibular area.

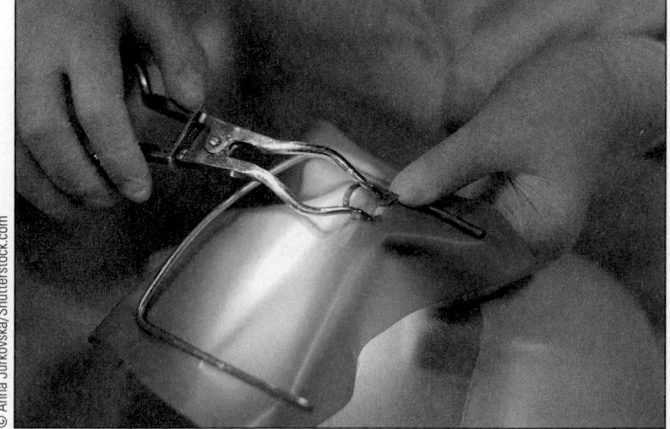

FIGURE 21-45
Dental dam being placed as a single unit.

Pharmacological Methods

Occasionally, traditional moisture control methods are not enough, and medications are needed. Some patients produce an excessive amount of saliva, or it may be very thick and difficult to control. There are also times when the patient's gingival tissue is so inflamed that the slightest touch will result in bleeding. Some surgical procedures which cut into soft tissue also create a bleeding control management challenge.

Controlling Excess Salivation

The use of medications in operative dentistry to control salivation is rare and generally limited to atropine. Atropine blocks the glands' sensory receptors, preventing the glands from being stimulated to produce saliva. The patient takes atropine 1–2 hours prior to the procedure. As with almost all drugs, there are potential disadvantages, side effects, and contraindications. Dentists rarely use medications to control saliva unless all other methods are ineffective.

Controlling Excessive Bleeding

The use of a local anesthetic containing a **vasoconstrictor** helps to control bleeding. Epinephrine is a common vasoconstrictor used in varying amounts in the anesthetic solution. The vasoconstrictor acts to narrow the blood vessels, which decreases hemorrhage and blood loss around the site of the injection.

Occasionally, gingival bleeding cannot be controlled. There are many ways to cut the gingiva inadvertently. This may occur from a dental dam clamp placed into the gingiva, slippage from an instrument, a patient biting the lip, or preparing a tooth for a crown. A solution referred to as a **hemostatic** agent can be placed topically on the gingival area using a cotton pellet or cotton roll. A hemostatic stops the bleeding by contracting the tissue to seal injured blood vessels. To help stop bleeding around the margins of a crown prep, a retraction cord coated with a hemostatic agent is often used.

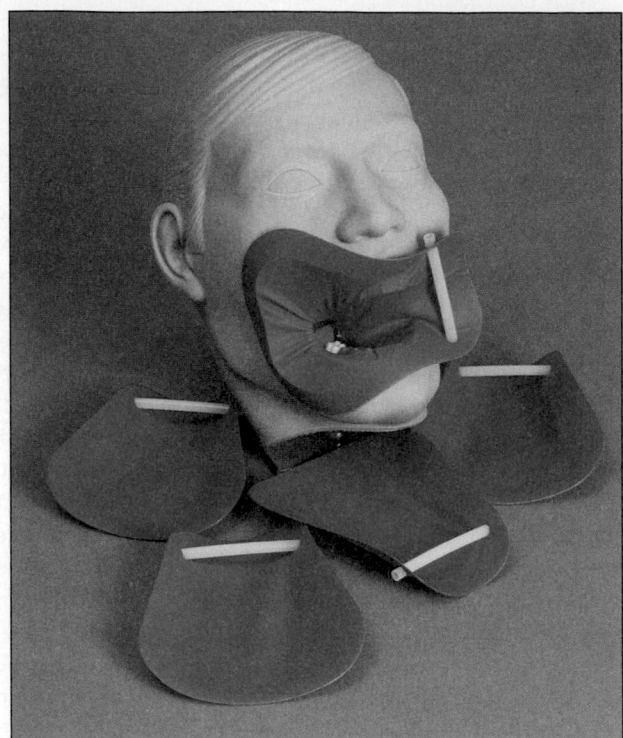

FIGURE 21-46
An alternative for a full dental dam placement.

The dam must be fitted around the teeth to be isolated; sometimes, a ligature or dental dam clamp is used to secure the dam (Figure 21-46).

There are a variety of anatomically shaped dental dams that can be placed using a clampless technique. Some types have a plastic anatomical frame attached to the dental dam. Others use flexible rings to hold the dam in place. Some of these dental dams are prestamped for use with the dental dam punch. Others have a nipple design. The nipples are cut off with scissors, leaving a hole beneath; there is no need for a punch or metal frame with this design.

Chapter Summary

It is the dental assistant's responsibility to maintain moisture control, keep the working area clean, and make certain the operator has visibility of the operating field at all times. This is accomplished by the assistant's using aspiration techniques discussed in this chapter. Many dental procedures require the added benefit of isolation of the field of operation using isolation techniques. A proficient dental assistant will be able to assist with or place a variety of isolation materials including the dental dam. The placement of the dental dam is an expanded function. Before performing this duty make certain it is legal in your state.

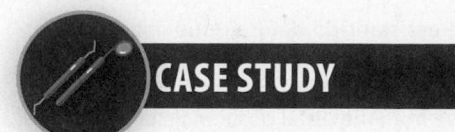

CASE STUDY

A 68-year-old male patient is scheduled for an endodontic procedure using the dental dam. The patient has a history of cardiac problems, is overdue for their prophylaxis, and is complaining about gingival bleeding.

Case Study Review

1. What should be the assistant's first concern?

2. What should the assistant do before seating the patient?

3. What might the dentist recommend?

Review Questions

Multiple Choice

1. All of the following are true statements about moisture control EXCEPT:
   a. It is important for the patient's safety.
   b. The interference of moisture with dental materials is prevented.
   c. It allows for better visibility and more efficient performance of procedures.
   d. It is a regulation of the CDC.

2. Which may be placed in a stationary position while performing a prophylaxis?
   a. oral evacuator tip
   b. saliva ejector
   c. dry angle
   d. cotton rolls and holder

3. The bevel of the HVE should face toward the _____ and the closed end toward the _____.
   a. cheek; tooth
   b. tooth; tongue
   c. operator; assistant
   d. assistant; operator

4. Which grasp is used to hold the HVE for suctioning and retracting the cheek?
   a. pen
   b. modified pen
   c. palm
   d. palm–thumb

5. When the dentist is preparing tooth #3, where does the assistant place the HVE bevel of the tip?
   a. toward the facial of tooth #3
   b. toward the lingual of tooth #3
   c. toward the cervix of tooth #3
   d. against the tongue for retraction

6. which isolation technique completely isolates the work area for placement of a restoration?
   a. dry angles
   b. cotton rolls and holder
   c. dental dam
   d. gauze squares

7. Which isolation technique is typically used in placing sealant and fluoride application?
   a. dry angles
   b. cotton rolls and holder
   c. dental dam
   d. gauze squares

8. Which device provides a clear, dry field; isolation; and light all at the same time?
   a. air-water syringe
   b. high-speed handpiece
   c. obturation unit
   d. isolite system

9. Which dental dam instrument has a working end that is a sharp projection and is used to provide holes in the dam?
   a. clamp
   b. punch
   c. forceps
   d. pliers

10. Tooth #19 is partially erupted and needs to be the anchor tooth. Which method of dental dam placement should be used?
    a. Place the dental dam as a single unit.
    b. Place the dental dam before the clamp.
    c. Place the dental dam after the clamp.
    d. Place clamp after the dental dam.

11. Tooth #30 is fully erupted and needs to be the anchor tooth. Which clamp is the best choice?
    a. #2
    b. #3
    c. #7
    d. #8

12. Which symbol is used on a clamp that is selected for a partially erupted tooth?
    a. A
    b. T
    c. D
    d. W
    e. PE

13. Tooth #12 has a Class I cavity. How many holes need to be punched?
    a. 1
    b. 2
    c. 3
    d. 4

14. What hole size on the adult punch plate is used for tooth #30 when used as an anchor tooth?
    a. 2nd
    b. 3rd
    c. 4th
    d. 5th

15. Which part of the dental clamp is placed toward the posterior to help extend the dental dam to the distal?
    a. prongs
    b. bow
    c. wings
    d. jaws

16. If the assistant needs to dry the inside of a large and deep cavity, what technique would be recommended?
    a. water from air/water syringe
    b. gauze square
    c. cotton pellet
    d. saliva ejector tip

17. Patients having what condition may be at medium risk when a dental dam is used during treatment?
    a. respiratory
    b. diabetic
    c. renal
    d. cardiac

18. What should the assistant do before removing the absorbent material after isolation?
    a. Gently pull the patient's tissue from the material.
    b. Always remove from the distal position first.
    c. Moisten it with water from the air/water syringe.
    d. Dry the area using the air/water syringe.

19. What is the first step in removing the dental dam when the "placing the clamp before dental dam" technique is used?
    a. Remove dental dam material.
    b. Remove dental frame.
    c. Remove dental clamp.
    d. Cut the septal dam.

20. The dentist is preparing a crown prep, and the gingival margins begin to bleed. What can they do to stop the bleeding throughout the remainder of the procedure?
    a. Apply more topical anesthetic.
    b. Have patient take atropine.
    c. Apply a hemostatic agent.
    d. Have assistant apply direct pressure until the procedure is completed.

Critical Thinking

1. Why is it important that the assistant keeps the operative site free of moisture during procedures?

2. The assistant passes the dentist the handpiece to cut the tooth in preparation for the placement of an amalgam. What should the assistant use to aspirate the water spray from the handpiece and dry the tooth? In what hands should the assistant hold the equipment?

3. If the water bounces back when the assistant uses the A/W to rinse a tooth, getting the dentist and patient wet, what did the assistant do? How can this be corrected?

4. What may cause a dental dam clamp to pop off a tooth? What is the potential danger of having the clamp pop off? What can the assistant do to prevent any potential danger?

5. When would the dentist elect to use pharmacological methods in treating a patient?

Key Terms

Term and Pronunciation	Meaning of Root and Word Parts	Definition
abrade (*uh*-**breyd**)	**abrade** = to wear off or down by scraping or rubbing	the sharp projections of dental instruments can scrape and damage tooth structure and existing dental restorations and appliances
amalgam (*uh*-**mal**-g*uh*m)	**amalgam** = an alloy of mercury with another metal or metals	usually amalgam is referred to as mercury combined with an alloy of metals possibly including silver, tin, copper, and sometimes zinc; used as a silver filling
anesthetize (*uh*-**nes**-thi-tahyz)	**an-** = without, lacking **aesthetic** = relating to the sensations **-ize** = to convert into	to administer an anesthetic (drug) to deprive sense of feeling to an area
antibiotic prophylaxis (an-ti-bahy-**ot**-ik) (proh-f*uh*-**lak**-sis)	**anti-** against **bio** = life, living organisms **-tic** = pertaining to **pro-** = in favor of **phýlaxis** = watching, guarding	practice of prescribing limited antibiotic therapy to dental patient at risk of contracting microbial disease as a result of invasive dental procedures; premedication

Term and Pronunciation	Meaning of Root and Word Parts	Definition
aspirate (**as**-p*uh*-reyt)	**aspirate** = *noun*: to draw or remove by suction *verb*: breath something in	to remove a fluid from a body cavity by suction or inhale a foreign body into the bronchi and lungs
bacteremia (bak-t*uh*-**ree**-mee-*uh*)	**bacteria** = one-celled organisms capable of being involved in infectious diseases -**emia** = condition of the blood	the presence of elevated levels of bacteria in the bloodstream
blanch (blahnch)	**blanch** = to make white, turn pale	when an instrument is placed against the gingiva the blood supply is lessoned and turns white
bond (bond)	**bond** = to hold or be held together; adhesive	to use bonding materials to physically bind to the tooth and chemically bond restorative materials to bonding agents; agents used to improve the bond between the restorative material and the tooth
circumference (ser-**kuhm**-fer-*uh*ns)	**circum-** = round about, to go around **fer** = that which carries -**ence** = indicating action	measure of the distance around a circle
clamp-bearing (**klamp**-bair-ing)	**clamp** = device with movable jaws used to secure and fasten objects together **bearing** = to hold up or support	device used to secure the dental dam material around the tooth
claustrophobic (klaw-str*uh*-**foh**-bik)	**claustrum** = to close, shut in, enclosed area **phobe** = abnormal fear -**ic** = suffering from	the feeling of being unpleasantly cramped, confined, or closed in space
dental dam (**den**-tl) (dam)	**dent** = teeth -**al** = pertaining to **dam** = barrier to obstruct the flow of water	thin sheet of rubber stretched around a tooth to keep it dry during dental work
endocarditis (en-doh-kahr-**dahy**-tis)	**endo-** = inside **card** = heart -**itis** = inflammation	inflammation of the lining of the heart and its valves; will often need to be hospitalized to receive antibiotics through a vein (intravenously); long-term antibiotic therapy needed to get the bacteria out of the heart chambers and valves; early treatment improves the chances of a good outcome; valve destruction or strokes can result in death
endodontic (en-doh-**don**-tiks)	**end-** = inside **odont** = tooth -**ic** = pertaining to	treatment of pulpal disease; removal of nerve and pulp tissue and replacement of filling material
etch (ech)	**etch** = to eat away surface with acid	to use agents (phosphoric acid) to roughen the tooth surface and make micropores; to prepare tooth surface for bonding of dental materials
gauge (geyj)	**gauge** = thickness of a sheet	measure of thickness of the dental dam material
height of contour (hahyt) (kon-**toor**)	**height** = distance to which something has been raised or uplifted above a level; a bulge **contour** = an outline especially of a curving or irregular figure	line encircling a tooth at its greatest bulge or diameter
hemostatic (hee-m*uh*-**stat**-ik)	**hemo** = blood **stat** = something that inhibits; restrain, stop -**ic** = having characteristics of	agent used to stop bleeding
impinge (im-**pinj**)	**impinge** = drive into, strike against, violate, bear upon	to pinch soft tissue between two hard objects; may cause temporary damage and pain
invert (in-**vurt**)	**invert** = turn inward; upside down	to turn the dental dam inward around the tooth
lightening strip (lahyt-**n-ing**) (strip)	**lighten** = to become less cumbersome, burdensome -**ing** = process of **strip** = a narrow piece, comparatively long, flat, and usually of uniform width	a strip of steel with abrasive bonded on one side; used to open rough or improper contacts of proximal restorations preventing passage through interproximal space
malpositioned (mal-**pohz-d**)	**mal-** = bad, abnormal **pose** = position	when a tooth is out of the normal position in the dental arch
matrix band (**mey**-triks) (band)	**matrix** = a surrounding substance within which something else originates, develops, or is contained **band** = a thin flat strip used to encircle objects to confine and hold together	metal or plastic band secured around the crown of a tooth to confine the restorative material filling a cavity

(Continues)

Term and Pronunciation	Meaning of Root and Word Parts	Definition
micropores (**mahy**-kr*uh*-pawr)	**micro** = too small to be seen with the unaided eye **pores** = tiny openings	microscopic openings in tooth structure produced by etching agents; created for physical bond with bonding agents
mucinous (**myoo**-sin-*uhs*)	**mucin** = secretion of mucous membranes; component of mucus **-ous** = possessing	any of a class of glycoproteins (sugar and protein) found in saliva; adhesive properties that acts as lubricants or protectants of the soft tissues of the oral cavity
occlusion (*uh*-**kloo**-zh*uh*n)	**occlus** = to close **-ion** = denoting action	closing of upper and lower jaws; fitting teeth of the lower jaw with corresponding teeth of the upper jaw
operative site (**op**-er-*uh*-tiv) (sahyt)	**operate** = a surgical procedure **-ive** = relating to **site** = location	location in the mouth where treatment is being performed
preparation (prep-*uh*-**rey**-sh*uh*n)	**prepare** = to put in proper condition or readiness **-tion** = an act of	a procedure to remove diseased hard tissues of a tooth and the shaping of the remaining tooth structure to an acceptable form necessary to receive and retain a restoration; also referred to as cavity prep (n) once the structure has been shaped
prepared (pri-**paird**)	**prepare** = to put in proper condition or readiness **-ed** = possessing or having the characteristics	cut and shaped to receive a dental restoration
prophylaxis (proh-f*uh*-**lak**-sis)	**pro-** = in favor of **phylaxis** =watching, guarding	preventing of dental disease by means of cleaning and polishing the teeth by a dentist or dental hygienist
prongs (**prawngz**)	**prongs** = pointed, projected part	pointed part of the clamp jaws; used to help secure clamp around neck of tooth
resin (**rez**-in)	**resin** = used in medicine and in the making of varnishes and plastics	types of synthetic resins (plastic) which are used in dentistry as adhesives and as restorative materials (tooth colored fillings)
restoration (res-t*uh*-**rey**-sh*uh*n)	**restore** = to return of something to a former, original, normal, or unimpaired condition **-ation** = indicating a result	a dental filling; a dental restorative material used to restore the function and shape of missing tooth structure
retracting (ri-**trakt**)	**retract** = to draw something back **-ing** = result of	pulling back tissue for better access and/or view
rubber dam (**ruhb**-er) (**dam**)	**rubber** = elastic material resistant to moisture **dam** = barrier to obstruct the flow of water	the term *rubber dam* has been replaced by *dental dam*
secondary caries (**sek**-*uh*n-der-ee) (**kair**-eez)	**second** = being the latter or next of a series **-ary** = connected with or pertaining to **caries** = progressive decay of a tooth	occurrence of dental decay that occurs on the tooth after the filling has been placed for a period of time; main reason to replace a dental restoration
septum (sep-**t*uh*m**) septae; plural form	**septum** = thin partition that divides two parts	thin piece of dental dam material between punched holes
sprung (spruhng)	**spring** = being suddenly released from a constrained position **sprung** = past tense	when a clamp does not have a secure grip around a tooth, the stainless steel acts like a spring and pops of the tooth
taut (tawt)	**taut** = tightly drawn, tense, not slack	stretched tight, without slack
template (**tem**-plit)	**template** = anything that serves as a pattern	a pattern on a thin piece of plastic that serve as a guide for punching holes in the dental dam
tenacious (t*uh*-**ney**-sh*uh*s)	**tenacity** = the act of holding fast **-ous** = possessing	ability of material to stick to; adhere; difficult to remove
universal (yoo-n*uh*-**vur**-s*uh*l)	**universe** = something considered collectively **-al** = pertaining to	general or widely known by all
vasoconstrictor (vas-oh-k*uh*n-**strik**-ter)	**vaso-** = vessel **constrict** = cause to contract or squeeze; to narrow **-or** = state or condition	a drug, agent, or nerve that causes narrowing of the walls of blood vessels

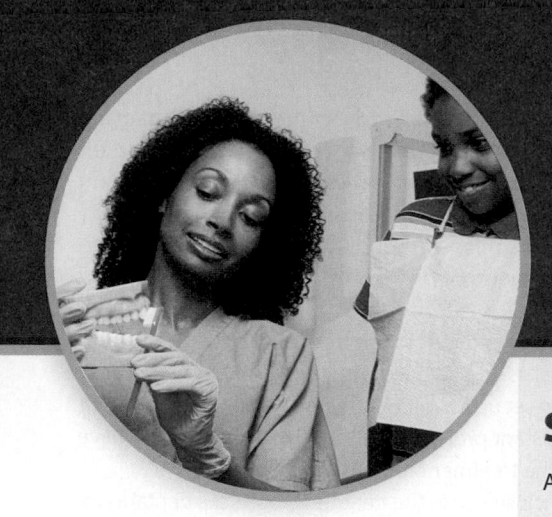

Specific Instructional Objectives

At the completion of this chapter, you will be able to meet these objectives:

1. Use terms presented in this chapter.
2. Differentiate between a limited/emergency examination and a comprehensive examination.
3. State the armamentarium necessary for a limited/emergency examination and new patient examination.
4. Discuss the role of the dental assistant during a limited/emergency examination and a new patient examination.
5. Describe forms included in patient's records.
6. Take patient's vitals.
7. Describe dental radiographs taken during examinations.
8. Explain purpose of the extraoral and intraoral soft tissue examination.
9. Describe recording of patient's occlusion and oral habits.
10. Recognize various types of dental charts.
11. Utilize tooth numbering and identification systems.
12. Interpret charting symbols and abbreviations.
13. Discuss the significance of the dental diagnosis.
14. Explain the importance of establishing patient goals when treatment planning.
15. Summarize steps in financial planning.

Introduction

Every patient treated in the dental office must undergo a new patient examination. The examination allows the dentist to systematically collect information about the patient's oral health in order to determine the patient's oral health needs. One of the most important parts of the exam is communicating effectively so each patient fully understands their oral health needs and the importance of having those needs met. The assistant plays an integral part during the new patient examination by observing the patient, obtaining important patient information, assisting the dentist during the procedure, and recording the conditions observed in the patient's oral cavity.

Types of Patient Examinations

There are two types of new patient examinations.

1. Limited/emergency oral examination
2. Comprehensive examination

Limited/Emergency Oral Examination

Patients who do not have a dentist of record will contact a dental office when they experience a dental emergency such as a toothache, broken tooth, or broken restoration. The patient usually wants to make an appointment to have the immediate problem treated by the dentist.

During the limited/emergency oral examination, the dental team will take a patient's medical history and complete vital signs, obtain consent from the patient, complete HIPAA forms, and generally acquire radiographs of the tooth or teeth that need to be treated. Intraoral images are particularly valuable because they allow the patient to see the problem so they can be used for patient education and post-treatment comparison. The dentist will also complete an oral examination of the specific area in the patient's mouth and may complete periodontal charting of the specific area.

Based upon these findings, the dentist will develop a dental diagnosis, and the treatment plan will be discussed in detail with the patient. At this point, it may be necessary for a dental staff member to speak with the patient regarding financial planning for the appointment. It is important that all new patients who come to the dental office for a limited/emergency examination understand that this is not a comprehensive examination. The patient should schedule a separate appointment for a comprehensive examination.

When the patient requires treatment that the dentist feels is beyond their capability, the dentist will refer the patient to a dental specialist. If the patient has been referred to the dentist's office, it is also considered a limited oral examination. A referral occurs when a patient is sent to another dentist, usually a dental specialist, for a consult or treatment. The referral should be reviewed carefully to ensure that the recommended examination or treatment is followed. The referring dentist may send radiographs to be reviewed, or the consulting dentist may need to take dental radiographs. After the consult is completed, the referring dentist should be contacted and the diagnosis or treatment should be shared. Ethically, the patient should be sent back to referring dentist and not become a new patient in the consulting office.

Comprehensive New Patient Examination

The dentist should perform a comprehensive new patient examination on all patients who are first time patients to the dental practice (see Procedure 22-5). Information collected during the comprehensive new patient examination is considered baseline information. All information gathered subsequently is compared to the baseline information to determine if the patient has had a change in their oral health.

Components of the New Patient Examination

The primary role of the dental assistant during the new patient examination is to record information obtained by the dentist for dental and periodontal charting. Therefore good communication

skills and attention to detail on the part of the dental assistant are absolutely essential. The dental assistant plays another important role during the new patient examination as the first clinical team member with whom the patient often interacts. The patient may be apprehensive regarding the appointment, so it is very important that the dental assistant be friendly and display a caring and empathetic attitude.

Prior to bringing the patient to the treatment room, it is important that the dental assistant make sure the room has been properly disinfected and set up for patient treatment. It is also important that the dental assistant properly sterilize all instruments and have them available in the treatment room for the dentist.

Once the patient is seated in the treatment room, the dental assistant will gather important information and make sure all legal documents have been properly completed. The dental assistant also may be required to take vital signs and to acquire radiographs during the new patient examination, so competence in radiography is essential. (Radiographs are discussed in Chapters 27-29) They will assist the dentist during the patient examination and chart all findings.

Patient Records

Since all patient forms are considered legal documents, they may only be completed by individuals age 18 and over. A parent or legal guardian must be present at the dental appointment to complete and sign the forms for any patient under the age of 18. In addition, some patients with impaired cognitive ability may require a court appointed legal guardian to be present at the appointment and to complete and sign all forms.

Patient Registration Form One of the first steps is to have the patient complete a patient registration form. It can be either electronic or paper. The paper form consists of a file folder that is identified with the patient's first and last name. The standard folder is 8½ × 11 inches with a system that fastens the patient forms in place within the folder. Many come with pockets or areas to hold the radiographs. The American Dental Association (ADA) has a form that can be purchased for use in the dental office and that covers the medical and dental health history information thoroughly (Figure 22-1). The electronic file mirrors the paper folder in content. However, accessing the information is achieved through a computer search using the patient's name.

The registration form includes information on demographics, which is a personal history including the following: full name, address, phone number, work number, Social Security number, marital status, sex, insurance, emergency contacts, and

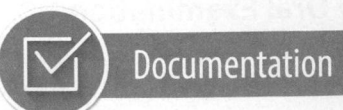

Documentation

Every dental employee should remember that the patient's record is the primary source of information about the patient and the dentist will use it for developing the diagnosis to provide the patient with the highest standard of dental care. It should be kept extremely accurate and up to date. It could be used in litigation, the act or process of seeking or contesting a lawsuit. This patient record could be brought forth in a lawsuit and will reflect on the dental office and employees as well as the patient care that was provided. It could also be used in forensics, where the identity of the patient is established though scientific methods by using the charting and radiographs. The record can be either in paper copy or on the computer.

Date _____

PATIENT NAME	SOCIAL SECURITY NUMBER	HOME PHONE ( )
Home Address	City, State, Zip	Birthdate / /
Marital Status ☐ Single ☐ Married ☐ Divorced ☐ Separated	☐ M ☐ F	Driver's License and State

Primary Insurance Company _____ Group _____ Subscriber _____

Secondary Insurance Company _____ Group _____ Subscriber _____

Responsible Party

NAME	SOCIAL SECURITY NUMBER	HOME PHONE ( )
Home Address	City, State, Zip	Birthdate / /
Marital Status ☐ Single ☐ Married ☐ Divorced ☐ Separated	Relationship to Patient	Driver's License and State
Responsible Person's Employer	Occupation	Work Phone ( )
Business Address	City	State Zip
Spouse's Name	Social Security Number	Birthdate / /
Spouse's Employer	Spouse's Occupation	Spouse's Work Phone ( )
Spouse's Business Address	City	State Zip

How did you hear about our Office?
(check only one)

Who selected this Office? ☐ Self ☐ Spouse ☐ Parent ☐ Employer

Where did you find the Phone Number to this Office?_____

☐ Referred by a friend	☐ Yellow Pages	☐ Relative	☐ Insurance Plan	☐ Welcome Wagon
☐ Other _____	☐ TV/Radio Ad	☐ Newspaper Ad	☐ Direct Mailing	☐ Sign by Building

If you were referred, whom may we thank for referring you?_____

CONSENT

• I will answer all health questions to the best of my knowledge _____
  Initial

After explanation by the doctor, I hereby authorize the performance of dental services upon the above named patients and whatever procedures that the judgments of the doctor may decide in order to carry out these procedures. I also authorize and request the administration of any anesthetics and x-rays as may be deemed necessary and advisable by the doctor.

Signature _____ Date _____ Relationship to Patient _____

TERMS AND CONDITIONS

This office depends upon reimbursement from the patient for the costs incurred in their case. The financial responsibility of each patient must be determined before treatment.
As a condition of treatment by this office. I understand financial arrangements must be made in advance. All emergency dental services, or any dental service performed without prior financial arrangements, must be paid for at the time the services are performed.
I understand that dental services furnished to me are charged directly to me and that I am personally responsible for payment. If I carry insurance, I understand that this office will help prepare my insurance forms to assist in making collections from insurance companies and will credit such collections to my account. However, this dental office cannot render services on the assumption that charges will be paid by an insurance company.

Assignment of Insurance: I hereby authorize releases of any information needed and also authorize my insurance company to pay directly to this Office benefits accruing to me under my policy. I understand that the fee estimate listed for this dental care can only be extended for a period of 90 days from the date of the patient's examination. I also understand that in order to collect my debt, my credit history may be checked through the use of my Social Security Number or any other information I have given you. I agree that in the event that either this office or I institute any legal proceedings with respect to amount owed by me for services rendered, the prevailing party in such proceedings shall be entitled to recover all costs incurred including reasonable attorney's fees. I grant my permission to you, or your assignee, to telephone me at home or at my work to discuss matters related to this form. I have read the above conditions and agree to their content.

Signed _____ **Date** _____

There may be a charge for any missed appointments or appointments not cancelled 48 hours before the appointment time.

FIGURE 22-1
Patient registration form.

Documentation

Transgender Patient Documentation

Transgender individuals face unique challenges when it comes to the health care system and which also extend into patient documentation. Medical records are often ill-equipped to document nonbinary values or for patients who have transitioned from a previous identity. Most records have "M," "F," and occasionally "U" for unknown. There needs to be a way to include sexual identity and gender identity in patient documentation. The office can modify the patient registration form with merely a question, "What is your gender identity?" followed by a blank for the patient to complete. The next step would be to ask, "What sex were you assigned at birth?" followed by a blank. Transgender patients find the direct question, "Have you had the surgery?" rude and intrusive. Medical forms typically ask about past surgeries where the patient could designate gender surgery. Until medical forms include the information needed about sex and gender identity, the doctor needs to inform the dental team where this information can be added. Some teams document it in areas like the doctor notes.

physician's name and phone number. The registration form also provides financial information about the patient and identifies the individual responsible for payment of the dental services. The dental auxiliary is responsible for ensuring that all information is completed by the patient before any treatment occurs.

Consent Form

The consent form is a legal document that must be completed by the patient or the patient's legal guardian before any treatment can be performed. The consent form gives the dental team members permission to treat the patient. The consent form often includes the office's mission statement and infection control policy, and it outlines office policies regarding payment, missed or cancelled appointments, and patient records. The consent form may also include a list of patient rights. Refer to Figure 22-2 for example of patient rights. The patient's consent form should periodically be updated according to the office policy.

HIPAA Forms

The Health Information Portability and Accountability Act (HIPAA) requires dental offices to develop, implement, and follow policies related to patient privacy and how patient information is shared with other dental professionals. As a result of this act, all dental offices must have standard practices for protecting patient privacy and sharing patient information (notice of privacy practices).

The notice of privacy practices must be shared with all patients prior to any dental treatment being provided. The patient should be given a copy of the office's privacy practices policy, and it should

be noted in the patient's chart that they received it, or the patient may sign a statement that they received the information. In addition, all dental offices must allow patients to specify what information can be shared and with whom that information can be shared. This information is typically shared with the dental office through a document entitled "Authorization for Release of Identifying Health Information." This document is only valid for one (1) year, so it is important that the dental team regularly check and update this document as needed. Also, the patient can retract or change the authorization at any time. Any changes require that the patient complete a new HIPAA Authorization for Release of Identifying Health Information form. Refer to Figure 22-3, "HIPAA Authorization Form."

HIPAA guidelines also require that all dental offices properly protect and store all dental records. All dental records must be stored out of the sight of other patients and properly secured at all times—even when the office is closed. HIPAA guidelines also require the electronic transmission of dental records. Therefore, dental offices must ensure that all electronic transmission of dental records is to a secure location and that all computer stations within a dental office are properly secured.

> It is very important that all dental team members properly follow all HIPAA guidelines. Violation of HIPAA policies can result in criminal or civil penalties against the individual and the office.

Patient's Rights

As a patient in our clinic, you are entitled to:

1. Considerate, respectful, and confidential treatment;
2. Continuity and completion of treatment;
3. Access to complete and current information about your condition;
4. Advance knowledge of the cost of treatment;
5. A full explanation of all service to be provided;
6. An explanation of recommended treatment, treatment alternatives, the option to refuse treatment, the risks of no treatment, and expected outcomes of various treatments; and
7. Treatment that meets the standard of care in the profession.

FIGURE 22-2
Example of Patient's Rights.

Patient name _____

Patient address _____

Patient phone number_____

I authorize the professional office of my dentist named above to release health information identifying me under the following terms and conditions:

1. Detailed description of the information to be released:
2. To whom may the information be released [name(s) or class(es) of recipients]:
3. The purpose(s) for the release (if the authorization is initiated by the individual, it is permissible to state "at the request of the individual" as the purpose, if desired by the individual):
4. Expiration date or event relating to the individual or purpose for the release: *No later than one year from the date the authorization is signed.*

FIGURE 22-3
HIPAA Authorization Form.

Medical History The patient is also requested to fill out a medical history. The medical history contains questions about past surgeries, systemic diseases, injuries, and allergies (Figure 22-4).

The purpose of the medical history is to collect information that may impact dental treatment, require the dentist to alter treatment, or require the patient to take an antibiotic **premedication**

PATIENT'S DENTAL HEALTH

Why have you come in to see us today? (e.g.: pain, checkup) _____

Previous Dentist _____ Last Visit _____ Date of last cleaning _____

Reasons for changing dentists: _____

What problems have you had with past dental treatment? _____

Are you nervous about seeing a dentist? ❑ Yes! ❑ No If yes, please tell us why: _____

How often do you brush? _____ Do you floss? ❑ Yes ❑ No How often? _____

(please circle each)

Y N I clench or grind my teeth during the day or while sleeping.
Y N My gums bleed while brushing or flossing.
Y N I like my smile.
Y N I prefer tooth-colored fillings.
Y N I avoid brushing part of my mouth due to pain.

Y N My gums feel tender or swollen.
Y N I have problems eating.
Y N I have had orthodontics.
Y N I have had a facial or jaw injury.
Y N I want my teeth straight.
Y N I want my teeth whiter.

What are your dental priorities? _____
(e.g.: apprentice, dental health, financial considerations)

PATIENT'S MEDICAL HISTORY

I consider my health to be (please check one) ❑ Excellent ❑ Good ❑ Fair ❑ Poor
Do you or have you had any of the following? Please circle Y for yes or N for no.

1.	Y	N	Heart Disease	22.	Y	N	Liver Disease				
2.	Y	N	Heart Murmur/Mitral Valve Prolapse	23.	Y	N	Jaundice				
3.	Y	N	Stroke	24.	Y	N	Hepatitis Type _____				
4.	Y	N	Congenital Heart Lesions	25.	Y	N	Diabetes				
5.	Y	N	Rheumatic Fever	26.	Y	N	Excessive Urination and/or Thirst				
6.	Y	N	Abnormal Blood Pressure	27.	Y	N	Infectious Mononucleosis (Mono)				
7.	Y	N	Anemia	28.	Y	N	Herpes				
8.	Y	N	Prolonged Bleeding Disorder	29.	Y	N	Arthritis	36.	Y	N	AIDS
9.	Y	N	Tuberculosis or Lung Disease	30.	Y	N	Sexually Transmitted/Venereal Disease	37.	Y	N	Immune Suppressed Disorder
10.	Y	N	Asthma	31.	Y	N	Kidney Disease	38.	Y	N	Hearing Loss
11.	Y	N	Hay Fever	32.	Y	N	Tumor or Malignancy	39.	Y	N	Fainting Spells
12.	Y	N	Sinus Trouble	33.	Y	N	Cancer/Chemotherapy	40.	Y	N	Glaucoma
13.	Y	N	Epilepsy/Seizures	34.	Y	N	Radiation Treatment	41.	Y	N	History of Emotional or
14.	Y	N	Ulcers	35.	Y	N	History of Drug Addiction				Nervous Disorders

Doctor Notes Only:

15. Y N Implants/Artificial Joints: ❑ Hip ❑ Knee ❑ Other

WOMEN

16. Y N I smoke or use tobacco. If yes, how much per day? _____ How many years? _____
17. Y N I have consumed alcohol within the last 24 hours.
18. Y N I usually take an antibiotic prior to dental treatment.
19. Y N Have you ever taken Fen-Phen or Redux?
20. Y N I have had major surgery: Year _____ Type of operation: _____ Year _____ Type of operation: _____

42. Y N Are you taking birth control medication?
43. Y N Are you or could you be pregnant or nursing?

21. Y N Do you have any other medical problem or medical history NOT listed on this form? _____

Are you allergic to any of the following?
Please circle Y for yes or N for no:

44. Y N Aspirin
45. Y N Ibuprofen
46. Y N Sulfa Drugs/Sulfites/Sulfides
47. Y N Penicillin
48. Y N Codeine
49. Y N Latex, Metals, Plastics
50. Y N Local Anesthetics (Novocaine)
51. Y N Other Medications - Which ones? _____

Please list all medications you are currently taking:

Medicine _____ Condition _____
Medicine _____ Condition _____
Medicine _____ Condition _____
Medicine _____ Condition _____
Physician's Name _____ Phone _____
Address _____ Fax _____

In the event of an emergency, please contact:

Name _____ Relationship _____ Phone _____
Name _____ Relationship _____ Phone _____

Initial medical/dental health reviewed by:
X _____ / ___ / ___ X _____ / ___ / ___
Doctor's Signature Date Patient's Signature Date

Periodic medical/dental health reviewed by:
X _____ / ___ / ___ X _____ / ___ / ___
Doctor's Signature Date If patient is a minor: Parent/Guardian's Signature Date

FIGURE 22-4
Patient's dental and medical history.

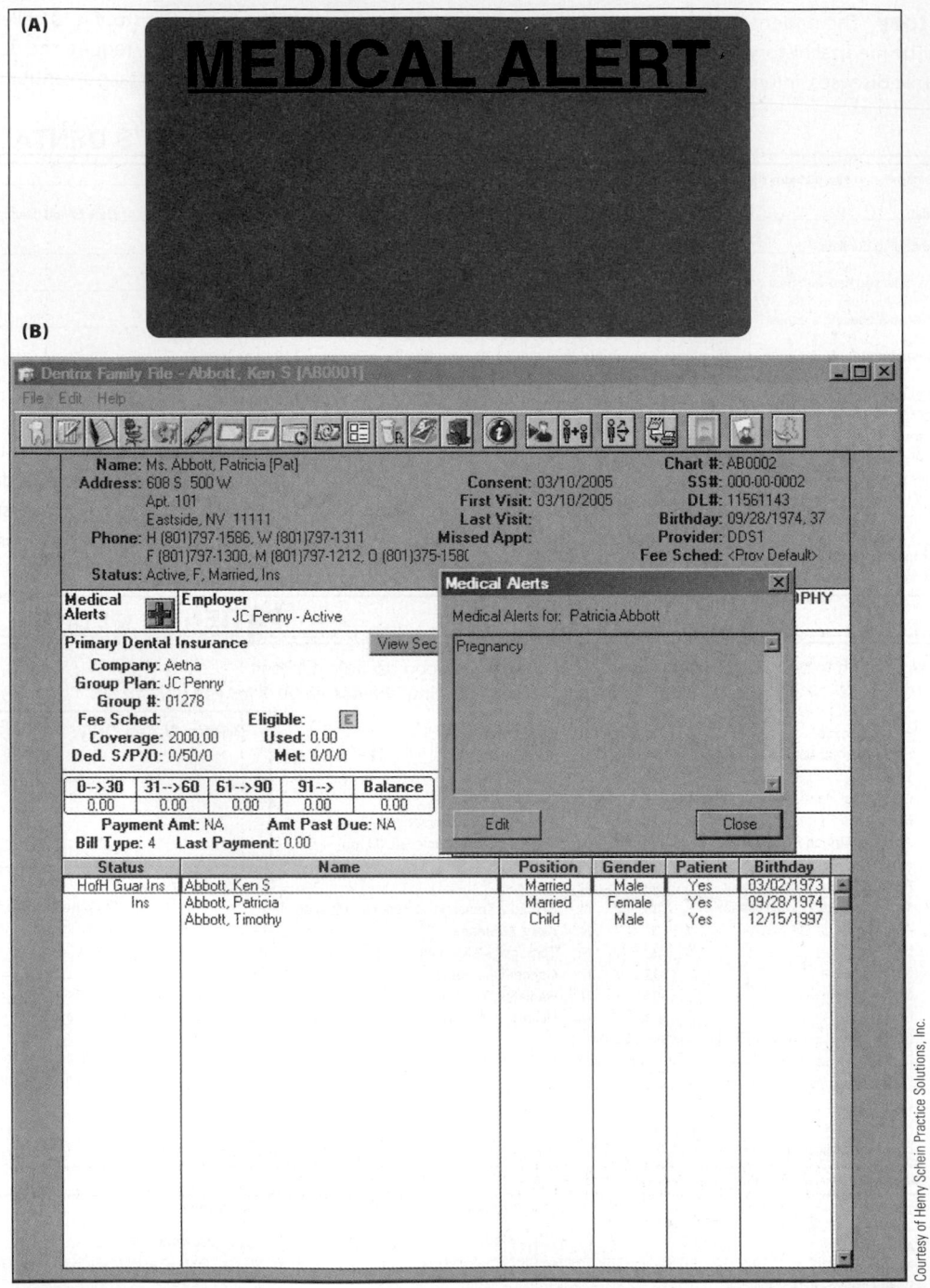

FIGURE 22-5
(A) Allergy and medical alert sticker. (B) Electronic medical alert.

prior to dental treatment; for example, a patient with artificial joints. It is critical for the dental team to know about any allergies that may affect treatment. Normally, the allergies of concern are related to anesthetics, latex, and antibiotics. Allergies and medical alerts are to be noted on the inside of the patient record to bring them to the attention of dental team members (Figure 22-5). The medical history should list all the patient's current and past medical conditions, and all current medications— both prescription and over the counter (OTC). It should also include the names and

contact information for the patient's current physician or physicians so the dental office can easily contact a physician if necessary.

Computerized software programs automatically print copies of the medical alert when the daily schedule prints. Numerous icons and colors are used on the medical history to identify concerns. This provides added notification of patients who may require special accommodations.

The dental assistant should carefully review the medical history with the patient and clarify any positive or yes responses.

It is important that the standard medical history questions are followed up by an interview or questioning session to ensure that all information is adequately covered. The standard medical history allows for consistency and prevents items from being overlooked or forgotten; the interview allows for further clarification.

The dentist may request a consultation with the patient's physician to clarify questions regarding the patient's medical history or to help make a determination regarding modifications in patient treatment or the need for antibiotic premedication. It is important that all conversations with the patient's physician be properly documented in the patient's note history.

Dental History Questions regarding the patient's dental history are included in the patient's record. (Refer to Figure 22-2.) This information alerts the dental assistant to any concerns the patient has regarding their current dental health. It also gives insight into any concerns the patient may have had regarding previous dental care. The last dental examination is noted, as well as the patient's last dental appointment and how often the patient seeks dental treatment. Some questions are asked regarding the patient's attitude toward dentistry and how they maintain their own personal oral health care. If the patient had a previous dentist, a patient is requested to sign a release of information form to be able to obtain their records of previous dental treatment.

Vital Signs

Proper documentation of the patient's vital signs is important to obtain baseline vital signs and to ensure that the patient can safely tolerate dental treatment. Baseline vital signs help the dentist compare subsequent measurements with the initial measurements. The measuring and recording of vital signs is an important part of the health evaluation and should be done with every patient before starting any dental treatment. Vital signs give the

dental operator specific information about the physical and emotional condition of the patient. They may point out previously undetected abnormalities. Vital signs, along with the overall patient health information and any pain that the patient reports to the dentist, aid in planning the patient's dental treatment and are essential during emergency treatment.

Vital signs include blood pressure, temperature, pulse, and respiration. Table 22-1 defines each vital sign, typical ranges for each, and implications of abnormal findings.

Blood Pressure Two measurements are always recorded when taking blood pressure. They are recorded as a fraction—the systolic pressure is the upper figure, and the diastolic pressure is the lower figure. They are always recorded in even numbers (the gauge has indications for even numbers only). There is no absolute number for normal blood pressure; it is recorded in ranges, much like other vital signs. Children normally have lower pressure; as adults age, the blood pressure goes up. Some, however, use 120 over 80 as an average for an adult. This means 120 systolic over 80 diastolic pressure, recorded as 120/80.

A higher-than-normal blood pressure is called **hypertension**, and a lower-than-normal blood pressure is called **hypotension**. An increase in the diastolic pressure is more significant than an increase in the systolic pressure, because it indicates that the heart is working harder. Blood pressure may be taken in the dental office using a stethoscope and sphygmomanometer as described in Chapter 15 or by using an automated wrist cuff (see Procedure 22-1).

Temperature Measurement of body temperature is an essential component of every patient's health evaluation. A thermometer is used to measure body temperature. Body temperature is compared to the normal body temperature range and, if higher or lower, it should be further investigated. A range is used when identifying the normal body temperature, because temperature varies from person to person and throughout the day. It is

TABLE 22-1 Vital Signs

Vital Sign	Equipment Needed	Typical Range—Adults	Typical Range—Children	Implication of Abnormal Findings
Temperature	Digital or mercury thermometer	97–99°F 36.1–37°C	98.5–99°F 36.94–37°C	Possible infection in the patient's body.
Pulse	Watch or clock with second hand, index finger of one hand	60–100 beats per minute	75–120 beats per minute	Rapid heart rate; may be caused by disease conditions or patient anxiety.
Blood pressure	Digital blood pressure cuff, or stethoscope and sphygmomanometer	>120 mmHg/ >80 mmHG		Pressure increases when blood is pumped through the blood vessels; may be caused by disease conditions or patient anxiety. For patients being treated for high blood pressure, dental visits may cause anxiety and further increase the blood pressure. May have implications when administering local anesthesia with a vasoconstrictor.
Respiration	Watch or clock with second hand	15–20 beats per minutes	18–35 beats per minutes	Patient breathing rapidly. May be caused by patient anxiety.

Procedure 22-1
Procedure Taking Blood Pressure Using Automated Wrist Cuff

This procedure is performed by the dental assistant in order to obtain the patient's blood pressure.

Equipment and Supplies
- hand sanitizer
- examination gloves
- patient
- blood pressure automated wrist cuff
- instructions for the wrist cuff. There are so many on the market that it is important to read the instructions before using the cuff that was purchased. Normally the following steps are used.

Procedure Steps

1. Wash hands and don examination gloves.

2. Seat patient in dental chair in upright position.

3. Have patient extend their arm and support arm on a flat surface.

4. Face dials of wrist cuff on palm side of the wrist (Figure 22-6).

5. Wrap the wrist cuff snugly around the patient's wrist.

6. Have patient hold their wrist at the same level as their heart.

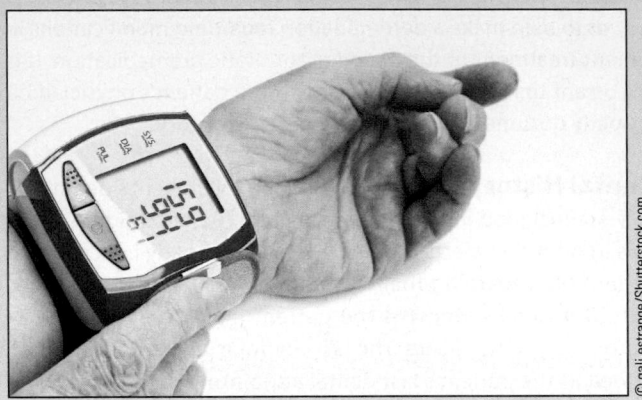

FIGURE 22-6
Placement of BP wrist cuff.

© gali estrange/Shutterstock.com

7. Turn on the BP monitor and follow the manufacturer's directions.

8. Write down the BP, date, time, and which arm was used to take the BP.

9. Take BP twice.

10. Remove gloves and wash hands.

11. Write down second reading.

---

well known that after exercise, emotional excitement, and even eating, temperature rises. A person's face may turn red and blush due to excitement, increasing body temperature. Temperature in young children and young infants will vary more than in adults.

Temperature can be measured using forehead temperature strips (described in Chapter 15) or a digital thermometer, **tympanic thermometer**, or noncontact thermometer. Procedure 22-2 presents an overview of how to measure temperature using a digital thermometer.

The tympanic thermometer (ear thermometer) has become popular for taking temperatures, especially on young children. It is placed gently in the ear canal, an infrared signal is bounced off the tympanic membrane or the ear drum, and the reading appears within a few seconds. This procedure (Procedure 22-3, "Taking a Tympanic Temperature") is easily performed because it does not involve an open mouth, congestion in the nasal cavity, difficulty breathing through the nose, length of time to obtain the reading, or the many other contraindications for taking an oral temperature. The only contraindication for the tympanic thermometer is that too much ear wax will not allow for a correct reading. Dental offices do not routinely take a temperature unless the situation arises where the information is needed; however, it

is always beneficial to have knowledge and an understanding of temperature, the role it plays in health, and the normal temperature ranges.

Pulse The pulse is the intermittent beating sensation felt when the fingers are pressed against an artery. A pulse rate is determined by palpation. Do not use the thumb to palpate, because it has a pulse of its own and could throw off the readings. Pulse may be palpated on one of several arteries: the radial, carotid, or temporal. The dental assistant most commonly uses the radial artery. The radial pulse site is located on the radial artery, on the thumb side of the wrist (refer to Chapter 15 for details). It can be found approximately one inch above the base of the thumb. This is the most common site used for obtaining pulses in the dental office.

When a pulse is taken and documented, there are several characteristics that can be noted. The *pulse rate*, or beats per minute, is always noted on the chart. The *pulse rhythm*, which notes the regular expansion and contraction of an artery caused by the heart pumping blood through the body, may also be described. It is often described as irregular, slow, or rapid. The term used when describing the strength of the pulse is the *pulse volume*.

Procedure 22-2

Taking an Oral Temperature Using a Digital Thermometer

This procedure is performed by the dental assistant in order to obtain the patient's body temperature.

Equipment and Supplies

- hand sanitizer
- examination gloves
- patient
- digital thermometer
- probe covers
- biohazard waste container

Procedure Steps *(Follow standard precautions)*

1. Wash hands and don examination gloves.

2. Assemble the thermometer and probe cover.

3. Seat the patient in the dental treatment room and position them comfortably in an upright position.

4. Verify that the patient has not had a hot or cold drink or smoked within the last half hour. (This may give a false temperature reading.)

5. Explain the procedure to the patient.

6. Verify that the thermometer is at 0. Position the new probe cover on the digital thermometer (Figure 22-7).

7. Insert the probe under the tongue to either side of the patient's mouth.

8. Instruct the patient to carefully close their lips around the probe without biting down on it (Figure 22-8).

9. Leave the probe in position until the digital thermometer beeps.

10. Remove the probe from the patient's mouth.

11. Read the results from the digital thermometer display window.

12. Dispose of the probe cover in a hazardous waste container.

13. Remove gloves and wash hands.

14. Document the procedure and record the results on the patient's chart.

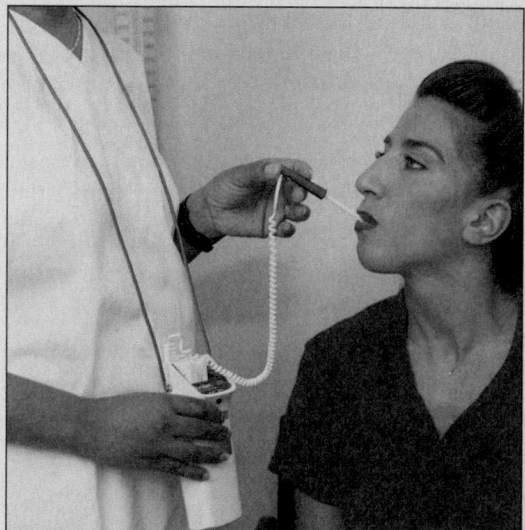

FIGURE 22-7
Slide the probe into the disposable cover, adjusting if necessary.

FIGURE 22-8
Insert the thermometer under the tongue and instruct the patient to close the lips around it.

The dental assistant would say that the pulse has either a strong or a weak beat.

After locating the pulse site, the dental assistant determines the number of beats per minute. This varies depending on the patient's age, sex, and physical and mental condition. It is expressed in a range without an absolute number.

Respiration Respiration is one breath taken in (inhalation) and one breath let out (exhalation) (refer to Chapter 15 for the procedure). Children have a more rapid respiration rate. Generally, as with the pulse rate, the younger the child, the faster the rate. Along with the rate of respirations, the dental assistant should record the respiratory rhythm, or the breathing pattern,

Procedure 22-3
Taking a Tympanic Temperature

This procedure is performed by the dental assistant in order to obtain the patient's body temperature.

Equipment and Supplies
- hand sanitizer
- examination gloves
- patient
- tympanic thermometer
- probe covers
- instructions for thermometer. There are so many on the market that it is important to read the instructions before using the thermometer that was purchased. Normally the following steps are used.

Procedure Steps (*Follow standard precautions*)
1. Take the thermometer out of its holder.

2. Place a new, disposable probe cover on the tip of the thermometer.

3. If taking a child's temperature, hold the head so it does not move; adults should hold their head stable.

4. For children, gently pull the ear straight back, and for an adult, gently pull the ear up and then back; gently place the probe of the thermometer in the canal of the ear (Figure 22-9). Do not force the probe, because it is not to touch the ear drum.

5. Press the button to turn on the thermometer. Most thermometers have the button held until it beeps. If this is

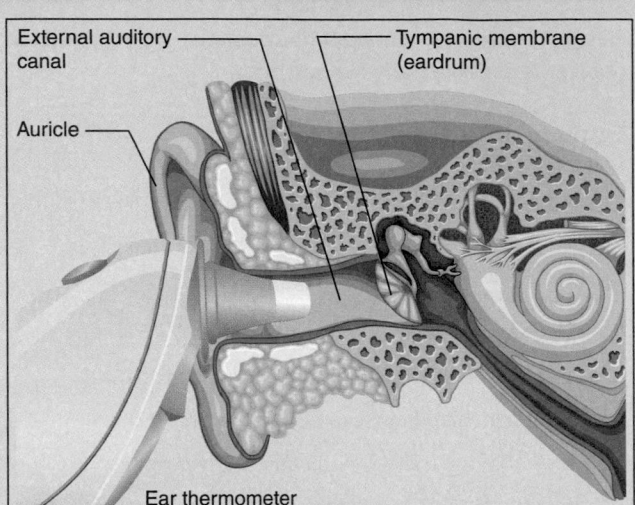

FIGURE 22-9
Gently enter the ear canal with tympanic thermometer.

not the direction on the thermometer that is being used, follow the manufacturer's directions.

6. After the beep, remove the thermometer from the ear opening. The temperature should be displayed in the window on the device.

7. Write down the temperature and note the time and date.

8. Dispose of the probe cover, and place the thermometer back into its holder.

---

and the respiration depth, the amount of air that is inhaled and exhaled, which is recorded as shallow, deep, and so on. Other notations about the breath sounds that are heard, such as raspy, wheezy, and so on, should be documented on the chart.

Dental Radiographs

It may be necessary for the dental assistant to obtain dental radiographs during both the limited/emergency new patient examination and the comprehensive new patient examination. The type of radiograph required will be dependent upon the type of exam. Since the limited/emergency new patient examination is a focused exam, the dental assistant may only need to obtain a PA (periapical radiograph examines the area around the apex of the tooth) and/or BWX (bitewing radiographs provide a view of the interproximal area of the teeth involved). However, during a comprehensive new patient examination, the dental assistant will typically need to obtain a FMX (full mouth set of radiographs)

and/or pano (panoramic radiograph provides a view of the entire mouth on one radiograph). Section VI provides details about dental radiography.

Extraoral and Intraoral Soft Tissue Examination

After the dental assistant has completed the patient's records, recorded vital signs, and taken all necessary radiographs, they inform the dentist that the patient is ready to be seen. The purpose of the extraoral and intraoral soft tissue exam is to identify lesions in the mouth, which may be atypical or pathologic. Atypical lesions are lesions that vary from normal but are not pathologic. Atypical lesions generally do not require treatment. Pathologic lesions are lesions that contain harmful cells and require specific treatment. A definite diagnosis of a pathologic lesion is made through a biopsy, during which the cells in the lesion are viewed under a microscope. Pathologic lesions require some type of definitive treatment. The role of the dental assistant during this process is to record all atypical and pathologic lesions observed by the dentist.

The first step in the extra and intraoral exam is to visually inspect the head and neck area as well as the oral cavity. The second step is to palpate all areas. During palpation the dentist will use the tips of one or two fingers to compress the tissue to either underlying bone or to a finger from the opposing hand; this allows the dentist to feel for and detect any lumps or bumps that may be present. All areas of the head and neck region and oral cavity should be thoroughly inspected and palpated, including the face, cheeks, lips, neck, throat, tongue, and gingiva.

The dentist will also evaluate the patient's temporomandibular joint (TMJ) using a combination of palpation and auscultation, listening for any popping or clicking in the joint. Popping or clicking are signs of possible joint damage that may require treatment by a dentist or specialist such as an orthodontist.

Examination of the Occlusion and Oral Habits

As part of the exam, the patient's occlusion is evaluated using the relationship between the maxillary and mandibular permanent first molars and the maxillary and mandibular permanent canines. In ideal occlusion, all teeth will occlude and the maxillary teeth will overlap the mandibular teeth. The patient's occlusion is evaluated and assigned to one of three classifications. Table 22-2 outlines the criteria for each occlusal classification of the permanent dentition. See Chapter 35 Orthodontics for more detail. Several additional tooth relationships also are documented in

most patient records. Refer to Table 22-3 for additional conditions that can occur with occlusion.

Dentists examine the oral cavity and the patient's hand for signs of bad oral habits that can negatively affect their teeth. The three most common bad oral habits are thumb sucking, bruxism, and nail biting. Thumb sucking happens in infants and young children, and if it occurs during a critical stage of tooth development, it may have long term effects: pressure pushes the teeth and might cause malocclusion such as an overbite, underbite, or open bite; a lisp may develop if the jaw bone position is affected; and the roof of the mouth can be altered or cause sensitivity. Thumb sucking is often identified by the patient's thumb or fingers showing wrinkling like being under water too long. Bruxism is recognized by excessive attrition on the incisal and occlusal surfaces. This can lead to brittle and sensitive teeth and the possibility of tooth fracture, tooth loss, severe jaw/muscle pain, and headaches. Nail biting is also first noted by examining the patient's hands. This habit can cause teeth to chip, erode, and become sensitive. It is important to note habits on the patient's chart, and these often form a part of their treatment plan.

Dental Charting

Each tooth is evaluated by the dentist, and the findings are noted and charted on the dental chart portion of the dental record. Recording the conditions in the patient's oral cavity on a document using symbols, numbers, and colors is a shorthand technique called charting. Charting, either manual or computer, is used in all dental offices. Dental charting must be completed on patients during a comprehensive new patient examination.

TABLE 22-2 Occlusal Classification

Occlusal Classification	Facial Profile	Molar Relationship	Canine Relationship	Other Conditions Present
Normal/ideal occlusion	Mesognathic	The mesiobuccal cusp of the maxillary first permanent molar occludes with the buccal grove of the mandibular first permanent molar.	The maxillary permanent canine occludes with the distal half of the maxillary canine and the mesial half of the mandibular first premolar.	NA
Class I malocclusion	Mesognathic	The mesiobuccal cusp of the maxillary first permanent molar occludes with the buccal grove of the mandibular first permanent molar.	The maxillary permanent canine occludes with the distal half of the maxillary canine and the mesial half of the mandibular first premolar.	Crowding in the maxillary or mandibular anterior teeth. Patient may also have an anterior crossbite or posterior crossbite.
Class II	Retrognathic—mandible is retruded	The mesiobuccal cusp of the maxillary first permanent molar occludes anterior to the buccal groove of the mandibular first molar. The width of this deviation must be at least the width of a premolar.	The distal surface of the mandibular canine is distal to the mesial surface of the maxillary canine. The width of this deviation must be at least the width of a premolar.	Class II, Division 1— The maxillary teeth are protruded. Class II, Division 11—The maxillary incisors are retruded.
Class III	Prognathic— mandible is protruded	The mesiobuccal cusp of the maxillary first permanent molar occludes posterior to the buccal groove of the mandibular molar. This width must be at least the width of a premolar.	The distal surface of the mandibular canine is mesial to the distal surface of the maxillary canine. The width of this deviation must be at least the width of a premolar.	

TABLE 22-3 Special Conditions That Can Occur with Occlusion

Condition	Localized or Generalized Throughout the Mouth	Area of the Mouth	Relationship of Teeth
Anterior crossbite	Localized	Anterior	Maxillary anterior teeth are lingual to the mandibular anterior teeth.
Posterior crossbite	Localized	Posterior	Maxillary posterior teeth are lingual to the mandibular posterior teeth. This may occur on one side of the mouth or both sides.
Edge-to-edge	Localized	Anterior	One or more anterior teeth meet incisal edge to incisal edge as opposed to the maxillary teeth overlapping the mandibular teeth.
End-to-end	Localized	Posterior	Molars meet cusp to cusp. With this relationship, the maxillary teeth do not overlap the mandibular teeth.
Open bite	Localized	Anterior	Lack of occlusion between the maxillary incisors.
Overjet	Localized	Anterior	The distance between the maxillary and mandibular incisors. This distance is measured with a periodontal probe. In ideal occlusion, the maxillary incisor should overlap the mandibular incisors. However, even with the overlap, the teeth should be contacting.

This information will be necessary for the dentist to completely understand the needs of the patient and develop a plan to meet those needs. Two common types of charts that can be used for dental charting are anatomical charts and geometric charts.

Charting is part of the patient's legal record maintained in the office. As with all legal and medical records, each patient's chart should be complete and correct.

Anatomical Dental Chart Anatomical charts provide a visual representation of the facial (buccal/labial), lingual, and occlusal/incisal surfaces of the teeth. Each image on an anatomical chart is an accurate representation of each tooth. This chart allows the clinician to accurately depict each restoration on the chart as it appears in the mouth.

Figure 22-10 shows an anatomical dental chart. Notice how the anatomy of each tooth is accurately represented. The drawing closest to the line dividing the arches represents the lingual

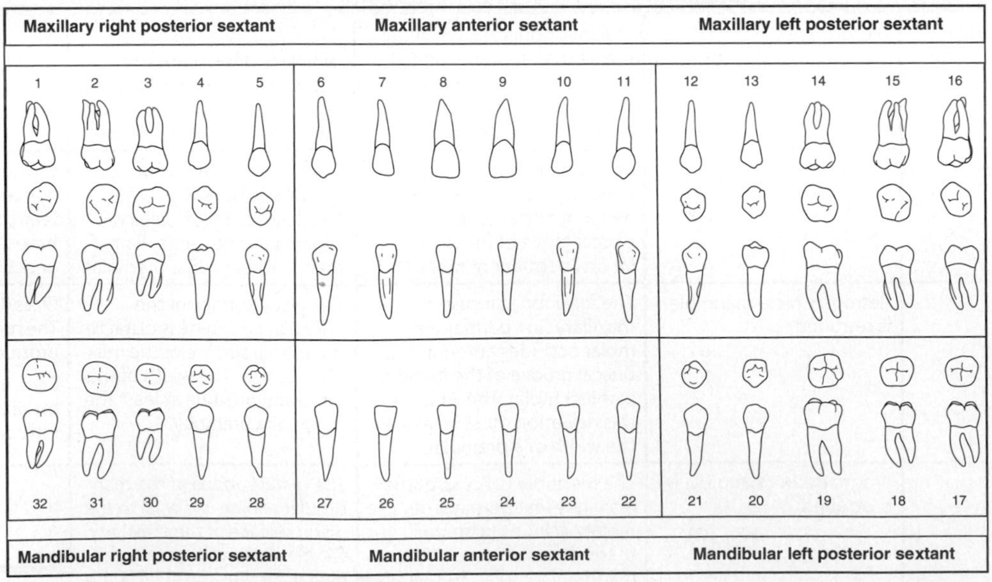

FIGURE 22-10
Anatomical dental chart divided into sextants. Teeth identified using universal numbering system.

surface, and the drawing farthest from the line is the buccal/labial surface. The drawing in the middle of the posterior teeth represents the occlusal surface.

Geometric Dental Chart

A geometric chart is a representation of the tooth using a geometric format (the symbol most commonly used is a circle). A geometric chart depicts the distal, mesial, facial, lingual, and occlusal/incisal surfaces of the tooth. A geometric chart allows the clinician to color in the surfaces to be charted.

Figure 22-11 shows a geometric dental chart. Notice how the mesial, distal, facial, lingual, and incisal/occlusal surfaces of each tooth are represented by shape. The portion of the symbol closest to the line dividing the arches represents the lingual surface, and the portion farthest from the line is the buccal/labial surface. The drawing in the middle represents the occlusal surface on the posterior teeth and the incisal on anterior teeth. The portion closest to the midline is the mesial surface, and the surface facing away from the midline is the distal.

Dental Chart Designs

The teeth shown on the chart can be divided into groups that are identified as either quadrants or sextants. Quadrants divide the mouth into four groups: the maxillary right, maxillary left, mandibular right, and mandibular left. Sextants divide the mouth into six groups: the maxillary right posterior, maxillary anterior, maxillary left posterior, mandibular left posterior, mandibular anterior, and mandibular right posterior. Figure 22-10 shows an anatomical dental chart divided into sextants. Figure 22-11 shows a geometric dental chart divided into quadrants.

Numbering Systems

Both anatomical and geometric charts use tooth numbering systems to identify teeth easily and efficiently. The three common numbering systems are the universal, international, and Palmer systems. Each system uses numbers to identify permanent teeth and numbers or letters to identify primary teeth. Different dental offices may use different numbering systems, so it is important that the dental assistant be familiar with each system (Table 22-4).

The universal numbering system uses numbers 1–32 to represent the adult teeth. The maxillary right third molar is tooth #1, and the numbers continue clockwise to end with the mandibular right third molar as tooth #32. Letters A through T are used to designate primary teeth. The primary maxillary right second molar is designated "#A," and the lettering continues clockwise to end with the primary mandibular right second as "#T." Figure 22-11 is a geometric chart showing the permanent and primary teeth identified using the universal numbering system.

The International Standards Organization system (also referred to as Federation Dentaire Internationale system) uses two numbers to identify each adult tooth. The first number represents the quadrant, and the second number is the order of the tooth from the midline. The adult teeth quadrants are numbered 1–4, with the maxillary right quadrant designated as quadrant 1. The numbering continues clockwise, ending with the mandibular right quadrant as quadrant 4. For example, tooth #18 is the 8th tooth in quadrant 1, which is the maxillary right third molar. By contrast, the primary teeth quadrants are numbered 5 through 8, with the maxillary right quadrant designated as quadrant 5. Tooth #51, therefore, would be the first tooth from the midline, or the maxillary right central incisor. Figure 22-12 identifies permanent and primary teeth using the international numbering system.

The Palmer numbering system uses a symbol (bracket) to represent the four quadrants. The crossed lines (+) represent the four quadrants with the symbol. For example, "⌐" represents the maxillary left quadrant. The number of the tooth from the midline is used to indicate the adult teeth (1–8) and is repeated in each quadrant with 1 being the central incisor. Letters are used for the primary teeth (a–e repeated in each quadrant with "a" being the central incisor). Figure 22-13 identifies permanent teeth using the Palmer numbering system.

Verbalizing Dental Charting

It is important that dental charting be properly verbalized to ensure accurate charting. The criteria and guidelines that must be followed when verbalizing dental charting are outlined in Table 22-5.

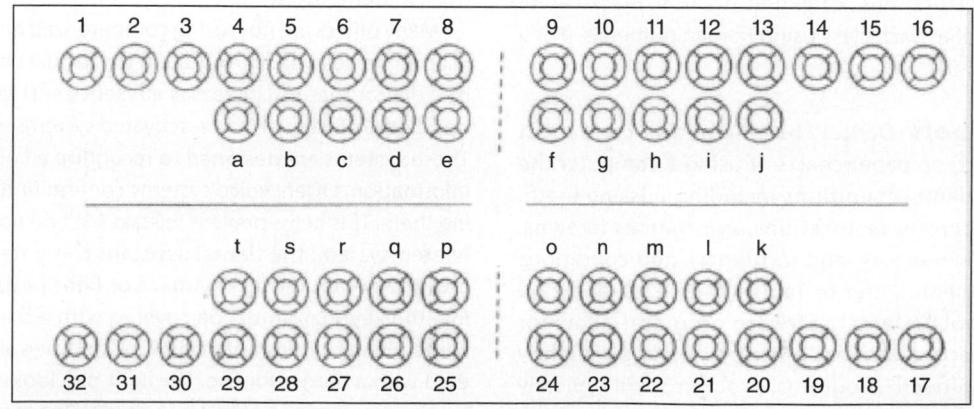

FIGURE 22-11
Geometric chart divided into quadrants identifying permanent and primary teeth using the universal number system.

TABLE 22-4 Tooth Numbering/Identification Systems

Numbering System	Numbers/Letters Used	Starting Point	Ending Point	How Information Is Verbalized
Universal numbering system—permanent dentition	1–32 Each tooth in the dentition is numbered based upon its location in the mouth.	Maxillary right 3rd molar—tooth #1	Mandibular right 3rd molar—tooth #32	Each tooth has a specific number. For example, the maxillary right first premolar is tooth #5.
Universal numbering system—primary teeth	A–T	Maxillary right 2nd primary molar— tooth #a	Mandibular right 2nd primary molar—tooth #t	Each tooth has a specific letter. For example, the maxillary left first primary molar is tooth #I.
International numbering system— permanent dentition	1–4 to represent the quadrant. The maxillary right quadrant is 1, maxillary left is 2, mandibular left is 3, and mandibular right is 4. Teeth in each quadrant are numbered 1–8. Tooth #1 is the central incisor, and tooth #8 is the 3rd molar. Teeth in between are numbered accordingly.	Central incisor in each quadrant	3rd molar in each quadrant	Each tooth is identified by a two-number identification. The first number is the quadrant, and the second number is the tooth. For example, the mandibular left 1st molar is tooth 36.
International numbering system— primary dentition	5–8 to represent the quadrant. The maxillary right quadrant is 5, maxillary left is 6, mandibular left is 7, and mandibular right is 8. Teeth in each quadrant are numbered 1–5. Tooth #1 is the primary central incisor, and tooth #5 is the primary second molar. Teeth in between are numbered accordingly.	Primary central incisor in each quadrant	Primary second molar	Each tooth is identified by a two-number identification. The first number is the quadrant, and the second number is the tooth. For example, the primary mandibular right canine is tooth 83.
Palmer—permanent dentition	Each tooth in the quadrant is numbered 1–8. Tooth #1 is the central incisor, and tooth #8 is the 3rd molar. A bracket is made around the tooth number to indicate the quadrant.	Central incisor in each quadrant	3rd molar in each quadrant	The quadrant is followed by the tooth number. For example, the maxillary left first molar would be identified as the lower left 6 and would be written 6L.
Palmer—primary dentition	Each tooth in the quadrant is numbered A–E. The primary central incisor is tooth #A, and the primary second molar is tooth #E. A bracket is made around the tooth to indicate the quadrant.	Primary central incisor	Primary second molar	The quadrant is followed by the tooth number. For example, the primary maxillary canine would be identified as the maxillary left cL and would be written cL.

Classifying Caries and Restorations Carious lesions and restorations on dental charting also are classified according to the surfaces involved. The system used to identify carious lesions and restorations, known at the G. V. Black Cavity Classification, identifies each class using Roman numerals. (For a review, see Table 22-6.)

Charting Symbols Dental charting allows the dentist to document (chart) on paper charts or using a computer the patient's existing dental conditions including missing teeth, **impacted** teeth, current restorations, **appliances** (crowns, **bridges, dentures, veneers**, and **implants**), and conditions that require treatment. (Refer to Tables 22-7, 22-8, and 22-9 for charting symbols). Dental software programs allow for efficient dental charting. While the symbols may vary slightly between dental software programs, programs will typically chart existing conditions in blue and conditions requiring treatment in red. This allows the clinician to easily visualize the dental needs of the patient. The chart is designed with the dental health care worker looking at the patient from the front with the patient's right on the left side of the chart. Therefore, the patient's right is the assistant's left, and the patient's left is the assistant's right.

Many offices are now using computerized or automated dental charting instead of, or in addition to, manual charting. Computerized dental charting increases efficiency and fosters standardization. Some offices use voice-activated systems with their software. These systems are designed to recognize a voice and record the information. Often, voice systems confirm findings before charting them. This helps prevent mistakes. When not using a voice-activated system, the dental assistant can enter the information into the computer by keyboard or light pen. When keyboarding, the keyboard must be covered with a barrier so that cross-contamination does not occur. The light pen should also be covered with a barrier for use. The light pen looks like a writing pen and is sometimes attached by a cord to the monitor. It is touched to the screen to activate a command. If, for example, the dental assistant wanted to note a composite restoration that was placed

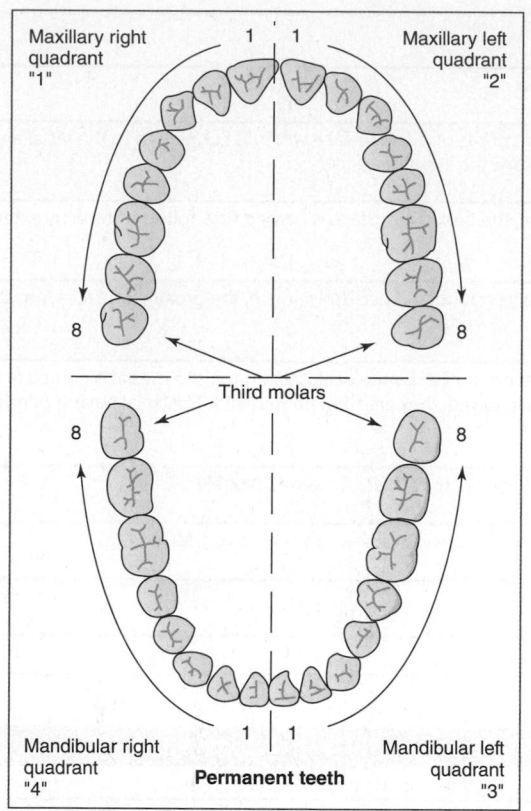

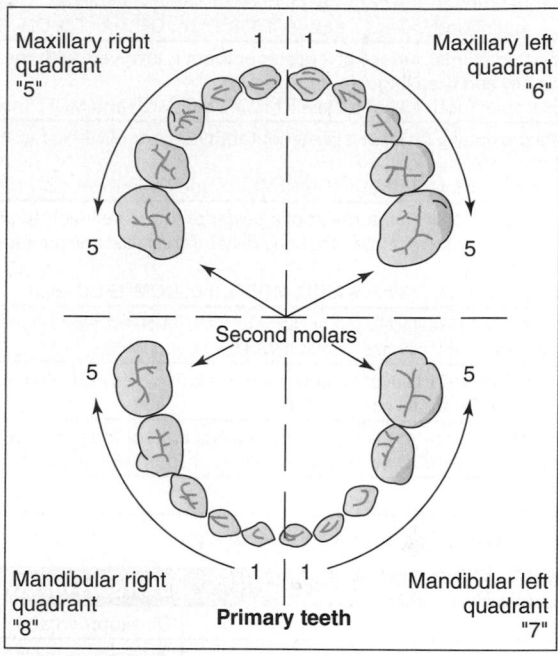

FIGURE 22-12
Permanent and primary dentition showing the International Standards Organization system.

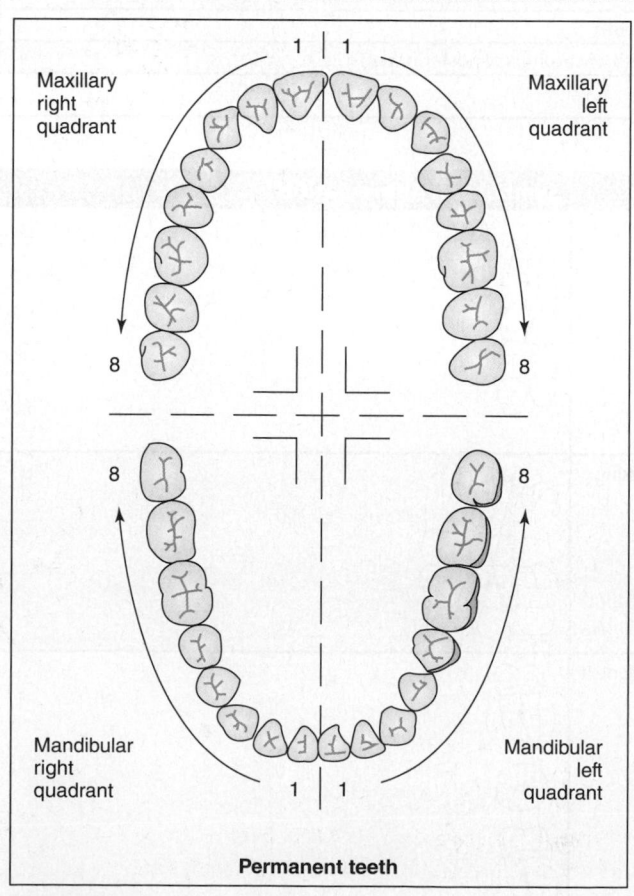

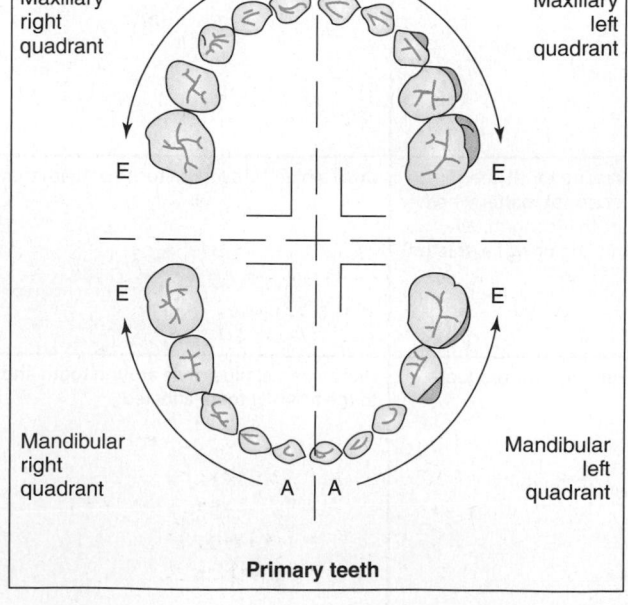

FIGURE 22-13
Permanent and primary dentition showing the Palmer system.

TABLE 22-5 Criteria for Naming Tooth Surfaces in Dental Charting

1.	If only one surface of an anterior or posterior tooth is involved, it alone is named. Example: Tooth #3 has a Class I occlusal, or Tooth #8 has a Class I lingual pit.
2.	If no proximal surfaces of a posterior tooth are involved but there is involvement of the occlusal surface which is connected to the facial and/or lingual surface, the occlusal is named first, followed by the facial, then, if necessary, the lingual surface. Example: Tooth #3 has a Class I OF, OB, OL, or OFL (not FO, OLF, BO, etc.)
3.	If one proximal surface of a posterior tooth is involved, with the occlusal surface, the proximal surface is named first, followed then by extensions facially and then lingually if necessary. Example: Tooth #3 has a Class II MI, DO, MO, MOF, and MOFL (not OD, OM, IM)
4.	If a proximal surface of a posterior tooth is involved with a facial or lingual surface, but not the occlusal surface, the proximal surface is named first. Example: Tooth # 3 has a Class II MF, DF, and DL (not FM, LD, etc.)
5.	If both the proximal surfaces of a posterior tooth are involved and connected to each other by the occlusal surface, the mesial is named first, followed by the occlusal, then the distal. If the facial and/or lingual surfaces are involved, they are then named with the facial having priority over the lingual. Example: Tooth #3 has a MOD, MODFL (not DOM, LFOD, etc.)
6.	If a proximal surface of an anterior tooth is involved, with no involvement of the incisal, the surface is named alone. Example: Tooth #8 has a Class III M, D.
7.	If the incisal surface of an anterior tooth is involved and when the incisal surface and proximal surfaces are involved, MI, DI, MID. Example: Tooth #8 has a Class IV MI.
8.	If an anterior or posterior has the gingival third of the tooth involved, it is named alone. Example: Tooth #3 has a Class V lingual, or Tooth #8 has a Class V facial.

TABLE 22-6 G. V. Black Cavity Classification

Classification	Surfaces Involved
Class 1	Developmental defects. Most commonly pits and fissures
Class II	Proximal surfaces of molars and premolars
Class III	Proximal surfaces of anterior teeth. Doesn't include the incisal edge
Class IV	Proximal surfaces of anterior teeth. Includes the incisal edge
Class V	Cervical (gingival third) of the tooth
Class VI	Incisal edge only of anterior teeth or cusp tips of posterior teeth

TABLE 22-7 Present and Missing Teeth and Existing Restorations

Condition	Charting Description	Symbol and Abbreviation
Present tooth/teeth	Nothing is noted.	
Missing tooth/teeth (does not matter whether tooth is congenitally missing or was extracted)	Draw a blue "X" over the tooth or teeth that are missing.	
Partially erupted tooth	Draw a partial blue circle around tooth and write PE next to the tooth or teeth affected.	PE

Condition	Charting Description	Symbol and Abbreviation
Exfoliated primary teeth	Draw a blue X over the entire tooth or teeth, including the root.	
Supernumerary tooth	Draw blue tooth at the location above the apices.	
Amalgam restoration	Color in the area(s) in blue on the tooth surfaces that is/are restored with an amalgam restoration.	Class I OCC amal
Amalgam restoration		Class II MO amal
Composite restoration	Outline the area(s) in blue on the tooth surface(s) that is/are restored with a composite or tooth colored restoration.	Class III M comp
Composite restoration		Class IV MI comp
Composite restoration		Class V LA comp

TABLE 22-7 *(Continued)*

Condition	Charting Description	Symbol and Abbreviation
Dental sealant	Draw a blue letter S on the surface(s) covered by a dental sealant. Write PFS beyond the root apex.	PFS PFS
Temporary restoration/ temporary crown	Outline in blue the area(s) on the tooth covered by the temporary restoration. Write TEMP beyond the root apex.	temp
Stainless steel crown	Outline in blue the tooth crown and write the letters SSC beyond the apex of the tooth.	SSC SSC SSC
Full noble metal crown/ full gold crown	Draw blue diagonal lines over the surfaces covered by the crown. Write FGC beyond the root apex.	FGC
Porcelain crown	Outline the entire crown in blue when the crown is all porcelain. Write PC beyond the root apex.	PC
Porcelain bonded to metal crown or porcelain fused to metal	Outline the entire crown in blue. Write the abbreviation PBM for crowns that are porcelain bonded to metal or PFM for crowns that are porcelain fused to metal beyond the root apex.	PBM or PFM
Inlay	Draw blue diagonal lines over the portion of the occlusal surface covered by the inlay. Write the abbreviation inl beyond the root apex.	inl

Condition	Charting Description	Symbol and Abbreviation
Onlay	Draw blue diagonal lines over the surfaces of the tooth covered by the onlay. Write onl at the apex of the tooth.	onl
Porcelain laminate veneer	Outline in blue the facial aspect of the tooth. Write PLV at the apex of the tooth.	PLV
Fixed bridge	Draw a blue "X" over the root surface of the tooth that has been extracted; this tooth is the pontic. Chart the pontic and teeth on either side of the pontic (abutment teeth) according to the type of crown used for each unit. All teeth are connected to represent one fixed appliance with each part representing a unit (3uBr) as shown in diagram. Write abbreviation of type of crown at the apex of the tooth. Premolar (anterior abutment) porcelain fused to metal; first molar is missing replaced by pontic in fuld gold; and second molar (posterior abutment) full gold crown is represented in symbol and abbreviation column.	PFM FGC FGC 3 u br
Endodontic treatment/ root canal therapy	Draw a blue line in the root of the tooth to symbolize the pulp being removed and a filling material placed in the pulp chambers of the tooth. Write abbreviation RCT at the apex of the tooth.	RCT
Dental implant	Draw horizontal blue lines through the root(s) and write IMPL below the tooth.	IMPL
Dental implant restored with crown	Draw horizontal blue lines through the root(s) and write IMPL below the tooth. Chart the crown according to the type of material used. Extracted molar replaced with an implant and restored with a full gold crown is shown in column symbol and abbreviation.	IMPL FGC

(Continues)

TABLE 22-7 (*Continued*)

Condition	Charting Description	Symbol and Abbreviation
Full denture	Draw a large blue X over all teeth in the arch. Write FUD (full upper denture) or FLD (full lower denture) at apices of central incisors roots.	FUD
Partial denture	Draw a blue X over the missing teeth. Join the teeth marked with an X to indicate the teeth placed with a removable partial denture.	PLD

TABLE 22-8 Conditions That Require Treatment

Condition	Charting Description	Symbol and Abbreviation
Dental caries	Color in red the surface(s) on the tooth that exhibit dental caries.	
Secondary or recurrent dental caries	Outline in red the existing restoration indicating secondary or recurrent dental caries.	
Fracture	Draw a red zig-zag line on the surface(s) of the tooth or root that are fractured.	
Impacted tooth/teeth	Circle in red the entire tooth including the root.	imp
Tooth to be extracted	Draw a single red diagonal line through the entire tooth and root.	

Condition	Charting Description	Symbol and Abbreviation
Tooth requiring root canal/endodontic treatment	Draw a red line in the root of the tooth to symbolize the tooth needs RCT.	RCT
Abscess	Draw a red circle at the apex of the tooth indicating an abscess and/or periapical **radiolucency**.	abs

TABLE 22-9 Periodontal Conditions and Tooth Positioning

Condition	Charting Description	Symbol
Calculus	Draw blue connecting marks resembling Cs.	
Periodontal pocket	Draw a blue arrow to area of the periodontal pocket and write the 4 mm depth below the arrow.	4
Gingival recession/furcation involvement	Draw a blue wavy line at the millimeter mark of the gingival recession and a solid red circle to indicate the area of furcation involvement.	
Mobility	Draw short blue parallel lines on the crown of the tooth that is mobile.	II
Rotated tooth	Draw a blue curved arrow in the direction of the rotation.	

(Continues)

TABLE 22-9 *(Continued)*

Drifting tooth	Draw a blue arrow pointing toward the mesial of the tooth that is drifting or inclined mesially.	
Drifting tooth *(continued)*	Draw a blue arrow pointing toward the distal of the tooth that is drifting or inclined distally.	
Overerupted	Draw a blue arrow pointing incisally/occlusally of the tooth overerupting.	
Open contacts	Draw short blue parallel lines between teeth where there is an open contact.	
Diastema	Draw long blue parallel lines between teeth where the diastema occurs.	

in the mouth, the assistant would touch the light pen to the screen over the tooth, highlighting the tooth. After highlighting the tooth, the assistant would move the light pen to the side of the screen and select "composite restoration" and the surfaces to be included. Finally, the dental assistant would touch the light pen to "existing" or "needs to be completed." The computer program would then put the color coding or symbol on the dental chart on the correct tooth and make a notation on the patient's chart under findings or treatment plan (Figure 22-14).

Dental software programs work differently but are learned easily. Offices evaluate which systems meet their needs before purchase. Many offices have computers or computer monitors in each operatory for the auxiliary to chart findings and complete the notations and services rendered. Dental assistants can become very proficient at computer charting (Figure 22-15). The software programs for computer charting can record conditions

of the dentition, tissue, occlusion, or any notations the dentist or auxiliary would like to make.

Periodontal Charting The periodontal examination is a thorough examination of the periodontium using periodontal charts. The periodontal charts depict the condition of the patient's periodontal tissues. The charting is completed either manually or on a computer. Periodontal probing is completed to determine the depth of the periodontal pocket by using a periodontal probe. The periodontal probe is a tapered instrument and is calibrated in millimeters to measure the gingival sulcus around each tooth. The dentist or hygienist uses the periodontal probe to take six (6) measurements on each tooth. There are three sites on the facial surface, including mesiofacial, midfacial, and distofacial, and three sites on the lingual surface, including mesiolingual, midlingual, and distolingual. The measurements are recorded on a periodontal chart (Figure 22-16).

Chart

Patient: Patricia Abbott
Birthdate: 09/30/1963

Chart #: ABB102

Date: 01/22/2021
SS#:

Provider: Dennis D. Smith D.D.S.
Phone: (801)763-9300
Office: 732 E. Utah Valley Drive # 500
American Fork, UT 84003

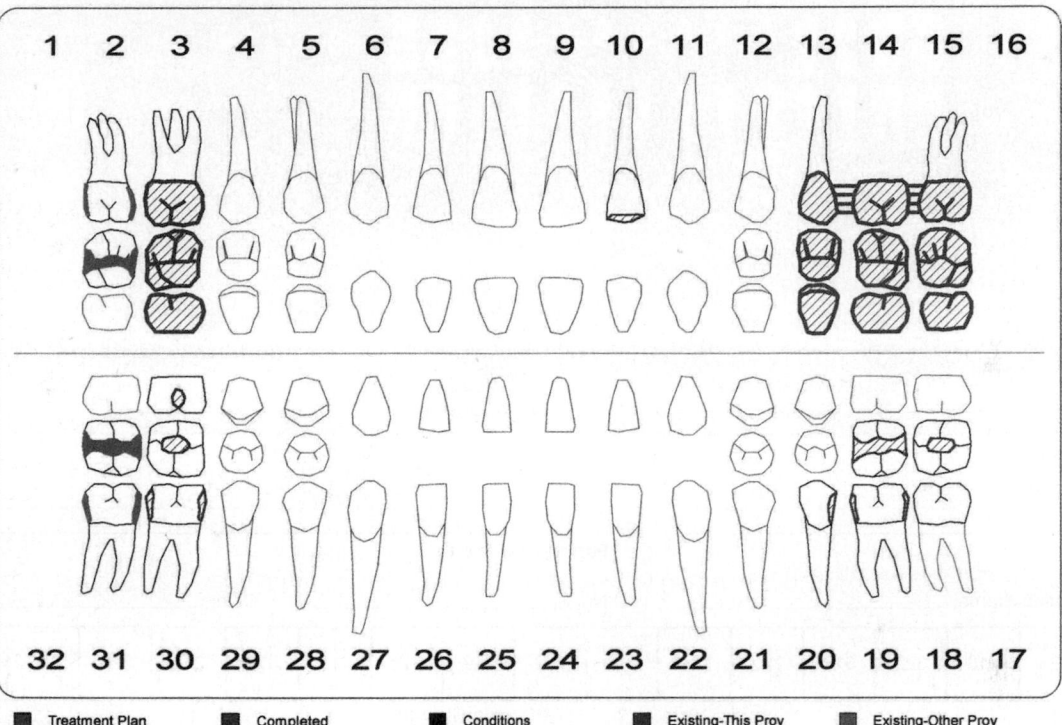

| | Treatment Plan | | Completed | | Conditions | | Existing-This Prov | | Existing-Other Prov |

Treatment Plan Estimate

Tooth	Description	Amount	Pat.	Dental Ins.
3	Crown-porc fuse high noble mtl	613.00	306.50	306.50
3	Crown buildup, includ any pins	149.00	29.80	119.20
3	Permanent Insert	0.00	0.00	0.00
10	Resin-one surface, anterior	71.00	14.20	56.80
13	Retainer crn-porc fused-hi nob	613.00	306.50	306.50
14	Pontic-porcelain fused to hnob	613.00	306.50	306.50
15	Retainer crn-porc fused-hi nob	613.00	306.50	306.50
18	Resin-1 surface, post-permanent	80.00	16.00	64.00
19	Resin-3 surface +, post-perm	146.00	29.20	116.80
20	Resin-1 surface, post-permanent	80.00	16.00	64.00
30	Resin-3 surface +, post-perm	146.00	29.20	116.80
	Treatment Plan Totals	3124.00	1360.40	1763.60

* Treatment Plans Are Estimates Only

Courtesy of Dentrix

FIGURE 22-14
Sample computer chart.

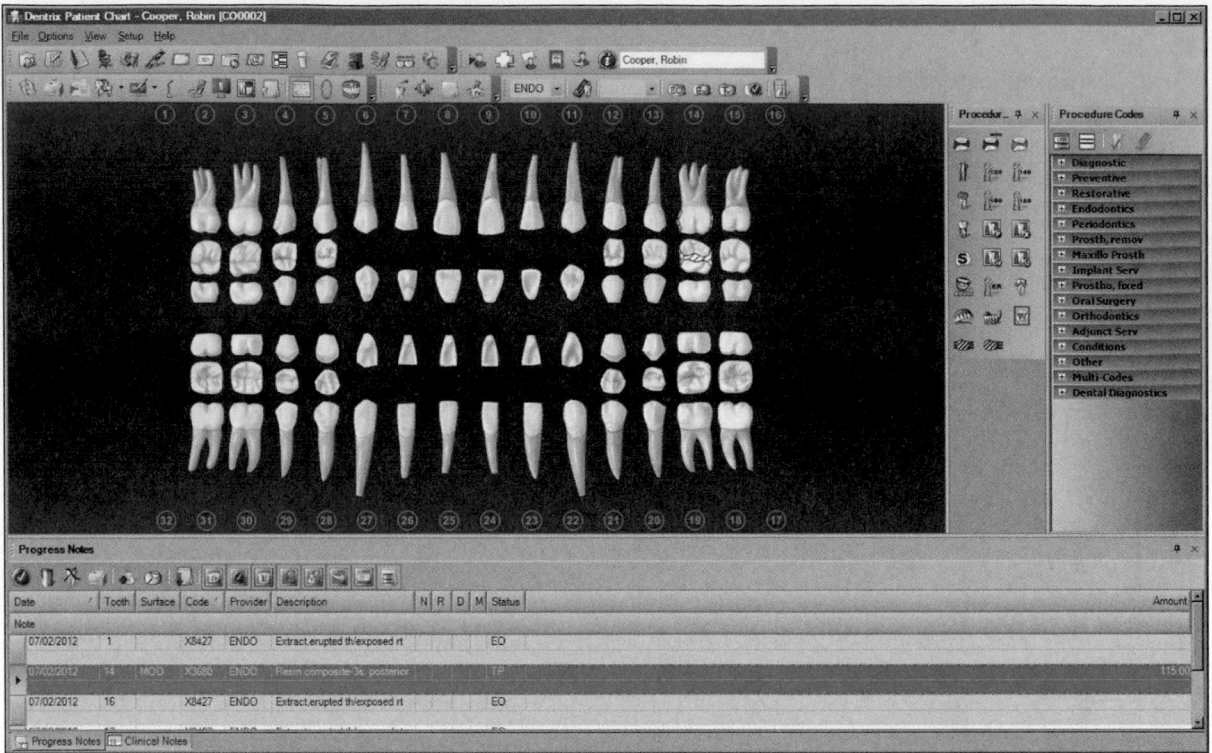

FIGURE 22-15
Sample computer chart.

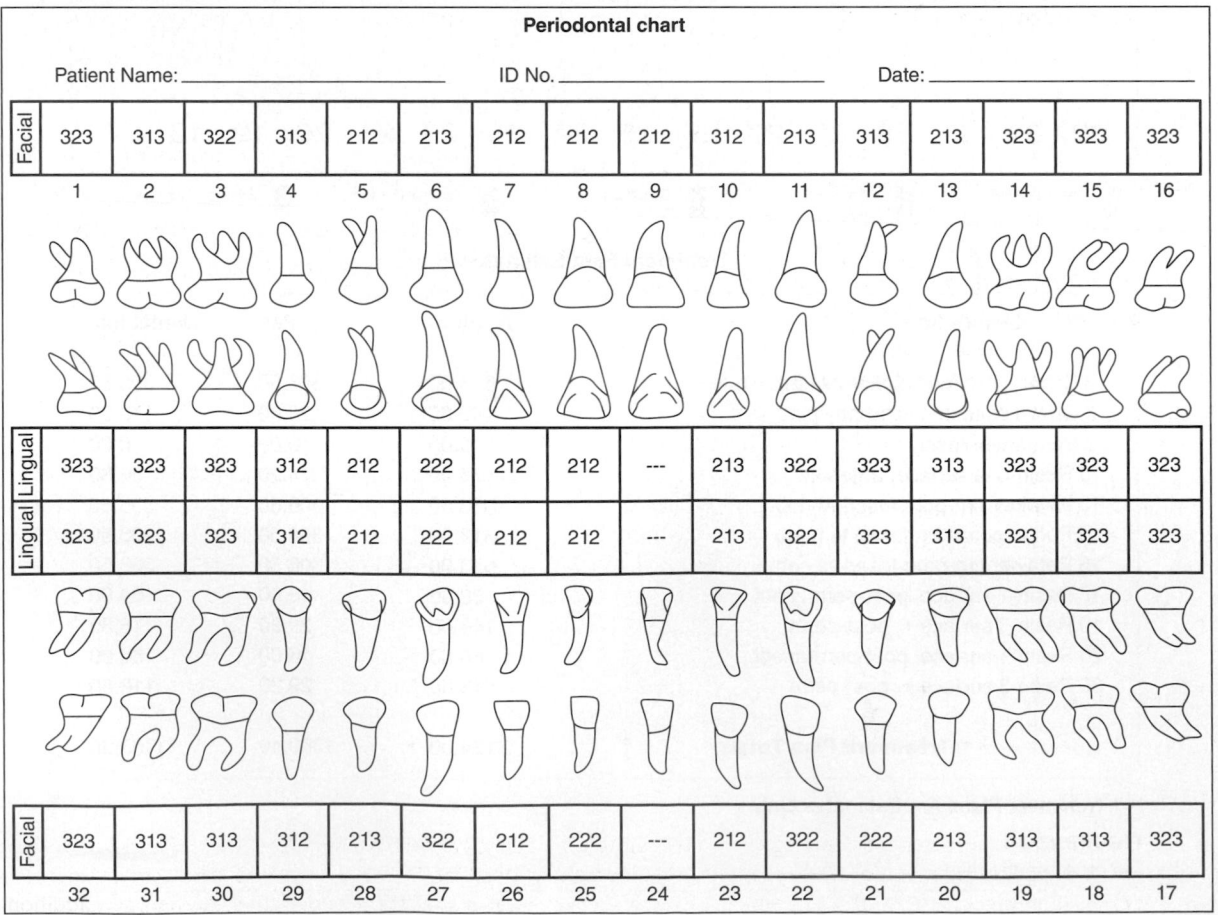

FIGURE 22-16
This is a sample periodontal chart for recording periodontal sulcus/pocket depths.

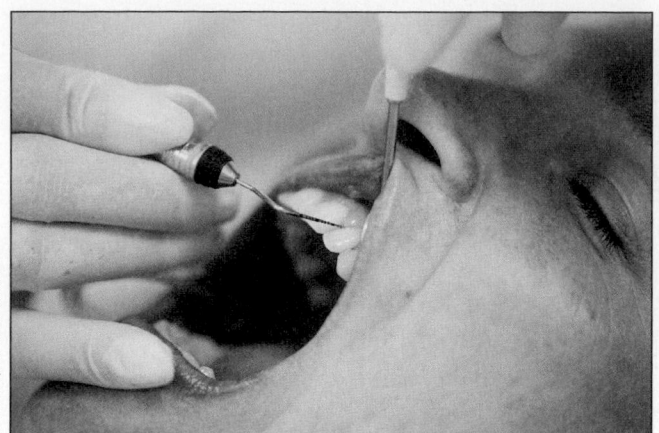

FIGURE 22-17
Periodontal probe used to measure pocket depth around the tooth to examine progression of periodontal disease.

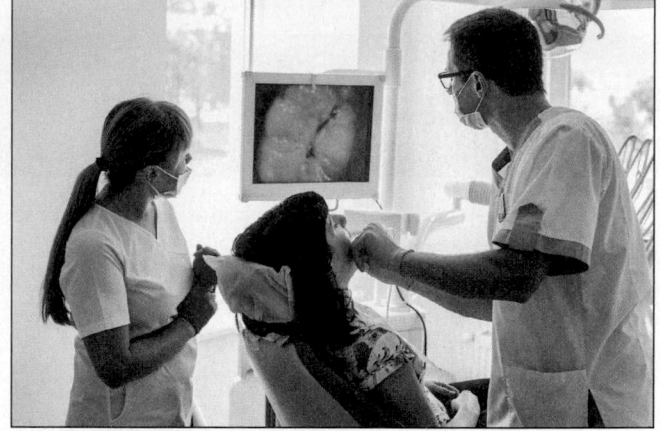

FIGURE 22-18
Intraoral image of carious lesion on the occlusal surface.

The periodontal probe is placed in the sulcus or periodontal pocket, and when the tip of the probe reaches the bottom of the sulcus, or epithelial attachment, a measurement is taken at the gingival margin. In health, periodontal probe depths range from 1 to 3 mm (Figure 22-17).

A full periodontal charting should be completed during each comprehensive new patient examination. Refer to Chapter 24, "Dental Prophylaxis and Recare Appointment," for an explanation of full periodontal charting.

Diagnosis

A diagnosis is a formal determination of the needs of the patient based upon information collected; it identifies all dental diseases and/or deficiencies in the oral cavity. The dentist is the dental team member who is responsible for making the dental diagnosis. Prior to communicating the diagnosis to the patient, it is important for the dental team to determine the goals of the patient and for the dentist to formally develop a dental treatment plan.

A very important part of dental treatment is to determine the goals of the patient: What does the patient desire as far as their oral health? Another way to state this is, why did the patient come to the dental office— what is the primary concern of the patient? While this information doesn't change the dental diagnosis, it will be important for the dentist to keep this information in mind when developing the dental treatment plan. It is important that the goals of the patient be considered during the treatment planning process.

The dentist may order additional diagnostic items such as intraoral images (described below), study models or bites (refer to Chapter 33 for details) that will aid in giving the patient a complete diagnosis, and visual aids.

Intraoral Images Intraoral images are electronic photographs of both intraoral and extraoral structures (Figure 22-18). Intraoral images are obtained using an intraoral camera that integrates with the dental office's software program. Intraoral images can be used for several purposes:

- Allow the patient to visualize their dental problems. This enables the patient to better understand their dental needs.

- Allow the patient to visualize the results of dental treatment. This is very often completed by examining before and after pictures side by side.

- Patient education. This allows the dental assistant or dental hygienist to show the patient various dental deposits as well as areas of disease caused by these deposits (i.e., dental caries, gingivitis, periodontitis).

- They can be submitted to dental insurance companies as documentation of need for treatment.
Procedure 22-4 provides instruction on steps for obtaining intraoral images.

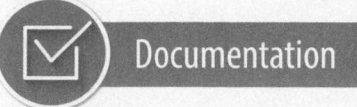 **Documentation**

Writing Service Rendered

The assistant documents all procedures completed in order during the patient's appointment on the Service Rendered form. For a comprehensive new patient examination, the assistant would record a list of all forms completed and signed by the patient, vital signs, radiographs (number and types of radiographs), extraoral and intraoral examination, periodontal charting, and additional diagnostic procedures. On last line, write the next return to clinic procedures.

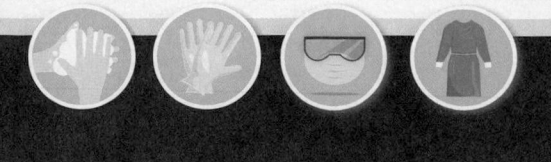

Procedure 22-4
Taking Intraoral Images

This procedure is performed by the dental assistant in order to obtain intraoral images.

Equipment and Supplies
- hand sanitizer
- PPE: Examination gloves, mask, protective clothing, and protective glasses
- patient
- dental chair
- patient bib and clip
- intraoral camera and protective sheath
- connections to computer software program
- gauze squares

Procedure Steps
1. Wash hands and don PPE.
2. Explain the procedure to the patient.
3. Obtain permission for obtaining the images.
4. Prepare the equipment, including connecting to the office software program and placing a protective sheath over the intraoral camera.
5. Position the patient for maximum visibility.
6. Adjust the lighting for maximum illumination.
7. Dry the area with gauze squares where the images will be obtained.
8. Position the intraoral camera for proper visualization (Figure 22-19).
9. Once the desired image is on the computer screen, capture the image.
10. Display the image for the doctor and patient to view.

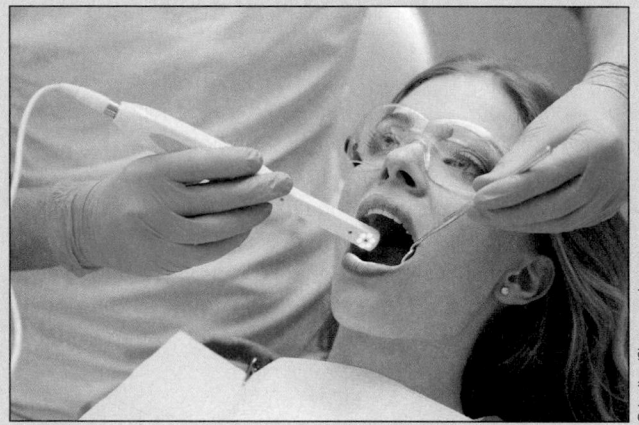

FIGURE 22-19
Positioning of intraoral camera.

© bezikus/Shutterstock.com

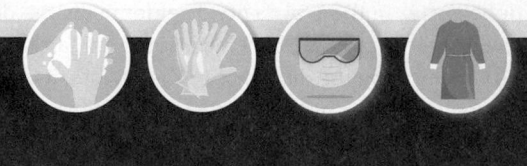

Procedure 22-5
Assist with New Patient Examination

The dental assistant transfers materials and instruments and records findings while the dentist completes the soft tissue and teeth and occlusion examination during the New Patient Examination procedure. A second assistant may be requested to record findings. This procedure can be legally performed by a certified dental assistant in some states.

Steps written in blue font are performed by the operator (dentist, hygienest or qualified dental assistant), and the chairside assistant's steps are written in black.

Prepare Patient for New Patient Examination
Equipment and Supplies
- PPE: examination gloves, mask, protective glasses, and protective clothing
- handwashing soap or hand sanitizer
- patient
- sanitized and barriers placed over equipment in dental treatment area
- patient seating setup (refer to Procedure 18-4)
- basic setup (refer to Procedure 19-1)
- patient forms to be completed
- paper, pen, and clipboard
- blood pressure equipment
- body temperature equipment
- clock with second hand

1. Request patient to complete the following forms in reception area:
   - ❏ Patient registration form
   - ❏ Consent form
   - ❏ HIPAA form
   - ❏ Medical history
   - ❏ Dental history

2. Escort and seat patient (refer to Procedure 18-4).
   ❏ Examine patient's appearance, speech, gait, and behavior to be called to the dentist's attention and noted in the patient's record.
   ❏ Seat patient in dental chair in upright position.
   ❏ Place patient napkin.
   ❏ Explain the procedure to the patient.
   ❏ Review medical and dental histories, and clarify any positive responses.

3. Take and record patient's vital signs, including:
   ❏ Blood pressure (refer to Procedure 22-1)
   ❏ Temperature (refer to Procedures 22-2 and 22-3)
   ❏ Pulse
   ❏ Respirations

4. Take dental radiographs requested by the dentist.

5. Inform the dentist that the patient is ready for the examination.

Assist with Extraoral Soft Tissue Examination Procedure

Equipment and Supplies
- PPE: examination gloves, mask, protective glasses, and protective clothing
- handwashing soap or hand sanitizer
- prepared dental treatment area
- patient seated in dental chair
- patient record to document findings (pen and paper or computer)

Procedure Steps

Operator examines and palpates the patient's extraoral tissues.

1. Assistant records findings throughout the procedure.

Visually examines the facial soft tissue and symmetry of the patient.

2. Assistant records:
   ❏ Any abnormal swelling or asymmetry
   ❏ Changes in tissue color and appearance of skin abrasions

Visually examines patient's lips (Figure 22-20).

3. Assistant records:
   ❏ Appearance of smile line, vermillion border, and the commissures of the lip

With patient's mouth in closed position, palpates the soft tissues beneath the mandible and floor of mouth with fingers (Figure 22-21).

4. Assistant records:
   ❏ Abnormalities of the external tissue of the mandible and floor of the mouth

Palpates the cervical lymph nodes by having the patient turn their head to the side. Gently feels the chain of lymph nodes from the ear to the collar bone and repeats on the opposite side of the neck (Figure 22-22).

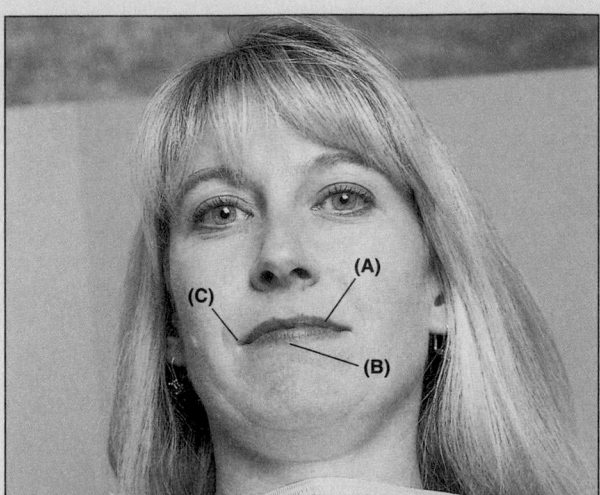

FIGURE 22-20
Visually examining (A) the smile line, (B) the vermillion border, and (C) the commissures of the lip.

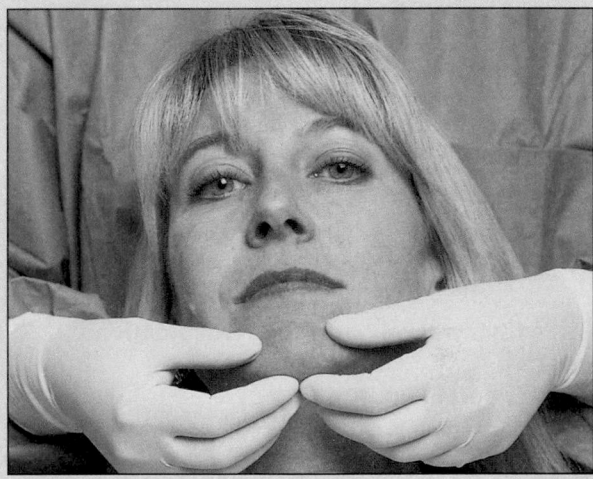

FIGURE 22-21
Examining the external tissues of the mandible and the floor of the mouth.

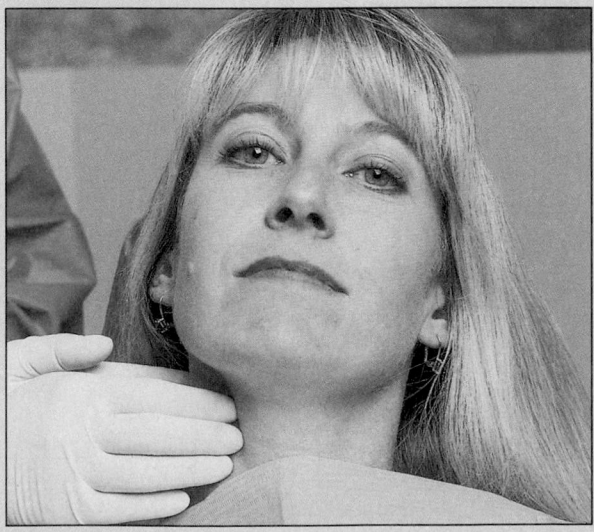

FIGURE 22-22
Examining the cervical lymph nodes.

(Continues)

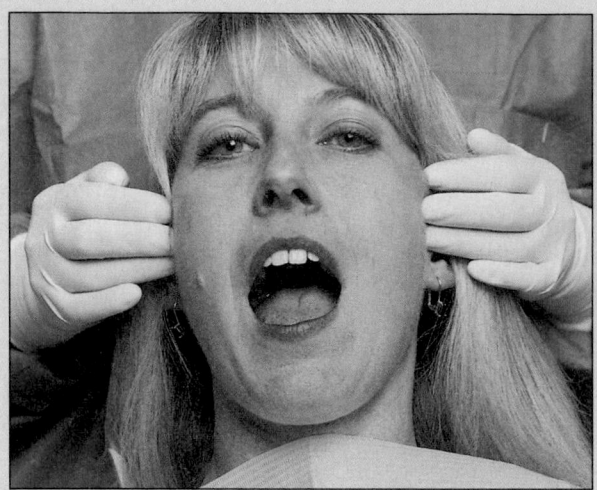

FIGURE 22-23
Examining the TMJ as the patient opens and closes their mouth.

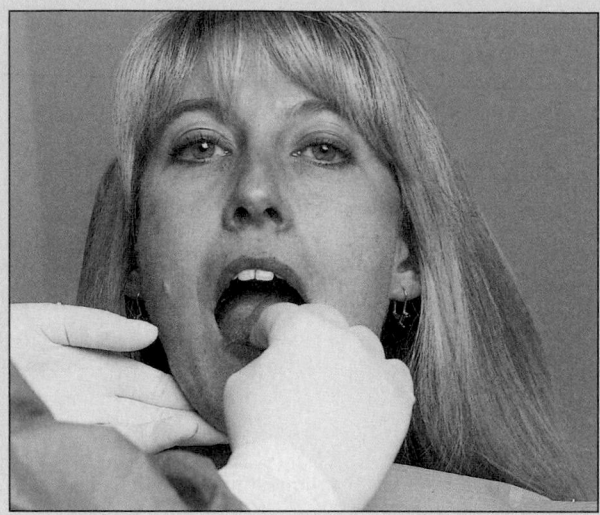

FIGURE 22-24
Examining the floor of the mouth.

5. Assistant records:
   ❏ Changes in cervical lymph nodes

   Palpates the temporomandibular joint by placing fingers on the joint as the patient opens and closes their mouth. The patient is asked to move their jaws in centric, lateral, protrusive, and retrusive positions (Figure 22-23).

6. Assistant records:
   ❏ Symptoms such as pain, tenderness, clicking, deviations in jaws position during opening and closing, and clicking and popping sounds

Assist with Intraoral Soft Tissue Examination Procedure
Equipment and Supplies
- PPE: examination gloves, mask, protective glasses, and protective clothing
- handwashing soap or hand sanitizer
- patient seated in dental chair
- prepared dental treatment area
- basic setup: Mouth mirror, explorer, and cotton pliers
- gauze squares
- tongue depressor (optional)
- patient record to document findings (pen and paper or computer)

Procedure Steps
1. Place patient in supine position for easier access, better intraoral visibility, and best position for transferring materials and instruments.

   Makes a visual assessment of the oral cavity for any obvious problems.

2. Assistant records:
   ❏ Oral lesions, abscessed teeth, and oral mucosa color changes

   Examines the tissues of the floor of the mouth. Supports the mandible with one hand while gently palpating with the fingers of the other hand on the ventral sides of the tongue and floor of mouth (Figure 22-24).

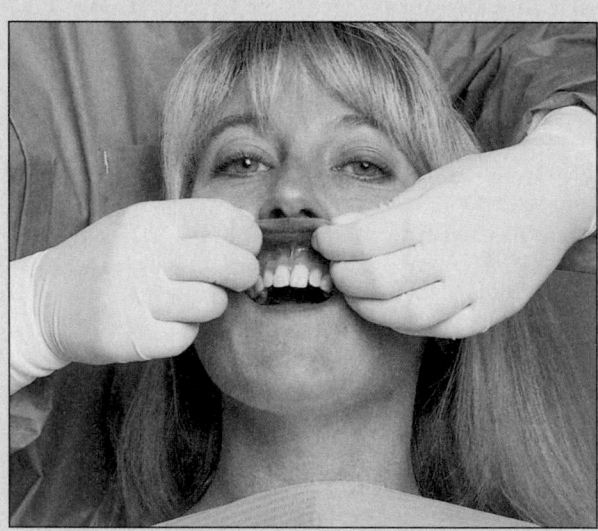

FIGURE 22-25
Examining the oral mucosa and the frenum.

3. Assistant records:
   ❏ Any swelling, tori, or other abnormalities

   Examines the oral mucosa and frena. Gently pull lips out using the thumbs and index fingers and inspects the oral mucosa and upper and lower frena. Palpates the oral mucosa in the lip and buccal areas for any abnormalities of the tissue (Figure 22-25).

4. Assistant records:
   ❏ Detection of lumps and attachment of the frena and flow of saliva

   Examines the tongue. Places a gauze square around the tip of the tongue and pulls the tongue to the side and visually inspects the posterior area on each side. Lifts tongue to examine the under portion of the tongue (Figure 22-26).

5. Assistant passes the dentist a gauze square and records:
   ❏ Appearance of any lesions or swelling and flow of saliva

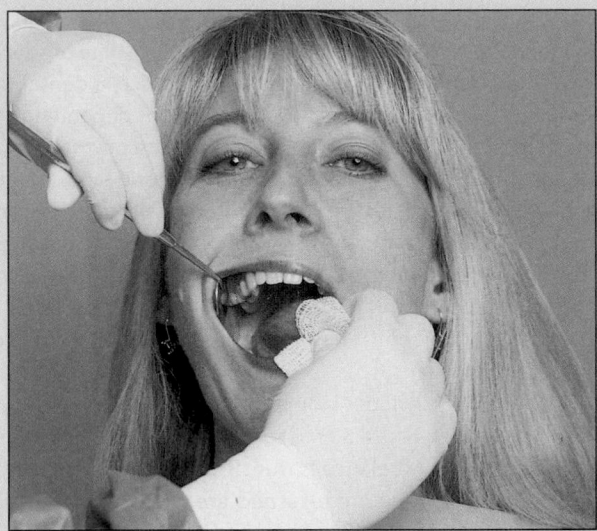

FIGURE 22-26
Examining the tongue using a gauze square on the tip of the tongue.

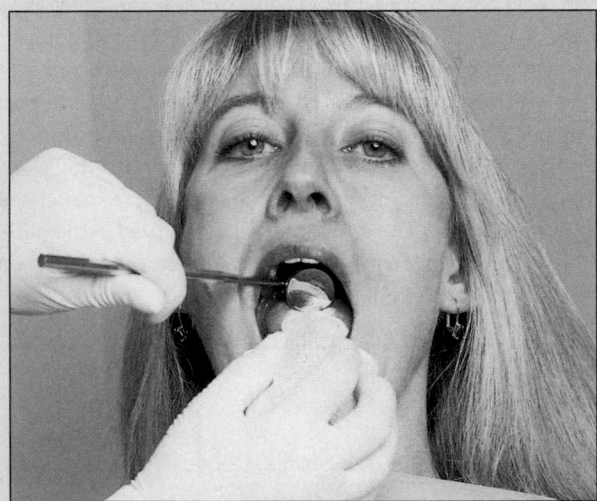

FIGURE 22-27
Examining the palate and the posterior of the tongue using a mouth mirror.

Examines the palate, uvula, oropharynx, and posterior of the tongue using the gauze square and mouth mirror. During this time, the patient is asked to "ahh" to expand the oropharynx to allow the operator to see clearly into the throat (Figure 22-27).

6. Assistant passes the mouth mirror and records:
   ❑ Color of the oral mucosa, papillae, anomalies, and presence or absence of coating on the tongue

Assist with Examination of the Occlusion and Teeth Procedure
Equipment and Supplies
- PPE: examination gloves, mask, protective glasses, and protective clothing
- handwashing soap or hand sanitizer

- patient seated in dental chair
- prepared dental treatment area
- air/water syringe tip
- HVE tip
- basic setup: Mouth mirror, explorer, and cotton pliers
- articulating holder and articulating paper
- clinical examination form to document findings (red/blue and black pencil or computer program)

Procedure Steps

Examines the patient's occlusion and for bad oral habits.

1. Assistant records findings on dental chart:
   ❑ Occlusal classification and special conditions occurring with occlusion
   ❑ Bad oral habits

Examines each tooth orally, confirms with radiographs, and verbalizes what needs to be charted.

2. Assistant passes mirror and explorer.
   ❑ Charts conditions of oral cavity using symbols on patient's dental chart
   ❑ Gently blows air from air/water syringe on tooth being examined as needed
   ❑ Blows air on mouth mirror when fogged from patient's breath

Examines periodontium and probes depths.

3. Assistant exchanges explorer and periodontal probe.
   ❑ Charts finding on periodontal chart
   ❑ Retrieves mirror and probes at completion of procedure

Completes additional diagnostic procedures as needed.

4. Assistant prepares and assists with requested procedures.
   ❑ Impressions and bite for study models (refer to Chapter 33 for material and procedure)
   ❑ Intraoral imaging equipment (refer to Procedure 22-4)

Explains to the patient that they will be scheduled for an appointment to return to clinic (RTC) for a dental prophylaxis and to discuss the treatment plan. Tells patient good bye and what a pleasure it was to meet them.

5. Assistant writes up procedure in Services Rendered.

Date	Services Rendered
02/12/XX	NP Ex, patient consent, HIPAA, medical/dental history, BP 120/80
	T=98.6F, P=80, R=18, fmx, extraoral and intraoral ex
	periodontal charting, intraoral images
	RTC: px and tx planning

6. Assistant dismisses and escorts patient to reception area (refer to Procedure 18-5).

Treatment Planning

The dental treatment (tx) plan is an organized approach to meeting all the dental needs of a patient. It allows the dentist to map out a plan for treating the patient that includes services needed, number of appointments necessary, the specific services to be provided at each appointment, and the patient's financial obligation. Effective communication of the plan to the patient is important if the patient is to understand their needs and the treatment plan. When discussing the treatment plan with the patient, incorporating dental radiographs and intraoral images enables the patient to have a better understanding of their needs. It is also important that the patient be presented with alternative treatment options as well as the implications of these options.

It is ultimately the decision of the patient to accept or reject all or part of the dental treatment plan. Dental team members should be available to answer all patient questions in a caring and empathetic manner. It is important that the patient feel that the dental team members are genuinely interested in them. The new patient is generally scheduled for prophylaxis (px) for their second appointment (refer to Chapter 24, "Dental Prophylaxis and Recare Appointment") if emergency care is not needed.

Financial Planning

At the conclusion of the dental treatment planning presentation, a dental team member should be present to discuss the financial implications of the dental treatment. For patients who have dental insurance, this will include discussion about the yearly deductible payment, copayments, and yearly limits. A pretreatment form can be submitted to the insurance company to find out in advance the patient's out-of-pocket costs. Many offices require all insurance copays and deductibles be paid at the time of service.

For those who do not have dental insurance, a dental team member may need to discuss financing options depending upon the needs of the patient. Some dentists require payment for service at the time services are rendered unless prior arrangements are made with the dentist or the business assistant. The dentist is not in the finance business and should not be expected to allow the patient to make payments. Many dental offices share information about dental financing programs that can assist the patient. Often the dentist has negotiated with a financing company for their patients.

Treatment that includes laboratory fabrication of dental appliances typically requires a 50% deposit at the time of the impression. The remaining balance is due at the time the appliance is delivered. Checks that are returned are subject to a returned check fee. Failed appointments may also be charged a fee and be included on the patient's treatment plan. It is important to have the patient examine all financial policies of the dental office at the new patient appointment and sign a financial agreement. Failure to pay for treatment and a history of failed appointments may result in the dentist refusing to continue treatment.

As with the dental treatment plan presentation, it is important that dental team members use effective communication during these conversations to avoid confusion and to portray a caring, empathetic attitude. All conversations regarding financial planning should include documentation that is stored in the patient's record for future reference, and also a hard copy should be signed and provided to the patient.

Chapter Summary

Dental charting provides legal documentation of the patient's oral cavity. The correct numbering system and charting symbols ensure proper documentation. Therefore, accuracy in charting is critical.

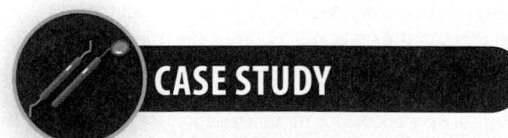

CASE STUDY

Dwayne Allen, a 50-year-old male, was in the dental office for a new patient dental examination. Upon taking his blood pressure, the dental assistant documented that Dwayne had a systolic pressure of 150 and a diastolic pressure of 90. A new patient examination and dental charting was completed on Mr. Allen. Interpret the charting using Figure 22-28.

Case Study Review

1. Which tooth (teeth) need(s) to be extracted?

2. Which teeth have dental caries?

3. What condition is charted between tooth #8 and #9?

4. Which tooth has periodontal pockets that are greater than the normal healthy depth?

5. Is Mr. Allen's BP within normal range? Should this reading be brought to the attention of the dentist?

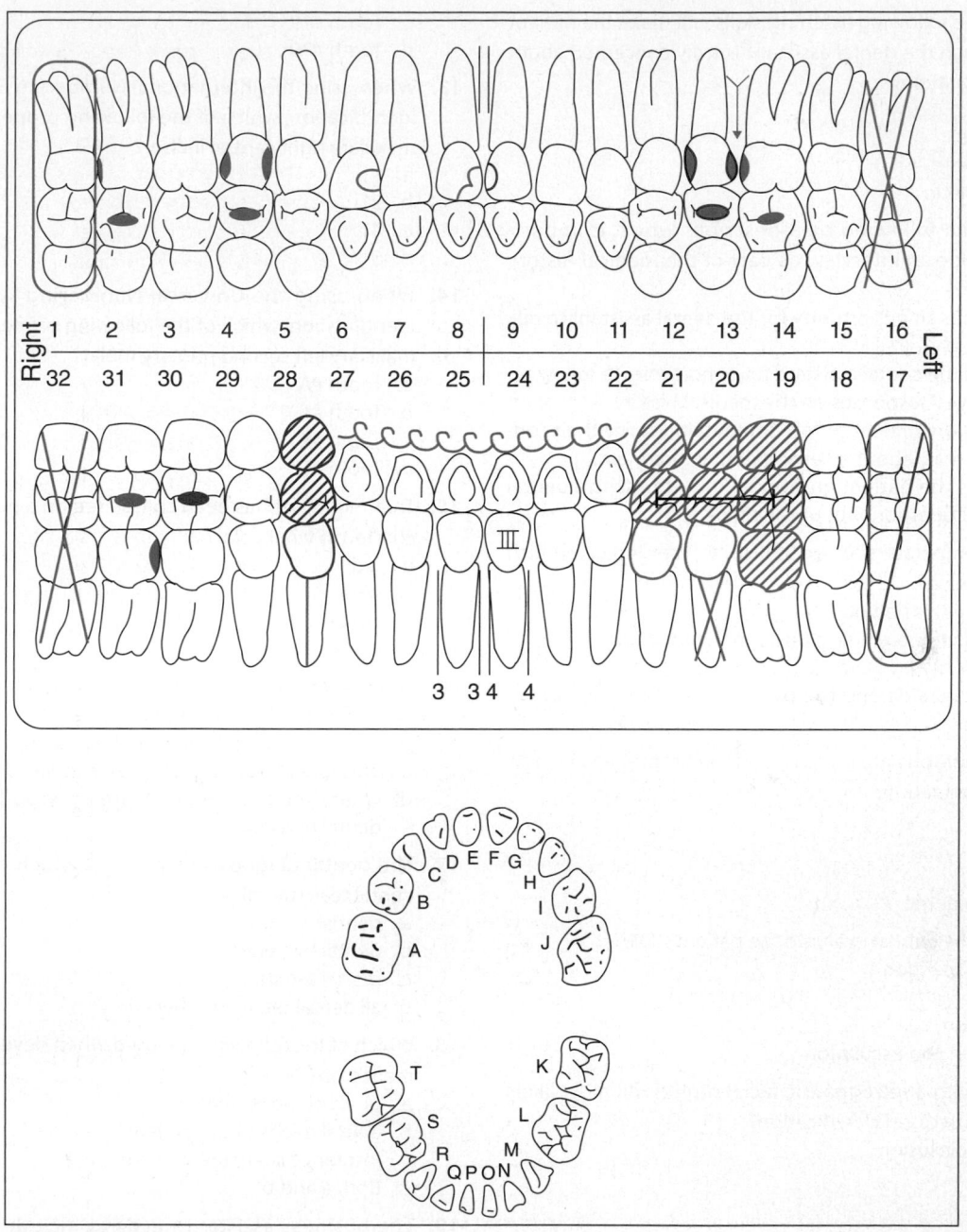

FIGURE 22-28
Charting using the anatomical chart and the universal system.

Review Questions

Multiple Choice

1. Which of the following procedures is generally not completed during a limited/emergency examination?
   a. medical history
   b. dental diagnosis
   c. financial planning
   d. full mouth dental charting

2. Information collected during a comprehensive new patient examination is known as the:
   a. baseline information.
   b. patient treatment plan.
   c. initial new patient information.
   d. individualized patient treatment plan.

3. Which of the following is not a part of the comprehensive new patient examination armamentarium?
   a. dental scaler
   b. mouth mirror
   c. saliva ejector
   d. periodontal probe

4. Which of the following listening skills will make the patient feel as though the dental assistant is truly concerned about his or her situation?
   a. friendly
   b. attentive
   c. empathetic
   d. sympathetic

5. Which of the following best describes why it is important to include an interview as part of the medical history procedure?
   a. It provides an opportunity for the dental assistant to talk with the patient.
   b. It allows the dental assistant an opportunity to follow up on any "yes" responses on the medical history.
   c. It allows the patient to talk and possibly voice their concerns or fears about receiving dental treatment.
   d. It allows the patient an opportunity to ask the dental assistant questions about the office.

6. A patient temperature above 99°F (37°C) may indicate which of the following?
   a. The patient is nervous.
   b. The patient is breathing through their mouth.
   c. The patient may have an infection in their body.
   d. It is hot outside and the patient is just hot from being outdoors.

7. What radiographs are indicated for a comprehensive new patient examination?
   a. BWX
   b. FMX
   c. PA
   d. cephalometric

8. How does the dentist evaluate the patient's TMJ?
   a. visual inspection
   b. palpation
   c. osculation
   d. palpation and osculation

9. A patient with a retrognathic facial profile will most likely have which occlusal classification?
   a. normal occlusion
   b. Class I
   c. Class II
   d. Class III

10. When the mouth is divided into quadrants, tooth #15 is located in which of the following quadrants?
    a. maxillary left quadrant
    b. maxillary right quadrant
    c. mandibular left quadrant
    d. mandibular right quadrant

11. In which sextant is tooth #25 located?
    a. mandibular left posterior
    b. mandibular anterior
    c. mandibular posterior
    d. maxillary anterior

12. When using the universal numbering system for tooth identification, which of the following properly identifies the mandibular left first permanent molar?
    a. Tooth #3
    b. Tooth #14

c. Tooth #19
d. Tooth #30

13. When using the International Numbering System for tooth identification, which of the following properly identifies the maxillary right central incisor?
    a. 11
    b. 21
    c. 41
    d. 51

14. When using the Universal Numbering system for tooth identification, which of the following properly identifies the maxillary left second primary molar?
    a. Tooth #A
    b. Tooth #J
    c. Tooth #K
    d. Tooth #T

15. Treatment that has been completed on a patient is typically charted in what color?
    a. red
    b. blue
    c. white
    d. black

16. The purpose of dental diagnosis is to identify:
    a. the wants/desires of the patient.
    b. the unmet dental needs of the patient.
    c. how quickly dental treatment can be completed.
    d. what dental procedures are covered by the patient's dental insurance.

17. The dental diagnosis is made by which of the following dental team members?
    a. dentist
    b. dental hygienist
    c. dental assistant
    d. all dental team members

18. Which of the following are used when developing the treatment plan?
    a. goals of the patient
    b. dental needs of the patient
    c. insurance coverage of the patient
    d. Both a and b

19. The business assistant needs to include a conversation about the patient's dental insurance during the financial planning appointment to include all EXCEPT:
    a. yearly deductible.
    b. copayments.
    c. monthly payments.
    d. yearly limits.

20. In treatment plans that include the fabrication of a dental appliance at a dental laboratory, the patient may be expected to:
    a. pay for the complete service when the impression is taken.
    b. pay for 50% of the total cost at the time the impression is taken.
    c. pay for the complete service when the appliance is delivered.
    d. make regular payments to the dentist.

Critical Thinking

1. A patient has had a negative experience with their teeth in the past. What impact could this have on the current treatment? What role can the dental assistant play in making this a positive experience for the patient?

2. If a dental assistant observes a patient walking with an unsteady gait to the dental treatment room but finds no indication of this symptom in the patient's medical and dental history, what should the assistant do?

3. A young adult broke their upper teeth at a drinking fountain, from the middle of the biting edge to the middle of each front tooth in an upside-down V pattern. Which surfaces, classifications, and teeth numbers would be involved if using the Universal System for numbering? The International System?

Key Terms

Term and Pronunciation	Meaning of Root and Word Parts	Definition
abutment (*uh*-**buht**-m*uh* nt)	**abut** = to adjoin on something at one end **ment** = a means	a tooth or tooth root that supports or stabilizes a bridge, denture, or other prosthetic appliance
appliance (*uh*-**plahy**-*uh*ns)	**apply** = to put to use **-ance** = indicating an action or quality	any device that helps with the patient treatment plan; help to repair damaged teeth, replace missing teeth and straighten crooked teeth
attrition (uh-**trish**-uhn)	**attrite** = worn by rubbing **-ion** = denoting action or condition	tooth wear caused by tooth-to-tooth contact resulting in loss of tooth tissue (incisal/occlusal surfaces)
atypical (ey-**tip**-i-k*uh* l)	**a** = not **typical** = normal, conforming to a particular type	not conforming to the normal types, irregular, abnormal
auscultation (aw-skuhl-**tey**-shuh n)	**auris** = ear **ausculate** = hear with attention	act of listening directly or through a stethescope
baseline (**beys**-lahyn)	**base** = a starting point, anything from a process as a point of measurement **line** = a course or method of action	a basic standard or level; guideline: *to establish a baseline for future studies*; a specific value or values that can serve as a comparison or control
bridge (brij)	**bridge** = connecting structure	appliance that connects the gap created by one or more missing teeth; made up of one or more crowns for the teeth on either side of the gap
bruxism (**bruhk**-siz-*uh*m)	**brux** = to clench and grind teeth **-ism** = denoting action or condition	involuntary habit of teeth grinding
cognitive (**kog**-ni-tiv)	**cognitive** = pertaining to the act or process of knowing	pertaining to the act or process of knowing, perceiving, remembering, and so on; of or relating to cognition: *cognitive development; cognitive functioning*
comprehensive (kom-pri-**hen**-siv)	**comprehend** = to understand the nature or meaning of **-ive** = expressing function	large scope; covering or involving much
demographics (dem-*uh*-**graf**-iks)	**demo-** = indicating people or population **graph** = record **-ics** = having characteristics of	patient demographics include patient name, date of birth, address, phone number, doctor information, SSN, sex, emergency contact, guarantor, insurance information
denture (**den**-cher)	**dent** = tooth **-ure** = indicating process or result	an artificial replacement of one or several of the teeth (partial) or all of the teeth (full denture)
diagnosis (dahy-*uh* g-**noh**-sis)	**diagnose** = to determine identity of a disease, illness **-osis** = indicating a process	the process of determining by examination the nature of a diseased condition
empathetic (em-p*uh*-**thet**-ik)	**empathy** = power of understanding another person's feelings **-etic** = pertaining to	of, pertaining to, or characterized by empathy: *a sensitive, empathetic school counselor*
examination (ig-zam-*uh*-**ney**-shuh n)	**exam** = to observe, test a person's body to evaluate general health or determine the cause of illness **-ine** = pertaining to **-tion** = expressing action	the act of examining; inspection; inquiry; investigation

(Continues)

Term and Pronunciation	Meaning of Root and Word Parts	Definition
forensic (f*uh*-**ren**-sik)	**forum** = a court of law **-ensis** = pertaining to	forensic dentistry; application of dental knowledge to the solution of legal issue in civil and criminal matters; dental radiographs and patient records can used in identifying a person
hypertension (hahy-per-**ten**-sh*uh*n)	**hyper** = over, above **tense** = stressed tightly **-ion** = denoting condition	abnormally high blood pressure that may eventually cause health problems like heart attack and stroke
hypotension (hahy-p*uh*-**ten**-shuhn)	**hypo** = decreased or lowered **tense** = stressed tightly **-ion** = denoting condition	abnormally low blood pressure; term used only when blood pressure has fallen so far that enough blood can no longer reach the brain causing dizziness and fainting
impacted (im-**pak**-tid)	**impact** = impinge; press closely into something **-ed** = indicating result from action	a tooth so confined in its socket it is incapable of normal eruption
implant (im-**plant**)	**im** = in **plant** = to place firmly in position	to insert or graft (tissue, organ or inert substance) into the body for repairing or replacement of a body part
intraoral images (in-tr*uh*-**awr**-*uh*l)	**intra** = within **oral** = mouth **image** = physical likeness or picture representation	an intraoral camera that takes an x-ray of the outside of the gum or tooth
litigation (lit-i-**gey**-shuhn)	**litigate** = to carry on a lawsuit **-ion** = denoting action	the process of taking legal action to determine a legal question or matter
palpation (**pal**-pey-sh*uh*n)	**palpate** = to examine by touch; purpose of diagnosing **-tion** = expressing action	a method of clinical examination using gentle pressure of the fingers to detect growths, changes in the size of underlying organs, and unusual tissue reactions to pressure
pathologic (path-*uh*-**loj**-ik)	**path** = disease **-ology** = study of **-ic** = pertaining to	of or pertaining to pathology; caused by or involving disease; morbid
periodontal charting (per-ee-*uh*-**don**-tl) (**chahrt**-ing)	**peri-** = about, around **odont** = tooth **-al** = pertaining to **chart** = a graphic representation **-ing** = expressing action	part of a dental chart where the measurements of the sulcus and periodontal pockets are taken around each tooth are charted
pontic (**pon**-tik)	**pons** = bridge like formation connecting two disjoined parts of a structure or organ **-ic** = pertaining to	an artificial tooth in a bridge
premedication (pree-med-i-**key**-sh*uh*n)	**pre** = before, in advance of **medicate** = to treat with medicine **-tion** = expressing action	the practice of giving drugs to a patient before anesthesia to relieve anxiety, diminish body reactions to pain, or improve postoperative comfort
radiolucency (rey-dee-oh-**loo**-s*uh*ncee)	**radio** = dealing with radiant energy **lucent** = translucent, clear	almost entirely transparent to radiation; almost entirely invisible in x-ray radiographs
tympanic thermometer (tim-**pan**-ik) (ther-**mom**-i-ter)	**tympanum** = middle ear **-ic** = pertaining to **thermo-** = heat, hot **-meter** = instrument measuring **degree,** quantity	digital ear thermometer uses an infrared ray to measure the temperature inside the ear canal; is +0.5°F (−17.5°C) than an oral temperature
veneer (v*uh*-**neer**)	**veneer** = to face or cover an object with a material that is more desirable	a layer of tooth colored material, usually porcelain or acrylic resin, attached to and covering the surface of a metal crown or natural tooth structure

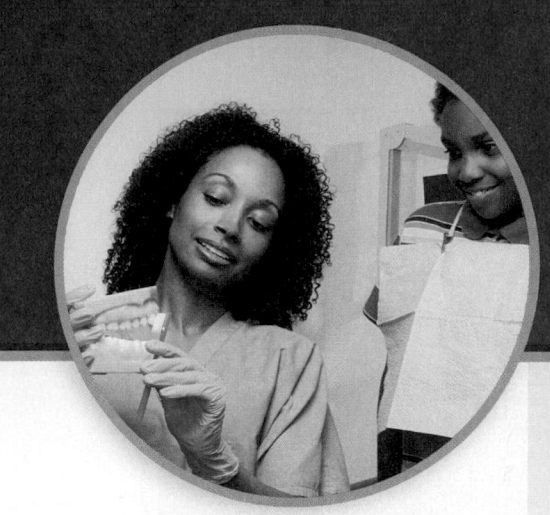

Anesthesia and Sedation

Specific Instructional Objectives

At the completion of this chapter, you will be able to meet these objectives:

1. Use terms presented in this chapter.
2. Defend the importance of pain control.
3. Compare and contrast local anesthetics and topical anesthetics.
4. Describe the purpose of non-injectable local anesthetics.
5. State the rationale for vasoconstrictors.
6. Compare and contrast the different concentrations vasoconstrictor in a local anesthetic cartridge.
7. Compare and contrast the three types of dental oral anesthetic techniques.
8. Identify the needle insertion site for the block injections discussed in the chapter.
9. Describe the supplemental local anesthetic techniques.
10. State the rationale for local anesthetic reversal agents.
11. Discuss the advantages of a computer controlled local anesthetic delivery system.
12. Discuss the complications that may occur due to local anesthesia administration.
13. Outline the steps in preventing a medical emergency related to local anesthesia administration.
14. Identify the signs and symptoms of a reaction to epinephrine from a local anesthetic cartridge.
15. List the armamentarium necessary for administration of dental anesthesia.
16. Identify the parts of the local anesthetic syringe.
17. Identify the parts of the local anesthetic cartridge.
18. Identify the parts of the local anesthetic needle.
19. State the correct sequence of steps in assembling a local anesthetic syringe.
20. State what should be included when making a chart entry for local anesthesia administration.
21. Discuss the specifics of the Needlestick Safety Act.
22. Outline the CDC recommendations for postexposure management.
23. Compare and contrast the different types of sedation.
24. State the beneficial effects of nitrous oxide on a patient.
25. List the signs and symptoms of Stage I analgesia.
26. Discuss nitrous oxide related safety measures.
27. Outline the steps in assisting with nitrous oxide administration.

Pain Management

Many people feel such anxiety or nervousness when visiting their dentist that they actually avoid being treated. Dentists want to make everyone feel comfortable and eliminate as much discomfort and anxiety from their patients as possible. There are several pain management options that help alleviate this problem. One of the most common is *anesthesia*. Anesthesia is the loss of bodily feeling due to receiving a type of medication called an *anesthetic*. This loss of feeling can be just in one area (local) or throughout the body (general) depending on the type(s) of anesthetic administered. Two main types are local anesthetics and general anesthetics.

Local Anesthetics

Local anesthetics are drugs used to produce a loss of feeling in only specified areas of the body. Dental local anesthesia is produced by applying or injecting the local anesthetic in a specific area of the oral cavity. The suffix "-caine" is used to indicate local anesthetic. All local anesthetics currently in use are synthetic. In dentistry, there are two commonly used types of anesthetics: anesthetics that are topically placed on the tissue (topical anesthetic) and anesthetics that are injected into specific nerve branches (injectable local anesthetic). When a local anesthetic is administered, sensory impulses, such as pain, touch, and thermal change, are temporarily blocked. Local anesthesia only works when it contacts the nerve fibers carrying impulses to the brain or the small nerve endings picking up sensations in the tissue. After the local anesthetic is injected into the tissue it *diffuses* (spreads) into the nerve fibers and *permeates* (spreads or covers throughout) the nerve fibers to then block the normal action of the nerves until the bloodstream carries the anesthetic away and the sensations return.

Topical Anesthetics

A topical anesthetic is placed directly on top of the mucous membrane. It anesthetizes the outer surface of mucosal tissues by blocking nerve transmission from tiny sensory nerve endings located near the surface. The purpose of **topical** anesthesia is to temporarily numb the soft tissue where the injection of the local anesthetic will be administered (injection site). The topical anesthetic makes the injection much more tolerable. It reduces or eliminates the stinging sensation felt when the needle of the syringe enters the oral mucosa. It also lessens pain from ulcers or injuries to mucosa and decreases the gag reflex in the soft palate during procedures touching the soft palate. To assist effectively or place the topical anesthetic correctly, the dental assistant must know the injection sites. Injection sites and placement of topical anesthesia will be discussed later in this chapter.

Topical anesthetic agents come in many forms; gels, ointments, patches, liquids, and sprays (Figures 23-1A, B, and C). The composition of topical anesthetics is classified as ester or amide local anesthetic. Benzocaine is an example of an ester topical anesthetic, and lidocaine is an example of an amide topical anesthetic. Which agent is used depends on the desired result and the dentist's preference. Topical gels and ointments are the most frequently used topical anesthetics in the dental office. They are

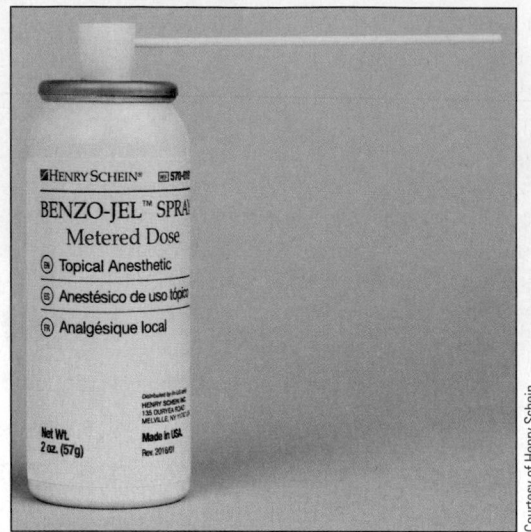

FIGURE 23-1A
Metered dose anesthetic spray.

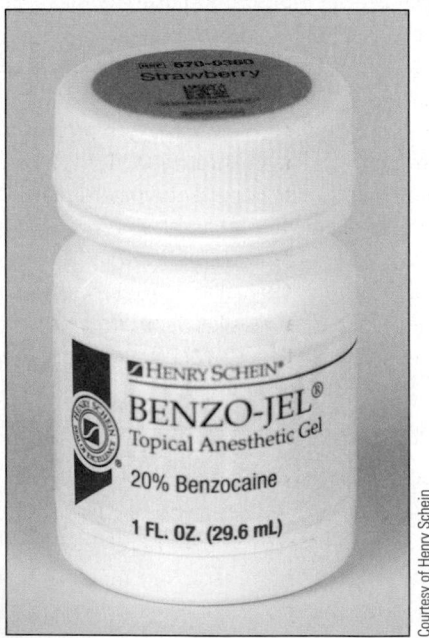

FIGURE 23-1B
Topical anesthetic gel.

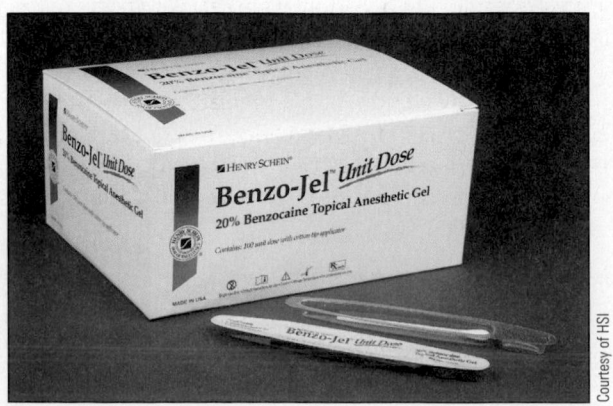

FIGURE 23-1C
Single dose topical anesthesia.

usually placed on the oral mucosa using a cotton tipped applicator. For the gel or ointment to have its full affect, the mucosa should be dried with a gauze square and the anesthetic must be left on the oral tissue for the time designated by the manufacturer's directions (generally 30–60 seconds).

Topical oral cavity patches are a newer product. When a patch is placed on the oral mucosa it provides anesthesia within 2 to 5 minutes depending on anesthetic concentration and location. This product adheres to the gingiva, delivers consistent release of anesthesia, and can be used for injection sites. It is also very effective in numbing sores from dentures and ulcers. Patches can be applied for 15 minutes, and the area may remain numb for up to 60 minutes.

Liquids and spray agents are generally applied to larger areas of the oral mucosa (Figure 23-1A). They can be used in the oropharynx to help control a strong gag reflex. This becomes particularly helpful when there is a need for an impression or intraoral radiographs.

The concentration of solution for topical anesthetics is greater than the concentration of solution used for local anesthetics. For example, lidocaine topical anesthetic is a 5 or 10% concentration, while the lidocaine used as a local anesthetic is a 2% concentration. Due to the higher concentrations of the topical anesthetics, there is a greater risk for allergic or toxic reactions to occur than there is with local or general anesthetics. Topical anesthetics may also contain flavorings that patients may be allergic to, such as banana, mint, or cherry. Dental assistants must know application sites and how to apply the anesthetic. In some states, the dental assistant can apply the topical anesthetic for the dentist before an injection. The dental assistant should be familiar with the scope of practice regulations in their state.

Noninjectable Anesthesia

Noninjectable anesthesia is needle-free and utilizes a topical anesthetic that combines lidocaine and prilocaine. It can put patients at ease by eliminating the needle, and it begins working in as little as 30 seconds. Oraqix® is a noninjectable anesthesia manufactured by Dentsply Pharmaceutical. The agent is supplied in individually packed cartridges, blunt tipped applicators, and its own autoclavable dispenser.

Oraqix® is used for subgingival anesthetic in areas requiring localized anesthesia in periodontal pockets during scaling or root planing procedures. At room temperature it is an oil solution that is easily applied into the periodontal pockets requiring treatment. At body temperature it turns into an elastic gel that remains in place while the anesthetic takes effect. The anesthetic effect has a duration of approximately 20 minutes. Up to five cartridges can be used in one dental appointment as the effect wears off.

Dental Local Anesthetics

Injectable local anesthetic is the most widely used method of pain control in dentistry. This method proves to be safe, reliable, and effective. Dental anesthetics temporarily numb the teeth, alveolar bone, and soft issues in the area anesthetized and do not travel throughout the body or cause unconsciousness. With the use of local anesthetics, the dentist can prevent the patient from feeling pain or discomfort at the surgical site during dental procedures.

Local anesthetics can be divided into two groups: esters and amides. Procaine, which was the first ester type of local anesthesia developed, became the most common anesthetic solution used for at least four decades. There was a high incidence of allergies to the preservative ingredients (para-aminobenzoic acid, or PABA) with the ester local anesthetics. Most people who had allergic reactions experienced temporary itching and a skin rash; on rare occasions asthma-like attacks occurred and in the most extreme cases anaphylaxis. For these reasons, procaine and other esters are no longer used as injectable dental anesthetics, and other types of anesthetics have been developed. There are many amide local anesthetics available for use in the dental office. Of the local anesthetics, lidocaine (Xylocaine) is one of the most commonly used amides by dentists. Lidocaine was introduced without PABA. Local injectable anesthetic solution is supplied in pre-measured sterile *cartridges* (Figure 23-2). Table 23-1 provides details on commonly used amide dental local anesthetics.

Currently, esters are only used for topical anesthesia in dentistry. Because they do not enter the bloodstream, they normally do not produce adverse reactions. Reactions to topical esters are extremely rare, and if they occur they remain as a localized reaction at the site of application. Amides very rarely cause allergic reactions and are used as injectable local anesthetic. Skin testing by an allergy specialist can confirm allergies to local anesthetics. For confirmed allergies, diphenhydramine may be recommended as a local anesthetic for procedures of short duration.

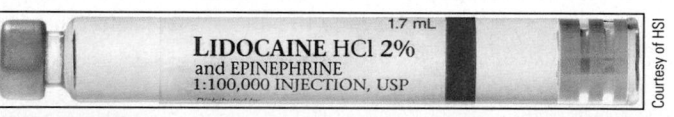

FIGURE 23-2
Local anesthetic cartridge.

TABLE 23-1 Commonly Used Dental Local Anesthetics

Generic Name	Brand Name	Vasoconstrictor Concentration
articaine 4%	Septocaine	1:100,000 and 1:200,00 epinephrine
bupivacaine 0.5%	Marcaine	1:200,000 epinephrine
lidocaine 2%	Xylocaine	Plain 1:50,000 epinephrine 1:100,000 epinephrine
prilocaine 4% plain	Citanest	None
prilocaine 4%	Citanest Forte	1:200,000 epinephrine
mepivacaine 3%	Carbocaine Polocaine Isocaine	None

Anesthesia is obtained by injecting the local anesthetic in close proximity of nerves near the site of treatment. The anesthetic spreads into the nerve and temporarily blocks the nerve membrane's ability to create an impulse and send the message that there is pain. The onset time is two to ten minutes depending on the type of local anesthetic used. The anesthetic effect will last 30–60 minutes in most cases depending on the type of local anesthetic used. The absorption of anesthetic is a consideration in the selection of the best solution in regards to onset and duration. All anesthetics are manufactured with weak bases (pK_a of 7.5 to 9.5) for optimal onset of blocking nerve conduction. The absorption of the anesthetic also depends on the particular anesthetic's solubility, which affects the ease of penetrating the nerve cell membranes and the duration of the blockage of nerve sensation. The local anesthetic solution is injected into the soft tissues. To be effective, it must contact the sensory nerve fibers. Once the anesthetic solution anesthetizes the nerve, sensations cannot pass through to register the feeling of pain in the brain. The tissues and teeth in the affected area can be operated on without the patient experiencing pain.

Vasodilation is one of the properties of local anesthetics. Vasodilation results in blood flow increasing at the site of the injection. As a result, the effect of "numbness" from the local anesthetic dissipates into the tissue space and the blood stream carries the solution away. The area will then regain normal function, and sensation will return. There are three categories of expected duration: short, intermediate, and long. Table 23-2 provides details about the duration of each commonly used dental local anesthetic.

Most dental treatment requires more than 30 minutes. Because this is longer than the effective duration of many anesthetics, vasoconstrictors may be added to the anesthetic solution to lengthen the time the anesthetic is effective for longer procedures. A vasoconstrictor constricts (decreases the size of) the blood vessels. Constricted blood vessels keep bleeding to a minimum and help keep the anesthetic from being carried away from the intended area at a slower pace. This allows the patient to stay numb for a longer period of time. Vasoconstrictors also increase the depth of the anesthetic effect.

The absorption and duration of the local anesthetic is also affected by the pH of the patient's tissue and vascularity of the tissue at the injection. When a localized infection is present, the tissue pH drops, decreasing absorption and duration of the local anesthetic. In cartridges that contain epinephrine, the amount of vasoconstrictor is written as a ratio of vasoconstrictor to anesthetic solution. The ratio of 1:100,000 is one of the more commonly used concentrations where there is one part epinephrine to 100,000 parts of solution. If a lower concentration of epinephrine is warranted, a 1:200,000 concentration in which half the amount of vasoconstrictor is present is often the anesthetic of choice. A 1:50,000 concentration of epinephrine is double that of 1:100,000 epinephrine concentration.

The most commonly used concentration of vasoconstrictor (1:100,000) will anesthetize the average pulp in less than 3 to 5 minutes; the pulp will stay numb for 60 minutes, and the soft tissue will remain anesthetized for 3 to 4 hours. Other vasoconstrictor concentrations are 1:50,000 and 1:200,000. Local anesthetics are also supplied plain (no epinephrine). The local anesthetic premeasured cartridges are presterilized and often come in sealed units called blister packs (Figure 23-3A).

Color Coding of Local Anesthetic Cartridges

Manufacturers of local anesthetics that want to carry the ADA Seal of Acceptance use a uniform cartridge colorcoding system (Figure 23-3B) for identifying local anesthetics and local anesthetic/vasoconstrictor combinations. This color coding, which standardizes local anesthetics and local anesthetic/vasoconstrictor combinations from manufacturer to manufacturer, includes a band near the stopper end of the cartridge. All caps on the cartridges are silver, and all stoppers are black regardless of type of

TABLE 23-2 Short, Intermediate, and Long-Acting Local Anesthetics

Category	Onset of Action	Pulpal and Soft Tissue Anesthesia Duration	Local Anesthetic Name
Short acting	Within 2 minutes	5–10 minutes pulpal anesthesia if given as an infiltration and 1 hour to 1.5 hours of soft tissue anesthesia	3% Mepivacaine
Intermediate acting	Within 2 minutes	1 hour to 1.5 hours pulpal anesthesia; 3 to 3.5 hours soft tissue anesthesia	4% Articaine 1:100,000 epinephrine
Intermediate acting	Within 4 minutes	45 minutes to 1 hour pulpal anesthesia; 3 to 4 hours soft tissue anesthesia	4% Articaine 1:200,00 epinephrine
Intermediate acting	Within 4 minutes	10 minutes pulpal anesthesia when administered as an infiltration; 45 minutes to 1 hour soft issue anesthesia. 1 to 2 hours pulpal anesthesia when administered as a block; 2 to 4 hours soft tissue anesthesia	4% Prilocaine 1:200,000 epinephrine
Intermediate acting	Within 2 minutes	Only to be used for infiltrations; no pulpal anesthesia	2% Lidocaine 1:50,000 epinephrine
Intermediate acting	Within 3 minutes	1 to 2 hours pulpal anesthesia as a block; 3 to 4 hours soft tissue anesthesia	2% Lidocaine 1:100,000 epinephrine
Long acting	Within 10 minutes	Long acting: pulpal anesthesia, 1.5 to 3 hours; up to 12 hours soft tissue anesthesia	.5% Bupivacaine 1:200,000 epinephrine

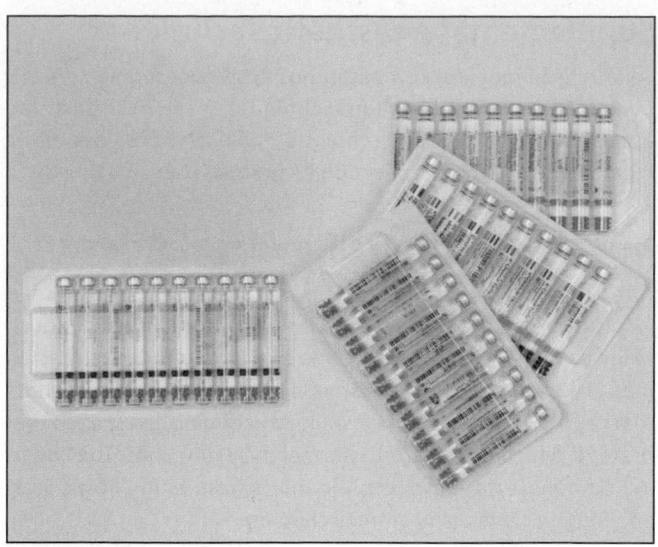

FIGURE 23-3A
Various anesthetic cartridges in blister packs.

Anesthesia Color Coding	
Anesthetic	**Color**
2% Lidocaine with epinephrine 1:100,000	
2% Lidocaine with epinephrine 1:50,000	
Lidocaine plain	
Mepivacaine 2% with levonordefrin 1:20,000	
Mepivacaine 3%	
Prilocaine 4% with epinephrine 1:200,000	
Prilocaine 4%	
Bupivacaine 4% with epinephrine	
Articaine 4% with epinephrine	

FIGURE 23-3B
Local anesthesia color coding.

local anesthetic or epinephrine concentration. The lettering on the cartridge is black and is durable print that is not removed with normal handling.

Currently, epinephrine is the only vasoconstrictor used in dental local anesthetic cartridges. It is extremely important to have an updated medical history on all patients as vasoconstrictors may cause an adverse reaction in some patients with heart disease, high blood pressure (hypertension), or hyperthyroidism. Some patients may be sensitive to exogenous epinephrine. The patient may have symptoms including tachycardia, shaking, cold sweat, tachypnea, dizziness, lightheadedness, and tingling in fingers, toes, and lips. These are all signs of an adrenaline rush. Epinephrine is the same as adrenaline that your body produces.

Your body naturally produces adrenaline to prepare you for fight-or-flight situations, which increase the heart rate and blood pressure so you can run faster. As a result, one cannot be allergic to epinephrine but may be sensitive to exogenous administration of epinephrine.

Injection Techniques

Three types of injections are given for dental procedures: (1) local infiltration (Figure 23-4), (2) field block (Figure 23-5), and (3) nerve block (Figure 23-6). The type of injection is determined by the injection site and the innervation of the area or specific tooth. The sites are divided between the maxillary and mandibular arches (Figures 23-7 and 23-8). The various injection techniques are provided in Tables 23-3 and 23-4. (Refer to Chapter 5 for divisions of the trigeminal nerve.)

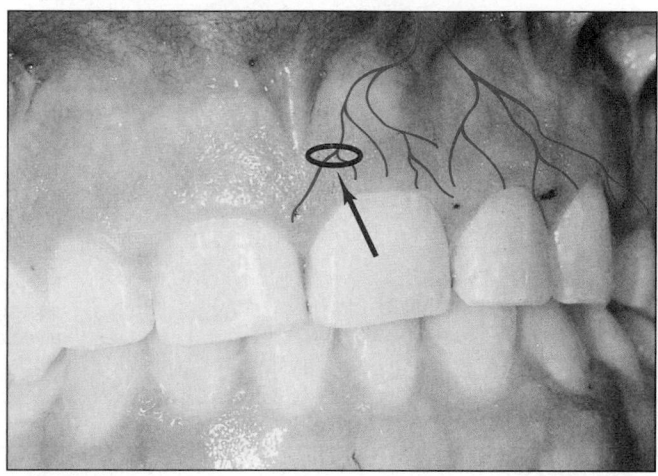

FIGURE 23-4
Area anesthetized with a local infiltration.

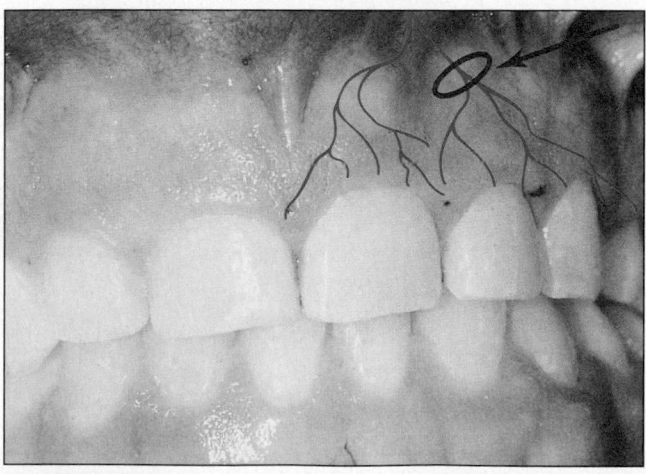

FIGURE 23-5
Area anesthetized with a field block injection.

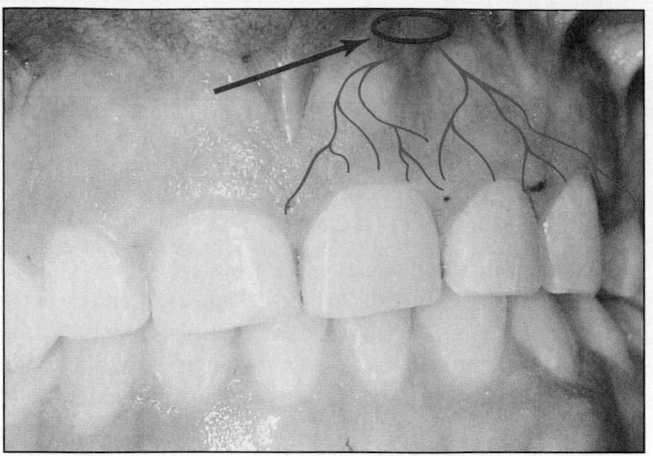

FIGURE 23-6
Area anesthetized with a nerve block injection.

Supplemental Anesthetic Techniques

Various techniques for administering anesthetics supplement the infiltration and block injection techniques or can be used as the only anesthetic injection technique. Table 23-5 provides detail regarding supplemental injection techniques used in dentistry.

Local Anesthetic Reversal Agent

After a patient's dental appointment, the patient is dismissed with postoperative numbness that may linger for several hours. Many patients must return to work, school, and other daily activities. The effects of a local anesthetic include lingering numbness that causes drooling, crooked smile, and diminished speech that makes it difficult to return to normal daily functions. The lingering numbness may also result in injury from biting lips, cheek, and tongue, particularly in small children.

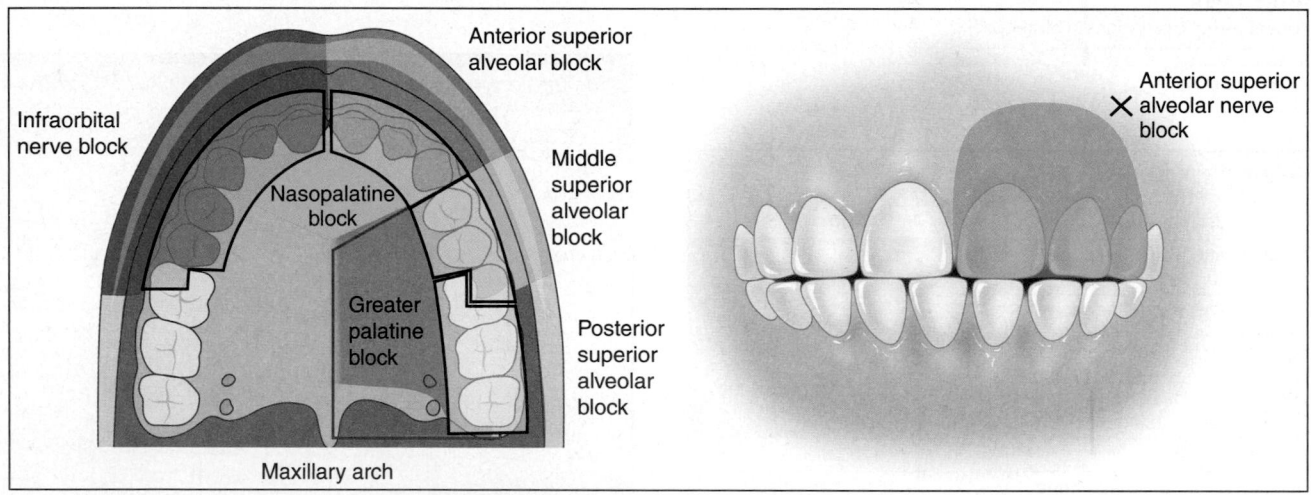

FIGURE 23-7
Maxillary nerve block areas anesthetized and insertion site for anterior superior nerve block.

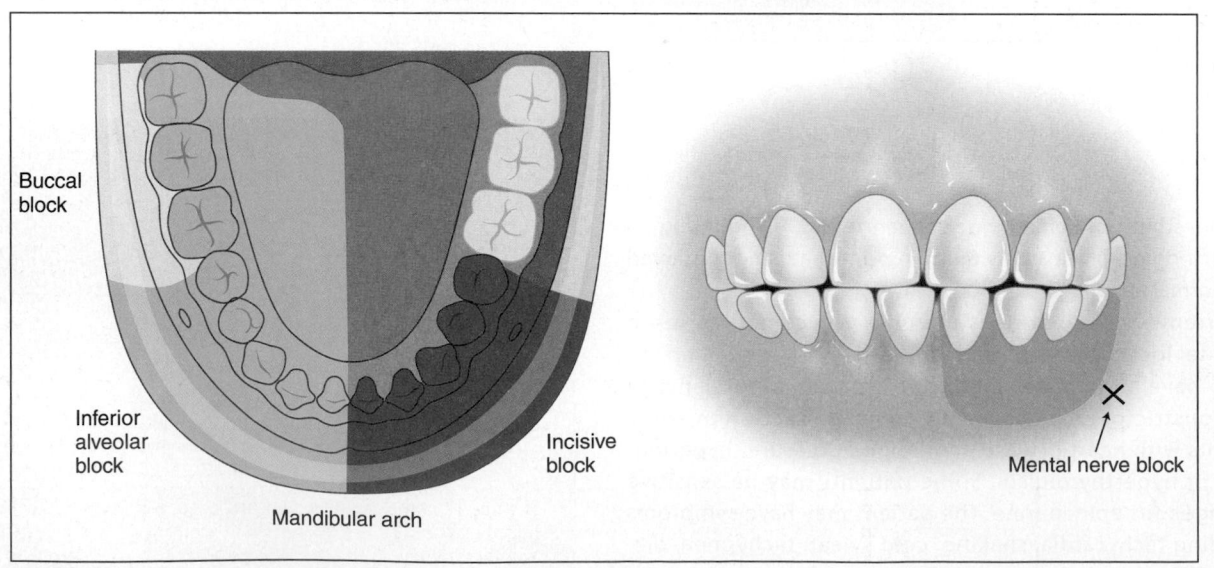

FIGURE 23-8
Mandibular nerve block areas anesthetized and insertion site for mental nerve block.

TABLE 23-3 Maxillary Local Anesthetic Injection Sites and Areas Anesthetized

Name of Injection	Affected Teeth/Tissues	Needle Insertion Site	Deposition Site of Local Anesthetic Solution
infiltration	Soft tissue anesthesia only of area injected—for example, the interdental papilla for scaling and root planing, soft tissue incision for a biopsy, gingivectomy, or frenectomy; porosity of maxillary bone allows for high success rate	Into soft tissue of area to be anesthetized	Soft tissue of area to be anesthetized using a 25 or 27 gauge short needle. Depth of insertion is 2–3 millimeters.
field block (also called supraperiosteal)	Pulp and soft tissue of an individual tooth	Height of the mucobuccal fold over tooth to be anesthetized	Near apex of individual tooth using a 25 or 27 gauge short needle
anterior superior alveolar (commonly referred to as infraorbital nerve block)	Pulps and soft tissue of maxillary incisors and canine in a quadrant	Height of the mucobuccal fold of the maxillary first premolar	At the bony contact of the infraorbital rim in the area of the infraorbital foramen with a 25 or 27 gauge long needle
middle superior alveolar	Pulps and soft tissue of maxillary premolars and the mesiobuccal root of the first maxillary molar in one quadrant	Height of the mucobuccal fold above the second premolar	Area between apices of maxillary first and second premolars 25 or 27 gauge short needle
posterior superior alveolar	Pulps and soft tissue of maxillary molars with the exception of the mesiobuccal root of the first maxillary molar in one quadrant	Height of the mucobuccal fold and distal to the last molar	Approximately ½ to ¾ of the length of a 25 or 27 gauge short needle
greater palatine nerve block	Soft tissue anesthesia only of the soft tissue on the hard palate from distal of canine to distal of last molar in one quadrant	Soft tissue just anterior to the greater palatine foramen	Soft tissue just anterior to the greater palatine foramen with a 25 or 27 gauge short needle
nasopalatine nerve block	Soft tissue anesthesia only of the soft tissue on the hard palate from distal of canine of one quadrant to distal of canine on the opposite quadrant	The lingual tissue adjacent to the incisive papilla	The lingual tissue adjacent to the incisive papilla 25 or 27 gauge short needle. Depth of insertion is 2–3 millimeters.

TABLE 23-4 Mandibular Local Anesthetic Injection Sites and Areas Anesthetized

Name of Injection	Affected Teeth/Tissues	Needle Insertion Site	Deposition Site of Local Anesthetic Solution
infiltration	Soft tissue anesthesia only of area injected—for example, the interdental papilla for scaling and root planing procedures; usually used only on mandibular incisors as posterior bone is too dense	Into soft tissue of area to be anesthetized	Soft tissue of area to be anesthetized using a 25 or 27 gauge short needle. Depth of insertion is 1–2 millimeters.
field block (also called supraperiosteal)	Pulp and soft tissue of an individual tooth.	Near apex of individual tooth in mandibular incisor area	Near apex of individual tooth in mandibular incisor area using a 25 or 27 gauge short needle
inferior alveolar nerve block (includes lingual nerve block anesthesia)	Pulps of all teeth in mandibular quadrant, buccal soft tissue from distal of premolar to midline, half of tongue on side that is injected, lingual soft tissues and of all teeth in quadrant, body of mandible	Soft tissues on the lingual aspect of the ramus of the mandible at the level of the coronoid notch of the mandible	Inside of the mandibular ramus, posterior to the retromolar pad, below and anterior to the mandibular foramen using a 27 gauge long needle; needle insertion is about ½ to ¾ of a long needle
buccal nerve block	Buccal soft tissue in the area of the mandibular molars	Buccal soft tissue distal and slightly buccal to the last mandibular molar	Buccal soft tissue distal and slightly buccal to the last mandibular molar at a depth of 1 to 3 millimeters with a long 25 or 27 gauge needle
mental nerve block	Buccal soft tissue anterior to the mental foramen to midline and skin of lower lip	The height of the mucobuccal fold anterior to the mental foramen	Anterior to the mental foramen, between the apices of the roots of the mandibular premolars and adjacent to the mandibular foramen; use a short 25 or 27 gauge needle
incisive nerve block	Pulps of the mandibular premolars, canine, and incisors in quadrant; skin of chin and lower lip on side anesthetized	The height of the mucobuccal fold anterior to the mental foramen	Anterior to the mental foramen, between the apices of the roots of the mandibular premolars and adjacent to the mandibular foramen; use a short 25 or 27 gauge needle

TABLE 23-5 Supplemental Dental Local Anesthetic Techniques

Intraosseous Anesthesia

Intraosseous anesthesia places local anesthetic directly into the cancellous bone (spongy bone). This injection is used for anesthesia in a single tooth or multiple teeth in a quadrant. The bone, soft tissue, and root of a tooth/teeth are anesthetized by the intraosseous injection. This type of anesthetic injection is useful for patients who do not like the feeling of a numb lip and tongue. It is immediate in action and is atraumatic for patients.

The intraosseous injection requires a special system for administration. A perforator, which is a solid needle that attaches to a low-speed handpiece, perforates the cortical plate of bone and leaves a very small hole for the anesthetic needle to be placed. An 8-mm, 27-gauge needle is inserted into the hole for administration of the anesthetic.

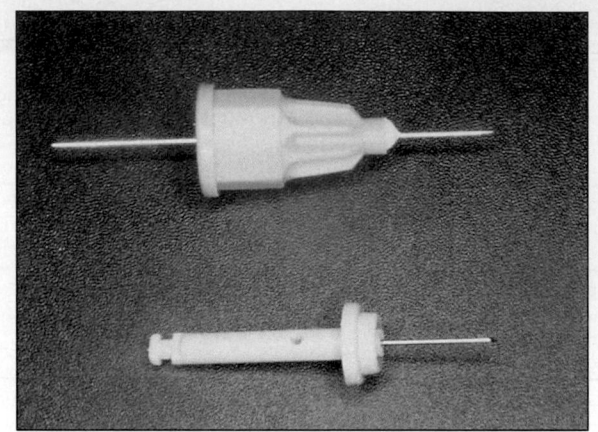

Periodontal Ligament Injection

The periodontal ligament injection, or *intraligamentary* injection, is used for pulpal anesthesia of one or two teeth in a quadrant and sometimes as an adjunct to another injection where the patient is only partially anesthetized. It also is used as an aid for diagnosing abscessed teeth and when a patient does not want the lip and tongue to be numb. This technique involves inserting the needle into the gingival sulcus along the long axis of the tooth to be treated on the mesial or distal or the root.

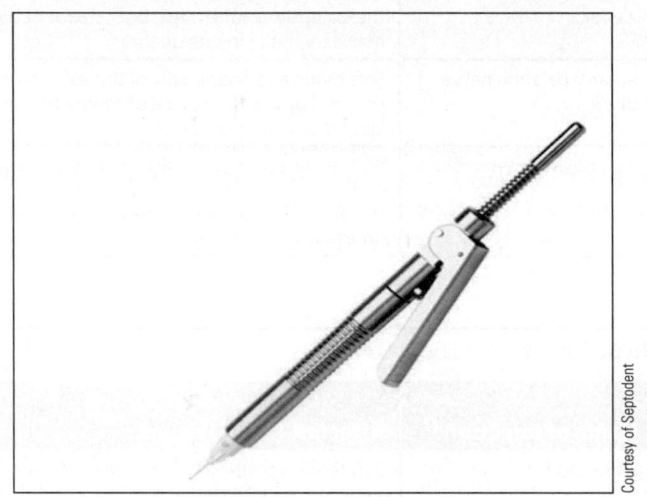

Courtesy of Septodont

Intrapulpal Injection

The intrapulpal injection technique deposits the anesthetic directly into the pulp chamber or root canal of the involved tooth. This injection may be used when there is difficulty in securing pain control. A 25- or 27-gauge short or long needle is used; sometimes, the needle is bent to access the pulp canal.

With the administration of Oraverse® (phentolamine mesylate) at the conclusion of the treatment, the residual soft tissue anesthesia can be reversed more quickly (Figure 23-9). The agent is injected into the same site as the local anesthetic in the same manner. The reversal agent is supplied in cartridges which may be loaded into the anesthetic syringe. Oraverse significantly decreases the time of residual soft tissue anesthesia from the local anesthetic injection. The reversal agent is most commonly used for the inferior alveolar nerve block as this injection results in anesthesia of the lower lip and tongue on the side of local anesthetic administration.

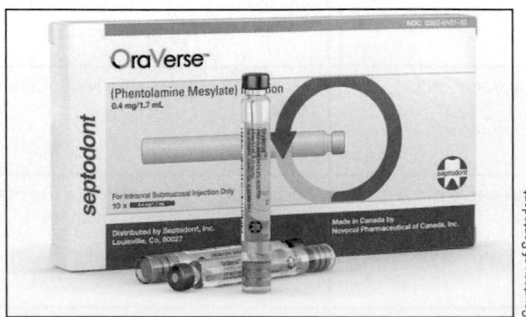

Courtesy of Septodont

FIGURE 23-9

Oraverse® local anesthetic reversal agent.

Computer Controlled Local Anesthesia

There are several computer controlled local anesthetic delivery (CCLAD) options available on the market. When a patient receives a local anesthetic injection, the needle is not the only thing that causes discomfort. Discomfort may also come from the pressure and volume of the fluid going into the tissues. These systems use a computer to control the flow rate of the anesthetic, providing a more comfortable and effective anesthetic delivery. The Wand® was developed for use with the CompuDent system (Figure 23-10). Another option is Dentapen® by Septodont (Figure 23-11). CCLAD systems utilize a standard dental local anesthetic cartridge and needle. They can be used to administer infiltrations, blocks, and supplemental injections.

Complications of Local Anesthesia Administration

The dentist has to deliver the injection without being able to see where the needle is going. The needle penetrates through tissues to deposit the anesthetic solution as close to the nerve as possible. To add to the complexity of a local anesthetic injection, a nerve, an artery, and a vein are commonly found together. Thus, there are

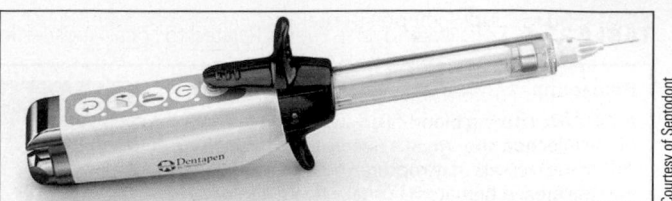

FIGURE 23-11
Dentapen® by Septodont.

numerous potential complications that may occur related to local anesthetic administration. Adverse effects from the administration of a local anesthetic can be due to the physical injection of the needle or from the anesthetic solution itself. Table 23-6 provides details regarding localized complications that may occur related to local anesthetic administration. Table 23-7 provides systemic reactions to local anesthetics.

Prevention and Management of a Local Anesthesia Related Emergency

As discussed in Chapter 15, prevention of a medical emergency is of the utmost importance. Prevention starts with a careful review of the patient's medical history. Having an updated medical history of your patients is vital in situations such as these.

Many existing conditions and medications the patient is taking may increase the chance of a complication with a local anesthetic. Anesthetics are metabolized in the liver. If a patient has liver impairment, the dose of the local anesthetic may need to be significantly reduced. The patient's physician should be contacted, and a medical consult should be obtained. Patients taking antidepressants may need a limited amount of epinephrine. Dentists often elect to consult with physicians for patients with documented cardiovascular disease and other systemic conditions in order to determine the physical status of the patient and whether or not local anesthesia can be safely administered to the patient.

Allergic reactions to amide local anesthetics are extremely rare. It is important to find out from the patient if they ever had an adverse reaction to a local anesthetic. If the patient states that they have had an adverse reaction to a local anesthetic, the dental assistant should ask the patient what type of reaction it was and document the reaction. Most reactions that patients experience are attributed to the epinephrine vasoconstrictor added to the anesthetic. Since epinephrine is involved in the natural fight-or-flight response for an emergency situation, patients who are sensitive to epinephrine experience the sensations associated with that response. This emergency response prepares the body to readily respond by accelerating the heart and lung action and increasing the blood flow to the extremities. After the epinephrine reaction subsides, the body feels shaky and weak for some time. This response is not expected by the patient, and they may be fearful as a result. The dental team should calm the patient and explain to the patient what caused the reaction. This reaction

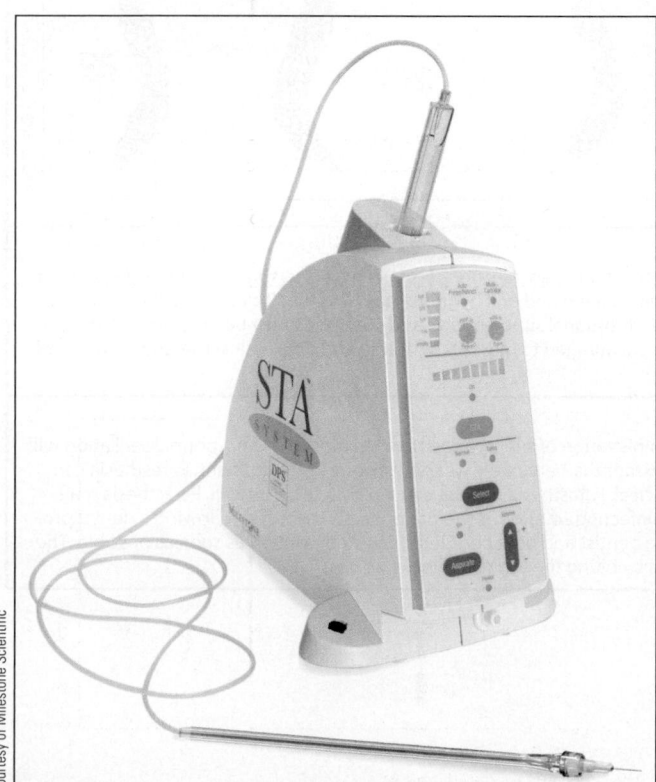

FIGURE 23-10
The Wand® by Compudent.

TABLE 23-6 Localized Adverse Events Related to Local Anesthetic Administration

Hematoma

A **hematoma** is a blood-filled swelling in the area of the injection site. When a needle goes through soft tissue, vessels may rupture and the blood flows into the area. A hematoma usually heals within 10–14 days. Hematomas most commonly occur during administration of a posterior superior alveolar nerve block, inferior alveolar nerve block, or anterior superior alveolar nerve block.

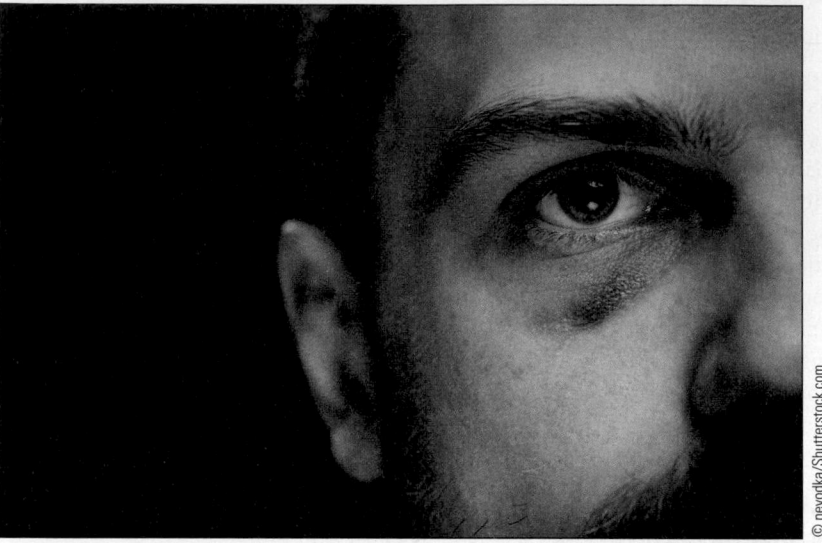

Inadvertent Anesthesia of Adjacent Areas

Unwanted anesthesia of adjacent areas usually is most common during the inferior alveolar nerve block and the anterior superior alveolar nerve block. This is due to the proximity of branches of the facial nerve. If these branches are inadvertently anesthetized, the patient experiences drooping of the facial muscles on the side of the anesthesia along with an inability to close the eye on the same side. The anesthesia will wear off and the muscles will resume function. Management includes removing contact lenses and closing the eye with a patch placed over it so the eye does not become dry.

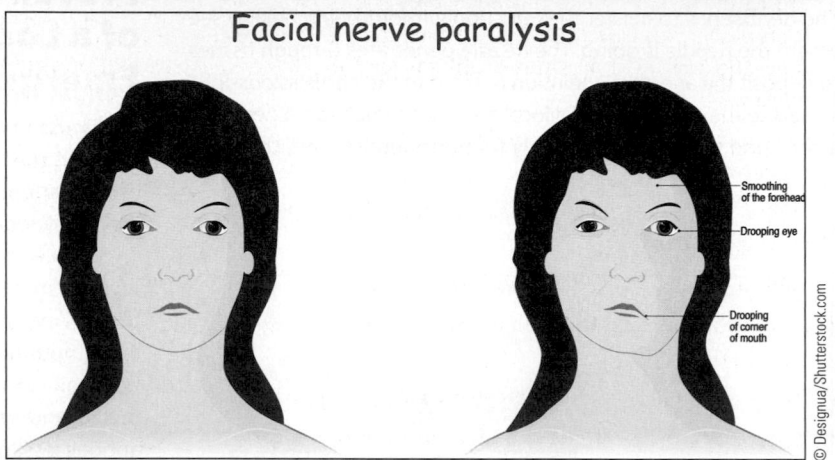

Trismus

Trismus is also known as lockjaw. Trismus is caused by trauma to the muscle fibers during an injection. Trismus results in soreness of the area and limited jaw opening. Trismus usually resolves in 10 days to 2 weeks as the area heals. Eating and oral hygiene may be difficult due to the limited opening. Patients may take nonsteroidal anti-inflammatory medications as needed. Nutritional supplements and soft foods may be recommended until the area heals and the patient is able to open fully. The patient should also be encouraged to massage the area and do physical therapy exercises of the jaw.

Parasthesia

Paresthesia is persistent numbness and pain for more than 24 hours after administration of a local anesthetic. In most patients, normal sensation will return in 10–14 days and virtually all temporary cases will be resolved within 6 months. Very rarely will paresthesia be permanent. Paresthesia can also be caused by a hematoma; the paresthesia will resolve as the hematoma heal. Paresthesia may be caused by edema as well. Paresthesia may also be caused by injection of local anesthetic contaminated by alcohol or disinfecting solution. If the patient calls the office following a dental procedure and complains of extended numbness, the patient should speak to the dentist and be scheduled or an examination as soon as possible. The major concern of short-term numbness is that patients may injure themselves by biting the tongue, cheeks, or lips.

TABLE 23-7 Systemic Adverse Events Related to Local Anesthetic Administration

Vasovagal Syncope One of the most common side effects of local anesthetic administration is vasovagal syncope. Such a reaction is caused by fear of the needle. Refer to Chapter 15 regarding the physiological response that leads to syncope as well as management of syncope. Syncope can be prevented by ensuring that the patient is supine while administering local anesthesia.
Systemic Toxicity A toxic reaction occurs due to an overdose from a local anesthetic. The first symptom is the stimulation of the central nervous system (CNS). The patient becomes more talkative, apprehensive, and excited, with an increased pulse rate and blood pressure. This is followed by depression of the CNS as the drug dissipates. Review of the medical history and updating at each visit is critical in preventing an overdose of a local anesthetic. The patient's medical history, the amount of anesthetic solution administered, as well as the rate at which the solution was injected determines the potential occurrence of a toxic local anesthetic reaction. It is important that the dentist aspirate prior to depositing the solution in order to confirm that the needle is not in a blood vessel. Inadvertent administration into a blood vessel will lead to rapid symptoms of systemic toxicity that must be managed. A significant overdose can lead to seizures and loss of consciousness. Refer to Chapter 15 regarding management of seizures and loss of consciousness.

needs to be noted in the patient's chart. The dentist may choose alternatives to manage the patient's pain in future appointments.

The dental assistant has a vital role in preventing and managing an emergency related to local anesthesia. Prevention of a local anesthesia related medical emergency includes:

- Thoroughly review the patient's medical history, which includes current medical conditions, medications, allergies, and history of previous problems with local or topical anesthetic.

- Ensure the appropriate anesthetic is prepared for the procedure.

- Observe for and address any fears or nervousness the patient may have.

- Place the patient in a supine position for the injection.

- Watch the patients throughout the administration of the anesthetic.

- Never leave a patient alone following an injection.

- Report any unusual patient reaction immediately to the dentist.

Armamentarium

It is important that the dental assistant has everything prepared prior to seating the patient so the dental procedure along with administration of local anesthesia is completed in a timely and

Safety

Dental health care workers must review the patient's medical history before every procedure (a patient's medical conditions can change between visits). Check the local anesthetic cartridge for type of local anesthetic and whether or not the cartridge contains epinephrine prior to syringe assembly.

seamless manner. This section covers the armamentarium necessary for the administration of anesthetic, how the equipment is assembled, and preparation of the work area.

Armamentarium for Topical and Local Anesthesia

As discussed earlier, the assistant should always read the patient's chart to check for contraindications and any notes regarding anesthetic prior to set up. The dental assistant should always consult with the dentist regarding the type of local anesthetic prior to loading the cartridge into the syringe. The amount of topical anesthetic that will be needed will be indicated by the number of teeth or quadrants that are being treated.

The syringe is the first item that should be placed on the tray. Next to the syringe is the local anesthetic cartridges of choice along with needles and a recapping device (Figures 23-12A, B, and C). The gel topical anesthetic as well as a cotton tip applicator to apply the topical should be next to the cartridges and the needles. The effect of the topical anesthetic is best achieved when the mucosa is dry. Gauze squares and cotton rolls are placed at the end of the tray to dry the area to be injected prior to the placement of the topical anesthetic (Figure 23-13). A sharps container should also be in the operatory for disposal of sharps and the local anesthetic cartridge.

Anesthetic Syringe The anesthetic syringe is the instrument used to administer the local anesthetic. Syringes may be metal (stainless steel) or non-metal (plastic). In the dental field syringes are usually not disposable. Metal syringes are autoclavable, while nonmetal syringes may be either disposable or autoclavable. There are two types of anesthetic syringes. Nonaspirating syringes do not have the ability to aspirate (suction). They are not used for dental local anesthetic injections and are often used for IV and IM injections. The aspirating anesthetic syringe is able to aspirate patient tissue fluid into the cartridge to confirm the tip of the needle is not in a blood vessel (Figure 23-14A). Once the needle is injected into the patient's oral mucosa, the dentist aspirates

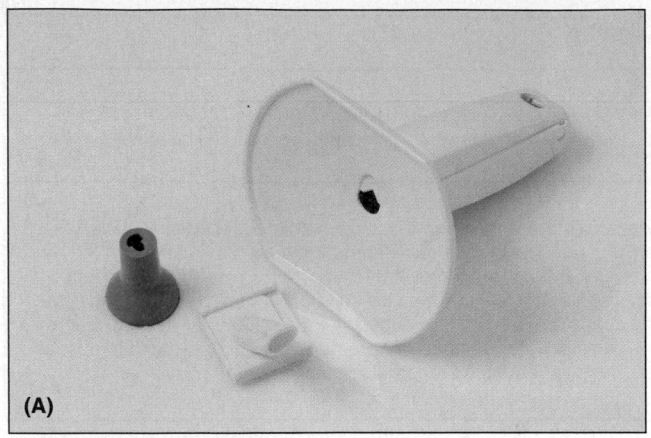

(A)

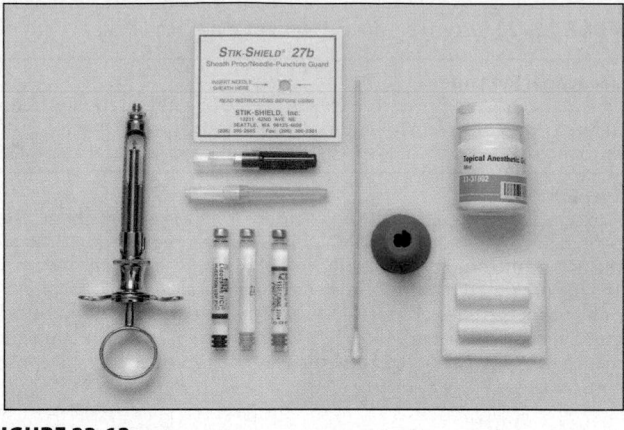

FIGURE 23-13
Armamentarium needed to assemble a local anesthetic syringe.

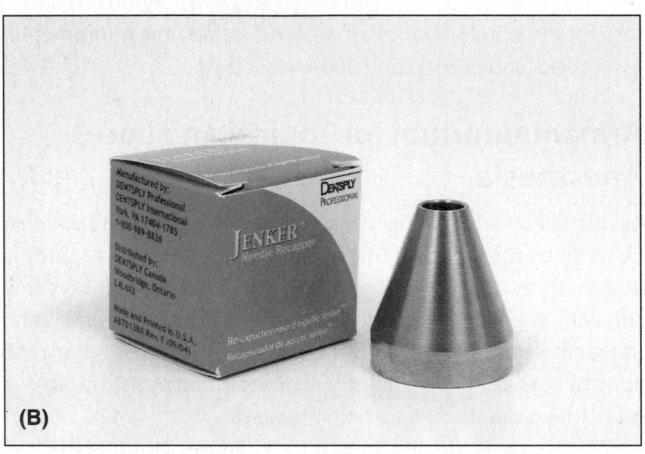

(B)

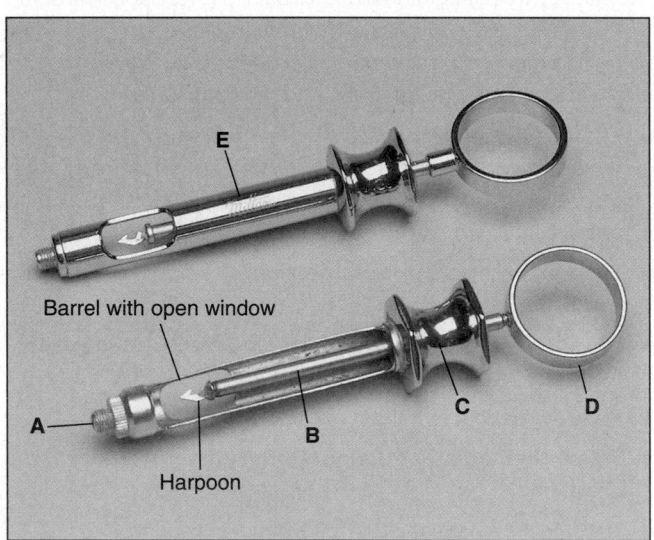

E

Barrel with open window

A

Harpoon

B

C

D

FIGURE 23-14A
Aspirating needle with parts labeled. (A) Needle adaptor. (B) Piston with harpoon. (C) Finger grip. (D) Thumb ring. (E) Syringe barrel.

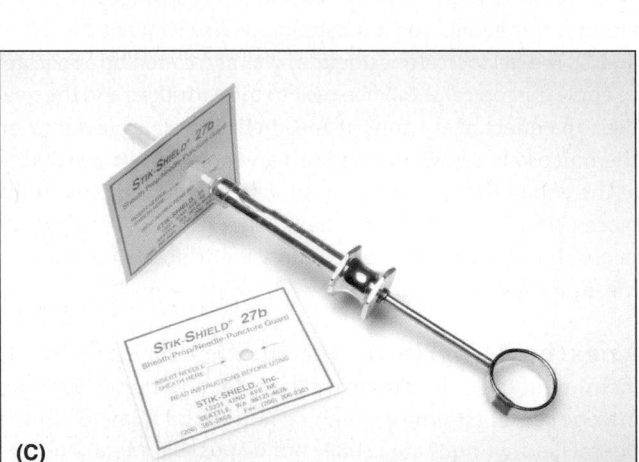

(C)

FIGURE 23-12A–C
Needlestick prevention device.

tissue fluid into the cartridge making certain that the needle has not penetrated a blood vessel. Signs of blood in the cartridge alert the dentist to reposition the needle. Safety syringes are also an option in a dental office. These are

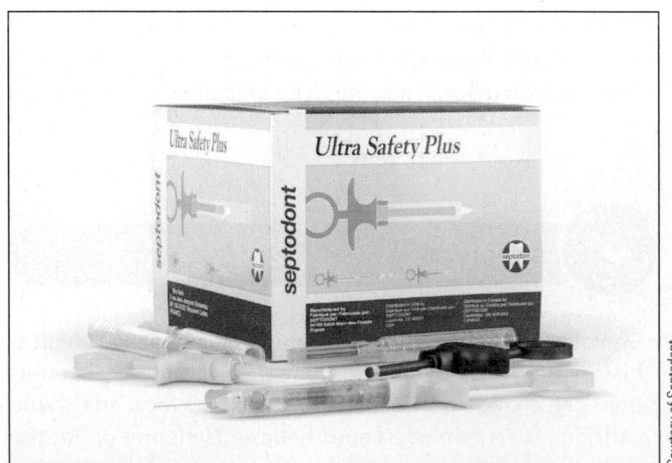

FIGURE 23-14B
Ultra Safety Plus safety syringe by Septodont.

Courtesy of Septodont

aspirating syringes, which have a built-in sheath that covers the needle when the needle is not in use (Figure 23-14B).

The assistant loads the anesthetic syringe once the patient is seated. The assistant needs to know the parts of the syringe, its proper function, maintenance, and sterilizing techniques to ensure patient safety and prolong the life of the syringe.

Parts of Aspirating Anesthetic Syringe   The *needle adapter* is the threaded tip for the attachment for the injection needle. The hub can loosen with use and should be checked prior to loading the syringe. Care should also be taken when removing the needle that the needle adapter has not become loose and is not accidently disposed of in the sharps container along with the needle (Figure 23-14A).

The *barrel* is the compartment for holding the anesthetic cartridge. The closed portion of the barrel, called the safeguard, protects the patient and assistant from injury in case of cartridge breakage. The opposite side, called the loading side, is open for the insertion of the cartridge. The window is the open portion of the safeguard that allows the dentist to observe the aspiration of tissue fluid into the cartridge (Figure 23-14A).

The piston is a metal rod that exerts pressure on the anesthetic cartridge loaded in the barrel to push the solution out through the needle (Figure 23-14A). At one end of the plunger is the *harpoon* (Figure 23-14A). The harpoon pierces the rubber portion of the anesthetic cartridge. When the plunger is pulled back, the harpoon pulls the rubber stopper, causing pressure to aspirate tissue fluid. If the needle is in the vessel, blood will be aspirated into the cartridge. At the other end of the plunger is the thumb ring for the placement of the operator's thumb. Attached to the barrel is the finger grip (rest), which is a grooved area for the dentist to hold the syringe with the index and middle finger.

Follow the manufacturer's recommendations for the care and handling of autoclavable syringes. After each use, the harpoon is cleaned with a brush and the syringe is prepared for sterilization like other autoclavable instruments. Some syringes need periodic lubrication in the threaded joints and where the thumb ring meets the finger bar. The harpoon may need to be replaced if it becomes bent or dull and does not remain embedded in the rubber stopper.

Anesthetic Cartridge   The anesthetic cartridge is composed of glass and contains premeasured amounts of anesthetic solution (Figure 23-15). There are many anesthetic solutions available. Two common anesthetics are lidocaine and mepivacaine. The amount of anesthetic, expiration date, presence of vasoconstrictor, and batch number are labeled on the cartridge. The batch number is used to track when and where the anesthetic was manufactured. This number is used in quality management and analysis. Today, the standard anesthetic cartridge contains 1.7 milliliters. Each cartridge has an expiration date until which

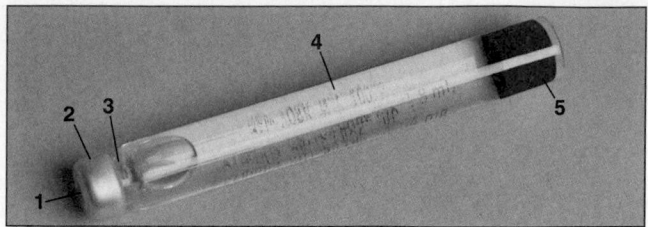

FIGURE 23-15
Anesthetic cartridge with parts labeled. (1) latex rubber diaphragm. (2) aluminum cap. (3) neck of cartridge. (4) glass cartridge with mylar label. (5) rubber stopper.

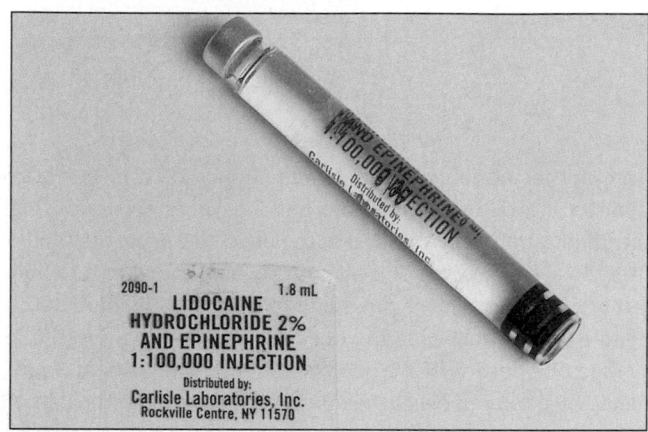

FIGURE 23-16
Anesthetic cartridge and mylar label with information identified.

the solution is still effective. The expiration date should be closely monitored. The cartridges should be stored at room temperature and in a dark place. The cartridge need not be heated before use (Figure 23-16).

One end of the cartridge is hermetically sealed by a metal cap surrounding a latex rubber membrane known as a *diaphragm*. The diaphragm is penetrated by the needle to expel the anesthetic solution from the cartridge. The diaphragm is made of latex rubber. To date there has never been an allergic reaction related to the latex diaphragm of a local anesthetic cartridge. There is a *rubber stopper* at the other end of the cartridge. The harpoon of the syringe is embedded in the rubber stopper when the syringe is loaded (Figure 23-15).

Dental Injection Needle   The cartridge penetrating end of the needle enters the diaphragm of the anesthetic cartridge and connects to the syringe via the needle adapter. The opposite end of the needle penetrates the patient tissues to inject the solution into the desired area. Most needles are composed of stainless steel. An injection needle has a lumen or hole that runs through the needle that is the passageway for anesthetic

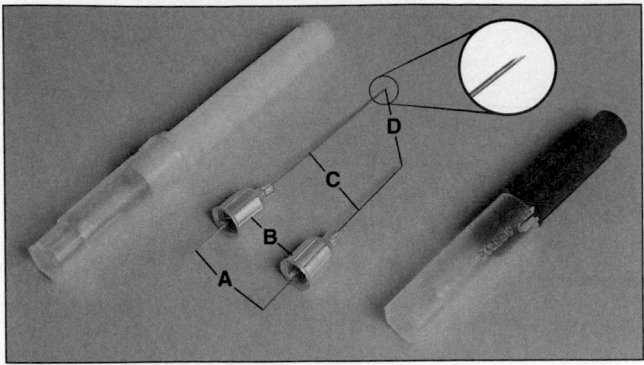

FIGURE 23-17
Needle parts labeled; short and long needles. (A) Syringe end. (B). Hub.
(C) Shank. (D) Bevel.

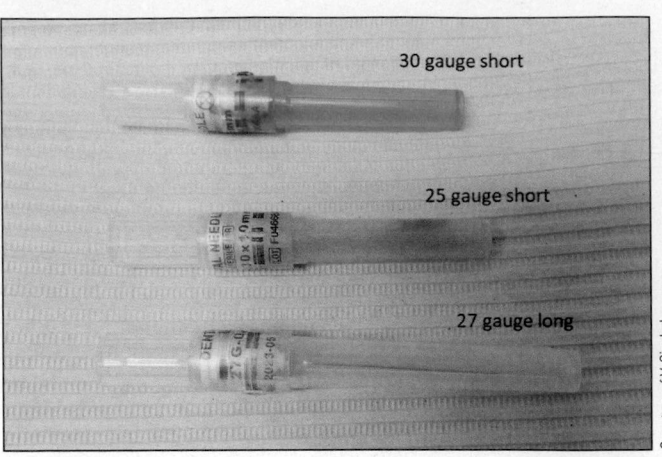

FIGURE 23-18
Dental needle gauges.

from the cartridge to patient tissue (Figure 23-17). The tissue penetrating end of the needle has a *bevel* or angle. During the administration of anesthesia, the bevel of the needle should face the alveolar bone. This allows the local anesthesia to flow out of the bevel in close proximity to the bone. The hub of the needle firmly attaches to the needle adapter of the anesthetic syringe. The portion of the needle that enters the patient is protected by a colored plastic needle cover (guard), and the part of the needle entering the cartridge is protected by a clear plastic protective cap. The needle guard and plastic cap are sealed together at the needle hub to ensure sterility (Figure 23-17). When opening a new needle, a seal must be broken; if the seal is already broken, do not use the needle, and dispose of the needle as if it had been used previously.

Needles are sized by length and *gauge* (diameter). The common dental lengths are short and long. The short needles are 1 inch in length and are generally used in maxillary injections and most children injections. The long needles are 1 ½ inches and are generally used in certain mandibular injections. Anesthetic manufacturers make different colored needle guards indicating the gauge of the needle (Figure 23-18). The common dental gauges are 25, 27, and 30. The higher numbers indicate the smaller gauge needles, and the lower numbers are larger gauges. The needles used in dental anesthetic are single use disposable needles, which ensures the sterility of the needles. If the operator penetrates the tissue with the needle more than four times during a procedure, the needle should be changed, because the needle becomes dull.

Sharps Container

As discussed in Chapter 11, needles and anesthetic cartridges must be discarded in a sharps container after use. The container must be

OSHA compliant: puncture and leakproof, disposable, securely sealed, and marked with the biohazard symbol (refer to Chapter 11). Some sharps containers have a needle remover to assist in safe removal of the needle from the syringe. The needle should be recapped with a needle recapping device after use and prior to removal from the aspirating syringe for disposal.

Assembling the Anesthetic Syringe

The syringe should be assembled once the patient is seated so the patient can see that all instruments were removed from sterile packages. The first step in loading the anesthetic syringe is to read the patient chart to determine which type of local anesthetic is recommended for the patient and what area is being anesthetized. Once the type of anesthetic has been selected, the cartridge should be inspected for the following:

- Expired shelf-life dates
- Large bubbles inside cartridge (may indicate contamination)
- Extruded stopper (caused by the solution being frozen)
- Corrosion (caused by immersion in disinfecting solutions)
- Cracks around the neck region and the rubber stopper
- Rust on the aluminum caps (caused by a broken or leaking anesthetic cartridge)

If you find any of these conditions, the cartridges should be discarded.

Preparing the Aspirating Syringe

Procedure 23-1 describes the steps in preparing the local anesthetic syringe by a right-handed operator.

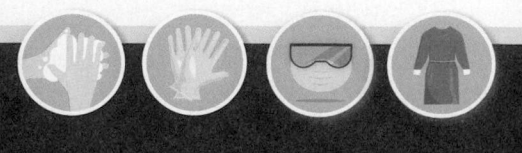

Procedure 23-1
Assembling the Local Anesthetic Syringe

This procedure is completed by a qualified dental assistant.

Equipment and Supplies
- Sterile aspirating syringe
- Local anesthetic
- Topical anesthetic plus cotton tip applicator
- Needle recapping device
- Selected dental needle

Procedure Steps

1. Read the patient chart to determine type of local anesthetic recommended for the patient. Consult with the dentist to confirm.

2. Remove the sterilized syringe from its autoclave bag or pouch. Inspect the syringe to be sure it is ready for use. Examine the syringe to ensure the hub and thumb ring are secure and the plunger moves freely before loading the syringe.

3. Inspect anesthetic (Figure 23-19) cartridge to ensure:
   - ❏ rubber stopper is even with the end of the cartridge
   - ❏ diaphragm and stopper are free of puncture marks
   - ❏ expiration date has not passed and solution is clear and free of large bubbles
   - ❏ no cracks or chips on the cartridge

4. Grasp syringe in one hand and use thumb ring to pull back on plunger (Figure 23-20).

5. Place cartridge in barrel with rubber end toward harpoon with the other hand. To prevent contamination, do not place a finger over the diaphragm while placing the cartridge in the syringe (Figure 23-21). Once the cartridge is in place, release the piston rod.

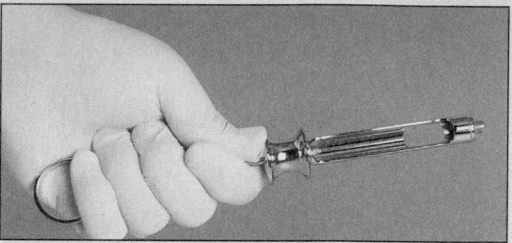

FIGURE 23-20
Left hand retraction of the piston of aspirating syringe.

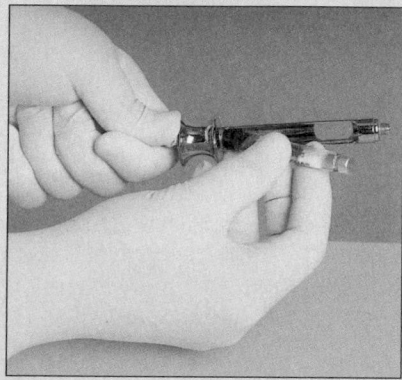

FIGURE 23-21
Inserting local anesthetic cartridge into aspirating dental syringe.

6. Release thumb ring to allow the harpoon to engage the rubber diaphragm of the cartridge. With moderate pressure, push the piston rod into the rubber stopper until it is engaged fully (Figure 23-22). Do not hit the piston rod to engage the harpoon, and do not hold your hand over the cartridge while engaging the harpoon.

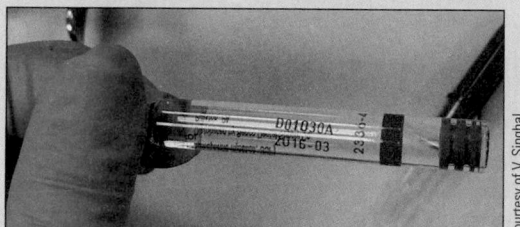

Courtesy of V. Singhal

FIGURE 23-19
Inspecting local anesthetic cartridge.

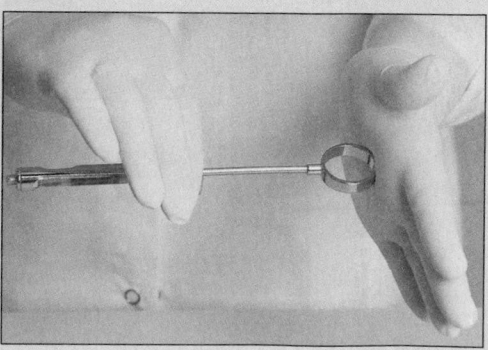

FIGURE 23-22
Engage the harpoon with pressure on the finger ring (bar).

(Continues)

7. Pull back on thumb ring to make certain the harpoon is engaged (Figure 23-23).

8. Remove protective cap from needle and penetrate rubber diaphragm with needle (Figure 23-24A). Screw needle to the syringe (Figure 23-24B). Make sure that the needle is secure but not too tight. A disposable needle guard is placed on the protective cap covering the needle (Figure 23-24C).

9. Remove needle cover (Figure 23-25).

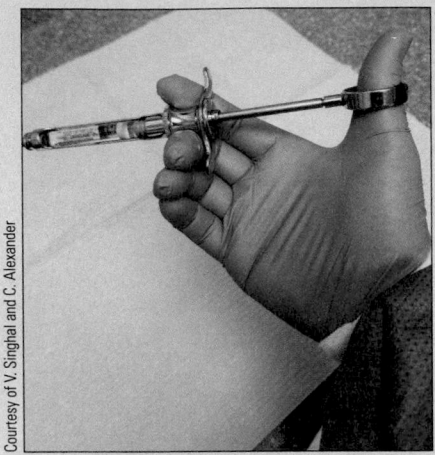

Courtesy of V. Singhal and C. Alexander

FIGURE 23-23
Pulling back on thumb ring.

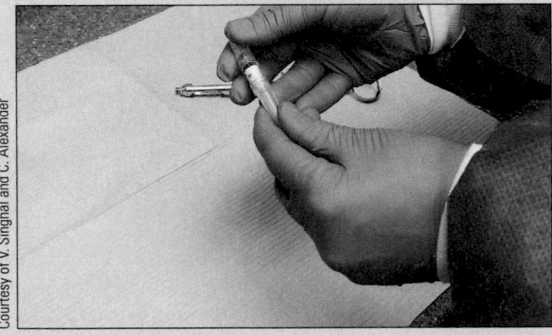

Courtesy of V. Singhal and C. Alexander

FIGURE 23-24A
Removing protective cap from needle.

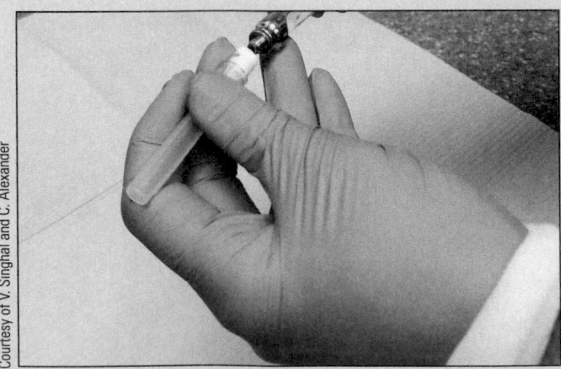

Courtesy of V. Singhal and C. Alexander

FIGURE 23-24B
Screw needle to the syringe.

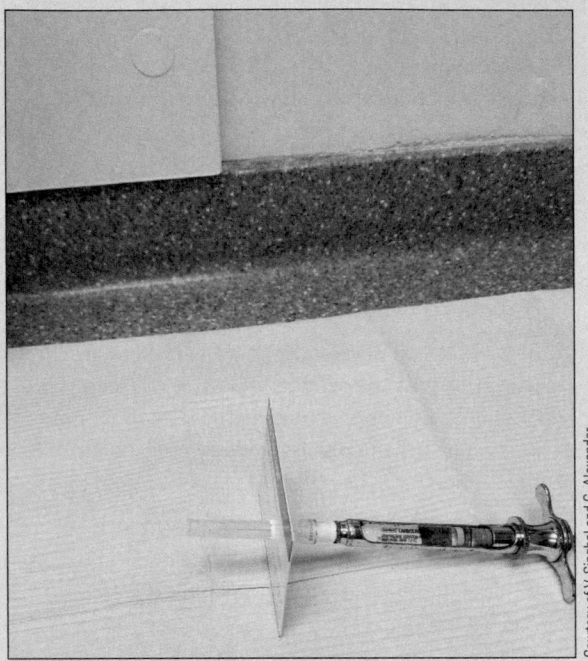

Courtesy of V. Singhal and C. Alexander

FIGURE 23-24C
Assembled needle with needle guard.

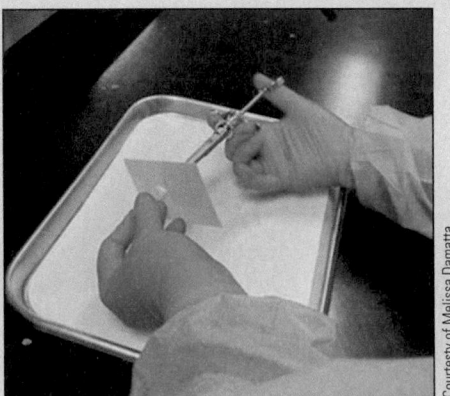

Courtesy of Melissa Damatta

FIGURE 23-25
Removing needle cover.

10. Push lightly on thumb ring to expel a few drops of solution to confirm proper assembly of the syringe (Figure 23-26).

11. Recap needle with use of needle guard (Figure 23-27).

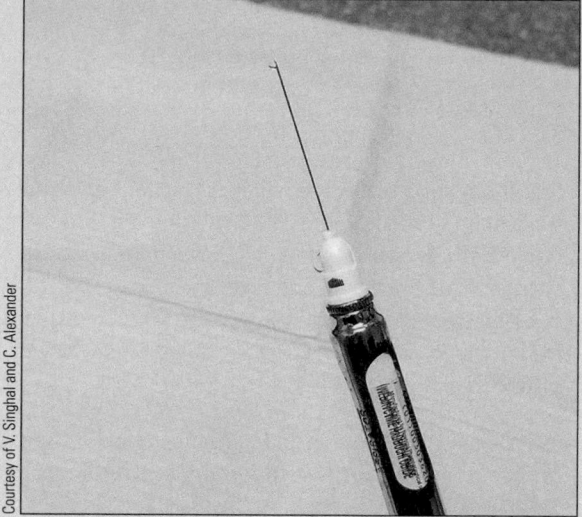

Courtesy of V. Singhal and C. Alexander

FIGURE 23-26
Expelling a few drops of local anesthetic solution.

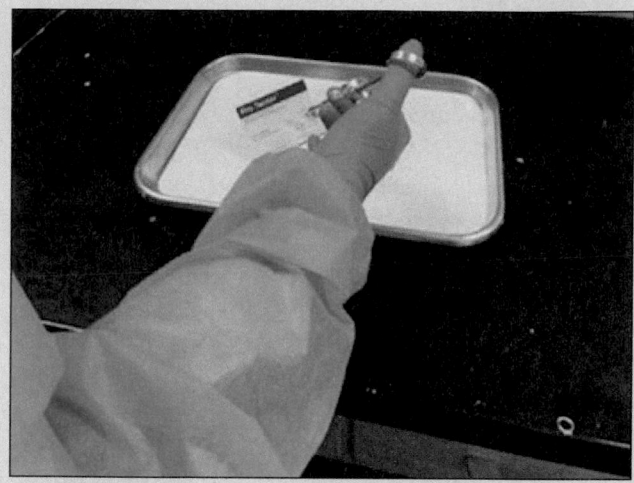

Courtesy of Melissa Damatta

FIGURE 23-27
Recap needle with use of needleguard.

Procedure 23-2
Assisting with the Administration of Topical and Local Anesthesia

This procedure is performed by the dentist. The dental assistant prepares the materials and the patient. Steps written in **blue** font are performed by the dentist, and the chairside assistant's steps are written in black.

Equipment and Supplies
- Patient seating setup (refer to Procedure 18-4)
- Anesthetic setup as described in Procedure 23-1 (Figure 23-28)
- Air–water syringe tip and evacuation tips
- Cotton rolls, cotton tip applicator, 2 × 2 gauze squares

Procedure Steps

Placement of Topical Anesthetic
1. Escort and seat patient (refer to Procedure 18-4).

Dentist greets the patient and takes position at the dental chair.

   ❑ *Signals for the procedure to begin (refer to Procedure 20-1).*

2. Pass mouth mirror and explorer at operator's signal.

Dentist examines procedure area with mirror and explorer.

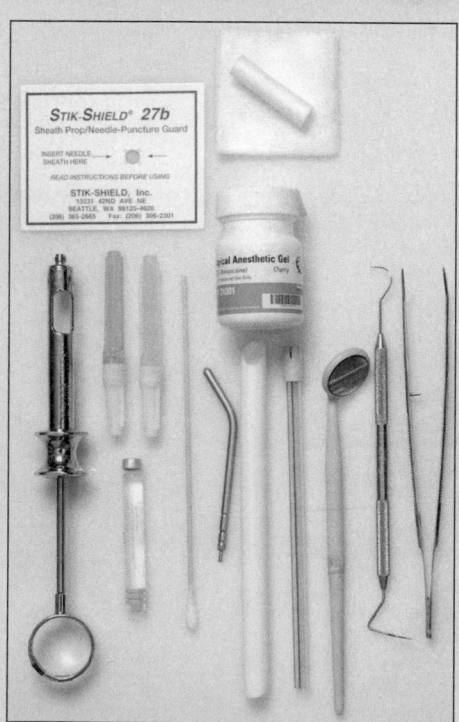

FIGURE 23-28
Anesthetic setup.

(Continues)

3. Prepare patient for the procedure by explaining what will be done.

4. Avoid words such as "hurt" and "shot." Explain that topical anesthetic will make the tissue numb and make the injection more comfortable for the patient.

5. Place a small amount of topical anesthetic on the tip of the cotton tip applicator.

   Operator retracts the tissues and uses a 2 × 2 gauze square to dry the oral mucosa at the site of injection (Figure 23-29).

   Operator keeps the tissue retracted and places the topical anesthetic at the injection site. Leaves cotton tip applicator with topical anesthetic in place for the amount of time recommended by the manufacturer (Figure 23-30).

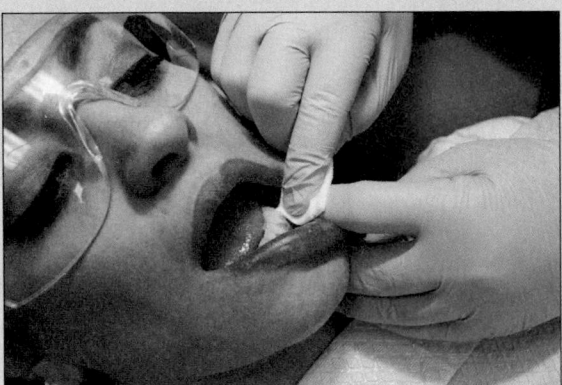

FIGURE 23-29
Dry tissue at site of local anesthetic administration with a 2 × 2 gauze.

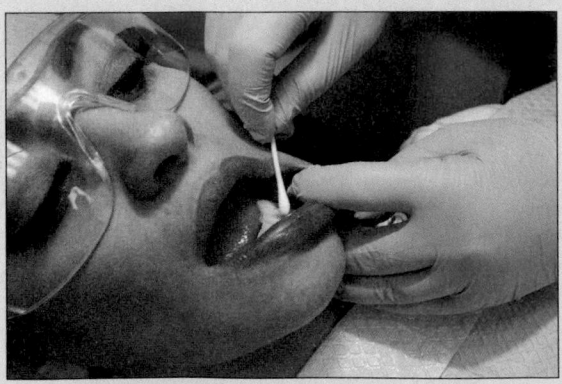

FIGURE 23-30
Place the topical anesthetic on the mandibular injection site.

Administering the Local Anesthetic

Operator assembles local anesthetic syringe while waiting for the topical anesthetic to take effect if not already assembled. Use the steps outlined in Procedure 23-1.

Operator checks the needle bevel so that it is directed toward the arch indicated for treatment (Figure 23-31) and then loosely replaces the cap on the needle. The protective cap is placed on the hub of the needle so that it is secure but can be removed easily.

1. Pass the syringe below the patient's chin (or behind the patient's head) (Figure 23-32), placing the thumb ring over the operator's thumb (the operator grasps the syringe at the finger rest and takes the syringe). As the operator takes the syringe, remove the protective guard. During the injection, observe the patient for any adverse signs or reactions.

Note: There are different methods to safely remove the cap and complete the transfer. It is important for the dentist and the assistant to establish a routine. The assistant can hold the operator's hand until they have cleared the needle.

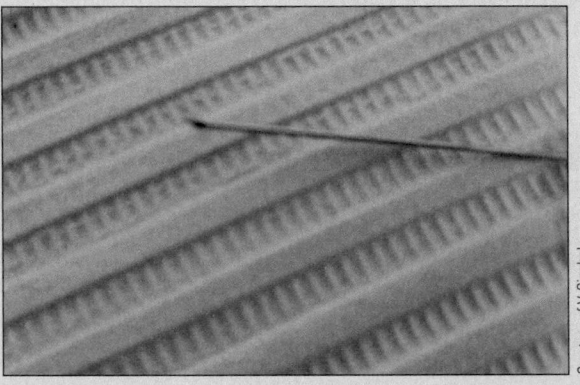

Courtesy of V. Singhal

FIGURE 23-31
Needle bevel.

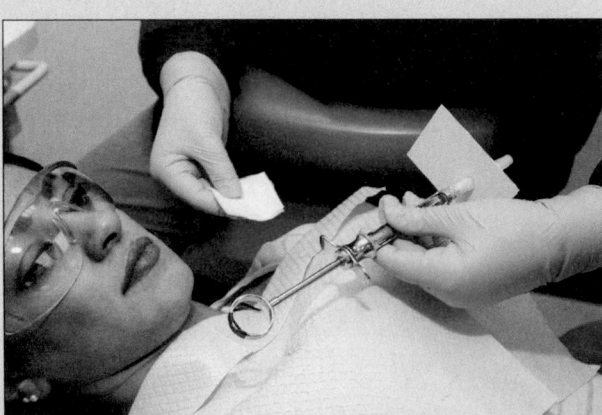

FIGURE 23-32
Pass the prepared anesthetic syringe.

Operator recaps the syringe with the use of a mechanical recapping device.

NOTE: After local anesthetic administration, the syringe is contaminated. Most needlesticks occur during recapping. To prevent this from happening, the dentist should recap the needle and retrieve it after the assistant has replaced the cartridge and has repositioned the syringe on the tray or counter. A variety of needle holders are available. These devices hold the needle cap so that the needle can be recapped while protecting the hands.

Operator places recapped syringe on the tray, out of the way for the rest of the procedure but close in case more anesthetic is needed.

2. Rinse the patient's oral cavity with the air–water syringe and evacuate to remove the water, saliva, and taste of anesthetic solution.

3. Remain with the patient after anesthetic in case the patient has a reaction or causes injury to the anesthetized area. Any unusual occurrence such as increased apprehension, breathing problems, chest pains, and excess perspiration should be reported to the dentist immediately and documented in services rendered.

Procedure 23-3
Disassembling a Dental Local Anesthetic Needle

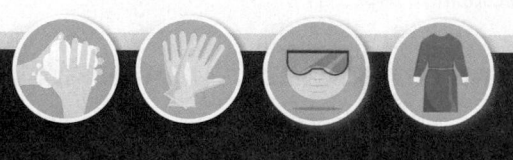

After the procedure is completed and the patient is dismissed, don utility gloves, take the syringe apart, and prepare it for sterilization. This procedure can be performed by the qualified dental assistant, dental hygienist or dentist.

Equipment and Supplies
- Utility gloves
- Syringe
- Sharps container

Procedure Steps

1. Carefully unscrew the needle and remove from the syringe. A hemostat can be used to hold the needle while it is being removed from the syringe. Also, there are mechanical devices that cut the needle from the hub; after being cut, the needle falls into a closed container. The needle is discarded in the sharps container.

2. Retract the piston to release the harpoon from the cartridge (Figure 23-33).

3. Remove the cartridge from the syringe by retracting the thumb ring enough to release the cartridge (Figure 23-34).

4. Place cartridge in the sharps container.

5. Prepare the syringe for sterilization.

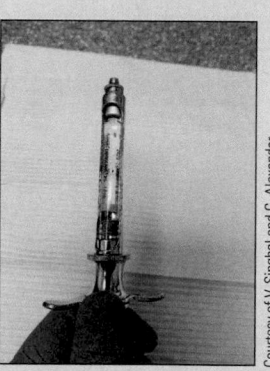

Courtesy of V. Singhal and C. Alexander

FIGURE 23-33
Retracting piston to release harpoon from cartridge.

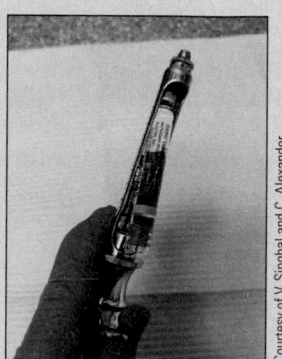

Courtesy of V. Singhal and C. Alexander

FIGURE 23-34
Removal of cartridge from syringe.

Reloading the Aspirating Syringe

Often the dentist will give the patient more than one injection for a procedure, requiring the assistant to reload the syringe chairside. Also during a procedure, the anesthetic may begin to wear off and the patient may begin to feel the discomfort of the procedure. The dentist may elect to inject additional anesthetic to help eliminate the discomfort until the procedure is complete. The assistant will need to reload the syringe with another anesthetic cartridge. The needle must be capped, and the harpoon should be disengaged from the cartridge by pulling back on the thumb ring of the syringe. The cartridge should then be removed. Be careful to not bend the cartridge penetrating end of the needle when removing the cartridge. A new cartridge should then be inserted and the harpoon engaged into the rubber stopper. Expel a few drops to ensure that the assembly is correct. The loaded syringe is ready to be passed to the dentist. Once the patient has been given the additional local anesthetic, the dentist should replace the needle cover by using a needle recapping device.

Charting Anesthetic Administration

Like other aspects of dental treatment, anesthetic administration should be entered in the patient record carefully and in detail once the patient is dismissed. The charting may be completed by the dentist, or by the hygienist or the qualified dental assistant under the dentist's supervision. Most dentists will want a comprehensive description of the anesthetic given to the patient. Include the following in the charting:

- The type of injection given
- Type of topical and local anesthetic administered
- If the local anesthetic contains vasoconstrictor
- Percentage of solution and concentration of vasoconstrictor
- Number of cartridges used
- Any adverse reactions by the patient

Many accidental needlesticks occur when the assistant recaps a contaminated needle. OSHA does not recommend recapping by using the "scoop technique" or recapping with two hands. If recapping is necessary, a needle recapping device must be used.

Some dentists also want to record the needle(s) used and the amount (in milligrams) of the solutions used.

Needlestick Safety

Dental offices are required to have a management plan related to an exposure incident such as a needlestick incident. The plan should include standard protocol such as first aid that is appropriate for the exposure type and who the incident should be reported to. The plan should also include the name and location of the medical facility that will conduct postexposure testing, counseling of the employee, and treatment if needed.

Needlesticks can occur during the transferring of the syringe or during the recapping procedure. Because occupational exposure of the health care worker to bloodborne pathogens from accidental sharps is a serious problem, the Needlestick Safety and Prevention Act was signed into law in 2000. The purpose of the act is to reduce the exposure of the health care worker to bloodborne pathogens. The act places additional requirements on employers related to sharps. The act mandated OSHA to revise the Bloodborne Pathogens Standard in 2001 to include greater detail for the employers to identify, evaluate, and implement safer medical devices. Safer medical devices to avoid percutaneous injuries from contaminated sharps

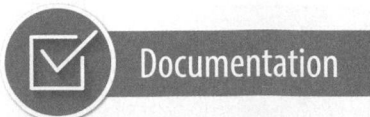 Documentation

Chart Entry for Local Anesthesia Administration
Administered 1 cartridge (1.7 ml) lidocaine (36 mg) with 1:100,000 epinephrine right posterior superior alveolar nerve block. Patient did not experience complications related to local anesthesia administration. Postoperative instructions provided prior to dismissal.

include sharps disposal containers, needle removal on sharps containers, recapping devices, and self-sheathing needles.

The act also required that nonmanagerial health care workers be involved in evaluating and choosing safer devices and required a sharps injury log. Dental offices with less than 10 employees are exempt from maintaining the log. A log, however, can be beneficial in providing valuable information on products and work practices most commonly involved in occupational injuries and can help in reducing or eliminating needlestick risks. OSHA Form 301: Injury and Illness Incident Report can be used to record circumstances of sharps injuries. The report asks questions about the employee, physician, and the incident, including what the employee was doing before the incident, what happened, a description of the injury, and what directly harmed the employee. In states that require a log, the log must be completed within 7 days of the incident and kept for 5 years following the end of the calendar year of the records.

Postexposure Management

Even when safer medical devices have been adopted, accidents happen. All occupational sharps injuries are considered medical emergencies. Immediately following the injury the CDC recommends that the health care worker take these steps:

- Wash area of injury with soap and water.
- Flush splashes to the nose, mouth, or skin with water.
- Irrigate eyes with clean water, saline or sterile irrigants.

The health care worker must report the incident to the supervisor and be evaluated by a qualified medical health care provider to reduce the risk of a bloodborne pathogen infection: hepatitis B virus, hepatitis C virus, or HIV. The CDC "Guidelines for Infection Control in the Dental Health-Care Setting, 2003" provides detailed information on postexposure management. Visit the CDC website for detailed information.

Procedure in the Event of a Sharps Injury

1. Wash the wound area thoroughly with soap and water.
2. In the event of a splash exposure to the nose, mouth, skin, flush the area with water.
3. Irrigate eyes with clean water, saline, or sterile irrigating solution.
4. Notify the dentist and find out which patient the instrument was used on.
5. Review the patient's chart and medical history.
6. Seek medical treatment per the office standard operating procedure.
7. Follow CDC and OSHA protocol for occupational exposure to bloodborne pathogens. (Refer to Chapter 12)

Postexposure Prophylaxis

If the exposure is work related, the health care insurance of the office or worker's compensation insurance will usually pay for the postexposure prophylaxis (PEP). The CDC provides postexposure management and PEP recommendations for medical providers. When a health care worker has been potentially exposed to HBV, the vaccination and vaccine-response status is examined. The hepatitis surface antigen status of the source (patient) should also be evaluated. After evaluation, it may be recommended that dental health care workers who are not immune to HBV need to begin the hepatitis B vaccine series.

As with the HBV exposure, when a worker is exposed to HCV, the status of both the source and exposed healthcare worker should be determined. Continued follow-up HCV testing should be performed to monitor if infection develops. If infection develops, a physician would determine the best course of treatment.

The HIV PEP includes a basic 4-week program. For most HIV exposures the regimen consists of two drugs, zidovudine (ZDV) and lamivudine (3TC). The PEP for HIV must be started within 72 hours of exposure, the sooner the better. If the source person's virus is known, the selection of drugs is dependent on what drugs are working for the source patient's virus.

Sedation

The formal education a dentist has received determines the type of sedation that can be administered. Guidelines are set by the American Dental Association for various levels of training and clinical experience required. Some specialties include the necessary training to administer conscious sedation, deep sedation, and general anesthesia (e.g., oral and maxillofacial surgery and periodontics). If a general dentist wishes to use conscious sedation, deep sedation, or general anesthesia, they must complete specific courses and programs to achieve this credential. Some dentists hire an anesthesiologist to administer general anesthetic to their patients while they complete the dental work. The types of sedation and anesthesia in dentistry are provided in detail in Table 23-8.

Safety

Patient and Staff Safety

The dental assistant plays a critical role to ensure the safety of patients receiving local anesthesia and the dental staff. Needlesticks and occupational sharps injuries are considered medical emergencies and must be evaluated promptly by a qualified health care provider to best decrease the risk of infection with hepatitis B virus, hepatitis C virus, or HIV. The CDC provides detailed information on postexposure management.

Nitrous Oxide Inhalation Sedation

Nitrous oxide gas was first discovered by Joseph Priestly in the early 1770s. Horace Wells (1815–1848) (Figure 23-35), a Connecticut dentist, was the first to use nitrous oxide as an anesthetic during dental surgery. He immediately recognized that it could be used to reduce pain during dental procedures. The use of nitrous oxide and oxygen gases combined provides relaxation and relieves apprehension for patients during dental treatment. These two gases used together allow a safe method of inhalation sedation for patients who experience anxiety during dental care. This gas allows patients to maintain consciousness while allowing the patient to relax. Nitrous oxide maintains the patient in Stage I or analgesia according to Geudel's signs and symptoms of anesthesia. Patients report a floating sensation, warmth, tingling fingers, and the feeling that time is passing quickly. However, oversedation can lead to unwanted symptoms such as an out-of-body experience or feeling excessively hot. Nausea and vomiting can occur if the patient becomes oversedated with nitrous oxide. In order to avoid oversedation, nitrous oxide should be titrated until an optimal sedation level is achieved. Used safely, nitrous oxide can be a wonderful aid to allow patients to be comfortable and relaxed while receiving dental treatment.

Nitrous oxide is a stable, nonflammable gas. When used with oxygen, nitrous oxide is one of the safest anesthetic agents available. It is administered through a nasal hood and has a sweet smell. As the patient breathes in the gas, it travels into the right and left bronchi and then the bronchioles and alveoli. The gases are then transferred across the alveoli in the lungs into the red blood cells of the circulatory system. The blood carries the gas in the blood plasma and red cells to the brain, where the nitrous oxide analgesic agent takes effect. This process is much the same as breathing atmospheric air, in which the body takes oxygen through the lungs and into the blood, and the blood carries the oxygen to the brain and throughout the body. Nitrous oxide relieves anxiety and also raises the pain threshold without the loss of consciousness. The patient is able to respond and follow instructions while being administered nitrous oxide sedation.

TABLE 23-8 Types of Sedation and Anesthesia Available in Dentistry

Oral sedation	Medication for oral sedation is taken before the dental appointment to relieve anxiety about the dental procedure. How long the drug lasts determines when the prescribed medication should be taken. For example, Valium lasts for more than 24 hours. As a result, it is best taken the night before the appointment. Valium has anti-anxiety properties in small doses. Slightly larger doses have a sedative-hypnotic effect, so the patient becomes drowsy. The patient must be driven to the appointment by a friend or family member and then must be taken home.
Intramuscular (IM) sedation	With intramuscular (IM) sedation a needle is used to inject the sedative drug in the office into the muscle of the upper arm or thigh or gluteal region. This is not a common form of sedation as the effect is not predictable. It is usually used when it is not possible to use other methods such as inhalation sedation or intravenous sedation. The effect of intramuscular sedation is to ease a fearful or anxious patient's concerns or apprehension when visiting the dentist. Intramuscular drugs take about 20 to 30 to start working. The dentist needs additional training and a special permit for IM sedation.
Intravenous sedation (IV sedation)	An intravenous (IV) conscious sedation occurs when sedative drugs are administered directly into the patient's blood system. An IV is set up in the vein and remains throughout the procedure. A specially trained person monitors the patient's pulse and oxygen levels. IV sedation allows the patient to be conscious but in a deep relaxed state. Often the patient does not remember what took place from the time the IV drug was started until the drug starts to wear off. Since IV medications can be titrated, the dentist has good control over the level of anesthesia. The dentist needs additional training and a special permit to administer IV sedatives. Additionally, reversal drugs and adjunct airway equipment should be in the office in the event of oversedation of the patient.
General anesthesia	When general anesthesia is administered, the patient goes into an unconscious state that is carefully controlled by an anesthesiologist. The anesthetic temporarily alters the central nervous system so that sensation or feeling is lost. General anesthesia is ideal for some patients for various dental surgeries and treatments. During general anesthesia, the patient's vital signs and fluids are closely monitored and a ventilator breathes for the patient while the patient is unconscious. The ventilator remains on until after the surgery and the patient recovers enough to breathe on their own. Usually general anesthesia is given in a hospital setting, but some oral and maxillofacial surgeons have "mini" operating rooms that are fully equipped to administer general anesthesia. Some dentists have received the necessary training to administer general anesthesia, but often an anesthesiologist performs this task so the dentist can concentrate on the surgery. The dental assistant is not involved with the administration of the general anesthetic but does assist during the surgery and is responsible for dismissing and monitoring the patient during recovery.
Inhalation sedation	In the dental office, inhalation sedation is synonymous with nitrous oxide and oxygen sedation. The next section of this chapter will focus on the use of nitrous oxide in the dental office.

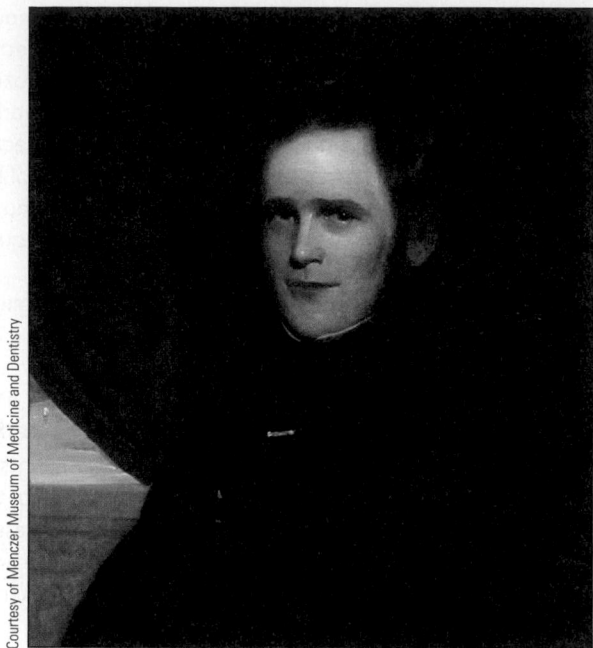

FIGURE 23-35
Horace Wells (1815–1848), artist unknown, c. 1838, oil.

Courtesy of Menczer Museum of Medicine and Dentistry

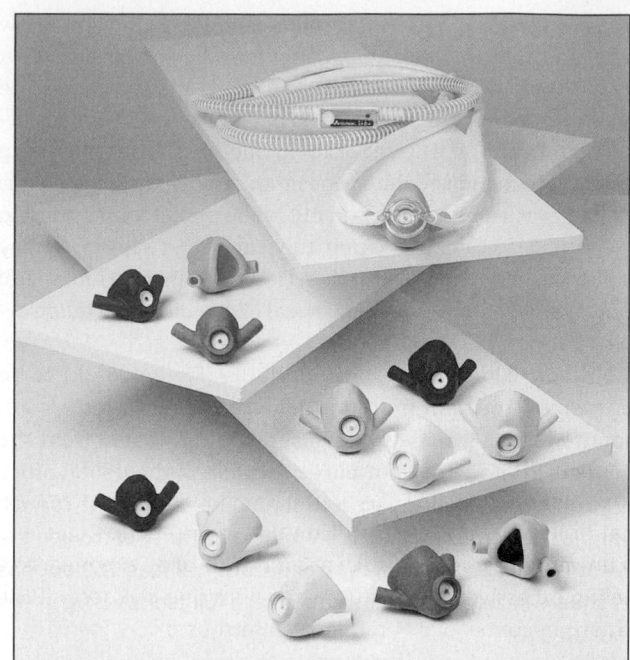

FIGURE 23-36
Nitrous oxide nasal hoods with scavenging circuit.

Safety and Precautions

The dental assistant should be aware of the safety concerns regarding nitrous oxide.

Dental Office Personnel Safety Studies demonstrate that long term chronic exposure to nitrous oxide may cause fertility problems as well as permanent neurological damage. Thus, the American Dental Association (ADA) has been monitoring and pursuing information about the safe use of nitrous oxide for many years. They convened an expert panel and made a number of recommendations to ensure safe usage of nitrous oxide for dental personnel. In addition, the National Institute of Occupational Safety and Health (NIOSH), which has continued activities relating to safe nitrous oxide concentrations in the dental office, reported that the recommended exposure limit of 25 ppm can be controlled by minimizing trace gases in the dental operatory, properly fitting nasal hoods (Figure 23-36), proper evacuation rates, and increasing the ventilation in the dental office. OSHA protocol for personal exposure monitoring is to complete two tests more than one week apart. If both test results are low, then periodic testing should be completed at least once a year. Chairside personnel exposed to nitrous oxide should be checked with diffusive samplers (dosimeters) at least annually.

Patient Safety To ensure patient safety, the patient's health history should be kept current, and all known allergies and past adverse drug reactions should be noted. Women in the first trimester of pregnancy, females undergoing pregnancy fertility treatment, immunocompromised people at risk of bone marrow

suppression, and people with neurological complaints need special consideration. Indications and contraindications for nitrous oxide use are outlined in Table 23-9.

Equipment Nitrous oxide is delivered to the patient through tubing connected to a nosepiece and tanks of nitrous oxide and

TABLE 23-9 Indications and Contraindications for Nitrous Oxide Use

Indications for Nitrous Oxide Use	Absolute Contraindications for Nitrous Oxide Use
• Anxiety related to dental treatment • A very sensitive gag reflex • Long appointment	• Patients unable to breathe through their nose • Patients using illicit drugs • Women in the first trimester of pregnancy • Females undergoing fertility treatments • Patients with chronic obstructive pulmonary disease (COPD) • Consult psychiatrist for patient under psychiatric care • Conditions that do not allow for good communication such as severe intellectual disability of the patient or advanced dementia

oxygen (Figure 23-37). The gases flow through a unit with a flow meter and adjustment controls. After the adjustments are made, the gas flows through the breathing tubes to the nasal hood. The excess gas and air exhaled from the patient flows through a scavenging nasal hood. The scavenging hood has tubes that bring the gas into it and separate tubes that remove the exhaled gas into the evacuation system and out of the operatory. Depending on the manufacturer of the unit, the scavenging nasal hood may be just one nasal hood as shown in Figure 23-36 or a double nasal hood as shown in Figure 23-37. Nasal hoods are either autoclavable or disposable.

Nitrous oxide units can be portable (Figure 23-38) or be centralized and wall mounted (Figure 23-39). When a wall-mounted nitrous oxide unit is used, the gas is sent from the cylinders located in a centralized location in the dental office through pressure lines to outlets in the treatment rooms. Cylinders of nitrous oxide gas are blue, and those of oxygen are green. The gauge on a full tank of nitrous will read 750 pounds per square inch (psi), and the gauge on a full tank of oxygen will read 2,000 psi.

At the start of each day, the nitrous oxide equipment should be monitored for safe operation. The tubing should be inspected for tears and kinks. Tears can lead to leakage of the nitrous oxide gas and unnecessary exposure of the dental health care worker (DHCW). The reservoir bag (Figure 23-37) should also be inspected for tears. Tears in the reservoir bag will also lead to leakage of the nitrous oxide gas. Any damaged hoses and reservoir bags should be immediately replaced. The nitrous oxide and oxygen equipment should be calibrated annually by a trained technician.

Procedure 23-4 outlines the steps for assisting in the administration of nitrous oxide.

Assisting in the Administration and Monitoring of Nitrous Oxide Sedation
Some states allow dental assistants to perform this task under the supervision of the dentist; in other states, dental auxiliaries assist the dentist in administering nitrous oxide and/or monitoring nitrous oxide. The dental assistant should be familiar with the scope of practice in their state.

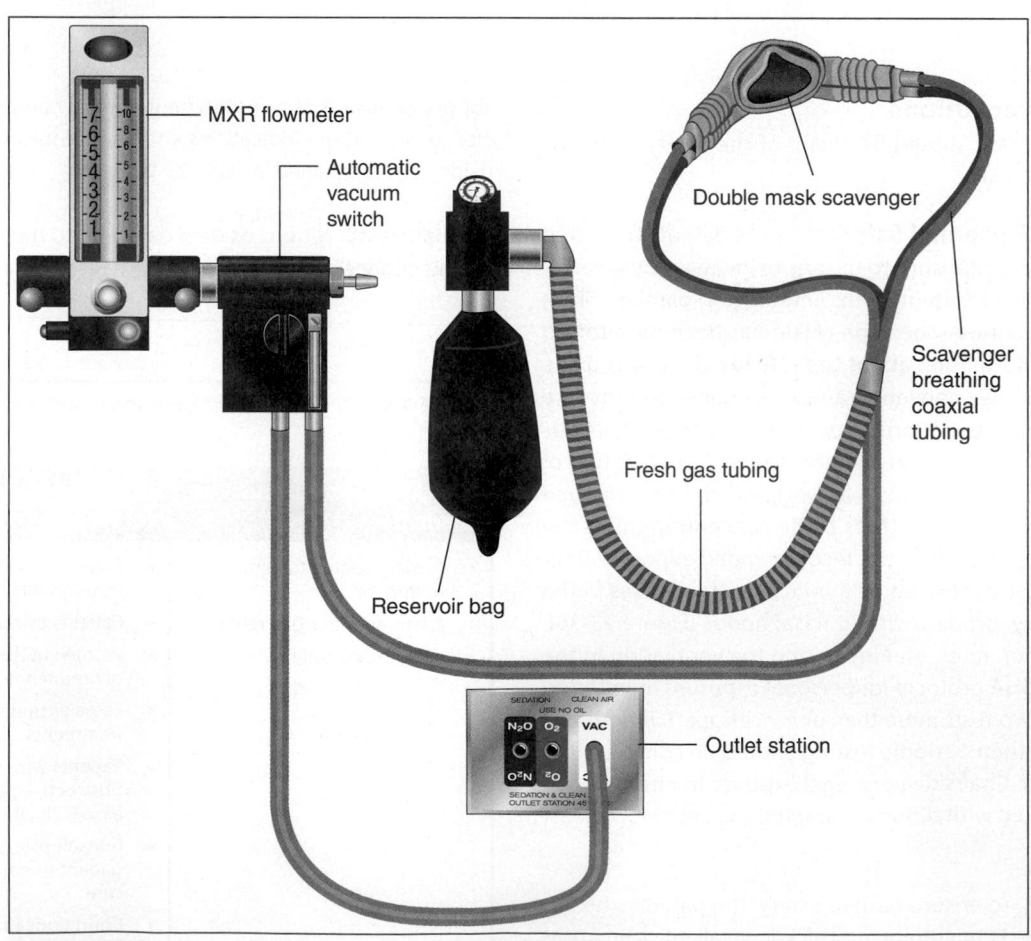

FIGURE 23-37
Components of a nitrous oxide system.

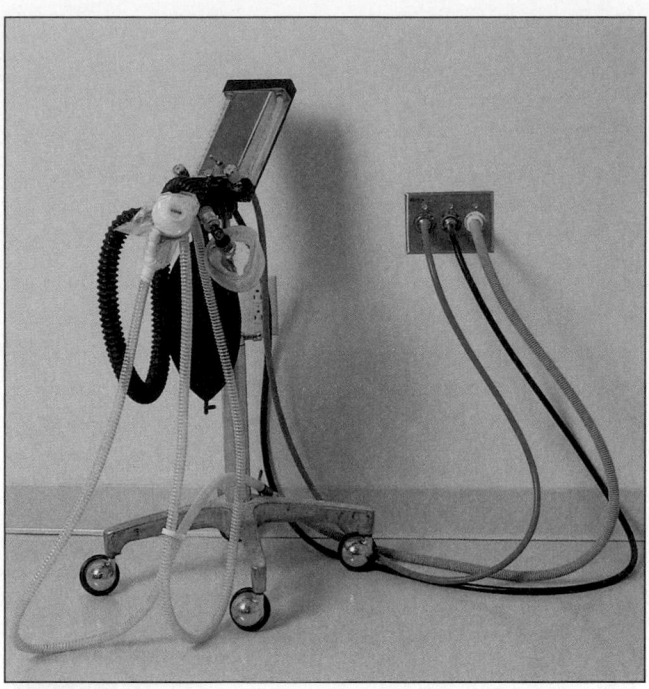

FIGURE 23-38
Portable nitrous oxide–oxygen unit.

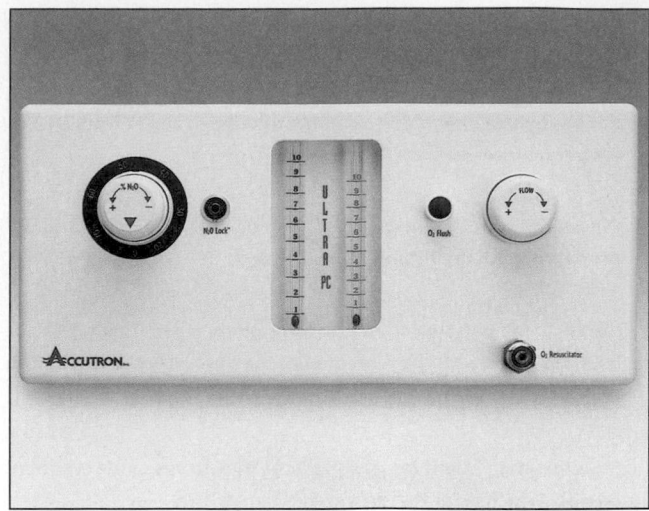

FIGURE 23-39
Example of a wall-mounted nitrous oxide–oxygen unit with gas cylinders in remote storage area.

Procedure 23-4
Assisting with the Administration of Nitrous Oxide

This procedure is performed by the dentist (or qualified dental assistant or dental hygienist based on the state scope of practice). Steps written in blue font are performed by the dentist, qualified dental assistant or dental hygienist, and the chairside assistant's steps are written in black.

Equipment and Supplies
- Patient Seating Setup (refer to Procedure 18-4)
- Nitrous Oxide Setup
  - ❏ Nitrous oxide unit
  - ❏ Nitrous oxide and oxygen tanks
  - ❏ Patient nasal hoods
  - ❏ Equipment and supplies for administration of local anesthetic (refer to Procedure 23-1)

Procedure Steps
1. Check all equipment as described earlier.

2. Check the levels of gases to determine that the tanks are full.

3. Escort and seat patient (refer to Procedure 18-4).

Dentist greets the patient and takes position at the dental chair.

❏ Signals for the procedure to begin (refer to Procedure 20-1).

4. Explain the procedure to the patient including the signs and symptoms the patient may experience from the nitrous oxide. Also explain the potential hazards of nitrous oxide to the patient.

5. Obtain written informed consent from the patient, allowing administration of nitrous oxide. An informed consent specifically for nitrous oxide must be obtained for nitrous oxide sedation at each administration visit.

Attaches a properly fitting sterile nitrous scavenger nasal hood to the tubing (see Figure 23-37).

(Continues)

Begins the flow of oxygen at 7 liters per minute to determine tidal flow. Tidal flow is the amount of liters that is exchanged each minute by a healthy adult. Average tidal flow ranges from 5–7 liters per minute in an adult.

Places the nasal hood over the nose of the patient, ensuring a proper fit, with the tubing draped to each side (Figure 23-40).

Instructs the patient to breathe through the nose slowly. Nitrous is titrated slowly to the patient until the desired level of sedation is reached.

Monitors the patient for any effects as the nitrous oxide is administered. Watches for Guedel's stage I anesthesia.

Watches the patient's chest and the reservoir bag expand and contract during the breathing.

Dentist administers local anesthetic solution within a few minutes of nitrous oxide optimal effect.

When the dental procedure is nearing completion, turns off the nitrous oxide and leaves oxygen flowing to prevent diffusion hypoxia. Diffusion hypoxia can result in confusion, shortness of breath and headache.

Removes the nasal hood from the patient's nose after 5 minutes or until all signs of the nitrous oxide sedation have disappeared. Turns off the oxygen at the unit. The flow meters for the nitrous oxide and oxygen will be at zero.

6. Seat the patient upright and ask how they feel. Record postoperative vital signs (blood pressure, pulse, and respiration).

7. Dismiss and escort patient to reception area when they no longer feel the effect of nitrous oxide (refer to Procedure 18-5).

8. Dispose of or autoclave the nasal hood depending on the type of nasal hoods utilized in the dental office.

9. Disinfect the tubing and the unit. Be careful not to spray the controls directly as moisture will enter into the area of the wiring. Use the saturate, wipe, saturate technique.

10. Complete all documentation on the patient's chart, including notation about the administration of nitrous oxide.

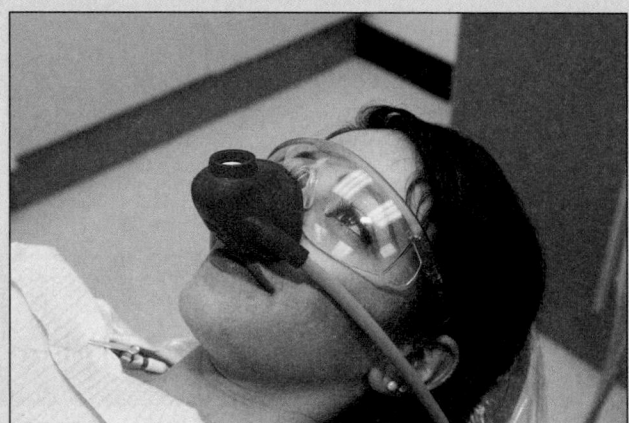

FIGURE 23-40
Nitrous oxide unit assembled and in place on patient.

Date	Services Rendered
02/18/XX	Updated medical and dental history, no changes noted. BP = 120/80; T = 98.6°F, P = 80, R = 18
	Administered 30% nitrous oxide with 70% oxygen for 30 minutes. Placed 20% benzocaine gel to injection sites for 2 minutes. Administered 2 cartridges (3.6 ml) of 2% lidocaine with 1:100,000 epi to mandibular left. No adverse reaction.
	Patient placed on 100% oxygen for 5 minutes at end of procedure. Patient stated she felt fine and was dismissed.
	#19 MOD amalgam completed
	RTC: #31 MO amalgam
	Assistant's initials

Chapter Summary

Because most procedures require some form of anesthesia, the dentist may select one or a combination of methods to control pain, depending on the patient and the procedure. The dental assistant is responsible for preparing, safely transferring, and caring for the anesthetic syringe and accessories. During this time, the assistant must be aware of the various topical solutions, the application sites, how to apply the topical anesthetic, and possible patient reactions. In addition, the assistant follows the dentist's directions for the administration of sedation and monitoring requirements.

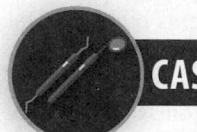 **CASE STUDY**

Chuck Thompson, 45 years old, was scheduled for a crown preparation. Topical anesthetic was placed and local anesthesia with 1:100,000 epinephrine was administered. Chuck became very talkative and excited. His pulse rate also increased.

Case Study Review

1. What kind of reaction is Chuck experiencing?

2. Are there any other symptoms to watch for?

3. What should be changed for the next visit?

Review Questions

Multiple Choice

1. Injectable local anesthetics permeate the nerve fiber to block sensations such as pain. The local anesthetics effect decreases as the anesthetic is carried away from the site of injection via the bloodstream.
Select the correct response based on the statements above.
a. Both statements are true.
b. Both statements are false.
c. The first statement is true, the second statement is false.
d. The first statement is false, the second statement is true.

2. Which of the following is correct regarding topical anesthetics?
a. Topical anesthetics are injected in order to produce local anesthesia for a dental procedure.
b. Topical anesthetics are available only as gel formulations.
c. The risk of an allergic reaction is higher with a topical anesthetic as compared to an injectable local anesthetic.
d. Topical anesthetics are always ester formulations.

3. Oraqix® is a noninjectable anesthetic that may be used for scaling and root planing appointments. A maximum of seven cartridges may be used during each appointment.
Select the correct response based on the statements above.
a. Both statements are true.
b. Both statements are false.
c. The first statement is true; the second statement is false.
d. The first statement is false; the second statement is true.

4. Which of the following is not correct regarding vaso-constrictors?
a. Vasoconstrictors constrict the blood vessels in the area of injection.
b. Vasoconstrictors increase the depth of anesthesia.
c. Vasoconstrictors increase the duration of anesthesia.
d. Vasoconstrictors allow the anesthetic to leave the site of administration quickly.

5. A patient presents to the office for treatment and the dentist determines that although epinephrine is needed, a lower dose of epinephrine would be beneficial to the patient. The treatment will last for about 30 minutes with no expected postoperative discomfort. Which of the following would provide the lowest dose of epinephrine?
a. 2% lidocaine 1:100,000 epinephrine
b. 4% prilocaine 1:200,000 epinephrine
c. 2% lidocaine 1:50,000 epinephrine
d. 3% mepivacaine

6. A nerve block anesthetizes only the soft tissues of the area injected. An infiltration injection anesthetizes the pulp of the tooth and soft tissues in the area injected.
Select the correct response based on the statements above.
a. Both statements are true.
b. Both statements are false.
c. The first statement is true; the second statement is false.
d. The first statement is false; the second statement is true.

7. Oraverse® is beneficial as it decreases the time of residual soft tissue anesthesia. Oraverse® is most commonly used after administration of the inferior alveolar nerve block.
   Select the correct response based on the statements above.
   a. Both statements are true.
   b. Both statements are false.
   c. The first statement is true; the second statement is false.
   d. The first statement is false; the second statement is true.

8. Which of the following is correct regarding trismus?
   a. Trismus occurs due to inadvertent anesthesia of the facial nerve.
   b. Trismus usually improves as the anesthetic effect wears off.
   c. Trismus is a blood filled swelling at the injection site.
   d. Trismus results in soreness of the area and limited jaw opening.

9. Facial nerve paralysis most commonly occurs during administration of the inferior alveolar nerve block. Facial nerve paralysis reverses as the local anesthetic wears off.
   Select the correct response based on the statements above.
   a. Both statements are true.
   b. Both statements are false.
   c. The first statement is true; the second statement is false.
   d. The first statement is false; the second statement is true.

10. Which of the following is not correct regarding the local anesthetic cartridge?
    a. The standard anesthetic cartridge is 1.7 milliliters.
    b. The local anesthetic cartridge is made of glass.
    c. The cartridges must be heated before use.
    d. The cartridges should be stored at room temperature in a dark place.

11. The tissue penetrating end of the needle has a bevel or angle. During the administration of anesthesia, the bevel of the needle should face the soft tissues.
    Select the correct response based on the statements above.
    a. Both statements are true.
    b. Both statements are false.
    c. The first statement is true; the second statement is false.
    d. The first statement is false; the second statement is true.

12. When completing a chart entry for local anesthesia administration, which of the following should be included?
    a. type of injection given
    b. percentage of local anesthetic
    c. concentration of epinephrine
    d. All of these

13. Which of the following is correct regarding the Needlestick Safety Act?
    a. The Needlestick Safety Act exempts nonmanagerial employees from evaluating and choosing safer devices.
    b. Dental offices with less than 20 employees are exempt from maintaining the log.
    c. The act mandated OSHA to revise the Bloodborne Pathogens Standard to include greater detail for the employers to identify, evaluate, and implement safer medical devices.
    d. States that require a sharps injury log require that the log must be completed within 2 days of the incident and kept for 5 years following the end of the calendar year of the records.

14. Oral sedative medications are taken prior to the dental appointment. Since the effects of the sedative will wear off, the patient is able to drive themselves home after the appointment.
    Select the correct response based on the statements above.
    a. Both statements are true.
    b. Both statements are false.
    c. The first statement is true; the second statement is false.
    d. The first statement is false; the second statement is true.

15. Which of the following is correct regarding nitrous oxide?
    a. Nitrous oxide may be used alone to provide relaxation and to relieve apprehension for patients during dental treatment.
    b. Nitrous oxide maintains the patient in Stage II anesthesia according to Geudel's signs and symptoms of anesthesia.
    c. Nitrous oxide can be titrated until an optimal sedation level is achieved.
    d. Oversedation with nitrous oxide results in a feeling of warmth and tingling fingers.

16. Which of the following is a sign or symptom of Stage I analgesia with nitrous oxide?
    a. feeling that time passes quickly
    b. vomiting
    c. out-of-body experience
    d. feeling excessively hot

17. National Institute of Occupational Safety and Health (NIOSH) recommends an exposure limit of 50 ppm of nitrous oxide gas. One way this can be achieved is through the use of properly fitting patient nasal hoods.
    Select the correct response based on the statements above.
    a. Both statements are true.
    b. Both statements are false.
    c. The first statement is true; the second statement is false.
    d. The first statement is false; the second statement is true.

18. Which of the following is not correct regarding parasthesia?
    a. Parasthesia is persistent numbness and pain for more than 24 hours after administration of local anesthesia.
    b. Parasthesia may be caused by a hematoma.
    c. Most parasthesias will resolve within 6 months.
    d. A patient who calls the office stating there is extended numbness after a procedure should be told that "it will go away."

19. One of the most common reactions to administration of local anesthesia is vasovagal syncope. Vasovagal syncope can be avoided by placing the patient in the upright position while administering the local anesthetic.
    Select the correct response based on the statements above.
    a. Both statements are true.
    b. Both statements are false.
    c. The first statement is true; the second statement is false.
    d. The first statement is false; the second statement is true.

20. Which of the following injections would provide anesthesia to only soft tissue in either the maxillary arch or the mandibular arch?
    a. nerve block
    b. infiltration
    c. field block
    d. supraperiosteal

Critical Thinking

1. What are the steps in preventing a medical emergency related to local anesthesia administration?

2. What is the body's response to epinephrine?

3. What is the armamentarium needed for administration of dental topical and local anesthesia?

Key Terms

Term and Pronunciation	Meaning of Root and Word Parts	Definition
hematoma (hee-ma-**toh**-m*uh*)	**hema** = blood **-oma** = marked growth, tumor	a mass of usually clotted blood that forms in a tissue, organ, or body space as a result of a broken blood vessel
pK_a	**pKa** = symbol of the acid dissociation; the closer the pKa of a drug is to the local tissue, the faster the onset of the action	a scale used to measure absorbability and acidity of hydrogen atom; allows for comparison of products
topical (**top**-i-k*uh*l)	**topo-** = place, local **-ic** = resembling **-al** = of the kind	applied externally to a particular part of the body (on top of); local; *a topical anesthetic*

## CHAPTER 24

Oral Prophylaxis and Recare Appointment

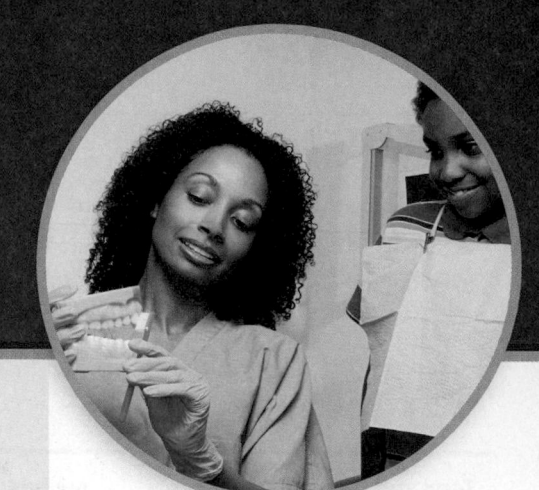

Specific Instructional Objectives

At the completion of this chapter, you will be able to meet these objectives:

1. Use terms presented in this chapter.
2. List the six dental hygiene standards of care.
3. Describe the steps of the assessment phase.
4. Identify data collected during periodontal charting.
5. Discuss the role of the dental assistant during comprehensive periodontal charting.
6. Discuss the importance of the dental hygiene diagnosis.
7. List the components of the dental hygiene care plan.
8. Explain the different types of dental hygiene treatment.
9. Identify the functions of the different types of dental hygiene instrumentation.
10. Differentiate between the various types of hand instruments that are used for dental hygiene treatment.
11. Identify a dental hygiene hand instrument by its design for use.
12. Differentiate between the various types of powered instruments that are used for dental hygiene treatment.
13. Recognize contraindications to powered scalers.
14. Determine the method of treatment for sensitivity based off the patient's symptoms
15. Discuss the role of the dental assistant during dental hygiene instrumentation.
16. Compose postoperative instructions following nonsurgical periodontal therapy.
17. Discuss the importance of the evaluation visit.
18. Document treatment.

Introduction

The dental hygiene visit appointment generally follows the new patient exam (refer to Chapter 22). If the patient presented with an emergency and received a limited exam, a comprehensive exam would need to be completed first before the patient is scheduled for their dental hygiene visit.

The dental hygiene visit is much more than a "cleaning." It plays an important role in preventing and arresting the progression of gingival and periodontal diseases. The dental assistant will play an important role in helping the patient recognize the value of the dental hygiene care visit.

Depending upon the dental office, the dental assistant's role during dental hygiene treatment can vary from limited to quite significant. Some dental offices practice assisted dental hygiene or accelerated dental hygiene. In such offices, the dental assistant typically sets up the operatory, seats the patient, completes required forms including updating medical and dental history, takes vitals, acquires the necessary radiographs, provides oral hygiene instructions, assists the dentist or dental hygienist (operator) during instrumentation, and when trained and qualified may perform the coronal polishing and fluoride treatments. The dental assistant may also provide other services that fall into the scope of their state law. Upon completion of the appointment, the dental assistant documents treatment in the services rendered form in the patient's chart, dismisses the patient, and breakdowns and sanitizes or disinfects the operatory.

The dental assistant should follow the criteria discussed in Chapter 22 when collecting information, having the patient complete legal documents, acquiring radiographs, and recording information. For offices that do not practice assisted dental hygiene, the dental assistant may still be responsible for assisting in the mentioned procedures during the dental hygiene visit from time to time. For these reasons, it is important to understand the procedures and steps during the dental hygiene appointment.

In order to provide guidance and help to ensure that the patient receives the best quality care possible, there are a list of standards developed by the American Dental Hygiene Association (ADHA). These standards were developed in 1985 (Figure 24-1). The dental hygiene standards for clinical dental hygiene practice break down the dental hygiene care visit into phases. There are six standards for clinical dental hygiene practice. These include assessment, dental hygiene diagnosis, planning, implementation, evaluation, and documentation. This chapter will review each component of the dental hygiene visit and the dental assistant's role in each component, if applicable.

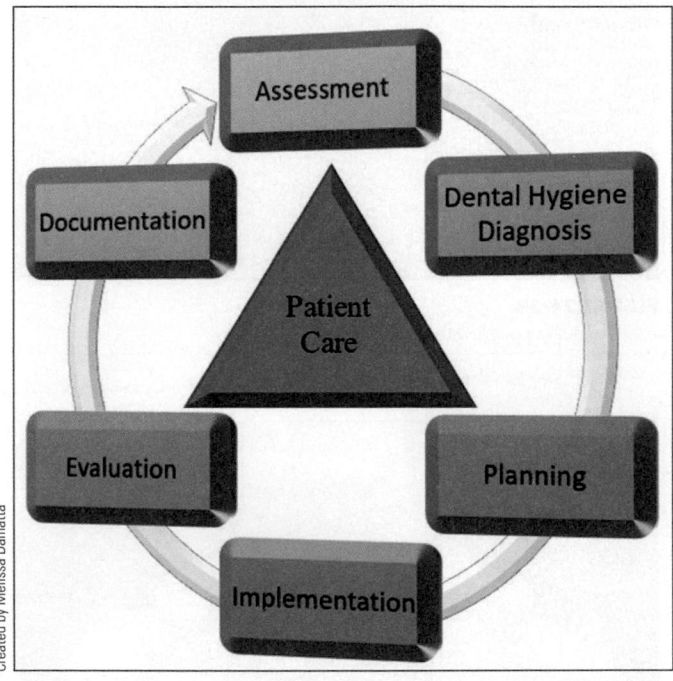

FIGURE 24-1
Dental hygiene standards of care.

Created by Melissa Damatta

Assessment

Assessment is a crucial part of the dental hygiene visit. This is the first step, where the operator collects and analyzes all of the oral health data from the patient. Without this step, the unique individual treatment needs of the patient cannot be identified adequately.

Many components of the assessment phase of dental hygiene treatment also are included in a comprehensive dental exam (see Chapter 22 for more detail):

- Health history: Including vital signs, social history, physical characteristics, medical health, and medication history
- Radiographs

- Extra and intraoral exam
- Intraoral images
- Completing or updating dental charting
- Completing or updating a comprehensive periodontal charting
- Determining patient goals

Additional procedures that must be completed during the assessment phase of dental hygiene treatment include determining the amount and location of hard and soft dental deposits, identification of risk factors that may contribute to disease, and measuring the level of periodontal disease.

The dental assistant can contribute to the assessment phase by updating the medical/dental histories, taking the blood pressure, acquiring any necessary radiographs and intraoral images, recording findings during the intraoral and extraoral examination, and completing periodontal and dental charting.

Hard and Soft Deposits

It is very important that the presence, amount, and distribution of both hard and soft deposits be recorded during the assessment phase in order to properly develop a dental hygiene care and treatment plan for the patient. Hard and soft dental deposits that can form in the oral cavity include dental biofilm and dental calculus (both discussed in Chapter 16).

Dental biofilm is considered a soft deposit and can be removed with a toothbrush and floss. Nevertheless, the operator should remove any soft deposits that are present during the dental hygiene appointment. Biofilm is removed during home care instructions with the patient and during instrumentation and polishing.

To assess dental biofilm, a biofilm control record (BCR) is performed, followed by home care instructions (refer to Chapter 16). Prior to instrumentation, the dental assistant can perform the BCR and provide the home care instructions to the patient, along with education on the cause of oral diseases. Performing instruction prior to instrumentation allows the patient to visually see

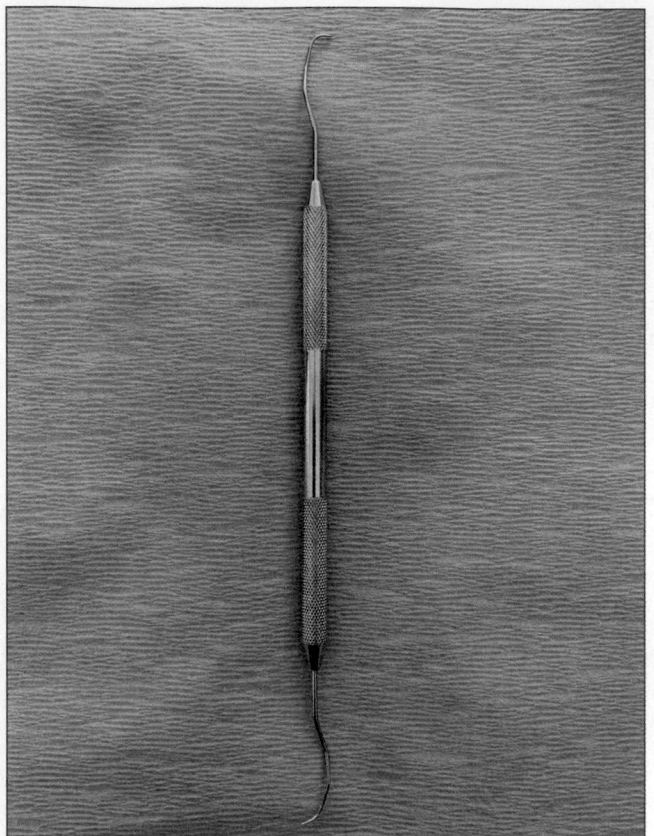

FIGURE 24-2A
ODU 11/12 explorer.

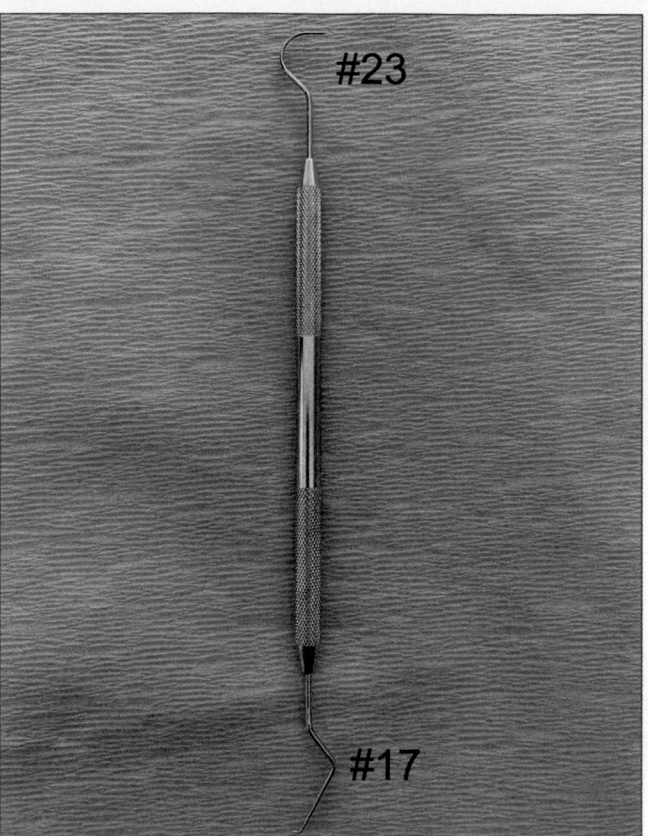

FIGURE 24-2B
A #17 explorer paired with a #23 explorer.

any biofilm remaining on their teeth following their home care procedures that day. Another advantage of providing home care instruction prior to instrumentation is the removal of the biofilm, reducing the need for unnecessary coronal polishing.

Dental calculus is considered a hard deposit. It begins as a soft deposit biofilm and becomes mineralized with calcium and phosphorus. Patients can't remove dental calculus at home; it can only be removed professionally using hand or powered instruments. To assess calculus, the operator will use a calculus detection explorer. The two most common types are the ODU 11/12 explorer (Figure 24-2A) and the #17 explorer, often paired with a #23 explorer (Figure 24-2B).

Dental deposits can be classified as supragingival or subgingival. **Supragingival** deposits are located on the tooth above the gingival margin; **subgingival** deposits are located on the tooth below the gingival margin. Figure 24-3 shows a patient with supragingival calculus, and Figure 24-4 shows a patient with subgingival calculus visible on a radiograph.

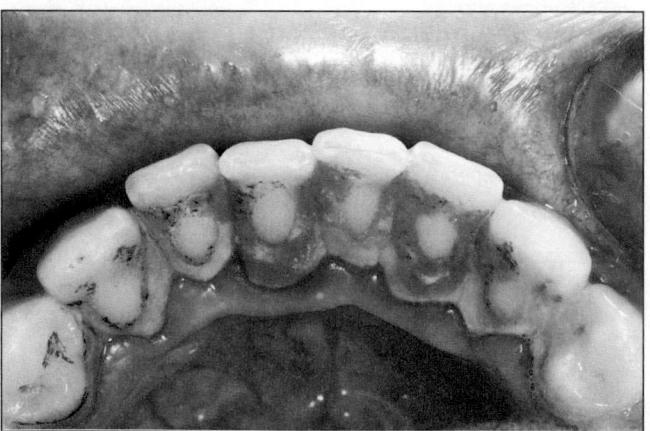

FIGURE 24-3
Supragingival calculus with stain.

Risk Assessment

Risk assessment is based on the health and clinical assessment. It identifies any oral or general health risks the patient may have. There are several risk factors for developing both dental caries and periodontal disease. Table 24-1 identifies risk factors for dental caries and for periodontal disease.

Measuring Periodontal Disease

Periodontal disease begins with gingivitis (no loss of attachment) and if left untreated will progress to periodontitis (loss of attachment). To assist in measuring the presence or absence of periodontal disease, a comprehensive periodontal charting will be completed. Figure 24-5A–C shows an example of a completed digital and paper comprehensive periodontal charting.

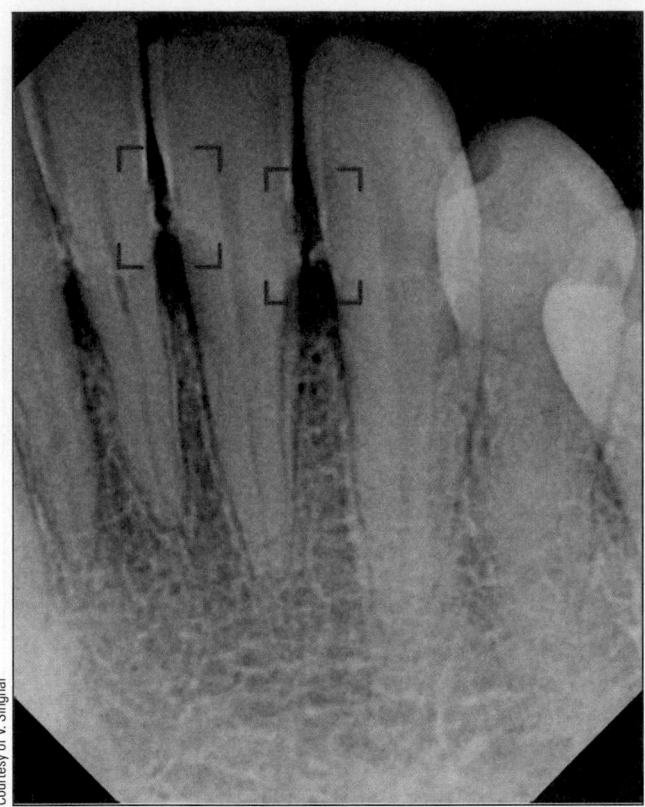

Courtesy of V. Singhal

FIGURE 24-4
Subgingival calculus located on a radiograph.

TABLE 24-1 Risk Factors

Risk Factors for Dental Caries	Risk Factors for Periodontal Disease
Decrease in saliva	Smoking
Diet high in fermentable carbohydrates	Diabetes
Inadequate sources of topical fluoride	HIV and AIDS
Poor oral hygiene	Poor oral hygiene
	Local contributing factors
	History of previous periodontal disease

The periodontal charting is started during the new patient exam with the periodontal probing measurements. The probing measurements are taken during the initial evaluation to screen for the type of hygiene appointment necessary for the patient. During the dental hygiene visit, the dental assistant will record the findings for the operator while they collect the remainder of the data needed for the periodontal charting. Be sure all missing teeth are recorded prior to beginning the periodontal charting. Inaccurately charting missing teeth will cause an error in the charting path. See Table 24-2 for descriptions of data collected during the comprehensive periodontal charting. See Chapter 38 for more information regarding the stages of periodontal disease.

TABLE 24-2 Data Collected During Comprehensive Periodontal Charting

Conditions	Description	Recording
Probing depths	Measured in millimeters (mm) using a periodontal probe. 0–3 mm is considered healthy. Anything above 3 mm could be a sign of disease.	Six measurements on each tooth are recorded. Distobuccal/facial, midbuccal/facial, mesiobuccal/facial, distolingual/palatal, midlingual/palatal, mesiolingual/palatal Paper charting: The operator will often tell the assistant which location to begin charting and which path to follow. Digital charting: Periodontal probing pathway may be pre entered as a template. Check with operator to ensure correct pathway is followed.
Bleeding points	Bleeding that occurs with mild manipulation of the periodontal sulcus/pocket.	Paper charting: Probing depth that elicits bleeding is circled in red. Digital charting: Varied entry depending on software. Can be charted as present/not present or represented by a numeric value.
Suppuration	The presence of inflammation and periodontal tissue breakdown causing a pus formation.	Paper charting: "S" in appropriate box Digital charting: Varied entry depending on software. Can be charted as present/not present or represented by a numeric value.
Gingival margin	Recession: Loss of gingival tissue exposing the underlying cementum. Measured in millimeters. If the margin is above the CEJ, notation is needed in order to calculate clinical attachment level (CAL).	Paper charting: Represented by a numerical value in appropriate box for the same six surfaces as probing depths. Digital charting: Varied entry depending on software. Charted same as on paper.

(Continues)

TABLE 24-2 *(Continued)*

Conditions	Description	Recording
Clinical Attachment Level (or loss) CAL	Measured from the CEJ (an unchanged point on tooth) to the base of the sulcus/pocket. This will necessitate addition or subtraction. If the tissue is overgrown over the CEJ, subtraction is needed. Subtract the probing depth and the tissue measurement above the CEJ. If there is recession present, addition is needed. Add recession measurement with probing depth.	Paper charting: Represented by a numerical value in appropriate box for the same six surfaces as probing depths and recession. Digital charting: Varied entry depending on software. Charted same as on paper. Most software auto calculates.
Mucogingival junction	Measures amount of attached gingiva remaining. A line that denotes the junction of the mucosa and the attached gingiva.	Paper charting: Represented by a numerical value in appropriate box. Usually represented by one measurement on each tooth for the maxillary and mandibular buccal/facials and mandibular linguals. Digital charting: Varied entry depending on software. Charted same as on paper.
Furcation	The dividing point of a multirooted tooth. Measured in Grades I, II, III, IV. Max and mandibular buccal and mandibular lingual have one recording, Maxillary palatal has two recordings (mesial and distal). Use of a furcation probe such as a Nabers probe is common. Note the curve of the working end to access the furcation. Furcation grades will be discussed in more detail in Chapter 38.	Paper charting: Drawing to represent the Furcation grade <ul><li>Grade I</li><li>Grade II</li><li>Grade III</li><li>Grade IV</li></ul>Digital charting: Numerical value representing grade is entered in appropriate box.
Mobility	Movement of the tooth in its socket. Scored as an N (normal), 1, 2, 3. On paper chart, can be recorded in half degrees.	Paper charting: – 1/2 degree I 1 degree + 1 1/2 degree II 2 degree + 2 1/2 degree III 3 degree Digital charting: Numerical value representing score is entered in appropriate box.
Fremitus	Vibration of the tooth that is palpable. Scored as an N, +, ++, +++.	Represented by the symbol "+".

Dental Hygiene Diagnosis

In 2016, the ADHA updated their standards of clinical dental hygiene practice to include the dental hygiene diagnosis (DHDx). They state that dental hygienists do in fact make multiple diagnoses for the patient's oral health care needs that fall into their scope of practice and services they are educationally qualified and licensed to provide. In 2018, dental hygienists made the jump from "Health Care Technologist and Technicians" to "Health Care Diagnosing or Treating Practitioners" on the Standard Occupational Classification put forth by the United States Office of Management and Budget. All the information gathered in the assessment stage, as well as the operator's own clinical expertise, are used to formulate a dental hygiene diagnosis or diagnoses. A determination would be made as to what treatment would benefit the patient. From there, a dental hygiene care plan would be developed.

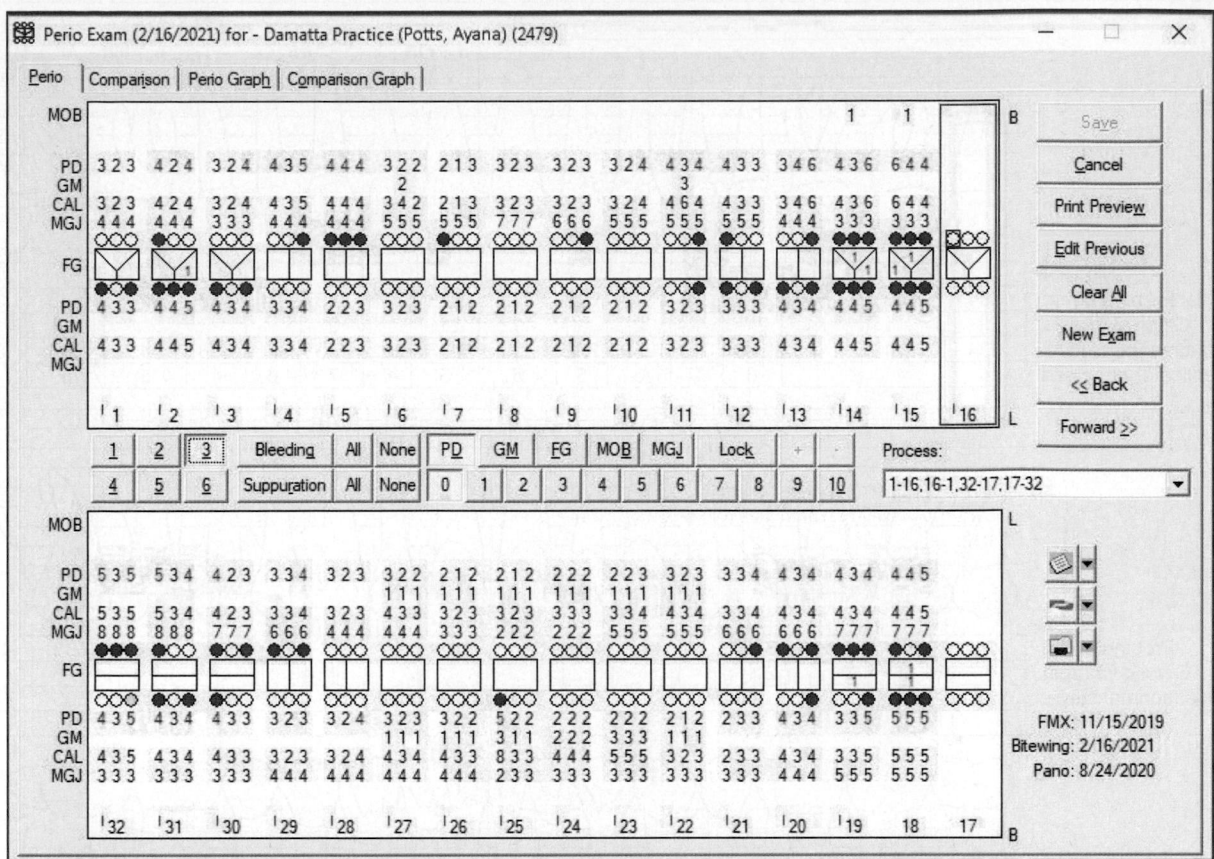

FIGURE 24-5A
Digital periodontal charting. Shows the probing depths, gingival margin, masticatory mucosa (MGJ), mobilities, clinical attachment levels, bleeding on probing, and furcations.

FINDINGS	USE BUTTON
Mobility Grade	MOB
Pocket Depth Measurement	PD
Gingival Margin Measurement	GM
Clinical Attachment Level	*Automatically Calculated*
Mucogingival Junction	MGJ
Furcation Grade	FG
Bleeding	Bleeding
Bleeding All	Bleeding all pockets
Suppuration	Suppuration
Suppuration All	Suppuration all pockets
Bleeding and Suppuration	Bleeding and Suppuration

Courtesy of Patterson Dental

FIGURE 24-5B
Key to Periodontal charting: Digital.

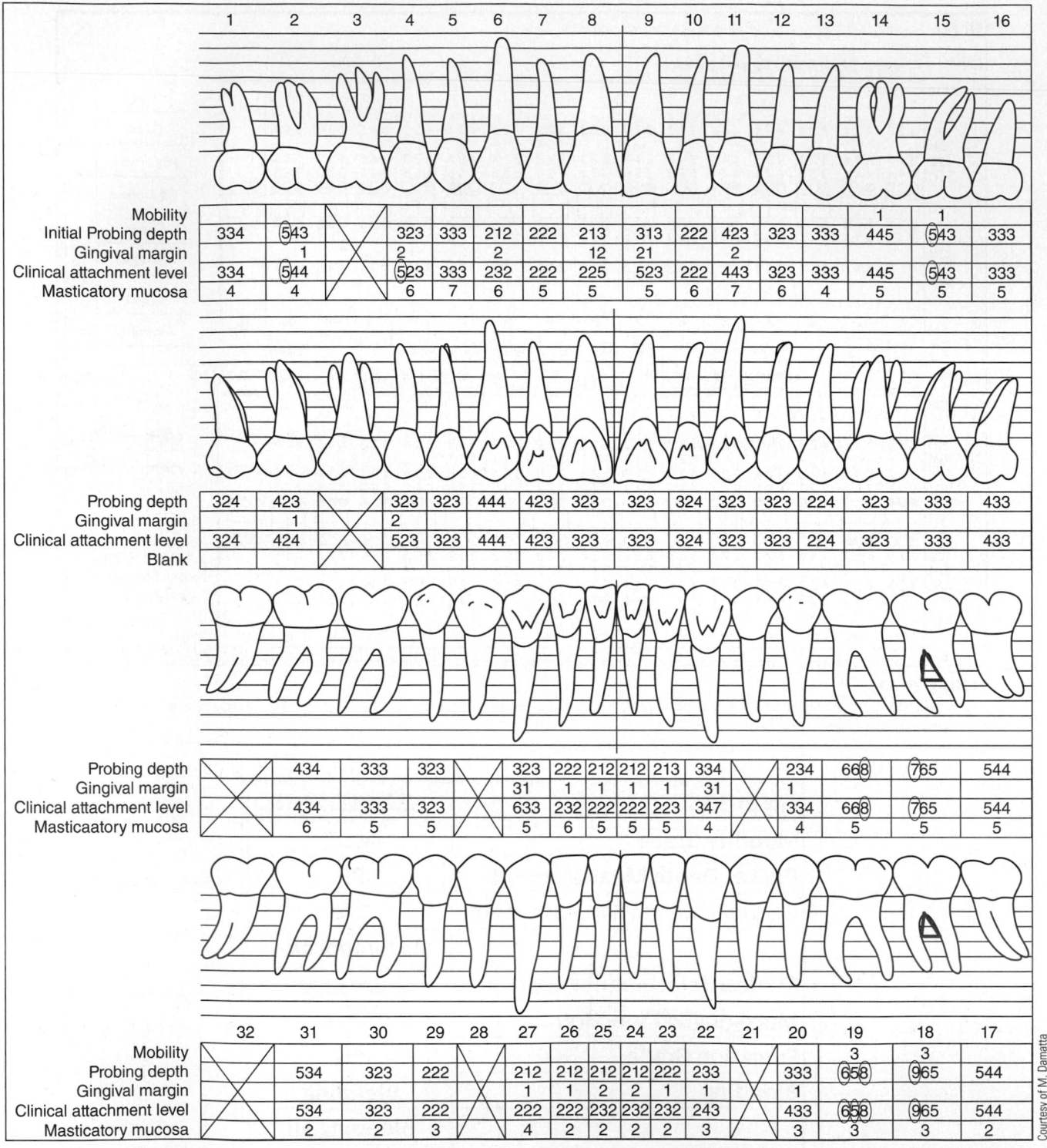

FIGURE 24-5C

Paper periodontal charting. Shows probing depths, gingival margin, clinical attachment levels, masticatory mucosa, mobilities, and bleeding on probing. Note furcation on teeth #2 and #18.

Planning

After assessment and the dental hygiene diagnosis, the information collected is used to develop the dental hygiene care plan. The plan should include all procedures needed to treat the needs of the patient and help prevent disease as well as the goals for those interventions. This includes any necessary treatment, behavioral changes, and referrals. Table 24-3 lists what should be included in the dental hygiene care plan. The dental hygienist should work closely with the dentist and any other health professionals to ensure the individual needs of the patient.

An important part of the dental hygiene care plan is obtaining informed consent. The patient or their guardian should be educated and counseled on all the services recommended before they give consent.

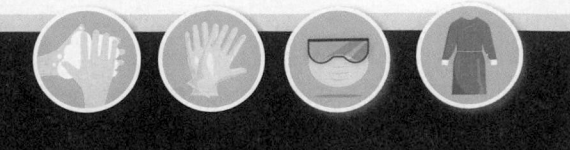

Procedure 24-1
Comprehensive Periodontal Charting

The chairside dental assistant will transfer and exchange instruments to the operator and will record all collected data for the operator.

Steps written in **blue** font are performed by the operator (dentist or dental hygienist), and the chairside assistant's steps are written in black.

Equipment and Supplies

Patient Seating Setup (refer to Procedure 18-4)

Instrument Setup (Figure 24-6)
- Basic setup: mouth mirror, explorer, and cotton forceps
- Periodontal probe (A)
- Nabers probe (B)

Procedure Steps

1. Escort and seat patient (refer to Procedure 18-4).

2. Prepare in advance for steps in periodontal charting.
   - ❏ Open patient's chart in dental software.
   - ❏ Navigate to the periodontal charting screen.
   - ❏ Begin a new exam or add to an existing exam.
   - ❏ Check with operator to ensure correct pathway is selected in the dental software.

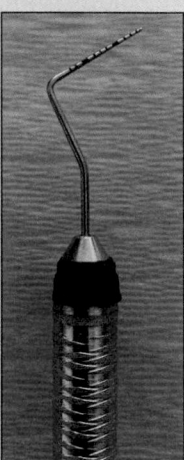 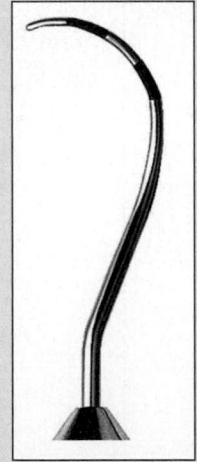

(A)   (B)

FIGURE 24-6
Periodontal probe and Nabers probe. Note the curve of the Nabers probe to access the furcation areas.

   - ❏ Introduce operator as they enter the treatment area.

   Greets the patient and takes position at the dental chair.

   - ❏ Signals for the procedure to begin (refer to Procedure 20-1).

3. Pass mouth mirror and periodontal probe at operator's signal.

   Examines for any missing teeth to be charted.

4. Confirm missing teeth charted. Record any missing teeth not already charted.

   Examines probe depths and notes bleeding points.

5. Record findings into the dental management software or in the patient record.

   Examines for suppuration.

6. Record findings into the dental management software or in the patient record.

   Examines the gingival margin.

7. Record findings into the dental management software or in the patient record.
   - ❏ Note if there is recession or gingival overgrowth.

   Examines the mucogingival junction.

8. Record findings into the dental management software or in the patient record.

9. Exchange periodontal probe for Nabers probe.

   Examines furcation.

10. Record findings into the dental management software or in the patient record.

11. Exchange Nabers probe for any single ended instrument (e.g., dental explorer).

   Examines mobility with two blunt ended instruments.

12. Record findings into the dental management software or in the patient record.

13. Retrieve all instruments.

   Examines fremitus.

14. Record findings into the dental management software or in the patient record.

(Continues)

15. Write up procedure in Services Rendered.

Date	Services Rendered
02/18/XX	Updated medical and dental history, no changes noted. BP = 120/80 T = 98.6F, P = 80, R = 18
	Comprehensive periodontal charting
	Assistant's initials

16. Dismiss and escort patient to reception area (refer to procedure 18-5).

TABLE 24-3 Dental Hygiene Care Plan

Demographic data
Periodontal and caries risk assessments
Goals set for patient
Number of appointments necessary to provide the treatment to the patient
Specific procedures to be provided at each appointment
Oral health education to be given to each patient during each appointment
Expected outcomes
Evaluation method

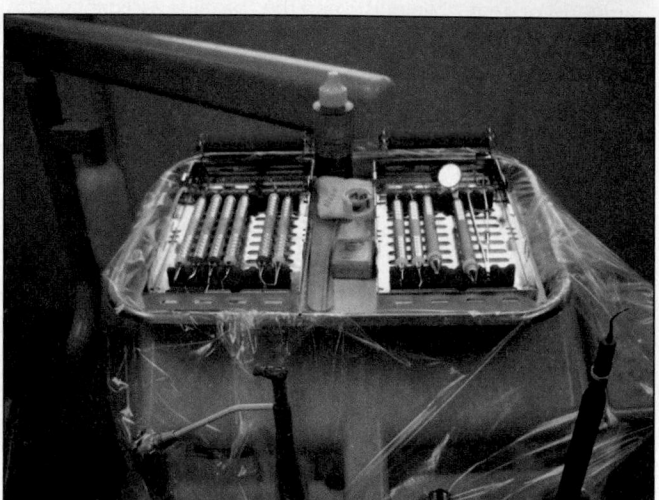

FIGURE 24-7
Dental hygiene armamentarium.

Implementation

Following the care plan is implementation. This is the phase where the treatment needs that were planned for the patient are completed. Depending on the type of plan or intervention that was agreed upon, this can be carried out in one appointment or multiple appointments. Regardless of the type of treatment needed, patient comfort is a big part of the appointment and should be considered in every aspect.

Armamentarium

The armamentarium needed for the dental hygiene visit will depend on the procedure. In addition to the basic tray setup, the dental hygiene tray will include a variety of instruments. Figure 24-7 shows common armamentarium needed for the dental hygiene appointment. Depending on the practice and type of treatment being completed, the setup will include both powered instruments and hand instruments. The instruments can be stored in either sterilization bags as shown in Figure 24-8 or in metal cassettes wrapped with a sterilization wrap (Figure 24-9). In addition to the instruments needed, an anesthetic setup may be necessary to enhance patient comfort. Table 24-4 lists the common dental hygiene armamentarium.

In assisted dental hygiene, the dental assistant will have their own tray setup on the assistant cart. When setting up the assistant tray, place the handles of the instruments facing in the direction of the hand being used to pass. For instance, for

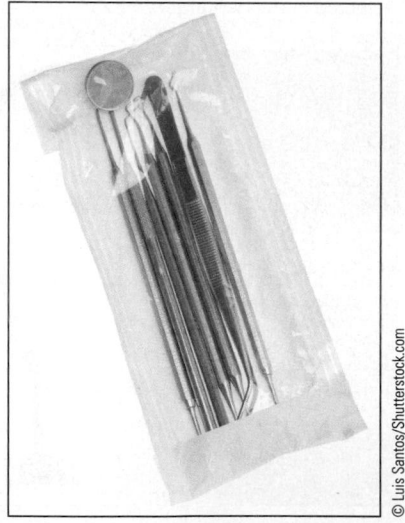

FIGURE 24-8
Bagged instruments.

© Luis Santos/Shutterstock.com

a right-handed operator, when passing the dental mirror, the assistant will use their right hand. Place the handle of the mirror to the right on the tray. When passing a curette, the assistant will use their left hand. Placement of the curette handle should be toward the left.

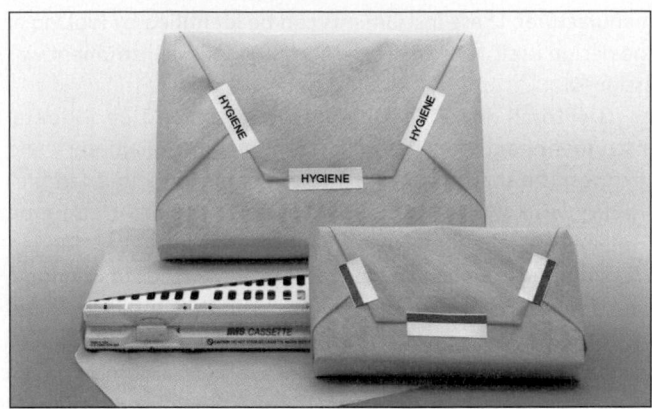

FIGURE 24-9
Cassette wrapped in blue wrap.

TABLE 24-4 Dental Hygiene Armamentarium

Prophylaxis
Dental mirror
Dental explorer—caries detection
Dental explorer—calculus detection
2 × 2 gauze squares
Dental floss
Saliva ejector
High volume evacuator
Sickle scalers
Universal curettes
Power scaler inserts or tips/wrench
Low-speed handpiece
Prophy angle attachment (cups and brushes)
Prophy paste in selected grit
Finger ring to hold prophy paste cup
Selected topical fluoride items (see Chapter 25)

Scaling and Root Planing
Dental mirror
Dental explorer—caries detection
Dental explorer—calculus detection
2 × 2 gauze squares
Dental floss
Saliva ejector
High-volume evacuator
Selected topical anesthetic
cotton tip applicator
Sterile self-aspirating syringe
Selected disposable needle
Selected anesthetic cartridge
Needlestick protectors
Sickle scalers
Universal curettes
Area-specific curettes (Gracey)
Power scaler inserts or tips/wrench
Topical fluoride items, if needed (see Chapter 25)

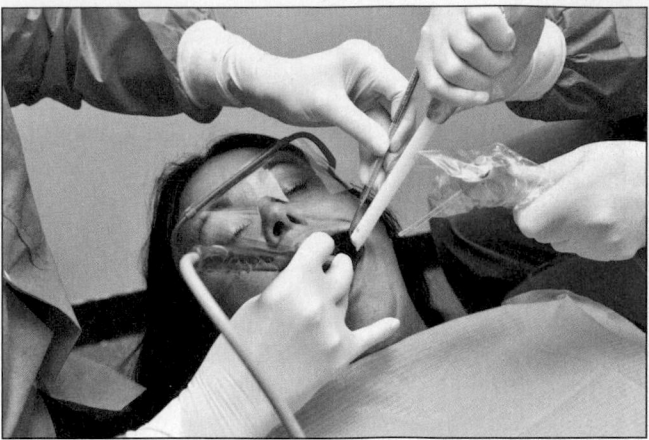

FIGURE 24-10
Assisting during ultrasonic instrumentation.

During treatment, the assistant will use the high-volume evacuation (HVE) during any procedures that produce aerosols. The assistant will also pass and exchange instruments and retract when needed. For retraction, when the operator is working on the patient's side toward themselves, the dental assistant will want to retract the tongue. When the operator is working on the patient's side away from themselves, the dental assistant will want to retract the cheek. Figure 24-10 shows a dental assistant assisting during a dental hygiene visit.

Hand Instruments The operator will complete various instrumentation procedures during the dental hygiene appointment. Types of instrumentation can include **scaling** and/or **root planing**, or a combination of both (SRP). Root planing is defined as the deliberate removal of diseased cementum and surface irregularities from the root surface. It was once thought that the toxins were strongly attached to the cementum, requiring deliberate removal of the cementum. Today, it is known that the bond of the toxins to the cementum is quite weak, necessitating a gentler approach and conserving as much cementum as possible.

Scaling involves removing biofilm and calculus from the tooth surface. Supragingival scaling or subgingival scaling may be performed, depending on where the deposits are. In most cases, however, a combination of supragingival and subgingival scaling is used.

Each of these procedures can be completed with hand instruments, power scalers, or a combination of both. There is a wide variety of hand instruments that can be utilized during the dental hygiene appointment. Each instrument will be carefully selected depending upon location and size of the deposit. This section will discuss the most commonly used instruments and their uses. Figure 24-11 shows some common hygiene instruments set up in a cassette.

Instrument Design All hand instruments have a basic identification and design. Scaling and root planing instruments are known as hygiene or periodontal instruments, depending on the

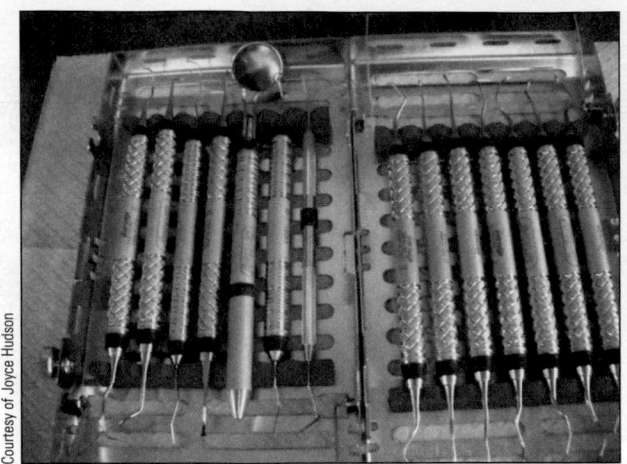

FIGURE 24-11
Common dental hygiene setup in a cassette.

manufacturer. These instruments can be identified by looking at the design itself or by the name and number the instrument was assigned.

As with all dental instruments, hygiene and periodontal instrument handles come in different weights, diameters, and textures. The shank of the instrument come in various lengths, rigidity, and shapes. Table 24-5 reviews the most common hygiene and periodontal instruments and their use and designs. Working ends of instruments can be single or double ended, with double ended instruments being paired or unpaired. Paired instruments are mirrored, which allows the use of one instrument to access the buccal and lingual without having to change instruments. Figure 24-12 shows a cross section of three different hand instruments.

Scalers Scalers are designed mainly to remove calculus supragingivally with very limited access subgingivally. Design

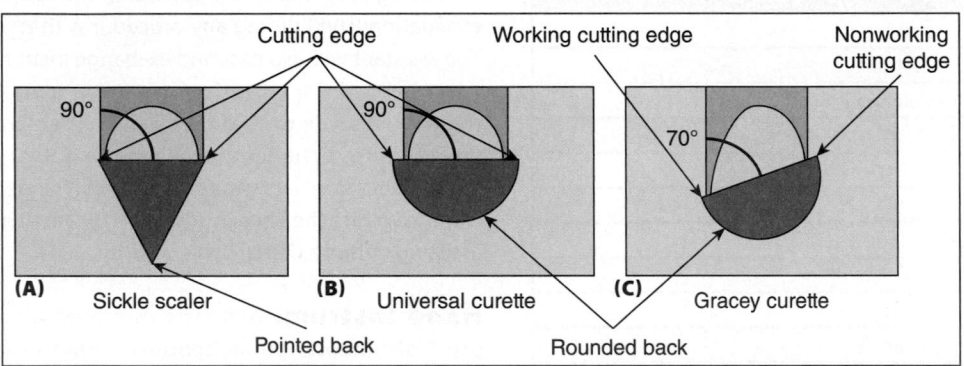

FIGURE 24-12
Cross sections of three common dental hygiene instruments. (A) Shows a triangular cross section (supragingival).
(B) Shows a semicircular cross section with two even cutting edges (Universal subgingival).
(C) Shows a semicircular cross section with one lower cutting edge (area-specific subgingival).

characteristics of the sickle scaler do not allow use of the instrument on recession, as it is quite rigid and can gouge the root surface. They have a pointed back and are triangular in cross section. Scalers have two cutting edges on each end that meet at a pointed tip (see Figure 24-13) and can be used posterior or anterior, depending on the design. Anterior sickle scalers have a short, simple shank, while posterior sickle scalers have a longer, complex shank. Figure 24-14 shows various scalers.

Universal Curettes A **Curette** can be either universal or area-specific. A universal curette is designed to allow use on both the anterior and posterior portions of the mouth with one instrument. They can be used to remove deposits both supragingival and subgingival; however, its design makes it ideal to use subgingivally without causing tissue trauma. They have a rounded back and are semicircular in cross section. Universal curettes also have two working cutting edges on each end but they differ from scalers by meeting into a rounded toe (Figure 24-13). They can be

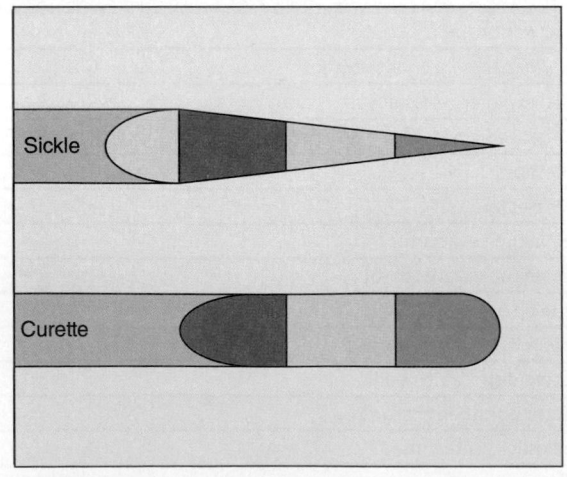

FIGURE 24-13
Leading, middle, and heel third of a scaler and curette.

TABLE 24-5 Design and Use of Common Instruments Used for Dental Hygiene Procedures

Scaler		Universal Curette		Area Specific Curette	
Instrument	Design and Use	Instrument	Design and Use	Instrument	Design and Use
Anterior sickle scaler H5 Anterior Jacquette scaler 33	• Simple shank • Use on crowns only • Pointed back, restricting subgingival access	Columbia 13/14	• Complex shank • Anterior and posterior use (truly universal) • Rounded back allowing subgingival use • Standard shank flexibility • Shorter shank	Gracey 1/2	• Simple shank • Anterior use • Rounded back allowing subgingival use • One working cutting edge • Rounded back allowing subgingival use • Standard and rigid shank flexibilities • Longer shank
Posterior sickle scaler 204s	• Complex shank • Use on crowns only • Pointed back, restricting subgingival access	Barnhart 5/6 *Courtesy of H. Schein*	• Complex shank • Anterior and posterior use (truly universal) • Rounded back allowing subgingival use • Standard shank flexibility • Longer shank	Gracey 11/12	• Complex shank • Posterior use • Rounded back allowing subgingival use • One working cutting edge • For mesial, buccal, and lingual surfaces • Standard and rigid shank flexibilities • Longer shank
		Columbia 4r/4l	• Complex shank • posterior use • Rounded back allowing subgingival use • Rigid shank flexibility • Longer shank	Gracey 13/14	• Complex shank • Posterior use • Rounded back allowing subgingival use • One working cutting edge • For distal surfaces • Standard and rigid shank flexibilities • Longer shank
		Columbia 2r/2l	• Complex shank • Anterior use • Rounded back allowing subgingival use • Rigid shank flexibility • Longer shank		

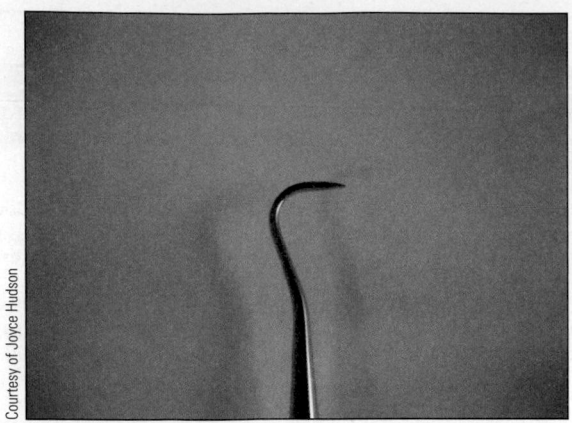

FIGURE 24-14A
Anterior sickle scaler.

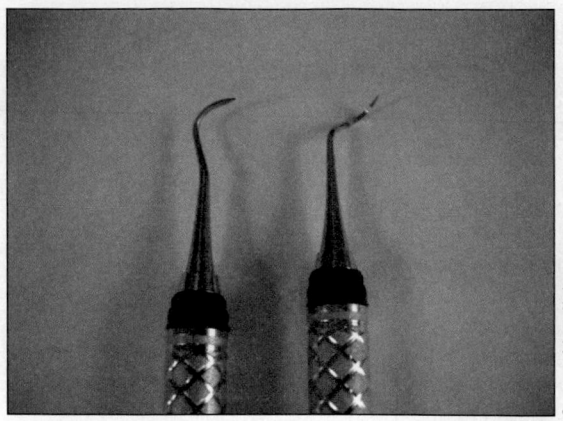

FIGURE 24-14B
Anterior (left) and posterior (right) sickle scaler. Notice the curve in the posterior shank to allow access to the posterior.

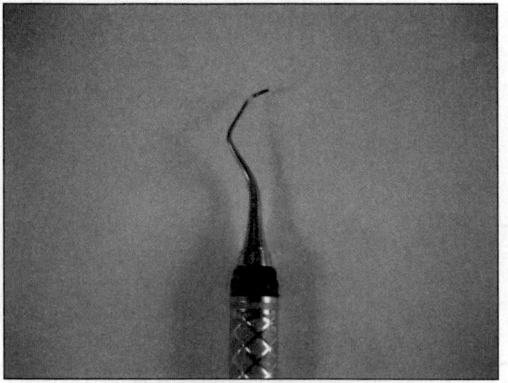

FIGURE 24-15
Universal curette.

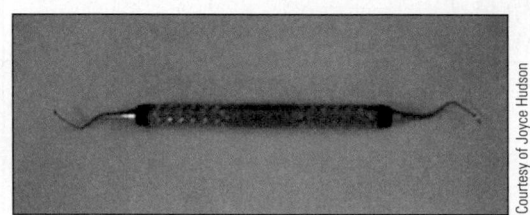

used posterior or anterior, depending on the design. Figure 24-15 shows a type of universal curette.

Area-Specific Curettes Area-specific curettes are periodontal instruments with longer shanks designed to reach deeper in periodontal pockets. They only have one working cutting edge per end. For this reason, area-specific curettes are designed to be used in specific areas of the mouth. For instance, some are used on the distal surfaces of molars, while others are designed to be used on the buccal, lingual, and mesial surfaces of molars. This will require the use of two area-specific curettes to complete instrumentation on the entire mandibular right first molar, versus one universal curette. The face of the instrument differs from a universal curette as it has an offset blade to 70°, making the working cutting edges lower than the nonworking cutting edge (Figure 24-16). The lower cutting edge is the working cutting edge and the edge that is used for calculus removal. Figure 24-17 shows a variety of area-specific curettes.

Powered Instruments Powered instruments/scalers can be either **sonic** or **ultrasonic**. They use different levels of frequencies measured by cycles per second and can be sourced

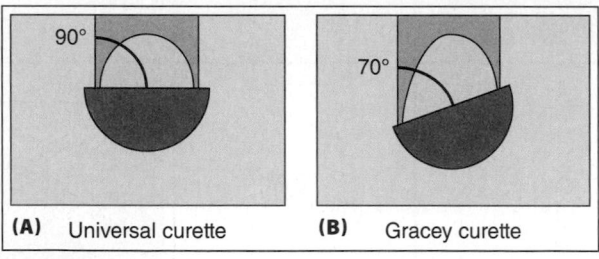

FIGURE 24-16
(A) Universal curette with two even cutting edges and (B) area-specific curette with a lower working cutting edge and a higher nonworking cutting edge.

by an air turbine (attached to the dental unit) or through a powered electronic generator that converts energy to ultrasonic vibrations (Figure 24-18). Both types require a handpiece to be attached to the unit and an insert or tip that attaches to the handpiece. Powered scalers work through a combination of mechanical vibration, **cavitation**, and **irrigation**. These actions fracture the calculus, disrupt the biofilm, and flush bacteria from the periodontal pocket. Powered scalers are also indicated for **extrinsic stain** removal. Interchangeable tips are available for

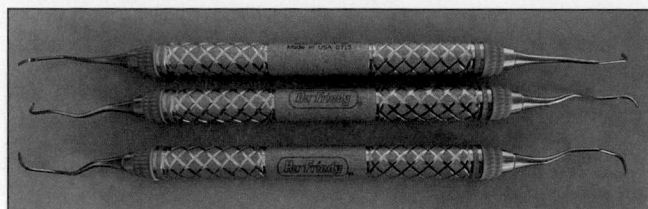

FIGURE 24-17
Various area-specific curettes.

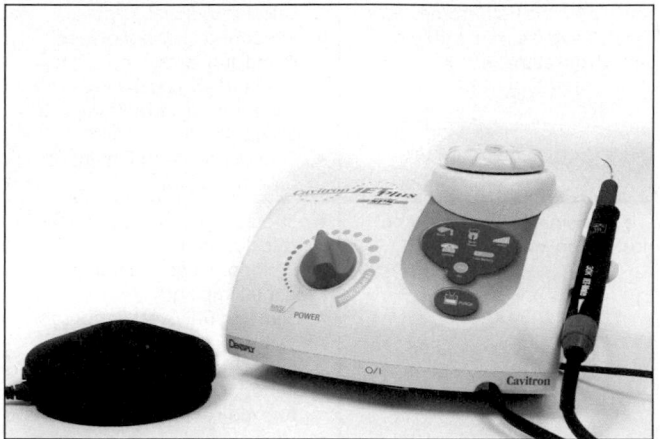

FIGURE 24-18A
Ultrasonic unit.

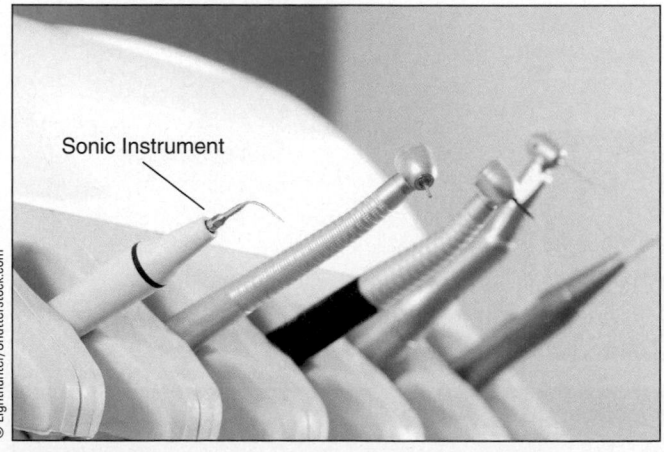

Sonic Instrument

© Lighthunter/Shutterstock.com

FIGURE 24-18B
Sonic unit attached to the dental unit using air turbine.

each unit varying from thinner tips, used for biofilm and light calculus removal and to access tighter deeper areas, to thicker tips used for more moderate to heavy calculus. Table 24-6A outlines the types of powered scalers that are available for use during dental hygiene treatment as well as the characteristics of each. Table 24-6B illustrates the steps for setting up both sonic and ultrasonic instrument units.

Water lines for powered instruments should be flushed 2 minutes at the beginning of each work day and 20–30 seconds in between each patient to flush any possible microbial buildup in the water lines.

Powered scalers produce spatter and aerosols that can be suspended in the air for 30 minutes to 2 hours. It is important to apply stringent infection control procedures. In addition to a mask, gloves, and protective clothing and eyewear, a face shield is required for the operator and the assistant. In assisted dental hygiene, the use of HVE is necessary to control aerosol production. To reduce the bacterial load that may be released in the aerosols and spatter, the patient should be given a preprocedural rinse prior to treatment.

There are certain contraindications to the use of a powered instrument. These include patients with a communicable disease, immunocompromised patients, respiratory diseases, **dysphagia**, and use of a **cardiac device.** A **piezoelectric** powered scaler may be less likely to cause a interference with a cardiac device than a **magnetostrictive** powered scaler. Studies show that interference is possible if the dental device is within 15 inches of the implanted cardiac device. Care should be taken not to wave the powered instrument or drag the cord over the patient's chest. Units should also be turned off when not in use. Patients who have newer shielded cardiac devices may be less susceptible to interference and be cleared for use; however, a medical consult with the patient's cardiologist is necessary due to the conflicting evidence.

Pain Control

There are various needs for pain management, and for each of those needs there are many options. The pain management must be matched to the specific needs of the patient. A patient may have tooth or gingival sensitivity or a combination of both. A patient who experiences tooth sensitivity during their dental hygiene appointment is likely to have **dentinal hypersensitivity**. This type of sensitivity is caused by exposed dentin due to some sort of damaging habit the patient has and can be extremely uncomfortable. Habits can include but are not limited to grinding, hard toothbrushing habits, using a toothbrush with harder filaments, high acid diet, and periodontitis. With this type of sensitivity, the discomfort is usually felt upon instrumentation or exposure to colder temperatures. In addition to instrumentation, care should be taken when the air/water syringe or HVE is used during the appointment. It is common for the dental professional to first identify the hypersensitivity during a dental hygiene appointment. Depending on the prevalence and locations of the hypersensitivity, a professional chairside desensitizing agent may be applied pretreatment. This seals off the dentinal tubules and allows the treatment that day to be more comfortable. Desensitizing agents can be gels, creams, liquids, pastes, or varnishes.

For post treatment, a fluoride varnish may also be applied to the sensitive areas along with patient education on behavioral changes. Fluoride varnish is applied to the root surface where there is exposed dentin. A trained and qualified dental assistant may

TABLE 24-6A Types of Power Scalers

Type of Power Scaler, Classification, and Frequency	Characteristics	Precautions	Types of Inserts Available
Type: Sonic *Classification:* Sonic *Frequency:* 2,500-7,000 cycles per second (CPS)	Elliptical motion. All sides of the insert are active and can be used for instrumentation.	Limited inserts available. Not for heavy calculus. Low range of vibrations, limits cavitation if any. Therefore, not designed for definitive root treatment.	• Supragingival and subgingival calculus removal. • Periodontal debridement of dental implants. • Slim and universal designs for various hard and soft deposit levels
Type: Magnetostrictive *Classification:* Ultrasonic *Frequency:* 18,000-45,000 cycles per second (CPS)	Elliptical motion. All sides of the insert are active and can be used for instrumentation	Unit uses water to cool tip. Without water, the tip becomes very heated and can cause pulp or soft tissue damage.	• Supragingival and subgingival calculus removal. • Periodontal debridement of dental implants. • Slim and universal designs for various hard and soft deposit levels. • Periodontal debridement of furcation areas.
Type: Piezoelectric *Classification:* Ultrasonic *Frequency:* 25,000-50,000 cycles per second (CPS)	Linear motion. Only the two sides of the tip are active.	Tips are small, can typically be lost. Need a wrench.	• Supragingival and subgingival calculus removal. • Periodontal debridement of dental implants. • Slim and universal designs for various hard and soft deposit levels • Periodontal debridement of furcation areas.

TABLE 24-6B Instrument Setup for Power Scalers

Instrument Setup for Sonic Scalers

1. Power dental unit on
2. Attach handpiece.
3. Flush water lines.
4. Attach tip to handpiece using designated wrench.

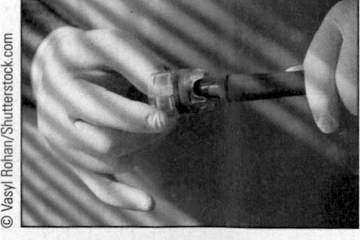
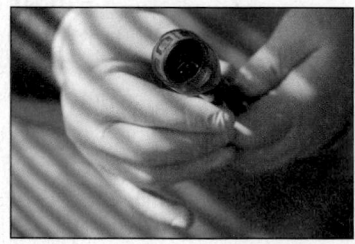

Instrument Setup for Magnetostrictive Scalers

1. Power unit on.

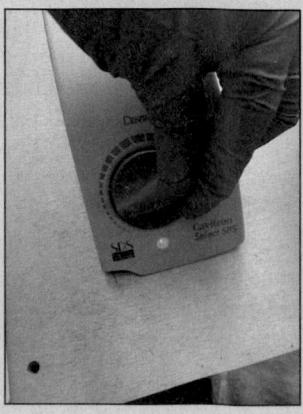

2. Attach handpiece.

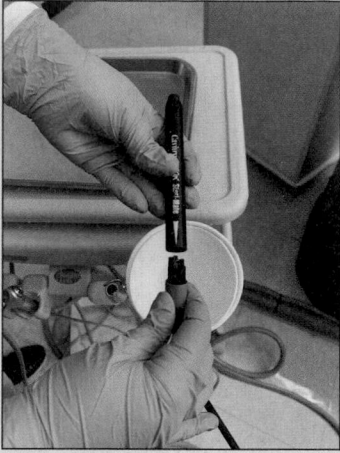

3. Flush water lines with power on lowest setting and water on highest setting.

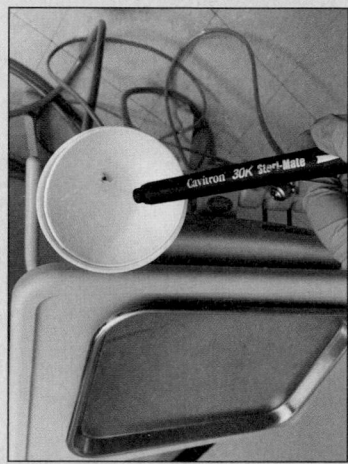

4. Hold handle upright and fill with water until a bubble is seen on top.

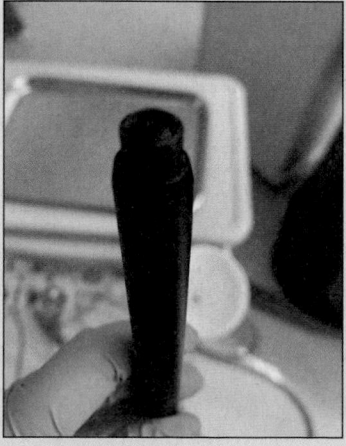

5. Guide insert into handle and push down until it snaps in.

6. Adjust water and power to desired level.

(Continues)

TABLE 24-6 *(Continued)*

Instrument Setup for Piezoelectric Scalers

1. Power unit on.

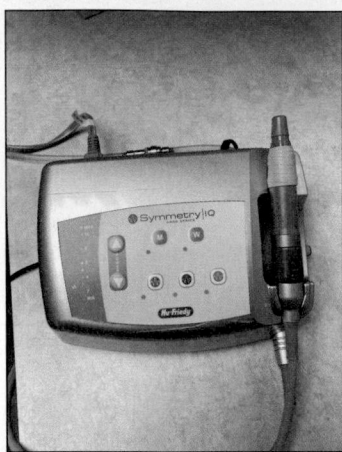

2. Flush water lines.
3. Place chosen tip onto handle with designated wrench.

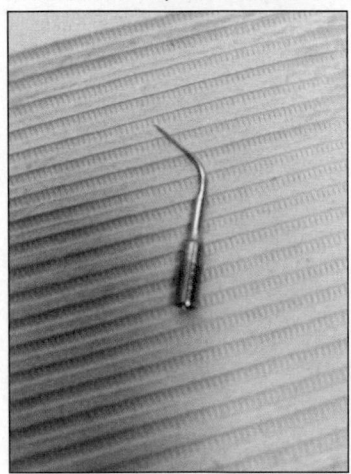 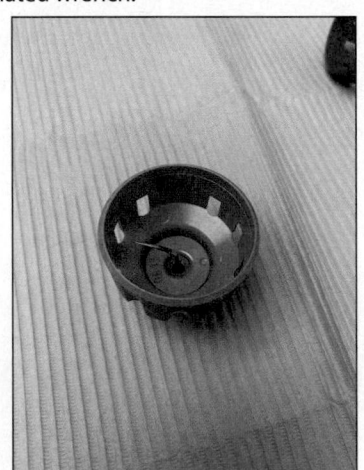

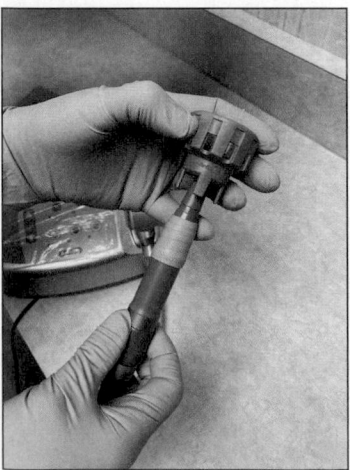

4. Adjust water and power to desired level.

apply the desensitizing agent if needed. Fluoride application is discussed more in Chapter 25. It is vital the patient understand the mechanism of their hypersensitivity and methods to reduce further destruction. These can include adjustments in dietary habits, recommendation of an at home desensitizing toothpaste such as an over-the-counter dentifrice with 5% potassium nitrate, appropriate toothbrushing habits, at home fluoride use, and reduction of parafunctional habits by use of a nightguard, if needed.

A patient can also experience gingival sensitivity. Gingival sensitivity can be addressed in several different ways. The method that is selected will depend on the amount of discomfort the patient feels as well as the **invasiveness** of the treatment needed. Something as simple as a topical gel or cream could be applied for mild sensitivity or for a basic preventative visit. For more moderate sensitivity, a noninjectable liquid topical anesthetic can be applied using a blunt tip cannula subgingivally. For patients who present with extreme sensitivity, or patients who require a more therapeutic treatment, a local anesthetic can be administered for complete patient comfort. A trained and qualified dental assistant may apply the topical anesthetic for generalized sensitivity or in a localized area prior to local anesthetic administration. For a patient who is experiencing anxiety or a dental phobia, other options such as nitrous oxide–oxygen sedation could be used either alone or in conjunction with other local or topical anesthetics. Refer to Chapter 23 for anesthetic delivery in more detail.

Oral Prophylaxis

The best approach to oral health is prevention. An oral **prophylaxis**, which is part of the dental hygiene visit, is considered preventative and is completed on a patient who has an intact periodontium or gingivitis. It includes the removal of supragingival and subgingival hard and soft deposits. Most often a blended approach of hand and powered instruments is used. While stain removal is a part of the oral prophylaxis, it is considered cosmetic due to lack of documented therapeutic value. A dental assistant who is trained and qualified may perform the coronal polishing. Coronal polishing is discussed in more detail in Chapter 25.

Nonsurgical Periodontal Therapy A patient who has a reduced periodontium, moderate to heavy calculus, periodontal pocketing, bleeding, and inflammation may require a more therapeutic visit such as **nonsurgical periodontal therapy** (NSPT). This is considered a phase I or initial treatment and a precursor to any periodontal surgical procedure. NSPT includes risk identification, patient behavior modification, adjunctive therapy, scaling and root planing, and reevaluation. **Adjunctive therapy** such as local or oral **chemotherapeutics** has been shown to enhance the treatment outcomes when provided the same day as initial therapy. Refer to Chapter 38 for more information on periodontal procedures, including chemotherapeutics.

During the initiation of therapy, scaling and root planing are typically completed in quadrants. During scaling and root planing, calculus, biofilm, and bacterial toxins are removed from a periodontal pocket to promote healing and to restore periodontal health. For a patient with a moderate periodontal disease,

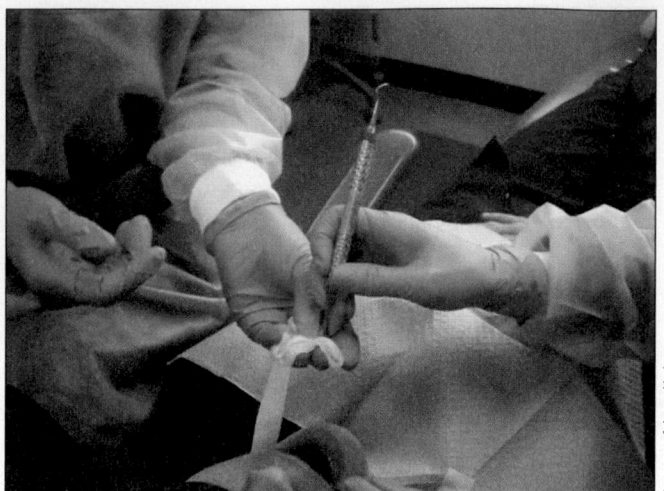

FIGURE 24-19
The dental assistant is cautiously cleaning and wiping the working end of the dental hygienist's instrument.

the operator may decide to start with two quadrants on the same side of the mouth, followed by a second appointment to complete the other half. For a patient with a more severe case of periodontal disease, the operator may decide to complete the treatment in single quadrants. If the patient does not respond to treatment, the next phase would be to refer to a periodontist for surgical treatment.

Periodontal **debridement** is a comprehensive procedure that encompasses removal of biofilm, toxins, and calculus from a root surface in a single visit. The goal of periodontal debridement is to remove all hard and soft deposits and gingival irritants in order to promote periodontal health while preserving the cementum. Periodontal debridement is most commonly completed using a combination of both hand instruments and power instruments.

The coronal polishing is not advised at the same appointment as the NSPT due to the possibility of embedding particles of the paste into the tissue, causing irritation and delaying the healing process. Coronal polishing is completed at the evaluation appointment. Evaluation visits are discussed later in this chapter. Figure 24-19 shows a dental assistant who is assisting a dental hygienist performing dental hygiene treatment. The dental assistant is cleaning and wiping the working end of the dental hygienist's instrument.

Safety

Care should be taken when wiping dental hygiene instruments for the operator. The instruments have cutting edges or blades that are sharp. Since instruments are almost always contaminated with blood while in use, a cut or puncture in the skin could be a possible risk of an infectious pathogen exposure. If this should happen, the office's OSHA Bloodborne Pathogen postexposure protocol should be followed.

Documentation

For NSPT, the following postoperative instructions should be given:

- When local anesthesia is administered, wait for anesthesia to wear off before eating/chewing or drinking any hot liquids. This will prevent the patient from chewing their lip or burning themselves without being aware of it.
- For soreness or tenderness, take OTC analgesics safe for patient to take, if necessary.
- Soft diet for the day.
- Resume normal or newly introduced home care routine.
- Chlorhexidine rinses may be indicated: Use as directed.
- Smoking interrupts the healing process: Should be avoided especially during the first 24 hours.
- Warm saltwater rinses
  - 1 tsp salt in 8 oz of warm water

Infection Control

For both the prophylaxis and NSPT, the patient always begins the appointment with a preprocedural rinse. Many hygiene procedures create aerosols that can cause contamination concerns within the dental environment. A preprocedural rinse with antimicrobial mouth rinse can reduce the number of bacteria in aerosols created during dental hygiene treatment. Some common procedures that can create an increased number of aerosols are powered instrumentation, air-powder polishing, rotary polishing, and utilizing the air/water syringe.

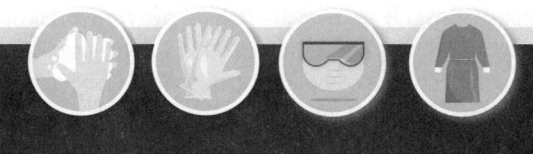

Procedure 24-2
Assisting During Oral Prophylaxis

This procedure is set up for a right-handed operator. An oral prophylaxis is completed by a dentist or a dental hygienist. The chairside dental assistant will transfer and exchange instruments to the operator, retract and use HVE, and remove debris from the instrument when necessary. Coronal polishing will follow and is discussed in Chapter 25.

Steps written in blue font are performed by the operator (dentist or dental hygienist), and the chairside assistant's steps are written in black.

Equipment and Supplies

Patient Seating Setup (refer to Procedure 18-4)

Hygiene Instrumentation Setup (Figure 24-20)
- Basic setup: mouth mirror, explorer, and cotton pliers (A)
- Periodontal probe (B)
- Calculus detection explorer (C)
- Power scaler inserts (D)
- Scalers—anterior and posterior (E)
- Universal Curette (F)

- Sharpening stone (G)
- Air/water syringe tip (H)
- Gauze squares (I)

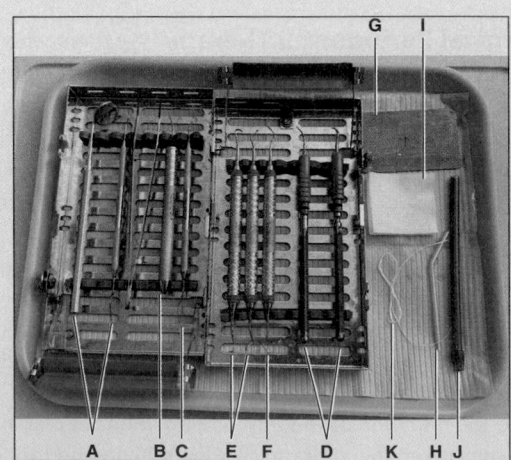

FIGURE 24-20
Tray setup for an oral prophylaxis.

- Saliva ejector (J)
- Dental floss (K)

Procedure Steps

1. Escort and seat patient (refer to Procedure 18-4).

2. Prepare in advance.
   - ❏ Open patient's chart.
   - ❏ Navigate to the dental charting screen.
   - ❏ Open patient's latest radiographic history on the computer monitor.
   - ❏ Introduce operator as they enter the treatment area.

   Greets the patient and takes position at the dental chair.

   - ❏ **Signals for the procedure to begin (refer to Procedure 20-1).**

3. Pass mouth mirror with right hand and explorer with left hand using a pen grasp.

   Examines for hard deposits.

4. Set up powered scaler insert as requested by operator.

5. Exchange explorer for powered scaler insert as requested by operator.
   - ❏ Pass powered scaler with left hand behind the patient's head, being careful not to drag the cord over the patient's chest.

   Begins powered instrumentation.

6. Use HVE with the left hand when clinician is using a power scaler.
   - ❏ Retraction of tongue or cheek using mouth mirror with right hand.

7. Exchanges powered scaler for calculus detection explorer.

   Examines for hard deposits.

8. Exchange calculus detection explorer for instruments as requested by operator with left hand.

9. Hold gauze square over patient's chest with left hand.

10. Suction debris removed during instrumentation.

11. Clean instrument as needed.

12. Use air and water syringe in the right hand to keep dental mirror clean of water.

13. Retrieve hand instrument from operator at the completion of instrumentation.

14. Rinse and evacuate mouth following instrumentation procedures.

15. Pass calculus detection explorer.

   Examines for completion of hard deposit removal.

16. Retrieve calculus detection explorer from operator.

   Prepares for coronal polishing (refer to Procedure 25-1).

   NOTE: A trained and qualified dental assistant can complete coronal polishing in some states.

17. Suction debris removed during coronal polishing.

18. Rinse and evacuate the patient's mouth to remove polishing agent debris.

   NOTE: Some practices use an air-powder polisher as an alternative or in conjunction with rubber cup polishing, discussed in Chapter 25.

19. Floss patient.

   Prepares for fluoride treatment (refer to Procedure 25-4).

   NOTE: A trained and qualified dental assistant can complete fluoride treatments in some states.

20. Write up procedure in Services Rendered.

Date	Services Rendered
02/18/XX	Updated medical and dental history, no changes noted. BP = 120/80 T = 98.6F, P = 80, R = 18
	Scaled full mouth using hand and powered instrumentation. Rubber cup polished full mouth with medium grit prophy paste in cherry flavor. Flossed all contacts. Placed 5% neutral sodium fluoride varnish in mint flavor full mouth. Post fluoride instructions given orally and written. Pt tolerated procedure well.
	Assistant's initials

21. Dismiss and escort patient to reception area (refer to Procedure 18-5).

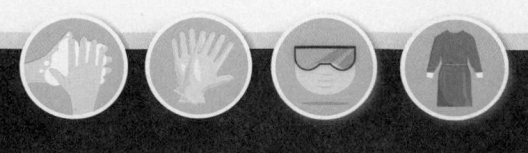

Procedure 24-3
Assisting During Scaling and Root Planing

This procedure is set up for a right-handed operator. This procedure is performed by a dentist or a dental hygienist. The chairside dental assistant will transfer and exchange instruments to the operator, retract and use HVE, and remove debris from instrument when necessary.

Steps written in blue font are performed by the operator (dentist or dental hygienist) and the chairside assistant's steps are written in black.

Equipment and Supplies

Patient Seating Setup (refer to Procedure 18-4)

Anesthetic Setup (refer to Procedure 23-2)

Hygiene Instrumentation Setup (Figure 24-21)
- basic setup: mouth mirror, explorer, and cotton pliers (A)
- periodontal probe (B)
- calculus detection explorer (C)
- power scaler inserts (D)
- scalers—anterior and posterior (E)
- universal curette (F)
- area-specific curettes (G)
- sharpening stone (H)
- air/water syringe tip (I)
- gauze squares (J)

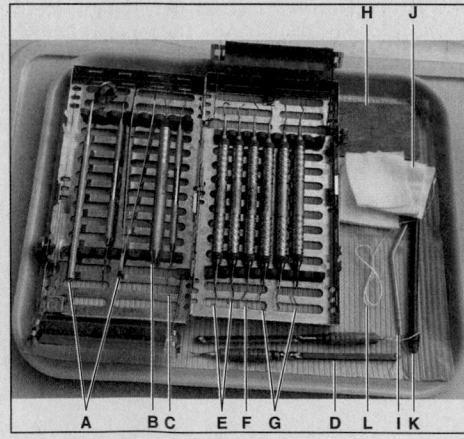

FIGURE 24-21
Tray setup for scaling and root planing.

- saliva ejector (K)
- dental floss (L)

Procedure Steps

1. Escort and seat patient (refer to Procedure 18-4).

2. Prepare in advance.
   - ❏ Open patient's digital chart.
   - ❏ Navigate to the dental charting screen.
   - ❏ Open patient's latest radiographic history on the computer monitor.
   - ❏ Introduce operator as they enter the treatment area.

   Greets the patient and takes position at the dental chair.

   - ❏ Signals for the procedure to begin (refer to Procedure 20-1).
   Administers local anesthesia (see Procedure 23-1).

3. Pass mouth mirror with right hand and explorer with left hand using a pen grasp.
   Examines for hard deposits.

4. Set up powered scaler insert as requested by operator.

5. Exchange explorer for powered scaler insert as requested by operator.
   - ❏ Pass powered scaler with left hand behind the patient's head, being careful not to drag the cord over the patient's chest.

   Begins powered instrumentation.

6. Use HVE with the left hand when clinician is using a power scaler.
   - ❏ Retraction of tongue or cheek using mouth mirror with right hand.

7. Exchange powered scaler for calculus detection explorer.
   Examines for hard deposits.

8. Exchange calculus detection explorer for instruments as requested by operator with left hand.
   Begins hand instrumentation.

9. Hold gauze square over patient's chest with left hand.

10. Suction debris removed during instrumentation.

11. Clean instrument as needed.

12. Use air and water syringe in the right hand to keep dental mirror clean of water.

13. Retrieve hand instrument from operator at the completion of instrumentation.

14. Rinse and evacuate mouth following instrumentation procedures.

15. Pass calculus detection explorer.

    Examines for completion of hard deposit removal.

16. Retrieve calculus detection explorer.

17. Floss patient.

18. Provide postoperative instructions.

19. Explain to the patient that they will be scheduled for an appointment to return to clinic (RTC) to complete treatment on opposite side.

20. Write up procedure in Services Rendered.

Date	Services Rendered
02/18/XX	Updated medical and dental history, no changes noted. BP = 120/80 T = 98.6F, P = 80, R = 18
	Placed 20% benzocaine gel to injection sites for 2 minutes. Administered two cartridges (3.6 ml) of 2% lidocaine with 1:100,000 epi to Maxillary Right PSA, MSA, ASA and Mandibular Right IANB, LB. No reaction.
	SRP to URQ and LRQ, with hand and powered instrumentation. Flossed all contacts. Pt tolerated procedure well.
	RTC: Left side SRP Assistant's initials

21. Dismiss and escort patient to reception area (refer to Procedure 18-5).

Home Care Instructions

Individualized oral hygiene instructions are an essential part of the dental hygiene appointment. Without a thorough understanding of the causes and prevention of dental disease, as well as how to effectively remove biofilm at home, the patient will not be successful at controlling their oral disease. This can be performed by the dental assistant prior to the dental hygiene treatment. Figure 24-22 shows a variety of materials needed for patient education during the dental hygiene appointment. Refer to Chapter 16 for information related to types of toothbrushes, toothbrushing technique, and adjunctive oral aids.

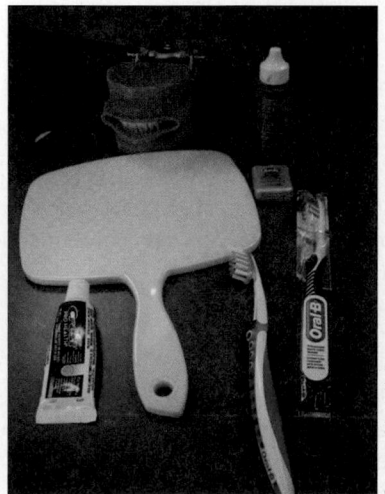

Courtesy of Joyce Hudson

FIGURE 24-22
Materials needed for home care instruction.

Evaluation

The purpose of the evaluation phase is to determine if the dental hygiene treatment goals were reached after following the proposed treatment in the dental hygiene care plan. This includes making plans for areas that need additional attention, whether in office or referred out. The timing of the evaluation phase depends upon the level of disease diagnosed initially at the dental hygiene appointment. For patients who present without active periodontitis, evaluation will be completed at a subsequent recare, or recall, appointment. For patients who present with active periodontitis, evaluation will be completed throughout the process of care if there are multiple appointments and approximately 4 to 6 weeks following completion of periodontal therapy. Refer to Chapter 38 for additional information about periodontal therapy. At the evaluation visit, the operator will evaluate the tissue response, such as changes to texture, bleeding, color, consistency, and shape. Home care will also be evaluated using the BCR and remediated as needed. Comparison to the baseline BCR is a great motivation tool to use during patient education. It is at the evaluation visit following completion of therapy that the recare or maintenance interval will be decided. The patient is determined to need a recare when they have an intact periodontium and low risk for caries and periodontitis. While the recare schedule is individualized to each patient, for a low risk, generally healthy patient, it is typically every 6 months. When the patient has a reduced periodontium or is more at risk for periodontitis, they will be placed on a maintenance interval, which will include localized subgingival root planing if necessary. For this type of patient, maintenance visits are completed typically every 3 to 4 months. At the recare and maintenance appointment, all six phases of the dental hygiene standards are completed from the start again, beginning with assessment.

Documentation

The dental assistant may be responsible for writing the Services Rendered at the completion of the appointment. It is important to include all procedures and be specific. The chart is a legal document that can be considered evidence of care that was provided on that day. When filling in the services rendered form, begin with an update and review of medical and dental histories and the patient's blood pressure. Then continue in the order of the dental hygiene standards. Continue with any assessment data completed, such as periodontal charting, presence of disease, hard and soft deposits, radiographs, oral cancer screenings, and so on, followed by a dental hygiene diagnosis, any treatment that was recommended, hygiene services provided (prophylaxis vs. NSPT, areas of mouth receiving instrumentation, if powered instrumentation was used, type of polishing, paste grit). If fluoride was administered, documentation is needed for type of fluoride, concentration, mode of delivery (tray, paint on, varnish), and flavor. Also included is home care instructions provided to the patient or guardian and the recare schedule assigned. If any postoperative instructions (POI) were administered, they need to be written as explained to the patient, and the entry must be signed or initialed by the assistant.

Chapter Summary

The dental assistant plays an important role in the dental hygiene care visit. Often, there are procedures such as the periodontal charting or home care instructions that may be eliminated or rushed through due to a lack of time. In fact, many of the services that are included in the dental hygiene care visit can be performed by a qualified and trained assistant. Assisted dental hygiene helps eliminate the stress to get all procedures completed and allows for a more comprehensive hygiene visit as required and recommended without sacrificing time.

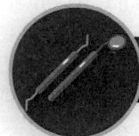

CASE STUDY

Mrs. Nguyen comes in for her first hygiene appointment at the office. She came in about a week prior for her comprehensive new patient examination. She is scheduled for the first side of her NSPT visit. As you seat Mrs. Nguyen, she mentions to you that she notices some sensitivity to cold lately by her gum recession and some bleeding in her gums.

Case Study Review

1. When should the BCR and home care instructions be completed for Mrs. Nguyen?

2. What type of instrumentation does Mrs. Nguyen need?

3. What would you recommend to help treat Mrs. Nguyen's sensitivity to cold?

Review Questions

Multiple Choice

1. In what order are the dental hygiene standards of care completed?
   a. diagnosis, assessment, planning, implementation, evaluation, and documentation
   b. planning, assessment, implementation, diagnosis, documentation, and evaluation
   c. assessment, diagnosis, planning, implementation, evaluation, and documentation
   d. assessment, diagnosis, planning, documentation, implementation, and evaluation

2. The dental hygienist assesses oral hard and soft deposits. Hard deposits located above the gingival margin would be recorded as:
   a. subgingival calculus.
   b. subgingival biofilm.
   c. supragingival biofilm.
   d. supragingival calculus.

3. When the dental hygienist locates inflammation of periodontal tissue and the formation of pus, what would be marked on the periodontal chart?
   a. gingival recession
   b. presence of furcation
   c. fremitus
   d. suppuration

4. All of these conditions are marked during periodontal charting EXCEPT:
   a. tooth mobility.
   b. gingival overgrowth.
   c. dental caries.
   d. bleeding points.

5. What can the chairside dental assistant do to assist the hygienist during comprehensive periodontal charting?
   a. transfer instruments
   b. record collected data
   c. write up services rendered
   d. All of these

6. Which dental team member can make the diagnosis of the patient's oral health care needs during the dental hygiene appointment?
   a. dentist
   b. dental hygienist
   c. expanded dental assistant
   d. All of these
   e. Both a and b

7. All the patient's care is discussed with the hygienist during the dental hygiene appointment EXCEPT:
   a. goals determined by hygienist and patient.
   b. oral hygiene education.
   c. number of appointments to provide treatment.
   d. cost of hygiene appointments.

8. In what standard are the soft and hard deposits removed?
   a. assessment
   b. planning
   c. diagnosis
   d. implementation

9. The hygienist needs to remove supragingival calculus. What instrument would the assistant transfer?
   a. universal curette
   b. area-specific curette
   c. scaler
   d. Naber's explorer

10. Which hygiene instrument is described as having a simple shank and is only used on crowns?
    a. Columbia curette
    b. Gracey curette 11/12
    c. anterior sickle scaler
    d. posterior jacquette scaler

11. Which instrument has a rounded back and can be used both supragingivally and subgingivally and on the anterior and posterior of the mouth?
    a. Jacquette scaler
    b. Barnhart 5/6 curette
    c. Gracey 1/2 curette
    d. Gracey 13/14 curette

12. Which type(s) of power scaler has small tips that operate in a linear motion to remove supra- and subgingival calculus?
    a. piezoelectric
    b. magnetostrictive
    c. sonic
    d. All of these

13. All of these are contraindications to using a powered scaler EXCEPT:
    a. immunocompromised patient.
    b. patient with cardiac device.
    c. patient with excessive amounts of calculus.
    d. patient who has difficulty swallowing.

14. Your patient states they are sensitive when drinking ice water, and they use a hard bristled toothbrush. This patient is most likely experiencing which type of sensitivity?
    a. gingival
    b. dentinal
    c. crown
    d. cementum

15. What can the chairside assistant do while assisting the hygienist during hygiene instrumentation?
    a. retract tissue
    b. rinse and evacuate
    c. set up powered scaler
    d. All of these

16. A qualified trained assistant can perform all of these tasks EXCEPT:
    a. apply desensitizing agent.
    b. remove light calculus.
    c. discuss postoperative instructions with patient.
    d. retract tissue.

17. All of these postoperative instructions should be written and discussed with the patient EXCEPT:
    a. avoid eating or drinking hot liquids until anesthesia has worn off.
    b. resume oral hygiene care.
    c. eat a soft diet for 3 days.
    d. begin using warm saltwater rinses.

18. When is the recare appointment generally scheduled for a patient at risk for periodontitis?
    a. once a year
    b. every 6 months
    c. 3–4 months
    d. 4–6 weeks after periodontal therapy

19. The patient is generally healthy and has a low risk for periodontitis. When would this patient be typically scheduled for their recare appointment?
    a. once a year
    b. every 6 months
    c. 3–4 months
    d. 4–6 weeks after periodontal therapy

20. What should the dental assistant include when writing up the services rendered?
    a. all procedures performed
    b. write procedure in order of dental hygiene standards
    c. patient's blood pressure
    d. All of this information

Critical Thinking

1. While assisting the dental hygienist with a comprehensive periodontal charting, the dental assistant records all the probing depths for the maxillary buccal/facial teeth. The dental hygienist is finished calling out their numbers, but the dental assistant notices they are short recordings for two teeth. What could they conclude? How could they prevent this error?

2. The patient presents for their 3:00 pm appointment with the dental hygienist. The dental assistant looks at the schedule and sees they are scheduled for NSPT on the right side. What type of instrumentation is needed to complete this appointment?

3. The dental hygienist is completing a prophylaxis appointment. They drop their anterior sickle scaler and ask the dental assistant to get them another one out of sterilization. How would you describe the instrument they are looking for?

Key Terms

Term and Pronunciation	Meaning of Root and Word Parts	Definition
adjunctive therapy (*uh*-**juhngk**-tive) (**ther**-*uh*-pee)	**adjunct** = something added to another thing **-ive** = expressing connection **therapy** = treatment of disease or disorders	therapy that is given in addition to a primary therapy which helps to make the primary therapy more effective
assessment (*uh*-**ses**-m*uh*nt)	**assess** = evaluate or judge value, character **-ment** = denoting action	an examiner's visual and physical evaluation of conditions and overall state of the patient
cardiac device (**kahr**-dee-ak) (dih-**vahys**)	**card-** = heart **-ic** = of or relating to **device** = something made for a particular purpose	a device which is implanted to help control irregular heartbeats or measure heart rhythms
cavitation (kav-i-**tey**-sh*uh*n)	**cavity** = any hollow space **-ation** = indication a process	bubbles formed in a fluid through vibrations formed from an ultrasonic instrument; these acoustic turbulences disrupt the bacterial cell wall
chemotherapeutics (kee-moh-ther-*uh*-**pyoo**-tiks)	**chemo-** = chemicals **therapeut** = treating or curing of disease **-ic** = of or relating to	a locally or systemically delivered chemical antimicrobial agent that supports the reduction of microorganisms
curette (ky*oo*-**ret**)	**curette** = to scrape or clean with an instrument	a spoon-shaped instrument with two cutting edges used to remove hard and soft debris from the crown and root of a tooth
debridement (dih-**breed**-m*uh*nt)	**debris** = the remains of anything broken down or destroyed **-ment** = result of an action	therapeutic instrumentations of the crown and root of the tooth which include scaling and root planing
dentinal hypersensitivity (**den**-tn-*uhl*) (hahy-per-**sen**-si-tiv-uhtee)	**dentin** = hard tissue forming major portion of the tooth surrounding the pulp cavity **-al** = pertaining to **hyper-** = excessive **sensitive** = easily pained **-ity** = expressing state or condition	tooth pain caused by exposure of the dentinal tubules of the root surface; resulting from exposure to cold temperatures and osmotic agents
dysphagia (dis-**fey**-jee-*uh*)	**dys-** = bad **-phage** = a thing that eats or devours **-ia** = denoting condition	difficulty in swallowing
extrinsic stain (ik-**strin**-sik) (steyn)	**extrins-** = exterior, outside **-ic** = of, relating to **stain** = a discoloration produced by a foreign matter; chemical	staining of the tooth surface; caused by food, drink, or bacteria that adheres to the pellicle on the tooth
invasiveness (in-**vey**-siv-ness)	**invade** = to enter and affect injuriously **-ive** = expressing tendency **-ness** = denoting state	infiltration into surrounding tissue causing destruction
irrigation (ir-i-**gey**-sh*uh*n)	**irrigate** = to supply with a spray or flow of some liquid **-ion** = denoting action	to flush with water or another agent

Term and Pronunciation	Meaning of Root and Word Parts	Definition
magnetostrictive (mag-nee-toh-**strik**-liv)	**magneto** = an object that possesses the property of attracting certain substances **constrict** = cause to contract or shrink **-ive** = expressing function	a material that changes shape and dimensions and is used to convert mechanical energy into electromagnetic energy and vice versa
nonsurgical periodontal therapy (non-**sur**-ji-kuhl) (per-ee-uh-**don**-tl) (**ther**-uh-pee)	**non-** = not **surgery** = treating disease by operative means; esp incision into the body **-ic** = relating to **-al** = pertaining to **peri-** = around **-odont** = teeth **-al** = pertaining to **therapy** = treatment of disease or disorders	to remove toxins or hard and soft debris from the periodontal pocket and root surfaces; including use of adjunctive therapy if necessary
piezoelectric (pahy-ee-zoh-i-lek-**trik**)	**piezo-** = pressure **electric** = involving electricity	crystals subject to mechanical stress producing an electric charge
prophylaxis (proh-fuh-**lak**-sis)	**prophylaxis** = the preventing of disease	removal of biofilm, calculus, and stains from the crown and root surfaces with manual and powered instruments as a preventative measure against oral diseases
root planing (root) (pleyn-ing)	**root** = portion tooth within the bone **plane** = smooth by blade moved along surface **-ing** = denoting action	the smoothing of the root surface of a tooth to promote gingival health
scaler (**skey**-ler)	**scale** = to remove inlayers **-er** = person or thing that performs a specified action	a dental instrument used for removal of calculus from teeth
scaling (**skey**-ling)	**scale** = to remove inlayers **-ing** = denoting action	the removal of calculus, biofilm, and stain on the teeth by means of instruments
sonic (**son**-ik)	**soni-** = sound **-ic** = pertaining to	use of vibrations and waves creating a high frequency that is audible to the human ear
subgingival (suhb-jin-**jahy**-vuhl)	**sub** = under, beneath **gingiva** = gums, soft tissue surrounding the tooth **-al** = pertaining to	occurring or located under the gingival margin
supragingival (**soo**-pruh- jin-**jahy**-vuhl)	**supra** = above **gingiva** = gums, soft tissue surrounding the tooth **-al** = pertaining to	occurring or located above the gingival margin
ultrasonic (uhl-truh-**son**-ik)	**ultra-** = surpass customary norms; beyond **soni-** = sound **-ic** = pertaining to	energy waves of higher frequency in relation to sonic waves

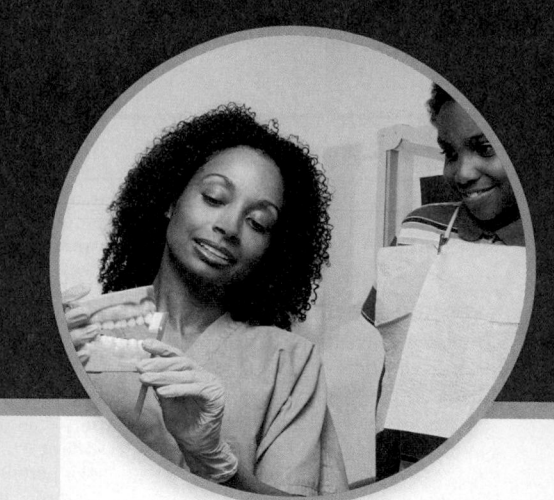

CHAPTER 25
Coronal Polishing and Topical Fluoride Application

Specific Instructional Objectives

At the completion of this chapter, you will be able to meet these objectives:

1. Use terms presented in this chapter.
2. State the rationale for coronal polishing.
3. Explain the contraindications for coronal polish.
4. Differentiate between intrinsic and extrinsic stain and state the cause of each.
5. Indicate the appropriate type of polishing method.
6. State the rationale for selective polishing.
7. Describe the rationale for each step in the coronal polish procedure.
8. Identify proper ergonomics while coronal polishing.
9. Choose the correct attachment for coronal polishing.
10. Determine the type of abrasive necessary based on individual need.
11. Describe the technique for air-powder polishing.
12. Explain the types of equipment and materials used to perform a coronal polish.
13. Describe the indications for professional topical fluoride.
14. State the types of topical fluoride available for a professional applied fluoride treatment.
15. Summarize the steps in the fluoride tray application.
16. Describe the characteristics of an ideal fluoride tray.
17. Summarize the steps in the fluoride varnish application.
18. Justify use of fluoride varnish over fluoride tray application.
19. Discuss indications for use of silver diamine fluoride.
20. Recognize the formulation of SDF and distinguish the purpose of each ingredient.
21. List steps in application of silver diamine fluoride.

Introduction

According to the American Academy of Periodontology, oral prophylaxis is the removal of biofilm, calculus, and stains by both scaling and polishing. Coronal polishing is a part of the oral prophylaxis, takes place following the removal of hard deposits (calculus) by the dentist or dental hygienist, and has been known to play a part in patient motivation. Patients tend to be more motivated to maintain their oral health due to the pleasurable smooth feeling the polishing leaves. This will help the patient understand what a biofilm and stain free surface feels like. Following the **coronal polishing**, fluoride is applied to the crown and/or root surface to promote remineralization and assist in the prevention of decay and hypersensitivity.

Fluoride has been shown to reduce decay, promote remineralization, and decrease hypersensitivity. Chapter 16 reviewed the history of fluoride use, benefits of use, its mechanism of action, and systemic versus topical application. This chapter will discuss the different fluoride options for professional topical use as well as the technique on delivery.

In some states, a trained and qualified dental assistant can perform these two parts of the oral prophylaxis, in addition to the dentist and the dental hygienist. The dental assistant must research the dental practice act for the state where they live to determine if a dental assistant is allowed to perform coronal polishing and/or administer topical fluoride applications to patients in a dental office, and the educational requirements the dental assistant must meet in order to legally perform this task in a dental office. Procedures that can be performed by a dental assistant in a dental office as well as the educational requirements can vary greatly between states. It is important for all dental professionals to be familiar with the scope of practice for the state in which they practice.

Coronal Polishing

The coronal polish is a cosmetic procedure that involves removing soft deposits and **extrinsic stains** (i.e., stains removed by polishing) from the surfaces of the teeth and restorations. This is accomplished with an **abrasive**, dental handpiece, rubber cup (sometimes this procedure is called a "rubber cup" polish), brush, and floss. The coronal polish may also be completed by **air-powder polishing**, which would require an air polishing unit along with an abrasive powder. It is important to note that coronal polishing does not take the place of instrumentation and is not considered an oral prophylaxis.

The coronal polish is the polishing of the **clinical crown** of the tooth. The clinical crown on a newly erupted tooth would involve polishing the enamel surface, while the clinical crown on a tooth with some gingival recession may involve the enamel and the dentin (Figure 25-1). Often, exposed dentin is not polished because of the possibility of increased sensitivity. Care should also be taken with composite restorations, acrylic veneers, and porcelain-filled surfaces because of the possibility of removing the finish and decreasing surface hardness, all of which will impact the selection of an abrasive.

Rationale for Coronal Polishing

After the teeth have been scaled to remove the hard deposits, the polishing is completed to remove any residual stain following instrumentation and to provide a smooth, polished surface. Additional benefits and indications include the following:

- Polished surfaces are easier for the patient to keep clean.
- The tooth surface absorbs fluoride better.
- The process of accumulation of new deposits is slowed.
- A clean tooth surface motivates the patient to maintain good oral hygiene habits.
- The teeth are prepared for placement of dental sealant.
- The teeth are prepared for orthodontic bracket and band placement.

Contraindications and Modifications

There are certain contraindications to coronal polishing, for some of which polishing will need to be modified, while for others it should be avoided altogether. In some cases, a **selective polish** may be performed. Selective polishing is the practice of limiting coronal

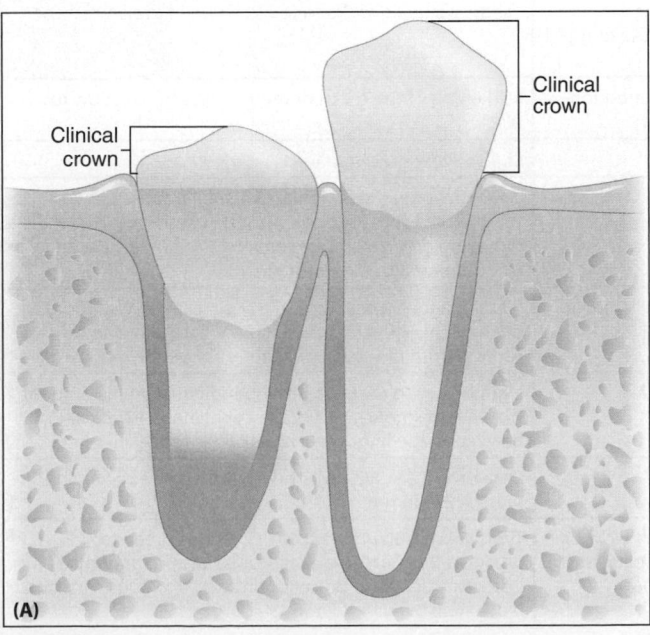
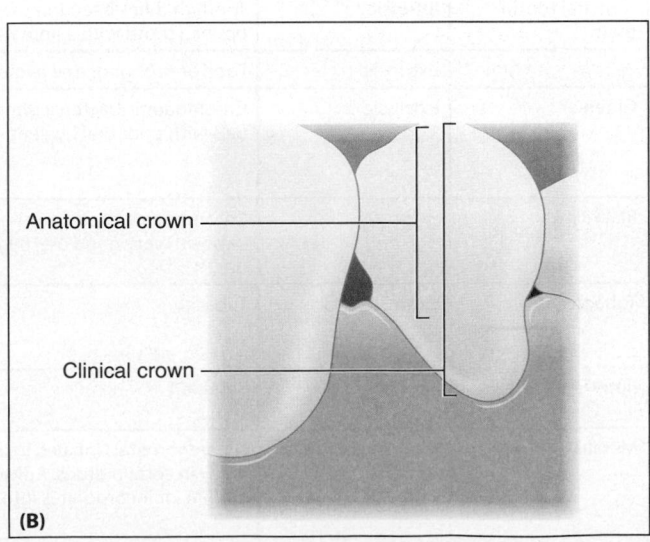

FIGURE 25-1
(A) Clinical crown shown on a partially erupted tooth and an erupted tooth. (B) Comparison of anatomical crown to clinical crown on mandibular left first bicuspid that has gingival recession.

polishing to only those tooth surfaces with extrinsic stain, as well as choosing the least abrasive paste necessary to perform the task. The goal of selective polishing is to remove the extrinsic stain from the tooth with as little trauma to the tooth surface as possible.

The following are contraindications where polishing should be avoided altogether:

- **Acute gingival infection:** The abrasive agents used in the coronal polish may cause delay in healing, and the polish technique could traumatize the already irritated tissues. Polishing should be postponed until the condition of the tissue improves. With mild inflammation, on the other hand, the polish removes the source of irritation.

- **Communicable disease:** Coronal polishing creates an aerosol that can remain suspended in the air for extended periods of time. This can increase the likelihood of disease transmission.

The following conditions may require modification of coronal polishing techniques:

- **Orthodontic appliances:** Use of a small rubber cup and a pointed or tapered brush, especially around the brackets.

- **Hypersensitive teeth:** Use a minimally abrasive agent with a light, intermittent stroke. Use a cotton roll or cotton swab to dry the area instead of the air/water syringe.

- **Green chromogenic bacterial stain:** Before beginning the coronal polish, use a solution of equal parts of 3% hydrogen peroxide and water. Apply to the stained areas with a cotton-tip applicator for a few seconds, and then rinse.

- **Minor oral irritations:** Avoid the areas when polishing and retracting the tissues or establishing a *fulcrum* (position of stabilization). Apply a protective coating of lubricant.

- **Respiratory conditions:** Avoid air/water syringe use, creating spatter, and air-powder polish use.

- **Restorations:** Use only approved paste for restorative material.

- **Newly erupted teeth:** Fluoride rich layer removed during coronal polishing. Newly erupted teeth are most vulnerable and should be avoided.

Dental Stains

Dental stains are significant because of their unattractive appearance. They also may provide rough surfaces for deposits to adhere to. Stains may indicate past or present physical habits or conditions, which aid the dental assistant in determining oral hygiene information and instructions to be given to the patient. Stains are discolorations of the teeth and are caused by foods, bacteria, tobacco, metals, drugs, imperfect tooth development, and excess fluoride, among other things. Stains adhere to the tooth structure, biofilm, and calculus or may be part of the internal structure of the tooth.

Stains are classified according to location, either **intrinsic** or extrinsic, and by their origin, either **exogenous** or **endogenous**.

TABLE 25-1 Types of Dental Stain

Type of Stain	Classification	Cause	Appearance
Dental fluorosis	Intrinsic	Ingestion of excess fluoride systemically during tooth development	Small white areas, to brown stains with pitting. Appearance depends upon extent of fluorosis. A tooth affected depends upon the teeth that were calcifying when the excess fluoride was ingested.
Tetracycline	Intrinsic	High concentrations of tetracycline antibiotics taken during the time the tooth was developing	Teeth appear light green to gray or light brown in color.
Nonvital tooth/teeth	Intrinsic	Tooth that has been treated with endodontics or a tooth with a nonvital pulp	Darkening of the tooth or teeth. Varies from yellow to black.
Yellow	Extrinsic	Food and/or poor oral hygiene	Light yellow in appearance.
Green	Extrinsic	Chromogenic bacteria; often seen in individuals with poor oral hygiene	Green in appearance. Typically appears at the cervical third of the tooth. Caution must be used when removing green stain. The enamel under the stain is overdemineralized and fragile.
Black line	Extrinsic	Chromogenic bacteria; often seen in individuals with very good oral hygiene	Black in appearance. Typically generalized throughout the mouth. Appears as a thin black line following the cervical third of the tooth slightly above the gingiva.
Tobacco	Extrinsic	Tobacco	Light brown to dark brown depending upon the amount the patient smokes and oral hygiene habits. Typically heavier on the lingual surfaces of the teeth.
Betel leaf	Extrinsic	Betel nut	Dark brown to black in appearance. May be generalized or localized in the mouth.
Metallic	Intrinsic/Extrinsic	Different metals inhaled in industry work or orally in certain drugs. Adheres to pellicle or biofilm, or incorporates into the tooth	Typically dark in appearance. Copper is green to greenish-blue. Amalgam can cause gray to gray-black. Iron dust can cause brown stain and iron drugs can cause black stain.
Chlorhexidine	Extrinsic	Prolonged use of chlorhexidine	Yellowish-green to brown in color. Not permanent and can be removed with brushing and/or coronal polish.

It is important for the dental assistant to be able to distinguish between intrinsic and extrinsic stains and to know what stains can and cannot be removed. Table 25-1 reviews the common types of dental stains. The dental assistant can explain to the patient the cause of the stains and what their options are for removal if possible or for further treatment if they are not removable. These options may include professional whitening, **enamel micro-abrasion**, and cosmetic restorative procedures. Coronal polishing is indicated to remove extrinsic dental stains; however, not all extrinsic stain can be removed by coronal polishing. Some extrinsic stain requires instrumentation by a licensed dentist or licensed dental hygienist to completely remove.

Intrinsic Stains

Intrinsic stains are inside the tooth structure and are mostly permanent (in some cases, whitening is successful). The origin of intrinsic stains can be both endogenous (originating from inside the tooth) and exogenous (originating from outside the tooth). Common types of intrinsic stain are dental fluorosis (Figure 25-2), tetracycline stain (Figure 25-3), darkening

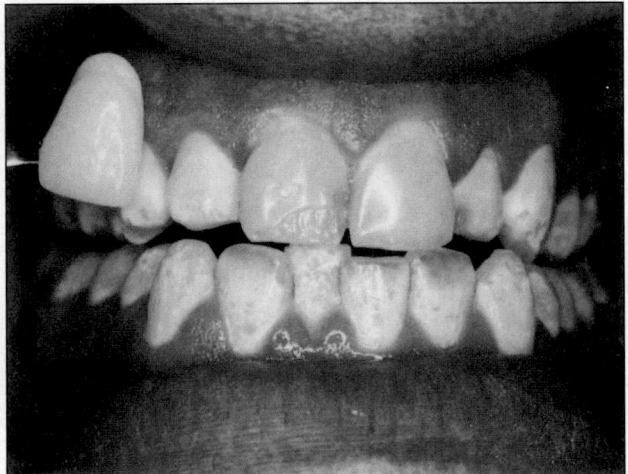

FIGURE 25-2A
Severe fluorosis.

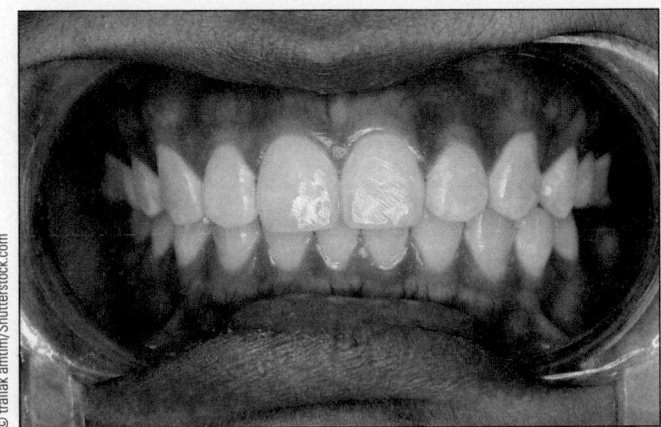

FIGURE 25-2B
Mild fluorosis.

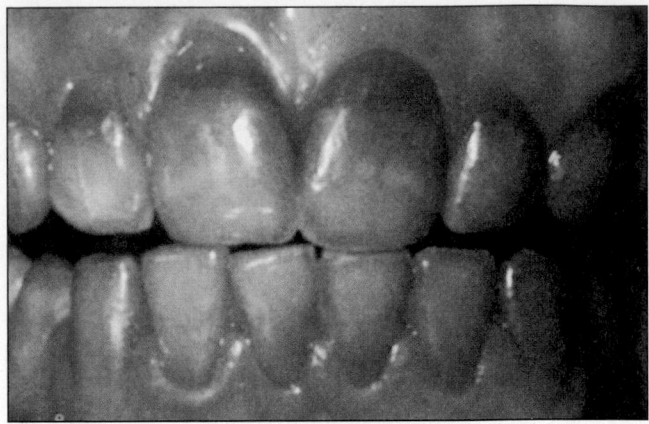

FIGURE 25-3
Tetracycline stain.

as the result of a nonvital tooth, and disruptions in tooth development.

Extrinsic Stains

Extrinsic stains are on the outside of the tooth structure and can be removed by instrumentation and polishing. Extrinsic stains are exogenous only. Common types of extrinsic stain are yellow stain (Figure 25-4), green stain, black line stain, tobacco (Figure 25-5), betel leaf, and metallic stain.

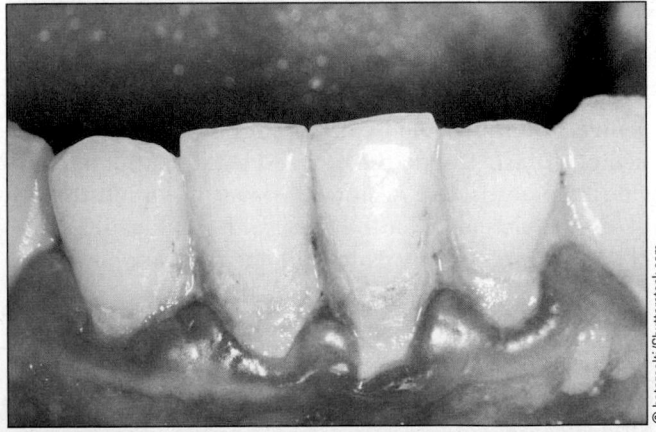

FIGURE 25-4
Yellow stained biofilm.

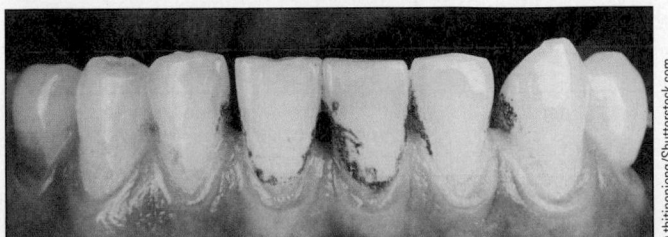

FIGURE 25-5
Tobacco stain.

Types of Coronal Polishing

Coronal polishing can be achieved by either using rubber cup polishing or air-powder polishing.

Rubber Cup Polishing

Rubber cup polishing polishes the tooth using a low-speed handpiece with a rubber cup attachment. The cup is mainly used on the smooth surfaces of the teeth, such as the buccal and lingual surfaces. Polishing paste is applied to the teeth with the rubber cup to remove biofilm and extrinsic stains. To polish the pits and grooves of the occlusal surfaces and palatal of the maxillary anteriors of the tooth, a brush attachment is used.

Equipment and Supplies The dental assistant will need to gather all necessary items prior to seating the patient for coronal polishing. All items used for coronal polishing are listed in Procedure 25-1 and must be either sterilized or disposable. The following equipment supplies are explained in more detail: low-speed handpiece, rubber prophy cup, prophy brush, and polishing agents.

Handpiece For the rubber cup coronal polish procedure, a low-speed dental handpiece is used with corresponding attachments. The handpiece is held in a modified pen grasp. A proper grasp will best enable to clinician to polish properly without causing harm to the patient and will reduce the risk of repetitive strain disorder. The fingers should close up on the prophy angle attachment, and the body of the handpiece should rest in the "V" of the hand. The operator will use their ring finger as a **fulcrum** while coronal polishing. A proper fulcrum will provide stability and assists the operator in maintaining a neutral wrist position. Figure 25-6 shows the neutral wrist position and a modified pen grasp. During the procedure, tooth structure provides the most stable fulcrum. However, if the soft tissue is used as a fulcrum, cover the tissue with a 2×2 gauze first to prevent slipping. The clinician holds the handpiece with

their dominant hand when using the modified pen grasp. Each finger on the dominant hand has a specific role in the modified pen grasp. Table 25-2 provides a basic outline of the placement and role or purpose of each finger. However, the exact placement may vary slightly among clinicians due to variation in hand size.

The speed of the handpiece is controlled by steady foot pressure on the rheostat. Keeping the speed even takes practice. An even, slow speed is desired, with just enough pressure to keep the cups and brushes rotating. The handpiece should be started when it is in the mouth, near the tooth to be polished. This establishes the speed of the handpiece before placing the cup and brush on the tooth. Apply the handpiece to the tooth with light to moderate pressure. When the handpiece is removed from the tooth for more than a moment, release the pressure on the rheostat so that the handpiece stops before being removed from the mouth. This prevents debris from splattering outside the mouth. Table 25-3 lists key points for using a dental handpiece.

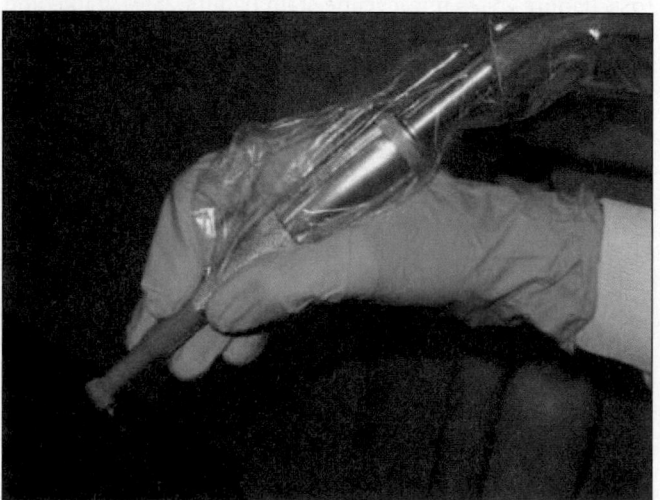

FIGURE 25-6
Modified pen grasp for low-speed handpiece with a neutral wrist position.

TABLE 25-2 Placement and Role/Purpose of Each Finger

Finger	Placement	Role/Purpose
Thumb	On the handpiece directly across from the index finger. There should be a space between the thumb and index finger.	Along with the index finger, the thumb securely holds the handpiece.
Index finger	On the handpiece directly across from the thumb. There should be a space between the index finger and thumb.	Along with the thumb, the index finger securely holds the handpiece.
Middle finger	Resting lightly the prophy angle.	The middle finger resting lightly on the prophy angle helps guide the handpiece and allows the clinician to control the handpiece.
Ring finger	Is the fulcrum finger. Should be placed on solid tooth structure. Should not be any further than 1–2 teeth away from tooth being polished.	Adds stability and prevents injury to the patient or clinician.
Pinky finger	Held closely to the other fingers but not on the handpiece or tooth structure.	NA

TABLE 25-3 Key Points of Using a Dental Handpiece

- Use a slow, even speed.
- Use light-to-moderate pressure. Just enough to flare the cup on the tooth.
- Always use a fulcrum.
- Start and stop handpiece inside patient's mouth.

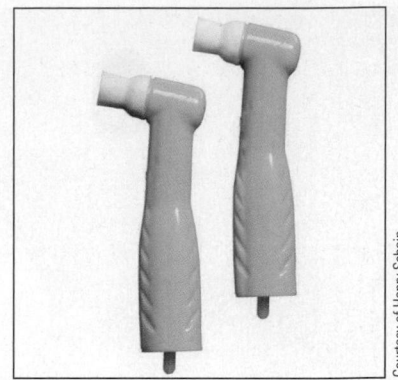

FIGURE 25-8
Disposable rubber cup prophy angles.

Rubber Prophy Cup The rubber prophy cup is used with an abrasive agent to polish the teeth and dental appliances (Procedure 25-1). Rubber prophy cups are available in several designs to fit the prophy angle heads. On the back of the prophy cup there may be a snap-on cup or a small metal screw attachment that is screwed into the corresponding prophy angle and a latch that slips over a knob on the contra-angle (Figure 25-7). Disposable prophy angles with attached prophy cups are also available (Figure 25-8).

Rubber prophy cups are made of either natural or synthetic rubber. Natural rubber cups are resilient and will not stain the teeth. Synthetic rubber cups are stiffer than the natural rubber, and the black cups may stain the teeth during the polish.

The rubber cup should be soft and flexible to adapt to the contours of the teeth. Edges should not be rough or frayed, which could irritate the tissues. The number of cups needed for the polishing depends on the number of abrasives used. One cup is used for each polishing agent. The edge of the cup is the part that actually does the polishing. The center of the cup holds and transports

the abrasive agent. The cup is flexed to adapt to the tooth surface by applying slight pressure to one edge (Figure 25-9). The cup is most efficient on the facial and lingual surfaces of the teeth and fixed appliances, along the gingival margin, and 1–2 mm into the sulcus.

The hand and wrist are used to move the handpiece to adapt the cup to the tooth surface. When working on the lingual or facial surfaces, flare the rubber cup as far as possible into the proximal and manipulate the cup into the sulcus, *not* on the gingival margin. Start from the gingival third with the edge of the cups flaring close to the sulcus area, and then move the cup toward the incisal/occlusal surface. Use a short, intermittent, overlapping stroke with a slow-revolving rubber

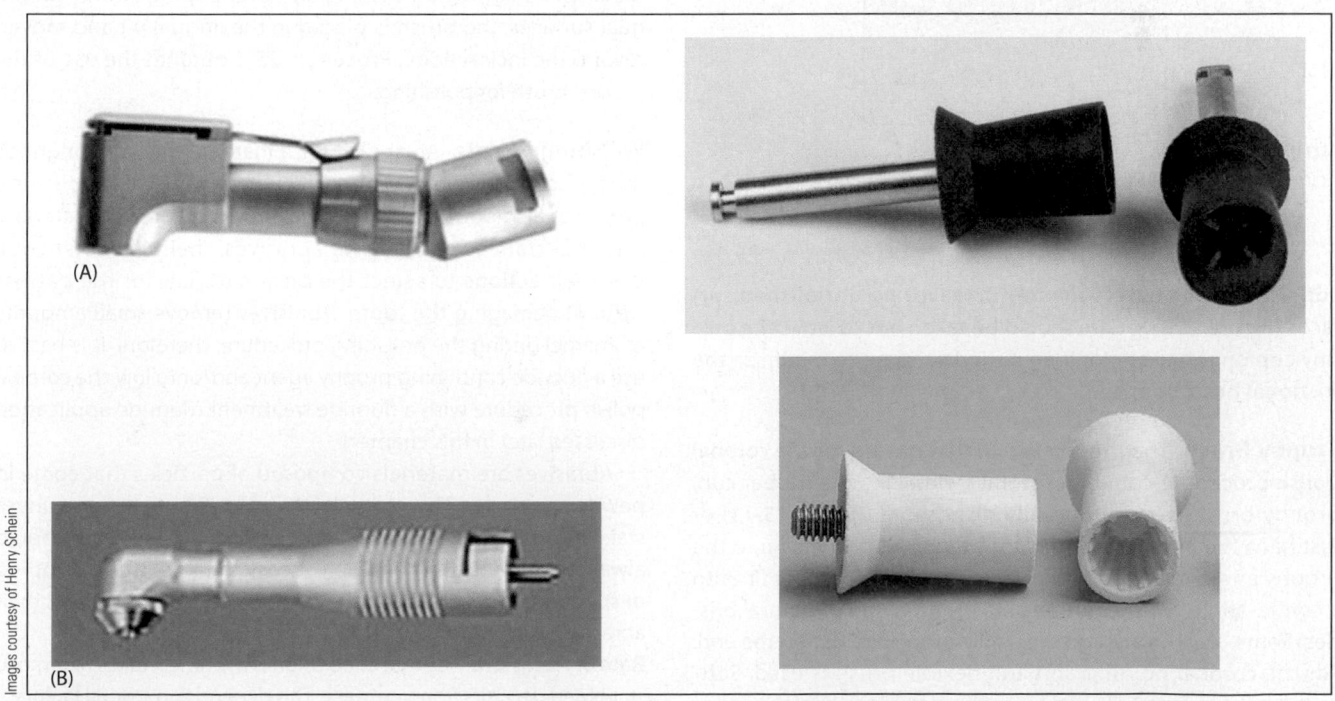

FIGURE 25-7
(A) Contra-angle head with latch type rubber cup. (B) Prophy angle head with screw-on prophy cup.

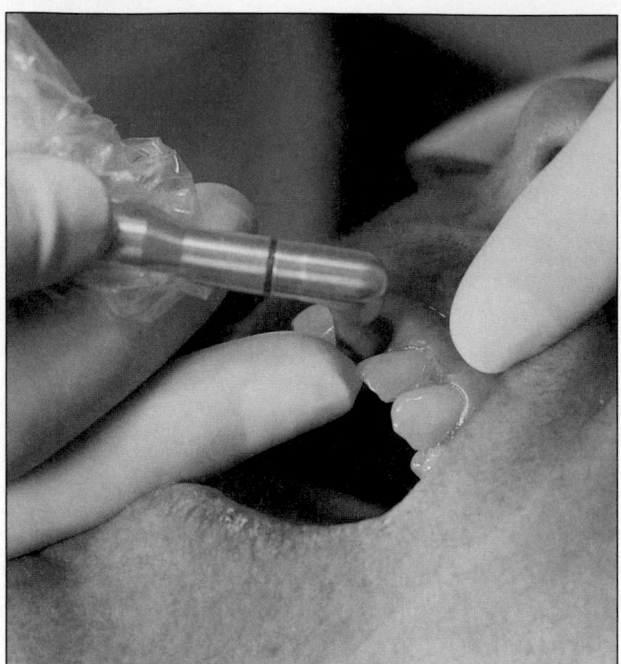

FIGURE 25-9
Adapting the rubber cup to flare into the proximal surfaces.

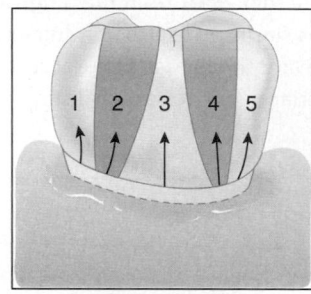

FIGURE 25-10
Examples of overlapping polishing strokes.

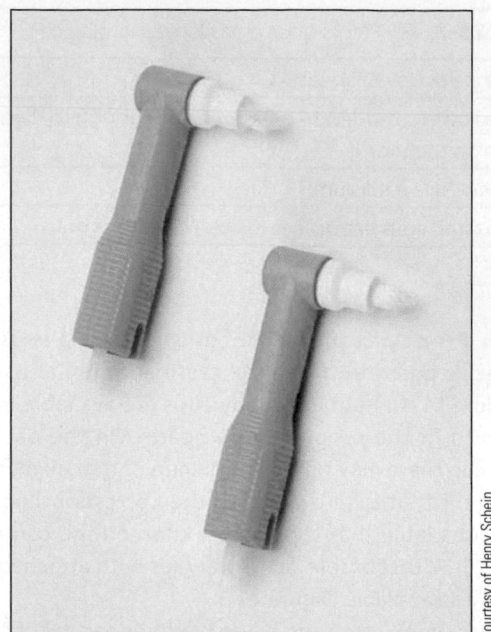

FIGURE 25-11
Disposable prophy brushes.

cup. This stroke covers the tooth, leaves no unpolished surfaces (Figure 25-10). Care should be taken not to leave the prophy cup on the tooth for long periods of time to minimize the frictional heat produced.

Prophy Brush The **prophy brush** that is used for the coronal polish procedure comes in several styles. Like the rubber cup, prophy brushes are either fully disposable (Figure 25-11) or just have the brush attachment that screws or snaps on to the prophy angle head. Latch types are also available that fit onto a contra-angle. Brushes are available with nylon or natural bristles. Some brushes are tapered, while others are flat on the end. For the coronal polish, a soft and flexible brush is used. Softening can be accomplished by soaking the brush in hot water before using it.

Prophy brushes are used on the occlusal surfaces to effectively clean the deep pits and fissures and also for the pits on the

lingual of the anterior teeth, but the bristles should *never* contact the gingival tissues and should be positioned only above the gingival third of the tooth. The prophy brush is not meant to be used on the flat surfaces of the tooth as it may slip and cause trauma to the tissue. This brush is used only on the enamel surface. Used in the same manner as the cup, the brush is flexed in the central fossa with a light, intermittent, and overlapping stroke. On lingual surfaces, the brush is placed in the lingual pit and moved toward the incisal edge. Procedure 25-1 outlines the use of the prophy brush for polishing.

Polishing Agents An abrasive is a material that cuts or grinds the surface, leaving grooves and a rough surface, while **polishing** produces a smooth, glossy surface with fine abrasive materials. It is important to understand abrasives, their characteristics, and their actions to select the best materials for the patient without damaging the tooth. Abrasives remove small amounts of enamel during the polishing procedure; therefore, it is best to use a fluoride containing prophy agent and/or follow the coronal polish procedure with a fluoride treatment (fluoride application discussed later in this chapter).

Abrasives are materials composed of particles that come in powders or pastes. They are selected according to the amount of stain and soft deposits that are to be removed. Abrasives should always be as moist as possible yet easy to use without dripping or spattering. These particles have characteristics that affect their abrasiveness. See Table 25-4.

Rate of Abrasion. The rate of abrasion is the time it takes to remove stains and deposits from a surface. This depends on several factors:

- By *increasing the speed of the handpiece*, the rate of abrasion is increased accordingly. This also increases the heat production.

TABLE 25-4 Characteristics of Abrasives

Characteristic	Effect on Abrasive
Particle shape	Sharp-edged particles are more abrasive than dull, rounded particles.
Particle hardness	Harder particles abrade faster. Particles must be harder than the surfaces they are used on.
Particle strength	Resistance of particles to break up during the polish; therefore, less material is used.
Particle size	The larger the particle, the more abrasive it is.
Grit or grade of abrasive particles	Materials are sifted through standardized sieves to grade fineness. Fine abrasives are called powders or flours and are graded F, FF, and FFF for increasing fineness.
Particle attrition resistance	Particles that do not dull or become embedded in the surface being polished are the most effective.

- The *pressure* can control the rate of abrasion. The firmer the pressure, the more abrasive. Also, frictional heat increases.
- The *amount of abrasive* material used affects the rate of abrasion. The more material that is used, the faster the abrasive works.
- The *type of abrasive* used determines the rate of abrasion. The larger and harder the particles, the faster the abrasion. Also, the rate of heat production increases.
- The *dryer the abrasive* materials, the more abrasive they are.

Select an abrasive material that is coarse enough to cut through the stains and polish until the surfaces are as smooth as possible. Then, select a finer material, if needed, to polish the surface until it is smooth and free of stain. Usually, one abrasive is enough to complete the task, but if the patient has a lot of stain, a coarser abrasive should be used. When using two types of abrasives, completely finish with one abrasive, and then rinse the patient's mouth thoroughly before beginning with another abrasive. Also, use separate dappen dishes, rubber cups, and brushes for each abrasive.

Types of Abrasives. The abrasives come in bulk form or individually packaged. Besides the abrasive, most commercial preparations contain water, a binder, **humectant** (retains moisture), color, and a flavoring. Prophy pastes can contain materials that stimulate the remineralization of tooth enamel, prevent the loss of enamel, have desensitizing agents, remove stains, and polish the tooth surface. The pastes come in a variety of grits including super fine, fine, medium, and coarse. Paste selection will depend on the amount of stain present. They also come in many flavors, and some are nonsplattering formulas. The prophy pastes come with a finger holder for easy access to the paste during the polishing procedure. See Figure 25-12. Table 25-5 reviews the common abrasives for both rubber cup polishing and air-powder polishing.

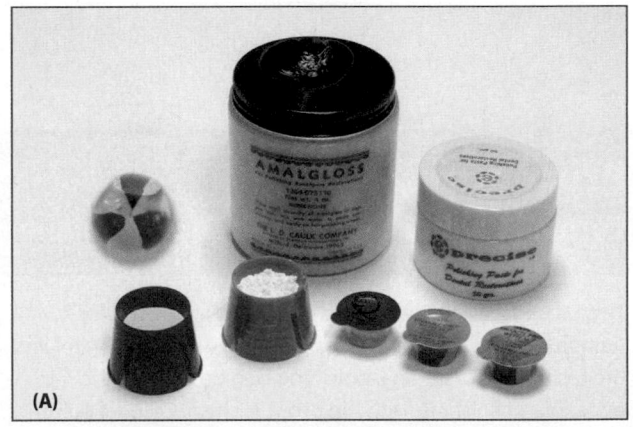

(A)

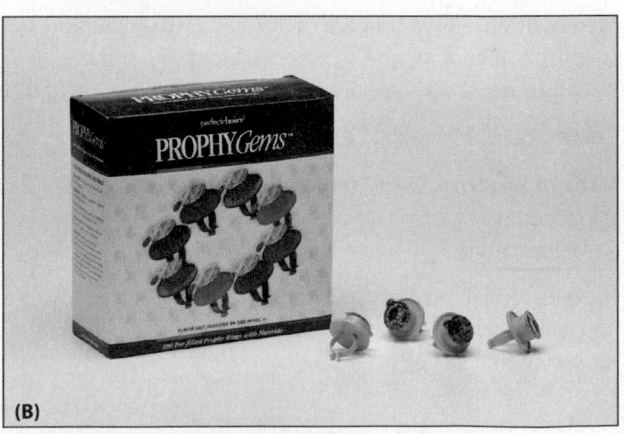

(B)

FIGURE 25-12

(A) Various types of abrasives, including powders and pastes. (B) Polishing agent in finger holder for easier application.

Safety

The clinician should utilize the proper personal protective equipment including protective eyewear, facemask, gloves, and protective clothing with barriers placed on the dental unit. The patient should also have protective eyewear during this procedure. When performing air-powder polish, provide the patient with a protective gown; the operator will wear a face shield and should consider a hair covering (Figure 25-15).

TABLE 25-5 Common Types of Abrasives

Type of Coronal Polishing	Paste	Characteristics
Rubber Cup	Zirconium silicate	Used for stain removal and polishing. This material may be used on gold restorations, exposed dentin, and tooth-colored restorations, as well as enamel.
	Silica/fine silica	Used to remove stains, as a high-powered cleaning agent and a fine polishing agent. Course silica particles break down during the application and become a fine grit to polish.
	Tin oxide	A very fine polishing agent used on enamel and metallic restorations. Used in a paste form, it is mixed with water, alcohol, or glycerin.
	Flour of pumice	Used to remove stains from the enamel. It is relatively coarse and should be followed by a fine polishing agent. It is not used on exposed dentin, tooth-colored restorations, or gold restorations because of its high abrasiveness.
	Chalk	(Also known as whiting)—a mild abrasive, it is used in some prophylactic pastes.
	Fluoride prophylaxis pastes	Available and very popular. Fluoride is added to commercially prepared prophylaxis pastes to replace the fluoride lost in the enamel surface during the polishing procedure due to abrasion. Fluoride prophylaxis pastes should not be used if the teeth are to receive enamel sealants after the coronal polish.
Air-Powder	Sodium bicarbonate	Biofilm and stain removal on enamel surfaces only. Not for use on restorations. Contraindicated for use on patients with sodium restricted diets (high blood pressure). Water soluble.
	Aluminum trihydroxide	Biofilm and stain removal on enamel surfaces only. Particles harder than sodium bicarbonate, but similar in size. Not for use on restorations. Indicated for use on patients with sodium restricted diets (high blood pressure). Non water soluble.
	Glycine	Safe for use on cementum, dentin, and restorations (including implants). Commonly used for subgingival use. Shows the least amount of gingival erosion.

Procedure 25-1
Coronal Polishing—Rubber Cup Technique

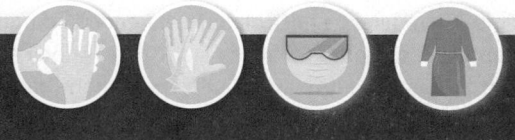

This procedure is done by a dentist, dental hygienist, or trained and qualified dental assistant. This procedure explains the technique for coronal polishing beginning with the rubber cup and finishing with the prophy brush. Coronal polishing is followed by a fluoride treatment

Steps written in blue font are performed by the operator (dentist, hygienist, or qualified dental assistant), and the chairside assistant's steps are written in black.

Equipment and Supplies

Patient Seating Setup (refer to Procedure 18-4)
- face shield
- hair covering

Instrumentation Setup (Figure 25-13)
- basic setup: mouth mirror, explorer, and cotton pliers (A)
- periodontal probe (A)
- air/water syringe tip (B)
- place on low-speed handpiece (K)
- finger ring to hold prophy paste cup (C)

- assortment of disposable rubber cups and brushes (D)
- lip lubricant (J)
- disclosing solution (optional)
- dental floss (E)
- prophy paste in various grits (F)
- dappen dish (G)
- gauze squares (H)
- saliva ejector (I)

Procedure Steps (Figure 25-14)

1. Escort and seat patient (refer to Procedure 18-4).

2. Prepare in advance.
   - ❑ Open patient's chart in dental software.
   - ❑ Navigate to the dental charting screen.
   - ❑ Open patient's latest radiographic history on the computer monitor.
   - ❑ Attach low-speed handpiece to dental unit.
   - ❑ Offer lip lubricant for the patient's comfort.
   - ❑ Introduce operator as they enter the treatment area.

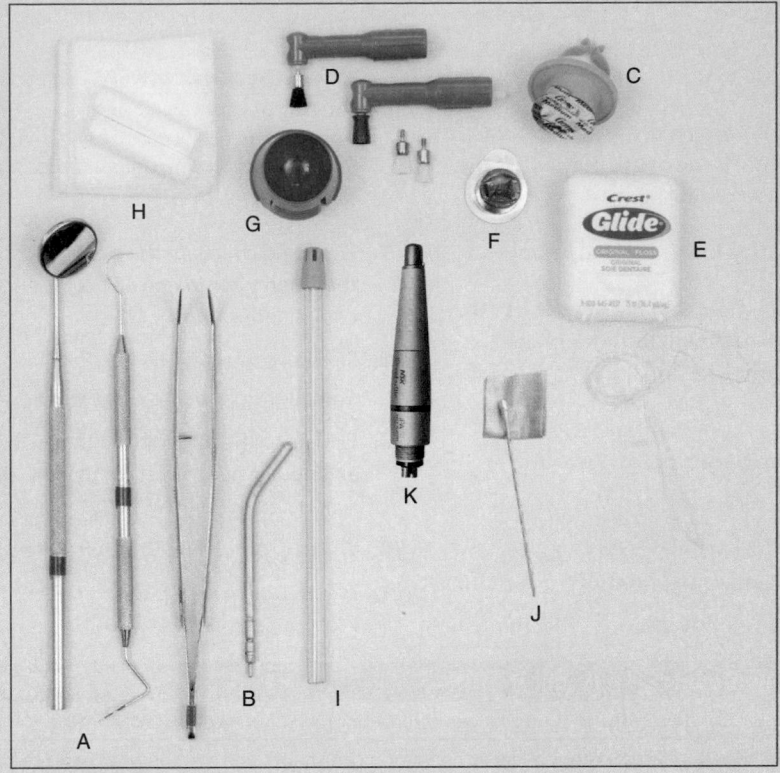

FIGURE 25-13
Tray setup for coronal polishing procedure.

Greets the patient and takes position at the dental chair.

Assembles handpiece with rubber cup attachment.

Determines what grit prophy paste to use by evaluating stain levels.

❏ Signals for the procedure to begin (refer to Procedure 20-1).

3. Dry the teeth and place disclosing solution (optional), to easily evaluate biofilm levels.

4. Prepare prophy paste in dappen dish.

5. Hold dappen dish at chest level for operator to replenish when needed.

Places abrasive polishing agent in the cup, places the handpiece in the patient's mouth and close to the tooth, but not on the tooth, and activates it.

Establishes a fulcrum as close to the tooth being polished as possible.

Places the cup at a 90-degree angle on the smooth surface of the tooth near the gingival sulcus and as far into the mesial or distal surface as possible.

Applies light pressure to flex the cup and flare it into the sulcus 1-2 mm.

Sweeps the rubber cup toward the incisal or occlusal edge.

Lifts the cup slightly off the tooth at the incisal or occlusal edge and repositions it near the gingiva to repeat the stroke, moving toward the opposite side of the tooth.

Repeats the stroke, overlapping each time, until the entire tooth surface is polished.

Moves to the adjacent tooth using the same steps until the surfaces of all teeth have been polished.

Replenishes paste as needed.

6. Rinse the mouth frequently, at least after polishing each quadrant, for patient comfort.

Removes rubber prophy cup from handpiece.

Assembles handpiece with prophy brush attachment.

Softens prophy brush in warm water.

(Continues)

Applies prophy paste to the brush, and replenishes when needed.

Establishes a fulcrum close to the tooth to be polished.

Moves the brush bristles toward the mesial buccal cusp tip and continues until the brush comes off the occlusal surface of posterior teeth.

Replaces the brush bristles in the central fossa.

Applies slight pressure again, and moves the brush up toward the distal buccal cusp until the brush comes off the occlusal surface.

Repeats this procedure on the occlusal surface of each posterior tooth until all of the occlusal surfaces are cleaned.

Places the prophy brush in the lingual pit, above the cingulum when polishing the lingual surfaces of the anterior teeth.

Applies light pressure to flex and spread the brush bristles.

Moves the brush toward the incisal edge to polish the lingual surface.

Repeats on all lingual surfaces that have deep pits and grooves.

7. Rinse and evacuate the patient's mouth thoroughly, removing all debris once polishing is completed.

8. Floss all contacts.

   Completes fluoride treatment (see Procedure 25-4).

9. Explain to the patient that they will be scheduled for an appointment to return to clinic (RTC) for their next scheduled hygiene visit.

10. Write up procedure in Services Rendered.

11. Dismiss and escort patient to reception area (refer to Procedure 18-5).

Date	Services Rendered
02/18/XX	Updated medical and dental history, no changes noted. BP = 120/80 T = 98.6F, P = 80, R = 18
	Coronal polished all surfaces using rubber cup and prophy brush with fine mint prophy paste. Used Medium grit paste on tooth #'s 3 and 14 Buccal for moderate brown stain. 2% Neutral Sodium Fluoride gel applied with hinged tray to both arches for 4-minute application. Post-op instructions given orally and written. Cherry flavor. No reactions, patient tolerated procedure well.
	RTC: 6mrc Assistant's initials

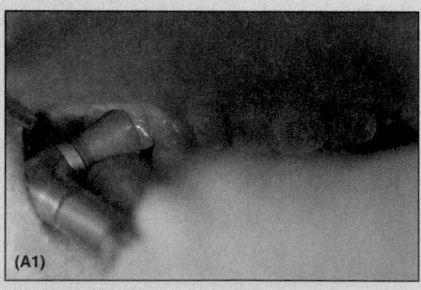
(A1)

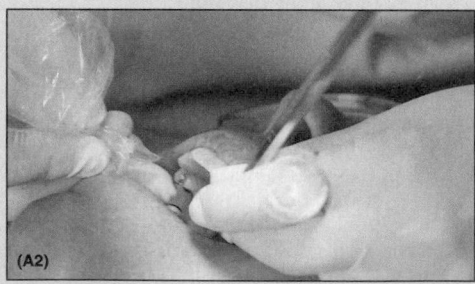
(A2)

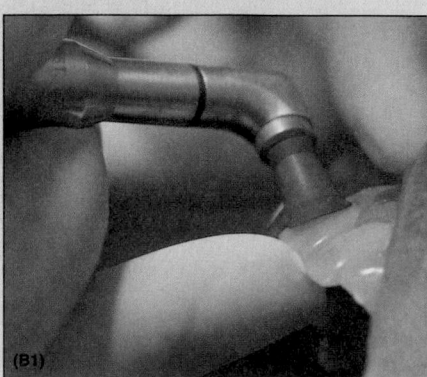
(B1)

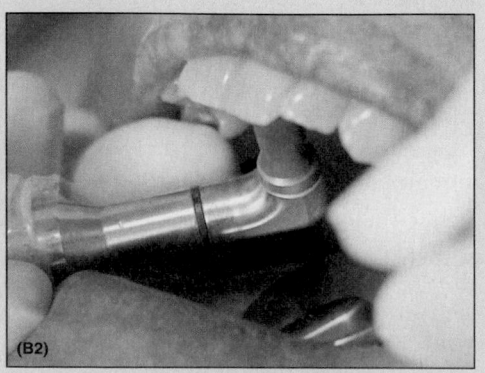
(B2)

FIGURE 25-14
(A1) Cheek is retracted to position cup on tooth. Fulcrum on same arch. (A2) Use indirect vision and fulcrum on same arch. (B) Maxillary anteriors, facial surface and lingual surface. (B1) Retract lip and fulcrum on incisal edge. (B2) Use a mouth mirror for indirect vision.

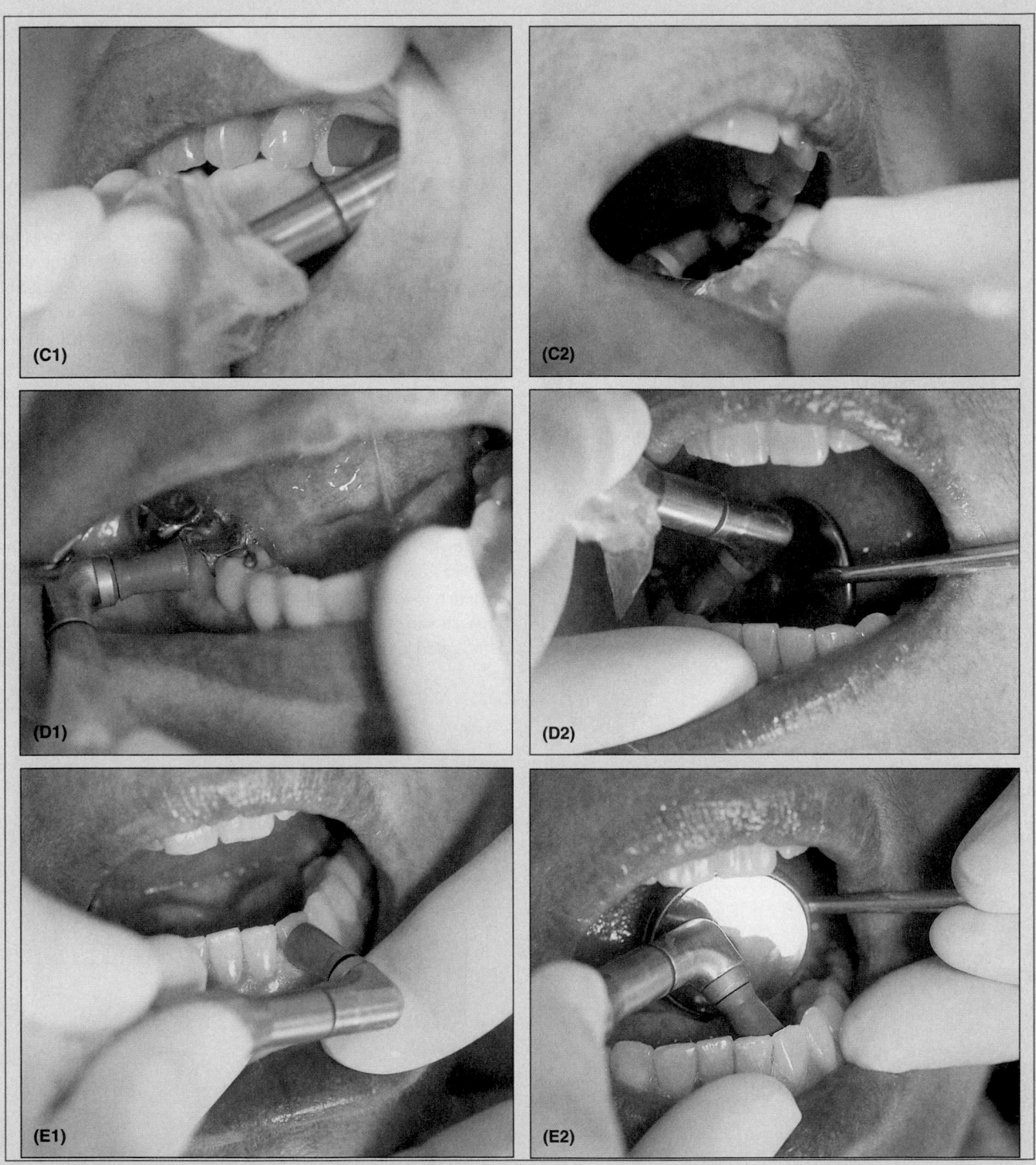

FIGURE 25-14

(C1) Retract cheek to position prophy angle and have patient close slightly. Fulcrum on same arch. (C2) Adapt cup to lingual surface. (D) Mandibular right posterior, buccal surface and lingual surface. (D1) Retract tissue to place prophy angle and have patient close slightly. (D2) Retract tongue with mouth mirror. (E) Mandibular anteriors, facial and lingual surface. (E1) Retract lip with a finger. (E2) Use mouth mirror for indirect vision and retraction of the tongue.

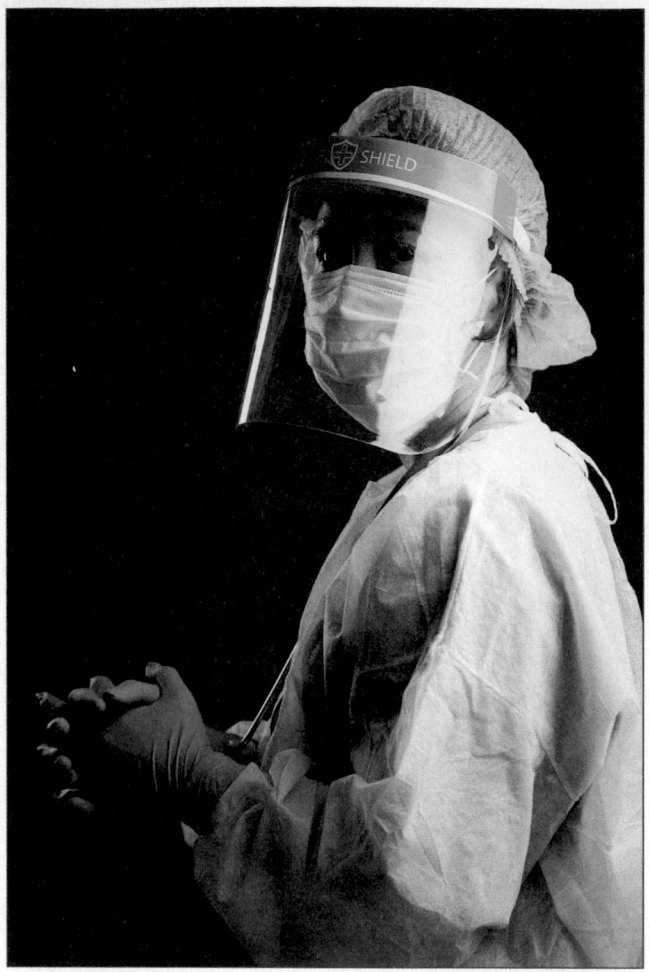

FIGURE 25-15
Face shield and hair covering.

Air-Powder Polishing

Air-powder polishing requires special equipment. An office could purchase a whole system that is a combination of an ultrasonic unit and air powder unit, or an air polishing unit alone. Also available is a separate unit that attaches to a dental unit using the air and water tubing (see Figures 25-16A, B, and C). For each of these units, a handpiece/nozzle and air powder are necessary. See Table 25-5 for different abrasive powders used during air-powder polishing.

Air-powder polish uses a fine powder, air under pressure, and water through a handpiece with a nozzle attachment. The handpiece is rather light when compared to the low-speed handpiece used when rubber cup polishing. The abrasive is usually a fine powdered sodium bicarbonate or nonsodium powder as the slurry. Nonsodium powder is indicated for use in patients with a sodium-restricted diet, such as those with high blood pressure.

The removal of biofilm and extrinsic stain is accomplished in a reasonable amount of time, and there is minimal loss of tooth structure when the air polishing system is used as directed by the manufacturer, which is one of the air-powder polishers' advantages. Air-powder polishing is a proper choice for a patient who requires heavier stain removal and presents with no contraindications. This system is used for crown surfaces, as any prolonged use on recession areas should be avoided. The exception is when using glycine, which is indicated for subgingival use up to 5 mm.

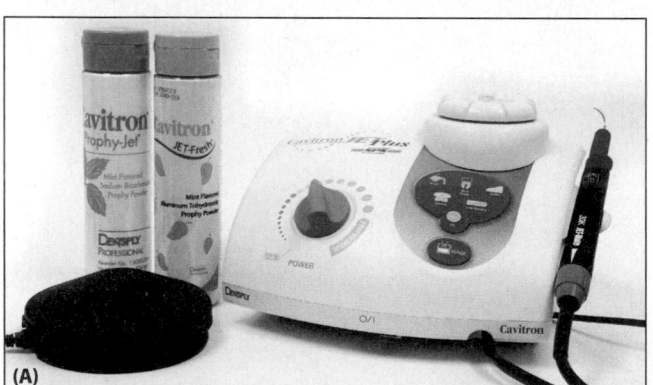

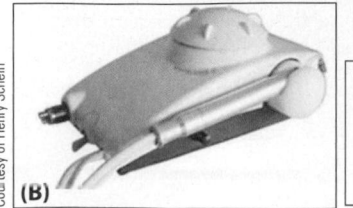

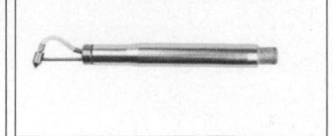

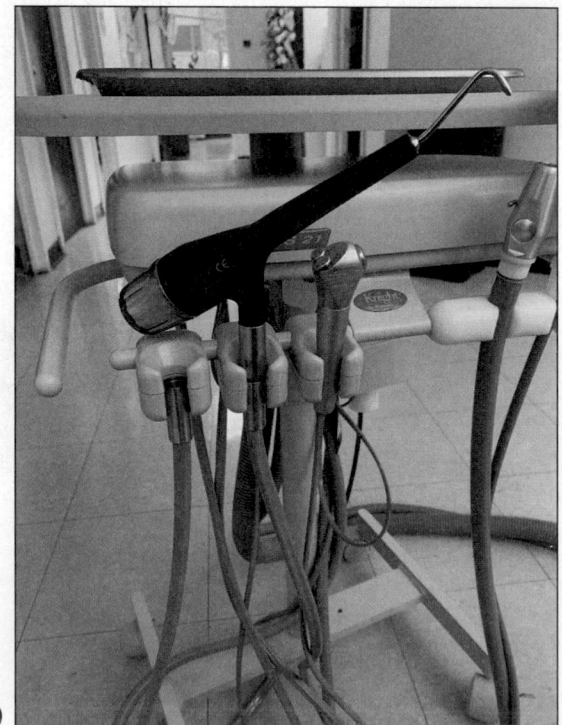

FIGURE 25-16
Various air polishing units. (A) Combination air polishing unit with ultrasonic unit. (B) Independent air polishing unit with a coordinating handpiece. (C) Air polishing unit that is attached to the air and water tubing directly on the dental unit.

Some disadvantages of the air polishing systems include significant aerosol spray; may cause mild stinging in other areas of the mouth due to the deflected spray; contraindicated for patients with respiratory illness; and are not used on composite restorations, demineralized enamel, or the margins of porcelain or cast restorations.

When using the air-powder polisher, the handpiece tip is held 3–5 mm away from the tooth surface and is kept in constant motion.

Procedure 25-2
Polishing with Air-Powder Polish

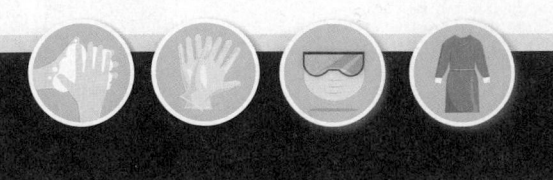

This procedure is done by a dentist, dental hygienist, or trained and qualified dental assistant. This procedure reviews the steps for air-powder polishing to remove coronal stain.

Steps written in **blue** font are performed by the operator (dentist, hygienist, or trained and qualified dental assistant), and the chairside assistant's steps are written in black.

Equipment and Supplies

Patient Seating Setup (refer to Procedure 18-4)
- face shield
- hair covering

Instrumentation Setup (Figure 25-17)
- basic setup: mouth mirror, explorer, and cotton pliers (A)
- air/water syringe tip (B)
- air-powder polisher nozzle and handpiece (C)
- lip lubricant (D)
- disclosing solution (optional)
- dental floss (E)
- appropriate abrasive powder (F)
- gauze squares and cotton rolls (G)
- saliva ejector (H)
- wide tip high evacuation tip (I)

Procedure Steps

1. Escort and seat patient (refer to Procedure 18-4).

2. Prepare in advance.
   - ❏ Open patient's chart in dental software.
   - ❏ Navigate to the dental charting screen.
   - ❏ Open patient's latest radiographic history on the computer monitor.

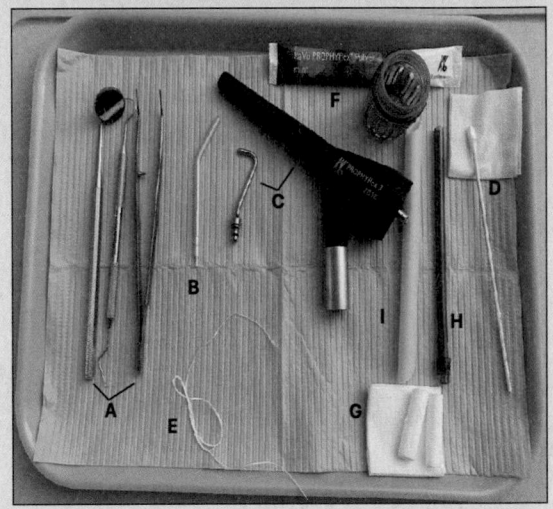

FIGURE 25-17
Tray setup for air-powder polishing procedure.

- ❏ Determine appropriate powder to be used based on patient's medical history and task to be performed (supragingival or subgingival).
- ❏ Set up air-powder polisher unit following manufacturer's guidelines (Figure 25-18).
  - ❏ Place nozzle.
  - ❏ Place powder prior to each use in appropriate reservoir, test the flow of the air-powder and water, and adjust if needed according to manufacturer's directions.
- ❏ Offer lip lubricant for the patient's comfort.
- ❏ Introduce operator as they enter the treatment area.

Greets the patient and takes position at the dental chair.

- ❏ **Signals for the procedure to begin (refer to Procedure 20-1).**

(Continues)

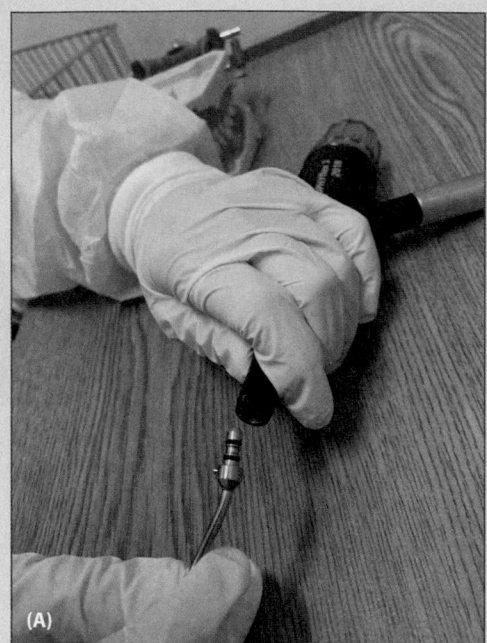

FIGURE 25-18
Air-powder polishing unit setup. (A) Place nozzle onto handpiece; (B) Place powder in reservoir.

3. Hold HVE at the occlusal or incisal of the tooth being polished and retract tongue or cheek as needed.

   Cups patient's lip/cheek to help control aerosols during procedure.

   Places nozzle 3–5 mm away from the tooth surface and away from the gingiva (Figure 25-19A).

   ❏ For anterior teeth, angles nozzle 30–60 degrees (Figure 25-19B).
   ❏ For posterior teeth, angles nozzle 80 degrees (Figure 25-19C).
   ❏ For occlusal surfaces, angles the nozzle 90 degrees (Figure 25-19D).

   Depresses foot pedal all the way to discharge powder and water in a spray for 4–5 seconds.

   Uses a consistent circular movement along the tooth, being careful not to contact restorations or dentin.

   Rinses area frequently.

   Continues to polish and rinse until all surfaces are polished.

4. Floss all contacts.

5. Explain to the patient that they will be scheduled for an appointment to return to clinic (RTC) for their next scheduled hygiene visit.

6. Write up procedure in Services Rendered.

7. Dismiss and escort patient to reception area (refer to Procedure 18-5).

Date	Services Rendered
02/18/XX	Updated medical and dental history, no changes noted. BP = 120/80 T = 98.6F, P = 80, R = 18
	Air-powder polish with sodium bicarbonate all surfaces with the exception of tooth #4 and 5 buccal restorations. Patient tolerated procedure well.
	RTC: 6mrc Assistant's initials

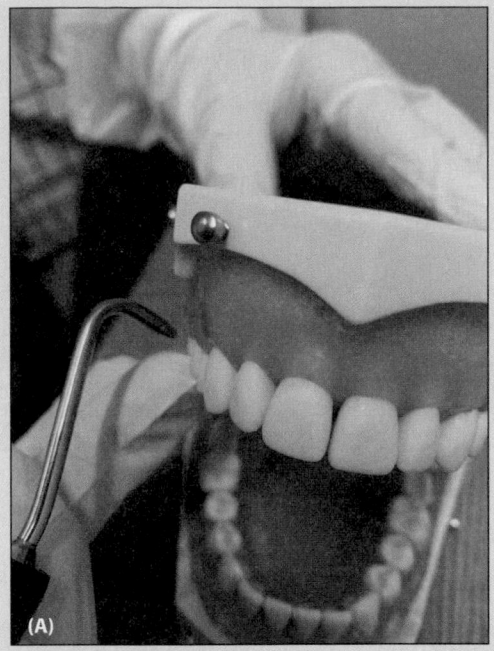
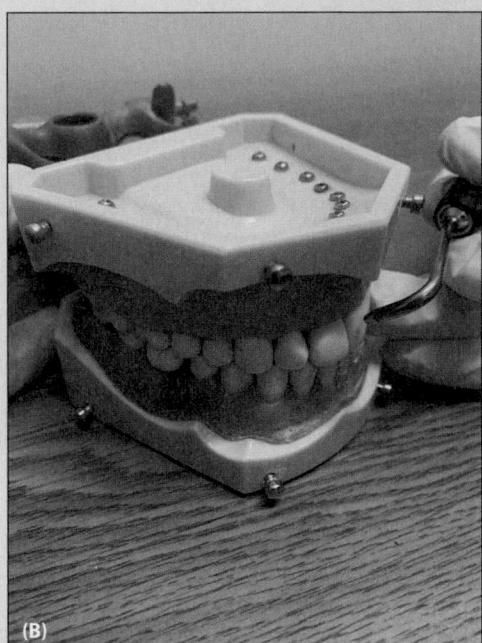
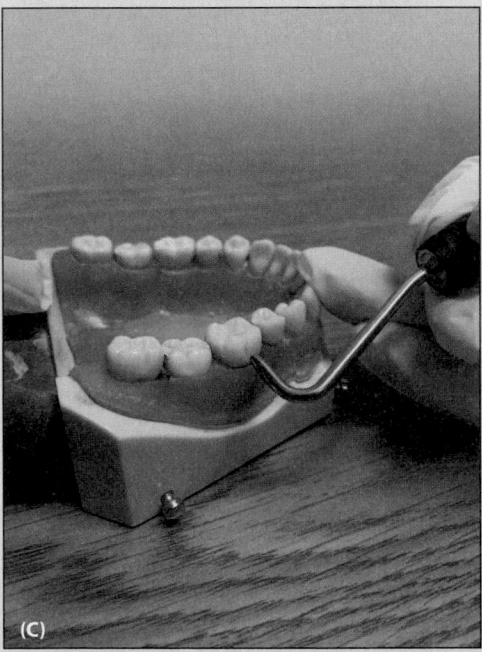
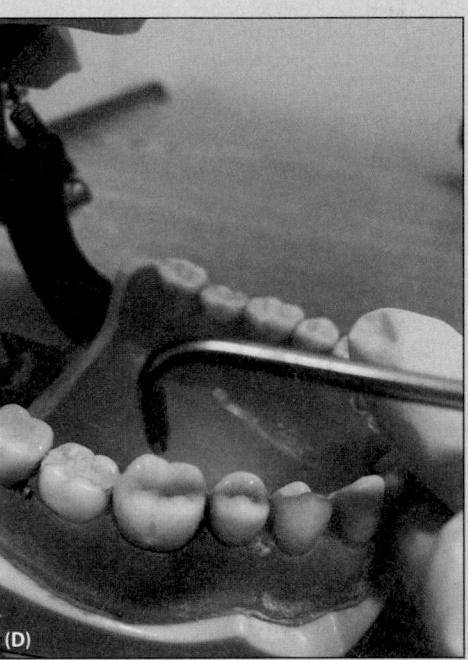

FIGURE 25-19
Procedure for air-powder polish. (A) Nozzle placed 3–5 mm away from tooth surface. (B) For anterior teeth, angle nozzle at 30–60 degrees. (C) For posterior teeth, angle nozzle at 80 degrees. (D) For occlusal surfaces, angle nozzle at 90 degrees.

Ergonomics During Coronal Polishing

Dental personal are at risk for developing repetitive strain disorders that affect the neck, back, shoulders, arms, and wrists. The development of repetitive strain disorders can negatively impact the ability of dental personal to work. The use of proper ergonomics can decrease the development of repetitive strain disorders in dental personal.

Proper ergonomics during coronal polishing requires the patient to be placed in a supine position (Figures 25-20A and B) and the operator to be in the neutral position. The neutral position allows the operator to work while maintaining a proper body alignment. This prevents stresses and strains on the body. Table 25-6 reviews the neutral position.

For maximum visibility, the patient should adjust their head position according to the arch you are working on. For the mandibular arch, ask the patient to put their chin down toward their

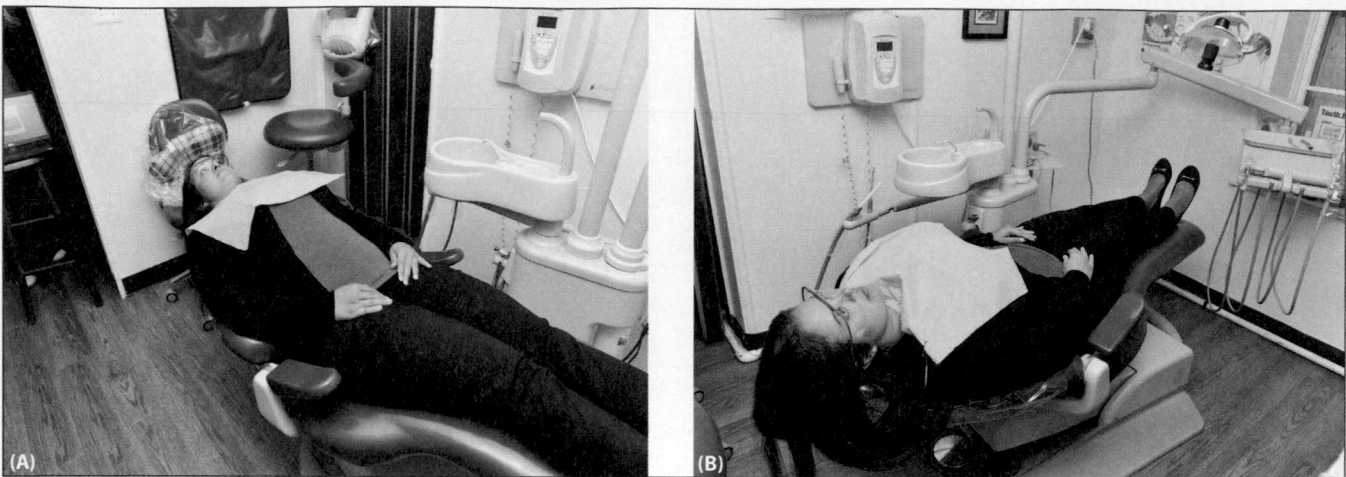

FIGURE 25-20
Supine position.

TABLE 25-6 Neutral Position

Characteristics of the Neutral Clinician Position	
• Feet flat on floor with thighs parallel to the floor or at a slight angle. • Body weight supported by operator stool.	
• Adjust base of patient chair so that clinician's elbows are at waist level when fingers touch teeth of treatment area.	
• Wrist kept in a neutral or straight position. The clinician should avoid flexing or extending the wrist in such a way to stress the muscles and tendons.	

chest. When working on the maxillary arch, ask the patient to put their chin up toward the ceiling. It is also helpful to have the patient move their head toward the operator while working on surfaces away from the operator and vice versa. The dental light should be positioned directly over the patient's mouth pointed down for the mandibular arch and over the patient's chest angled 45 degrees toward the mouth for the maxillary arch for maximum visibility. Refer to Figures 25-21A and B.

The operator should use a dental mouth mirror when polishing. The mirror will enable the clinician to retract tissue, reflect light, and use **indirect vision** to see areas in the mouth that are not directly visible (Table 25-7). Proper use of the dental mouth mirror will enable the clinician to better maintain ergonomics. Often the clinician will utilize the dental mirror for many purposes at the same time. For example, when working on the lingual surfaces of the mandibular right teeth, the right-handed clinician will use the mirror to retract the tongue, reflect light on the area, and use indirect vision to the area since they clinician can't directly see this area of the mouth.

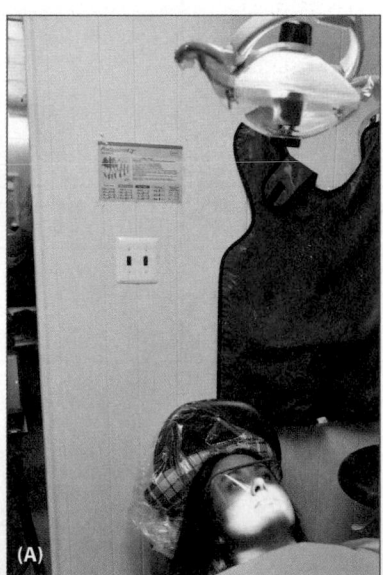

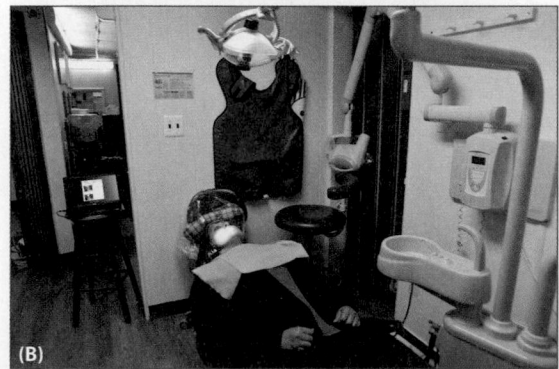

FIGURE 25-21
Dental light position. (A) Working on mandibular arch; notice the light placement directly above arch. (B) Working on maxillary arch; notice light placement over the patient's chest and tilted up toward the oral cavity.

TABLE 25-7 Use of a Dental Mirror

Use	Purpose
Retraction	To move soft tissue (cheeks, tongue, etc.) so the clinician can better visualize and access the area
Reflection	To reflect light from the dental light to a specific area of the mouth
Indirect vision	To visualize an area of the mouth that is not directly visible

Topical Fluoride Application

Fluoride application is a therapeutic procedure that can reduce a patient's risk of developing dental caries. It is incorporated into the hygiene treatment plan based upon caries risk, regardless of the patient's age.

Topical fluoride application involves applying a high concentration of fluoride to the outer tooth surface. In the presence of this high concentration of topical fluoride, a calcium fluoride compound forms on the enamel's surface. This compound releases fluoride and promotes remineralization of the tooth surface thereby making the tooth less susceptible to decay as well as reducing hypersensitivity. After eruption, exposure of the tooth to fluoride will result in high levels of fluoride at the surface layer and less fluoride in the deeper layers. Chapter 16 discusses the mechanism of fluoride and patient assessment in more detail.

Fluoride Tray Application

In the dental office, fluoride gels, foams, and rinses are commonly applied. The gel and foam solutions are convenient to use and remain in the fluoride tray. Both fluoride gels and foams are effective in reducing dental caries. However, there are more clinical trials demonstrating the effectiveness of fluoride gel in reducing dental caries than there are clinical trials demonstrating the effectiveness of fluoride foam in reducing dental caries. Research also indicates that there is no significant difference in fluoride uptake between sodium fluoride (NaF) and acidulated phosphate fluoride (APF).

Fluoride trays are available in various sizes, mainly small, medium, and large. It is important that the dental assistant select the proper size tray for each patient to ensure maximum coverage of each tooth surface and to allow for maximum patient comfort. Trays that are too large can be uncomfortable for patients and contribute to the patient gagging. Fluoride trays are also available in hinged and unhinged styles. Figure 25-22 shows hinged and unhinged fluoride trays. Using a hinged or unhinged tray is based upon clinician preference only. Fluoride trays are a disposable item and are not meant to be reused.

Fluoride trays should have a distal dam. The distal dam maintains fluoride in the tray and prevents the fluoride from seeping from the distal side of the tray into the patient's throat. This can contribute to patient gagging and cause the patient to ingest the fluoride, which can increase the changes of the patient developing fluoride toxicity.

Fluorides come in many flavors, and usually the dental office will have several flavors for the patient to choose from. The dental

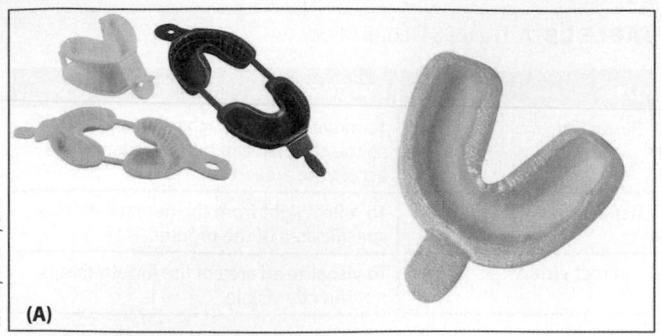

Courtesy of Henry Schein

(A)

FIGURE 25-22
(A) Hinged and (B) unhinged tray.

assistant should read and follow the directions for the type of fluoride being applied in order to determine the length of application and helpful hints. The most common agents are 2% sodium fluoride and 1.23% acidulated phosphate fluoride (see Chapter 16).

It is recommended that a tray fluoride application be applied to the teeth for 4 minutes for both NaF and APF. While there are laboratory studies indicating that a 1-minute treatment is effective when using APF, the uptake is not 100% when compared to a 4-minute application. The use of a 1-minute application should only be used for patients who cannot tolerate the trays in their mouth for extended periods of time (such as a sensitive gag reflex). It is important to note that APF is contraindicated on restorations.

Fluoride has **substantivity**, which means it will continue to work even after the trays are removed from the oral cavity and the fluoride is no longer in contact with the teeth. Therefore, patients should refrain from eating, drinking, smoking, or chewing gum for 30 minutes following treatment. This will allow the patient to receive maximum benefit from the fluoride application. See Table 25-8 for characteristics of the different types of fluoride that can be used for a tray fluoride application.

TABLE 25-8 Fluoride Solutions Available for Tray Use (Foam or Gel)

Type of Fluoride	Percentage	PPM (parts per million)	pH	General Information	Frequency of Application
Sodium fluoride (neutral sodium fluoride)	2%	9,050 ppm	7.0	• Preferred fluoride for patients with cosmetic restorations (porcelain or composite resins). • Can be recommended to patients with reduced salivary flow. • Can be used to treat dentinal hypersensitivity.	2 or 3 times per year based on caries risk level
Acidulated phosphate fluoride	1.23% sodium fluoride	12,300 ppm	3.0–4.0	• Contraindicated for patients with cosmetic resins or porcelain	2 or 3 times per year based on caries risk level
Stannous fluoride	8%	19,300 ppm		• Must be mixed immediately prior to application • Short shelf life • Very bitter and can cause staining	2 or 3 times per year based on caries risk level

Procedure 25-3
Topical Fluoride Application—Tray Technique

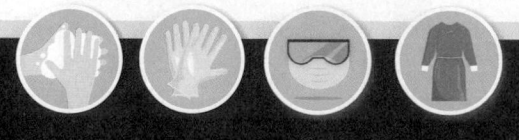

This procedure is done by a dentist, dental hygienist, or trained and qualified dental assistant after the coronal polishing is completed or pit and fissure sealants have been applied.

Steps written in blue font are performed by the operator (dentist, hygienist, or qualified dental assistant), and the chairside assistant's steps are written in black.

Equipment and Supplies

Patient Seating Setup (refer to Procedure 18-4)

Instrumentation Setup (Figure 25-23)
- air/water syringe tip (A)
- saliva ejector (B)
- cotton rolls, gauze sponges (F)
- chosen fluoride solution (C)
- appropriately sized trays (D)
- timer (for 1 or 4 minutes) (E)

Procedure Steps

1. Escort and seat patient (refer to Procedure 18-4).

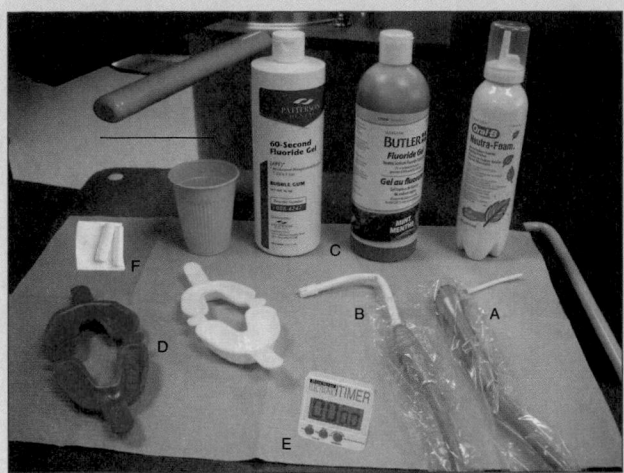

FIGURE 25-23
Fluoride tray setup.

reaching for the tray, keeps finger in the patient's mouth and tells them to keep the mouth open.

Places the tray over the dried teeth (Figure 25-24D). The maxillary and mandibular arches can be done at the same time or individually.

Pushes finger alongside teeth to dispense the fluoride solution around the teeth or asks patient to bite on the trays (Figures 25-24E and F).

Places the saliva ejector between the arches and has the patient close gently (Figure 25-24G). Ensures the saliva ejector does not engage the floor of the mouth.

Asks patient to tip their chin slightly toward their chest to avoid dripping fluoride in the back of the throat.

2. Prepare in advance.
   - ❏ Open patient's chart in dental software.
   - ❏ Navigate to the dental charting screen.
   - ❏ Open patient's latest radiographic history on the computer monitor.
   - ❏ Select appropriate fluoride solution.
   - ❏ Introduce operator as they enter the treatment area.

3. Explain that, in order for the fluoride to be most effective, the patient should not eat, drink, or rinse for at least 30 minutes after the fluoride treatment.

4. Select the trays and try them in the patient's mouth to ensure coverage of all the exposed teeth.

5. Place the selected fluoride solution in the tray. The tray should be about one-third full (2 ml per tray) (Figure 25-24A).

   Greets the patient and takes position at the dental chair.

   Signals for the procedure to begin (refer to Procedure 20-1).

   Dries all the teeth with the air syringe (Figure 25-24C). In order to keep the teeth dry while

6. Set the timer for the designated amount of time.

   Stays with patient entire length of treatment.

   Removes the saliva ejector and the trays from the patient's mouth when the timer goes off (Figure 25-24H).

   Informs patient not to swallow or close their mouth.

7. Quickly evacuate the mouth with the saliva ejector to completely remove any excess fluoride.

8. Have the patient expectorate for 1 minute.

9. Remind the patient not to eat, drink, or rinse for 30 minutes.

10. Explain to the patient that they will be scheduled for an appointment to return to clinic (RTC) for their next scheduled hygiene visit.

11. Write up procedure in Services Rendered.

12. Dismiss and escort patient to reception area (refer to Procedure 18-5).

Date	Services Rendered
02/18/XX	Updated medical and dental history, no changes noted. BP = 120/80 T=98.6F, P=80, R=18
	2% Neutral Sodium Fluoride gel applied with hinged tray to both arches for 4-minute application. Post-op instructions given orally and written. Cherry flavor. No reactions, patient tolerated procedure well.
	RTC: 6mrc Assistant's initials

(Continues)

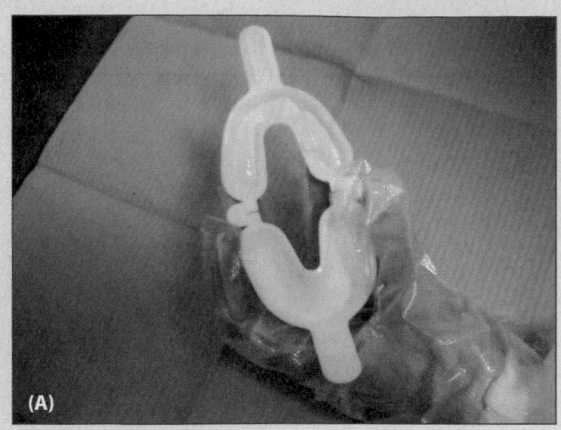

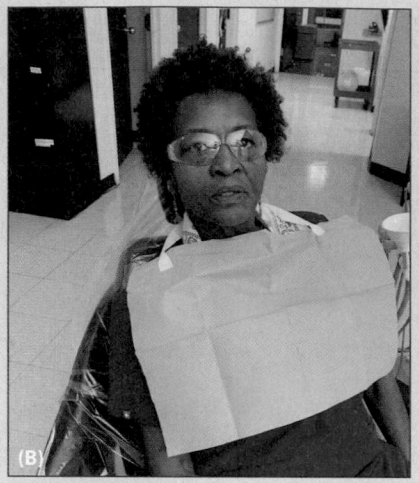

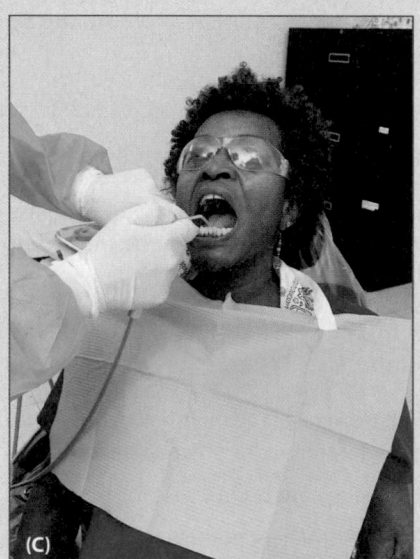

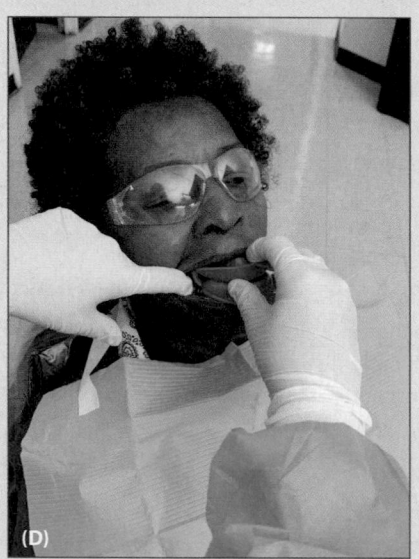

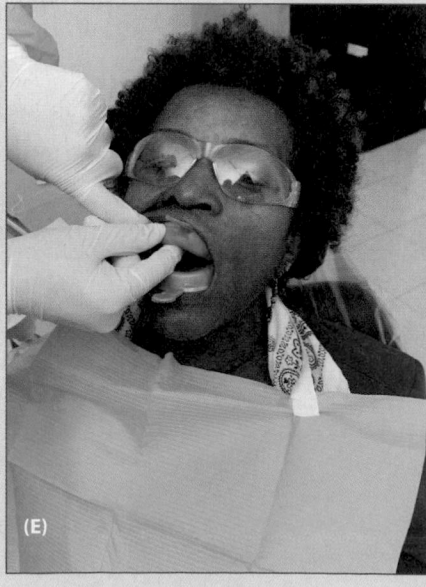

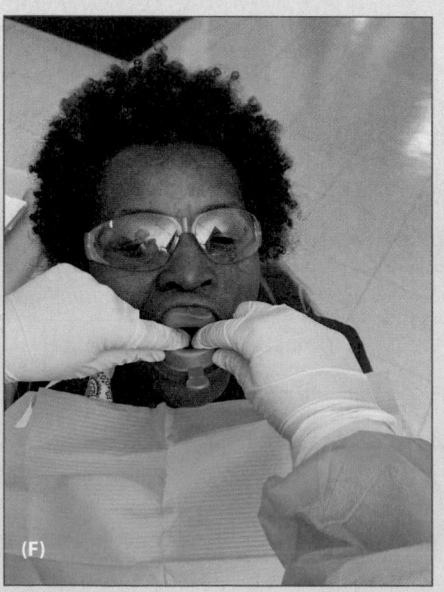

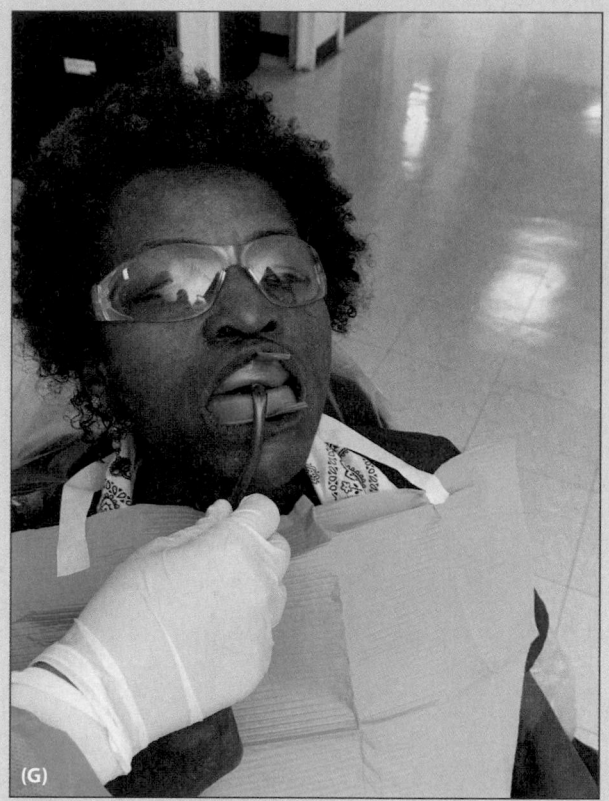
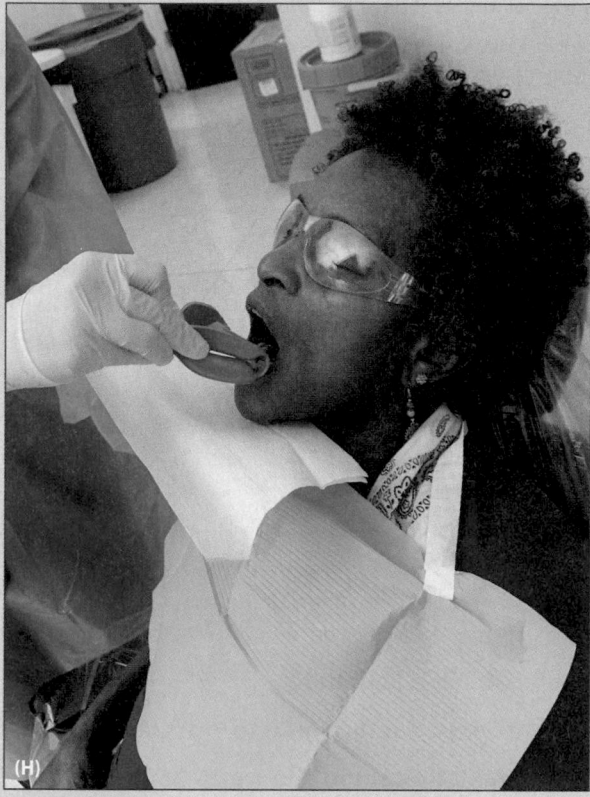

FIGURE 25-24
Fluoride procedure tray steps. (A) Choose proper tray size and fill 1/3 with fluoride solution. (B) Patient is sitting upright. (C) Dry all teeth. (D) Place fluoride tray. (E) Use fingers to force fluoride interproximal on maxillary, (F) and mandibular. (G) Have patient sit for allotted time of application with saliva ejector between arches. (H) Remove trays and have patient expectorate.

Fluoride Varnish Application

Fluoride varnish is a 5% neutral sodium fluoride that delivers approximately 22,600 ppm (parts per million) of fluoride to the tooth surface. A total of 0.3–0.5 ml of varnish is needed to cover an entire dentition depending on if the dentition is primary, permanent, or mixed. Unlike topical tray fluoride applications, the tooth does not have to be dried prior to applying fluoride varnish. Fluoride varnish sets in the presence of moisture, so the oral cavity should never be completely dried prior to application, nor should it be saturated with saliva.

Fluoride varnishes were first introduced to the dental community as a cavity liner and desensitizer. Fluoride varnishes are not yet approved for cavity reduction by the FDA. Using fluoride varnish in this way is considered an **off-label use**. Originally, the varnishes left a yellow appearance when applied to the tooth. The yellow stain would remain on the tooth for as long as 24 hours. Many fluoride varnishes on the market today are available in "white" or "clear." These are certainly more acceptable to most patients.

Typically following an oral prophylaxis, a patient's teeth feel very smooth and slick, a feeling patients often like. Fluoride varnish, however, leaves a coating on the teeth so the patient's teeth feel quite different when they leave the dental office following an oral prophylaxis. Fluoride varnish will leave the teeth feeling a bit rough. It is important that patients understand that while their teeth may not feel smooth, the fluoride varnish results in the maximum amount of topical fluoride being applied to their teeth, which is beneficial to patients who are at risk for developing dental caries.

Once applied to the tooth surface, the fluoride varnish needs to stay in contact with the tooth for many hours. Therefore, the patient should be instructed to avoid brushing and flossing, hot foods or beverages, alcoholic beverages, or eating anything hard or crunchy. The amount of time to refrain from these activities depends on the manufacturer, but the average range is 2–6 hours. Each manufacturer is different in how they explain the postoperative instructions, so all instructions should follow the specific manufacturer's recommendations.

Unlike topical fluoride gels or foams, there is very little systemic uptake of fluoride varnish, so the chance of systemic toxicity is negligible. For this reason, it is the perfect choice to apply to the teeth of young children, especially those who are at risk for developing dental caries.

Topical fluoride varnish application has many advantages over topical tray fluoride application:

- Fluoride varnish delivers the maximum amount of topical fluoride to the tooth surface.

- Application takes approximately 1–3 minutes.
- The procedure provides for greater patient comfort.
- Patient find the taste more desirable.

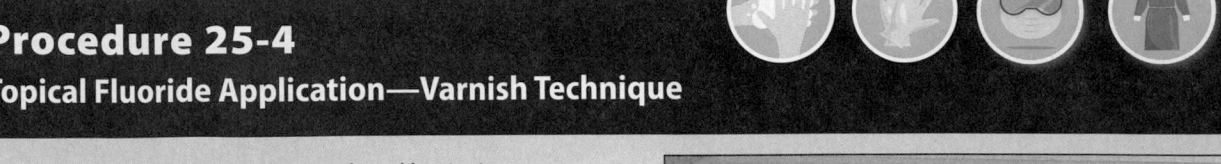

Procedure 25-4
Topical Fluoride Application—Varnish Technique

This procedure is done by a dentist, dental hygienist, or trained and qualified dental assistant after the coronal polishing is completed or pit and fissure sealants have been applied. The dental assistant should be familiar with their state's regulations.

Steps written in blue font are performed by the operator (dentist, hygienist, or qualified dental assistant), and the chairside assistant's steps are written in black.

Equipment and Supplies

Patient Seating Setup (refer to Procedure 18-4)

Instrumentation Setup (Figure 25-25)
- basic setup: mouth mirror, explorer, and cotton pliers (A)
- air/water syringe tip (B)
- saliva ejector, evacuator tip (HVE) (C)
- cotton rolls, gauze sponges (D)
- fluoride varnish (premeasured unit doses or individual applications with applicator brushes and tubes) (E)

Procedure Steps

1. Escort and seat patient (refer to Procedure 18-4).

2. Prepare in advance.
   - ❏ Open patient's chart in dental software.
   - ❏ Navigate to the dental charting screen.
   - ❏ Open patient's latest radiographic history on the computer monitor.
   - ❏ Introduce operator as they enter the treatment area.

   Greets the patient and takes position at the dental chair.
   - ❏ Signals for the procedure to begin (refer to Procedure 20-1)

3. Review postoperative instructions with patient and caregiver.

   Seats patient in supine position.

   Dries the tooth or teeth with air and isolates the area.

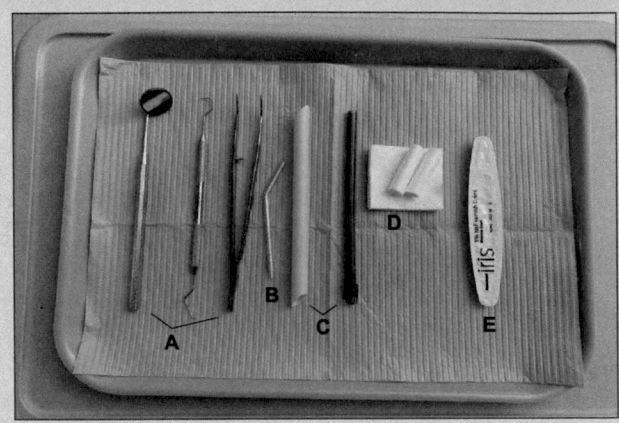

FIGURE 25-25
Fluoride varnish tray setup.

Applies varnish to the teeth using an applicator (Figure 25-26).
- ❏ Paints from the gingival margin to the occlusal/incisal part of the tooth on the buccal and lingual surfaces.
- ❏ Evenly dispenses on teeth.
- ❏ Wipes brush with a 2 × 2 gauze before refilling varnish on brush applicator.
- ❏ Dental floss can be used to apply the varnish to the proximal surfaces.
- ❏ Fluoride varnish will set in the presence of saliva.

Repeats steps until all surfaces are covered.
Follows manufacturer's postoperative instructions.
- ❏ Patient may rinse immediately.

4. Explain to the patient that they will be scheduled for an appointment to return to clinic (RTC) for their next scheduled hygiene visit.

5. Write up procedure in Services Rendered.

6. Dismiss and escort patient to reception area (refer to Procedure 18-5).

Date	Services Rendered
02/18/XX	Updated medical and dental history, no changes noted. BP = 120/80 T = 98.6F, P = 80, R = 18
	5% Neutral Sodium Fluoride varnish applied to all surfaces. Post-op instructions given orally and written. Mint flavor. No reactions, patient tolerated procedure well.
	RTC: 6mrc Assistant's initials

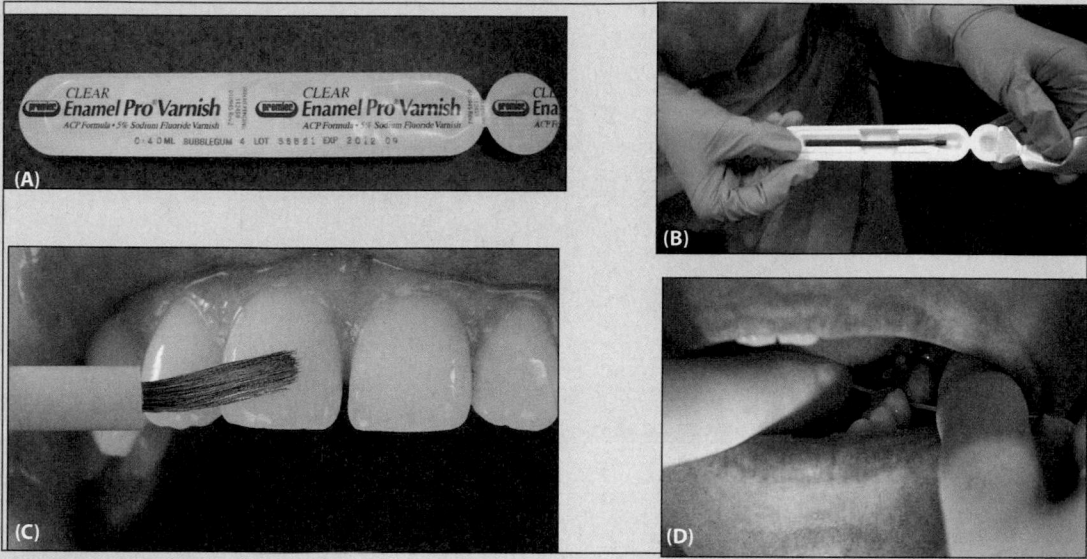

FIGURE 25-26
Fluoride varnish procedure. (A) Fluoride varnish. (B) Applicator with fluoride varnish. (C) Placement of fluoride varnish. (D) Floss to manipulate varnish interproximal.

Silver Diamine Fluoride

Silver diamine fluoride (SDF) has been used for decades internationally. In 2014, it was approved for use in the United States for treatment of hypersensitivity and has since been approved as a breakthrough therapy to arrest dental caries. While the idea of arresting decay in this noninvasive way could seem ideal, there are a few items that must be considered.

SDF is a liquid and comes in a formulation of 38% SDF (25% silver ion, 5% fluoride ion, 8% ammonia) and 32% water. The silver ion acts as an antimicrobial and has substantivity, the fluoride assists in the remineralization, and the ammonia is a stabilizer. It contains 44,800 ppm of fluoride, which is about double the concentration of varnish.

SDF is beneficial to those patients who have decay and may be unable to access dental treatment, such as the elderly or those who are medically compromised. It is also beneficial to those who cannot tolerate certain dental procedures, such as infants, those with intellectual disabilities, or those with extreme dental phobia. One may consider the use of SDF for patients who have multiple carious lesions or for those carious lesions that may be difficult to access.

SDF comes in a dropper bottle. An 8-ml bottle of SDF contains about 160 drops, with each drop treating four to six lesions. Placement of a lip lubricant is beneficial, ensuring no lubricant contaminates the area to be treated. To mask the smell of the SDF, the lip lubricant could be scented. The treatment area should be isolated and dried. The SDF should be placed in a glass dappen dish and is applied with a microbrush. After dipping the microbrush into the solution, the microbrush is rubbed with a scrubbing motion into the carious lesion for about 1 minute. To access the interproximal surface, use a "spongy" type floss. Place the floss interproximally, saturate one side of the floss with the SDF, and then pull it through. After the placement of SDF, place a fluoride varnish in order to seal the SDF in place.

For caries arrest, SDF should be applied one to two times per year. Table 25-9 reviews the advantages and disadvantages to its use. It is important to discuss the effects as the SDF will stain the carious lesion black (Figure 25-27). While this may not be concerning when involving posterior teeth, it may be of some concern when involving anterior teeth.

TABLE 25-9 Advantages and Disadvantages of Silver Diamine Fluoride

Advantages	Disadvantages
Cost-effective	Does not restore form or function of tooth
Low risk of spreading infection	Causes black stain of lesion
No local anesthesia required	Cannot be used in the presence of canker sores or oral ulcerations
Reduced treatment time versus restoration	

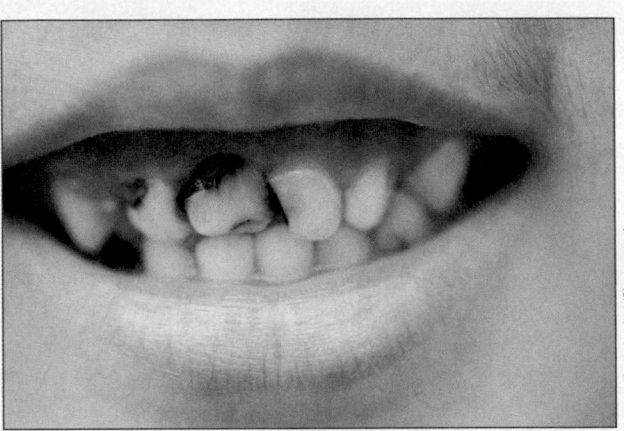

Source: Treetree2016/Shutterstock.com

FIGURE 25-27
Carious lesions stained black from SDF application.

Chapter Summary

While not an oral prophylaxis in itself, coronal polishing and fluoride placement is an important part of the oral prophylaxis. The extent of patient motivation it can provide by producing a smooth surface and reduction of stains can be vital in the success of the patient's home care. In cases where the patient presents with decay that cannot be treated, while still rather new and evolving, SDF could be a potential option for arresting the decay.

Coronal polishing and fluoride placement are also crucial steps for the placement of enamel sealants. While the coronal polishing will prepare the tooth for the placement of the sealant, the fluoride will help to remineralize any areas that were exposed to the etchant. With various options for polishing techniques and a vast selection of attachments and abrasives, the patient is sure to have a suitable end result with minimal trauma to the tooth surface.

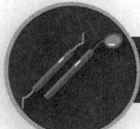

CASE STUDY

Mrs. Barnes comes to her regularly scheduled prophylaxis visit. When reviewing her medical history, you note that she is now taking amlodipine for her newly diagnosed high blood pressure. Her blood pressure today was 123/78. While the dental hygienist was scaling, they noted that Mrs. Barnes had some staining, mainly on the anterior teeth. Mrs. Barnes states that she has been drinking coffee and still has not "kicked her smoking habit" yet.

Case Study Review

1. What is most likely causing Mrs. Barnes' staining?

2. What type of dental stain does Mrs. Barnes have, and is it removable with coronal polishing?

3. If the air-powder polisher is used on Mrs. Barnes, which powder would be most suitable and why?

Review Questions

Multiple Choice

1. Coronal polishing is a _____ procedure.
   a. cosmetic
   b. therapeutic
   c. neither cosmetic nor therapeutic
   d. both cosmetic and therapeutic

2. Which of the following is considered a contraindication to coronal polishing?
   a. the presence of extrinsic stain
   b. acute gingival infection
   c. communicable disease
   d. There are no contraindications to coronal polishing.

3. All extrinsic staining can be removed by coronal polishing alone.
   a. True
   b. False

4. Air-powder polishing would be the technique of choice for which patient?
   a. A patient with no stain
   b. A patient who has heavier stain
   c. A patient who requires subgingival biofilm removal
   d. Both b and c

5. Which of the following teeth should the dental assistant polish, if using the concept of selective polishing?
   a. All teeth
   b. All teeth with extrinsic stain
   c. All teeth with restorations
   d. All teeth with intrinsic stain

6. Flossing is not considered part of the coronal polishing procedure.
   a. True
   b. False

7. The following is true of a prophy brush EXCEPT:
   a. it only comes in disposable attachment.
   b. to soften the bristles, place in hot water.
   c. it is only used on occlusal surfaces.
   d. it normally follows the rubber cup during coronal polish.

8. When air-powder polishing, place the nozzle _____ away from the tooth.
   a. 1–2 mm
   b. 2–3 mm
   c. 3–5 mm
   d. 10 mm

9. Which of the following personal protective equipment (PPE) should a dental assistant use when performing coronal polishing?
   a. masks
   b. gloves
   c. protective gown
   d. protective eyewear
   e. All of these

10. What is the approximate concentration of fluoride in parts per million (ppm) in a fluoride varnish?
    a. 230 ppm
    b. 9,000 ppm
    c. 12,300 ppm
    d. 22,000 ppm

11. To receive optimum benefit, office applied fluoride gels should be applied for:
    a. 30 seconds.
    b. 1 minute.
    c. 3 minutes.
    d. 4 minutes.

12. Patients should be instructed not to eat or drink for approximately 30 minutes following a tray fluoride application because gel fluoride has:
    a. substantivity.
    b. a long shelf life.
    c. the ability to inactivate nutrients in foods.
    d. the potential to become not effective when mixed for food or beverages.

13. Research shows that hinged fluoride trays are more effective than unhinged trays when administering a tray topical fluoride treatment.
    a. True
    b. False

14. The purpose of the distal dam on a fluoride tray is to:
    a. allow the fluoride to flow better interproximally.
    b. allow for better uptake of the fluoride by the teeth.
    c. prevent the fluoride from irritating the gingival tissues.
    d. prevent fluoride from flowing from the tray into the patient's throat.

15. Suction should not be used when administering fluoride varnish because fluoride varnish sets in the presence of:
    a. air.
    b. moisture.
    c. cold temperatures.
    d. warm temperatures.

16. Which of the following types of topical fluorides results in the least amount of *systemic* fluoride uptake?
    a. 2% neutral sodium fluoride gel
    b. 1.23% acidulated phosphate fluoride gel
    c. 5% fluoride varnish
    d. 8% stannous fluoride gel

17. When may SDF be the preferred topical fluoride?
    a. Patient unable to tolerate dental treatment for caries
    b. Caries that are difficult to access for treatment
    c. Medically compromised patients
    d. All of these

18. Which is a disadvantage in using SDF?
    a. higher cost
    b. increased chance of spreading infection
    c. stains lesion black
    d. local anesthesia is not required

19. What is the purpose of silver ion in SDF?
   a. antimicrobial and substantivity
   b. assists in remineralization
   c. stabilizer
   d. All of these

20. SDF should be scrubbed into the carious lesion with a micro-brush for 1 minute. A fluoride varnish is placed next to seal the SDF in place. *Select the correct answer based on these statements.*
   a. The first statement is true, and the second is false.
   b. The first statement is false, and the second is true.
   c. Both statements are true.
   d. Both statements are false.

Critical Thinking

Mrs. Jones just completed her oral prophylaxis and is ready for her fluoride treatment. She presents with a history of past decay and two areas of new decay that require treatment. She has restorations present throughout her mouth, including crowns.

1. Which fluoride solution would be best for Mrs. Jones?
   a. neutral sodium fluoride
   b. acidulated phosphate fluoride
   c. stannous fluoride
   d. a or b

2. What is the percentage of fluoride ion available in acidulated phosphate fluoride?
   a. 1.23%
   b. 2%
   c. 8%
   d. 10%

3. The appropriate fluoride placement time for Mrs. Jones is:
   a. 1 minute.
   b. 2 minutes.
   c. 4 minutes.
   d. 6 minutes.

Key Terms

Term and Pronunciation	Meaning of Root and Word Parts	Definition
abrasive (*uh*-brey-siv)	**abrade** = to wear off or down by scraping or rubbing **-ive** = expressing function	a substance (as emery or pumice) used for abrading, smoothing, or polishing
air-powder polishing (air-pou-der) (**pol**-ish-ing)	**air-** = compressed (under pressure) air to power dental instruments **powder** = solid substance reduced to fine, loose particles by crushing, grinding **polish** = to make smooth and glossy by rubbing or friction **-ing** = expressing action	combination of air and water pressure to deliver a controlled stream of abrasive through the handpiece nozzle to roughen or polish a tooth surface, depending on coarseness of agent
chromogenic (kroh-m*uh*-jen-ik)	**chromo-** = indicating color or pigment **-gen** = that which produces **-ic** = having characteristics of	producing color or pigment
clinical crown (**klin**-i-k*uh* l) (kroun)	**clinic** = area where study and perform procedures on teeth **-al** = pertaining to **crown** = part of tooth that is visible beyond the gum line	a part of the crown of a tooth visible in the oral cavity
coronal polish (k*uh*-**rohn**-l) (**pol**-ish)	**coron** = crown **-al** = pertaining to **polish** = to make smooth and glossy by rubbing or friction	burnishing of the anatomic crowns of the teeth to remove dental biofilm and extrinsic stains; process does not involve calculus removal, however
enamel micro-abrasion (ih-**nam**-uh l) (mahy-kroh-*uh*-**brey**-zh*uh*n)	**enamel** = hard calcified structure of the tooth's crown **micro-** = extremely small **abrade** = to wear off or down by scraping or rubbing **-ion** = denoting action	use of chemical and mechanical means to remove slight tooth structure to reduce superficial discoloration

Term and Pronunciation	Meaning of Root and Word Parts	Definition
endogenous (en-**doj**-*uh*-n**uh** s)	**endo-** = within **-gen** = that which produces **-ous** = possessing a quality	produced within or caused by factors within the organism
exogenous (ek-**soj**-*uh*-n**uh** s)	**exo-** = outside, external **-gen** = that which produces **-ous** = possessing a quality	originating or produced outside of the organism
extrinsic stain (ik-**strin**-sik) (steyn)	**extrinsic** = originating or acting from outside **stain** = discoloration produced by foreign matter not easily removed	adherence of bacteria or discoloring agents to dental enamel that cause the tooth to assume an unusual color or tint; it varies in shade according to the agent: coffee, tea, and tobacco cause brownish-black stains; chromogenic bacteria green to brown; and leaks from amalgam restorations bluish-gray to black
fulcrum (**fuhl**-kr*uh* m)	**fulcrum** = the support, or point of rest	point of stabilization for instrumentation with the ring finger
humectant (hyoo-**mek**-t*uh* nt)	**humid** = noticeably moist **-ant** = characterized by	an agent that promotes retention of moisture; a substance added to a powder, such as a dentifrice, to prevent hardening on exposure to air
indirect vision (in-d*uh*-**rekt**) (**vizh**-uhn)	**in-** = not, non **direct** = by the shortest course **vision** = act of perceiving with the eye	visualization afforded by use of a mouth mirror for viewing intraoral structures during dental treatment
intrinsic (in-**trin**-sik)	**intrinsic** = originating or acting from inside	originating or due to causes within a body, organ, or part
off-label use (**awf-ley**-b*uh* l) (yoos)	**off** = deviating from **label** = a word descriptive of belonging in a particular category **use** = to apply for some purpose	a drug used to treat a condition for which it has not been officially approved
polishing (**pol**-ish-ing)	**polish** = to make smooth and glossy by rubbing or friction **-ing** = expressing action	to make smooth and glossy usually by friction
ppm (parts per million)	**parts** = a portion or division of a whole **per** = for each or every **million** = 1,000,000 in number	commonly used unit of concentration for small values; one part per million is one part of a solution for each million parts of another solution
prophy brush (**proh**-fee) (bruhsh)	**prophy** = is short for prophylaxis **brush** = bristles attached to a handle for cleaning	made with nylon bristles to fit into the dental grooves and pits
selective polish (si-**lek**-tiv) (**pol**-ish)	**select** = chosen in preference of another **-ive** = expressing function **polish** = to make smooth and glossy by rubbing or friction	cleaning only aesthetically objectionable tooth surfaces; stresses daily patient self-care for the removal of plaque biofilms
substantivity (**suhb**-st*uh* n-tiv-i-tee)	**substance** = quality **-ive** = expressing tendency **-ity** = expressing state or condition	property of continuing therapeutic action despite removal of vehicle; the ability of an agent to retain its effectiveness
topical fluoride application (**top**-i-k*uh* l) (**floor**-ahyd) (ap-li-**key**-sh*uh*n)	**topo-** = to place **-ic** = characterized by **-al** = pertaining to **fluoride** = mineral used to remineralize tooth surfaces **apply** = put onto **-ion** = denoting action	a fluoride applied directly to the teeth

## CHAPTER 26

Dental Sealants

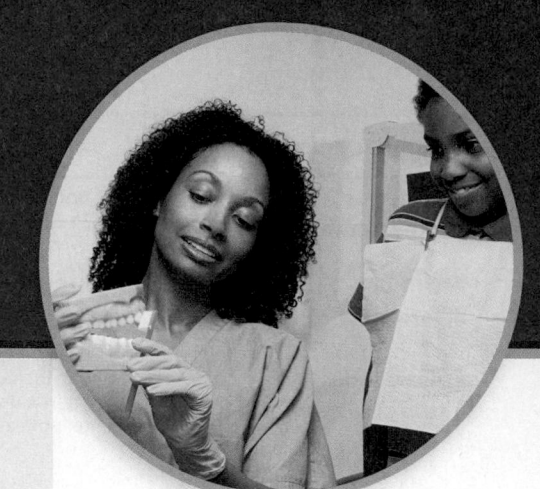

Specific Instructional Objectives

At the completion of this chapter, you will be able to meet these objectives:

1. Use terms presented in this chapter.
2. Explain how dental sealants are an important part of a preventive program.
3. List indications and contraindications for dental sealants.
4. Compare and contrast the types of sealant materials.
5. Discuss safety concerns during placement of dental sealants.
6. Recall steps in placing a dental sealant.
7. Determine the cause of sealant failure.

Introduction

Toothbrushing, flossing, fluoride, and the natural cleansing of saliva have the greatest benefit for reducing caries formation on smooth surfaces of the enamel. Bacteria and food particles collect in the pits and fissures (grooves) of posterior teeth and often cannot be removed by toothbrushing. A single toothbrush bristle is larger than the pits and fissures of a tooth and is unable to remove debris that may be in the grooves of the posterior teeth (Figure 26-1). Saliva, which is beneficial in cleansing the mouth, does not flush away the disease producing microorganisms from pits and fissures, leaving these areas much more susceptible to caries.

Dental **sealants** (also known as "pit and fissure sealants") are an effective means to prevent cavities and to prevent the initiation and progression of early carious lesions in pits and fissure. A dental sealant is a resin material that is applied and mechanically bonded to an acid etched enamel surface to seal existing pit and fissures from the oral environment. They provide a plastic coating over the chewing surfaces of the premolars and molars where decay most often occurs. The CDC reports that 80% of occlusal caries can be prevented by applying dental sealants. Studies demonstrate that sealants that are properly placed on teeth and teeth that remain sealed are 100% protected against decay. The ADA recommends that pit and fissure sealants should be used as a part of total caries preventive programs. Sealants as an integral part of a complete preventive program are a major factor in preventing dental caries. In several states, the placement of dental sealants may be delegated to dental assistants who have specific training.

Indications for Dental Sealants

Dental sealants are resin-based materials that are placed in the pits and fissures of permanent or primary teeth. When a dental sealant is placed, it forms a barrier in the pits and fissures, keeping food debris and bacteria from collecting and reducing dental decay in those hard to clean crevices. Sealants that are placed correctly are effective in protecting the pits and fissures of posterior teeth from decay. This is beneficial as most children and teenagers suffer from dental decay in the pits and fissures of posterior teeth.

Permanent molars are the most susceptible and most likely to benefit from dental sealants, but there may be times when the dental provider feels it necessary and beneficial to place dental sealants on primary molars as well. The primary teeth are placeholders for the permanent teeth so keeping these teeth healthy is important until the permanent teeth erupt. According to the National Institute of Health (NIH), children should get sealants as soon as the first permanent molars have erupted and the occlusal surface is visible. This usually occurs between the ages of 5 years

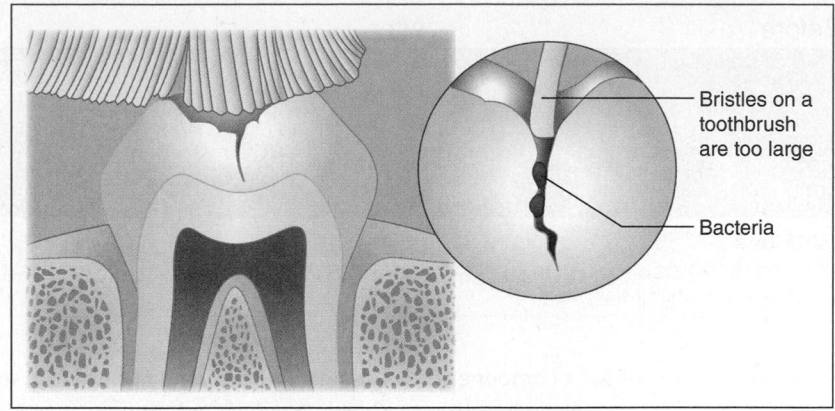

FIGURE 26-1
Toothbrush bristle is too large to get into the pits and fissure of a tooth.

and 7 years. The second permanent molars erupt between 11 years of age and 14 years of age; these too should receive sealants upon eruption. Premolars may need to be sealed as well in order to prevent decay; this is determined by the dentist after examination of the teeth. If the premolars have deep groves, sealants may be prescribed. Some central and lateral incisors may have deep pits that would benefit from sealants as well. Additionally, patients who are susceptible to caries or who have a history of a high caries rate are good candidates for sealants, including adults.

If a tooth has a very small incipient carious lesion when the sealant is placed, any remaining bacteria will no longer cause decay and will not continue to grow. Bacteria cannot survive under a properly placed dental sealant. Therefore, it is crucial that each dental sealant is properly placed. Some sealants contain fluoride that is released after the material is **polymerized** to further aid in prevention of caries.

Contraindications for Dental Sealants

Dental sealants are not recommended for a tooth that already has extensive dental decay present, has an open restoration, or if there is interproximal decay present. Molars and premolars with well joined pits and fissures may not require sealants. A patient who has teeth with pits and fissures that have been present in the oral cavity for several years and are caries free may not require sealants. Patients who may not cooperate for successful completion of this procedure may also not be good candidates for this procedure. Patients who are known to have allergies to components of dental sealants should not have dental sealants. Some sealants contain **methacrylate**, which may result in allergies. The packaging material should be read in order to determine the composition of the sealant material.

Types of Sealant Materials

There are many types of dental sealants available, and the sealant material may vary slightly among manufacturers. The dental assistant needs to become familiar with various compositions, appearances, and methods of polymerization.

Resin-Based Sealants

The most commonly used are **dental composite resins (BIS-GMA)** or resin based. These composites are diluted making them less **viscous**, which enhances the flow that is typically required for the placement of the sealant into the pits and fissures. Dental composites can last up to 10 years, are inexpensive, and come in kits with everything needed for application. They are quick and easy to use, which is important when working on active children.

Some sealant materials contain fluoride and continue to release fluoride after the material has been applied. This creates a fluoride layer that helps with the remineralization process and makes the tooth more resistant to decay. Although some sealants contain fluoride, the manufacturer may state that contact with fluoride, oil, or moisture during the placement of the sealant may negatively affect the set of the sealant. Be sure to check the manufacturer's directions with each material used.

Filled and Unfilled Resins Sealants may be filled resins or unfilled resins. The filled composite sealant contains a small amount of quartz and silica particles. The more filler that is added, the greater the viscosity, the harder the sealant material, and the more likely it will need adjustment after it is placed. The unfilled sealant materials are less viscous and usually do not require an occlusal adjustment after the sealant placement is complete. It will wear down naturally with normal chewing.

Sealant Colors Sealants may be available as clear, tooth colored, lightly tinted colors, or white **opaque**. The white opaque and tinted sealants are easier for the clinician to evaluate once placed on the tooth. There are some sealants that are opaque or tinted during the placement and then set clear (Figure 26-2). This allows the operator to visualize the application of the material and once set is cosmetically acceptable to the patient.

Method of Polymerization Sealants can also be **autopolymerized** or **photopolymerized**; one main difference between the two is the amount of working time that material will allow.

Autopolymerizing Sealant System Autopolymerizing sealant systems are **self-curing**; these include two (2) components, a

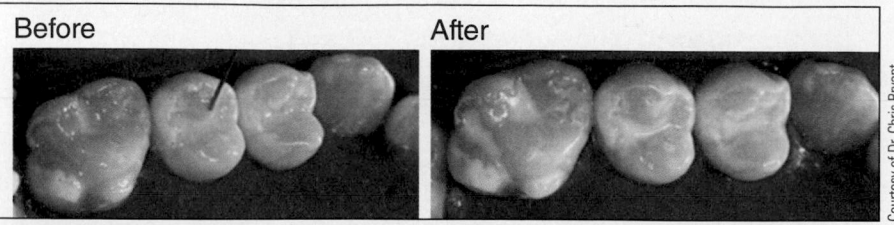

FIGURE 26-2
Color-changing composite resin sealant. The sealant is pink when placed on an etched surface (before) and becomes clear when it sets (after).

base and a catalyst. When equal amounts of each component are mixed together, a chemical reaction takes place and the material begins to polymerize. Working conditions may alter the rate of polymerization. For example, a warmer office temperature will result in a faster polymerization rate. It generally takes one minute for the initial set to begin, so the material must be placed immediately before initial setting begins. The material tends to become more viscous as time progresses, so placement of the material into the pits and fissures may become increasingly difficult as the material polymerizes. Thus, a new mix may be required for any remaining teeth that require sealing. Complete polymerization (final set) occurs within two minutes. An experienced clinician may be able to seal more than one tooth at a time prior to material polymerization.

Photopolymerized Sealant Systems The photopolymerizing (also referred to as light-cured) sealant systems use a special light (**curing light**) to cure the sealant materials with photoinitiators. The photoinitiator is a substance added to a dental material that reacts to light and acts as a catalyst to initiate the setting (polymerization) process. This system is advantageous in that there is no mixing involved and longer working times. The resin is positioned in the pit and fissures and then polymerized (hardened) by photoinitiators in the resin that are sensitive to visible blue light spectrums. This is mainly done in a one-step delivery system; the material is supplied in a light protected syringe that will allow the operator to easily dispense the material to the tooth. Once the material is in place, the curing light will set the resin, allowing the operator to place and cure the material in a manner in which the clinician is able to control the working time. For many operators this is a great advantage over the autopolymerizing system. It is important that the operator and patient wear protective eyeglasses when using the curing light as the light can cause damage to the retina of the eyes.

Dental Curing Light A dental **curing light** is used to cure (set) light-cured materials. Many dental products are now light cured. There are various types of curing lights dentists may choose from depending on the types of materials they use and their preferences. Curing light technology is rapidly changing to improve curing intensities and speed. Dentists evaluate the characteristics of curing lights needed according to the intensity and spectrum of the light, the speed of the cure, the heat that is generated, and whether they are lightweight and ergonomic in design, quiet, portable, durable, and reliable. Most curing lights have small motors,

or sometimes fans, and tips (wands); some have filters, protective shields, handles, and triggers to activate the light (Figure 26-3). Some have digital display countdown timers and preset curing times. In some offices, curing lights are mounted on the sides of counters or integrated into dental units to conserve counter space.

Light curing units have advanced a great deal over the years and continue to do so as the technology and materials evolve. Curing light technologies include tungsten halogen, light emitting diode (LED), argon laser, and plasma arc (PAC).

The traditional curing light uses a tungsten halogen bulb as the source of light. This curing light has been around for a while and is durable, less expensive, and cures all resin-based materials relatively quickly. It does give off some heat, uses a filter to remove useless energy emitted by the halogen bulb, and provides an audible beeper at 5- or 10-second intervals. The halogen curing lights have a fan to cool the unit; thus it is important to remember not to turn off the unit until the fan has stopped. Light intensities can vary and change with use. To determine if the light is working at full capacity, the curing light should be tested monthly. Some lights come with a built-in **radiometer** which adjusts to compensate for any light deterioration.

The LED curing lights are lightweight; some are small and ergonomically designed and have cordless portability. Some curing lights are mounted on the sides of counters or integrated into the dental unit to conserve counter space. These units are durable, produce minimal heat, have no bulbs, and are quiet because there is no need for a fan. This technology is rapidly changing to

Eye Protection Against Curing Light

A high-irradiance blue light is used in the curing light to polymerize resins. Back-reflection of the blue light of the curing light can affect the eyes of the operator, assistant, and patient, all of whom should wear radiation-filtering protection (orange- or green-colored lens) glasses. (Figure 26-4). Chronic exposure can cause retinal damage, leading to degeneration of the macula and eventual vision loss. Even when wearing the tinted glasses, it is recommended to avoid looking at the blue light directly; the glasses only reduce short-term effects. The protective shield should also be placed on the resin light tip to avoid personnel in the area from being affected by the blue light.

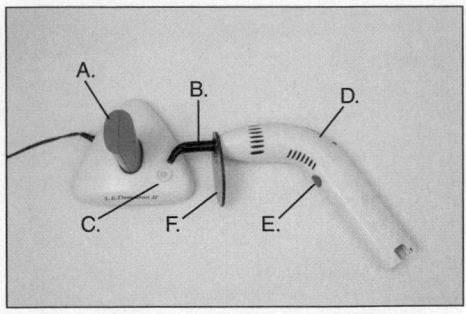

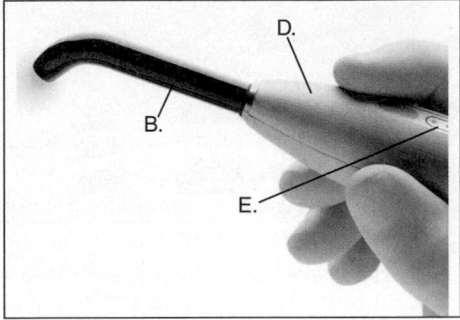

FIGURE 26-3
Curing light system. (A) Battery pack. (B) Wand or tip. (C) Radiometer. (D) Motor. (E) Trigger to activate the light. (F) Protective shield.

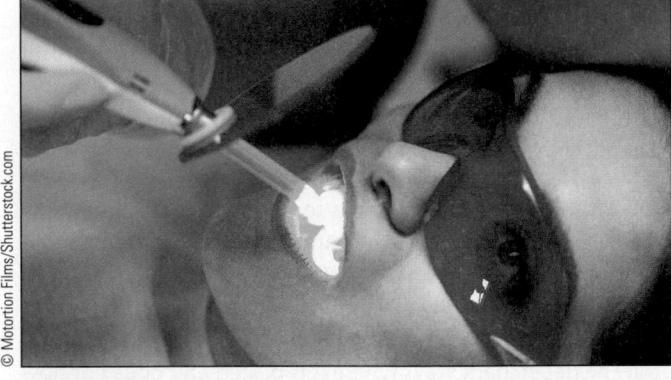

FIGURE 26-4
Patient, operator, and assistant should wear tinted radiation-filtering protective glasses. A protective shield should be on curing list when curing the dental sealant.

© Motortion Films/Shutterstock.com

improve light performance. It is not as important to check the corded LED light units with a radiometer as it is with the halogen lights. But the cordless LEDs that are battery powered need to be checked according to the manufacturer's recommendations. The batteries wear down, and the light output decreases. Some curing light units now have radiometers built in, so the light can be tested more conveniently. The LED lights are still changing and improving. These lights are so convenient that more and more dental offices are purchasing them. As with all the other curing lights there are pros and cons. The LED may shut down due to overheating during long curing intervals and may not cure all materials. Before purchasing a new light, the personnel responsible for ordering should check the manufacturer for the procedures and materials that the lights are most effective.

The argon laser technology generates light by using electricity and argon gas. It produces a relatively high-intensity light that does not generate noticeable heat. The speed of curing ranges from moderate to very fast (5 second curing time). The argon laser lights are not compatible and will not cure some materials due to the type of photoinitiator used in the materials. The argon laser curing lights are much more expensive than other types of curing lights and require a cord.

The ultrafast and powerful plasma arc curing (PAC) lights are used for curing resin-based composites and bleaching teeth. The light tips filter the light to match that of the photoinitiator in the dental material, and in some units the curing is completed in less than 5 seconds. Some models have a built-in radiometer to insure optimum energy usage. PAC units are expensive, require a cord, and may not cure all materials.

Curing Light Radiometer Curing lights should be tested periodically with a radiometer (light meter) because the light bulbs will deteriorate over time and not produce an adequate cure. Small handheld meters are available to test the halogen curing lights (Figure 26-5). The light tip is positioned over a small area on the meter and then turned on. A reading is given to determine the intensity of the light and the need to replace the bulb.

Steps in Placing a Resin Dental Sealant There are few dental procedures that are as easy, quick, and painless as having sealants placed. The basic steps in the placement of dental sealants include preparation of tooth surface, isolation, drying of the surfaces, applying **etchant** to the surfaces, rinsing and drying, placement and polymerization of dental sealant material,

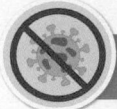 **Infection Control**

The first step in cleaning and disinfecting a curing light is to thoroughly read the manufacturer's directions. All lights must be cool before cleaning or disinfecting. The dental assistant should place barrier sleeve covers over the resin light and wands or tips for infection control but also to prevent resin from adhering to the end. If the tip comes in contact with any resin materials during the curing process, immediately wipe it with the manufacturer's recommended solution on a gauze square to remove any residue. Never scrape residue off with a metal instrument as scratching the tip will affect the light's curing ability. A new barrier should be placed for each patient, and if the area under the barrier becomes contaminated, follow the manufacturer's recommendation for disinfection and sterilization.

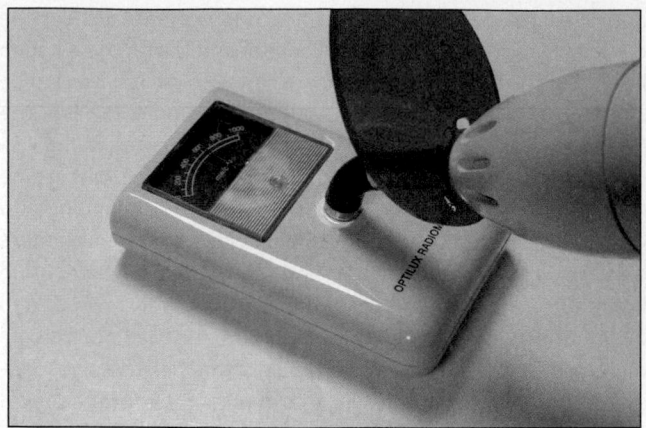

FIGURE 26-5
Halogen curing light tested for accuracy with a radiometer.

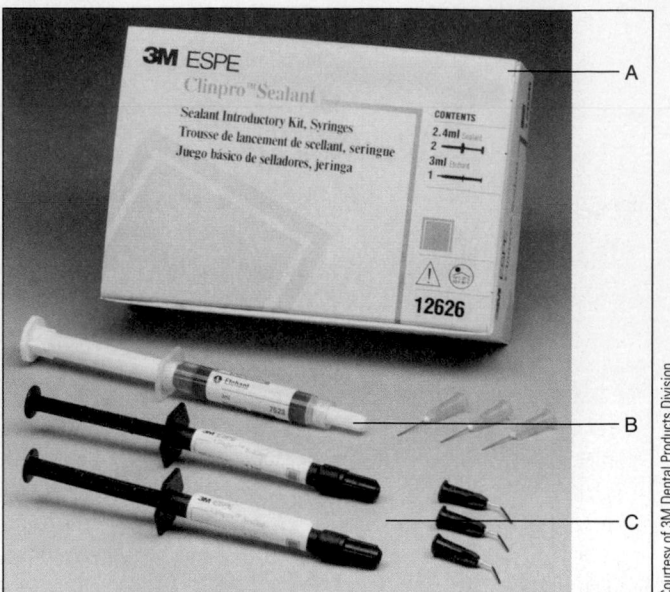

FIGURE 26-6
(A) Sealant kit, (B) etchant syringe and etchant tips, and (C) two sealant syringes and tips.

and occlusal evaluation. Dental sealants are supplied in kits with **compatible** materials (Figure 26-6).

Preparing the Tooth Surface For a successful dental sealant, the surface of the tooth must first be cleaned. Plain flour of pumice is used to clean the tooth and ensure that all pits and fissures are debris free. Pumice is free of flavoring agents, oils, or fluorides and leaves no residue. Flavoring, oils, and fluorides interfere with the mechanical bonding and the set of some sealants; read manufacturer's directions closely. It is mixed to a **slurry** and placed into a dappen dish. A slurry is a 1:4 ratio of flour of pumice to water, similar to the consistency for making a sand castle. The operator scoops up pumice in a rubber cup or prophy brush and cleans the tooth surface. The grittiness of the slurry easily removes any debris. The tooth is then rinsed thoroughly for at least 30 seconds to remove remaining debris and residual pumice.

Microabrasion (air abrasion) can be used by the dentist prior to placing dental sealants in place of cleaning the surface with pumice. This is a very safe procedure that uses an instrument that works like a mini sandblaster; by spraying away any minute decay, this thoroughly cleans out the grooves. The patient should wear protective eyewear to prevent eye irritation from the spray.

Isolation The area should then be isolated to allow for a dry working field; a dry field is necessary for the **retention** of the sealant. The placement of a sealant should be painless; thus a dry field may be established by use of cotton rolls or dri angles. (Refer

to Procedure 26-1, Figure 26-9.) If the area needing sealants also needs restorative work, the placement of a dental dam provides the best isolation. Although the dental dam provides the best moisture control, it is painful without an anesthetic injection, and one of the greatest benefits of a sealant is that it is painless, making it a great introductory procedure with small children. After isolation is complete, the surfaces should be dried thoroughly with the air/water syringe, removing all moisture that would interfere with the bonding of the resin.

Etch and Rinse The next step is to apply the etchant material (also called conditioner). The etchant is supplied as a gel or liquid that is usually composed of 30–50% **phosphoric acid** or a similar acid. The etchant is generally applied with a microbrush or resin brush (Figure 26-7). The gel is recommended for the novice operator. The gel etchant stays where it is placed and does not flow like the liquid etchant and is colored blue, allowing the operator to see where the etchant has been applied. The etchant should be carefully applied 2 mm beyond those areas that are to be sealed to ensure a good seal at the margins, reducing marginal

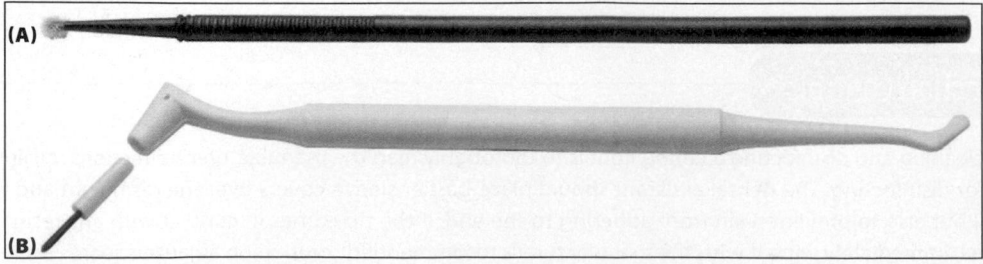

FIGURE 26-7
(A) Microbrush is a one-piece disposable applicator. Available in many colors to note materials being used. The working end bends for better access. (B) Resin brush handle and disposable brush.

fracturing and possible **microleakage**. The etchant should remain in contact with the surface for 20–60 seconds. Always be sure to read the manufacturer's directions for each type of etchant. Etching the tooth allows the sealant material to flow into the microscopic areas of the tooth, which will help permit a **bond** (mechanical retention) of the sealant material. This also has the benefit of killing bacteria at the bottom of the tooth groove.

The acid should be rinsed completely for 20–40 seconds and then the area should be dried. This will leave the surface that has been etched and ready for the sealant with a white "chalky" appearance (white, frosty, and dull). (Refer to Procedure 26-1, Figure 26-10.) At a microscopic level, the acidic etchant dissolves some of the tooth's mineral content from the enamel. The enamel is now rough rather than smooth. It is important not to allow the etchant to come into contact with the gingival tissue or oral mucosa; the acid etchant will burn this sensitive tissue. Making sure that the surfaces to be sealed are completely rinsed and dried is an integral aspect of the placement process. Contamination of the tooth surface with saliva will cause sealant failure; the etchant must be reapplied prior to sealant application should this saliva come in contact with the surfaces to be sealed. The tooth surface that is etched but not sealed will begin to remineralize after it is covered with saliva and will have no permanent damage.

Apply Primer Some sealant systems are supplied with a **primer** that may be applied to the tooth after cleaning, etching, rinsing, and drying the tooth. This is an optional step; primers are believed to enhance bonding and sealant retention.

One-step etching and bonding materials are also available. These materials combine the acid etchants, primers, and adhesives in an all-in-one system. These materials are placed on the tooth and dried but not rinsed; the tooth is then ready for sealant placement.

Place Sealant The sealant material may be placed directly on the tooth surface from the sealant syringe tip, or place the sealant in a resin well (or on a mixing pad) and apply with a brush (refer to Procedure 26-1, Figure 26-8.) It is important to not overfill the pits and fissures. Overfilling results in wasting of

Preventing Etchant Damage

Care must be given during the etching process because most etching agents contain phosphoric acid that burns soft tissue. The patient, operator, and assistant should wear protective glasses when etchants are used. In addition, the patient should be asked to close their eyes. If the etchant gets into the eye, immediately flush with water and check with a doctor. If the etching agent accidently contacts the soft tissues, immediately rinse the area with large amounts of water and explain to the patient what happened and that the area may be sensitive.

material and may also interfere with occlusion. Occlusal adjustment is discussed below. The curing light should be applied for at least 20–30 seconds. The self-curing material will polymerize in approximately 60–90 seconds.

Evaluate Sealant and Adjust Occlusion Once the polymerization has been completed, the sealant should be evaluated with the tooth or teeth still isolated and dry. As long as the area remains dry, any addition of sealant can occur without starting the procedure back at the etchant step. The sealant is checked for voids using an explorer; if voids are present, additional material may be added to fill voids. Voids or cracks may cause leakage under the sealant, allow penetration of debris, and cause decay to form under the sealant. The operator should also evaluate the sealant to ensure that all areas of the tooth are covered and check sealant for retention. If the sealant fails to mechanically adhere to the tooth, the process should be repeated.

If the sealant is sound, the isolation materials can be removed and the occlusal bite of the patient should be evaluated. Occlusion can be checked easily with the use of articulating paper in a holder. The paper will leave marks on the areas that are interfering with occlusion. (Refer to Procedure 26-1, Figure 26-12.) These specific areas can be adjusted with a large round bur or a white stone and contra angle handpiece.

Sealant Maintenance Dental sealants should last at least 5–10 years. Sealants can fail. Sealant failure would be detected upon routine dental during the recare visits for cracks, chips, or the loss of the sealant; sealants can be reapplied as needed.

Glass Ionomer Sealants

The use of **glass ionomers** is another option for a pit and fissure sealant material. It is popular in some offices because the purchase of separate material for sealant procedures is not needed. Glass ionomers are available in powder or liquid form, in capsules with a cannula for dispensing the material, and in a syringe with disposable applicator tips. The glass ionomer sealant materials bond to the tooth chemically, so an etching step is not needed. An acid in the glass ionomer material breaks down the enamel and then fuses with it. This is a very strong bond with less chance of marginal chipping or poor bonding.

Glass ionomer sealants are used with patients who have a high rate of caries or xerostomia. They contain fluoride, which is released continually for about two years. Glass ionomers have some appealing properties:

- They are generally easier to place than resin-based sealants.
- They require no etching or bonding agent.
- They can be used on smooth surfaces of the tooth because they are less fluid than composites.
- They do not require that the area be completely dry for placement because they are not moisture sensitive.
- They bond directly with the enamel.

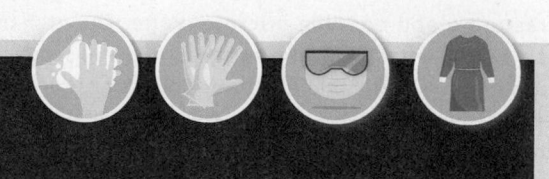

Procedure 26-1
Placing Photopolymerized Dental Sealants

The chairside dental assistant prepares material and transfers materials and instruments while the operator places the dental sealant. This procedure can be legally performed by a trained dental assistant in some states.

Steps written in **blue** font are performed by the operator (dentist, hygienist, or qualified dental assistant), and the chairside assistant's steps are written in black.

Equipment and Supplies

Patient Seating Setup
- PPE: examination gloves, mask, protective glasses, and protective clothing
- handwashing soap or hand sanitizer
- sanitized dental treatment area and barriers placed over equipment
- patient's medical and dental records
- patient seating setup (refer to Procedure 18-4)
- articulating paper in articulating paper holder
- blood pressure equipment
- patient

Basic Setup (Figure 26-8)
- mouth mirror (A)
- explorer (B)
- cotton pliers (C)

Dental Sealant Setup (Figure 26-8)
- etchant syringe and syringe tip (D)
- sealant material syringe and syringe tip (E)
- microbrush (F)
- resin brush (G)
- resin well (H)
- flour of pumice in dappen dish (I)
- articulating paper (J)
- 2-inch cotton rolls (K)
- cement spatula (L)
- primer (optional) (M)
- contra angle handpiece (N)
- disposable prophy angle and rubber cup (O)
- finishing burs in bur block (P)
- curing light with shield and tip barrier cover
- tinted resin protective glasses (three pairs: patient, operator, and assistant)

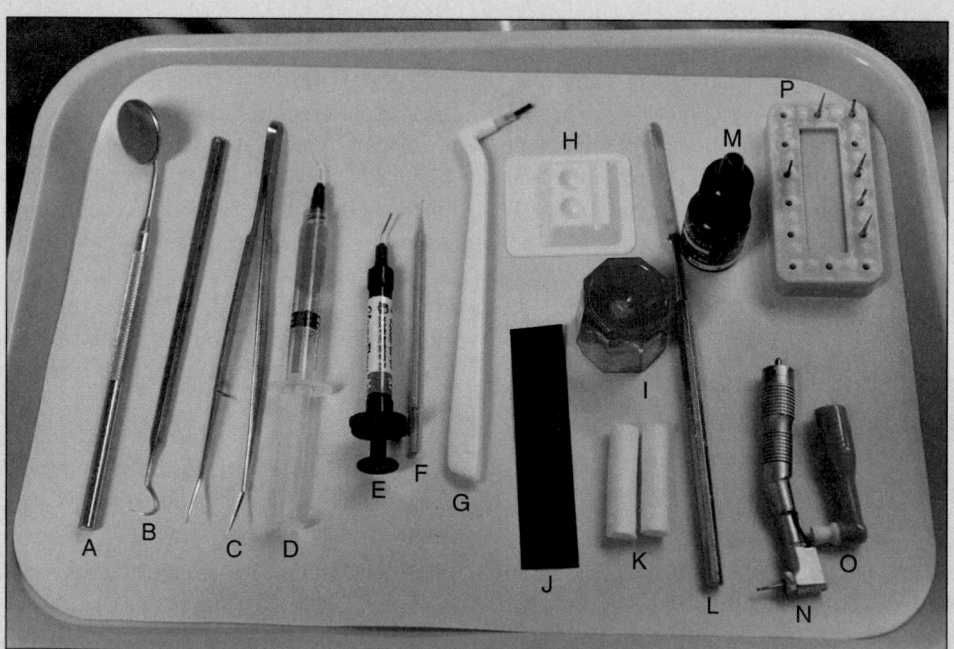

FIGURE 26-8
Dental sealant tray setup.

Procedure Steps

1. Escort and seat patient (refer to Procedure 18-4).

2. Prepare in advance for steps in placing dental sealant.
   - ❏ Make pumice slurry at a 1:4 ratio of pumice and water.
   - ❏ Add water from the air/water syringe into the dappen dish.
   - ❏ Use cement spatula to add pumice to the water.
   - ❏ Mix pumice and water using cement spatula.
   - ❏ If too dry, add a little more water. If there is standing water, place an end of a cotton roll into the mix to absorb excess water.
   - ❏ Insert prophy cup into prophy angle.
   - ❏ Place cotton rolls in cotton roll holder prongs.
   - ❏ Inform the operator that the patient is ready.
   - ❏ Introduce operator as they enter the treatment area.

   Greets the patient and takes position at the dental chair.

   - ❏ Signals for the procedure to begin (refer to Procedure 20-1).

3. Pass mouth mirror and explorer at operator's signal.

   Examines tooth or teeth for sealant placement with mirror and explorer.

   - ❏ Teeth must have deep pits and fissures and be sufficiently erupted.
   - ❏ Teeth should not have carious lesions.

4. Exchange explorer for prophy angle.

5. Hold dappen dish with pumice at patient chin level in left hand.

   Scoops slurry of pumice into prophy cups and cleans the pits and fissures.

6. Rinse the area with air/water syringe and HVE for 20–30 seconds when operator has completed cleaning the surfaces.

7. Exchange prophy angle for explorer.

   Reevaluates for debris or residual pumice.

   - ❏ Uses an explorer to remove any debris remaining in pits and fissures.

8. Retrieve mirror and explorer.

9. Rinse as needed.

10. Pass cotton roll holder loaded with cotton rolls.

    Isolates tooth/teeth with cotton rolls (Figure 26-9).

11. Dry tooth/teeth surfaces for 20–30 seconds with air from air/water syringe.

12. Pass etchant syringe with tip inserted or place etchant onto microbrush and pass to operator (operator preference).

    Etches the tooth/teeth surfaces.

   - ❏ Applies etchant following manufacturer's directions.
   - ❏ Uses a gentle dabbing motion while applying the etchant for the designated amount of time (usually 15–30 seconds).
   - ❏ Leaves etchant on surface for 30–60 seconds as directed by manufacturer.

13. Rinse the tooth surfaces for 60 seconds and dry.

    Evaluates tooth surface—should appear chalky if etched properly (Figure 26-10).

   - ❏ Repeats etch if surface is not chalky.
   - ❏ Does not allow the surface to be contaminated by saliva after etchant is placed.
   - ❏ Replaces cotton rolls if necessary in order to ensure moisture control.

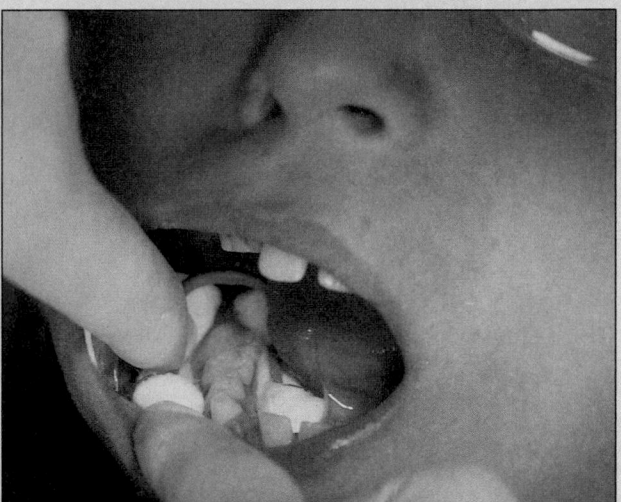

FIGURE 26-9
Isolation of area with cotton holders and 2 inch cotton rolls on each side.

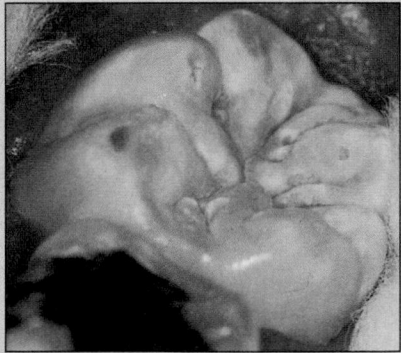

FIGURE 26-10
White chalky tooth surface of a properly etched tooth.

(Continues)

14. Anticipate next step to operator's preference:
    - ❏ Put on tinted resin protective glasses.
    - ❏ Hand a pair of tinted resin protective glasses to patient and operator.
    - ❏ Pass sealant syringe with syringe tip inserted, OR
    - ❏ Place sealant into resin well and pass resin brush.

    Applies dental sealant material.

    - ❏ **Flows sealant into the pits and fissure and reaches the desired thickness (Figure 26-11).**
    - ❏ **Places the sealant on the mesial side of the tooth and allows it to flow toward the distal side of the tooth.**
    - ❏ **Uses the tip or resin brush to carefully move the sealant and prevent air bubbles.**
    - ❏ **Uses explorer to gently work in sealant as needed.**

15. Retrieve resin application instruments and pass resin light.

    Cures resin for time recommended by manufacturer (20–60 seconds).

    - ❏ **Stabilizes light with finger rest when curing.**
    - ❏ **Begins curing 1 mm away from the tooth for first second.**
    - ❏ **Brings tip as close as possible to tooth for remaining time.**
    - ❏ **Increases time for resins more than 2 mm deep.**

16. Retrieve resin light and pass mirror and explorer.

    Evaluates sealant for voids and retention problems using mirror and explorer.

    - ❏ **Maintains isolation and keeps area free of moisture.**
    - ❏ **Checks to see whether the sealant is hardened and smooth.**
    - ❏ **Adds sealant material and cures if there are voids as required.**
    - ❏ **Repeats the entire process if the sealant is not retentive and pays close attention to proper moisture control.**

17. Assist as needed if operator needs to add sealant or repeat the entire process.

18. Pass moistened gauze square and articulating paper in articulating paper holder while retrieving the cotton holders.

    Wipes the surface with a moistened gauze square to remove the air-inhibited layer.

    Checks occlusion with articulating paper (Figure 26-12).

    Adjusts occlusion as needed using contra angle and preference of finishing burs.

19. Pass contra-angle with operator's preference of finishing bur inserted as needed.

    Tells patient good bye and what a pleasure it was to see them.

20. Provide patient with postoperative instructions.
    - ❏ Explain how chewing on ice and hard, chewy candy can damage the sealant.
    - ❏ Educate patient or primary caregiver about need for reevaluation of sealants on follow up visits.

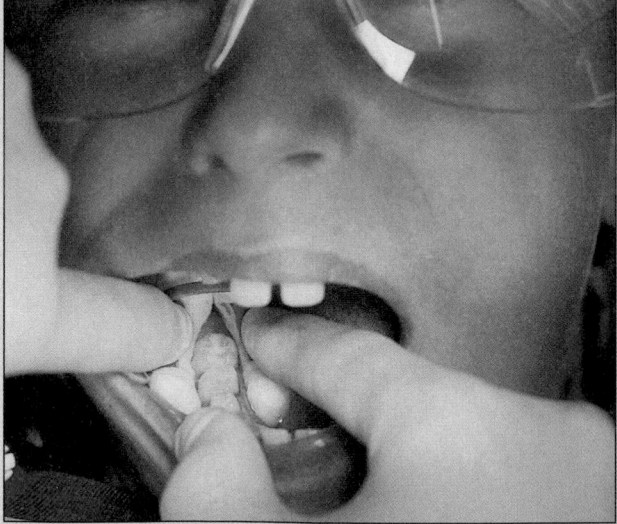

FIGURE 26-11
Sealant placed into the pits and fissures of the tooth.

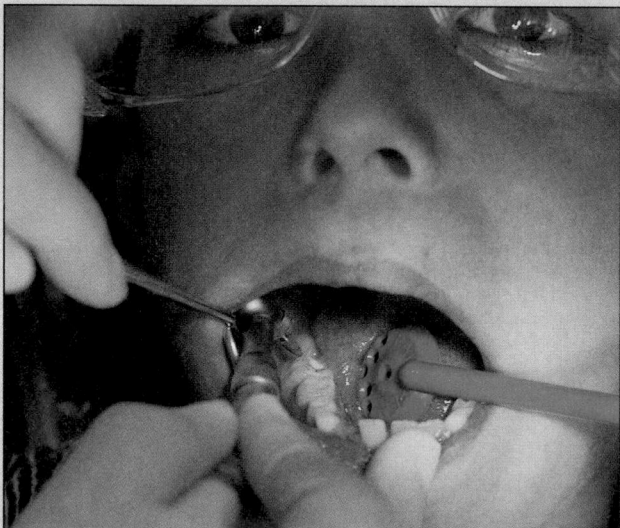

FIGURE 26-12
Articulating paper marks indicated high spots on the sealant.

21. Write up procedure in Services Rendered.

22. Dismiss and escort patient to reception area (refer to Procedure 18-5).

Date	Services Rendered
02/18/XX	Reviewed medical and dental history, BP 120/80
	#18 PFS
	#19 PFS
	#20 PFS
	POI do not chew ice or hard, chewy candy and follow up with evaluation of PFS
	RTC: RC and evaluation of sealants assistant's initials

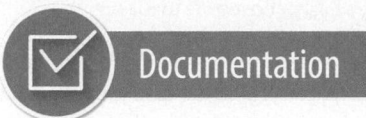

Documentation

Writing Services Rendered for a Dental Sealant Appointment

When writing the services rendered after an appointment, all procedures completed must be included. Each service rendered should begin with an update and review of medical and dental histories and the patient's blood pressure. Some dentists request that the specific materials used be included: cleaning agent, etchant, and sealant. The postoperative instructions (POI) need to be written as explained to the patient, and the entry must be signed or initialed by the assistant.

Enameloplasty Sealant Technique

Another retention method for sealants is modifying the enamel with a bur (enameloplasty). The dentist will use a fissurotomy bur to open the pits and fissures for better retention of the sealant material (Figure 26-13). When a fissure has a narrow slit opening with a large base and when the fissure has a narrow short opening with a broad base, the enameloplasty technique is advisable. The enamel does not have nerves, so there is no pain. Teeth that have a deep V shaped fissure do not need enameloplasty, and the standard sealant procedure is advised.

Cause of Sealant Failures

When applied correctly, failures of dental sealants are rare. If a failure does occur, most happen within the first 3–6 months of placement. Not getting a good bond between the tooth surfaces and the sealant due to improper application is the primary cause of dental sealant failure. The causes of sealant failure are operator error, time, and patient habits. (Refer to Table 26-1.)

TABLE 26-1 Evaluation of Light-Cured Sealants

Observation	Operator Error	Correction
Sealant comes off when retention is checked with explorer after being light cured.	Leading cause: moisture contamination due to saliva after the tooth has been etched	Remove all sealant, isolate, reetch, rinse, dry, and apply new sealant.
	Use of cleaning agent containing flavoring, fluoride, or oil	Read directions for recommended cleaning agents and use slurry of pumice as needed.
	Inadequate etching, rinsing, and drying	Allow etchant to remain on tooth for time specified by manufacturer, rinse and dry, check for opaqueness, and reapply etchant if surface lacks dull, frosty appearance.
	Inadequate curing	Cure resin for time recommended by manufacturer. Hold light close to resin. Low light intensity. Reetch, rinse and dry, and reapply sealant.

(Continues)

TABLE 26-1 *(Continued)*

Voids in sealant after being light cured	Improper application of sealant resulting in formation of air bubbles	Flow sealant into pits/fissures evenly when first applying. Add fresh sealant material to holes and cure.
Marks from articulating paper on sealant after checking occlusion	Overfilling of dental sealant	Remove high spots with finishing burs and contra angle handpiece. Recheck with articulating paper and adjust until sealant is out of occlusion.
Open margins	Underfilling of dental sealant	Add sealant to cover margins and cure.
Observation	**Patient Habits**	**Correction**
Cracks and open margins	Chewing ice and hard, sticky candy	Reinforce patient's need to follow dietary recommendations. Remove and place new sealant.
Observation	**Aging of Sealant**	**Correction**
Dry, brittle, and cracked sealant	Sealant reached maximum life	Remove and place new sealant
Formation of decay under sealant	Operator error, patient habits, or aging of sealant	Remove sealant and restore tooth with restoration. Reinforce need to check sealant every 6 months.

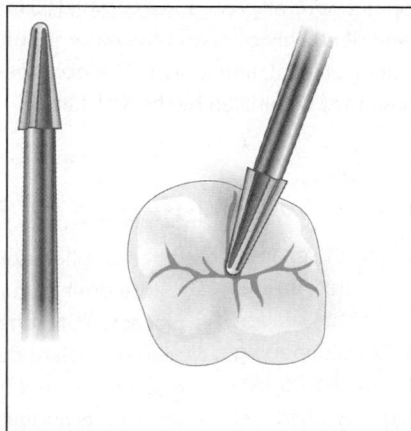

FIGURE 26-13
(A) Fissurotomy bur. (B) A fissurotomy bur being used to open up deep pits and fissures.

Chapter Summary

Dental sealants are an excellent means of preventing and reducing tooth decay in pits and fissures. Sealants are placed mainly on permanent teeth, preferably just after they erupt in the mouth. There are several types of sealants, including composite resins and glass ionomers. Depending on the individual state's Dental Practice Act, the dental assistant may or may not place sealants. If dental assistants are allowed to place sealants, they must obtain the needed additional education and skills. The technique for placing sealants requires practice to become proficient. The dental assistant can place successful dental sealants by following manufacturer's directions on the materials used and use detailed best practices on the techniques, such as good isolation, knowledge on use of materials, and technique skills.

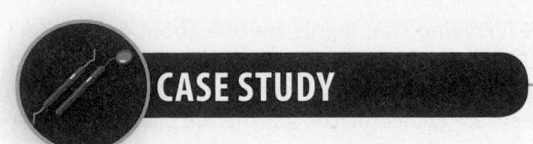

CASE STUDY

Pricha is 7 years old, and teeth #3, #14, #19, and #30 have newly erupted in her mouth. On her recent visit to the pediatric dentist, they suggested Pricha have sealants placed on teeth #19 and #30. Of the other two teeth, #3 has shallow open grooves, and #14 has occlusal decay.

Case Study Review

1. Why is it important to place dental sealants on the newly erupted molars?

2. Why would it be contraindicated to place sealants on tooth #3?

3. What should be placed on tooth #14 and why?

Review Questions

Multiple Choice

1. Which of the following is best practice in preventing caries in pits and fissures of newly erupted molars?
   a. daily toothbrushing
   b. routine flossing
   c. dental sealants
   d. increase carbohydrates

2. Which of the dental professionals are legally allowed to place dental sealants?
   a. dentist
   b. dentist and dental hygienist
   c. dentist, dental hygienist, and chairside assistant
   d. dentist, dental hygienist, and state-qualified dental assistant

3. What percent of dental sealants that are properly placed remain sealed protect against caries?
   a. 50
   b. 75
   c. 80
   d. 100

4. Dental sealants are indicated for all of the following EXCEPT:
   a. recently erupted teeth.
   b. teeth that have been caries free for four or more years.
   c. on occlusal pits and fissures of noncarious primary teeth.
   d. on deep occlusal fissures.

5. All of these are contraindications for placing a sealant EXCEPT:
   a. patient allergic to sealant material.
   b. lack of patient cooperation.
   c. patient is between 11 and 14 years of age.
   d. extensive dental decay.

6. What are the two methods of polymerization?
   a. chemically cured and light cured
   b. water cured and chemically cured
   c. light cured and heat cured
   d. heat cured and water cured

7. All the following statements are true about the opaque or tinted sealants EXCEPT:
   a. they are easier to place due to their ability to flow easily.
   b. the placement is easier because of good visibility.
   c. these sealants are less difficult to identify.
   d. patients prefer clear sealants.

8. What type of material is used for sealants?
   a. glass ionomers
   b. composite resins (BIS-GMA)
   c. filled resins
   d. All of these

9. All of the following statements about fluoride are true EXCEPT:
   a. fluoride is released after polymerization and creates a fluoride layer.
   b. there is no fluoride in any dental sealant materials.
   c. the fluoride in the glass ionomer material is released for about 2 years.
   d. check with the manufacturer's directions to see if fluoride prophy pastes are compatible with the sealant materials.

10. Why would the dentist choose a glass ionomer sealant?
    a. does not require a completely dry area for resin placement
    b. requires no etching or bonding
    c. works well with patients with high rate of caries
    d. All of these

11. Unfilled resins would be selected if the dentist wanted _____.
    a. a stronger sealant
    b. a sealant that had greater viscosity
    c. a sealant that flowed easily into pits and fissures
    d. a sealant that would not wear down with chewing

12. Which curing lights are purchased more often by dental offices because they are lightweight, ergonomically designed, and cordless?
    a. halogen
    b. LED
    c. argon laser
    d. PAC

13. Which curing lights have built in radiometers?
    a. halogen
    b. LED
    c. PAC
    d. All of these

14. All the following statements are true EXCEPT:
    a. most etchants contain phosphoric acid.
    b. the patient, operator, and assistant should wear tinted protective glasses during the placement of the sealant.
    c. the etched area of the tooth surface will never remineralize.
    d. if the etchant contacts soft tissues, rinse with a large amount of water.

15. Which of the following is a false statement about light-curing safety?
    a. Only looking directly at the blue-light will cause damage to the eyes.
    b. Chronic exposure can cause vision loss.
    c. The operator should avoid looking at light even when wearing tinted glasses.
    d. Back reflection of the light can cause eye damage.

16. All of the following statements are true about dental sealants EXCEPT:
    a. sealants bond mechanically to the tooth surface.
    b. the teeth are etched before sealants are placed.
    c. sealants are light cured only.
    d. sealants are placed on caries-free occlusal surfaces.

17. The air abrasion units and the fissurotomy burs are_____.
    a. used to prepare the tooth for sealants
    b. used to finish the sealant material
    c. used to begin the polymerization of the sealant
    d. not used in the sealant procedure

18. Which is the order of steps when placing a light-cured sealant?
    a. etch, pumice, isolate, place sealant, cure
    b. isolate, pumice, etch, place sealant, cure
    c. pumice, etch, isolate, place sealant, cure
    d. pumice, etch, isolate, mix sealant, place sealant

19. Which may be a cause of caries forming under a dental sealant?
    a. The operator failed to place the sealant properly.
    b. The patient failed to follow the POI given at the sealant appointment.
    c. The dental sealant aged.
    d. All of these

20. Which is the leading cause of the dental sealant coming off and not being retained after it is first placed?
    a. inadequate etching
    b. inadequate curing
    c. inadequate application of sealant
    d. inadequate moisture control

Critical Thinking

1. When should dental sealants be placed on a patient? Are sealants only placed on children?
2. On a 6-month recall appointment for a child patient, you notice that a sealant is missing on tooth #30. Should the sealant be replaced? If so, can the sealant be replaced without etching the tooth first?
3. Discuss the various methods for keeping the area dry when placing a sealant.

Key Terms

Term and Pronunciation	Meaning of Root and Word Parts	Definition
autopolymerize (aw-toh-puh-lim-uh-rahyz)	auto = self, by oneself poly = many parts -ize = to convert into, to make	to react or cause to react to form a larger number of parts by combining parts by addition of activator and catalyst within the materials
BIS-GMA	BIS = acronym for bisphenol GMA = acronym for A-glycidyl methacrylate	resin commonly used in dental composites, sealants, and dental cements

Term and Pronunciation	Meaning of Root and Word Parts	Definition
bond (bond)	**bond** = bind, holds together	process that holds/adheres a material to the natural tooth surface
compatible (kuhm-**pat**-uh-buhl)	**compatible** = capable of existing in agreeable combination	capable of forming a chemically stable system; materials that do not affect the properties of another material
curing light (**kyoor**-ing) (lahyt)	**cure** = process to toughen or harden a material **-ing** = expressing action **light** = visible radiation; illumination	dental equipment light source used to harden or set a resin material
dental composite resin (**den**-tl) (kuhm-**poz**-it)(**rez**-in)	**dent** = teeth **-al** = relating to **composite** = made of separate parts or elements **resin** = synthetic materials that have a polymeric structure; plastic	synthetic resin with good mechanical retention used in dentistry as restorative material, adhesives, or sealant
etchant (**ech**-uh nt)	**etch** = to wear away the surface in furrows by chemical action of an acid **-ant** = physical agent	an acid or corrosive chemical used to eat away the tooth surface to make small openings to increase the retention of resin materials
glass ionomer (glas) (ahy-**on**-uh-mer)	**glass** = a translucent material made by melting silicate **ionomer** = class of plastics with bonding action	only dental restorative material that forms a durable chemical bond to dentin; formed by reaction of aluminosilicate glass with polyacrylic acid
methacrylate (meth-**ak**-ruh-leyt)	**meth-** = chemical compound derived from methane **acrylic** = derived from acrylic acid **-ate** = indicates an acid	a thermoplastic acrylic resin (plastic) material made from methacrylic acid used in dental resin restoration
microleakage (mahy-kroh-**lee**-kij)	**micro-** = too small to be seen with unaided eye **leak** = unintended crack through which liquid enters **-age** = process	minute amounts of fluids, debris, and microorganisms enters the microscopic space between a dental restoration and the tooth surface
opaque (oh-**peyk**)	**opaque** = prevents light passing through; bodies situated behind cannot be distinctly seen	opaque material does not reflect light and is not transparent
phosphoric acid (fos-**fawr**-ik) (**as**-id)	**phosphor-** = representing phosphorus **-ic** = relating to **acid** = neutralizes alkalis, dissolves materials	an acid when comes in contact with teeth begins to soften and dissolve enamel; used as an etching solution
photopolymerize (**foh**-toh- puh-**lim**-uh-rahyz)	**photo** = light **poly** = many parts **-ize** = to convert into, to make	to react or cause to react to form a larger number of parts by combining parts under the influence of light, radiant energy, or ultraviolet light
polymerize (puh-**lim**-uh-rahyz)	**poly-** = many **mer** = molecule **-ize** = to convert into	process of chaining together simple molecules to form a more complex molecule with different properties; curing composites by heat, light, or chemical action
primer (**prim**-er)	**prime** = to prepare, make ready **-er** = denoting action or process	first coat given to a surface as a base or sealer
radiometer (rey-dee-**om**-i-ter)	**radio-** = dealing with radiant energy **meter** = measure	an instrument for detecting and measuring small amounts of radiant energy
retention (ri-**ten**-shuh n)	**retain** = to hold in place or position **-tion** =	the power to hold material in place
sealant (**see**-luh nt)	**seal** = anything that tightly or completely closes or secures something **-ant** = agent, serving in the capacity of	transparent synthetic resin applied to surfaces of molars and premolars to seal out decay; preventive measure against tooth decay

(*Continues*)

Term and Pronunciation	Meaning of Root and Word Parts	Definition
self-curing (self) (**kyoor**-ing)	**self** = being of one piece of the same material **cure** = process to toughen or harden a material **-ing** = expressing action	any plastic resin that can be polymerized by the addition of an activator and a catalyst without the use of external heat
slurry (**slur**-ee)	**slurry** = a thin mixture of an insoluble substance, as water and sand	pumice and water mixed to a slurry to clean the tooth surface
viscous (**vis**-kuhs)	**viscous** = has the consistency of being sticky, thick adhesive	the property of a fluid that resists the force tending to cause the fluid to flow

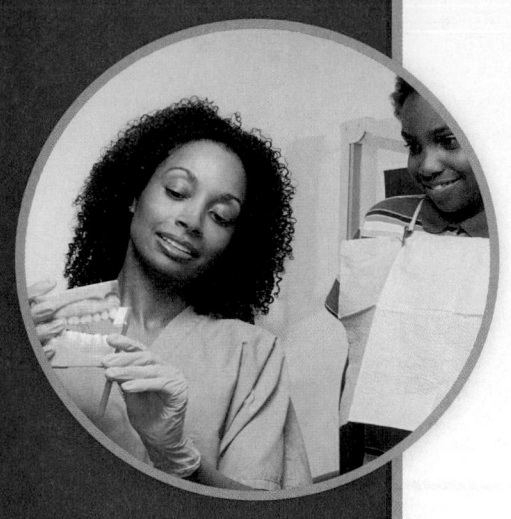

Introduction to Dental Radiography, Radiographic Equipment, and Radiation Safety

Specific Instructional Objectives

At the completion of this chapter, you will be able to meet these objectives:

1. Use terms presented in this chapter.
2. Discuss the purpose of dental radiographs.
3. Identify the person who discovered the x-ray.
4. Define radiation.
5. List the characteristics of electromagnetic radiation.
6. Compare and contrast x-rays with long wavelengths and short wavelengths.
7. Discuss ionization.
8. Compare and contrast the indirect theory of injury and the direct theory of injury.
9. Compare and contrast the different types of interaction that can take place with x-rays.
10. Discuss the components of the dental x-ray machine.
11. State the steps in the production of dental radiographs.
12. Compare and contrast the impact of each of the machine settings on x-ray production.
13. Differentiate among the four types of radiation produced.
14. Define the qualities of a diagnostic image.
15. Discuss the five principles of shadow casting.
16. Describe the principles of ALARA.
17. Differentiate among the units of radiation measurement.
18. Differentiate between the somatic effects and genetic effects of radiation.
19. Compare and contrast between radiosensitive and radioresistant cells.
20. Compare and contrast the occupational exposure and nonoccupational exposure maximum permissible dose.
21. Discuss the nonlinear, nonthreshold curve.
22. State the purpose of intraoral dental images.

23. Discuss the composition of intraoral dental film.
24. Differentiate between radiolucent and radiopaque areas.
25. Define film speed.
26. State the purpose of each intraoral image receptor size.
27. Describe the components of the intraoral film packet.
28. Identify the purposes of extraoral images.
29. Identify the purposes of duplicating film.

Introduction

The science or study of radiation as it is used in medicine is called *radiology*. It provides the foundation for obtaining images that allow the dentist to view conditions of the oral cavity that would not otherwise be seen. The images referred to as *radiographs* can be captured on film or digital sensors. In this section, both will be referred to as image receptors. Dental radiographs are an important element of patient treatment and diagnosis. Dental radiographs are used to:

- Identify dental decay and diseases in the oral cavity.
- View the health of the teeth and surrounding areas.
- Identify and diagnose suspicious areas of concern.
- Locate abnormalities in the hard and soft tissue.
- Identify foreign objects and lesions.
- Record changes in trauma or periodontal health.
- Obtain further information from trauma incidents.
- Provide continued information during and after treatment for implants, root canals, orthodontic treatment, oral surgery, and other dental procedures.
- Examine growth and development patterns.
- Provide information for the preparation of treatment planning.
- Provide a baseline record of the condition of the patient's oral cavity and dentition.
- Identify patients, such as in forensics, abductions, and other investigations.

The History of Radiology

Wilhelm Conrad Roentgen discovered x-rays in 1895 (Figure 27-1). Roentgen was a professor of physics at the University of Wurzburg in Germany. During this time, he was performing experiments with a cathode ray tube called the Crookes-Hittorf tube. This glass vacuum tube had an electrical circuit connected to each end. Roentgen, as well as a number of other physicists at this time, was interested in the stream of bluish-colored light that passed from one end of the tube to the other when the electrical circuit was connected. The colored light was later discovered to be a stream of electrons that traveled from the *cathode* (negative) end to the *anode* (positive) end of the tube. The electromagnetic energies used in dentistry have wavelengths short enough to penetrate solid objects. Roentgen found that they could go through objects as thick as a book. After months of experimentation, he found a way to create photographic images of objects exposed to these unknown rays, or "X" rays. Wilhelm Roentgen thus gave birth to the science of radiography, which has developed into one of the most important tools in modern dentistry. He was awarded the Nobel Prize for Physics in 1901 for his discovery of x-radiation as well as the characteristics of x-radiation.

Radiation Physics

Radiation is the release of energy through space in the form of waves or particles. Dentists use radiation, also referred to as radiant energy, to penetrate anatomical structures and produce images needed to diagnose existing conditions. These images are produced on either **dental film** or a **digital sensor** and the images are called radiographs. The energy used to produce radiographs is called x- radiation, or x-rays for short. X-rays are a form of energy called *electromagnetic radiation*,

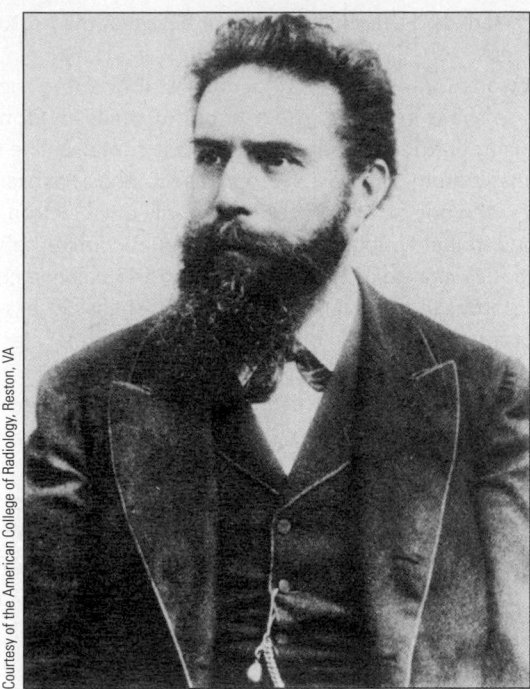

FIGURE 27-1
Wilhelm Conrad Roentgen (1845–1923) discovered x-rays in 1895.

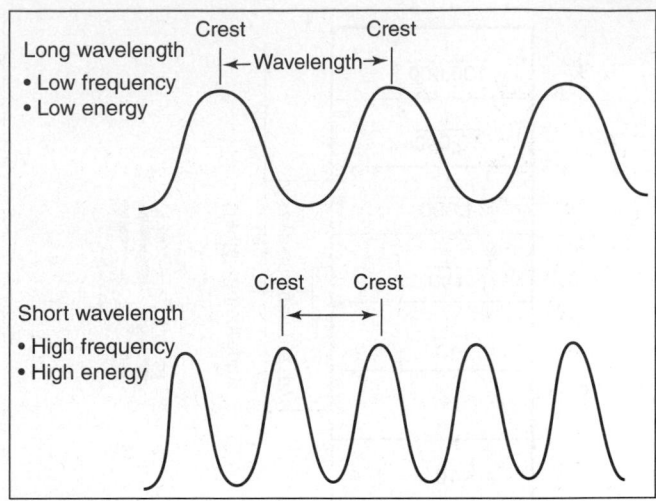

FIGURE 27-2
Wavelengths as they relate to energy, frequency, and x-rays. In dentistry, the shortest wavelength, with high frequency and energy, is used to expose image receptors.

which is emitted by particles that are accelerated. This form of radiation exhibits wavelike behavior as it travels through space.

The most familiar forms of electromagnetic energy are radio and television waves, and visible light. All electromagnetic energy has some similar properties. First, energy travels in waves, which move in straight lines at the speed of light (186,000 miles per second). Second, the waves only consist of energy. Therefore, energy can be sent through lines to a receiver, such as a television. No mass is involved, only energy. Third, electromagnetic energy travels through space in the form of transverse waves. The wavelength, the distance between the peaks of adjacent waves, is called a cycle.

Electromagnetic Energy

Electromagnetic energy is characterized by *wavelength*. The wavelength is the distance between the peaks of the waves (Figure 27-2). Examples of electromagnetic radiation with longer wavelengths are visible light, television, and radio waves. Forms of electromagnetic radiation with shorter wavelengths are x-rays and gamma rays. The electromagnetic scale identifies the relationship between the type of energy and the length of its wave (Figure 27-3). The more cycles that pass a point in a given time, the higher the frequency. Therefore:

● short wavelengths with high frequency equals more energy.

● long wavelengths with low frequency equals less energy.

It is important that individuals working with radiation understand the behavior and nature of x-rays. Visible light is the only wavelength that is detectable with human senses. Invisible x-rays, used for diagnosis in dentistry, carry 10,000 times more energy than visible light. X-rays travel in a straight line and can be deflected off an object and scatter. They can penetrate matter, whereas visible light is absorbed or reflected. X-rays have the ability to cause ionization. Ionization is discussed in the next section.

The wavelengths desired to expose dental radiographs are *short wavelengths*. These have high frequency, high energy, and high penetrating power. On the other hand, *long wavelengths* have low energy, low frequency, and low penetrating power. They are unsuitable for exposing dental radiographs as they are absorbed by the patient.

The Structure of an Atom and Ionization

Understanding the composition of an atom helps the dental assistant understand the process of *ionization*, in which atoms change into negatively or positively charged ions during radiation exposure (Figure 27-4A). Ionization by an x-ray photon can cause cellular damage through direct means or indirect means. These are discussed later in this section. *Atoms* make up all matter. An *atom* is composed of a nucleus, the inner core that is positively charged; and *electrons*, negatively charged particles that orbit the nucleus. The nucleus is composed of *protons* (positively charged) and *neutrons* (not charged). The electrons are bound to the nucleus by an electromagnetic force. Electromagnetic forces are created by the negative charge between

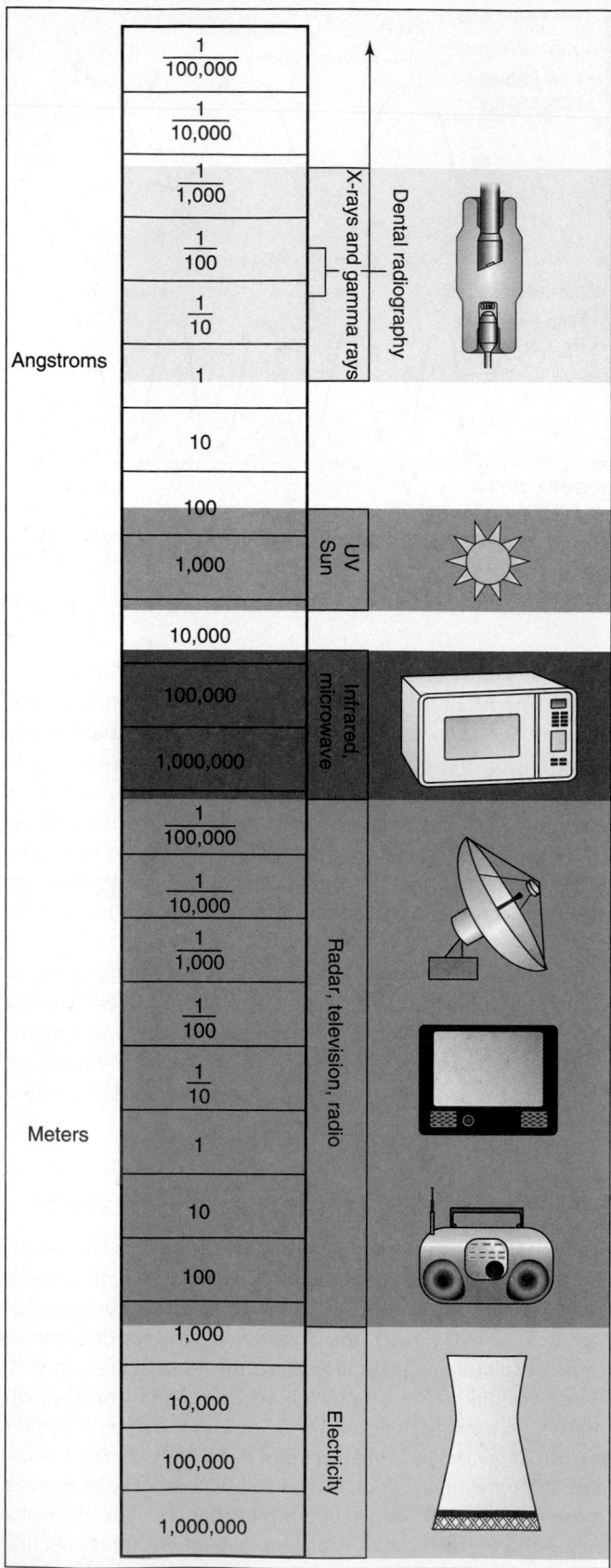

FIGURE 27-3
Electromagnetic energy spectrum and in applications.

the electrons and the positive charge between the protons in the nucleus.

Electrons in an atom may occupy stable energy levels, known as shells or orbits. The number of shells an atom has depends upon the number of electrons it contains. The more electrons an atom contains; the more shells it has. For example, an atom with one or two electrons has only one electron shell. Electrons are held in place by electromagnetic forces between the negative charge of the electrons and the positive charge of the protons in the nucleus. Electrons in shells closer to the nucleus are more strongly bound to the nucleus than electrons in the outer shells.

If an atom is disturbed such as when an x-ray photon collides with the atom, electrons are lost, and the atoms that have lost their electrons become positively charged ions (Figure 27-4A). These positively charged ions are now able to react with atoms in tissues and other matter. This process can alter living cells and tissues and even cause permanent damage. Much stronger x-ray photons are required to dislodge an inner shell electron as opposed to an electron in an outer shell of an atom.

In the human body damage may occur through ionization as well. Injury related to ionization can occur through direct means or indirect means. The *direct theory of injury* states that the cell may be damaged if an x-ray photon directly hits the nucleus of a cell, resulting in ionization (Figure 27-4B). The *indirect theory of injury* states that a cell may be damaged if an x-ray photon causes ionization of water molecules within the cell (Figure 27-4C). This is more likely to occur as compared to the direct theory because the body is composed of mostly water. The water molecule bond is broken to form OH^- and H+. These two ions may recombine to form water again; however, they can also combine to form H_2O_2 or hydrogen peroxide, which is toxic to the cells.

Types of Interaction The x-ray beam can interact with the body's tissues in different ways. One way that was just discussed is ionization. The x-ray beam may also pass through the matter and not interact or cause ionization. Table 27-1 provides details about each type of interaction that can occur during patient radiographic procedures.

Producing X-Rays

Qualified dental professionals produce x-rays using a machine that consists of an x-ray head mounted on an extension arm that is connected to a control panel that the radiographer uses to operate the machine (Figures 27-5 and 27-6). The x-ray head contains the x-ray tube, which generates the x-rays (Figure 27-7). The x-rays can penetrate structures and capture images on either traditional dental film or a digital sensor. Traditional film must be chemically processed in order to view the image. Processing is similar to using chemicals to develop

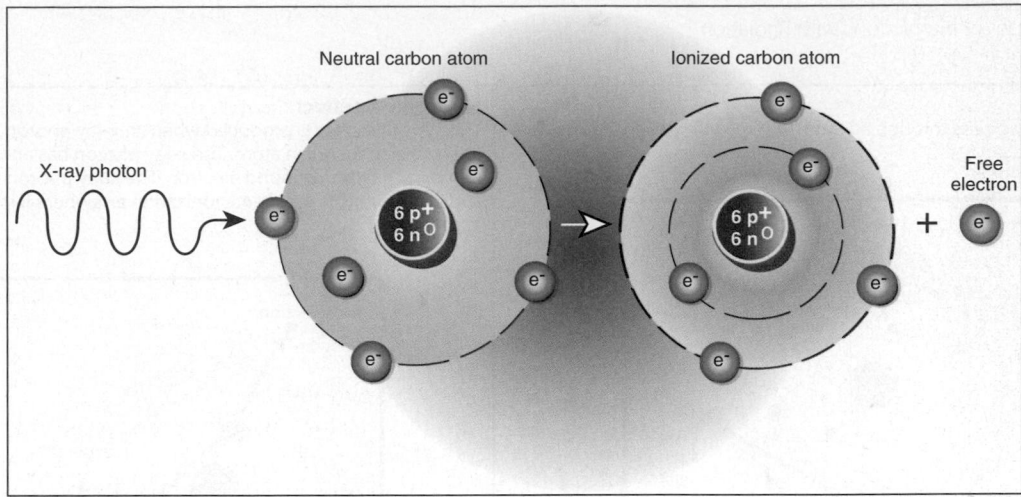

FIGURE 27-4A
The process of ionization. Protons (+ charge) and neutrons (no charge) comprise the nuclei of atoms. Clouds of electrons (− charge) orbit nuclei at different energy levels (sometimes called "shells"). When an x-ray beam interacts with electron clouds, the ionization of atoms occurs.

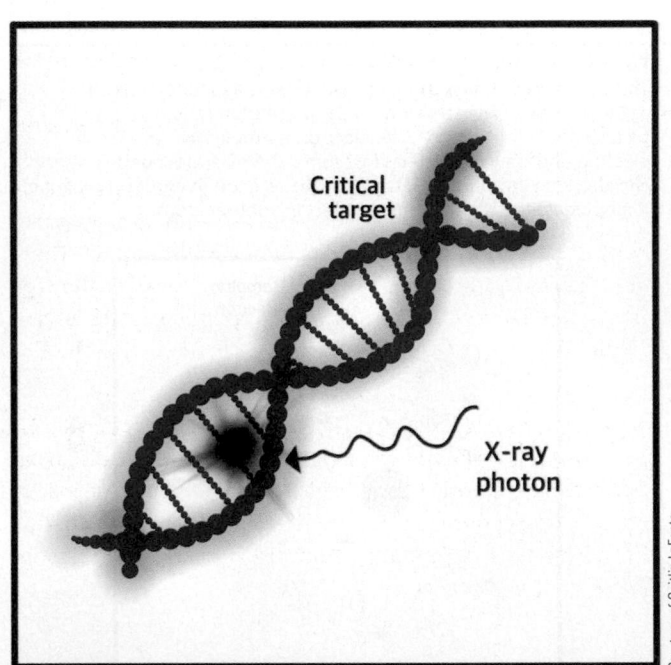

FIGURE 27-4B
Direct damage by an x-ray photon.

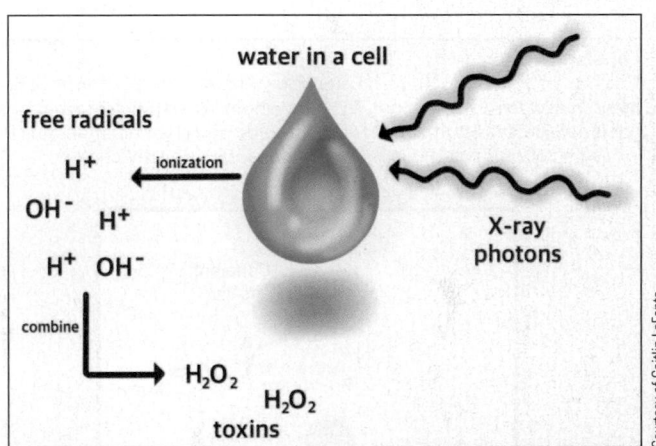

FIGURE 27-4C
Indirect damage by an x-ray photon.

photographs. Digital sensors allow viewing of the image on a computer screen without chemical processing. Chemical processing and digital imaging are discussed in detail in Chapters 28 and 29 respectively.

Components of the Dental X-Ray Unit

In a dental practice, x-ray units can be either wall mounted or portable. Wall mounted x-ray units are the most common (Figures 27-5 and 27-6). Portable x-ray units can be mobile on wheels or handheld like a KaVo NOMAD Pro 2 Handheld X-ray System (Figure 27-8). Whether wall mounted or portable, the majority of dental radiology machines are now digital. Some states may have restrictions regarding who may operate a

TABLE 27-1 Types of Interactions with Radiation

No interaction
An x-ray photon can pass through an atom with no interaction and no ionization.

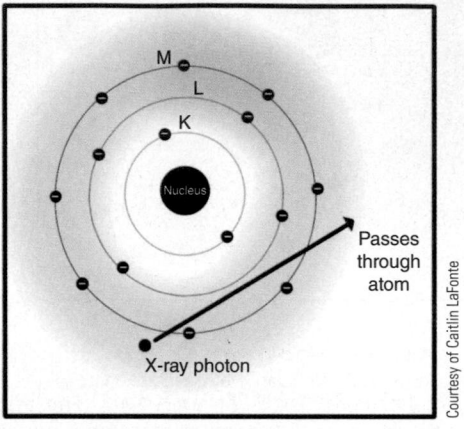

Courtesy of Caitlin LaFonte

Photoelectric effect
This type of scatter is produced when an x-ray photon hits an inner (K-shell) electron in an atom. The x-ray photon has enough energy to dislodge the tightly bound electron. The x-ray photon loses energy and is deflected. It can create ionization elsewhere if it hits another atom.

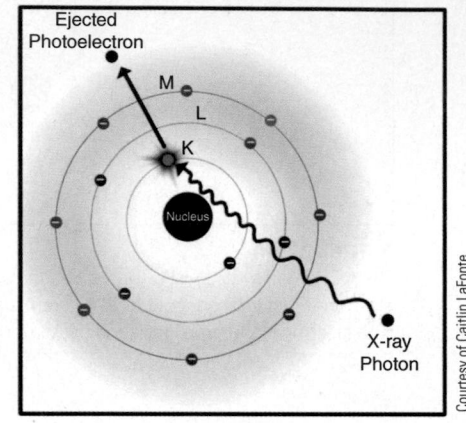

Courtesy of Caitlin LaFonte

Coherent scatter
This type of scatter is produced when a low energy x-ray photon hits an outer shell electron in an atom. The x-ray photon does not cause ionization but is deflected in another direction. This type of scatter radiation can result in fogging of an image. Fogging will be discussed in a later chapter.

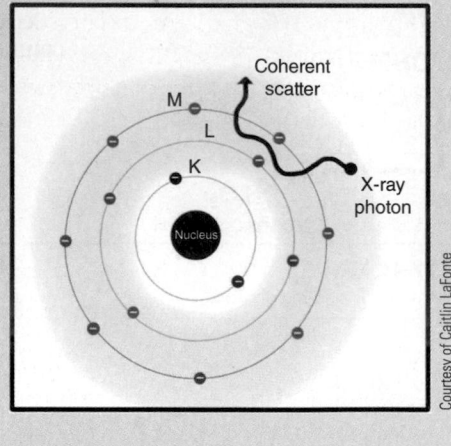

Courtesy of Caitlin LaFonte

Compton scatter
This type of radiation is produced when an x-ray photon hits an outer shell electron in an atom. The x-ray photon causes ionization by dislodging the electron. The electron is now known as a recoil electron; the x-ray photon has lost some energy and is now a longer wavelength x-ray photon. If the photon has enough energy remaining, it may create the same Compton effect in another atom.

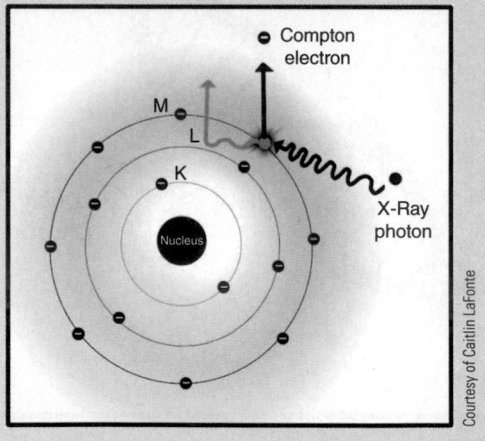

Courtesy of Caitlin LaFonte

dental radiology unit. The dental assistant should check the state scope of practice regulations prior to operating a dental radiology unit.

The dental assistant should know and understand the components within a dental x-ray unit. The assistant may be responsible for obtaining radiographs, as well as for the care and maintenance of equipment used to obtain patient radiographs.

Control Panel The *control panel* is where the circuit board and controls are. These allow the operator to adjust the correct

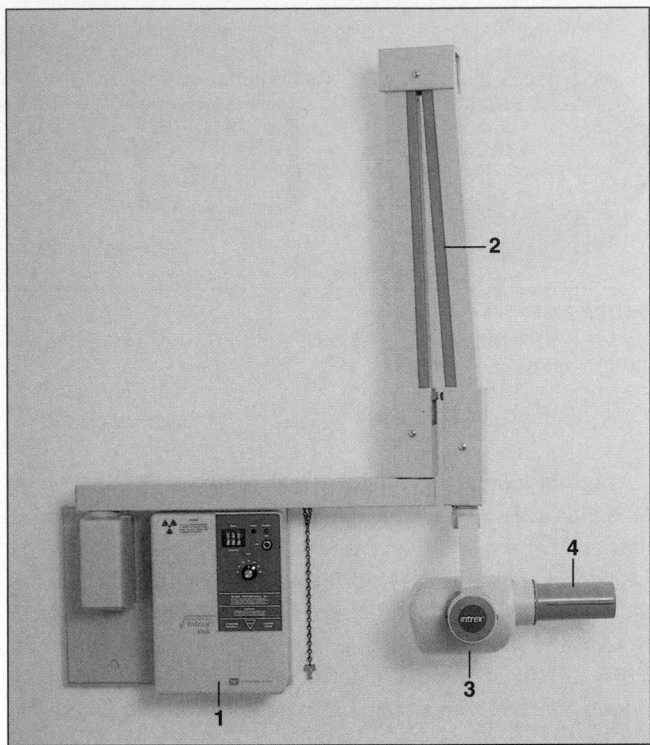

FIGURE 27-5
Wall mounted x-ray machine. (1) Control panel. (2) Extension arm.
(3) Tubehead. (4) Position indicator device (PID).

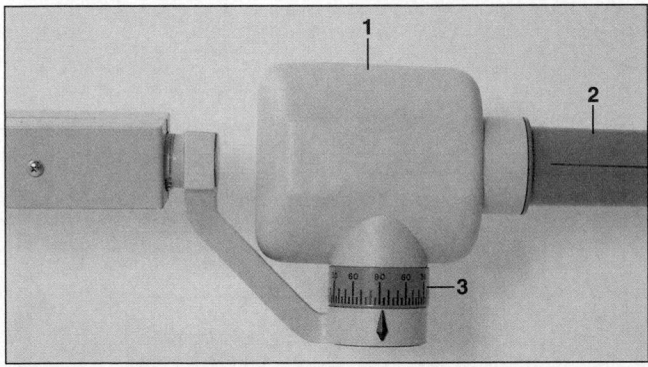

FIGURE 27-6
Parts of the dental arm assembly. (1) Tubehead. (2) PID. (3) Vertical indicator
scale.

setting for each patient (Figure 27-9). It is also where the on/off
switch is located, as well as the controls for the milliamperage
(mA), kilovoltage (kV), and the electronic timer. The operator
chooses settings according to the individual (e.g., children need
less radiation), the area of the oral cavity needing diagnostic
x-rays, exposure technique, and film speed. Film speed is defined
as the measure of film's sensitivity to light. Film speed will be discussed later in this section.

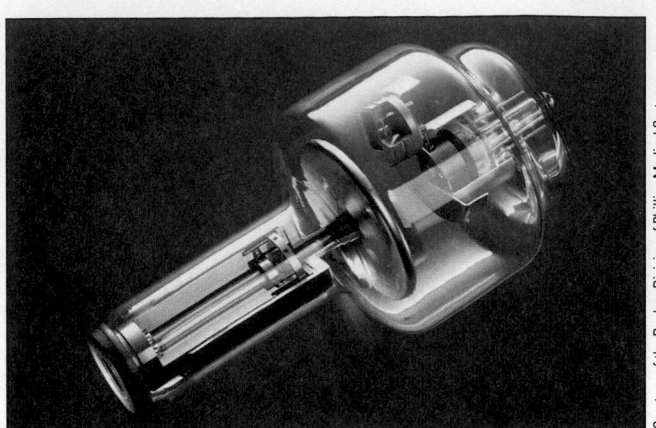

FIGURE 27-7
X-ray tube.

Arm Assembly and Tubehead The arm assembly
is attached firmly to the wall in the x-ray room. The flexible
extension of the arm allows the operator to freely position the
tubehead for the various positions required for dental radiography exposures. Attached to the x-ray tubehead is the positioning indicator device (PID). The PID directs the primary beam of
radiation toward the object to be radiographed. The PID may
be either circular or rectangular (Figure 27-10). The rectangular collimator reduces radiation exposure by 50% as it absorbs
any excess radiation not needed to expose the image receptor
(Figure 27-11). The beam exits the PID toward the image receptor, which will capture the images created when radiation is
absorbed by hard tissues and passes through soft tissue. The PID
is available in 8 inches or 16 inches. The purpose of each will be
discussed later in this chapter.

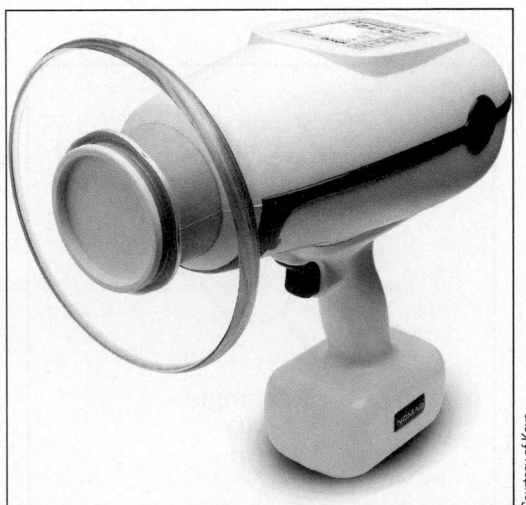

FIGURE 27-8
Nomad® handheld radiology machine.

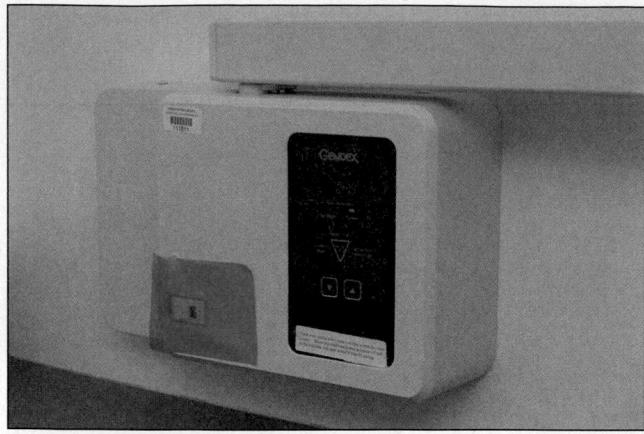

FIGURE 27-9
Control panel.

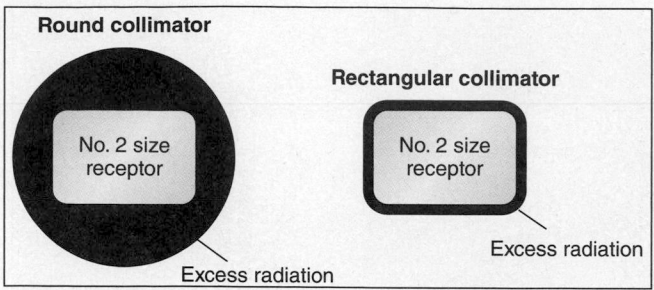

FIGURE 27-11
Compared to the rectangle collimator, the round collimator exposes the patient to greater excess radiation.

Radiation Production

The *tubehead* is where the x-ray vacuum tube and the step-up and step-down *transformers* are located. The step-down transformer takes the 110 volts that come from the wall outlet and brings the voltage down to approximately 10 volts. This allows the filament in the x-ray tube to heat up and produce the electrons (Figure 27-12A). The high voltage (step-up transformer) provides the kilovolts needed to propel the electrons from the cathode end of the x-ray tube to the anode end of the x-ray tube (Figure 27-13). The tubehead is made of a metal casing that is lead lined or made of lead to limit the amount of radiation leakage. An oil bath surrounds the components in the tubehead to absorb the heat that is produced. The heat is derived from the production of the cloud of electrons and the production of the x-rays.

The *x-ray tube*, approximately 6 inches long and 0.5 in diameter, is often called a Coolidge tube. The tube is made from leaded glass and has a window (aperture window) of unleaded glass on the side where the x-rays exit. The tube is in vacuum (all air has been removed from the tube), so that the electrons are free to travel at the speed of light and not collide with air or gas molecules. On the cathode side of the tube is a *focusing cup* made of molybdenum with a filament of tungsten. This is where the electrons originate. Tungsten, a natural element, is used because it has a high melting point, high ductility so it can be made into a fine wire, and a high atomic number so that a large number of electrons are ejected when it is heated. The focusing cup is designed to direct the stream of electrons to the anode. The anode (+), which is opposite the cathode (−), is made of a tungsten target. The tungsten target is set at an angle to direct the

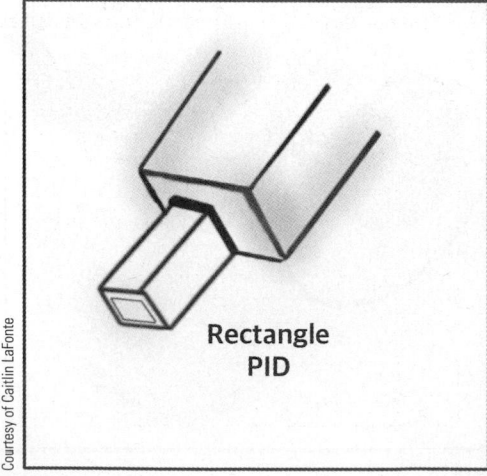

FIGURE 27-10
Rectangle shaped PID.

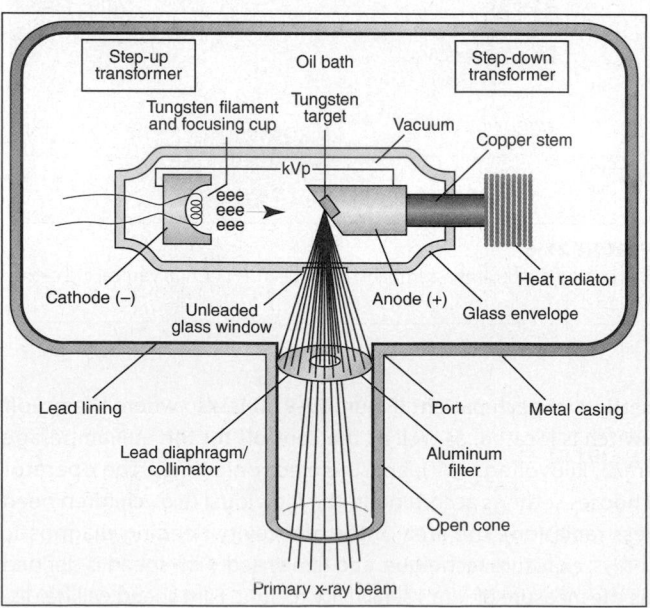

FIGURE 27-12A
X-ray production in the tubehead.

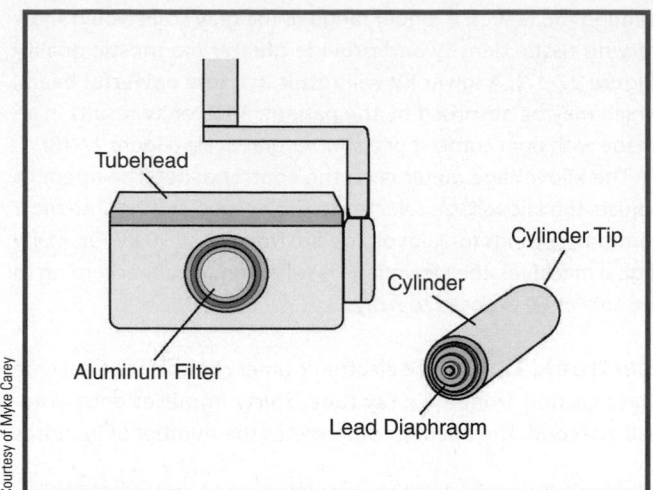

FIGURE 27-12B
Aluminum filter and lead collimator.

Courtesy of Myke Carey

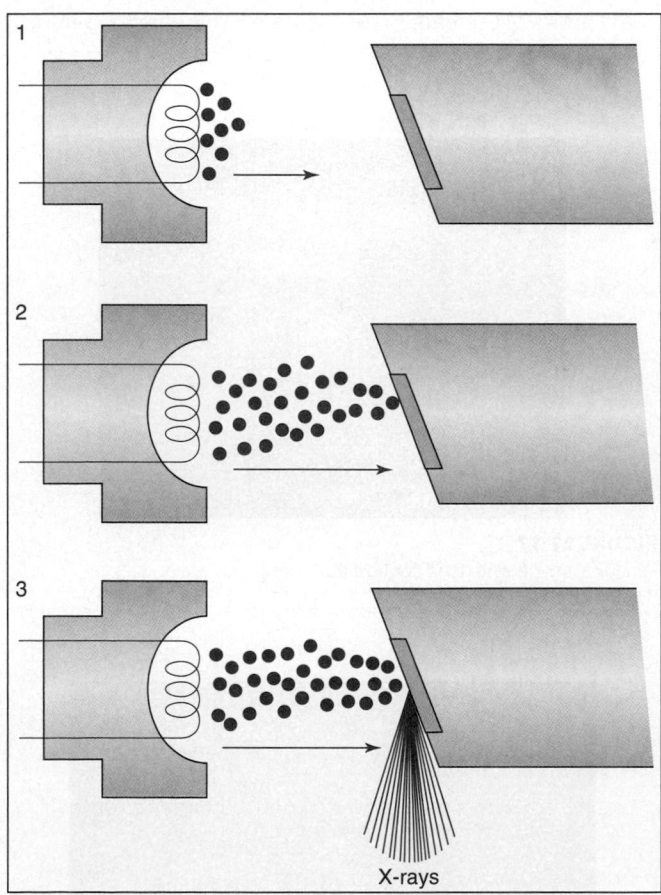

FIGURE 27-13
The production of dental images occurs in the x-ray tube. First, the filament circuit is activated, and the filament heats up, causing thermionic emission to occur. Second, when the filament reaches a certain temperature, electrons rapidly travel from the cathode to the anode. Third, the electrons contact the tungsten target, and their kinetic energy is converted into x-rays and heat.

flow of the x-rays. The small spot on the tungsten target where the electrons hit is called the *focal spot*. After the electrons hit the target, a great deal of heat is generated. The tungsten target is attached to a copper stem, which is then attached to a heat radiator that conducts the heat away from the focal spot. The heat dissipates through the copper stem and is absorbed by the surrounding oil.

After leaving the anode, the x-rays go through the aperture, or unleaded window, and encounter a solid metal filter, usually made of aluminum (Figures 27-12A and B). This *aluminum filter* is placed in the path of the x-rays to eliminate the low energy or long wavelength x-rays **photons** (those with low penetrating power). This filter is added to the *inherent filters* of the machine. Inherent filters include permanent components of the x-ray tube such as the glass window. The inherent filtration is not enough to ensure that only the high energy photons reach the patient and the image receptor. Thus, aluminum filters are added to the machine. Filtration and the regulations related to it will be discussed later in this chapter. The high energy or hard x-rays with short wavelengths, called the *central beam*, continue through the filter to the *collimator*, or lead diaphragm (Figure 27-12 B). The collimator is a lead disc with an opening in the middle that restructures the beam and filters out additional weak rays with long wavelengths. The opening limits the size of the x-ray beam that is allowed to pass through the open cone and out the PID. The x-ray beam cannot exceed 2.75 inches in diameter (Figure 27-14). Approximately 1% of the energy created during the x-ray process is converted into useful x-rays. The remaining 99% of the energy is dissipated as heat.

Bremsstrahlung radiation is the primary type of radiation in the x-ray beam exiting from the tubehead. *Bremsstrahlung* originates from a German word meaning "braking." This braking action takes place when the electrons strike the anode target, resulting in a production of x-rays.

Milliamperage
The *milliamperage (mA)* determines the quantity of electrons. Milli (1/1,000) amperage is a measurement unit for electrical current—the higher the mA, the greater the

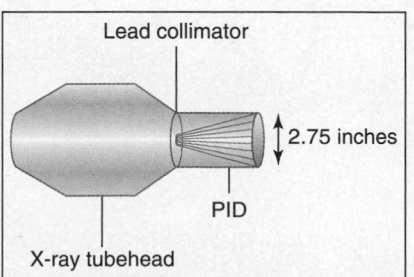

FIGURE 27-14
The collimator diameter is 2.75 inches at the end of the PID.

quantity of electrons and x-ray photons and the darker (more dense) the image (Figure 27-15). The lower the mA setting, the lower the quantity of electrons and the lower the quantity of x-ray photons, resulting in a lighter (less dense) image (Figure 27-16). Some dental x-ray machines use 10 or 15 mA. Many machines are set up with selectors for 10 or 15 mA on the control panel. Some newer units are preset at 7 mA for all x-rays.

Kilovoltage

The *kilovoltage (kV)* determines the quality or penetrating power of the central beam. The higher the kV, the greater the penetration power of the x-rays, and the less required exposure time. Therefore, there is less patient radiation. Higher quality of radiographs (showing a longer range of the gray scale) are the results of higher speeds of radiation going through the tissues. A longer range of the gray scale would show varying tissue density and provide greater diagnostic quality (Figure 27-17). A lower kV will result in a less powerful beam, which may be absorbed by the patient. A lower kV results in an image with poor contrast or a shorter gray scale (Figure 27-18).

The kilovoltage meter is on the control panel. The operator adjusts the kilovoltage selector to the desired setting. The most common settings for kilovoltage are from 70 to 90 kV. On many digital machines, the kilovoltage is set automatically according to the area to be exposed to x-rays.

Electronic Timer

The electronic timer controls the total time that rays flow from the x-ray tube. Thirty impulses equal one-half a second. The operator determines the number of impulses

---

Milliamperage X-Ray Beam Factors

Increased milliamperage = increased density = darker images
Decreased milliamperage = decreased density = lighter images

Kilovoltage X-Ray Beam Factors

Increased kilovoltage = low contrast = longer gray scale
Decreased kilovoltage = high contrast = shorter gray scale

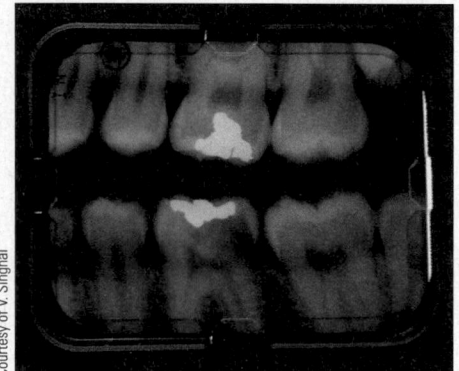

FIGURE 27-15
Bitewing image with high density.

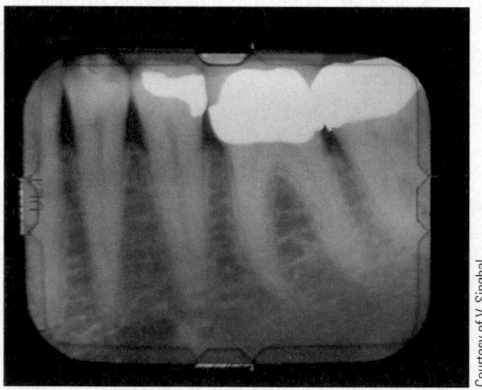

FIGURE 27-17
Periapical image with good contrast and a long gray scale.

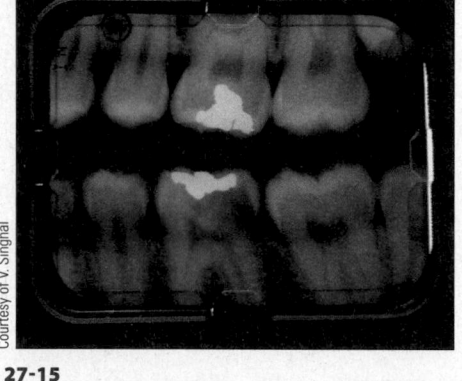

FIGURE 27-16
Bitewing image that lacks density.

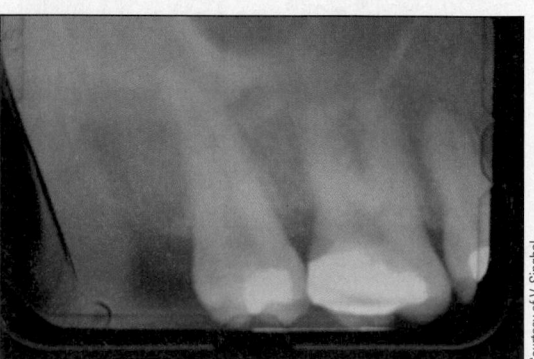

FIGURE 27-18
Periapical image with poor contrast and a short gray scale.

or exposure time after evaluating the technique to be used, the type of radiographic receptor, the target (tooth) to image receptor distance, and which tissues are going to be radiographed. The digital machines have touch pads and/or switches with simple drawings of adults or children on which to select patient size. After the operator indicates patient size, the amount of kV, and the area to be radiographed, the machine sets the timer automatically.

The exposure switch is outside the room or behind a lead barrier. The operator pushes the switch, and the electrons flow from the x-ray tube for the indicated time. The milliamperage, kilovoltage, and electronic timer components control the image quality factors of milliamperage seconds, contrast, and density. Increased time will increase the density of the image, and decreased time will decrease the density of the image.

Milliamperage Seconds The *milliamperage seconds (mAs)* determines the amount of radiation exposure the patient receives. To determine mAs, the dental assistant calculates the milliamperage times the exposure time. Once set, most offices do not change the kVp (peak kilovolts) and mAs, except for child and adult variations.

Radiation Types

There are four types of radiation that are encountered during radiographic exposures. Each type is discussed below in this section.

Primary Radiation

Primary radiation is the central beam that comes from the x-ray tubehead. It consists of high energy, short wavelength x-rays that travel in a straight line. Primary radiation, often called the primary beam, is the useful beam that produces the diagnostic image on the image receptor (Figure 27-19).

Secondary Radiation

Secondary radiation forms when primary x-rays strike the patient or contact matter. The waves are often transformed into longer wavelengths that lose their energy.

Scatter Radiation

Scatter radiation is deflected from its path as it strikes matter. Often, secondary and scatter radiation are used interchangeably. This radiation scatters in all directions, and therefore presents the most serious danger to the operator. Due to scatter radiation, the operator must stand at least 6 feet from the patient while exposing x-ray image receptors, or stand behind structural shielding and out of the path of the primary beam (Figure 27-19).

Leakage Radiation

Leakage escapes in all directions from the tube or tubehead. The x-ray machine must be checked for leakage and should not be used until the problem is addressed. Leakage radiation is not useful for the diagnostic process; the long wavelengths only cause harm.

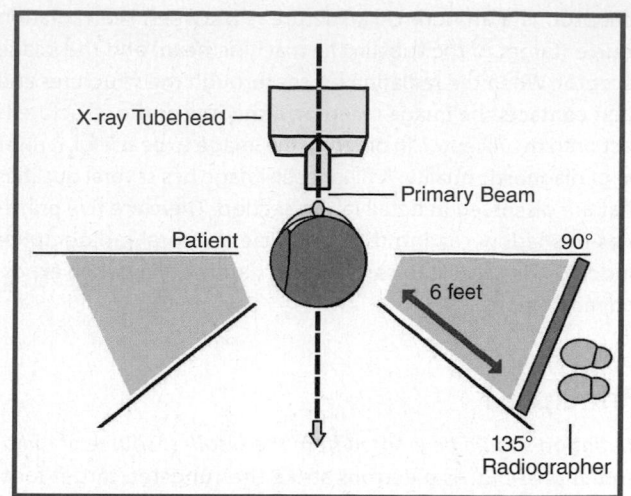

FIGURE 27-19
Operator should stand a minimum of 6 feet from primary beam and out of path of primary beam.

Taking Quality Radiographs

Quality radiographs are those that are of a diagnostic quality. Contrast and density are two important factors that affect the quality of a radiograph.

Contrast

A radiographic image is a black-and-white picture that also shows shades of gray. The *contrast* is the difference between shades of gray. The black, white, and shades of gray on an image reflect the densities of the subject and the receptor. Contrast is controlled by the kilovoltage setting, the developing process for traditional films (if the developing solution is old or exhausted it will cause poor contrast), film fog (possibly caused by a light leak in the darkroom), and distortion (caused by patient or cone moving). The developing process and the impact that it can have on the quality of the images will be discussed in Chapter 28.

Density

The *density* is the degree of darkness on a radiographic image. Contrast is basically the difference between the densities of adjacent areas on an image. Several factors affect the density of an image, including the distance from the x-ray tube to the patient, patient tissue thickness, and the amount of radiation reaching the receptor. Density is controlled by mAs, developing techniques, kilovoltage, and film fog. Film fog will be discussed in Chapter 28.

Shadow Casting

One of the most important concepts in dental radiography is the concept of shadow casting. Shadow casting produces an image of the desired anatomical structures on the image receptor. The anatomical structure is between the radiation source (target of the tube in the machine head) and the image receptor. When the radiation passes through the structures and then contacts the image receptor, a shadow of the structure is cast onto the receptor. In order for the image to be useful, it must be of diagnostic quality. A diagnostic image has several qualities that are discussed in detail in this section. There are five principles of shadow casting that a proficient dental radiographer understands, takes into consideration, and applies when exposing radiographs.

Principle 1

Radiation should be emitted from the smallest source of radiation as possible. As electrons strike the tungsten target focal spot of the tungsten target, x-rays are emitted. The smaller the focal spot inside the x-ray tube, the greater the detail on the image (Figure 27-20A). A large focal spot results in a less sharp image with a **penumbra** (Figure 27-20B). As the electrons strike the focal spot, this area becomes extremely hot. As discussed earlier, approximately 99% of the energy generated by the electrons striking the focal spot of the tungsten target is produced as heat; only 1% of the energy produced by the electrons striking the tungsten target is produced as x-ray photons. To prevent damage to the x-ray generating apparatus, the focal spot cannot be kept as a pinpoint area and must be slightly larger. The slightly larger focal spot results in a minimal loss of sharpness caused by a penumbra around the edges of the image. Sharpness of an image is also affected by composition of traditional films and patient movement during exposure. These will be discussed later.

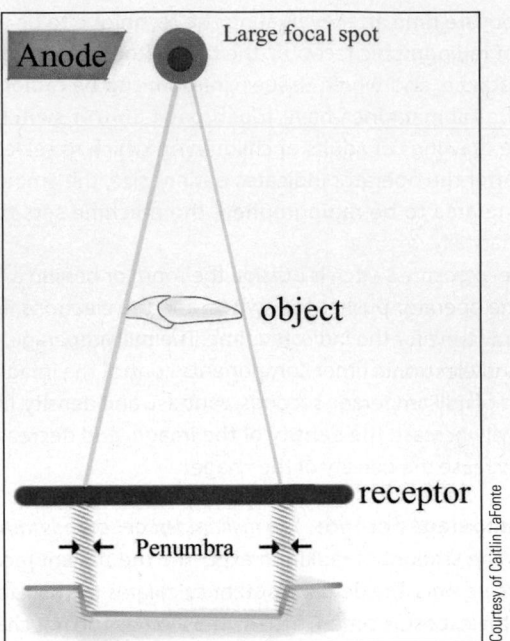

FIGURE 27-20B
Large focal spot and large penumbra.

Principle 2

The x-ray source-to-object distance should be as long as possible. The x-ray source-to-object distance refers to the distance between the focal spot and the receptor (Figure 27-21). The use of a long position indicating device (PID or cone) will enable the x-ray photons to emerge in a more parallel line, therefore producing an image that is similar in size and shape to the actual object.

Principle 3

The distance between the object and the image receptor should be as short as possible. The object in this principle refers to the tooth or structures being radiographed. Placing the object close to the receptor reduces magnification and increases image sharpness. The *bisecting angle technique* uses a short 8 inch PID (discussed in Chapter 28) and follows this principle more so than the *paralleling technique*, which uses a long 16 inch PID (discussed in Chapter 28). However, the bisecting angle technique is more prone to image distortion due to beam angulation errors and is not recommended as a primary technique. The increased object

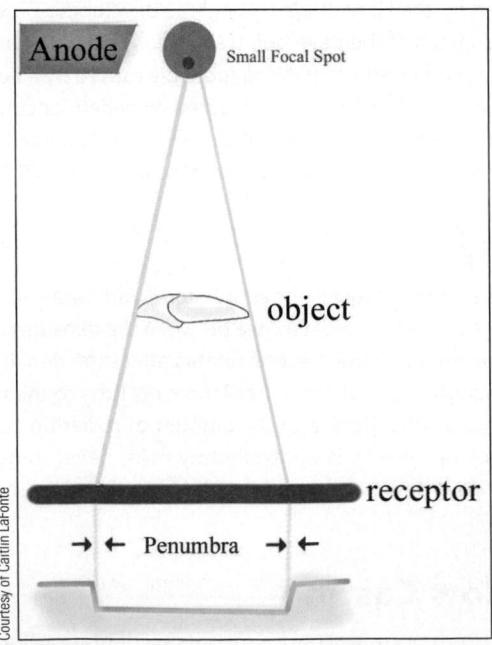

FIGURE 27-20A
Small focal spot and minimum penumbra.

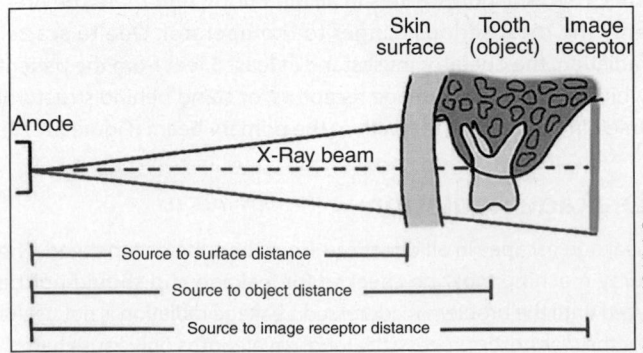

FIGURE 27-21
Distances in the paralleling technique.

to receptor distance of the paralleling technique results in magnification of the image. However, the parallel beams of the long 16 inch PID used in the paralleling technique negate this effect, resulting in an image that is more true in size and shape to the actual object than would result from the bisecting technique.

Principle 4

The receptor should be placed parallel to the long axis of the tooth. When the receptor and the long axis of the tooth are parallel (as in the paralleling technique), the distortion of the radiographed image is decreased.

Principle 5

The x-ray beam should be directed perpendicular to the image receptor and the tooth. The x-ray beam must be directed perpendicular to the long axis of the tooth. If the tooth and the image receptor are placed parallel to each other as in the paralleling technique, the x-ray beam is also perpendicular to the image receptor.

Entry of the x-ray at a 90 degree angle to the long axis of the tooth and the image receptor improves anatomic accuracy and reduces shape distortion or magnification. The central ray (CR) is the center of the x-ray beam and is often used to indicate the beam entry as well as centering the image.

Distance and the Inverse Square Rule

When the x-ray beam exits from the unleaded window in the x-ray generating apparatus, it enters the PID. The beam diverges to the size of the PID. As it exits the opening of the PID, it widens as it travels away from the opening. The beam also loses intensity as it travels away from the PID (Figure 27-22). The inverse square law explains how the distance at which the x-ray beam exits the PID affects the intensity of the beam. The inverse square law states that the intensity of radiation is inversely proportional to the square of the distance from the source of radiation. As the x-rays travel away from the source, they become less intense. Therefore, with an 8 inch PID (short PID), a beam that is four times more intense reaches the image receptor as compared to a 16 inch (long PID). This is because the x-rays have further to travel with a 16 inch PID. When the PID length goes from 8 inches to 16 inches, the beam is one fourth as intense. The formula used to calculate beam intensity is the inverse square law:

We will apply this concept to the paralleling technique discussed in detail in Chapter 28.

$$\frac{Original\ intensity}{Intensity\ 2} = \frac{New\ distance^2}{Original\ distance^2}$$

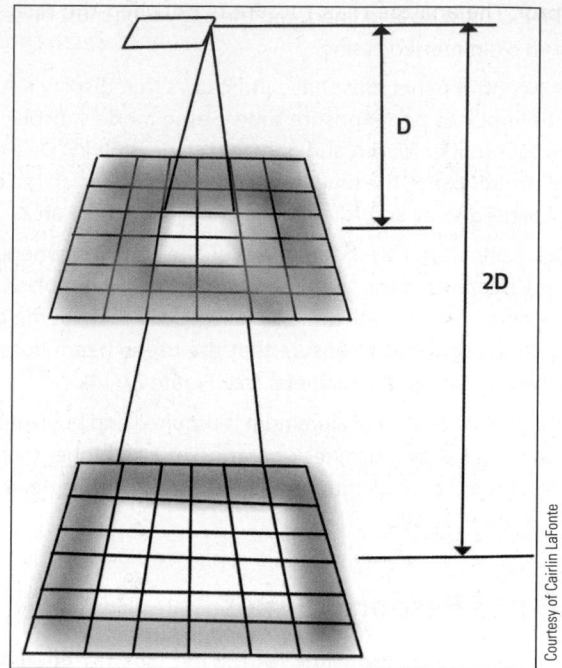

FIGURE 27-22
Inverse square law.

Courtesy of Caitlin LaFonte

Safety and Precautions

The Patient and Consumer Radiation Health and Safety Act was signed into law by President Ronald Reagan in August 1981. This act established what is known as the ALARA standards. ALARA is an acronym for As Low As Reasonably Achievable. The United States Nuclear Regulatory Commission states that ALARA "means making every reasonable effort to maintain exposures to ionizing radiation as far below the dose limits as practical." In simple terms ALARA refers to the use of the lowest amount of radiation needed to obtain a diagnostic image. All dental personnel use the ALARA concept for radiation protection before, during, and after exposure. Some ALARA concepts are discussed in this chapter, and other factors will be discussed in Chapter 28.

Manufacturer's Responsibilities

The federal government has set up safety specifications that all manufacturers of dental x-ray units must meet, as follows:

● The machine must have a separate control switch to cut off electricity to the machine. The exposure switch must have an electronic timer to stop the electricity automatically when the control switch is released. This "deadman" switch ensures that the exposure ends when the preset time has passed and not when the button is released.

- The PID must be lead lined, and the x-ray tube must be sealed in an oil-immersed casing.

- The control panel must have indicators that display mA, kV, and impulses per exposure time. Some models display the preset number for mA and only two choices for kV. On a digital control panel, the timer is preset, and changes on the digital panel display according to the chosen exposure area.

- The collimator, fitted directly over the opening where the x-ray beam exits the tubehead, is made of a lead plate. The opening, or hole, in the middle of the lead plate of the collimator is regulated to ensure that the useful beam does not exceed 2.75 inches in diameter (see Figure 27-14).

- Filtration of 2.5 mm of aluminum is required and built into the head of all x-ray machines operating at a kV higher than 70. Total filtration of 1.5 mm is required for x-ray units operating at or below 70 kVp.

Dentist's Responsibilities

- The dentist is responsible for having all x-ray equipment installed safely and maintaining it properly. Many states require that the machines be inspected and tested annually by a qualified technician. The office is required to follow the state regulations for x-ray generating machines. Records of maintenance and testing must be maintained in the office. Some states require that the test results be submitted to the state. The office design must provide occupants protection from radiation through the use of lead filtration. The location of the x-ray room and the protective lead barriers must meet specific requirements for safety, allowing at least 6 feet in the opposite direction of the primary ray.

- The dentist must prescribe radiographs for patients responsibly, remembering that only radiographs for a proper diagnosis are necessary. The dentist is responsible for adhering to the "Recommendations for Patient Selection and Limiting Radiographic Exposure." See the ADA website, *https://www.ada .org/~/media/ADA/Member%20Center/FIles/Dental _Radiographic_Examinations_2012.ashx*, to download the chart. These guidelines indicate that the dentist is responsible for ensuring treatment of each patient for her or his individual radiographic needs, thus avoiding overprescription of routine radiographs for every patient. The chart is a guide—it is important that radiographs should be prescribed based on the need of the patient.

- The protocol for suspected x-ray machine malfunction is to stop usage immediately when a problem is apparent. It is the dentist's responsibility to repair x-ray equipment and to ensure ongoing safety and compliance.

- The dentist is responsible for having dental assistants properly credentialed and trained for exposing and processing radiographs. The dentist is also responsible for supervising dental assistants in these tasks.

Dental Assistant's Responsibilities

- The dental assistant must be trained in aseptic techniques, radiation hygiene, and maintenance of quality assurance and safety.

- Dental assistants must obtain proper education in exposure and processing techniques. They must understand the physics and biological effects of ionizing radiation and use their knowledge during every radiographic exposure.

- The dental assistant must understand the ALARA principle and use a lead apron with a thyroid cervical collar for the patient's safety every time a radiographic image is obtained (Figure 27-23).

- Dental assistants must properly label and store patient radiographs to prevent loss.

- Dental assistants must be aware of their state regulations related to operation of a dental radiology unit.

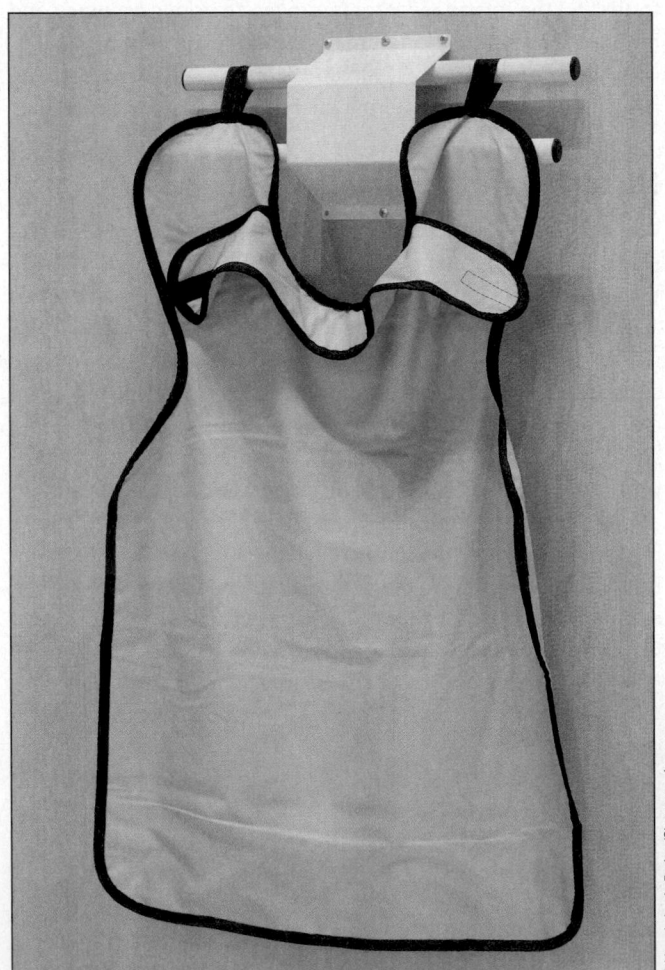

FIGURE 27-23
Lead apron with a thyroid collar.

© Vereshchagin Dmitry/Shutterstock.com

Patient's Responsibilities

The patient is responsible for notifying the office of any changes in health (pregnancy, for instance). Patients are also responsible for presenting, to the best of their abilities, radiation histories as part of their dental records.

Radiation Units of Measurement

The terminology for the measurement of radiation has changed. Several new terms are replacing older, more familiar ones. Table 27-2 provides the radiation units of measurements.

In 1937, the International Committee for Radiological Units established the official definition of radiation quantity. A *Roentgen (R)* equals the amount of radiation that ionizes one cubic centimeter of air. A *radiation absorbed dose (rad)* or *gray (GY)* is the amount of ionizing radiation absorbed in a substance. A *Roentgen equivalent man (rem)* or *sievert (Sv)* is the dose of radiation to which the body tissues are exposed, which is measured in terms of the estimated biological effects in relation to an exposure dose of one *R* of "x" or gamma radiation. A *milliroentgen (mr)* is one one-thousandth (1/1,000) of an *R*.

The *relative biological effectiveness (RBE)* is the measurement unit used to compare the biological effects on various tissues irradiated by different forms of energy. Dental x-rays have arbitrarily been assigned an RBE unit of one.

The rem is determined by multiplying the rad by the RBE. Therefore, 100 rads times one RBE equals 100 rems. The rad and the rem are considered equal for dental radiographs; a rad is an absorbed dose, not the amount coming from the machine or the rem.

Biological Effects of Radiation

X-rays can damage body tissues. Some of these injuries heal, but some do not. If the cell is affected by direct radiation, the cell may die immediately, change in structure and/or function, change at *mitosis*, or remain unaffected.

Somatic and Genetic Effects of Radiation

The cells in the body are divided into two groups: *somatic* and *genetic*. The somatic group includes all cells except the reproductive cells. The genetic group includes all the reproductive cells, such as the ova and the sperm. The biological effects of radiation

are classified according to the type of cell affected by the radiation, that is, somatic or genetic.

The somatic effects of radiation leave the individual in poor health and with cataracts, cancer, or leukemia. The effects are not passed to the next generation; the consequence of the radiation exposure remains with the primary individual. The *genetic effects*, in contrast, may not involve the primary individual exposed to the radiation. Genetic effects cannot be repaired and are passed to future generations.

Radiosensitive Cells Some cells are more *radiosensitive* than others. The more radiosensitive cells are immature cells, rapidly dividing cells, and cells that do not perform specialized functions. Examples of rapidly dividing cells are the *basal cells* of the skin. They are sloughed off and continuously replaced. Therefore, a person may develop skin cancer due to prolonged exposure to sunlight, a high dosage of radiation, or frequent radiation exposure.

Today, people are more informed about the effects of radiation. All patients must receive protection from x-ray radiation with the use of a *lead apron* with a thyroid collar during radiographic exposure (Figure 27-23).

Mature cells that rarely undergo cell divisions are *radioresistant*, or less sensitive to radiation. Examples of radioresistant cells are nerve and muscle cells. Table 27-3 shows the levels of sensitivity of different cells.

TABLE 27-3 Tissue and Organ Radiation Sensitivity

Most sensitive	Lymphoid Reproductive cells Bone marrow Intestinal epithelium Thyroid
Moderately sensitive	Skin Intestinal tract Oral mucosa
Sensitive	Connective tissue Growing bone
Less sensitive	Mature bone Salivary glands Liver
Least sensitive	Kidney Muscle Nerves

TABLE 27-2 Radiation Measurement Terms

Measurement Terms	Standard System (Traditional)	Metric Equivalent or Système Internationale (SI)
Exposure (C/kg)	Roentgen (R) 3.88 × 10 R =	Coulomb per kilogram 1 C/kg
Dose	Radiation absorbed dose (RAD) 100 rads =	Gray (GY) 1 GY
Dose equivalent	Radiation equivalent man (REM) 100 rems =	Sievert (Sv) 1 Sv

Low-level radiation normally does not cause damage that cannot be repaired within cells. Tissues that are radiosensitive in the dental region are the lens of the eye and the thyroid gland. Because of their location near the oral cavity, these tissues may be exposed to the primary beam (central ray) of the x-ray. Very high radiation dosages (not used in dentistry) have been known to cause cataracts in the eye and thyroid carcinoma. It is unlikely that dental x-rays cause one of these serious effects, but it is always necessary to use the least amount of radiation possible. Dental offices use a thyroid shield extension on the lead apron to further protect patients.

Occupational Exposure

Individuals who routinely use ionizing radiation in their occupations are regulated by dose limitations defined by the National Council on Radiation Protection and Measurements. The *maximum permissible dose (MPD)* is the maximum dose of radiation that, in light of present knowledge, would not be expected to produce any significant radiation effects in a lifetime. The MPD calls for the dose limit of occupational exposure to be at 0.05 Sv (5.0 rems) per year or 100 mrem per week for radiation workers. Nonoccupational exposure and pregnant workers are regulated at one-tenth this limit. Most resources recognize the 0.05 Sv per year maximum; however, recommendations by the International Commission on Radiological Protection call for the occupational exposure dose limits to be 20 mSv (2.0 rems).

Daily Radiation Exposure The general population is exposed to two major categories of radiation daily: natural and artificial. Annually, a person encounters an average of 6.2 mSv (620 mrems) of radiation from all sources. Natural sources make up a large percent of radiation exposure. Radiation comes from the earth (radon, for instance), the sun, and the atmosphere. The rest of radiation exposure comes from artificial radiation, such as x-rays used for diagnosis, as well as from consumer products, such as television, airline travel, tobacco, and smoke alarms.

Accumulation of Radiation The effects of radiation are cumulative, meaning that the effects of exposure increase every time the individual is exposed to radiation. This is often called the long-term effect.

The normal aging process tends to accelerate due to radiation accumulation. Most adults know that the skin of individuals who have (or had) high exposure to the sun ages at an increased rate—the higher the doses, the more rapid the effects. This period between direct exposure and the development of biological effects (or symptoms) is called the latent period.

The response to radiation is believed to be a nonlinear, nonthreshold dose response curve (Figure 27-24). This curve basically states that there is no safe dose for radiation exposure. However, at low doses, the body is able to repair itself. As the dose

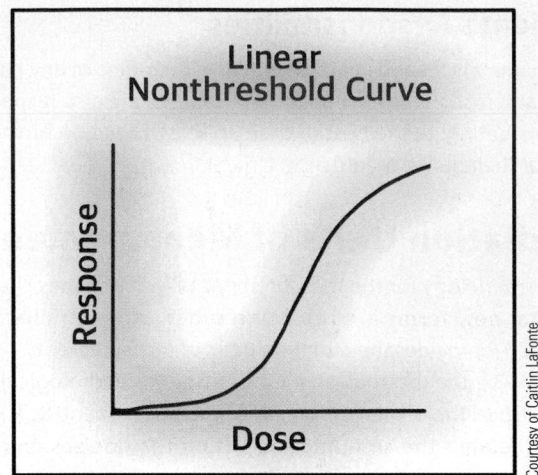

FIGURE 27-24
Nonlinear nonthreshold curve.

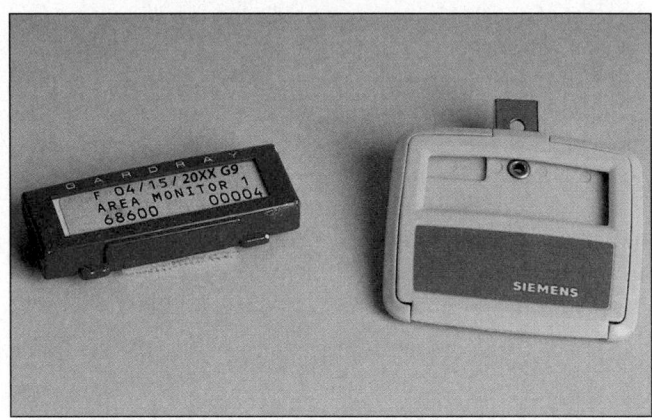

FIGURE 27-25
Dosimetry badges for radiation monitoring.

increases, the response (damage) significantly increases, and the body may not be able to repair the damage.

Any dental assistant producing radiographs should wear a *radiation monitoring device* or *dosimeter* badge (Figure 27-25) at the waist or neck level outside of the clothing at all times while in the dental office. This badge monitors an individual's radiation exposure and accumulated dosage in the office. It is important that the badge is not to be worn outside of the office, because it will produce an inaccurate reading. The badges are normally read monthly; and each employee should be apprised of the outcome immediately. Corrective measures should be taken if needed.

A quality assurance (QA) program should be developed for the exposure, production, and processing of radiographs in the dental office. Quality assurance will be discussed in Chapter 29.

Intraoral Dental Film

Intraoral dental film is film placed inside the oral cavity. Intraoral films are used to obtain *periapical images* (Figure 27-17), *bitewing images* (Figure 27-16), and *occlusal images*. These image types will be specifically discussed in the paralleling and bisecting technique lessons of this section.

Composition of Dental Film

It is important to understand the qualities of intraoral film. A sound understanding of the quality and characteristics of the film will allow the dental assistant to maintain high-quality radiographs. The film used in dental radiography is composed of a flexible, thin, polyester plastic base that is about 0.2 mm thick (Figure 27-26). This semiclear base (cellulose acetate) has a slightly bluish tint to enhance the quality of the image. It permits easy handling during the processing and makes viewing the image easier. The base is coated on each side with an adhesive. The adhesive ensures that the *emulsion* is distributed uniformly over the base. The emulsion is placed on both sides of the base to reduce the amount of radiation needed. The emulsion is made of a homogeneous mixture of silver halide crystals suspended in a gelatin. Halides are halogen compounds, such as chlorine, bromine, and iodine, that combine with another element, such as silver. In dental films, silver is combined most frequently with bromine. During radiation exposure, the silver halide crystals store the energy to which they have been exposed, and react with the chemicals in the processing tank to form a black or *radiolucent* region on the film. The silver halide crystals that have not been struck by the radiation are not energized. These appear as white or *radiopaque* areas on the image. The unenergized crystals are removed from the film during processing.

The radiopaque and radiolucent areas are created based on the structures that the beam goes through before it strikes the film. Structures such as compact bone, enamel, and dentin are dense and do not allow the beam to go through. In these areas

on the film, the crystals do not receive the energy from the x-ray photons, and those areas appear radiopaque. Soft tissue like the dental pulp, gingival tissue, periodontal ligament, and lips and muscles do not block radiation. The x-ray photons strike the silver halide crystals on the film in these areas and energize the crystals. As a result, these structures appear dark or radiolucent on the radiograph. When dental decay is present, the tooth has lost its mineralization in the area of the decay. Tissues that are slightly less dense, such as cancellous bone, dentin, and cementum, will appear in varying shades of gray but are still considered to be radiopaque structures. Dental materials such as amalgam, gold, porcelain, cements, and some resins appear radiopaque. These materials are discussed in later chapters. Refer to Figure 27-27 for the appearance of structures and material on a radiograph.

This energy is stored in the silver halide crystals as a *latent image* that does not become visible until the film has been exposed to chemicals for a given time at a given temperature. If a film has been exposed to visible light, it appears black after the processing. If the film was not exposed to light or radiation, the film appears clear after processing. The emulsion washes off and appears as a semiclear blue base. On top of the emulsion is a protective coating that is used to protect the emulsion, especially from the rollers in an automatic processor. Film processing and the chemicals used in processing will be discussed in detail in Chapter 28.

It should be noted that the film base has a small raised dot on one corner of the film. This dot is used for identification and mounting of the dental radiographs after processing. Mounting of films will be discussed in Chapter 28.

Dental Film Speed

Film speed is defined as the amount of radiation to expose a film of diagnostic quality. The size of the silver halide crystals in the emulsion regulates the speed of the film; normally, the larger the crystals, the faster the film. Larger crystals result in a less sharp image; however, the diminished sharpness is minimal when compared to smaller crystals in slower speed film. The

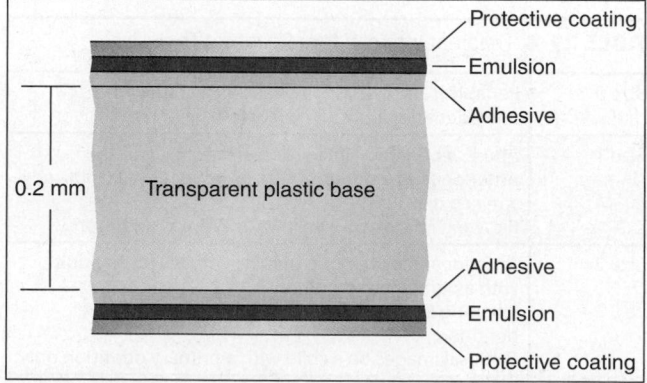

FIGURE 27-26
Composition of dental x-ray film. Transparent plastic base.

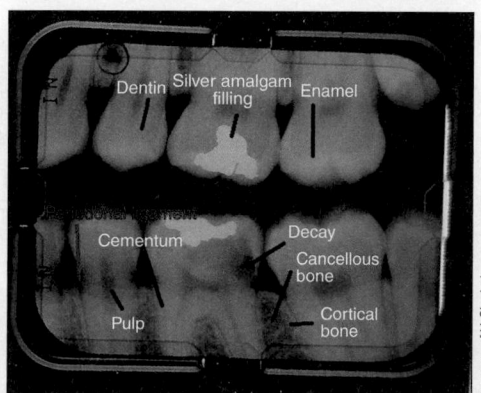

FIGURE 27-27
Appearance of anatomical structures and silver amalgam on a radiograph.

reduction in radiation in fast speed film with larger crystals is significantly less than with slow speed film and smaller crystals. Dentists typically use one of the three dental radiographic films: D-speed film, called Ultraspeed; E-speed film, called Ektaspeed; or F-speed film, called InSight (Figure 27-28). Ektaspeed film requires approximately 40% less exposure time than Ultraspeed; and InSight requires 60% less exposure time than D-speed film and 20% less exposure time than E-speed film. InSight/F-speed film is the highest-speed dental film, allowing for the greatest reduction in radiation exposure for the patient. The American National Standards Institute (ANSI) is the organization that classifies dental radiographic film. The current classifications are the letters A–F.

● Kodak InSight dental film is an F-speed film, developed in 2000, that reduces radiation exposure up to 20% compared to Kodak Ektaspeed Plus intraoral dental film, and up to 60% compared to D speed films.

● A patient having an 18-film series (full mouth) using a long, round PID without a lead apron results in a genetic exposure of 0.5 mrad; with a lead apron, the genetic exposure is approximately 0.01 mrad. If a thyroid collar is used, a 50% reduction is noted in the thyroid area.

● A patient having an 18-film series using a rectangular PID, instead of a round PID, reduces the radiation exposure to the patient by approximately 60% as compared to exposure with a round PID.

● The *best* way to reduce a patient's radiation exposure is to use F-speed film and rectangular collimation. Many manufacturers offer rectangular cone attachments for the dental PID.

● The National Council on Radiation Protection and Measurements (NCRP) makes recommendations on radiation protection and measurements, and disseminates information and guidance. In a report titled "Radiation Protection in Dentistry" (Report 145), the Council stated that a lead apron is not necessary if a dental office is using F-speed film and rectangular collimation. Staying current on changes and recommendations via the ADA and NCRP is critical for a dental team using ionizing radiation. The NCRP works with the Centers for Disease Control and Prevention.

Dental Film Sizes

Dental intraoral film packets come in five basic sizes (Figure 27-29). Each size is used for a specific radiographic exposure, depending on the size of the patient's oral cavity and the area to be radiographed (Table 27-4). The film is selected to produce the best radiographic results with the least radiation exposure for the patient.

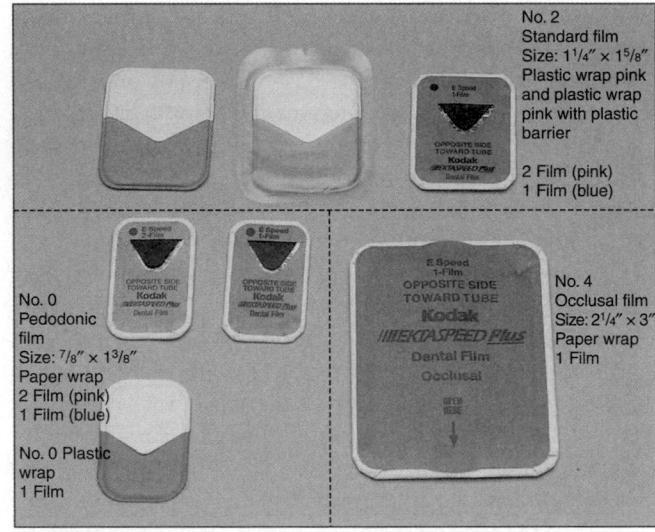

FIGURE 27-29
Sample dental x-ray films showing sizes and numbers. (Size No. 1, narrow anterior film size, and Size No. 3, long bitewing film size, are not shown.)

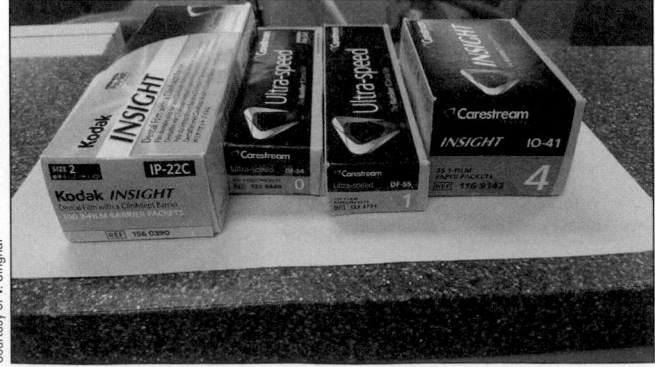

FIGURE 27-28
Kodak Ultraspeed and Kodak Insight film boxes.

TABLE 27-4 Different Intraoral Film Sizes and Their Uses

Size 0	Periapical and bitewing images on a child with a primary dentition only
Size 1	Anterior periapical images on an adult Anterior and posterior periapical images on a child with a mixed dentition Bitewing images on a child with a mixed dentition
Size 2	Anterior and posterior periapical images on an adult with a permanent dentition Bitewing images on an adult with a permanent dentition Occlusal images on a child with a primary dentition only
Size 3	Bitewing images on an adult (1 on each side)
Size 4	Adult occlusal images

Dental Film Packet

Dental film is available in dental film packets that are designed to protect it from moisture and light. The intraoral film comes in boxes of 50 to 150 film packets. The boxes are labeled with the type of film, quantity of film packets, film speed, number of films in each film packet, expiration date, and if packets have barriers. Some film packets have two films inside. During exposure, both films will obtain the same image so a duplicate film is available. This is beneficial in the event the patient needs a copy

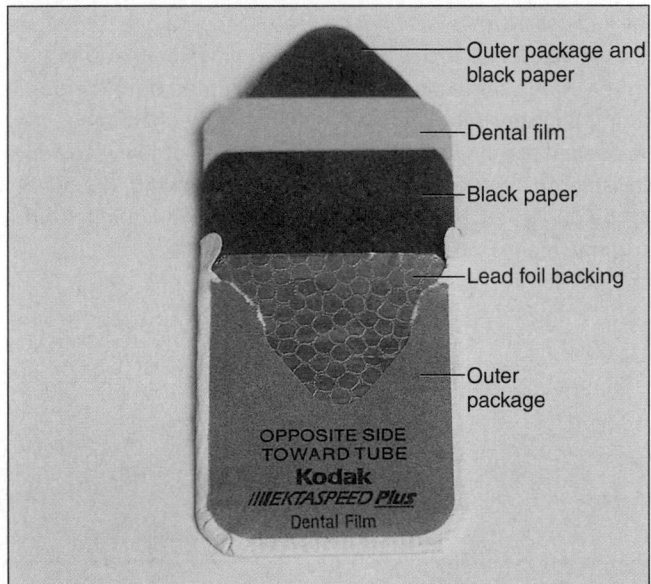

FIGURE 27-30A
Parts of a dental film packet.

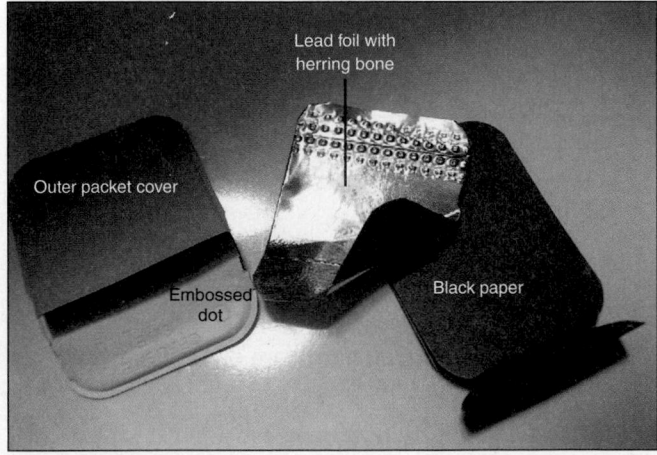

FIGURE 27-30B
Components of a film packet.

of the image or if a film has to be sent to the patient's insurance company. Barriers are an advantage for infection control purposes. Infection control specific to radiology will be discussed in Chapter 28.

The intraoral film packet has a sealed outer paper or plastic wrap. Some packets come with plastic barriers, which are beneficial in infection control. Inside the wrapper, black paper is folded around the film, and a lead foil backing is placed on the backside of the film or the side of the film that will be placed away from the x-ray tube (Figures 27-30A and 27-30B). The lead foil has a herringbone pattern on it and absorbs any unused radiation and the scattering of secondary radiation, and helps prevent film fogging. If the film is placed in the oral cavity with the lead foil toward the PID, the herringbone pattern will be visible on the image and the image will be lack density. The outer plastic, or paper wrap, is completely sealed to prevent moisture from getting to the film. The outside film package shows where the identification dot is located. The dot is convex on the white side of the film package. If the embossed dot on the film packet is placed at the apex of the roots of the teeth and is not located at the incisal or occlusal surfaces during exposure, the dot may affect the diagnostic quality of the radiograph. If the dot is at the apical area of the processed film, the dot can obscure the apical area on the image and make it difficult to view for diagnosis of diseases. Package color and numbering may differ from one manufacturer to another.

Dental Film Storage

Before use, dental radiographic film should be stored carefully. It is sensitive to stray radiation, high temperatures, and chemicals. Dental film should not be stored in the areas where patient exposures are completed or in the dark room where the processing chemicals may affect the films. Ideally, unexposed film should be stored at 10°C to 20°C (50°F to 70°F) with relative humidity levels that range from 30 to 50%. Follow manufacturer's directions for film storage and care. Many dental offices store the film in the refrigerator. The dental assistant should pay careful attention to the expiration date on the boxes of film. Placing the boxes of film in the storage area so that the oldest film is used first to prevent any film from expiring. Using expired film for a patient's radiographs may inhibit diagnostic quality.

After the film has been exposed and processed, it should be mounted and placed in a protective envelope. All radiographs should be handled with care so that the integrity of the radiograph is not compromised, and they are not scratched. Radiographs are records of the patient's conditions at that time and may be used as legal documents. Processing and mounting and storing of films will be discussed in Chapter 28.

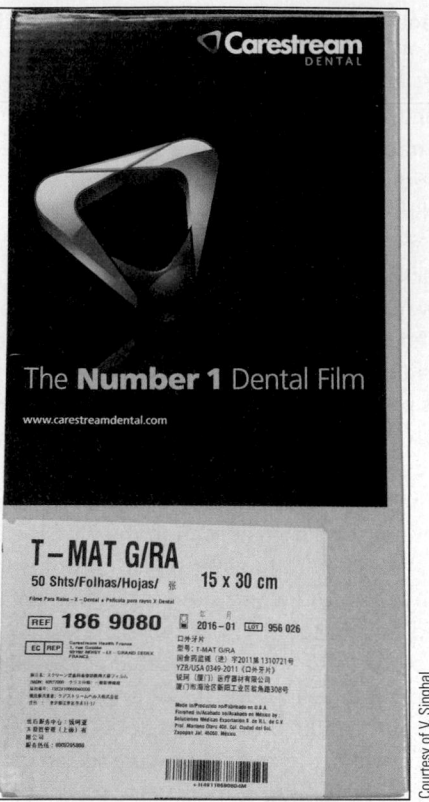

Courtesy of V. Singhal

FIGURE 27-31
Duplicating film.

Traditional Extraoral Film and Duplicating Film

When exposing the extraoral film, the film is placed outside of the patient's oral cavity. The film size is larger than the largest intraoral film and is held in a cassette during exposure. There are a variety of extraoral film sizes and patient exposure positions to expose specific areas of the maxilla, mandible, and head. Extraoral techniques will be discussed in Chapter 29.

Duplicating film is designed to make a copy of an existing patient image on traditional film (Figure 27-31). Duplicating film looks exactly like regular radiographic film but does not capture the x-ray beam; thus it cannot be used to expose patient images. It must be used in a special duplicating machine that transmits light through the radiograph you wish copied onto the duplicating film thus producing an image. A copy of an image may be needed to send to the patient's insurance company, to a specialist, or to another office if the patient is moving. The quality of the duplicated images is as important as the quality of the original images. Steps in film duplication will be discussed in Chapter 28.

Chapter Summary

This chapter examines the discovery of x-rays. It is important for dental assistants to understand the physics and biological effects of ionization radiation, use their understanding of the principles of shadowcasting during every radiographic exposure, understand the ALARA principle, and use the lead apron with cervical collar for the patient's safety every time a radiograph is obtained. The dental assistant should understand the role of dental film in radiation exposure. The assistant must label and store patient radiographs properly to prevent loss and avoid the need for radiographs to be retaken.

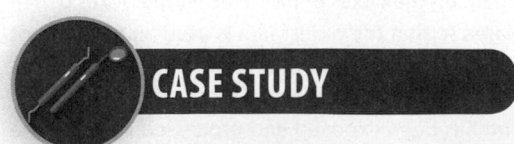

CASE STUDY

You are preparing to take radiographs on a patient using traditional film. You are aware of ALARA and want to do everything possible to reduce radiation exposure to you and your patient.

Case Study Review

1. What is one way you can reduce radiation exposure to your patient prior to obtaining images?

2. What is one way you can reduce radiation exposure to your patient during exposure?

3. What is one way you can reduce radiation exposure to your patient after exposure?

4. What is one way that you as the operator can ensure you do not receive unnecessary radiation?

Review Questions

Multiple Choice

1. Dental radiographs can aid in the diagnosis of disease such as dental decay. Dental radiographs are not considered to be an important part of the patient's treatment.
   Select the correct response based on the statement above.
   a. Both statements are true.
   b. Both statements are false.
   c. The first statement is true, the second statement is false.
   d. The first statement is false, the second statement is true.

2. William Conrad Roengten discovered the x-ray. William Conrad Roentgen was awarded the Nobel Prize for Physics for his discovery of x-radiation as well as the characteristics of x-radiation.
   Select the correct response based on the statement above.
   a. Both statements are true.
   b. Both statements are false.
   c. The first statement is true, the second statement is false.
   d. The first statement is false, the second statement is true.

3. Which of the following is not correct regarding radiation?
   a. Radiation is the release of energy.
   b. Radiation has the form of waves.
   c. Radiation has the form of particles.
   d. Radiation does not have the ability to penetrate structures.

4. Electromagnetic energy has the characteristics of waves and particles. Electromagnetic energy travels through space in waves.
   Select the correct response based on the statement above.
   a. Both statements are true.
   b. Both statements are false.
   c. The first statement is true, the second statement is false.
   d. The first statement is false, the second statement is true.

5. X-rays with low energy are desirable for radiographic exposures as they have the high penetrating power. X-rays with high energy are not desirable for radiographic exposures as they have the low penetrating power.
   Select the correct response based on the statement above.
   a. Both statements are true.
   b. Both statements are false.
   c. The first statement is true, the second statement is false.
   d. The first statement is false, the second statement is true.

6. An x-ray photon may dislodge an inner shell proton resulting in ionization. Ionization results in a positively charged ion, which can react with other atoms.
   Select the correct response based on the statement above.
   a. Both statements are true.
   b. Both statements are false.
   c. The first statement is true, the second statement is false.
   d. The first statement is false, the second statement is true.

7. Which of the following is correct regarding the Indirect Theory of Injury?
   a. In the Indirect Theory of Injury, the DNA of a cell is injured by an x-ray photon.
   b. In the Indirect Theory of Injury, ionization does not occur.

c. In the Indirect Theory of Injury, hydrogen peroxide may form resulting in toxicity to the cell.
   d. All of these are correct.

8. Which of the following components of the x-ray machine focuses the electrons toward the anode?
   a. focusing cup
   b. tungsten filament
   c. step-up transformer
   d. copper stem

9. Which of the following is correct regarding the milliamperage (mA) setting of the standard dental x-ray machine?
   a. Most standard dental x-ray machines operate at 20 mA.
   b. The mA setting controls the quantity of electrons produced.
   c. An increase in mA results in a denser image.
   d. An increase in mA results in a lighter image.

10. Which of the following is not correct regarding the timer on the standard dental x-ray machine?
    a. The timer controls the duration of time the x-rays flow from the x-ray tube.
    b. The time is measured in impulses; there are 60 impulses per second.
    c. An increase in time will result in a lighter image.
    d. All of these are correct.

11. Which of the following is correct regarding density of a dental radiographic image?
    a. Density is controlled by the milliamperage (mA) setting.
    b. Density is the differences in adjacent gray areas on a radiographic image.
    c. The kilovoltage (kVp) setting does not impact density.
    d. Developing techniques do not impact density of a radiographic image.

12. Principle 1 of shadow casting states that radiation should be emitted from the smallest possible radiation source. A small radiation source results in a larger penumbra on the image.
    Select the correct response based on the statement above.
    a. Both statements are true.
    b. Both statements are false.
    c. The first statement is true, the second statement is false.
    d. The first statement is false, the second statement is true.

13. Which of the following is correct regarding the inverse square rule?
    a. The x-ray beam converges as it exits the position-indicating device (PID).
    b. The x-ray beam becomes more intense as the distance it travels increases.
    c. With an 8 inch PID, the beam is four times as intense at the receptor as compared to a 16 inch PID.
    d. All of these are correct.

14. Which of the following is not correct regarding the cellular effects of radiation?
    a. Genetic cells are those involved in reproduction.
    b. The effect of radiation on somatic cells results in poor health.
    c. Damage to somatic cells may be passed on to the next generation.
    d. Genetic damage from radiation can be repaired by the body.

15. The MPD calls for the dose limit of occupational exposure to be at 0.05 Sv or 5.0 rems per year for radiation workers. Non-occupational exposure and pregnant workers are regulated at 0.005 Sv or 0.5 rem per year.
    Select the correct response based on the statement above.
    a. Both statements are true.
    b. Both statements are false.
    c. The first statement is true, the second statement is false.
    d. The first statement is false, the second statement is true.

16. Which of the following is not correct regarding accumulation of radiation?
    a. The latent period is the period of time between injury and the appearance of symptoms.
    b. The effects of radiation are accumulative over time.
    c. The lower the radiation dose, the higher the effect.
    d. The body is able to repair itself after exposure to lower doses of radiation.

17. Which of the following images are not obtained from the use of intraoral film?
    a. periapical
    b. bitewing
    c. occlusal
    d. panoramic

18. Which of the following is not correct regarding film speed?
    a. Smaller crystals mean faster film.
    b. Smaller crystals result in a less sharp image.
    c. Slow speed film results in reduced radiation as compared to fast speed film.
    d. F-speed film is the fastest traditional dental film.

19. Extraoral film is used for exposures outside of the oral cavity. Extraoral film sizes are larger than the largest intraoral film.
    Select the correct response based on the statement above.
    a. Both statements are true.
    b. Both statements are false.
    c. The first statement is true, the second statement is false.
    d. The first statement is false, the second statement is true.

20. Duplicating film can be used to capture intraoral and extraoral patient images. Films may be duplicated to send to the patient's insurance company or to another practitioner.
    Select the correct response based on the statement above.
    a. Both statements are true.
    b. Both statements are false.
    c. The first statement is true, the second statement is false.
    d. The first statement is false, the second statement is true.

Critical Thinking

1. What are the steps in the production of x-rays?
2. What are the responsibilities of the dental assistant in relation to ALARA?

Key Terms

Term and Pronunciation	Meaning of Root and Word Parts	Definition
dental film (**den**-tl) (film)	**dent-** = teeth **-al** = pertaining to **film** = x-ray sensitive material used in taking radiographs	thin sheet of acetate specially treated for use in radiography; must be chemically processed in darkroom to produce image
digital sensor (**dij**-i-tl) (**sen**-sawr)	**digit** = number; displaying image as numbers **-al** = pertaining to **sensor** = device sensitive to radiation	replaces film with an electronic sensor; viewed on computer without needed for darkroom processing
latent (**leyt**-nt)	**late** = after delay **-ent** = causing an action	not yet revealed or manifest; present itself later
penumbra (pi-**nuhm**-br*uh*)	**penumbra** = a shadowy, marginal area	something that surrounds and obscures the shadow of an opaque object
photon (**foh**-ton)	**photo-** = light **-on** = used in names of subatomic particles	a particle representing light or other electromagnetic radiation

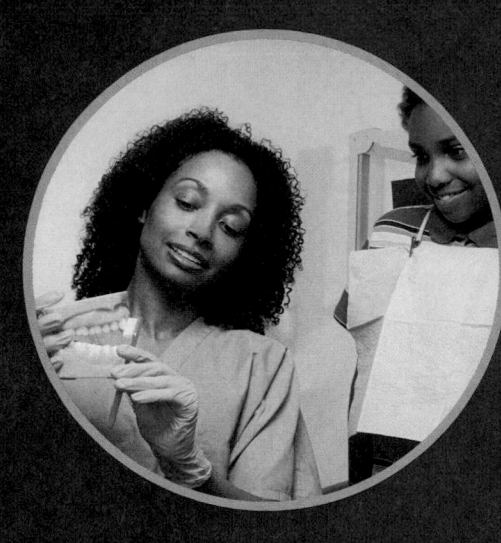

Dental Radiology Infection Control, Exposure, Processing and Evaluation of Dental Radiographs, and Mounting of Dental Radiographs

Specific Instructional Objectives

At the completion of this chapter, you will be able to meet these objectives:

1. Use terms presented in this chapter.
2. Discuss the infection control protocol related to dental radiography.
3. Compare and contrast the sequence of exposures in the bisecting technique and the paralleling technique.
4. Compare and contrast patient position during the bisecting technique and the paralleling technique.
5. Compare and contrast the image receptor holders in the bisecting technique and the paralleling technique.
6. Discuss image receptor placement for bitewing images.
7. Discuss image receptor placement for periapical images.
8. Discuss the importance of angulation during intraoral exposures.
9. State the cause of a conecut image.
10. Explain the errors caused by image receptor placement.
11. Differentiate between elongation and foreshortening.
12. Discuss interproximal overlap.
13. Describe the errors that may be caused during exposure.
14. State the purpose of occlusal images.
15. State the procedure for exposing adult occlusal images.
16. Discuss image receptor placement during modified exposure techniques.
17. List the steps in exposing a pediatric full set of images.
18. Explain the protocol for management of patients with special needs.
19. Discuss the protocol for maintaining radiographic records.
20. Compare and contrast the developer and fixer solutions.

21. Compare and contrast the manual processing technique and the autoprocessing technique.
22. Describe the components of the darkroom.
23. Describe the manual processing tank.
24. Explain the importance of checking the temperature of the manual processing solutions.
25. Outline the steps in the manual processing technique.
26. Outline the steps in the automatic processing technique.
27. Compare and contrast solutions for automatic processors and manual processors.
28. Discuss the maintenance of processing equipment.
29. Identify film processing errors.
30. Outline the steps in mounting traditional films.
31. Compare and contrast the lingual mounting view and the labial mounting view.
32. State the sequence of viewing mounted radiographs in a full mouth series.
33. Outline the steps in film duplication.

Introduction

Taking a quality radiograph is a skill that takes practice and patience. The dental assistant will take many different radiographic images on patients of all ages. These images must be of the quality the dentist needs to provide an accurate diagnosis. The techniques for exposing periapical and bitewing images are discussed and demonstrated in this chapter. The occlusal technique is also discussed in this chapter. It is important for the dental assistant to know how to expose images on special needs patients. This chapter also reviews infection control in dental radiology before, during, and after exposure. Once the radiographs are exposed, the dental assistant needs to understand how they are processed and mounted. Common radiographic exposure and processing errors are identified and discussed so that the dental assistant can use the correct techniques to prevent these errors in the future. This chapter also discusses how and why radiographs are duplicated, and that radiographs are part of the patient's permanent record and must be properly stored and maintained.

Infection Control in Dental Radiographic Procedures

Maintaining infection control is an important component in dentistry and the dental radiographic exposure procedure. Infection control and the chain of transmission were discussed in detail in Chapter 11. This chapter will discuss the aspects of infection control maintenance as well as the rationale for infection control during radiographic exposure.

There are several ways that disease can be transmitted from the patient to the dental professional, from the dental professional to the patient, or from one patient to another patient. The student should review the modes of transmission covered in Chapter 11. There are many factors involved in maintaining infection control during dental radiographic procedures. Some instruments used in radiographic exposures may require sterilization. Equipment that cannot be sterilized must be disinfected.

Barrier versus Disinfection versus Sterilization

The student should refer to Chapter 11 regarding personal protective equipment (PPE), barriers, disinfection, and sterilization. Cross contamination can occur in many ways while exposing dental radiographs. For example, when the image receptor (traditional film or a digital sensor) is placed in the oral cavity and is then placed on the work surface that is not appropriately covered, the surface may become contaminated. Another instance is when the operator presses the exposure button or moves the machine head in order to place it for exposure while wearing gloves that were just in the patient's oral cavity. If these areas are not appropriately covered, they may become contaminated. If using a digital system, there is a risk of contamination of the digital sensor, the computer screen, the computer mouse, and the computer keyboard. Since the exposure button, the machine head/position-indicating device (PID), computer keyboard, mouse, and sensor cannot be autoclaved,

CHAPTER 28 Dental Radiology Infection Control, Exposure, Processing and Evaluation of
Dental Radiographs, and Mounting of Dental Radiographs

845

these noncritical instruments must be either disinfected or covered with a barrier (Figures 28-1A, B, C, and D). Additional surfaces that can be potentially contaminated are the dental chair and the lead apron. Care must be taken not to cross contaminate other surfaces, including other patients or even yourself.

When using a disinfectant on surfaces, care should be exercised regarding the electrical switches of the x-ray machine or the light switch and light handle and machine head. The assistant should spray the disinfectant on a paper towel and use the paper towel to wipe these areas (Figure 28-2). Many offices choose to use the barrier technique and cover the x-ray unit instead of exposing the electronic unit to moisture from wet disinfectants (Figure 28-1B). If using a digital sensor, it should also be covered with a special plastic sheath to prevent contamination as the sensor cannot be autoclaved (Figure 28-3). The manufacturer's instructions should be followed for disinfection of the sensor.

Some other items that are used while exposing radiographs can undergo sterilization. Image receptor holders and other instruments such as a mouth mirror used in the oral cavity are considered semicritical instruments and must be properly sterilized between patients. These include the holders for the image receptors such as XCP kits. These will be discussed in detail later in this chapter. Critical instruments are not

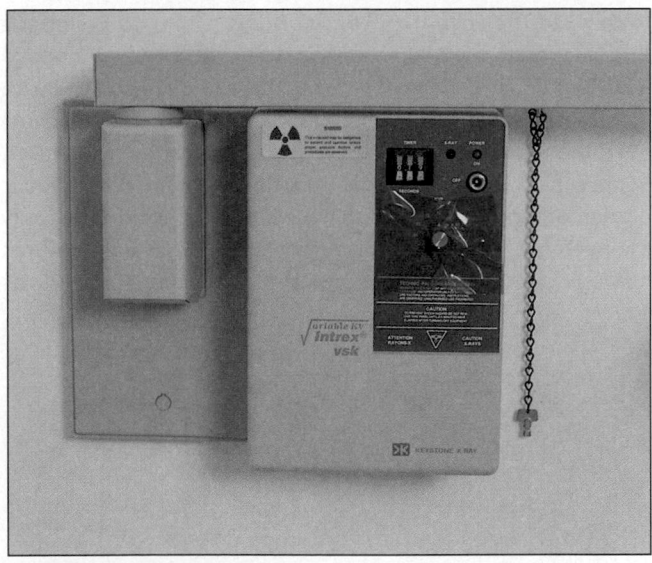

FIGURE 28-1A
Control panel.

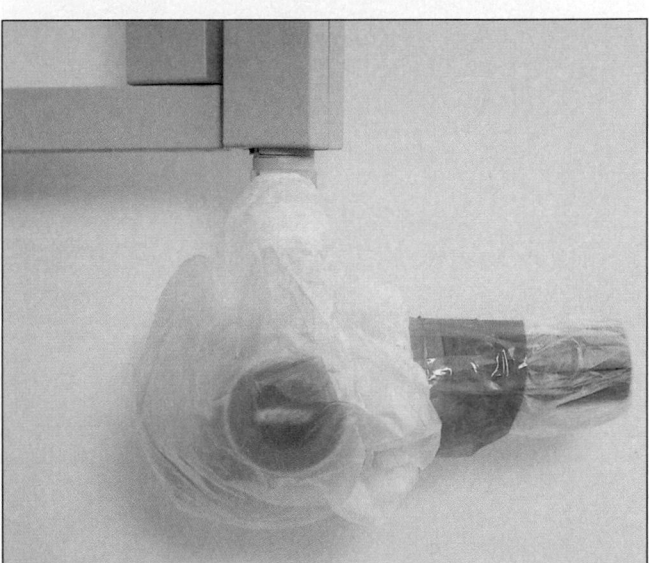

FIGURE 28-1B
Tubehead with barriers.

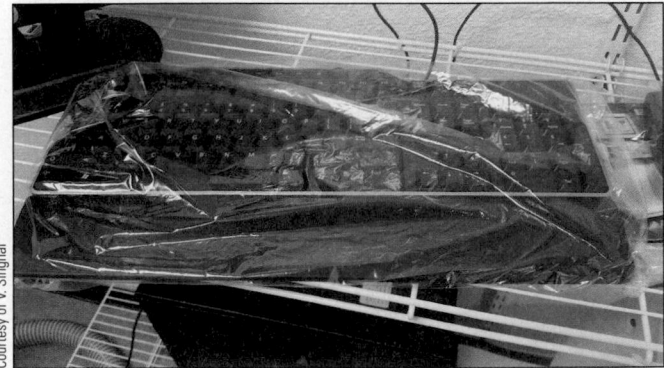

Courtesy of V. Singhal

FIGURE 28-1C
Computer keyboard for digital imaging covered with plastic barrier.

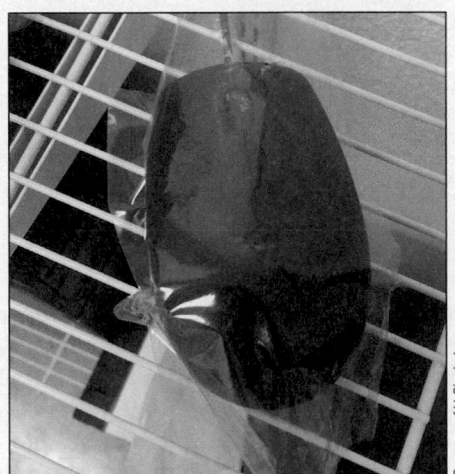

Courtesy of V. Singhal

FIGURE 28-1D
Computer mouse covered with barrier.

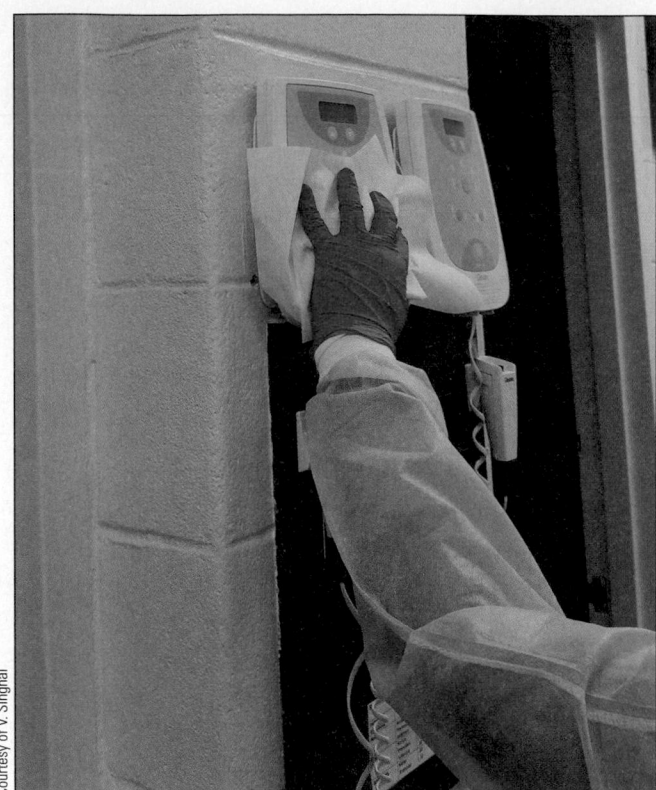

FIGURE 28-2
Using a paper towel sprayed with disinfectant to wipe radiology machine control panel.

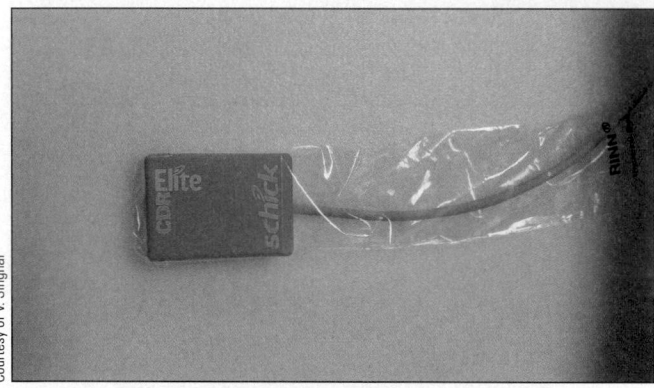

FIGURE 28-3
Digital sensor with barrier cover.

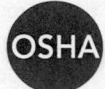

Infection Control before Exposure The exposure area and equipment need to be prepared before exposing radiographs to prevent cross contamination.

Exposure Area Preparation The use of gloves while handling contaminated image receptors is required. Be sure to follow the infection control protocol for handwashing and donning and doffing of PPE outlined in Chapter 11. While wearing utility gloves, wipe all surfaces with a disinfectant including the countertop workspace, dental chair, dental light, and lead apron. Disinfection of surfaces is outlined in Chapter 11.

The operator should be sure to cover the control panel including the exposure button to protect it from contamination (Figure 28-1A). You will be touching this every time you need to expose the receptor. Some offices prefer to cover the tubehead with a plastic barrier; other offices may choose to wipe it after use with a paper towel that has been sprayed with a disinfectant (Figure 28-1B). You will be touching the machine head many times while completing radiographic exposures. Some offices may opt to cover the dental chair with a plastic barrier; others may choose to wipe it after use and cover only the headrest with a plastic barrier (Figure 28-4). Some offices may opt to cover the lead apron with a plastic barrier once it has

usually used in dental radiologic procedures. Proper disinfection of the work area must be completed before and after each patient. Noncritical equipment that may be touched during the procedure should be properly disinfected or covered with barriers. These include surfaces that may become contaminated and the machine head. Infection control is an important responsibility of the dental assistant before, during, and after exposure.

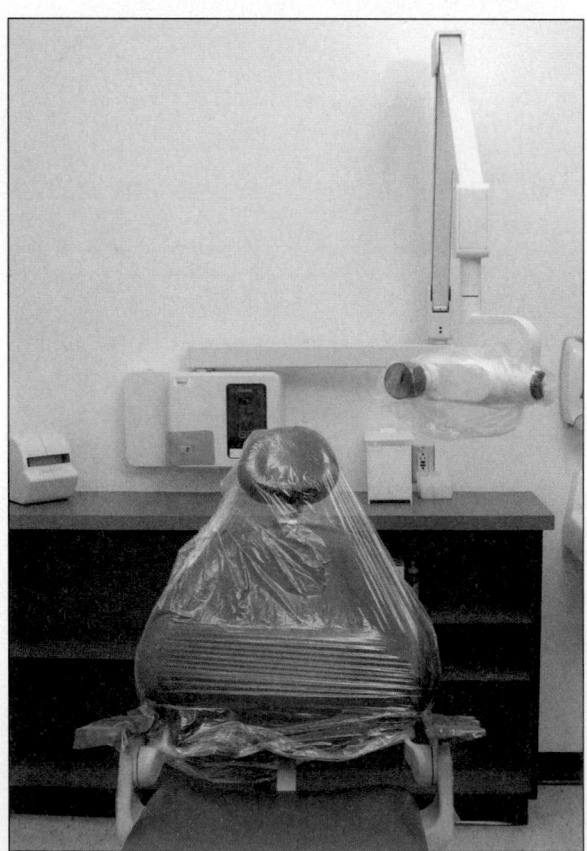

FIGURE 28-4
Barrier on exposure area chair.

CHAPTER 28 Dental Radiology Infection Control, Exposure, Processing and Evaluation of Dental Radiographs, and Mounting of Dental Radiographs

847

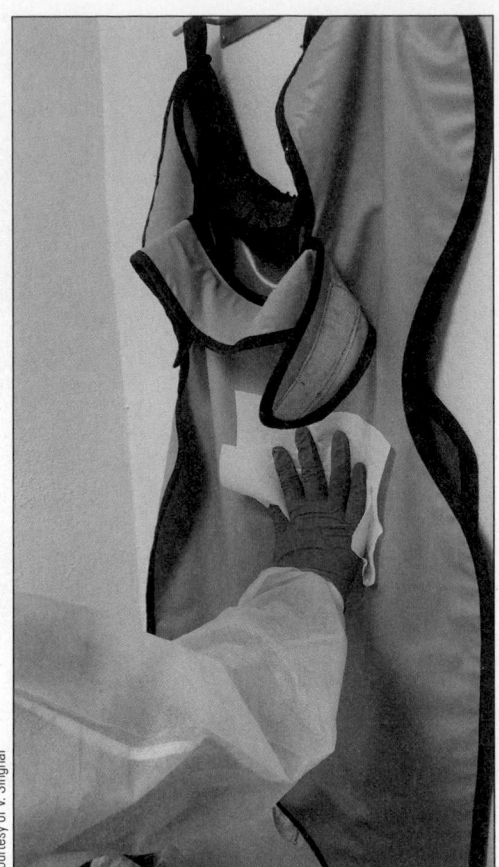

Courtesy of V. Singhal

FIGURE 28-5
Wiping lead apron with towel after disinfection spray.

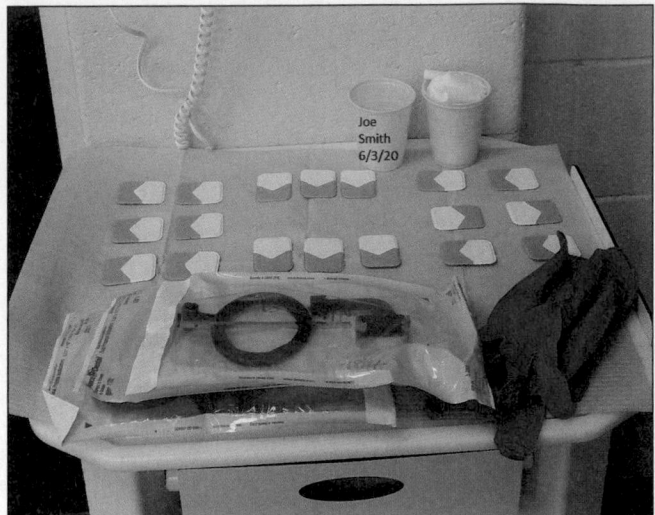

Courtesy of V. Singhal

FIGURE 28-6
Traditional films and supplies needed for radiographic exposures.

been placed on the patient; other may choose to wipe the lead apron with disinfectant after use (Figure 28-5). Preventing cross contamination is one of your most important duties as a dental assistant.

Equipment Preparation Prepare your area by placing all the needed materials on a covered surface. This includes any needed receptor holders, cotton rolls and rubber bands, and disposable cups for used traditional films and for contaminated disposables such as cotton rolls (Figure 28-6). The disposable cup for the traditional films should be labeled with the patient's name. If using a digital sensor, obtain the sensor and sheath to protect the sensor while exposing images (Figure 28-6).

If the radiographer is using sensors, the patient's computer chart must be opened in the software and ready for capturing the images that will be processed by the computer into the proper chart section. Digital radiography will be discussed in Chapter 29. A barrier should be placed over the keyboard and mouse to protect against contamination during the exposure procedure (Figures 28-1C and 28-1D). Gather all needed image receptors and equipment before you begin exposing the required areas (Figure 28-6). By collecting everything before starting, you will minimize the potential for cross contamination.

Patient Preparation Seat and prepare the patient for radiographic exposure before donning gloves. Review the patient's chart and the prescription the dentist has written for the number and type of radiographs to be taken. Adjust the chair to the appropriate height for the operator; position the patient so the midsagittal plane is perpendicular to the floor and the maxilla is parallel to the floor. The need for radiograph(s) and the safety provided for the patient from the dangers of radiation should be explained to the patient and the previously disinfected lead apron placed over the patient (Figure 28-7). The patient should be requested to remove eyeglasses and any intraoral removable appliances prior to exposure of intraoral images. Explain that these items will block the radiation, show up as an *artifact* on the radiograph, and interfere with the image that the dentist needs for diagnosis.

Once handwashing is completed and PPE is donned as outlined in Chapter 11, the sterilization bags containing the receptor holding devices should be opened (Figure 28-8A). The devices need to be assembled and placed on the covered designated area (Figure 28-8B). Proper image receptor holder assembly will be discussed later in this chapter. If using traditional films, the films should be placed on the work surface (Figure 28-6). The correct sequence of exposure will be discussed later in this chapter.

Digital sensors need to be placed inside supplied plastic sheaths (Figure 28-3). When using a phosphor plate digital system, care needs to be taken in placing the plate into the protective barrier (Figure 28-9). Digital imaging with the use of digital sensors and phosphor plates will be discussed in detail in Chapter 29.

Infection Control during Exposure After the traditional film has been exposed, the receptor holding devices should be placed on the cover in the designated area. The radiographer should never place any contaminated items on an uncovered surface.

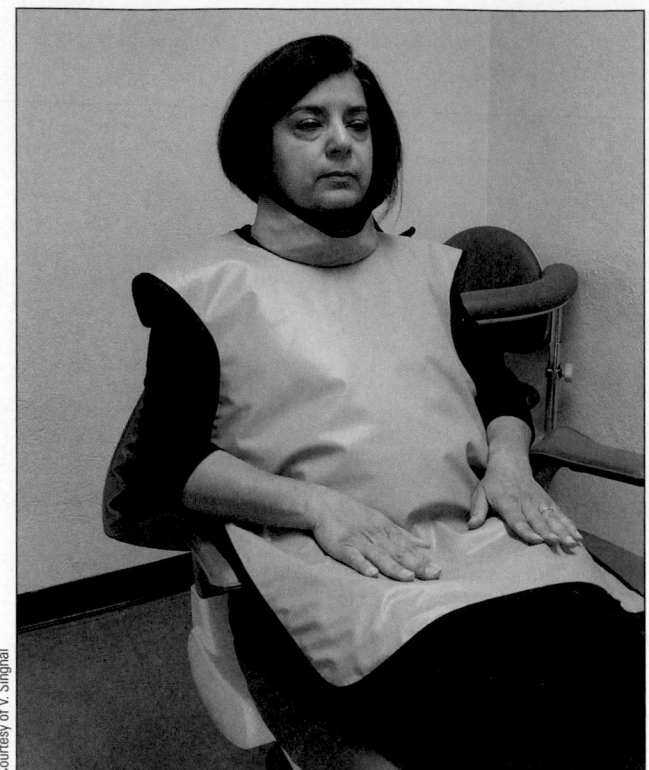

Courtesy of V. Singhal

FIGURE 28-7
Lead apron placed on seated patient.

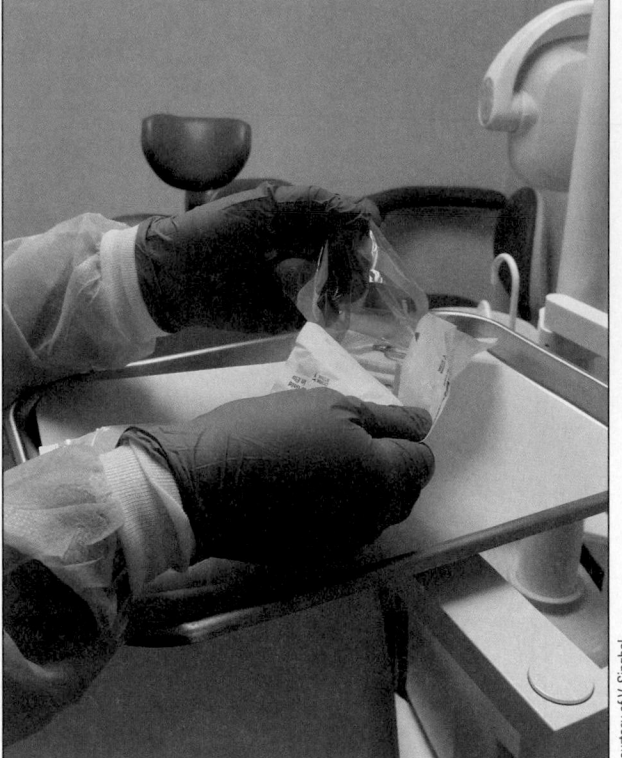

Courtesy of V. Singhal

FIGURE 28-8A
Opening of sterile pouches with XCP kits.

The instruments, holding devices, and receptors should only be placed on the designated covered work surface in order to avoid contamination of unprotected areas. During exposure, excess saliva should be removed from the film with paper toweling (Figure 28-10). The contaminated films are placed into a disposable plastic cup, taking care to avoid contaminating the outside of the cup (Figure 28-11).

If the operator is using films with protective barriers, the outer plastic covering should be opened and the film packet from inside should be dropped without any contact from contaminated gloves into a clean plastic disposable cup (Figure 28-11). Care must be taken to not contaminate the film as the barrier is peeled away from the film and dropped into the cup. These film packets are considered uncontaminated as they were protected from saliva and blood, and may be processed as uncontaminated packets. The outside of the cup should also not be contaminated from gloves that have been in the patient's oral cavity. The film packets, once inside the clean cup, can be processed without concern about contamination of the processing workspace or equipment.

Most digital sensors sheaths will maintain intact through the entire procedures. Continually check that the sheath does not become torn, and replace as needed. If a sheath becomes torn, the sensor will need to be disinfected using a paper towel that has been sprayed with a disinfectant or per manufacturer's directions.

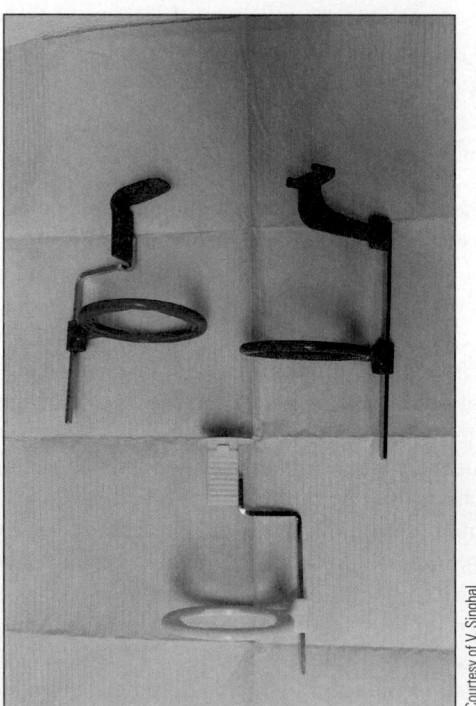

Courtesy of V. Singhal

FIGURE 28-8B
Assembled image receptor holders.

CHAPTER 28 Dental Radiology Infection Control, Exposure, Processing and Evaluation of Dental Radiographs, and Mounting of Dental Radiographs

849

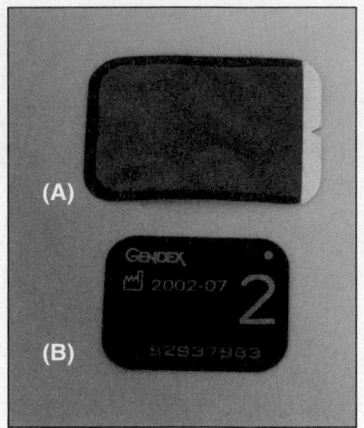

FIGURE 28-9
(A) Barrier. (B) Imaging plate.

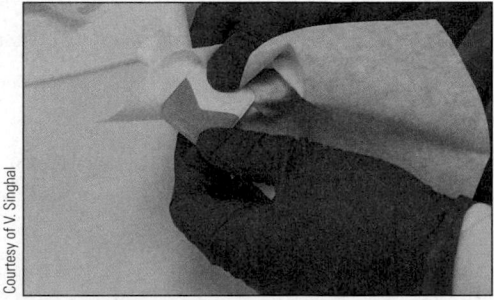

Courtesy of V. Singhal

FIGURE 28-10
Drying an exposed film packet.

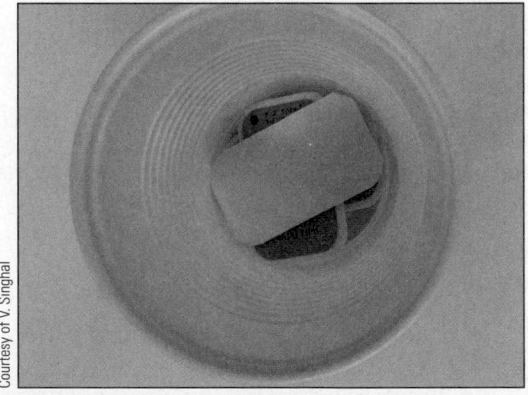

Courtesy of V. Singhal

FIGURE 28-11
Exposed films in cup ready for processing.

Infection Control after Radiographic Exposure Once all the radiographs have been exposed, the contaminated films remain in the labeled cup until they are taken to the darkroom or the autoprocessor to be processed. The lead apron is removed and placed onto a hanger. The lead apron should never be folded as the lead can crack, resulting in excess radiation not being absorbed by the lead and entering the patient. The protective sheaths are removed from sensors and disposed of. Patient exam gloves are removed, hands are washed, and utility gloves are donned. All contaminated products are disposed of, and the countertops and work

area are disinfected. The lead apron is disinfected with a paper towel that has been sprayed with a disinfectant (Figure 28-5). The dental assistant removes utility gloves, washes hands, documents the patient's chart, takes traditional films to the processing area, or completes computer entries for digital radiographs.

Infection Control during Traditional Film Processing During traditional film processing, there is also a risk of cross contamination of work surfaces as well as automatic processors. When using traditional film processing methods, the dental auxiliary must take care to prevent contamination of many areas in the darkroom. These areas include the work area where films will be opened, the film hanger used to secure and process the films during manual processing technique, and the darkroom autoprocessor during autoprocessing. Additionally, cross contamination can occur when an autoprocessor with a daylight loader is utilized outside of the darkroom. This section will cover infection related to either method of processing.

Infection Control Related to Automatic Processing Automatic processing methods may vary slightly depending on the machine used. If a Peri-Pro is being utilized (Figure 28-12), the operator should gather the cup with the patient's name and film packets, an empty cup for trash and clean disposable gloves (Figure 28-13). These items should be placed inside the Peri-Pro through the opening of the daylight loader. The lid of the daylight loader should then be closed, and the operator should insert hands donned with clean gloves into the machine through the side openings. Once the hands are inside, the operator should wear the gloves and process the films as discussed later in this chapter. All trash should be placed in the empty disposable cup. Once all films have been processed, the operator should remove the gloves and place in the cup designated for trash. The operator should remove the hands through the side openings with clean hands to avoid contamination of this area. Wearing another pair of gloves, the trash should be removed through the daylight loader (Figure 28-14). With gloves, the operator should separate the lead foil from the trash and place in the lead recycling container (Figure 28-15). The outer wrapping and black paper and gloves and cup can be disposed of in the regular trash. The films can be collected with clean hands in a clean cup as they exit the Peri-Pro.

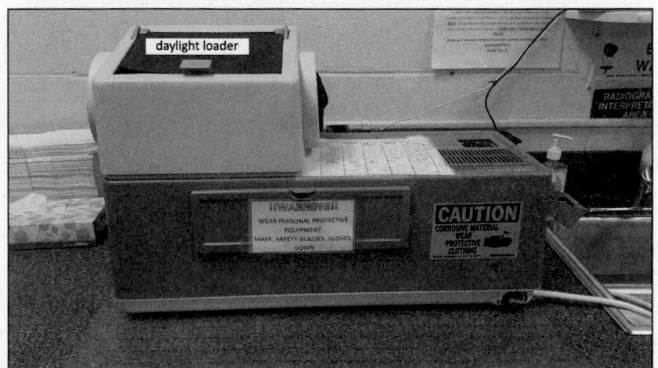

Courtesy of V. Singhal

FIGURE 28-12
Peri-Pro automatic film processor with daylight loader.

Procedure 28-1
Infection Control Before, During, and After Exposure

Items to be Disinfected:
- x-ray machine head, control panel
- dental chair and the buttons/knobs used to position the patient
- work area including countertops and trays
- patient lead apron
- computer keyboard and mouse

Before the Patient Arrives
1. Assess the treatment area for potential surface that may be touched during the procedure.
2. Wash and dry hands and don PPE. Refer to Chapter 11. Disinfect and cover the surfaces of the items listed above.
3. Remove gloves and wash hands. Don clean gloves. Open the patient's chart in the software program when using a digital sensor.
4. Assemble and organize all supplies that will be needed while obtaining radiographs.

Equipment and Supplies
- tray or counter cover for holding supplies
- the number of traditional films required for procedure or digital sensor
- if using digital sensors, sheaths used to cover the digital sensor
- image receptor-holding devices
- cotton rolls
- paper towel for wiping contaminated film
- cup with patient's name to hold traditional films if being used
- cup for trash such as used cotton rolls
- gloves

Procedure Steps

Patient Preparation
1. Remove gloves and wash hands. Seat and prepare patient before donning clean gloves.
2. Position patient in dental chair.
3. Adjust headrest so that maxilla is parallel to the floor and the midsagittal plane is perpendicular to the floor.
4. Explain to patient the need for radiographs and steps taken for radiation safety.
5. Ask patient to remove jewelry, removable dental appliances, lip rings, tongue rings, and all metal artifacts that may show in the image.
6. Place the lead apron on patient and secure the thyroid collar.
7. Adjust the height of chair appropriately for the height of radiographer.

Equipment Preparation

Prepare equipment for radiographic exposure before beginning exposure.

1. Wash hands according to standard protocol, and don clean treatment gloves.
2. Open sterilization bags and prepare receptor holding devices.
3. Turn on machine and adjust settings.

During Exposure

Be aware of potential contamination of equipment while exposing images.

1. Expose radiographs.
2. Dry traditional films with paper towel to remove excessive saliva and place in cup with patient's name; remove outer plastic barrier from film packet as needed.
3. Transfer receptor holding device from work area to oral cavity.
4. Never place receptor holding device on an uncovered surface.
5. Change torn sheaths on sensors as needed.
6. Ensure that the computer keyboard and mouse are covered with barriers throughout the procedure.

After Exposure
1. Remove gloves, wash hands, and escort patient to the treatment area after removing lead apron.
2. Wash hands and don clean treatment gloves.
3. If using traditional films, take films to processing area in cup.
4. If using digital sensor, remove sensor sheath and dispose.
5. If using digital system, remove computer keyboard cover and mouse cover and dispose.
6. Remove treatment gloves, wash hands, and don utility gloves.
7. Dispose of all contaminated products and disinfect work area.
8. Place film holders in area of contaminated instruments to be sanitized and sterilized.
9. Disinfect and store lead apron on hanger.
10. Remove gloves and wash hands.
11. Complete all required documentation.
12. Document paper chart or complete computer entries for digital radiographs.

CHAPTER 28 Dental Radiology Infection Control, Exposure, Processing and Evaluation of
Dental Radiographs, and Mounting of Dental Radiographs

851

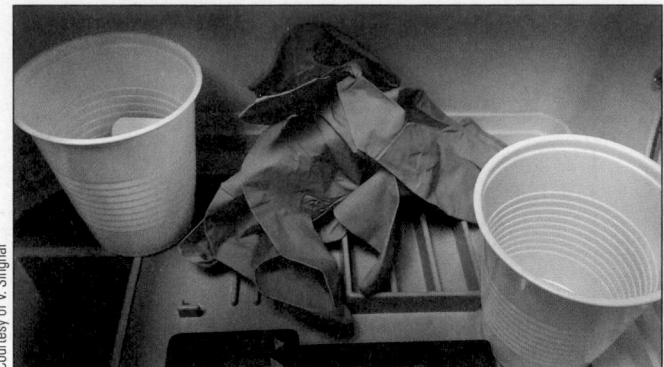

FIGURE 28-13
Supplies for film processing inside daylight loader of Peri-Pro.

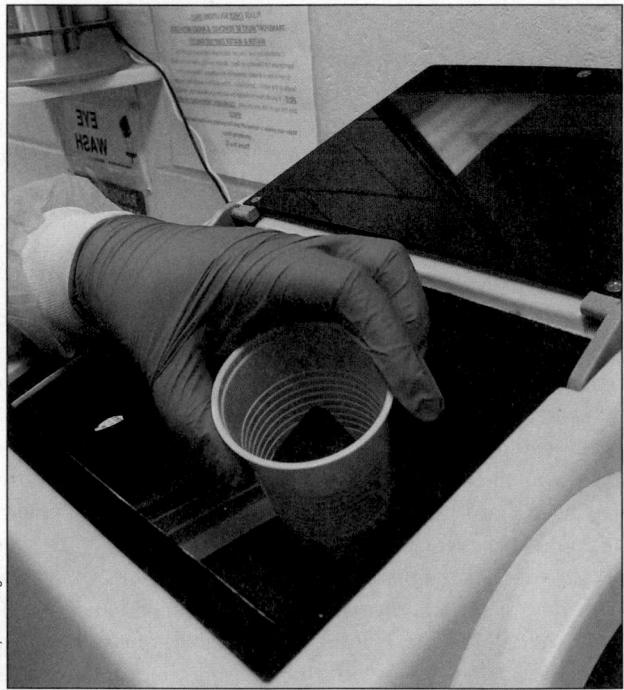

FIGURE 28-14
Removing trash through daylight loader of Peri-Pro.

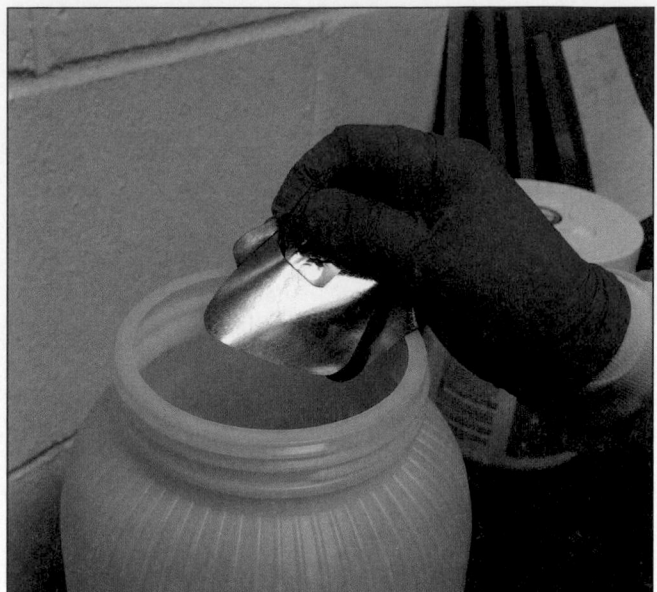

FIGURE 28-15
Lead foil being placed into lead foil recycling container.

Paralleling Technique

Two lines are parallel if they always remain the same distance apart and never intersect (Figure 28-16). Two lines intersect if they cross each other at some point (Figure 28-17) and two

FIGURE 28-16
Parallel lines.

Techniques for Exposing Intraoral Radiographs

There are two basic techniques used to expose intraoral radiographs, the paralleling technique and bisecting angle technique (BAT). The paralleling technique uses devices known as extension cone paralleling (XCP) kits that assist in the placement of the image receptor and the PID (Figure 28-8B). Both procedures will be discussed in this chapter. Since digital radiography is becoming more common, the term used will be image receptor. This term includes the traditional film and digital sensors.

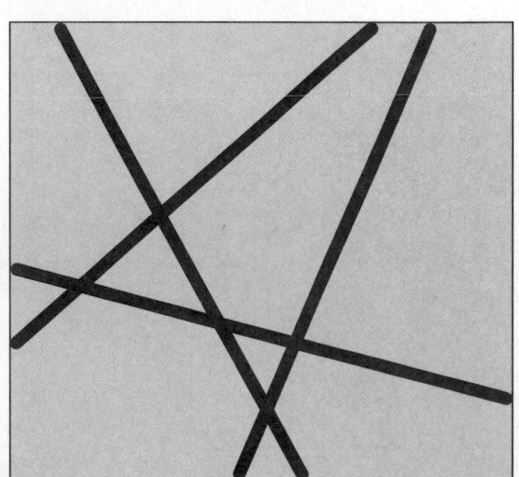

FIGURE 28-17
Intersecting lines.

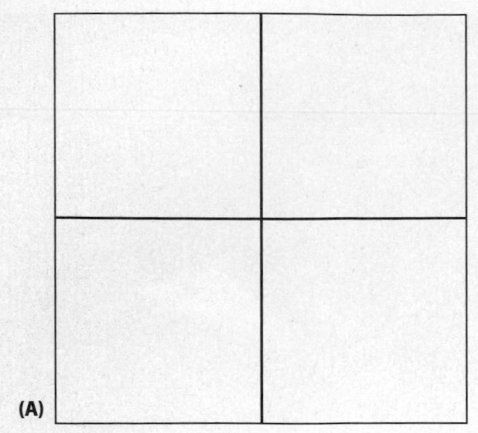

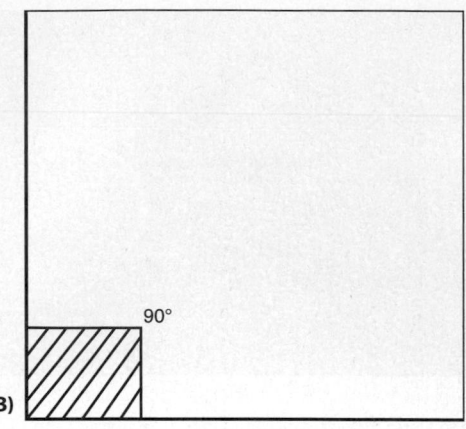

FIGURE 28-18
(A) Perpendicular lines. (B) Right angle.

lines are perpendicular if they cross each other and form a 90° angle (Figure 28-18). The paralleling technique begins with placing the image receptor parallel to the long axis of the tooth (Figure 28-19). The central ray of the x-ray beam is directed perpendicular to both the image receptor and the long axis of the tooth (Figure 28-19). To obtain parallelism between the image receptor and the long axis of the tooth, the receptor must be placed at a distance from the tooth (object) and toward the center of the oral cavity. This is referred to as the object-receptor distance. Principle 3 in Chapter 27 states that an increase in object-receptor distance results in the loss of image sharpness and increased magnification. To compensate for this, a longer PID (16 inches) is used when using the paralleling technique. The longer PID provides an increased source (target) to receptor distance as described in Principle 4 in Chapter 27. The XCP kits are used to maintain parallelism between the image receptor and the object and are discussed below (Figure 28-8B).

Extension Cone Paralleling (XCP) Devices The extension cone paralleling (XCP) kit devices are commonly used for the paralleling technique. The use of these devices aids in acquiring high-quality images with fewer retakes. The XCP has bite blocks (receptor holders) for anterior periapical, posterior periapical as well as vertical and horizontal bitewings, a metal arm (indicator rod), and an aiming ring (Figure 28-20A–C). Universal kits have a universal arm for all exposures (Figures 28-20D and 28-20E).

The bite blocks secure the image receptor in position parallel to the long axis of the tooth as the patient bites on the block to hold the device in place. There are a variety of bite block sizes for adult and pediatric patients. The arms are metal rods that attach to the bite block. The arm indicates where the vertical angulation of the cone needs to be set to have the central ray (CR) of the x-ray beam perpendicular to both the image receptor and tooth. The correct placement of vertical angulation prevents distortion and provides a more diagnostic image (Figure 28-21). The dial on the machine head provides the vertical angulation of the PID (Figure 28-22). This dial is primarily used in the bisecting technique. The aiming ring guides the radiographer for the proper placement of the PID to completely cover the receptor reducing the chance of partial exposure of the receptor.

Factors That Affect the Paralleling Technique There are several factors that must be considered in exposing radiographs using the paralleling technique:

- patient head position
- receptor placement and position
- vertical angulation
- horizontal angulation
- central beam or central ray point of entry

Patient Head Position The patient should be positioned upright with the midsagittal plane perpendicular to the floor and maxilla parallel to the floor (Figures 28-7 and 28-23).

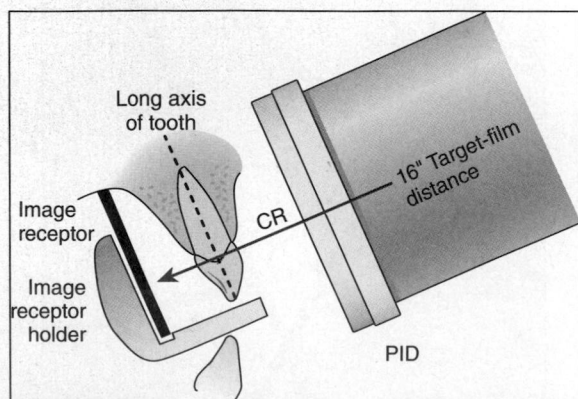

FIGURE 28-19
Position of image receptor and central ray in paralleling technique.

CHAPTER 28 Dental Radiology Infection Control, Exposure, Processing and Evaluation of Dental Radiographs, and Mounting of Dental Radiographs

853

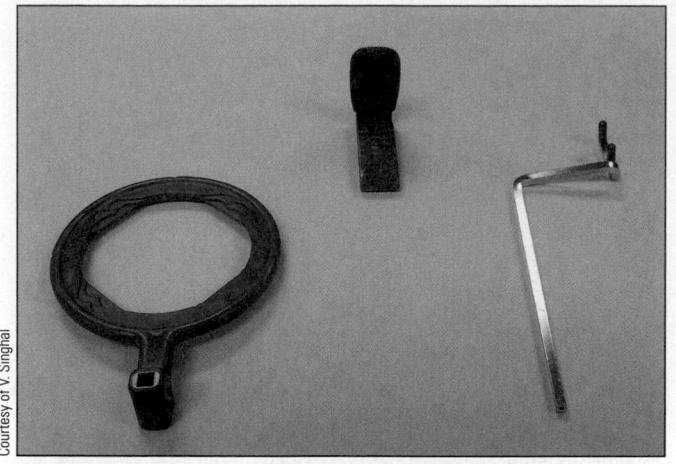

Courtesy of V. Singhal

FIGURE 28-20A
Anterior XCP rod, ring, and bite block.

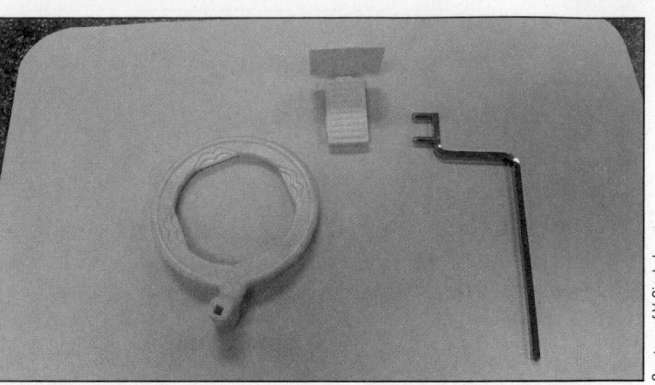

Courtesy of V. Singhal

FIGURE 28-20B
Posterior XCP rod, ring, and bite block.

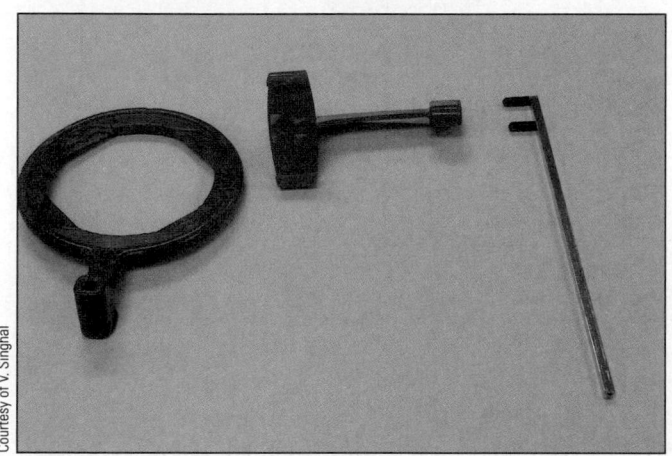

Courtesy of V. Singhal

FIGURE 28-20C
Horizontal bitewing XCP rod, ring, and bite block.

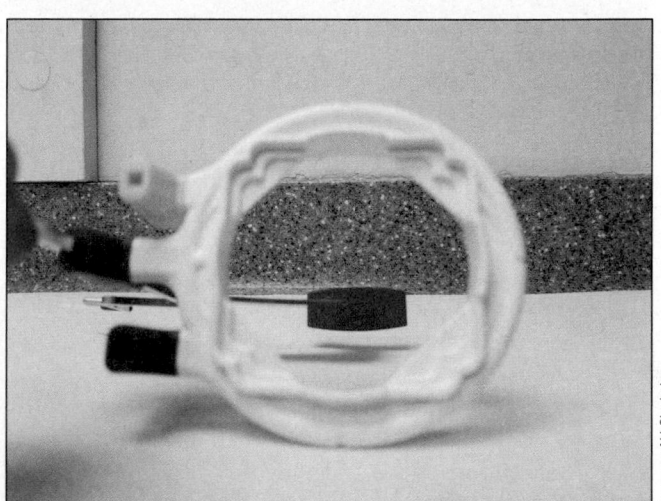

Courtesy of V. Singhal

FIGURE 28-20D
Universal XCP kit with vertical bitewing bite block.

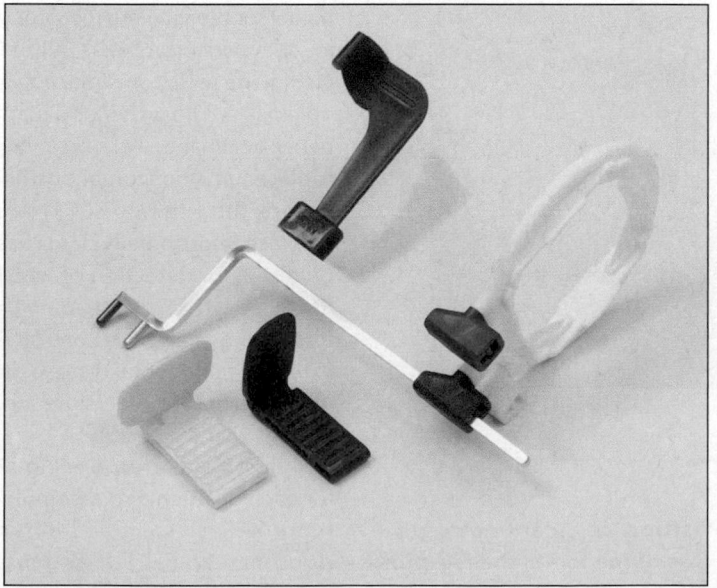

FIGURE 28-20E
Universal XCP kit.

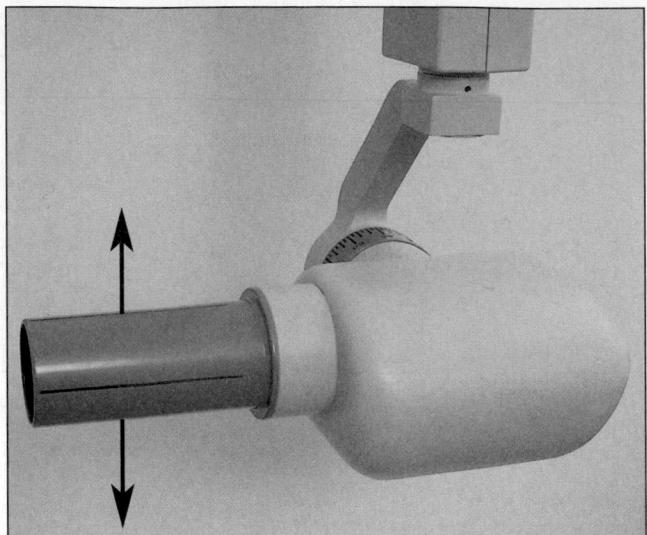

FIGURE 28-21
Example of cone positioning for vertical angulation (up and down rotation).

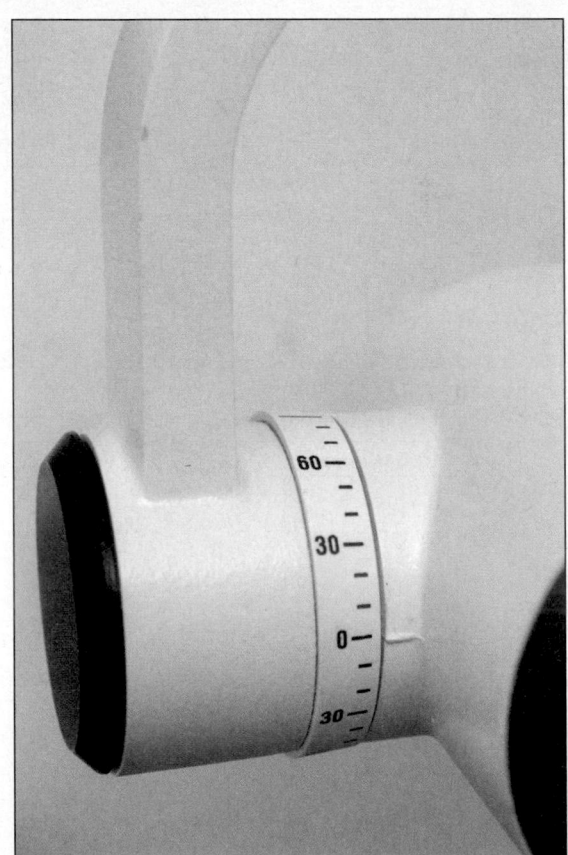

FIGURE 28-22
The numerical degree guide on the side of the tubehead.

Receptor Placement and Position In order to place the receptor parallel to the long axis of the tooth, the receptor should be placed more toward the center of the oral cavity.

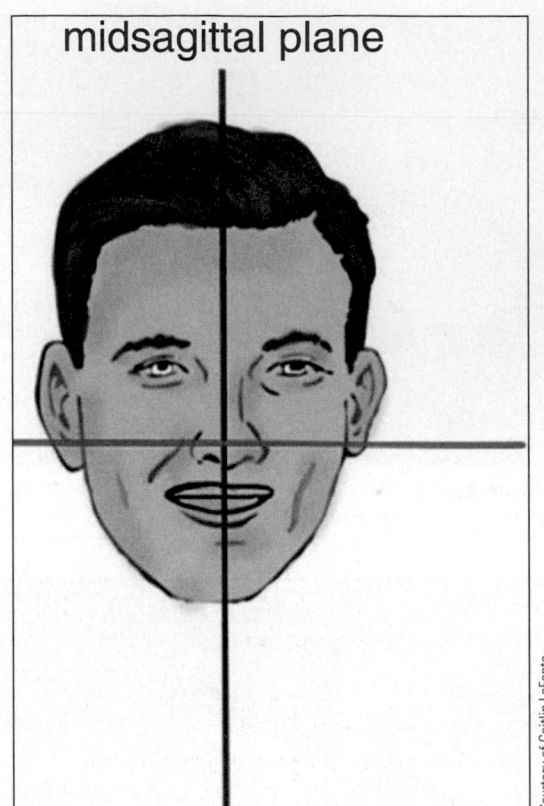

midsagittal plane

Courtesy of Caitlin LaFonte

FIGURE 28-23
Midsagittal plane.

This placement will also allow the patient to bite completely on the bite block and obtain the apices of the teeth for periapical images (Figure 28-19).

The radiographer needs to select the corresponding receptor holder for the required receptor placement in the oral cavity. The anterior periapical XCP is utilized for anterior periapical images. The image receptor is placed vertically in the holder for anterior images. The posterior periapical XCP is utilized for posterior periapical images. For posterior placement, the image receptor is placed in a horizontal position (Figure 28-24). For bitewing images, the bitewing XCP is selected. Bitewing receptors may be placed horizontally or vertically. The horizontal bitewing is preferred for detection of interproximal decay. Decay will be discussed later in this chapter. The vertical bitewing is preferred for viewing of alveolar bone levels, as it aids in the diagnosis of extent of periodontal disease. Horizontal and vertical bitewing image receptor holders are available for bitewing exposures (Figures 28-20C and 28-26).

Select the corresponding aiming ring and indicator arm for each position and assemble the XCP instrument. The posterior XCP is assembled in two positions for the maxillary right/mandibular left and maxillary left/mandibular right (Figure 28-27A and B).It is assembled for the maxillary left/

CHAPTER 28 Dental Radiology Infection Control, Exposure, Processing and Evaluation of Dental Radiographs, and Mounting of Dental Radiographs

855

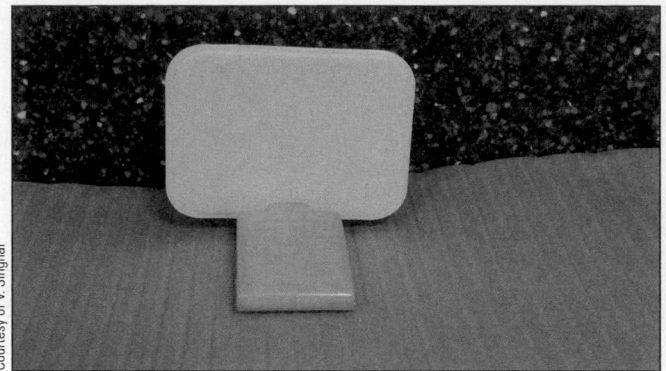

FIGURE 28-24
Posterior XCP bite block with horizontal image receptor.

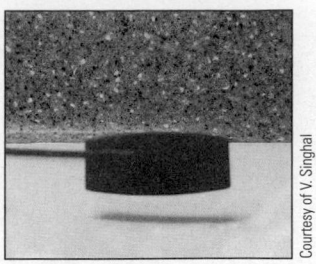

FIGURE 28-26
Image of vertical bitewing holder for traditional film.

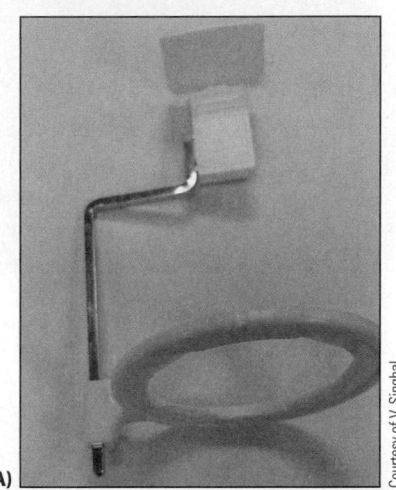

(A)

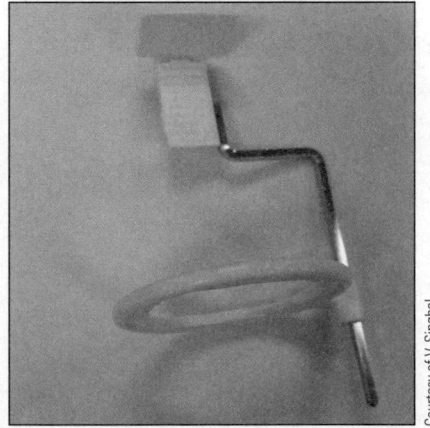

(B)

FIGURE 28-27
(A) Posterior XCP assembled for maxillary left and mandibular right quadrants. (B) Posterior XCP assembled for maxillary right and mandibular left quadrants.

mandibular right with the indicator rod positioned to left side of the receptor holder; for the maxillary right/mandibular left, the rod is attached to the right of the receptor holder The universal XCP kits are color-coded to make this step much easier (Figure 28-20D).

Placement of Image Receptor into Holder Once the exposure area and patient have been prepared using the infection control protocol as discussed earlier in this chapter, the operator may begin the exposure process. When using traditional intraoral dental films, the films should be laid out on a template for the FMX which is placed onto the work space (Figures 28-6 and 28-28). This allows the operator to pick up a packet for each area. When the packet is exposed and the film packet is placed into the cup with the patient's name, that spot on the template is empty. This allows the operator to expose an FMX without the risks of a double exposure of an area and a missing exposure of another area.

Each film packet should be placed into the holder of the XCP kit with the embossed dot in the slot so that it will be at the occlusal surfaces of the teeth. The white side (tube side) of the film packet is facing the operator so that it will also be facing the PID when placed in the oral cavity (Figure 28-29A). For bitewings, the dot orientation does not matter, as it will be located near the cervical areas of the teeth on the bitewing image (Figure 28-29B).

FIGURE 28-25
Radiographic image of vertical bitewing.

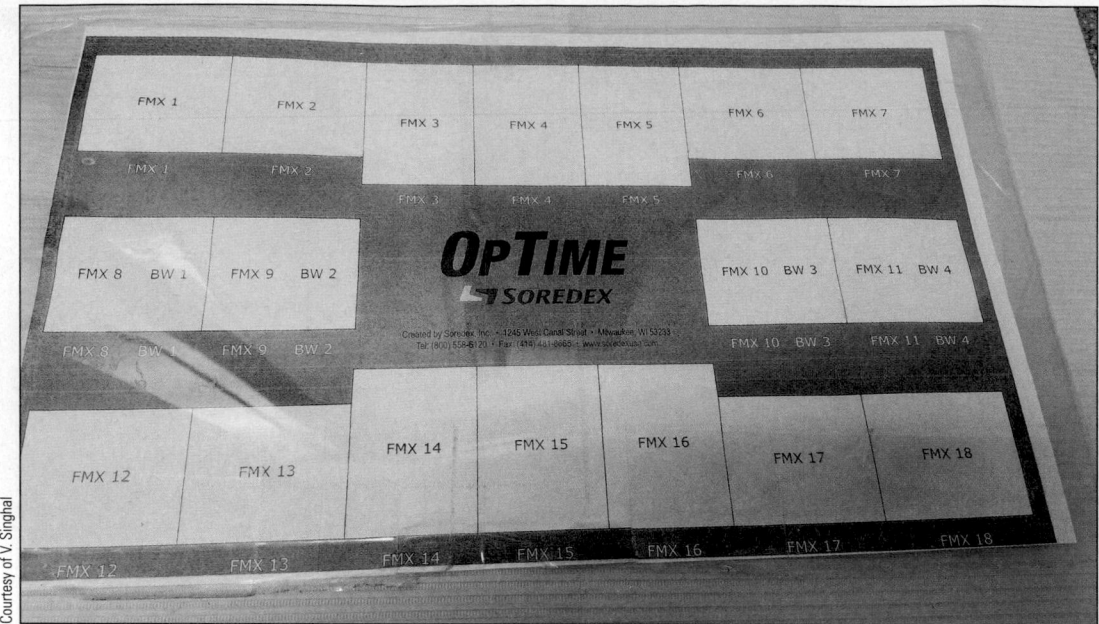

Courtesy of V. Singhal

FIGURE 28-28
Template for traditional films for adult full set of radiographs.

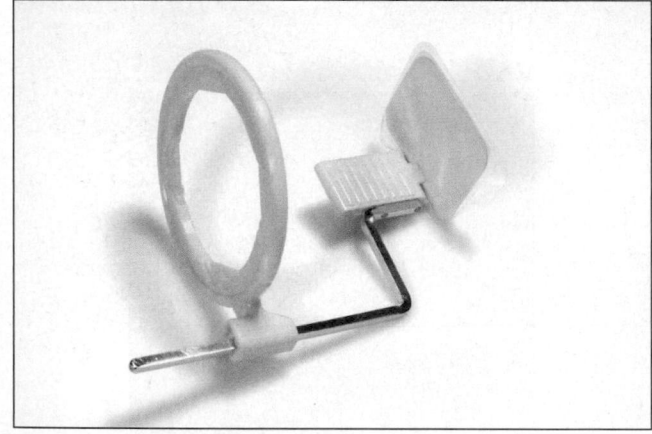

FIGURE 28-29A
Posterior traditional film XCP with horizontal film placed with white side facing operator and PID.

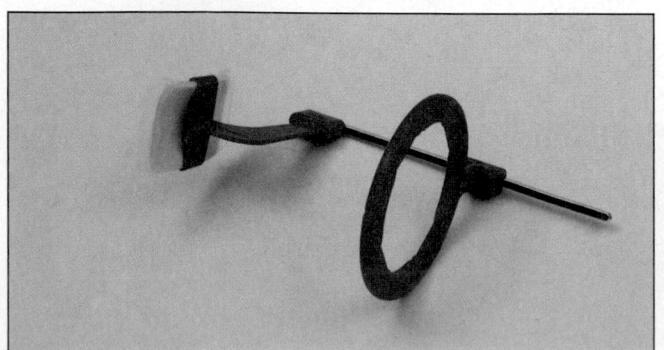

FIGURE 28-29B
Horizontal traditional bitewing XCP with film placed with white side toward operator and PID.

Placement of Receptor Holder in Oral Cavity Gently rotate the XCP and image receptor into the patient's oral cavity and position for the desired exposure. Place the image receptor parallel to the long axis of the tooth. Place the biting surface of the holder against the tooth and have the patient close their teeth to hold the image receptor in place. Do not slide the bite block or have the patient bite the holder into position. The edge of the receptor can cause trauma to the patient's soft tissue. If the patient is unable to bite completely because it is painful, reposition the receptor further from the tooth (more toward the midline of the oral cavity) and request that the patient close (Figure 28-30). The edge of the receptor needs

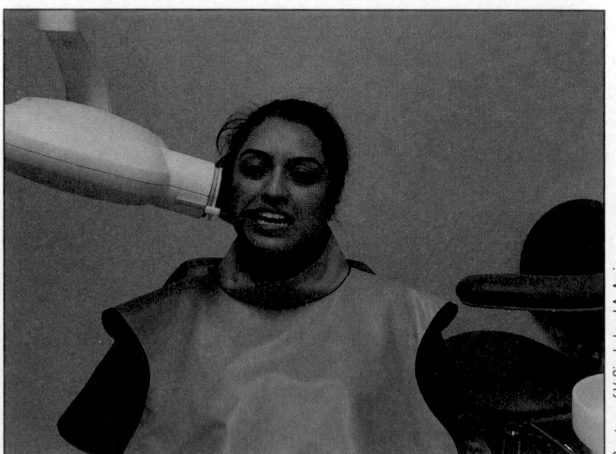

Courtesy of V. Singhal and A. Amin

FIGURE 28-30
Image receptor in place and patient biting down fully for exposure of maxillary right molar periapical image.

CHAPTER 28 Dental Radiology Infection Control, Exposure, Processing and Evaluation of Dental Radiographs, and Mounting of Dental Radiographs

857

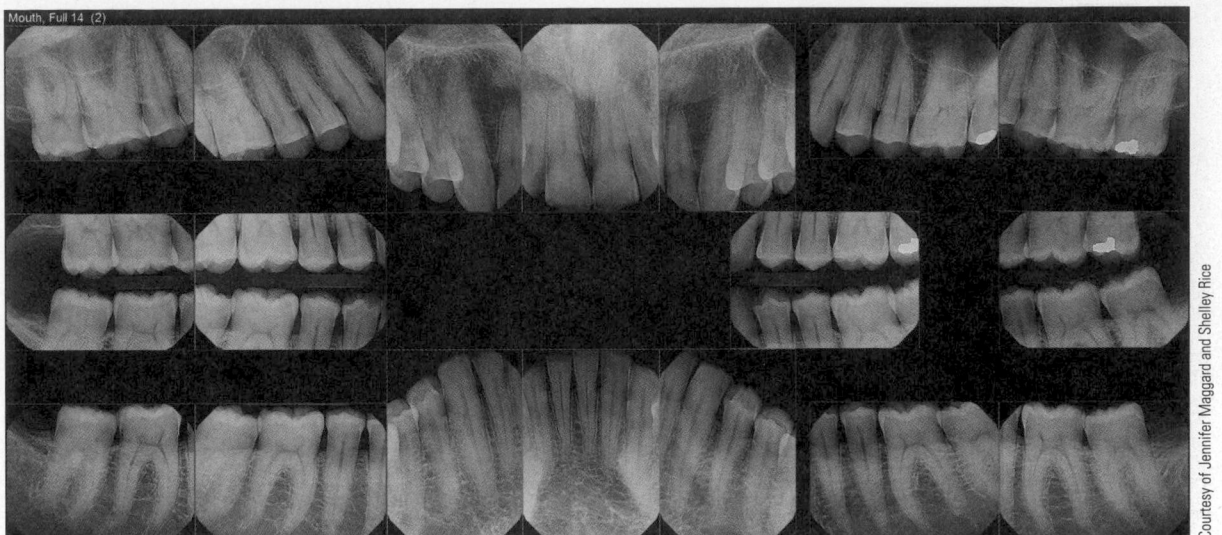

Courtesy of Jennifer Maggard and Shelley Rice

FIGURE 28-31
Full set of 18 images with horizontal bitewings.

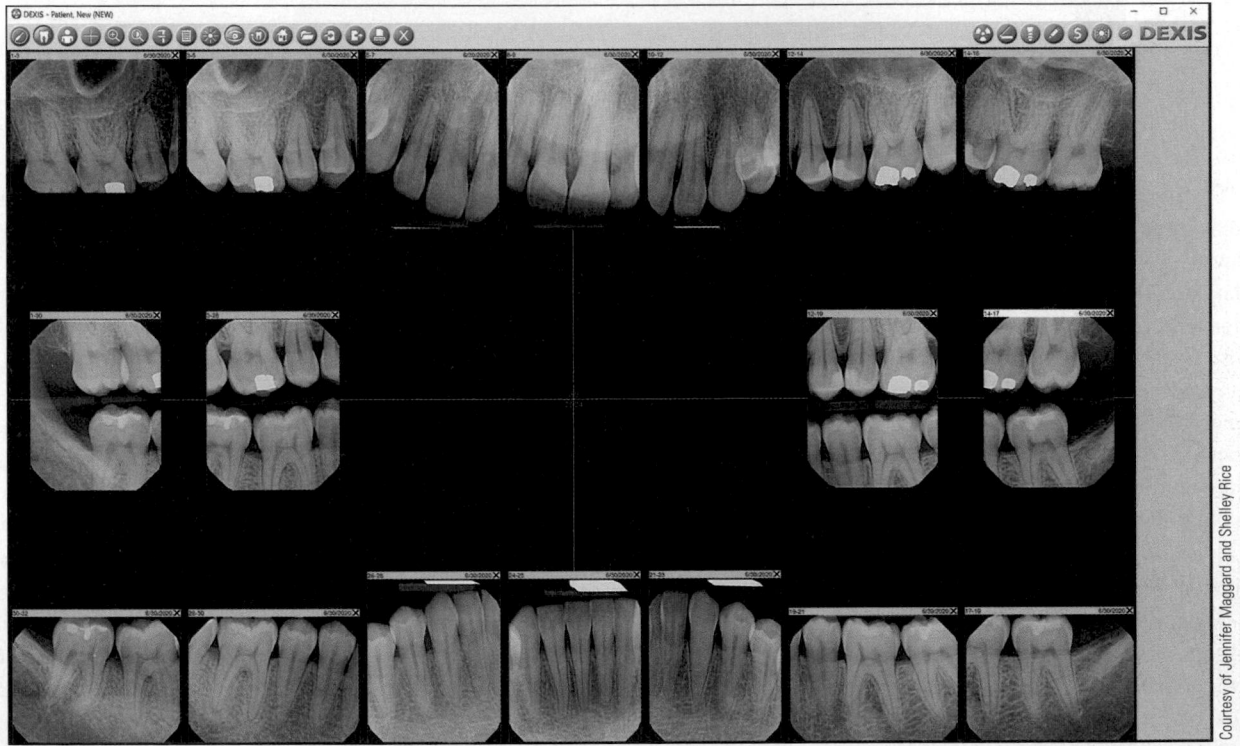

Courtesy of Jennifer Maggard and Shelley Rice

FIGURE 28-32
Full set of 18 images with vertical bitewings.

to extend evenly beyond the occlusal plane allowing for the entire tooth to be exposed as well as 2–3 mm beyond the apices (Figure 28-19). Three to four teeth are obtained on each image depending on the area being exposed and the size of the receptor being used.

Adult Full Mouth Survey of Radiographs

An adult full mouth survey (FMS) may consist of 18 images (Figures 28-31 and 28-32) or 20 images (Figure 28-33). An adult full mouth survey of radiographs is usually taken every 3–5 years. The bitewing images are taken annually. This variation

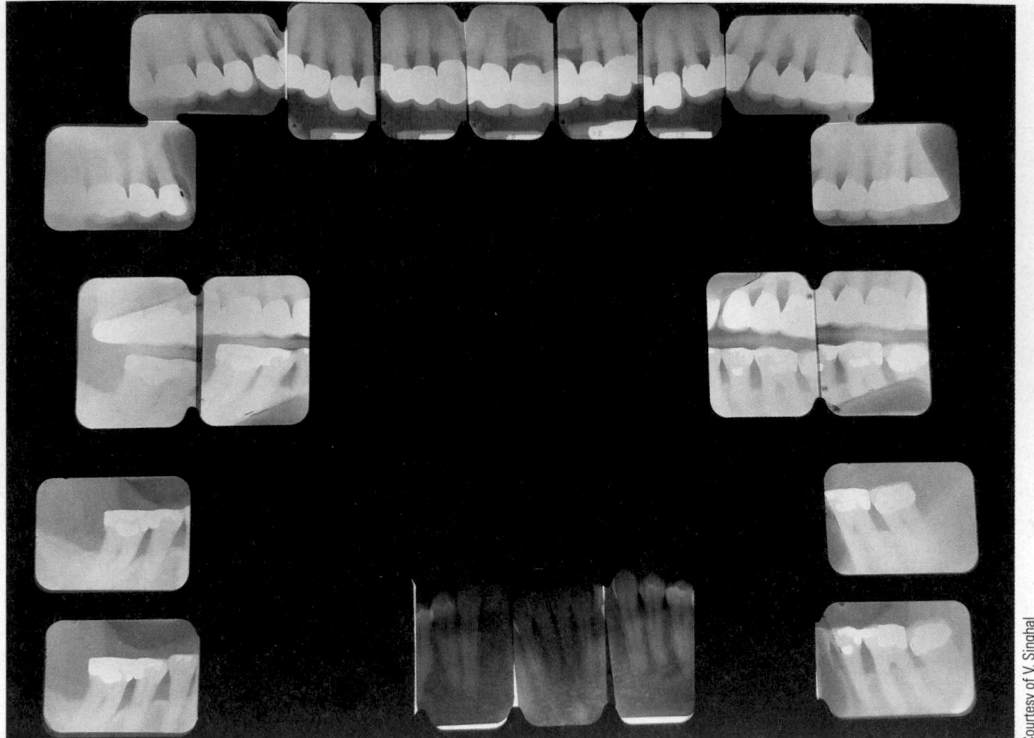

Courtesy of V. Singhal

FIGURE 28-33
Full set of traditional films with 20 images.

is due to the number of images exposed in the maxillary anterior area. Some practitioners prefer to use a size 1 receptor for all maxillary anterior exposures and may have four images in the maxillary anterior area and three images in the mandibular anterior area (Figure 28-33). If needed, a maxillary midline exposure may also be taken for a total of five maxillary anterior images and three mandibular anterior images (Figure 28-33). Two images will be obtained in each posterior quadrant (premolar periapical and molar periapical). Additionally, two bitewing images will be obtained on the right side and left side (premolar and molar bitewings on each side).

Receptor Position for Periapical Images   Placement of the image receptor is critical to obtain the desired teeth on the image and to avoid retakes that would result in unnecessary radiation to the patient. Following a sequence allows the operator to work in an efficient manner without the risk of double exposing an area or not exposing an area.

Cotton rolls are often placed between the teeth and the bite block of the arch that is not being exposed. The cotton rolls would be secured to the bite block with a rubberband. This technique makes it easier for the patient to close on the bite block and stabilize it to prevent movement. The cotton roll is placed over the teeth in the arch that is not going to be exposed, and then the bite block is placed on top of it. The patient is asked to close and secure the Rinn in place. This is an optional technique and may be

used for all exposures, or only for those in areas where the patient is having difficulty closing.

Bisecting Technique

Although the paralleling technique is the method of choice, it is not always possible to use. Anatomy of the oral cavity and some dental procedures do not always allow for ideal image receptor positioning. This may make obtaining diagnostic radiographic images challenging. Anatomy of the oral cavity that sometimes makes the paralleling technique difficult includes a shallow, flat palate; a shallow floor of the mouth; patients who are edentulous; patients with limited opening; and very small children. Some surgical procedures like root canal therapy require that radiographs be exposed during the procedure to examine the location of files and materials in the root canals. Using the paralleling method is difficult if exposures are required when the endodontic file or *gutta percha* filling material is in the canal during root canal therapy.

In an attempt to overcome these situations, another technique may be used for intraoral radiographic exposures. The *bisection of angle technique* (BAT) is an alternative method that may be used when the paralleling technique is not possible. Knowledge of both techniques enables the radiographer to make modifications to suit the individual needs of the patient.

CHAPTER 28 Dental Radiology Infection Control, Exposure, Processing and Evaluation of Dental Radiographs, and Mounting of Dental Radiographs

859

TABLE 28-1 Exposure Sequence for Paralleling Technique for an Adult Full Mouth Series of Radiographs If Using All Size 2 Image Receptors

Maxillary right canine periapical
Maxillary incisor periapical
Maxillary left canine periapical
Mandibular left canine periapical
Mandibular incisor periapical
Mandibular right canine periapical
Maxillary right posterior quadrant premolar periapical
Maxillary right posterior quadrant molar periapical
Mandibular left posterior quadrant premolar periapical
Mandibular left posterior quadrant molar periapical
Maxillary left posterior quadrant premolar periapical
Maxillary left posterior quadrant molar periapical
Mandibular right posterior quadrant premolar periapical
Mandibular right posterior quadrant molar periapical
Right premolar bitewing
Right molar bitewing
Left premolar bitewing
Left molar bitewing

TABLE 28-2 Exposure Sequence for Paralleling Technique for an Adult Full Mouth Series of Radiographs If Using Size 2 Image Receptors for Posterior Periapical Images and Bitewings and Size 1 Image Receptor for Anterior Periapical Images

Maxillary right canine periapical
Maxillary right central/lateral incisor periapical
Maxillary midline image (if requested by dentist)
Maxillary left central/lateral incisor periapical
Maxillary left canine periapical
Mandibular left canine periapical
Mandibular incisor periapical
Mandibular right canine periapical
Maxillary right posterior quadrant premolar periapical
Maxillary right posterior quadrant molar periapical
Mandibular left posterior quadrant premolar periapical
Mandibular left posterior quadrant molar periapical
Maxillary left posterior quadrant premolar periapical
Maxillary left posterior quadrant molar periapical
Mandibular right posterior quadrant premolar periapical
Mandibular right posterior quadrant molar periapical
Right premolar bitewing
Right molar bitewing
Left premolar bitewing
Left molar bitewing

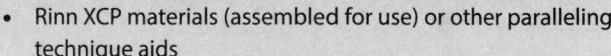

Procedure 28-2

Exposure of a Full Mouth Series of Radiographs Using the Paralleling Technique

This procedure is performed by the qualified dental assistant. The dentist requests a full-mouth set of radiographs. The dental assistant prepares the equipment (Rinn XCP instruments), the area, and the patient; takes the radiographs; and processes and mounts the traditional films (if being used) for viewing.

This procedure explains receptor placement and exposure for the central incisors in each arch, one-half of the maxillary arch, and one-half of the mandibular arch. The same technique is used to expose the opposite side.

Equipment and Supplies

- patient's chart
- barriers for the radiography room and equipment (refer to Procedure 28-1)
- image receptor (appropriate size); if using traditional film, the appropriate number of film packets is needed
- protective sheaths if using sensors; plastic barriers for keyboard and mouse if using a digital system
- cotton rolls (optional)

- Rinn XCP materials (assembled for use) or other paralleling technique aids
- lead apron with thyroid collar
- container for exposed traditional film
- paper towel or tissue

Procedure Steps

1. Review the patient's chart and follow aseptic procedures as outlined in Procedure 28-1.

Maxillary Arch Exposures

Maxillary Canines (Figure 28-34, vertical image receptor)

1. Tilt and rotate the image receptor in the holder, place it in the patient's oral cavity, and position it away from the lingual surfaces. The receptor is placed in the oral cavity directly behind the center of the canine and toward the midline of the oral cavity.

(Continues)

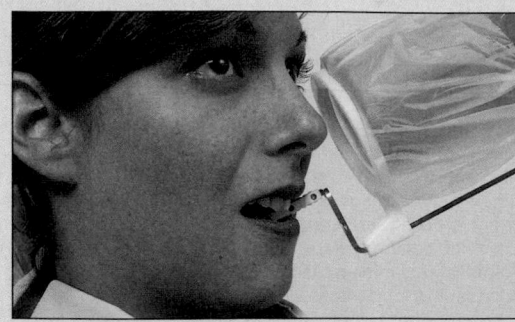

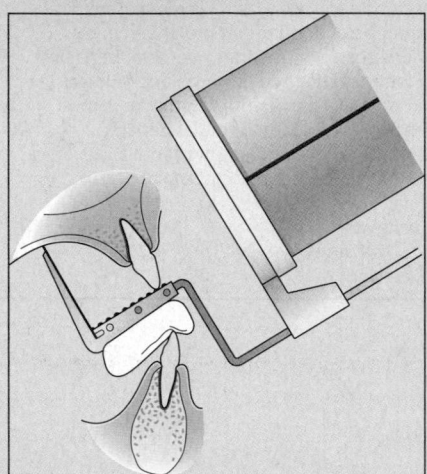

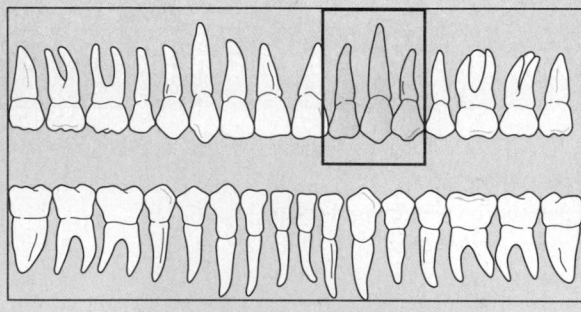

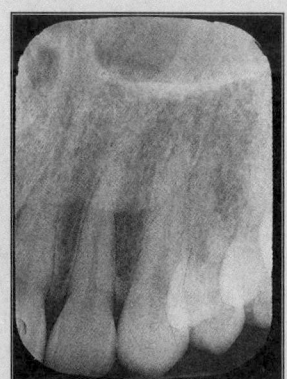

FIGURE 28-34
Maxillary canines.

2. Ask the patient to close slowly and center the canine on the bite block. Holding the metal rod, slide the positioning ring toward the patient's face.

3. Position the PID parallel to the metal indicating rod and place it flush with the positioning ring. This directs the central ray perpendicular to the image receptor.

4. The receptor and the long axis of the tooth are parallel so that the central ray will be directed perpendicular to the image receptor. Because of the curvature of the maxillary arch, the distal sides of the canine are overlapping the first premolar on many canine radiographs. The central ray is directed at the center of the canine.

Maxillary Incisors (Figure 28-35, vertical image receptor)

1. Bring the tubehead near the area of exposure.

2. Tilt the holder and rotate it into the patient's oral cavity. Position it in the oral cavity away from the lingual surfaces and center it behind the central incisors. Ask the patient to close slowly and evenly on the bite block.

3. Holding on to the metal rod, slide the positioning ring close to the patient's face. Position the PID parallel to the metal indicating rod and place it flush with the positioning ring. This directs the central ray perpendicular to the image receptor.

4. The incisal edges rest on the flat portion of the bite block.

5. The diagram shows the receptor, tooth, positioning ring, and open end of the cone parallel to each other. The central ray will be perpendicular to the image receptor. A size 2 receptor will capture all four incisors. The teeth are centered on the radiograph, showing the apices, roots, and crowns. The bite block may be seen as a radiopaque area on the image near the incisal edge of the teeth.

CHAPTER 28 Dental Radiology Infection Control, Exposure, Processing and Evaluation of
Dental Radiographs, and Mounting of Dental Radiographs

861

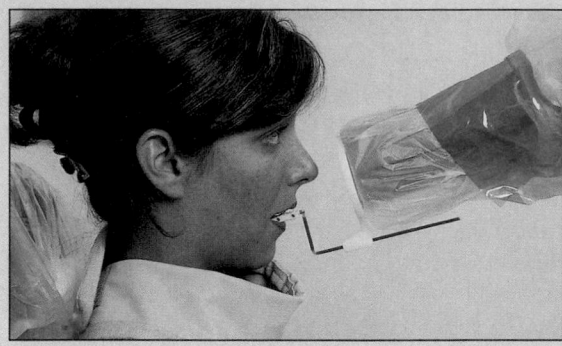

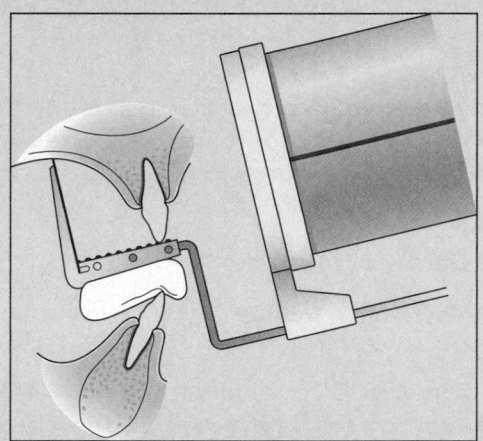

Maxillary Premolars (Figure 28-36, horizontal image receptor)

1. For the maxillary premolars, rotate the image receptor into the patient's oral cavity and position it away from the lingual surfaces, toward the middle of the palate.

2. Place the anterior edge of the receptor behind the middle of the canine to ensure that the receptor will cover the area of the two premolars as well as the distal of the canine.

3. While keeping the holder in place, have the patient close slowly on the bite block. Hold the metal rod and slide the positioning ring toward the patient's face.

4. Position the PID parallel to the metal indicating rod and place it flush with the positioning ring. This directs the central ray perpendicular to the image receptor. Note that the angle of the receptor and the holder is positioned so that the central ray will pass through the contact point of the first and second premolars.

5. The bite block is centered on the premolars. On this radiograph, the distal side of the cuspid is visible, and the first and second premolars show that the contact between them is open.

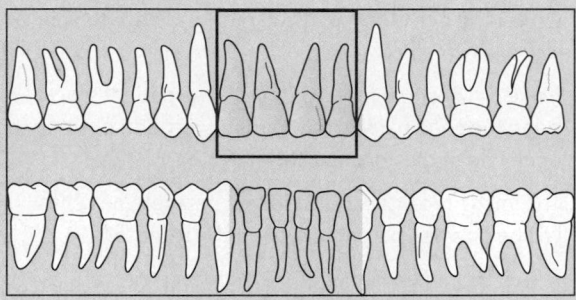

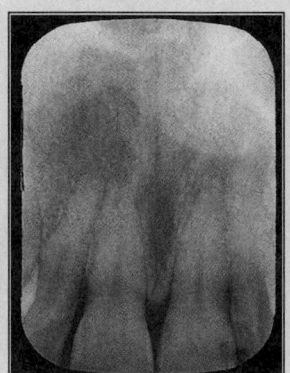

FIGURE 28-35
Maxillary incisors.

(Continues)

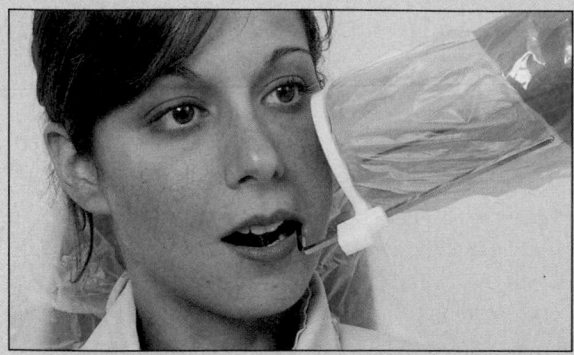

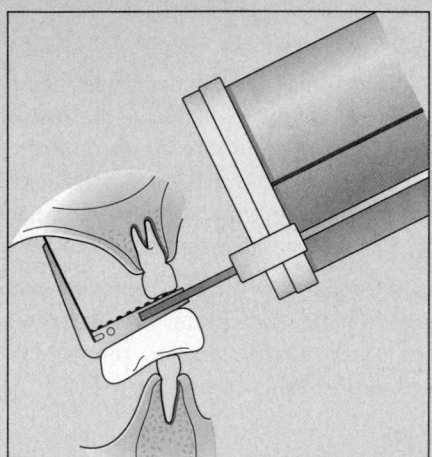

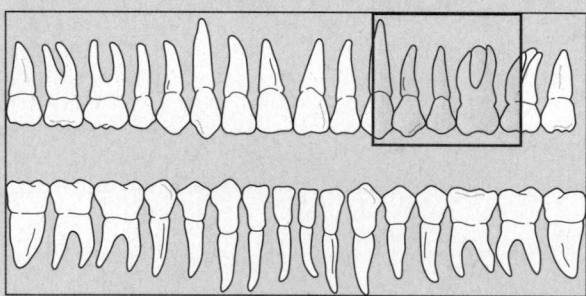

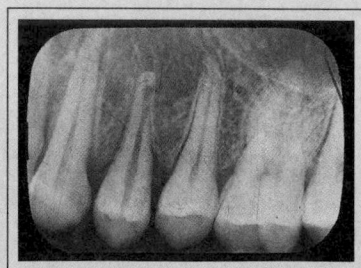

FIGURE 28-36
Maxillary premolars.

Maxillary Molars (Figure 28-37, horizontal image receptor)

1. For the maxillary molars, rotate the image receptor holder into the patient's oral cavity. Place the image receptor in the patient's surfaces of the molars.

2. Center the bite block on the second molar. Have the patient close slowly on the bite block. Hold the metal rod and slide the positioning ring toward the patient's face.

3. Position the PID parallel to the metal indicating rod and place it flush with the positioning ring. This directs the central ray perpendicular to the image receptor.

4. Figure 28-37 shows the receptor, tooth, and cone lined up for the correct direction of the central ray. This radiograph shows the open contact between the first and second molars. The distal surface of the second premolar is visible on the image.

Mandibular Arch Exposures

Mandibular Canines (Figure 28-38, vertical image receptor)

1. For the mandibular canine, rotate the receptor holder into the patient's oral cavity and position the image receptor away from the lingual surfaces.

2. Center the bite block on the canine and have the patient slowly close.

3. Move the positioning ring close to the patient's face, bring the cone parallel to the metal rod, and position the open end of the cone flat with the ring.

4. The image receptor and tooth are parallel. The central ray will be directed perpendicular to the receptor.

5. In the diagram in Figure 28-38, the receptor is angled on the center of the canine. Place the receptor in the floor of the oral cavity; the tongue should be behind the image receptor. The receptor should be between the tongue and the lingual alveolar bone.

CHAPTER 28 Dental Radiology Infection Control, Exposure, Processing and Evaluation of
Dental Radiographs, and Mounting of Dental Radiographs

863

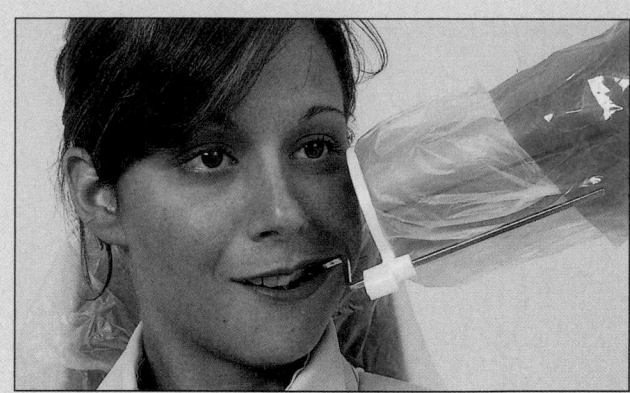

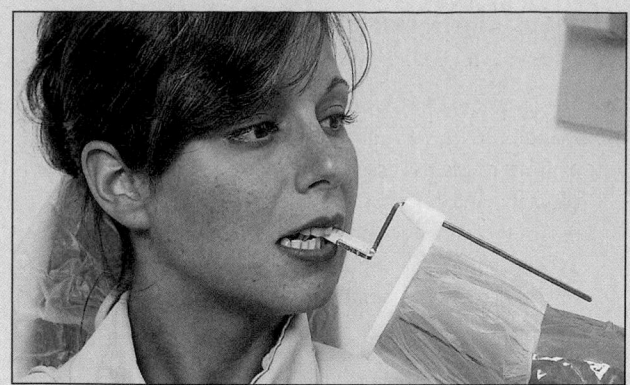

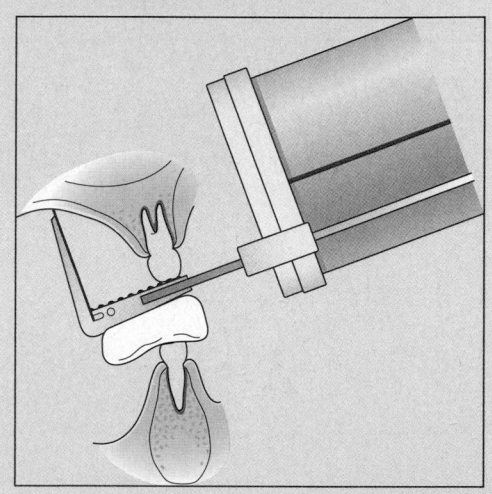

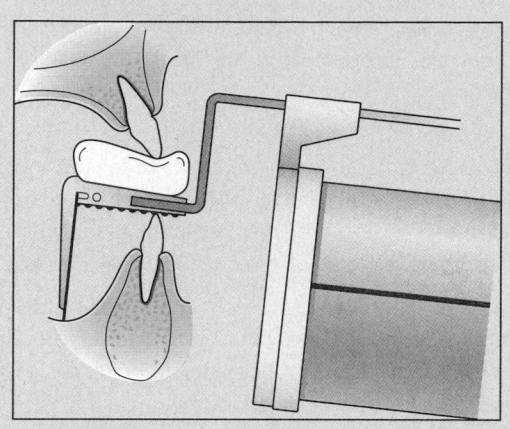

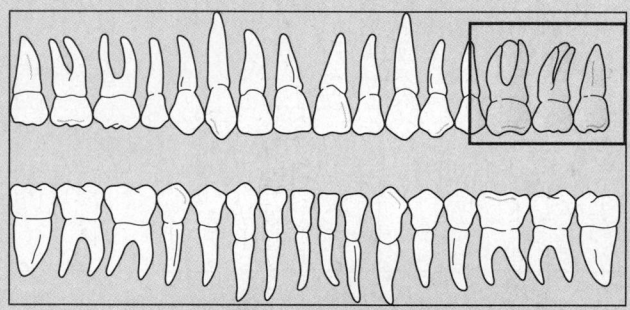

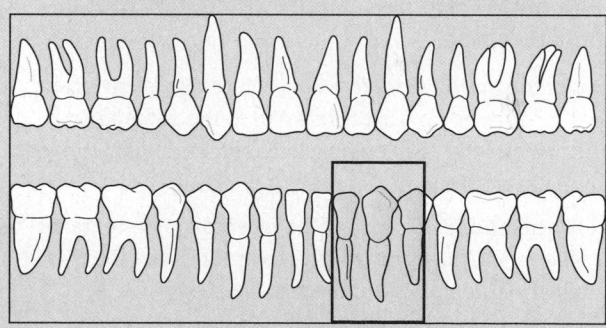

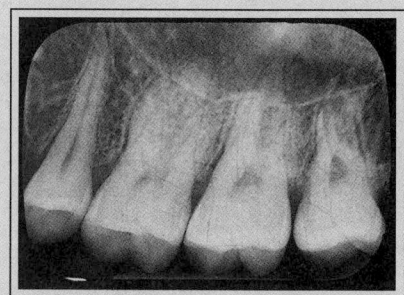

FIGURE 28-37
Maxillary molars.

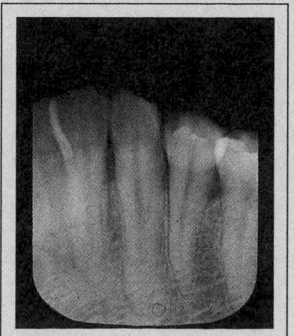

FIGURE 28-38
Mandibular canines.

(Continues)

Mandibular Incisors (Figure 28-39, vertical image receptor)

1. The anterior XCP is assembled in the same way for mandibular and maxillary positions. For the mandibular incisors, rotate the assembled image receptor holder and place it in the patient's oral cavity, gently pressing the receptor on the floor of the oral cavity behind the incisors and away from the lingual surface. The receptor should be between the tongue and the lingual alveolar bone.

2. Ask the patient to close slowly on the bite block. Holding the metal rod, slide the positioning ring close to the patient's face.

3. Bring the PID close and place the cone parallel to the metal rod. The open end of the PID should be flush with the ring.

4. The diagram in Figure 28-39 shows how far the receptor needs to be placed in the oral cavity to see the entire length of the tooth. The tongue is moved posteriorly when the receptor is being placed. The mandibular incisors are centered on the bite block.

5. The central ray is directed between the two central incisors through open contact areas. The curve of the arch will cause some overlapping on the distal sides of the lateral incisors.

Mandibular Premolars (Figure 28-40, horizontal image receptor)

1. For the mandibular premolars, rotate the image receptor holder and place the receptor in the patient's oral cavity, gently positioning it between the lingual surface of the teeth and the tongue.

2. Place the anterior edge of the receptor at the center of the canine to ensure that the receptor covers the area of the two premolars and the distal of the canine.

3. Ask the patient to close on the bite block.

4. Note the position of the receptor as it is placed in the space between the tongue and the mandibular arch.

5. The receptor and teeth are parallel. The first and second premolars are seen on the image with the contact points open along with the distal of the canine.

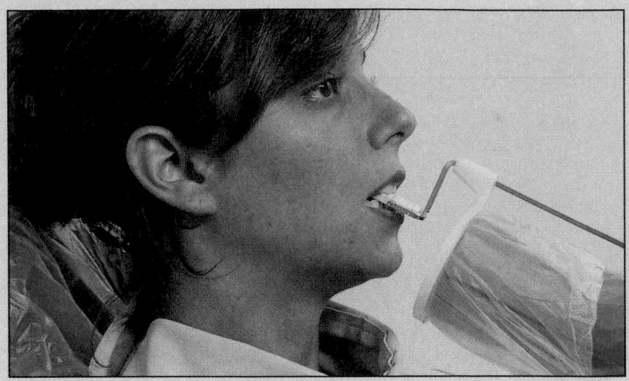

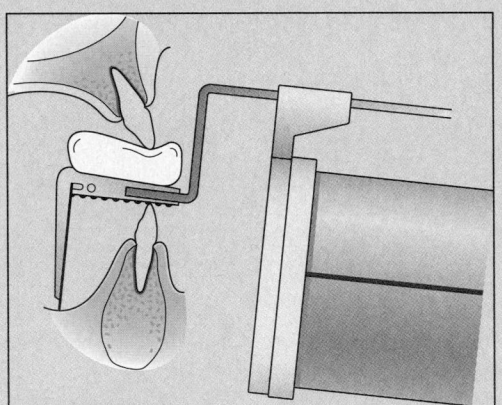

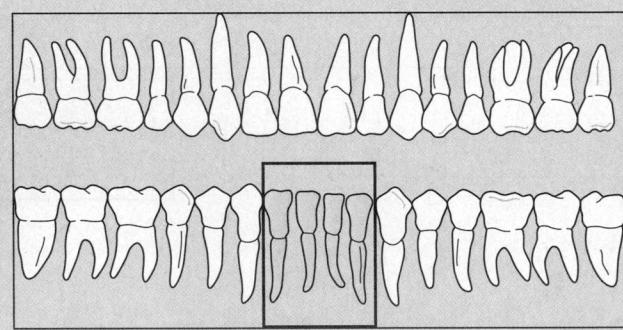

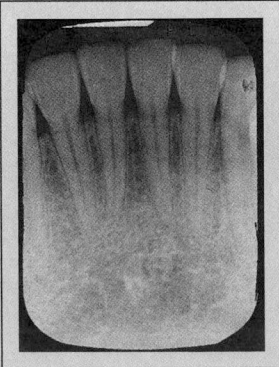

FIGURE 28-39
Mandibular incisors.

CHAPTER 28 Dental Radiology Infection Control, Exposure, Processing and Evaluation of
Dental Radiographs, and Mounting of Dental Radiographs

865

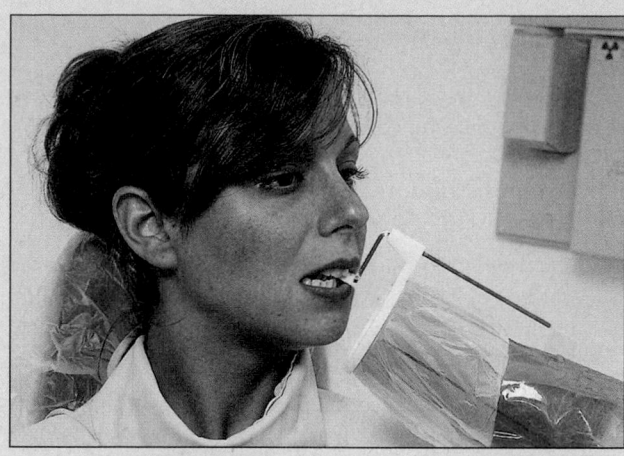

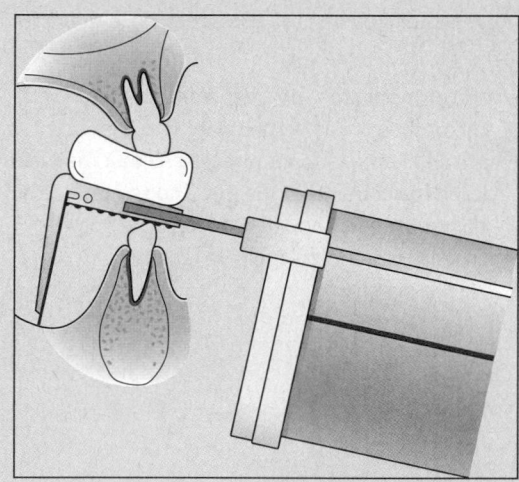

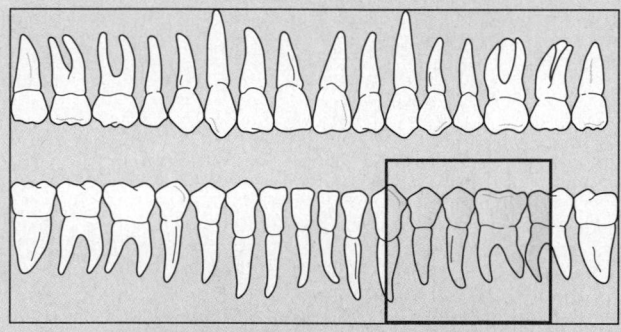

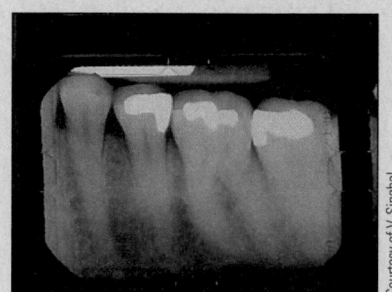

FIGURE 28-40
Mandibular premolars.

Courtesy of V. Singhal

Mandibular Molars (Figure 28-41, horizontal image receptor)

1. For the mandibular molars, rotate the image receptor holder into the patient's oral cavity, positioning it between the tongue and the lingual surfaces of the teeth.

2. Center the bite block over the second molar. Hold it in the desired position, and ask the patient to gently close.

3. Gently place the patient's cheek over the bite block.

4. Align the positioning ring flush to the patient's face. Align the PID flush with the ring of the XCP and ensure that it is parallel to the rod of the XCP.

5. Note how close the image receptor is to the lingual surface. The image receptor should be between the tongue and the lingual surfaces of the teeth.

6. The first, second, and third molars are seen on this image with the contacts open. The third molar may not be erupted into the oral cavity, but it will be visible on the image.

7. During placement, to prevent the receptor and receptor holder from moving forward, hold the bite block in position until the patient closes firmly on it.

Bitewing Exposures

To position bitewing radiographs when using the paralleling technique, a bitewing XCP instrument is used (Figure 28-29B).

Horizontal Premolar Bitewing Exposures (Figure 28-42)

1. Be sure the image receptor is centered in the bitewing holder.

2. The drawing and radiograph in Figure 28-42 illustrates the position of the image receptor covering the premolars, with the front edge of the receptor aligned with the middle of the mandibular second premolar.

3. Rotate the image receptor into the oral cavity and place the receptor near the lingual surface of the teeth. Position the receptor to center the mandibular premolars in the receptor. Request the patient to close their teeth together.

4. Move the ring of the XCP close to the patient's face. Position the PID so it is flush with the ring. The cone positioning for the premolar bitewing begins with the vertical angulation set between +10° and +15°, depending on the slant of the receptor as it is positioned in the patient's oral cavity.

5. The horizontal angulation is 0°, and the PID is positioned so that the beam is aimed directly between the contacts of the premolars, and the cone is perpendicular to the receptor.

(Continues)

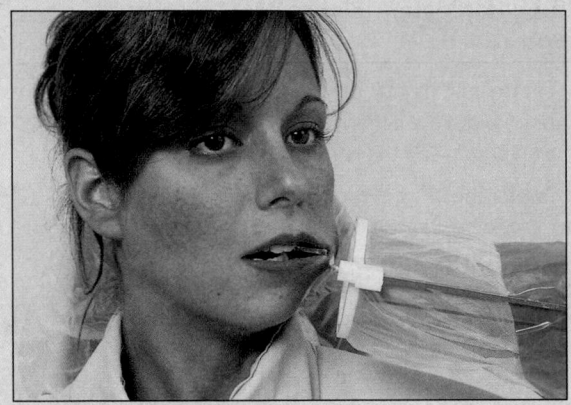

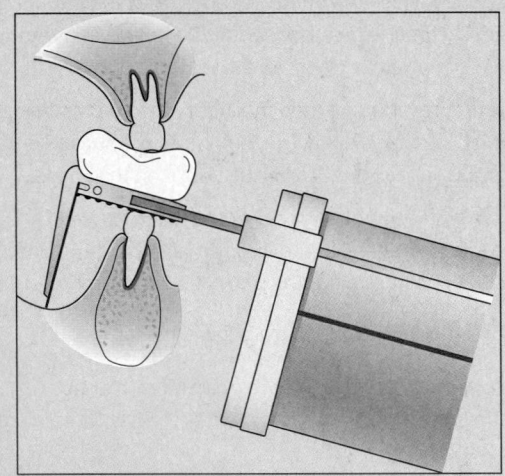

Molar Bitewing (Figure 28-47)

To position bitewing radiographs when using the paralleling technique, a bitewing XCP instrument is used (Figure 28-29B).

1. Be sure the image receptor is centered in the bitewing holder.

2. The drawing and radiograph in Figure 28-43 illustrate the position of the image receptor covering the molars, with the front edge of the receptor aligned with the middle of the second premolar.

3. Rotate the image receptor into the oral cavity and place the receptor near the lingual surface of the teeth. Position the receptor to center the mandibular second molar in the receptor. Request the patient to close their teeth together.

4. The vertical angulation for the molar bitewing is set at 0° so that the cone is perpendicular to the receptor. The horizontal angulation is directed so that the beam is between the contacts of the first and second molars. Place the cone near the patient's face, covering the receptor and perpendicular to the receptor.

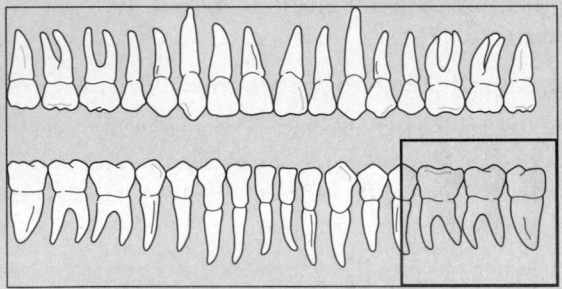

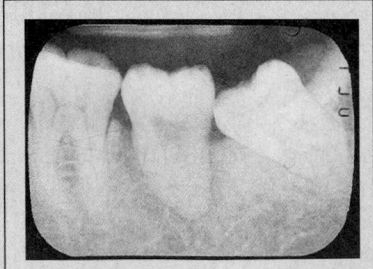

FIGURE 28-41
Mandibular molars.

CHAPTER 28 Dental Radiology Infection Control, Exposure, Processing and Evaluation of
Dental Radiographs, and Mounting of Dental Radiographs

867

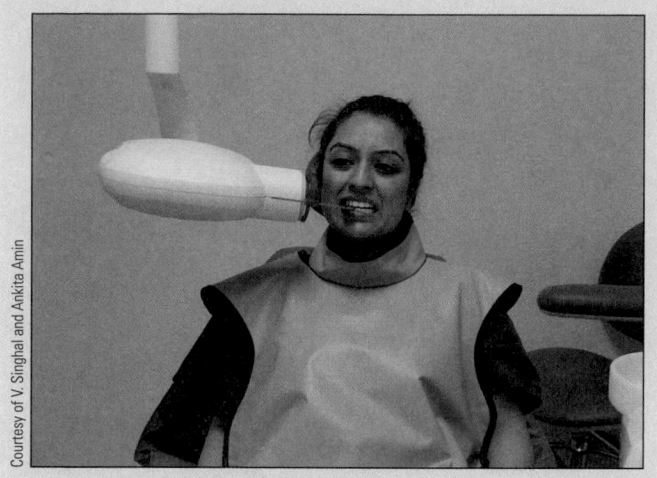

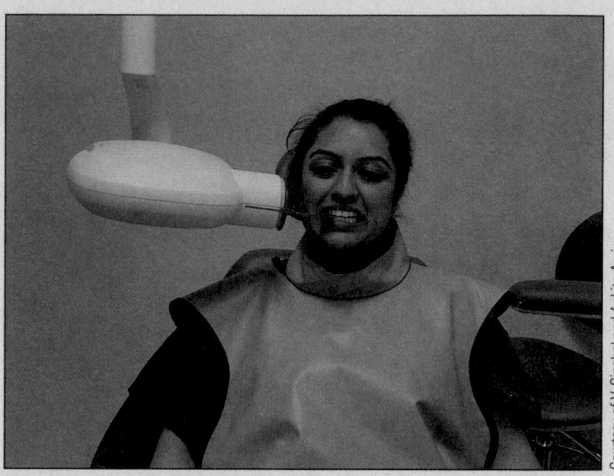

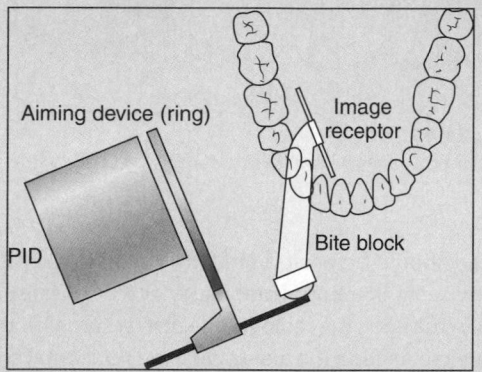

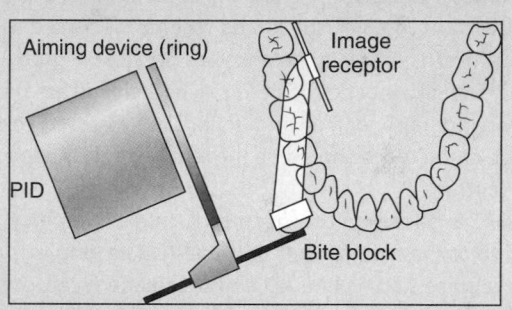

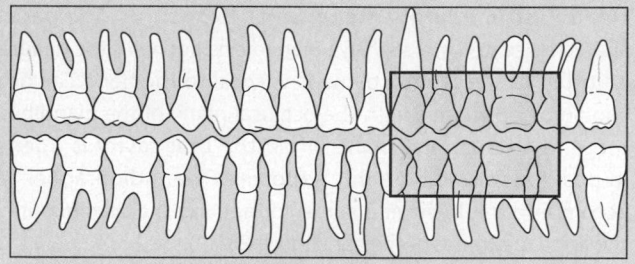

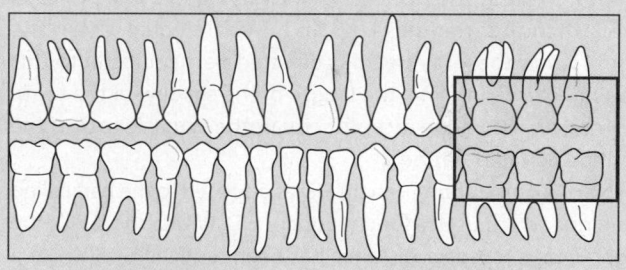

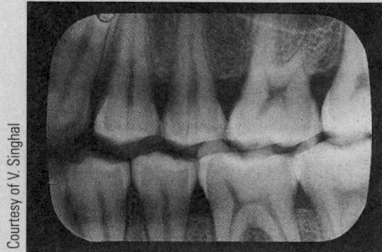

FIGURE 28-42
Horizontal premolar bitewing exposure.

FIGURE 28-43
Horizontal molar bitewing exposure.

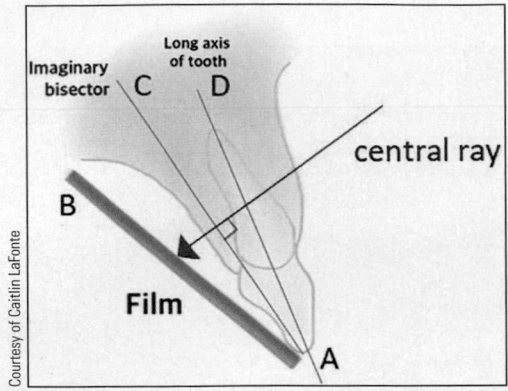

FIGURE 28-44
Position of image receptor and central ray to imaginary bisector

One difference between the paralleling and bisecting techniques is that in the BAT, the image receptor is placed as close to the tooth and area being exposed as possible (Figure 28-44). With BAT even the most difficult to reach teeth and areas can be properly radiographed. If all angulations are assessed correctly, the image of the tooth should be the same size and shape as the original tooth.

The BAT is based on the geometric rule of isometry—also referred to as *Cieszynski's Rule of Isometry*. The long axis of the tooth is represented as line AD and the image receptor as line AB (Figure 28-44). Angle A is the point where the tooth and receptor meet at the occlusal or incisal. If angle A is bisected by AC, then the triangles DAC and CAB are equal. When the central ray of the x-ray beam is directed perpendicular to this imaginary bisecting line, the length of the shadow of the tooth recorded on the image receptor equals the actual length of the tooth being radiographed.

The BAT uses a short (8-inch) PID as opposed to the paralleling technique which uses a long (16-inch) PID. With a short PID, the target–image receptor distance has been reduced by 50%. As a result, the image is magnified because the beam diverges more as it exits the 8-inch PID (Figure 28-45).

Factors Affecting Bisecting the Angle Technique

Several factors must be considered in exposing radiographs using the BAT technique: head position, exposure time, image receptor position and placement, vertical angulation, horizontal angulation, and central ray point of entry.

Head Position The head position is critical when using the BAT; PID vertical angulations ranges have been established using proper head position and image receptor placement. There are precise head positions for the maxillary and mandibular periapical exposures and bitewings.

Head Position during Maxillary Exposures The patient should be seated in the upright position with the headrest adjusted so the midsagittal plane is vertical and perpendicular to the floor.

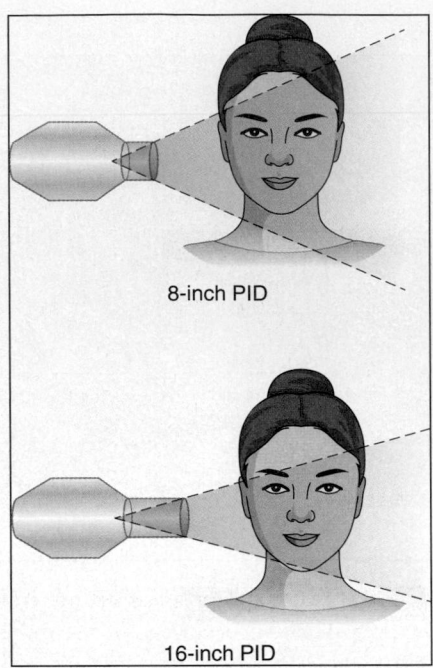

FIGURE 28-45
Magnification of image with an 8-inch PID due to beam divergence.

The head should be positioned with the occlusal plane of the maxillary teeth in a horizontal plane; the occlusal surfaces are parallel to the floor. The radiographer can accomplish this by having a line connecting the ala–tragus line horizontal and parallel to the floor (Figure 28-46).

Head Position during Mandibular Exposures The patient should be seated in a slightly reclined position with the headrest adjusted so the sagittal plane is vertical to the floor. The head should be positioned with the occlusal plane of the mandibular teeth in a horizontal plane when the oral cavity is opened in position for radiographic exposure. The radiographer can accomplish this by having a line connecting the commissure of the lip to the tragus of the ear (Figure 28-47).

Exposure Time The exposure time is dependent on the area being radiographed, image receptor speed, kVp, mA, and

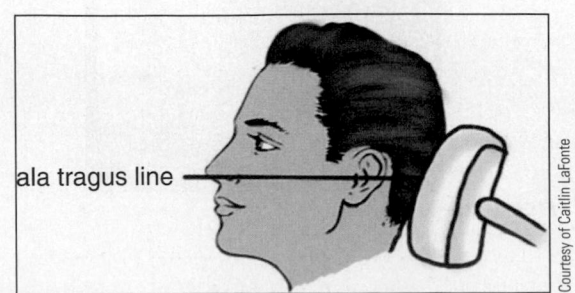

FIGURE 28-46
Head position for maxillary exposures when using the bisecting technique.

CHAPTER 28 Dental Radiology Infection Control, Exposure, Processing and Evaluation of
Dental Radiographs, and Mounting of Dental Radiographs

869

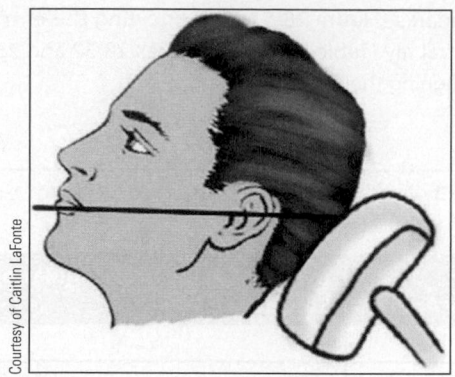

FIGURE 28-47
Head position for mandibular exposures when using the bisecting
technique.

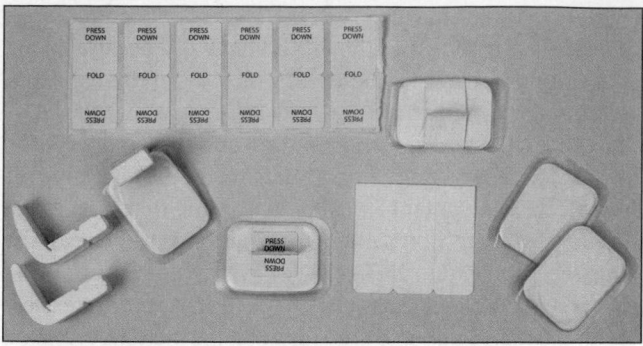

FIGURE 28-48A
Bitewing loops and tabs and disposable bite blocks.

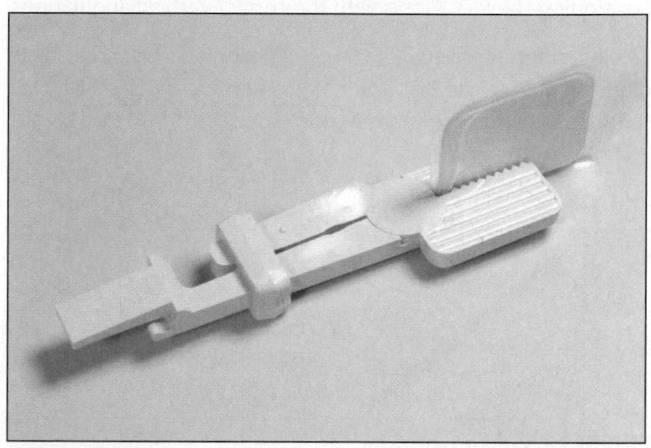

FIGURE 28-48B
Snap-A-Ray.

source to receptor distance. The times are generally shorter
with BAT than with the paralleling technique to compensate for
the decreased source to image receptor distance. The radiographer should always refer to exposure times chart established
for the specific x-ray machine determined by a radiation physicist. The timer should be set prior to placing the image receptor to limit the time the receptor must remain in the patient's
oral cavity.

Receptor Position and Placement The radiographer needs to
select the receptor necessary to expose the images prescribed by
the dentist. The proper receptor position is difficult to obtain and
maintain without a holder.

Select Receptor Holder There are many receptor holding
devices that may be used to hold the receptor using the
bisection of angle technique including disposable bite blocks,
stick-on or loop-type tabs for bitewings (Figure 28-48A), and
BAT autoclavable bite blocks that may be used with an XCP
kit or a Snap-A-Ray holder (Figure 28-48B). Similar to the
paralleling technique, the image receptor is placed vertically
in the holder for anterior placement. For posterior placement
the receptor is placed in a horizontal position. There are
receptor holders that correspond to the vertical and horizontal
placements.

Place Receptor into Holder If using a traditional image
receptor, the tube side of the packet needs to face the tooth
with the shaded side away from the source of radiation. The
embossed dot of the periapical image receptor packet should
be placed toward the occlusal/incisal surfaces for periapical
images.

Place Holder into Patient's Oral Cavity Gently place and position
the image receptor and holder in the patient's oral cavity. Place the
holder with the receptor in the oral cavity so the receptor contacts
the occlusal/incisal of the tooth. If using a bisecting bite block, place

the biting surface of the bite block against the occlusal/incisal surfaces of the teeth of interest and ask the patient to close their teeth
to hold the receptor in place. The edge of the receptor needs to
extend evenly beyond the occlusal plane by ⅛ inch to allow for
the entire tooth to be exposed along with 2–3 mm beyond the
apices of the teeth (Figure 28-49).

When using the BAT, only size 2 receptors should be used for
an adult. The adult full mouth survey (FMX) consists of 14 periapical images (7 in each arch) and four bitewings (Figures 28-31
and 28-32). The seven periapical images in each arch consist of:

- two right and left molars images
- two right and left premolars images
- two right and left canine images
- one central/lateral incisor image

Vertical Angulation When the PID is positioned parallel to
the occlusal plane, it is on the 0 reading on the angle meter.
The suggested angulation for each area in the oral cavity is
determined by the angle of the long axis of the teeth in the

alveolar bone. For maxillary exposures, positive angulations are used. This means that the PID is above the occlusal plane and pointing downward (Figure 28-50). For mandibular exposures, negative angulations are used. This means that the PID is below the occlusal plane and pointing upward (Figure 28-50). The correct vertical angulation exists when the central ray is directed perpendicular to the imaginary line that bisects the angle formed by the long axis of the tooth and the plane of the image receptor (Figure 28-44).

Charts of the average angulation for each exposure are available for the radiographer to use in establishing the correct vertical angulation (Table 28-3). Provided the head and image receptor placement is accurate, these angulations are within a 5° range of accuracy. The radiographer should verify that this angle is perpendicular to the imaginary bisecting line and adjust as needed while positioning the PID. Along with the correct vertical angulations,

facial landmarks (Figure 28-51) and knowing the entry points for the central ray (Table 28-4 and Figures 28-52 and 28-53) are helpful in aligning the PID.

TABLE 28-3 Vertical Angulation Chart for Maxillary and Mandibular Exposures

Maxillary Arch	Average (+) Vertical Angulation Settings
incisor	+50°
canine	+45°
premolar	+30°
molar	+20°
Mandibular Arch	**Average (−) Vertical Angulation Settings**
incisor	−15°
canine	−20°
premolar	−10°
molar	−5°
Bitewings	**Average (+) Vertical Angulation Settings**
premolar	+5° to +10°
molar	+5° to +10°

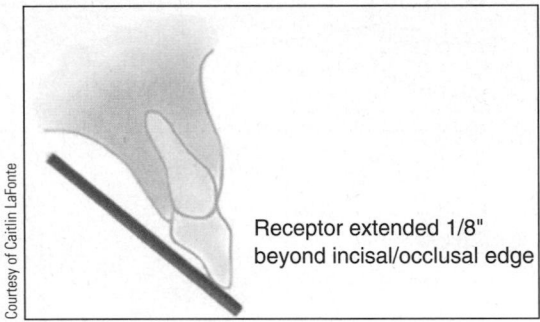

FIGURE 28-49
Image receptor should extend 1/8 inch beyond the occlusal or incisal surface of tooth being imaged.

Receptor extended 1/8" beyond incisal/occlusal edge

Courtesy of Caitlin LaFonte

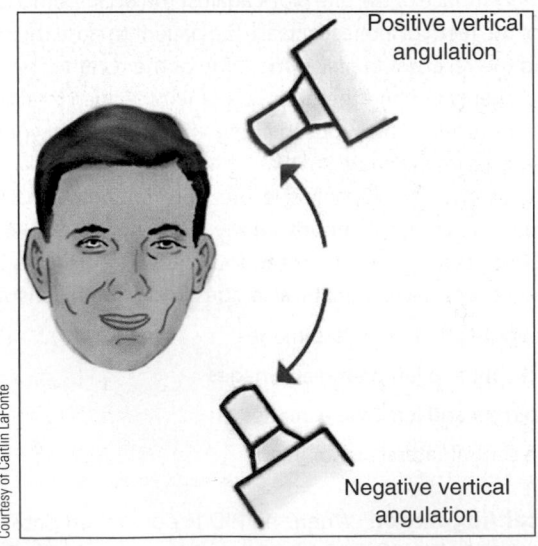

Positive vertical angulation

Negative vertical angulation

Courtesy of Caitlin LaFonte

FIGURE 28-50
Positive and negative vertical angulation of PID.

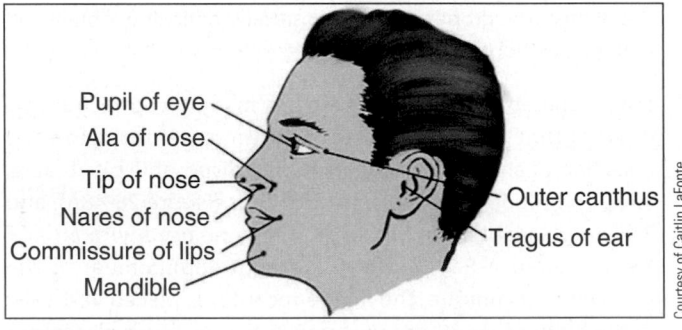

Pupil of eye
Ala of nose
Tip of nose
Nares of nose
Commissure of lips
Mandible
Outer canthus
Tragus of ear

Courtesy of Caitlin LaFonte

FIGURE 28-51
Anatomical landmarks to use during bisecting the angle exposures.

Common vertical angulation errors are elongation (Figure 28-54) and foreshortening (Figure 28-55). Elongation occurs when the CR is directed at a less-than-recommended angle. This can occur when the radiographer does not visualize the bisecting line and instead directs the CR perpendicular to the long axis of the tooth (Figure 28-54A). Foreshortening occurs when the CR is directed at too steep of an angle and/or perpendicular to the receptor (Figure 28-55). The radiographer must develop the skill of visualizing the imaginary bisecting line of the angle formed by the tooth and receptor and directing the CR perpendicular to the imaginary bisector.

CHAPTER 28 Dental Radiology Infection Control, Exposure, Processing and Evaluation of
Dental Radiographs, and Mounting of Dental Radiographs

871

TABLE 28-4 Entry Points for Maxillary and Mandibular Bisecting Images

maxillary canine	Just below the ala of the nose
maxillary incisor	Tip of the nose
maxillary premolar	Inner canthus of the eye or pupil
maxillary molar	Outer canthus of the eye
mandibular canine	A point located on the corner of the chin when a line is dropped down from the ala of the nose
mandibular incisor	Mandibular symphysis
mandibular premolar	A point on the mid-mandible area when a line is dropped down from the pupil of the eye
mandibular molar	A point on the mid-mandible area when a line is dropped down from the outer canthus of the eye
premolar bitewings	A point on the occlusal plane when a line is dropped down from the pupil of the eye
molar bitewings	A point on the occlusal plane when a line is dropped down from the outer canthus of the eye

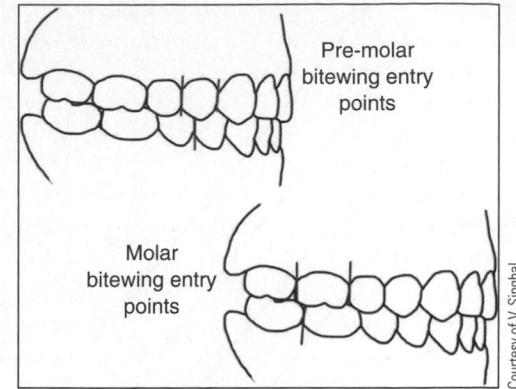

FIGURE 28-53
Central ray entry points for premolar and molar bitewings.

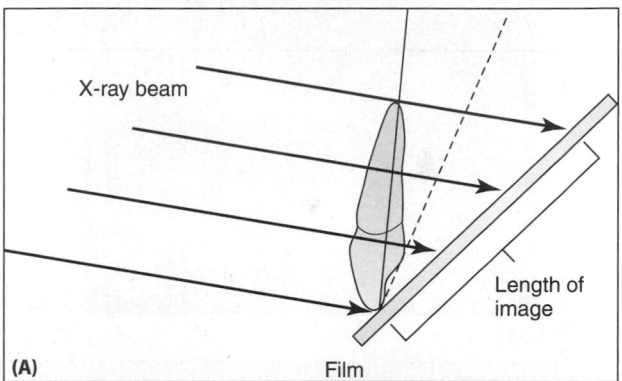

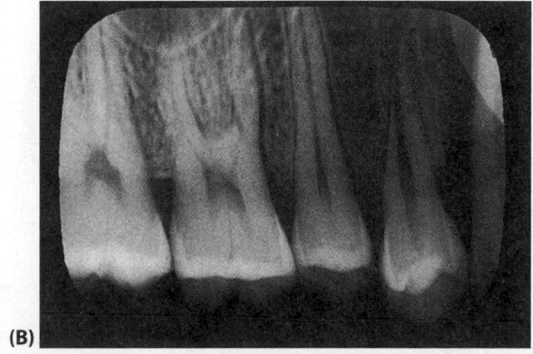

FIGURE 28-54
(A) The diagram shows how a film is elongated. (B) Elongation on a radiograph.

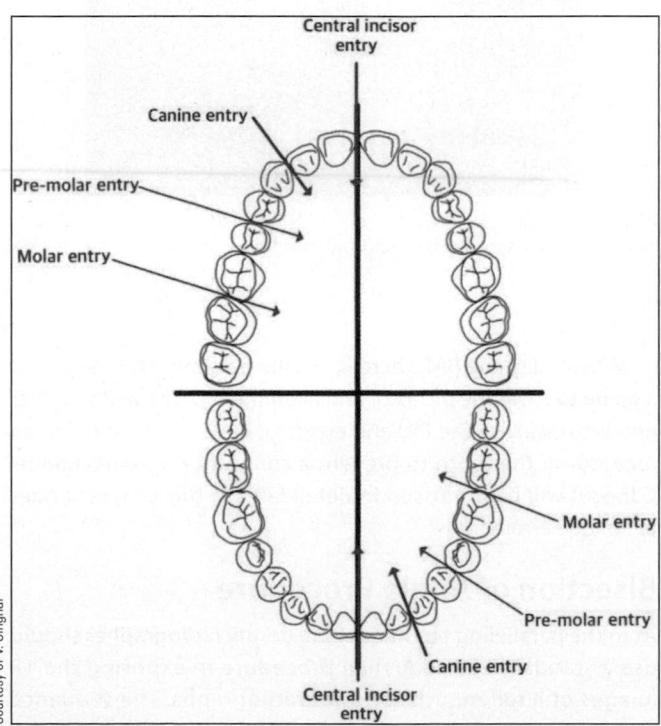

FIGURE 28-52
Central ray entry points for anterior and posterior periapical images.

Horizontal Angulation As with the paralleling technique, the PID also needs to be placed with the central ray directed perpendicular to the horizontal plane of the image receptor and teeth.

The horizontal angulation is the side-to-side movement of the machine head (Figure 28-56). The central ray must be perpendicular to the curvature of the arch and image receptor. When the horizontal angulation is correct, "open contacts" or a thin black line between the teeth will be visible (Figure 28-57). This allows viewing of the interproximal areas and existing decay without overlap. Overlap occurs when the surfaces of adjacent teeth are superimposed over one another when the radiographer fails to

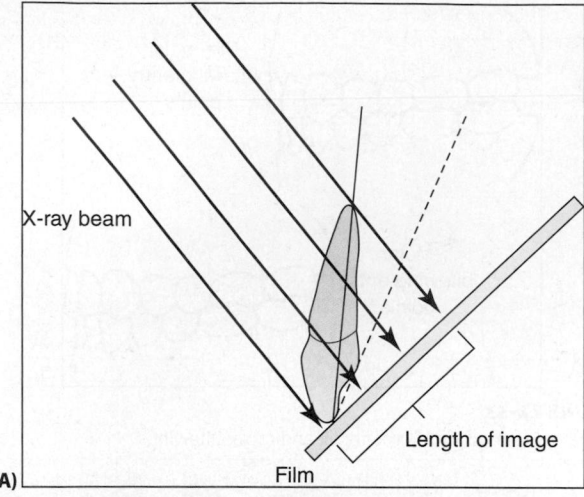

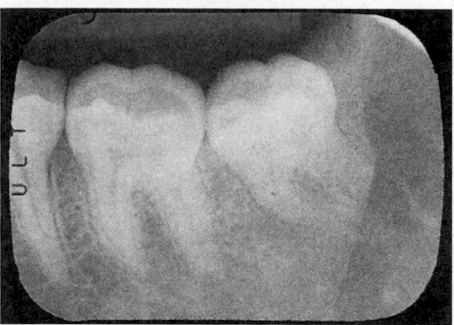

FIGURE 28-55
(A) The diagram shows how a film is foreshortened. (B) Foreshortening on a radiograph.

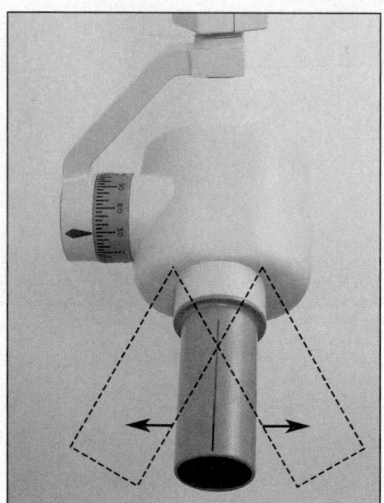

FIGURE 28-56
Example of cone positioning for horizontal angulation (left and right rotation).

place the horizontal line perpendicular to the arch curvature and the image receptor (Figure 28-58). Open contacts are critical for horizontal bitewing images. Overlapped interproximal areas on horizontal bitewing images result in a nondiagnostic image.

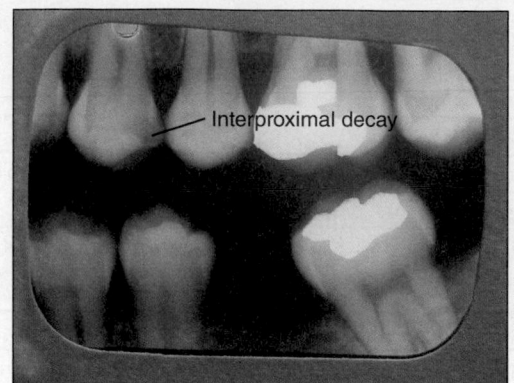

FIGURE 28-57
Horizontal bitewing with open contacts and interproximal decay visible.

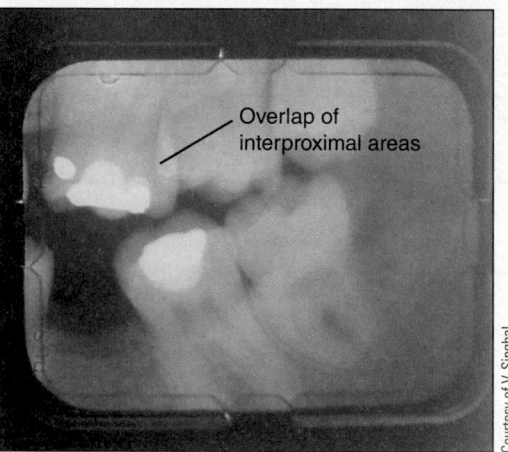

FIGURE 28-58
Nondiagnostic horizontal bitewing with overlap in interproximal areas.

When using the BAT, there is usually no aiming ring to use as a guide to cover the receptor and align the PID. The radiographer needs to visualize the PID and ensure it covers the entire image receptor of the tooth to prevent a *conecut* or a partial image. Conecut will be discussed in detail later in this chapter under technique errors.

Bisection of Angle Procedure

As in the paralleling technique, the dental radiographer should use a standardized sequence procedure in exposing the 18 images of a full mouth series of radiographs. The sequence of exposures is slightly different than that used for exposure of a full mouth series of radiographs when the paralleling technique is used. This is because there is no XCP, and as a result, disassembly and reassembly of the XCP for the posterior areas are not required. Table 28-5 outlines the sequence to be used for exposure of an FMX using the BAT. If done correctly, the images that are produced by the BAT technique should appear the same as those that are produced by the paralleling technique. Refer to Procedure 28-2 for radiographic images for each of the areas described below in Procedure 28-3.

CHAPTER 28 Dental Radiology Infection Control, Exposure, Processing and Evaluation of Dental Radiographs, and Mounting of Dental Radiographs

873

TABLE 28-5 Exposure Sequence for an Adult Full Mouth Series When Using the Bisecting Technique

Maxillary right canine periapical
Maxillary incisor periapical
Maxilary left canine periapical
Mandibular left canine periapical
Mandibular incisor periapical
Mandibular right canine periapical
Maxillary right premolar and molar periapical
Mandibular right premolar and molar periapical
Maxillary left premolar and molar periapical
Mandibular left premolar and molar periapical
Left premolar and molar bitewings
Right premolar and molar bitewings

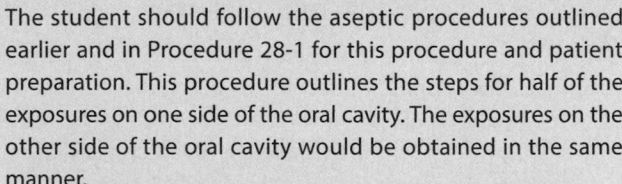

Procedure 28-3
Full Mouth Series Exposure with Bisecting-the-Angle Technique

The student should follow the aseptic procedures outlined earlier and in Procedure 28-1 for this procedure and patient preparation. This procedure outlines the steps for half of the exposures on one side of the oral cavity. The exposures on the other side of the oral cavity would be obtained in the same manner.

Maxillary and Mandibular Periapical Exposures

For maxillary periapical exposures, the patient should be seated with the maxilla parallel to the floor and the midsagittal plane perpendicular to the floor (refer to Figure 28-46). For mandibular periapical exposures, the patient should be positioned so the occlusal plane of the mandibular teeth are parallel to the floor when the oral cavity is opened (refer to Figure 28-47).

Equipment and Supplies
- patient's chart
- barriers for the radiography room and equipment
- image receptor (appropriate size); if using traditional film, the appropriate number of film packets is needed
- protective sheaths if using sensors; plastic barriers for keyboard and mouse if using a digital system
- cotton rolls (optional)
- bisecting bite blocks and tabs (refer to Figures 28-48A and B)
- lead apron with thyroid collar
- container for exposed traditional film
- paper towel or tissue

Maxillary Canine Exposure
1. The receptor is placed in the vertical position in the patient's oral cavity for the anterior periapical images. The receptor is placed with the canine centered on the receptor. The incisal border of the receptor is parallel to and 1/8 inch extended past the incisal surface. The

radiographer adjusts the cone to the average vertical angulation of +45° (Figure 28-59).

2. The horizontal angulation line is directed parallel to the interproximal spaces and between the lateral incisor and the canine (see Figure 28-52). The radiographer moves the anterior of the PID to cover the mesial of the receptor and checks that the CR enters in line with the ala of the nose (see Figure 28-51).

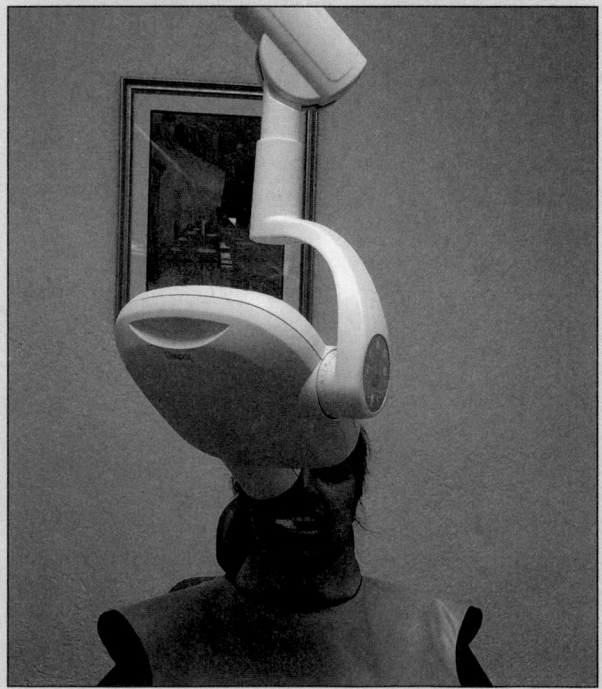

Courtesy of V. Singhal and Ankita Amin

FIGURE 28-59
Maxillary canine exposure using BAT.

(Continues)

Maxillary Incisor Exposure

1. The receptor is placed in the vertical position in the patient's oral cavity for the maxillary incisors. The receptor is placed with the central incisors centered on the receptor. The incisal border of the receptor is parallel to and ⅛ inch extended past the incisal surface. The radiographer adjusts the cone to the average vertical angulation of +50° (Figure 28-60).

2. The horizontal angulation line is directed parallel to the interproximal spaces and between the central incisors (see Figure 28-52). The radiographer moves the anterior of the PID to cover the mesial of the receptor and checks that the CR enters in line with the tip of the nose (see Figure 28-51).

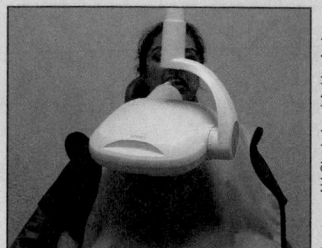

FIGURE 28-61
Mandibular canine exposure using BAT.

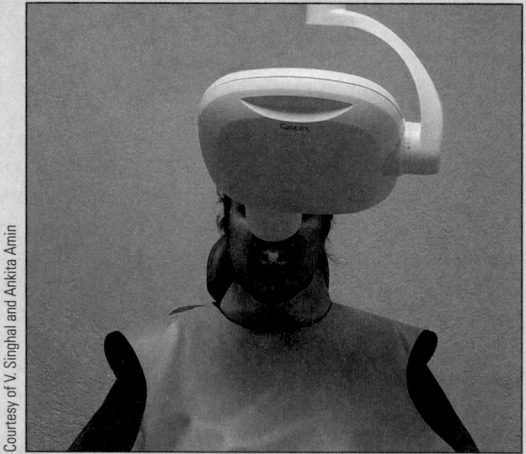

FIGURE 28-60
Maxillary incisor exposure using BAT.

Mandibular Canine Exposure

1. The image receptor is placed in the vertical position in the patient's oral cavity for the anterior periapicals. The receptor is placed with the canine centered on the receptor. The incisal border of the receptor is parallel to and ⅛ inch extended past the incisal surface. The radiographer adjusts the PID to the average vertical angulation of −20° (Figure 28-61).

2. The horizontal angulation line is directed parallel to the interproximal spaces and between the lateral incisor and the canine (see Figure 28-52). The radiographer moves the anterior of the PID to cover the mesial of the receptor and checks that the CR enters in line with a point located on the corner of the chin when a line is dropped down from the ala of the nose (see Figure 28-51). The PID is placed just apical to the CEJ, and the vertical angulation is rechecked and adjusted as needed.

Mandibular Central/Lateral Exposure

1. The image receptor is placed vertically in the patient's oral cavity. The receptor is centered over the contact points of the centrals. The incisal border of the receptor is parallel to and extends ⅛ inch beyond the incisal surface. The radiographer adjusts the PID to the average vertical angulation of −15° (Figure 28-62).

2. The horizontal angulation line is directed parallel to the interproximal spaces and between the central incisors (see Figure 28-52). The radiographer moves the anterior of the PID to cover the mesial of the receptor and checks that the CR enters in line with the tip of the center of the chin on the mandible (see Figure 28-51).

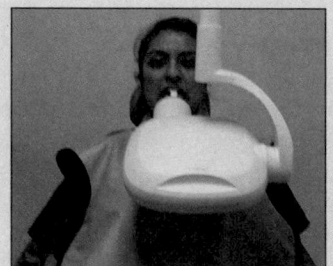

FIGURE 28-62
Mandibular incisor exposure using BAT.

Maxillary Bicuspid Exposure

1. The receptor is placed horizontally in the patient's oral cavity covering the distal half of the canine. The contact point of the first molar and the second bicuspid is in the center of the receptor. The occlusal border of the receptor is parallel to and ⅛ inch extended beyond the occlusal surface. The radiographer adjusts the cone to the average vertical angulation of +30° (Figure 28-63).

CHAPTER 28 Dental Radiology Infection Control, Exposure, Processing and Evaluation of
Dental Radiographs, and Mounting of Dental Radiographs

875

2. The horizontal angulation line is directed parallel to the interproximal spaces and between the first and second premolars (see Figure 28-52). The radiographer moves the anterior of the PID to cover the mesial of the receptor and checks that the CR enters in line with the inner canthus of the eye (see Figure 28-51).

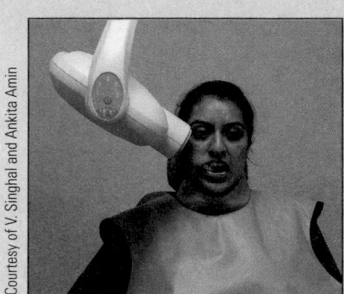

FIGURE 28-63
Maxillary premolar exposure using BAT.

Maxillary Molar Exposure

1. The image receptor is placed in the horizontal position in the patient's oral cavity for the posterior periapicals. The anterior of the receptor should cover the distal half of the second premolar to ensure exposing the mesial of the first molar. The second molar is in the center of the receptor. The occlusal border of the receptor is parallel to and ⅛ inch beyond the occlusal surface. The radiographer adjusts the PID to the average vertical angulation of +20° (Figure 28-64).

2. The horizontal angulation line is directed parallel to the interproximal spaces and between the first and second molars (see Figure 28-52). The radiographer moves the anterior of the PID to cover the mesial of the receptor and checks that the CR enters in line with the outer canthus of the eye (see Figure 28-51).

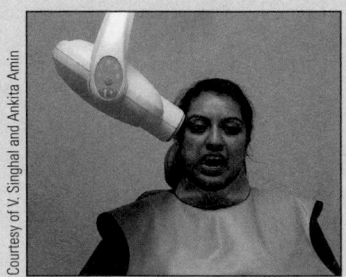

FIGURE 28-64
Maxillary molar exposure using BAT.

Mandibular Premolar Exposure

1. The receptor is placed horizontally in the patient's oral cavity covering the distal half of the canine. The contact point of the first molar and the second premolar is in the center of the receptor. The occlusal border of the receptor is parallel and ¼ inch beyond the occlusal surface. The radiographer adjusts the PID to the average vertical angulation of −10° (Figure 28-65).

2. The horizontal angulation line is directed parallel to the interproximal spaces and between the first and second premolars (see Figure 28-52). The radiographer moves the anterior of the PID to cover the mesial of the image receptor and verifies that the CR enters in line with a point on the mid-mandible area when a line is dropped down from the pupil of the eye (see Figure 28-51).

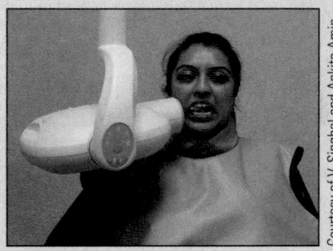

FIGURE 28-65
Mandibular premolar exposure using BAT.

Mandibular Molar Exposure

1. The receptor is placed in the horizontal position in the patient's oral cavity for the posterior periapical images. The anterior of the receptor should cover the distal half of the second premolar to ensure exposing the mesial of the first molar. The second molar is in the center of the image receptor. The occlusal border of the receptor is parallel to and ⅛ inch beyond the occlusal surface. The radiographer adjusts the PID to the average vertical angulation of −5° (Figure 28-66).

2. The horizontal angulation line is directed parallel to the interproximal spaces and between the first and second molars (see Figure 28-52). The radiographer moves the anterior of the PID to cover the mesial of the receptor and checks that the CR enters in line with a point on the mid-mandible area when a line is dropped down from the outer canthus of the eye (see Figure 28-51).

(Continues)

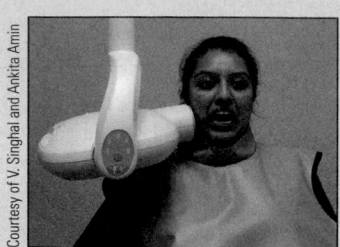

FIGURE 28-66
Mandibular premolar exposure using BAT.

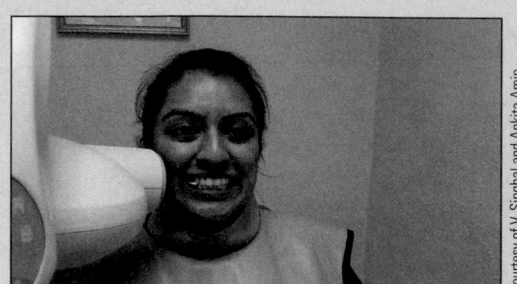

FIGURE 28-68
Premolar bitewing exposure with tabs using BAT.

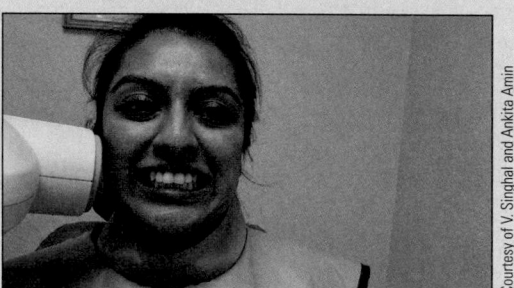

FIGURE 28-69
Molar bitewing exposure with tabs using BAT.

Bitewing Exposures

1. When using the bisection of angle technique to expose bitewings, a bitewing tab attached to the traditional film is used to position and hold the tooth in place during exposure (see Figure 28-48A). The patient is placed in the same position for maxillary periapical images with the patient sitting in the upright position with the ala–tragus line parallel to the floor (see Figure 28-46). The receptor is placed parallel to the teeth, and the central ray (CR) is directed perpendicular to the teeth and image receptor as with the paralleling technique (Figure 28-67). The vertical angulation is set at +10°.

2. The radiographer aligns the CR of the primary beam parallel to the interproximal of the premolars for the premolar bitewing (see Figures 28-53, 28-67, and 28-68) and parallel to the interproximal to either side of the second molar (see Figures 28-53, 28-67, and 28-69). The PID is placed just mesial to the edge of the receptor making certain the receptor is completely covered by the cone.

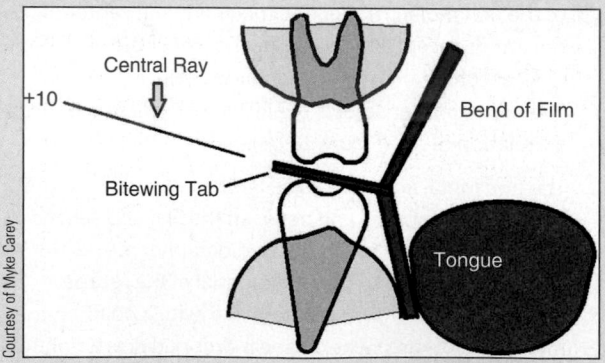

FIGURE 28-67
Bitewing exposure, central ray angulation, and placement of tab using BAT.

CHAPTER 28 Dental Radiology Infection Control, Exposure, Processing and Evaluation of Dental Radiographs, and Mounting of Dental Radiographs

877

Comparison of BAT and Paralleling Techniques

The BAT and paralleling techniques are two very different methods the radiographer can use to obtain images under a variety of conditions. Both techniques give the radiographer a larger tool box to choose from when presented with challenges in obtaining an accurate image.

The paralleling method is preferred and should be used unless contraindicated. The paralleling technique can produce an image with significantly less distortion and can be repeated for future comparison of a particular area. The paralleling technique can produce a more accurate image in terms of the size and shape of the tooth and other anatomical structures.

Theoretically, the BAT should be able to produce images that are equal in quality to those produced by the paralleling method. However, the BAT produces inferior images due to the distortion and magnification inherent in this technique. Additionally, it is difficult to duplicate the procedure exactly for a particular area for future comparison. Although the bisection of the angle is more difficult for the radiographer because the imaginary bisector is difficult to assess, there is still a need for the radiographer to become skilled in this technique for situations when an image cannot be obtained using the paralleling technique. The XCP instruments are uncomfortable for some patients and may contraindicate the use of the paralleling technique. The BAT may also be needed to expose a third molar that has not fully erupted. In many cases, the image receptor and paralleling XCP cannot be positioned distal enough in the oral cavity to capture the area in the image. A successful radiographer is a skilled technician in both dental radiography techniques.

Critique of Radiographs

When a radiographer obtains an image, the images are a reflection on the quality of care given to a patient. Without quality images a dentist cannot prescribe the correct treatment for the patient; poor quality radiographs may result in retaking the image and unnecessary exposure of the patient to radiation. The radiographer must focus on producing the best quality image with the least amount of exposure to the patient and make the first exposure the best exposure.

In order to produce quality diagnostic radiographs, the dental radiographer needs to be able to evaluate the images and recognize radiographs that meet criteria and those that contain errors. The radiographer should be able to identify the cause of the errors, correct the errors, and improve the exposing technique. A good quality image is based on:

- proper exposure technique
- patient cooperation
- proper processing procedure
- radiology equipment that is functioning properly
- image receptor quality

This section will focus on technique errors. Processing errors will be discussed later in this chapter.

Common Technique Errors

The exposure errors made by the radiographer may be due to improper use of the XCP instruments, incorrect receptor placement, or errors in angulation.

Errors in Assembling XCP Instruments There are several errors that may occur that are due to incorrect assembly of the XCP instruments and/or placement of the receptor into the bite block. The radiographer must ensure that for each XCP kit, the proper ring, arm, and bite block have been selected. Use of one incorrect component will result in improper assembly and nondiagnostic images. When assembling the XCP kits, the radiographer must also check to ensure that the bite block is completely visible through the ring. If it is only partially visible, a conecut will result.

Conecut The radiographer should always look through the ring and make certain that the receptor holder and receptor are in the center of the ring. If the ring is not covering the receptor, the PID placed in line with the ring will not expose all of the receptor and result in a *conecut*. In the paralleling technique, this is more common with the posterior XCP assembly because the handle on the aiming ring is off center (Figure 28-70A). The operator must be sure to hold the XCP straight out in front to ensure that the bite block is completely visible through the aiming ring. If the XCP is not assembled properly and the bite block is only partially visible, part of the image will be cut off. This is also referred to as conecutting (Figure 28-70B). Conecutting can also be caused by exposing procedure. This may also occur if the PID is not lined up completely flush with the aiming ring, the ring is not flush to the face, or the PID drifts once the operator leaves the exposure area.

Errors in Image Receptor Placement Improper placement of the image receptor using the XCP receptor devices can result in nondiagnostic images.

Parallelism In the paralleling technique, the image receptor must be parallel to the tooth in order to place the vertical angulation parallel to the long axis of the tooth and the receptor (Figure 28-19). In order to achieve this, the image receptor and bite block must be placed at a distance from the tooth or teeth to be exposed. Without parallelism, distortion such as elongation or foreshortening will result (Figures 28-54 and 28-55).

Embossed Dot of Traditional Film Not Properly Oriented The embossed dot on a traditional film packet is primarily used for ease in mounting of traditional films. Improper placement of the dot may also block important structures on the images. The dot should be placed toward the occlusal/incisal for all periapical images. If the dot is placed so that it appears at the apices of the teeth in the image, it may block the apical area of a tooth and make diagnosis difficult (Figure 28-71).

Reversed Placement of Traditional Film This error occurs when the traditional film is exposed with the wrong side of the packet facing the tube. In this position, the lead foil backing

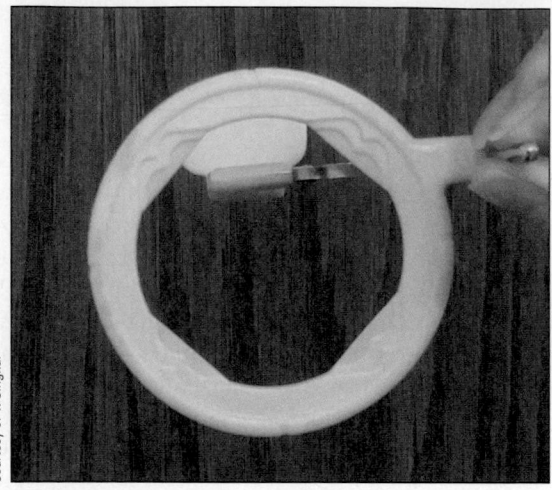

Courtesy of V. Singhal

FIGURE 28-70A
Incorrectly assembled XCP would result in conecut, or bite block not fully visible through aiming ring.

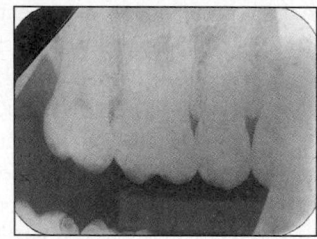

FIGURE 28-70B
Image of conecut film as well as cut off of apical areas.

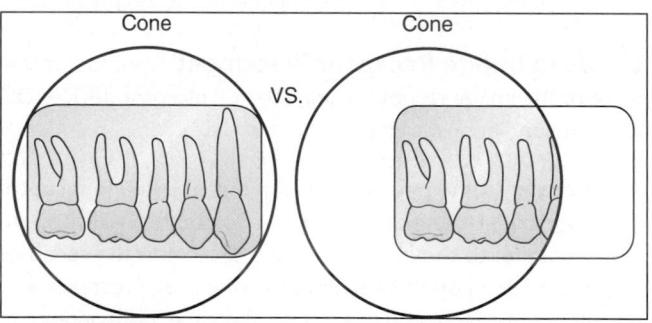

FIGURE 28-70C
Correct and incorrect placement of PID resulting in conecut.

prevents some rays from reaching the film. The image appears lighter than normal, and the embossed dot is concave from the labial view. Some images show a pattern of dark marks called a *herringbone pattern* due to a pattern imprinted on the lead foil (Figure 28-72).

Vertical Angulation Errors
The vertical angulation is the up and down positioning of the PID. When using the paralleling technique, the image receptor and tooth are parallel in the patient's oral cavity and the vertical angulation is directed at a right angle to the image receptor and tooth. With the correct image receptor placement and vertical angulation, the

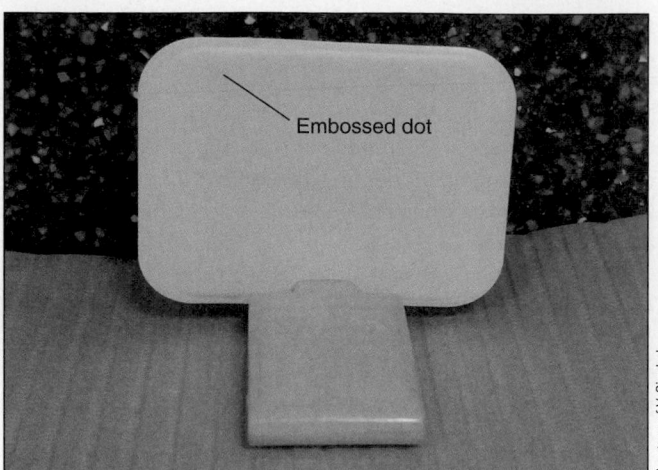

Embossed dot

Courtesy of V. Singhal

FIGURE 28-71
Embossed dot of traditional film not placed in slot of bite block.

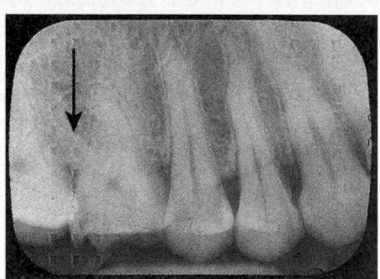

FIGURE 28-72
Reversed film with herringbone pattern of lead foil.

radiographer can obtain an image that is equal in size and shape to the structure being exposed.

The image receptor holder with the bite block is designed to maintain the receptor in the oral cavity parallel to the long axis of the tooth. The indicator rod is attached to the holder and indicates at what position the vertical angulation is at a right angle to the image receptor and the tooth. The vertical angulation of the x-ray beam is designated by the grooved lines on the side of the PID. The radiographer can easily direct the vertical angulation at a right angle to the image receptor and tooth by placing the side lines of the PID parallel to the indicator rod. Improper image receptor placement and vertical angulation may result in a distortion of the object. Distortion occurs when a part of the object in the image is larger or smaller than it should be but the remainder of the image is correct in proportion (Figure 28-73). Distortion usually occurs when the traditional film is used and it bends when placed in the oral cavity.

Elongation Occurs when the PID is placed at a lower angle than the indicator rod (angulation is decreased). The image is longer than the actual object. This is more common in the bisecting technique (Figure 28-54).

Foreshortening Occurs when the PID is placed at a greater angle than the indicator rod. The image is shorter than the actual object, like the shadow when the sun is high noon. This is more common in the bisecting angle technique (Figure 28-55).

CHAPTER 28 Dental Radiology Infection Control, Exposure, Processing and Evaluation of
Dental Radiographs, and Mounting of Dental Radiographs

879

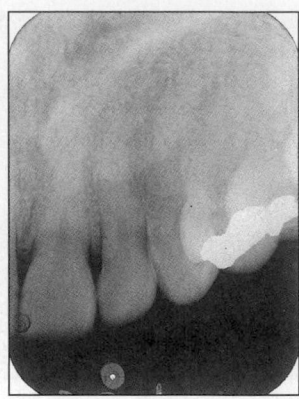

FIGURE 28-73
A curved film distorts radiograph images.

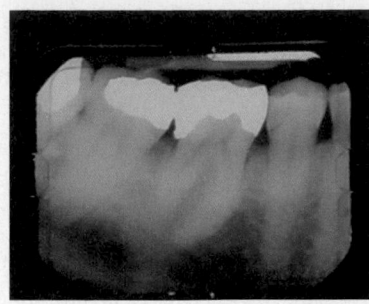

FIGURE 28-74
Poor placement of image receptor resulting in a nondiagnostic premolar periapical image.

Courtesy of V. Singhal

Horizontal Angulation Errors The *horizontal* angulation is the side-to-side positioning of the PID. When using the paralleling technique, the aiming ring helps in directing the PID into the proper position to completely cover and expose the receptor.

The horizontal angulation is designated by the lines on the top and bottom of the PID (Figure 28-56). The horizontal angulation needs to be parallel to the interproximal surfaces to show all of the proximal surfaces. A diagnostic radiograph will show a thin radiolucent line between the teeth; this is particularly important for horizontal bitewings (Figure 28-57). The aiming ring is helpful in preventing this error, but the radiographer needs to set the horizontal angle parallel to the interproximals to ensure that the interproximals are not superimposed over each other, causing overlapping. For bitewings the horizontal angulation is zero. Overlapping will appear as a radiopaque area between the teeth from having the horizontal angulation placed too far mesial or distal (Figure 28-58).

Errors during Exposure

There are several additional errors that may occur during exposure including patient cooperation.

Saliva Leak (Traditional Film) This may happen when the traditional film is bent while placing the film into the film holder, which breaks the seal of the film packet. Saliva is able to reach the inside of the packet, causing the black paper envelope to become wet and adhere to the film. The paper may stick to the traditional film through processing, which causes irregular black areas on the processed film, or you may even see visible paper remains.

Improper Placement of Image Receptor The image receptor needs to be placed with the desired teeth to be exposed centered on the receptor. Look through the aiming ring and make certain the mesial of the receptor covers at least one half of the tooth anterior to the tooth being exposed (Figure 28-74).

Cutoff of Apices If the maxillary receptor is not high enough in the palate, and the mandibular receptor is not deep in the floor of the mouth, the apices of the teeth may be cut off from the image (Figure 28-70B). This may occur if the patient is not biting completely on the bite block; thus, the image receptor is not placed into the location completely and securely. A radiolucent area is also visible on the image in the area of the crowns when the patient does not bite down completely (Figure 28-70B). Check to ensure that the patient is biting fully on the bite block with their teeth. Some patients close their lips but do not fully bite. This may be because the image receptor is hurting the patient in that particular area. Slightly repositioning the receptor will allow the patient to bite fully and more comfortably.

Bent Traditional Film Packet If the patient bites too hard, pressure may cause the film to bend at the corners. The processed film will show black lines where the film was bent (Figure 28-75). Asking the patient to gently bite or placing a cotton roll between the teeth and the film holder may eliminate this problem. This may also happen if the operator bends the film packet prior to placing the film in the oral cavity. The film packet should never be bent as this may crack the emulsion and result in a nondiagnostic image when the film is processed.

Double Exposure Double exposure occurs when the traditional film was accidently placed back into the oral cavity and exposed a second time. The processed image shows teeth

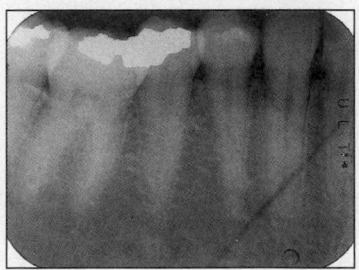

FIGURE 28-75
A bent film appears as a black crease or a thin, dark, radiolucent line.

and anatomical areas from two areas superimposed over each other on one film (Figure 28-76). To avoid this, always follow the sequence discussed in this chapter.

Artifacts in Image
Failure to remove eyeglasses, jewelry such as nose rings and tongue rings, and removable oral appliances (partials, retainers) covers areas of the image. The appliances are visible, and anatomic structures may not be visible. It is important to ask the patient to remove these items before obtaining radiographic images (Figure 28-77).

Tilted Image
The receptor is not placed parallel to the occlusal plane. Make certain the receptor is placed straight behind the area being exposed and is not tilted (Figure 28-78). This error occurs mostly when using the BAT.

Blurred Image
This error may occur when the receptor or patient moves slightly during exposure. As a result, a blurred image is visible (Figure 28-79). Instruct the patient to remain still during exposure, and watch the patient during exposure to make certain they do not move.

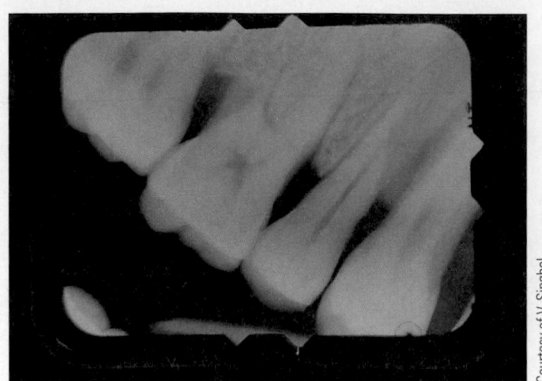

FIGURE 28-78
Tilted occlusal plane.

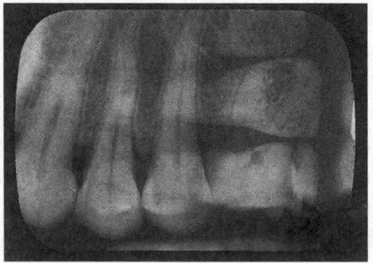

FIGURE 28-76
Double exposure. A film was exposed twice, with each exposure shown on the x-ray film.

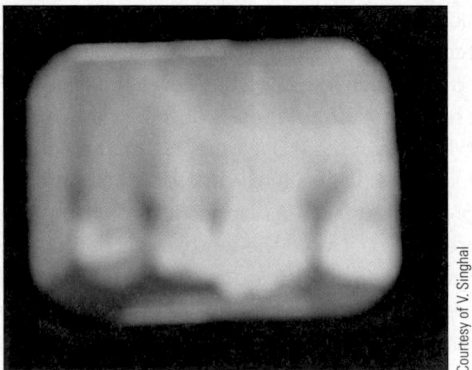

FIGURE 28-79
Blurred image.

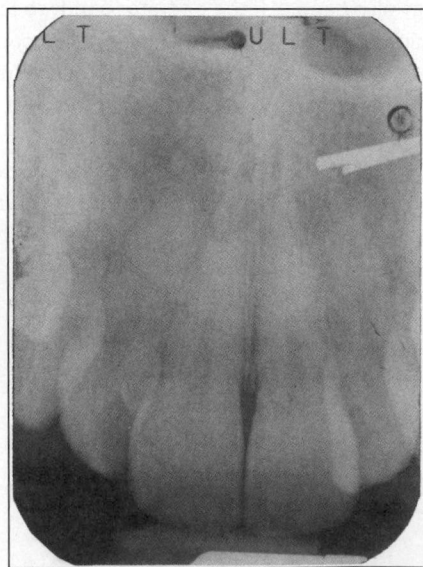

FIGURE 28-77
A radiographic image with artifact.

Occlusal Techniques

The occlusal technique gets its name from the placement of the image receptor between the occlusal surfaces of the maxillary and mandibular teeth while the patient bites or "occludes" to hold the receptor in place during exposure. Occlusal images are prescribed to view large areas in an arch with a single exposure. They are used to diagnose and examine larger areas of the maxillary or mandibular arches that other intraoral images such as periapicals and bitewings cannot detect. There are many reasons a dentist may prescribe an occlusal dental radiograph. These include a desire to:

- view large areas of the oral cavity, palate, jaw, or floor of the mouth
- view and locate impacted teeth
- view positioning of the teeth in the arches
- identify the location of salivary gland stones
- view and locate supernumerary teeth

CHAPTER 28 Dental Radiology Infection Control, Exposure, Processing and Evaluation of Dental Radiographs, and Mounting of Dental Radiographs

881

- locate objects, pathologic conditions, cleft palates, cysts, tumors, or root fragments
- evaluate fractures in the maxilla or mandible

The occlusal exposure is the projection of choice when other extraoral radiographs may not be possible. Other extraoral images will be discussed in Chapter 29. Easy placement of the image receptor makes it an exposure of choice for children and special needs patients. There are several occlusal techniques that can be used to view the maxillary and mandibular arches. The two most commonly used are the maxillary *topographical* view and the mandibular *cross-sectional* view. Occlusal projections are also obtained in pediatric patients. This section will discuss the adult occlusal exposures. Pediatric occlusal exposures will be discussed later in this chapter. Procedure 28-4 provides the steps in obtaining occlusal images in an adult patient.

Procedure 28-4
Adult Occlusal Exposures

Equipment and Supplies
- barriers for the x-ray room
- occlusal film (size 4 for adults)
- lead apron with thyroid collar
- container or barrier for exposed film

Procedure Steps

1. Follow aseptic procedures as outlined in Procedure 28-1.

Maxillary Anterior Topographic Technique

The maxillary anterior topographic view is preferred when a view of the anterior portion of the palate is needed.

1. The patient's head is positioned with maxilla parallel to the floor; this can be achieved by positioning the ala–tragus line parallel to the floor. The midsagittal plane of the patient must be perpendicular to the floor (see Figure 28-46).

2. The size 4 image receptor for adults is used to expose an entire arch on one image. The traditional film is placed with the white side of the film toward the palate and the embossed dot toward the anterior. The receptor is positioned with the long dimension of the receptor going from right to left in the oral cavity. The anterior edge of the receptor should extend ¼ inch (2–3 mm) beyond the labial surfaces of the maxillary teeth (Figure 28-80). The patient holds the receptor in place by gently biting the image receptor (Figure 28-80). Once the image receptor has been placed, the radiographer should set the vertical angulation at +65° (Figures 28-80 and 28-81).

3. The vertical angulation is determined using the bisecting angle technique. The average angulation is set at +60° to +65° (Figure 28-81). The top of the PID is placed at the bridge of the nose. The central ray should be ½ inch above the tip of the nose and directed toward the center of the film. The resulting image will give a topographical view of the maxillary arch.

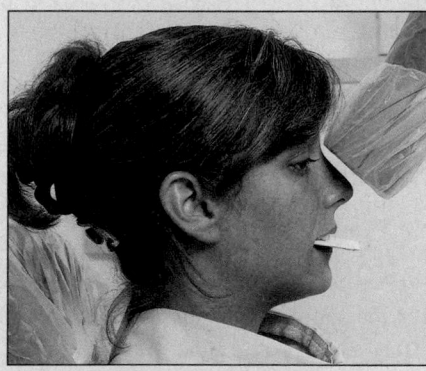

FIGURE 28-80
Maxillary topographical occlusal image exposure.

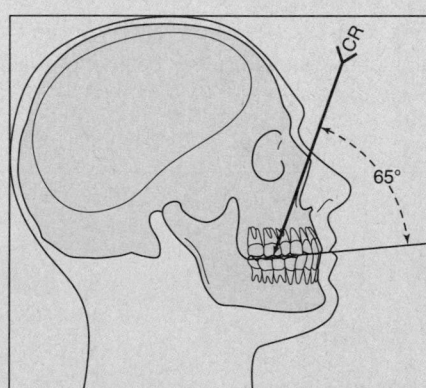

FIGURE 28-81
Vertical angulation for maxillary anterior topographic technique.

(Continues)

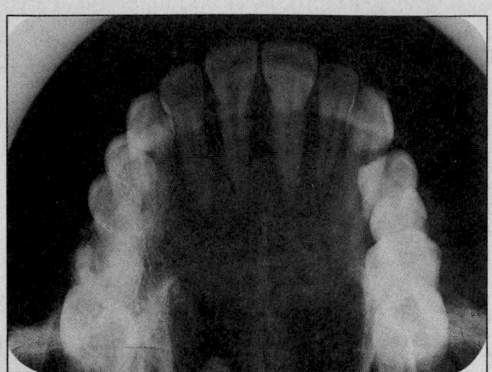

FIGURE 28-82
Maxillary anterior topographical exposure.

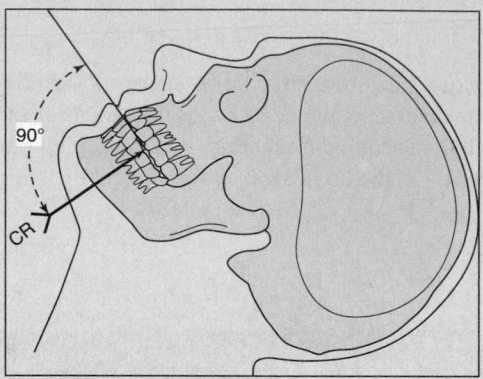

FIGURE 28-84
Central ray angulation for mandibular cross-sectional exposure.

Mandibular Occlusal: Cross-Sectional Projection

The cross-sectional projection is also known as the mandibular right-angle projection. This radiograph shows the buccal and lingual aspects of the mandible as well as the floor of the mouth. The dentist can get a better view of the salivary glands and ducts and the floor of the mouth. The patient's head position and occlusal are critical to exposing a diagnostic radiograph.

1. The patient is positioned supine, and the patient's head is tilted back so the mandible is perpendicular to the floor (Figure 28-83).

2. The traditional size 4 film is placed with the white side of the film toward the mandible. The image receptor is placed long from right to left with just ¼ inch beyond the labial surfaces of the incisors (Figure 28-83).

3. The vertical angulation is at a right angle to the receptor. The PID is set with the central ray at 90° to the image receptor. The point of entry is just below the chin and toward the center of the receptor (Figure 28-84). The resulting image provides a view of the anterior portion of the mandible and the floor of the oral cavity (Figure 28-85).

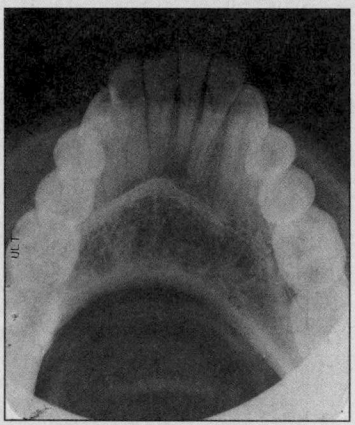

FIGURE 28-85
Cross-sectional occlusal radiograph of the mandibular arch.

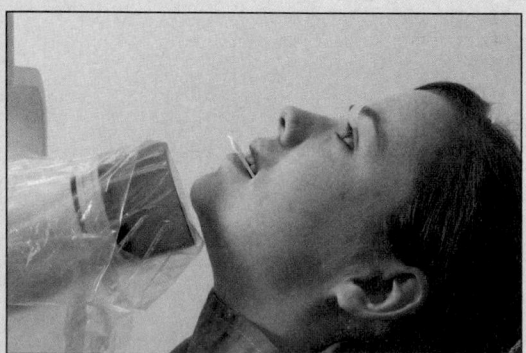

FIGURE 28-83
PID placement for mandibular cross-sectional projection.

CHAPTER 28 Dental Radiology Infection Control, Exposure, Processing and Evaluation of
Dental Radiographs, and Mounting of Dental Radiographs

883

Localization Techniques

One limitation of standard dental radiology techniques is that the image is flat, though the object being imaged is three-dimensional. In a radiographic image, the dimensions that are known are the anterior–posterior dimension and the inferior–superior dimension. However, the dimension of depth is lost. At times, it is necessary to utilize localization techniques in dentistry to obtain information regarding object location in all three dimensions. This may be necessary to determine where an impacted maxillary canine may be located (buccal or lingual) so that orthodontic treatment can be utilized to bring the tooth into position. This may also be necessary if an instrument tip breaks off and is lodged in the gingiva. Removal will require that the exact location be identified to ensure removal is completed in the least invasive manner possible. There are two methods that can provide three-dimensional information: the right angle technique and the tube shift technique.

Right Angle Technique

The right angle technique is usually used in the mandible and utilizes two images in order to determine the exact location of an object. One image is a mandibular cross-sectional occlusal projection. The second image is a standard periapical or bitewing image. If an object is visible on a periapical image taken in the mandibular right canine area, it is not known if that object is on the buccal or the lingual. The location of the object is known in an anterior–posterior dimension and a mesial–distal dimension (Figure 28-86). A second image, mandibular occlusal cross-sectional, may be obtained. This image provides information about the object in a buccal–lingual dimension (Figure 28-86). Comparison of the two images will provide information about the object and whether or not is located on the buccal or the lingual aspect of the area.

Tube Shift Technique (SLOB rule)

The "same lingual, opposite buccal" (SLOB) rule is utilized to identify the location of an object. This technique utilizes periapical or bitewing images in order to determine the location

of an object. If an object is seen on one image, a second image can be obtained of that area after shifting the beam either mesially or distally. For example, in Figure 28-87A, the amalgam identified by the arrow can be on the buccal or the lingual surface of the tooth. Figure 28-87A is a premolar periapical exposure. Figure 28-87B is a molar periapical image; the beam was shifted distally. The object appears to have moved to the mesial. Thus, the object moved opposite the direction of the PID. Thus, the object (amalgam) is on the buccal side.

This technique is used in endodontic therapy to determine the location of the canals in the teeth. In Figure 28-88A, the arrow identifies an endodontic filling. However, it is not known if that filling is in the palatal canal or in the buccal canal. Figure 28-88A is a premolar periapical image. Figure 28-88B is a molar periapical image. The filling material has shifted distally. This shift is in the same direction as the PID. Thus, the canal is identified as the lingual or palatal canal.

Modified Exposure Techniques

Not all radiographic techniques previously explained will apply to all patients. There are some patients who will require the dental assistant to modify the technique or the number of images exposed. Examples of patients who may require modifications include pediatric and edentulous patients and those with a gag reflex. Those with anatomical variations might also present a challenge to the radiographer. Patients with maxillary or mandibular tori will also require a slight alteration in the exposure technique.

Edentulous Patients

An *edentulous* patient, one without teeth, still requires radiographs for a variety of reasons. Exposures may be taken to evaluate bone levels or to examine for retained root tips or disease processes. Similar to the pediatric patient, exposure settings may need to be reduced. The type of images taken may range from a full mouth series (14 periapical images), a panoramic image, occlusal images, or a combination of those listed (Figure 28-89). The type of images may vary based on the procedure that the patient needs as well as what the dentist may feel is necessary. The technique may vary slightly

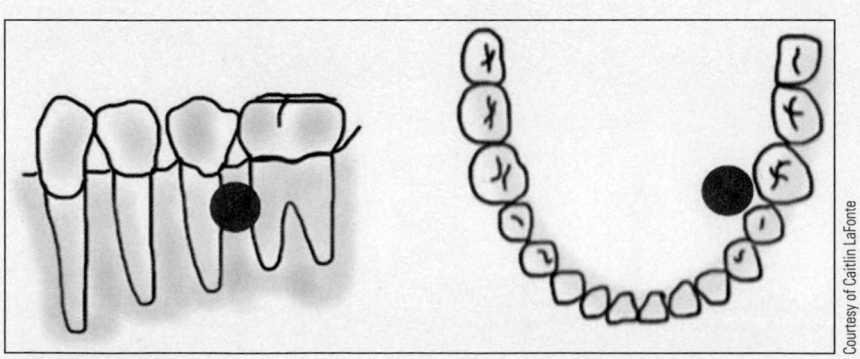

FIGURE 28-86
Right angle technique.

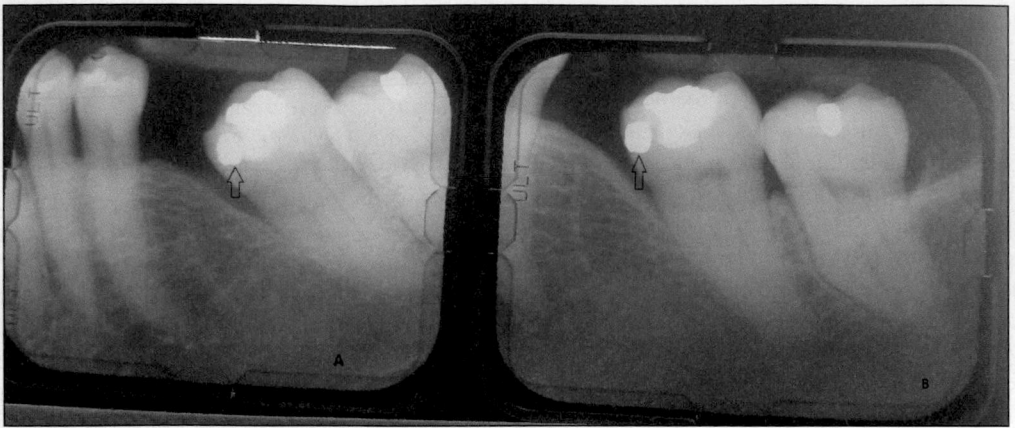

Courtesy of V. Singhal

FIGURE 28-87
Use of SLOB rule.

as well. For example, due to the absence of teeth, cotton rolls may be needed, and the bisecting angle will be slightly different. In an edentulous patient, the ridge of the alveolar bone forms the angle with the image receptor; the beam would be perpendicular to this angle (Figure 28-90). A panoramic image can also be obtained to examine edentulous arches. A supplemental periapical image can be exposed if needed in an area in question.

Tori

A patient with anatomical variations, such as tori, will also need special consideration. This will require the dental assistant to slightly alter the placement of the receptor holder in the patient's oral cavity (Figures 28-91 and 28-92). The image receptor should be placed between the tongue and the mandibular torus and more toward the center of the floor of the oral cavity. In the maxillary arch, the image receptor should be placed behind the maxillary torus. Placing the image receptor on the torus itself in either arch will cause significant discomfort to the patient.

Pediatric Patients

Pediatric patients present with many components of treatment that will require a different approach. They have much smaller

oral cavities than adults, which require fewer images and a smaller image receptor. Children also require more explanation of the procedure. The radiographs ordered for pediatric exposures are prescribed based on each patient's needs, but especially important for the pediatric patient is the age of the child. This will also be a determining factor in the number of images prescribed and the type of radiograph (bitewing, occlusal, etc.). For a new patient exam on a child who has a primary dentition, the dentist may prescribe only occlusal images or only bitewing images or a combination. For a new patient exam on a child who has a mixed dentition, the dentist may prescribe bitewings with an extraoral panoramic image and selected posterior periapical images. A new patient exam on a child with a permanent dentition usually warrants a full set of images. For all three types, bitewing images are obtained every 6–12 months as determined by the dentist. The main differences when taking exposures on children include:

- the size of the image receptor
- the number of images required
- decreased exposure time due to decreased bone density of the pediatric patient
- the technique—on younger children, the bisecting angle technique may be more acceptable to the child

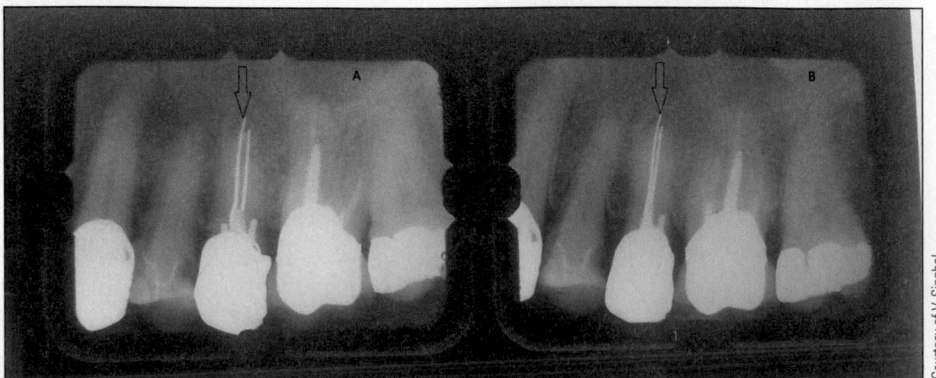

Courtesy of V. Singhal

FIGURE 28-88
Use of SLOB rule in endodontics.

CHAPTER 28 Dental Radiology Infection Control, Exposure, Processing and Evaluation of
Dental Radiographs, and Mounting of Dental Radiographs

885

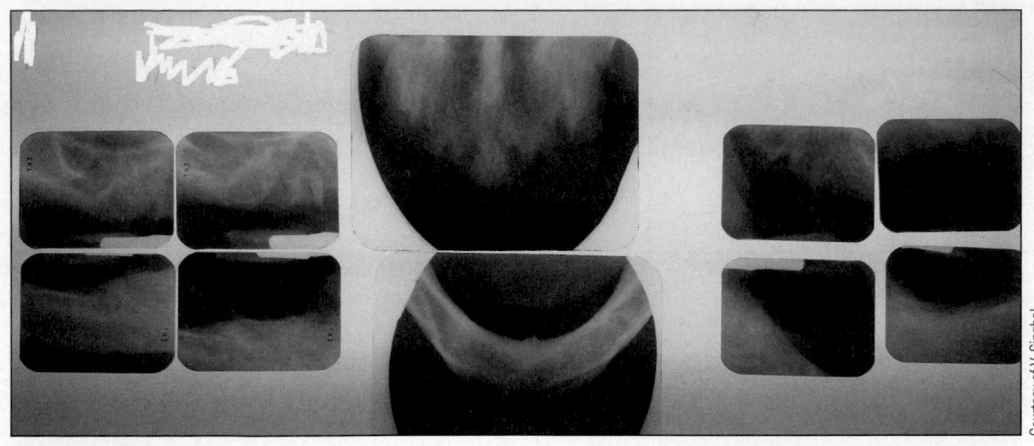

Courtesy of V. Singhal

FIGURE 28-89
Combination of occlusal and posterior periapical images of an edentulous patient.

- placement modifications which may be required if the child cannot tolerate the receptor due to higher sensitivity

Pediatric Image Receptor Size and Number of Images The receptor size should be determined clinically based on the teeth that are present and individual arch size of

the child. Select periapical images may be needed on a child if decay is suspected and the teeth cannot be viewed clinically. Size 0 receptors are used when the child has no permanent teeth present in the dentition (less than 6 years of age). Size 1 image receptors are used when a mixed dentition is present (usually age 6–12 years). Size 2 image receptors are used on a very young

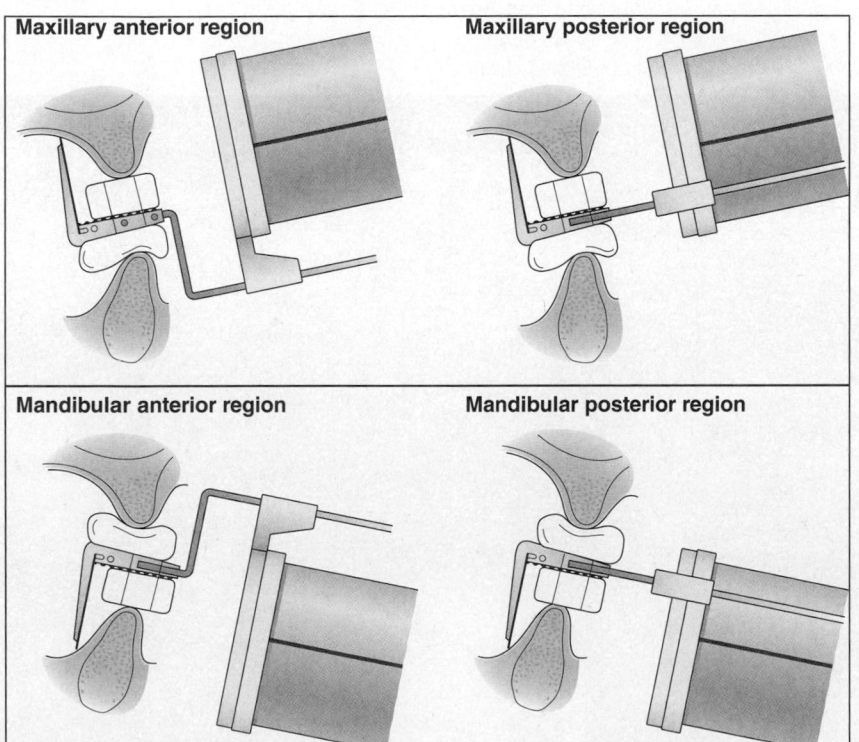

FIGURE 28-90
Radiographs of a full mouth series of an edentulous patient. Cone and receptor-holding device are positioned in four areas. Note: an additional bite block is secured to the Rinn bite block to provide the height that the teeth would normally provide. A cotton roll is placed on the opposite side to assist the patient in holding the bite block securely.

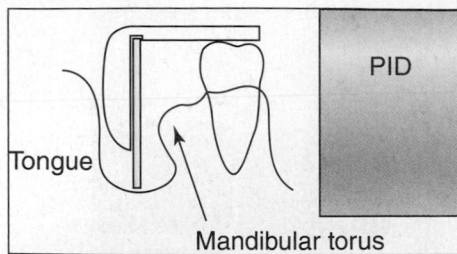

FIGURE 28-91
Image receptor placement with a mandibular torus.

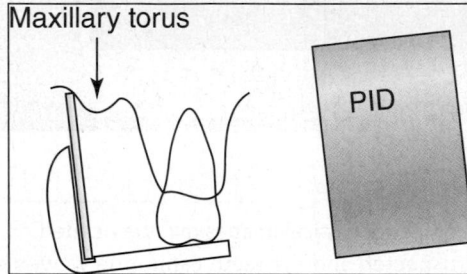

FIGURE 28-92
Image receptor placement with a maxillary torus.

child (less than 6 years of age) in order to obtain two occlusal images. Generally, a full mouth series of eight images is exposed when type 0 and 1 receptors are used on a child with a mixed dentition (Figure 28-93):

- Two bitewings—one on each side
- Four periapical images—one on each side
- Two occlusal images—one on each arch using a size 2 image receptor

Pediatric Occlusal Images A size 2 image receptor is usually used for periapical and bitewing exposures in a child who has all permanent teeth present or is in the later stages of the mixed dentition (over the age of 12 years). The size should still be determined clinically based on the child's arch size. Generally 12 images are obtained when size 2 receptors are used (Figure 28-94). Some children under the age of 18 may require a standard adult full mouth series of images. This would be determined by the size of the child and the size of the oral cavity.

- Two bitewing images (one on each side)
- Three maxillary anterior periapical images
- Three mandibular anterior periapical images
- Two maxillary molar periapical images (one on each side)
- Two mandibular molar periapical images (one on each side)

Pediatric Periapical and Bitewing Exposures In addition to the pediatric occlusal images described in Procedure 28-5, the dentist may order two deciduous bitewings and four periapical images. Procedure 28-6 provides the technique for obtaining these exposures.

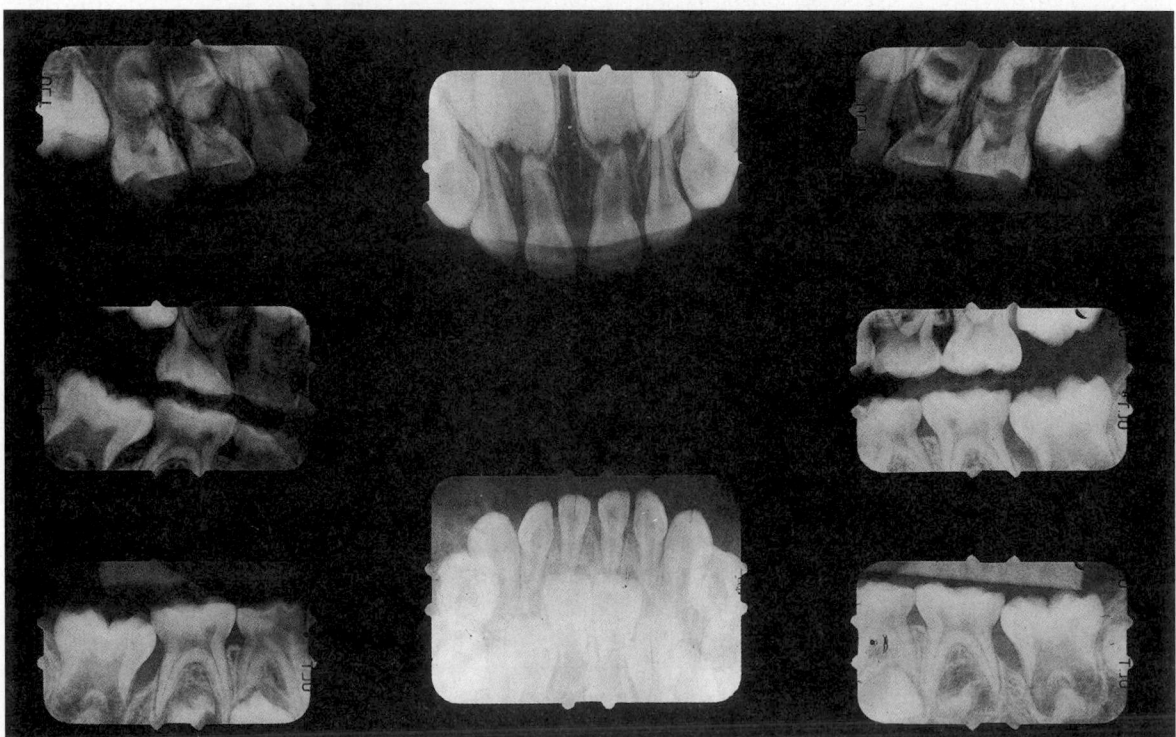

FIGURE 28-93
Pedodontic survey on child 3–6 years old includes two bitewing, two occlusal, and four periapical images.

CHAPTER 28 Dental Radiology Infection Control, Exposure, Processing and Evaluation of
Dental Radiographs, and Mounting of Dental Radiographs

887

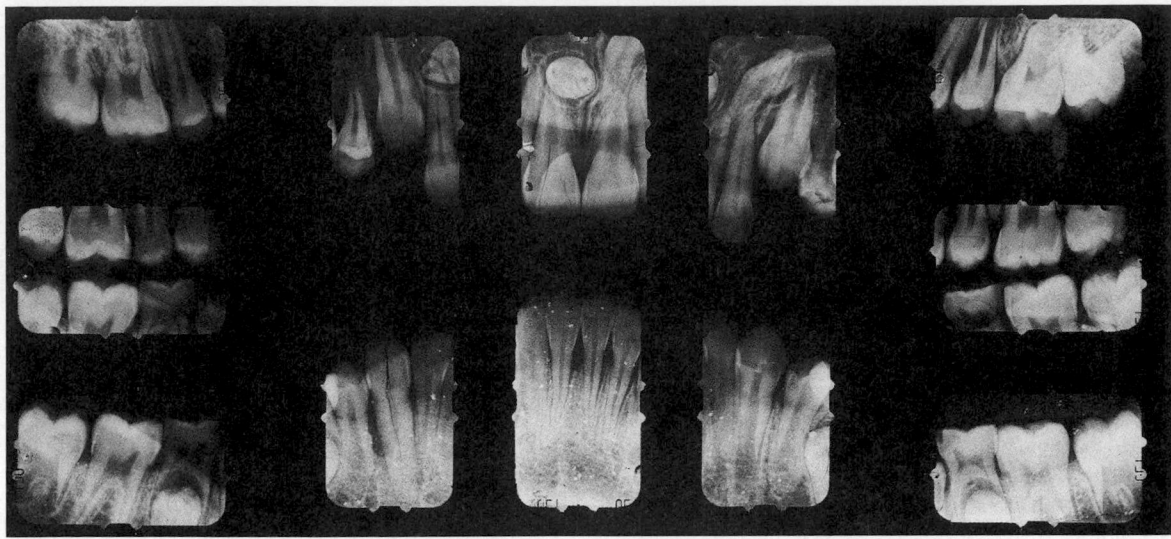

FIGURE 28-94
Full mouth series on a child with a mixed dentition.

Procedure 28-5
Pediatric Occlusal Images

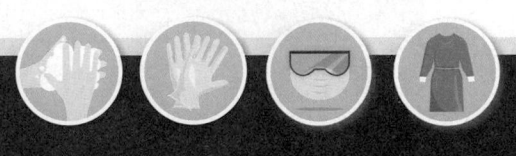

Pediatric occlusal techniques are similar to adult occlusal techniques. The pediatric maxillary topographical technique uses a size 2 image receptor. The student should follow the aseptic procedures outlined earlier and in Procedure 28-1.

Equipment and Supplies
- barriers for the x-ray room
- size 2 image receptor
- pediatric size lead apron with thyroid collar
- if using traditional film, a container or barrier for exposed film

Procedure Steps

Maxillary Occlusal Topographical Image
1. Position the patient so the maxillary arch is parallel to the floor.

2. Place the image receptor in the oral cavity with the long side from right to left. The anterior edge of the receptor should extend ¼ inch (2–3 mm) beyond labial surfaces of the maxillary teeth. The PID should be aligned so that the top of the PID is aligned with the bridge of the

nose (Figure 28-95). The PID should be at a +60° angle (Figure 28-96). The resulting image provides a view of the anterior portion of the palate (Figure 28-97). Impacted permanent teeth and developing permanent teeth would be visible in this image.

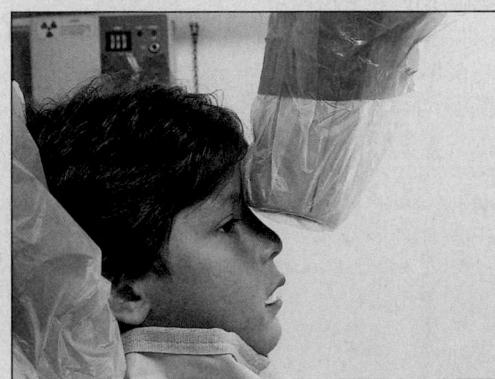

FIGURE 28-95
PID aligned for pediatric maxillary topographical occlusal image.

(Continues)

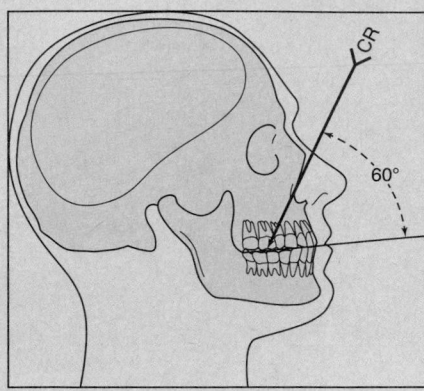

FIGURE 28-96
Central ray angle for pediatric maxillary topographical exposure.

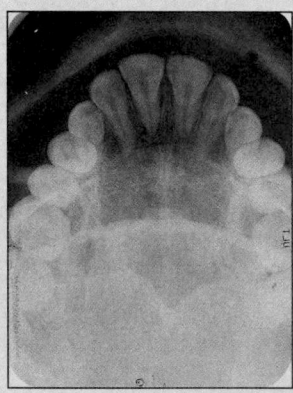

FIGURE 28-97
Pediatric maxillary anterior topographical image.

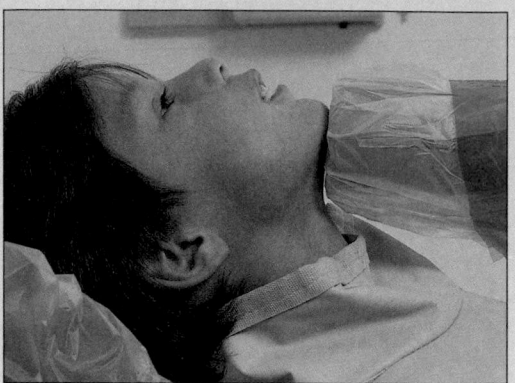

FIGURE 28-98
PID position for pediatric mandibular cross-sectional projection.

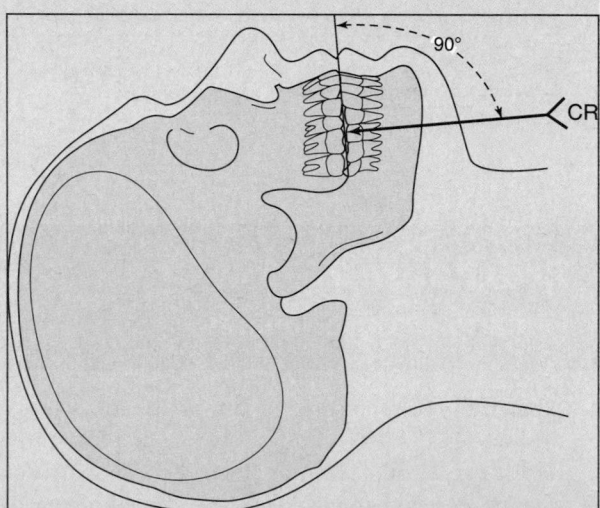

FIGURE 28-99
Central ray entry for pediatric mandibular cross-sectional projection.

Mandibular Cross-Sectional Occlusal Image

1. The patient is positioned supine (Figure 28-98).

2. If using a traditional size 2 film, it is placed with the white side of the film toward the mandible. The image receptor is placed long from side to side with just ¼ inch beyond the labial of incisors. The center of the chin is centered in the opening of the PID. The central ray comes in at a 90° angle to the image receptor (Figure 28-99). The resulting image provides a view of the anterior portion of the mandible and the floor of the oral cavity (Figure 28-100).

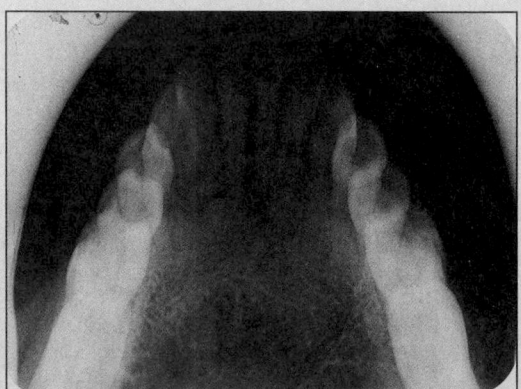

FIGURE 28-100
Pediatric mandibular cross-sectional image.

CHAPTER 28 Dental Radiology Infection Control, Exposure, Processing and Evaluation of
Dental Radiographs, and Mounting of Dental Radiographs

889

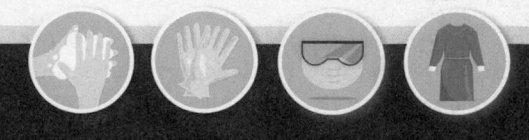

Procedure 28-6
Pediatric Periapical and Bitewing Exposures

The student should follow the aseptic procedures outlined in Procedure 28-1.

Equipment and Supplies

- barriers for the x-ray room and equipment
- image receptor, six size 0 image receptors for bitewings and periapical images (in addition to size 2 receptor for occlusal images)
- protective sheath if using digital sensors
- cotton rolls
- Rinn XCP holders (assembled for use) or other paralleling technique aids and bitewing tabs
- pediatric lead apron with thyroid collar
- labeled disposable cup for exposed traditional film (if using)
- paper towel or tissue

Deciduous Bitewings

1. To position bitewing radiographs, a tab or positioning instrument is used. Tabs come with adhesive backs or with loops to surround the film (see Figure 28-48A). Tabs are used on traditional films. The positioning instrument comes with a bitewing holder, an indicator rod, and a positioning ring (see Figure 28-29B). Pediatric Rinn holders are available for traditional films and digital sensors.

2. While holding the traditional film horizontally, place the tab in the center of the film or, if using a positioning instrument, make sure the receptor is centered in the bitewing holder. The white side of the traditional film should be directed toward the positioning ring.

3. Position the image receptor covering the deciduous first and second molars, with the front edge of the receptor to the middle of the canine.

4. Hold the tab and place the receptor near the lingual surface of the teeth in the patient's oral cavity, positioning the receptor so it covers the mandibular deciduous molars.

5. While holding the tab in place, have the patient close and slowly rotate the fingers out of the way.

6. When using a positioning instrument, place the bitewing holder in the patient's oral cavity, away from the lingual surface of the teeth. Position the receptor to cover the deciduous molars. Have the patient close slowly on the bitewing holder and hold it in place.

7. The cone positioning for the molar bitewing with vertical angulation is set to +10°.

Maxillary Deciduous Molar Periapical Image

1. For the maxillary deciduous molars, rotate the image receptor holder into the patient's oral cavity, and position it away from the lingual surfaces, toward the middle of the palate.

2. Place the anterior edge of the receptor behind the center of the canine to ensure that the receptor will cover the area of the two molars.

3. While holding the image receptor in place, have the patient close slowly on the bite block. Hold the metal rod and slide the positioning ring toward the patient's face.

4. Bring the tubehead toward the ring, placing the PID flush against the ring. Note the angle of the receptor and the receptor holder, which is positioned so that the central ray passes through the contact point of the first and second deciduous molars.

5. Center the bite block on the deciduous molars. On this image, the distal side of the canine is seen and the first and second deciduous molars have the contact between them open (see Figure 28-93).

Mandibular Deciduous Molars

1. For the mandibular deciduous molars, rotate the image receptor holder into the patient's oral cavity and gently position it between the lingual surface of the teeth and the tongue.

2. Place the anterior edge of the receptor at the center of the canine to ensure that the receptor covers the area of the two deciduous molars.

3. Ask the patient to close on the bite block.

4. Note the position of the receptor as it is placed in the space between the tongue and the mandibular arch. The receptor and teeth are parallel. The first and second deciduous molars are seen on this image with the contact points open (see Figure 28-93).

Pediatric Patient Management Managing a pediatric patient is usually different from managing an adult patient when taking radiographs. When working with a pediatric patient, it is important to keep in mind the age of the child and relate to them the best you can when explaining the procedure. Using terms the child understands to explain what you will be doing may help gain the child's cooperation. You may refer to the x-ray machine as a "camera" and tell the patient you will use it to take a picture of their teeth. The lead apron is of pediatric size and could be referred to as a blanket. It may also be helpful to show them exactly what you will be doing in order to allay fears of the unexpected. Do not forget to have confidence in yourself as well. If you are calm and patient, you will be able to gain the trust of the child and further their cooperation. If the child does not cooperate after you have tried various methods, you may ask the parent or caregiver for assistance to stabilize the child during the exposure. It is important to note that the parent or caregiver should also be wearing a lead apron while the child is on the caregiver's lap during exposures (Figure 28-101). Most importantly, do not force the child to undergo dental radiographs unless it is an emergency situation. Forcing the child to have radiographs taken may result in traumatizing the child. This could cause a fear of future visits to the dentist. If radiographs are not absolutely required, postponing the radiographs until the next visit can help keep the child calm and unafraid of returning to the office.

Patients with a Gag Reflex

Some patients will exhibit a gag reflex upon trying to capture dental radiographs. This is usually caused by stimulating the tissues of the soft palate. This can happen when the dental assistant is trying to expose a posterior image and the receptor holder is dragged along the soft palate. As a dental radiographer, it is important to alter your exposure technique to avoid this reflex if possible. It is again helpful to be confident and calm when working with a hypersensitive gag reflex patient. If the patient is comfortable with the operator they will feel at ease, and hopefully their reflex will be reduced. It is critical to relax the patient as much as possible.

Once the dental assistant has gained the trust of the patient, it is advised to work as quickly and efficiently as possible. The assistant will want to gather all armamentarium before beginning exposures. This will expedite the procedure. It is also helpful to double-check all settings on the x-ray unit are preset before placing the sensor. This will help limit the amount of time the sensor is in the patient's oral cavity. Care should be taken to expose the desired image quickly, as this will also limit the time the receptor is in the patient's oral cavity. This will decrease the chance of the patient gagging.

The order in which the dental radiographs are obtained is also important. It is best to start with anterior exposures and end with the maxillary molar exposure. The anterior exposures will be easier for the patient and will help them feel more comfortable and confident before exposing the posterior areas. The maxillary molar exposure is saved for last due to the fact that it is the most likely exposure to elicit the gag reflex.

Distraction techniques also may be beneficial. Asking the patient to breathe through their nose or asking them to raise one leg and focus on the leg may help to take the attention off the exposure. Some patients, no matter the actions the dental assistant takes, will have a gag reflex. For these patients it is uncontrollable. A panoramic radiograph is usually prescribed in this situation.

Endodontic Exposures

Radiographs are taken periodically during the endodontic procedure (Figure 28-102). The radiographs allow the dentist to check the progress of the procedure and take the necessary measurements. Technique suggestions associated with endodontic procedures are as follows:

- Use the paralleling technique to reduce distortion whenever possible.

- Place the receptor in a hemostat, Snap-A-Ray, or XCP instrument endodontic positioning device. The endodontic receptor-holding device is made of plastic and aids in positioning the receptor while keeping the patient's oral cavity open. The patient needs to hold the oral cavity open during this time, because there is a reamer in the root canal that extends beyond the tooth. The endodontic receptor holder is like the Rinn receptor holder in that there is also a ring to line up the cone (Figure 28-103).

- Loosen the dental dam from the frame on one side and position the image receptor on the lingual surface, parallel to the tooth. If a plastic frame is not used, the metal dental dam frame may have to be removed to prevent the frame from being exposed on the radiograph and possibly distorting the image.

- The receptor should cover the entire length of the tooth and the surrounding area at the apex of the root.

- Center the tooth on the receptor and direct the central ray perpendicular to the long axis of the tooth. The patient must keep the oral cavity open because of protruding endodontic instruments and materials, so work quickly (Figure 28-103).

Special Needs Patients/Compromised Patients

Patients come to the office with a wide variety of special needs. Consideration and creativity often are required to obtain the

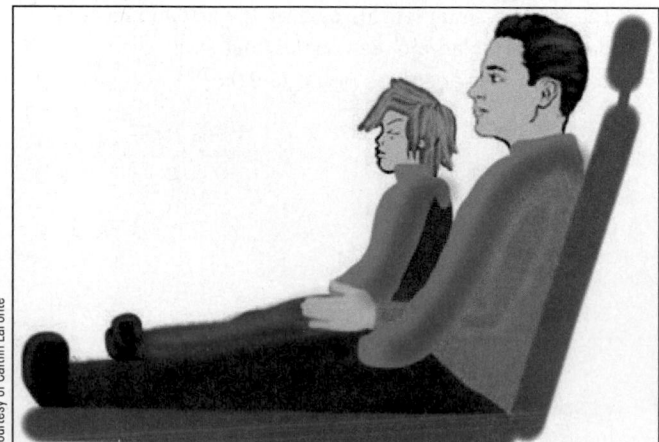

FIGURE 28-101
Parent and child covered with lead apron during exposures.

CHAPTER 28 Dental Radiology Infection Control, Exposure, Processing and Evaluation of
Dental Radiographs, and Mounting of Dental Radiographs

891

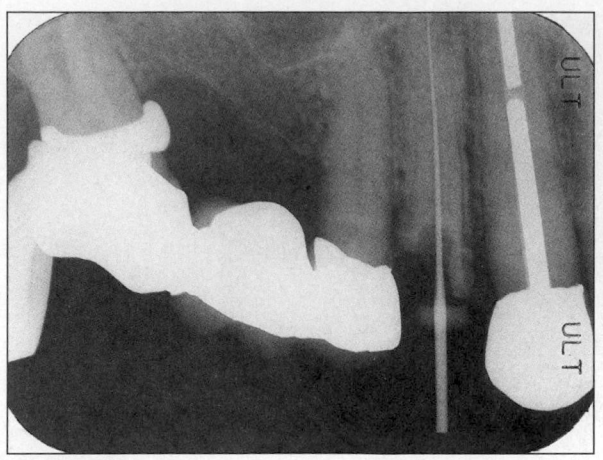

FIGURE 28-102
When an x-ray is positioned for an endodontic radiograph, the patient does not close on the film holder because the reamer in the root canal is beyond the line of occlusion. The radiograph shows the reamer in place.

desired radiographs. The wheelchair patient is one example where advance preparation is needed in order to have the treatment room ready (Figure 28-104). When there is a plan in place to expose the images, the procedure is much easier for everyone involved. With other special needs patients, a parent or guardian may be asked to assist in holding the patient or the image receptor steady; however, every attempt should be made to obtain the images by other means. Work as quickly as possible. Technique suggestions associated with treatment for special needs patients are as follows:

● Before treating special needs patients, discuss how to best handle them with the entire office. A good time to do this is during office meetings. The entire staff needs to work

together to make the patient's visit as simple and comprehensive as possible.

● Prepare all areas in the office that the patient will be in before the appointment, including the reception and treatment rooms. For example, have extra radiation protection in the treatment room for the parent or guardian in case they have to hold the image receptor in the patient's oral cavity.

● Call the patient, caregiver, or guardian in advance and ask for suggestions on how to best accommodate the patient's needs.

● Read about patients' conditions to better understand and communicate with them. For example, when working with a deaf patient, learn a few words in sign language.

Vision Impaired Patient Patients who have vision impairment require clear verbal communications. Carefully explain exactly what is involved in the procedure and what you are doing before you begin. Let them know anything they might feel or taste when possible. Check with them to see if they have any questions or concerns.

Deaf or Hard of Hearing Patient Patients who have a hearing loss may be able to lip read. If they can, remove your mask and speak slowly and clearly so that they can read your lips as you give them information. Written communication is another means for informing the patient about the procedure. Have the steps of the procedure listed for them to review, and ask if they have any questions. Learning a few terms in sign language is an excellent way to show the patient that you really care and you want to communicate something about the treatment he or she is receiving.

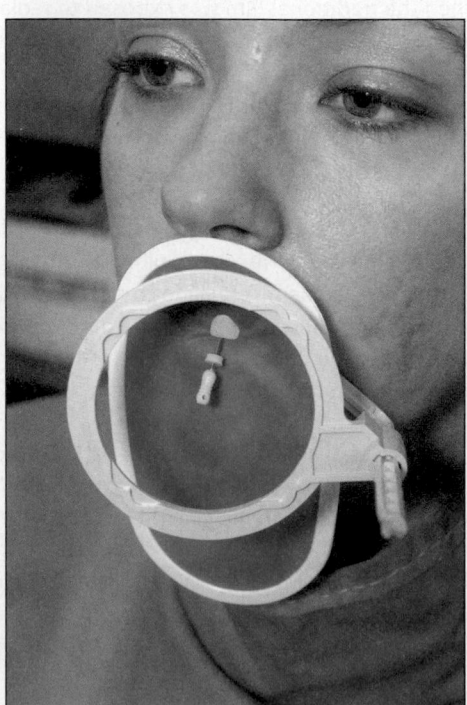

FIGURE 28-103
Patient with endodontic film holder positioned for exposure.

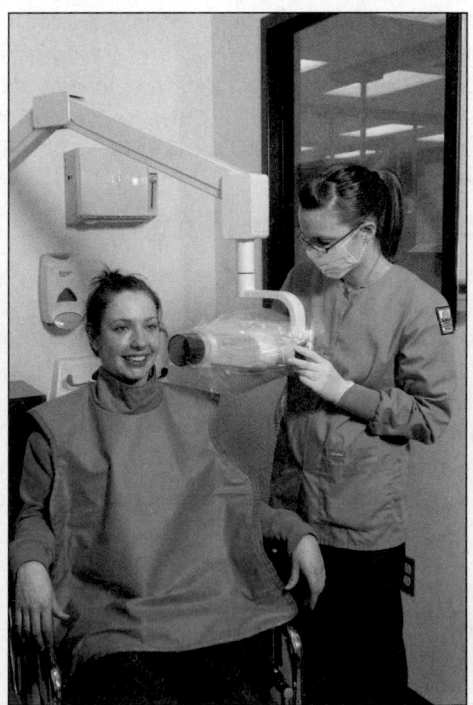

FIGURE 28-104
Wheelchair patient having intraoral radiographs taken.

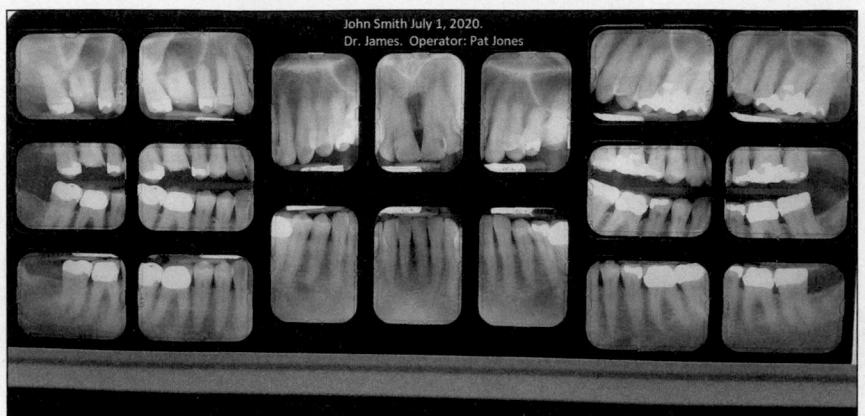

FIGURE 28-105A
Full mouth set of radiographs in mount labeled with patient's name, date, and radiographer's name.

Radiography Record Keeping

Radiographs are a part of the patient's legal records and are crucial for proper diagnosis and treatment. Traditional films in the dental office are easy to lose when there is a failure to identify the radiographs through each step of exposing and processing. Traditional films need to be properly identified from labeling the cup holding the contaminated exposed films, to the film hanger when using the manual processor, to the mount with the patient's name, date, and radiographer's initials (Figure 28-105A). The films need to be mounted immediately upon completion of processing. Processing and mounting will be discussed later in this chapter.

LEGAL

The radiographer must enter the type and number of images exposed on the patient's services rendered, the date images were exposed, and the radiographer's initials. Records must be documented accurately. Film envelopes for traditional films may also be used to help in reducing the loss and abrasion of films. The envelope should be labeled with the patient's name, operator name, dentist name, and date films were exposed (Figure 28-105B).

Processing Dental Film

Only traditional dental films need to be chemically processed. Digital exposures do not undergo processing by chemicals. Digital imaging is discussed in Chapter 29. Proper exposure of the film is only part of what results in a diagnostic radiographic image. Chemical processing of traditional films plays an important role in obtaining quality radiographs. To understand what happens during the processing of the dental film, it is important for the assistant to know the specific components of each processing

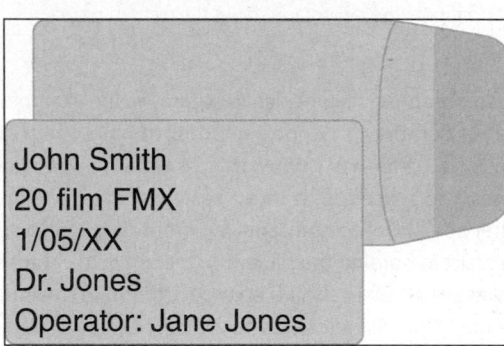

John Smith
20 film FMX
1/05/XX
Dr. Jones
Operator: Jane Jones

FIGURE 28-105B
Traditional film envelopes with patient's name and date of birth, dentist's name, and operator's name.

solution and how each component works to produce the visible image. When the traditional film was exposed to radiation, the crystals in the emulsion stored the radiation energy that they were exposed to and formed a latent image. Chemical processing will convert the latent image into a permanent, visible image the clinician can utilize to interpret and diagnose.

Developing Process

The films are first placed in the developing solution. The developing solution reduces the silver halide crystals into black metal silver. The black metal silver produces the dark or radiolucent areas on the image. The developing solution, also referred to as the *developer*, is the first solution in processing that the exposed films will be placed into.

Some of the crystals are incompletely or partially exposed by the x-ray beam. These crystals will also be changed by the developer, resulting in gray tones on the film. The variation in exposures is determined by the structure that the x-rays pass through before they reach the film. Crystals that received no radiation will remain

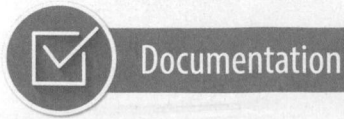
Documentation

July 17, 20XX
Exposed full mouth set of radiographs using paralleling technique. A total of 20 exposures using size 1 image receptor in the anterior areas and size 2 image receptor for the posterior and bitewing exposures.

CHAPTER 28 Dental Radiology Infection Control, Exposure, Processing and Evaluation of
Dental Radiographs, and Mounting of Dental Radiographs

893

unchanged by the radiation and the developer. The unchanged areas appear white or clear on the completely processed film. When the film is correctly processed, the developing solution allows for the light (radiopaque) and dark (radiolucent) areas to be processed on the film. Thus, the developer is able to differentiate between the exposed and unexposed silver halide crystals. The exposed silver halide crystals are reduced to black metal silver through a process called *selective reduction*. The developing solution is composed of several chemicals as outlined in Table 28-6.

Fixing Process

Fixing is needed to complete the processing of the film. The developed film must be cleared of undeveloped crystals. The fixing solution removes these crystals. The *fixer* also hardens the emulsion on the film base and increases its resistance to abrasion. The fixing process also prevents the film from discoloring or darkening with age or exposure to white light. The fixing solution is also composed of several chemicals as outlined in Table 28-7.

Processing Techniques

The trend now is toward digital dental radiography. However, there are offices that still use traditional films. It is important that the dental assistant understand how films are processed.

The fundamental requirements for good processing are adequate equipment and a standardized method. There are two primary methods to process films: manual and automatic processing. Although the manual technique is not frequently used in the dental office, it still remains the backup system for times when the automatic processor is not operating properly. This technique is also used in processing the larger extraoral films that do not fit into some automatic processors. By studying the manual method first, it helps the new dental assistant understand each step in processing. The manual processing technique is available online on the Student Companion Website.

Automatic Processing

There are a variety of automatic processors available for purchase. The machine that is purchased is based on the needs of the office. Some needs include space available for equipment and also quantity of films that will be processed. The processing machines are designed with an automatic roller transport that moves films through the developer, fixer, and wash tanks. The first rinsing step is eliminated when using the automatic processor. The rollers squeeze out any residual developing solution before the film is immersed into the fixer solutions (Figure 28-106). Once the films leave the wash tank, the rollers transport the films through the dryer unit, which completely dries the film before it emerges ready for mounting and viewing (Figure 28-106).

Some processing machines have heating devices to control the temperature of the solutions. Machines with this feature have a light which shows when the appropriate chemical temperature has been reached (Figure 28-107). Processors may be attached to plumbing to keep running water throughout the wash tank, or tanks may be contained and the radiographer changes the water on a daily basis. Some processors may require manual replenishing or may auto replenish processing solutions (Figure 28-108).

Solutions are specially formulated for the automatic processor for the higher chemical temperature (83°F/28.3°C) and shortened processing time of 5–7 minutes. The processing solutions should

TABLE 28-6 Chemical Components of the Developing Solution

Developing Agent (hydroquinone)
The developing agent is the chemical compound capable of changing exposed grains of silver halide to metallic silver. The developing agent is composed of hydroquinone and elon. Hydroquinone is the reducing agent and completes the selective reduction process. Elon generates the gray tones. The agent produces no noticeable effect on unexposed grains of the emulsion. Hydroquinone is very temperature sensitive: overactive if warm and underactive or not active if cold. Ideal temperature for developing of films is 68°F (20°C).

Antioxidant Preservative (sodium sulfite)
The antioxidant prevents developing solution from oxidizing in the presence of air.

Accelerator (sodium hydroxide)
Activates the developer and maintains its alkalinity. It also softens the emulsion on the film.

Restrainer (potassium bromide)
The restrainer controls the action of the developer. The restrainer stops the developer from affecting the unexposed silver halide with the time frame established by the manufacturer's directions. If the action of the developer is not restrained, the film will darken and the result will be fogging.

TABLE 28-7 Chemical Components of the Fixing Solution

Clearing Agent (ammonium thiosulfate)
The clearing agent or fixing agent (also known as hypo) dissolves and removes undeveloped silver halide from the emulsion. The clearing agent clears and produces the white or radiopaque areas on the image.

Preservative (sodium sulfite)
The preservative inhibits the decomposition of the fixer.

Acidifier (acetic acid)
The fixer works best in an acidic environment. The acid neutralizes the alkaline environment created by the developer that may be carried over by the film from the developer solution.

Hardener (potassium alum)
The hardening agent shrinks and hardens the gelatin in the film emulsion. The hardener shortens the drying time, protects the emulsion, and makes the image permanent.

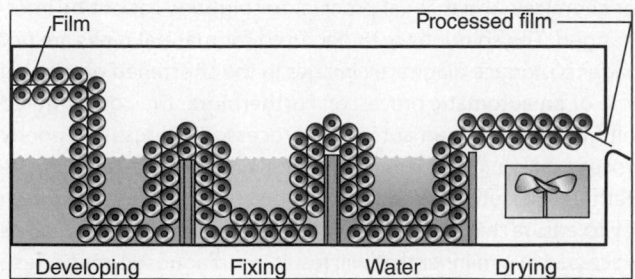

FIGURE 28-106
Drawing of the inside of a typical automatic film processor.

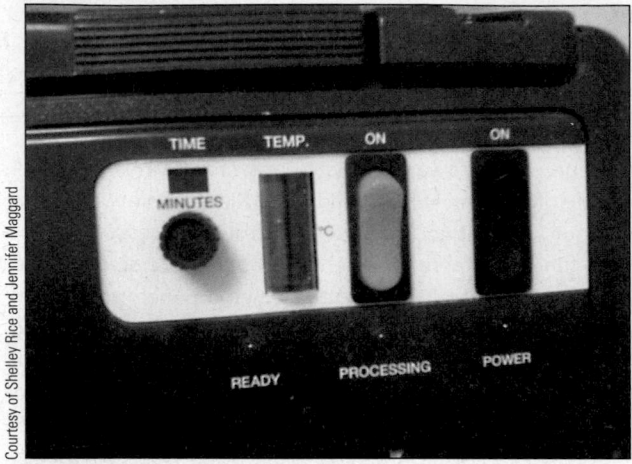

Courtesy of Shelley Rice and Jennifer Maggard

FIGURE 28-107
Ready light turns red when processing solutions are at the correct temperature.

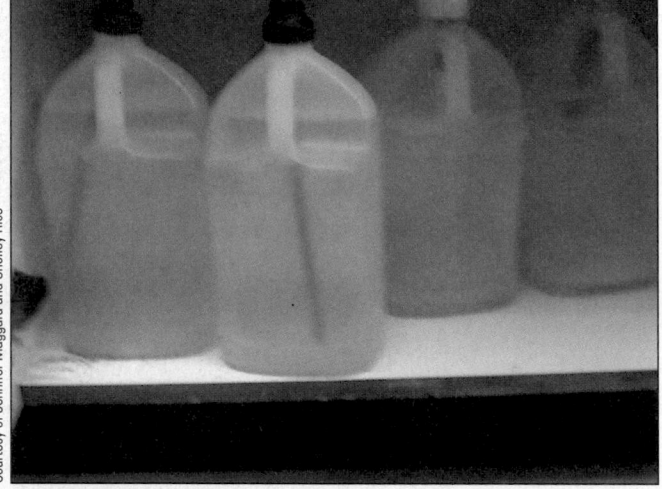

Courtesy of Jennifer Maggard and Shelley Rice

FIGURE 28-108
Replenishing bottles with developer and fixer connected to automatic processor.

be replenished daily with solution and not with water. Water will dilute the solutions and result in poorly processed films. The manufacturers of the processing solutions recommend changing the solutions every 3–4 weeks in offices that have an average daily run of 20–30 intraoral films per day. In high-volume offices, solutions may need to be changed every 1–2 weeks. Automatic processor chemicals and manual processing solutions cannot be interchanged. The solutions manufactured for manual tanks are not made to produce diagnostic images in the shortened processing time of an automatic processor. Furthermore, the concentrated solutions made for an automatic processor will result in poorly processed films if used in manual tanks with the time–temperature method. The autoprocessors should be tested at the start of each day to ensure that the solutions are fresh and that the films will be processed in a manner that will result in a diagnostic image. Testing the solutions and films is discussed in Chapter 29.

Some processors do not have daylight loaders that allow the operator to safely insert films under standard room lighting conditions. These types of machines require the use of a safelight while processing, and they must be placed in a darkroom (Figure 28-111). Other autoprocessors are designed with daylight loaders (Figure 28-12). The daylight loaders have a safelight window or lid that allows the radiographer to view the opening of the film packet and insert the film into the processor with the white light still on. Opening the film packet at first may be more difficult for the new radiographer; however, it is important that only the film is placed into the film feed slots in the processor (Figure 28-109). The radiographer needs to make certain only one film at a time is placed into each film feed slot. The packet and black paper should be placed into the contaminated waste and the lead foil in the designated regulated waste (Figure 28-15).

Some smaller processors are made for the type 2 size film. All other sized films require adjustment in the procedure or use of carriers (Figure 28-110). There are ports for size 0 and 1 and occlusal ports for size 4 films. These carriers must be used for the size 0 or size 1 films or the films, if placed directly into the film feed slot, will fall into the developing solution and become overdeveloped. They are too small to be transported via the roller system into the fixer and the water tanks. The size 4 film is too large and will not fit into the smaller autoprocessors without a special carrier (Figure 28-110).

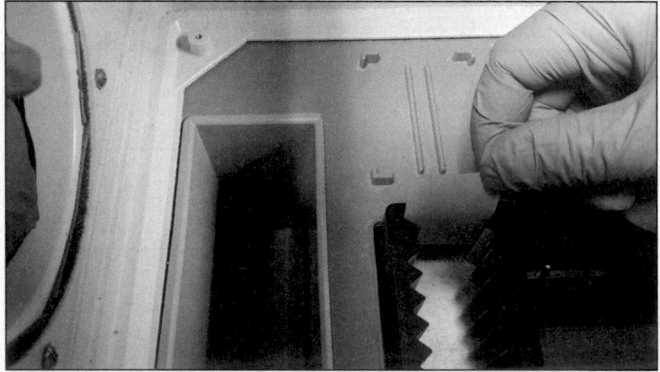

Courtesy of V. Singhal

FIGURE 28-109
Film being placed into the film feed slot of a Peri-Pro, which has a daylight loader.

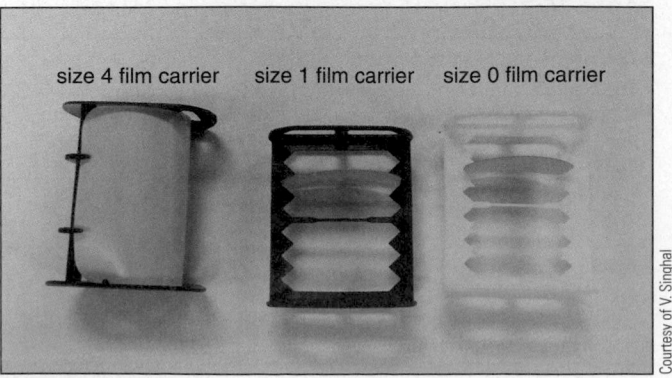

size 4 film carrier   size 1 film carrier   size 0 film carrier

Courtesy of V. Singhal

FIGURE 28-110
Carriers for size 0, 1, and 4 films.

CHAPTER 28 Dental Radiology Infection Control, Exposure, Processing and Evaluation of
Dental Radiographs, and Mounting of Dental Radiographs

895

Some of the larger processors accept the insertion of all sizes of intraoral and extraoral films. There is a ledge on the processor with lines to indicate where the film should be placed (Figure 28-111). It is also designed so multiple films can be processed simultaneously without touching each other during processing.

Some automatic processors have a rapid processing function, also referred to as the "endo function" (Figure 28-112). When the dentist is performing endodontic root canal therapy, he or she needs to see exactly where the endodontic file is placed. By using the endo function, the processing of film quickly helps guide the endo procedure. The endo function processes the film without the same contrast as with the regular settings; however, this allows the dentist to see the contrast between the steel endodontic file and the tooth being prepared. Processing films using the endo setting is not ideal for diagnosing except when needed in a hurry. The film also can be a little damp because the film goes through the dryer faster, and it should be placed on a film hanger until it is completely dry before mounting. Procedure 28-8 provides the steps in automatic processing in a processor with a daylight loader.

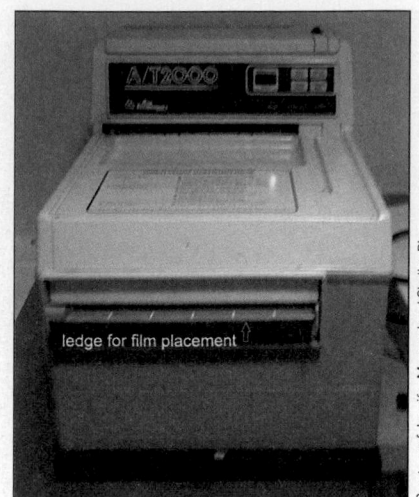

Courtesy of Jennifer Maggard and Shelley Rice

FIGURE 28-111
Ledge on autoprocessor for placing films for processing.

Procedure 28-7
Automatic Processing of Films in an Autoprocessor with a Daylight Loader (Peri-Pro)

This procedure is performed by the dental assistant. The dental assistant prepares the equipment, supplies, and work area. The exposed radiographs are taken to the automatic processor by the dental assistant to process.

Equipment and Supplies
- exposed radiographs in labeled cup
- automatic Peri-Pro processor with daylight loader (see Figure 28-12)
- gloves
- disposable cup

Procedure Steps (*Follow Aseptic Procedures*)
1. Turn on the automatic film processor at the beginning of each day. This ensures that it is warmed up and ready to process after the radiographs are exposed. The chemicals must be heated to the correct temperatures or the images will appear light, and the diagnostic quality will be diminished.

2. Don protective gown and protective eyewear. Wash and dry hands.

3. Place exposed radiographs in labeled cup in the daylight loader with one additional empty cup and gloves (see Figure 28-13).

4. Position hands through the sleeves of the daylight loader and don gloves.

5. Remove each radiograph from its packet, and place each film individually into a slot in the processor (see Figure 28-109). Hold the films by the edges so they are not contaminated. As the films are dropped into the processor, continue to unwrap each film and place in a slot. Place the empty packets in the empty cup.

6. After all films are unwrapped, remove the gloves and place them in the contaminated container with the empty packets. Remove your hands from the sleeves of the daylight loader. Wash and dry hands.

7. Don clean gloves. Open the top of the daylight loader and carefully gather the cups with film wrappers and gloves for disposal (see Figure 28-14).

8. Separate the film packets and gloves and dispose of them in trash. Dispose of the lead foils in the lead foil recycling container (see Figure 28-15). Remove gloves, and wash and dry hands.

9. Remove processed films from the outlet area with clean hands, and prepare for placement in a labeled film mount (discussed later in this chapter).

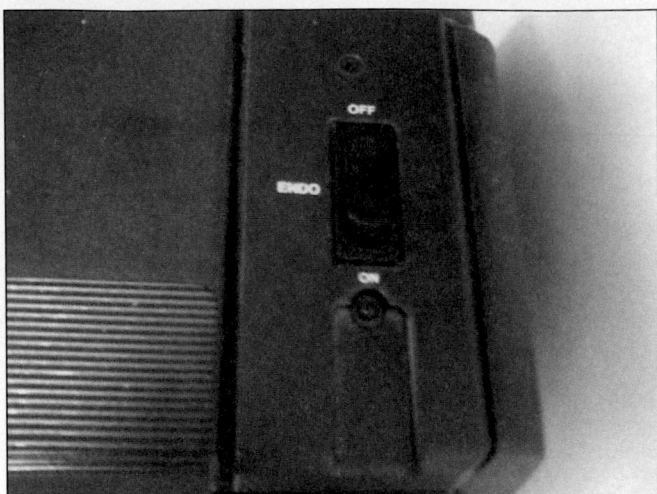

FIGURE 28-112
Rapid processing option.

Care and Maintenance of Automatic Processor The automatic processor manufacturer recommendations should be meticulously followed. The manufacturer provides a cleaning and replenishment schedule. Many recommend running a cleaning film at the beginning of each day to remove residual gelatin and dirt from the rollers. The cleaning film will also tell the operator if the rollers are clean enough to process films. The manufacturer has recommended cleaning solutions and procedures for thoroughly cleaning the processor. The processor and the roller transport system should be cleaned before the changing of processing solutions.

Handling Processing Solutions

It is important to closely follow manufacturer's directions when preparing and storing the solutions. The manufacturer provides recommendations for handling the processing solutions, which may include:

- store chemicals in a cool, dry area
- check expirations dates of processing solutions
- cover chemicals immediately when in the tanks or autoprocessors to prevent oxidization
- change water daily
- check solutions daily and replenish as needed
- check solutions daily and change as needed based on the volume of radiographs processed in the office and based on the manufacturer's recommendations
- dispose of solutions as per state law guidelines; in most states the solutions are collected and cannot be disposed of in the sink drain

Comparison of Processing Techniques

The greatest advantage in using the automatic processor when compared to the manual processing technique is that less

processing time is required for automatic processing. Other advantages include:

- no need for darkroom when using a daylight loader
- less equipment and less space required for autoprocessing techniques
- time and temperature are controlled; thus, better quality radiographs are produced
- consistent results for all intraoral and extraoral radiographs

There are a few disadvantages in using an automatic processor:

- Breakdown of machine resulting in damage and loss of films
- Less films can be processed at a time

Common Film Processing Errors

Common film processing errors result from how the film was handled during the processing stage, and the maintenance and setup of the film processing equipment. Dental radiographic film is sensitive to the temperature of the processing solutions, and films must be handled carefully when they are being unwrapped and placed in the processing machine. Maintenance of the processing machine is necessary to ensure clean films without streaks or stains. This section will discuss processing errors that may occur with films, what may cause them, and how to prevent them.

Film with Light Image

Light and dark film images can occur not only while exposing the film but also during processing (Figure 28-113). A light film is considered to be underprocessed. If the film is underprocessed, the developing time was too short, the developer temperature was lower than recommended, or the developing solution was exhausted (i.e., too weak from overuse and needing to be changed).

Film with Dark Image

Dark film images are overdeveloped, caused by the developing solution temperature being too high or the solution being too concentrated, or the film being left in the developer too long (Figure 28-114). Routinely check solutions and adjust

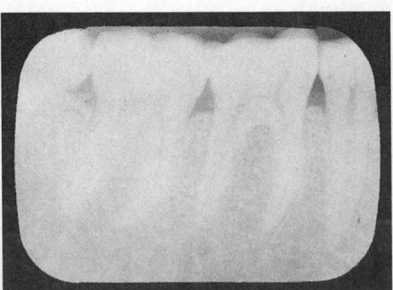

FIGURE 28-113
A light image due to a film processing error.

CHAPTER 28 Dental Radiology Infection Control, Exposure, Processing and Evaluation of
Dental Radiographs, and Mounting of Dental Radiographs

897

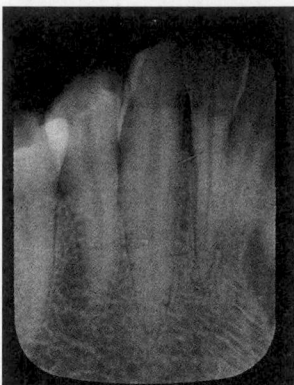

FIGURE 28-114
A dark image due to a film processing error.

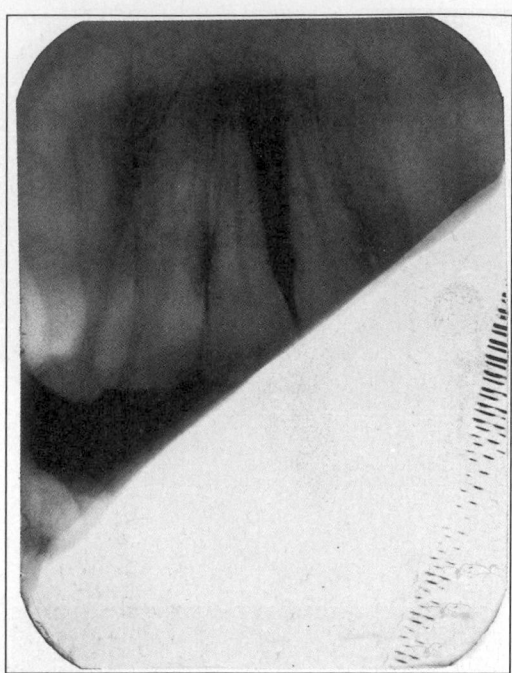

FIGURE 28-115
Partial image due to low processing solution.

processing times accordingly. Refer to the film processing section earlier in this chapter for more detail on how to check the temperature of processing solutions. Several methods for monitoring film quality are discussed later in this chapter.

Fogged Film

A fogged film error has a gray appearance, and there is lost image detail and contrast. It is like viewing a film image through a dense fog. Fog on films can be caused by improper storage conditions, using outdated films, light leaks in the processing room, or light leaks from loose fittings on the automatic processors and daylight loaders. Also, safelights may need to be adjusted or changed; for example, they may be too close to the processing area, too bright, or faulty.

Partial Image

A partial image on the film is the result of film placement in the processing tanks when the solution levels are low. The film is not completely immersed, and a partial image results (Figure 28-115). Always check the levels of the processing solutions. Some evaporation takes place daily, and the films absorb some of the developer as well, so replenish the developer regularly. To avoid the chance of a partial image when using manual processing, do not use the top clips on the manual processing film racks. Refer to the online platform for manual processing.

Spotted Films

Spots on the film result from not handling the films carefully or not keeping the area around the processing tanks clean. As a result of these actions, the following might occur:

● Water touching unprocessed film will leave a clear area(s) on the film.

● White spots on the film may be caused by contact with the fixer before the film is placed into the developer. This is caused by drops of fixer, which may splash onto the counter around the processor when refilling or replenishing the solutions (Figure 28-116).

● Dark spots on the film may be caused by contact with the developer. If the unprocessed film comes in contact with the developer before the film is placed into the developer solution, it will leave dark spots on the film (Figure 28-117).

● Yellow-brownish stains on films are usually caused by improper or insufficient washing or rinsing of the film during the processing sequence. Use of exhausted developer and fixer or insufficient fixing time may also cause a yellow-brownish stain on the films (Figure 28-118).

● Static electricity can cause black branching lines on the film. Opening a film packet too quickly can cause a small charge of electricity during times of low humidity (Figure 28-119).

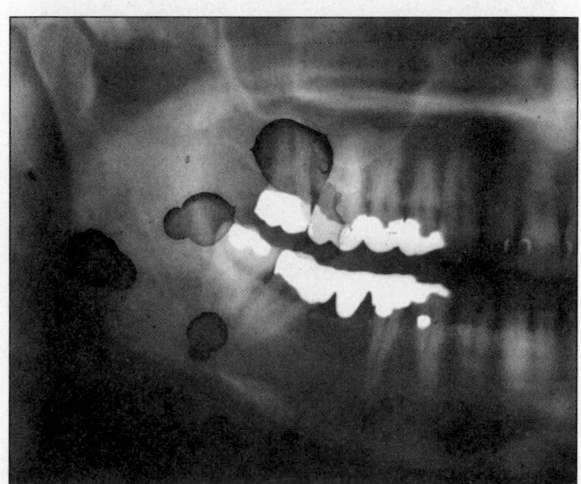

FIGURE 28-116
An image with white (fixer) spots.

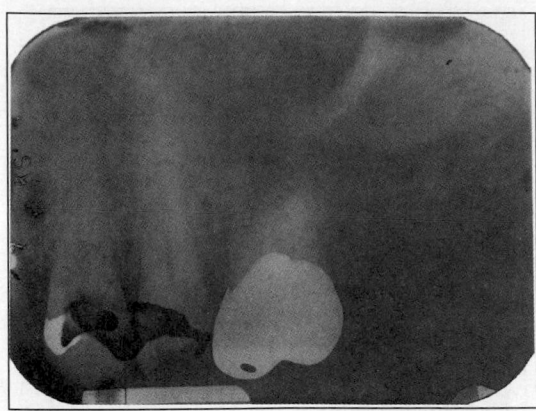

FIGURE 28-117
An image with dark (developer) spots.

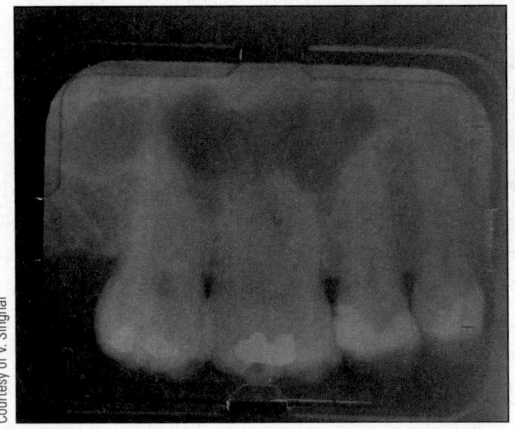

FIGURE 28-118
Yellow/brown film.

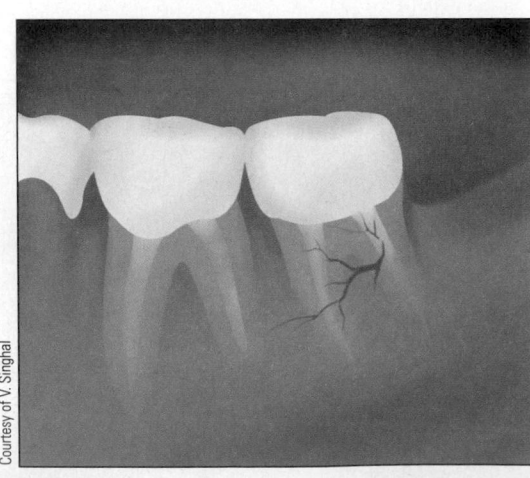

FIGURE 28-119
Static electricity.

Torn or Scratched Film

Rough handling of the film can lead to the emulsion on the film being torn or scratched, leaving a white area or mark on the processed film. Films can be scratched and torn if they are not handled carefully in overcrowded tanks, or during retrieval, if the film is lost off the film racks. The emulsion can also be scratched through the glove by a long fingernail (Figure 28-120).

Air Bubbles on the Film

Air bubbles are trapped on the film if it is not agitated when placed in the processing solutions. The air bubbles leave round, white spots where they were attached to the film (Figure 28-121).

Reticulation

Reticulation occurs when a film has been exposed to a high temperature followed by a low temperature. The film emulsion swells and then shrinks. The film looks like it has been dried and has tiny cracks. The temperature of the solutions and the water should be monitored to ensure that they are within the recommended temperature ranges.

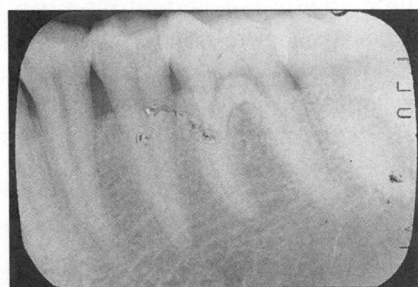

FIGURE 28-120
A radiograph with a torn or scratched emulsion.

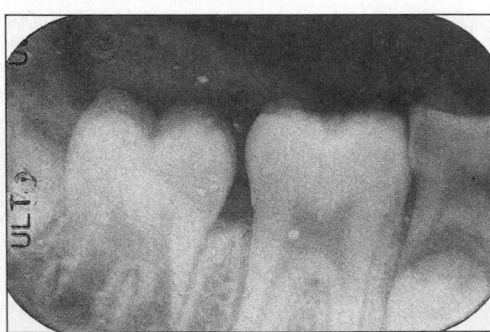

FIGURE 28-121
Films that are agitated poorly when placed in the processing solutions leave air-bubble artifacts on the processed film.

CHAPTER 28 Dental Radiology Infection Control, Exposure, Processing and Evaluation of Dental Radiographs, and Mounting of Dental Radiographs

899

Streaks

Streaks on films may result from unclean rollers when using automatic processors or from unclean film racks. Debris is picked up as the films pass through the rollers, leaving a streaked appearance on the film. Streaks from unclean film racks occur during the manual processing procedure; debris, including processing solutions, runs from the racks onto the film.

Film Mounts and Film Mounting

Film mounts are used to maintain the images in anatomical order, protect the radiographs, and aid in ease of viewing. There are a variety of film mounts available to suit the various intraoral film sizes (#0–#4), number of films, and types of radiographic surveys to be mounted. Some of the most popular mounts are:

- Single mounts for single films as shown in Figure 28-122A. Single films may also be placed into a coin envelope (see Figure 28-105B)

- Film full mouth series mounts (Figure 28-122B)

- Two film bitewing mounts for pediatric bitewings (Figure 28-122C)

- Four film bitewing mounts for adult bitewings (Figure 28-122C)

Mounts are made of many different materials including cardboard, black plastic, or clear vinyl plastic. Some mounts have slots for films, and some have pockets that the films slide into and the entire film is encased and protected.

Mounting Views

Films are placed in the mount for the dentist's preference for viewing. There are two views used for the placement of the films into the mount: the labial view and the lingual view. *Labial mounting* is viewed as if the dentist is seeing the patient from the front of the face (Figure 28-123). This is the same manner of viewing the radiographs on the viewbox where they are placed with the patient's right on the viewer's left (Figure 28-124). The films are placed in the mount with the convex side of the embossed dot toward the dentist (Figure 28-123). The labial view is the most preferred by dentists and is the American Dental Association (ADA) standard.

The lingual view is viewed as if the dentist is viewing the patient from the lingual side as if standing on the tongue and looking out (Figure 28-125). The films are placed with the concave side of the embossed dot toward the dentist (Figure 28-125). The film is flipped backward compared to the ADA standard recommended labial view. From this view the patient's right side is to the right of the dentist when viewing the mounted films (Figure 28-125). Since the labial method of mounting is the preferred method, it will be discussed in detail in Procedure 28-8 and Figures 28-126 to 28-130.

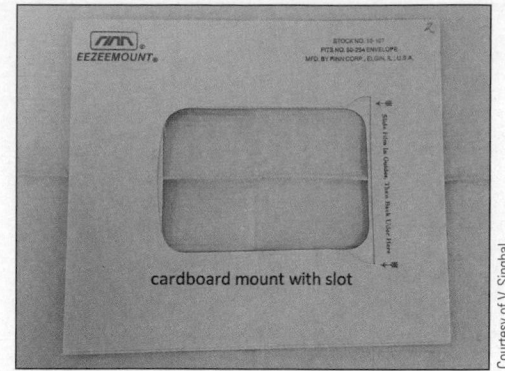

FIGURE 28-122A
Single film mount.

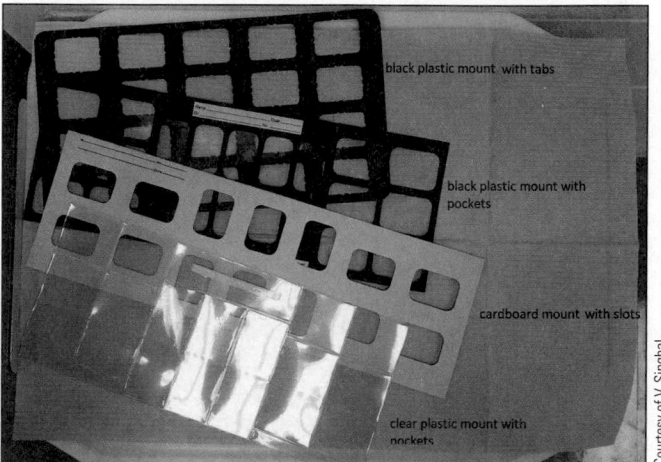

FIGURE 28-122B
Assorted full mouth series mounts.

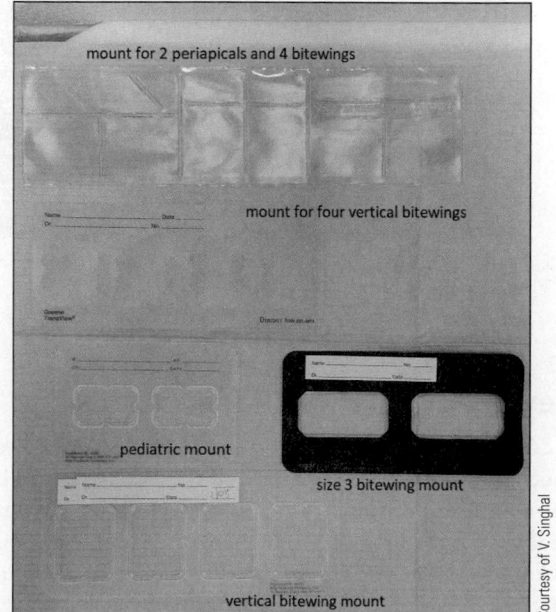

FIGURE 28-122C
Assorted bitewing mounts.

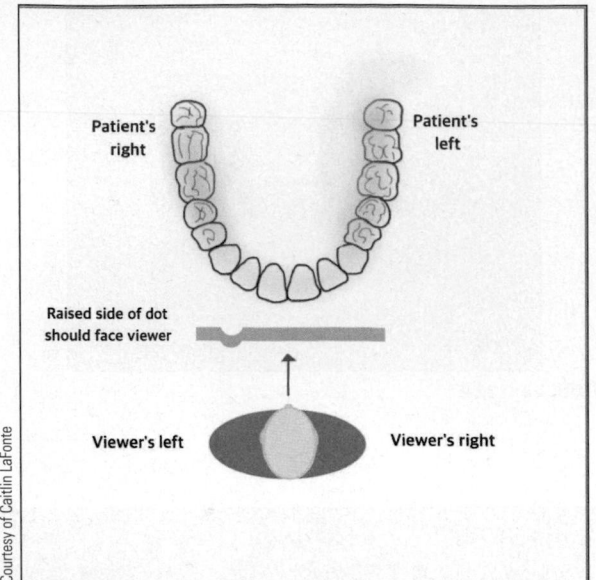

FIGURE 28-123
Labial mounting view.

Courtesy of Caitlin LaFonte

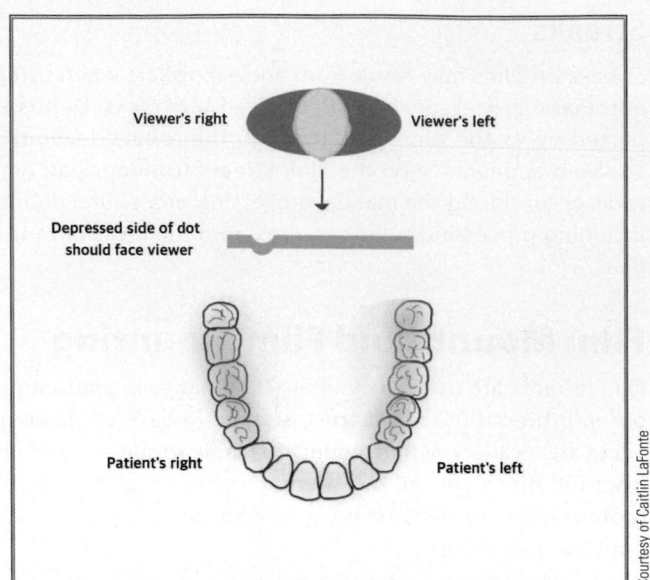

FIGURE 28-125
Lingual mounting view.

Courtesy of Caitlin LaFonte

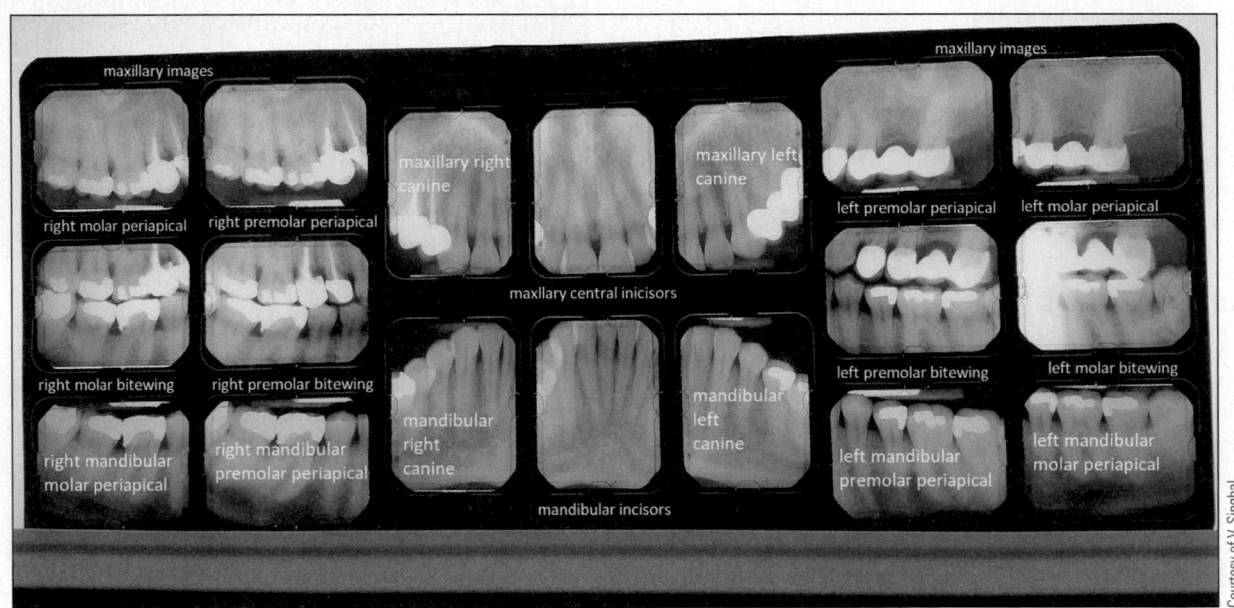

FIGURE 28-124
Full mouth series of radiographs on viewbox.

Courtesy of V. Singhal

Viewing of Mounted Radiographs

Once the radiographs are mounted in anatomical order, whether traditional or digital, they should be viewed by the operator. Traditional images should be viewed on a viewbox. Ideally a black opaque mount is best as it blocks out the background light and allows for easier viewing of traditional films. The dental radiographer should view each image for any deviations from normal. On each periapical image, the operator should look at the teeth including pulps, roots, and periapical areas as well as alveolar bone. Any deviations from normal should be reported to the dentist. Radiographic anatomy and radiographic pathologies will be discussed in Chapter 29. Images should be viewed in sequence to ensure that all images are viewed completely and that any abnormalities are noted and reported to the dentist. The viewing sequence is shown in Figure 28-131.

CHAPTER 28 Dental Radiology Infection Control, Exposure, Processing and Evaluation of
Dental Radiographs, and Mounting of Dental Radiographs

901

Procedure 28-8
Mounting Traditional Films

This procedure is performed by the dental assistant. A view-box may be utilized when mounting the radiographs.

Equipment and Supplies (Figure 28-126)
- radiographs
- lighted viewbox
- radiograph mount for 18-film full mouth series and pen for labeling
- clean, dry surface

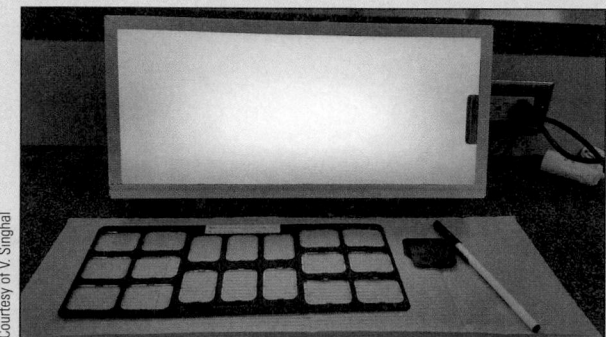

FIGURE 28-126
Supplies needed for traditional film mounting.

Procedure Steps
1. Wash and dry hands.

2. Label the radiograph mount with the patient's name, the date of the exposure, and the operator's name (see Figure 28-105A).

3. Turn on the viewbox and place all radiographs on the mount with the convex side of the dots facing up (Figures 28-127 and 28-128).

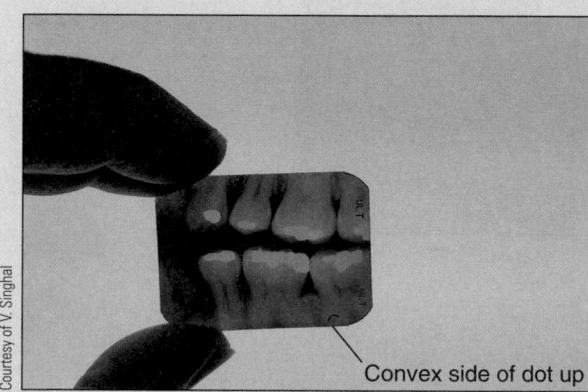

Convex side of dot up

FIGURE 28-127
Film with convex side of dot facing the operator.

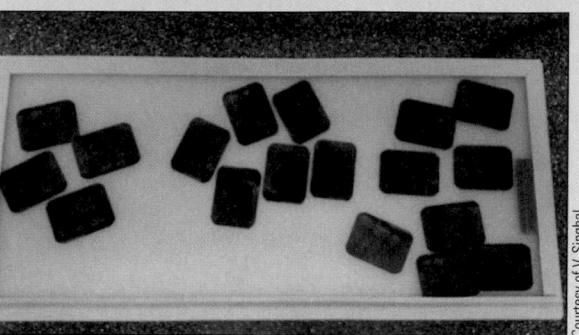

FIGURE 28-128
Films on viewbox with convex side of dot facing operator.

4. Using the viewbox, categorize all radiographs into three groups: bitewings (four in number), anterior (six in number), and posterior (eight in number) (Figure 28-129).

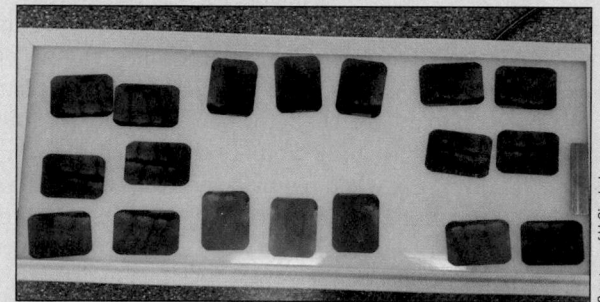

FIGURE 28-129
Films with convex side of dot facing operator, oriented properly and grouped together.

5. Place the bitewing radiographs in the mount, making sure the dots remain convex, the molars are toward the outside, and the bicuspids (premolars) are toward the inside. Make sure that the radiographs are mounted according to the curve of Spee (Figure 28-130).

6. Put the anterior radiographs in place, with the maxillary above and the mandibular below. The incisal edges should be closest to each other in the mount, and the roots positioned as they grow. The centrals are placed in the middle with the canines on the outer sides. The maxillary centrals are much larger than the mandibular central incisors (see Figure 28-124).

7. Place the remaining posterior radiographs. The molars should be placed toward the outside and the bicuspids (premolars) toward the inside. The maxillary molars

(Continues)

have three roots, and the mandibular molars have two roots. Both should be placed according to their position in the oral cavity, with the roots opposite each other and the biting surfaces more closely positioned (see Figure 28-124).

8. Review the mounted radiographs to verify that they have been placed properly.

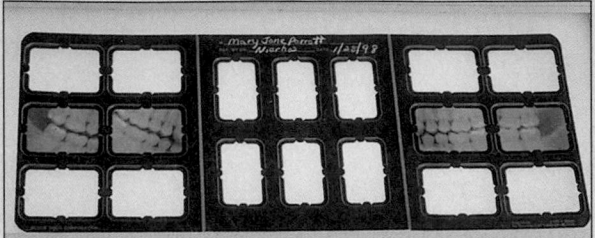

FIGURE 28-130
Full mouth series mount with bitewing radiographs in place.

Duplicating Radiographs

The duplication of radiographs is performed in the darkroom using a duplicating film and a film duplicating machine. The duplicating film is stored in a box similar to the panoramic film box. Make certain to double-check the box to confirm that it is a duplicating film before turning off the white light. Only the safelight should be on, when removing the duplicating film from the box and positioning it onto the duplicating machine.

Some smaller autoprocessors have built-in duplicators that utilize size 2 duplicating film. Each individual film needs to be duplicated independently and then processed in the autoprocessor just like an original traditional film would be. The duplicate films are then mounted as traditional intraoral films are. The operator must always remember that the original films should never be given to another practitioner as they are part of the legal record. Also remember that the quality of the duplicates is never as good as the original films. Some offices may use film packets with two films inside. Use of double film packets allows exposure of two sets at once so that one is available to send to another practitioner if the need arises. Digital images can be printed and mailed or sent electronically to another practitioner.

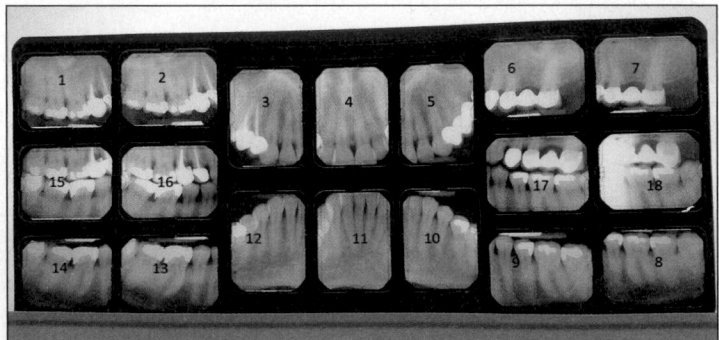

FIGURE 28-131
Viewing sequence of a full set of radiographs.

CHAPTER 28 Dental Radiology Infection Control, Exposure, Processing and Evaluation of
Dental Radiographs, and Mounting of Dental Radiographs

903

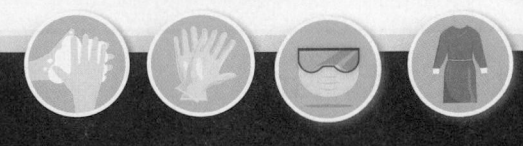

Procedure 28-9
Steps in Film Duplication

Equipment and Supplies
- film to be duplicated
- duplicating machine
- manual processor or autoprocessor
- patient's chart

Procedure Steps
1. Wash and dry hands.

2. Position the film being duplicated onto the duplicating machine in the same orientation as when the operator views the mounted images; the convex side of the dot should be facing up (Figure 28-132).

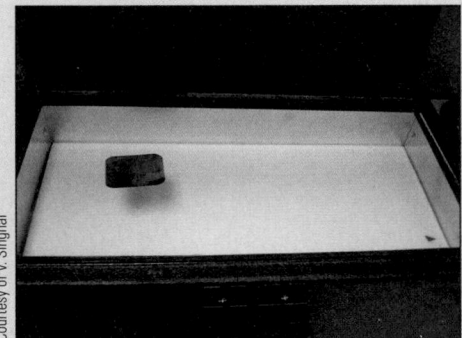

FIGURE 28-132
Film placed on duplicator with convex side of dot facing up.

3. The emulsion side or dull side of the duplicating film is placed directly onto the film. There is a notch on the duplicating film sheet, and the notch should be oriented in the top right corner of the duplicator surface (Figure 28-133). It is easier to feel the notch rather than see the emulsion. Orientation of the notch

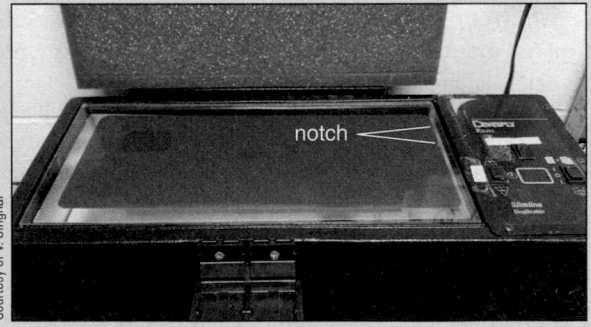

notch

FIGURE 28-133
Duplicating film with emulsion side down and notch in upper right corner placed on original film.

will ensure that the emulsion side is facing down and touching the films.

4. The timer for the duplicator light is set per manufacturer's directions (Figure 28-134); the standard time is usually 10 seconds. The longer the time the light is on, the lighter the duplicated image will be; shorter times result in darker duplicated images. If the original images are dark or dense, use an increased duplication time to lighten the copies. Close the duplicator lid and start the duplication process.

5. The next step is to manually process the duplicated image like the original film. This can be with the use of manual processing or with a large autoprocessor (see Figure 28-111).

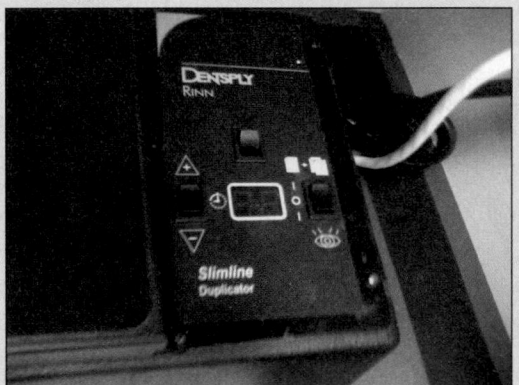

FIGURE 28-134
Timer on film duplication machine.

6. The duplicated film is labeled with the patient's name, date the original film was taken, and that the film being provided is a duplicate (Figure 28-135). The dental auxiliary should document in the patient's chart that the film was duplicated, the date the duplication was performed and who will be receiving the duplicated film.

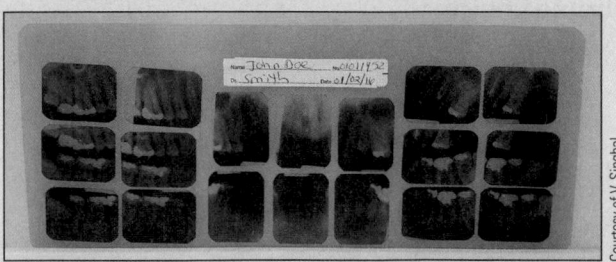

FIGURE 28-135
Duplicated full set of radiographs.

Chapter Summary

The dentist uses quality radiographs as an important component of formulating a dental diagnosis. The two techniques used to expose intraoral radiographs are bisecting and paralleling. Both techniques are described in this chapter, but the most widely used is the paralleling technique. It is important for the dental assistant to know how to use both of these techniques properly in order to obtain quality images.

Once the film-based radiographs have been exposed, they must be processed. Manual and automatic processing equipment and techniques are described and compared. Chemical components of the developing and fixing solutions are listed, and the role they play in converting the latent image into a visible permanent radiograph is discussed.

Radiographs are then accurately mounted for viewing. There are various types of dental radiographic mounts to choose from. Helpful hints provided are important to use in the accurate mounting of radiographs.

Common radiographic errors during the processing and exposing of images are listed with examples. Careful attention to positioning during exposure and detailed step-by-step procedures for processing can assist in the elimination of errors.

Patient radiographs are needed for many reasons. For instance, insurance companies require copies of the patient's radiographs to determine insurance coverage, and other dental offices require a copy of the patient's images for their own diagnoses. Radiographs can be duplicated so that the original radiographs never have to leave the office. The special film and equipment needed for this process are discussed. Dental offices are required to properly store final radiographs to prevent losses, thereby avoiding the need for retakes of radiographs.

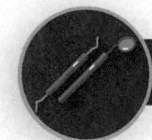 **CASE STUDY**

You have just completed exposing a full set of 18 radiographs on a new patient using traditional films. You are now ready to process the films. The autoprocessor is running and ready for the films. Once all the films are in the film feed slot and in the machine, you clean up the area. As the films emerge, you notice that part of each of the films remained unprocessed.

Case Study Review

1. What may have gone wrong?

2. What should have been done before processing the films?

3. Since the films are not diagnostic, what needs to be done now?

Review Questions

Multiple Choice

1. Instruments/surfaces used in dental radiography may require a barrier, disinfection, or sterilization. The digital sensor may be autoclaved, whereas the x-ray machine head should have a barrier.

   Select the correct response based on the statement above.

   a. Both statements are true.
   b. Both statements are false.
   c. The first statement is true, and the second statement is false.
   d. The first statement is false, and the second statement is true.

2. Which of the following is the correct sequence for exposing a full mouth series using size 2 image receptors with the paralleling technique?
   a. maxillary right canine, maxillary incisors, maxillary left canine, mandibular left canine, mandibular incisors, mandibular right canine, maxillary right premolars, maxillary right molars, mandibular left premolars, mandibular left molars, maxillary left premolars, maxillary left molars, mandibular right premolars, mandibular right molars
   b. maxillary right canine, maxillary incisors, maxillary left canine, mandibular right canine, mandibular incisors, mandibular left canine, maxillary right premolars, maxillary right molars, mandibular left premolars, mandibular left molars, maxillary left premolars, maxillary left molars, mandibular right premolars, mandibular right molars

c. maxillary right canine, maxillary incisors, maxillary left canine, mandibular left canine, mandibular incisors, mandibular right canine, maxillary left premolars, maxillary left molars, maxillary right premolars, maxillary right molars, mandibular left premolars, mandibular left molars, mandibular right premolars, mandibular right molars

d. maxillary right canine, maxillary incisors, maxillary left canine, mandibular left canine, mandibular incisors, mandibular right canine, maxillary right premolars, maxillary right molars, mandibular right premolars, mandibular right molars, mandibular left premolars, maxillary left premolars, maxillary left molars

3. Which of the following is not correct regarding patient positioning during exposures?
   a. For the paralleling technique, the maxilla should be parallel to the floor.
   b. For the paralleling technique, the midsagittal plane should be perpendicular to the floor.
   c. For maxillary exposures using the bisecting technique, the ala–tragus line should be parallel to the floor.
   d. For mandibular exposures using the bisecting technique, the mandibular teeth should be perpendicular to the floor.

4. Which of the following is not correct regarding image receptor holders for the paralleling technique?
   a. The bite block for the paralleling technique allows the patient to bite and hold the device in place during exposures.
   b. Disposable bite blocks may be used to obtain exposures in the paralleling technique.
   c. The aiming ring allows the operator to align the position-indicating device (PID) to reduce the risk of partial exposure.
   d. The metal arms in the paralleling extension cone kits allow the operator to set the vertical angulation for the exposure.

5. When obtaining the premolar bitewing image, the image receptor should be centered on the premolars. The front edge of the receptor should be aligned with the distal edge of the mandibular canine in order to capture contact between the canines and the first premolars in both arches.

   Select the correct response based on the statement above.

   a. Both statements are true.
   b. Both statements are false.
   c. The first statement is true, and the second statement is false.
   d. The first statement is false, and the second statement is true.

6. Which of the following is not correct regarding errors in vertical angulation?
   a. Elongation and foreshortening are errors that occur related to vertical angulation.
   b. Elongation occurs when the angle is not sufficient.
   c. Foreshortening occurs when the angle is too steep.
   d. Elongation and foreshortening occur more commonly with the paralleling technique.

7. Conecut images most commonly occur due to improper assembly of the anterior extension cone paralleling (XCP) kit. Conecut may also occur if the position-indicating device (PID) drifts during exposure.

   Select the correct response based on the statement above.

   a. Both statements are true.
   b. Both statements are false.
   c. The first statement is true, and the second statement is false.
   d. The first statement is false, and the second statement is true.

8. Which of the following image receptor placement errors occurs when the image receptor is not parallel to the tooth?
   a. elongation
   b. conecut
   c. herring bone
   d. dot of film at apex

9. Which of the following is not a purpose for occlusal images?
   a. diagnose dental decay
   b. locate salivary gland stones
   c. locate supernumerary teeth
   d. evaluate fractures

10. Which of the following is not correct regarding the placement of the maxillary occlusal topographical exposure?
    a. The white side of the film should be toward the palate and the embossed dot toward the anterior.
    b. The receptor is positioned with the long dimension of the receptor vertical, lengthwise in the oral cavity.
    c. The patient holds the receptor in place by gently biting the image receptor.
    d. Once the film has been placed, the radiographer should set the vertical angulation at positive 65°.

11. Which of the following is correct regarding modified exposure techniques related to an edentulous patient?
    a. Edentulous patients do not need radiographs.
    b. Bitewings should be included in a full set of radiographs on an edentulous patient.
    c. When using the bisecting angle technique in an edentulous patient, the angle is formed by the image receptor and the alveolar bone.
    d. Cotton rolls are not beneficial when completing exposures in an edentulous patient.

12. For maxillary occlusal topographical procedures on a child, the maxilla should be positioned parallel to the floor. The position-indicating device (PID) should be positioned at +60° with the top of the PID at the bridge of the nose.

    Select the correct response based on the statement above.

    a. Both statements are true.
    b. Both statements are false.
    c. The first statement is true, and the second statement is false.
    d. The first statement is false, and the second statement is true.

13. Which of the following is correct regarding the management of a pediatric patient during radiographic exposures?
    a. Pediatric patients do not need to use a lead apron.
    b. Use terms the pediatric patients will understand such as "camera."
    c. Pediatric patients should be managed in the same manner as adults.
    d. Pediatric patients should be forced to have radiographs if needed.

14. Which of the following is correct regarding radiographic record keeping?
    a. Dental radiographs are separate and therefore not considered to be a part of the dental record.
    b. Traditional films do not need to be identified during exposure and processing since they will be mounted and labeled.
    c. The chart entry should include the type of radiograph, but the number of radiographs is not required.
    d. The radiographer must sign the chart entry for radiographs.

15. The developer is able to differentiate between the exposed and unexposed silver halide crystals. The exposed silver halide crystals are reduced to black metal silver through a process called selective reduction.

    Select the correct response based on the statement above.

    a. Both statements are true.
    b. Both statements are false.
    c. The first statement is true, and the second statement is false.
    d. The first statement is false, and the second statement is true.

16. Which of the following is the correct sequence of steps for the manual processing tank?
    a. developer, water bath rinse, fixer, water bath wash
    b. developer, fixer, water bath wash
    c. fixer, water bath rinse, developer, water bath wash
    d. fixer, developer, water bath wash

17. The darkroom should have room lighting for times when processing is not taking place. The darkroom should also have safelighting, which filters out the red-orange spectrum of light.

    Select the correct response based on the statement above.

    a. Both statements are true.
    b. Both statements are false.
    c. The first statement is true, and the second statement is false.
    d. The first statement is false, and the second statement is true.

18. Which of the following is correct regarding the manual processing tank?
    a. The manual processing tank has two insert tanks, both of which are placed on the left side of the main water tank.
    b. The manual processing tank has an overflow pipe so water can flow into the pipe and drain out in case the tank overfills.
    c. The manual processing tank has a standard plumbing connection to allow water to flow into the main water tank.
    d. The manual processing tank has a cover to prevent oxidation of chemicals.

19. As the dental assistant, you come in each morning and fill the manual processing tank with water after checking the solution levels and testing them for strength. While processing a set of films one morning, you noticed that several had cracks on them. Which of the following may have resulted in the cracked emulsion?
    a. developer and water at the same temperature
    b. low levels of developer
    c. low levels of fixer
    d. cold water bath temperature as compared to the developer temperature

20. Which of the following is correct regarding maintaining processing solutions in a manual tank?
    a. Solutions should be changed every 8 weeks based on 20–30 intraoral films per day.
    b. The solutions should be tested weekly.
    c. The solutions for autoprocessors should not be used in manual processing tanks.
    d. If solution levels become low from use, add water to increase the volume and levels.

Critical Thinking

1. How does the dental assistant maintain infection control while processing films in a Peri-Pro with a daylight loader?

2. How does the dental assistant maintain infection control while processing films in the darkroom?

3. What are the steps the dental assistant should follow when manually processing films?

Key Terms

Term and Pronunciation	Meaning of Root and Word Parts	Definition
oxidation (ok-si-**dey**-shuhn)	**oxider** = to combine with oxygen **-ation** = denoting action or process	chemical solutions lose freshness after prolonged exposure to the oxygen in the air; often have a coating of oxide, darken in color

## CHAPTER 29

Extraoral Radiography, Digital Radiography, and Radiographic Interpretation

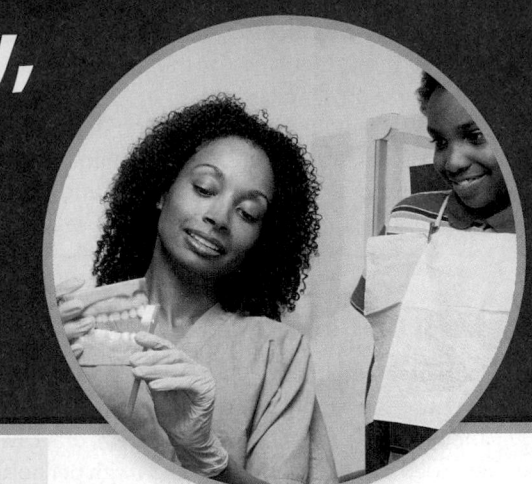

Specific Instructional Objectives

At the completion of this chapter, you will be able to meet these objectives:

1. Use terms presented in this chapter.
2. State the purpose of extraoral radiographs.
3. Discuss panoramic radiography.
4. Describe the panoramic machine.
5. List the steps in a patient panoramic exposure.
6. Compare and contrast common panoramic radiographic errors.
7. Discuss other extraoral images used in dentistry.
8. Compare and contrast digital radiography and traditional film-based radiography.
9. Differentiate between indirect digital and direct digital dental radiography.
10. Compare and contrast the advantages and disadvantages of digital radiography.
11. List the steps in obtaining intraoral digital dental images.
12. Discuss three-dimensional imaging in dentistry.
13. Discuss the benefits of hand-held/portable intraoral radiology units.
14. Identify the normal anatomical structures on a dental radiograph.
15. Identify dental pathologies on a radiographic image.
16. Identify periodontal pathologies on a radiographic image.
17. Discuss dental anomalies that may be seen on a dental radiograph.
18. Identify various commonly used dental materials as they appear on a dental radiograph.
19. Discuss quality management protocol related to dental radiology.
20. Discuss the laws related to dental radiology.
21. State the responsibilities of the dental assistant as the radiographer.
22. Discuss the steps in risk management.
23. Discuss the relationship of HIPAA to dental radiographs.

Introduction

Extraoral radiography is standard practice in the dental office, and extra oral radiographs are taken routinely as part of patient records. Types of extraoral imaging include panoramic radiographs, used in general and specialty dental offices, and cephalometric radiographs that are mainly taken by orthodontists. The lateral jaw radiograph and the transcranial temporomandibular joint radiograph are the other extraoral radiographs discussed in this chapter. Three-dimensional digital dental imaging is also discussed in this chapter.

The dental assistant should become familiar with radiograph interpretation, because it will help them take quality radiographs and be more prepared for the selected treatment. Interpretation involves learning the terminology and then identifying the landmarks on a radiograph.

Digital radiography is becoming standard in many dental offices, and it is likely that all dental offices in the future will take and store digital radiographs. Digital equipment and techniques, and their advantages and disadvantages, will be discussed. Digital radiography equipment is changing and improving, while the technique is being made easier for the dentist and dental staff to learn and incorporate into their office routine.

Extraoral Radiographs

Extraoral radiographs are used by the dentist to identify large areas of the skull on one radiograph. These radiographs give the dentist an overall view of the teeth, oral cavity, and skull and are used most often in conjunction with periapical, bitewing, and occlusal radiographs. Orthodontists and oral maxillofacial surgeons routinely use extraoral radiographs, especially panoramic and cephalometric exposures.

Panoramic Radiography

Many dental offices have *panoramic radiography* machines (Figures 29-1A, B, and C). Panoramic machines take a radiograph that shows the entire maxilla and mandible on one image (Figure 29-2). Panoramic radiography is commonly known by the brand name of the first panoramic x-ray machine, Panorex. There are many types of panoramic machines, including film-based units and digital imaging units. The film-based machine has a *cassette* that houses the panoramic film. With both the film-based and the digital unit, the image receptor and the x-ray head rotate opposite each other around the patient's head. Because they are connected by bars extending from the top of the machines, they rotate at the same speed. The result is an image that extends from the condyle on one side of the patient's head to the condyle on the other side. There is some overlapping and loss of detail, but panoramic radiographs are valuable when an overall assessment of the patient is needed. Panoramic images can be taken on adults, children, edentulous patients, patients who have trismus, and patients in wheelchairs.

Panoramic images give the dentist a general view of the following:

- the entire dentition
- nasal and orbital areas
- alveolar bone
- carious lesions
- fractures, cysts, and tumors
- malocclusion
- maxilla and mandible
- sinuses
- unerupted teeth
- dental appliances and restorations
- periodontal disease
- temporomandibular joint

Fundamentals of Panoramic Radiography When using film-based panoramic machines, it is necessary for the film to be correctly placed into the cassette under safelight conditions prior to exposure. Direct digital units use digital sensors, inserted directly into the cassette; therefore, there is no need for film placement. Indirect digital units must have the phosphor imaging plate placed inside the cassette prior to exposure. Panoramic radiography is based on the principle of *tomography* (meaning part). Tomography shows the imaging of one layer or section of the body while blurring images from other areas. In panoramic radiography, the image conforms to the curve of the dental arches. The patient is positioned, and when the panoramic exposure button is pushed, the tubehead rotates in one direction around the patient while the image receptor rotates in the opposite direction (Figure 29-3). Some machines require that the patient stand during the exposure, and other machines allow the patient to sit during the exposure. The rotation is synchronized from *rotational centers*. The rotational center is basically the axis around which the tubehead and receptor rotate. Rotational centers vary in number and location, depending on the manufacturer of the panoramic machine. Rotational centers also influence the shape and size of the focal trough. The *focal trough* (Figure 29-4), also known as the image layer or zone of sharpness, is a three-dimensional (3D) curved zone in which the dental arches are positioned to achieve the sharpest image. The panoramic machine will expose this selected plane of tissue, while the areas outside the selected plane will be blurred. The size and shape of the focal trough vary from one panoramic machine to another, but each machine is designed to accommodate the average person. The quality of the panoramic radiograph depends on the precise positioning of the patient's teeth within the focal trough, and the degree to which the patient resembles the average-person design of that specific machine. The manufacturer provides specific instructions for positioning the patient.

Panoramic Unit Panoramic units are constantly being updated and improved (Figure 29-1). They differ by the size and shape of the focal trough, the number and location of the rotational centers, and the type of cassette (holder) used for the x-ray film. All units, however, include the following basic components:

- exposure controls
- head positioner (Figure 29-1A and B)

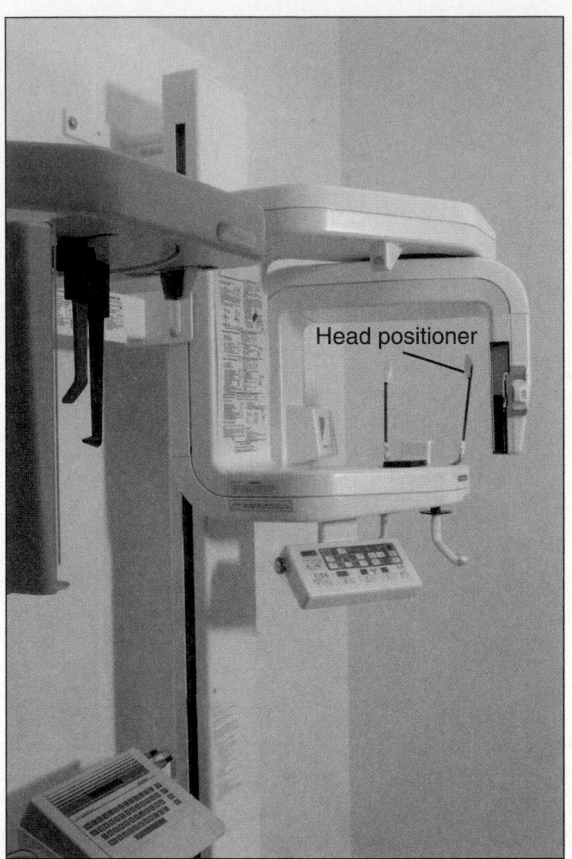

FIGURE 29-1A
A panoramic unit.

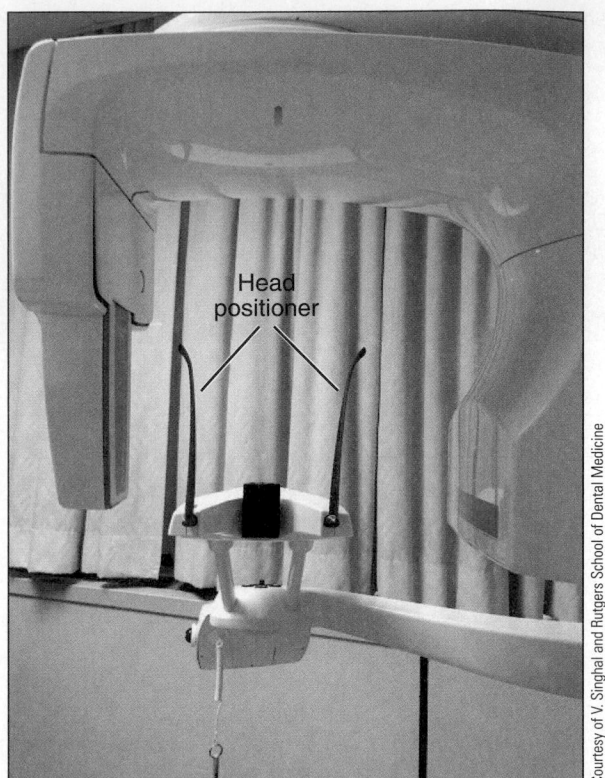

FIGURE 29-1B
A panoramic unit.

Courtesy of V. Singhal and Rutgers School of Dental Medicine

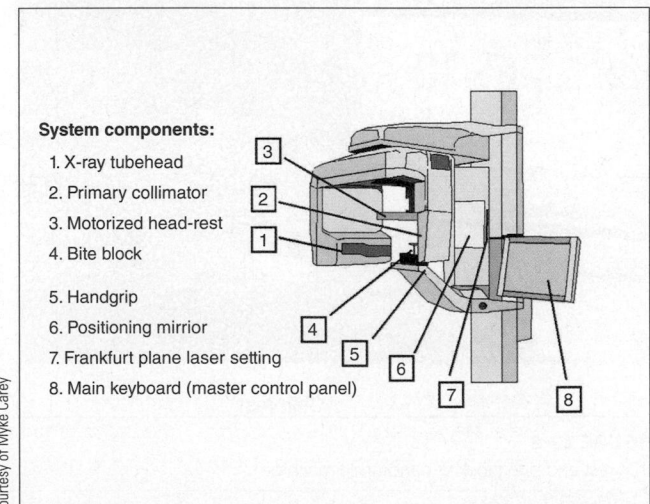

System components:

1. X-ray tubehead
2. Primary collimator
3. Motorized head-rest
4. Bite block
5. Handgrip
6. Positioning mirror
7. Frankfurt plane laser setting
8. Main keyboard (master control panel)

Courtesy of Myke Carey

FIGURE 29-1C
A panoramic unit.

- x-ray tubehead (Figure 29-1C)
- cassette holder

Exposure Controls The exposure controls are usually located outside the x-ray room. In cases where the controls are part of the unit, the exposure control button itself is located outside

the room. The master control panel (Figure 29-1C) allows the radiographer to make the necessary adjustment to expose the prescribed radiograph. The exposure settings are recommended by the manufacturer; however, the kVp and the mA can be adjusted based on size of patient or density of the patient's tissues. The instruction manual provides information on variations for different exposures. Other controls include the following:

- The on/off button, when pressed, turns on the power to the master control and the panoramic stand. The red light in the on/off button will illuminate along with the kVp digital readout. Pressing the button again will turn off the power to the master control and panoramic stand.

- Preprogrammed exposure factors are selected by pressing buttons for pediatric patients, small adults, average adults, and large adults.

- TMJ selection enables a 3 second exposure when the hand switch is pressed, allowing timed TMJ exposures in either the open mouth or the closed mouth position.

- The kVp digital readout displays selected kilovoltage setting.

- The kVp selector adjusts the amount of kVp emitted.

- A hand switch initiates panoramic or TMJ exposures. The button must be pressed until panoramic or TMJ exposure is terminated.

- The x-ray exposure lamp glows and an audible tone sounds during an exposure.

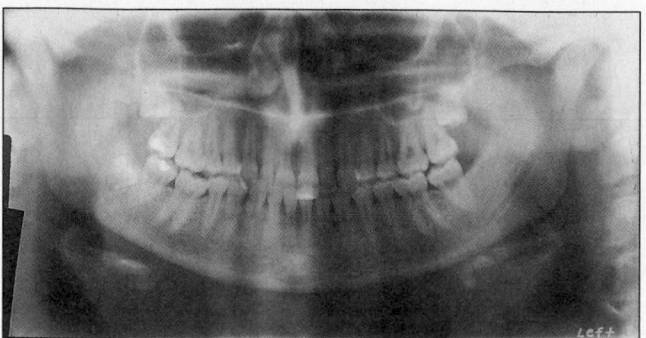

FIGURE 29-2
A panoramic radiograph.

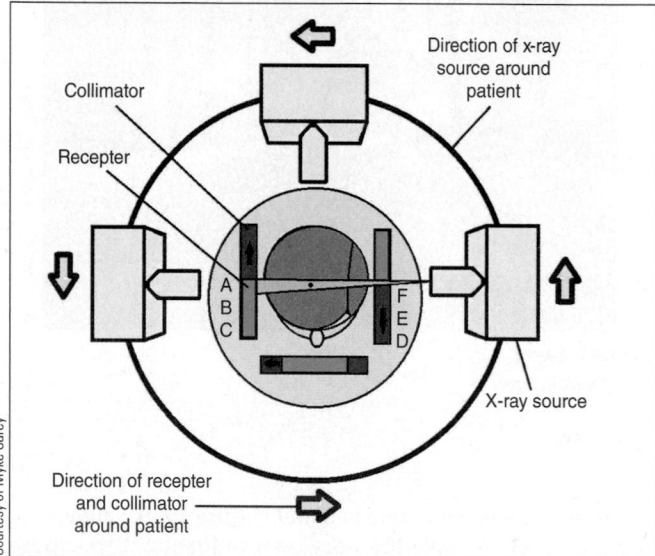

Courtesy of Myke Carey

FIGURE 29-3
Direction of tubehead and image receptor around patient.

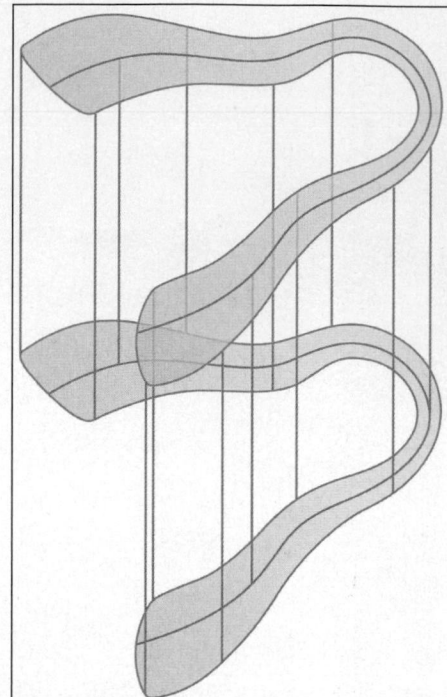

FIGURE 29-4
Focal trough or image layer.

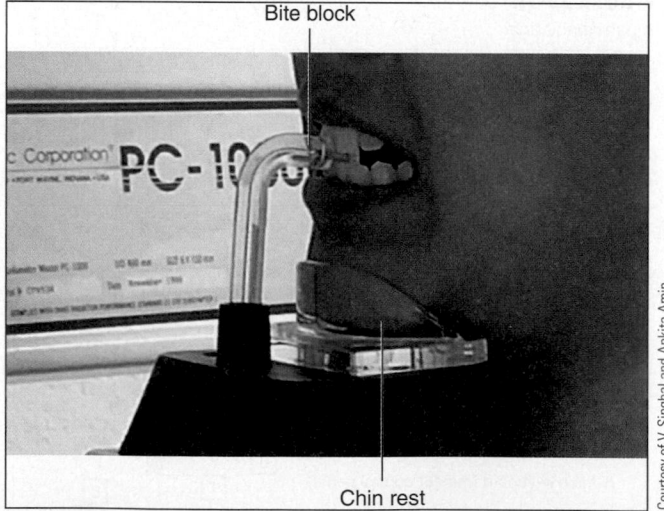

Courtesy of V. Singhal and Ankita Amin

FIGURE 29-5
Chin rest and bite block of panoramic machine.

Head Positioner The head positioner (Figures 29-1A and B) consists of lateral head supports or guides, a chin rest (Figure 29-5), a notched bite block (Figure 29-5), and a forehead rest. There are also handles for the patient to hold on to for support located near this area. Each panoramic machine is slightly different, and the operator must follow the manufacturer's instructions on how to correctly position the patient.

X-Ray Tubehead The extraoral x-ray tubehead (Figures 29-1C and 29-3) is similar to an intraoral x-ray tubehead; however, the collimator shape is different. The collimator used in panoramic machines has a narrow vertical slit, in contrast to the small round or rectangular shape of intraoral machines. The x-ray beam is emitted from the panoramic tubehead through the narrow slit, forming a vertical band of x-rays, which pass through the patient and expose the image receptor through a vertical slit. The patient receives minimal radiation exposure due to the collimator shape and the amount of x-rays emitted from the x-ray tubehead (Figure 29-6).

Cassette Film Holders Cassettes are used to hold the film or phosphor plates during exposure (Figure 29-7). Cassettes are either flat, hard containers that open on the back or flexible, thin sleeves that open on one end (Figure 29-7). Both prevent light from entering while allowing the x-rays to pass through. The cassettes must be marked in order to distinguish left from right because there is no raised dot on the film. With some

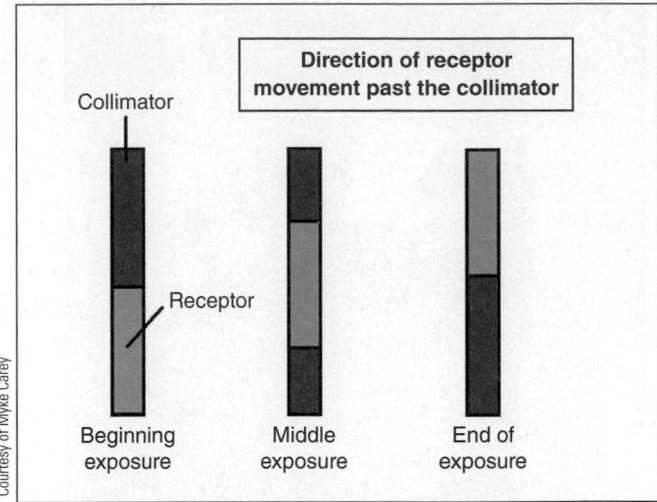

FIGURE 29-6
Direction of panoramic receptor movement past the collimator.

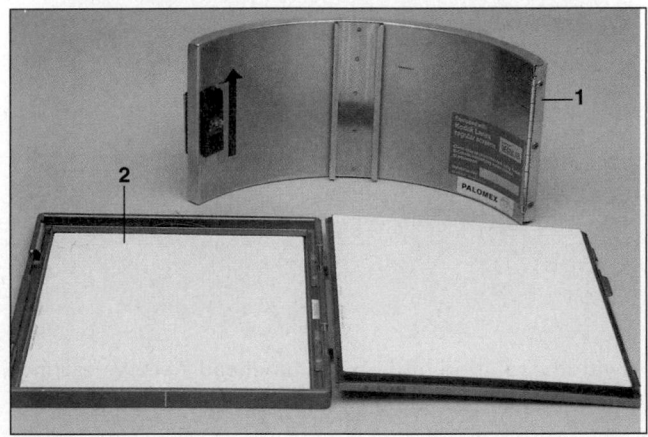

FIGURE 29-7A
1. A hard cassette for a panoramic x-ray. 2. Intensifying screens on the inside of a cephalometric cassette.

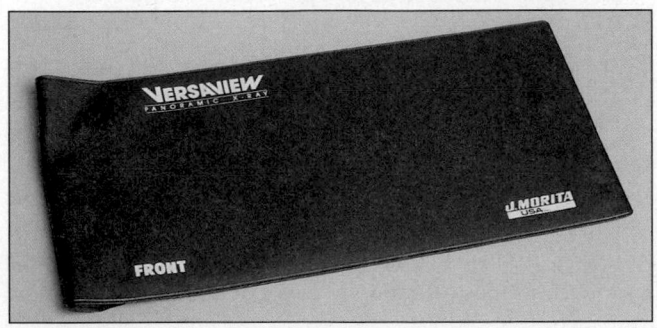

FIGURE 29-7B
Soft cassette.

panoramic machines, the films are labeled with the patient's name, dentist's name, and date of exposure. The assistant enters the information digitally before exposure. After exposure of a film-based panoramic radiograph, and under safelight conditions, the film is run through a marking device. The film is then processed, and the information appears on the film. There is no need to load the film into the cassette when using a direct digital technique, because the sensor is already embedded into the cassette. If using the indirect digital technique, the operator must load the phosphor plate prior to exposure. Open the patient's chart on the computer screen, select the correct radiograph to be taken, and then expose the radiograph; the image will appear on the monitor and will need to be saved in the appropriate patient's computer chart.

Traditional film-based cassettes are usually lined with *intensifying screens* (Figure 29-7). Care must be taken to avoid scratching the screens and to keep them free of stains and debris. The action of the x-rays on the film is increased, or intensified, by the screens; therefore, the required exposure to the patient is decreased. A substance called phosphor is used on the screens. The phosphor emits light when struck by x-rays. Some phosphors emit blue light, and others emit green light. It is important to use film that is sensitive to the kind of light the phosphor emits. The green-light phosphors are known as *rare earth phosphors* and are faster; thus, the patient receives fewer x-rays during exposure. *Calcium tungstate* phosphors emit blue light. These screens are not as fast and require more x-ray photons to expose a radiograph than the rare earth screens.

Extraoral Film The traditional extraoral film comes in a variety of large sizes, ranging from 5 × 12 inches for the panoramic to 8 × 10 inches for the cephalometric exposure. The film is not wrapped individually; it comes in a box of 50 or more sheets (Figure 29-8). Therefore, the film must be loaded into the cassettes in the darkroom under safelight conditions. The box must be closed carefully to prevent light exposure to the remaining film in the box. Extraoral film is screen film, requiring the use of screens for exposure. The film is placed between two intensifying screens in the cassette holder.

Film-Holding Devices Panoramic machines have cassette holders attached to them. With other extraoral exposures, the cassette holder may be attached to a wall, or the patient may hold the cassette. For some extraoral exposures, the cassette is placed on a flat surface, and the patient rests her or his face on it.

Panoramic Exposure Technique Suggestions There are many types of panoramic machines, and each machine has specific instructions provided by the manufacturer for successful exposures on a variety of patients. Be sure to read and follow these instructions. A few guidelines for all panoramic exposures follow:

● The patient should always wear a double-sided lead apron *without* a thyroid collar (Figure 29-9). The collar interferes with the x-ray beam and causes an artifact on the image. Because the x-ray beam is directed upward, the x-ray exposure to the thyroid gland is minimal.

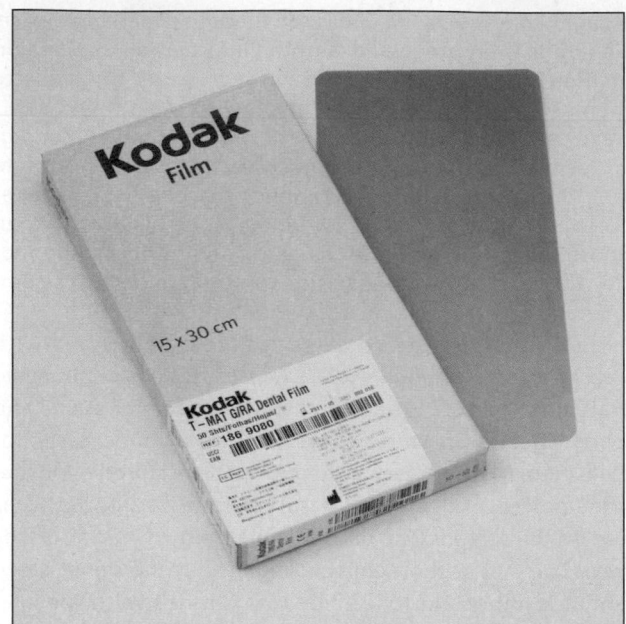

FIGURE 29-8A
Extraoral film: Panoramic film.

FIGURE 29-8B
Extraoral film: Cephalometric film.

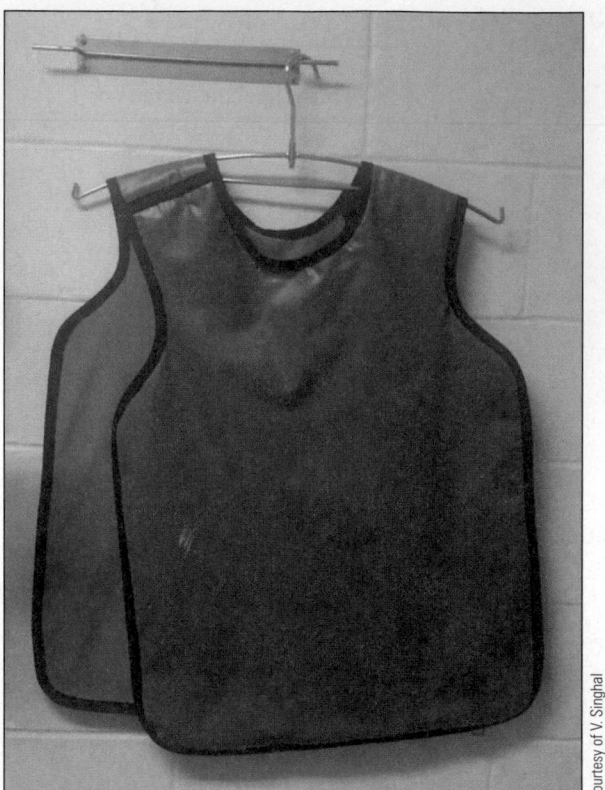

FIGURE 29-9
Double-sided lead apron without thyroid collar.

- The patient needs to be still during the entire exposure. Every machine is equipped with some type of chin rest, bite block, and head positioner to prevent movement.

- Explain the procedure to the patient, including the rotation of the machine and what to do during the exposure. Remove bulky sweaters, coats, hair clips, or anything that may interfere with the rotation of the x-ray tubehead. Remove earrings, necklaces, and dental appliances as well.

- Place the cassette in the machine, prepare the patient, carefully position the patient following the procedure steps of the panoramic unit, using the guidelines set the machine, and take the exposure. Procedure 29-1 (Figures 29-10 through 29-14) provides the steps for a panoramic exposure.

Common Panoramic Radiography Errors Table 29-1 provides details regarding common panoramic radiography errors related to patient preparation and positioning. The patient must be positioned correctly to expose the clearest and most accurate image possible (Figure 29-12). Panoramic radiographs show the dentist the entire dentition and related structures, from one condyle to the other condyle. The dental assistant must pay attention to every detail while positioning the patient.

Other Extraoral Images

There are several other extraoral images that may be obtained for dental purposes. Table 29-2 outlines those images and their specific uses.

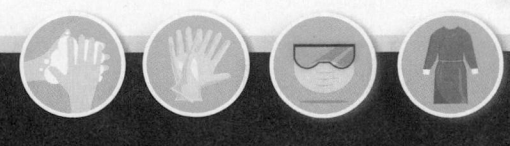

Procedure 29-1
Panoramic Exposure

This procedure is performed by the dental assistant at the direction of the dentist. The assistant prepares the cassette (if required), panoramic machine, and patient for exposure. Follow all infection control guidelines as discussed in Chapter 28.

Equipment and Supplies

- mouth mirror
- cassette and panoramic film if using a film-based machine
- casette and phosphor plate if using indirect digital unit
- cassette and phosphor plates
- bite block
- barrier for the nondisposable bite block
- lead apron without thyroid collar
- panoramic machine

Preparation for Film-Based Panoramic Radiographic Exposure

1. Under safelight conditions, load the cassette in the darkroom. The cassettes are lined with two intensifying screens, and the panoramic film is placed between them. The cassette must be securely closed to prevent light leaks. With some cassettes, information can be added, such as left and right, the patient's name, the date, and the dentist's name.

2. Place the cassette into the cassette holder of the panoramic machine (Figure 29-10).

3. Prepare the bite block. A protective barrier such as plastic wrap should be placed on the bite block. The bite blocks should be sterilized between patients. Some bite blocks are disposable.

4. Adjust the machine to the patient's approximate height, and set the kilovoltage and milliamperage according to the manufacturer's guidelines.

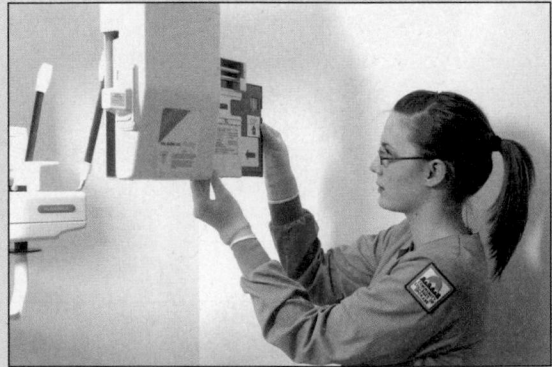

FIGURE 29-10
Placing a cassette into the panoramic machine.

Preparation for Digital Panoramic Radiographic Exposure

1. Turn on the computer and load software to enter the patient's identification information, and select the type of radiograph to be exposed.

2a. **Indirect Digital Technique:** Load the phosphor plate into the cassette. This is similar to the traditional film method but the phosphor plates do not require intensifying screens. The cassette must be securely closed to prevent light leaks. Place the cassette into the cassette holder of the panoramic machine (Figure 29-10).

2b. **Direct Digital Technique:** There is no need to load a cassette because the sensor is already part of the machine. The sensors are similar technology to those used for intraoral exposures.

3. Prepare the bite block. A protective barrier such as plastic wrap can be placed on the bite block. The bite block, if not disposable, must be sterilized between patients.

4. Adjust the machine to the patient's approximate height and set the kilovoltage and milliamperage according to the manufacturer's guidelines.

Preparing the Patient for Panoramic Exposure

1. Explain the procedure to the patient, and answer any questions.

2. Ask the patient to remove eyeglasses, earrings, tongue bars, facial piercing, hairpins and clips, necklaces, hearing aids, partial and full dentures, and anything else that may interfere with the image exposure or cast a shadow on the image.

3. Place and secure the lead apron on the patient. The lead apron used for the panoramic exposures is double-sided *without* a thyroid collar (Figure 29-11). This apron is placed with one side on the front of the patient and one side on the back to protect the patient as the machine rotates around during the exposure.

4. Guide the patient into position, whether sitting or standing. Ask the patient to stand or sit up as straight as possible so that the spine is perfectly straight (Figure 29-12). If the spinal column is not straight, it will cast a white shadow in the middle of the radiograph.

5. Raise the machine to the appropriate level so that the patient can easily bite on the bite block. Have the patient move forward until the upper and lower teeth are secured in the groove on the bite block (see Figure 29-5). The groove aligns the teeth in the focal trough. If the

(Continues)

patient is edentulous, the alveolar ridges should be positioned over the grooves of the bite block. Cotton rolls can also be used to assist in positioning. Some machines have chin rests that are specifically designed for the edentulous patient (Figure 29-13).

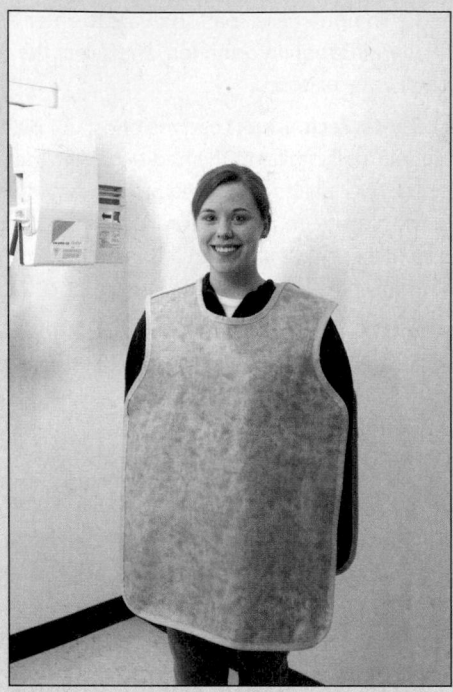

FIGURE 29-11
A patient wearing a lead apron, ready to be positioned in the panoramic machine.

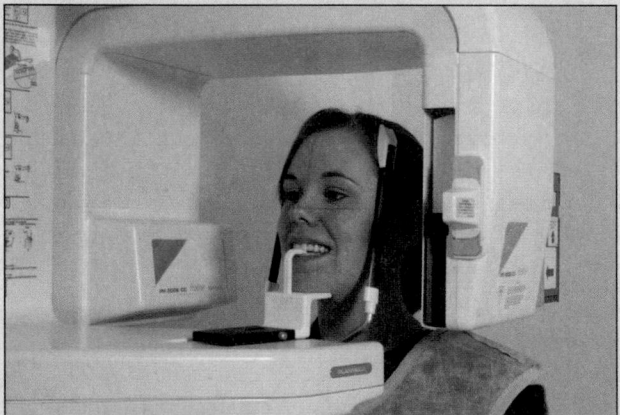

FIGURE 29-12
A patient biting on the bite block and correctly positioned for panoramic exposure. The horizontal line highlighted on the patient's face indicates the midsagittal plane, and the vertical line shows the Frankfort plane.

6. The Frankfort plane is the imaginary line drawn from the middle of the ear to just below the eye socket across the bridge of the nose. This line must be parallel with the floor, so that the occlusal plane is at the correct angle (Figure 29-14).

7. The midsagittal plane is the imaginary line that evenly divides the face into right and left halves. This midsagittal plane must be perpendicular to the floor so that the head is not tilted; otherwise, the image will be distorted (refer to Figure 28-23).

8. Some panoramic machines have lights to assist with the positioning of the Frankfort plane and the midsagittal plane (Figure 29-12). At this point, turn the light on and adjust the patient accordingly.

9. Before taking the exposure, have the patient swallow, place the tongue at the roof of the mouth, and close the lips around the bite block. Reassure the patient and instruct them to remain still during the exposure.

10. Expose the image from a location at least six feet from the patient or behind a shield. Position yourself to view the patient at all times.

11. Depress the hand switch exposure button until the exposure button terminates automatically. A whistle-like tone will sound, and the x-ray light will glow during the exposure.

12. Release the exposure button after the arm rotation has stopped. (*Note:* Releasing the button during exposure will cause the emission of radiation and motion of the arm to cease immediately. The exposure cannot be restored. The unit will need to be returned to start position with the manual rotation button, the exposed

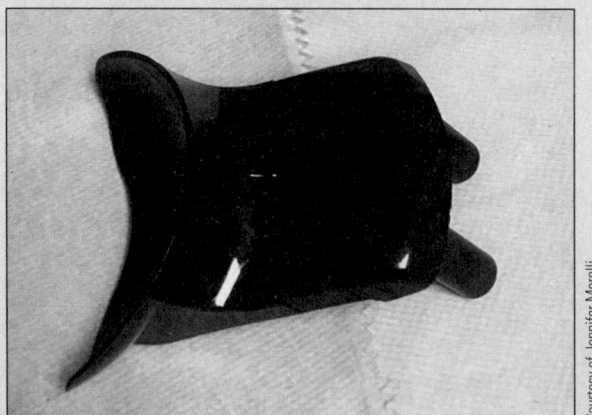

Courtesy of Jennifer Morelli

FIGURE 29-13
Edentulous chin rest.

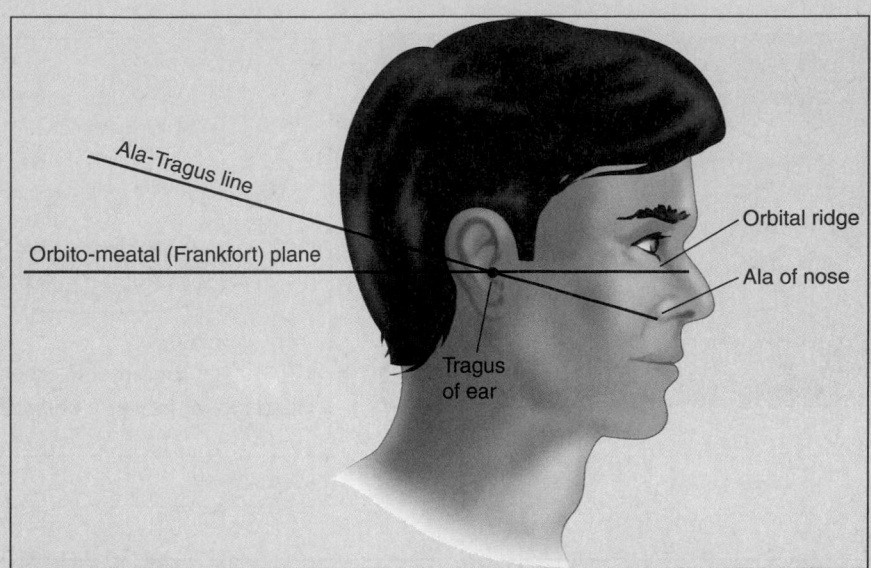

FIGURE 29-14
Frankfort plane.

traditional film will need to be replaced with a new unexposed film, and the procedure will need to be started over again.)

13. After the exposure is completed, open the positioner guide knob and ask the patient to step out of the unit.

14. Return the tubehead to the start position by pressing the manual rotation switch. Place the drum into locked position and remove the traditional film cassette. Return any special settings that were made for the exposure to the normal setting established by the office.

15. Deliver the cassette with the exposed film to the darkroom for immediate processing as described in Chapter 28. Direct digital exposures do not need processing and may be viewed on the computer screen immediately. Indirect digital exposures will need to be scanned before viewing on the computer.

TABLE 29-1 Common Errors Related to Panoramic Exposures

Common Error: The patient's head is positioned too far forward, and as a result, they are positioned too far forward on the bite block (Figure 29-15). The anterior teeth are not in the grooves on the bite block but are biting in front of the grooves. The anterior teeth will be out of the focal trough, so they will be blurred. The spine is superimposed on the ramus areas of the mandible, and the bicuspids appear overlapped (Figures 29-16 and 29-17). *Correct Position:* Have the patient bite in the grooves of the bite block and hold in this position (see Figure 29-5). The head supports might need to be adjusted to prevent the head from moving forward.

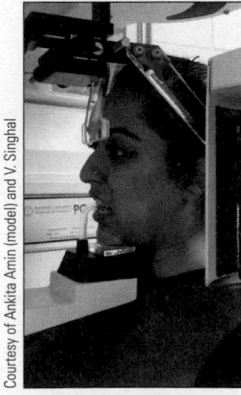

Courtesy of Ankita Amin (model) and V. Singhal

FIGURE 29-15

(Continues)

TABLE 29-1 *(Continued)*

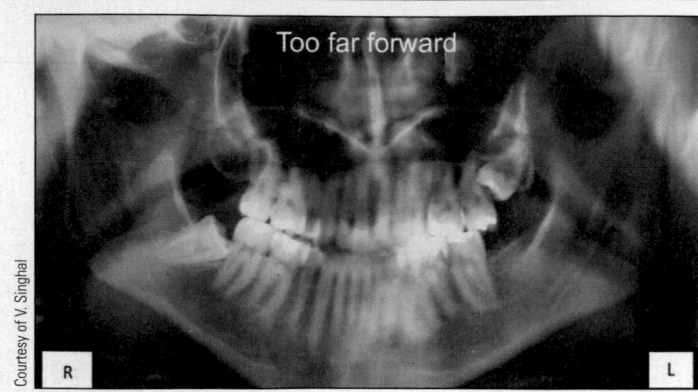

Too far forward

R   L

Courtesy of V. Singhal

FIGURE 29-16

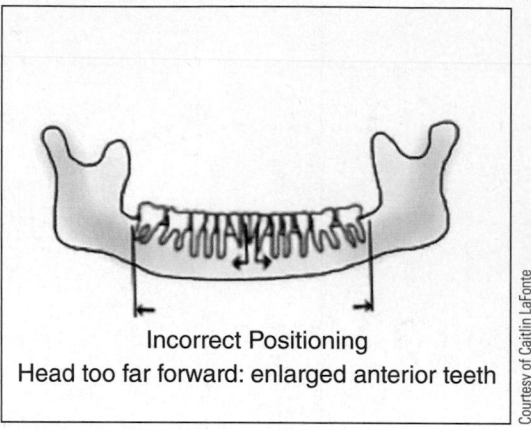

Incorrect Positioning
Head too far forward: enlarged anterior teeth

Courtesy of Caitlin LaFonte

FIGURE 29-17

Common Error: The patient's head is positioned too far back (Figure 29-18). The anterior teeth are not in the grooves on the bite block but are biting behind the grooves. The maxillary and mandibular anterior teeth will be out of the focal trough and, thus, will be blurred and appear wide. Ghost images of the mandible and spine will also appear (Figures 29-19 and 29-20).
Correct Position: Have the patient bite in the grooves of the bite block and hold in this position. The head supports might need to be adjusted to prevent the head from moving backward.

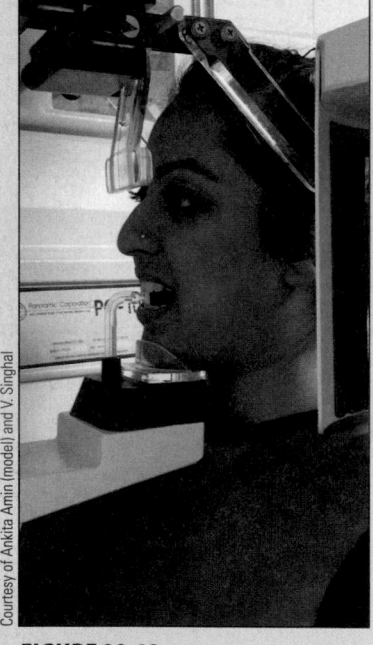

Courtesy of Ankita Amin (model) and V. Singhal

FIGURE 29-18

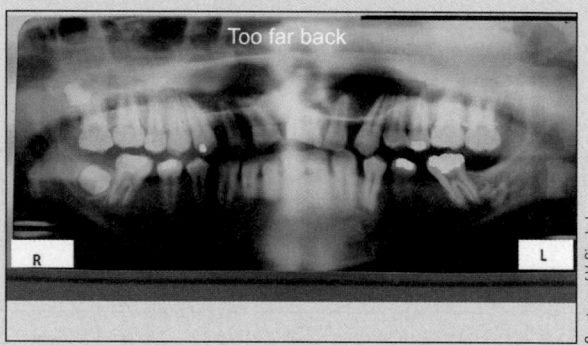

Too far back

R   L

Courtesy of V. Singhal

FIGURE 29-19

TABLE 29-1 *(Continued)*

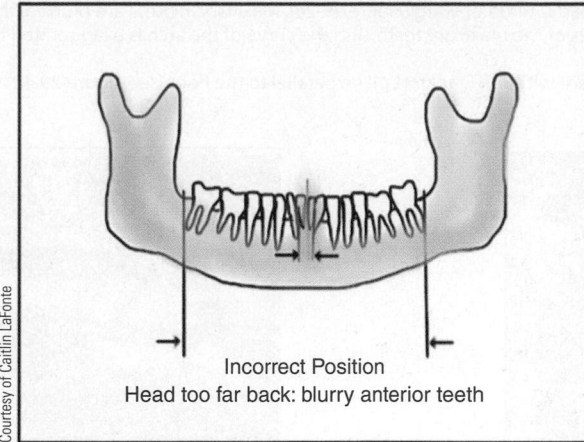

Courtesy of Caitlin LaFonte

Incorrect Position
Head too far back: blurry anterior teeth

FIGURE 29-20

Common Error: Frankfort plane: Patient's head is tilted downward (Figure 29-21). Apices of the lower incisors are blurred, mandibular condyles may not be seen, a shadow of the hyoid bone is superimposed over the center of the mandible, and the curve of the arch is exaggerated in an upward direction (Figures 29-22 and 29-23).

Correct Position: Carefully position the patient with the Frankfort plane parallel to the floor (see Figure 29-12).

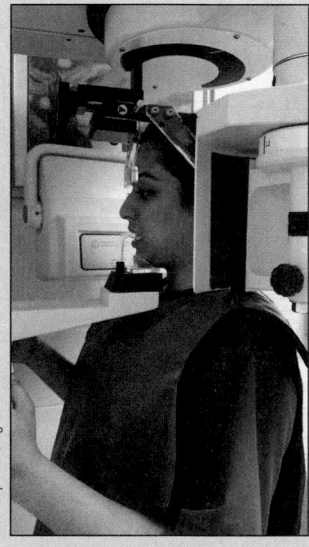

Courtesy of V. Singhal

FIGURE 29-21

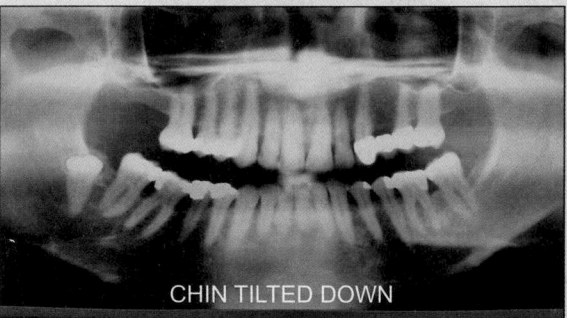

CHIN TILTED DOWN

Courtesy of V. Singhal

FIGURE 29-22

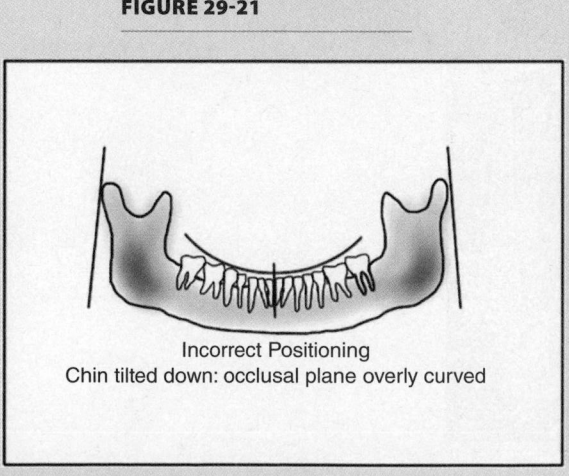

Courtesy of Caitlin LaFonte

Incorrect Positioning
Chin tilted down: occlusal plane overly curved

FIGURE 29-23

TABLE 29-1 *(Continued)*

Common Error: Frankfort plane: Patient's head is tilted upward (Figure 29-24). Maxillary incisors are blurred, the hard palate and floor of the nasal cavity appear superimposed over the apices of the maxillary teeth, and the curve of the arch is exaggerated in a downward direction (Figures 29-25 and 29-26).
Correct Position: Carefully position the patient with the Frankfort plane parallel to the floor (see Figure 29-12).

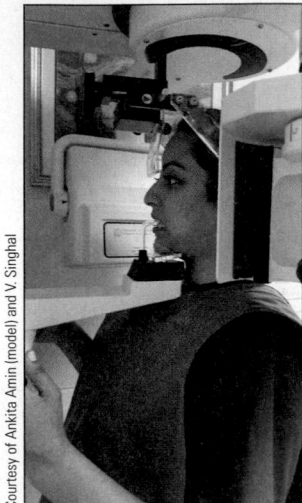

FIGURE 29-24

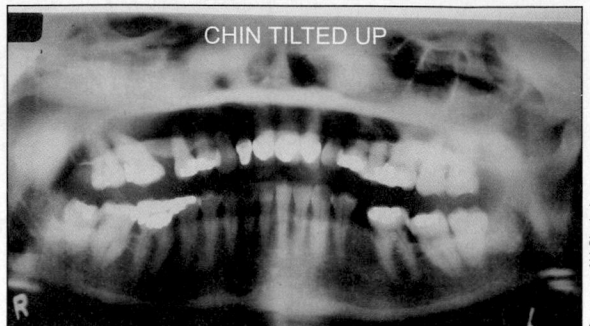

FIGURE 29-25

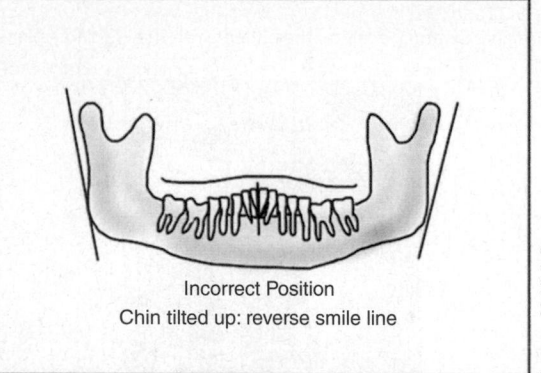

Incorrect Position
Chin tilted up: reverse smile line

FIGURE 29-26

Common Error: Head tilted to one side (Figure 29-27). When the head is tilted to one side, there is unequal left and right magnification between the two sides (Figures 29-28 and 29-29).
Correct Position: Carefully position the patient with the Frankfort plane parallel to the floor (see Figure 29-12).

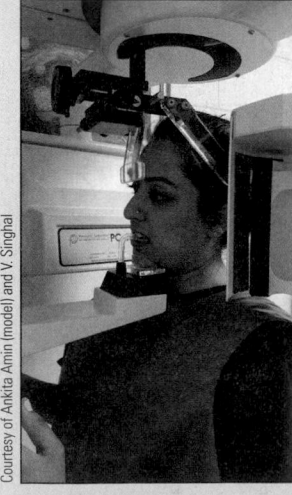

FIGURE 29-27

TABLE 29-1 *(Continued)*

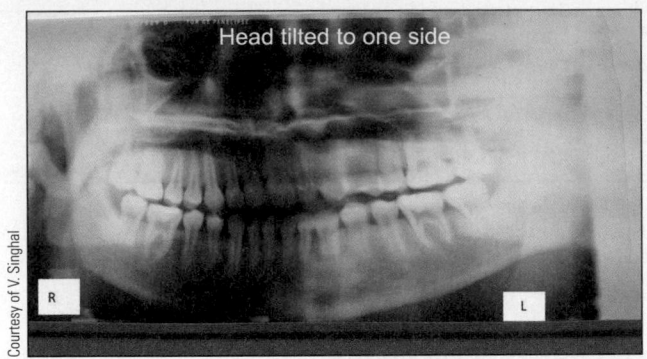

Courtesy of V. Singhal

FIGURE 29-28

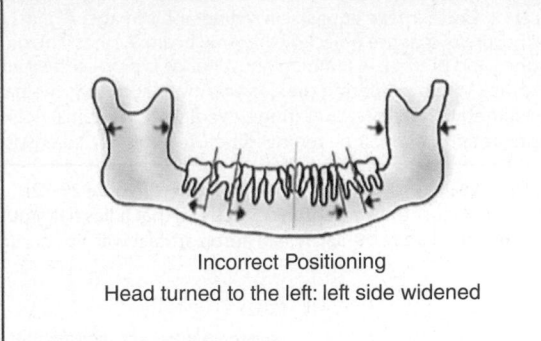

Incorrect Positioning
Head turned to the left: left side widened

Courtesy of Caitlin LaFonte

FIGURE 29-29

Common Error: Patient's tongue was not resting on the roof of the mouth during exposure. This will cause a dark radiolucent area above the apices of the maxillary teeth (Figure 29-30).
Correct Practice: Instruct and watch the patient as they swallow, and then raise the tongue to the roof of their mouth and hold it there during the exposure.

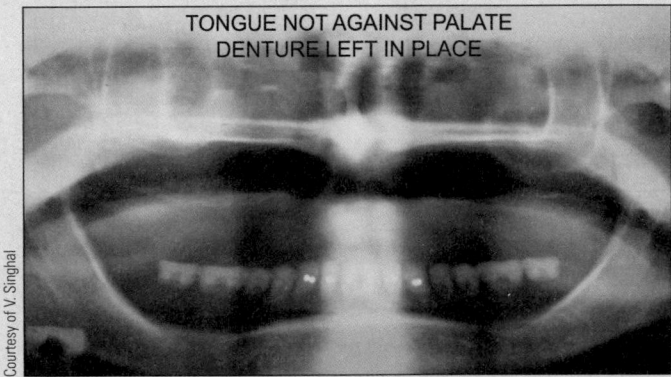

Courtesy of V. Singhal

FIGURE 29-30

Common Error: Patient was not standing or sitting up straight, resulting in a ghost image of the spine superimposed on the center of the image (Figure 29-31).
Correct Position: Position the patient so that the midsagittal plane is perpendicular to the floor and the midline is centered on the bite block (see Figure 29-12).

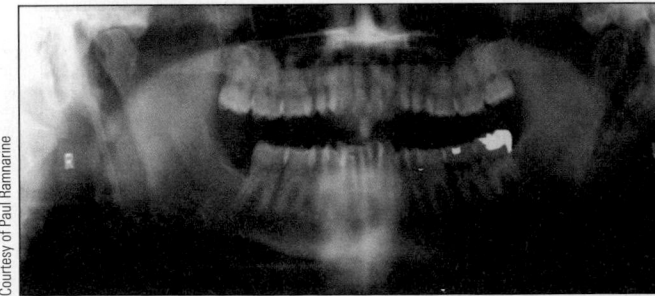

Courtesy of Paul Ramnarine

FIGURE 29-31

(Continues)

TABLE 29-1 *(Continued)*

Common Error: Ghost image appears on radiographic image. A *ghost image* is a radiopaque artifact seen on the panoramic film that is caused by double exposure of a dense object by the x-ray beam. A ghost image is similar to the real image but is cast on the opposite side of the x-ray and is larger, higher, and blurred. A common ghost image is produced by an earring left in one ear.
Correct Practice: When preparing the patient, make sure that the patient has removed all metal objects that might cast a ghost image on the film. All metal objects (e.g., earrings, eyeglasses, hairpins, necklaces, facial piercing, partial or removable dentures, hearing aids, and orthodontic retainers) must be removed before exposure to ensure that the radiograph is of adequate quality for diagnosis.

Common Error: Lead apron artifact is visible in image (Figure 29-32).
Correct Practice: Adjust the lead apron correctly so that it lies flat around the patient and below the cassette and x-ray tubehead as they rotate around the patient (Figure 29-33). A lead apron artifact will also occur if a lead apron with a thyroid collar is used.

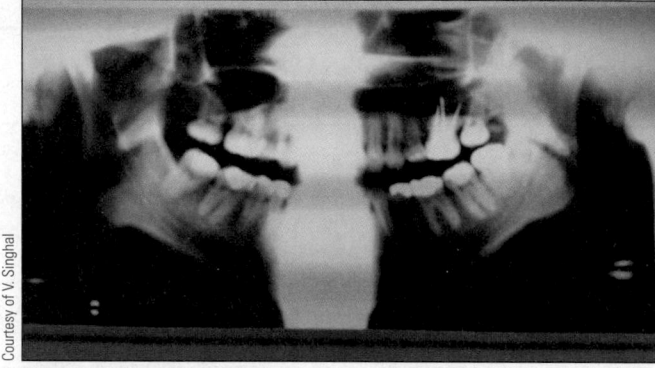

Courtesy of V. Singhal

FIGURE 29-32

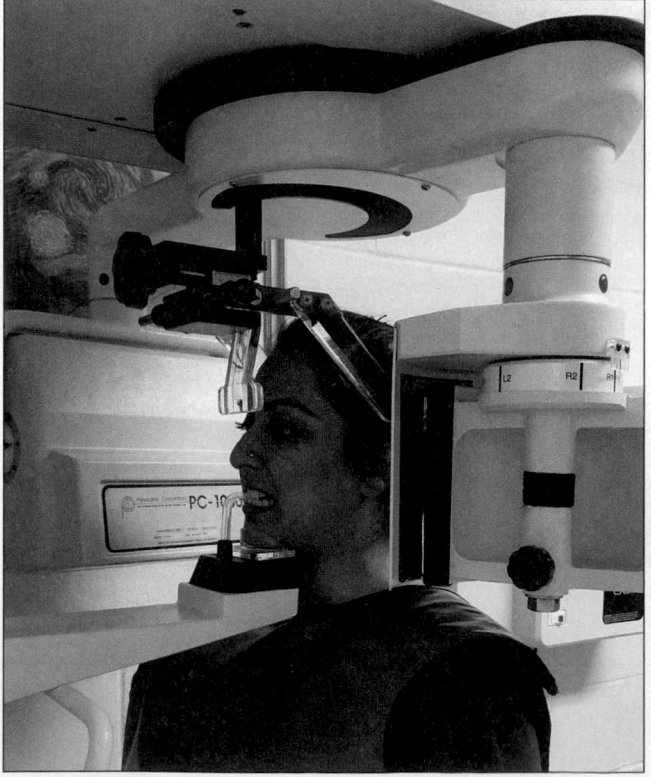

Courtesy of Ankita Amin (model) and V. Singhal

FIGURE 29-33
Correct position for a panoramic exposure

TABLE 29-2 Other Extraoral Dental Images

A *cephalometric radiograph* (*cephalo* means "head" and *metric* means "measurement") is used to assess the patient's skeletal structure and profile (Figures 29-34 and 29-35). The cephalometric radiographs are used mainly by orthodontists for treatment planning of their patients, but some oral maxillofacial surgeons and general practitioners include these radiographs for patient assessment. The patient's bony structure and soft tissues are recorded on the cephalometric radiograph. Lateral (side) or posterior anterior (back to front) views are used for orthodontic measurements, examination of the sinuses, implant evaluation, and TMJ assessment (Figure 29-35). A cephalometric unit provides a way to ensure that the patient is accurately positioned in a manner that can be duplicated as the patient grows and as repeated radiographs are needed for comparison. The unit consists of a *cephalostat*, or head-holding device; a cassette holder for an 8 × 10 inch cassette; and an x-ray tubehead.

For lateral views, position the patient by placing the left side of their head against the cassette, positioned so that the midsagittal plane is parallel to the cassette. The Frankfort plane of the patient, or line from the tragus of the ear to the floor of the orbit, is parallel to the floor. The x-ray beam is directed perpendicular to the cassette.

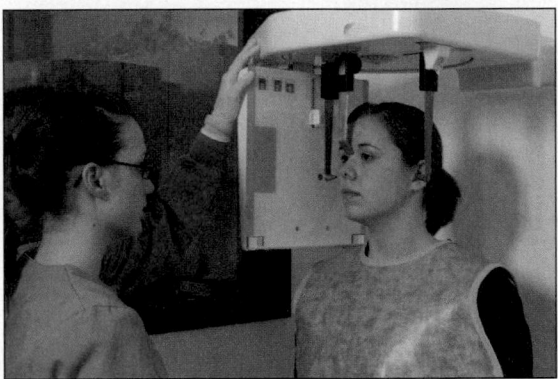

FIGURE 29-34
Patient positioned for a lateral cephalometric radiograph.

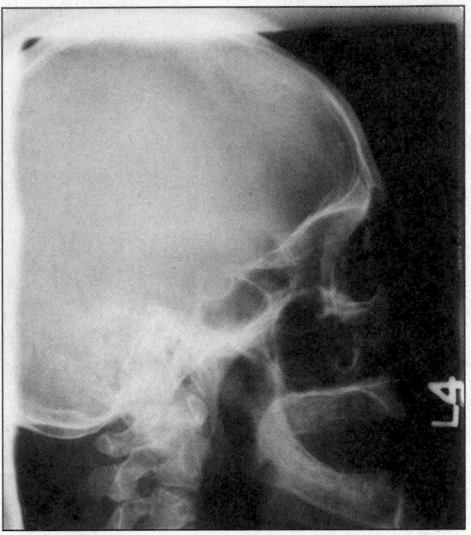

FIGURE 29-35
A lateral cephalometric radiograph.

For *posterior anterior* radiograph views, the patient faces the cassette with the Frankfort plane parallel to the floor and the x-ray beam directed at the occipital bone and perpendicular to the cassette (Figures 29-36 and 29-37). This image is used to identify disease, trauma, growth and development.

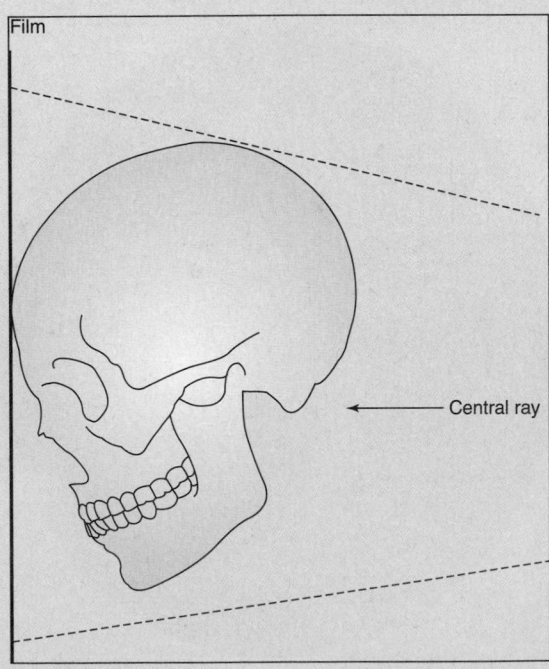

FIGURE 29-36
Direction of central ray for a posterior anterior image.

(*Continues*)

TABLE 29-2 *(Continued)*

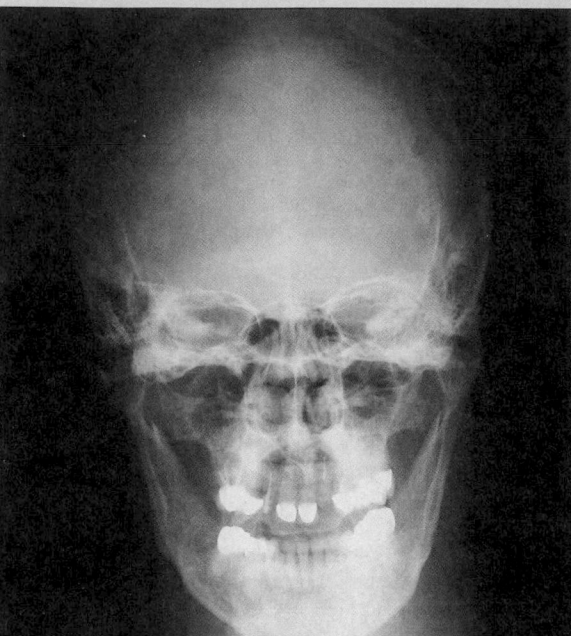

FIGURE 29-37
Posterior anterior radiograph.

The *lateral jaw* radiograph can be used if the dental office does not have a panoramic x-ray machine. Large areas of the jaw can be radiographed by using a 5 × 7 or an 8 × 10 inch film cassette and instructing the seated patient to hold the cassette next to their face and rest it on their shoulder. The x-ray tubehead is positioned on the opposite side and directed so that the central ray is perpendicular to the patient's head and the cassette. The x-ray exposure time is increased because of the layers of tissue and bone. The patient's head is positioned differently depending on the area the dentist needs to view.

The *transcranial temporomandibular joint radiograph* is taken with the patient holding a cassette against the side of the head and the cone/central x-ray positioned on the opposite side of the patient's head, slightly above and behind the external auditory meatus. Positioning devices assist in correctly aligning the head for the exposure (Figure 29-38). The radiograph can be taken with the patient's mouth open or closed.

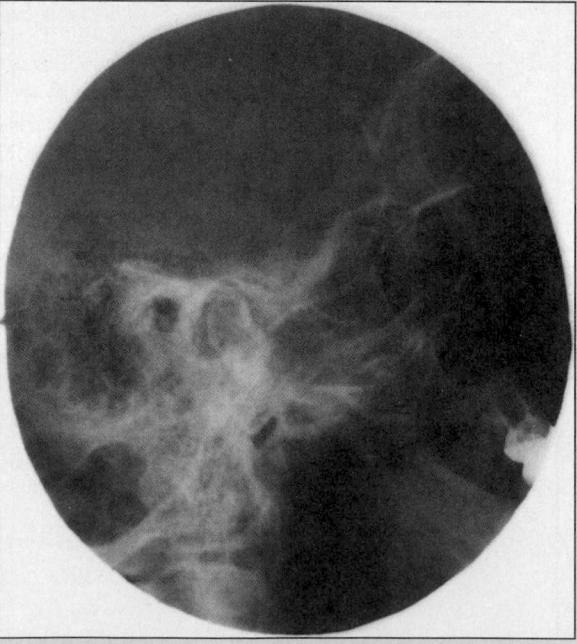

FIGURE 29-38
Transcranial TMJ radiograph with the mouth closed, showing the relationship of the condyle to the glenoid fossa.

Digital Radiography in the Dental Office

Digital intraoral imaging (digital radiology) is one of the many changes in dentistry that continues to develop and become the standard of practice. Digital radiography is expected to eventually replace all conventional film exposure. Digital radiology is a computerized system that allows the dentist to take an intraoral or extraoral radiograph and then display the image on a computer screen without processing the dental film (Figure 29-39). Table 29-3 provides definitions of terminology related to digital radiography.

The Fundamental Concepts of Digital Radiography

Digital radiography breaks the radiographic image into electronic pieces called *pixels* and then displays them on the computer. The image can be digitized, enhanced, printed, stored, or sent to another office by email, Internet transmission modes, or portable digital storage media. In digital radiography systems, the *image* is the term used to describe the picture produced, instead of *radiograph* or *dental film*. Digital radiography is not limited to intraoral images; extraoral images, such as panoramic and cephalometric images, can be taken with digital imaging systems.

In the traditional system, when the x-rays strike the film the information is recorded on the film. This is known as an *analog*

image. Analog images depict a continuous spectrum of gray shades between black and white. The analog image is a smooth transition from one color or shade to another. In digital imaging, the sensor receives the analog information and converts it into a digital image within the computer. The digital image is like a mosaic, comprised of many small pieces known as *pixels*. Pixel is short for "picture elements." Each pixel is a small dot within a digital image—more pixels equal a higher resolution and a sharper image. Each pixel has a distinct shade of gray, black, or white. The gray scale of the image is important for diagnosing the condition of the teeth, tissues, and surrounding bone. The dentist relies on the contrast—radiolucency and radiopacity—to determine the presence of disease. The computer monitor can display over 200 shades of gray, but the human eye can only detect around 32 shades of gray. Therefore, computer software is used to enhance gray shades to improve detailing and comparison.

A sensor or image receptor takes the place of traditional radiographic film (Figure 29-40). This sensor is an electronic or specially coated plate that is positioned in the oral cavity and then exposed to x-rays. When the x-ray beam contacts the sensor, an electronic charge is produced on the surface of the sensor. This electronic form or signal is digitized, or converted into data that can be read and stored by the computer. Depending on the type of imaging system, the sensor may connect directly to the computer through a fiber optic cable, or the sensor may be wireless.

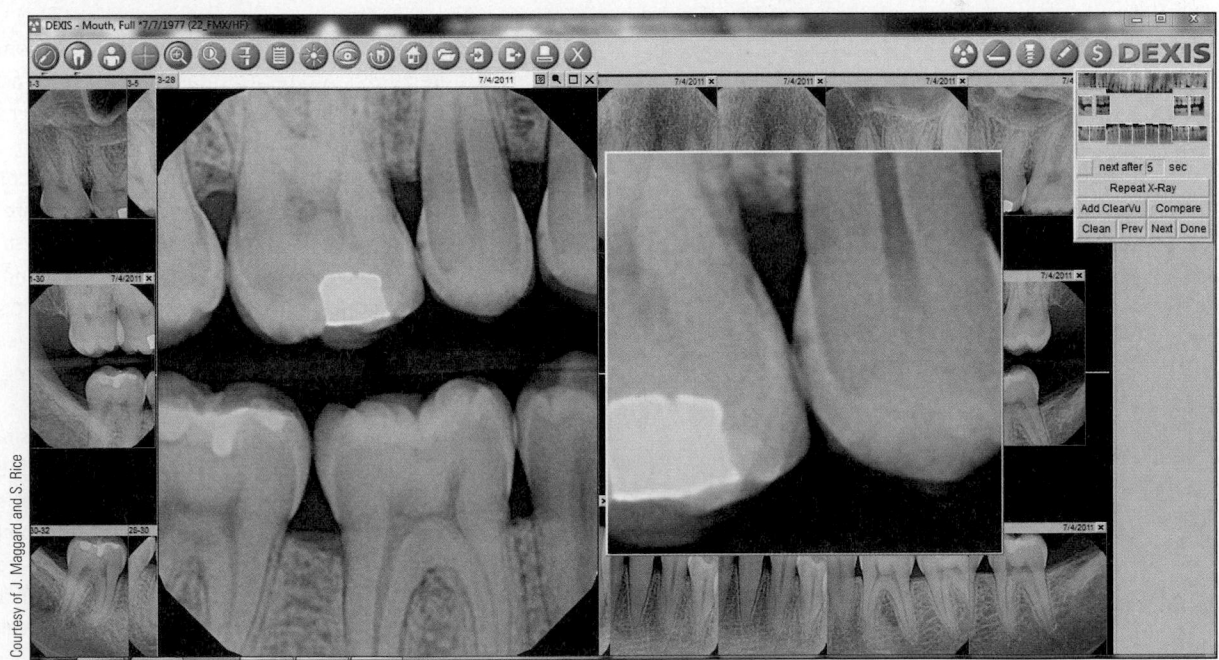

Courtesy of J. Maggard and S. Rice

FIGURE 29-39
Digital dental software.

TABLE 29-3 Digital Radiology Terminology

Term	Definition
analog image	An image produced by traditional film, in which there is a continuous spectrum of gray shades between black and white.
charge-coupled device (CCD)	A solid-state detector used in many common electronic devices, such as video cameras, fax machines, and surgical microscopes. In digital radiography, the CCD is the image receptor in the intraoral sensor. This receptor converts x-rays into electrical charges, the intensity of which is related to a color (gray scale).
digital radiography	A filmless imaging system that uses a sensor and computer to capture an image and convert it into pixels (electronic data). This image is enhanced, presented, and then stored as part of the patient's record.
digital subtraction	This feature allows images that were taken at different times to be compared. The images are electronically merged with images that did not change, thereby canceling each other out. The images that did change will stand out. Another feature of digital subtraction is the ability to reverse the gray scale of the image. The *radiolucent* areas on an image (normally black) are now white, and the *radiopaque* areas on an image (normally white) are now black.
digitize	The conversion of an x-ray film image into a digital image that can be processed by a computer.
direct digital imaging	A technique of exposing an intraoral sensor to radiation in order to obtain a digital radiographic image that can be viewed on a computer. This method uses an intraoral sensor, x-ray machine, computer monitor, and computer software program.
gray scale	Shades of gray visible in an image.
indirect digital imaging	A technique used for scanning radiographic images on pre-existing traditional dental films into digital images before moving on to storage phosphor imaging. This method uses an intraoral sensor, x-ray machine, scanner, computer monitor, and computer software program.
pixel	Derived from the plural of *picture* (pix) and the word *element* (el), pixels are discrete units of information that comprise an image.
sensor	A small electronic or specially coated plate that is sensitive to x-rays. When placed intraorally and exposed to radiation, the sensor captures the radiographic image.
storage phosphor imaging	An indirect digital imaging method of obtaining a digital image. The image is recorded on a special phosphor-coated plate and then placed in an electron scanner. A laser scans the plate and produces an image on the computer monitor.

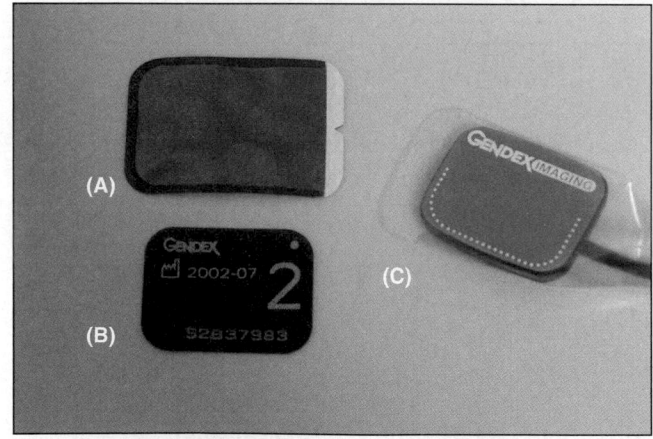

FIGURE 29-40
(A) Phosphor storage plate barrier. (B) Phosphor storage plate. (C) Direct digital sensor.

Types of Digital Imaging

Currently there are both direct and indirect methods of obtaining a digital image.

Direct Digital Imaging A *direct digital imaging* system includes the following components: x-ray machine, digital sensor (refer to Figure 28-3), computer monitor, and computer software (Figure 29-39). A direct digital imaging system allows the image to appear almost immediately on the computer screen once the sensor is exposed. This digital imaging system uses a solid-state sensor that contains an x-ray sensitive silicon chip with an electronic circuit (Figure 29-40C). These sensors are either a *charge-coupled device (CCD)* or *complementary metal oxide semiconductor (CMOS)* technology. CCD and CMOS technologies work equally well in converting x-rays into an electronic signal, which is then sent to the computer. The difference between the two is the design of the electronic chip. The manufacturer of the sensors determines which technology to use.

The CCD is one of the most common image receptors used in dental digital radiography. Developed in the 1960s, the CCD is used in many devices, such as fax machines, home video cameras, microscopes, and telescopes. The CCD is a solid-state detector comprised of a grid of small transistor elements that convert x-rays to electrons. The electrons produced by the x-ray are deposited in a small box or "well" known as a pixel. A pixel is the digital equivalent of a silver halide crystal used in traditional radiology. However, the arrangement of the silver halide crystals is random, unlike the pixels in digital radiography, which are structured in an ordered arrangement. Once the elements are exposed to x-rays, they are read and the electron charges are converted to form the digital image.

With direct digital imaging the sensor is placed in the patient's oral cavity and exposed to x-rays; the image is produced on the surface of the sensor, digitized, and then transmitted to the computer. Software is then used to enhance the image and store the image as part of the patient's records.

Indirect Digital Imaging An indirect digital imaging system contains the following components: phosphor image plates (Figure 29-40), either a scanner with a carousel inserted (Figures 29-41A and B) or a small plate scanner (Figure 29-41C), and a computer and computer software (Figure 29-39).

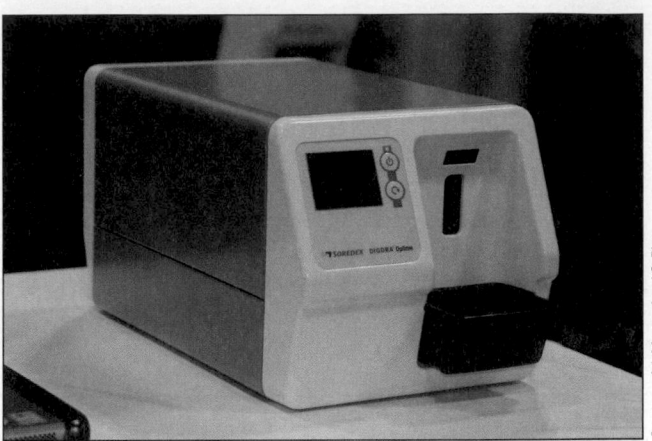

FIGURE 29-41C
Small phosphor plate scanner.

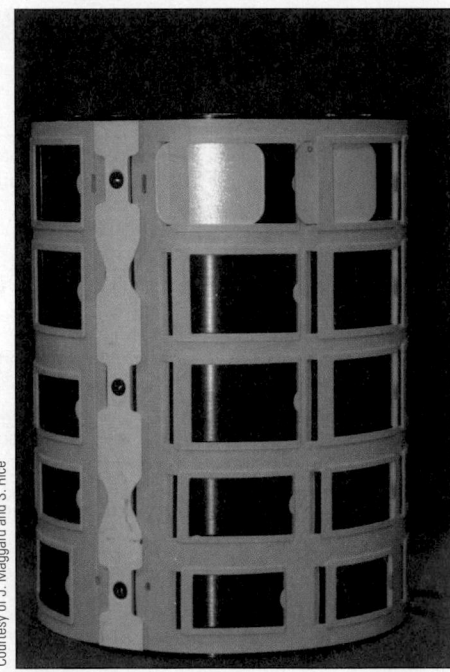

FIGURE 29-41A
Carousel for scanning of phosphor storage plates.

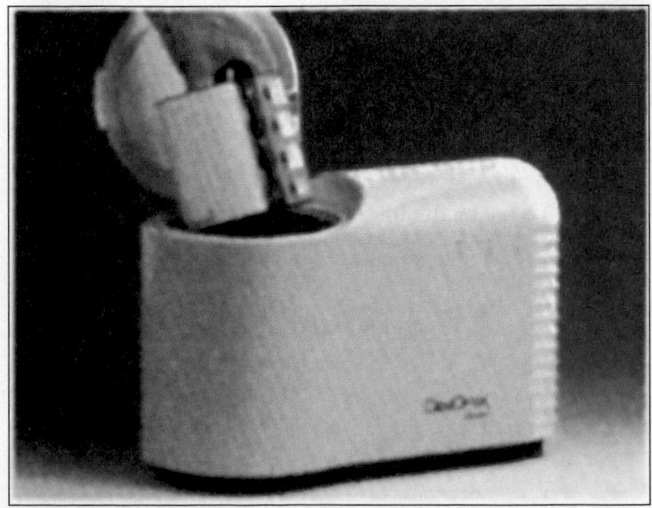

FIGURE 29-41B
Placing phosphor plate carousel into scanner.

The *photostimulable phosphor (PSP)* plate sensor technology, also called phosphor storage imaging, is a wireless system that uses specially coated imaging plates instead of sensors to record the image. This system is very different from the direct digital imaging system. PSP sensors are similar to film in the way they look. However, PSP technology uses plates that are coated with a phosphor layer, which, when exposed to x-rays, stores the energy as a latent image, similar to the way silver halide crystals within the film emulsion store the latent image. The image plates are covered with a barrier (Figure 29-40) and then placed in the oral cavity using a film-holding device. They are flexible and much like intraoral film. Unlike the direct digital imaging sensors, there is no cable attached. Once the plate is exposed to x-rays, they are placed on a carousel (Figure 28-41A) and then a high-speed laser scanner (Figure 29-41B) or a small plate scanner (Figure 29-18C) to release the energy stored on the plates, converting the information into a digital image. The computer uses the digital values to reconstruct the image on the computer. Laser scanning processing makes the PSP technology similar to film-based radiology in that both the dental film and the image plate must be "developed" later. Because of this extra step, which ranges from seconds to minutes, this type of digital radiography is more time consuming than direct digital imaging. After the image plates have been scanned, they must be cleared between each use by exposing them to bright light, such as room light, for several minutes. Similar to direct digital sensors, PSP plates cannot be autoclaved and must be covered with a plastic barrier to prevent the spread of disease.

The software for both types of systems is provided by the manufacturers that offer digital imaging systems. They offer a variety of features to enhance and manipulate the images for better detection and for improved patient understanding. Some of the features offered by software systems include the following:

- charting
- density and contrast
- digital subtraction
- embossing
- magnification
- measuring tools

- reversing the gray scale
- side-by-side displays of images

Advantages and Disadvantages of Digital Radiography

Although digital radiography is continually advancing, there are advantages and disadvantages to this technology. Table 29-4 provides details on some of these advantages and disadvantages.

Digital Radiology Techniques

This procedure serves as a general guideline when using digital radiology. Digital exposures should be conducted under aseptic conditions as discussed in Chapter 28. Manufacturers of digital radiography systems provide detailed instructions on preparation of the equipment and the patient, taking the exposure, and using the software. Procedure 29-2 provides the steps in obtaining digital dental radiographs.

TABLE 29-4 Advantages and Disadvantages of Digital Radiology

Advantages	Disadvantages
Less exposure to radiation for the patient. Sensors are more sensitive and require less radiation, falling by 50% compared to using F-speed films.	The initial expense of the equipment and software. Prices vary according to manufacturer and system quality.
Results appear on the computer monitor almost immediately after exposure to x-rays. The dentist can then enhance, contrast, zoom, take exact measurements, make notes about the image, and alter the color and brightness/contrast of the image, right at chairside to better evaluate the patient's condition.	Training is required to become proficient in using the digital imaging hardware and software. Correctly positioning the sensor or imaging plate is still a prerequisite for a detailed, quality radiograph. Positioning technique errors are similar to traditional x-ray exposure positioning errors.
Patients can view images when the dentist is discussing areas of concern.	Direct digital sensors are usually thicker than x-ray film packets. Placement is often uncomfortable for the patient. However, sensor design is continuously improving.
Since digital images are stored on computer media, much less space is required for storage.	There are concerns about rapid and costly updating, computer viruses, and system failures.
The darkroom, processing equipment, and solutions are eliminated, thereby eliminating the maintenance of this equipment and the need to deal with the storage of used chemicals.	Infection control is a concern with digital radiography. The sensors are covered with barriers that can tear and are not always totally aseptic. The keyboard and mouse must also be covered, and the covers changed with each patient. Follow manufacturer's instructions for cleaning and disinfecting the sensor and keyboard.
Digital images are quickly and easily sent via an email attachment to other dental offices, insurance companies, patients, and so on. This allows, for example, faster processing of insurance claims.	Security concerns regarding electronic transmission of images exist.

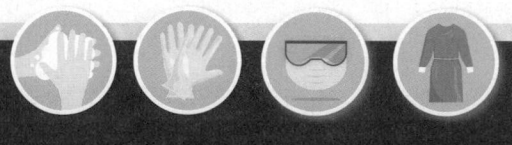

Procedure 29-2
Digital Radiography Techniques

Equipment and Supplies

The student should follow the aseptic procedures outlined in Chapter 28 for this procedure and patient preparation.

- barriers for the x-ray room
- sensor or phosphor imaging plates (see Figure 29-40)
- barriers for the sensors or phosphor imaging plates (see Figure 29-40)
- cotton rolls (optional)
- appropriate and assembled image receptor holders (see Figure 28-8B)
- lead apron with thyroid collar (see Figure 27-23)

Procedure Steps

1. Turn on the computer and load the software to select the patient chart or identification (Figure 29-42).

2. Select the radiology icon of the chart and select the type of radiographic series to be exposed.

3. Prepare the x-ray machine and adjust the settings. For most digital systems, the exposure settings are half those used for F-speed dental film exposures. For suggestions on exposure settings, always follow the manufacturer's instructions.

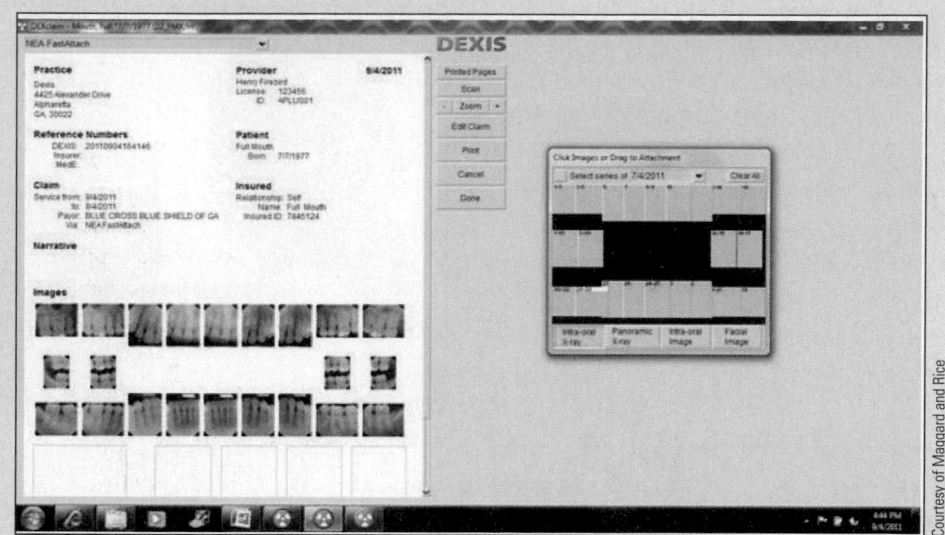

FIGURE 29-42
Digital patient chart.

Courtesy of Maggard and Rice

4. Select a receptor (sensor or phosphor plate) that has been disinfected and then prepare it by placing an approved barrier over image receptor. Place receptor in an appropriate receptor holder (Figures 29-43 and 29-44).

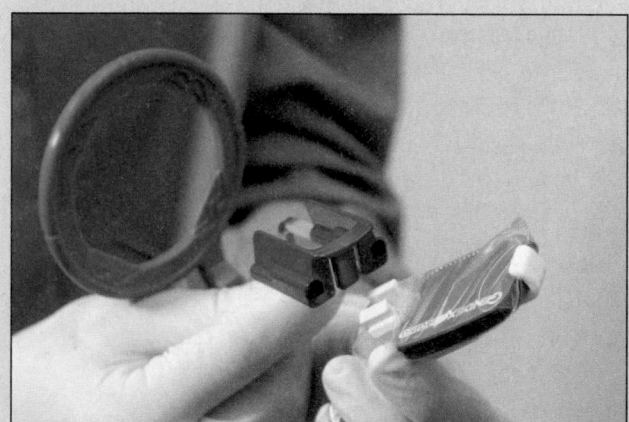

FIGURE 29-43
A sensor that has been prepared with a barrier prior to placement in the patient's mouth.

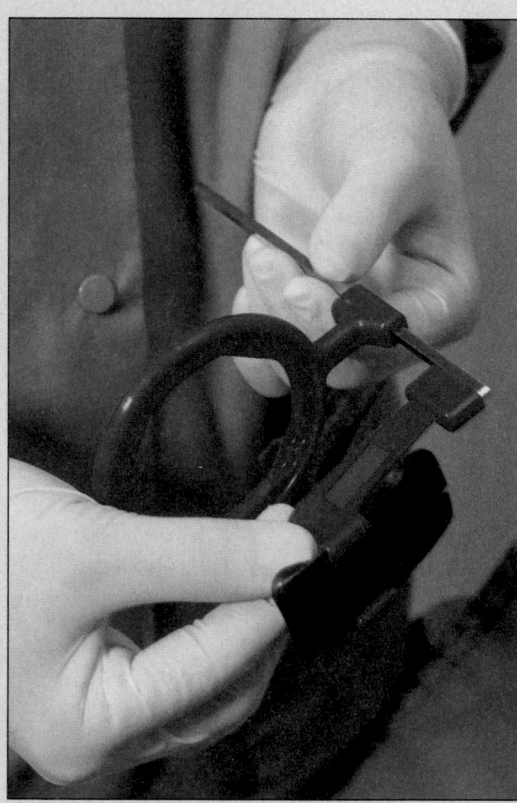

FIGURE 29-44
Phosphor storage plate being placed into Rinn XCP holder.

Preparation of Patient

1. Patient preparation should be the same as for traditional film exposures.

(Continues)

Taking the Exposure

1. Place the receptor in the patient's oral cavity (Figure 29-45), and carefully move into position for desired exposure. Refer to Chapter 28 for exposure techniques.

2. Align the x-ray cone and PID to direct the central rays, using the same technique for film exposure (refer to Procedure 28-2).

3. Using the keyboard or mouse, activate the sensor for exposure.

4. Press the exposure button to expose the sensor.

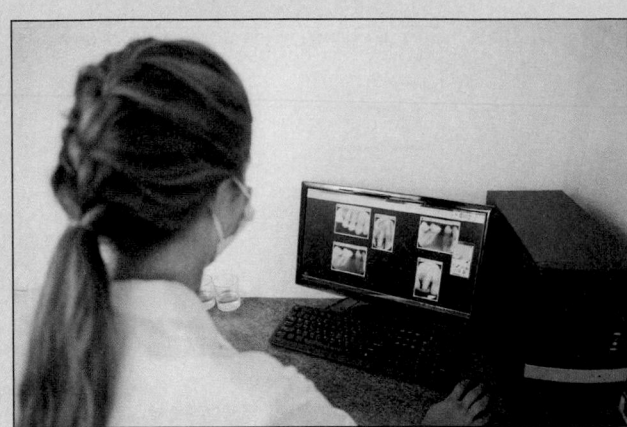

FIGURE 29-46
A dental assistant reviewing digital radiographs on the computer.

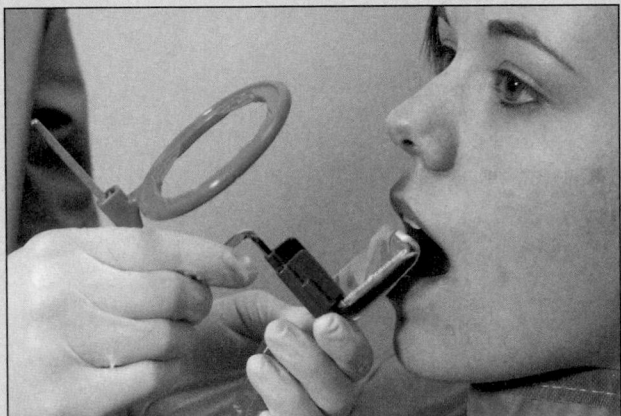

FIGURE 29-45
A sensor being placed in the patient's oral cavity for correct alignment.

Direct Digital Imaging System

1. Wait until the image appears on the monitor and evaluate it (Figure 29-46). If the image is what the dentist needs for a quality diagnosis, continue with the next image to be exposed. If a positioning error has occurred, do not remove the sensor from the patient's oral cavity; determine what caused the error, and correct the sensor position or realign the PID. (*Note:* Even though the amount of radiation that the patient is exposed to is reduced, retakes should be limited, just as they are when taking traditional radiographs.)

2. When the image is satisfactory, remove the sensor or reposition it for additional exposures. Repeat until all prescribed exposures are acquired.

Indirect Digital Imaging System

1. Remove the image receptor from the patient's oral cavity.

2. Remove the imaging plate from the film holder, and remove the plastic barrier.

3. Place the covered imaging plate in a container until all exposures have been taken.

4. After all exposures are complete, in a semi-dark room place the imaging plates in the carousel and then in the scanner and activate (see Figures 29-41A and B).

5. The images will begin to appear on the monitor (Figure 29-46). Evaluate the images according to the requirements for quality diagnostic images. If the image does not meet diagnostic standards, erase the image from the plates by exposing them to room light and disinfect them according to the manufacturer's instructions, and then follow the same technique listed previously. Retake of images must be completed upon a dentist's prescription after evaluation of the images.

After Exposure

1. Images may be sent to the patient's insurance company or a specialist if further treatment is needed (Figure 29-47).

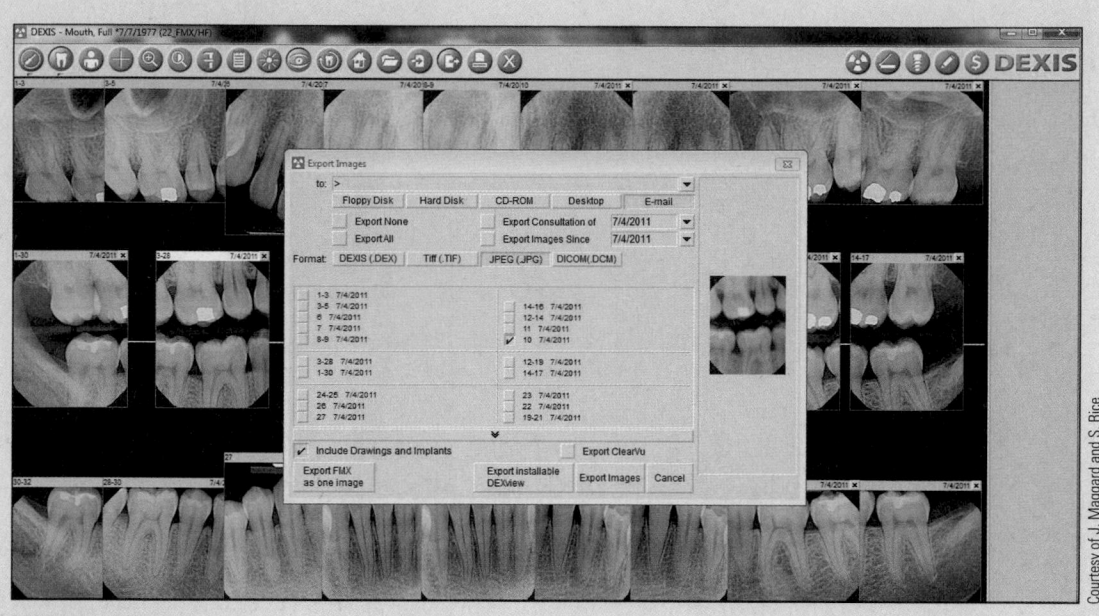

Courtesy of J. Maggard and S. Rice

FIGURE 29-47
Exporting of images through digital imaging system.

Three-Dimensional Imaging in Dentistry

Dentistry has entered into the world of 3D dental imaging and diagnosis. The 3D imaging unit, also known as a *cone beam computed tomography (CBCT)* unit, is about the size of a panoramic unit (Figures 29-48 and 29-49). It can be placed in the dental office for dental applications. Additional regulations regarding lead shielding of walls apply as the 3D imaging machines operate at a significantly higher kVp as compared to standard dental radiology machines. Additionally, many states do not allow the dental assistant to operate a CBCT machine. It is important that the dental assistant be aware of their state regulations regarding CBCT machines.

This technology offers dentists and dental specialists comprehensive diagnosis data, improves information and interpretation for various treatment-related procedures, and enables the design of treatment plans with more predictable results. It shows more information than traditional dental films or CT scans. However, CBCT is used in specific instances such as implant placement, removal of third molars, and other invasive procedures. It is not considered a routine practice in dentistry.

The 3D dental image scan shows an immediate 3D reconstruction of a patient's oral cavity, face, maxilla, and mandible, including the condyles and surrounding structures. Tooth positions are visualized to show impactions in the alveolar bone, the location of adjacent teeth, and their proximity to vital structures, such as the mandibular nerve canal and sinus walls.

With the 3D imaging device, the x-ray beam is cone-beam shaped and aimed at a flat image receptor. Depending on the imaging device, the image is usually captured in a single rotation around the patient's head. The cone beam shows hundreds of images of the patient from different positions around the scan rotation. The information is transferred to the computer, which reconstructs it into three different views. The images provide three different views: an *axial* view begins below the chin and moves to the top of the head (Figure 29-50), the *sagittal* view allows for side-to-side viewing of the patient (Figure 29-51), and the *coronal* view begins behind the patient's head and moves to the front of the face (Figure 29-52). The measurements and information gathered are dimensionally accurate and detailed.

Once the data is reconstructed, imaging software is used for the multilayer viewing of the anatomical volume (Figure 29-50). The CBCT machine uses units known as voxels. A voxel is a 3D measurement of volume. It is similar to a two-dimensional pixel in traditional radiology. The voxel absorbs the radiation upon exposure. The data in the voxel is converted into the image by the computer system. This information is then saved on a designated system in a format that specialists, dentists, and other imaging-related services can access.

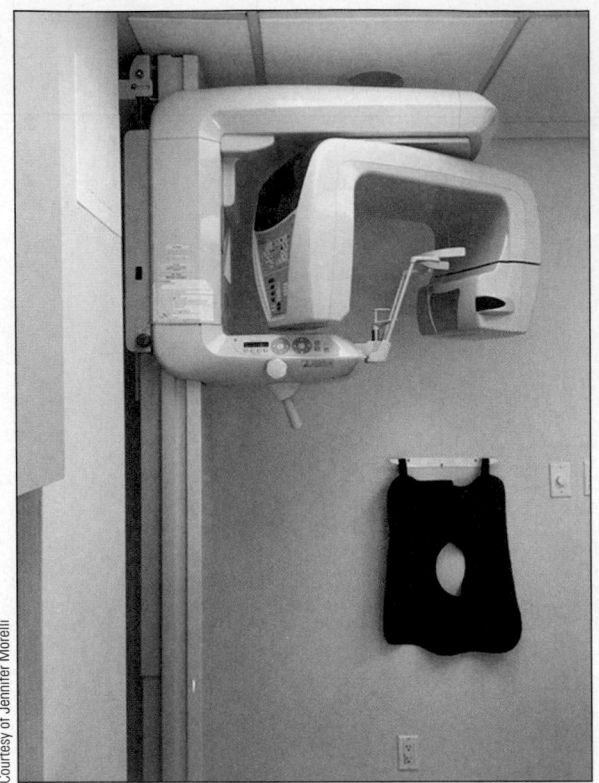

FIGURE 29-48
CBCT machine.

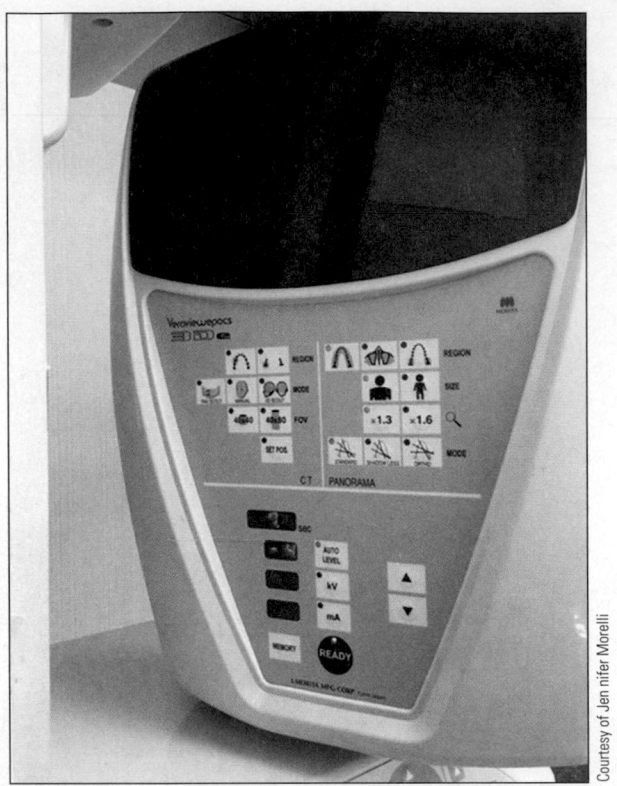

FIGURE 29-49
CBCT machine control panel.

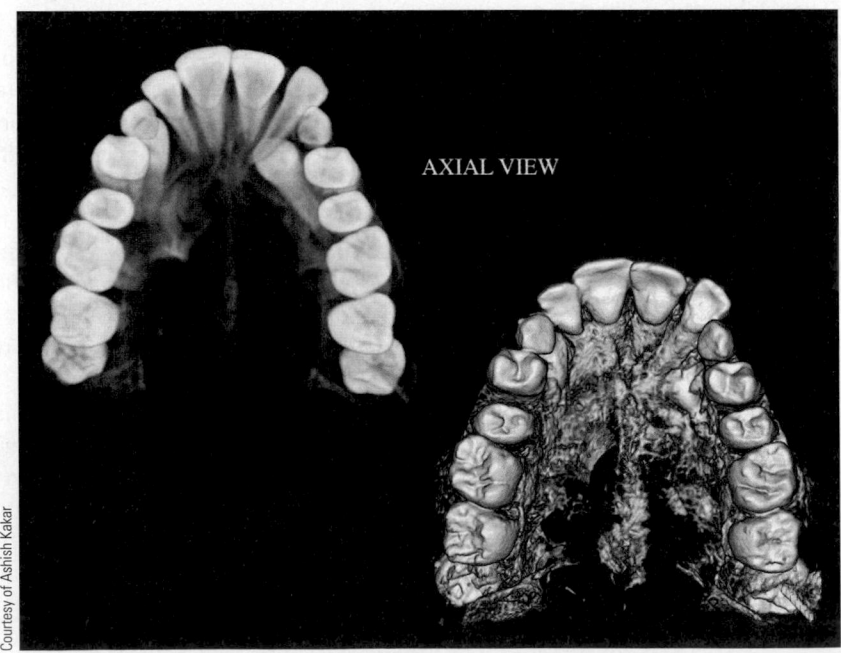

AXIAL VIEW

FIGURE 29-50
Axial view of a CBCT scan.

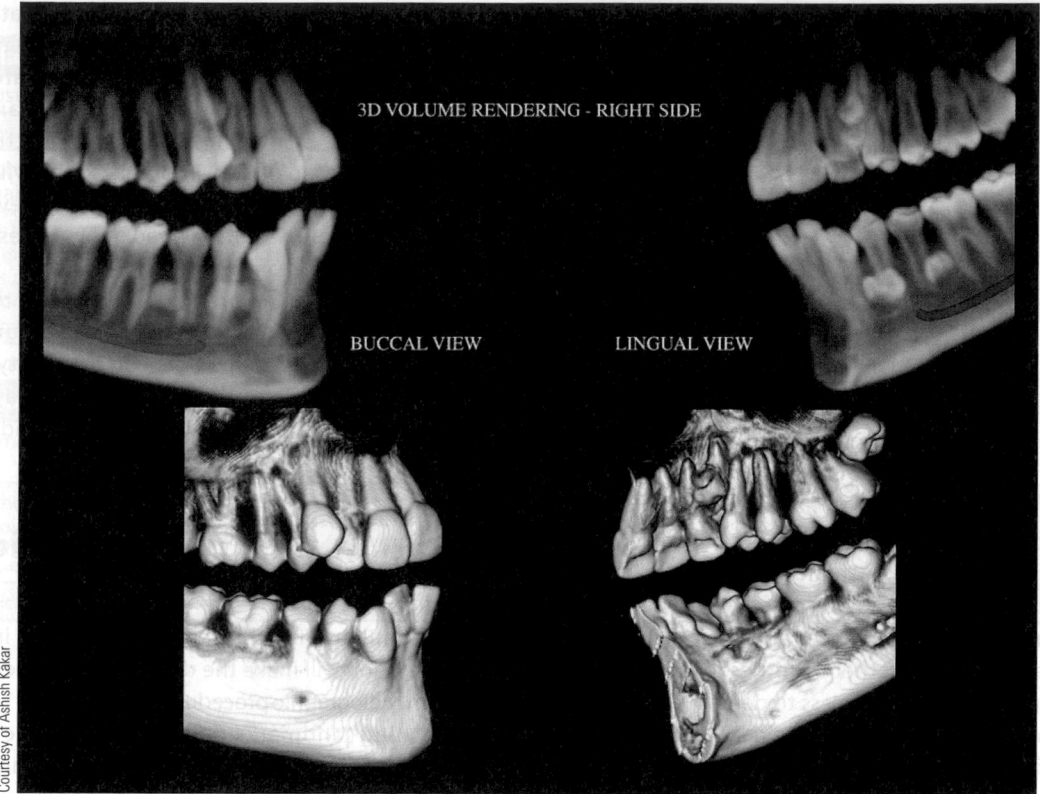

3D VOLUME RENDERING - RIGHT SIDE

BUCCAL VIEW   LINGUAL VIEW

Courtesy of Ashish Kakar

FIGURE 29-51
Sagittal view and volume rendering of a CBCT image.

Uses and Benefits of Three-Dimensional Imaging

There are many applications for this technology in all aspects of dentistry. Three-dimensional dental images are recommended for the following:

- To provide data to determine bone quality and quantity
- To obtain anatomical details
- To locate pathology, such as cysts, tumors, and bone lesions
- To evaluate deformities and pathologies
- To view critical landmarks and show minute detail
- To allow for early detection and evaluation
- To allow accurate planning and measuring for dental implants
- To plan orthognathic surgery
- To evaluate the TMJ
- To show the entire dentition and the whole maxillofacial and mandibular regions
- To produce complete and partial 3D face photos
- To allow use of precise measuring tools for improved general dental imaging
- To locate and evaluate impactions and many other dental conditions

- For advance treatment planning and assisted delivery abilities, software has been designed to make custom precision surgical guides, virtual models, and laser-generated resin models

Patient Preparation

With the 3D dental imaging machine, the patient can have the scan completed right in the dental office. With the 3D dental imaging equipment, the patient either stands or is seated comfortably in an open scanner. Once the patient is seated, images are scanned in a short period of time that varies with each machine, usually from 8 to 20 seconds. Once the scan is complete, the information is transferred to the computer through different software programs. Software is quick and effective, reconstructing critical anatomy in less than 30 seconds. The software is designed to solve dental problems through perceptive integration of diagnosis, computer-aided therapy planning, and detailed intraoperative implementation.

Once the information has been successfully scanned, the dentist can show the patient the images and then discuss the diagnosis and give the patient an understanding of their treatment options.

TABLE 29-7   (Continued)

The lateral fossa, also called canine fossa, is a fossa or depressed area above the lateral incisor. On a radiograph it appears as a radiolucency above the apex of the lateral incisor or between the lateral incisor of the maxilla and the adjacent canine. The dental assistant must be able to differentiate between this normal anatomical structure and a periapical pathology that also appears radiolucent and at the apex of the tooth. Periapical pathologies will be discussed later in this chapter. This structure is visible in the maxillary incisor periapical image and maxillary canine periapical image (Figure 29-54).
The nasal fossae (cavity) are the radiolucent round areas above incisors outlined in radiopaque cortical bone. The nasal fossa is a space and thus appears radiolucent. It is visible in the maxillary incisor periapical image and the maxillary canine periapical image and may be visible in the maxillary premolar periapical image (Figure 29-54).
The maxillary sinus appears as a radiolucent round area outlined by radiopaque cortical bone and is visible in maxillary posterior periapical images and on panoramic images (Figures 29-55 and 29-56).
The infraorbital foramen is a radiolucent area inferior to the inferior border of the orbit. It is usually seen on panoramic images (Figure 29-56).
The orbits are the openings for the eyes. They are usually seen on panoramic images (Figure 29-56).
The external auditory meatus is a radiolucent area in the temporal bone for the auditory canal. It is visible in panoramic images (Figure 29-56).

Radiopaque Landmarks

The nasal conchae project from the lateral walls of the nasal cavity and are thin, radiopaque bony projections. They are visible in the maxillary incisor periapical image and panoramic images (Figures 29-56 and 29-57).
The floor of the nasal fossa is the radiopaque line along the lower border of the nasal fossae. The floor of the nasal fossa is the roof of the oral cavity or the hard palate. It is cortical bone and thus appears radiopaque. It is visible in the maxillary incisor periapical image and the maxillary canine periapical image as well as panoramic images (Figures 29-56 and 29-57).
The anterior nasal spine appears as a radiopaque projection below the nasal cavity. It is visible in the maxillary incisor periapical image (Figure 29-58).
The nasal septum appears as a radiopaque line continuing from the nasal spine separating the entire nasal fossa vertically. Anatomically, the septum is a thin cortical bone that divides the nasal fossa in half. It is visible in the maxillary incisor periapical image and in panoramic images (Figures 29-56 and 29-58).
The shadow of the nose may also appear on the maxillary incisor image as a radiopaque outline. It is visible in the maxillary incisor periapical image.
The floor of the maxillary sinus appears as a radiopaque line of cortical bone at the lower border of the maxillary sinus. It is visible in maxillary posterior periapical images and the maxillary canine periapical image and in panoramic images (Figures 29-56 and 29-59).
The septa of the sinus are the radiopaque cortical bony structures separating the maxillary sinus into compartments. These are visible in the maxillary periapical premolar and molar images (Figure 29-59).
The inverted Y appears as an upside down Y in the canine periapical images of the maxillary arch. It is composed of the radiopaque floor of the nasal cavity and floor of the maxillary sinus plus the nasal cavity and the sinus cavity (Figure 29-60).
The maxillary tuberosity appears as the radiopaque bony protuberance posterior to the last molar. It is visible in the maxillary molar periapical image and on panoramic images (Figures 29-56 and 29-61).
The hamulus appears as a radiopaque, small, hook-like projection distal to the maxillary tuberosity. It is physically located at the end of the sphenoid bone for tendon attachment (Figure 29-56).
The hamular notch is radiopaque concavity between the maxillary tuberosity and hamulus (Figure 29-56).
The zygomatic process may appear as a radiopaque U-shaped opacity overlapping the molar roots (Figures 29-56 and 29-61).
The zygoma or cheekbone forms the cheekbone. It is seen on maxillary molar periapical images and also panoramic images (Figures 29-56 and 29-61).
The coronoid process of the mandible appears as a radiopaque area in the distal aspect of the maxillary molar periapical image and panoramic images (Figures 29-62 and 29-70).
The mastoid process of the temporal bone lies just posterior to the ear (auditory canal). It is visible in panoramic images (Figure 29-56).
The styloid process is a projection of bone that comes from the temporal bone and lies posterior to the glenoid fossa. It is visible in panoramic images (Figure 29-56).

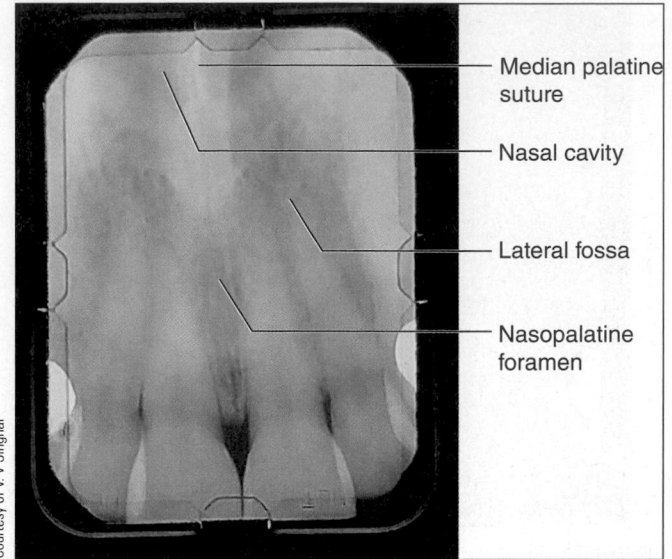

FIGURE 29-54
Nasal cavity, medial palatine suture, and lateral fossa on maxillary incisor periapical image.

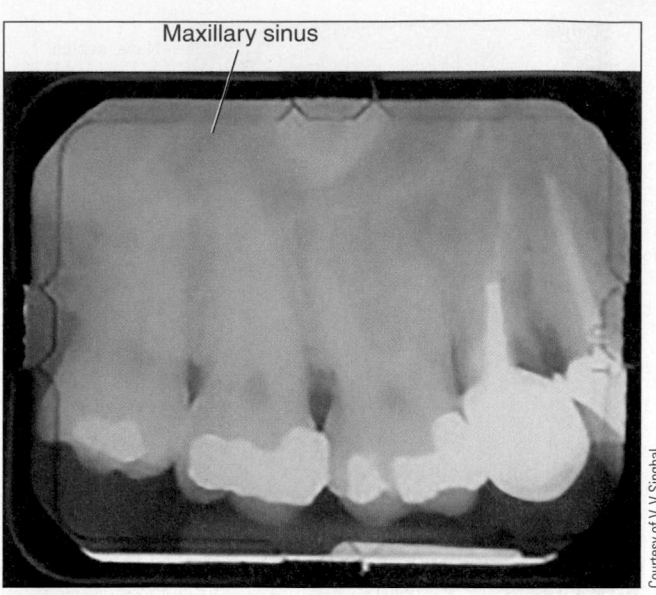

FIGURE 29-55
Maxillary molar periapical image with maxillary sinus.

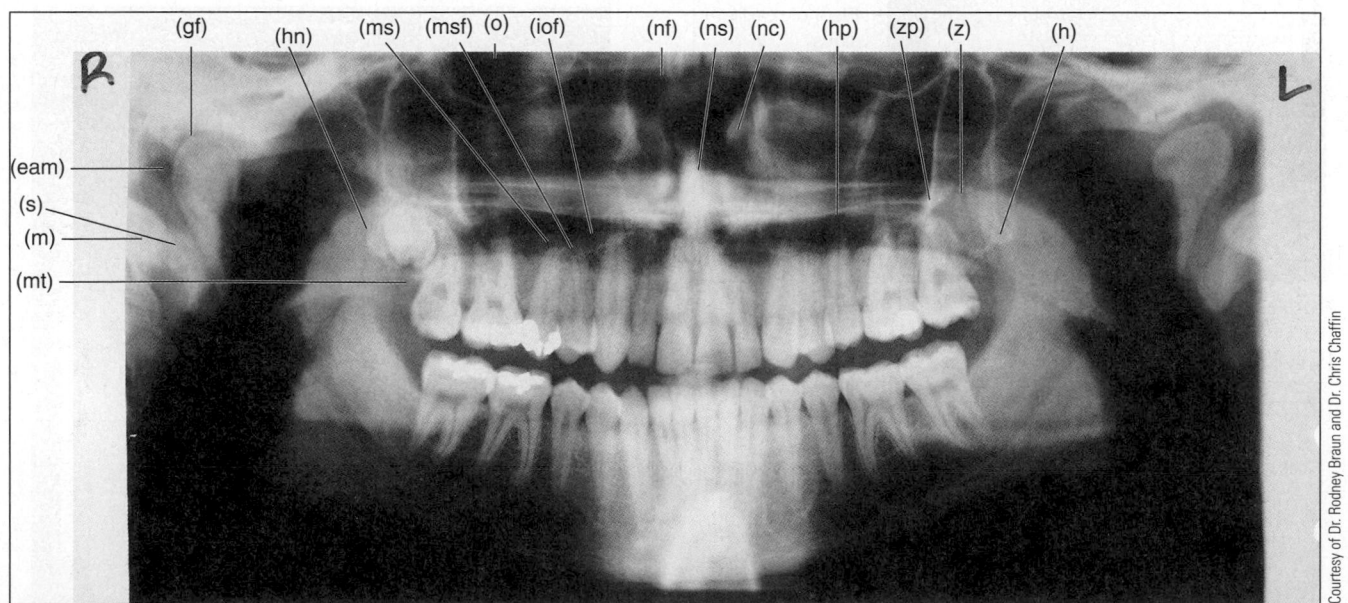

FIGURE 29-56
A panoramic and periapical radiograph identifying the maxillary landmarks. (mt) maxillary tuberosity. (m) mastoid process. (s) styloid process. (eam) external auditory meatus. (gf) glenoid fossa. (hn) hamular notch. (ms) maxillary sinus. (msf) maxillary sinus floor. (o) orbit. (iof) infraorbital foramen. (nf) nasal fossa. (ns) nasal septum. (nc) nasal conchae. (hp) hard palate. (zp) zygomatic process. (z) zygoma. (h) hamulus.

Radiographic Interpretation: Radiographic Pathologies

Once the dental assistant is familiar with normal radiographic anatomy, they should be able to recognize pathologies. This section discusses diseases that affect the tooth.

Dental Caries

Caries may occur on the occlusal, interproximal, buccal, or lingual surfaces of a tooth. Caries may be considered incipient, moderate, advanced, or severe depending on the depth and extent of decay. Clinical and radiographic exams are important in determining the location and extent of decay.

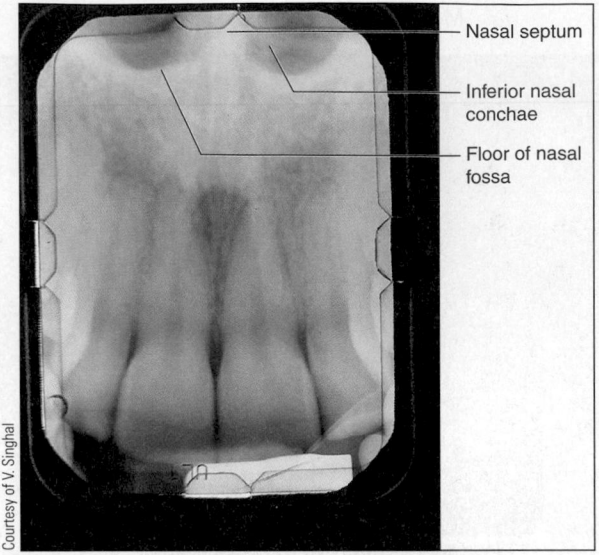

Courtesy of V. Singhal

- Nasal septum
- Inferior nasal conchae
- Floor of nasal fossa

FIGURE 29-57
Maxillary central incisor periapical image showing nasal septum, floor of nasal fossa, and inferior nasal conchae.

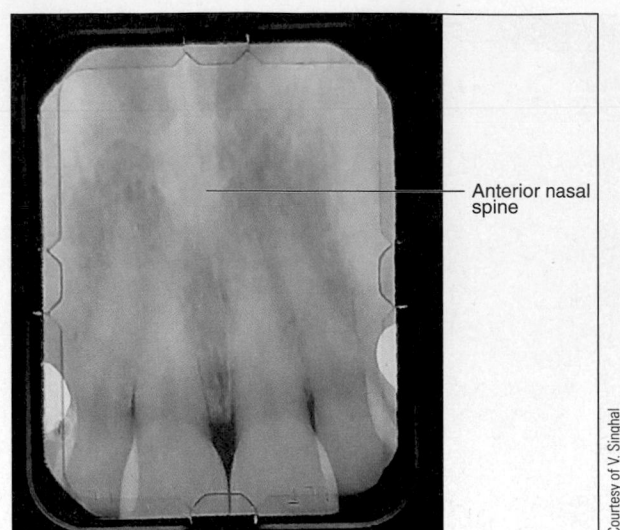

Courtesy of V. Singhal

- Anterior nasal spine

FIGURE 29-58
Maxillary central incisor periapical image showing anterior nasal spine.

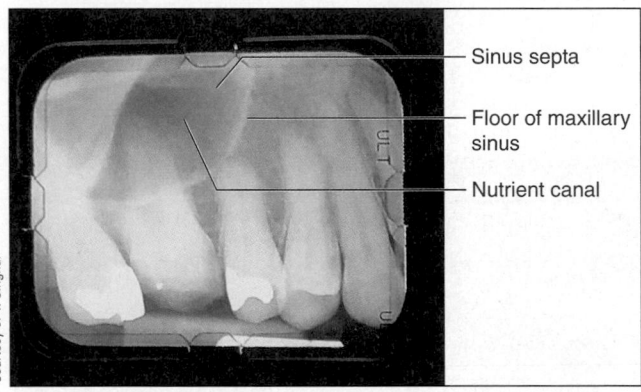

Courtesy of V. Singhal

- Sinus septa
- Floor of maxillary sinus
- Nutrient canal

FIGURE 29-59
Maxillary molar periapical image showing nutrient canal, sinus septa and floor of maxillary sinus.

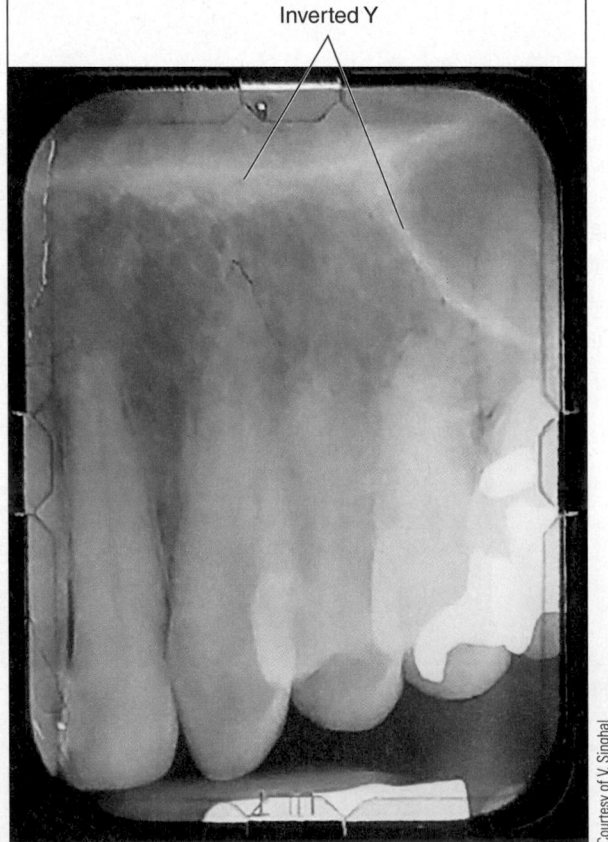

Inverted Y

Courtesy of V. Singhal

FIGURE 29-60
Maxillary canine periapical image showing inverted Y.

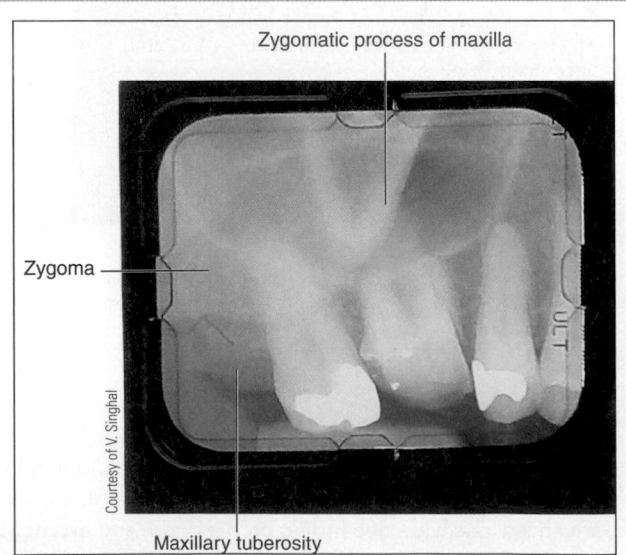

Zygomatic process of maxilla

Zygoma

Courtesy of V. Singhal

Maxillary tuberosity

FIGURE 29-61
Maxillary molar periapical image showing zygoma, zygomatic process of the maxilla, and maxillary tuberosity.

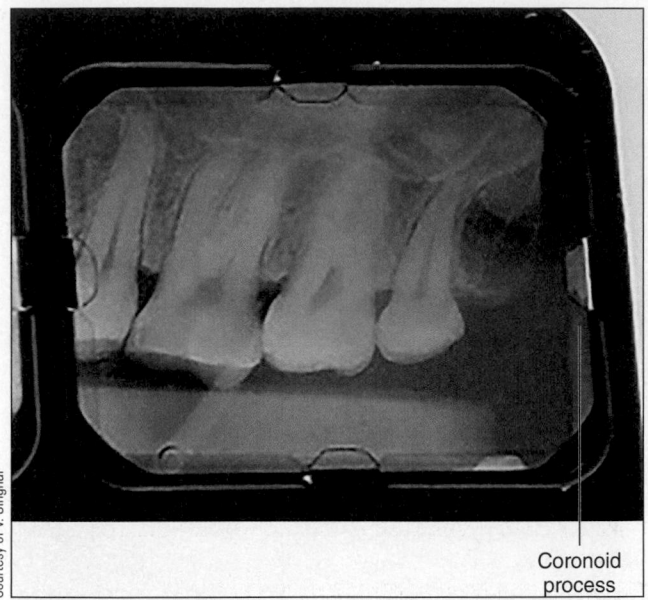

Courtesy of V. Singhal

Coronoid
process

FIGURE 29-62

Maxillary molar periapical image showing the coronoid process of the mandible.

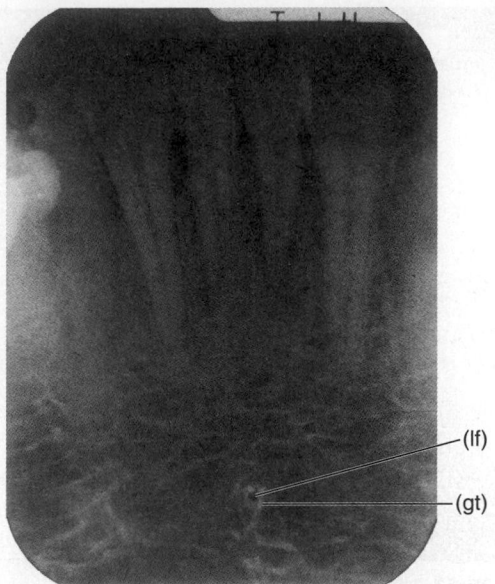

(lf)

(gt)

FIGURE 29-63

(lf) Lingual foramen. (gt) Genial tubercles.

TABLE 29-8 Mandibular Radiographic Structures

Radiolucent Structures
The lingual foramen is the radiolucent oval between and below the apices of the mandibular central incisors. This structure is found on the mandibular incisor periapical image (Figure 29-63).
The mental foramen is the small round radiolucent area usually located beneath the bicuspid apices. This structure is found on the mandibular premolar periapical image and panoramic images (Figures 29-64 and 29-70).
The submandibular fossa is the radiolucent area beneath the mylohyoid ridge. This structure is found on the mandibular molar periapical image (Figure 29-65).
The mandibular canal is a radiolucent passageway for the mandibular nerve and associated blood vessels. It is found in the mandibular molar periapical image and panoramic images (Figures 29-66 and 29-70).
The glenoid fossa is a depression on the lower border of the temporal bone where the condyloid process of the mandible articulates as the temporomandibular joint. This structure is visible on panoramic images (Figure 29-56).
Nutrient canals are radiolucent paths that extend toward the alveolar crest. They can be found anywhere including in the sinuses but are most commonly seen in the mandibular anterior region (Figure 29-59).

Radiopaque Structures
The genial tubercles are the radiopaque projections just below the mandibular central incisor root apexes (Figure 29-63).
The mental ridge is the radiopaque band of cortical bone that extends from the center front of the mandible to the premolar area. This structure is found on the mandibular incisor periapical image and the mandibular canine periapical image (Figure 29-67).
The Curve of Spee is the radiopaque cortical bone extending upward from the incisor region to the most posterior molars (Figure 29-68).
The internal oblique ridge of the mandible is a radiopaque band of cortical bone that extends down from the ramus of the mandible and ends in the area of the mandibular molars where it blends in with the mylohyoid ridge. This structure is found on the mandibular molar periapical image (Figure 29-65), molar bitewing images (Figure 29-69) and panoramic images (Figure 29-70).
The mylohyoid ridge is continuous with the internal oblique ridge of the mandible. The internal oblique ridge becomes the mylohyoid ridge in the area of the molars. It is a radiopaque line on the image and is physiologically located on the buccal aspect of the mandible in the molar area. This structure is found on the mandibular molar periapical image (Figure 29-65) and panoramic images (Figure 29-70).
The external oblique ridge of the mandible is a radiopaque band of cortical bone that angles from the retromolar area to the bicuspid area. Physiologically it is located on the external surfaced of the mandible. This structure is found on the mandibular molar periapical image (Figure 29-69) and panoramic images (Figure 29-70).
The inferior border of the mandible appears as the radiopaque band of cortical bone at lower edge of mandible. This structure is found on the mandibular periapical image and panoramic images (Figures 29-67 and 29-70).
The condyle is a projection on the top of the ramus, which rests in the glenoid fossa. This structure is visible on panoramic images (Figure 29-70).
The medial sigmoid notch or mandibular notch is the indented area between the condyle and coronoid processes on the ramus; also known as the coronoid notch or the mandibular notch. This structure is visible on panoramic images (Figure 29-70).
The ramus of the mandible is the portion that runs vertically. This structure is visible on panoramic images (Figure 29-70).
The angle of the mandible is the corner where the body of the mandible and the ramus of mandible meet. It is visible on panoramic images (Figure 29-70).
The hyoid bone is a U-shaped bone suspended by ligaments below the mandible but anterior to the larynx. This structure is visible on panoramic images (Figure 29-70).

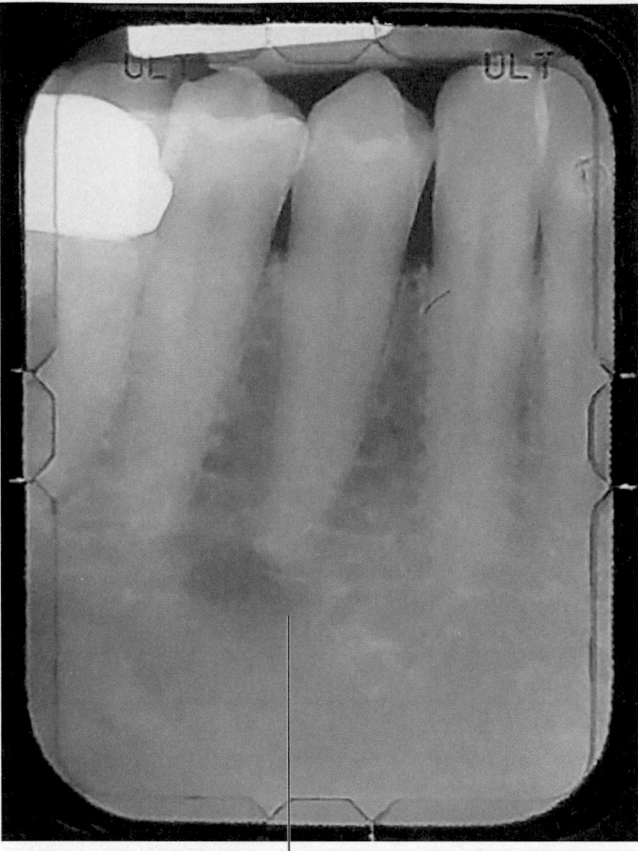

Courtesy of V. Singhal

Mental foramen

FIGURE 29-64
Mandibular premolar periapical image showing mental foramen.

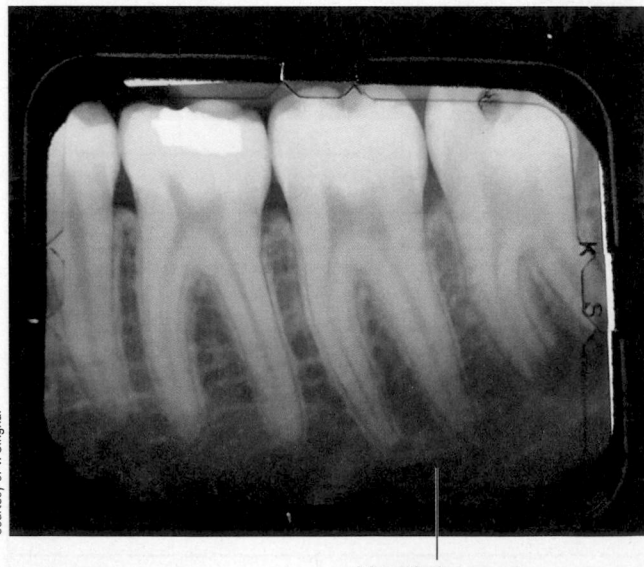

Courtesy of V. Singhal

Mandibular canal

FIGURE 29-66
Mandibular molar periapical image showing mandibular canal.

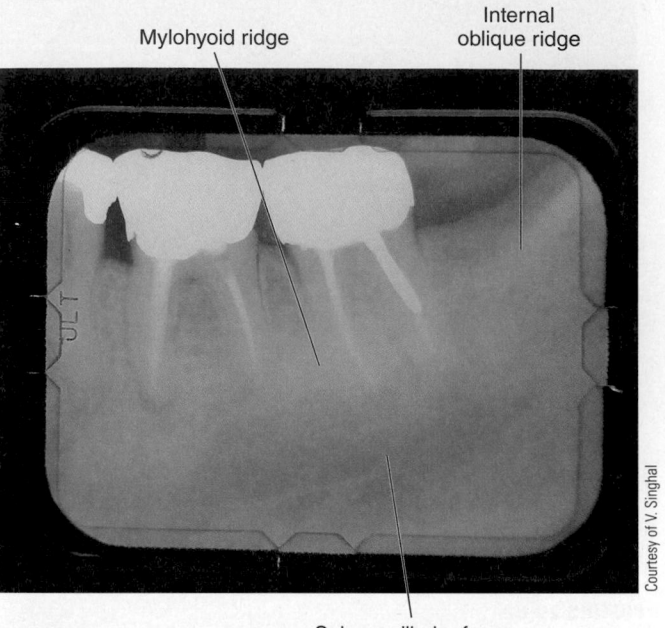

Mylohyoid ridge

Internal oblique ridge

Submandibular fossa

Courtesy of V. Singhal

FIGURE 29-65
Mandibular molar periapical image showing mylohyoid ridge and internal oblique ridge.

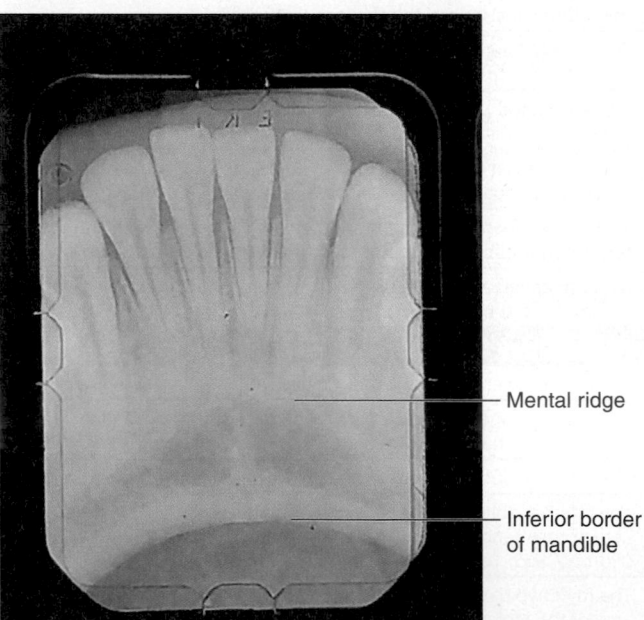

Mental ridge

Inferior border of mandible

Courtesy of V. Singhal

FIGURE 29-67
Mandibular incisor periapical image showing mental ridge and inferior border of mandible.

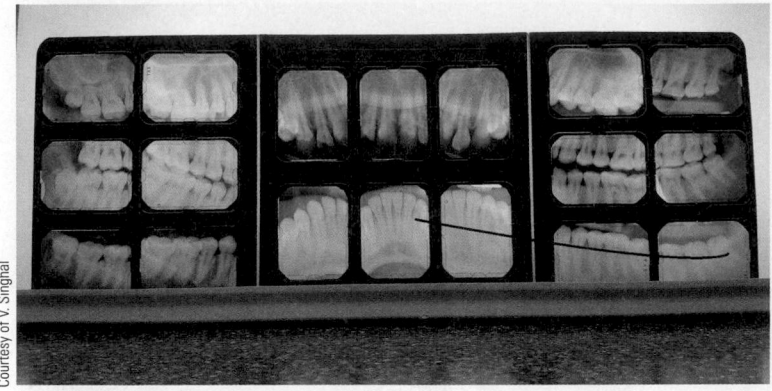

FIGURE 29-68
Curve of Spee.

Courtesy of V. Singhal

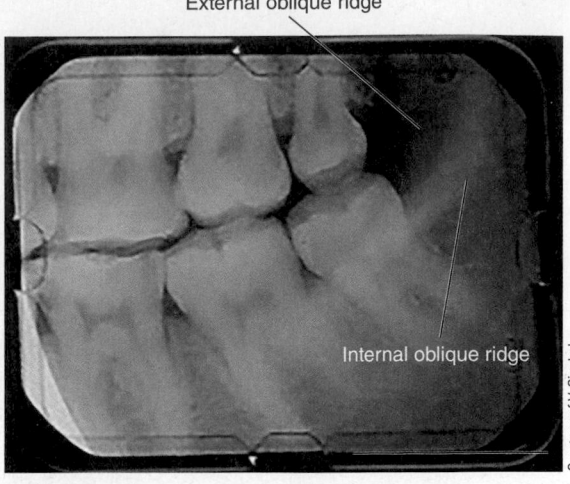

External oblique ridge

Internal oblique ridge

Courtesy of V. Singhal

FIGURE 29-69
Molar bitewing showing the external oblique ridge.

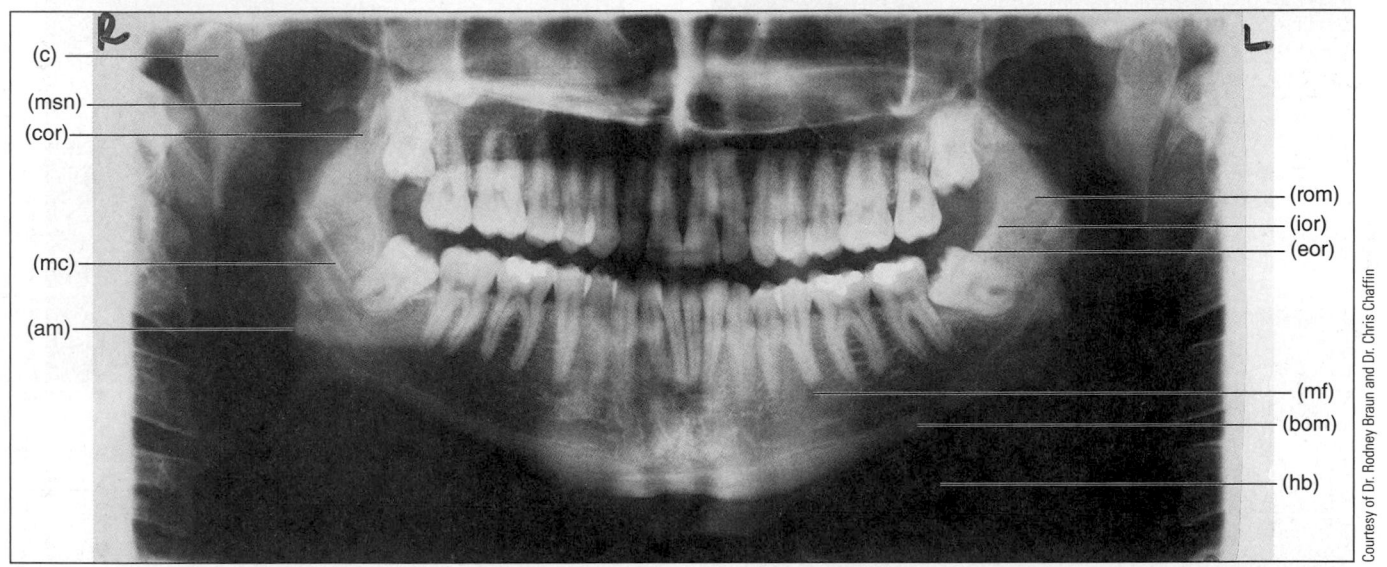

(c)
(msn)
(cor)
(mc)
(am)

(rom)
(ior)
(eor)
(mf)
(bom)
(hb)

Courtesy of Dr. Rodney Braun and Dr. Chris Chaffin

FIGURE 29-70
Panoramic radiograph identifying mandibular landmarks. (am) angle of the mandible. (mc) mandibular canal. (cor) coronoid process. (msn) medial sigmoid notch or mandibular notch. (c) condyle. (eor) external oblique ridge. (ior) internal oblique ridge. (rom) ramus of the mandible. (mf) mental foramen. (bom) border of mandible. (hb) hyoid bone.

Incipient Decay *Incipient* means beginning, and incipient decay is present only in the enamel of the occlusal surfaces of posterior teeth and is not visible radiographically. A clinical exam is critical in the detection of incipient occlusal lesions. The pits and fissures of the occlusal surfaces may have dark staining and may be "sticky" when an explorer is used (Figure 29-71).

Incipient decay on the proximal surfaces is present only in the enamel and is less than halfway through the enamel toward the DEJ (Figure 29-72). Radiographically the decay appears as a triangle with the apex pointing toward the DEJ (Figure 29-72). Incipient decay on proximal surfaces of teeth cannot be detected by a clinical exam. Diagnostic quality bitewings that show open spaces between the contacts are an important part of diagnosing incipient decay.

Moderate Decay Moderate decay on occlusal surfaces is not visible radiographically as the cusps of the posterior teeth will obscure the areas of decay on the image. A clinical exam is an important component of detecting moderate occlusal decay (Figure 29-71). Moderate interproximal decay is in enamel only. The decay extends more than 50% through the enamel but has not yet invaded the DEJ (Figure 29-73A). An artifact known as cervical burnout appears on many radiographs. It is due to the position of the x-ray beam as it passes through the CEJ in the interproximal areas. This causes a radiolucency that can be mistaken for interproximal decay (Figure 29-73B). The experienced clinician can usually differentiate between cervical burnout and interproximal decay. A clinical exam can confirm the presence of decay in this area.

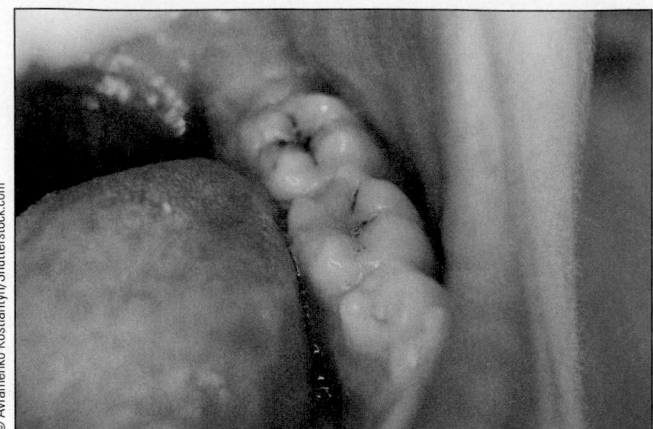

FIGURE 29-71
Incipient decay on mandibular left first molar, moderate decay on mandibular left second molar.

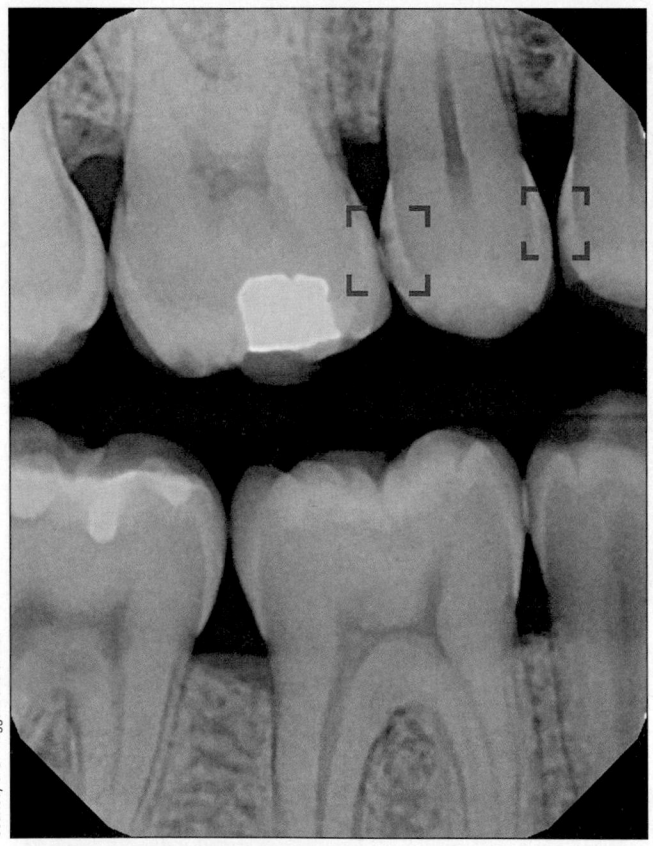

FIGURE 29-72
Radiograph of incipient decay on mesial surface of maxillary first molar and interproximal surfaces of maxillary premolars.

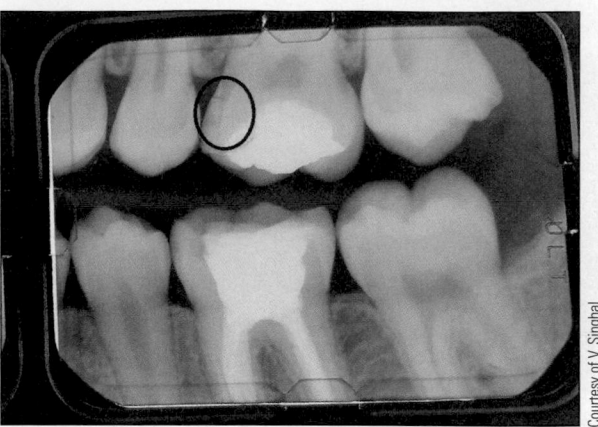

FIGURE 29-73A
Moderate interproximal decay encircled on molar bitewing.

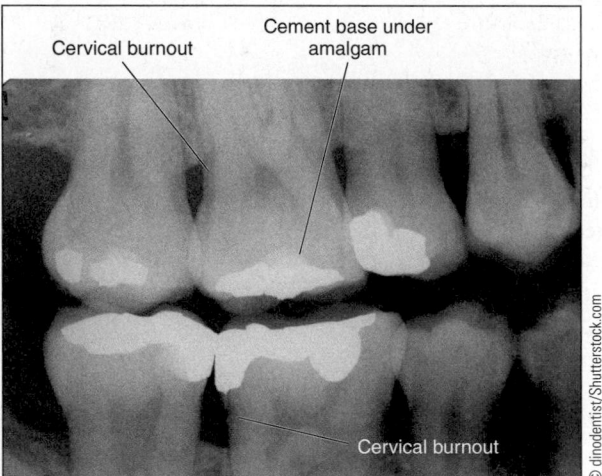

FIGURE 29-73B
Radiolucencies that may be mistaken for decay.

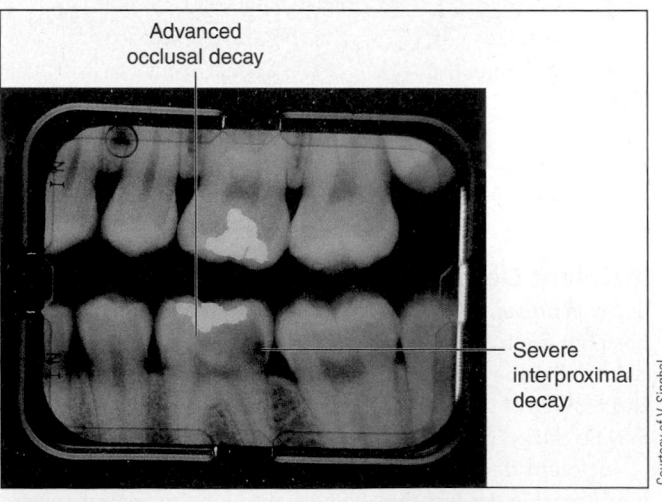

FIGURE 29-74
Advanced occlusal decay and severe interproximal decay.

Advanced Decay Advanced occlusal decay is visible radiographically. It appears as an oval-shaped radiolucency under the enamel on the occlusal surface. Advanced occlusal decay is less than halfway through the dentin toward the pulp (Figure 29-74). Advanced interproximal decay appears as two triangles. The first triangle is in the enamel. The second triangle appears in the dentin once the decay invaded the dentin. Advanced interproximal decay is less than halfway through the dentin toward the pulp (Figure 29-75).

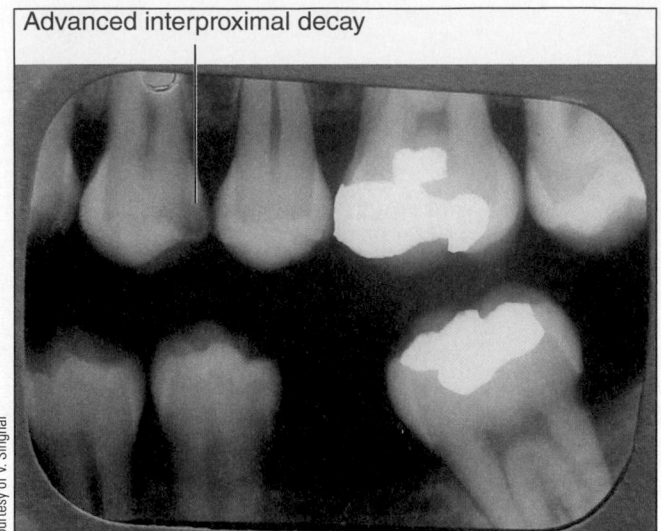

Advanced interproximal decay

Courtesy of V. Singhal

FIGURE 29-75
Advanced interproximal decay.

Severe Decay Severe occlusal decay appears as a large radiolucency under the occlusal surface of the tooth. Severe occlusal decay is more than halfway through the dentin toward the pulp of the tooth (Figure 29-76). Severe interproximal decay is also more than halfway through the dentin toward the pulp (Figure 29-74).

Smooth Surface Decay Decay can also occur on the buccal and lingual surfaces of teeth (Figure 29-77A). These are smooth surfaces and should be diagnosed via a clinical exam. On a radiograph, buccal or lingual decay will appear as a radiolucent circular area in the middle of the tooth (Figure 29-77B). Since a radiograph is two-dimensional, it is difficult to determine if the decay is on the buccal surface or lingual surface only based on the image. It is also difficult to determine the depth of the lesion from a radiographic image. Buccal or lingual decay can also occur on the exposed root surfaces of teeth.

Root Caries Root surface caries may occur on the cementum of exposed root surfaces. On radiographs the lesion appears as a scooped-out or saucer-shaped area along the interproximal root surface of the tooth.

Recurrent Decay Recurrent decay occurs under an existing restoration (Figure 29-78). This may be due to leakage of the margins of the restoration that allows food and bacteria to enter the tooth, or it may be due to decayed tooth material being left behind when the restoration was placed. This may also be caused by poor contouring of the restoration when placed (Figure 29-79). Overhangs allow food to get trapped and cause decay on the proximal margin of the restoration. If the restoration does not mimic natural tooth structure, food can become impacted between the restoration and the adjacent tooth, resulting in recurrent decay. Recurrent decay appears as a radiolucency under the existing restoration.

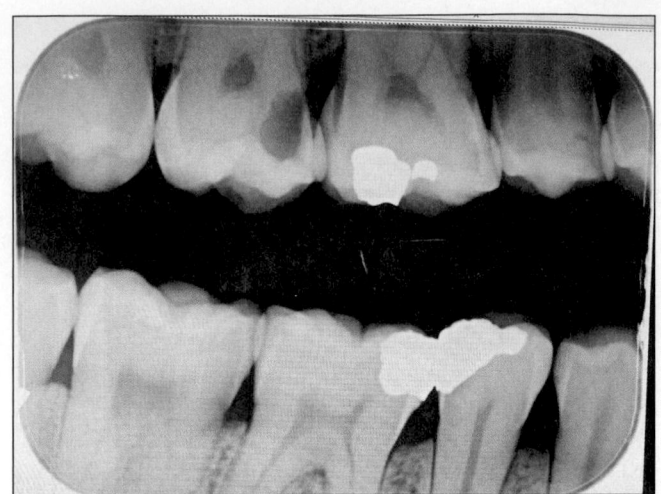

© Good Image Studio/Shutterstock.com

FIGURE 29-76
Severe occlusal decay.

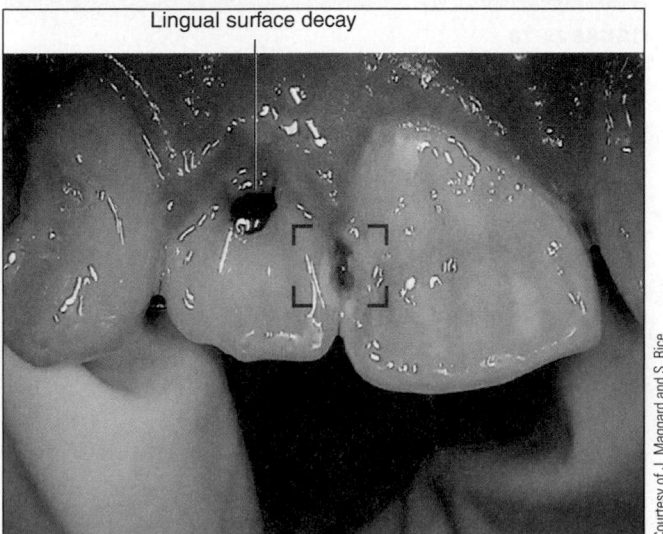

Lingual surface decay

Courtesy of J. Maggard and S. Rice

FIGURE 29-77A
Lingual decay on maxillary lateral incisor.

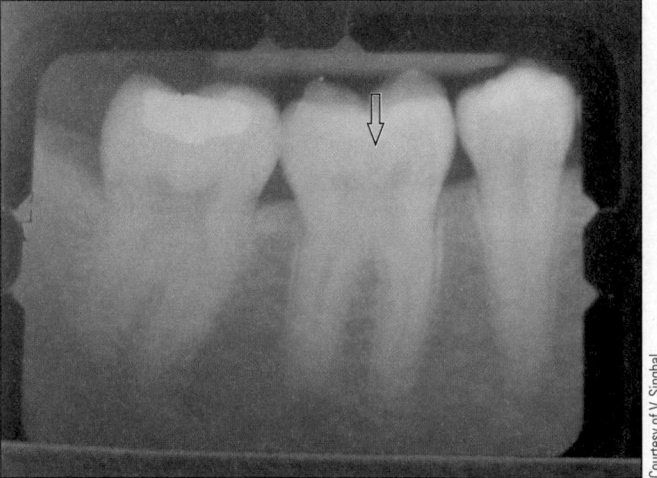

Courtesy of V. Singhal

FIGURE 29-77B
Buccal or lingual decay.

Recurrent decay

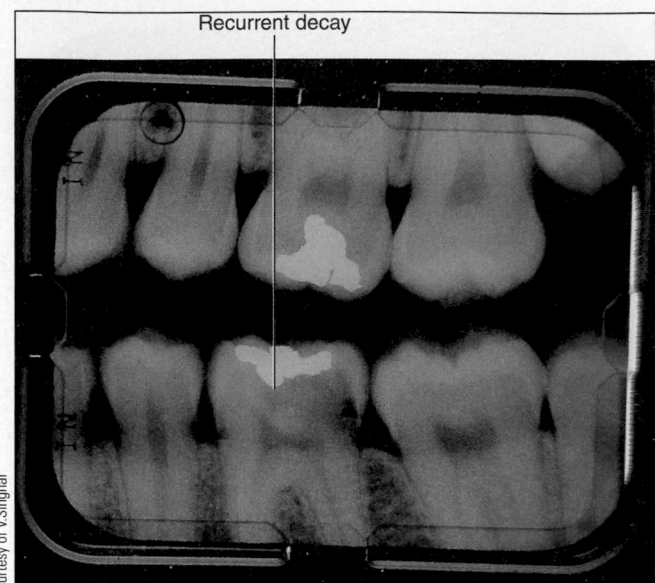

Courtesy of V.Singhal

FIGURE 29-78
Recurrent decay.

Poorly contoured crown

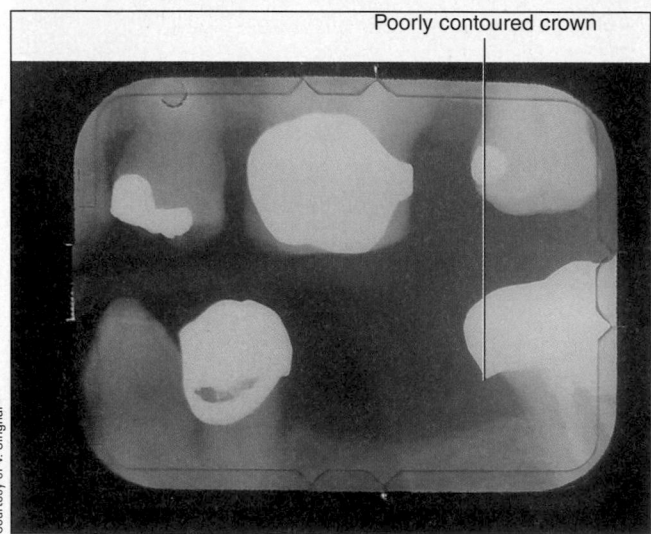

Courtesy of V. Singhal

FIGURE 29-79
Overhang on poorly contoured crown.

Rampant Decay Rampant decay occurs on multiple teeth and also spreads rapidly (Figure 29-80). It is considered to be severe decay. Rampant caries is seen in children with poor diets or in young children who sleep with a milk or juice bottle. The sugar content of the fluids remains in contact with the teeth, resulting in caries on multiple teeth. Rampant caries may also be seen in adults who are experiencing xerostomia either due to medications or to head and neck radiation therapy. Radiographically, rampant caries appears as radiolucencies on multiple teeth.

Pulpal and Periapical Lesions

If carious lesions are not treated, they will progress. This section discusses diseases of the pulp and the apical areas of teeth.

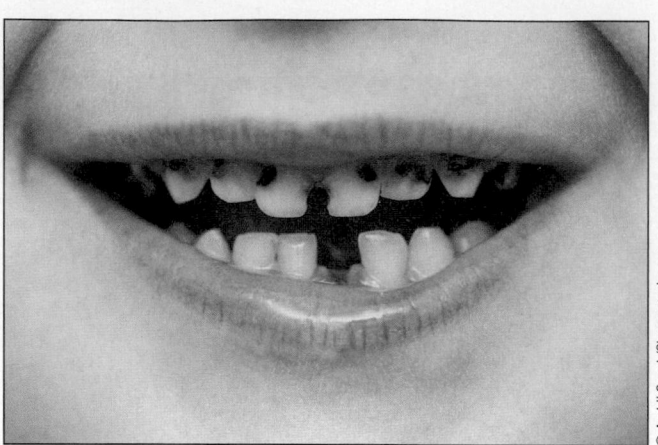

© Andrii Spy_k/Shutterstock.com

FIGURE 29-80
Clinical appearance of rampant decay.

Pulpitis *Pulpitis*, or inflammation of the pulp, does not show radiographic changes in the pulp. It is generally diagnosed radiographically by the presence of deep caries or tooth fractures and by subjective signs and symptoms. Signs and symptoms include pain or sensitivity when cold or sweets contact the tooth, but the sensitivity goes away when the cold or sweet substance is removed. Pulpitis may be reversible or irreversible. Reversible pulpitis resolves when the decay is removed and the tooth is treated with a restoration. Irreversible pulpitis demonstrates sensitivity to a stimulus such as cold or sweets that lingers even after the stimulus is removed. Irreversible pulpitis is treated by endodontic therapy. The patient may also complain of the presence of a constant low-grade ache. Pulpal tests may be conducted to determine pulpal status.

Widened Periodontal Ligament Membrane A widened periodontal ligament (PDL) membrane occurs as the exudate from the pulpitis inflames the membrane making it wider. A widened PDL space is visible on a radiograph as a wider radiolucent area around the root of the tooth. The normal width of the periodontal ligament space is 0.5 millimeters or less (Figure 29-81).

Breakdown of Lamina Dura The breakdown of the lamina dura occurs from the pressure from the inflamed periodontal membrane (Figure 29-82). The pressure causes the lamina dura, or the cortical lining of the bony socket, to break down. This is evidenced on the radiograph as disappearance of lamina dura and widening of periodontal membrane space.

Periapical Abscess A periapical abscess is an infection that develops at the tip of the root of a tooth. A periapical abscess may be acute or chronic and appears as a radiolucent lesion at the apex of the infected root(s) (Figure 29-83). The acute abscess is painful as the pus collects in the area affected and causes gingival swelling. Swelling and fever may result. The acute periapical abscess may become a chronic abscess if the infection is able to escape through an opening in the gingiva. This opening is called a fistula; patients may call refer to it as a gumboil (Figure 29-84).

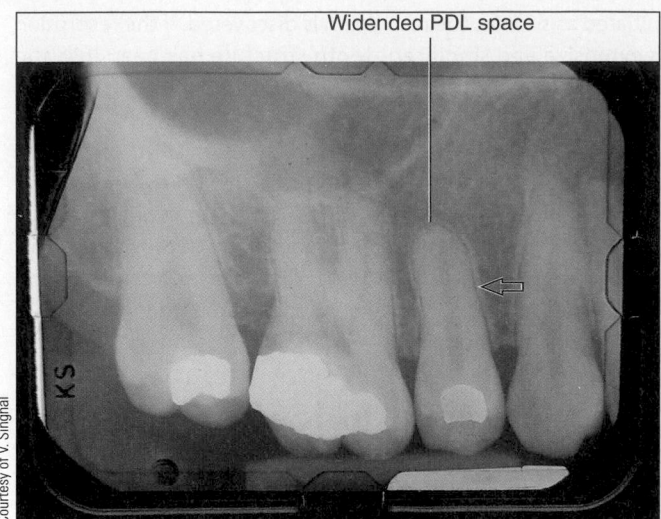

FIGURE 29-81
Widened periodontal ligament (PDL) space.

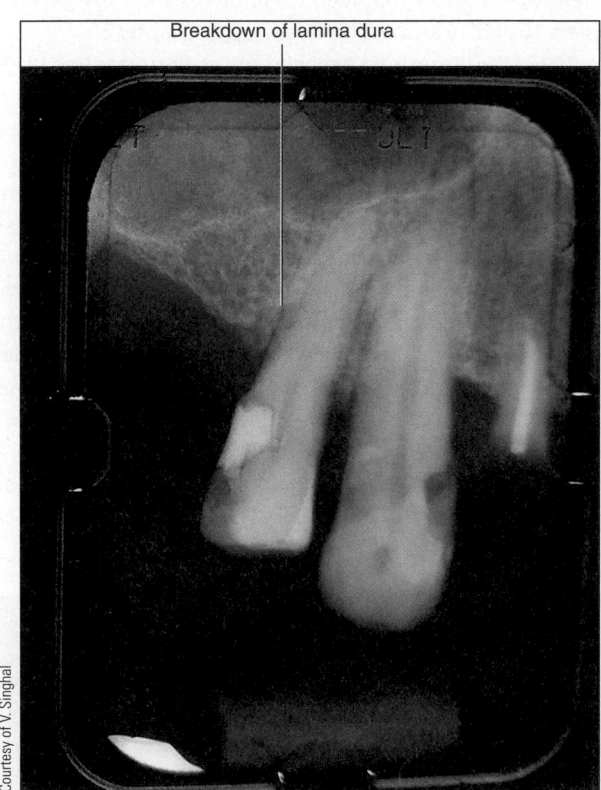

FIGURE 29-82
Breakdown of the lamina dura.

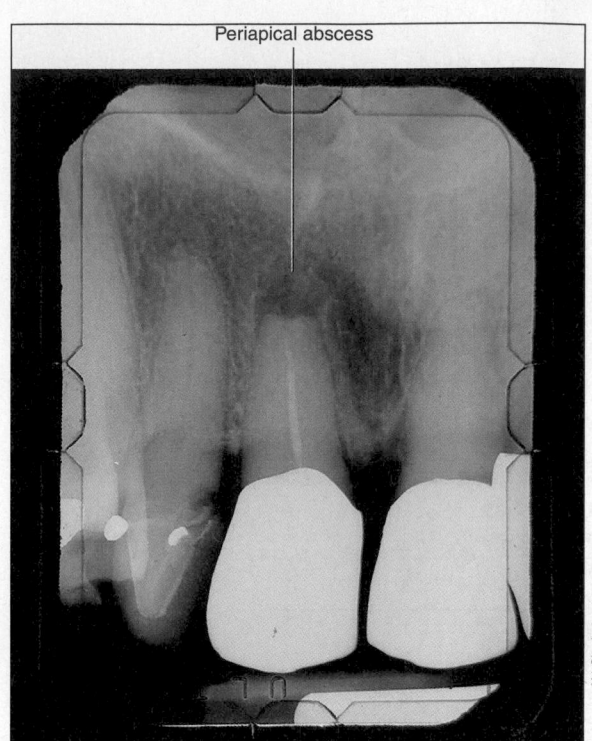

FIGURE 29-83
Periapical abscess.

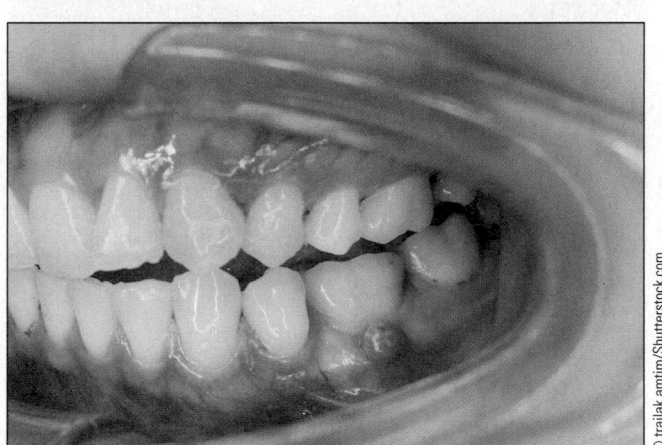

FIGURE 29-84
Fistula.

The tiny opening on the gingival surface has a small tract or trail that leads to the periapical abscess. The pus collecting in the periapical area is draining out through this tract and fistula into the oral cavity. The patient may say that sometimes that get a bad taste; this is due to the draining pus. Since the infection is able to drain, a chronic periapical abscess is generally not painful.

Radiopaque Lesions

Some areas that are visible on a dental radiograph may appear as radiopaque lesions.

Condensing Osteitis   *Condensing osteitis*, also known as *chronic focal sclerotic osteomyelitis*, is dense bone that develops periapically in response to chronic pulpal involvement or necrosis. It appears as a radiopaque area around the apex of a tooth. The molar and premolar periapical areas are the most common area where this occurs. Endodontic therapy should be performed if the pulp is infected.

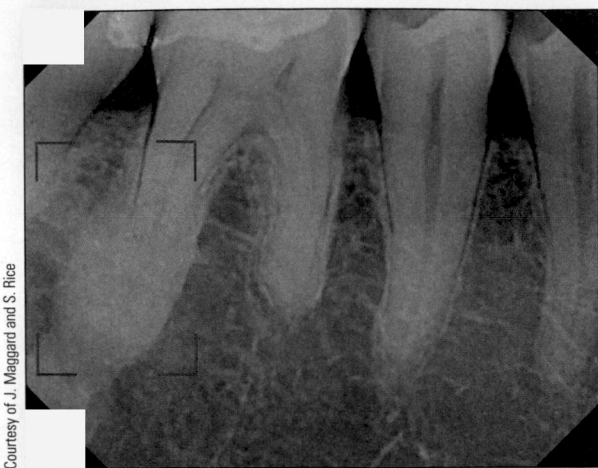

FIGURE 29-85
Condensing osteitis.

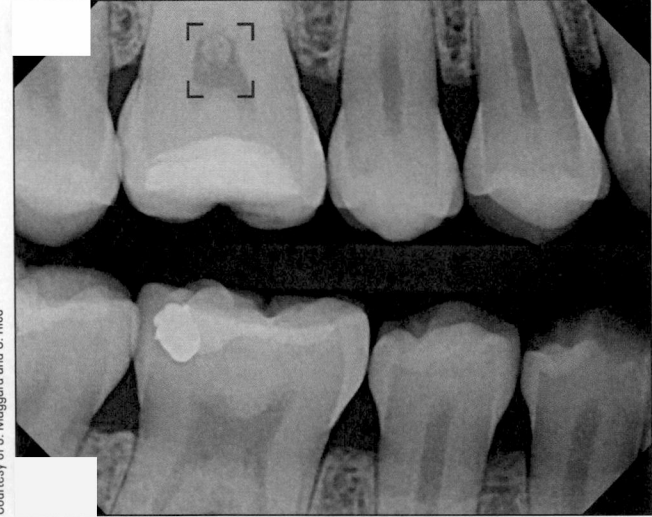

FIGURE 29-86
Pulp stones.

Pulp Stones Pulp stones have an unknown cause and are calcified structures that appear as radiopacities in the pulp of the tooth. They may be found in either the crown or the root. Pulp stones are asymptomatic and do not require treatment (Figure 29-86).

Resorption

Resorption may occur in various manners. Resorption may be normal, such as when the roots of the primary teeth resorb to allow the permanent teeth to erupt. Resorption may also be caused by a pathological process such as in internal and external resorption.

Physiological Root Resorption Physiological root resorption occurs during normal exfoliation due to the pressure of the erupting tooth (Figure 29-87).

Internal Resorption Internal resorption occurs within the pulp tissue of the tooth (Figure 29-88). In many cases this is due to trauma or injury to the pulp. Endodontic therapy should be

initiated as soon as the resorption is discovered. If the resorption is extensive and significant tooth structure has been lost, the tooth may need to be extracted.

External Resorption External resorption starts of the outside surface of a tooth and progresses inward (Figure 29-89). External resorption may also occur due to trauma or if extensive orthodontic forces are placed on a tooth during movement. This is most frequently seen in the maxillary anterior teeth or the mandibular molars. Extensive external resorption may require extraction of the tooth.

Periodontal Pathologies: Radiographic Interpretation of Periodontal Disease

Since radiographs are used to view hard tissues such as bone or the tooth, gingivitis cannot be differentiated on a radiographic image. Gingivitis is inflammation of the soft tissues surrounding the dentition. Factors that lead to gingivitis were discussed in Chapters 10 and 16 and will be discussed in Chapter 38.

In 2018, the American Association of Periodontics (AAP) updated the classifications from the original classifications of 1999. Periodontal disease is now classified as chronic, aggressive (localized and generalized), necrotizing, and as a manifestation of systemic disease. The AAP guidelines identify ways of staging and grading a patient to determine the extent of periodontal disease. The first step includes assessing the extent of disease via a clinical exam, obtaining probing depths and radiographs. Determining the extent of missing teeth is also part of the assessment. Based on the information gained, it is determined if the patient has mild, moderate, severe, or very severe periodontal disease. The AAP guidelines consider several factors to determine the extent of periodontal disease. However, this section will focus only on the radiographic bone loss (RBL) as a determining factor for periodontal disease. Table 29-9 provides the guidelines for stages of periodontal

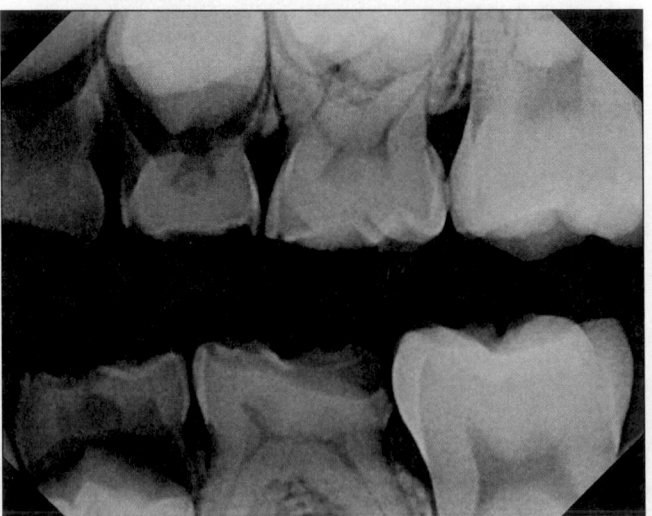

FIGURE 29-87
Physiologic resorption.

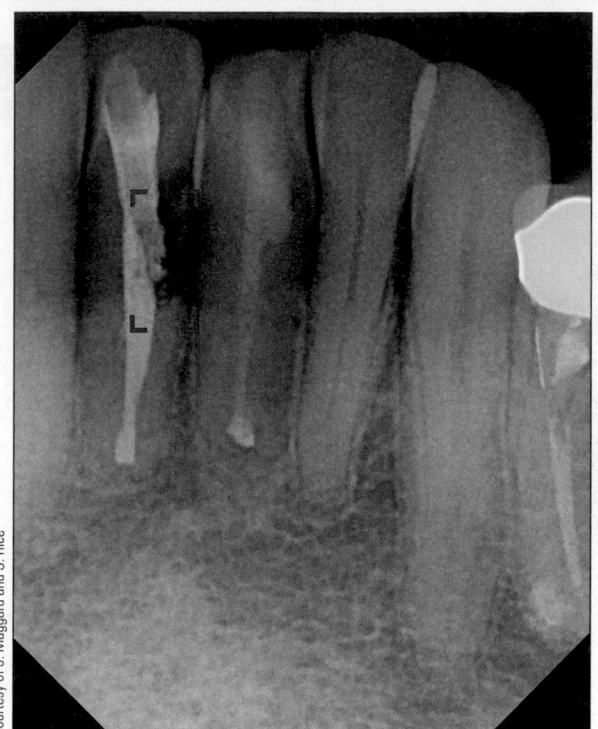

Courtesy of J. Maggard and S. Rice

FIGURE 29-88
Internal resorption.

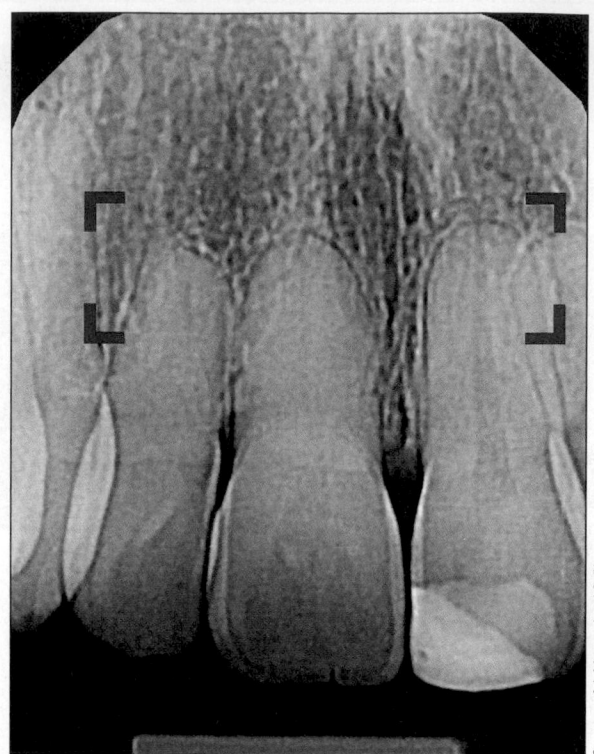

Courtesy of J. Maggard and S. Rice

FIGURE 29-89
External resorption.

disease based on RBL and loss of teeth due to periodontal disease. Additionally, bone loss can be localized or generalized. For example, a patient may have 15% bone loss generally throughout the dentition but may have localized 30% bone loss around the mandibular left first molar. A patient may also have generalized bone loss and have vertical bone loss in a specific area.

Radiographic Dental Anomalies

This section discusses the radiographic appearance of dental anomalies. It is important for the dental assistant to be able to differentiate between what is considered to be normal and what is abnormal. The clinical appearance of some of the anomalies in Table 29-10 is also discussed in Chapter 9.

Radiographic Appearance of Dental Materials

The dental assistant should be able to recognize the appearance of dental materials on a radiograph. Depending on the composition and density of the dental material, it will appear radiolucent or radiopaque. Table 29-11 summarizes the various radiolucent materials used in dentistry and their radiographic appearance. Some nonmetallic materials with less density will appear radiolucent on the radiograph. It may be difficult to distinguish the radiolucent area of a restoration and decayed area. One way to distinguish radiographically is by looking at the margins around the radiolucent area. A restoration has fine even

lines of the preparation, and a decayed area will have irregular lines. Additionally, a clinical exam can help distinguish whether or not the radiographic radiolucent area is decay or a nonmetallic restoration.

Table 29-12 provides the types of radiopaque dental materials visible on a radiograph. Some dental materials that generally appear radiolucent such as unfilled resins now have radiopaque materials added to the dental material so they appear radiopaque on the image.

Quality Assurance in Dental Radiology

Quality assurance in dental radiology refers to the monitoring of procedures and equipment used to safely produce diagnostic radiographs. There are many different quality control tests that are used to keep track of x-ray machines, films, screens, cassettes, the dark room, and processing equipment. It is important to be sure that all of these aspects are functioning properly to ensure the radiographs that are being exposed are of proper diagnostic quality. These quality control tests are also important to avoid any repeat images or processing errors for traditional films.

X-Ray Machine Tests

The x-ray machine itself should be calibrated annually by a qualified trained technician. There are several other tests that are performed on the x-ray machine. Table 29-13 provides a description of each of these tests.

TABLE 29-9 Stages of Periodontal Disease

American Association of Periodontology Stages	Extent of Bone Loss and Loss of Teeth
Stage I mild periodontitis Less than 15% bone loss and generalized horizontal bone loss 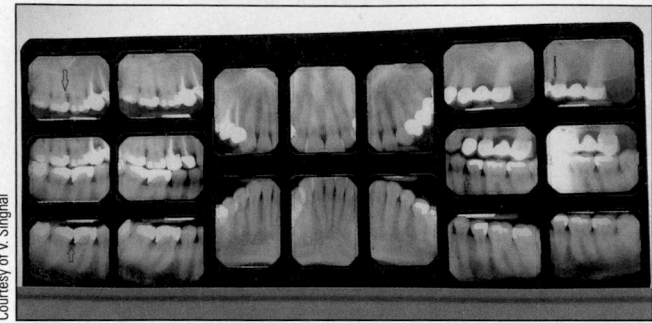 **FIGURE 29-90A** Generalized Stage I bone loss. 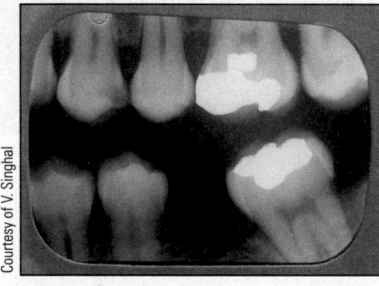 **FIGURE 29-90B** Generalized horizontal bone loss.	Less than 15% bone loss at the coronal one-third (Figure 29-90) No tooth loss
Stage II moderate periodontitis 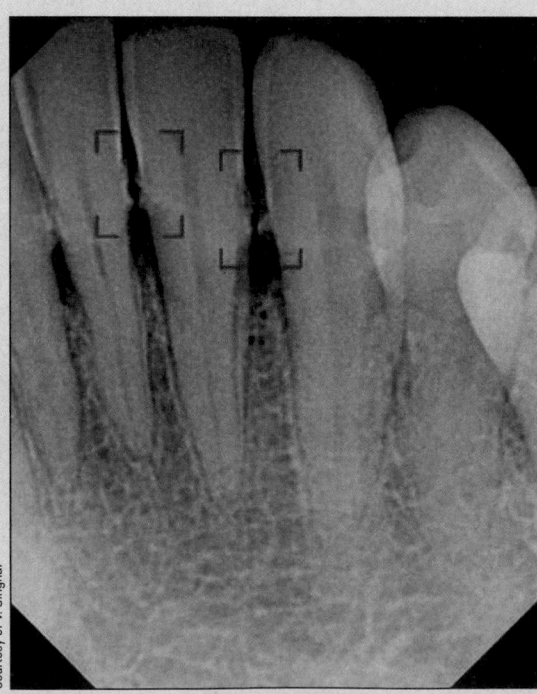 **FIGURE 29-91** Stage II moderate bone loss.	15% to 33% bone loss at the coronal one-third (Figure 29-91) No tooth loss

Courtesy of V. Singhal

TABLE 29-9 *(Continued)*

American Association of Periodontology Stages	Extent of Bone Loss and Loss of Teeth
Stage III advanced periodontitis 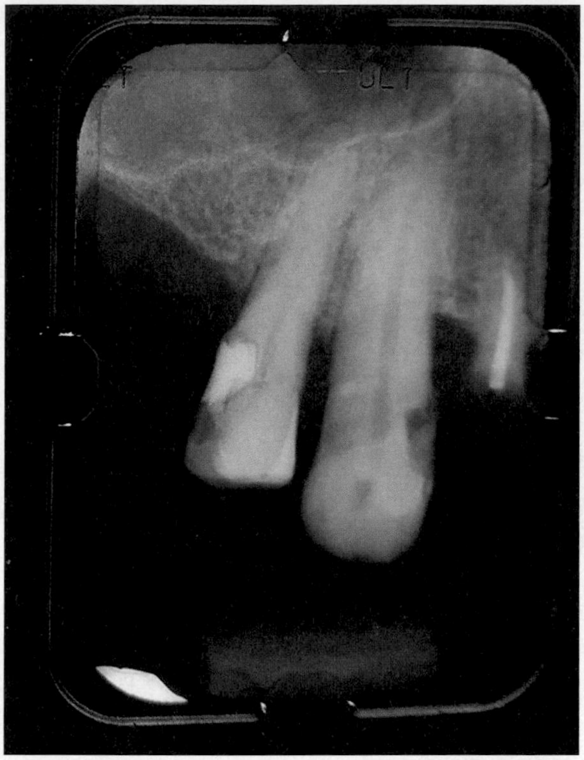 Courtesy of V. Singhal **FIGURE 29-92** Stage III advanced periodontitis.	Middle one-third of tooth and beyond (Figure 29-92) Less than or equal to four teeth missing
Stage IV severe periodontitis 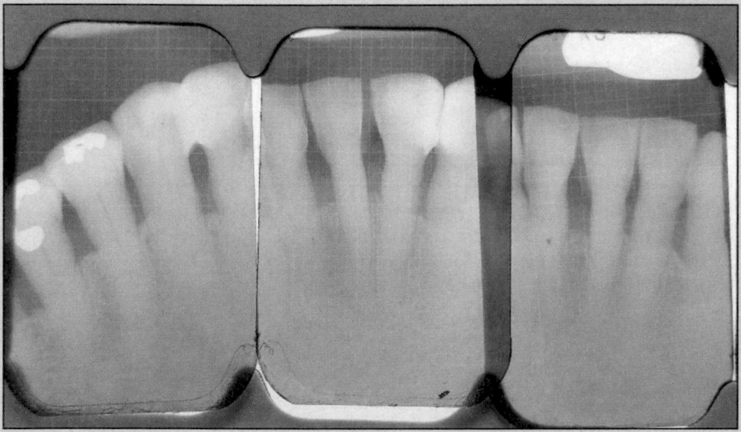 Courtesy of V. Singhal **FIGURE 29-93** Stage IV severe periodontitis.	Middle one-third of tooth and beyond (Figure 29-93) Missing five or more teeth

(Continues)

TABLE 29-10 Tooth Anomalies

The normal development of a tooth can be interrupted by many factors including infection spreading to the developing tooth, fever, trauma, and genetics. This table includes normal developing stages that can be mistaken as anomalies as well as radiographs depicting some abnormal development.

Developing teeth are visible on a radiograph (Figures 29-94 and 29-95). The tooth germ appears as a round radiolucency before the appearance of the calcified dental papilla (Figure 29-95).

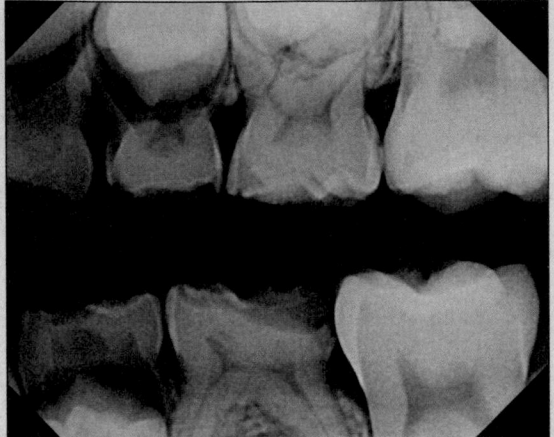

FIGURE 29-94
Bitewing showing physiological resorption of deciduous teeth.

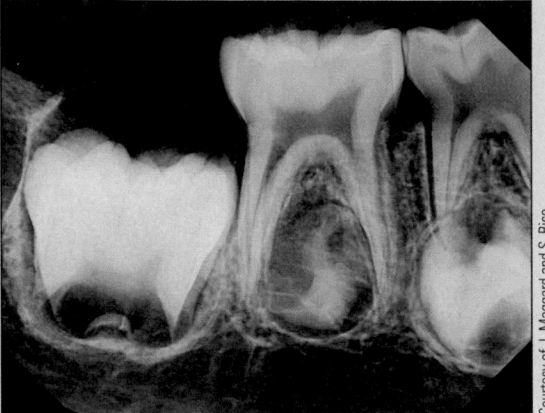

FIGURE 29-95
Tooth germ of developing teeth.

Mixed dentition on radiographs shows erupted deciduous and developing permanent teeth located apically to the primary teeth ready to replace them. Root resorption can be seen on the primary teeth (Figure 29-96).

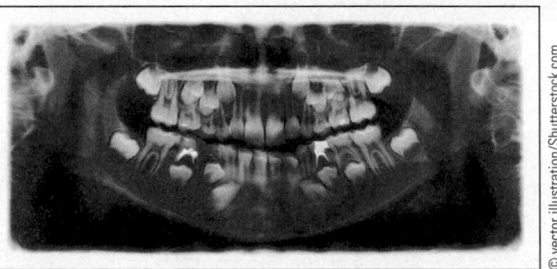

FIGURE 29-96
Mixed dentition.

Images of impacted teeth (Figure 29-97) can help the dentist determine if the tooth can be directed into proper position or if it needs to be extracted. Soft tissue and hard tissue impaction and positioning of the impacted tooth are shown on the radiograph. Third molar and maxillary cuspids are the teeth most often impacted. Depending on the stage of development, the impacted tooth may have a dental sac, but until the tooth contacts the opposing the tooth, apices remain open (Figure 29-96).

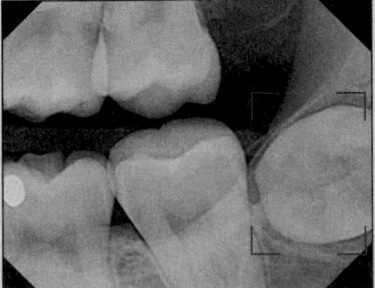

FIGURE 29-97
Impacted third molar.

TABLE 29-10 (*Continued*)

Supernumerary teeth are also referred to as hyperdonts and are underdeveloped extra teeth. The most common are mandibular bicuspids, maxillary incisors, and a fourth molar behind the third molars. A mesiodens is a supernumerary tooth specifically between the maxillary incisors (Figure 29-98). A distodens is a fourth molar behind the third molar.

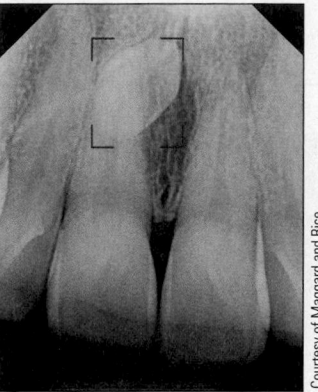

Courtesy of Maggard and Rice

FIGURE 29-98
Supernumerary tooth.

Congenitally missing teeth is an anomaly also referred to as hypodontia and is the failure of a tooth to develop. The teeth most often missing are maxillary third molars, mandibular third molars, and maxillary lateral incisors (Figure 29-99). Oligodontia is when many teeth are missing, and anodontia is when there is a complete absence of teeth.

Canine moved into position of congenitally missing lateral incisor

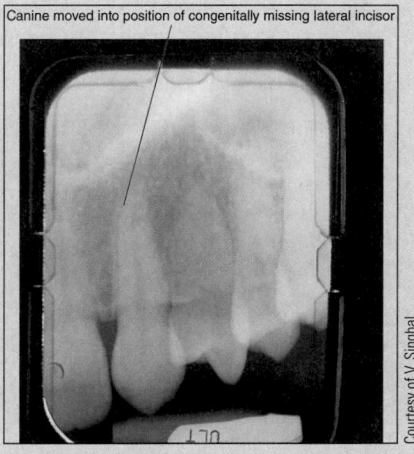

Courtesy of V. Singhal

FIGURE 29-99
Hypodontiacongenitally missing lateral incisor.

Dilaceration is a developmental disturbance that causes the root of the tooth to be distorted or bent (Figure 29-100). It is most common in the posterior teeth. Dilaceration can occur at the crown or the root of the tooth. A dilacerated root is more commonly seen than a dilacerated crown.

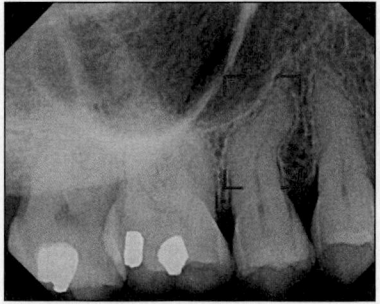

Courtesy of J. Maggard and S. Rice

FIGURE 29-100
Dilaceration.

Concrescence occurs when the cementum of teeth fuses together. Trauma or severe crowding may be a cause of concrescence. The teeth most commonly affected are the second and third molars.

(Continues)

TABLE 29-10 *(Continued)*

Hypercementosis is an excess buildup of cementum on the root of a tooth, giving it a bulbous appearance. Hypercementosis may be caused by trauma or by lack of an opposing tooth.

Bone Anomalies
Bone anomalies may occur during development due to genetic or environmental condition. They may also occur due to chronic infection and acquired infections after birth.

A cleft palate is a radiolucent area between the right and left maxilla where the bones fail to fuse during development (Figure 29-101).

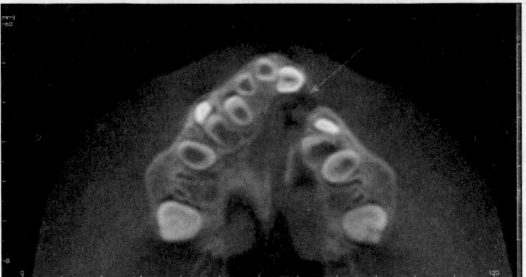

FIGURE 29-101
CT scan of cleft palate.

A dentigerous cyst is a radiolucent area around a developing tooth (Figure 29-97). The most common dentigerous cyst develops around third molars that have late eruption or difficulty in eruption.

Tumors can appear radiolucent, radiopaque, or mixed. Radiolucent tumors occur when the lesion destroys normal bone and is replaced with tumor tissue. A radiopaque tumor tissue has greater density than the original tissue. An odontoma is a tumor of the tooth that has a variety of appearances ranging from radiolucent to radiopaque due to the varying tissue densities (Figure 29-102).

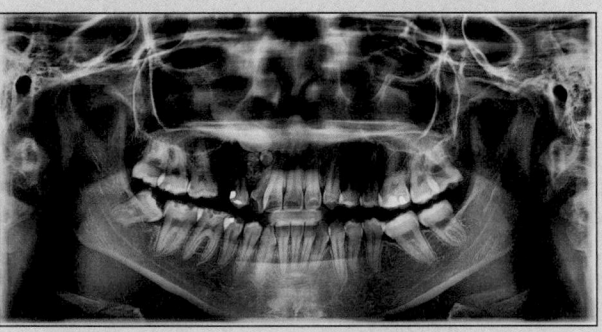

FIGURE 29-102
Odontoma.

A fracture will appear as a radiolucent line where the fracture occurred (Figure 29-103). It may show a displacement of the fractured part.

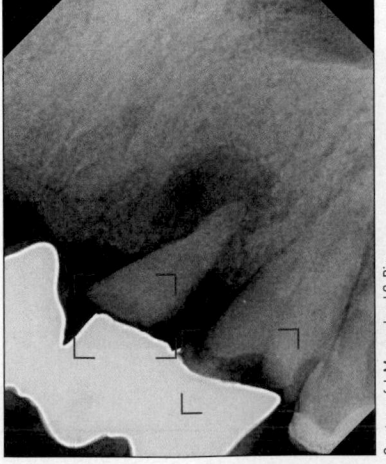

FIGURE 29-103
Fractured root.

TABLE 29-10 *(Continued)*

Extraction sockets appear as radiolucent areas for up to six months after an extraction (Figure 29-104). Bone will eventually fill in the area where the tooth was removed.

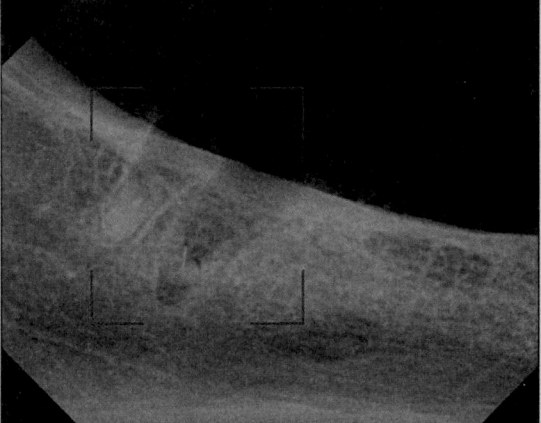

Courtesy of J. Maggard and S. Rice

FIGURE 29-104
Extraction socket.

Salivary stones (sialolith) appear as small, round radiopaque areas. When a duct is blocked or injured, saliva may become calcified and form a stone (Figure 29-105).

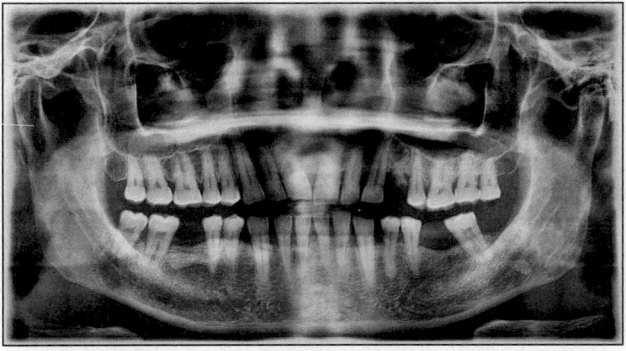

© Rames Khusakul/Shutterstock.com

FIGURE 29-105
Salivary gland stone in left mandible.

TABLE 29-11 Dental Materials That Appear Radiolucent on Images

Unfilled resin materials are made of a synthetic plastic and appear radiolucent on the radiograph (Figure 29-106). The synthetic resin can be distinguished from caries by a defined cavity preparation outline; however, it may be difficult in distinguishing recurrent caries. A clinical exam aids in the determination of decay or a restoration in the area of the radiolucency.

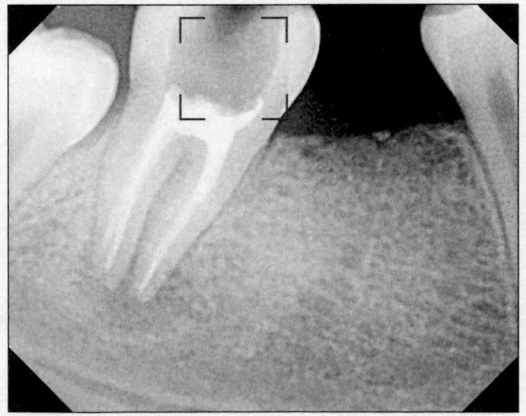

Courtesy of J. Maggard and S. Rice

FIGURE 29-106

(Continues)

TABLE 29-12 *(Continued)*

Acrylic crowns appear completely radiolucent and will not be visible on the image (Figure 29-107). They are used as temporary crowns after preparation of a tooth for a permanent crown and prior to cementation of a permanent crown. The prepared tooth structure is visible on the image.

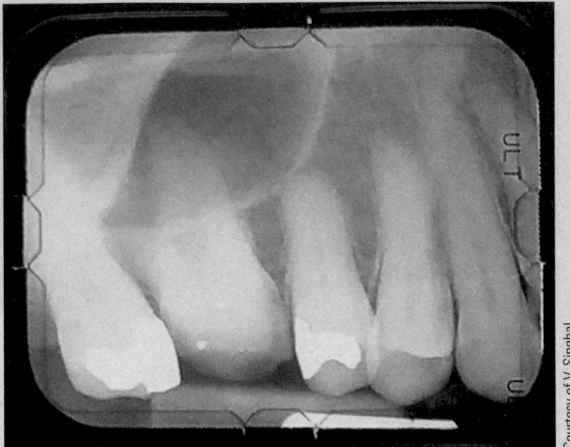

Courtesy of V. Singhal

FIGURE 29-107

Full dentures are acrylic, so they do not show on the radiograph. However, if the teeth are porcelain, they will appear radiopaque (see Figure 29-30).

TABLE 29-12 Dental Materials That Appear Radiopaque on Images

Filled resins have radiopaque materials added to make them appear radiopaque on the radiograph (Figures 29-108 and 29-110).

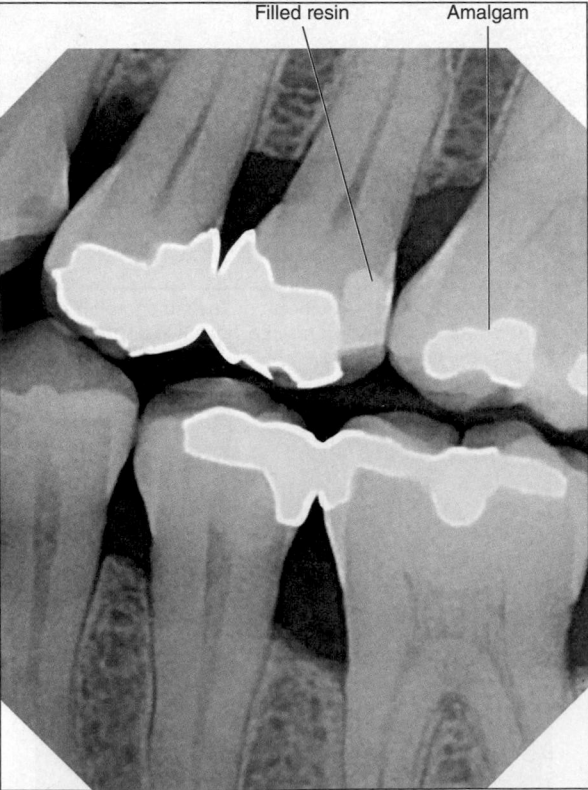

Filled resin   Amalgam

FIGURE 29-108

TABLE 29-12 (*Continued*)

The thickness of radiopaque cements used under all porcelain restorations is visible, allowing the clinician to differentiate between veneers and porcelain jacket crowns and the tooth structure/cement line on the radiographic image (Figure 29-109). Cements placed as bases under large and deep restorations will also appear as radiopacities under an amalgam or a composite restoration (see Figure 29-73B).

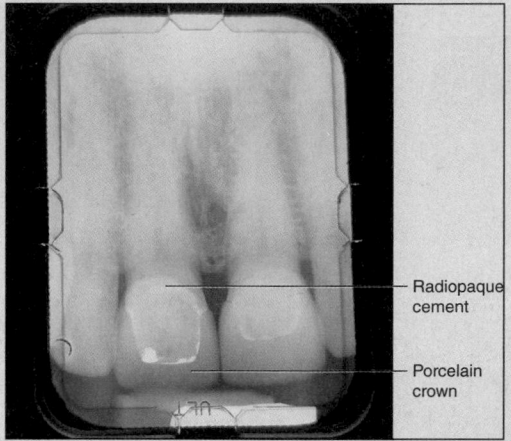

Radiopaque cement

Porcelain crown

Courtesy of V. Singhal

FIGURE 29-109

Metal restorations and appliances appear radiopaque. Metal restorations include dental amalgam (Figure 29-108), stainless steel crowns, gold crowns (Figure 29-110), metal onlays and inlays, porcelain fused to metal crowns (Figure 29-110), bridges (Figure 29-111), implants (Figure 29-112), orthodontic appliances (bands, brackets, and wire), wires holding fractures, and implants as well as post and core restorations (Figure 29-113). Amalgam restorations may be differentiated from metal crowns based on margins. Cast metal crowns have smooth margins as compared to amalgams. Additionally, crowns are usually larger than amalgam restorations.

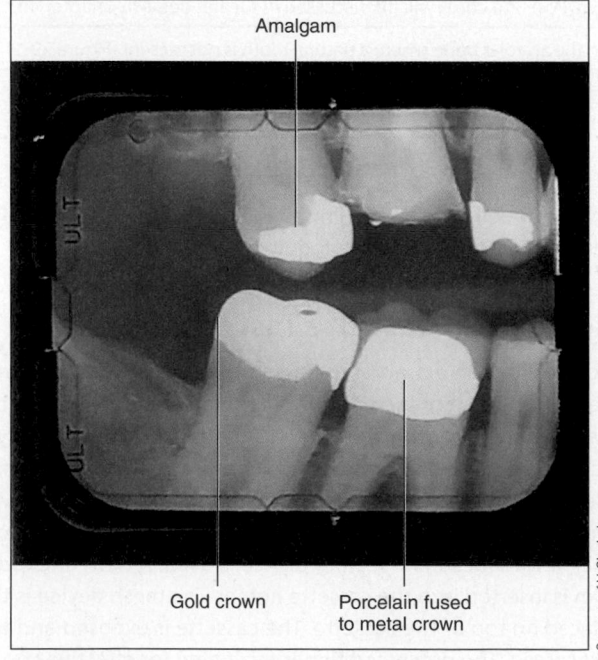

Amalgam

Gold crown

Porcelain fused to metal crown

Courtesy of V. Singhal

FIGURE 29-110

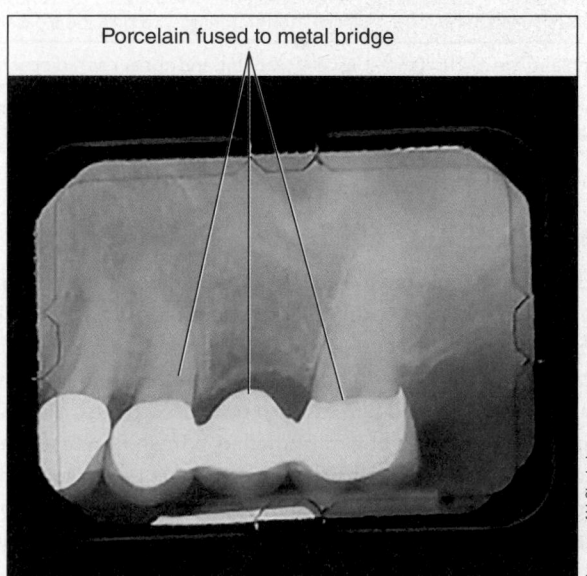

Porcelain fused to metal bridge

Courtesy of V. Singhal

FIGURE 29-111

(*Continues*)

TABLE 29-12 (Continued)

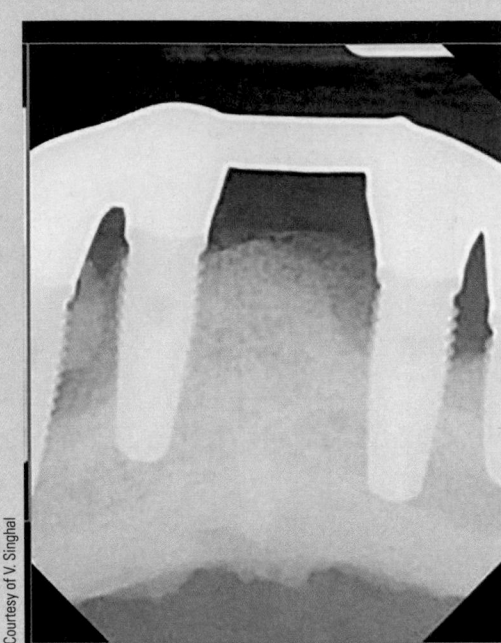

Courtesy of V. Singhal

FIGURE 29-112

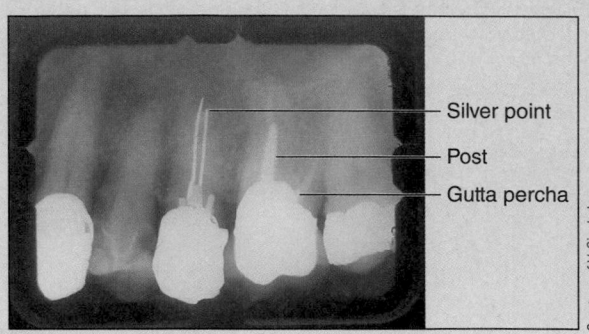

Silver point
Post
Gutta percha

Courtesy of V. Singhal

FIGURE 29-113

Removable partial dentures have an acrylic base for the teeth that is fixed to a metal framework. If the partial denture is not removed during expo-sures, the radiopaque metal will be visible in the images. Removable partial dentures will be discussed further in Chapter 43.
Endodontic treatment material appears radiopaque. The gutta-percha is a dense rubber material that fills the root canal (Figure 29-113). Many end-odontic procedures require the use of metal dental materials such as silver points and retrograde fillings for apicoectomy procedures.
Post and core buildups are metallic materials (Figure 29-113). A post is placed into a tooth that has a root canal in order to provide support to the tooth. The core buildup is placed around the post to provide a base for the crown. Post and cores will be discussed in further detail in Chapter 40.
Implants are made of metal, usually titanium, and appear as radiopaque "screws" in the alveolar bone where a natural tooth is not present (Figure 29-112).
Retention pins are pins that are placed within the dentin of a tooth to aid in the retention of a large restoration. The use of retention pins has decreased over time.

Radiographic Film Test

Radiographic films must also be properly cared for and stored properly in order to obtain diagnostic radiographs. The films should be stored in a cool, dry place. They should not be stored in the same operatory that radiographs are taken in as this can cause film fog. Fogged film can also be caused by use of expired film. Once a new box of film is opened, a fresh film test should be done to determine if the film is acceptable to use to create a diagnostic quality radiograph. A film from the new box should be processed in fresh chemicals. Ideally, it should result in a clear, blue tint, which shows that it was properly stored (Figure 29-114). In order to monitor an automatic processor, an unexposed film and a film exposed to white light should be processed each day. The two films will reveal the strength of the processing chemicals and ensure the equipment is working properly. The film that is not exposed to white light should ideally appear clear and dry when it emerges from the automatic processor, while the film exposed to light should emerge black and dry. If the films do not appear this way, the processor needs to be checked for any malfunctions. If the test film is fogged (Figure 29-115), the box

should not be used as the films in the box have been affected in a manner that has resulted in fogging.

Screen and Cassette Test

Screens used in extraoral radiography also need special care to keep them functioning properly. The screens and cassette should be examined monthly for scratches or defects. The intensifying screens should be cleaned every month using a recommended cleaner. There should always be an appropriate contact between the screens of the cassette and film. In order to test this con-tact, a wire mesh-like testing device is used. A new, unexposed film is inserted into the cassette holder. The mesh device is then placed on top of the cassette. The cassette is exposed and then processed. The processed film is evaluated for effective contact between the screen and the film. If there is significant contact, there will be an even image of the wire mesh on the film. If there is poor contact, then there will be darker areas on the film, and the mesh image will not be even (Figure 29-116). If this occurs, the cassette should be replaced as the uneven contact is usually the result of a warped cassette.

TABLE 29-13 X-ray Machine Quality Assurance Tests

Quality Assurance Test	Description
x-ray output test	Evaluates output and beam quality. It also evaluates patient safety of the beam.
tubehead stability test	Checks for any movement of the tubehead while exposing radiographs.
kilovoltage test	Measures the kilovoltage during exposures to make sure it is within normal limits.
milliamperage test	Evaluates the milliamperage during exposures to check for correct settings and densities.
collimation beam alignment test	Used to determine the dimensions of the beam in order to tell whether or not the collimator is restricting the beam to the appropriate size.
focal spot test	Tests the size of the focal spot.
timer test	Used to evaluate the length of the exposure in time.
half value layer test	Ensures the half value layer is preventing against low energy and is enough to protect patients.

The cassettes should be examined each month. Evaluate cassettes for any damage such as warping and damaged closures that could lead to light leaks and result in nondiagnostic images.

Viewbox Test

Viewboxes are used to view traditional radiographs after they are processed. When turned on and working properly, they will cast light through the radiographs illuminating them (Figure 29-117). The view boxes should be kept free of dirt and dust so that radiographs can be clearly viewed. If the clear viewing surface becomes discolored, it should be replaced. The dental assistant should also be sure to replace any bulbs that may be out or not functioning properly.

Darkroom Test

The radiographer needs to continually strive to reach adequate standards in processing the radiographs, including checking the safelight distance and strength, checking for any white light leakage, and using overall techniques that provide quality radiographs. One of the ways to check for darkroom fog is the coin test. Following are the steps in performing a coin test:

- Turn off safelight.
- Remove film from package and place coin on the film (Figure 29-118).
- Turn on safelight and let film sit for 2 minutes.
- Process film and look for light leaks around the room.
- Evaluate film; if outline of coin is visible, a fog problem exists that needs to be corrected (Figure 29-119).

Determining source of fogging:

- Perform another coin test; this time leave the safelight off.
- If the fog is reduced, it is a safelight problem. The safelight may be too close to the work area, or the safelight is too strong and is affecting the film.

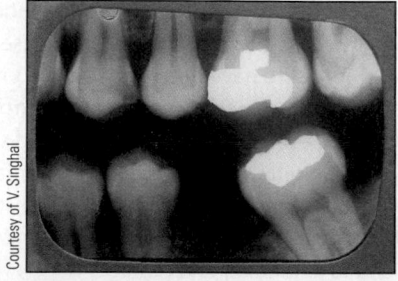

Courtesy of V. Singhal

FIGURE 29-114
Clear film. This film has not been exposed to x-rays.

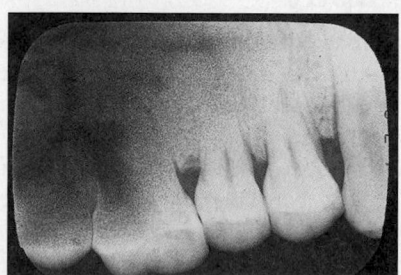

FIGURE 29-115
Fogged film.

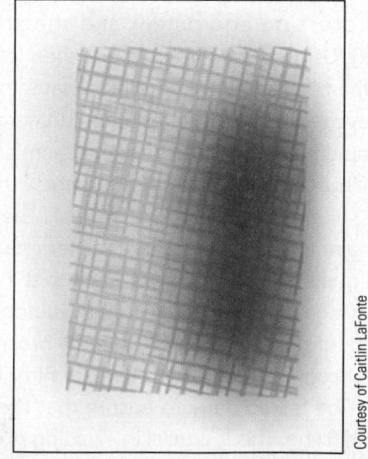

Courtesy of Caitlin LaFonte

FIGURE 29-116
Poor screen to film contact.

Courtesy of V. Singhal

FIGURE 29-117
Clean and evenly lit viewbox.

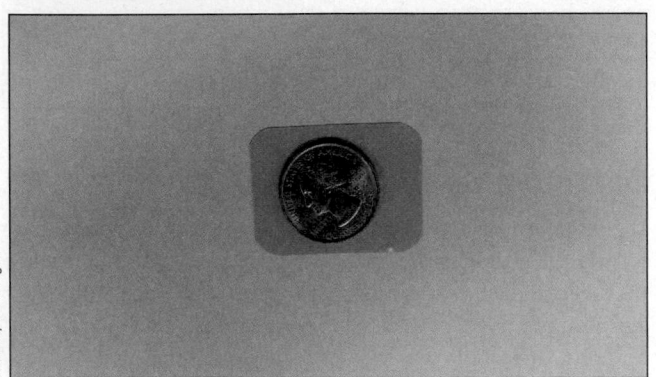

Courtesy of V. Singhal

FIGURE 29-118
Coin test to evaluate for film fog in darkroom.

- If the fog is not reduced, there is most likely white light leakage.
- Once white light leakage is identified, those areas should be sealed with black tape.

The dark room should be evaluated monthly for any light leaks.

Processing Equipment Test

It is critical to be sure that all equipment involved in processing radiographs is working efficiently. If the quality control of the processing equipment is compromised, this can lead to undiagnostic radiographs, causing patients to be re-exposed to more radiation. It is important to monitor the manual and automatic processing equipment and the strength of the chemicals daily. Using a test film to check chemical strength and proper equipment functioning is discussed later in this section.

Chemical levels should allow films to be submerged completely. Low levels should be replenished with the chemical made for the equipment (manual or autoprocessing) and not with water as water will dilute the solutions and make them weak. The autoprocessor needs to be maintained at the appropriate temperature to ensure production of quality diagnostic films. Refer to the manufacturer's documentation regarding maintenance of the autoprocessor.

The strength of the chemicals is tested by processing an unexposed film and comparing it to a reference film. The processing solutions must be tested daily to ensure that they are properly developing and fixing. This is crucial in avoiding processing errors, which will be discussed later as well. Developing solutions can be tested by processing a reference film exposed with a step wedge (Figure 29-120). The operator should expose several reference films

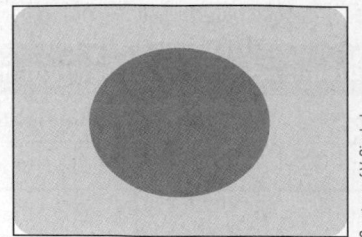

Courtesy of V. Singhal

FIGURE 29-119
Image of coin on film.

for processing at the start of each day. One step wedge reference film is processed using fresh developer and fixer solutions after a film is exposed. A step wedge is a tool that is used to test various densities created by the developer for quality control. It consists of aluminum steps that increase in density as the steps get higher. The step wedge is placed on top of a film and then exposed. Multiple films should be exposed and then saved for daily quality control. Process just one of the films with fresh chemicals. It is kept to compare the daily step wedge films processed thereafter. If the reference film with long scale contrast matches the film taken for quality control each subsequent day, then the developer maintains its strength (Figure 29-121A). If subsequent films are lighter than the reference film and the scale of contrast is short, the developer solution may be too weak and needs replacement (Figure 29-121B).

The fixer strength should also be monitored. To test the fixer, place an unexposed film directly into the fixer. The film should clear in about 2 minutes. If it takes longer to clear, then the solution must be replaced.

Dental Radiographic Equipment Test

Digital radiography is becoming much more popular and common. With less equipment needed for processing radiographs, the amount of quality assurance procedures is decreased but not eliminated. It is still critical to have quality assurance procedures for digital systems. There are many components in the system that need to be monitored, such as wires, plates, and sensors. It is important to inspect digital sensors for scratches or faulty wire connections. If a phosphor plate system is being used, it is necessary to inspect the plates for scratches or bends. Scratched and bent plates can lead to a nondiagnostic image.

Laws Regulating Dental Radiography

There are both federal and state laws regulating the practice of dental radiography. These regulations are in place to ensure that the radiation equipment is operating safely and effectively and that both dental operators and dental patients are protected from excess unnecessary radiation. It is imperative that the dental radiographer is knowledgeable of the legal and ethical aspects to perform their duties at their highest abilities.

Federal regulation for dental radiography equipment began in the early 1970s setting standards for operating accuracy, minimum filtration for radiation produced by machines, and specific machine settings. Most states require that all dental radiation-producing

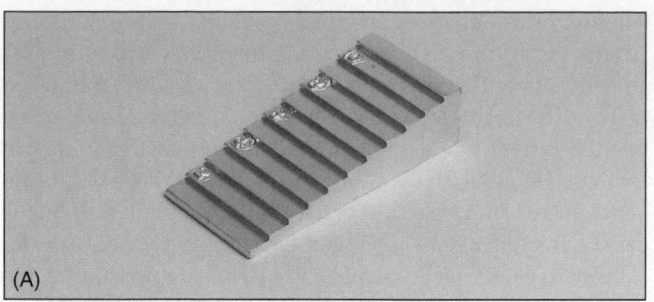

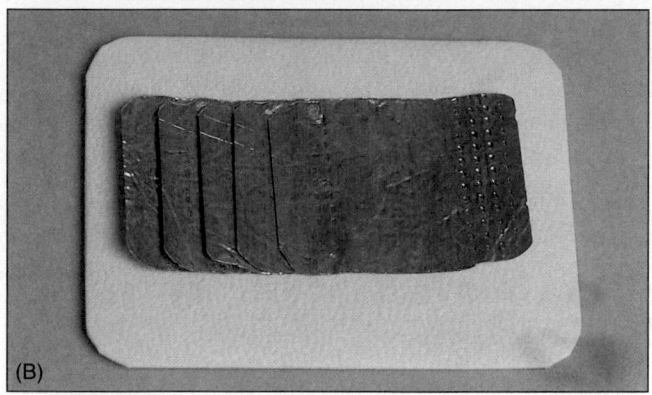

FIGURE 29-120
(A) Manufactured step wedge. (B) Step wedge made from the lead foil from x-ray film packets.

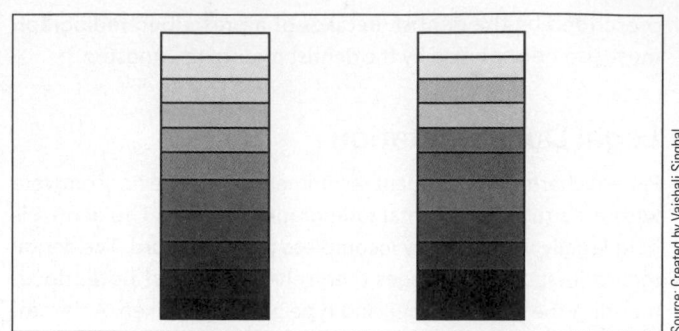

Source: Created by Vaishali Singhal

FIGURE 29-121
(A) Long scale contrast. (B) Short scale contrast.

equipment be registered and inspected at the time of installation. Inspection is performed by an approved physicist that provides quality assurance (QA) of dental radiation exposures. Upon meeting the regulations, the dentist is provided a certificate that must be posted on the equipment. Many states require annual inspections of dental radiology equipment. The proof of inspection must then be submitted to the state's regulatory agency. Upon meeting all the regulations set forth by federal and state agencies, a certificate is sent to the dental facility to be posted in the radiography area.

Requirements of the Dental Assistant as the Radiographer

As dental radiographers, the duty of obtaining quality images should not be taken lightly. Keep in mind that the radiation has the ability to cause ionization in the human body. The radiation exposure can be harmful to both the patient and the practitioner. Image quality is an important aspect of dental radiography; however, operator and patient protection are most critical. When the quality

of an image decreases, so does the ability to effectively diagnose dental disease. The first exposure should be of ideal quality so that unnecessary retakes are avoided.

The requirement to become a dental radiographer often begins with completion of a state-approved dental radiology course and passing a certification test to prove competency. Specific requirements vary by state, so the dental assistant should be aware of state requirements. In states that require certification or licensure, the dental radiographer's state certificate must be displayed in a conspicuous location in the office in which the dental radiographer is employed. Even if your state does not require a certificate, most states require the operator perform dental radiographic procedures under the direct supervision of a dentist. Direct supervision means that the dentist must be present in the office to authorize radiographs and remain present while radiographs are being taken on a patient. Approved dental assisting programs provide a curriculum that usually covers the topics discussed in Chapters 27, 28, and 29 of this text.

Responsibilities of the Dental Assistant

The dental auxiliary may assist the dentist in fulfilling the dentist's legal obligation to inform the patient of the need for radiographs in relation to the recommended treatment. The patient should be informed of the type of radiograph required, how many, and what the dentist can expect to learn from taking the radiograph. The radiograph would provide the dentist with needed information to make an informed diagnosis.

While the dentist prescribes the radiograph, the auxiliary takes the time to educate the patient as to the importance of the request. The patient must approve the continuation of treatment and radiographic exposure.

An authorized and qualified dental auxiliary should move forward by obtaining the necessary radiographic exposure as

 Documentation

2/2/XX
Mr. Garcia presents for a routine exam. Four horizontal bitewings are obtained. Clinical exam and radiographic exam reveal no pathologies. Oral prophylaxis completed.
NV-recare visit 8/2/XX.
Radiographs exposed by (*dental assistant name*)

prescribed by the dentist. Retakes of a prescribed radiograph must also be approved by the dentist prior to re-exposure.

Legal Documentation

Patient charts and treatment recommendations are not complete without a full set of dental radiographic images. The dentist is held legally liable for any incomplete patient record. The dental record includes the images themselves and chart notes documenting the date, number, and type of images taken. An example of this would be a chart entry.

Risk Management

As discussed in Chapter 3, in the health profession, *respondeat superior*. Legally the dentist is responsible for the actions of all dental auxiliaries in the office. Usually, if a malpractice lawsuit is filed, it is done so against the dentist. However, lawsuits may be filed against the dental auxiliary as well. A dental office must follow a standard of care that minimizes the risk of a lawsuit being brought forth by a patient. All patients must sign an informed consent before they are treated. This is usually part of the dental record that the patient completes during the first visit to the office. The informed consent is obtained by the dental office after the office provides information about standard treatment that the patient will receive. The informed consent for radiology purposes includes the diagnosis, recommended radiographs (including number and who will expose), alternative treatment, risk of the procedure (radiographs), and risk of not having the procedure (radiographs). Any other questions that the patient may have should also be answered prior to exposing any radiographs. After the disclosure of all information to the patient, the patient signs the informed consent authorizing treatment. All states require that the patient sign the informed consent before dental treatment is started.

Occasionally a patient refuses to allow radiographs even after hearing the importance and necessity of radiographs. It is important to record this refusal in the patient's chart along with written documentation containing the patient's signature that they were informed and given treatment options and the opportunity to ask questions. In this situation, the dentist would need to decide whether or not any treatment can take place. If radiographs are necessary to make an accurate diagnosis and formulate an appropriate treatment plan, treatment should not proceed without the necessary radiographs. Some offices may request that the patient sign a waiver for radiographs so treatment can continue. However, this is asking the patient to consent to negligence and will not hold up if a malpractice lawsuit is filed by the patient. Treating a patient without the radiographs necessary for a diagnosis can result in a malpractice lawsuit for negligence. The patient should be dismissed as treatment without the necessary diagnostic information results in a breach of standard of care that can result in legal action. Remember that there is a statute of limitation during which a patient can file a lawsuit as discussed in Chapter 3. Most medical malpractice cases are tried in a civil court as they are considered to be accidental and therefore are a type of tort. Most medical malpractice cases are not tried in a criminal court, as usually the practitioner did not have any criminal intent toward the patient.

HIPAA and Patient Privacy for Radiographs

Health Insurance Portability and Accountability Act (HIPAA) and the Patient Privacy Act extend to radiographs as well. The dental auxiliary must be prudent in protecting the privacy of this patient information. The dental auxiliary must remove any radiographs from the view box or computer monitor before seating the next patient. Take care not to leave the previous patient's radiographs visible to the next patient or in clear view of any patient passing in the hallway or anywhere else in the office.

Dental radiographs are labeled with a patient's name and have specific anatomical identifiers unique to that individual. This information is confidential. Consideration to HIPAA compliance and the Patient Privacy Act is also necessary when transferring radiographs to a dental specialist for consultation and when a patient moves records to another dental office. All dental facilities should have a protocol for transferring and receiving dental records that is compliant with HIPAA.

Chapter Summary

Extraoral radiographs are used by the dentist to identify large areas of the skull in one radiograph. It is important for the dental assistant to know how to prepare for extraoral exposures in order to obtain diagnostic quality images. Digital radiography is one of the recent advancements in dentistry. The dental assistant should be familiar with both direct digital imaging and indirect digital imaging for intraoral exposures. Three-dimensional imaging has now entered the profession of dentistry. The 3D dental image scan shows immediate 3D reconstruction of a patient's mouth, face, and jaw areas. This technology shows an excellent image quality with the finest details in three dimensions and with the lowest possible radiation dose. It is important for the dental assistant to be familiar with the radiographic appearance of normal anatomy, anomalies, and dental materials as well as decay and periodontal disease. The dental assistant plays an important role in radiographic quality assurance in the dental office. In order to maintain quality assurance, the dental assistant should be aware of how to maintain processing equipment and films as well as how to test for strength of processing chemicals. Maintaining equipment needed for digital exposures is an important role of the dental assistant. The dental assistant must always keep in mind the legal and ethical implications related to dental radiographic exposures.

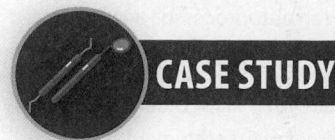

CASE STUDY

Dr. Danton is considering changing the way his office takes radiographs. His patients have been asking about reducing radiation exposure during radiographic exposures. Dr. Danton has been practicing for about 10 years and is comfortable with traditional film exposures for both intraoral and extraoral radiographs, but he also wants to keep up with technology and current trends in dentistry.

Case Study Review

1. Describe alternatives to traditional film exposures that Dr. Danton can explore.

2. Enumerate the advantages and disadvantages of digital technology.

3. What factors must be considered by the dental team deciding to use a digital radiography system?

Review Questions

Multiple Choice

1. Extraoral radiographs are used to evaluate large areas of the skull on one radiograph. Extraoral radiographs are usually used in conjunction with periapical, bitewing, and occlusal images.

   Select the correct response based on the statement above.

   a. Both statements are true.
   b. Both statements are false.
   c. The first statement is true; the second statement is false.
   d. The first statement is false; the second statement is true.

2. Which of the following is not correct regarding panoramic exposure technique?
   a. Remove bulky sweaters, coats, and hair clips that may interfere with the rotation of the x-ray tubehead.
   b. The patient should always wear a lead apron without a thyroid collar.
   c. The image receptor is placed in the patient's oral cavity, and the patient gently closes on the film.
   d. The patient is positioned in the chin rest, biting on a bite block, with the head properly positioned for the exposure.

3. Which of the following is correct regarding focal trough?
   a. It is also known as the zone of sharpness.
   b. The size and shape of the focal trough are the same in all panoramic machines.
   c. The patient's teeth should be positioned outside the focal trough in order to obtain diagnostic images.
   d. The focal trough is a two-dimensional curved zone.

4. Cephalometric images are used by orthodontists for treatment planning purposes. Cephalometric images provide a soft tissue outline of the patient on the image.

   Select the correct response based on the statement above.

   a. Both statements are true.
   b. Both statements are false.
   c. The first statement is true; the second statement is false.
   d. The first statement is false; the second statement is true.

5. Digital imaging systems use a sensor in place of traditional film. The positioning of the sensor is similar to the positioning of traditional film in the oral cavity during exposures.

   Select the correct response based on the statement above.

   a. Both statements are true.
   b. Both statements are false.
   c. The first statement is true; the second statement is false.
   d. The first statement is false; the second statement is true.

6. Indirect digital imaging sensors are phosphor storage plates. Phosphor storage plates may be wired or unwired.

   Select the correct response based on the statement above.

   a. Both statements are true.
   b. Both statements are false.
   c. The first statement is true; the second statement is false.
   d. The first statement is false; the second statement is true.

7. Which of the following is an advantage of digital dental radiology?
   a. There is less radiation exposure to the patient.
   b. Initial setup costs are high.
   c. Thickness of digital sensors may cause discomfort.
   d. There are security concerns during electronic record transmission.

8. Which of the following is not a plane of view in three-dimensional imaging?
   a. axial
   b. transverse
   c. coronal
   d. sagittal

9. Which of the following is not correct regarding hand-held intraoral radiology units?
   a. They have been helpful in areas that face access to care issues.
   b. The units are preset at 60 kVp but can be adjusted.
   c. They will not work in a power outage since they need an electrical source.
   d. They have additional shielding around the x-ray tube that allows the operator to stay in the room during exposures.

10. Which of the following structures is the cortical bone that appears as the radiopaque peaks between the teeth?
    a. lamina dura
    b. periodontal ligament membrane
    c. dentinoenamel junction
    d. alveolar crest

11. Which of the following structures is a radiopaque bony protuberance posterior to the last maxillary molar?
    a. hamulus
    b. zygomatic process
    c. tuberosity
    d. coronoid process

12. Which of the following is a mandibular radiopaque structure?
    a. mandibular canal
    b. lingual foramen
    c. nutrient canals
    d. mylohyoid ridge

13. A mesiodens is a supernumerary tooth specifically between the maxillary incisors. A distodens is a fourth molar behind the third molar.
    Select the correct response based on the statement above.
    a. Both statements are true.
    b. Both statements are false.
    c. The first statement is true; the second statement is false.
    d. The first statement is false; the second statement is true.

14. Concrescence occurs when the cementum of teeth fuses together. Excessive spacing between teeth may be a cause of concrescence.
    Select the correct response based on the statement above.
    a. Both statements are true.
    b. Both statements are false.
    c. The first statement is true; the second statement is false.
    d. The first statement is false; the second statement is true.

15. Which of the following dental materials appear radiolucent?
    a. amalgam
    b. gold crowns
    c. porcelain jacket crowns
    d. unfilled resins

16. Unfilled resins appear radiolucent on radiographic images. Filled resins appear radiopaque on radiographic images.
    Select the correct response based on the statement above.
    a. Both statements are true.
    b. Both statements are false.
    c. The first statement is true; the second statement is false.
    d. The first statement is false; the second statement is true.

17. When testing the chemicals in an autoprocessor, an unexposed film and a film exposed to white light should be processed. The film exposed to room light should appear black, and the unexposed film should appear clear with a slight blue tint.
    Select the correct response based on the statement above.
    a. Both statements are true.
    b. Both statements are false.
    c. The first statement is true; the second statement is false.
    d. The first statement is false; the second statement is true.

18. Most states require that all dental radiation-producing equipment be registered and inspected at the time of installation. Upon meeting the regulations, the dentist is provided a certificate that must be posted on the equipment.
    Select the correct response based on the statement above.
    a. Both statements are true.
    b. Both statements are false.
    c. The first statement is true; the second statement is false.
    d. The first statement is false; the second statement is true.

19. Which of the following is not correct regarding the responsibilities of the dental assistant as the radiographer?
    a. The first exposure should be ideal in order to prevent unnecessary radiation exposure to the patient.
    b. The dental assistant should be familiar with the regulations in their state as some states require radiology certification.
    c. In states that require certification and licensure, the dental assistant should ensure that the documents are visibly displayed in the office.
    d. Radiographs may be taken by the dental assistant without direct supervision by the dentist.

20. Which of the following is correct regarding HIPAA and dental radiographs?
    a. It is acceptable to leave radiographs of the prior patient in the operatory when seating the next patient.
    b. It is acceptable to leave patient radiographs in view of anyone who may be passing by in the hallway.
    c. To ensure patient privacy, the office should have protocol in place when transferring radiographs to a specialist or the patient's insurance company.
    d. HIPAA does not apply to dental radiographs.

Critical Thinking

1. As the dental assistant, it is your job to maintain quality assurance of the darkroom. You decide to test for film fog. Upon processing of the film that had the coin on it under safelight condition, you notice that the film emerged with the image of the coin. What is your next step to determine the cause of the film fog?

2. A patient appears to have a fractured mandible. The dentist requests a radiograph. What type of radiograph would be most beneficial for diagnosing a fractured mandible?

3. Name the types of radiographs in which all of the following can be seen: alveolar crest, coronoid process, maxillary tuberosity, and the mental foramen.

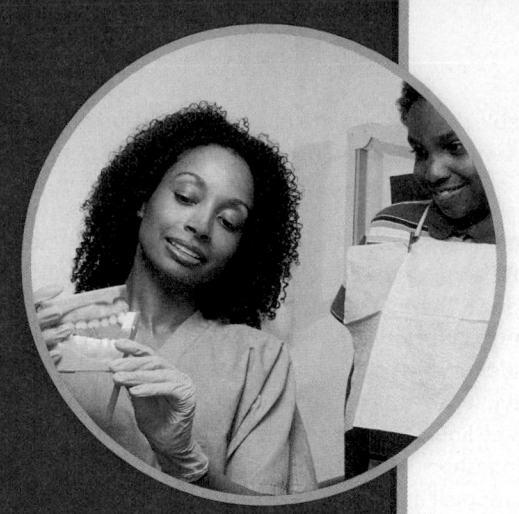

## CHAPTER 30

Dental Emergency Procedures and Dental Cements

Specific Instructional Objectives

At the completion of this chapter, you will be able to meet these objectives:

1. Use terms presented in this chapter.
2. Discuss emergency treatment for soft tissue oral trauma.
3. Recall the cause and emergency treatment for oral lesions.
4. Describe the appearance and treatment of periodontal tissue injuries.
5. Differentiate between classifications of tooth fractures.
6. Recall signs, symptoms, and treatment of the progression of dental caries.
7. Describe cavity preparation form and structure.
8. State the guidelines for mixing dental cements.
9. Describe the use, composition, properties, and manipulation considerations of dental cements.
10. Describe the steps in preparing for and placing temporary cement restorations.

Introduction

Patients call the dental office about any number of dental emergencies. Some of these emergencies can be treated temporarily the same day in the dental office, and others require that the patient be referred to a dental specialist. The majority of dental emergencies are due to patients suffering from dental decay and can be treated with a temporary restoration. When the dentist restores a patient's tooth, there are many dental materials that are used depending on how deep the cavity is, how much tooth structure is left, and the type of temporary material that is needed. In this chapter, dental cements will be discussed: what they are; when they are used; and how each material is prepared, manipulated, and placed.

Dental Emergencies

A dental emergency involves pain experienced by a patient from their soft tissue, teeth, or a nondental problem that mimic dental pain (sinus infection and TMJ disorder, both of which cause pain in the maxilla and mandible). Most offices reserve time in the daily schedule for emergencies. When the patient calls the dental office, the receptionist asks pertinent questions to determine what kind of dental emergency the dental team should expect.

Soft Tissue Emergencies

Some patients present for dental emergency appointment with oral trauma, painful oral lesions, or periodontal tissue injuries.

Oral Trauma

Trauma to the lips, tongue, and intraoral soft tissues is a common occurrence. Since the lips are exposed, they are prone to injury. Trauma to the face can cause the cheeks or tongue to suffer from a bite as the tissues may become lodged between teeth.

Children are especially prone to mouth injuries. These occur because children may be eating while walking or playing and may fall with the food in the oral cavity. Children may also be walking or running with a toy or sharp object. A fall while carrying an object may result in injury to the oral cavity.

Injuries to the oral cavity may bleed heavily and, as a result, look worse than they actually are. Because the head, neck, and oral cavity are highly **vascular**, even a small cut may bleed quite a bit. However, this vascularity also allows for rapid healing of the oral cavity.

Lip, Tongue, and Cheek Bites Accidental biting of the tongue or cheek mucosa while eating is the most common event that results in a cut on the tongue. These usually do not need sutures and heal on their own. If the bite occurs during eating, rinse the mouth to remove any food particles. If the area is bleeding, apply pressure to stop the bleeding. The bitten area will be swollen and irritated and, as a result, more prone to being bitten again. A conscious effort must be made to ensure that the area does not suffer from injury again when eating.

At times, a fall may cause the tongue to become lodged between the teeth, resulting in a bite injury. This may be more severe than a bite that is caused accidentally while eating. If the bite is due to a fall, the injured area should be evaluated for debris, and any evident debris should be removed with the use of a clean piece of gauze. A fall may also cause injury to the upper lip if the lower teeth traumatize the upper lip during the fall. Additionally, a fall may injure the lower lip if the lower lip gets caught between the teeth.

Lip and cheek injuries may also occur during contact sports. This is because the lips are exposed and any trauma or impact may cause the lips to get caught between the teeth; the cheeks may also get caught between the teeth due to impact during sports. A mouthguard will aid in minimizing lip injuries by creating a barrier between the teeth and the lips. If the lips do suffer from impact during contact sports, the lips will not get caught between the teeth and injuries will be less severe. Additionally, the mouthguard will protect the teeth from being damaged. Mouthguards are usually made to cover the maxillary teeth since they are more prominent and more likely to suffer from injury; however, for heavier contact sports such as boxing, a mouthguard may be fabricated for both maxillary and mandibular teeth.

Any bleeding due to injury should be controlled by applying pressure with a clean piece of gauze. Once the bleeding stops, a cold compress may be applied to the area to minimize the swelling. If the bleeding continues despite the application of pressure, the patient should be advised to come into the office or seek help at the nearest hospital for care as sutures may be required to control the bleeding. Additionally, professional help may be required in the event debris is embedded in the wound. A follow-up visit within three to four (3–4) days of the incident may be necessary to ensure that an infection has not resulted. Antibiotics may be prescribed at the initial visit in order to prevent an infection.

A teaspoon of table salt dissolved in a glass of warm water may be used for rinsing several times a day. This will help to minimize swelling and also kill infection causing bacteria that may be present.

Palatal Burns Palatal burns (thermal burns) occur when hot food is eaten and adheres to the palate. A common such food is hot cheese on pizza. Thermal burns may also appear on the posterior area of the palate. Hot liquids such as coffee can also cause palatal burns. Additionally, liquids that are heated in a microwave oven may result in uneven heating and can cause palatal burns. This is because the liquid has hot and cold areas that may not be mixed prior to ingestion.

Palatal burns appear as **erythematous** areas that are partially **eroded**. The patient will usually be able to tell the clinician the cause of the burn. Thus, diagnosis is based upon clinical appearance of the burn as well as clinical history.

Treatment is dependent upon the extent of the burn. In case of pain, analgesics may be prescribed. Topical **benzocaine** ointments may also be applied as they will form a barrier which covers the lesion. This barrier will protect the injured area from further trauma when eating. Thermal burns usually become less painful within a couple of days and heal within seven (7) to fourteen (14) days.

Lodged Objects At times, food or other debris may get caught in the gingival sulcus or between the teeth; common objects include poppy seeds, popcorn kernels, or pieces of broken floss. The patient can attempt removal by using a clean, new, and undamaged piece of floss to remove the object from between the teeth. If this does not dislodge the object, a small knot may be made in the floss and the floss inserted between the teeth. The patient may pull the knot through the teeth to allow the object to catch onto the knot. If this also does not result in successful removal, the patient should schedule an appointment to see the dentist as soon as possible. The dentist will be able to use professional instruments to attempt to remove the lodged object. Objects can become lodged frequently due to gaps between teeth. If this occurs, the patient can be educated about restorative work that can help to minimize gaps and the occurrence of lodged objects.

Oral Lesions

Bacterial, viral, and fungal infections are the main causes of oral lesions (mouth sores). Mouth sores are painful or aching and sometimes scary if it is the first time a patient has experienced a sore. Patients call for immediate attention for the pain and to find out what is wrong. Refer to Chapter 9, "Oral Pathology," for descriptions and images of oral lesions and Table 30-1 for dental emergency treatment for oral lesions.

Periodontal Abscess A periodontal abscess is a collection of pus from a bacterial infection that occurs in the gingiva. It is generally caused by chronic periodontal disease; if only the gingiva is affected, it is termed a *gingival abscess*. An abscess can lead to serious complications. Refer to Table 29-1 for dental emergency treatment.

TABLE 30-1 Periodontal Lesions (refer to Chapter 9 for images of lesions)

Periodontal Lesions	Symptoms	Emergency Treatment
Periodontal abscess	Local inflammation affecting periodontal tissue Longstanding periodontal disease Preexisting periodontal pockets Rapid onset, stimulated by touch and spontaneous pain Can visibly be confused with periapical abscess	Curettage to establish drainage Prescribe antibiotics Warm saline rinses and soft diet Scaling and root planing and referral: may require further consultation with periodontist
Pericoronitis	Inflamed and swollen tissue surrounding the crown of a partially erupted tooth Acute and severe pain, discharge of pus, trismus Patient complains of bad taste or halitosis	Irrigate with saline Prescribe antibiotics, warm saline rinses, gentle massage with toothbrush Referral for possible tissue excision or tooth removal
Primary herpetic gingivostomatitis	Highly contagious virus Tingling and painful gingival ulceration Fever, headache, malaise, irritability	Appointment should be rescheduled if vesicles (blisters) are present Recommended: Rest, diluted mouthwashes, increased fluid intake, soft diet Topical analgesics Initial lesion may last for 2–6 weeks; recurrent lesion for up to 10 days
Aphthous ulcers	Ulceration on soft tissues of mouth or base of gingival tissue Not contagious, no known cause Painful and makes eating difficult	Prescribe palliative medication; generally a gel to cover the lesion and prevent irritation Some contain steroids to minimize inflammation
Thrush	Fungus appearing as soft white lesion on tongue, oral mucosa and/or oropharynx Occurs in patients who are immunocompromised, have certain systemic conditions (diabetes mellitus), taking corticosteroids or long-term antibiotics	Prescribe antifungal medications Refer patient to contact physician about medical conditions

Pericoronitis Pericoronitis usually occurs in relation to the eruption of third (3rd) molars (wisdom teeth) during late adolescence. In some instances, there may be limited room for these teeth to erupt, and as a result, they may not be able to emerge or erupt only partially. When the teeth partially erupt, a flap of gingival tissue or operculum may partially cover the tooth. Food particles may become trapped under the operculum, resulting in inflammation and infection. Pericoronitis can also occur if the tooth is unable to erupt due to lack of space.

Oral Herpetic Lesions Oral herpetic lesions, commonly known as cold sores or fever blisters, may bring patients to the dental office. These usually appear on the lips but can also occur intraorally. These lesions are caused by a virus and are contagious. Once introduced, the virus remains within the nerve tissue of that region. The virus remains dormant until activated. Activation may occur due to manipulation of that area, exposure to sun, or hormonal changes such as during menstruation or stress. Once the virus becomes active, the patient initially feels a tingling sensation, followed shortly by the formation of fluid filled vesicles in the infected area that form a large blister. The vesicles may rupture, releasing the fluid and virus. This is the infectious stage of the oral herpetic lesions. Infection may be transmitted from person to person through contact with the infected area. Once the blistering phase is complete, the vesicles become encrusted and dry and are no longer infectious. The area then heals, and the virus returns to its dormant state until it is activated again.

Apthous Ulcers Apthous ulcers are ulcerated areas that occur on the soft tissues of the mouth or at the base of the gingival tissues. They are not contagious but can be painful and can make eating difficult. There is no known cause for these ulcerations to occur, and they usually heal within seven (7) to fourteen (14) days.

Thrush Thrush is a fungal infection of the oral cavity. The fungus, candida albicans, appears as a soft white lesion on the tongue and oral mucosa; it may also be present in the oropharynx. Candida albicans can occur in anyone but is more likely to occur in those who are immunocompromised or who have certain systemic conditions such as diabetes mellitus. Patients who are taking medications such as corticosteroids to manage a disorder may also suffer from candida albicans.

Periodontal Tissue Injuries

Injuries to the mouth can affect the periodontal tissues. These injuries can lead to mobility of the tooth. Refer to Table 30-2 for dental emergency treatment.

Concussion A concussion is caused from a heavy blow. The force injures the tooth-supporting structures (periodontium) without abnormal loosening or displacement of the tooth.

Subluxation Subluxation is a partial dislocation of a tooth. It is one of the most common dental traumatic injuries to the periodontium. The tooth has increased mobility but is displaced from the alveolar bone.

TABLE 30-2 Periodontal Tissues Injuries

Injury	Symptoms	Emergency Treatment
Concussion	No visual displacement or mobility May be bleeding at gingival crevice Tender to percussion due to injured and inflamed periodontal ligament Radiograph no abnormalities	Stabilize tooth with composite if necessary Follow-up: monitor pulp condition for a year
Subluxation	Tender to percussion Increased mobility with no displacement due to damage to the periodontal tissues Bleeding at gingival crevice	No immediate treatment needed but may splint tooth for 2 weeks if needed. Follow-up: monitor pulp condition for a year
Intrusive luxation	Tooth pushed into the alveolus causing fracture of alveolar bone Crown appears shorter or not visible in severe cases	May allow for spontaneous eruption Gently brush area and soft foods for 7 days Orthodontic or surgical repositioning may be needed if tooth does not erupt in 2–3 weeks Potential RCT if vessels are severed
Lateral luxation	Displacement of tooth in labial, lingual, distal, or mesial position Sulcular bleeding Sensitive to touch Usually results in bony plate fracturing	Administer local anesthetic Reposition using finger pressure Splint for 4 weeks May result in necrosis and future RCT
Extrusion	Tooth loose and elongated Sensitive to percussion Partial displacement of tooth out of alveolus	Clean tooth and surrounding area with saline Reposition with light finger pressure within 48 hours Splint tooth into alveolus Follow-up: PO 2 weeks RCT if pulp necrotic

Intrusive Luxation Intrusion of a tooth is displacement further into the alveolar bone. In many cases, the supporting alveolar bone may be fractured. Intrusion results in the poorest tooth prognosis when compared to other periodontal tissue injuries. The pulp may suffer from necrosis, the root may suffer from resorption, and the tooth may also **ankylose** to the bone. Intrusion is most common with the primary incisors. Posterior teeth are seldom intruded due to their anatomic location; permanent anterior teeth are more likely to suffer from a fracture.

Lateral Luxation Lateral **luxation** is the displacement of a tooth that is nonaxial in direction. Lateral luxation usually results in fracture of the buccal or palatal bony plate. The tooth is usually displaced into the area of the fracture and is not mobile. Lateral luxation is usually due to a traumatic event resulting in the nerve supply and periodontal ligaments being severed and the apex of the tooth being trapped in the area of the fracture.

Extrusion Extrusion of a tooth is partial displacement of the tooth out of the alveolar bone; this usually occurs due to trauma. In extrusion, the periodontal ligament may or may not remain intact. Additionally, the blood supply to the tooth may be severed and the root surface will be exposed. Upon examination, the tooth appears longer than the others, is sensitive to **percussion**, and is mobile. A radiograph will reveal a tooth that exhibits an enlarged periodontal ligament space.

Avulsion Avulsion is the complete displacement of a tooth in its entirety from its location in the socket. Upon examination, the socket is empty or may have a blood clot present (Figure 30-1). A radiograph should be exposed to confirm that there has been no alveolar or root fracture. The tooth is usually dislodged due to trauma, resulting in severance of the nerve supply as well as the supporting periodontal ligaments.

In the event that a phone call is received from a patient or a caregiver of a child regarding a tooth that has been avulsed, the patient or caregiver should be advised to locate the tooth, rinse for approximately ten (10) seconds under cool running water, and attempt to reimplant it if possible (only permanent teeth should be reimplanted). This may be done by reinserting the tooth into the socket and asking the patient to bite on a clean washcloth or handkerchief to keep it in position. The patient should be requested to come immediately to the dental office.

If reimplantation is not possible, the tooth should be kept moist. This may be done by placing the tooth in the mucobuccal fold between the mandibular molars and the buccal mucosa. If the child is young and swallowing of the tooth is a concern, the tooth may be placed in a glass of milk (not water as the chemicals in water may damage the fibers and prevent successful reimplantation). The patient may also **expectorate** into a container and the tooth may be placed in the patient's saliva. Containers that contain a special medium that will keep the tooth vital for a short time are also available. Many schools and childcare centers now keep these available in case a child experiences trauma that causes a tooth to avulse. One such medium is Hank's storage medium.

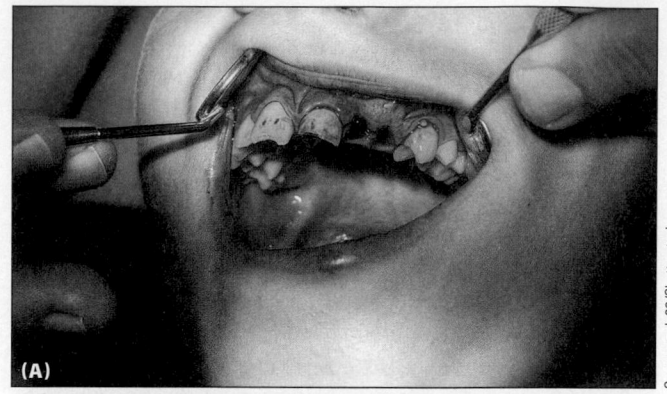

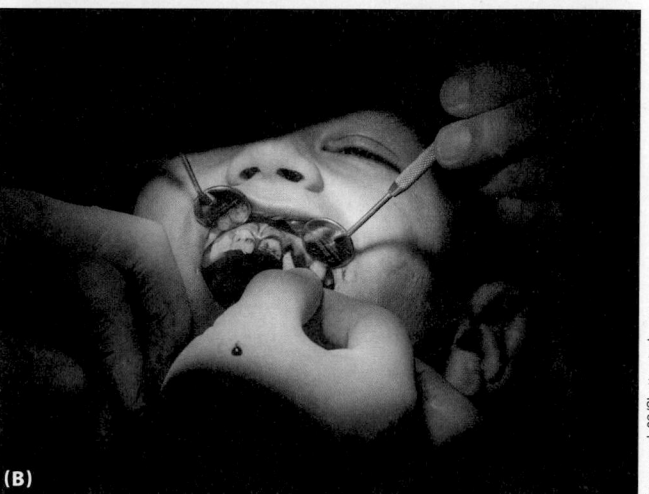

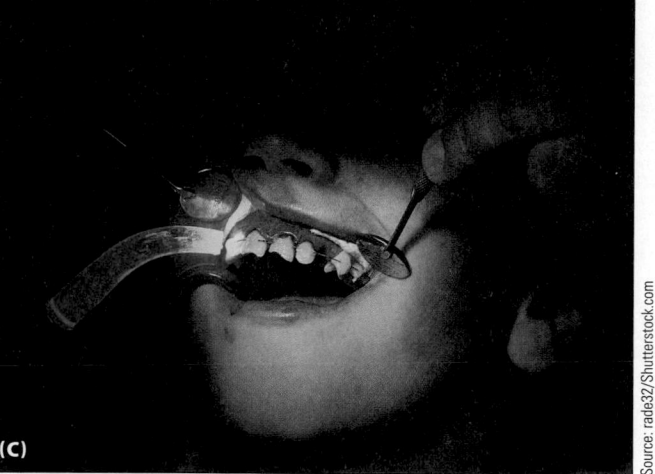

FIGURE 30-1

Avulsed tooth. (A) Teeth #8 and #9 Class II and Class III fracture and Teeth #10 and #11 knocked out. (B) Avulsed tooth #10 is placed into the empty sulcus using gentle finger pressure. (C) Teeth are splinted in place using light-cured resin and wire.

Once the patient arrives at the dental office and the evaluation has been completed, rinse the area with saline. If the tooth has been reimplanted, the dentist should ensure that it is in the proper position, this can be accomplished by a clinical exam and a radiographic exam. Any present lacerations should be sutured, and a flexible splint should be placed to keep the tooth stable. Antibiotics should be prescribed to prevent an infection, and the patient should be instructed to eat soft foods and to not participate in any contact sports. A prescription for a **chlorhexidine** rinse may be provided to the patient with instructions to use twice per day for 7 days. The chlorhexidine will provide a topical antimicrobial effect and minimize the risk of an infection. A tetanus booster may also be necessary if the tooth was in dirt and if the patient is not sure of immunity against tetanus; refer the patient to the physician for a booster shot.

The patient should return to the office within 7–10 days of the incident, and endodontic therapy should be completed with the splint left in place. The splint may be removed after two (2) weeks, and the patient should return for follow-up visits at four (4) weeks, twelve (12) weeks, six (6) months, and one (1) year after the incident.

The prognosis of an avulsed tooth varies significantly. Ideally, for optimum results and success, the tooth should be reimplanted within an hour of avulsion. Rapid reimplantation will prevent the ligaments from **desiccation**, resulting in a greater rate of reattachment of the fibers and greater chance of retaining the tooth. Additionally, a tooth with a fully formed root system has a greater chance of success when reimplanted as opposed to one that is not yet fully mature. Endodontic therapy is a must on avulsed teeth. Those that do not undergo root canal treatment have a poor prognosis. Complications after reimplantation include ankylosis, resorption, pulpal necrosis, and tooth loss.

Hard Tissue Emergencies

Dental pain is an unpleasant event that is experienced by many at some point in time. Dental pain is at times difficult to diagnose because it may be due to one of many causes. Some of the most common emergencies are cracked or fractured teeth, and a fractured or dislocated jaw.

Hard Tissue Trauma

Hard tissue trauma occurs when injury results to the hard tissues of the body such as the bones or teeth. Hard tissue trauma may result in dislocation or fracture of the affected area.

Fractured Tooth and/or Roots
Trauma can lead to a fractured tooth. Fractures are most likely to occur on maxillary anterior teeth (Table 30-3). The fracture may be limited to the enamel only, may involve the dentin and enamel, or may be severe and involve the pulp, dentin, and enamel.

Trauma can also result in the fracture of the root of a tooth. A root fracture is not visible and also may not be visible on a dental radiograph. A patient may present with pain; an exam

TABLE 30-3 Ellis Tooth Fracture Classification

Classification	Appearance	Emergency Treatment
Class I	Enamel fracture Crown fractures that extend through enamel only Tooth has rough edges, without visible color changes and unusually not tender	No immediate treatment required Smooth sharp edges with rotary instrument and handpiece
Class II	Enamel and dentin fracture without pulp exposure A yellow layer of dentin may be visible; tooth is tender to touch and air exposure	Smooth sharp edges and/or repair tooth with composite material Follow-up: may require future porcelain veneer or crown
Class III	Crown fracture with pulp exposure; involve the enamel, dentin, and pulp layers. There is a visible area of pink, red, or blood at center of the tooth and tooth is tender to touch and air exposure.	**Pulp capping, partial pulpotomy** Repair tooth with composite Refer to endodontist for follow-up endodontic therapy and crown

TABLE 30-3 (*Continued*)

Classification	Appearance	Emergency Treatment
Class IV	Traumatized nonvital tooth with or without loss of tooth structure	RCT if the tooth has a closed apex Apexification if the tooth has an open apex
Class V	Luxation; tends to dislocate tooth from alveolus	Tooth repositioned into its original location and splinted
Class VI	Avulsion; complete separation of tooth from alveolus Fracture of root with or without loss of crown structure	Reimplantation of tooth if kept in favorable condition by patient to the dental office Place flexible splint Prescribe antibiotics and chlorhexidine rinse Refer patient to physician for potential tetanus booster Primary tooth not replanted to avoid damaging developing permanent tooth Follow-up: RCT with splint in place and future crown
Class VII	Displacement of tooth with contusion or fracture of alveolar bone	Reposition tooth and the fractured segment and splint Stabilize for 4 weeks. After splint removal at 4 weeks, radiographic and clinical examination at 8 weeks, 4 months, 1 year, and 5 years
Class VIII	Fracture of crown and its replacement	RCT, post and core, and crown
Class IX	Fracture of primary teeth	Pulpotomy or extraction

and radiograph reveal no abnormalities. In such an event, a root fracture should be considered, particularly if a history of trauma exists. In the event of a root fracture, the tooth would need to be extracted.

Dislocated Jaw A dislocated jaw is where the lower part of the mandible moves out of position and becomes detached from the TMJ. This is generally thought to occur in sports and accidents, but it may also occur from stretching the jaw too much such as when yawning or biting. A dislocated jaw can often be treated by manually repositioning the mandible into place (manual reduction). A bandage may be placed around the head and jaw. Analgesics and the use of ice is prescribed.

Fractured Jaw In the event of trauma leading to the fracture of a tooth or root, radiographs must be taken to ensure that the trauma did not also cause a fracture of the maxilla or the mandible. If a bony fracture is found to have occurred, that too must be treated. Fractures of the mandible are more common than the maxilla. Ice is applied immediately to decrease swelling and pain, and analgesics and antibiotics are prescribed. The patient is generally referred to an oral surgeon for treatment of a bony fracture. Minor jaw fractures may be treated by wrapping a bandage around the patient's head and under their chin to keep them from opening their jaw wide. The surgeon may perform a **closed reduction** to move the broken jawbone back to its normal position and may need to place screw metal plates or wires onto the sides of the jaw to support it while it heals. The jaws may need to be wired to hold them in place and prevent movement to help the bones heal properly. The patient is shown how to use a small pair of cutters and when to use them in the case of an emergency. The patient is provided a pair of cutters to take home.

It may take weeks or months for the jawbone to heal. Patients are directed to eat foods blended with liquids and to clean their mouth 4–6 times a day using a pedo soft toothbrush and water flosser to help prevent infection.

Progression of Dental Caries

One of the most common causes of dental pain is decay. Decay is also called dental caries or dental cavities. If caries are left untreated, they can progress, resulting in pulpitis and a periapical abscess.

Dental Caries Dental caries (dental decay) results from the destruction of tooth enamel. Enamel protects the dentin and the pulp of the tooth. If a patient has decay, an appointment may be requested because of sensitivity of that tooth. The patient may feel pain when eating something sweet or cold. Some patients may not have any sensitivity yet notice that there is "a hole" in the tooth.

Caries, once diagnosed, must be treated to stop the progress of the decay. This is accomplished by removal of the decay until solid healthy tooth structure is evident. Since the tooth now has an opening where the decay was once present and has been removed, that area must be restored to prevent leakage of fluid and food into the tooth. Since time scheduled for dental emergencies is limited, the dentist may place a **dental cement** as a **temporary restoration** until the patient returns for a future appointment. If time allows, the dentist may restore the area using an amalgam or composite material.

Pulpitis If the carious lesion is deep, pulpitis may occur. Pulpitis is defined as an inflammation of the dental pulp. Pulpitis can be reversible or irreversible (Table 30-4).

TABLE 30-4 Progression of Dental Caries

Pulp Status	Symptoms	Emergency Treatment
Healthy pulp	No inflammation present Asymptomatic Mild response to hot, cold, pressure stimulus	None needed
Reversible pulpitis	Inflammation present No spontaneous or nocturnal pain Mild to sharp pain of short duration to sharp shooting pain well localized Stimulated by hot, cold, sweet, touch, biting Radiograph shows exposed dentin or pathway to expose dentin	Avoid thermal stimuli Prescribe analgesics and antibiotic Remove decay Indirect pulp cap Referral to endodontist
Irreversible pulpitis	Severe inflammatory response and vital pulp Spontaneous and nocturnal pain Moderate to severe pain that lingers and poorly localized Stimulated by hot, cold, sweet, touch, biting; increases when lay down Radiographs show exposed pulp	Remove decay Direct pulp cap Prescribe analgesic and antibiotics Referral for RCT or extraction of tooth

TABLE 30-4 (*Continued*)

Pulp Status	Symptoms	Emergency Treatment
Pulpal **necrosis**	Presence of bacteria and nonvital pulp Asymptomatic due to destruction of pulpal sensory nerves Pulp exposed to oral environment	Prescribe antibiotic Referral for RCT or extraction of tooth
Pulp **necrobiosis**	Pulp canals of multirooted teeth varying degree of inflammation One canal vital, one irreversibly inflamed, and one necrotic	Prescribe antibiotic Referral for RCT with each root treated individually dependent on diagnosis or extraction of tooth
Apical periodontitis	Inflammation of periodontal ligament Presence of irreversibly inflamed pulp Acute response moderate to severe pain; stimulated by touch, pressure; may have spontaneous pain Chronic response asymptomatic; may have pain from surrounding tissues when stimulated Radiograph shows widening of the periodontal ligament space	Prescribe antibiotics if warranted RCT or extraction
Periapical abscess	Severe inflammatory response and swollen lymph nodes Acute abscess: facial swelling, high fever, and **malaise**; constant throbbing pain; sensitive to percussion, heat, and pressure Chronic abscess: asymptomatic when inflammation is naturally draining Radiograph shows round/oval **radiolucency** at apex of infected tooth	Incision and drainage of abscess Prescribe analgesic and antibiotics Warm water rinses Referral for RCT or tooth extraction
Cellulitis	Bacterial infection leading to rapid spread of infection through connective tissue spaces Painful swelling, red and shiny skin	Immediate attention required Number of treatment options: Localized periapical abscess treated by intraoral drainage May need opening of root canals Prescribe antibiotics Follow-up for potential RCT

Reversible Pulpitis Reversible pulpitis can occur due to decay that has not yet reached the pulp but is causing inflammation. Reversible pulpitis also may occur when there is abrasion present and the dentin is exposed. Reversible pulpitis results in sensitivity when the tooth is exposed to something cold. The sensation of sensitivity goes away once the source of the cold is removed. Removal of the decay and placing a restoration should resolve the pulpitis. When the decay is removed, prior to placing the final restoration, a cement base material may be placed into the prepared tooth. This **base** material is an **indirect pulp cap** and protects the pulp from outside stimulants such as cold foods and drinks or sweets.

Irreversible Pulpitis Irreversible pulpitis is a severe inflammation of the pulp. Irreversible pulpitis may occur due to deep decay that has invaded the pulp. Irreversible pulpitis may also occur in the event that much of the decayed dentin had to be removed; as a result, there is little dentin protecting the pulp from outside stimulation. The patient may call stating that they

are in constant pain and that the pain becomes worse when they lie down at night. The patient may also state that the pain keeps them up at night. In such an event, a base material may be placed during the emergency appointment to protect the pulp from outside stimulation. The base material acts as a **direct pulp cap** or barrier between the pulp and the permanent restoration. In some instances the base material may be used as a temporary restoration for approximately 2 weeks. Once the temporary restoration is placed, the dentist can monitor the tooth for occurrence of sensitivity. If the tooth remains sensitivity free, some of the base material is removed and the permanent restoration is placed on top of it.

If sensitivity persists, referral to an endodontist and endodontic therapy (**RCT**) may be required. Refer to Chapter 37, "Endodontics," for detail about RCT. In cases of severe decay where extensive tooth structure has been lost, an extraction may be necessary.

In the event that extensive tooth structure is lost after removal of decay, a **post and core** buildup may be necessary. A post adds strength to the tooth, and the core will allow for rebuilding of the lost tooth structure. The final permanent restoration has greater stability once the post and core has been completed.

Periapical Abscess A periapical abscess can result from decay that is left untreated and progresses to invade the pulp of the tooth. An abscess may form around the apex of the tooth. This occurs because bacteria enter through the decayed area of the tooth and have access to the apex of the tooth. The bacteria travel to the apical area, and an infection results. An abscess is a localized collection of pus that is a result of the death of the pulp of a tooth. An abscess may be acute or chronic.

An emergency patient with an acute periapical abscess usually presents with pain that is throbbing and constant. When tested, the tooth is sensitive to percussion, heat, and pressure. The tooth is also **nonvital** when **vitality tests** are performed. An acute periapical abscess may not be obviously visible radiographically. Evidence of an acute abscess is based on clinical symptoms upon presentation to the dental office. Radiographically, a widening of the periodontal ligament (PDL) space may be visible.

A chronic periapical abscess can develop from an acute periapical abscess. A chronic abscess is usually not painful because the pus is able to drain from the infected area. The infection drains through a **fistula** (a passageway from the apex of the tooth to the surface of the oral mucous membranes) that allows the pus to escape where a gum boil forms. Since the pus is able to leave the periapical area and the pressure does not build up around the apical area of the tooth, chronic periapical infections do not result in pain.

Loose or Dislodged Restorations

Some patients may present with a restoration that has become loose and may have also dislodged from the tooth. These may be amalgams, composites, crowns, or bridges. If a restoration loosens or dislodges, there is usually an underlying reason. The tooth may have decayed under the restoration, causing the supporting tooth structure to become soft and the restoration to fail. Decay can occur under a restoration for several reasons:

- When preparing the tooth for a restoration, not all the decayed tooth structure was removed and the restoration was placed on top of it. This allowed the decay to continue to progress under the restoration.

- The patient was not able access those areas of the oral cavity during oral home care, resulting in food buildup. This led to decay of the tooth structure which supports the restoration.

- The decay may have been extensive, and when it was removed, much of the natural tooth structure was lost. As a result, if a large composite or amalgam is placed, it may fracture or dislodge because there is no supporting tooth structure to keep it in place.

- The restoration may not have been fabricated properly. For example, a crown must have retention in order for it to remain secure on the tooth. As a result, the tooth must be prepared in a manner that allows for retention of the crown.

In the event that the patient presents with a restoration that has completely dislodged, an exam and possible radiographs would be necessary to diagnose the reason for the dislodged restoration. The tooth would then need to be prepared based on the diagnosis. If the reason for the lost restoration was the presence of decay, the decay would need to be completely removed, leaving a cavity in the tooth that would need to be prepared to receive a restoration (cavity preparation). If the patient presents on an emergency basis due to a dislodged restoration and time does not allow complete treatment, the decay would be removed and a temporary cement restoration placed (refer to Procedure 30-1). A follow-up appointment is scheduled to place a permanent restoration. If the restoration is too large and much of the supporting tooth structure is missing due to extensive decay, the tooth may need a crown for greater retention and coverage.

If a restoration such as a crown is loose but has not dislodged, the crown is gently removed, and a temporary cement is mixed and placed in the crown. The crown is reseated onto the existing prepared tooth. Sometimes the crown cannot be removed with gentle attempts. In this instance, it would be beneficial to wait until the crown dislodges and request that the patient return to the office when it does. Excessive force should not be used to remove the crown as this may cause greater damage of the natural tooth structure underneath. A diagnosis and treatment plan can then be formulated for the affected area, which may result in adjusting the crown preparation and fabrication of a new crown for the patient.

Cavity Preparation

The procedure to remove decay and shape the cavity is referred to as **cavity preparation**. Cavity preparation is one of the more common procedures performed by the dentist and assisted by the chairside dental assistant in a general dentistry office. During this procedure, the diseased tissue is removed, and the remaining healthy tooth structure is shaped to receive and retain a restoration. The tooth structure that is shaped to receive the restoration is also referred to as the cavity preparation. This procedure is performed before the placement of a dental cement, dental amalgam, or a composite resin restoration. The cavity preparation involves:

- The removal of caries and existing restorations if present

- The cutting and shaping of the remaining tooth structure into the desired form necessary for receiving a restoration

Most cutting during the cavity preparation is performed with burs in low and high-speed handpieces. Handcutting instruments (hatchets and chisels) may also be needed for refining details of the cavity preparation after using cutting burs or before using the burs to remove soft decay.

Cavity Preparation Form The shape of the cavity preparation is designed to protect the remaining tooth structures, reestablish normal form, function and a healthy state for the tooth. Cavity preparation includes the following considerations (Figure 30-2).

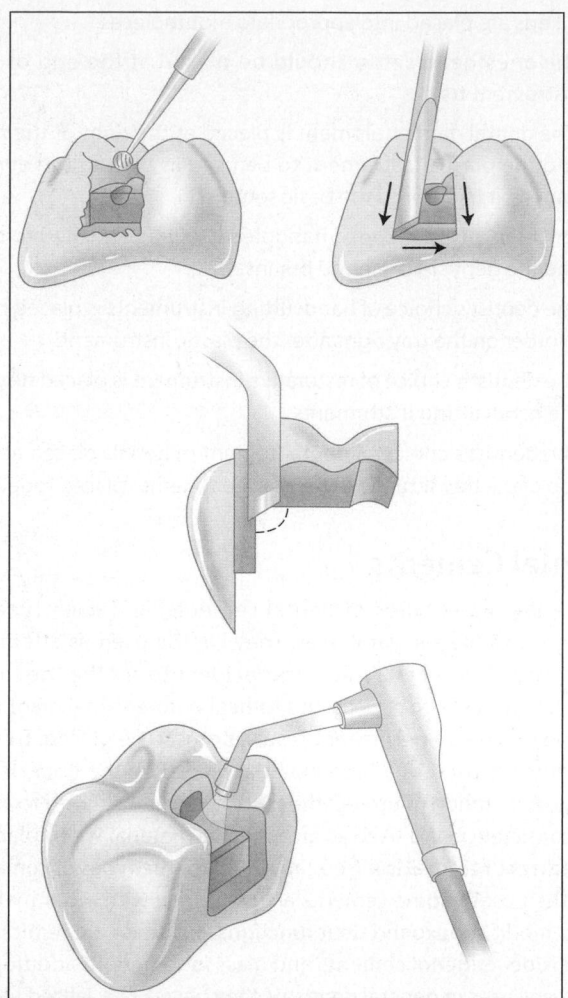

FIGURE 30-2
The steps of cavity preparation: opening the cavity with a bur, outlining the cavity, refining, and then finishing the cavity preparation.

Cavity Structure Once the tooth is prepared, there are terms used to describe the inside of the cavity preparation. Knowledge of these terms helps the dental assistant to communicate better with the dentist and also understand the details of the cavity preparation.

The preparation of the tooth forms walls, lines, and angles. A wall is the side or floor of the cavity preparation. The *wall* is named according to the surface of the tooth it is nearest to, such as the buccal wall or distal wall. The internal wall that runs parallel to the long axis of the tooth is the **axial wall**. The wall that overlies the pulp is the **pulpal wall** or floor. The wall nearest the gingiva that is perpendicular to the long axis of the tooth is the **gingival wall**.

Lines are formed when two surfaces meet and form a line angle. The *line angles* are named according to the two surfaces, such as the distopulpal line angle or the axiogingival line angle (Figure 30-3). Note that the names of the two surfaces are usually joined with an "o" between the words. At the corners of the cavity preparation, three lines (surfaces) come together to form *point angles*. The point angles are named by joining the names of the walls, such as the mesiolinguopulpal point angle or the distobuccopulpal point angle (Figure 30-4).

The **cavosurface margin** is the angle that is formed by the junction of the wall of the preparation and the untouched surface

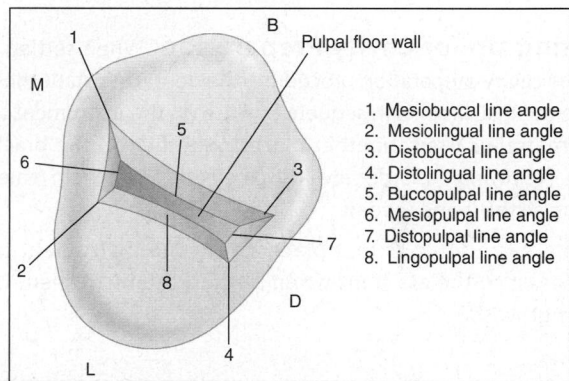

1. Mesiobuccal line angle
2. Mesiolingual line angle
3. Distobuccal line angle
4. Distolingual line angle
5. Buccopulpal line angle
6. Mesiopulpal line angle
7. Distopulpal line angle
8. Lingopulpal line angle

FIGURE 30-3
Cavity preparation line angles (looking down on an occlusal view of a premolar).

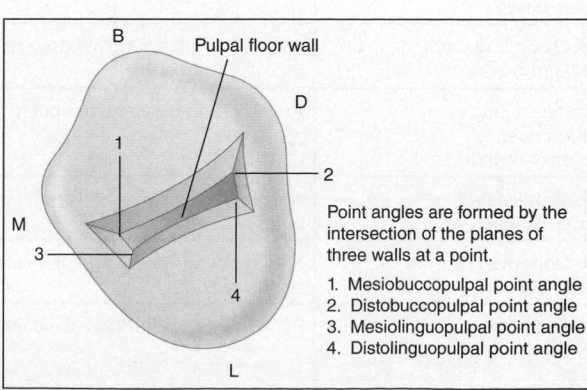

Point angles are formed by the intersection of the planes of three walls at a point.

1. Mesiobuccopulpal point angle
2. Distobuccopulpal point angle
3. Mesiolinguopulpal point angle
4. Distolinguopulpal point angle

FIGURE 30-4
Cavity preparation point angles.

- **Outline form**—designates overall shape of the cavity preparation. This form is determined by the extent of the decay, the type of restorative material, and the retention of this material.

- **Resistance form**—the internal shape of the cavity that protects the tooth and restoration from the stresses of mastication.

- **Retention form**—the internal shape of the cavity walls that retains the restoration. In an amalgam preparation, the walls of the preparation are often slightly undercut for mechanical locking of the amalgam and the cavity preparation.

- **Convenience form**—an alteration to the cavity preparation that is necessary for instrumentation during the preparation and insertion of restorative materials. This is usually beyond the outline form and opens the tooth for the dentist to have enough space to prepare the cavity properly.

- **Finishing or refinement of the cavity preparation**—the final planing of the cavity walls before the placement of the restoration.

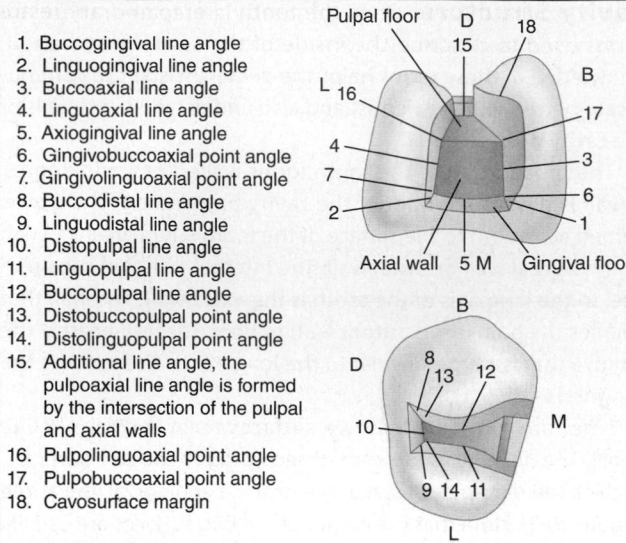

1. Buccogingival line angle
2. Linguogingival line angle
3. Buccoaxial line angle
4. Linguoaxial line angle
5. Axiogingival line angle
6. Gingivobuccoaxial point angle
7. Gingivolinguoaxial point angle
8. Buccodistal line angle
9. Linguodistal line angle
10. Distopulpal line angle
11. Linguopulpal line angle
12. Buccopulpal line angle
13. Distobuccopulpal point angle
14. Distolinguopulpal point angle
15. Additional line angle, the pulpoaxial line angle is formed by the intersection of the pulpal and axial walls
16. Pulpolinguoaxial point angle
17. Pulpobuccoaxial point angle
18. Cavosurface margin

FIGURE 30-5
Cavity preparation line angles, point angles, and cavosurface margins. (The top figure is a mesial view; the bottom figure is an occlusal view.)

of the tooth (Figure 30-5). The sealing of this margin is critical to prevent marginal leakage. Sometimes, this margin is beveled (slanted) during the preparation.

Setting Up for Cavity Preparation When setting up for the cavity preparation procedure, the dental assistant should place the instruments in sequence of use on the instrument tray and materials used together placed together on the bracket table. Following this order, it will also help the assistant in remembering all the items needed.

- The basic setup is first placed onto the instrument tray closest to the assistant when placing the instrument tray lengthwise.

- All tips are placed into appropriate mouthpieces.
- The anesthetic setup should be placed at the end of the instrument tray.
- The dental dam equipment is placed at the right of the tray, and the plastic instrument to be used in placing the dental dam next in order to the basic setup.
- The high and low-speed handpieces will be attached to unit and the dentist's preferred bur inserted.
- The dentist's choice of handcutting instruments is placed next in order on the tray right after the plastic instrument.
- The dentist's choice of restorative instrument is placed next to the handcutting instruments.
- The dentist's choice of dental cement materials placed at the top of the tray setup with items used together placed together.

Dental Cements

There are many types of dental cements, and each type of cement can have several uses. They can be used as a temporary restoration after a traumatic incident to soothe the tooth and provide time for the tissues to heal before a final diagnosis can be made and permanent restoration can be placed. Dental cements are used as a base material placed on the floor of the cavity preparation to protect the pulp. They can be mixed to a luting consistency and used as an adhesive material when placing an **indirect restoration** (see Table 30-5 for the types of cements and their uses). Some cements are combined with other materials to modify or expand their functions. Examples are reinforced zinc oxide–eugenol cements and glass ionomers. In addition to the many uses in general dentistry, they have a specialized use in most dental specialties.

The ADA and the International Standards Organization (ISO) have classified dental cements into three types according to their use and properties:

TABLE 30-5 Types of Cements and Their Uses

Type of Cement	Uses
Zinc Phosphate (water-based)	An insulating base. Permanent cementation of indirect restorations and orthodontic bands and brackets
Zinc Oxide-Eugenol (eugenol-based)	A low-strength palliative base and temporary restoration. Temporary cementation of indirect restorations
Reinforced Zinc Oxide-Eugenol (eugenol-based)	An insulating base and temporary restoration. Permanent cementation of indirect restorations
Polycarboxylate (water-based)	A high-strength base and temporary restoration. Permanent restoration of indirect restorations and orthodontic band/brackets
Glass Ionomer (water-based)	A high-strength base and permanent restoration. Permanent cementation of indirect restorations and orthodontic band/brackets
Resin Cement (Composite or Composite Resin) (resin-based)	Permanent cementation of indirect restorations of ceramic or composite and orthodontic bands
Resin-Modified Glass Ionomer (water based)	Cementation of metallic restorations or porcelain-fused-to-metal restorations

- Type I materials include cements or **luting** agents. They may be permanent or temporary materials. These cements may be used as an adhesive for indirect restorations, as a temporary adhesive for provisional restorations, or as an adhesive for orthodontic appliances.

- Type II materials include which may be permanent restorative materials (glass ionomer cement) or temporary restorative materials, such as intermediate restorative materials (IRM).

- Type III materials include liners and bases, which are placed in the cavity preparation before the placement of the permanent restoration.

Mixing Dental Cements Dental cements are mixed at chairside by the dental assistant as indicated by the dentist, following the manufacturer's instructions and the dentist's preferences. It is the dental assistant's responsibility to maintain the materials and the mixing equipment.

Dental cements are supplied in a powder/liquid form, two-paste system, capsule, or dispensing syringe. Most of these materials are mixed manually, but a few of the powder/liquid cements come in capsules that are mixed mechanically. Cements are mixed in a precise ratio to attain a specific consistency, ranging from a liquid glue-like solution for placing crowns to a putty consistency for bases and temporary restorations.

Dental cements can be set, or cured, by self-curing (chemical reaction between two materials), by means of a curing light (light cured), or by dual curing. Light-cured materials are becoming popular because the operator has more time to place and manipulate the materials before curing them. These materials are sensitive to overhead lights, however, and must be protected from light if dispensed ahead of time. A dual-cured material combines self-curing properties with light-curing techniques.

Guidelines for Mixing Dental Cements The most common cause for a cement to fail is the assistant's improper mixing technique. Each cement is supplied with the manufacturer's directions, which should be strictly followed. There are basic guidelines that are important in mixing cements supplied as a powder and liquid:

- Read manufacturer's directions thoroughly.
- Check expiration of dental cement.
- Examine materials. The liquid has a shelf life. If the liquid discolors and thickens, it should be discarded.

- Determine the use of the cement: base, temporary restoration, or luting consistency.

- Use instruments and mixing surfaces recommended by the manufacturer.

- Fluff the powder before dispensing. Measure out the powder and liquid using supplied measuring device included with packaging; too much or too little powder will affect the consistency of the cement and setting time. Too much powder results in thicker, faster setting that may crumble, and too little powder results in a thin mix and sets slower.

- Level powder level with the measurer using cement spatula to dispense accurate amounts. Place powder on one end of the mixing surface.

- Divide powder into increments recommended by manufacturer. When there are larger and smaller increments, the smaller increment is generally mixed first.

- Place the recommended number of drops of liquid on the opposite end of the mixing surface just before mixing to minimize the loss of water from evaporation. The space between prevents the powder and liquid from touching and start setting until mixed and for room for mixing. Hold the bottle or vial upright and allow a full drop to be released; do not allow liquid to touch the mixing surface while dispensing; touching the surface will affect the full measure of liquid.

- Incorporate one powder increment at a time into the liquid. Mix each increment for the time recommended by the manufacturer.

- Mix the entire amount within the time recommended. Mixing too slow or too fast will affect the material's setting time.

Cement Composition and Manipulation There are many types of dental cements available. Dental cements are typically water-based, eugenol-based, or resin-based. Traditional water-based cements are often referred to as crown and bridge cements. They include polycarboxylate, zinc phosphate glass ionomer, and resin-modified glass ionomer cements. These cements provide adequate retention for metal restorations. Zinc oxide–eugenol (ZOE) cements have been used for many years in dentistry as bases, temporary fillings, and luting of restorations. Modified ZOE cements contain ingredients that result in stronger cements. Eugenol-containing cements are only used for metallic restorations and are not suitable for bonded

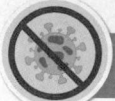

Infection Control

Dental cements are usually mixed on a supplied paper pad. Although the paper pads are easy to use and cleanup, they present a disinfection problem. After mixing, the top sheet of the paper pad is discarded, and the rest of the pad is placed on the tray. Once in the sterilizing area, the paper pad should be wiped with a disinfectant around the edges where the assistant may have held the pad. While this method works, after a while the edges of the paper pad begin to curl, and the pad becomes difficult to use. An alternative to using paper pads is a Teflon slab.

restorations because the eugenol interferes with the curing of bonding agents and resin-based materials. Categories of resin cements include resin and self-adhesive resin cements. These cements are especially suitable for bonded all-ceramic indirect restorations. These cements are light-cured or dual-cured and are available in multiple shades for high esthetic results. Adhesive and self-adhesive resin cements are formulated to bond to ceramic and metal substrates.

The dentist will select specific cements based of the particular use intended, physical properties, ease of use, and personal preference. Following is a description of common dental cement's composition, properties, and recommended manipulation techniques.

Zinc Phosphate Cement Zinc phosphate cement is one of the oldest cements, and while it does have some disadvantages, it is still a reliable choice for a permanent luting (Type I) cement and a base (Type II) cement. It comes in a powder/liquid form, and several brands are available. (Refer to Table 30-5 for the various uses of zinc phosphate cement.)

Composition The zinc phosphate powder is primarily zinc oxide with a small amount of magnesium oxide and pigments. The powder is available in shades of white, yellow, and gray. The liquid is a solution of phosphoric acid in water buffered by agents to slow down the setting reaction. Because the liquid is acidic and irritating to the pulp, the tooth must be protected with a base, **sealer**, **desensitizer**, or **liner** before the cement is placed.

When the powder and liquid are mixed together, a chemical reaction occurs and heat is released. This reaction is called **exothermic**. As heat is produced, the reaction speeds up even more. There are specific guidelines to follow when mixing zinc phosphate cement in order to minimize the temperature rise and slow down the reaction process. This provides reasonable working time and allows for maximum incorporation of the powder.

Properties When mixed, the zinc phosphate cement is high in strength and reaches two-thirds of this strength in less than an hour. Zinc phosphate sets (hardens) in 5–9 minutes and has a long mixing time of up to 2 minutes. **Viscosity** is affected by mixing time and temperature. Zinc phosphate bonds to the tooth by means of mechanical interlocking.

Manipulation Considerations When the zinc phosphate powder is mixed with the liquid, an exothermic reaction occurs. The cement is mixed on a cool glass slab in order to *dissipate* (spread) the heat of the mix. The slab is cooled in cold water and then dried completely. Do not rub when drying as this will cause the slab to get warm. Any moisture left on the slab affects the properties of the cement. The glass slab should be clean and free of scratches and dried cement. A stainless steel cement

spatula is used to mix the powder into the liquid. The spatula should also be cool.

The powder and liquid should be the same brand and type of cement. The powder and liquid may come in dispensing bottles, or a scoop for the powder and a dropper for the liquid may be required. The bottle of powder is fluffed, or lightly shaken. The powder is placed on one side of the slab and then divided for mixing. Then the liquid is dispensed on the slab (Figure 30-6). The powder is usually divided into differently sized increments for easier mixing. Follow the manufacturer's instructions.

As mentioned previously, one objective in mixing the cement is to dissipate the heat from the exothermic reaction. If the heat is dissipated, the setting reaction is slowed and more powder can be incorporated to make the cement stronger. To accomplish this goal, several mixing techniques are used:

- The glass slab is cooled.
- The first increment of powder is mixed into the liquid for 10 to 15 seconds before more powder is brought into the mix.
- **Spatulate** the mix slowly when incorporating the powder into the liquid.
- Mix slowly over a large area of the slab, wiping both sides of the spatula.

Of all the cements, mixing zinc phosphate is the most critical, and each procedural step must be followed (see Procedure 30-1). When zinc phosphate cement is mixed into a base consistency, the cement resembles thick putty. When zinc phosphate cement is mixed into a luting consistency, the cement is creamy and follows the spatula about 1 inch above the mixing slab.

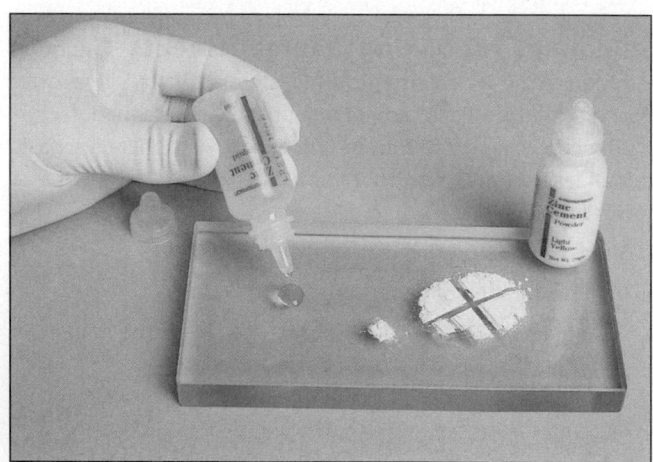

FIGURE 30-6
Zinc phosphate powder dispensed and divided into increments on one end of the cooled glass slab and the liquid being dispensed on the opposite end of the slab.

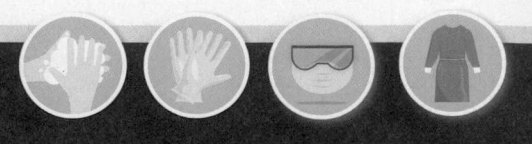

Procedure 30-1
Mixing Zinc Phosphate Cement

The dental assistant prepares the material and mixes the cement to a base or luting consistency following the manufacturer's direction for specific information on proportions, incorporation technique, and mixing and setting times. After the cement is mixed to the base consistency, the dentist places the cement into the cavity preparation. When the cement is mixed to the luting consistency, the cast restoration and cement are passed to the dentist. Sometimes the dental assistant places the cement in the cast restoration and passes the filled restoration to the dentist to place on the prepared tooth. These procedures can be legally performed by a trained dental assistant in some states.

Equipment and Supplies (Figure 30-7)
- PPE: examination gloves, mask, protective glasses, and protective clothing
- handwashing soap or hand sanitizer
- sanitized dental treatment area and barrier on working surface
- zinc phosphate powder and liquid (dispensers, if needed)
- cooled glass slab
- cooled flexible stainless steel cement spatula
- 2 × 2 inch gauze sponge
- timer
- plastic filling instrument

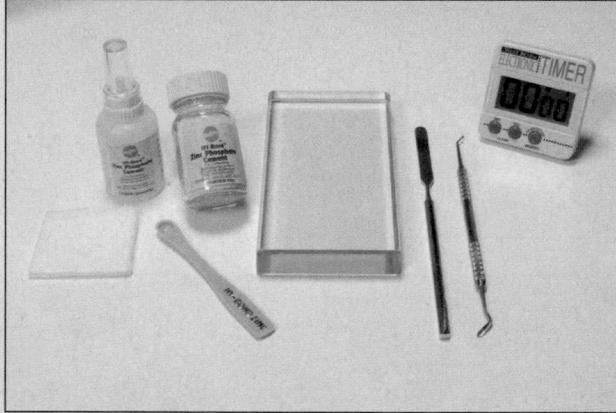

FIGURE 30-7
Zinc phosphate tray setup.

Procedure Steps *(Follow aseptic procedures)*

1. Shake the powder before removing the cap.

2. Place an appropriate amount of powder on one end of the slab. The amount of powder to be used is determined by the powder–liquid ratio, and the amount of cement required for the procedure.

3. Level the powder with the flat side of the spatula blade into a layer of about 1 mm thick.

4. Divide the powder into small increments according to the manufacturer's directions.

5. Gently shake the liquid. Dispense the liquid from a dropper bottle onto the opposite side of the glass slab. Hold the liquid vertical (perpendicular to the slab) above and without touching the slab while dispensing in order to produce uniform drops.

6. Incorporate a small portion of powder into the liquid, following the specific manufacturer's directions on mixing times.

7. Using a *wide sweeping or a figure 8 motion*, spatulate the powder and liquid over a *large area of the glass slab* (Figure 30-8).

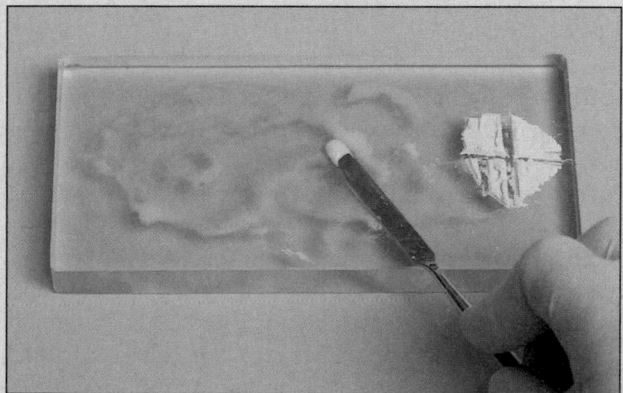

FIGURE 30-8
Mixing zinc phosphate powder and liquid. As the powder is incorporated, a larger area of the glass slab is used.

8. Incorporate each increment of powder thoroughly into the mix before adding more powder. Adding small amounts of powder will help neutralize the acid, control the setting time, and achieve a smooth consistency of the mix. The mix will appear watery at first, and then, as more powder is incorporated, the mix will become creamy.

9. Continue to add additional increments to the mix within the prescribed time until the desired consistency is reached.

10. The consistency for luting (cementing) will be creamy. It will follow the spatula for about 1 inch as it is lifted off the glass slab (Figure 30-9A).

11. The consistency for a base should be putty-like, and you should be able to roll the base into a ball or cylinder with the flat side of the spatula (Figure 30-9B).

(Continues)

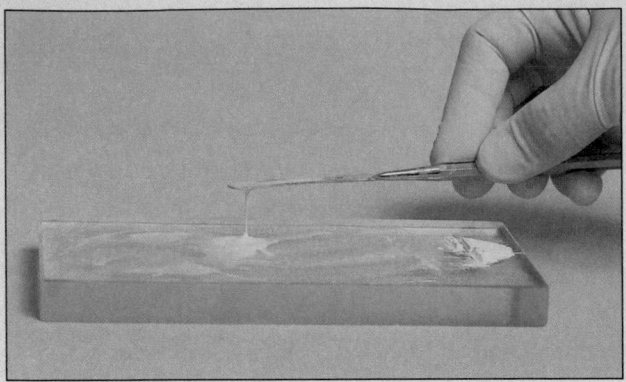

FIGURE 30-9A
Demonstration of luting consistency—the cement is creamy and the
spatula lifts the cement 1 inch from the glass slab.

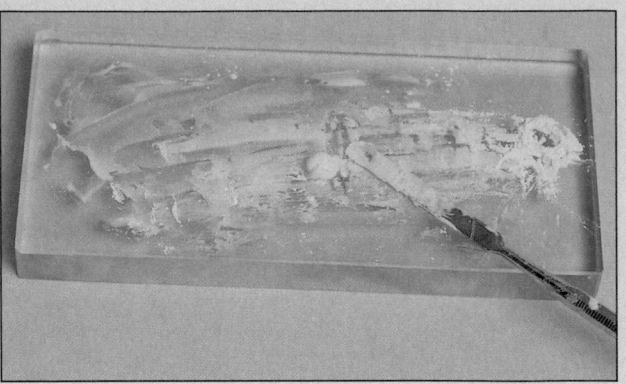

FIGURE 30-9B
Base consistency— thick putty. *Note:* Most of the glass slab was used,
and there is excess powder with which to pick up and manipulate the
base material.

12. Once the cement has been mixed to the desired consistency, wipe off the spatula with 2 × 2 inch gauze. Hold
the glass slab under the patient's chin in right hand and
pass the plastic filling instrument to the dentist with
the left hand. Hold gauze square to wipe plastic filling
instrument as needed.

13. When the dentist has finished with the mixed cement,
retrieve the plastic instrument and wipe the spatula and
glass slab with a moistened 2 × 2 inch gauze.

14. Clean the glass slab and spatula. Soak them in water or
a solution of soda bicarbonate to loosen the hardened
cement, and then sterilize or disinfect.

Zinc Oxide–Eugenol Cement Zinc oxide–eugenol cement,
often referred to as ZOE, is another cement that has been used
for many years. It is noted for its sedative or soothing effect on
the dental pulp (refer to Table 30-5 for the various uses of zinc
oxide–eugenol). The functions of this cement are diverse because
of additives that enhance its properties. There are two types of
this cement. Type I is not as strong and is used for bases and
cementation of preformed temporary restorations. Preformed
temporary crowns are tooth-shaped caps that protects a natural
tooth until a permanent crown can be placed. They are made of
an acrylic-based material or stainless steel and are available in a
variety of sizes and tooth forms (Figure 30-10). The luting consistency is placed into the crown and then cemented in place over
the prepared tooth.

Type II has been reinforced and is stronger and can be used
for permanent cementation. One type II zinc oxide–eugenol
cement is different from the rest in function. It is called an intermediate restorative material (IRM). This material is placed in
the patient's mouth and lasts up to 1 year. This material comes
both in a powder/liquid form and in capsules (Figure 30-11).
It is used when a tooth cannot be restored immediately, such as
a dental emergency appointment is limited time, during illness,
when the patient is moving, or because of economic reasons.

Composition ZOE is available in several forms, including
powder/liquid, two-paste systems, capsules, and syringes. The
powder for the conventional (type I) ZOE cement consists of
zinc oxide, resin, zinc acetate, and an accelerator. The liquid is
eugenol, which is sometimes mixed with other oils, such as clove
oil. The reinforced (type II) ZOE cement includes the addition of
alumina and polymers (resins) to the powder, and the addition
of ethoxybenzoic acid to the eugenol. Non-eugenol zinc oxide

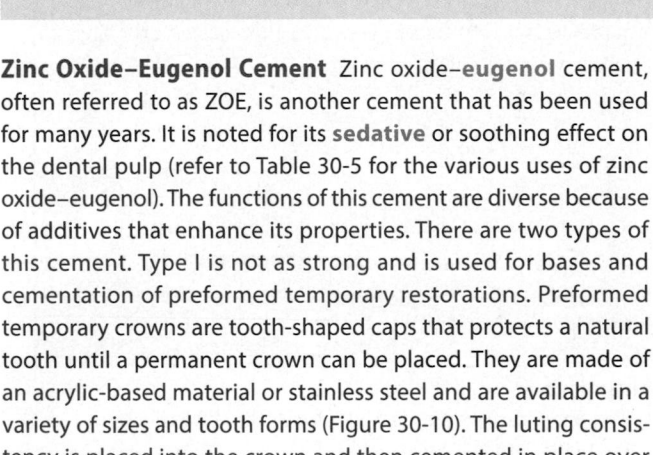

(A)

Source: Krezodent/Shutterstock.com

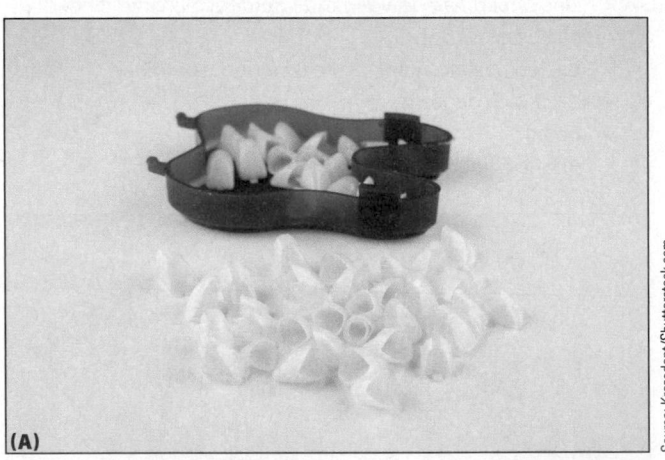

Source: aodaodaodaod/Shutterstock.com

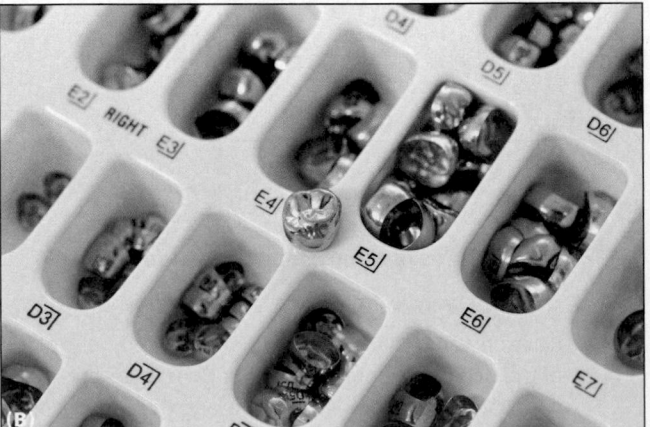

FIGURE 30-10
Temporary crowns. (A) preformed acrylic dental crowns (B) stainless steel
crowns

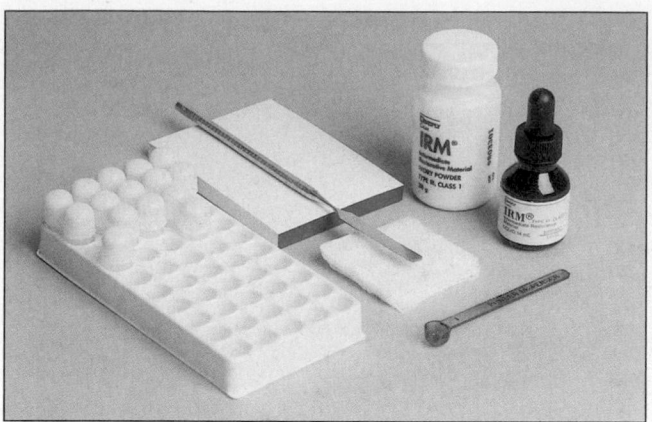

FIGURE 30-11
IRM type II (ZOE) comes supplied in powder/liquid form and in premeasured capsules.

cements are available for patients who are sensitive to eugenol. The non-eugenol cements (type I) are formulated with other oils.

Properties   ZOE has several properties that affect the selection of this material. ZOE is very soluble in the mouth and dissolves quickly. Reinforced ZOE has the strength required for permanent cementation and retention, but it is not as strong as zinc phosphate. The pH of zinc oxide–eugenol cements is neutral. With their sedative effect on the tooth, these materials do not require a protective base or liner.

Eugenol is not compatible with composites or acrylic restorations and retards their setting process. ZON (non-eugenol) materials are not used.

Manipulation Considerations   Most ZOE materials are mixed on a paper pad with a stainless steel cement spatula. A glass slab may be used to control the setting time. Gently shake the powder before dispensing and swirl the liquid. Usually these materials

Safety

Eugenol

Although eugenol has long been known for its sedative effect on the pulp, it can also be irritating to the gingival tissues and the pulp when applied directly to these tissues. Sometimes, when a product containing eugenol contacts the oral mucosa, the patient feels a burning sensation, and the tissues become red and irritated. The tissues will sometimes slough off and are tender to the touch, thereby making eating and brushing uncomfortable. Several days may be necessary for the tissues to heal and become less sensitive. Eugenol also has a strong odor, which may be offensive to some patients.

Manufacturers of eugenol containing products, such as zinc oxide–eugenol cements and periodontal dressing, now offer products containing a eugenol substitute, called non-eugenol products.

have specific powder dispensers and liquid droppers. Care should be taken not to allow the eugenol into the rubber bulb of the dropper. The eugenol breaks down the rubber, thereby contaminating the liquid.

The type of material being mixed determines whether the powder is incorporated into the liquid in increments or brought in all at once. Usually, the mixing time is 30–60 seconds. All of the powder is mixed into the liquid to produce a uniform, smooth, creamy mix. ZOE cements set quickly in the mouth because of the moisture and the warmth (see Procedure 30-2).

Some ZOE cements are two-paste systems comprised of an accelerator and a base. They are dispensed in equal lengths on a paper pad. The two pastes have different colors and are mixed until a uniform color is achieved, which takes about 10–15 seconds (see Procedure 30-3).

Procedure 30-2
Mixing Zinc Oxide–Eugenol Cement—Powder/Liquid Form

The dental assistant prepares the material and mixes the cement to a base or luting consistency following the manufacturer's direction for specific information on proportions, incorporation technique, and mixing and setting times. After the cement is mixed to the base consistency, the dentist places the cement into the cavity preparation. When the cement is mixed to the luting consistency, the preformed temporary restoration and cement are passed to the dentist. Sometimes the dental assistant places the cement in the cast restoration and passes the filled restoration to the dentist to place on the prepared tooth. These procedures can be legally performed by a trained dental assistant in some states.

Equipment and Supplies (Figure 30-12)
- PPE: examination gloves, mask, protective glasses, and protective clothing
- handwashing soap or hand sanitizer
- sanitized dental treatment area and barrier on working surface
- zinc oxide–eugenol cement
- dispensers for specific material
- paper pad or glass slab
- cement spatula
- timer
- plastic filling instrument
- 2 × 2 inch gauze sponges
- alcohol or orange solvent

(Continues)

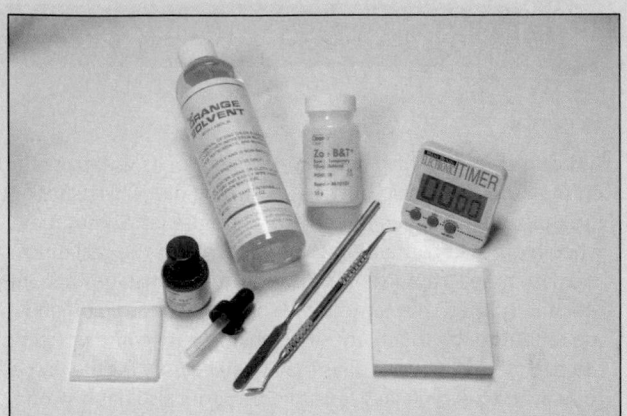

FIGURE 30-12
Tray setup for zinc oxide-eugenol cement in powder/liquid form.

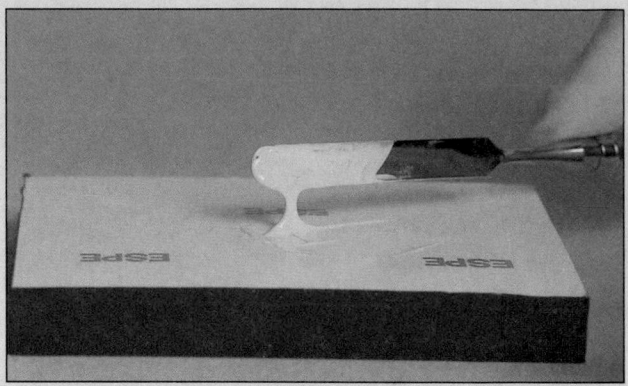

FIGURE 30-13
Consistency of ZOE temporary luting cement.

Procedure Steps *(Follow aseptic procedures)*

1. Fluff the powder before removing the cap.

2. Place the powder on the mixing pad according to the manufacturer's directions. Replace the cap to avoid spilling and contamination.

3. After swirling, place the liquid on the paper pad. Hold the dispensing dropper perpendicular to the mixing pad and dispense the drops without touching the mixing surface. Dispense near the powder but not touching it. Replace the cap to avoid spilling and contamination.

4. Incorporate the powder into the liquid in divided increments or all at once, according to the manufacturer's directions.

5. Spatulate with the flat part of the blade, use a swirling and folding motion with an even pressure to wet all particles of the powder. With some cements, a firm pressure is required to accomplish this.

6. Gather up the powder and liquid from the edges of the mix.

7. Gather up the entire mass into one unit on the slab to test its consistency.

8. The consistency for temporary luting will be creamy, like frosting (Figure 30-13).

9. The consistency for an insulating base or IRM will be putty-like and can be rolled into a ball or cylinder.

10. Once the material has been mixed to the desired consistency, wipe the spatula with a 2 × 2 inch gauze. Pass the temporary crown to dentist with right hand and plastic filling instrument with the left hand. Hold the pad close to the crown while the dentist fills the crown.

11. Hold the pad under the patient's chin in the right hand, and pass the plastic filling instrument with the left hand to the dentist to place the base/IRM material.

12. Receive the plastic filling instrument and wipe it off.

13. Remove the top page of the paper pad and fold to prevent accidental contact with the cement.

14. Clean material that has hardened on the spatula or glass slab. Wipe it with alcohol or orange solvent.

The setting time ranges from 3–5 minutes in the oral cavity for most ZOE materials. They are mixed to either a luting or base consistency depending on their use and the specific material.

Polycarboxylate Cement Polycarboxylate cement, also known as zinc polycarboxylate, is used for permanent cementation of crowns and as an insulating base. This cement is said to be kind to the pulp and was the first cement that had the ability to chemically bond to the tooth structure. There are several brands of polycarboxylate cement, and this cement comes both in a powder/liquid form and in capsules.

Composition The powder of the polycarboxylate cement is similar to the zinc phosphate powder, with zinc oxide as the main component and a small amount of magnesium oxide. Some stannous fluoride is added to most polycarboxylates to improve their strength and reduce film thickness, not necessarily for its anticarious effect. The liquid is what makes this cement different; it is a viscous solution of polyacrylic acid copolymer in water. The powder comes in a bottle with a specific dispenser, and the liquid comes in a squeeze bottle or a calibrated syringe. Polycarboxylate cement also comes in a capsule delivery system (Figures 30-15A and B).

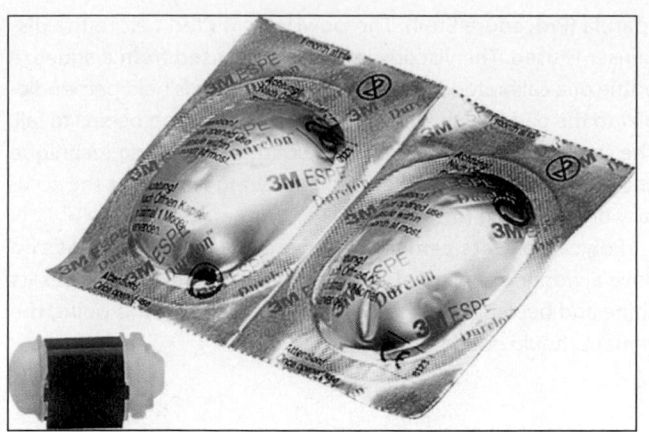

FIGURE 30-15A
Polycarboxylate capsule.

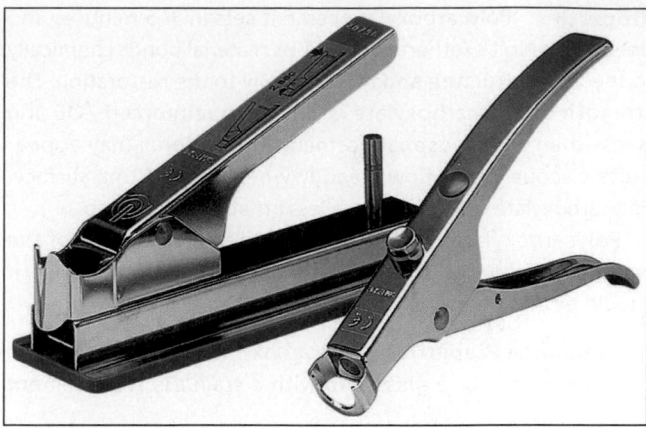

FIGURE 30-15B
Activator/applier set.

Procedure 30-3
Mixing Zinc Oxide–Eugenol Cement—Two-Paste System

The dental assistant prepares the material to luting consistency and passes it to the dentist. Sometimes the dental assistant places the cement in the temporary crown and passes the filled restoration to the dentist to place on the prepared tooth. The dental assistant assists the dentist during the placement of the temporary crown. The placement of the crown on the tooth can be legally performed by a trained dental assistant in some states.

Equipment and Supplies (Figure 30-14)
- PPE: examination gloves, mask, protective glasses, and protective clothing
- handwashing soap or hand sanitizer
- sanitized dental treatment area and barrier on working surface
- two-paste zinc oxide–eugenol (accelerator and base)
- paper pad
- cement spatula
- 2 × 2 inch gauze sponge (moistened)
- plastic filling instrument

Procedure Steps (*Follow aseptic procedures*)

1. Dispense the amount of material required for the procedure. Equal lengths of the accelerator and the base are usually placed parallel to each other on the paper pad.

2. Gather the materials and mix using swirling and **stropping** motion into a **homogeneous** mass. Spread over a small area, and then gather. Repeat the process. The material should be a creamy mix that follows the spatula up for an inch (luting consistency).

3. Wipe both sides of the spatula to remove any unmixed material and then gather all the material into one area.

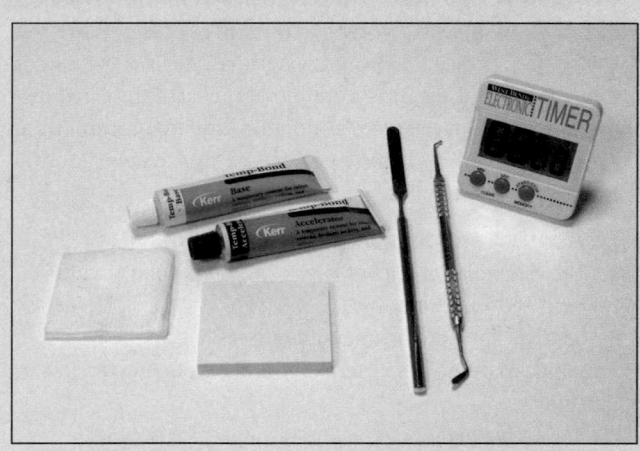

FIGURE 30-14
Tray setup for the zinc oxide–eugenol cement two-paste system.

4. Wipe off the cement spatula with the moist 2 × 2 inch gauze sponge. Hold the glass slab or paper pad under the patient's chin in the right hand, and pass the plastic filling instrument to the dentist with the left hand. The dentist fills the temporary with the luting cement.

5. Hold gauze square while the dentist fills the temporary with the luting cement and wipe the plastic filling instrument as needed.

6. When the dentist has finished with the mixed cement, retrieve the plastic instrument, and wipe the spatula and plastic instrument with a moistened 2 × 2 inch gauze. The paper pad sheet is removed, folded to prevent touching the cement and spreading it onto instruments or the patient's face, and disposed of in a container. Disinfect pad on sides before returning to storage.

Properties   Polycarboxylate cement sets in 3–5 minutes and does not exhibit exothermic heat. This material bonds chemically to the tooth structure and mechanically to the restoration. The strength of polycarboxylate is similar to reinforced ZOE and is less than zinc phosphate cement. The material may appear quite viscous, but it flows readily when applied to a surface. Polycarboxylate cement is much less irritating to the pulp.

Polycarboxylate materials have a shelf life because of the water in the liquid. If the liquid discolors and becomes thick, it should be discarded.

Manipulation Properties   Polycarboxylate cements are mixed on a paper pad or a glass slab with a stainless steel cement spatula (Procedure 30-4). The powder is fluffed before the dispenser is used. The viscous liquid is dispensed from a squeeze bottle or a calibrated syringe. The liquid bottle is held perpendicular to the pad or slab and is squeezed until a drop begins to fall. The size of the drop varies because of this dispensing technique and the viscosity of the liquid. Using a syringe improves the accuracy of dispensing the liquid.

Polycarboxylate cements are mixed in 30–60 seconds and have a working time of about 3 minutes. The material loses its shine and becomes stringy or forms cobwebs. At this point, the cement should not be used.

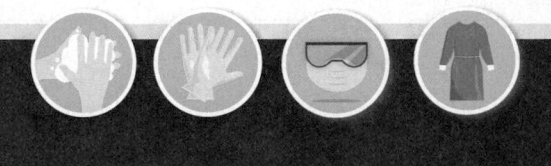

Procedure 30-4
Mixing Polycarboxylate Cement

The dental assistant prepares the material to base or luting consistency and passes it to the dentist. After the cement is mixed to the base consistency, the dentist places it into the cavity preparation. Sometimes the dental assistant places the cement in the cast restoration and passes the filled restoration to the dentist to place on the prepared tooth. These procedures can be legally performed by a trained dental assistant in some states.

Equipment and Supplies (Figure 30-16)
* PPE: examination gloves, mask, protective glasses, and protective clothing
* handwashing soap or hand sanitizer
* sanitized dental treatment area and barrier on working surface
* polycarboxylate powder and dispenser for powder
* polycarboxylate liquid (in squeeze bottle or calibrated syringe)
* paper pad or glass slab
* flexible stainless steel spatula
* 2 × 2 inch gauze sponge (moistened)
* timer
* plastic filling instrument

Procedure Steps (*Follow aseptic procedures*)
1. The powder is fluffed before dispensing with the dispensing scoop.

2. The powder is measured and dispensed on one side of a paper pad or a glass slab. Replace the cap to avoid spilling and contamination.

3. Uniform drops of liquid are placed toward the opposite side of the powder. Follow the manufacturer's directions for the appropriate number of drops per scoop of powder. Replace cap to avoid spilling and contamination.

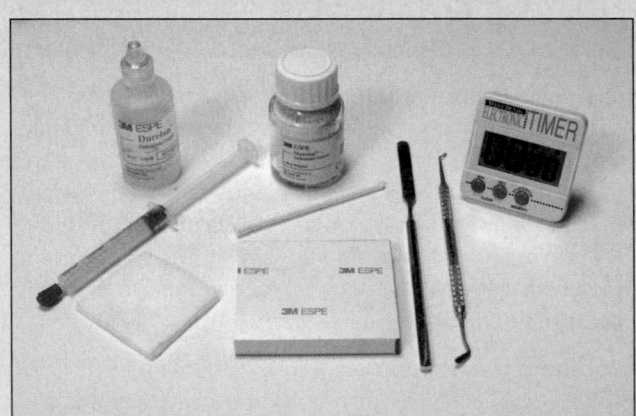

FIGURE 30-16
Mixing polycarboxylate cement tray setup. Note liquid is shown in both dispenser bottle and calibrated syringe forms.

4. Incorporate amount of the powder into the liquid as recommended by the manufacturer, using a swirling motion while adding powder, and using a folding motion while applying some pressure to wet all the powder. Mix the powder and liquid together quickly until all the powder is incorporated. Because the liquid is thick, it is harder to incorporate it into the powder.

5. The mix will be glossy and slightly more viscous than zinc phosphate cement. Gather all the cement, wiping both sides of the spatula.

6. For luting consistency, the mix should follow the spatula up 1 inch. Pass the crown and plastic filling instrument to the dentist and hold mix in position near crown as the dentist fills the crown.

7. For a base consistency, the same amount of powder is used, but the liquid ratio is decreased. The mix for the

base should be glossy, but the consistency is tacky and stiff. Hold the glass slab under the patient's chin in the right hand, and pass the plastic filling instrument to the dentist with the left hand. Hold a gauze square to wipe the plastic filling instrument as needed.

8. The mix must be used immediately before it becomes dull and stringy and forms cobwebs (Figure 30-17).

9. The cleanup is done immediately by wiping the spatula with a wet 2 × 2 inch gauze or by soaking the spatula with the dried cement in a 10 percent sodium hydroxide solution. The paper pad sheet is removed, folded to prevent touching the cement and spreading it onto instruments or the patient's face, and disposed of in a container. Disinfect pad on sides before returning to storage.

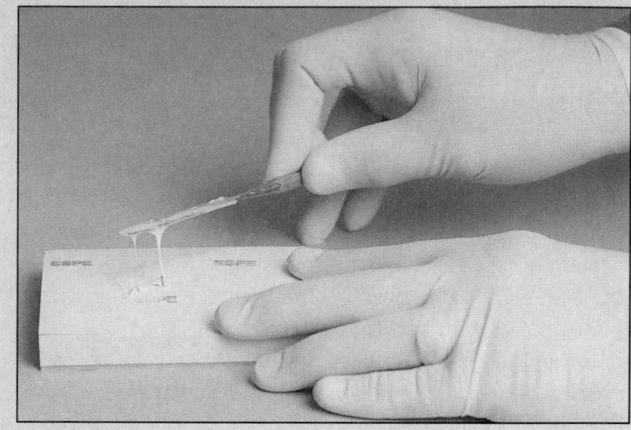

FIGURE 30-17
When cement is mixed for too long, the mix becomes thick and cobwebs form.

Glass Ionomer Cement Glass ionomer cement is one of the most popular systems. The glass ionomer cements are a combination of the silicate and polycarboxylate cements. Their applications are very diverse and have been modified for many uses. Thus, there is more than one type of glass ionomer material. Some of these are as follows:

● Type I—a fine-grain glass ionomer for use in the cementation of crowns and bridges because it chemically bonds to the tooth structure

● Type II—a coarser-grain glass ionomer available in various shades for use in selected restorations, such as Class III and V, and pediatric restorations

● Type III—a liner and dentin bonding agent

● Type IV—pit and fissure sealants

● Type V—used for the bonding of orthodontic bands and brackets

● Type VI—silver or amalgam fillings are combined with glass ionomer material and are used for crown and core buildups

● Type IX—designed to be used for some posterior restorations, especially for children

Glass ionomer cements are available in powder/liquid, paste systems, syringes, and premeasured capsule forms. The glass ionomers come in self-curing, light-curing, and dual-curing materials.

Composition Glass ionomer powder is a silicate glass powder containing calcium, aluminum, and fluoride (calcium–fluoroaluminosilicate glass). The liquid is an aqueous solution (the solution contains water) of polyacrylic acid. The water is important for the setting of the cement; therefore do not dispense it until just before mixing.

Properties Glass ionomer material is strong enough to act as a supportive base and is similar to zinc phosphate cement in strength. It mechanically and chemically bonds to the enamel, dentin, and metallic materials and releases fluoride ions, which prevent secondary decay by strengthening the tooth structure. Glass ionomer cement has low solubility in the mouth. Glass ionomers have nonirritating qualities similar to polycarboxylate cements. They, therefore, will be tolerated by the pulp and are free from phosphoric acid. The complete setting reaction of glass ionomers takes up to 24 hours. After it is set, the cement has reached its maximum strength and resistance to the oral cavity environment.

Manipulation Considerations It is important to read the manufacturer's instructions. Mixing and setting times will vary by manufacturer and the type of glass ionomer. Glass ionomer cements are mixed on a paper pad or a cool glass slab (Procedure 30-5). The paper pads are preferred for easy cleanup, but glass slabs may be used to retard the setting action. Because of the water content, the materials should be mixed quickly, following the manufacturer's directions. Water evaporation affects the properties of the cement.

Although many properties of the glass ionomers are the same as those of the polycarboxylate cements, the liquid of the glass ionomers is not as viscous (thin film thickness) and is, therefore, easier to dispense and mix. The powder is dispensed first, using the scoop and the amount indicated in the manufacturer's instructions, and the liquid is dispensed just prior to manipulation. Mixing time is usually 30–60 seconds, and working time for the material is about 2 minutes.

The tooth is isolated, cleaned, and dried before the cement is placed. The tooth does not have to be completely dry because this cement sticks to a slightly moist tooth surface. The glass ionomer cement sets in the mouth in about 5 minutes. The excess cement is allowed to stay on the margins until the cement is set. Then an explorer or excavator is used to remove the excess cement. This is different than polycarboxylate cement, which is removed before it is set.

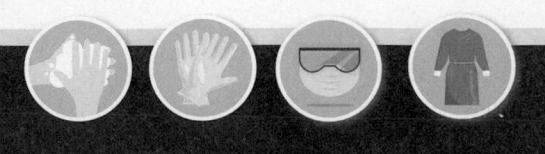

Procedure 30-5
Mixing Glass Ionomer Cement

The dental assistant prepares the cement setup, mixes the material to base or luting consistency, and assists the dentist in the placement into the cavity preparation. After the cement is mixed to the luting consistency, the dentist places the cement into the crown. Sometimes the dental assistant places the cement in the crown and passes the filled restoration to the dentist to place on the prepared tooth. These procedures can be legally performed by a trained dental assistant in some states.

Equipment and Supplies (Figure 30-18)

- PPE: examination, gloves, mask, protective glasses, and protective clothing
- handwashing soap or hand sanitizer
- sanitized/disinfected dental treatment area and barrier or working surface
- glass ionomer materials and appropriate dispensers
- paper pad or cool glass slab
- flexible stainless steel spatula
- 2 × 2 inch gauze sponges (moistened)
- timer
- plastic filling instrument

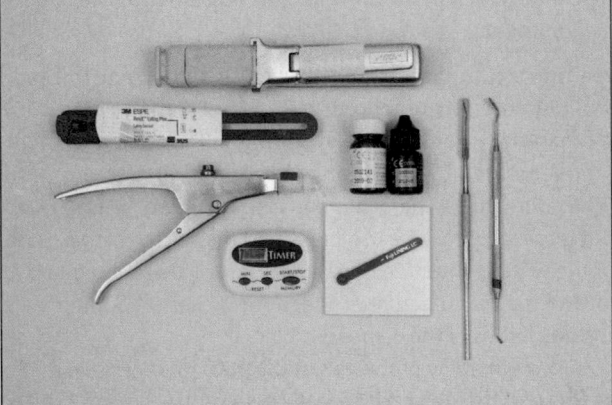

FIGURE 30-18
Tray setup for mixing the glass ionomer cement.

Procedure Steps *(Follow aseptic procedures)*

1. Carefully read the manufacturer's direction for specific use, ratios, mixing times, manipulation technique, and consistency.

2. Fluff the powder, use the recommended scoops, and place the recommended number of scoops on the paper pad or glass slab. Replace the cap to avoid spilling and contamination.

3. Swirl the liquid and then place the specified number of drops on the pad near the powder. DO NOT squeeze the bottle; let liquid drop from the bottle, or dispense material using the syringe technique. Replace the caps immediately to prevent evaporation (Figure 30-19).

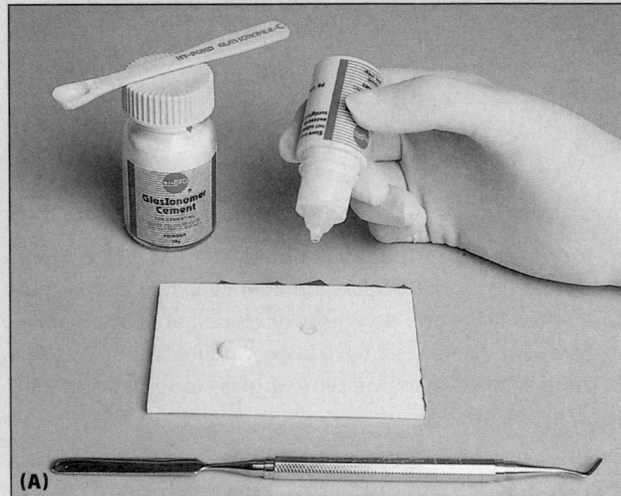

(A)

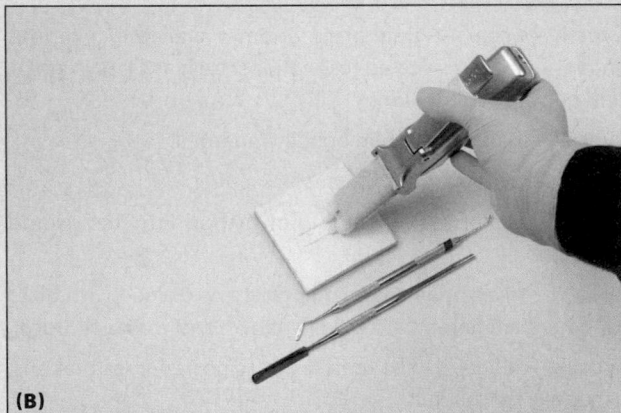

(B)

FIGURE 30-19
(A) Dispensed glass ionomer powder and liquid. (B) Dispensed glass ionomer using the syringe material.

4. Divide the powder into halves or thirds, and then draw the sections into the liquid one at a time per manufacturer's directions.

5. Mix to base or temporary consistency. Spatulate using a swirling motion over a small area until all the powder is incorporated and it is tacky and stiff. Once the cement has been mixed to the desired consistency, wipe off

the spatula with a 2 × 2 inch gauze. Hold the glass slab under the patient's chin in the right hand, and pass the plastic filling instrument to the dentist with the left hand. Hold a gauze square in the left hand to wipe the plastic filling instrument as needed.

6. Mix to luting consistency when cementing a crown. The consistency for luting (cementing) is creamy and glossy. Pass the crown and plastic filling instrument to the dentist, and hold the mix in position in the right hand near the crown as the dentist fills the crown. Hold a gauze square in the left hand to wipe the plastic filling instrument as needed.

7. To clean up, remove the top paper, fold it, and dispose of it. The instruments are wiped after use for easier

cleanup. The sides of the mixing pad are wiped with disinfectant.

8. Glass ionomer capsules are also available. They are activated by placement in an activator or dispenser to break the seal between the powder and liquid in the capsule. The capsules are then placed in an amalgamator to be mixed (triturated) for a specific amount of time, usually 10 seconds. Follow the manufacturer's directions. Insert the capsule in the appropriate dispenser and pass it to the dentist for dispensing the material needed.

9. To clean up, the capsule is discarded, and the activator and dispenser are disinfected.

Resin-Modified Glass Ionomer Cement   The composition of the resin-modified (reinforced) glass ionomer cement is modified to include a light-curing resin component in addition to the traditional glass ionomer setting reactions. The material is supplied in protective containers because both components are light sensitive. Resin-modified glass ionomer cements are stronger, more water insoluble, and more adhesive to tooth structures than conventional glass ionomer cement. Resin-modified glass ionomer cement comes in a variety of forms including powder/liquid form and capsules. Like glass ionomer cement, the resin-modified glass ionomer cement releases fluoride to protect the enamel against decalcification and demineralization.

Cement Strength   A cement's strength is measured by is flexural strength and bond strength. The flexural strength of cement must resist fracture when the restoration is loaded during chewing. Zinc oxide–eugenol cements are the weakest cements, followed by polycarboxylate and zinc phosphate cements, whereas resin cements are the strongest.

Water-based (zinc phosphate, polycarboxylate, and glass ionomer) and eugenol-based cements have low bond strengths to enamel and dentin. Resin cements used with bonding agents (see Chapter 32) have the highest bond strengths to tooth structure. Self-adhesive resin cements do not require a separate bonding agent.

Procedure 30-6
Assisting with a Temporary Cement Restoration

The chairside dental assistant prepares material and transfers materials and instruments while the dentist completes the cavity preparation procedure. The operator (dentist, dental hygienist, or qualified assistant) places the dental dam and cement, and carves the temporary.

Steps written in blue font are performed by the operator (dental hygienist or trained dental assistant in some states), and the chairside assistant's steps are written in black.

Equipment and Supplies

Patient Seating Setup
- PPE: examination gloves, mask, protective glasses, and protective clothing
- handwashing soap or hand sanitizer

- sanitized dental treatment area and barriers placed over equipment
- patient's medical and dental records
- patient seating setup (refer to Procedure 18-4)
- blood pressure equipment
- patient

Local anesthetic setup (refer to Procedure 23-2)

Dental dam setup (refer to Procedure 21-2)

Cavity preparation setup
- low-speed and high-speed handpieces
- assortment of burs (doctor's preference)
- handcutting instruments (doctor's preference)

(Continues)

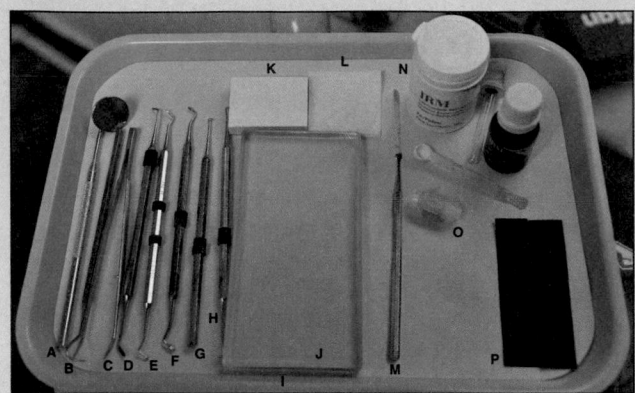

FIGURE 30-20
Temporary cement restoration setup.

Dental cement restoration setup (Figure 30-20)

- mouth mirror (A)
- dental explorer (B)
- cotton pliers (C)
- plastic instrument (D)
- spoon excavator (E)
- amalgam condenser (F)
- burnisher (G)
- carver (H)
- instrument tray (I)
- glass slab (J)
- mixing paper pad (K)
- gauze square (L)
- cement spatula (M)
- IRM liquid and powder, measuring devices (N)
- IRM capsule (O)
- articulating paper (P)
- amalgamator with barrier in place (not shown)

Procedure Steps

1. Escort and seat patient (refer to Procedure 18-4).

2. Prepare in advance for steps in cavity preparation procedure.
   - ❏ Attach handpieces to dental unit.
   - ❏ Insert burs into handpieces.
   - ❏ Expose one (1) periapical radiograph of the area.
   - ❏ Inform dentist that the patient is ready.
   - ❏ Introduce dentist as they enter the treatment area.

   Dentist greets the patient and takes position at the dental chair.
   - ❏ **Signals for the procedure to begin (refer to Procedure 20-1).**

3. Pass mouth mirror and explorer at dentist's signal.

   Dentist examines tooth or teeth with mirror and explorer.

   Dentist administers local anesthetic.

4. Assist in administration of local anesthetic (refer to Procedure 23-2).

   Operator places dental dam.

5. Assist in placement of dental dam (refer to Procedure 21-3).

   Dentist examines area after placement of dental dam.

6. Transfer mirror and explorer.

   Dentist removes caries and cuts tooth structure to form cavity preparation.

7. Assist with removal of dental caries and tooth structure.
   - ❏ Retrieve explorer and transfer handpiece.
   - ❏ Hold HVE near handpiece head during cutting to evacuate dental spray.
   - ❏ Rinse and aspirate as needed.
   - ❏ Keep mirror clean during procedure by gently blowing air on mirror.
   - ❏ Use air and HVE to remove debris as needed.
   - ❏ Rinse and dry area after dentist has prepared the tooth.
   - ❏ Do not over dry; over drying may damage the pulp.

   Dentist refines the cavity preparation as needed.

8. Retrieve handpiece and pass handcutting instruments as needed by dentist to refine cavity preparation.

   Dentist examines preparation prior to placing dental materials.

9. Retrieve handpiece and pass explorer.

10. Retrieve mirror and explorer.

11. Rinse and dry area after dentist refines cavity preparation.

12. Mix reinforced zinc oxide–eugenol dental cement manually (refer to Procedure 30-2).
    - ❏ Or mix using a premeasured IRM capsule
    - ❏ Set amalgamator time to manufacturer's directions.
    - ❏ Activate capsule (firmly twist or press on capsule until you feel a snap as the membrane separating is broken and the liquid is released) at operator's signal.
    - ❏ Place capsule in ears of amalgamator and press to begin trituration.
    - ❏ Remove capsule from amalgamator after trituration.
    - ❏ Open capsule by removing cap and place mixed cement onto mixing surface (pad/glass slab).
    - ❏ Adjust consistency to operator's preference if needed using powder/liquid from bulk package; add powder to thicken mix or add liquid if mix is too thick.
    - ❏ Remove the top page of the paper pad and fold to prevent accidental contact with the cement.

    Operator places and condenses cement into cavity preparation.

13. Assist in placing the cement.
    - ❏ Pass mirror and plastic filling instrument.
    - ❏ Hold the glass slab in right hand under the patient's chin in right hand.

❑ Hold gauze square in left hand to wipe plastic filling instrument as needed.

❑ Retrieve plastic filling instrument and pass operator's preference of amalgam condenser.

Operator carves the dental cement to reestablish anatomy and function.

14. Assist operator in carving the cement.

❑ Retrieve amalgam condenser and pass operator's preference of carver.

❑ Exchange carvers as needed.

❑ Rinse and dry area after operator has carved the cement.

❑ Retrieve carver after restoration is carved.

Operator removes the dental dam and examines the occlusion of the temporary restoration.

15. Assist in removal of dental dam and pass articulating paper in holder.

Operator places the articulating paper between the patient's teeth and asks the patient to gently bite down.

Examines for any markings on the restoration from the articulating paper.

16. Pass carver if occlusion needs to be adjusted.

Operator reexamines the occlusion.

17. Retrieve carver and pass gauze square to remove markings.

Operator removes markings with gauze square.

18. Retrieve gauze square and pass articulating paper in holder.

Operator places the articulating paper between the patient's teeth and asks the patient to gently bite down.

Examines for any markings on the restoration from the articulating paper.

Once there are no markings the occlusion has been established.

In some states the dentist must perform a final examination of a placed restoration.

19. Retrieve articulating paper in holder and pass gauze square.

Operator removes articulating paper markings.

20. Retrieve gauze square.

21. Provide patient with postoperative instructions.

❑ Explain how chewing on ice and hard, chewy candy can damage the cement restoration.

❑ Educate patient that this is only a temporary restoration and that they need to have a permanent restoration placed.

22. Write up procedure in Services Rendered.

23. Dismiss and escort patient to reception area (refer to Procedure 18-5).

Date	Services Rendered
02/18/XX	Emg appt, patient called about intermittent pain that has progressed to more severe
	and constant pain in lower rt quad BP = 120/80, 1PA of area
	#19 IRM temporary restoration
	POI do not chew ice, gum or hard, chewy candy on the side of the temporary and
	Follow-up with evaluation. If temporary comes out call office immediately
	RTC: Follow-up examination for possible pulpitis
	Assistant's initials

Chapter Summary

Dental emergencies are commonplace in the dental office. They range from soft tissue trauma to lesions and hard tissue injuries. The dental assistant needs to know the signs, symptoms, and treatment for dental emergencies. Dental cements are often needed in the treatment of dental emergencies. The chairside assistant prepares, mixes, and transfers the material and instruments, while the dentist places the cement material in the oral cavity. Some states allow the assistant to also place some of the dental cement materials in the oral cavity. Knowledge of dental cements' properties is necessary for the dental assistant to properly prepare and manipulate the materials. The assistant's knowledge of these dental materials is beneficial for patient education and protection.

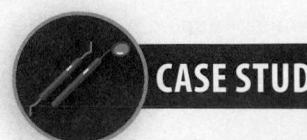

CASE STUDY

Garrett Greenwood is having a large filling placed in tooth #30. He has experienced sensitivity in the past after restorations and is concerned he will have the same problem with this filling.

Case Study Review

1. Discuss the steps that can be taken to reduce or eliminate sensitivity.

2. What information could the dental assistant give the patient about his concerns?

Review Questions

Multiple Choice

1. All of these treatments for treating oral injuries are true EXCEPT:
   a. apply pressure with clean gauze.
   b. apply cold compress to swelling.
   c. rush to hospital for sutures.
   d. rinse mouth to see extent of injury.

2. All of these statements are true about palatal burns EXCEPT:
   a. patient does not know how it happened.
   b. analgesics may be prescribed.
   c. topical ointment can be used to cover the lesion.
   d. generally heal in 7–14 days depending on the severity.

3. Which oral lesion is highly contagious, and direct contact should be avoided?
   a. aphthous ulcer
   b. periocoronitis
   c. oral herpetic lesion
   d. thrush

4. Which oral lesion may need to be treated by surgical excision?
   a. aphthous ulcer
   b. periocoronitis
   c. oral herpetic lesion
   d. thrush

5. When observing the area of the injury, there is minimal bleeding and the crown is barely visible. What type of injury may this be?
   a. concussion
   b. extrusion
   c. intrusion
   d. avulsion

6. The area of the injury has an empty, bleeding sulcus. What type of injury may this be?
   a. concussion
   b. extrusion
   c. intrusion
   d. avulsion

7. Which injury would require that the tooth be reimplanted within an hour?
   a. concussion
   b. extrusion
   c. intrusion
   d. avulsion

8. Which Ellis classification is described as a crown fracture with a pulp exposure?
   a. Class I
   b. Class II
   c. Class III
   d. Class IV

9. Which would require an immediate pulp capping or partial pulpotomy?
   a. Class I
   b. Class II
   c. Class III
   d. Class IV

10. A patient call into the office complaining a toothache. They state that there is severe pain that increases when they lay down. That the pain literally kept them up all night. What condition may cause these symptoms?
    a. reversible pulpitis
    b. irreversible pulpitis
    c. pulpal necrosis
    d. chronic abscess

11. Which condition may require RCT or extraction as a treatment?
    a. periapical abscess
    b. apical periodontitis
    c. pulpal necrosis
    d. All of these

12. Which form when prepared during the cavity preparation procedure provides the overall shape of the cavity preparation?
    a. retention form
    b. resistance form
    c. convenience form
    d. outline form

13. What term is given to the angle formed by the junction of the wall of the cavity preparation and the unprepared surface of the tooth?
    a. axial wall
    b. pulpal wall
    c. axiogingival line angle
    d. cavosurface margin

14. All of these statements about mixing dental cements are true EXCEPT:
    a. Place the powder and liquid on the mixing surface at the start of the procedure.
    b. Place power and liquid at opposite ends of the mixing surface.
    c. Mixing the cement too quickly will affect the material's setting time.
    d. Dental cements have expiration dates.

15. When is a dental cement mixed to a luting consistency?
    a. placing a base
    b. placing a temporary restoration
    c. placing a temporary crown
    d. All of these

16. Which cement(s) can be used as a temporary restoration?
    a. zinc oxide–eugenol
    b. polycarboxylate
    c. reinforced zinc oxide–eugenol
    d. All of these

17. With which cement is it important to closely follow mixing directions because of its exothermic properties?
    a. zinc phosphate
    b. ZOE
    c. glass ionomer
    d. polycarboxylate

18. A patient presents for an emergency appointment with a Class III fracture. Which cement would provide a soothing, palliative affect when placed?
    a. zinc phosphate
    b. ZOE
    c. glass ionomer
    d. composite resin

19. Which cement cannot be placed beneath a resin material as it affects it properties and set?
    a. zinc phosphate
    b. ZOE
    c. glass ionomer
    d. composite resin

20. Which is the correct order in preparing for and placing a temporary cement restoration?
    1. Place dental dam.
    2. Fill the cavity preparation with cement.
    3. Check occlusion with articulating paper.
    4. Administer anesthetic.
    5. Cut cavity preparation.
    6. Restore anatomy and function using carvers.

    Answer choices:

    a. 1, 5, 6, 3, 4, 2
    b. 1, 4, 5. 2, 6, 3
    c. 4, 1, 5, 2, 6, 3
    d. 4, 1, 5, 2, 3, 6

Critical Thinking

1. A parent calls the office and explains that their 4-year-old child has had their tooth knocked out. What should the assistant tell the parent?

2. Explain how the correct amount of powder and liquid to be dispensed is determined. What may happen if too much liquid is dispensed? If too little liquid is dispensed?

3. The dentist needs to cement a stainless steel crown temporarily for an emergency. What cements could be used? What consistency would be needed?

Key Terms

Term and Pronunciation	Meaning of Root and Word Parts	Definition
ankylose (**ang**-kuh-lohs)	**ankyl/o** = to unite or grow together -**ose** = possessing	consolidation of the tooth with the bone
apexification (ey-peksi-fi-**key**-shuhn)	**apex** = tip of the root -**ate** = denotes function -**ion** = denotes action, condition	a process that promotes the closure of the root apex; calcium hydroxide is placed in the root canal after the apex is removed (apicoectomy)
avulsion (uh-**vuhl**-shuh n)	**avulse** = to pull off or tear away forcibly -**ion** = action or condition	complete displacement of a tooth in its entirety from its location in the socket

(Continues)

Term and Pronunciation	Meaning of Root and Word Parts	Definition
axial wall (**ak**-see-*uh* l)	**axis** = the central line of any body **-al** = pertaining to, forming	relating to the internal long axis of the tooth in the cavity preparation
base (beys)	**base** = the bottom layer or coating	foundation for restoration, often a replacement for dentin
benzocaine (**ben**-zoh-keyn)	**benzo** = chemical compound of benzoic acid and phenyl group **-caine** = a medical coinage for drug used as a local anesthetic	topical local anesthetic
cast restoration (kast) (res-t*uh*-**rey**-shuhn)	**cast** = to receive form in a die/mold **restore** = reestablish to former condition **-ate** = denotes function **-ion** = denotes action, condition	a restoration made in a lab from models of tooth for replacement of lost tooth structures and cemented onto the remaining tooth structure; gold alloy crown
cavity preparation (**kav**-i-tee) (prep-*uh*-**rey**-shuh n)	**cavity** = a hollow place in the tooth produced by caries **prepare** = to make ready for something **-tion** = expressing action	used as a verb; the process of using dental instruments to mechanically remove caries and diseased and unsupported tooth structures
cavity preparation (**kav**-i-tee) (prep-*uh*-**rey**-shuh n)	**cavity** = area in tooth caused by dental instruments **preparation** = something that is prepared	used as a noun; the remaining tooth structure shaped to support a dental restoration or prosthesis
cavosurface margin (key-**voh**-surfis) (**mahr**-jin)	**cave** = cavity **surface** = exterior face of an object **margin** = a border or edge	wall of a cavity preparation and the exterior surface of a tooth; outline of the cavity preparation
chlorhexidine (klor-**hex**-ih-deen)	**chlor/o** = chlorine **hexane** = hydrocarbon of alkane series **amine** = compound derived from ammonia	antibacterial rinse used in the oral cavity
closed reduction (klohzd) (ri-**duhk**-shuhn)	**closed** = not open; self-contained **reduce** = bring into a certain state or condition **-ion** = denoting action	procedure that sets (reduces) a fractured bone within the skin; skin is not opened
concussion (k*uh*n-**kuhsh**-*uh*n)	**concuss** = injure by a violent blow or fall **-ion** = denoting action	injury to the periodontal ligament and blood vessels at the apex of the tooth caused by a forceful impact to the tooth
contusion (k*uh*n-**too**-zh*uh*n)	**contuse** = tissue injury without breaking the skin; bruise **-ion** = denoting action	injury that causes blood vessel(s) to leak blood; a bruised tooth from too much pressure
curettage (kyoor-i-**tahzh**)	**curette** = scoop-shaped surgical instrument used to remove tissue from cavities **-age** = process	surgical procedure performed by dentist to clean/remove tissue by scraping or scooping a cavity contained in the mouth
dental cement (**den**-tl) (si-**ment**)	**dent** = teeth **-al** = relating to **cement** = soft, sticky substances that dry hard and used to mend broken object or for making things adhere	dental material used as bases, temporary restorations and to cement indirect restorations
desensitize (dee-**sen**-si-tahyz)	**de** = to lessen **sensitive** = easily pained **-ive** = expressing tendency	reduce pulpal pain by application of coating of soothing dental material
desiccation (**des**-i-key-shuhn)	**desiccate** = dried up **-tion** = expressing action	to dry by removing water
direct pulp cap (dih-**rekt**) (puhlp) (kap)	**direct** = straight, without intervention **pulp** = soft innermost part of a tooth; contains nerves and blood vessels **cap** = to provide or cover with	a palliative cement is placed on top of a traumatic pulp exposure to stimulate secondary dentin formation
eroded (ih-**rohd**-ed)	**erode** = to eat into or away **-ed** = result	worn away as if by abrasion
erythematous (er-*uh*-**thee**-m*uh*-tus)	**erythema** = abnormal redness of the skin or mucous membrane **-ous** = possessing	abnormal red appearance of skin or mucous membranes caused by dilation of superficial blood vessels

Term and Pronunciation	Meaning of Root and Word Parts	Definition
excision (ek-**sizh**-*uhn*)	**excise** = to cut out or off **-ion** = denoting action	surgical removal
exothermic (ek-soh-**thur**-mik)	**exo-** = external, outside **therm-** = heat **-ic** = relating to	a chemical change that releases heat
expectorate (ik-**spek**-t*uh*-reyt)	**ex-** = out **pectoris** = chest, anterior wall **-ate** = denotes function	to clear out the chest or lungs; to spit
extrusion (ik-**stroo**-zh*uh* n)	**extrude** = to thrust, expel **-ion** = denoting action or condition	partial displacement of the tooth out of the alveolar bone
eugenol (**yoo**-j*uh*-nawl)	**eugenol** = a colorless, oily, spicy aromatic liquid; extracted as oil of cloves	dental analgesic and antiseptic, which is derived from clove oil
fistula (**fis**-choo-luh)	**fistula** = passage formed by disease to lead from an abscess	abnormal passageway between an organ and the outside of the body
gingival wall (jin-**jahy**-v*uhl*) (wawl)	**gingiv(a)** = gums of the mouth **-al** = pertaining to **wall** = upright structure	cavity preparation wall closest to the gingiva
halitosis (hal-i-**toh**-sis)	**halitus** = breath **-osis** = denotes a condition	a condition of having bad-smelling breath
homogeneous (hoh-m*uh*-**jee**-nee-*uhs*)	**homo** = same **-gen** = that which produces **-eous** = composed of	a mixture to two materials having a uniform composition and properties once mixed
indirect pulp cap (in-dih-**rekt**) (puhlp) (kap)	**in-** not in **direct** = straight, without intervention **pulp** = soft innermost part of a tooth; contains nerves and blood vessels **cap** = to provide or cover with	a palliative cement is placed on top of a thin layer of dentin overlying a near pulp exposure to stimulate secondary dentin formation
indirect restoration (in-d*uh*-**rekt**) (res-t*uh*-**rey**-sh*uh*n)	**in** = not **direct** = made on natural structures **restoration** = return to original form	restoration such as a crown or bridge prepared in the dental laboratory
intrusion (in-**troo**-zh*uh* n)	**intrude** = to thrust or force into **-ion** = denoting action or condition	displacement of a tooth further into the alveolar bone
liner (**lahy**-ner)	**line** = to cover the surface **-er** = something that serves	material applied in a thin layer over pulpal floor
luting (**loo**-ting)	**luting** = cementing objects together	cementing restoration to tooth structure using a cement
luxation (**luhk**-sey-zh*uh*n)	**luxate** = to put out of joint; dislocate **-ion** = denoting action or condition	displacement of a tooth that is nonaxial in direction
malaise (ma-**leyz**)	**mal-** = bad, ill **ease** = comfort	a condition often indicates the onset of a disease or a general body weakness or discomfort
necrobiosis (nek-roh-bahy-**oh**-sis)	**necro-** = dead tissue **bio-** = life **-osis** = condition	gradual degeneration and death of cells
necrosis (*nuh*-**kroh**-sis)	**necr/o** = dead tissue **-osis** = condition, state	cell/tissue death
nonvital (non-**vahyt**-l)	**vital** = relating to life **non-** = not	a dead tooth; has no access to blood flow
operculum (oh-**pur**-ky*uh*-luh m)	**operculum** = cover, lid	mucosal flap partially or completely covering an unerupted or partially erupted tooth

(Continues)

Term and Pronunciation	Meaning of Root and Word Parts	Definition
palliative (**pal**-ee-ey-tiv)	**palliate** = to lesson severity of pain without curing **-ive** = expressing function	relieves symptoms without curing
partial pulpotomy (**pahr**-shuhl) (puhl-**pot**-uh-mee)	**part** = a portion of a whole **-al** = pertaining to **pulp** = inner substance of the tooth **-o-** = connecting vowel **-tomy** = surgical cutting of a specific part or tissue	procedure to remove inflamed pulp tissue beneath an exposure to reach healthy pulp tissue
percussion (per-**kuhsh**-uh n)	**percuss** = to strike or tap for diagnostic **-ion** = action or condition	method of diagnosis which uses short taps on a tooth to determine a condition based on sound and patient sensitivity
pericoronitis (per-ee- kawr-uh-**nahy**-tis)	**peri-** = encircling, around **coron** = crown of tooth **-itis** = inflammation	gingival inflammation of soft tissue surrounding a tooth
post and core (pohst) (kohr)	**post** = strong piece of metal set upright as a support **core** = central, innermost, most essential part of anything	dental restoration that is placed when there is inadequate tooth structure remaining to support a traditional restoration; a small metal rod (post), is inserted into the root canal space of the tooth; a filling, or core, is placed around the post; a post and core is covered with a crown if deemed necessary by the clinician
pulp capping (puhlp) (**kap**-ing)	**pulp** = inner substance of the tooth **capping** = to cover as if with a cap	the covering of an exposed or nearly exposed dental pulp with medicament to protect pulp and encourage healing
pulpal wall (**puhlp**-uhl) (wawl)	**pulp** = inner substance of the tooth **-al** = pertaining to **wall** = upright structure	internal wall of cavity preparation in a horizontal plane above the pulp
radiolucent (rey-dee-oh-**loo**-suh nt)	**radio** = dealing with radiation **lucent** = clear	structure such as soft tissue that allows passage of the x-ray beam and appears dark or radiolucent on a radiograph
RCT	**R** = root **C** = canal **T** = therapy	procedure to treat disease of the pulp by removing the nerve and tissue from the pulp cavity and placing a filling material in the root canals
sealer (**see**-ler)	**seal** = to block completely to prevent entrance or escape **-er** = denoting action or process	material placed in the cavity preparation to protect sensitive tooth tissues and pulp
sedative (**sed**-uh-tiv)	**sedate** = to calm or quiet **-ive** = expressing function	anesthetic placed near the pulp to sooth the pulp nerves
spatulate (**spach**-uh-leyt)	**spatula** = broad, flat instrument used for mixing **-ate** = denotes function	mix a dental material using a cement spatula
stropping (**strop**-ing)	**strop** = press firmly **-ing** = expressing action	mixing technique that uses a back and forth pressing and swiping motion against the mixing surface
temporary restoration (**tem**-puh-rer-ee) (res-tuh-**rey**-shuhn)	**temporary** = for a short period of time **restoration** = return to original form	a filling placed for a limited period of time (days to months) to seal and soothe tooth until a permanent restoration can placed
trismus (**triz**-muhs)	**trismus** = unable to open mouth	painful condition of not being able to fully open mouth due to severe contraction of the chewing muscles of the jaw
vascular (**vas**-kyuh-ler)	**vas/o** = vessels **-ar** = of or relating to	relating to vessels providing abundant blood supply
vesicle (**ves**-i-kuh l)	**vesica** = a bladder, sac **-ule** = indicating smallness	small fluid containing sac; blister
viscous (**vis**-kuh s)	**viscous** = sticky, thick, adhesive consistency	use of dental materials that are sticky and thick to improve adhesive qualities
vitality test (vahy-**tal**-i-tee) (test)	**vital** = relating to life **-ty** = denoting state **test** = an examination procedure	the health of the pulp is tested using hot, cold, pressure, and an electric current from an instrument (pulp tester/vitalometer)

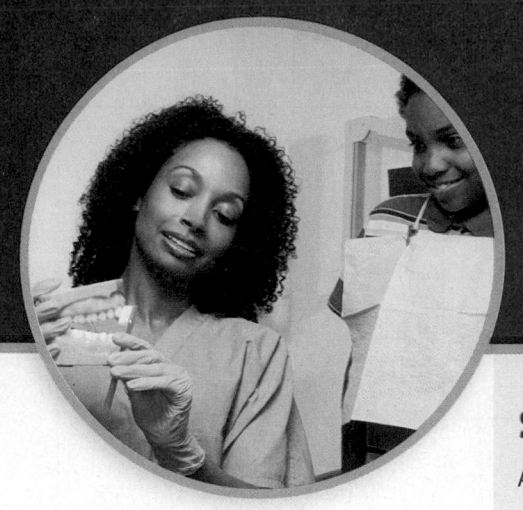

## CHAPTER 31

Amalgam Procedures and Materials

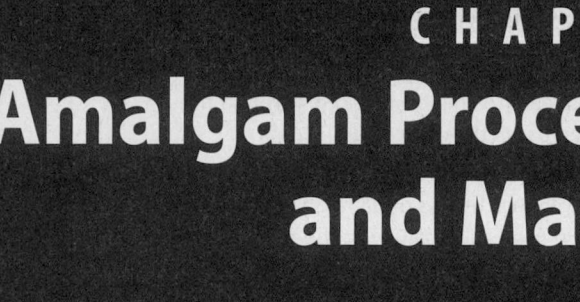

Specific Instructional Objectives

At the completion of this chapter, you will be able to meet these objectives:

1. Use terms presented in this chapter.
2. Discuss dental material properties.
3. Recall agencies and organizations regulating dental materials.
4. Describe treatment of cavity preparation for placement of dental amalgam.
5. Identify the different matrix band systems and their uses.
6. List advantages and disadvantages in using dental amalgam as a direct restoration.
7. Explain the clinical importance of the properties of amalgam.
8. Discuss mercury hygiene for patients and for dental workers.
9. Describe the steps in completing an amalgam restoration.
10. Discuss the indications and contraindications for finishing and polishing amalgam restorations.
11. Describe the steps in finishing and polishing an amalgam restoration.

Introduction

Dental amalgam has been used successfully for filling posterior teeth for many years. Composition, types, and safety concerns are discussed, as well as proper handling, mixing techniques, and placement of an amalgam restoration. There are some concerns about the mercury in the dental amalgam, and the dental assistant should keep up to date on current information to stay informed.

The chairside dental assistant generally prepares and mixes the material, while the dentist completes the cavity preparation and places the material in the oral cavity. The dental assistant's role when working with dental restorative materials depends on the expanded functions of individual state practice acts, which regulate dentistry. Some states allow the dental assistant to perform these basic responsibilities, as well as placing the materials in the oral cavity.

Knowledge of dental material properties is necessary for the dental assistant to properly prepare and manipulate the materials and is also beneficial for patient education and protection. Expanded-function dental assistants must understand and be competent with placing and finishing such materials.

Properties of Dental Materials

Replacing the natural tooth structure has presented a number of challenges. The oral cavity environment and functions create complex situations. Properties that are considered for dental materials include the following: acidity, adhesion, biting force, corrosion, dimensional change, elasticity, flow, galvanism, hardness, microleakage, retention, bonding, solubility, thermal conductivity, viscosity, and wettability.

Acidity

Acidity is viewed in terms of its effect on a given material and on the tissues in the mouth.

- The normal pH of the oral cavity is about neutral (pH 7.0). Some foods, such as citrus fruits, and some bacteria found in the biofilm are acidic. Saliva aids in reducing the acidity of the mouth, but dental materials are subject to varying amounts of acid. How materials react to changing acidity levels in the mouth determines their use in the oral cavity.

- Another consideration is that the acidity of the materials may cause irritation to the gingival tissues or damage to the pulp. These materials can be used successfully in the mouth, but care is taken to prepare and/or place them following the manufacturer's directions to minimize their affect.

pH Scale

The pH scale, which ranges from 0 to 14, measures the level of acidity or alkalinity of a substance. A pH of 7 is neutral, a pH less than 7 is acidic, and a pH greater than 7 is basic.

Adhesion

Adhesion is the force of attraction that holds unlike substances together. Adhesion involves physical or chemical forces. Chemical adhesion is quite strong and preferable, but physical adhesion is more common. Adhesion is a way to attach solid structures to each other. An example of physical adhesion is biofilm adhering to a tooth. Certain dental cements function on the basis of a chemical reaction, which results in chemical adhesion.

Biting Forces

Dental materials are subject to various types of biting forces. Natural dentition can withstand much more force than prostheses, such as dentures and bridges. A *force* is defined as any push or pull on an object. The result of force on an object is resistance. *Stress* is defined as the force per unit area of a material. As force is applied the reaction of the object to resist the external force is stress. Forces can cause stress over a large area, such as a quadrant, or over a small area, such as the occlusal surface of a tooth. The average biting force for a person with natural dentition varies from 130 to 170 pounds on the molars and progresses downward to about 40 pounds on the incisors. When force is applied on an individual tooth, this represents about 25,000 pounds per square inch (psi) on a single cusp or a molar. Enough stress can be placed on an object to cause a change. This change, or deformation, is known as *strain*.

- Types of stress and strain are described in the following (Figure 31-1): *Tensile*—pulls and stretches a material. Under tensile stress and strain, the structure tends to be elongated. An example of tensile stress and strain are wires that are pulled in opposite directions or elastic, rubber bands used in orthodontics. The ability of a material to withstand forces of tensile stress without failing is known as **ductility**.

- *Compressive*—pushes, or compresses, a material. An example of compressive stress and strain is chewing or biting. The ability of a material to withstand compressive stresses without fracturing is known as **malleability**.

- *Shearing*—slides one part of a material parallel to another part in a back-and-forth motion. An example of shearing stress and strain is bruxism, or grinding of the teeth.

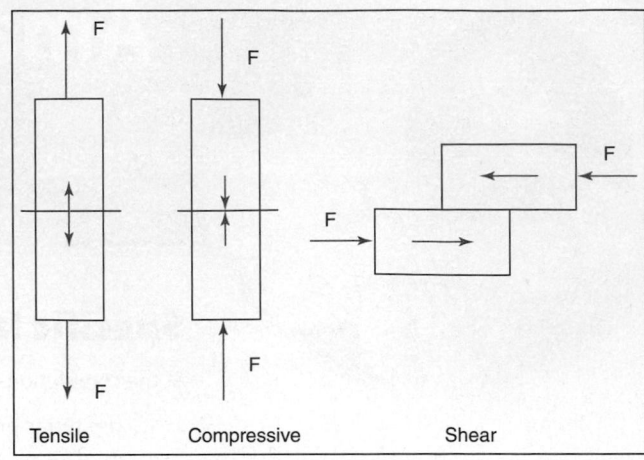

FIGURE 31-1
Tensile, compressive, and shearing stress and strain.

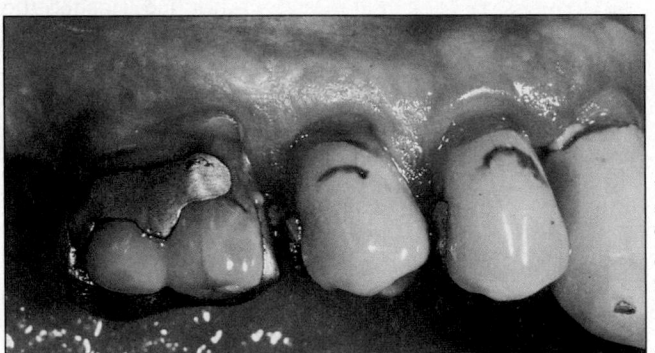

Courtesy of Dr. Gary Shellerud

FIGURE 31-2
An amalgam restoration showing corrosion and tarnish.

Corrosion

Corrosion is the result of chemical or electrochemical attacks by the oral environment on pure metal, such as gold, or on an alloy, such as amalgam. Components of food or saliva react with the metals and cause deep pitting and roughness. Sometimes the metals become dull and discolored. This effect is referred to as **tarnish** (Figure 31-2).

Dimensional Change

Dimensional change in a material can occur from a variety of causes, such as the setting process of a material or exposure to heat or cold. The change in a material is usually measured as a percentage of the original length or volume. If dental amalgam containing zinc is contaminated with water from saliva during condensing, it produces a hydrogen gas. This gas becomes incorporated in the amalgam and leads to delayed expansion. This may cause pain and even tooth fracture.

Elasticity

Some materials have the property of elasticity, which is the ability of a material to return to its original shape, after being distorted or deformed by an applied force, once that force is removed. Rubber bands exhibit this property; but if they are stretched for too long or too far, they reach their *elastic limit* and will not return to their original shape.

The *elastic modulus*, or modulus of elasticity, is a measure of the stiffness of a material below the elastic limit. This is a measure of how a material can resist deformation or change.

Flow

A flow, or creep and slump, is a continuing deformation of a solid. Under a constant force, certain materials change and deform. Amalgam is subject to flow under constant compressive forces.

Galvanism

When two different metals are present in the mouth, there is a potential for the creation of small electrical shocks. This is known as **galvanism**. The oral fluids act as a carrier between the two metals to cause an electrical shock. This can occur when a gold restoration in one arch contacts an amalgam restoration in an opposing tooth on the opposite arch. The same shock happens if an individual bites a piece of tin foil and it contacts a tooth with metallic restoration.

Hardness

The resistance of a material to scratching or indentation is known as the material's hardness. A material's sufficient hardness makes the restoration resistant to scratching and wear from mastication and abrasion. There are various ways to measure the hardness of a material. The Brinell hardness test uses an indenter (steel ball), presses it into the material, and measures the indentation in the material being tested.

Microleakage

When saliva and debris from the oral cavity seep between the tooth structure and restorative materials, this is known as **microleakage**. The dentist prepares the cavity and places materials to prevent microleakage, but some microleakage still occurs. Recurrent decay and tooth sensitivity are some of the problems resulting from microleakage (Figure 31-3).

Retention

In dentistry, retention is the means by which materials are held in place. Different types of retention methods are used with the various types of restorative materials. Materials placed directly into the cavity preparation (direct restorative materials), such as amalgam and composites. Direct restorative materials are mixed and then placed directly in the cavity preparation in a single appointment and are retained in place by mechanical means. A **mechanical retention** includes preparing the walls of the cavity preparation to be convergent (slanted in), roughening the tooth surface with etchant, or placing retentive grooves into the cavity walls.

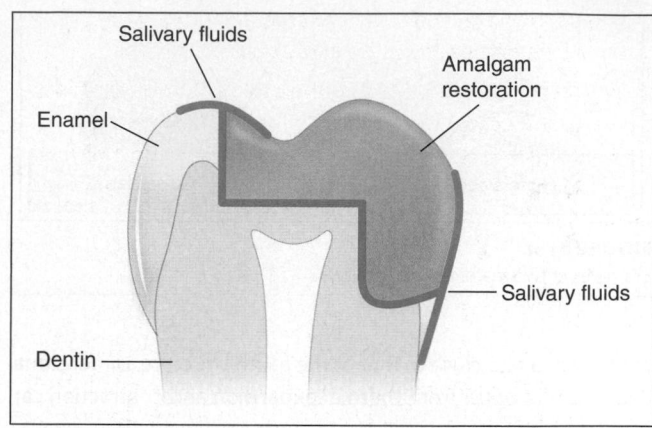

FIGURE 31-3
Microleakage can occur around the margins of an amalgam restoration.

Retention for indirect restorations, such as gold inlays or crowns, is accomplished with bonding agents and cements. Cements and bonding agents may be retained to the tooth surface by mechanical or chemical means. A **chemical retention** involves a chemical reaction between the tooth surface and the material.

Bonding

Bonding is the process by which materials adhere firmly or hold together. In dentistry, a bonding agent is used to bond the dentin and enamel with restorative materials.

Solubility

When a material is soluble, it dissolves in fluid. The solubility of a dental material is one factor used to determine its success in the oral cavity. A material that is soluble may be useful as a base or liner where it is not exposed to oral fluids. However, if the material is exposed to saliva, it dissolves and exposes the tooth structure.

Thermal Properties

Thermal conductivity is the ability of a material to transmit heat. With some materials heat transmits rapidly, while with others the process is very slow. The thermal conductivity of a material is a consideration when it is placed near the dental pulp, because a material that has a low rate of thermal conductivity offers more protection. Materials are placed in layers over the pulp to protect it from thermal changes. For example, the patient with a denture can drink hotter coffee because the denture base material has low thermal conductivity; thus, it protects the tissues under the denture. A metallic restoration placed near the pulp will have a high thermal conductivity and cause pain when drinking hot beverages.

Thermal expansion is another consideration for dental materials. With temperature changes, materials expand and contract. When materials are used in the oral cavity, they must expand and

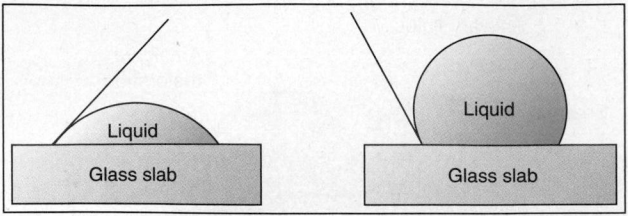

FIGURE 31-4
Examples of two materials' wettability.

contract at a rate close to that of the tooth structure. Dimensional changes that occur from thermal expansion and contraction can lead to microleakage, small cracks, and sensitive teeth.

Viscosity

The viscosity of a material is related to its ability to flow. The thicker the material, the less it flows; therefore, a thin material is less viscous and flows easily. Honey that is cool is thick and viscous, but when heated, it becomes thinner and less viscous. Materials that are more viscous do not spread easily over a surface. For example, if cement is too viscous, it will not flow over the tooth surface to produce adequate retention.

Wettability

The ability of a material to flow over a surface is wettability. This is an important property when applying certain dental materials. Wettability can be demonstrated by observing the shape of a drop on a solid material (Figure 31-4). If the drop spreads out (forming a low contact angle), the solid is readily wetted by the liquid. If the drop beads (forming a high contact angle), there is poor wetting of the solid. For instance, pit and fissure sealants should have good wettability in order to cover the grooves of the occlusal surface.

Regulations of Dental Materials

Dental materials are regulated and tested for function and safety before they become available for use. The ADA and the Food and Drug Administration (FDA) regulate dental materials. The ADA Council on Scientific Affairs is responsible for the testing of dental materials and periodically publishes a listing of certified dental materials in the *Journal of the American Dental Association* and in *Clinical Products in Dentistry: A Desktop Reference*.

In addition, the following international organizations develop standards for materials, instruments, and equipment produced around the world: the Fédération Dentaire Internationale and the International Standards Organization (ISO).

Although some materials used in dentistry have been around for a long time, there are constant changes and new products that are always being introduced. The dental team should be updated by attending seminars and dental conferences, reading books and professional magazines, and through local sales representatives.

The ADA Seal of Acceptance

The ADA, in cooperation with the government, sponsors research on more than 50 types of dental materials. From this research, specifications and standards are established. These standards are updated continually and are used to evaluate new materials. If a material meets specification requirements, the *ADA Seal of Certification* is awarded. This certifies that the material meets the criteria established by the ADA and the government, and that it is safe and effective.

For new types of dental materials, the ADA Council on Scientific Affairs conducts the program for evaluation and acceptance. Before these products are eligible to apply for the ADA Seal, they must be cleared by the U.S. Food and Drug Administration to be marketed directly to the consumer. These products may be marketed for over-the-counter sales or solely for oral health care professionals. The Council utilizes published technical standards, including ADA guidelines and specifications. There are guidelines to follow for companies and manufacturers that want to be in the acceptance program. Once the company or manufacturer has applied and been granted the Seal of Acceptance by the Council of Scientific Affairs, and after a license agreement has been signed, they can use the ADA Seal of Acceptance on their products. The *Seal of Acceptance of the ADA* indicates that the material has been proven to be safe and effective through biological, laboratory, and clinical evaluation. The following types of products may be included: therapeutic agents, drugs, chemicals, materials, instruments, and equipment used in the prevention of dental diseases. Cosmetic products may also be eligible for the seal. The ADA Seal of Acceptance is recognized by the public as a product endorsement by the dental profession; this assists them in making an informed decision when purchasing over-the-counter dental products.

Preparation for Placement of Dental Amalgam

After the patient has been anesthetized and the dental dam has been placed, the dentist performs the cavity preparation procedure and removes the decay using burs and handcutting instruments. The dentist is able to diagnose tooth decay through a variety of cavity detection methods. Cavities can be detected with radiographs, by probing with an explorer, or with the use of a special dye. This dye detects caries by distinguishing between good, sound, hard dentin, and dentin that is infected with bacteria and softened. The dye is placed in the preparation early in the procedure to avoid removing too much tooth structure. The dye is applied for about 10 seconds and then rinsed off. Burs and spoon excavators usually remove all the stained dentin. This process is repeated until no caries remain. This material can also be used to identify cracks and root canals.

Another noninvasive diagnostic tool, called the DIAGNOdent caries detection, is a Class II laser that measures fluorescence levels in the tooth structure to quantify caries progression.

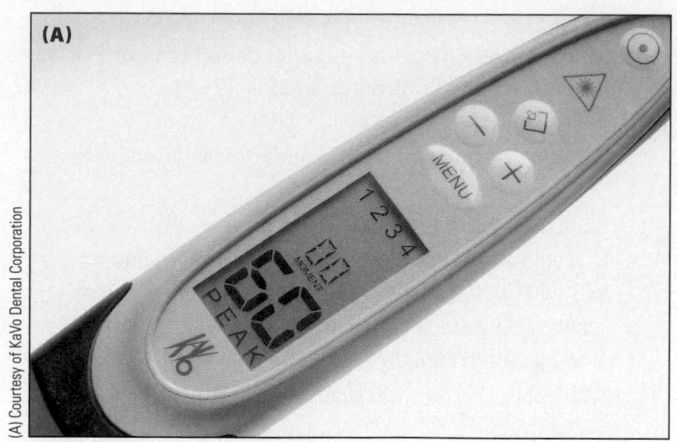

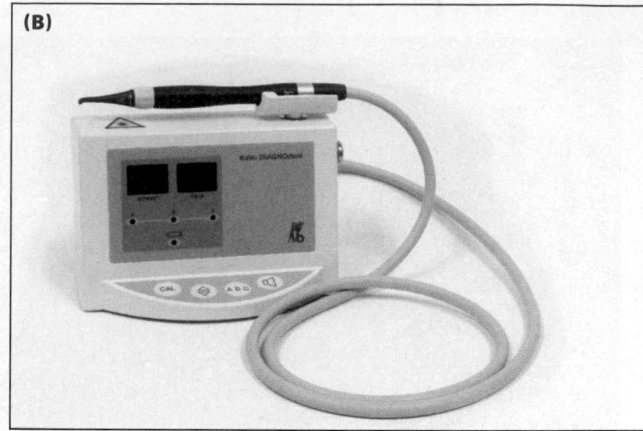

FIGURE 31-5
(A) DIAGNOdent pen. (B) DIAGNOdent unit.

The DIAGNOdent comes in a battery-operated, microprocessor-controlled display unit with handpiece and tips or a handheld pen unit for easier handling and greater mobility. Several tips are packaged with the units, and the tips can be sterilized (Figures 31-5A and B). Altered tooth structures and bacteria fluoresce (give off light) when exposed to specific wavelengths of light. A clean, healthy tooth structure exhibits little or no fluorescence, while a tooth with decay fluoresces according to the extent of the caries. The pen has a 90% detection rate of caries without cavitation (hidden cavities), proximal, and secondary caries. Healthy teeth register a low reading, while teeth with decay register higher readings. Laser units may also emit audio signals, which allow the dentist to hear as well as see display changes.

Benefits of using a laser caries detection unit include the following:

● Accurate diagnosis of hidden tooth decay
● Simple, fast, and painless
● Quantification of caries over time
● Early detection of initial caries
● Can be used by hygienist to detect suspicious areas requiring further examination (calculus and early periodontitis)
● Provides accurate visual and audio representation of the measured tooth structure

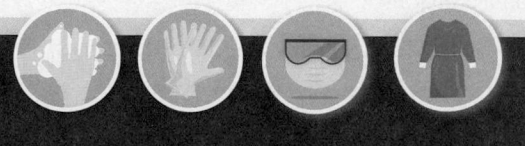

Safety

Laser Beam

Do not look into the laser beam. This unit may interfere with pacemakers.

Bases, Liners, and Varnishes

Treatment of cavity preparations varies with the amount of enamel and dentin removed, and how near the prep is to the pulp. A base, liner, and/or varnish may need to be placed prior to the amalgam material.

Cement Bases A cement base is mixed to a thick putty consistency and placed in the cavity preparation to protect the pulp and provide mechanical support for the restoration. These cement bases are placed on the floor of the cavity preparation to raise the level of the floor of the preparation to the ideal height (Procedure 31-1). There are several different types of cements that can be used for bases. These include glass ionomers, hybrid ionomers, reinforced ZOE, zinc phosphate, and polycarboxylate.

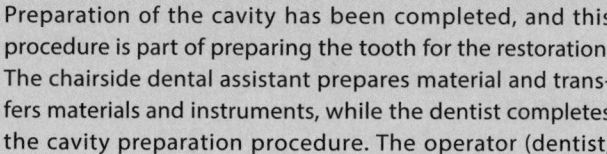

Procedure 31-1
Placing Cement Bases

Preparation of the cavity has been completed, and this procedure is part of preparing the tooth for the restoration. The chairside dental assistant prepares material and transfers materials and instruments, while the dentist completes the cavity preparation procedure. The operator (dentist,

dental hygienist, or qualified assistant) places the cement base.

Steps written in **blue** font are performed by the operator, and the chairside assistant's steps are written in black.

(Continues)

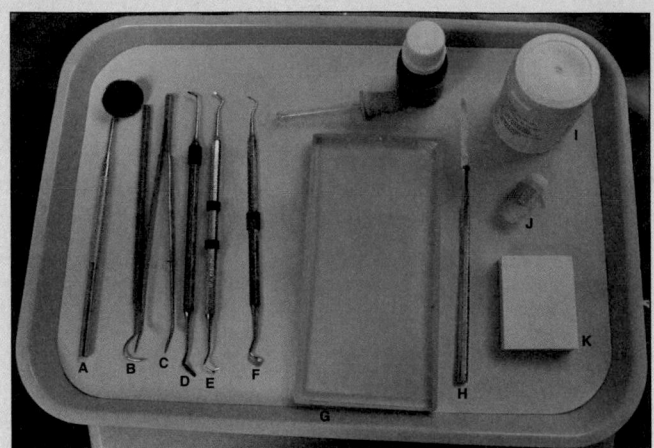

FIGURE 31-6
Cement base setup.

Equipment and Supplies (Figure 31-6)
Basic Setup
- mirror (A)
- explorer (B)
- cotton pliers (C)
- air/water syringe tip
- HVE tips

Cavity Preparation Setup
- plastic filling instrument (D)
- handcutting instruments (doctor's preference)
    - ❑ spoon excavator (E)
- low-speed and high-speed handpieces
- assortment of burs (doctor's preference)

Cement Base Setup
- amalgam condenser (F)
- glass slab (G)
- cement spatula (H)
- IRM powder, liquid, measurers and manufacturer's directions (I)
- IRM capsules and manufacturer's directions (J)
- mixing paper pad (K)
- amalgamator

Procedure Steps *(Follow aseptic procedures)*

Dentist completes cavity preparation procedure.

1. Use air/water syringe and HVE to remove debris as needed.
    - ❑ Rinse and dry area after dentist has prepared the tooth.
        - ❑ Do not overdry; overdrying may damage the pulp.

    Operator determines where to place the base and the size of the area.

    - ❑ Evaluates access and visibility.

2. Pass mirror and explorer.

3. Mix reinforced zinc oxide–eugenol dental cement manually (refer to Procedures 30-2).
    Or mix using a premeasured IRM capsule.
    - ❑ Set amalgamator time to manufacturer's directions for base consistency.
    - ❑ Activate capsule (firmly twist or press on capsule until you feel a snap as the membrane separating is broken and the liquid is released) at operator's signal.
    - ❑ Place capsule in ears of amalgamator and press to begin trituration.
    - ❑ Remove capsule from amalgamator after trituration.
    - ❑ Open capsule by removing cap and place mixed cement onto mixing surface (pad/glass slab).
    - ❑ Adjust consistency to operator's preference if needed using powder/liquid from bulk package; add powder to thicken mix or add liquid if mix is too thick.
    - ❑ Leave a small amount of powder on the slab.
    - ❑ Collect the base on the blade of the plastic filling instrument.

4. Assist in placing the cement.
    - ❑ Exchange explorer and plastic filling instrument.
    - ❑ Hold the glass slab in right hand under the patient's chin.
    - ❑ Hold gauze square in left hand to wipe plastic filling instrument as needed.

    Places the cement in the cavity preparation (Figure 31-7).

    - ❑ Condenses the cement into place on the floor of the cavity prep using the small condensing end of the plastic filling instrument or amalgam condenser.
    - ❑ If the material is sticky, places a small amount of the cement powder on the mixing pad and dips the end of the condenser as needed.
    - ❑ Continues until a sufficient base layer is placed.

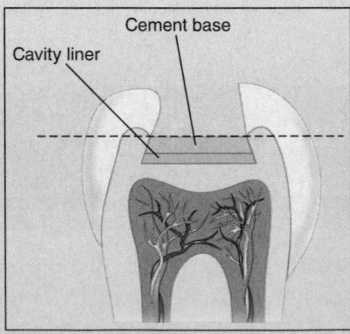

FIGURE 31-7
Placement of the cement base in a cavity preparation.

Evaluates the placement.
- ❏ Base should cover the floor of the cavity preparation.
- ❏ Leaves enough room for the restorative materials.
- ❏ Base is not on pins or in retentive grooves.

5. Exchange plastic filling instrument and explorer.

Removes any excess materials with an explorer.

6. Retrieve mirror and explorer.

7. Clean up the mixing materials.
- ❏ Remove cement from the spatula as soon as possible.
- ❏ Remove the paper from the pad or clean glass slab.

The preparation, sensitivity of the pulp, and type of restoration indicates which cement to use. These materials are often referred to as a high-strength base.

Cavity Liners
Calcium hydroxide cement is used as a low-strength base or liner under any restoration, such as in indirect or direct pulp capping procedures. This material has a therapeutic effect on the pulp. Calcium hydroxide is not necessary to form secondary dentin, but its slightly irritating effect provides the mild irritant that encourages secondary dentin to form. Also, calcium hydroxide has antibacterial properties that keep bacteria from actively spreading.

Calcium hydroxide comes in a powder/liquid form, a two-paste system, or a one-paste system. The form many offices use is the two-paste system: catalyst and base. Calcium hydroxide comes in a self-curing and a light-curing formula (Figure 31-8).

Composition
Calcium hydroxide has a complicated formula, with several ingredients in addition to calcium hydroxide. Some liners are radiolucent so they can be seen on a radiograph. The light-cured calcium hydroxide formula also contains a polymer resin.

Properties
Calcium hydroxide is low in strength and is placed in a thin layer near or over the pulp. It is easy to mix and place. The cement has low thermal conductivity but is usually not used in a thick enough layer to provide thermal protection. An insulating base may be placed over the thin layer of calcium hydroxide.

Manipulation Considerations
The two-paste system is mixed on a small paper pad with a metal spatula, an explorer, or a small ball-ended instrument (liner applicator; refer to Procedure 31-2).

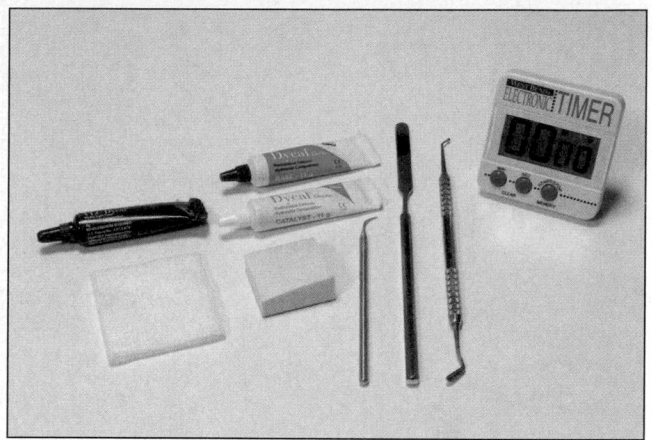

FIGURE 31-8
Various forms of calcium hydroxide, including the light-cured material (in the dark tube) and the two-paste materials.

The base and the catalyst of the two-paste system come as a set and cannot be interchanged with those of other calcium hydroxide paste systems.

This material is dispensed in equal portions and mixed for about 10–15 seconds. Setting times vary from 2–7 minutes.

Placement
A cavity liner is placed in the deepest portion of the cavity preparation on the axial walls or pulpal walls (Procedure 31-2). After the liner hardens, it forms a cement layer with minimum strength. It is placed on the dentin or on an exposed pulp. Liners protect the pulp from chemical irritations as well as provide a therapeutic effect to the tooth. Examples of cavity liners are calcium hydroxide, ZOE, and glass ionomer.

Procedure 31-2
Placing Calcium Hydroxide Cement Liner—Two-Paste System

The chairside dental assistant prepares material, and transfers materials and instruments, while the dentist completes the cavity preparation procedure. The operator (dentist, dental hygienist, or qualified assistant) can place the liner.

Steps written in **blue** font are performed by the dentist/operator, and the chairside assistant's steps are written in black.

Equipment and Supplies

Preprocedural Setup
- mirror and explorer
- air/water syringe tip
- HVE tips

(Continues)

Calcium Hydroxide Cement Liner Setup (Figure 31-9)

- manufacturer's directions
- calcium hydroxide two-paste system
- small paper pad
- small ball-ended instrument (liner applicator) or explorer
- 2 × 2 inch gauze sponge

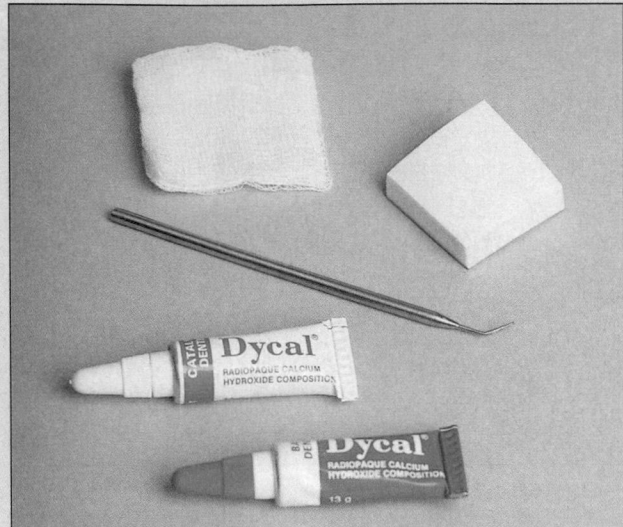

FIGURE 31-9
A two-paste calcium hydroxide tray setup.

Procedure Steps *(Follow aseptic procedures)*

Dentist completes cavity preparation procedure.

1. Use air/water syringe and HVE to remove debris as needed.
   - ❑ Rinse and dry area after dentist has prepared the tooth.
     - ❑ Do not overdry; overdrying may damage the pulp.

   Operator determines where to place the base and the size of the area.
   - ❑ **Evaluates access and visibility.**

2. Pass mirror and explorer.

3. Dispense small and equal amounts of both the base and catalyst onto the paper pad.
   - ❑ Base and catalyst should be close but not touching.
   - ❑ Wipe off the ends of the tubes and replace the caps.
   - ❑ Mix the two materials together using the liner applicator in a circular motion.

- ❑ Mix until the materials are a uniform color within the 10- to 15-second mixing time.
- ❑ Use a 2 × 2 inch gauze to remove excess material from the mixing instrument.

4. Assist in placing the liner.
   - ❑ Retrieve explorer.
   - ❑ Pass the liner applicator to the operator and hold the paper pad close to the patient's chin.
   - ❑ Between applications, wipe off the instrument with gauze for the operator.

   Places the liner on the floor of the preparation (Figure 31-10).
   - ❑ **Places the liner applicator into the mixed liner.**
   - ❑ **Places the liner in the deepest portion of the cavity preparation in a thin layer; the liner will flow into the area.**
   - ❑ **Be careful not to touch the instrument to the sides of the preparation.**
   - ❑ **Spreads the liner in the direction desired by pushing with the liner applicator.**
   - ❑ **Repeats this procedure until the liner covers the deepest portion of the cavity preparation.**
   - ❑ **Removes any liner from the enamel walls using an explorer.**

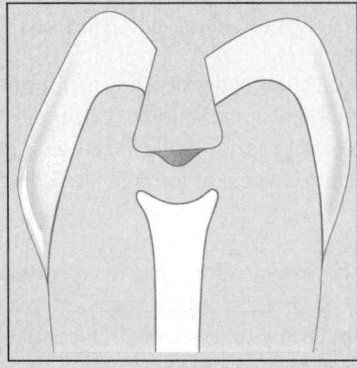

FIGURE 31-10
Placement of a cavity liner in preparation.

5. Exchange liner applicator and explorer.
   - ❑ Wipe off liner applicator.
   - ❑ Tear and fold the top page of the paper pad and dispose of it.
   - ❑ Disinfect the paper pad.

6. Retrieve mirror and explorer.

Cavity Varnish A cavity **varnish** is a material used to seal the dentin tubules that are exposed during an amalgam cavity preparation. The varnish prevents acids, saliva, and debris from reaching the pulp. Cavity varnish is used under amalgam restorations to prevent microleakage and under zinc phosphate cements to prevent penetration of acids to the pulp. If cavity liners or medicated bases are used, varnish is placed after or on top of these materials. This thin liquid is placed on the surface of the dentin only. There are various types of varnish, and some come with **solvents**.

Composition Cavity varnishes are resin solutions of different compositions. The copal varnish contains organic solvents (ether, acetone, or chloroform) and is used only under metal restorations because the solvent material in the varnish may interfere with the setting action of composite and resins. A universal varnish does not have organic solvents and may be used under all restorations.

Properties Varnishes are placed in a thin layer over the dentin tubules. The varnishes do not exhibit any strength and do not provide any thermal insulation. Cavity varnishes are insoluble in oral fluids and reduce leakage around the margins of restorations, thereby preventing microleakage. Varnish also prevents the penetration of acids from some cements into the dentin. These materials are nonacidic and nonirritating.

Manipulation Properties Cavity varnishes are often placed in two layers for greater protection and to prevent voids. Recap the varnish immediately to minimize its evaporation. The cavity varnish comes with a separate bottle of solvent. If the varnish becomes too thick, solvent can be added. The solvent can also be used to clean the applicator and to remove any varnish on the external tooth surfaces.

Cavity varnish is not mixed; it is placed over the liner, or it is placed directly on the tooth with various types of applicators, such as small cotton pellets or brushes (Procedure 31-3).

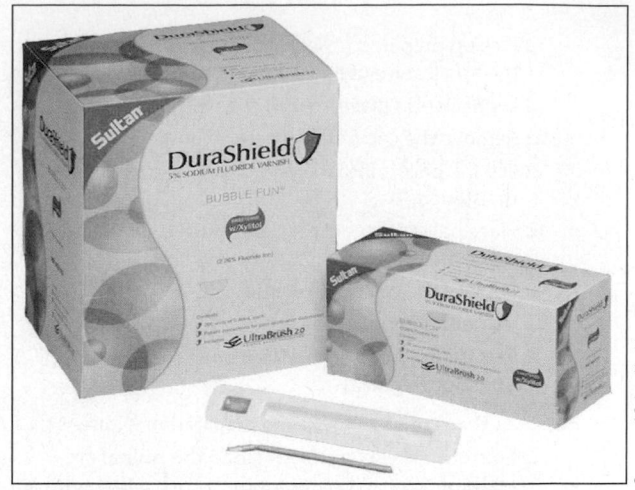

FIGURE 31-11
Fluoride varnish with disposable brush.

Courtesy of Sultan Healthcare

Fluoride Varnish Fluoride varnish is used to prevent dental decay. It is also a cavity varnish and desensitizer. This natural resin contains fluoride, which is slowly released once applied to the tooth surface (Figure 31-11).

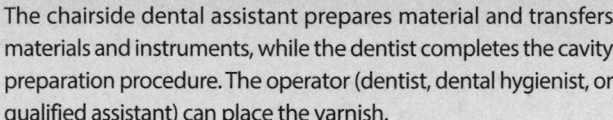

Procedure 31-3
Placing a Cavity Varnish

The chairside dental assistant prepares material and transfers materials and instruments, while the dentist completes the cavity preparation procedure. The operator (dentist, dental hygienist, or qualified assistant) can place the varnish.

Steps written in **blue** font are performed by the dentist/operator, and the chairside assistant's steps are written in black.

Preprocedural Setup
- mirror and explorer
- air/water syringe tip
- HVE tip

Equipment and Supplies (Figure 31-12)
- manufacturer's directions
- cavity varnish and solvent
- two cotton pliers
- small brushes or cotton pellets; some dentists may use cotton pellets rolled into small, football-shaped balls
- gauze squares

Procedure Steps *(Follow aseptic procedures)*

Dentist completes cavity preparation procedure.

1. Use air/water syringe and HVE to remove debris as needed.
   - ❏ Rinse and dry area after dentist has prepared the tooth.
   - ❏ Do not overdry; overdrying may damage the pulp.

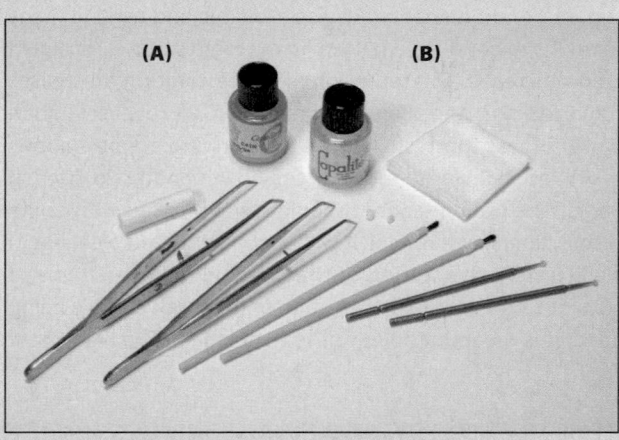

FIGURE 31-12
(A) Varnish and (B) solvent with an assortment of materials that can be used in the placement of the varnish: cotton pellets and cotton pliers, resin brushes, and microbrushes.

Operator evaluates the cavity preparation to determine access, visibility, and placement of the liner.

2. Pass mirror and explorer.

3. Prepare varnish.
   - ❏ Shape two very small cotton pellets about 2 mm in size to look like small footballs; roll pellet between thumb and middle finger.

(Continues)

❏ Pick up prepared pellets with the two cotton pliers for the application of two layers of varnish.

❏ Lock pliers in place holding the pellets.

❏ Remove the cap from the varnish bottle.

❏ Dip the pellets into the varnish until they are moistened.

❏ Place pellets on gauze square and dab off the excess varnish.

❏ Replace the cap on the varnish.

❏ Retrieve explorer.

❏ Pass cotton pliers with pellets one at a time at operator's signal.

Applies the varnish to the cavity preparation (Figure 31-13).

❏ **Paints a thin layer of varnish to the pulpal area, walls of the cavity preparation, and to the edge of the margins; do not place on enamel or flood the cavity prep.**

❏ **Allows the first coat to dry for 30 seconds.**

❏ **Applies the second coat using the second pellet to thoroughly coat the surface and fill in any voids.**

Evaluates the varnish placement.

4. Exchange cotton pellet and explorer.

Removes excess varnish with fresh cotton pellet or pellet dipped into solvent.

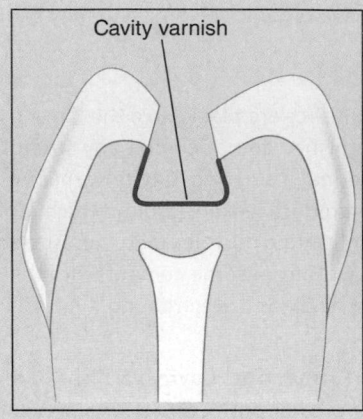

FIGURE 31-13
Placement of cavity varnish in preparation.

5. Pass fresh pellet in new sterile cotton pliers as needed to remove excess varnish.

❏ Never place anything that has been used in the mouth back in the bottle of varnish.

❏ Retrieve mirror and cotton pliers.

❏ Dispose of the cotton pellets.

❏ Clean the cotton pliers with solvent before sterilizing them.

6. Retrieve mirror and explorer.

Amalgam Bonding

Amalgam bonding agents are also available and used in many restorations to bond the amalgam to the tooth surface. Amalgam bonding increases the retention of the restoration, decreases marginal leakage, and allows for a more conservative restoration (removal of less tooth structure). The bonding agent is a low-viscosity resin similar to those discussed in Chapter 26, "Dental Sealants." The bonding agent should never be used with cavity varnishes, liners, or eugenol. It will be contaminated by eugenol and will inhibit the setting of the bonding material. It is also important to prevent contamination of the tooth surface being bonded; it is recommended to use dental dam. The placement

Sensitivity to Methacrylate and HEMA

Do not use amalgam bonding materials with persons who are sensitive to methacrylate or HEMA.

of the amalgam follows immediately, before the bonding agent sets (Procedure 31-4). Other retention methods, including the placement of retention pins and core buildups as covered in Chapter 30, can be used.

Procedure 31-4
Placing a Self-Curing Amalgam Bonding Agent

The chairside dental assistant prepares material and transfers materials and instruments, while the dentist completes the cavity preparation procedure. The operator (dentist, dental hygienist, or qualified assistant) can place the amalgam bonding agent (Figure 31-14).

Steps written in **blue** font are performed by the operator (dentist or qualified dental assistant), and the chairside assistant's steps are written in black.

Equipment and Supplies

Preprocedural Setup

- mirror and explorer
- air/water syringe tip
- HVE tip

Amalgam Bonding Setup

- manufacturer's directions

- dentin activation liquid
- adhesive agent
- bonding base bottle
- bonding catalyst bottle
- resin mixing wells
- resin brush
- suppled pellets
- gauze squares

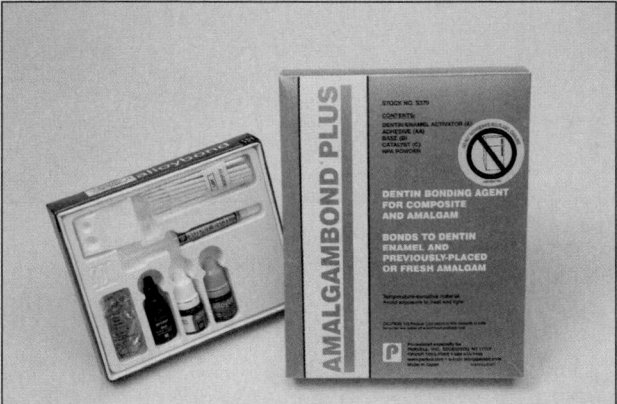

FIGURE 31-14
Amalgam bonding materials.

Procedure Steps *(Follow aseptic procedures)*

Dentist completes cavity preparation procedure.

1. Use air/water syringe and HVE to remove debris as needed.
   - ❑ Rinse and lightly dry area after dentist has prepared the tooth.
     - ❑ Do not overdry; overdrying may damage the pulp.
2. Prepare activator per manufacturer's directions.
   - ❑ Dispense 1 or 2 drops of activator into mixing well.
   - ❑ Pass mirror and brush.

- ❑ Hold mixing well with activator at patient's chin level with right hand.

Operator applies activator to exposed dentin for 10 seconds.

3. Rinse the tooth thoroughly to remove activator and lightly dry.
4. Prepare adhesive agent.
   - ❑ Dispense 1 or 2 drops of adhesive agent into mixing well.
   - ❑ Exchange brush with fresh brush.
   - ❑ Hold mixing well with adhesive agent at patient's chin level with right hand.

Operator applies adhesive agent.
   - ❑ **Brushes a thin layer of adhesive agent onto activated dentin surfaces.**

5. Exchange air/water syringe and brush.

Operator blows away puddles of agent with a gentle air stream to achieve an even, thin layer of coverage.
   - ❑ **Leaves undisturbed for 30 seconds.**

6. Begin trituration so alloy is ready to condense as soon as the amalgam and resin mixture of base/catalyst has been applied (alloy needs to be condensed while mix is wet).

7. Prepare resin mixture.
   - ❑ Dispense 2 drops of base and 1 drop of catalyst into a clean, dry mixing well.
   - ❑ Mix thoroughly with gentle stirring for 3–5 seconds.
   - ❑ Exchange air/water syringe and a fresh brush.
   - ❑ Hold mixing well with resin mix at patient's chin level with right hand.

Operator brushes a thin, even layer of resin mix onto dentin and enamel of cavity preparation.

8. Prepare to pass amalgam to operator.

Operator begins placement and condensation of amalgam immediately before the resin dries.

Treatment of Cavity Preparations

The cavity preparation for a restoration depends on the amount of decay, the location of the decay, and the type of materials used to restore the tooth. The operator examines the cavity preparation to assess pulpal involvement in order to determine when a liner, base, or varnish should be placed. Treatment of cavity preparations varies with the amount of enamel and dentin removed and how near the prep is to the pulp. Using the categories from Table 31-1, possible treatments are summarized as follows:

1. Treatment for an ideal cavity preparation:
   - A base is not required because only a minimal amount of enamel and dentin has been removed. Some dentists place only the restoration, while others prefer to place liner. If an amalgam restoration is going to be placed, two thin layers of cavity varnish are often placed over the dentin.

2. Treatment for a beyond-ideal cavity preparation:
   - With a beyond-ideal preparation, the level of the dentin is restored with a cement base.
   - With an amalgam restoration, there are several options. One option is to place two thin layers of varnish to seal the dentin tubules, and then place a layer of a cement base, such as zinc phosphate.
   - Another option is a reinforced ZOE base, which has a soothing effect on the pulp. Varnish is not used with this material.
   - Other options include a polycarboxylate or glass ionomer base, which also do not require a varnish.

3. Treatment for a near-exposure cavity preparation:
   - The closer the cavity preparation comes to the pulp, the more precautions are needed. There are also several options for treatment of the near-exposure preparation.

TABLE 31-1 Depth of Cavity Preparations and Pulpal Relation

Pulpal Involvement	Illustration
1. Ideal level This preparation does not involve the pulp but is through the enamel and just into the dentin. It is large enough to retain a restoration.	
2. Beyond ideal More enamel and dentin are removed, but the preparation is not close to the pulp.	
3. Near exposure This cavity preparation involves a large amount of enamel and dentin being removed, but the pulp is not exposed. The floor of the preparation may be slightly pink due to proximity to the pulp.	
4. Pulp exposure Enough enamel and dentin have been removed to expose a portion of the pulp. There will be blood in the cavity preparation.	

- With preparations that are going to be restored with amalgam, a liner of calcium hydroxide, glass ionomer, or ZOE is first placed over the deepest portion of the prep in the dentin. Once this layer is placed, two thin layers of varnish may be inserted over the exposed dentin. Then, a layer of cement base can be applied. Zinc phosphate, polycarboxylate, or glass ionomer cements can be used for this layer.

- Another option for amalgam restorations is to place a liner over the deepest portion of the preparation, then a layer of reinforced ZOE, polycarboxylate, or glass ionomer cement. This is then sealed with a cavity varnish.

- With some preparations, the dentist may choose not to place a cavity varnish.

- When a cavity liner is placed on a near exposure, the procedure is often referred to as an indirect pulp capping.

4. Treatment for an exposed-pulp cavity preparation:

- With an exposed pulp, the dentist must decide whether endodontic treatment is indicated or if an attempt should be made to save the vitality of the tooth. If the treatment of choice is to save the pulp, a procedure called a direct pulp capping (DPC) is performed.

- One treatment involves the placement of calcium hydroxide or a glass ionomer liner, which is then reinforced by ZOE as a temporary restoration. This gives the dentist time to see whether the pulp is going to heal.

- Another treatment involves the placement of a liner, followed by a layer of ZOE cement, two thin layers of varnish, and a cement base.

- Some dentists prefer to place a liner and then a layer of polycarboxylate or glass ionomer cement base.

Matrix Systems for Dental Amalgam

During the preparation of a tooth for an amalgam restoration, one or more axial surfaces may need to be removed (Class II cavity preparation). Once these surfaces are removed, the only way to restore the tooth is to have an artificial wall in place of the missing wall or surface. This wall holds the restorative materials in the preparation during the filling of the cavity. A **matrix** replaces the surface and acts as the artificial wall. A matrix is not needed when all the axial wall remain (Class I cavity preparation).

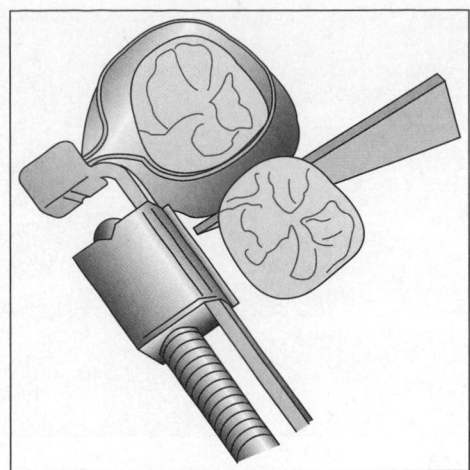

FIGURE 31-15
Occlusal aspect of the universal retainer, matrix band, and wooden wedge placed around the tooth.

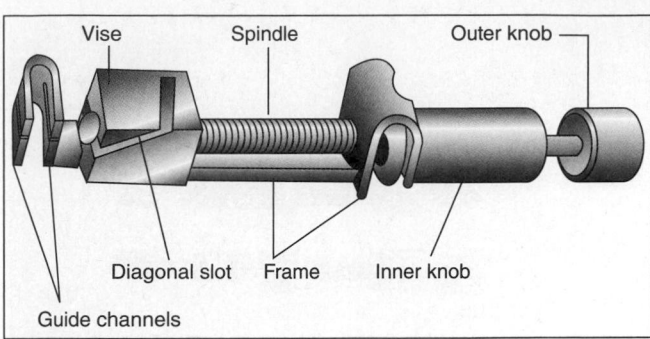

FIGURE 31-16
Parts of a straight universal retainer.

TABLE 31-2 Components of the Universal Retainer

Part	Function
Frame	Main body of retainer
Guide channels	Slots on the end of the retainer that hold the matrix band. The slots direct the band to the right or left of the retainer.
Vise (locking)	Holds the ends of the matrix band in place, in the diagonal slot
Spindle	A screw-like rod used to secure the band in the vise
Inner knob (adjusting knob)	Adjusts the size of the matrix band loop by moving the vise along the retainer frame
Outer knob (locking knob)	Tightens and loosens the spindle against the band in the vise

Several different matrix systems are available, and the type of matrix selected depends on the location of the preparation and type of restorative materials being used. For amalgam restorations, the universal matrix, the AutoMatrix, sectional matrix systems, or the T-band matrix is used.

Universal Matrix Retainer

The *matrix* is a collective term used to refer to the matrix band and the **retainer** (Figure 31-15). The matrix band forms the missing surface or wall and reestablishes the normal contour of the prepared tooth while the tooth is being filled with the restorative material. The matrix band is inserted into the retainer and then placed on the tooth. The retainer is the device that holds the band. It is tightened on the tooth and secures the band in place.

The universal retainer, also referred to as the Tofflemire retainer, is the most common matrix and retainer system used for amalgam restorations. A stainless steel matrix band is placed into the universal retainer and placed onto the prepared tooth. Wedges are used to secure the matrix band and to the keep the gingival portion tightly in place against the tooth.

Parts of the Universal Matrix Retainer This

retainer has a top (occlusal) side and a bottom (gingival) side (Figure 31-16). The occlusal side is the smooth side of the guide channels and the vise and is directed toward the occlusal surface. The gingival side is directed toward the gingival tissues and has the diagonal slot on the vise and the open ends of the guide channels. Table 31-2 describes the parts and functions of the universal matrix retainer.

Universal Retainer Styles The universal retainer is avail-

able in several styles so that it can be positioned from either the lingual or the facial surfaces. The straight universal retainer is the most commonly used, and it is placed on the buccal or facial side, while the *contra-angle* universal retainer is placed on the lingual surface. It is angled slightly to accommodate the clearance of the anterior teeth (Figure 31-17).

Matrix Bands Matrix bands are made of stainless steel and

are approximately all the same length. They differ in the shape of one edge and their widths (Figure 31-18). The size and shape of the cavity prep indicate which band is used. The more the prep extends toward the gingiva, the wider the matrix band needs to be. The matrix band is slightly curved, and when it is looped over so that both ends meet, the small **circumference** edge faces toward the gingiva and the larger circumference edge faces toward the occlusal surface when placed in the universal retainer. (See Procedure 31-5 for steps in assembling and placing the universal matrix band and retainer.)

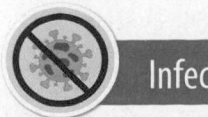 **Infection Control**

The retainer can be sterilized and reused. The bands and wedges are sharp and must be disposed of in the sharps container after the procedure.

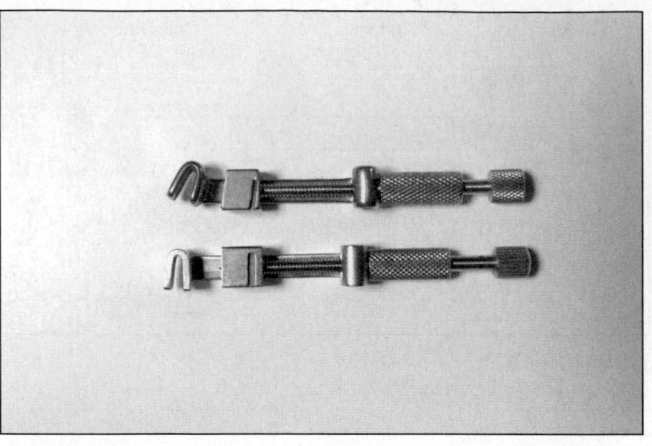

FIGURE 31-17
Top: contra-angle universal retainer (note the angle of the guide channel section). Bottom: straight universal retainer.

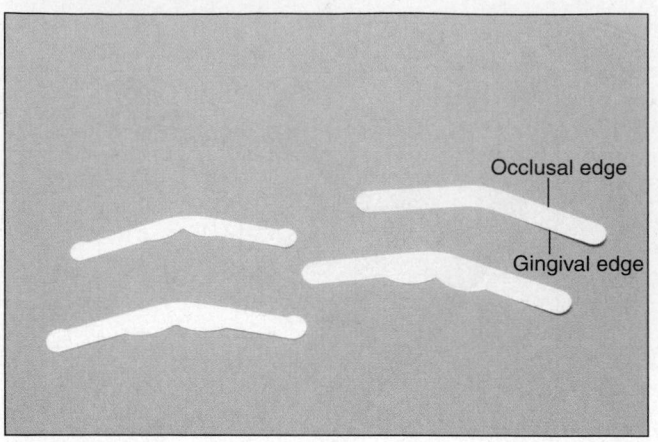

FIGURE 31-18
Examples of various matrix bands. The extension of cavity preparation determines the width of the band selection. The gingival and occlusal edge of the matrix band should extend the cavosurface margin of the cavity preparation.

Procedure 31-5
Assembly of the Universal Matrix and Retainer

This procedure is performed by the dentist or the dental assistant. Assembly of the matrix and retainer is completed by the assistant before the procedure begins. The operator (dentist, dental hygienist, or qualified assistant) places the universal matrix and retainer.

Equipment and Supplies
- universal retainer
- assortment of matrix bands

Procedure Steps (*Follow aseptic procedures*)

1. Hold the retainer with the guide channels and the diagonal slot on the vise facing up.

2. While holding the frame of the retainer, rotate the inner knob (adjustment knob) until the vise is within ¼ inch of the guide channels.

3. Turn the outer knob (locking knob) until the pointed end of the spindle is clear (below) of the slot in the vise.

4. Prepare the matrix band for placement in the retainer by holding the band to look like a smile (matrix band curves upward), with the gingival edge on the top and the occlusal edge on the bottom.

5. Bring the ends together to form a teardrop-shaped loop (Figure 31-19). Be careful not to crease the band at any time. The larger circumference of the band, the occlusal edge will be on the bottom, and the smaller circumference, the gingival edge, will be on the top.

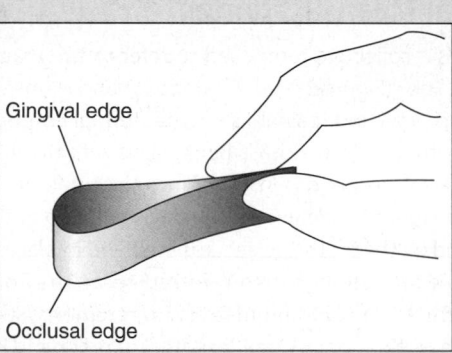

FIGURE 31-19
Hold the matrix band in a smile and loop the ends of the band together. The smaller circumference, the gingival edge, will be on the top, and the larger circumference, the occlusal edge, will be on the bottom.

6. With the gingival edge still on the top, place the occlusal edge of the band in the diagonal slot of the vise. The loop is extended toward the guide channels.

7. Place the matrix band in the facing to the left or right of the guide channels (Figure 31-20).
   - ❏ Place the matrix band in the guide channels toward the right if the matrix is to be placed on the maxillary right or mandibular left quadrant (Figure 31-21).
   - ❏ Place the matrix band in the guide channels toward the left if the matrix is to be placed on the maxillary left or mandibular right quadrant.

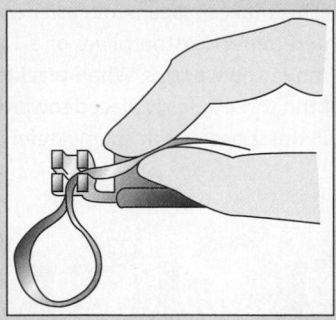

FIGURE 31-20
Hold the universal retainer with the guide channels and slot facing up and insert the matrix band into the vise slot and guide channels.

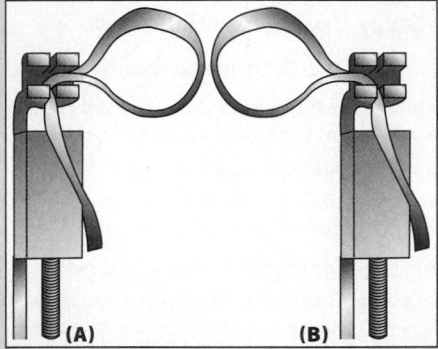

FIGURE 31-21
(A) Placement of matrix band in retainer for maxillary right/mandibular left.
(B) Placement of matrix band in retainer for maxillary left/mandibular right.

8. Once the band is placed in the vise slot with the guide channels, turn the outer knob until the tip of the spindle is tight against the band in the vise slot (Figure 31-22).

9. Move the inner knob to increase or decrease the size of the loop to match the diameter of the tooth.

10. If the band becomes creased or bent during the assembly, it can be smoothed out by inserting the handle of the mouth mirror into the loop and running it around the inside of the loop (similar to curling ribbon when wrapping a gift).

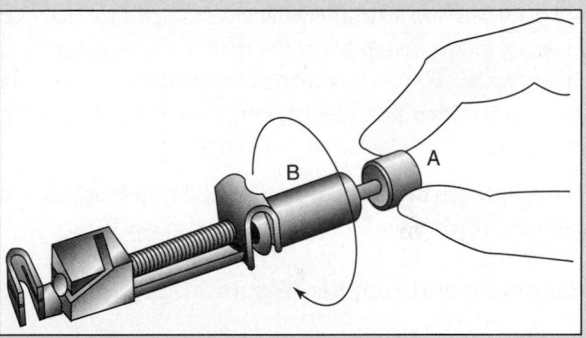

FIGURE 31-22
(A) By turning the outer knob of the universal retainer, the band will be secured. (B) By turning the inner knob of the universal retainer, the matrix band loop increases and decreases in size.

Wedges In addition to replacing the missing tooth surface of the cavity preparation, the matrix restores the natural contours of the tooth and the proximal contact with the adjacent tooth. The matrix must be stable enough to withstand the pressure of the restorative material being condensed in the cavity preparation. A matrix needs to be placed securely to contain the amalgam material within the walls to prevent any excess material from getting near the gingiva. Placing a wedge can help in securing the placement of the matrix band.

Once the matrix is in place around the tooth, a wedge (a small, triangular piece of wood or plastic) is inserted interproximally against the matrix band near the gingival margin of the preparation. This **wedge** holds the band securely in place and also prevents excess filling material from escaping between the tooth and the matrix band. This excess is called an **overhang**. An overhang can be damaging to the gingival tissues if left in place, so the correct positioning of the wedge is important in order to prevent this from occurring. The wedge also slightly separates the teeth to compensate for the thickness of the band. This ensures good contact with the adjacent tooth after the band has been removed.

Wedge Types Wedges are supplied in different sizes and are either natural wood, clear, or colored. They usually come in an

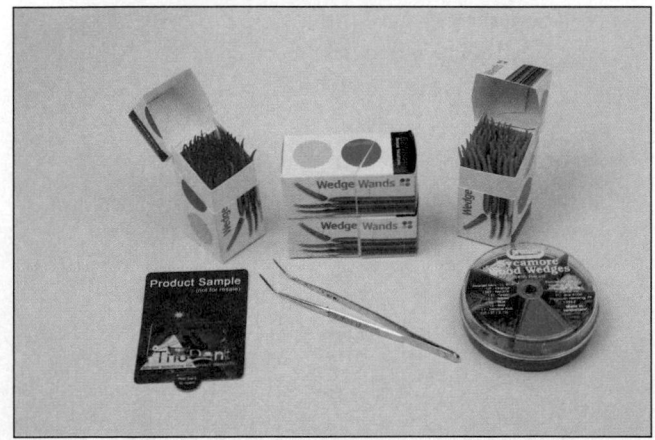

FIGURE 31-23
Assortment of wedges showing different sizes and types.

assortment kit with various sizes, with colors marking the different sizes (Figure 31-23). Some wedges can be altered in shape with a knife, if needed. Once the procedure is complete, the wedges are discarded.

Wedge Placement Wedges are only used when the preparation includes a proximal surface(s). For example, if the tooth had a mesio-occlusal (MO) cavity preparation, only one wedge would be needed on the mesial. For a MOD cavity preparation, a wedge would be needed on both the mesial and distal. On the posterior teeth, either the wooden or plastic wedges can be used.

The wedges are usually placed from the lingual side on the posterior teeth. This makes placement easier and prevents interference with the retainer. Cotton pliers or a 110 plier can used to place and remove the wedges. When placing the wedge, the base (largest) of the three sides is placed toward the gingiva. The wedge should fill the space and fit snugly (refer to Figure 31-15).

Procedure 31-6
Placement and Removal of the Universal Matrix

The chairside dental assistant prepares materials and transfers materials and instruments while the operator places the universal matrix. Assembly of the matrix and retainer is completed by the assistant before the procedure begins. The operator (dentist, dental hygienist, or qualified assistant) places and removes the universal matrix and retainer.

Steps written in **blue** font are performed by the operator and the chairside assistant's steps are written in black.

Equipment and Supplies (Figure 31-24)

Preprocedural Setup
- mirror and explorer
- air/water syringe tip
- HVE syringe tip

Universal Matrix Setup
- assembled universal retainer and matrix band
- cotton pliers or 110 pliers
- ball burnisher
- 2 × 2 inch gauze sponges
- assortment of wedges

Placement of the Wedge and Universal Matrix

Procedure Steps *(Follow aseptic procedures)*

1. Pass assembled matrix band and retainer.

   Places the matrix band over the prepared tooth with the smaller opening of the band toward the gingiva.
   - ❏ **Directs the slot on the vise toward the gingiva.**
   - ❏ **Keeps the retainer parallel to the buccal surface as the loop is placed around the tooth.**

   Eases the loop through the interproximal surface.
   - ❏ **Places one finger over the loop to stabilize the loop and the retainer.**
   - ❏ **Gently presses the matrix below the gingival cavo-surface margin.**
   - ❏ **Uses a wedge to widen the space if there is difficulty in getting the matrix through the contact area.**
   - ❏ **Adjusts the guide channel to center the retainer on the buccal surface of the tooth once the matrix band is around the tooth (Figure 31-25).**

   Turns the inner knob to tighten the band around the tooth.
   - ❏ **Band should be secure around the tooth.**

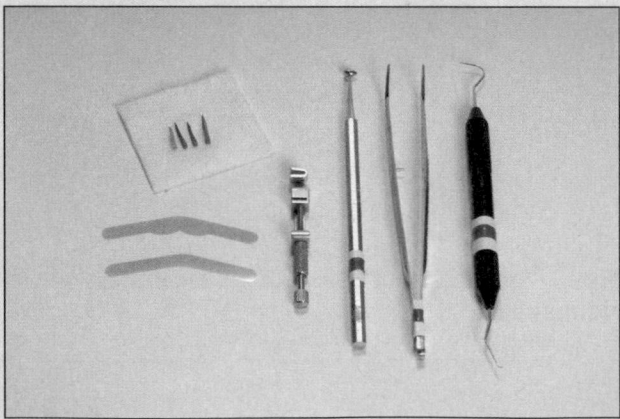

FIGURE 31-24
The materials needed for the placement of the universal matrix.

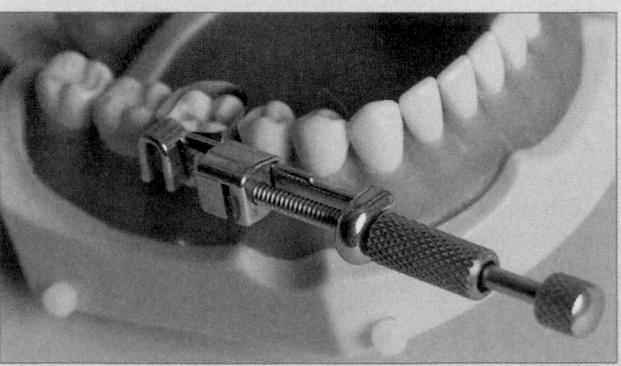

FIGURE 31-25
Placing the universal retainer with a matrix on a tooth, and centering the retainer on the buccal surface of the tooth.

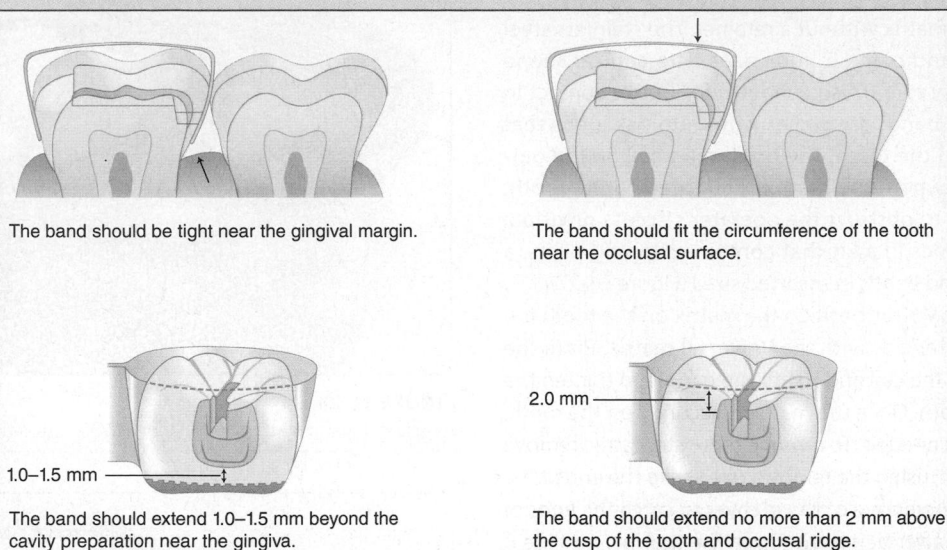

The band should be tight near the gingival margin.

The band should fit the circumference of the tooth near the occlusal surface.

1.0–1.5 mm

The band should extend 1.0–1.5 mm beyond the cavity preparation near the gingiva.

2.0 mm

The band should extend no more than 2 mm above the cusp of the tooth and occlusal ridge.

FIGURE 31-26
Criteria for correctly placed matrix band.

❏ **Retainer should be snug to the tooth. If the band is too tight or too loose, the contour of the restoration may change the contours of the tooth and the proximal contact.**

2. Pass mirror and explorer.

   Checks the margins of the matrix band using mirror and explorer.
   ❏ **Band should extend no more than 1–1.5 mm beyond the gingival cavosurface margin.**
   ❏ **Occlusal edge should extend no more than 2 mm above the highest cusp (Figure 31-26).**

3. Exchange explorer and ball burnisher.

   Uses a ball burnisher to contour the band and ensure contact with the adjacent teeth.
   ❏ **Places the burnisher on the inner surface of the band.**
   ❏ **Applies pressure until the band becomes slightly concave at the contact area.**

4. Retrieve mirror and burnisher.

5. Pass cotton pliers with right hand and hold wedge in palm of right hand.

   Picks up wedge with the base toward the gingiva.

   Places the base wedge(s) toward the gingiva.

   Gently presses the wedge into the interproximal space to stabilize the band at the gingival margin of the preparation.

6. Retrieve cotton pliers and pass mirror and explorer.

   Checks the seal at the gingival margin of the preparation with an explorer. There should be no gap between the band and the preparation.

Removal of the Wedge and Matrix

This procedure is performed by the operator with assistance by the dental assistant. Once the tooth has been filled with restorative material, the matrix and wedge are removed to finish carving the anatomy of the tooth.

Procedure Steps *(Follow aseptic procedures)*

1. Pass cotton pliers or 110 forceps.

   Removes wedge.
   ❏ **Grasps the wedge at the base with the pliers and pulls in the opposite direction of the insertion.**

2. Retrieve pliers and wedge.

   Removes the retainer.
   ❏ **Holds the matrix in place with a finger on the occlusal surface.**
   ❏ **Turns the outer knob of the retainer to loosen the spindle in the vise.**
   ❏ **Separates the retainer from the band by lifting the retainer toward the occlusal surface.**

3. Retrieve retainer and pass cotton pliers.

   Removes the band.
   ❏ **Grasps band with cotton pliers.**
   ❏ **Gently frees the band from around the tooth.**
   ❏ **Lifts one end of the band in a linguo–occlusal direction.**
   ❏ **Lifts the band from the proximal surface.**
   ❏ **Repeats with the other end of the band. The tooth is ready for the final carving.**

4. Retrieve cotton pliers and pass operator's choice of carver.

AutoMatrix

The AutoMatrix is a matrix without a retainer. The stainless steel bands are conical and come in four sizes. The conical shape makes the band easy to burnish (smooth) for better contact in proximal areas. The bands are circles with autolock loops that lock the matrices on the teeth. The tightening coil on the outside of the band is where the matrix is adapted to the tooth. There is no retainer to obstruct the operator's access or vision. The AutoMatrix comes in a kit that contains clipping pliers, a tightening device, and bands in assorted sizes (Figure 31-27).

To place the AutoMatrix, position the matrix on the tooth following the same criteria as with the universal matrix. Place the tightening device in the coil and rotate the handle to tighten the band around the tooth. Once the matrix is securely on the tooth, place the wedges as needed. To remove the AutoMatrix, remove the wedges and then, using the removal pliers, clip the end of the autolock loop. The pliers have a plastic cover to catch the ends of the loop as they fall after being cut. Open the matrix and slide it toward the buccal or lingual sides while pulling it occlusally.

Sectional Matrix Systems

A sectional matrix system is most often used on Class II restorations to restore anatomical contacts. The matrix is stable and produces a tight contact with no overhangs. The system consists of oval matrix bands, rings to hold the matrix bands, and forceps to place the rings. The oval-shaped matrix bands are contoured and come in different sizes. They are slightly thicker than the universal matrix bands. The rings are used to hold the matrix bands in place and usually come in two different sizes. The forceps are designed to open the rings for placement and removal. They are like dental dam forceps except the ends are shorter, broader, and angled slightly for better retention.

A separate matrix band/ring is used for each surface, so on a mesio-occluso-distal (MOD) two-matrix bands/rings would be used. Placing the sectional matrix takes some practice, but once the procedure is learned it can be done quickly to produce a

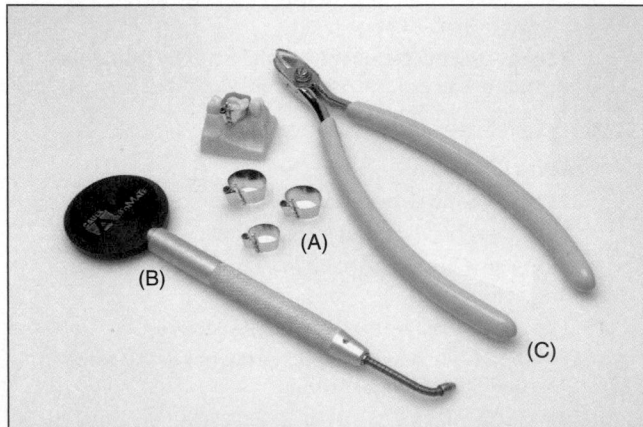

FIGURE 31-27
AutoMatrix kit including (A) matrix with coil, (B) tightening device, (C) removal pliers.

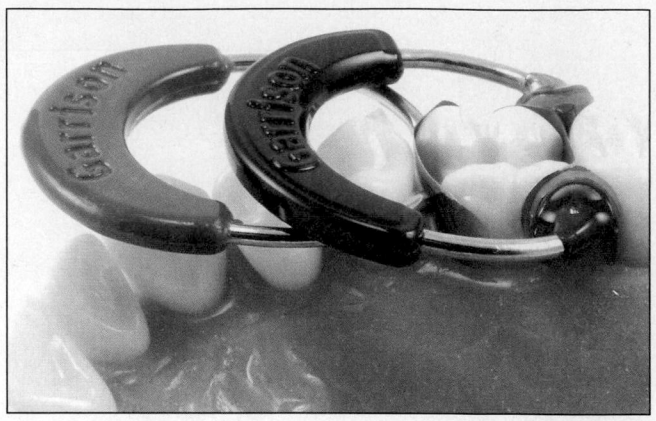

FIGURE 31-28
A sectional matrix system in place for a MOD restoration placement.

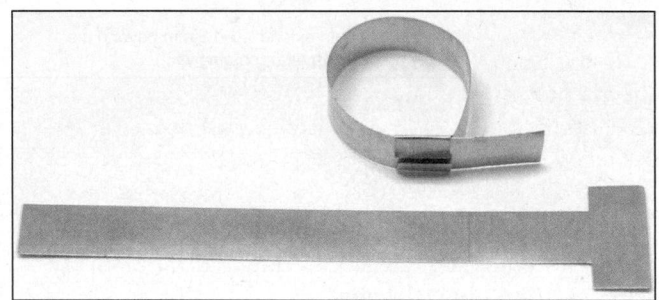

FIGURE 31-29
T-band as supplied (bottom image) and T-band prepared for placement (top image).

functional matrix. Wedges are used with this matrix system. They are usually placed after the band is placed and before the ring is positioned. The main function of the wedge with this system is to prevent gingival overhangs (Figure 31-28).

T-band Matrices

T-bands are made of pliable, thin brass in the shape of the capital letter T (Figure 31-29). T-bands are a preformed matrix. When looped into a circle, the extensions can be secured and adjusted to the size of the tooth. They do not require the use of a retainer. When placing a Class II restoration in a primary tooth, a T-band can be used instead of the larger adult matrix band. They may also be needed where a retainer will not fit into the preparation area of an adult. (Details of the placement of the T-band are covered in Chapter 34, "Pediatric Dentistry.")

Dental Amalgam

One of the most common restorative materials is **dental amalgam**, which has been used for many years (Figure 31-30). Dental amalgam is an effective, long-lasting, and comparatively inexpensive restorative material. Amalgam is a combination of an **alloy** with **mercury**. An alloy is the combination of two or more metals, and mercury bind the alloy particles together to form a uniform and workable mass.

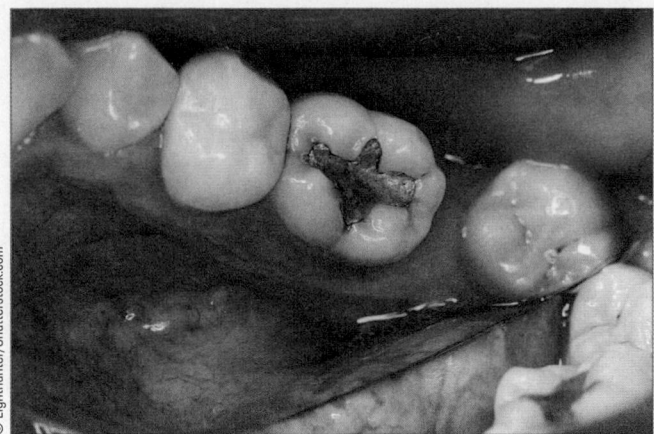

FIGURE 31-30
Occlusal amalgam restoration on a mandibular molar.

© Lighthunter/Shutterstock.com

The indications for placing amalgam fillings include the following:

- A long success record
- Working well in areas that are difficult to keep dry (moisture control)
- Can be used on both primary and permanent teeth
- Less technique sensitive
- Poor patient oral hygiene
- Less expensive restorative material

The contraindications include the following:

- Poor esthetics, as amalgam is a silver material
- Controversy about the mercury content and allergies
- Used only on the posterior teeth
- Occasional discoloration around the margins of the restoration

Dental amalgam is pliable when first mixed, so it is easily placed in the cavity preparation. It is carved before hardening to resemble the tooth structure and regain function. This material is used only on the posterior teeth because of its strength and because it is not **esthetically** pleasing.

Composition

Dental amalgam is composed of silver, tin, copper, and zinc (optional) to form an alloy. This alloy is mixed with mercury to form the amalgam. The ADA has specifications that regulate the composition of dental amalgam (Table 31-3) for the characteristics of each of the alloy components).

TABLE 31-3 Dental Amalgam Composition

Silver	**40–70%** **High-copper amalgam** **68–72%** **Low-copper mix** • Used to form a metallic compound with mercury (Hg), which determines the dimensional changes that occur during hardening • Increases restoration strength • Increases expansion • Is slow to amalgamate • Hardens rapidly • Tarnishes easily • Decreases setting time
Tin	**22–30%** **High-copper amalgam** **26–37%** **Low-copper amalgam** • Aids in amalgamation (chemical combining) of alloy with Hg because of its strong Hg affinity • Reduces expansion during setting • Reduces strength • Setting time is slower • Is more susceptible to corrosion (conventional alloy) • Tends to weaken amalgam
Copper	**12–30%** **High-copper amalgam** **4–5%** **Low-copper amalgam** • Increases strength and hardness • Increases expansion of amalgam during hardening • Reduces the flow of finished restoration • Resists corrosion (high copper) • Reduces marginal failure (high copper)
Zinc	**0–1%** **For high- and low-copper amalgams** • Minimizes the oxidation of other metals in the alloy during manufacturing. Zinc is a scavenger and reacts with oxygen, preventing it from combining with silver, tin, or copper. Note: Should moisture contamination occur during the manipulation or condensation of the amalgam, delayed expansion might occur. zinc-containing dental amalgams are particularly sensitive to moisture. Zinc reacts with water to form zinc oxide and hydrogen gas, which may cause the unwanted and excessive expansion of the set amalgam restoration.

Types of Dental Amalgam

Dental amalgam consists of a low- and a high-copper and a zinc and zinc-free alloy. Metals for the alloys are prepared in several ways to produce the lathe cut (**comminuted** particles) and **spherically** shaped particles. The way these metals are prepared affects their properties. Low-copper alloys are available with comminuted and spherical particles. High-copper alloys are supplied as comminuted, spherical, or combination particles (*admix*).

Spherical alloys have smoother surfaces that require less mercury when mixed. These alloys are also easier to condense and have improved carving and polishing properties. Combination alloys adapt better to the cavity preparation and produce better contacts with the adjacent teeth.

Although zinc in the dental amalgam acts as a scavenger of oxygen and prevents oxidation, when it comes in contact with moisture, it produces hydrogen gas and causes a delayed expansion, pain, deterioration, and eventual tooth fracture. When the working area cannot remain moisture free during placement, the dentist will select a zinc-free amalgam. Zinc-free amalgam tends to be less pliable and has a higher incidence of marginal breakdown of the restoration.

Forms of Dental Alloy

Dental alloy is purchased in a disposable **capsule** form. The capsule contains a premeasured amount of alloy and mercury and sometimes a pestle. The pestle is made of metal or plastic and aids in the mixing of the alloy and mercury. In the capsule, a thin membrane separates the alloy and the mercury until they are mixed. Some capsules come with activators to break the membrane, while others are twisted or compressed before being mixed. The capsules are most often plastic and come with screw-type or friction-fit caps. Disposable capsules are color coded to distinguish single, double, and triple mixes (also called spills). A single mix makes a small amount of amalgam with a 1:1 weight ratio of alloy to mercury, double mix is a 2:2 ratio, and the largest mix is the triple mix with a 3: 3 ratio (Figure 31-31).

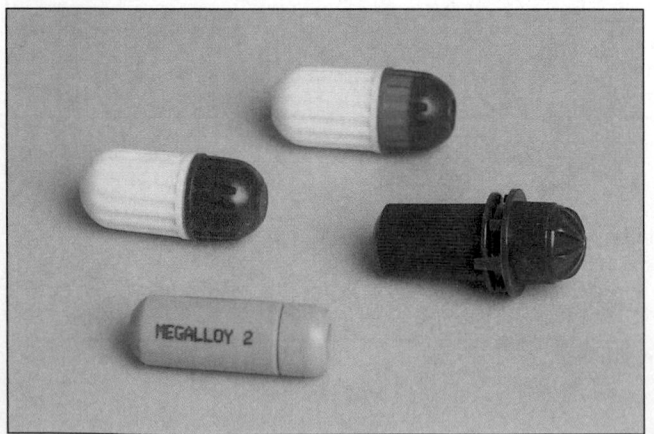

FIGURE 31-31
Samples of amalgam capsules.

Mercury Used in Dental Amalgam

Dental mercury is a very toxic chemical and must meet the specifications listed by the ADA. Dental professionals are aware of the hazards and safety measures when working with dental mercury to prevent problems from occurring.

Mercury is the only metal that is in a liquid state and vaporizes (particles of mercury scatter and float freely in the air) at a relatively low room temperature. Mercury is absorbed through the pores of the skin and through inhalation. Some potential sources of mercury contamination in the dental office are as follows:

- Mercury leaking out of a capsule during trituration
- Mercury vapor occurring during triturating and dispensing
- Polishing an amalgam restoration
- Removal of a hardened amalgam restoration
- Contact with the amalgam during the procedure
- Carpeting in the treatment rooms that retains amalgam particles; vacuuming these surfaces disperses the mercury through the air
- Scraps of amalgam left in an open container

Studies have revealed that in most dental offices, the level of mercury vapor is well below the maximum safe environmental concentration levels. Another study testing the blood mercury level in dentists displayed a reading well below the level at which symptoms begin to show.

There has been some concern about the level of mercury in patients with numerous amalgam restorations. Recent studies have shown that these patients ingest a very low amount of mercury from the amalgam fillings, well below what they would ingest from food, water, and the atmosphere. A small number of people have a possible risk for an allergic reaction to mercury. The response manifests as a skin reaction that appears after the placement of an amalgam restoration. Including questions on the medical history is a prevention step. Because of these concerns, the dentist and dental assistant should stay current with research and ADA recommendations.

Amalgam Properties

Proper manipulation of the amalgam is important in the overall strength and success of the restoration. The strength of the amalgam is not adequate to withstand occlusal forces alone. The preparation is designed so that the remaining tooth structure sustains the forces to the amalgam.

Amalgam is subject to dimensional change, such as expansion and contraction. The amount of expansion and contraction is controlled by the composition of the alloy and the manipulation techniques.

Another property of amalgam is the ability of the material to *creep*. Creeping is a change in the material when under a constant load.

Amalgam restorations are subject to *corrosion* and *tarnish* in the oral cavity. Tarnish is the discoloration of the surface, and corrosion is the deterioration of the surface (Figure 31-33). The

Safety

Mercury Hygiene

The ADA recommends that a program of mercury hygiene be established at every dental practice. Potential office hazards involving mercury can be eliminated by practicing appropriate mercury hygiene. Guidelines include the following:

- Wear disposable gloves, a facemask, and protective glasses when working with the amalgam.
- Educate all personnel regarding the potential hazards of mercury, as well as good mercury hygiene practices.
- A no-touch technique should be used when handling mercury. If the skin is exposed, wash with soap and water, and rinse under running water.
- Use capsules containing a measured amount of mercury and alloy.
- Use an amalgamator with a protective cover both to reduce the chance of any mercury vapor being released and to confine any mercury that might be sprayed from an ill-fitting capsule.
- Store mercury and amalgam scraps in capped, wide-mouthed, unbreakable jars containing used x-ray fixer, finely divided sulfur, glycerin, or mineral oil (amalgam scrap container).
- Carpeting in dental treatment rooms is not recommended. Carpeting retains mercury, which is difficult to retrieve.
- Use water spray and high-volume evacuation when cutting old amalgams or polishing new restorations. Wear a mask during these procedures.
- Avoid working with mercury or amalgam near a heat source, such as the autoclave.
- Handle mercury only over **impervious** surfaces. The area should have a continuous lip to retain any spillage.
- The office should have proper ventilation to reduce the possibility of mercury vapor inhalation. Change the air filter frequently.
- Change the chairside traps by placing the disposable traps into a container that is marked "Contact Amalgam Waste for Recycling." For the reusable traps, remove the trap from the dental unit and empty contents in the marked container.
- Office personnel should have periodic urinalyses to check for any mercury in the body.
- Monitor the dental office to determine mercury levels.
- Keep a mercury spill kit if the office uses large quantities of mercury. Clean up any mercury scraps or spills immediately, following OSHA recommendations (Figure 31-32).

combination (admixed) and the spherical high-copper amalgams are less susceptible to corrosion. Careful finishing and polishing of the amalgams reduces tarnish and corrosion.

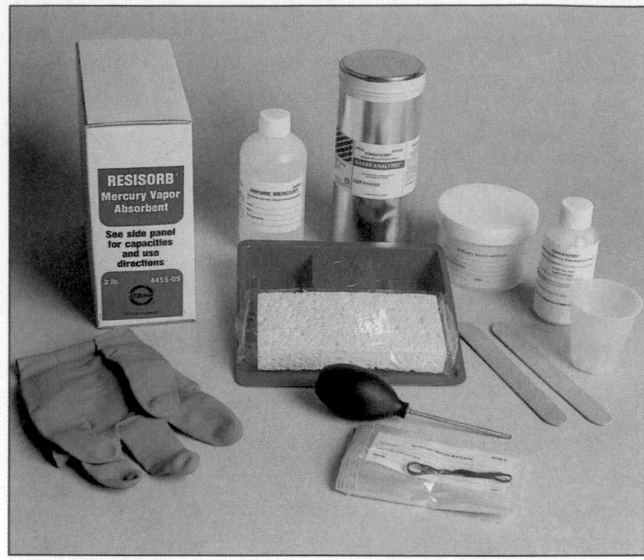

FIGURE 31-32
Mercury spill kit.

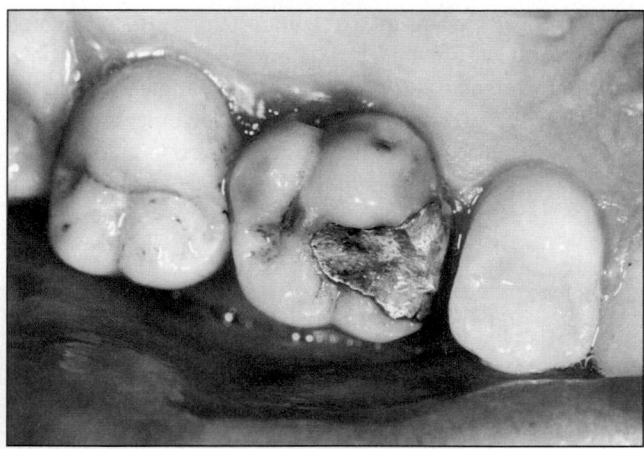

FIGURE 31-33
Tarnished and corroded amalgam restoration and secondary decay are present.

Amalgam Manipulation

The process of **trituration** is the mechanical combining (mixing) of the dental alloy and mercury. The process of **amalgamation** is the actual chemical reaction that occurs between the alloy and the mercury that forms the silver amalgam. A specially designed machine is used to triturate (amalgamate) the alloy and mercury; it's called a dental **amalgamator** or **triturator**. These machines have holders (also called clips or arms) to hold the capsules, holder cover, timers, variable speed controls, and start button (Figure 31-34). General steps for use of the amalgamator are outlined in Procedure 31-7. Read and follow the manufacturer's directions and alloy specifications. Each amalgamator must be set for the type of dental alloy used. Usually, trituration of the alloy and mercury is 10–15 seconds. This produces a homogeneous and uniform mix.

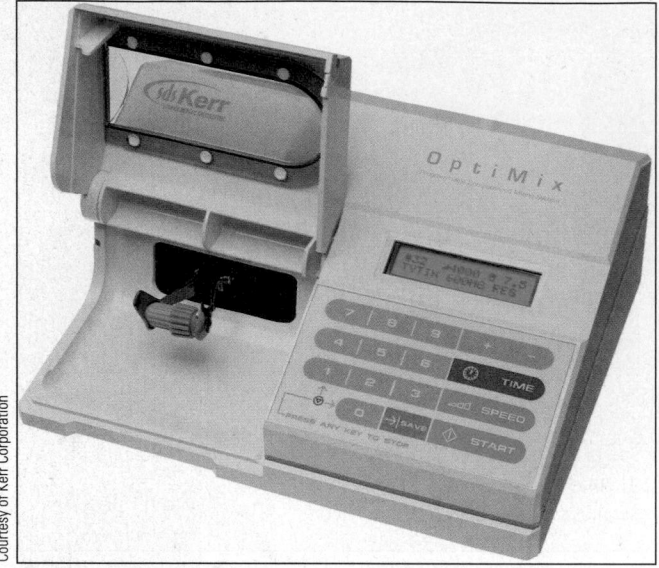

FIGURE 31-34
A dental amalgamator.

Courtesy of Kerr Corporation

Trituration of the amalgam is an important step for restoration success. The quality of the mix is determined by the mixing time, speed of the amalgamator, and force being applied during the trituration. Varying conditions in the trituration process can cause certain problems. If the amalgam is mixed too long (over triturated), it will be crumbly and dull in appearance, and the strength of the amalgam will be reduced. If the amalgam is undermixed (under triturated), it will be soupy before hardening and difficult to remove from the capsule.

Safety

Mercury Exposure

Exposure to mercury can occur through contact of liquid mercury with the skin, through ingestion, or through the lungs with inhalation of mercury vapor. Good mercury hygiene (Clinical Tips) minimizes exposure of patients and dental personnel to liquid mercury and mercury vapor. Follow these Clinical Tips:

- Do not touch liquid mercury, even with gloved hands.
- Use precapsulated amalgam to reduce handling of liquid mercury and to reduce the possibility of spills of liquid mercury in the office.
- Use an amalgam carrier to transfer amalgam to the prepared cavity.
- Use high-volume evacuation during placement and removal of amalgam restorations.
- Store amalgam scrap in sealed containers containing x-ray fixer or commercial scrap container. Amalgam scraps are a regulated waste.
- Monitor the dental office for mercury vapor regularly.
- Monitor dental personnel for mercury exposure annually.

Procedure 31-7
Triturating Dental Amalgam

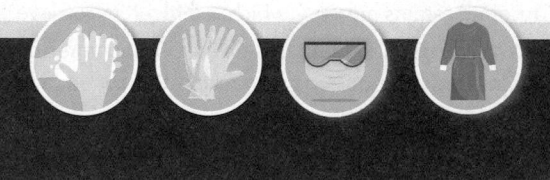

This procedure is completed by the dental assistant. The materials and equipment are prepared before the procedure begins. The types of amalgamator and capsules vary.

Equipment and Supplies
Preprocedural Setup
- PPE: examination gloves, mask, protective glasses, and protective clothing
- handwashing soap or hand sanitizer
- sanitized dental treatment area and barriers placed over equipment

Dental Amalgam Setup (Figure 31-35)
- amalgamator
- premeasured capsule of dental alloy and mercury
- dental amalgam manufacturer's directions
- amalgam well or squeeze cloth
- amalgam carrier
- amalgam condenser
- scrap container for excess amalgam

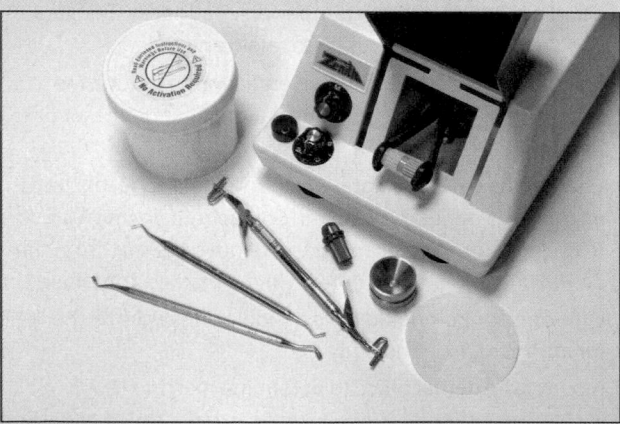

FIGURE 31-35
Items needed to mix and place an amalgam restoration, including an amalgamator, an amalgam capsule, an amalgam well and squeeze cloth, an amalgam carrier, two amalgam condensers (small and large), and an amalgam scrap container.

Procedure Steps *(Follow aseptic procedures)*

1. Wash or sanitize hands.

2. Don PPE (never handle amalgam materials without wearing examination gloves).

3. Place a barrier over the work area (bracket table cover).

4. Assemble and arrange the materials for the procedure.

5. Read the manufacturer's directions and select the trituration time and speed for the type of alloy and amalgamator.

6. At the signal of the dentist, prepare the capsule by twisting the cap, squeezing the capsule, or using an activator.

7. Insert the capsule into the holder of the amalgamator (Figure 31-36).
   - ❏ Place one end of the capsule into the holder first.
   - ❏ Slide the other end down into place.
   - ❏ Practice placing the capsules into the cradle with one hand.
   - ❏ Check to make certain the capsule is secure in the holder.

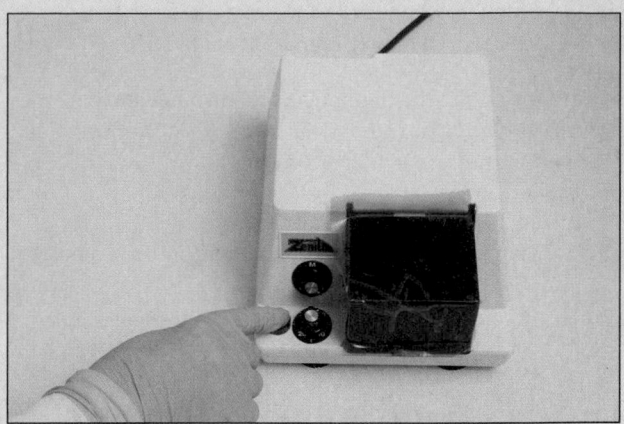

FIGURE 31-37
Press start button to begin amalgamation.

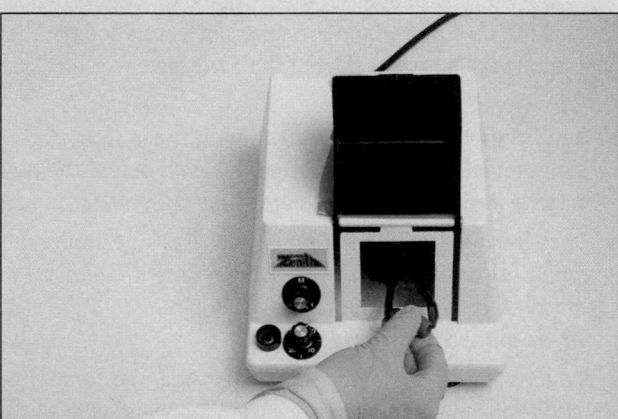

FIGURE 31-36
Placing a capsule in an amalgamator using one hand.

8. Close the cover of the amalgamator.

9. Press the start button on the amalgamator for the prescribed time and speed. The timer will automatically switch off after the prescribed trituration time (Figure 31-37).

10. Lift the cover and remove the capsule when amalgamator stops.

11. Open the capsule and empty the amalgam into an amalgam well.
    - ❏ Avoid touching the amalgam with gloved hands. Use cotton pliers, if necessary.
    - ❏ Examine the amalgam appearance. A well-mixed amalgam will have a glossy appearance with a smooth, velvety consistency.

12. Reassemble the capsule and place it to the side.

13. Load the amalgam carrier (Figure 31-38).
    - ❏ Place one end of the amalgam carrier into the amalgam.
    - ❏ Place index finger below the level of the carrier.
    - ❏ Pack the carrier by applying pressure so that the cylinder is packed lightly (overpacking reduces setting time).
    - ❏ Wipe excess material from the end of the carrier onto the sides of the amalgam well.
    - ❏ Load the other end of the carrier with amalgam.

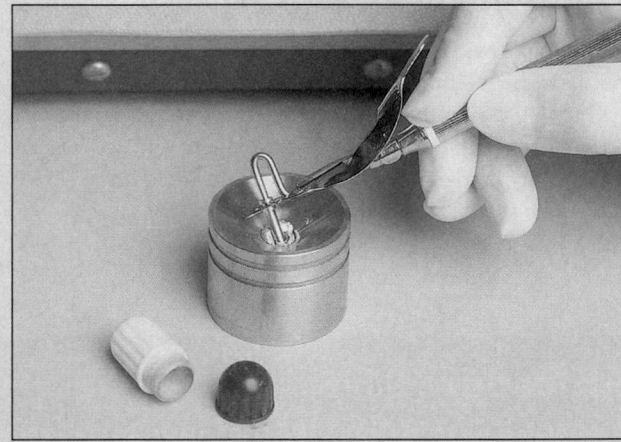

FIGURE 31-38
Loading the amalgam carrier.

14. Pass the amalgam carrier to the dentist.

15. Prepare to exchange a condenser for the carrier.

(Continues)

16. Repeat the loading until all the material has been dispensed or the cavity preparation is filled.

Toward the end of the manipulation, the amalgam becomes harder to load into the carrier because it begins to set. This is the stage that takes practice in order to become proficient.

17. To clean up, expel any excess amalgam into the amalgam well.
   ❏ Empty amalgam from the well into the amalgam scrap container and tightly close the lid (Figure 31-39).

18. The instruments are then cleaned and sterilized.

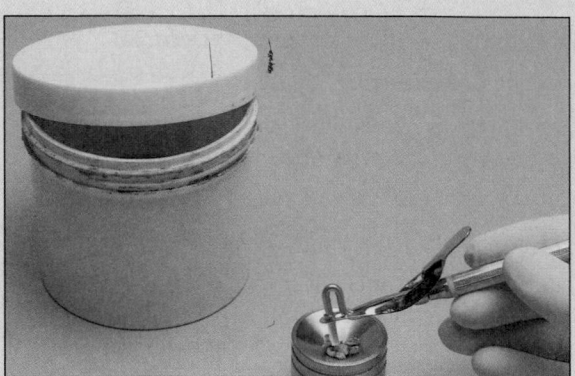

FIGURE 31-39
Placing excess amalgam into a sealed amalgam scrap container.

 **Safety**

Amalgam Capsule Safety

The dental assistant must check that the amalgam capsule is securely placed in the amalgam holder and the cover is closed. If the capsule is not secure during trituration, the capsule can fly out of the holder and open. This would spray alloy and mercury about the dental treatment room causing mercury contamination.

Amalgam Restoration

After the cavity has been prepared, the bases, liners, and/or varnishes have been applied and the matrices have been placed (Class II only), the tooth is ready to be restored. During the restoration phase of the procedure, the amalgam is mixed, placed into the cavity preparation, and carved. See Procedure 31-8 for the complete amalgam restoration sequence.

Amalgam Restoration Postoperative Instructions

Lastly, post-op instructions for the amalgam procedure are given. The patient is still numb, and the amalgam restoration has met its final setting strength. The patient should receive written and oral instructions for the following:

● No eating or drinking until the numbness wears off. The patient needs to be warned that doing so before the numbness wears off can result in injury to the patient's lip and face.

● Once the numbness has worn off, it is okay to eat but only on the opposite side of the mouth from where the restoration was placed. After 24 hours, the amalgam restoration should be set and can be chewed upon.

● If once the numbness wears off the amalgam restoration feels high to the bite, the patient needs to follow up with the dentist to have the restoration adjusted properly.

● The amalgam restoration could be sensitive for a few days to a month, but if sensitivity turns into discomfort or pain, the patient needs a follow-up appointment with the dentist.

Procedure 31-8
Assisting with a Class II Amalgam Restoration

The chairside dental assistant prepares material and transfers materials and instruments, while the dentist completes the amalgam restoration procedure. The dentist administers the local anesthetic and completes the cavity preparation. The operator (dentist, dental hygienist, or qualified assistant) places the topical anesthetic, dental dam, bases/liners/varnishes, matrices, and dental amalgam and carves the amalgam restoration.

Steps written in **blue** font are performed by the operator (dentist or qualified dental assistant), and the chairside assistant's steps are written in black.

Equipment and Supplies

Patient Seating Setup
- PPE: examination gloves, mask, protective glasses, and protective clothing

- Handwashing soap or hand sanitizer
- Sanitized dental treatment area and barriers placed over equipment
- Patient's medical and dental records
- Patient seating setup (refer to Procedure 18-4)
- Blood pressure equipment

Basic Setup (Figure 31-40A)

- mouth mirror (A)
- explorer (B)
- cotton pliers (C)

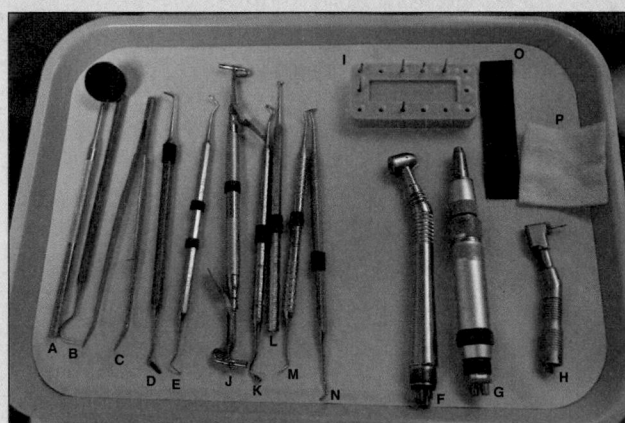

FIGURE 31-40A
Class II amalgam restoration setup.

Local Anesthetic Setup (refer to Procedure 23-2)

Dental Dam Setup (refer to Procedure 21-2) (Figure 31-40A)

- plastic instrument (D)

Cavity Preparation Setup (refer to Procedure 30-6) (Figure 31-40A)

- handcutting instruments (doctor's preference)
  - spoon excavator (E)
- high-speed handpieces (F)
- low-speed straight handpiece (G)
- contra-angle handpiece (H)
- assortment of burs (doctor's preference) (I)

Amalgam Restoration Setup (Figure 31-40A)

- amalgam carrier (J)
- amalgam condenser (K)
- burnisher (L)
- carvers (operator preference)
  - Hollenbeck carver (M)
  - cleoid–discoid carver (N)

- Expendables:
  - articulating paper (O)
  - 2 × 2 gauze square (P)

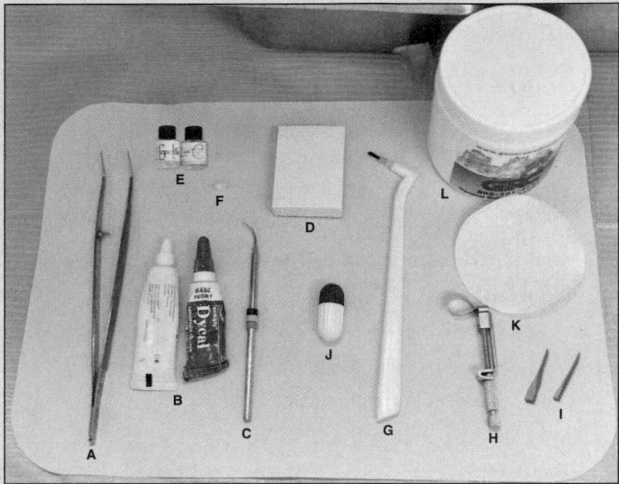

FIGURE 31-40B
Dental materials setup.

Dental Materials Setup (Figure 31-40B)

- cotton pliers (A)
- calcium hydroxide two-paste system (B)
- small ball-ended instrument (liner applicator) or explorer (C)
- small paper pad (D)
- cavity varnish and solvent (E)
- cotton pellets (F)
- resin brush (G)
- assembled universal retainer and matrix band (H)
- assortment of wedges (I)
- premeasured amalgam capsule (J)
- amalgam squeeze cloth (K)
- scrap container for excess amalgam (L)
- amalgamator (not shown)

Procedure Steps

1. Escort and seat patient (refer to Procedure 18-4).

2. Prepare in advance for steps in cavity preparation procedure.
   - Open patient's chart in dental software.
   - Navigate to the dental charting screen.
   - Open patient's latest radiographic history on the computer monitor, or place on view box.
   - Attach handpieces to dental unit.
   - Insert burs into handpieces.

(Continues)

❏ Inform dentist that the patient is ready.

❏ Introduce dentist as they enter the treatment area.

Dentist greets the patient and takes position at the dental chair.

❏ Signals for the procedure to begin (refer to Procedure 20-1).

3. Pass mouth mirror and explorer at operator's signal.

Dentist examines tooth or teeth with mirror and explorer.

Dentist administers local anesthetic.

4. Assist in administration of local anesthetic (refer to Procedure 23-2).

❏ Pass gauze square and applicator with topical anesthetic.

Operator dries area and applies topical to injection site.

❏ Retrieve gauze square.

❏ Retrieve applicator.

❏ Pass loaded anesthetic with shield in place.

❏ Keep needle cover in shield.

❏ Place left arm across patient.

Dentist injects patient and places needle/syringe into needle cover held in shield.

❏ Rinse and evacuate patient's mouth.

Operator places dental dam.

5. Assist in placement of dental dam (refer to Procedure 21-3).

❏ Select dental dam clamp based on patient's chart and observing patient's mouth.

❏ Tie safety ligature around the bow of the clamp.

❏ Engage clamp forceps into clamp and pass to operator.

Operator tries clamp over tooth to be clamped and examines the mouth for dental dam placement.

❏ Retrieve clamp in clamp forceps.

❏ Pass dental dam material attached to dental dam frame with right hand.

❏ Pass dental punch to operator with left hand.

Operator punches dental dam for Class II cavity preparation.

❏ Pass clamp for operator to place into dental dam.

❏ Pass clamp forceps.

Operator places the clamp, dental dam, and frame as a unit.

❏ Retrieve clamp forceps and pass plastic instrument.

Operator releases dental dam from wings of the clamp using plastic instrument.

❏ Rinse, evacuate, and dry the operation site.

❏ Pass floss.

Operator flosses septum of dental dam between the teeth being isolated.

❏ Retrieve floss and pass plastic instrument.

Operator inverts the dental dam around the cervix of the isolated teeth.

❏ Assist inversion by following the operator with air syringe.

Dentist examines area after placement of dental dam.

❏ Transfer mirror and explorer.

❏ Ask dentist's preference of bur for high-speed and low-speed handpieces.

❏ Insert burs into handpieces.

Dentist removes caries and cuts tooth structure to form cavity preparation.

6. Assist with removal of dental caries and tooth structure (Figure 31-41).

❏ Retrieve explorer and transfer handpiece.

❏ Hold HVE near handpiece head during cutting to evacuate dental spray.

❏ Rinse and aspirate as needed.

❏ Keep mirror clean during procedure by gently blowing air on mirror.

❏ Use air/water syringe and HVE to remove debris as needed.

❏ Rinse and dry area after dentist has prepared the tooth.

  ❏ Do not overdry; overdrying may damage the pulp.

Dentist refines the cavity preparation as needed.

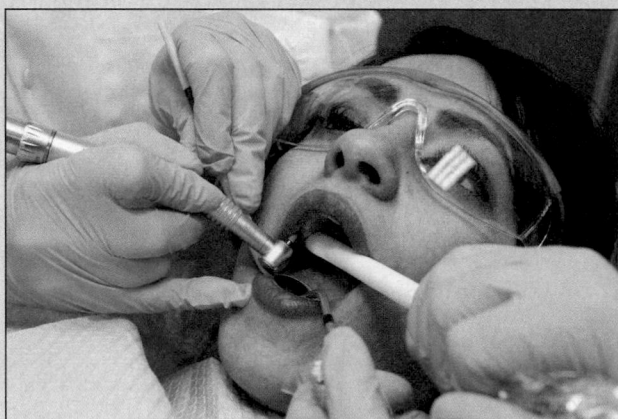

FIGURE 31-41
Cavity being prepared by the dentist with a dental assistant evacuating and keeping the mirror dry and clean.

7. Retrieve handpiece and pass handcutting instruments as needed by dentist to refine cavity preparation.

Dentist examines preparation prior to placing dental materials.

8. Retrieve handcutting instruments and pass explorer.

❏ Retrieve mirror and explorer.

❏ Rinse and dry area after dentist refines cavity preparation.

9. Assist in placement of liner.

❏ Place liner on mixing pad and mix to homogeneous consistency within 30 seconds using liner applicator.

❏ Clean applicator and pass to operator.

❏ Hold mixing pad and clean gauze in left hand to clean applicator between applications.

Operator applies liner to the floor of preparation.

10. Assist in application of varnish.
    ❏ Roll small cotton pellet to a point, dip pellet into varnish, and squeeze in gauze.
    ❏ Retrieve applicator.
    ❏ Pass prepared pellet using cotton pliers.

    Operator applies varnish to floor and walls of the preparation.

    ❏ Hold air/water syringe in right hand to blow air into preparation as requested.

11. Assist operator in placing the universal retainer and matrix.
    ❏ Load the universal retainer for the appropriate quadrant.
    ❏ Turn the inner knob to increase the diameter of the matrix band for ease in slipping over the tooth.
    ❏ Pass the loaded retainer to the operator.
    ❏ Retrieve cotton pliers.

    Operator places the matrix band around the prepared tooth with the retainer on the buccal side.

    ❏ **Turns the inner knob to tighten the band snuggle around the tooth.**
    ❏ **Examines the placement of the band.**
    ❏ Pass the mirror and explorer to examine placement.

    Operator marks area to be contoured with an explorer and modifies the shape of the matrix band with a burnisher as needed.

    ❏ Exchange explorer and burnisher as requested.

12. Assist in placement of the wedge.
    ❏ Hold the wedge in right hand with the base down.
    ❏ Exchange burnisher and cotton pliers with left hand.

    Operator grasps the wedge with the pliers.

    ❏ **Places the wedge interproximally between the band and the tooth adjacent to the missing wall with the base of the wedge toward the gingiva.**
    ❏ Pass the mirror and explorer.

    Operator examines that the matrix band placement:

    ❏ **Is below the gingival step.**
    ❏ **The wedge is tight against the band.**
    ❏ **There is not space between the band and the gingival step.**
    ❏ Retrieve the mirror and explorer.
    ❏ Rinse and dry the area as needed; there may be slight bleeding from the placement of the band and wedge.

    Operator signals for mix of dental amalgam.

13. Prepare dental amalgam.
    ❏ Read amalgam manufacturer's directions and set time and speed of triturator.
    ❏ Place a 2 spill capsule into the triturator holder, close the lid, and press the start button.
    ❏ Open the capsule and place the amalgam into the amalgam well.
    ❏ Load both ends of the amalgam carrier.

14. Assist in placing dental amalgam into cavity preparation (Figure 31-42).
    ❏ Pass loaded carrier to operator.

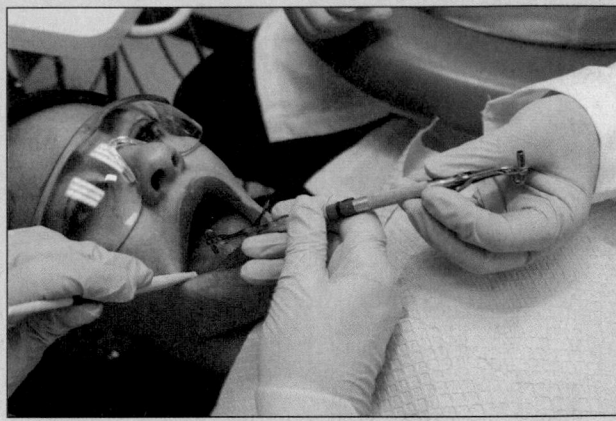

FIGURE 31-42
A loaded amalgam carrier ready for use.

Operator presses lever and places amalgam first into the step of the preparation.

❏ Retrieve carrier and pass condenser of choice and mirror.
❏ Hold HVE in right hand to evacuate debris as requested.

Operator condenses amalgam into the cavity preparation.

❏ Interchange carrier followed by the condenser until the cavity preparation is slightly overfilled.
❏ Retrieve condenser and pass burnisher as requested.

Operator burnishes the amalgam restoration as needed.

15. Assist in initial carving of amalgam restoration.
    ❏ Retrieve burnisher and pass explorer.

    Operator releases amalgam from the top of the matrix band with explorer.

    ❏ Retrieve explorer and pass operator's choice of carvers.

    Operator carves the amalgam to restore the primary anatomy of the tooth.

    ❏ **Operator leaves the band in place until the amalgam has been given sufficient time to begin to set; early removal will fracture the amalgam.**

16. Assist in removal of retainer, wedge, and matrix band.

    Operator loosens the outer knob and removes the retainer from the matrix band.

    ❏ Retrieve the retainer and pass the cotton pliers.

    Operator removes the wedge from the interproximal.

    ❏ Hold right palm up to retrieve the wedge and retrieve the cotton pliers with the left.

    Operator removes band by holding the ends and pressing the band against the adjacent tooth to not fracture the amalgam or destroy the contact.

17. Assist in final carving of amalgam restoration.

(Continues)

❏ Pass operator's choice of interproximal carver.

Operator carves the interproximal area of the restoration.

❏ Exchange interproximal carver for operator's choice of carver to carve the occlusal of the restoration.

Operator completes final carving to establish anatomy and function of the tooth.

❏ Retrieve mirror and carver.
❏ Rinse and evacuate the area.

18. Assist in removal of the dental dam.
❏ Pass clamp forceps.

Operator removes the clamp.

❏ Pass the crown and bridge scissors.

Operator cuts the dental dam septa to avoid fracturing the interproximal area of the restoration and for ease in removal.

❏ Rinse and evacuate the mouth.

Operator checks the dental dam to ensure that all material has been removed.

❏ Pass floss as needed to remove any remaining floss.

19. Assist in checking occlusion (Figure 31-43).
❏ Pass gauze square and articulating forceps holding articulation paper.

Operator checks the occlusion.
❏ Dries the area with gauze square.
❏ Places articulating paper against the teeth.

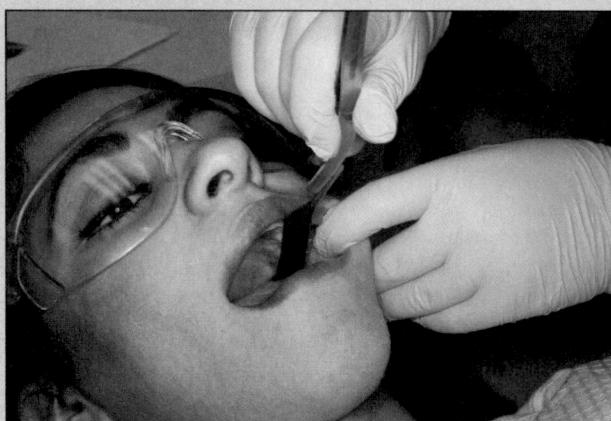

FIGURE 31-43
Articulating paper positioned against the teeth for the patient to gently close on to check the occlusion.

❏ Asks the patient to gently close on the paper; caution must be taken to avoid fracturing the amalgam margin.
❏ Pass mirror and carver of choice if restoration registers high spots.

Operator adjusts restoration with carver until it is absent of any articulation marks.

❏ Retrieve mirror and exchange carver and gauze square to remove markings.

Dentist makes a final check of all work of an expanded assistant. In some states the dentist must perform a final examination of a placed restoration.

20. Assist in final evaluation of amalgam restoration (Figure 31-44).

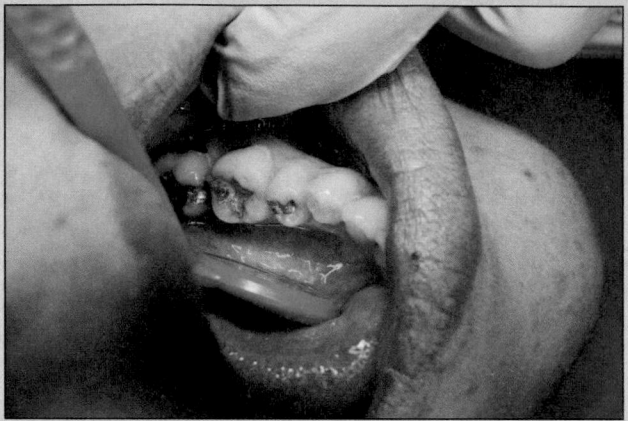

FIGURE 31-44
A finished amalgam restoration.

❏ Pass mirror and explorer.

Operator burnishes restoration and accentuates anatomy (optional).

❏ Pass moistened cotton pellet with cotton pliers and liner applicator.
❏ Retrieve cotton pliers and applicator.

21. Provide patient with postoperative instructions orally and in written form.

22. Write up procedure in Services Rendered.

Date	Services Rendered
02/18/XX	Updated medical and dental history, no changes noted. BP 120/80; T= 98.6F, P=80, R=18
	Placed 20% benzocaine gel to injection sites for 2 minutes. Administered 2 cartridges (3.6 ml) of 2% lidocaine with 1:100,000 epi to mandibular left. No reaction
#19	MOD amal restoration with calcium hydroxide liner and copal varnish
	POI do not bite on lip, no eating/drinking until numbness wears off, eat only on opposite side until numbness has worn off, can chew on restoration after 24 hours, call office if restoration feels high or if there is discomfort or pain; chewing on ice and hard, chewy candy can damage restorations
	Assistant's initials

23. Dismiss and escort patient to reception area (refer to Procedure 18-5).

Safety

Cautions when Using Dental Amalgam

The use of dental amalgam does come with several cautions. Dental health care workers should only handle amalgam or instruments used with amalgam with gloved hands. If the bare hand comes in contact with amalgam, the workers must wash hands in soap and water immediately. Amalgam that splashes in the eyes should be flushed out immediately. When amalgam is removed, the workers must wear a mask and protective glasses for protection from particles and mercury vapor. Unused amalgam after treatment is subject to strict disposal protocols for possible environmental reasons. NOTE: Amalgam will also clean the finish from other metals like jewelry.

Finishing and Polishing an Amalgam Restoration

The action of **finishing** an amalgam is to improve the abnormalities of the restoration's anatomy, remove any irregularities in the margins, and smooth roughness of the restoration. **Polishing** an amalgam ensures the surface of the restoration is smooth and shiny. The ultimate reason to polish an amalgam is to provide a smooth surface to reduce the amount of biofilm and debris that can adhere to the restoration and increase its longevity and health of the surrounding periodontium (Figure 31-45). The rationale for finishing and polishing an amalgam restoration is to improve:

- gingival health
- biocompatibility of amalgam
- integrity of junction of tooth surface and restoration
- maintenance by patient with easier biofilm removal with tooth brushing and flossing
- length of service of the restoration

The finishing and polishing procedure is completed for two different reasons. First, finishing and polishing is a final step in placing a new amalgam restoration. When an amalgam is placed, a dentist utilizes burnishers and carvers to ensure that the restoration is smooth and flush with the margins of the tooth. If completed correctly, many dentists believe that no further change to the new restoration is necessary. In some cases, the amalgam restoration needs more finishing than can be provided at the time of its placement. Large Class II restorations in stress-bearing locations are less durable and may need the articulation checked after the amalgam has set. Also, oral conditions may not be ideal for the placement of amalgam due to patient management challenges, difficulty in moisture control, and patient trauma with the presence of bleeding. It may be necessary to have the patient return 24 hours later to complete the final touches after the amalgam has established its final set.

Second, finishing and polishing restore functionality to older amalgam restorations. As an amalgam ages, a number of issues can occur. Tarnish, when the amalgam discolors over time, and corrosion, the action of acids on the restoration causing the surface to become pitted and rough, are the most common cosmetic issues (Figure 31-46). Recurrent decay, decay under an already placed restoration, occurs when the margins of the restoration and tooth separate and break down over time. Bacteria can seep into the space, otherwise known as microleakage, decaying the tooth. Irregularities in the margins of the restoration where the amalgam and tooth are not **flush**, like **flash**, **ditching**, or **open margins**, allows for the adherence of biofilm and acids in the rough areas. Smoothing of these areas reduces the opportunity for bacteria to cause decay around and under the existing restoration. Occlusal problems occur as the teeth slightly shift and move over time. Even the slightest irregularity in occlusion could cause the patient discomfort upon mastication or even cause the restoration to fracture. By removing these issues, the life of the amalgam restoration can be preserved and may not necessarily need to be replaced. Finishing and polishing of older, defective amalgam restorations are often completed during the routine prophylaxis procedure.

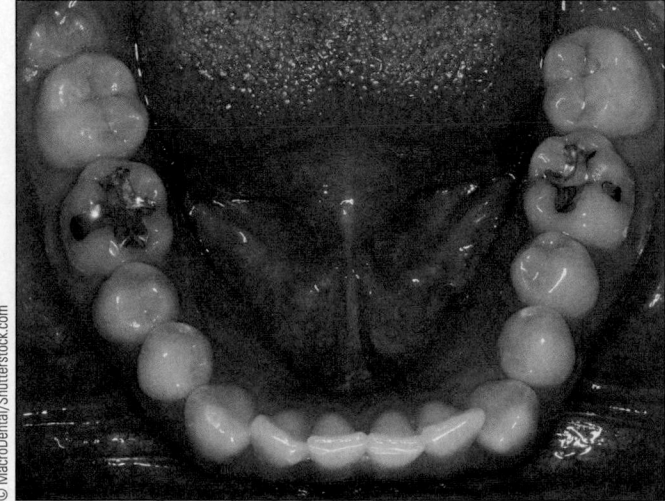

FIGURE 31-45
Finished and polished dental amalgam restorations.

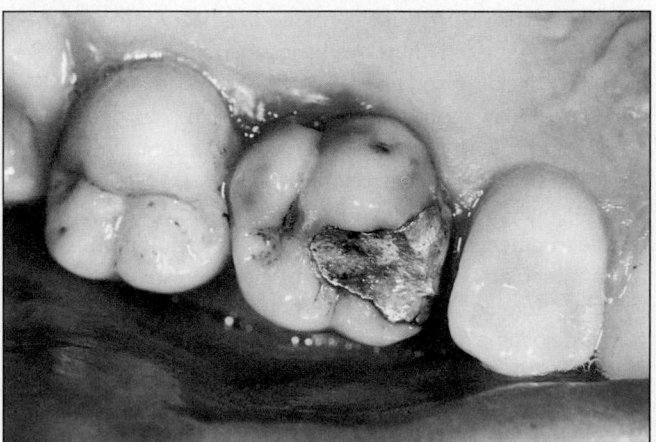

FIGURE 31-46
Old tarnished and corroded amalgam restoration.

Finishing and Polishing Amalgam Controversy

Finishing and polishing an amalgam restoration is a controversial subject in dentistry.

"Whether or not it is necessary to finish and polish an amalgam restoration remains to some a controversial subject. Some dentists will argue that a correctly carved amalgam does not require any more manipulation. Whereas, others state that an amalgam restoration that will contribute to the long-term dental health of a patient requires proper finishing and polishing procedures." (Scribd Polishing-Amalgam Restoration, Feb 19, 2012). Research has been completed to evaluate surface homogeneity, marginal adaptation, and loss of substance. The results of the clinical assessment of amalgam restorations at three years by Bryant showed that "polished restorations were found to have substantially superior surface texture and less likelihood of surface discoloration. No evidence was found to support the use of immediate finishing techniques."

Indications for Finishing and Polishing

Certain criteria must be indicated as not all amalgam restorations are a candidate for finishing and polishing in order for an amalgam to be polished. First, the amalgam restoration needs to be intact. There is no rationale to finish and polish a restoration that needs to be replaced due to decay or fracture. Second, the restoration has to have good interproximal contact if it is a Class II restoration. Open interproximal contacts in a Class II restoration are not optimal and need replacement. Next, irregularity in the margins of the restoration and tooth structure need to be apparent and require recontouring. Finally, if an amalgam restoration is interfering with a patient's gingival health and the problem can be removed by simple finishing or polishing the area, the procedure can be completed.

Contraindications for Finishing and Polishing

Even though an amalgam restoration may appear to be a candidate for finishing and polishing, there are other issues that can rule out the procedure. First, if the restoration has all the indications for finishing and polishing but has massive overhangs interproximally, it should be replaced. These overhangs are not able to be removed with only finishing and polishing. Next, if the amalgam restoration is located in a tooth with a need to be crowned or extracted, performing a finishing or polishing procedure is not indicated as the tooth and/or amalgam restoration will be removed in the near future. Finally, if recurrent decay under the amalgam restoration has been detected upon examination or on radiographs, it will need immediate replacement. Performing a finishing and polishing procedure on an amalgam restoration with contraindications is a waste of time management and clinical resources.

Differences Between Finishing and Polishing

Finishing and polishing an amalgam restoration is completed as one procedure but requires the use of different abrasiveness in their products. The finishing portion is always completed prior to the polishing portion. During the finishing portion of the procedure, #4 or #6 finishing burs are utilized on the amalgam restoration to remove the heavy and deep scratches and gouges. They are also used to reduce and smooth the uneven areas at the cavosurface margin of the tooth.

Once it has been determined that the finishing portion is complete, then polishing can occur. A series of less abrasive points are then used in decreasing (coarse, medium, and fine) order to smooth the topical scratches, which at this point should be lighter and less deep. A slurry of pumice or tin oxide assists in polishing the amalgam, provides a shiny and smooth appearance, and results in better resistance to tarnish and corrosion of the restoration.

Finishing and Polishing Procedure

After ensuring the patient is educated about an amalgam finishing and polishing procedure, make sure consent is gained for the procedure. The operator examines the restoration to be finished and polished and checks all cavosurface margin for any open margins, flashing, or ditching. If the restoration is also interproximal, the operator checks between the teeth with the explorer and floss to determine if there are any areas where the floss may catch or tear. With the articulating paper, the operator checks the occlusion for any high areas that need to be removed. Once the restoration has been carefully examined, the restoration is isolated to be finished and polished.

Explain Amalgam Finishing and Polishing Procedure

As with any procedure, it is important to thoroughly explain the procedure to the patient. An amalgam finishing and polishing is not a restorative procedure requiring replacement of the restoration. The patient must understand at the end of the procedure that the same existing amalgam restoration has been smoothed and recontoured, which in turn could extend the life of the restoration. Most dental insurance policies do not cover finishing and polishing procedures. Improper consent could result in legal action against the dentist and the dental assistant.

Isolating the Amalgam Restoration   The optimal way to isolate the areas in the procedure is with the use of a dental dam. Use of the dental dam will assist in catching any particles, dust, or possibly mercury vapors that can be produced in the procedure. This provides better protection to the patient by preventing inhalation or swallowing any byproducts of the procedure. Generally though, a patient receiving an amalgam finishing and polishing will not be anesthetized. Use of the dental dam in that situation can be uncomfortable. Instead, use of cotton rolls in the vestibule area or beneath the tongue is more commonly used. Dri-angles can be placed in the cheek area to protect the cheek from buildup of byproducts from the procedure.

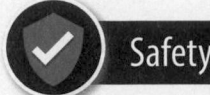 Safety

Finishing and Polishing Vapor

During the finishing and polishing procedure vapor and dust is released, which could contain some mercury particles. As in any procedure, all PPE (personal protective equipment) is to worn. Keep the area well ventilated. Use the HVE and water to capture as much of the particles as best as possible. Use a closed, dry, airtight container if any possible scraps of amalgam may detach from the restoration.

Finishing the Amalgam Restoration

The first step is to remove the irregularities of the cavosurface margin with round finishing burs in a low-speed handpiece. The size #4 or #6 round finishing bur is an average size bur used. The larger the bur the better, as it will cover more surface area, which will minimize uneven ditching and scratching. The operator should start at the cavosurface margin of the occlusal, use low to medium speed to avoid overheating the tooth and the restoration, and follow along the cavosurface margin line with light pressure. Make sure the bur is covering the tooth and restoration surface at the same time to ensure they are being adjusted evenly. By doing so, the irregularities between the tooth and restoration will result in a flush, blended surface. If the restoration extends to the facial or lingual portion of the tooth, follow the same instructions as the occlusal cavosurface margin. If the restoration approaches closely to the gingival margin, the use of thinner abrasive discs may be necessary to avoid contact with the gingival margin.

Once the margins are flush, any occlusal areas with high spots will need to be removed. Again, use the #4 or #6 round bur with light pressure at a low to medium speed and run the bur over the occlusal area in an even and constant sweeping motion. The use of this motion and speed will help prevent ditching, scratching, or overheating the restoration. Make sure to complete one area of the occlusal prior to moving onto another area. Once it appears the irregularities are removed, examine the restoration using an explorer and check the cavosurface margin for any irregularities. Use the articulating paper on the occlusal to identify any remaining high areas.

When the occlusal area is complete, the interproximal can be completed if necessary. Because it would be difficult to use a bur interproximally, a **finishing strip** needs to be utilized. It is important that the interproximal contact not be disrupted. In order to do so, it is necessary for the smooth section of the finishing strip to be placed at the contact to work it interproximally. Once below the contact, the abrasive portion of the finishing strip can be used to smooth the rough areas of the restoration. Wrapping the finishing strip around the contour of the tooth, use a gentle back and forth motion over the restoration to smooth. Care needs to be taken to ensure the finishing strip does not come in contact with the soft tissues of the oral cavity as trauma may result. Once completed with the finishing strip, use floss interproximal and an explorer to detect any rough areas possibly left behind.

 Safety

Amalgam Cautions

The use of dental amalgam does come with several cautions. Dental health care workers should only handle amalgam or instruments used with amalgam with gloved hands. If the bare hand comes in contact with amalgam, the workers must wash hands in soap and water immediately. Amalgam that splashes in the eyes should be flushed out immediately. When amalgam is removed, the workers must wear a mask and safety glasses for protection from particles and mercury vapor. Unused amalgam after treatment is subject to strict disposal protocols for possible environmental reasons. NOTE: Amalgam will also clean the finish from other metals like jewelry. Remove all jewelry when working with amalgam.

Polishing the Amalgam Restoration

The polishing of the amalgam restoration can be completed in one of two ways. One technique is to make a slurry of water and pumice or **tin oxide** in a dappen dish. The low-speed handpiece, prophy angle, and rubber cup are used to polish the amalgam. After placing some of the slurry in the prophy cup, apply it to all areas of the tooth that just were finished. Use a light sweeping pressure to the entire restoration. If the restoration is a Class II, attempt to go as far interproximal as possible. Prior to rinsing out the mouth of the slurry, use a piece of floss to spread the slurry interproximal and assist in polishing.

Another way to polish the amalgam restoration is with a series of abrasive points. The abrasive points are used in order of most abrasive to least abrasive (Figure 31-47). The abrasive points are placed in the contra-angle on the low-speed handpiece. The most abrasive Brownie is used first. Utilize a low to medium speed to avoid overheating the tooth and restoration. Just like the round carbide burs, the Brownie is first adapted to the cavosurface margin using light pressure and overlapping strokes. Once these areas are complete, then the Brownie is adapted to the other areas of the restoration, leaving the surface with a dull appearance. The Greenie is the next most abrasive and is used in the same manner as the Brownie. Because the Greenie is less abrasive, the larger scratches will be smoothed out a little more, generating a shinier restoration. Last to be used is the least abrasive Super Greenie. After its use, the restoration will have a very high shine or luster. In some cases, the tin oxide or pumice slurry is used after the abrasive points as a final polish. This is not always indicated if the abrasive points have worked appropriately.

Evaluating the Amalgam Restoration

After the finishing and polishing process is complete, it is important to thoroughly rinse the mouth of any debris that may have accumulated. The amalgam restoration then needs to be reassessed for scratches, rough areas, flush margins, occlusion, and correct contour of the restoration and tooth. If there appears to be an issue, some of the above steps may need to be completed again

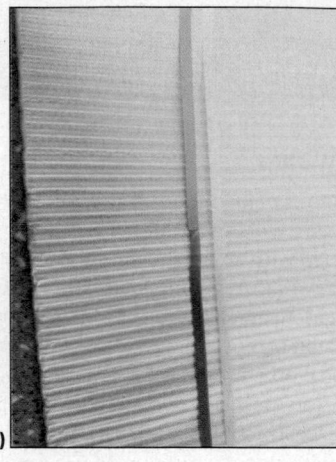
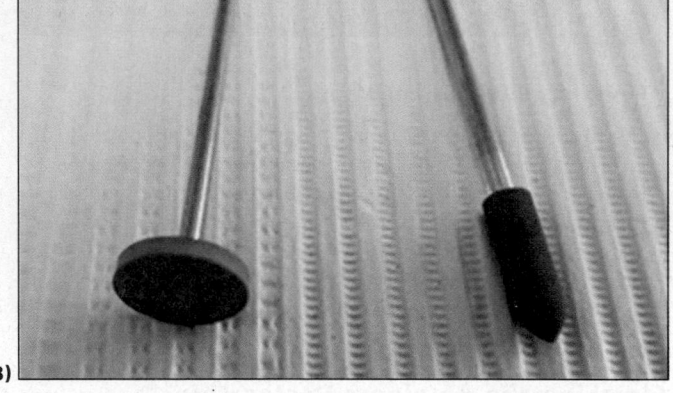

FIGURE 31-47
(A) Lightening strip and (B) abrasive points (Brownie and Greenie).

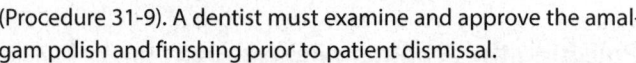

(Procedure 31-9). A dentist must examine and approve the amalgam polish and finishing prior to patient dismissal.

Characteristics of a well-polished amalgam restorations include:

- Smooth anatomic surfaces
- Intact contact areas
- Correctly spaced embrasures
- Refined margins
- Smooth resistant surfaces
- Functional effectiveness
- Acceptable appearance
- No biofilm-retaining irregularities
- Restored health of the gingival tissues

Procedure 31-9
Assisting with Finishing and Polishing an Amalgam Restoration

The chairside dental assistant prepares materials and transfers materials and instruments, while the operator finishes and polishes an amalgam restoration. The operator can be the dentist, dental hygienist, or qualified assistant. In some states the dentist must perform a final examination of a placed restoration.

Steps written in **blue** font are performed by the operator (dentist or qualified dental assistant), and the chairside assistant's steps are written in black.

Equipment and Supplies

Patient Seating Setup (refer to Procedure 18-4)

Finishing Amalgam Restoration Setup
- low-speed handpiece
- contra-angle attachment
- #4 and #6 finishing burs
- articulating paper
- articulating paper holder

Polishing Amalgam Restoration Setup
- abrasive points: Brownie, Greenie, Super Greenie

- finishing strips
- right angle attachment (prophy angle with rubber cup)
- dappen dish (2)
- flour of pumice
- tin oxide
- cement spatula

Procedure Steps

1. Escort and seat patient (refer to Procedure 18-4).

2. Prepare in advance for steps in cavity preparation procedure.
   - ❑ Open patient's chart in dental software.
   - ❑ Navigate to the dental charting screen.
   - ❑ Open patient's latest radiographic history on the computer monitor, or place on view box.
   - ❑ Attach handpieces to dental unit.
   - ❑ Insert burs into handpieces.
   - ❑ Inform dentist that the patient is ready.
   - ❑ Introduce dentist as they enter the treatment area.

   Dentist greets the patient and takes position at the dental chair.

❏ Signals for the procedure to begin (refer to Procedure 20-1).

3. Assist in examination of amalgam restoration.
   ❏ Pass mirror and explorer.

Operator examines the amalgam restoration.

   ❏ Retrieve mirror and explorer and pass floss.

Operator checks the interproximal area of the restoration.

   ❏ Pass articulating paper in articulation holder.

Operator checks the occlusion for any high areas.

4. Assist operator in isolating the amalgam restoration.
   ❏ Pass operator's preference of cotton rolls or dri-angles.

Operator places cotton rolls or dri-angles for moisture control and to protect the soft tissue.

5. Assist operator in finishing the amalgam restoration.
   ❏ Pass contra-angle handpiece with operator choice of finishing bur.
   ❏ Rinse, evacuate, and dry the operation site as needed throughout the procedure.

Operator finishes the cavosurface margin of the amalgam until it is flush with the tooth and removes irregularities to produce a smooth surface.

   ❏ Pass articulating paper with holder.

Operator reexamines for any remaining high area.

   ❏ Pass finishing strips if an interproximal area needs to be finished.

Operator uses a gentle back-and-forth motion with finishing strips until the surface is smooth.

   ❏ Pass dental floss.

Operator uses floss to detect any interproximal rough areas.

6. Assist operator in polishing the amalgam restoration.
   ❏ Pass contra-angle handpiece with operator choice of abrasive points.

Operator uses the points to produce a smooth surface with a high shine.

❏ Mix slurry of pumice in dappen dish.
❏ Pass prophy angle and hold dappen dish of pumice at chin level.

Operator polishes the amalgam surface with slurry of pumice.

   ❏ Rinse, evacuate and dry the operation site as needed throughout the procedure.
   ❏ Mix slurry of tin oxide in dappen dish.
   ❏ Pass prophy angle and hold dappen dish of tin oxide at chin level.

Operator polishes the amalgam surface with slurry of tin oxide.

   ❏ Pass dental floss.

Operator spreads slurry with floss to polish the interproximals.

   ❏ Rinse and dry area.

7. Assist in evaluation finished/polished amalgam.
   ❏ Pass mirror and explorer.

Dentist examines the restoration and approves of the amalgam finishing and polishing.

   ❏ Pass dental floss.

8. Write up procedure in Service Rendered.

Date	Services Rendered
02/18/XX	Updated medical and dental history, no changes noted. BP = 120/80; T = 98.6F, P = 80, R=18
#19	OCC finish and polish amalgam restoration; #4 finishing bur, abrasive points (brownie, greenie, super greenie), restoration free of gouges and scratches
	Polished amalgam with tin oxide slurry and prophy cup; flossed to ensure all tin oxide was removed; check occlusion with articulating
	POI can eat and drink at any time; if find rough spot or has discomfort while occluding contact office to have area examined
	Assistant's Initials

9. Dismiss and escort patient to reception area (refer to Procedure 18-5).

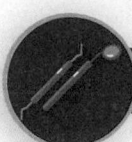

CASE STUDY

During a new patient examination, the patient, Sarah, tells the assistant that she is embarrassed about the condition of her silver fillings. She explains that they are very old, but she cannot afford to replace all her fillings. Upon examination, it is noted that tooth #18 is tarnished and corroded, #19 amalgam has a slight fracture along with being tarnished, #20 is tarnished and has an overhang, #30 has flash around the margins, and #31 has an open contact area next to #30.

Case Study Review
1. Which teeth can be finished and polished?
2. Which teeth cannot be finished and polished and need to be replaced?

Review Questions

Multiple Choice

1. If the pH of the dental material is less than 7, it has a high _____. This property must be considered before being used as a restoration. It can cause gingival tissue irritation and pulpal damage if care in not taken when preparing and placing the material.
   a. galvanism
   b. corrosion
   c. acidity
   d. bonding

2. The function and safety of dental materials is regulated by the _____.
   a. ADA
   b. FDA
   c. ISO
   d. All of these

3. Which is responsible for testing dental materials and listing certified dental materials?
   a. Council on Scientific Affairs
   b. Council on Dental Materials
   c. Council on Seal of Acceptance
   d. All of these

4. What material may be placed when a large amount of dentin is removed during the cavity preparation procedure?
   a. one layer of varnish
   b. cavity liner
   c. cement base
   d. amalgam bonding

5. The dentist removes a minimal amount of dentin during the cavity preparation. What materials are typically used prior to the placement of the dental amalgam?
   a. base, then liner
   b. liner, then varnish
   c. varnish, then base
   d. varnish, then liner

6. The bonding agent is a low viscosity resin and should never be used with:
   a. cavity varnish.
   b. liner.
   c. eugenol.
   d. All of these

7. Which of the following cavity preparations need a universal retainer and matrix?
   a. Class I
   b. Class II
   c. Class III
   d. Both b and c

8. What part of the universal retainer adjusts the size of the matrix band?
   a. outer knob
   b. inner knob
   c. vise
   d. spindle

9. Which matrix band system(s) may be used when a retainer will not fit into the area being restored and needs a matrix without a retainer?
   a. Tofflemire
   b. T-band
   c. Sectional
   d. Both b and c

10. When would a dental amalgam restoration be preferred over other direct restorations?
    a. patient has poor hygiene
    b. less expensive
    c. patient has a bruxing problem
    d. All of these

11. When may the dentist elect to NOT use dental amalgam as a restoration?
    a. restoring an anterior tooth
    b. cannot maintain moisture control
    c. patient has methacrylate allergies
    d. restoring a primary tooth

12. Which ingredient of dental amalgam allows for the material to be pliable when first mixed in order to place it easily into the cavity preparation?
    a. silver
    b. tin
    c. copper
    d. mercury

13. What metal is of the greatest percent in a dental alloy?
    a. silver
    b. tin
    c. copper
    d. zinc

14. What type of flooring should be avoided when using dental amalgam?
    a. tile
    b. concrete
    c. wood
    d. carpet

15. Which is the sequence for completing an amalgam restoration?
    a. anesthetic, cavity prep, dental dam, matrix, varnish, liner, trituration, carve, load carrier, and condense
    b. anesthetic, dental dam, matrix, cavity prep, liner, varnish, trituration, condense, load carrier, and carve
    c. anesthetic, dental dam, cavity prep, matrix, varnish, liner, trituration, load carrier, carve, and condense
    d. anesthetic, dental dam, cavity prep, liner, varnish, matrix, trituration, load carrier, condense, and carve

16. Which POI are given to the patient after an amalgam restoration has been placed?
    a. Do not eat while area is numb.
    b. Eat on side opposite of amalgam restoration.
    c. Chew on restoration after 24 hours.
    d. All of these

17. When should a Class II amalgam restoration be finished and polished for best results and longevity?
    a. right after the amalgam is placed
    b. 24 hours after placement
    c. one week
    d. one year

18. An amalgam restoration is recommended for finishing and polishing for all these reasons EXCEPT:
    a. presence of amalgam flash.
    b. restoration is tarnished.
    c. recurrent decay.
    d. restoration is corroded.

19. Which is the sequence for the finishing and polishing procedure of an amalgam restoration?
    a. cotton rolls, abrasive points, finishing burs, tin oxide, and pumice
    b. dental dam, abrasive points, finishing burs, pumice, and tin oxide
    c. cotton rolls, finishing burs, abrasive points, pumice, and tin oxide
    d. dental dam, finishing burs, abrasive points, tin oxide, and pumice

20. Which are the criteria of a well-finished and polished amalgam restoration?
    a. restoration of function
    b. restored health of gingival tissues
    c. smooth and shiny surface
    d. All of these

Critical Thinking

1. A patient complains that every time they bite down, they feel like they get an electrical shock in their mouth. The dental assistant notices that the mandibular molar has an amalgam and the opposing maxillary molar has a newly placed gold crown. What may be the cause of this patient's pain? How does the dental assistant explain this to the patient?

2. While placing the matrix band and wedge, the operator is not able to control the saliva and maintain a moisture free area. What type of dental alloy could be used, and why?

3. While triturating the amalgam capsule in the amalgamator, the capsule dislodges from the holder and is propelled from the amalgamator. The capsule is forced open, and amalgam spills onto the patient's face. What should the assistant do?

Key Terms

Term and Pronunciation	Meaning of Root and Word Parts	Definition
alloy (**al**-oi)	**alloy** = substance of two or more metals	dental alloy is a mixture of metallic elements; containing silver, tin, copper, and zinc to be used as a restoration
amalgamation (*uh*-mal-*guh*-**mey**-sh*uhn*)	**amalgamate** = to combine, unite **-tion** = act or process of	reaction between metal alloys and mercury to make dental amalgam
amalgamator (uh-**mal**-guh-mey-ter)	**amalgam** = an alloy of mercury with another metal **-ate** = denotes a function **-or** = denotes machines	equipment used to combine mercury with dental alloy to form a new alloy (amalgam)
calcium hydroxide (**kal**-see-*uhm*) (hahy-**drok**-sahd)	**calc-** = containing calcium **-ium** = indicating a metallic element **hydro-** = representing hydrogen; water **oxide** = compound of oxygen bonded to with another element	dental material used as a therapeutic dental liner that stimulates the formation of secondary dentin
capsule (**kap**-s*uhl*)	**cap** = case, container **-ule** = indicating smallness	amalgam capsules designed to contain and for mixing dental alloy and mercury to form dental amalgam
chemical retention (**kem**-i-*kuhl*) (ri-**ten**-sh*uhn*)	**chemic-** = relating to chemistry; producing substance having a specific molecular composition **-al** = pertaining to **retain** = to hold in place **-ion** = denoting action	when a chemical reaction between the tooth surface and material occurs, that holds the material in place; chemical or bonding adhesion
circumference (ser-**kuhm**-fer-*uhn*s)	**circum** = round about, around **-ence** = indicating a condition	when the boomerang shaped Tofflemire's ends are held together, a smaller and larger circumference is created: larger toward occlusal, smaller toward CEJ
comminute (**kom**-*uh*-noot)	**com-** = with, together **minor** = lesser as in size **-ute** = extremely small	dental alloy is pulverized into a fine powder

(Continues)

Term and Pronunciation	Meaning of Root and Word Parts	Definition
corrosion (k*uh*-**roh**-zh*uh*n)	**corrode** = to eat or wear away gradually by chemical action **-ion** = indicating a process	process where a metal is eaten away by a chemical action
dental amalgam (**den**-tl) (*uh*-**mal**-g*uh*m)	**dent** = teeth **-al** = pertaining to **amalgam** = an alloy of mercury with another metal(s)	a mixture of mercury, silver, tin, and copper triturated in a machine to create a restorative material
ditching (**dich**-ing)	**ditch** = to make a narrow channel **-ing** = the process of	creation of scratches or concave areas due to excessive finishing of the amalgam
ductility (**duhk**-tl-i-tee)	**duct** = any tube **-ile** = expressing capability **-ity** = expressing condition	physical property of a dental material that has the ability to be hammered thin or stretched into wire without breaking
esthetically (es-**thet**-ik-lee)	**esthete** = person who has appreciation of beauty **-ic** = having some characteristic of -al = pertaining to **-ly** = having qualities	especially concerned with the appearance of teeth as it is achieved by arrangement, form, and color of a dental restoration
finish (**fin**-ish)	**finish** = to bring to a desired condition	procedure used to reduce excess dental restorative material to establish appropriate occlusion and contour and remove surface blemishes and produce a smooth surface using rotary cutting instruments
finishing strip (**fin**-ish-ing) (strip)	**finish** = to bring to a desired condition **-ing** = expressing action **strip** = long narrow piece of material of uniform width	plastic or paper strips containing abrasives of varying grits to finish the interproximals of restorations
flash (flash)	**flash** = a ridge of thin excess material that squeezed out and left on an object	excess material that results from overfilling a restoration
flush (fluhsh)	**flush** = even or level surface	when the dental restoration is even with the surface of the tooth
galvanism (**gal**-v*uh*-niz-*uh*m)	**Galvani, Luigi** = physiologist who discovered electricity can be produced by chemical action **-ism** =denoting action or condition	electric current created by chemical reaction of dissimilar metals
impervious (im-**pur**-vee-*uh*s)	**im-** = not **pervious** = permeable; admitting of passage	a material's surface is impenetrable; does not permit penetration
malleability (mal-ee-*uh*-**bil**-i-tee)	**malleable** = capable of being shaped by hammer or pressure **-ile** = capability **-ity** = expressing state	a material that is capable of being shaped by hammering or pressing; property of materials such as silver and gold
matrix (**mey**-triks)	**matrix** = takes form, enclosed mold	a metal or plastic placed around a tooth to recreate missing walls in order for a restoration to be placed
mechanical retention (m*uh*-**kan**-i-kuhl) (ri-**ten**-sh*uh*n)	**mechanic** = person skilled in operating equipment **-al** = pertaining to **retain** = to hold in place **-ion** = denoting action	dental restoration is held in place by the shape of the cavity preparation and placing retentive grooves in the cavity walls
mercury (**mur**-ky*uh*-ree)	**mercury** = only metal liquid at room temperature; heavy toxic metal	liquid metal added to alloy to form dental amalgam (silver filling)
microleakage (**mahy**-kroh- **lee**-kij)	**micro** = small **leakage** = undesired flow	act of leaking saliva in between a restoration and tooth structure
open margins (**oh**-p*uh*n) (**mahr**-jin)	**open** = not closed; to permit passage through **margin** = a border	space left between a tooth and restoration due to inadequate burnishing or deterioration of the restoration
overhang (oh-ver-**hang**)	**over** = beyond the edge of something **hang** = to incline downward	excess restoration material that has leaked under and out of the matrix band
polish (**pol**-ish)	**polish** = smooth, shine	to make the surface of a material smooth and glossy by rubbing with a polishing instrument
retainer (ri-**tey**-ner)	**retain** = to hold in place or position **-er** = a person or thing	device used to hold a matrix band in place around the circumference of a tooth

Term and Pronunciation	Meaning of Root and Word Parts	Definition
solvent (**sol**-*vuh* nt)	**solute** = substance dissolved in another substance **-ent** = causing an action	the substance that is being dissolved by another substance, for example, salt water: salt is the solute and water is the solvent
spherical (**sfer**-i-*kuh* l)	**sphere** = ball shaped **-al** = pertaining to	dental alloy that is produced with a round body and all its points equidistant from center
tarnish (**tahr**-nish)	**tarnish** = destroy purity or stain metal surface by exposure to air or moisture	discolor or dull the luster of a metallic surface by oxidation
thermal conductivity (**thur**-m*uh* l) (kon-duhk-**tiv**-i-tee)	**therm** = heat **-al** = pertaining to **conduct** = to act as a medium for conveying something such as heat or electricity **-ive** = expressing function **-ity** = expressing state or condition	the measure of a dental material to transfer heat or cold
thermal expansion (**thur**-m*uh* l) (ik-**span**-sh*uh* n)	**therm** = heat **-al** = pertaining to **expand** = to increase in size **-ion** = process of	change in the dental material shape and size due to response to a change in temperature
tin oxide (tin) (**ok**-sahyd)	**tin** = a metallic element used to coat metals to prevent corrosion **oxide** = compound of oxygen with another element	material consisting of tin and oxygen used as the final step to finish and polish an amalgam restoration
trituration (trich-*uh*-**rey**-sh*uh*n)	**triturate** = to reduce to fine particles by rubbing, grinding **-tion** = the act of	the mixing of the amalgam mercury and the alloy powder in the amalgam capsule
triturator (trich-*uh*-**rey**-tohr)	**triturate** = to reduce to fin particles by rubbing, grinding **-tor** = a person or thing	a machine that is used to mix the capsule of amalgamator
varnish (**vahr**-nish)	**varnish** = preparation of resin matter in oil or alcohol; leaves a hard transparent coating on a surface	resin used historically to seal dentin beneath amalgam restorations
wedge (wej)	**wedge** = to pack or fix tightly, triangular in shape	a small triangular-shaped piece of plastic or wood placed between two teeth in order to hold a matrix in place and spread the contact open for restoration placement

## CHAPTER 32

Composite Procedures and Materials

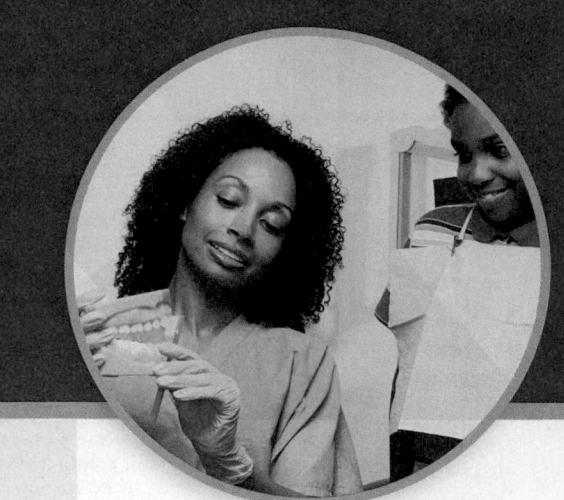

Specific Instructional Objectives

At the completion of this chapter, you will be able to meet these objectives:

1. Use terms presented in this chapter.
2. Differentiate among the types of composite resins.
3. Explain the purpose of etching and bonding.
4. Discuss matrix systems used with composite restorations.
5. Describe the composite restoration procedure.
6. Recall the types of direct esthetic dental restorations.

Introduction

Composite resins, tooth-colored restorative materials, are the most popular and most widely used, because patients want a more natural appearance for their teeth. There are several types and categories of materials used to fill both the anterior and posterior teeth. The various **composites** and combinations are discussed, as well as the placement techniques for them.

Composite Restorative Materials

Composite restorative materials, also referred to as universal resin composites, dominate the field of esthetic restorations. These materials have a natural appearance and can be matched to the patient's tooth color. They were originally used primarily for anterior restorations but have now developed as esthetic restorations for the posterior teeth. Composite restorative materials can be used for Class I, II, III, IV, V, and VI caries (Figures 32-1 and 32-2). Composite materials are also used for **veneers** on anterior teeth that have been stained or that have some erosion, to close a diastema, or to esthetically recontour teeth. These procedures are discussed in Chapter 40, "Fixed Prosthodontics."

Technology is expanding the types of materials available as alternatives to dental amalgam. With concerns over the mercury in amalgams and the desire for the natural appearance of teeth, there is ongoing research and development with composite restorative materials. Composites, glass ionomers, and porcelain materials, as well as combinations of these materials, are used for esthetic restorations.

These direct restorative materials are inserted into the cavity preparation and then self-cured, light cured, or dual cured. They come in disposable syringes and various unit-dose containers (single-application) called **compules** and have a variety of shades or shade modifiers. The location and the size of the cavity determine which material the dentist chooses.

Composition of Composites

The primary components in a composite are the resin matrix and filler particles. Secondary components are the **coupling agent**, initiator/accelerator system, and pigments.

- An organic resin polymer matrix, such as dimethacrylate resin, identified as BIS-GMA or urethane dimethacrylates.
- Some inorganic filler particles, such as quartz, silica, and lithium aluminum silicate. They provide strength and wear resistance.

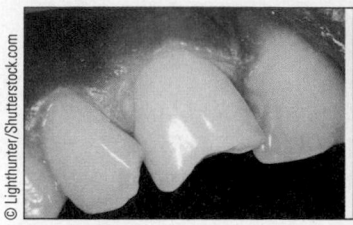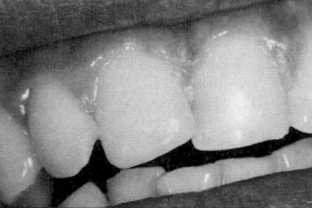

FIGURE 32-1
Before and after photos of a fractured anterior tooth (#8) that was restored with composite restorative material.

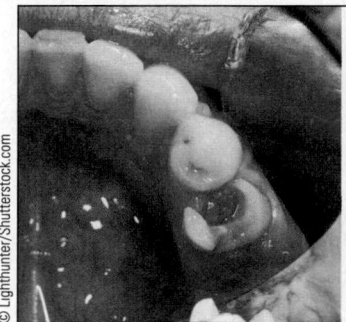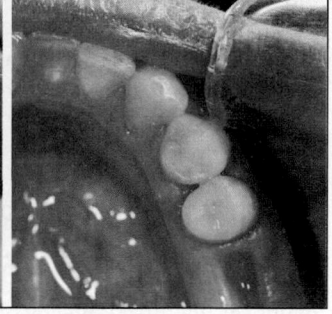

FIGURE 32-2
Before and after photos of a posterior tooth that was restored with composite restorative material.

- An organic silane-coupling agent. The inorganic filler particles are treated with an organic silane coupling agent to provide a bond between the inorganic fillers and the resin matrix.

- The initiator/accelerator system causes setting to occur when the composite is exposed to the blue curing light.

- Pigments provide color for shade matching and esthetics.

- Barium, strontium, zinc, or zirconium may be added to make the composite material more radiopaque.

Chemically cured and light-cured resins are available. The chemically cured composite resin comes as a two-paste system; equal parts of both pastes are mixed chairside until uniformly blended and then applied to the preparation. These types of systems do not require a light for curing.

Light-cured resin materials are most commonly used today in the dental office, do not need mixing, and are available in one tube or single dose cartridges. These resins will set once a curing light is shined upon the material. The light is in the blue spectrum. Direct viewing of the light can lead to retinal damage; both patient and operator should wear special eyewear to protect the retina. The curing light units also come with a special shield to allow viewing by the operator through the shield while keeping the eyes protected.

Light-cured resin material should be placed into the cavity preparation in small increments. Each increment should be cured with the light before placing the next increment. Placing large amounts of resin into the cavity preparation will result in incomplete curing of the material as the light is unable to penetrate the deeper layers; this may result in failure of the restoration.

Types of Composite Fillers

Composite resin restorative materials are classified according to the type, amount, and size of the **filler particles**. The filler particles can make up as much as 84% of the composite material by volume.

- The macrofill composite was the first type of composite introduced and contains filler particles that range in size from 1 to 3 microns. These materials are used for Class IV restorations because they are strong enough to resist fracture and are esthetically pleasing. They do not polish to the same high finish as the microfill and the hybrids and are not used clinically as often as the newer composites.

- The microfill composite contains fillers range in size from 0.01 to 0.1 microns. They are used as a cosmetic filling material for Class III and V restorations. Microfills are also used for direct veneers and diastema closures. Some microfills are reinforced for Class IV restorations and the occlusal portion of Class I and II restorations. Microfill composites are esthetic restorations that resist wear due to abrasion, and they polish well, leaving a high-luster finish.

- The **hybrid** composite is a combination of both macrofillers and microfillers. They contain more than one type of filler particles, usually glass and silica. The glass particles are in the 1- to 3-micron range, and the silica is around 0.04 microns. These composites are stronger and less likely to fracture in high-stress areas than the microfill composites. The hybrids combine the strength and esthetics of the other composites to make a restoration that is strong and polishable. They are used in both the anterior and the posterior areas of the mouth.

- The nanofill composites contain filler particles that are extremely small (0.05–0.10 microns). This allows for higher filler levels that results in improved physical properties and esthetics (they are highly polishable). Nanofill and nanohybrid composites are the most popular composite restorative material in use and have universal clinical applications.

Properties of Composite Restorative Materials

The properties of composite resin materials vary depending on the type and size of the filler. These aspects of the composites are constantly being improved for a strong, esthetic, long-lasting restoration. Overall, composites exhibit the following properties:

- Composites possess resistance to fracturing.
- Occlusal wear resistance is improving.
- Good esthetics allow matching the tooth structure.
- Some composites are radiopaque, making them more visible on radiographic film.
- Composites bond efficiently to dentin and enamel in the cavity preparation, unlike amalgam, where the cavity preparation is designed to hold or retain the amalgam in place.
- Composites are often placed in layers to reduce the effect of polymerization (setting) shrinkage.
- Composite resins have adequate strength for specific applications. The strength requirement varies for various classifications of cavities. For example, the anterior Class III and V cavities do not require great strength but do require color stability. The posterior Class I and II must exhibit enough strength to withstand occlusal stresses, but appearance is not as critical. All composite restorations require a smooth finish to reduce the potential for biofilm and debris accumulation and for staining.
- Expansion and contraction rates of composite materials are similar to the tooth structure.

Preparation for Placement of Composite

As with the dental amalgam restorative procedure, after the patient has been anesthetized and the dental dam has been placed, the dentist performs the cavity preparation procedure and removes the decay using burs and handcutting instruments. Treatment of cavity preparations varies with the amount of enamel and dentin removed and how near the prep is to the pulp. A liner and/or base may need to be placed prior to the composite material. When there is exposed dentin, calcium hydroxide liner or glass ionomer liner and/or glass ionomer base may be used under the composite restoration (Procedure 32-1). If there is a near pulp exposure, calcium hydroxide liner is placed first, then a layer of polycarboxylate cement or glass ionomer cement base may be placed before the composite restoration. Varnish or material containing eugenol CANNOT be used because they inhibit the set of the composite.

Treatment of Cavity Preparation for Composite Restoration

Before placing the composite restoration, the cavity prep needs to be **etched** and a **bonding agent** needs to be placed.

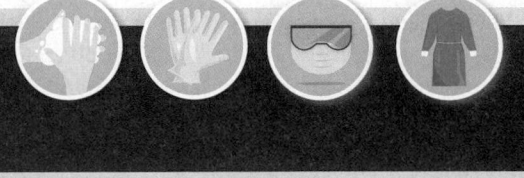

Procedure 32-1
Placing Light-Cured Glass Ionomer Cavity Liner

The chairside dental assistant prepares material and transfers materials and instruments, while the dentist completes the cavity preparation procedure. The operator (dentist, dental hygienist, or qualified assistant) can place the liner.

Steps written in blue font are performed by the operator (dentist or qualified dental assistant), and the chairside assistant's steps are written in black.

Equipment and Supplies

Basic Setup
- mirror and explorer
- air/water syringe tip
- HVE tips

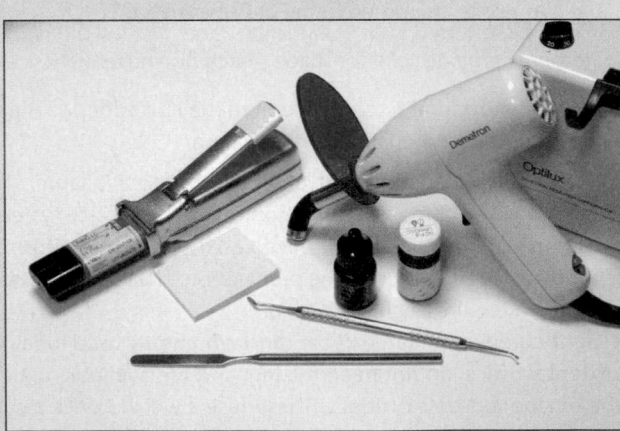

FIGURE 32-3
Light-cured glass ionomer liner setup.

Light-Cured Glass Ionomer Cavity Liner Setup (Figure 32-3)

- manufacturer's directions
- cavity liner—glass ionomer
- application instrument—small, ball-shaped instrument or explorer
- gauze sponges and cotton rolls
- curing light

Procedure Steps *(Follow aseptic procedures)*

Dentist completes cavity preparation procedure.

1. Use air/water syringe and HVE to remove debris as needed.
   - ❏ Rinse and dry area after dentist has prepared the tooth.
     - o Do not overdry; overdrying may damage the pulp.

   Operator determines where to place the liner and the size of the area.
   - ❏ **Evaluates access and visibility.**

2. Pass mirror and explorer.

3. Wash and dry the area with the air/water syringe and HVE.

4. Prepare the glass ionomer liner to be used.
   - ❏ Dispense and mix according to directions.
     NOTE: Usually, light-cured materials do not have to be mixed but are placed directly in the preparation.

5. Assist in placing the liner (Figure 32-4).
   - ❏ Exchange the liner applicator and explorer.
   - ❏ Hold the paper pad close to the patient's chin.
   - ❏ Between applications, wipe off the instrument with gauze for the operator.

   Places the liner on the floor of the preparation.
   - ❏ **Places the liner applicator into the mixed liner.**
   - ❏ **Places the liner in the deepest portion of the cavity preparation in a thin layer; the liner will flow into the area.**
   - ❏ **Be careful not to touch the instrument to the sides of the preparation.**

- ❏ **Spreads the liner in the direction desired by pushing with the liner applicator.**
- ❏ **Repeats this procedure until the liner covers the deepest portion of the cavity preparation.**
- ❏ **Removes any liner from the enamel walls using an explorer.**

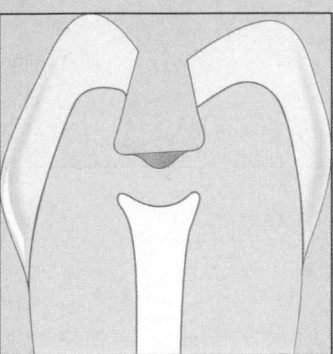

FIGURE 32-4
Placement of glass ionomer liner in preparation.

6. Retrieve mirror.
   - ❏ Exchange liner applicator and curing light.
   - ❏ Wipe off liner applicator.
   - ❏ Tear and fold the top page of the paper pad and dispose of it.
   - ❏ Disinfect the paper pad.

   Holds the light over the tooth.
   - ❏ **Activates the light for the time recommended by manufacturer (usually 10–20 seconds).**

7. Assist in the examination of the liner placement.
   - ❏ Pass mirror and exchange curing light and explorer.

   Examines the cavity preparation after the liner has cured.

8. Retrieve mirror and explorer.

Etchants Etchants enhance retention and bonding between the tooth surface and dental materials. Etching products are typically comprised of a 30–40% phosphoric acid solution. (Refer to Chapter 26, "Dental Sealants," if you need review about etchants.) The etchant comes in liquid or gel form and is packaged in bottles or syringes. Liquids are placed with microbrushes or small cotton pellets. Gel etchants placed with a syringe tip are the most common. Gels are packaged with a number of disposable tips (Figure 32-5).

Etchants are used both on enamel and dentin tooth surfaces and are tinted for more accurate placement. The etchant is usually left on for 30–60 seconds and rinsed thoroughly (Procedure 32-2). The acid etch makes microscopic space in the tooth surface, which increases the surface roughness. The bonding agent flows into these spaces and aids in the bonding process allowing for micromechanical retention.

Bonding Agents Bonding agents are also known as **adhesives** or bonding resins. These materials are used to improve

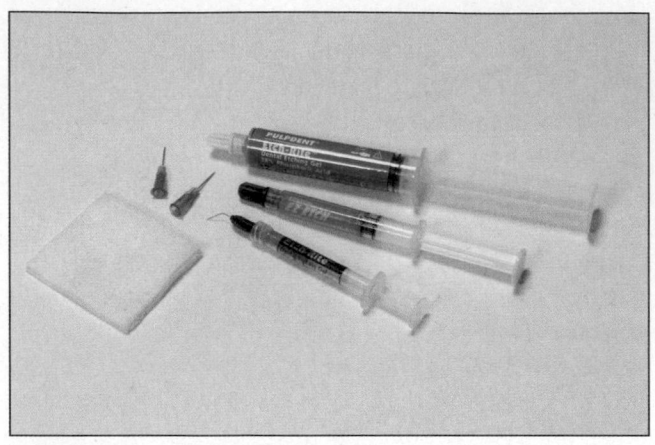

FIGURE 32-5
Various types of etchant materials.

Safety

Preventing Etchant Damage

Care must be given during the etching process because most etching agents contain phosphoric acid that burns soft tissue. The patient, operator, and assistant should wear protective glasses when etchants are used. In addition, the patient should be asked to close their eyes. If the etchant gets into the eye, immediately flush with water and check with a doctor. If the etching agent accidently contacts the soft tissues, immediately rinse the area with large amounts of water and explain to the patient what happened and that the area may be sensitive.

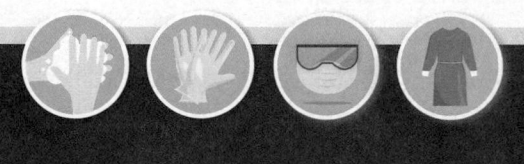

Procedure 32-2
Placing the Etchant

The chairside dental assistant prepares material and transfers materials and instruments while the operator places the isolation materials and the etchant. This procedure can be legally performed by a trained dental assistant in some states.

Steps written in blue font are performed by the operator (dentist, hygienist, or qualified dental assistant), and the chairside assistant's steps are written in black.

Equipment and Supplies

Basic Setup
- mirror and explorer
- air/water syringe tip
- HVE tips

Etchant Setup (Figure 32-6)
- manufacturer's directions
- acid etchant, usually a 30–40% phosphoric acid solution
- isolation materials (dental dam or cotton rolls)
- applicator (syringe, cotton pellets, or small applicator tips)
- dappen dish
- timer

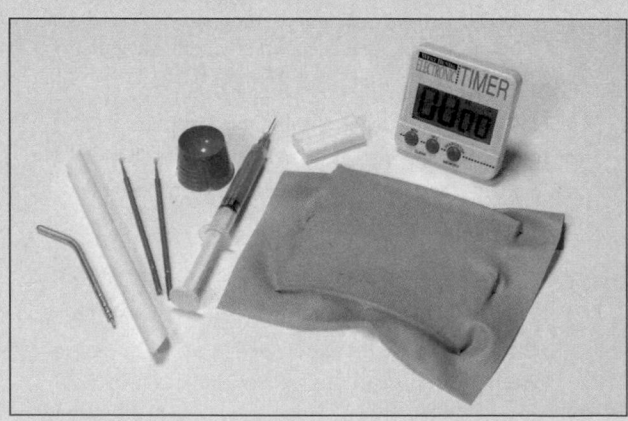

FIGURE 32-6
Tray setup for placing the etchant materials.

Procedure Steps (*Follow aseptic procedures*)

Tooth has been anesthetized and dental dam has been placed.

Dentist completes the cavity preparation and liners/bases have been placed as needed.

1. Rinse the area with air/water syringe and HVE when operator has completed the cavity preparation or liner/base has been placed.

2. Prepare the etchant applicator or syringe.
  ❏ Pass mirror and etchant syringe with tip inserted or place etchant onto microbrush and pass to operator (operator preference).

3. Dry cavity preparation surfaces for 20–30 seconds with air from air/water syringe.

Etches the tooth/teeth surfaces.

Applies etchant following manufacturer's directions. Usually, the etchant is placed on the enamel first and then the dentin, because the dentin is more sensitive to the etchant.
  ❏ Uses a gentle dabbing motion while applying the etchant for the designated amount of time (usually 15–30 seconds).

  ❏ Leaves etchant on surface for 30–60 seconds as directed by manufacturer.

4. Retrieve etchant applicator.

5. Rinse the tooth surfaces for 60 seconds and dry.

Evaluates tooth surface-should appear chalky if etched properly.
  ❏ Repeats etch if surface is not chalky.
  ❏ Does not allow the surface to be contaminated by saliva after etchant is placed.

If saliva or other fluids contact the surface, the etching process must be repeated.

6. Retrieve mirror and explorer.

---

the retention between the tooth structure (enamel and dentin) and the restoration. These materials come in many forms and are often complete systems (Figure 32-7). These materials bond enamel and dentin to porcelain, resins, precious and nonprecious metals, composites, and amalgam.

Bonding materials are low-viscosity resins that may or may not contain fillers. Some bonding agents contain additives with adhesive enhancers, and some contain fluoride. These materials are mainly light cured or dual cured. Procedure 32-3 outlines the steps for placing a bonding agent.

Bonding agents can be classified as total-etch (also called etch-and-rinse) and self-etch systems. Total-etch bonding agents utilize phosphoric acid to clean and etch enamel and dentin. Total-etch bonding agents remove the **smear layer** and replace it with resin.

Self-etch bonding agents utilize an acidic **primer** or primer-adhesive to prepare the enamel and dentin for bonding.

Self-etch bonding agents are used without phosphoric acid and without rinsing. Self-etch bonding agents modify the smear layer rather than remove it, so no rinsing is required. A new type of self-etch bonding agent is called universal bonding agent. These products can be used with or without phosphoric acid and have additional ingredients that can prime metals and ceramics.

Enamel Bonding Adhesion of dental materials to enamel is accomplished by etching with phosphoric acid. This solution alters the surface of the enamel and creates microscopic undercuts between the enamel rods (Figure 32-8). Low-viscosity, unfilled resin bonding agents then penetrate into these undercuts and mechanically lock into them. The restorative material then bonds to this layer and becomes a solid unit. Bonding to enamel is required before placement of composite restorations, pit and fissure sealants, veneers, resin-cemented crowns and bridges, and orthodontic brackets.

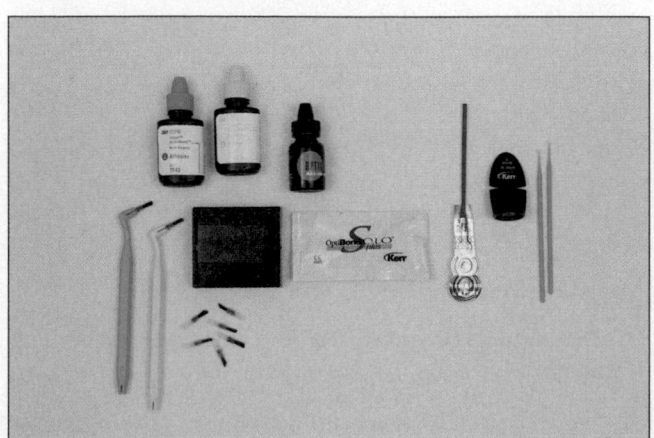

FIGURE 32-7
Bonding agents and systems.

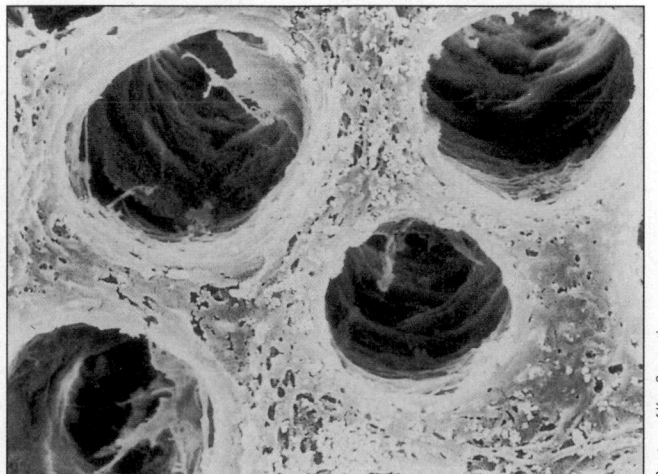

Courtesy of Kerr Corporation

FIGURE 32-8
Microscopic view of etched dentin.

Dentin Bonding Dentin bonding is more challenging than enamel bonding. Some of the obstacles are listed as follows:

- Dentin has a high water content, which can interfere with the bonding to the tooth.

- The composition of the dentin is more organic than inorganic.

- However, the dentin must maintain a small amount of moisture to prevent **desiccating**, or drying out, the tooth. If this happens the structure of the tooth could be damaged.

- Dentin is directly above the pulp, so the operator must take care not to injure the pulp.

- When the dentin is cut with a bur during cavity preparation, it forms a smear layer. This layer of debris lies on the cavity floor and walls and prevents contact between the intact dentin and the bonding agent or adhesive.

Current dentin bonding materials use an etchant to remove the smear layer, because the smear layer is not attached firmly and is unreliable. When the smear layer is removed, the adhesives achieve a mechanical bond with the dentin. Many of the bonding agents are suitable for both enamel and dentin surfaces because of the etchant application. There are some systems that contain acid etchant, primer or conditioner, and adhesive (bonding) material all manufactured to be used together. Primer wets the dentin and penetrates the dentinal tubules. It is applied after etching to the enamel and dentin and air-dried to cause evaporation of the solvent, and then the bonding agent is applied.

Safety

Eye Protection Against the Effect of Curing Light

The blue curing light can affect the eyes of the operator, assistant, and patient, who all should wear radiation-filtering protection (orange- or green-colored lenses) glasses. Avoid looking at the blue light directly even when wearing the tinted glasses. The protective shield should also be placed on the resin light tip to avoid personnel in the area being affected by the blue light.

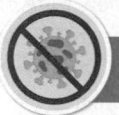

Infection Control

It is recommended to place barrier sleeve covers over the resin light and wands/tips for infection control. A new barrier should be placed for each patient, and if the area under the barrier becomes contaminated, follow the manufacturer's recommendation for disinfection or sterilization.

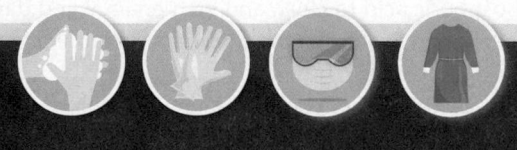

Procedure 32-3
Placing the Bonding Agent

The chairside dental assistant prepares material and transfers materials and instruments while the operator places the bonding agent. This procedure can be legally performed by a trained dental assistant in some states.

Steps written in blue font are performed by the operator (dentist, hygienist, or qualified dental assistant) and the chairside assistant's steps are written in black.

Equipment and Supplies

Basic Setup
- mirror and explorer
- air/water syringe tip
- HVE tips

Bonding Setup (Figure 32-9)
- manufacturer's direction
- bonding agent
- applicators (disposable tips or brushes)
- dappen dish
- isolation means
- air/water syringe
- curing light and shield
- timer

Procedure Steps (*Follow aseptic procedures*)

The tooth has been isolated and prepped, and the liner placed and etched.

1. Rinse the tooth as soon as the time is up.
   - ❏ Continue to rinse for at least 5–10 seconds.

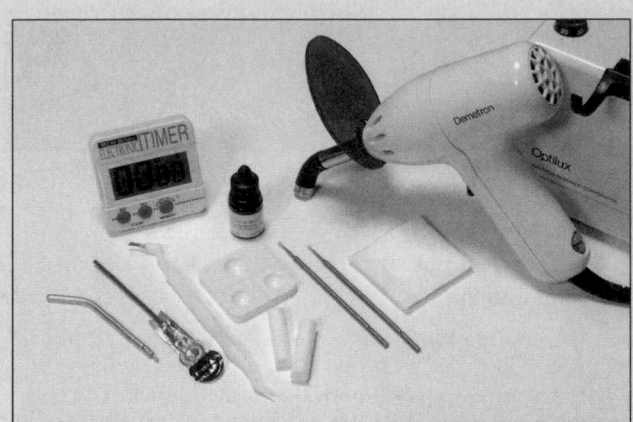

FIGURE 32-9
Tray setup and materials for placing bonding agents.

2. Place primer or conditioner on brush or applicator (operator preference).
   ❑ Pass mirror and applicator to operator.

   Applies bonding agent per manufacturer's directions.

3. Retrieve mirror and applicator and pass curing light.

   Sets bonding agent with curing light.
   ❑ **Holds the light over the tooth.**
   ❑ **Activates the light for the time recommended by manufacturer (usually 10–20 seconds).**

4. Assist in the examination of the bonding agent placement.
   ❑ Pass mirror and exchange curing light and explorer.

   Examines the cavity preparation after the bonding agent has cured.

5. Retrieve mirror and explorer.
6. Dispose of the applicator tips or brushes.

❑ Move quickly to prevent bacterial contamination of the dentin.

Operator places primer or conditioner if bonding involves both the enamel and dentin.

Matrix Systems for Composites

During the preparation of a tooth for composite restoration, one or more axial surfaces may need to be removed (Class II, III, IV cavity preparations). Once these surfaces are removed, the only way to restore the tooth is to use a matrix. A matrix is not needed when all the axial walls remain (Class I and V cavity preparations).

Matrix Strip

Two types of matrix systems are matrix strips and sectional matrices. A thin, clear plastic matrix strip is used with composite, glass ionomer, or **compomer** restorative materials on the anterior teeth (see Procedures 32-4). The clear matrix will allow the light to pass through to cure the material. The strip can be made of nylon, acetate, **celluloid**, or resin and is approximately three inches long and three-eighths inch wide. Clear wedges may also be used to allow passage of the light. A sectional matrix can provide anatomically correct and tight contacts.
The functions of the strip matrix are as follows:

● Provides an anatomical contour and proximal contact relation
● Prevents excess material at the gingival margin
● Confines the restorative material under pressure while the material is being cured
● Protects the restorative material from losing or gaining moisture during the setting time
● Allows the polymerizing light to reach the composite restorative material

Crown Matrix Form

The *crown matrix form (celluloid crown)* is a thin, plastic form that is shaped like the crown of a tooth. On anterior teeth, when the incisal edge is involved (Class IV restorations), a crown form is often used to restore the tooth. The crown forms come preformed in various designs and sizes. The restorative material is placed both in the cavity preparation and in the crown form. The crown form is then placed on the tooth. These crown forms are clear and can be used with light-cured materials. Once the restorative material is set, the crown form is removed and the tooth is ready for final contouring and finishing.

Composite Restoration

After the cavity preparation has been protected with a cavity liner, has been etched, a bonding agent applied and a matrix placed (if needed), the composite restorative material can be placed. Composites are mainly packaged as one-paste systems that are light cured. The paste may come in a syringe for multiple applications or in single-dose cartridges (compules) that are used with a syringe (Figure 32-11). Compules allow easy placement of the composite paste and protect the paste from exposure to **ambient light**, which can initiate curing and make placement of the composite more difficult.

The pastes also come in a variety of shades. A specific shade guide comes with composite systems to assist in the selection of a shade that matches the patient's natural dentition. A shade guide is always used when selecting the composite material.

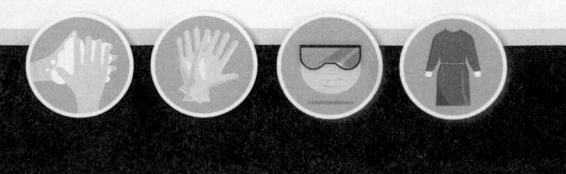

Procedure 32-4
Placement and Removal of the Matrix Strip

The chairside dental assistant prepares material and transfers materials and instruments. The operator (dentist, dental hygienist, or qualified assistant) places and removes the matrix strip.

Steps written in blue font are performed by the operator (dentist or qualified dental assistant), and the chairside assistant's steps are written in black.

Equipment and Supplies
- mirror and explorer
- cotton pliers
- matrix strip
- assortment of clear wedges
- 2 × 2 inch gauze sponges
- crown and bridge scissors

Procedure Steps (*Follow aseptic procedures*)

Placement of the Matrix Strip

1. Assist in the placement of the matrix strip.
   - ❑ Pass mirror and explorer.

   Operator examines the cavity prep prior to placing the matrix.

2. Exchange explorer and matrix strip.

   Contours the strip by drawing the strip over the rounded edge of the handle of the mouth mirror.

3. Retrieve mirror.

   Places the matrix strip between the teeth.
   - ❑ *Holds the strip tightly and slides toward the gingiva.*
   - ❑ *Adjusts the position of the strip so that the entire preparation is covered by the strip.*

4. Assist in placement of the wedge.
   - ❑ Hold the wedge with base down in right palm.
   - ❑ Pass cotton pliers with left hand.

   Operator grasps the wedge with the pliers.
   - ❑ *Places the wedge interproximally between the band and the tooth adjacent to the missing wall with the base of the wedge toward the gingiva.*

5. Retrieve pliers and pass the mirror and explorer.

   Operator examines that the matrix band placement:

- ❑ *is below the gingival step*
- ❑ *the wedge is tight against the band*
- ❑ *there is not space between the band and the gingival step*

6. Retrieve the mirror and explorer.

   Places restorative material and the matrix strip is pulled tightly around the tooth to adapt the material to the convex surface of the tooth.
   - ❑ *Holds the matrix strip in place by hand or with a clip retainer until the material has been cured (Figure 32-10).*

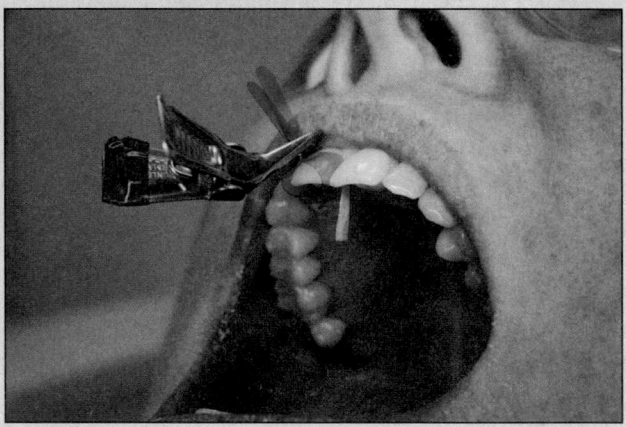

FIGURE 32-10
A strip matrix and wedge are placed. A clip retainer is being used to hold the strip in place.

Removal of Matrix Strip

Procedure Steps (*Follow aseptic procedures*)

1. Assist in removal of the matrix strip after the material has been cured.
   - ❑ Pass cotton pliers and retrieve the clip retainer.

   Operator first removes the clip retainer if one was used.

   Removes the wedge(s) with cotton pliers.

2. Retrieve the wedge and cotton pliers.

   Gently pulls the matrix strip away from the restorative material.

   Removes the matrix strip by pulling it in a lingual–incisal or facial–incisal direction.

3. Retrieve matrix strip.

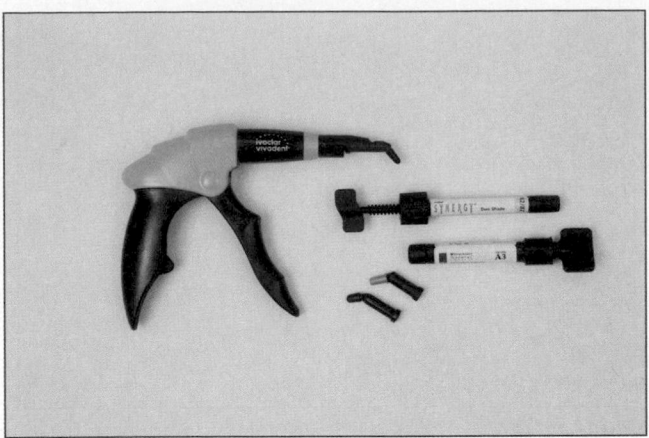

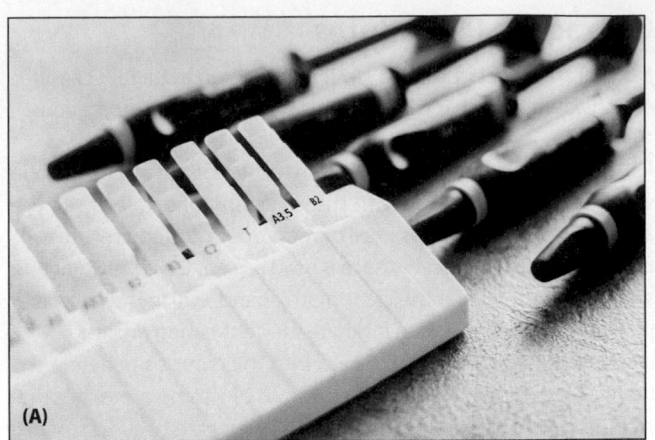

(A)

FIGURE 32-11
Composite material dispensing units including syringes and tips and individual cartridges and a dual-clicker dispenser.

Determine the shade on a clean tooth, with the patient in natural light and prior to placement of the dental dam (drying of a tooth will change the appearance of the color of the tooth). Use the designated shade guide for the material being placed, or use the VITA Shade Guide, which is a universally accepted shade guide (Figures 32-12A and B). Shades can be mixed to create an exact match for the patient. The shade guide has the various shades grouped together depending on **hue**. The A hue group is in the red–yellow range, the B group is more of a yellow range, the C group is in the gray range, and the D group is in the red–yellow–grey range. The **chroma** of the shade is designated with a number. For example, a chroma of 1 on group A is designated as A1. Once the hue is selected, the correct chroma from within the groups should be selected next. The shade tabs should be held next to the patient's existing natural teeth in order to make the final selection of shade. The dentist, assistant, and patient often assist in the selection of the final shade. Some kits may be available with pigments. Pigments are colors that are added to the resin to create an exact match to the patient's natural dentition.

Plastic or Teflon-tipped filling instruments are generally used to place and shape the composite. These instruments come in various sizes and shapes, which aid in adapting the composite material to the cavity preparation. After each layer is placed, it is light cured into a hardened form. Layering of the composite is also a method to modify the restoration shade. The layers can be composed of various types of composites with diverse properties

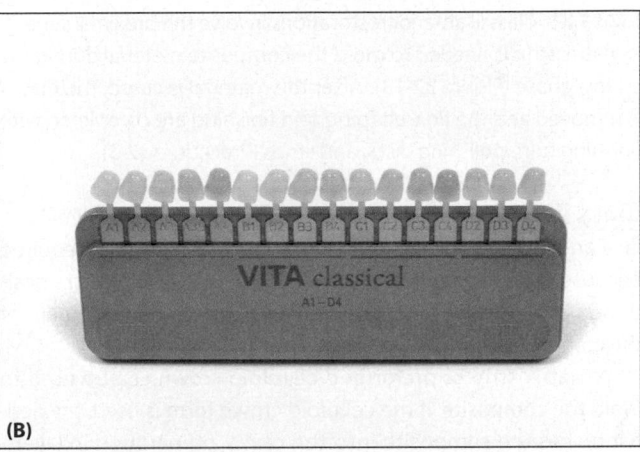

(B)

FIGURE 32-12
(A) A shade guide that came with the composite material. (B) The VITA Shade Guide.

to enhance the qualities of the material. Shrinkage of composites can also be minimized by placing the composite in small layers in the cavity preparation.

Finishing and polishing of composites are important steps to produce a smooth and glossy surface. A smooth, highly polished surface is desired to prevent biofilm retention, minimize the possibility of gingival irritation, and allow for good oral hygiene. Gross reduction of composites is accomplished with diamonds, carbide finishing burs, finishing disks, and strips of alumina. Polishing can be done with rubber cups and points and various polishing tools. One- and two-step polishers impregnated with diamonds or alumina are quick. Finishing and polishing are always done in a wet field.

 **Documentation**

Shade Selection

It is important that the dental assistant write in services rendered all materials and steps performed during the composite procedure, in particular, documenting details about the shade selection. The hue and chroma should be noted along with drawing a picture of how the chroma may be distributed on the tooth when a tooth has multiple shades of color. Documenting that the patient assisted in the shade selection can be helpful if there is a dispute later about restoration color.

Composite Procedures

Most of the procedures are similar, but there are a few changes or considerations change with the different cavity preparations.

Classes I and II Classes I and II are posterior restorations. Shade selection is not as critical with these restorations as it is with the anterior classes. The Class I restoration does not require a matrix, because only the occlusal surface is involved. For Class II restorations, some operators prefer the clear matrix band, which is used with a retainer and wedges, which facilitate the light-curing process.

Some anatomy may be carved into the composite before the final curing. Discs may be difficult to use in some areas, but diamonds, finishing burs, and polishing points are used to smooth and finish the restoration.

Class III Class III anterior restorations involve the proximal surface. A matrix strip is needed to mold the composite material during the curing phase (Figure 32-13). After the material is cured, the matrix is removed and the final shaping and finishing are completed with finishing burs, polishing discs, and strips (Procedure 32-5).

Class IV Class IV anterior restorations involve the proximal surface and incisal edge. In some cases, retention pins are required because of the amount of lost tooth structure. The pins are positioned once the tooth is prepared and before the placement of the composite material.

A matrix strip or preformed celluloid crown can be used to mold the composite. If the celluloid crown form is used, the dentist places the composite into the cavity preparation in layers, curing after each step. A crown form is partially filled and placed

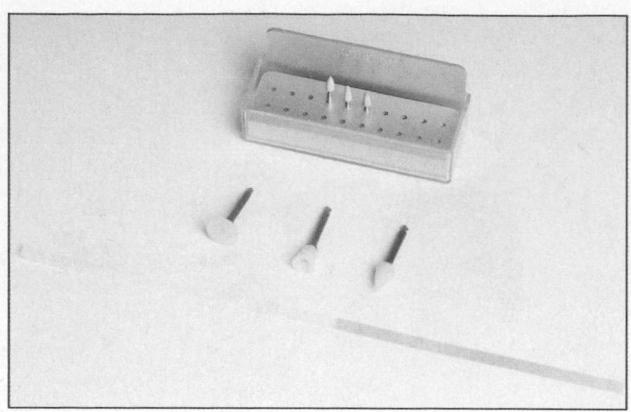

FIGURE 32-13
Polishing burs and an abrasive strip for composites.

over the cured resin in the preparation to form the incisal angle of the restoration. The crown form is prepared with a small hole placed into the incisal edge to prevent air from being trapped. Excess material is removed, and the curing light is used to harden the composite.

After the material is cured, the crown form is removed and the final shaping and finishing are completed with finishing burs, polishing discs, and strips.

Class V A Class V, gingival, one-third restoration may not require a matrix strip, or a precontoured matrix may be used. The restorative materials can be placed in the cavity preparation, shaped with a plastic or composite filling instrument, and then light cured. Finishing should be minimal with these restorations.

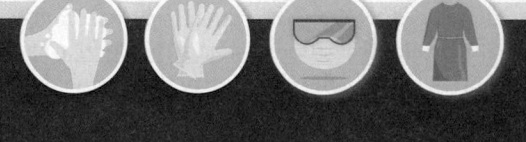

Procedure 32-5
Assisting with a Class III Composite Restoration

The chairside dental assistant prepares material and transfers materials and instruments, while the dentist completes the composite restoration procedure. The dentist administers the local anesthetic and completes the cavity preparation. The operator (dentist, dental hygienist, or qualified assistant) places the topical anesthetic, dental dam, bases/liners, etchant, bonding agent, matrices, and composite restorative material and finishes and polishes the composite restoration.

Steps written in **blue** font are performed by the operator (dentist or qualified dental assistant), and the chairside assistant's steps are written in black.

Equipment and Supplies

Patient Seating Setup (refer to Procedure 18-4)

Local Anesthetic Setup (refer to Procedure 23-2)

Dental Dam Setup (refer to Procedure 21-2)

Cavity Preparation Setup (refer to Procedure 30-6)

Cavity liner— Light-Cured Glass Ionomer (refer to Procedure 32-1)

Etchant Setup (refer to Procedure 32-2)

Bonding Setup (refer to Procedure 32-3)

Composite Matrix System Placement Setup (refer to Procedure 32-4)
- strip matrix
- assortment of clear wedges
- 2 × 2 inch gauze sponges
- crown and bridge scissors

Composite Restoration Setup (Figure 32-14)

- mouth mirror (A)
- explorer (B)
- cotton pliers (C)
- plastic filling instrument (D)
- spoon excavator (E)
- composite placement instrument (F)
- composite condensing instrument (G)
- bonding agent (H)
- resin brush (I)
- microbrush (J)
- etchant (K)
- composite syringe material (L)
- shade guide (M)
- matrix clip retainer (N)
- finishing strips (O)
- wedges (P)
- resin mixing well (Q)
- articulating paper (R)
- sandpaper discs (S)
- finishing burs (T)
- curing light and shield (not shown)
- protective curing glasses (not shown)

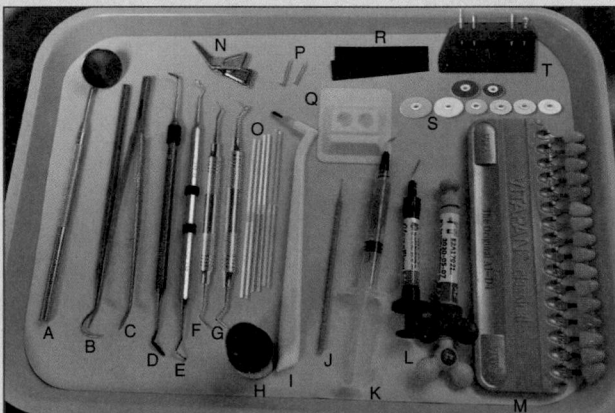

FIGURE 32-14
Class III composite restoration setup.

Procedure Steps

1. Escort and seat patient (refer to Procedure 18-4).

2. Prepare in advance for steps in cavity preparation procedure:
   - ❑ Open patient's chart in dental software.
   - ❑ Navigate to the dental charting screen.
   - ❑ Open patient's latest radiographic history on the computer monitor, or place on view box.
   - ❑ Attach handpieces to dental unit.
   - ❑ Insert burs into handpieces.

- ❑ Inform dentist that the patient is ready.
- ❑ Introduce dentist as they enter the treatment area.

Dentist greets the patient and takes position at the dental chair.

   ❑ **Signals for the procedure to begin (Procedure 20-1).**

3. Pass mouth mirror and explorer at operator's signal.

Dentist examines tooth or teeth with mirror and explorer.

Dentist administers local anesthetic.

4. Assist in administration of local anesthetic (refer to Procedure 23-2).

5. Assist in determining shade (Figure 32-15).
   - ❑ Pass shade guide.
   - ❑ Turn dental lamp off.
   - ❑ Record shade on patient's chart.

Dentist determines the composite material shade.
   ❑ **Uses natural light and compares shade guide to patient's teeth.**

Operator places dental dam.

6. Assist in placement of dental dam (refer to Procedure 21-3).

Operator tries clamp over tooth to be clamped and examines the mouth for dental dam placement.

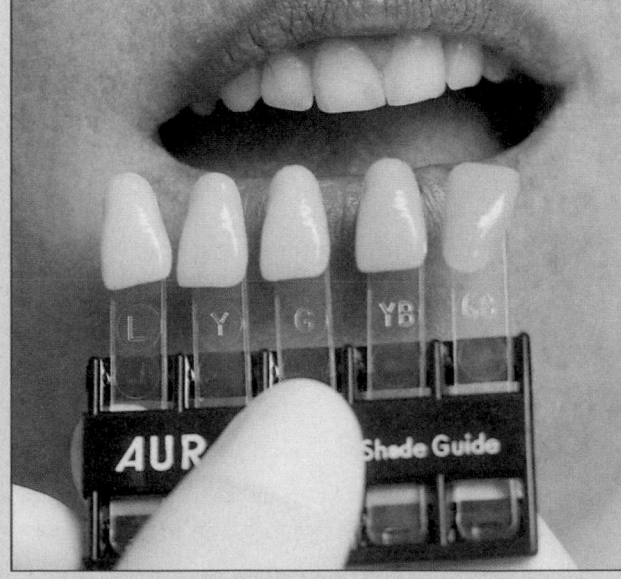

FIGURE 32-15
Determining a shade before the placement of the dental dam.

(Continues)

❏ Retrieve clamp in clamp forceps.

❏ Pass dental dam material attached to dental dam frame with right hand.

❏ Pass dental punch to operator with left hand.

Operator punches dental dam for Class III cavity preparation.

❏ Pass clamp for operator to place into dental dam.

❏ Pass clamp forceps.

Operator places the clamp, dental dam, and frame as a unit.

❏ Retrieve clamp forceps and pass plastic instrument.

Operator releases dental dam from wings of the clamp using plastic instrument.

❏ Rinse, evacuate, and dry the operation site.

❏ Pass floss.

Operator flosses septum of dental dam between the teeth being isolated.

❏ Retrieve floss and pass plastic instrument.

Operator inverts the dental dam around the cervix of the isolated teeth.

❏ Assist inversion by following the operator with air syringe.

Dentist examines area after placement of dental dam.

❏ Transfer mirror and explorer.

❏ Ask dentist's preference of bur for high-speed and low-speed handpieces.

❏ Insert burs into handpieces.

Dentist removes caries and cuts tooth structure to form cavity preparation.

7. Assist with removal of dental caries and tooth structure.

❏ Retrieve explorer and transfer handpiece.

❏ Hold HVE near handpiece head during cutting to evacuate dental spray.

❏ Rinse and aspirate as needed.

❏ Keep mirror clean during procedure by gently blowing air on mirror.

❏ Use air/water syringe and HVE to remove debris as needed.

❏ Rinse and dry area after dentist has prepared the tooth.

   o Do not overdry; overdrying may damage the pulp.

Dentist refines the cavity preparation as needed.

8. Retrieve handpiece and pass handcutting instruments as needed by dentist to refine cavity preparation.

Dentist examines preparation prior to placing dental materials.

9. Retrieve handpiece and pass explorer.

❏ Retrieve mirror and explorer.

❏ Rinse and dry area after dentist refines cavity preparation.

Operator determines where to place the liner and the size of the area.

❏ **Evaluates access and visibility.**

10. Pass mirror and explorer.

11. Wash and dry the area with the air/water syringe and HVE.

12. Prepare the glass ionomer liner to be used.

❏ Dispense and mix according to directions.

NOTE: Usually, light-cured materials do not have to be mixed but are placed directly in the preparation.

13. Assist in placing the liner.

❏ Exchange the liner applicator and explorer.

❏ Hold the paper pad close to the patient's chin.

❏ Between applications, wipe off the instrument with gauze for the operator.

Places the liner on the floor of the preparation.

❏ **Places the liner applicator into the mixed liner.**

❏ **Places the liner in the deepest portion of the cavity preparation in a thin layer; the liner will flow into the area.**

❏ **Be careful not to touch the instrument to the sides of the preparation.**

❏ **Spreads the liner in the direction desired by pushing with the liner applicator.**

❏ **Repeats this procedure until the liner covers the deepest portion of the cavity preparation.**

❏ **Removes any liner from the enamel walls using an explorer.**

14. Retrieve mirror.

❏ Exchange liner applicator and curing light.

❏ Wipe off liner applicator.

❏ Tear and fold the top page of the paper pad and dispose of it.

❏ Disinfect the paper pad.

Holds the light over the tooth.
- ❏ Activates the light for the time recommended by manufacturer (usually 10–20 seconds).

15. Assist in the examination of the liner placement.
- ❏ Pass mirror and exchange curing light and explorer.

Examines the cavity preparation after the liner has cured.

16. Retrieve mirror and explorer.
17. Prepare the etchant applicator or syringe.
- ❏ Pass mirror and etchant syringe with tip inserted or place etchant onto microbrush and pass to operator (operator preference).
- ❏ Some operators prefer placing a matrix strip prior to etching to prevent the etchant from being placed on the adjacent.
18. Dry cavity preparation surfaces for 20–30 seconds with air from air/water syringe.

Etches the tooth/teeth surfaces.

Applies etchant following manufacturer's directions. Usually, the etchant is placed on the enamel first, and then the dentin, because the dentin is more sensitive to the etchant.

- ❏ Uses a gentle dabbing motion while applying the etchant for the designated amount of time (usually 15–30 seconds).
- ❏ Leaves etchant on surface for 30–60 seconds as directed by manufacturer.
19. Retrieve etchant applicator.
20. Rinse the tooth surfaces for 60 seconds and dry.

Evaluates tooth surface-should appear chalky if etched properly.
- ❏ Repeats etch if surface is not chalky.
- ❏ Does not allow the surface to be contaminated by saliva after etchant is placed.

If saliva or other fluids contact the surface, the etching process must be repeated.

21. Retrieve mirror and explorer.
22. Rinse the tooth as soon as the time is up.
- ❏ Continue to rinse for at least 5–10 seconds.
- ❏ Move quickly to prevent bacterial contamination of the dentin.

Removes matrix strip if used.
- ❏ Retrieve matrix strip and wedge if used.

Operator places primer or conditioner if bonding involves both the enamel and dentin.

23. Place primer or conditioner on brush or applicator (operator preference).
- ❏ Pass mirror and applicator to operator.

Applies bonding agent per manufacturer's directions.

24. Retrieve mirror and applicator and pass curing light.

Sets bonding agent with curing light.

- ❏ Holds the light over the tooth.
- ❏ Activates the light for the time recommended by manufacturer (usually 10–20 seconds).
25. Assist in the examination of the bonding agent placement.
- ❏ Pass mirror and exchange curing light and explorer.

Examines the cavity preparation after the bonding agent has cured.

26. Retrieve mirror and explorer.
27. Dispose of the applicator tips or brushes.
28. Assist in the placement of the matrix strip.
- ❏ Pass mirror and explorer.

Operator examines the cavity prep prior to placing the matrix.

29. Exchange explorer and matrix strip.

Contours the strip by drawing the strip over the rounded edge of the handle of the mouth mirror.

30. Retrieve mirror.

Places the strip matrix between the teeth.
- ❏ Holds the strip tightly and slides toward the gingiva.
- ❏ Adjusts the position of the strip so that the entire preparation is covered by the strip.
31. Assist in placement of the wedge.
- ❏ Hold the wedge in right hand with the base down.
- ❏ Exchange mirror and cotton pliers with left hand.

(Continues)

Operator grasps the wedge with the pliers.

❏ Places the wedge interproximally between the band and the tooth adjacent to the missing wall with the base of the wedge toward the gingiva.
❏ Pass the mirror and explorer.

Operator examines the matrix band placement to ensure:

❏ it is below the gingival step.
❏ the wedge is tight against the band.
❏ there is not space between the band and the gingival step.
❏ Retrieve the mirror.

Operator signals for preparation of composite materials.

32. Pass single-application syringe.

Operator places a layer of the composite material directly into the cavity preparation.

33. Pass composite placement instrument.

Operator condenses and shapes composite.

34. Exchange composite placement instrument and curing light.

Operator continues to place incremental layers and then light cures after each layer is placed.

35. Continue exchanging composite application syringe, composite placement instrument, and curing light until the cavity prep is filled.

Holds matrix around the tooth to restore contour and maintain the composite in position after the prep is filled.

36. Assist in removal of the matrix strip after the material has been cured.
❏ Pass cotton pliers and retrieve the clip retainer.

Operator first removes the clip retainer if one was used.

Removes the wedge(s) with cotton pliers.

37. Retrieve the wedge and cotton pliers.

Gently pulls the matrix strip away from the restorative material.

Removes the matrix strip by pulling it in a lingual–incisal or facial–incisal direction.

38. Pass mirror and exchange cotton pliers and explorer.

Operator evaluates the composite placement and finishes the restoration.

39. Assist in finishing the composite restoration.
❏ Pass low-speed handpiece with operator's choice of finishing burs, diamonds, or abrasive discs.
❏ Use air/water syringe and HVE when the operator is using the handpiece.
❏ Pass abrasive strips to smooth the interproximal area at operator's signal.

Operator polishes the composite restoration.

40. Assist in polishing the composite restoration.
❏ Pass low-speed handpiece with operator's choice of polishing points, discs, and cups.
❏ Use air/water syringe and HVE when the operator is using the handpiece.

41. Assist in removal of the dental dam.
❏ Pass clamp forceps.

Operator removes the clamp.

❏ Pass the crown and bridge scissors.

Operator cuts the dental dam septa to avoid fracturing the interproximal area of the restoration and for ease in removal.

❏ Rinse and evacuate the mouth.

Operator checks the dental dam to ensure that all material has been removed.

❏ Pass floss as needed to remove any remaining floss.

42. Assist in checking occlusion.
❏ Pass gauze square and articulating forceps holding articulation paper.

Operator checks the occlusion.

❏ Dries the area with gauze square.
❏ Places articulating paper against the teeth.
❏ Asks the patient to gently close on the paper; caution must be taken to avoid fracturing the resin margin.
❏ Pass mirror and rotary finishing instrument of choice if restoration registers high spots.

Operator adjusts restoration with rotary finishing instruments in low-speed handpiece until it is absent of any articulation marks.

❏ Retrieve mirror and exchange handpiece and gauze square to remove markings.

Dentist makes a final check of all work of an expanded assistant. In some states the dentist must perform a final examination of a placed restoration.

43. Assist in final evaluation of composite restoration.
  ❏ Pass mirror and explorer.

44. Provide patient with postoperative instructions orally and in written form.

45. Write up procedure in Services Rendered.

46. Dismiss and escort patient to reception area (Procedure 18-5).

Date	Services Rendered
02/18/XX	Updated medical and dental history, no changes noted. BP = 120/80; T = 98.6F, P = 80, R = 18
	Placed 20% benzocaine gel to injection sites for 2 minutes. Administered 2 cartridges (3.6 ml) of 2% lidocaine with 1:100,000 epi to mandibular left. No reaction
#9	M composite restoration (shade #) with glass ionomer liner, etchant, and bonding agent
	POI do not bite on lip, no eating/drinking until numbness wear off, eat only on opposite side until numbness has worn off, can chew on restoration, call office if restoration feels high or if there is discomfort or pain; chewing on ice and hard, chewy candy can damage restorations
	Assistant's initials

Types of Direct Esthetic Dental Restorations

There are four types of materials used as direct esthetic dental restorations: composites, glass ionomer, hybrid glass ionomer, and compomers.

Composites

Besides the universal composite discussed previously, there is flowable and packable composite. These composites have been modified to provide additional applications and use.

Flowable Composites A flowable composite is similar to the microfill and hybrid composites in filler content and particle size. It has less filler material and a low viscosity that allows for an easy flow and direct application into cavity preparations by small syringe tips. Flowable composites can adapt to the irregularities of cavity walls and flow into narrow preparations of conservative dentistry. It has many uses, such as linings for large cavity preparations; as additives to temporaries; for filling voids in non-carious areas, including toothbrush abrasion areas, or areas of occlusal tooth loss due to bruxism; and, in some cases, as a pit and fissure sealant. There are several advantages of flowable composites: they are easy to place, can reach small areas, and are esthetic with many shades available. Disadvantages include a lack of strength, more shrinkage than hybrid composites, and that they cannot be used alone to fill large preparations (Figure 32-16).

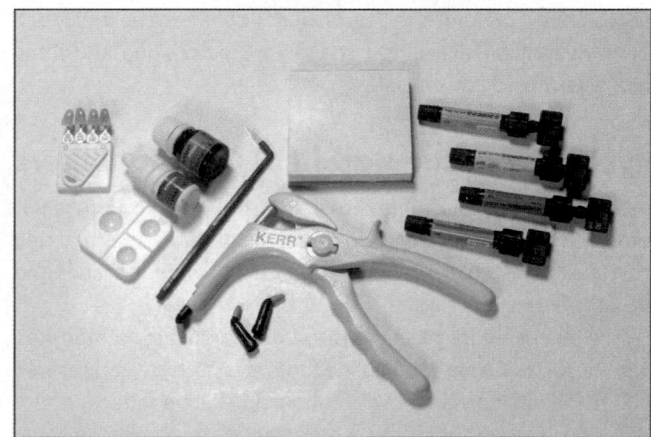

FIGURE 32-16
A flowable composite system.

Packable Composites The packable composite is sometimes called a condensable composite. They are more putty-like and stiffer in consistency than other composites, and they are highly viscous and contain large amounts of fillers. They are used in posterior areas for **core buildups** and in places requiring a resistant, stronger restoration. Packable composites can be pressed into the restoration in layers. Sometimes, various types of composite are layered for optimum results. Packable composites are not subject to as much shrinkage when polymerized as certain other composites because they contain less resin and more filler.

Glass Ionomer Restorations

Glass ionomer materials are used as an esthetic restoration most often in non-stress-bearing restorations (Figure 32-17). Examples include Classes I (both stress and non-stress-bearing areas), II (non-stress-bearing areas), and V (non-stress-bearing areas). Class V includes restoring the gingival one-third and root surface cavities. These materials are often used in pediatric and geriatric restorations, sealants, long-term temporaries, and core buildups. Glass ionomers bond well by adhering chemically to the tooth structure. Upon setting these materials, release fluoride on the finished preparation to resist recurrent decay. The materials have low solubility; therefore, the tooth does not have to be totally dry. They are available in multiple shades, are radiopaque, and come in powder/liquid and capsules.

Hybrid (or Resin-Modified) Glass Ionomers

The combination of composite resins and glass ionomers has improved the quality of glass ionomer restorations. They are used for Class III and V restorations. They come in various shades and are light-cured materials.

The technique for placement is similar to that for composites, with the following exceptions: The tooth is conservatively prepared with no need for mechanical retention or bevels. A retraction cord may be placed with the Class V preparations to expose the entire margin of the cavity preparation. The preparation is cleaned with a chlorhexidine soap solution. Follow the manufacturer's directions on finishing and polishing the restoration. Some need to be kept moist or have lubricants placed when polishing. A layer of light-cured enamel bonding agent is applied over the finished restoration.

Compomers

Compomers are a cross between composites and glass ionomers in characteristics and properties. They are single-paste, light-cured systems that release fluoride and are bonded to the walls of the cavity with dentin or enamel adhesives. Compomers are mostly used on all types of restorations for primary teeth and on Class III and V restorations for permanent teeth. They adhere to dentin without etching the tooth, but a primer or adhesive must be used (Figure 32-18).

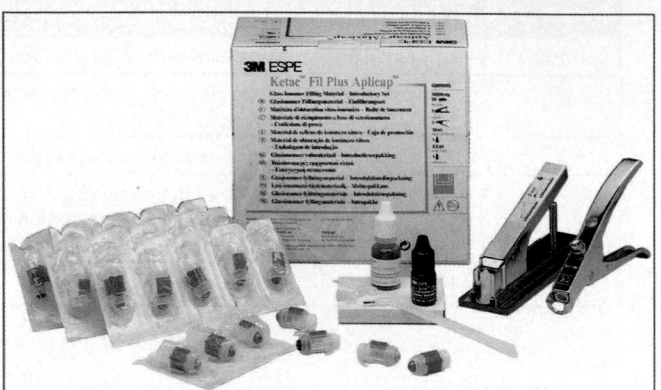

Courtesy of 3M ESPE

FIGURE 32-17
A glass ionomer restorative material kit.

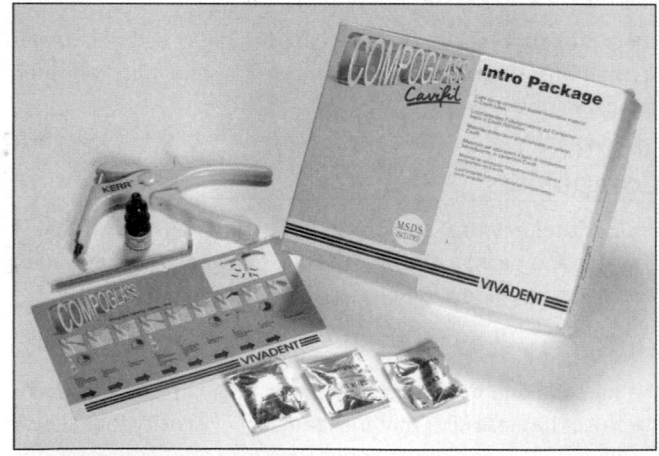

FIGURE 32-18
A compomer restorative material kit.

Chapter Summary

Knowledge of the properties of composite restorative materials is necessary for the dental assistant to properly prepare and manipulate the materials and also allows the dental assistant to be a step ahead of the dentist. The dental assistant gains knowledge of sequence and techniques used in placing the composite restoration in this chapter.

The general chairside assistant prepares restorative materials for the dentist to place in the prepared cavity. In some states dental assistants or hygienists are allowed to place matrices and restorative materials. The restorative dental assistant or restorative dental hygienist completes specific education including didactic and clinical training to become licensed to perform these skills.

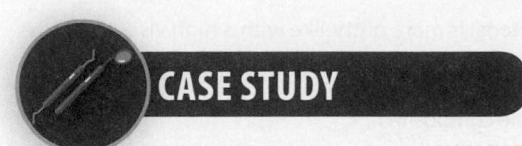

CASE STUDY

The dentist is running a little longer with a patient and asks Josiah, the dental assistant, to take Ms. Krishna's shade after she is seated. Josiah notices that the cervical area of the canine to be prepared is much yellower than the incisal third. The tooth is also partially covered by biofilm.

Case Study Review

1. What does Josiah need to do to the tooth prior to shade selection?

2. How can Josiah approach selecting a tooth of many shades?

3. Explain how Josiah could represent his selection to the dentist when the dentist examines the patient.

Review Questions

Multiple Choice

1. Which restorative material is the most popular and widely used?
   a. glass ionomers
   b. composites
   c. porcelain
   d. compomers

2. Which composite has the highest level of filler particles, is highly polishable, and is the most popular?
   a. macrofill
   b. microfill
   c. hybrid
   d. nanofill

3. Which of the following materials should NOT be used with a composite resin?
   a. material containing eugenol
   b. glass ionomer liner
   c. calcium hydroxide liner
   d. All of these

4. Which provides a bond between filler and resin matrix?
   a. dimethacrylate
   b. quartz and silica
   c. coupling agent
   d. initiator/accelerator

5. Hybrid composites are a combination of macrofillers and microfillers. The nanofill and nanohybrid have universal application and are the most popular.
   Select the correct response based on these statements.
   a. Both statements are true.
   b. Both statements are false.
   c. The first statement is true; the second statement is false.
   d. The first statement is false; the second statement is true.

6. All of these materials can be used as a liner/base when placing a composite restoration EXCEPT:
   a. calcium hydroxide liner.
   b. glass ionomer cement.
   c. zinc oxide–eugenol cement.
   d. polycarboxylate cement.

7. When dentin is exposed during the cavity preparation, calcium hydroxide may be placed under the composite restoration. Polycarboxylate cement is placed when there is a near pulp exposure.
   Select the correct response based on these statements.
   a. Both statements are true.
   b. Both statements are false.
   c. The first statement is true; the second statement is false.
   d. The first statement is false; the second statement is true.

8. What material is used to make microscopic spaces to allow for better retention?
   a. bonding agent
   b. composite
   c. etchant
   d. glass ionomer

9. An etchant is used to remove the smear layer left after the cavity preparation. Etchants provide a surface to achieve a mechanical bone with the dentin when using dentin bonding materials.
   Select the correct response based on these statements.
   a. Both statements are true.
   b. Both statements are false.
   c. The first statement is true; the second statement is false.
   d. The first statement is false; the second statement is true.

10. Which is the correct order of placing these materials?
    a. primer, etchant, bonding agent, and composite
    b. etchant, bonding agent, primer, and composite
    c. primer, etchant, composite, and bonding agent
    d. etchant, primer, bonding agent, and composite

11. Which matrix systems is preferred for Class III composites?
    a. celluloid matrix and clear wedge
    b. universal matrix and wooden wedge
    c. T-bands and plastic wedge
    d. celluloid crown

12. Which matrix systems is preferred for Class IV composites?
    a. celluloid matrix and clear wedge
    b. universal matrix and wooden wedge
    c. T-bands and plastic wedge
    d. celluloid crown

13. All of these are true when taking the shade EXCEPT:
    a. the assistant can use a designated shade guide or universal shade guide.
    b. the assistant should determine shade in natural light using shade tab next to the tooth.
    c. the assistant should check shade before dental dam placement.
    d. the tooth should be thoroughly dried before taking shade.

14. The dentist can minimize shrinkage of the composite by placing the resin _____.
    a. in small layers and curing until hardened
    b. quickly all at once into the cavity preparation and curing for longer times
    c. in crown forms before curing
    d. in matrix and holding it tight in place during curing

15. Which is the correct order in completing the composite restoration procedure?
    a. etchant, liner, primer, bonding agent composite, and finishing and polishing
    b. liner, etchant, primer, bonding agent, composite, and finishing and polishing
    c. liner, etchant, primer, bonding agent, composite, and polishing and finishing
    d. primer, etchant, liner, bonding agent, composite, and finishing and polishing

16. Which material has a low viscosity and would be selected to fill areas of tooth abrasion or for lining large cavity preparations?
    a. packable composites
    b. flowable composites
    c. glass ionomers
    d. compomers

17. Which material is more putty-like with a high viscosity and is often used for core buildups?
    a. packable composites
    b. flowable composites
    c. glass ionomers
    d. compomers

18. Which material may be selected for patients with high caries risk due to its release of fluoride after placement?
    a. packable composites
    b. flowable composites
    c. glass ionomers
    d. compomers

19. A hybrid glass ionomer is a combination of glass ionomer and _____.
    a. a compomer
    b. universal composite resin
    c. flowable composite
    d. packable composite

20. Which material adheres to the dentin without etching the tooth and releases fluoride?
    a. compomer
    b. universal composite resin
    c. flowable composite
    d. packable composite

Critical Thinking

1. The dental assistant documents that the shade selection is C2. What do the "C" and "2" represent?

2. The dental assistant has placed a Class V composite, and it is completely hard after being set with the curing light. What instrumentation can be used to finish the composite?

3. Which cavity preparations will require the use of a matrix strip during placement of a composite restoration?

Key Terms

Term and Pronunciation	Meaning of Root and Word Parts	Definition
adhesive (ad-**hee**-siv)	**adhere** = to stick or hold fast **-sion** = of or pertaining to	two or more dissimilar substances united by a molecular force acting in an area of contact
ambient light (**am**-bee-*uh*nt) (lahyt)	**ambient** = surrounding, encircling **light** = radiance, illuminated, makes things visible	outside light or light from lights in operatory
bonding agent (**bond**-ing) (**ey**-j*uh*nt)	**bond** = something that fastens, holds together **-ing** = expressing the action of **agent** = means by which something occurs or is achieved	material used to join resin composite or resin cement to tooth structure

Term and Pronunciation	Meaning of Root and Word Parts	Definition
celluloid (**sel**-yuh-loid)	**cellulose** = main constituent of plant cell walls used in making paper, rayon, and film **-ose** = resembling, like	clear plastic celluloid strips used as a matrix when inserting resin cement or resin materials in proximal cavities
chroma (**kroh**-muh)	**chroma** = quality or intensity of color	degree of color saturation
compomer (kuh m-**puh**-mer)	**comp** = composite **-omer** = glass ionomer	polyacid-modified composites; derives name from merging parts of composite and glass ionomer; also contains fluoride
composite (kuh m-**poz**-it)	**com** = together **position** = to place	dental composite resins are types of synthetic resins used in dentistry as a tooth-colored restoration
compules (**komp**-yool)	**compule** = plastic tip that supplies one dose of a material	plastic dispensing unit with one dose of material
core buildup (kohr) (**bild**-uhp)	**core** = central or innermost part **buildup** = process of strengthening	a missing portion of a the tooth is restored with a dental material to support a crown restoration
coupling agent (**kuhp**-ling) (**ey**-juhnt)	**coupling** = device or chemical joining two materials **agent** = a chemical that causes a change	usually silane removes moisture, improves the distribution of fillers in the composite matrix, and provides chemical bond between resin and filler
desiccating (**des**-i-keyt-ing)	**desiccate** = remove most of the water; dehydrate **-ing** = expressing action	the state of extreme dryness
etch (ech)	**etch** = to cut into a surface by dissolving it with acid	dissolve tooth structure or restorative material with acid
filler particles (**fil**-er) (**pahr**-ti-kuhlz)	**fill** = to put as much as can be held into **-er** = denoting action or process **part** = portion **-cle** = indicating smallness	silica, quartz, or various glasses added to composites to improve wear resistance, occupy volume, reduce shrinkage, and provide radiopacity
hue (hyoo)	**hue** = a graduation or variety of a color; tint	quality that distinguishes one family of color from another; yields perceived color
hybrid (**hahy**-brid)	**hybrid** = anything derived from different sources; produced through manipulation of unlike parts for specific characteristics	resins made from a combination of macrofill and microfill particles
primer (**prim**-er)	**prime** = to prepare or make ready for a particular purpose or operation **-er** = denoting action or process	chemical agent used to improve bonding of a material
smear layer (smeer)	**smear** = to stain or make dirty with something **layer** = a thickness of some material laid on or spread over a surface	layer of enamel or dentin produced by grinding with dental burs
veneer (vuh-**neer**)	**veneer** = to face or cover with a material that is more desirable as a surface material	custom-made shells of tooth-colored material bonded to the front surface of the teeth to improve their appearance

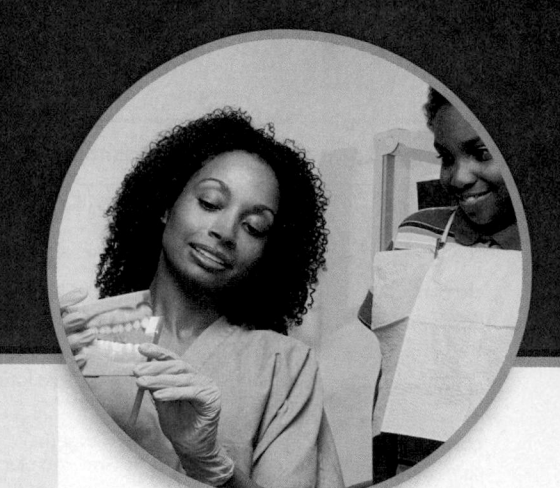

CHAPTER 33
Dental Laboratory Materials

Specific Instructional Objectives

At the completion of this chapter, you will be able to meet these objectives:

1. Use terms presented in this chapter.
2. Distinguish between alginates and alginate substitutes.
3. Describe factors that can influence working and setting times for alginates.
4. Demonstrate the knowledge and skills needed to prepare, take, and remove alginate impressions and wax bites.
5. Explain why an alginate impression must be stored properly.
6. Describe the uses of elastomeric impression materials.
7. Distinguish between polyvinyl siloxane and polyether impression materials.
8. Demonstrate the knowledge and skills necessary to prepare elastomeric impression materials such as polysulfide, silicone (polysiloxane and polyvinyl siloxanes), and polyether for the dentist.
9. Compare and contrast different types of gypsum materials.
10. Discuss the materials necessary for fabrication of diagnostic casts.
11. Explain how excess water affects the manipulation and properties of gypsum materials.
12. Demonstrate the knowledge and skills necessary to pour and trim a diagnostic cast.
13. Identify use of a dental articulator and facebow for dental casts or study models.
14. Demonstrate taking a facebow transfer and mounting models on an articulator.
15. Identify various classifications and uses of waxes used in dentistry.
16. Identify the differences and similarities in techniques of the common methods of fabricating custom-made impression trays.
17. Demonstrate the knowledge and skills necessary to fabricate and fit custom temporary restorations.
18. Identify the two types of provisional materials.
19. Identify properties of provisional materials and indicate their clinical importance.

Introduction

There are a number of ways that dental materials are used by a dental assistant. Some materials, specifically those in the dental laboratory, are not used in the dental treatment room. Other materials are used initially in the treatment room and then taken by the dental assistant to the laboratory, where a second procedure is completed. The models can be taken to an in-office dental laboratory, where the laboratory technician completes the procedures, or the models may be sent out to a commercial dental laboratory for additional procedures. As these materials are used in the oral cavity and exposed to contaminants, it is always important to ensure that cross-contamination does not occur. The dental assistant must pay special attention when transferring materials from the treatment room to the dental laboratory.

Any dental assistant who has skills in performing laboratory duties is an asset to their employer. The better cross-trained the dental team members are, the better the dental office functions. Many basic functions in the dental laboratory are routinely performed by the dental assistant, such as pouring and trimming **study models**, fabricating custom trays, and fabricating **provisional restorations**. To accomplish these procedures, the dental assistant must understand the materials that are used, the properties of each material, and the steps in each procedure.

Hydrocolloid Impression Materials

Impressions are taken to produce an accurate three-dimensional duplicate of an individual's teeth and surrounding tissues. The impression makes a negative reproduction in which **gypsum** material can be poured and therefore creates a completed positive model. Varying degrees of **accuracy** can be obtained depending on the type of impression material and gypsum used. The operator gives directions to the dental assistant on the type of model that is desired. Models can be used for many purposes. One of the most common models that the dental assistant will make is the study **cast** or primary model. Normally, the impression material used is irreversible hydrocolloid, which is commonly called alginate.

Alginate (Irreversible Hydrocolloid) Impression Material

Alginate is a generic name used for a group of **irreversible hydrocolloid** impression materials. Alginate is used when less accuracy is needed. One of the most common areas in which alginate is used is in making diagnostic casts or study models. **Alginate impression** material is also used routinely in making opposing models for fixed and removable prosthetics, orthodontic appliances, mouth guards, bleach trays, provisional restorations, and custom trays.

The three types of alginate material are traditional, extended storage, and alginate substitutes. The extended storage alginate lasts about 4 to 5 days after the impression is taken. Traditional alginate material and alginate substitutes are discussed later in this chapter. Alginate material's primary ingredient is either sodium or potassium alginate, therefore giving the material its generic name. Potassium alginate is extracted from seaweed and kelp, which is a marine growth found primarily off the coastline of Japan. This material readily dissolves in water to form a viscous sol (liquid). Added to this potassium alginate is a calcium sulfate which, through a chemical reaction, forms a gel (solid). To control the setting time and allow for the material to be placed in a tray and into the patient's mouth, trisodium phosphate is added. Without this retarder, the material would be set before it could be inserted into the patient's mouth. A retarder slows the setting of the material. To increase the strength and stiffness and make up the bulk of the material, fillers are used. Some of the fillers that may be in alginate are diatomaceous earth, zinc oxide, color, and flavoring. The fillers constitute from one-half to three-quarters of the total composition of the material. A small amount of potassium titanium fluoride is added to the material to counteract a specific action of the alginate whereby it tends to soften the

surface of the gypsum products and not allow them to fully set on the surface. Due to the particularly chalky taste, alginate may come in assorted flavors or liquid flavoring drops may be added during mixing. Table 33-1 lists some ideal features of alginate materials.

Advantages and Disadvantages of Alginate Alginate has a number of advantages that explain its extensive use in the dental office:

- Ease of manipulation
- Minimal equipment required
- Economical
- Meets the requirements for accuracy for a number of applications
- Rapid setting
- Comfort for the patient
- Can be used for both teeth and tissue impressions
- Withdraws over undercuts (recessed areas that are wider on the bottom than on the top) because of its elastic properties

The disadvantages of alginates primarily come from the loss of accuracy due to atmospheric conditions. If the impression is not the extended alginate and is stored prior to pouring, it is susceptible to **dimensional change** due to loss or gain of water. If the impression loses water content due to heat, dryness, or exposure to air, it causes shrinkage. This condition is known as **syneresis**. If the reverse happens and the impression takes on additional water and causes swelling, the impression will have a dimensional enlargement, known as **imbibition**. The material also can cause some tissue distortion or displacement

TABLE 33-1 Ideal Features of Alginate Impression Materials

Powder doesn't require agitation before dispensing.
Dustless powder—minimizes inhalation and controls messiness in mixing area.
Homogeneous, smooth, uniform mix—no clumps, bubbles, or voids
Alginate stacks in tray and flows during insertion in the mouth
Sets in 1 to 2 minutes for fast-set product
Good elastic recovery when removed from the mouth—minimal distortion
Flexible—easily removed from the mouth
Adequate tear strength
Acceptable taste, texture, and scent

due to its thickened consistency. Another disadvantage is that it is not as precise or accurate as some of the other materials on the market.

Setting Time for Alginate

The time from which the alginate powder material is mixed with water until it is completely set is called the gelatin time. The gelatin time is different depending on the type of material used. As mentioned previously, most of the materials come in two types: Type I is a fast-set alginate and Type II is a regular-set alginate. The gelatin time for both is broken into two different increments. The first is the working time, where the dental assistant mixes the material to the desired consistency, loads it into the tray, and inserts and positions the tray into the patient's mouth. The working time for the regular set is approximately 1 minute and even less than that for the fast set. The second phase is the setting time, where the material remains in the patient's mouth and sets until the chemical reaction is completed, the gel is formed completely, and the tray is removed from the patient's mouth. The Type I gelatin time including both the working and setting times ranges from 1 to 2 minutes. The Type II gelatin time normally ranges from 2 to 4½ minutes including both working and setting times. The setting times can be altered. The most convenient way to control the setting time is to adjust the temperature of the water. The suggested temperature of water to be used is room temperature. If the temperature of the water is higher, working and setting times are shorter. If the water is cooled, the working and setting times are longer. Warm weather causes the alginate to set more rapidly as well. Some offices refrigerate the water during hot, humid times.

The choice of whether to use Type I or Type II is made according to the preference of the operator and the conditions of the patient needing the impression. The outcome of both materials is the same. Cases in which the slower Type II material is beneficial would be where the operator is working alone, or the tray is going to be difficult to insert into the oral cavity in the correct position in the patient's mouth. The faster set, Type I, is beneficial where the patient is a child or where the patient has a problem with gagging and the tray needs to be removed as rapidly as possible for patient comfort.

Some alginates contain chromatic agents that cause the alginate to change color throughout the mixing and setting of the material. Once the powder is incorporated into the water, the alginate is a bright pink or purple. The color begins to fade to a lighter pink, signaling the amount of time left to load the tray and seat it in the patient's mouth. Once seated, the alginate will fade completely white, indicating the complete set time and removal from the patient's mouth.

Alginate Packaging, Storage, and Shelf Life

Normally, alginate is purchased in airtight plastic canisters the size of coffee cans (Figure 33-1). The powder may be inside, in a foil or plastic bag, to be placed in the mixing container when ready for use. Along with the powder are the measuring devices for the powder and the water. Some of the canisters have built-in areas

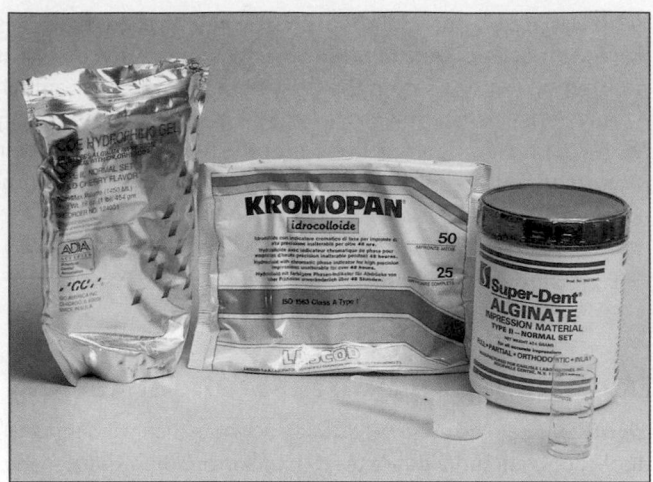

FIGURE 33-1
Foil bags and plastic canister of alginate with measuring devices.

on the outside for the water-measuring devices. This is convenient for the dental assistant. Alginate can be bought in premeasured sealed bags, but this is much more costly and normally unnecessary because measuring the powder is not a difficult procedure. Most dental offices currently use powder/water alginate.

It is important that alginate not be stored in an area that can have temperatures 72° F/23° C because it causes loss of strength and lower resistance to deformation. If kept in an area where moisture can contaminate it, the material will demonstrate erratic setting times. Optimum storage is in a cool, dry place. Keeping the lid screwed tightly in place while not in use aids in prevention of unintentional moisture contamination. The normal shelf life for alginate materials is not more than 1 year.

Alginate Powder/Water Ratio

All the alginate materials come with their own specific measuring devices for both the powder and the water. First, read the manufacturer's directions for dispensing the material. The dispensing of each material may be slightly different. For instance, some of the materials direct that the powder be fluffed with the lid on prior to putting it into the powder scoop, while others may indicate that the powder should be packed into the scoop. This makes a definite difference regarding the amount of powder that is used. The water measure is normally a plastic cylinder with lines on it to indicate the amount of water for each scoop of powder. Normally, it takes two scoops of powder to two increments of water for each mandibular impression. Three of each are normally needed for the maxillary impression. (These amounts can change depending on the size of the patient's arches.)

It is important that the correct amounts of both powder and water are used. If a lower water-to-powder ratio transpires, a stiffer, thicker mix is produced. Along with being more difficult to use, the material has decreased detail, decreased ability to pull from undercuts, decreased flexibility, increased tissue displacement, rapid setting time, increased strength, and a mix that is not as uniform in consistency. If a higher water-to-powder ratio is used, the impression has a decreased resistance to deformation, decreased strength, and increased setting time. Both increases and decreases in spatulation affect the setting time and decrease the strength of the material.

Bowls and Spatulas Used for Alginate Impressions

The operator can either use a flexible rubber bowl and a flexible spatula to mix the alginate or use a disposable bowl. The flexible rubber bowl allows easy mixing of the alginate but must be sterilized or disinfected after use. The disposable bowl comes with a disposable spatula that can be thrown away. They eliminate the aseptic procedures required after contamination of the rubber bowl and spatula (Figure 33-2).

Alginate Substitute

Alginate substitutes are silicone-based impression materials intended as an alternative to traditional alginate materials. One popular brand is available in a premixed package with a dispensing unit (Figure 33-3). This alginate unit can be mounted on the wall or placed on the counter. The premixed alginate is placed in the dispensing unit, and the assistant places a dispensing tip on the unit. The material is then dispensed directly into the tray (Figure 33-4). This unit is similar to, or the same as, the unit for dispensing some polysiloxane or polyether materials (final impression materials). It can also come in a cartridge with a mixing tip and a gun for dispensing. This extruder operation for mixing eliminates hand mixing. The mixing unit must be wiped down with surface disinfectant thoroughly after each use to prevent cross-contamination.

Trays Used for Alginate Impressions

Several trays are available for alginate impressions (Figure 33-5). Most commonly used are the perforated trays that come in metal and plastic. The trays have holes in them for the material to ooze through and lock the impression material in the tray. If not using the perforated

trays, the material may stay in the patient's mouth as the tray is removed. The impression then has to be retaken due to loss of accuracy from the flexible material coming loose from the rigid tray. Some operators use a rim lock tray in place of the perforated tray. The rim lock tray has a border around the top of it to aid in holding the material in place. This tray has no perforations in it. Alginate adhesive may also be applied to the impression tray to

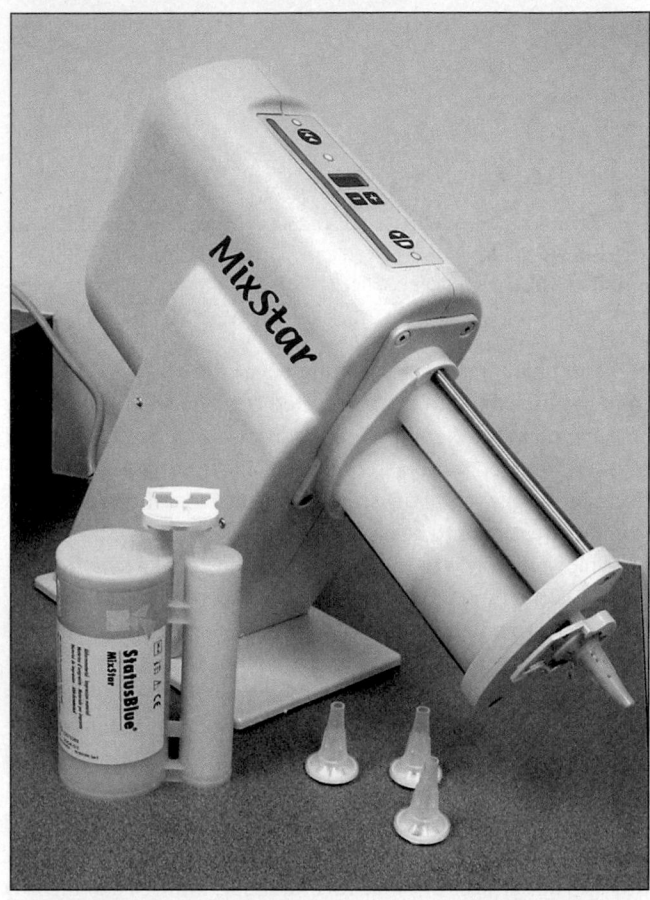

FIGURE 33-3
Unit for dispensing premixed alginate substitute.

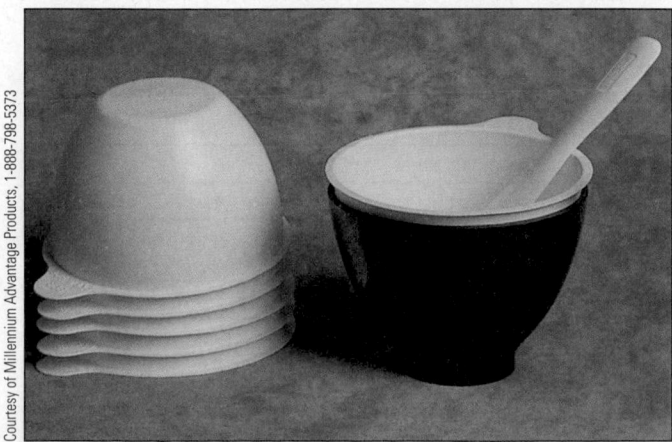

Courtesy of Millennium Advantage Products, 1-888-798-5373

FIGURE 33-2
Disposable bowl and spatula used for mixing alginate and plaster.

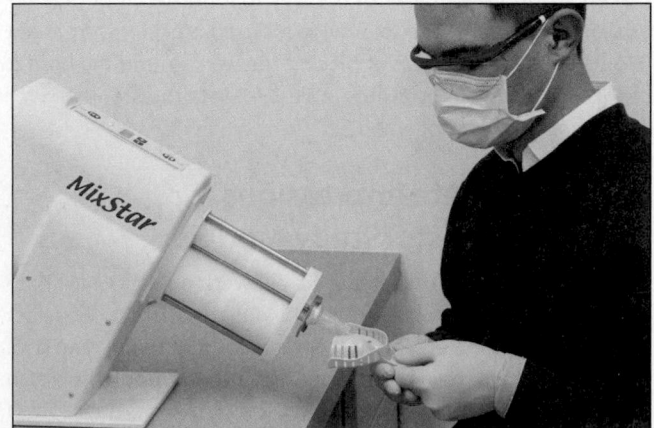

FIGURE 33-4
Dispense material directly in tray.

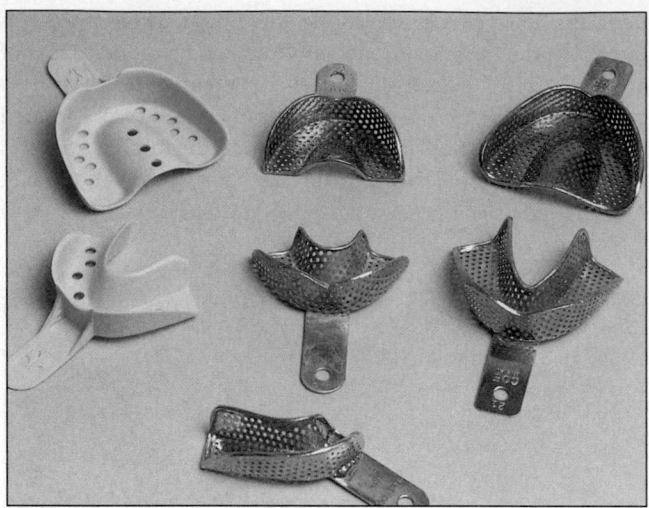

FIGURE 33-5
Assortment of alginate trays in different sizes.

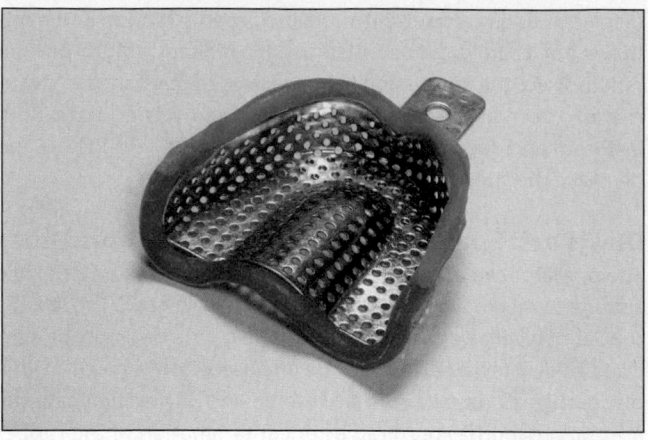

FIGURE 33-6
Alginate tray with beading wax on the periphery. The wax aids in tray extension and patient comfort.

prevent the impression from lifting out of the tray upon removal from the mouth. Both the perforated tray and the rim lock tray come in plastic and metal. The metal trays can be cleaned and reused after sterilization. In order to achieve complete sterilization of reusable metal trays, it is important to remove all debris from the trays prior to heat sterilization.

Whichever tray is used, the operator must make sure that the tray fits correctly in the patient's mouth. Selecting the correct tray is essential to obtaining an accurate impression. The trays come in several sizes. The operator first examines the patient's mouth and identifies a sterilized or disposable tray that he or she thinks will fit. The trays should be tried in the patient's mouth to ensure a correct fit and comfort for the patient. The tray should extend 2 or 3 mm beyond the last molar area and below both the lingual and facial tooth surfaces. Keep in mind that there should be enough room for 2 mm of the alginate material between the tray and all surfaces of the teeth and tissue. If the size of the tray seems appropriate but the tray does not extend over the last molar area, utility wax strips can be used. The wax is placed in layers until the desired length is achieved. The wax also can be placed around the border of the tray to lengthen it on the lingual and facial areas and to provide more comfort for the patient (Figure 33-6). The process of placing the wax around the border of the tray is called beading. Table 33-2 lists the standards for taking an alginate impression.

Taking Alginate Impressions for Diagnostic Casts (Study Models)

In some states, dental assistants are allowed to take the alginate impressions, while in other states, the dental assistant can select the tray, mix the material, load the material into the tray, and pass the tray for the dentist to place in the patient's mouth. It is also important to note that in some states, the assistant is not allowed to take a final impression for orthodontics and prosthetics.

The alginate material can be mixed using the Alginator II° method (Procedure 33-1) or the manual method (Procedure 33-2).

The material can also be mixed in a plastic bag: place powder in the bag, add water, and knead. The "bag procedure" is very effective in ensuring aseptic technique because the bag can easily be disposed of, but mixing in this manner incorporates more air bubbles if not done properly.

The Alginator II device makes mixing easier, as well as increasing the likelihood of a bubble-free mixture. Rather than the operator rotating the bowl, the device spins the bowl about 300 times a minute.

Wax Bite Registration

A wax bite registration is taken to establish the relationship between the maxillary and mandibular teeth (see Procedure 33-4). It can be used to verify the occlusal relationship when trimming the diagnostic casts (study models). Normally, wax that is formed in a horseshoe shape is used, but the flat sheets of utility wax can be used as well.

Other materials are also used in taking a bite registration. Polysiloxane impression material, specifically designed for occlusal registration, can be dispensed using a dispensing gun

TABLE 33-2 Accuracy of Alginate Impressions

Tray covers all necessary areas.
Tray is centered on central incisors.
Tray is not pushed down or up too far, allowing teeth to penetrate through material to tray.
Impression is not torn.
Impression is free of bubbles and voids.
Impression shows sharp anatomic detail of all teeth and tissues.
Impression has a good "peripheral roll" and includes all vestibule areas.
Mandibular impression shows good detail in retromolar area and shows lingual frenum and mylohyoid ridge area.
Maxillary impression shows good detail in tuberosities and palate areas.

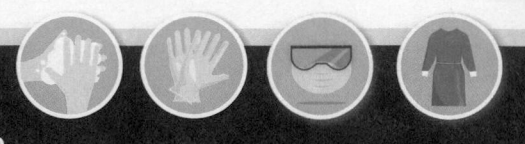

Procedure 33-1
Mixing Alginate with an Alginator II Mixing Device

This procedure is performed to mix alginate needed for an irreversible hydrocolloid impression. The materials are prepared, and the Alginator II mixing device is prepared and ready.

Equipment and Supplies
- PPE: examination gloves, mask, protective glasses, and protective clothing
- handwashing soap or hand sanitizer
- sanitized dental treatment area and barriers placed over equipment

Alginator II Mixing Setup (Figure 33-7A)
- alginator II (Figure 33-7B)
- flexible spatula/broad blade or disposable spatula (A)
- flexible rubber bowl(s) or Alginator II flexible bowl only (B)
- alginate material powder measuring devices (C)
- water measuring device with water (D)
- alginate flavoring (optional)

Procedure Steps

Material Preparation

1. Measure the impression water (room temperature) for the mandibular impression, normally two calibrations of the water measurement device supplied by the manufacturer.

2. Place water in the rubber bowl attached to the Alginator II. Some operators use an additional bowl in the Alginator II so that it can be cleaned easily. Leaving the bowl attached allows for more control; attach it by rotating slightly to the side and fitting into the grooves on the bottom of the bowl.

3. Fluff the powder before opening the powder canister, if indicated by the manufacturer's directions.

4. Fill the measure with powder by overfilling and then leveling off with the spatula (use the flat blade, not the edge blade of the spatula). Dispense two corresponding scoops (for mandibular impression) into the water in the rubber bowl.

5. Add drops of flavoring to the water, if being used.

6. Incorporate the mixture slightly.

7. Hold the spatula to the side of the bowl with the mixture and use slight pressure. Turn on the Alginator II; the material is mixed as the bowl rotates (300 times a minute). Use the side of the spatula blade during this process.

8. Collect material by using the edge of the spatula starting from the deepest area in the bowl. Upon completion, the material should be homogeneous and smooth, without bubbles.

9. Remove excess material from bowls with paper towels, and then clean thoroughly and disinfect.

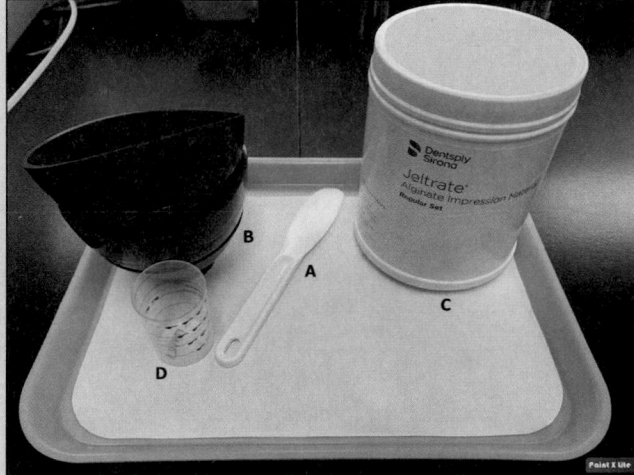

FIGURE 33-7A
Alginator II mixing setup.

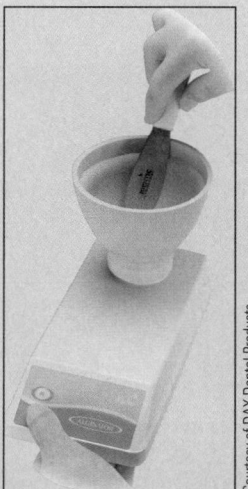

Courtesy of DAX Dental Products

FIGURE 33-7B
Alginator II used for mixing alginate.

Procedure 33-2
Mixing an Alginate Impression and Loading Impression Tray

This procedure is performed to mix alginate needed for an irreversible hydrocolloid impression. The materials are prepared, mixed and loaded into an appropriately fitted impression tray.

Equipment and Supplies

Patient Seating Setup (refer to Procedure 18-4)

Impression Setup (Figure 33-8)
- flexible spatula/broad blade or disposable spatula (A)
- flexible rubber bowl(s) or disposable bowl (B)
- alginate material with water and powder measuring devices (C)
- water
- alginate flavoring (optional)
- impression tray(s) (D)
- beading wax (if necessary) (E)

Procedure Steps

1. Escort and seat patient (refer to Procedure 18-4).

Material Preparation

2. Place wax around the borders of the impression trays, if necessary, to extend the borders of the trays or to provide additional patient comfort.

3. Measure the impression water (room temperature). For the mandibular impression, this is normally two calibrations of the water measurement device supplied by the manufacturer; the maxillary uses three.

4. Place water in the flexible mixing bowl.

NOTE: Place the water in the bowl first to ensure that all the powder is incorporated into the mixture.

5. Add flavoring, if it is being used.

6. Fluff the powder prior to opening the powder canister, if indicated by the manufacturer's directions.

7. Fill the measure of powder by overfilling and then leveling off with the spatula (use the flat blade, not the edge blade of the spatula) to get an accurate measure.

8. Dispense two corresponding scoops into a second flexible rubber bowl. (Three scoops for the maxillary impression.)

9. Place powder in water when ready.

10. Mix the water and powder first with a stirring motion.

11. Mix by holding the bowl in one hand, rotating the bowl occasionally, and using the flat side of the spatula to incorporate the material through pressure against the side of the bowl (Figure 33-9). The mixing time for Type I fast set is 30 to 45 seconds, and for Type II regular set, 1 minute.

12. Mix until homogeneous and creamy.

13. Load it into the impression tray. On the mandibular tray, the material should be loaded from both lingual sides (Figure 33-10). Use the flat side of the blade to condense the material firmly into the tray, pushing material from front to back. On the maxillary tray fill from the posterior part of the tray. (Figure 33-11A). Smooth impression material with a wet finger (Figure 33-11B).

14. Remove a small amount of material from palate portion (Figure 33-11C).

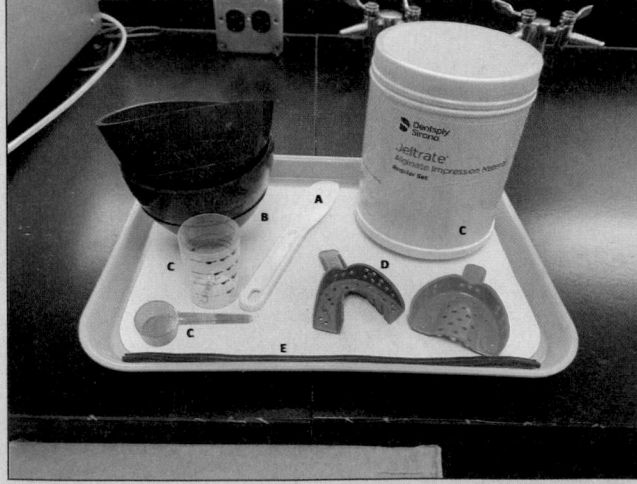

FIGURE 33-8
Impression setup.

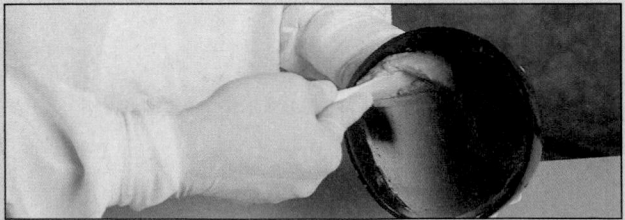

FIGURE 33-9
Mixing alginate material in a flexible rubber bowl, while pushing on sides of bowl to eliminate air bubbles.

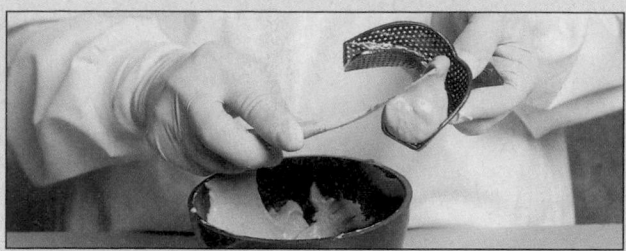

FIGURE 33-10
Loading mandibular alginate tray from lingual side to eliminate air spaces.

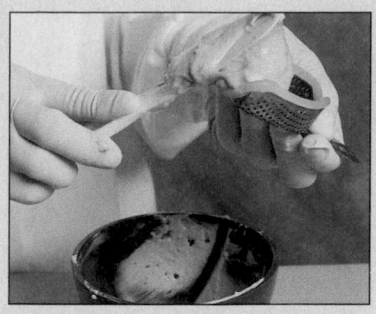

FIGURE 33-11A
Load impression tray from the posterior.

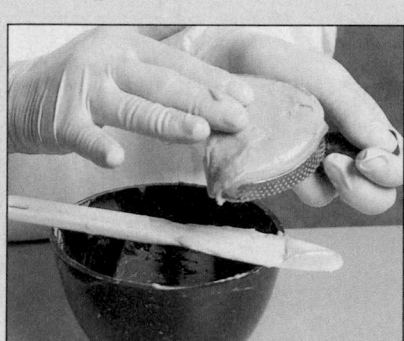

FIGURE 33-11B
Smooth material.

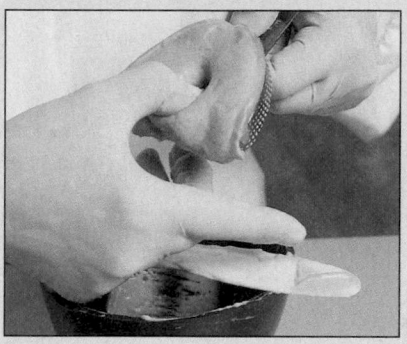

FIGURE 33-11C
Remove a small amount of material from the palate area.

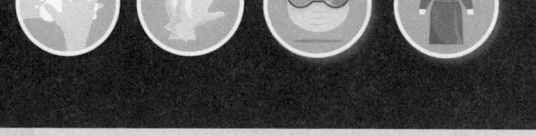

Procedure 33-3
Taking an Alginate Impression

Refer to Procedure 33-2, "Mixing an Alginate Impression and Loading Impression Tray," to identify PPE, patient setup, equipment, and supplies. Take the mandibular model first to allow the patient to build confidence and feel more secure before the maxillary impression, which often causes more gagging.

Steps written in **blue** font are performed by the operator (dentist or qualified dental assistant), and the chairside assistant's steps are written in black.

Procedure Steps

Operator signals for procedure to begin.

1. Pass prepared mandibular tray from Procedure 33-2 to operator.

   Faces the patient and retracts the right cheek slightly.

   Rubs the excess alginate material onto the occlusal surfaces of the teeth in order to obtain more accurate anatomy.

   Inverts the impression tray so that the material is toward the teeth.

   Turns the tray so that it passes through the lip opening with one side of the tray entering first, using the other hand to retract the opposite corner of the mouth.

Seats the heel of the left side of the tray, then proceeds to seat the anterior, then rolls to seat the right heel. Keeps the incisal edges of the teeth 1–2 mm from the tray.

Asks patient to raise the tongue and move it side to side to ensure that the lingual aspect of the alveolar process is defined in the impression.

Pulls out the lip from the center with the other hand.

Allows the lip to cover the tray. It should be close to the handle portion of the tray.

Holds it in the patient's mouth with two fingers on the back of the tray, one on the right side, one on the left side, until set.

Allows material to set. Checks the excess material around the edges of the impression tray, or in the bowl, to determine if the material is set. The material should feel firm and not change shape when pushed.

Removes alginate impression (see below).

2. Accept alginate impression from operator.

   Take maxillary impression by performing the following steps.

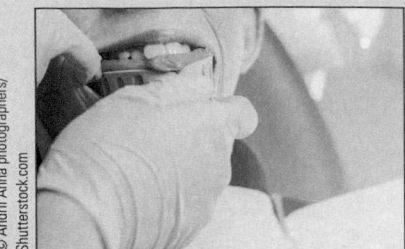

FIGURE 33-12
Placing the maxillary tray.

3. Pass prepared maxillary tray from Procedure 33-2 to operator.

Stands behind or to the side of the patient.

Places some alginate on the occlusal surfaces of the maxillary teeth.

Places the maxillary tray in the patient's mouth by turning the tray so that it passes through the lip opening with one side of the tray entering first, using the other hand to retract the opposite corner of the mouth (Figure 33-12).

Seats and centers the tray by positioning its posterior border and then continues forward. Leaves space between tray and teeth.

Holds it in position until the material is set in the bowl (Figure 33-13).

Removing the Alginate Impression
Procedure Steps

Ensures material is completely set by feeling the material in the mixing bowl or by feeling excess material in the mouth.

Loosens the tissue of the lips and cheek around the periphery with fingers to break the suction-like seal.

Places fingers of the opposing hand on the opposite arch to protect the adjacent arch as the tray is being removed.

Removes the tray in an upward or downward motion (depending on the arch) with a quick snap. Turns it to the side to allow it to be removed from the oral cavity.

Removes any excess alginate material from the patient's mouth with the evacuator and has the patient rinse. Checks the patient's face for any excess alginate material. If present, gives the patient a tissue and mirror to remove the material.

Checks the impression for accuracy (Figure 33-14)

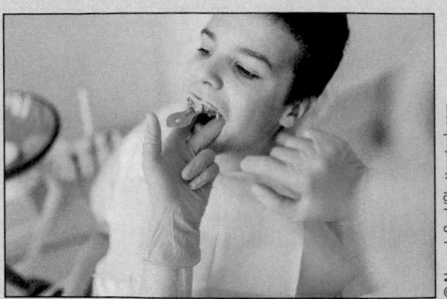

FIGURE 33-13
Holding tray in position as material sets.

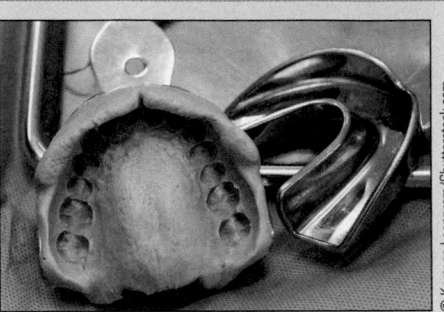

FIGURE 33-14
An accurate impression.

4. Rinse the impression gently with water to remove saliva, blood, or debris.

5. Disinfect impression according to manufacturer's instructions.

6. Wrap the alginate impression in an airtight container or a moist towel (not too wet) and place it in a plastic bag labeled with the patient's name if there is a time lapse (maximum of 20 minutes) before pouring. If the impression is placed in a wet towel for an extended period of time, imbibition (taking up extra moisture) may occur.

7. Write up procedure in Services Rendered.

Date	Services Rendered
02/18/XX	Reviewed medical and dental history, BP = 120/80
	Took 1 maxillary and 1 mandibular alginate impression for study casts. Patient tolerated procedure well.
	RTC: Recare Assistant's initials

8. Dismiss and escort patient to reception area (refer to Procedure 18-5).

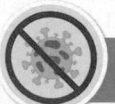 **Infection Control**

Disinfecting Alginate Impressions

This procedure is performed by the dental assistant immediately after removing the alginate impressions from the patient's mouth and caring for the patient. Since the impressions are transferred either to an in-office lab or a commercial lab off-site, they must be disinfected to prevent cross-contamination. Proper PPE such as examination gloves, mask, protective glasses and protective clothing must be worn. Only an approved disinfectant may be used. Rinse the impressions gently under tap water to remove any debris, blood, or saliva. Spray the impressions with an approved disinfectant. If not pouring immediately, place the impressions in a covered container. Label the container with the patient's name and date/time of impressions.

and cartridge tip (Figure 33-15). It is dispensed directly onto the occlusal surface, and the patient is asked to close in the normal biting position and remain closed until the material sets, normally within 2 minutes. The set material is removed, disinfected, stored, and used to establish the patient's occlusal relationship.

Reversible Hydrocolloid Impression Material (Agar-Agar)

One of the oldest impression materials that has good detail and is used for final impressions is **reversible hydrocolloid** impression material, sometimes referred to as agar-agar. The composition for this material is somewhat similar to alginate in that the main component is derived from seaweed and kelp. It also has fillers, additives, coloring, and flavoring. The unique difference between

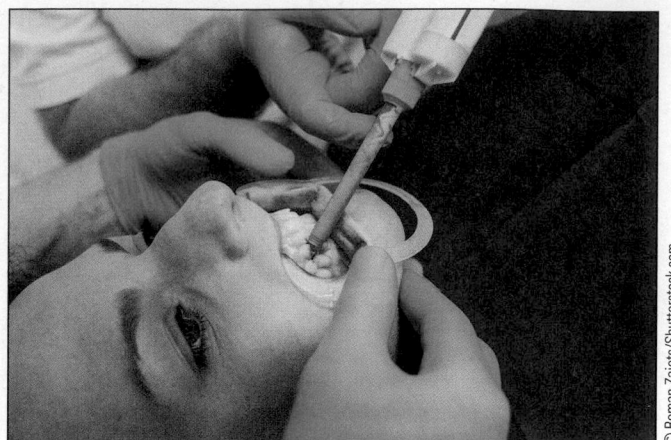

© Roman Zaiets/Shutterstock.com

FIGURE 33-15
Taking a bite registration polysiloxane material.

Procedure 33-4
Taking a Bite Registration

This procedure is performed to record the patient's bite in centric occlusion.

Steps written in blue font are performed by the operator (dentist or qualified dental assistant), and the chairside assistant's steps are written in black.

Equipment and Supplies
Patient Seating Setup (refer to Procedure 18-4)
Bite Registration Setup (Figure 33-16)
- bite registration wax (A) or wax horseshoe or polysiloxane and extruder gun and disposable tips
- laboratory knife (B)
- warm water (C) or torch

Procedure Steps
1. Escort and seat patient (refer to Procedure 18-4).

   Operator signals for procedure to begin

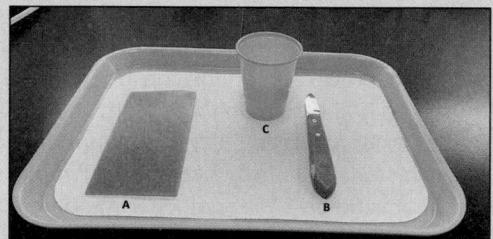

FIGURE 33-16
Bite registration setup.

2. Pass bite registration wax to operator.

   Tries the bite registration wax to determine correct length. If correction is needed, the laboratory knife is used to trim off the excess.

   Instructs the patient to practice biting to establish occlusion. You may have to instruct the patient in biting in occlusion.

3. Accept bite registration wax from operator.
4. Heat bite registration wax in warm water or with a torch to soften it.
5. Pass bite registration wax to operator.

   Places wax on the mandibular occlusal surface of the patient. If using polysiloxane, the bite registration material is extruded from the disposable tip directly onto the occlusal surface of the mandibular teeth (Figure 33-17A).

   Instructs the patient to bite together gently in the correct occlusion. You need to make sure the patient is in proper occlusion.

   Has patient keep teeth together in occlusion while the wax cools, approximately 1 to 2 minutes. If using polysiloxane, the patient gently occludes until the material sets (Figure 33-17B).

   Removes wax or polysiloxane bite without distortion.

6. Accept bite registration wax from operator.
7. Rinse and disinfect the wax or polysiloxane bite registration with appropriate surface disinfectant.

(Continues)

8. Label and store for use during trimming of the diagnostic casts (Figure 33-17C).

9. Write up procedure in Services Rendered.

Date	Services Rendered
02/18/XX	Reviewed medical and dental history, BP = 120/80
	Took polysiloxane bite registration
	RTC: Recare Assistant's initials

10. Dismiss and escort patient to reception area (refer to Procedure 18-5).

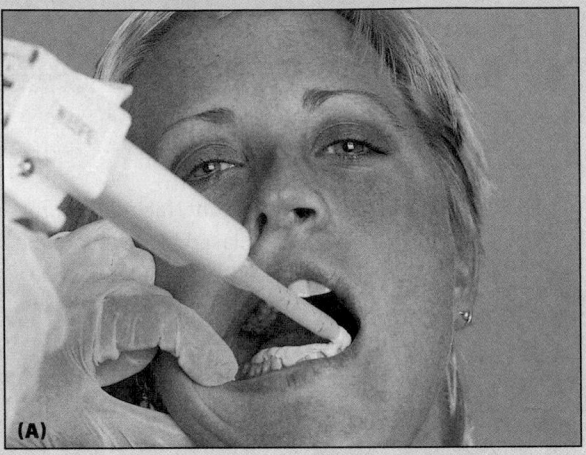
(A)

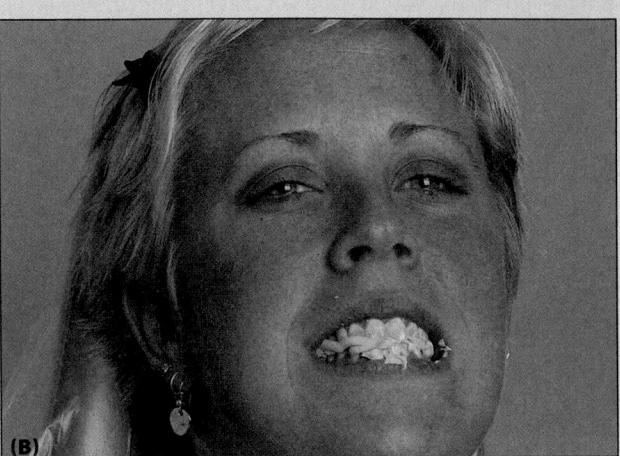
(B)

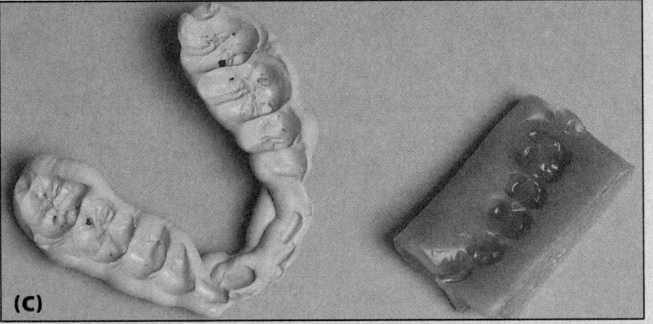
(C)

FIGURE 33-17
(A) Bite registration material is extruded from the tip directly onto the occlusal surface of the mandibular teeth. (B) Patient occludes gently until the material sets. (C) Polysiloxane or wax bite taken on a patient for use in establishing patient's occlusion.

reversible and irreversible hydrocolloid material is the setting reaction. The setting of the irreversible hydrocolloid (alginate) is accomplished by a chemical reaction. Reversible hydrocolloid changes from a gel to a sol and back again due to thermal reaction. The material begins in a gel (solid) state and, after boiling in a hydrocolloid conditioner unit for 10 minutes, it becomes liquid and remains in that state for hours if placed in a water storage bath of or until the operator is ready to use it. Five minutes before taking the impression, the tray material is moved into a water bath of 45°C (110°F). It is further cooled in the mouth as cool water flows through the water trays, connected to hoses at the dental unit. Most units have two water connectors where the hoses can be attached. Due to the equipment needed and sensitivity of the technique for tempering the alginate, many dental offices do not use or have discontinued the use of reversible hydrocolloid.

Advantages and Disadvantages of Reversible Hydrocolloid The primary advantage of using reversible hydrocolloid is the accuracy of the impression. Accuracy is more precise and more detailed than that for alginate (irreversible hydrocolloid), and reversible hydrocolloid can be used for impressions for crown and bridge construction. This material can be used for impressions for both teeth and tissue. After the initial equipment has been purchased, it is more economical than many materials on the market for final impressions.

The main disadvantage is the additional equipment needed to prepare the material. In addition, reversible hydrocolloid can lose accuracy due to atmospheric conditions. Also, the preparation and setting time is increased to 10 minutes. This material was used widely in earlier years and now has somewhat declined due to the emergence of a number of elastomeric impression materials available with similar accuracy.

Reversible Hydrocolloid Packaging and Equipment

The tray material is supplied in collapsible plastic tubes. The syringe material is supplied in either cylinders in a jar or syringe carpules. Both materials come in several colors and strengths. Special water-cooled trays and attachment hoses to circulate the water must be used with this material (Figure 33-18).

A hydrocolloid conditioner unit is used to prepare the material for use. This electric unit has three compartments (Figure 33-19). As with all equipment and material, read the manufacturer's directions and specific times for the material to be placed in each compartment. Normally, a timer is built into the conditioner. Each compartment in the conditioning unit is filled with clean water.

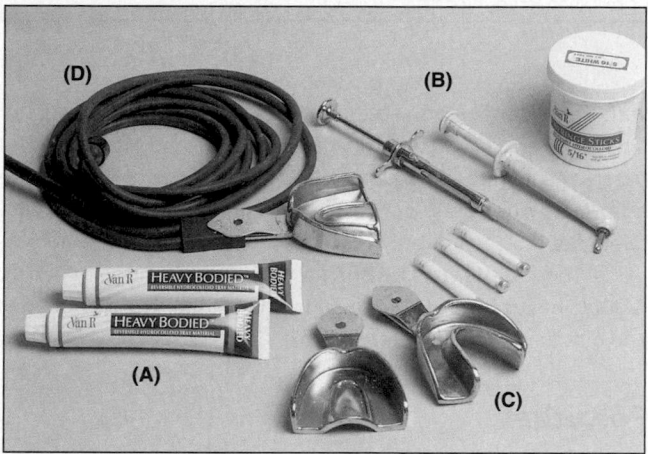

FIGURE 33-18
Hydrocolloid. (A) Tubes. (B) Syringes and cartridges. (C) Trays used with hydrocolloid conditioning unit to obtain final impressions. (D) Attachment hoses to circulate water.

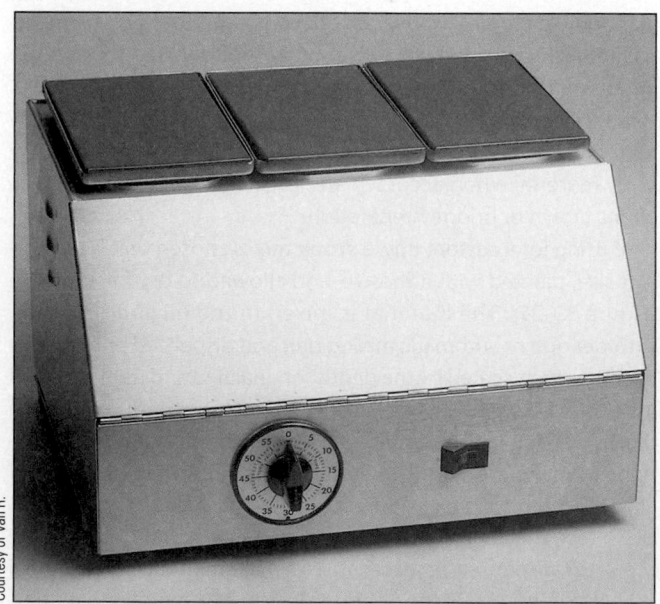

Courtesy of Van R.

FIGURE 33-19
Hydrocolloid conditioning unit with boiling bath, storage bath, and conditioning unit.

The first compartment on the left (facing the unit) is for boiling the material. The tubes are placed, with the lids tight and upside down, in the unit. The syringe material is placed in a holding case for the cartridges or inside the boiling syringes if cylinders are used. The material must stay in the syringes or tubes, or it will disperse throughout the water and be unusable. There, the material is boiled for 10 minutes. Digital machines can be set to start the timer for 10 minutes as soon as the boiling temperature is reached. If not using a digital machine, the dental assistant has to monitor the boiling temperature and time carefully. After the boiling process is complete, the temperature drops to the preset storage temperature.

After the tubes and syringe material are boiled, they are moved to the middle compartment for storage. In this compartment, the temperature is set to maintain the material in a liquid state. The material can stay in this compartment for hours or days before use.

The third compartment on the right, facing the unit, is for tray material only. The material is placed in a water-cooled tray and then in the compartment to be tempered for 5 minutes. This cools the material so that it does not burn the patient's mouth upon insertion. The syringe material remains in the fluid state to get into the crevices around the prepared tooth and obtain the necessary anatomy on the adjacent teeth. Because of the small opening in the syringe, the amount coming from the syringe cools rapidly as it is used.

The hydrocolloid conditioner unit requires little maintenance. The compartments should be emptied and rinsed out on a regular basis and then wiped with a soft cloth and refilled with clean water. A condition cleaner can be placed in the compartments and left for 1 hour to remove any buildup. The cleaner is then rinsed out prior to placing clean water in the compartments.

Elastomeric Impression Materials

Elastomeric impression materials have rubber-like qualities and are used for areas that require precise duplication. They provide better detail than alginate impressions and are more dimensionally stable. They are used for fixed restorations and fixed or removeable prosthetics and appliances. Materials in this classification are not as affected by atmospheric changes as are hydrocolloids. They are more elastic and rubber-like when set, and thus allow removal from the mouth to take place without tearing and distortion. A distortion is a dimensional change in shape. There are three primary groups of materials in this classification: polysulfide, **silicone** (polysiloxane and polyvinyl siloxanes), and polyether, with the latter two being the most popular. Each group has slightly different properties and characteristics, even though all have elastic qualities. All the materials have a **catalyst** and **base** that are mixed together to start the chemical self-curing process. The catalyst is the ingredient that accelerates or starts the process of setting the material. The process by which the catalyst and accelerator begin to cure and the material changes from a paste to an elastic, rubber-like material is called **polymerization**. The accelerator is dispensed as a paste from a small tube or in liquid form from a bottle with a dropper. The

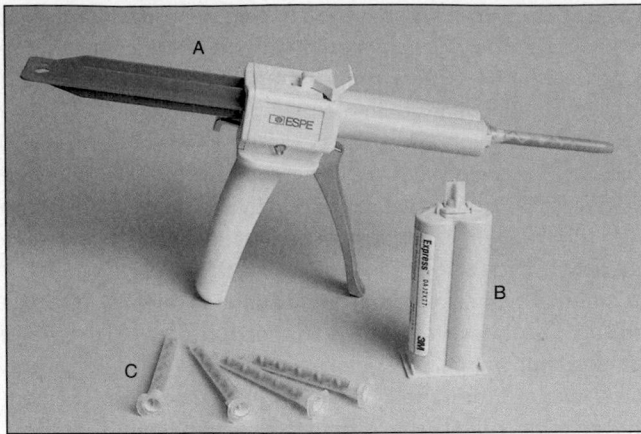

FIGURE 33-20
(A) Extruder gun. (B) Cartridge. (C) Mixing tips.

TABLE 33-4 Advantages and Disadvantages of Polysulfide

Advantages	Disadvantages
Relative stability after the final set has been achieved	Odor (it smells like sulfur because of the base)
Good accuracy	Taste
Sharpness of detail	Staining (it permanently stains clothes because of the accelerator)
Relatively long shelf life (several years)	Relatively long setting time (10 minutes is required from the start of the mix to the setting of the material prior to removal from the patient's mouth)
No noticeable change in dimension when left out for days	

base that makes up the volume of the material is normally dispensed in a paste. Often, the tube openings of base and catalyst are different sizes, with the catalyst tube opening being smaller. Today, many of the materials are dispensed in an "extruder gun" with a mixing tip (Figure 33-20). The mixing tip brings together the correct amount of the base and the catalyst material and dispenses it, premixed. If this technique is used, there is no need for a mixing pad and a spatula. A new tip is required for each application, and the material must be purchased in special cartridges (see Figure 33-20). Additionally, a fine tip may be added to the mixing tip for the light body elastomeric material to dispense around prepared teeth to ensure all details are captured in the impression. Dental offices that use a large volume of elastomeric impression material may use an automatic mixing unit which holds a bulk amount of base and catalyst that is mixed and then dispensed on to an impression tray. The benefits of the mixing unit are that there is minimal waste of material, and clean-up and cross-contamination are minimized. Light, medium, or heavy body material can be mixed in the unit. Table 33-3 lists examples of automatic mixing machines. As with the extruder gun technique, a new mixing tip must be used each time. The mixing unit must be wiped with a surface disinfectant after each use to prevent cross-contamination.

Polysulfide

The **polysulfide** impression materials have been around for a long time and may be called mercaptan or rubber-base materials. Due to the taste, staining and long setting time, polysulfide materials are not used as often anymore and have been replaced

TABLE 33-3 Automatic Mixing Machine Examples

Product	Company
3M ESPE Pentamix 3	3M Oral Care Solutions Division
Duomix	DENTSPLY Caulk
Dynamix speed	Heraeus
MixStar eMotion	DMG America

with the silicone or polyether materials which will be discussed later. They are supplied in two pastes: a base and a catalyst. The base is the larger tube and the whiter color of the two. It is made from liquid polysulfide **polymer** (thiokol polysulfide rubber) with filler added. The dark brown accelerator is made from lead peroxide. These pastes can be purchased as light (syringe material), regular, heavy, and extra heavy (tray material). The advantages and disadvantages are listed in Table 33-4.

Polyether

Polyether, an impression material used for crowns and bridges, has excellent accuracy and dimensional stability. It is supplied in tubes as pastes, the larger tube for the base and the smaller one for the catalyst. More commonly, they are packed in automixed cartridges or what is called a sausage pack (larger packaging) used for automized mixing. Polyethers come in light body, regular body and heavy body. Light body is used as a syringe material and is more flowing. Regular body is often used for denture impressions as it is stiffer than light body, however still flowable. Heavy body has the stiffest consistency and is often used as tray material. The light body material will bond nicely to the heavy body material when accuracy and precision is needed, such as after a crown or bridge preparation.

If using for a custom tray, a **stock** tray is chosen that is the correct size, painted with adhesive, and allowed to dry for 1 minute (Figure 33-21). The material is mixed in the mixing tip via an extruder gun or automatic mixing unit and dispensed onto a stock tray. The tray is seated by the dentist or qualified and trained dental assistant in the patient's mouth. After about 2 minutes of holding the impression in the patient's mouth, agitate the tray in all directions to make room for the final polyether impression material after the teeth are prepared. Remove the tray after 3 minutes.

To take the final impression with polyether after the teeth are prepared, dispense the material in a similar manner. Less material is needed because of the volume already in the preliminary tray. The material is loaded into an injection syringe, and the excess material is placed in the preliminary impression. The impression tray is then reinserted into the patient's mouth and held for

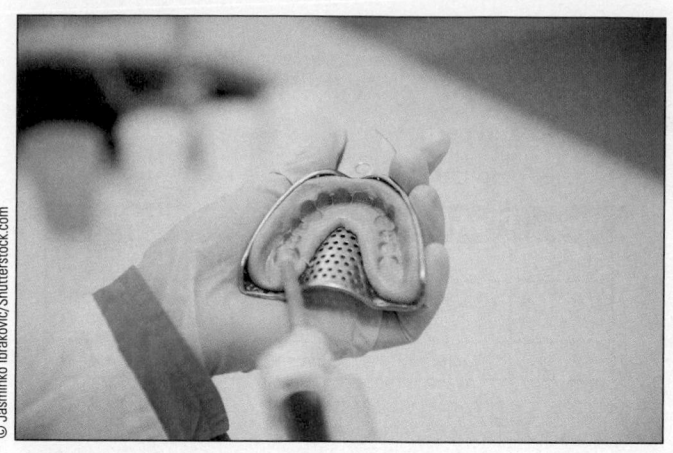

FIGURE 33-21
Custom impression tray.

4 minutes to obtain an accurate impression. This technique can be accomplished in a one-step technique as well, eliminating the preliminary tray.

After the tray is loosened from the mouth and removed with a quick snapping motion, protecting the opposing arch, it is rinsed with cold water and then completely air dried. The impression can be disinfected with a 2% solution of glutaraldehyde for 10 minutes.

Silicone (Polysiloxane and Polyvinyl Siloxanes)

A number of new silicone materials have been introduced in recent years. Silicone has the advantages of polysulfide without the disadvantages but is more expensive. Advantages of the material include high accuracy, no shrinkage, dimensional stability, high tear resistance, no taste, and no odor.

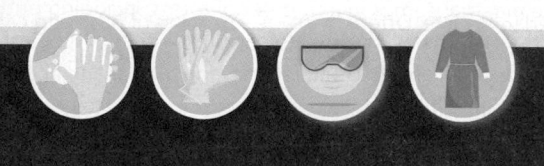

Procedure 33-5
Taking a Polyether Impression

Polyether is a material used in taking final impressions for which extreme accuracy is required. This procedure uses the extruder gun method to mix and dispense polyether material.

Steps written in **blue** font are performed by the operator (dentist or qualified dental assistant), and the chairside assistant's steps are written in black.

Equipment and Supplies

Patient Seating Setup (refer to Procedure 18-4)

Impression Material Setup (Figure 33-22)
- polyether base and catalyst cartridge in light body and heavy body (A)
- extruder guns (B)
- mixing tip (C)
- impression syringe mixing tip (D)
- triple tray that has been painted with corresponding adhesive and permitted to dry (E)

Procedure Steps

1. Escort and seat patient (refer to Procedure 18-4).

   After the tooth has been prepared, the area is cleaned and dried, the retraction cord is placed, and the doctor indicates that they are ready for the final impression.

2. Place impression syringe mixing tip onto extruder gun with light body material.

3. Place mixing tip on extruder gun with heavy body material.

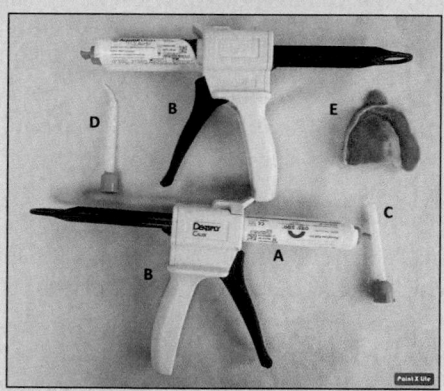

FIGURE 33-22
Polyether impression setup.

Operator signals to begin. Removes packing cord.

4. Pass extruder gun with light body material to operator.

   Syringes material around the tooth preparation and soft tissues. Keeps tip of syringe at the margin and continues around the edge slowly moving upward until the entire occlusal surface is covered.

   Passes extruder gun back to assistant.

5. Load triple tray impression tray with heavy body material from extruder gun with mixing tip while operator is syringing material around prepared tooth.

6. Transfer the tray to the operator. The mixing and loading (working time) must be completed within 4 minutes.

(Continues)

Places and seats tray into the oral cavity and asks patient to bite and hold until material sets, approximately 6 minutes from mixing in order to achieve a final set.

Removes impression from the oral cavity taking care to protect the opposing teeth.

7. Accept the impression from the operator.

8. Rinse the impression with water to remove saliva, blood, and debris.

9. Disinfect according to manufacturer's instructions.

10. Place the impression in a sealed container or bag that is labeled.

11. Remove mixing tips from extruder guns and dispose of tips.

12. Disinfect extruder guns.

13. Write up procedure in Services Rendered.

Date	Services Rendered
02/18/XX	Reviewed medical and dental history, BP = 120/80
	Took 1 full maxillary polyether impression for final impression.
	RTC: Insert PFM Crown #13 Assistant's initials

14. Dismiss and escort patient to reception area (refer to Procedure 18-5).

The material comes in a number of forms, including putty for making a custom tray for a preliminary impression, in tubes of base and accelerator (catalyst) for injection, and regular and heavy type for impressions. It is also available in cartridge form to be used with the mixing tip and extruding gun (automix cartridge system), and in bulk containers to be used in an automatic mixing unit.

The putty material comes in two colors and is for making custom trays. Each container of putty has a colored scoop that corresponds to the color of the putty of either the base or the catalyst (Figure 33-23). Do not mix up the scoops because doing so will contaminate the material and cause the polymerization process to start, making the material hard and useless. The material is dispensed with an equal volume of base and catalyst putties. Knead and mix the putty quickly until a homogeneous color is achieved. This mixing takes about 30 seconds. Mixing putty with latex gloves will adversely affect the set of some materials—read the directions. The silicone is placed in the tray, covered with a thin plastic sheet, and placed in the patient's mouth or over the model. The thin plastic sheet is placed to help add resistance when placing the tray, as well as void out any sharp anatomy detail such as cusps and grooves. This will allow for space when it is time to take the final impression. It takes about 3 minutes for the material to harden. Remove the plastic, and a custom tray is ready for the impression material. The putty material is not suitable for detailed impressions.

When ready for the impression, there are two options to syringe. The syringe material can be injected from the mixing tip into the impression syringe for use around the sulcus of the tooth. Another option is to use a syringe mixing tip (Procedure 33-5). The tray is loaded by the operator squeezing the dispenser handle of the extruding gun and engaging the plunger. The plunger enters the cartridge and extrudes the material through the mixing tip and into the putty material in the impression tray. When ready, the tray is placed in the patient's mouth and immobilized until set (3½ minutes for a fast set and 5 minutes for a regular set). The impression is removed after the seal is loosened and the opposing teeth are protected. The impression is run under cold water and sprayed with disinfectant. The impression is very stable and can be poured weeks

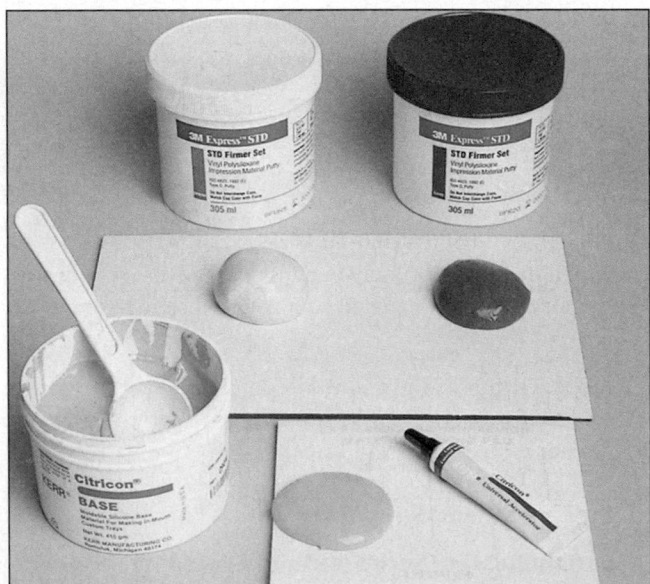

FIGURE 33-23
Silicone putty material.

later. The total time from mixing to the final set is from 4 to 6 minutes (see Procedure 33-6).

Light-cured impression material is also available. The advantage of this material is that the setting time is controlled by the operator. The disadvantage is that it is sometimes difficult to move the curing light over the complete surface of the material. A clear plastic impression tray must be used. The light must hit all areas in order to bring about the curing. The light acts as a catalyst to set up the material.

Gypsum Materials

Several different gypsum materials are used when pouring an impression to make a model. It is important to identify the application for the material before determining the type of gypsum product to use. Gypsum materials vary in strength, dimensional

Procedure 33-6
Taking a Silicone (Polysiloxane) Two-Step Impression

Silicone (polysiloxane) is a material used in taking final impressions for which extreme accuracy is required.

Steps written in **blue** font are performed by the operator (dentist or qualified dental assistant), and the chairside assistant's steps are written in black.

Equipment and Supplies

Patient Seating Setup (refer to Procedure 18-4)

Silicone Impression Setup (Figure 33-24)
- vinyl overgloves (see Figure 11-36)
- two containers of putty (one base and one catalyst) with color-coordinated scoops (see Figure 33-23)
- stock tray with adhesive painted on interior (see Figure 33-5)
- plastic sheet for use as a spacer (not shown)
- extruder gun, mixing tip with injection syringe (see Figure 33-20)
- cartridges of impression material, loaded in extruder gun (Figure 33-24)
- timer

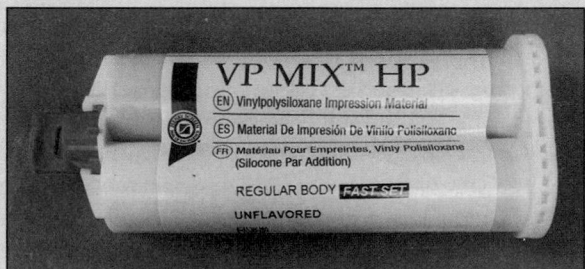

FIGURE 33-24
Polysiloxane cartridge for extruder gun.

Preliminary Putty Impression
Procedure Steps
1. Escort and seat patient (refer to Procedure 18-4).
2. Don vinyl gloves.
3. Mix equal scoops of the base and catalyst putty together.
4. Knead until a homogeneous mixture is obtained within the manufacturer's recommended timeframe (normally 30 seconds). The mixture must be a single color with no streaks.

5. Pat it into a patty and load it into the prepared tray. With a finger, make a slight indentation where the teeth are located.

   Places the plastic spacer sheet over the material and inserts it into the patient's mouth. The objective is to create 2 mm of space for the final syringeable viscous impression material.

6. Set timer for 3 minutes.

   Removes tray from the patient's mouth, removes the spacer, and checks the putty for accuracy and leaves to set further.

Final Impression
After the tooth has been prepared, the area is cleaned and dried, the retraction cord is placed, and the doctor indicates that they are ready for the final impression.

Procedure Steps
1. Prepare extruder gun by loading with cartridge containing light-body or wash material and syringe mixing tip.
2. Pass extruding gun to the operator.

   Removes cord.

   Syringes material around the tooth and soft tissue (refer to Procedure 40-2).

3. Accept extruding gun from operator.
4. Change tip from syringe tip to mixing tip.
5. Extrude the material (light-body) through the mixing tip and placed in the preliminary impression (Figure 33-25).
6. Pass tray to operator.

   Seats the tray immediately into place and holds it steady for 3 to 5 minutes, depending on the material used.

   Removes impression tray after the material has set. Releases the seal and takes care to protect the opposing teeth from the quick snap.

7. Accept the impression from operator.
8. Rinse the impression immediately under water and dry. Disinfect according to the manufacturer's directions.
9. Pour impression immediately, but can be poured up to weeks later and still remain dimensionally stable.
10. Write up procedure in Services Rendered.

(Continues)

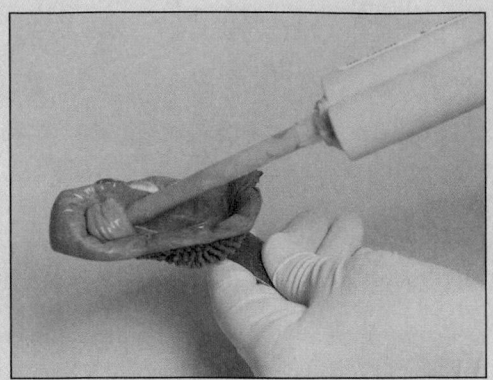

FIGURE 33-25
Extrude material through mixing tip onto customy tray.

Date	Services Rendered
02/18/XX	Reviewed medical and dental history, BP = 120/80
	Took 1 full preliminary impression and 1 quad maxillary polysiloxane impression for final impression.
	RTC: Insert Zirconia crown #14 Assistant's initials

11. Dismiss and escort patient to reception area (refer to Procedure 18-5).

accuracy, resistance, reproduction detail, water/powder ratio, and setting times. See Table 33-5 for water-to-powder ratios of gypsum materials.

Primary types of gypsum used in dentistry are as follows:

- Type I: Impression plaster
- Type II: Model or laboratory plaster
- Orthodontic stone/combination of Type II: Model or laboratory plaster, and Type III: Laboratory stone
- Type III: Laboratory stone
- Type IV: Die stone
- Type V: High-strength, high-expansion die stone

During the process of manufacturing the various types of plasters and stones, the gypsum product (which is mined as a hard rock) is ground to a fine powder. It is then heated in large, cylindrical kettles equipped with agitators. The heating is controlled accurately and is continued until a specific amount of water is driven out of the gypsum. This process is known as **calcination**. Several methods of calcination are used to derive various stones and investment die stones. During this process, the gypsum, which is calcium sulfate dihydrate (one molecule of calcium sulfate to two molecules of water), is changed to hemihydrate powder (one water molecule to every two molecules of calcium sulfate). Because both plaster and stone are white in color, yellow, blue, and pink **pigments** are added to the stone to make it easier to distinguish which material is being used.

Strengths of the gypsum products are determined by the calcination process and the water/powder ratio needed to incorporate the mixture. Plaster (beta hemihydrate) comprises gypsum particles that are larger and more irregular than the particles of stone (alpha hemihydrate), which have undergone further processing and were transformed into denser particles. It is important to follow the manufacturer's directions when mixing gypsum products. One of the chief obstacles to overcome when mixing these products is incorporating air and wetting each particle. Plaster particles are more irregular and require more water to wet each surface of each particle. The ratio of water to powder for plaster is 50 mL of water to 100 grams of powder; stone requires only 30 mL of water to 100 grams of powder. Die stones require even less water because the particles are smaller, less irregular, and denser.

Incorporating the water is an important step in mixing gypsum products. Using a flexible rubber bowl and a stiff spatula allows the operator to stir the viscous material and press against the sides of the bowl to eliminate air bubbles. Avoid whipping the powder and the water together, because doing so adds air to the mixture. It should be mixed to a creamy, putty-like consistency. A grainy mixture will not pour into the impression. The incorporating and spatulating procedure should take about 1 minute. Overspatulating causes a breakdown of crystals and soft spots in the model.

There are several different methods to pouring models. There is the double-pour, in which the anatomical portion of the cast is mixed and poured first. After this a second mix is made and the base (art) portion is poured. An inverted pour is when both the art and anatomical portions are poured at the same time. The anatomical portion is inverted onto the art portion immediately after pouring.

TABLE 33-5 Water-to-Powder Ratio Recommendations

Gypsum	Powder	Water
Type I: Impression plaster	100 grams	60 mL
Type II: Laboratory or model plaster	100 grams	50 mL
Type III: Laboratory stone	100 grams	30 mL
Type IV: Die stone	100 grams	24 mL
Type V: Die stone	100 grams	18–22 mL

Gypsum sets when the plaster or stone transforms back to the dihydrate through a chemical reaction. This process gives off heat, called an exothermic reaction. The temperature of the water increases or decreases the setting time. The hotter the water, the more rapidly the material sets. There are retarders such as borax and sodium citrate that can be added to the material to slow down the set. Potassium sulfate accelerates the setting time. The manufacturers add small concentrations of the retarders or accelerators to cause a decrease or an increase in the setting rate of the gypsum.

The gypsum powder is measured by weight, and the water is calibrated by volume. It is important to have the correct water-to-powder ratio. If less water is incorporated, the model can have greater setting expansion. It will have increased strength and hardness but may result in a thick mixture that becomes a dry, crumbly mass that cannot flow into the impression. At this stage, more water cannot be added to the mixture. It will need to be disposed of and a new mixture made. If too much water is incorporated into the mixture, the model will be weak, slow setting, and filled with air spaces. A plaster model will set in 10 to 20 minutes, which can be determined by feel. If the heat has dissipated, the model is set. It goes through a cycle and heats up and seems to perspire; then the heat diminishes and the model is cool and dry. The final set occurs after 24 hours when the model reaches the optimum hardness.

All gypsum products are packaged in some type of plastic bag or container to ensure that they do not become contaminated with moisture. If contaminated, the properties and the setting reaction may be altered. These plastic bags are normally further packaged in a cardboard box for easier handling.

All impressions should be disinfected prior to pouring models. In the event a model needs to be disinfected, it may be soaked in a 5% hypochlorite solution for 30 minutes.

Plaster

Plaster (plaster of Paris) is a white gypsum referred to as beta-hemihydrate. It was one of the first gypsum products available to dentistry. It is the weakest and least expensive of gypsum products. It is calcinated in an open kettle method, and the result is particles that are rough, irregular, and porous. The final product is a powder that, when mixed with water, reverts to a gypsum product or dihydrate. Plaster takes more water to incorporate the powder. After the model dries and the water evaporates, the areas where the water was become air bubbles. This is the primary reason that plaster is weaker than stone. Stone is more compact and requires less water, therefore making a stronger model. Plaster is used in areas where detail and strength are not as important. Plaster is used to pour up study models, for opposing models, in mounting study models and casts, and for repairing casts (see Procedures 33-7 through 33-10).

Type I: Impression Plaster
Impression plaster (modified Type II: laboratory or model plaster) was used to take impressions before the newer, easy-to-manipulate impression materials now on the market. This plaster (Type I), mixed with a water-to-powder ratio of 60 mL of water to 100 grams of powder, is placed in the mouth carefully on the area to be duplicated, and then the operator must wait for the plaster to set. After the set

(usually 4 to 5 minutes), the material is broken apart and reassembled in the laboratory. Because the material is so rigid, it fractures and breaks easily. Today, this material is rarely used for impressions; it is used primarily to mount casts on an **articulator** because of its quick setting time.

Type II: Laboratory or Model Plaster
Model plaster is used routinely in the dental office by the dental assistant to pour diagnostic casts or study models. It is normally white in color and is slightly stronger than the Type I: impression plaster, because it requires a water-to-powder ratio of 50 mL of water to 100 grams of powder, making the material less porous.

Type III: Laboratory Stone
Type III: Laboratory stone is stronger than plaster and is used where more strength is needed. It requires 30 mL of water to 100 grams of powder, making it denser, harder, and stronger. It is normally yellow in color due to the manufacturer's added pigments, more expensive than plaster, and referred to as alpha-hemihydrate. It is used for study models (diagnostic casts) that require greater strength, working casts, and models for partial and full dentures.

Orthodontic Stone
Orthodontic stone is a mixture of laboratory or model plaster and laboratory stone. This white stone allows for a stronger model to be used for the diagnosis and treatment of orthodontic cases.

Type IV: Die Stone
Type IV: Die stone is calcinated by autoclaving in the presence of calcium chloride. This modified alpha-hemihydrate is referred to as die stone. A die is a positive replica of the prepared tooth made from stone. It requires much less water (less than 24 mL to 100 grams of powder) to incorporate its small, uniform particles. More stone with less water and air makes the model strong and resistant to abrasion. It is used most often for dies or where a very strong model or cast is needed.

Type V: High-Strength, High-Expansion Die Stone
Recently, the ADA added a new material to its list of gypsum products. Type V: Die stone requires from 18 to 22 mL of water to 100 grams of powder, making it the strongest accepted gypsum product available for use in the dental office.

Trimming and Finishing Diagnostic Casts

Diagnostic casts (study models) are used to present the case to the patient. It is important that they have an attractive appearance. Not only are they part of the patient's permanent record, but they are also a direct reflection of the type of work the office performs for the patient. They can be trimmed in a geometric form that is pleasing in appearance. Standard guidelines are used in trimming the casts (see Procedure 33-11).

Two-thirds of the trimmed model are made from the anatomical portion of the cast (see Figure 33-38). The anatomical portion includes the teeth, the mucosa, and frenum attachments and is about 1 inch high. This area was duplicated from the oral cavity. The remaining one-third is the base or art portion of the cast. This portion is trimmed in a geometric form

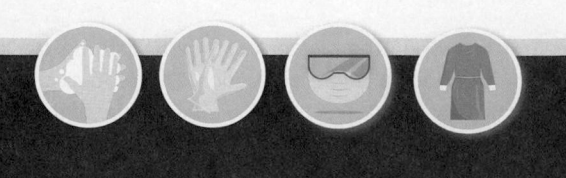

Procedure 33-7
Mixing Plaster for an Alginate Impression

This procedure is performed by the dental assistant in the dental laboratory.

Equipment and Supplies (Figure 33-26)
- PPE: examination gloves, mask, protective glasses, and protective clothing
- spatula, metal with rounded end and stiff, straight sides (A)
- two flexible rubber mixing bowls (B)
- scale (C)
- plaster (100 grams)
- water measuring device (calibrated syringe or vial) (D)
- room-temperature water (D)
- vibrator with paper or plastic cover on platform (E)
- alginate impression (disinfected) (F)

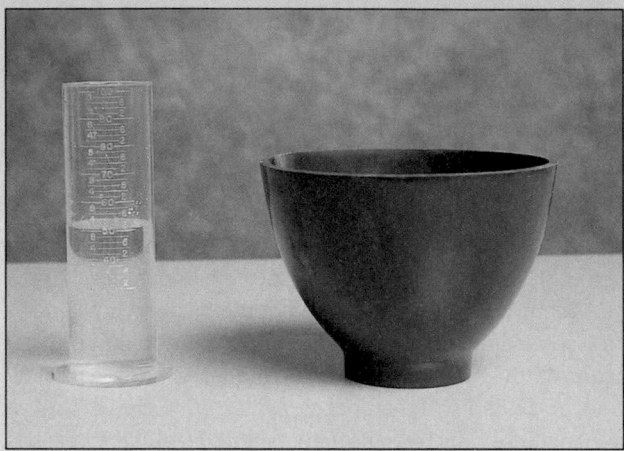

FIGURE 33-27
Measure 50 mL of water into a flexible mixing bowl.

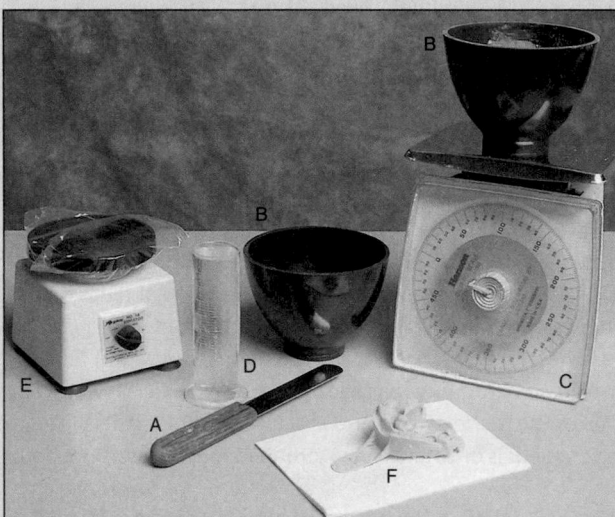

FIGURE 33-26
Equipment for mixing plaster.

Procedure Steps

Mixing the Plaster
1. Measure 50 mL of room-temperature water into one of the flexible mixing bowls (Figure 33-27).

2. Place the second flexible mixing bowl on the scale and set the dial to zero. This allows the plaster powder to be weighed (Figure 33-28).

3. Weigh out 100 grams of plaster in the second rubber bowl.

4. Add the powder from the second bowl to the water of the first bowl. (Placing the water in first allows for all the powder to become incorporated into the mixture.)

5. Allow several seconds for the powder to dissolve into the water.

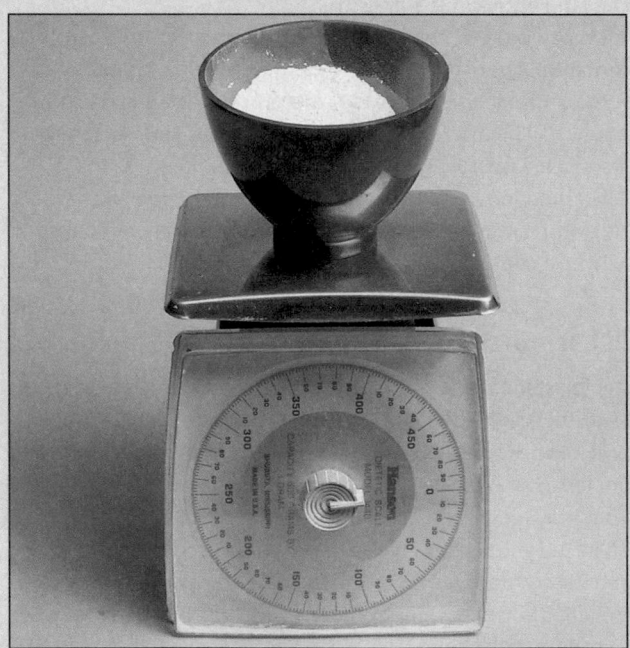

FIGURE 33-28
Measure 100 g of plaster into a bowl for pouring alginate impression.

6. Mix the particles together using the spatula. The initial mixing should be completed in 20 seconds. The total mixing procedure should take about 1 minute.

7. Turn on the vibrator to medium or low speed.

8. Place the rubber bowl on the vibrator platform, pressing lightly.

9. Rotate the bowl on the vibrator to allow the air bubbles to rise to the top surface (Figure 33-29). The mixing and vibrating should be completed within a couple of minutes. The mixture is ready if the spatula can cut through it and it stays to the sides without changing positions. It will appear like whipped cream with a smooth, creamy texture (Figure 33-30). Another way to check whether the powder/water is in correct ratio is to place a spoonful on the spatula and turn it upside down. If the material remains in place, the mixture is ready.

NOTE: When the spatula is held sideways, mixture will fall from it.

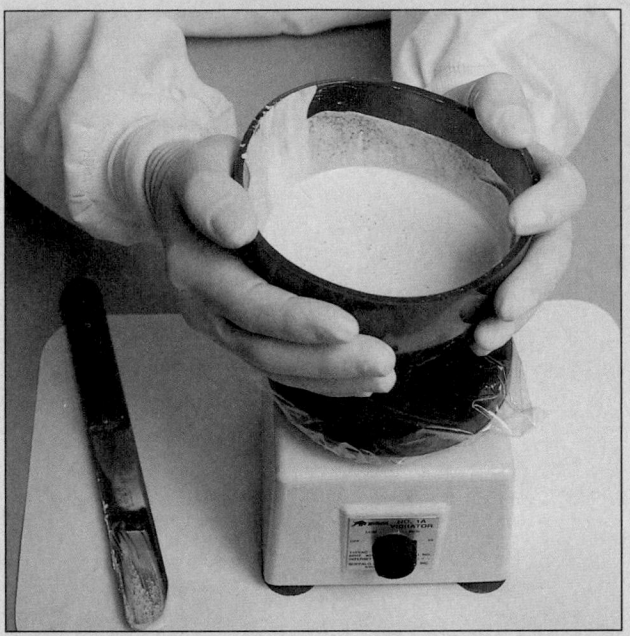

FIGURE 33-29
Vibrator brings air bubbles to surface of plaster mixture.

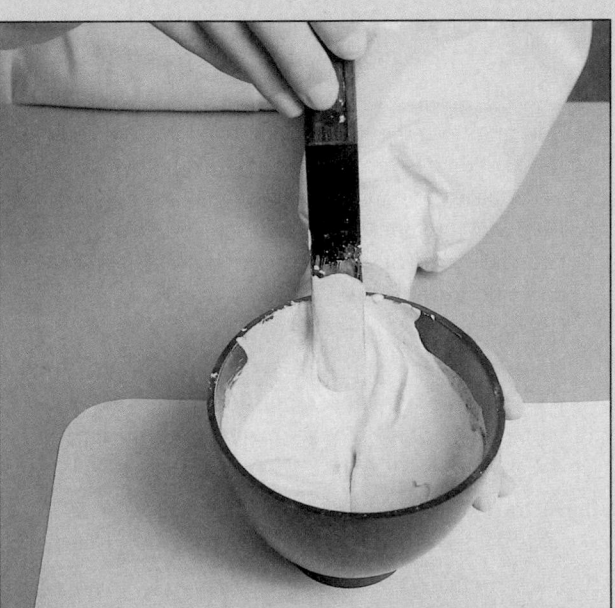

FIGURE 33-30
Plaster's consistency should allow it to retain position as spatula slides through it.

Procedure 33-8
Pouring Anatomic Portion of Plaster Study Model

The impression is ready to pour, the excess moisture is removed, and a laboratory knife has been used to eliminate any excess impression material that will hamper the pouring of the model. This procedure is performed by the dental assistant in the dental laboratory immediately after mixing the plaster.

Equipment and Supplies (Figure 33-31)
- PPE: examination gloves, mask, protective glasses, and protective clothing
- metal spatula (stiff blade with rounded end) or disposable spatula (A)
- mixed plaster from Procedure 33-7 (B)
- vibrator with paper towel or plastic cover on platform

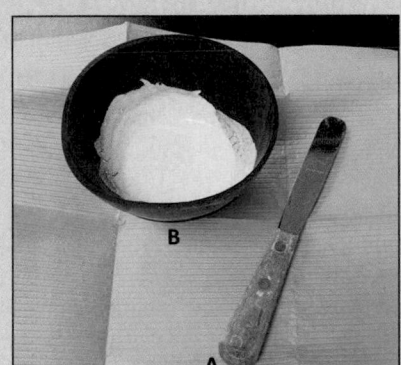

FIGURE 33-31
Equipment for pouring plaster study model.

(Continues)

Procedure Steps

1. Set the vibrator at low or medium speed.

2. Hold the impression by the handle with the tray portion on the platform of the vibrator.

3. Allow a small amount of plaster to touch the most distal surface of one side of the arch in the impression (Figure 33-32). When the plaster touches the impression that is on the vibrating platform, it flows down the back of the impression and into the anatomy of the teeth.

4. Add small increments of the plaster in the same area as the plaster flows around toward the anterior teeth and to the other side of the arch. (Using this technique allows the air to push ahead of the plaster material and eliminates bubbles. This produces a model that has detailed anatomic qualities.)

5. Add the plaster in this manner until it flows out the other side of the impression and fills the anatomic portion of the model. Rotating the impression around on the platform of the vibrator aids the material to travel around the arch.

6. Fill the entire impression (while off the vibrator) using larger increments after the anatomy portion is filled.

7. Place lightly on the vibrator to coalesce (combine) once tray is completely filled. Overvibration can cause bubbles to form.

8. Place small blobs of plaster on the top of the plaster so that it can attach to the art portion of the model if a double-pour method is to be used. (A flat surface may break apart at a later date.)

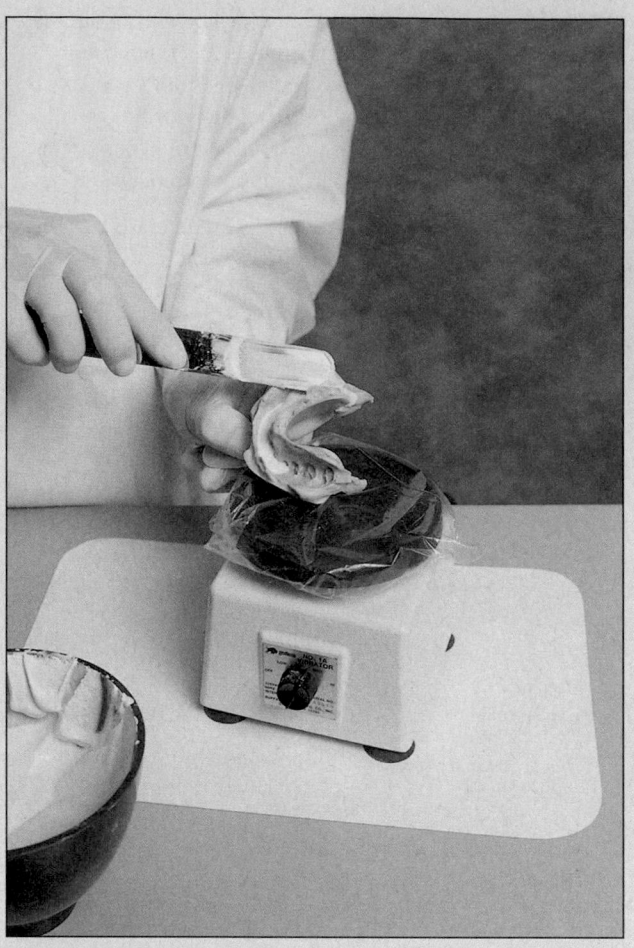

FIGURE 33-32
Mixed plaster is vibrated into alginate impression, starting at the posterior area of arch and continuing to fill from that area while material rotates around the opposite side of arch.

Procedure 33-9
Pouring Art Portion of Plaster Study Model Using Double-Pour Method

This procedure is performed by the dental assistant in the dental laboratory after the anatomic portion of the study model has set.

Equipment and Supplies (Figure 33-33)
- PPE: examination gloves, mask, protective glasses, and protective clothing
- metal spatula (stiff blade with rounded end) or disposable spatula (A)
- flexible rubber bowl or disposable bowl (B)
- plaster (B)
- vibrator with a paper towel or plastic cover on platform (see Figure 33-32)
- paper towels (C)
- water measuring device (D)
- calibration measurement device (not shown)
- room-temperature water

Procedure Steps

1. Allow anatomical portion of the impression to set for 5 to 10 minutes following pouring.

2. Wipe the rubber bowl and spatula with a paper towel and dispose of the material.

3. Wash, clean, and dry the rubber bowl and spatula for a second pour of plaster.

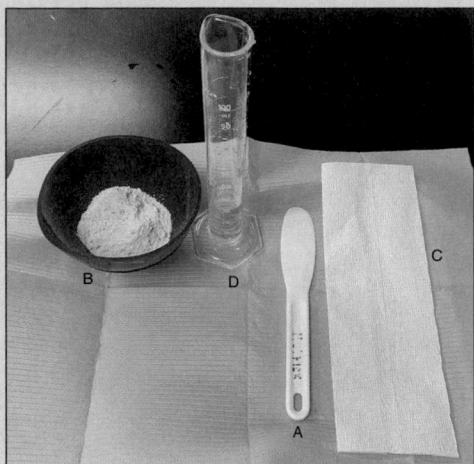

FIGURE 33-33
Equipment for pouring art portion of plaster study model.

4. Mix 100 grams of powder to 40 mL of water if pouring for a maxillary and mandibular base. If pouring only one model, mix half the amount of powder and water. The ratio of powder to water can be altered to create a thicker mix, which is desirable for bases.

5. Mix the plaster in the same manner as before. It will appear much thicker. This part of the model is not as crucial as the anatomical portion. Areas that have bubbles can be repaired easily.

6. Gather the plaster on the spatula and place it on a glass slab or a paper towel (Figure 33-34). It is important to allow the material to mass upward and not to spread out like a pancake.

7. Invert the poured anatomy portion onto the base material.

8. Hold the tray steady and situate the handle so that it is parallel to the paper surface or glass slab. It is important to get a base that is even and uniform in thickness. This makes it easier to trim the model later.

9. Drag the excess plaster carefully up over the edges of the cast, filling in any voided areas (Figure 33-35). Try not

to cover any margins of the impression tray while doing this. This locks the plaster onto the tray and may cause the cast to fracture when removing the impression material and the tray.

NOTE: If using a one- or single-pour method, the base is poured immediately after the anatomical portion is poured. The double-pour method allows the material to initially set in the anatomical portion prior to inverting it and ensures that the plaster does not flow from any crucial areas.

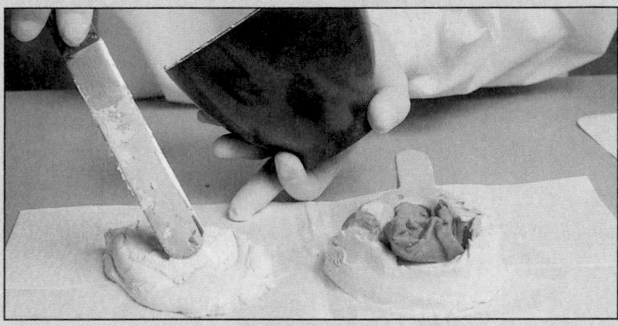

FIGURE 33-34
Plaster is gathered to make a base. The plaster must have enough body so that it does not flatten.

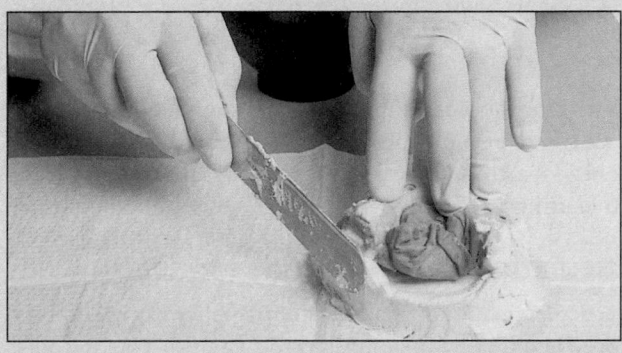

FIGURE 33-35
Operator must smooth plaster sides of base after inversion of filled impression.

Procedure 33-10
Removing Plaster Model from Alginate Impression

This procedure is performed by the dental assistant in the dental laboratory after the study model has set.

Equipment and Supplies (Figure 33-36)
- PPE: examination gloves, mask, protective glasses, and protective clothing
- laboratory knife (A)
- maxillary and mandibular plaster models, set in alginate impressions (B)

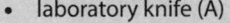

(Continues)

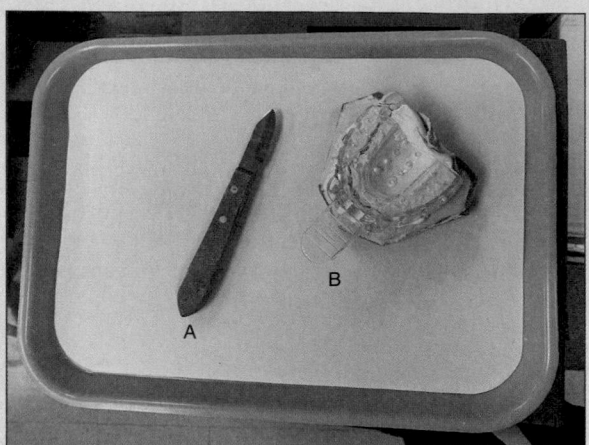

FIGURE 33-36
Equipment for removing plaster model from alginate impression.

Procedure Steps (*Follow aseptic procedures*)

1. Allow the plaster to set for 40 to 60 minutes before removing the impression material and the tray. The exothermic heat should be gone from the plaster material to indicate it is set. Feel the plaster material to ensure it is cooled.

2. Gently remove any plaster on the margin of the tray using a laboratory knife (Figure 33-37).

3. Holding the handle of the impression tray, lift the tray straight upward.

4. Remove any necessary plaster if the tray does not come off by identifying the area that is holding it back. Be sure to lift in an upward motion to remove the tray. Wiggling side to side or lifting sideways may fracture the teeth and anatomical portion of the cast.

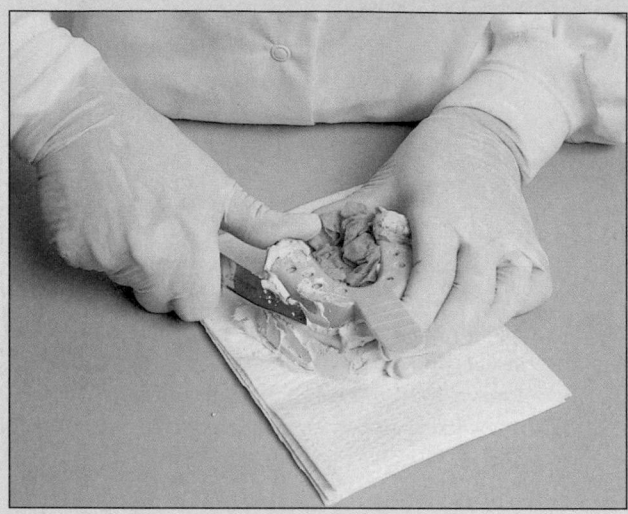

FIGURE 33-37
Before removing the impression from the model, use knife to remove remaining plaster from the impression.

with specific angles. When maxillary and mandibular models are trimmed and in occlusion, they should have an overall height of 3 inches. To evaluate if objectives for making study casts were met, see Table 33-6.

Articulating Casts or Study Models

An articulator is used to duplicate the patient's occlusion on models (Figure 33-39). An articulator is a frame that holds models

TABLE 33-6 Trimmed Diagnostic Casts (Study Models) Evaluation

Both maxillary and mandibular models are trimmed symmetrically following specific cut angles indicated.
All anatomic portions of the model are accurate.
Trimmed models sit on end and maintain occlusion.
Each model exhibits a ½-inch base and a 1-inch anatomic portion.
Final finishing is accomplished and the models present a professional appearance (see Figure 33-57D).

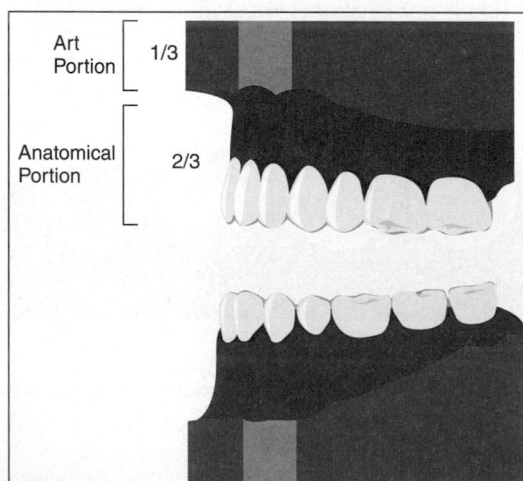

FIGURE 33-38
Anatomical and art portion of a trimmed model.

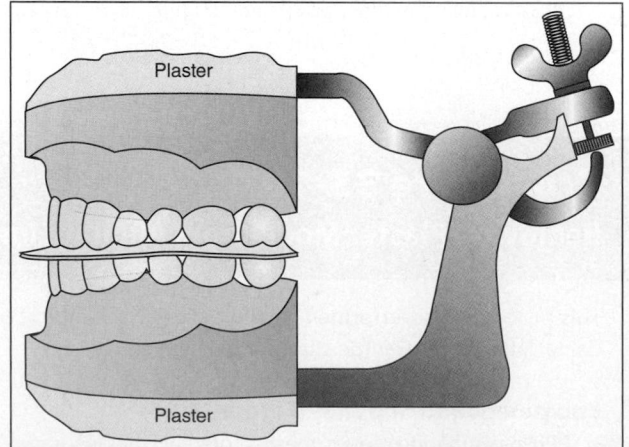

FIGURE 33-39
Articulator.

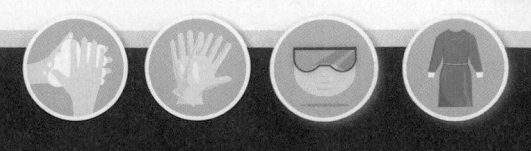

Procedure 33-11
Trimming Diagnostic Casts/Study Models

This procedure is performed by the dental assistant in the dental laboratory after the study model has set, been separated from the alginate impression, and prepared for trimming.

Equipment and Supplies (Figure 33-40)
- PPE: examination gloves, mask, protective glasses, and protective clothing
- maxillary and mandibular models (only maxillary model shown) (A)
- two flexible rubber mixing bowls (B)
- laboratory knife (C)
- pencil (D)
- measuring straight edge (E)

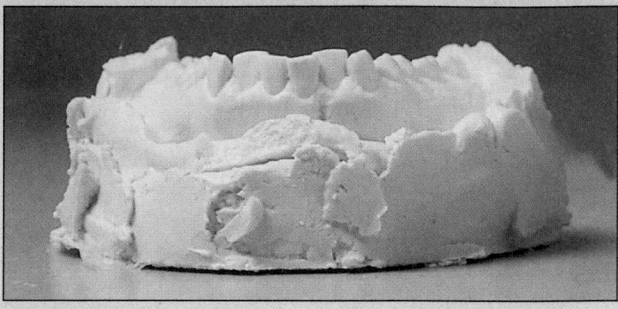

FIGURE 33-41
Before proceeding to trim study model, model base should be parallel to counter.

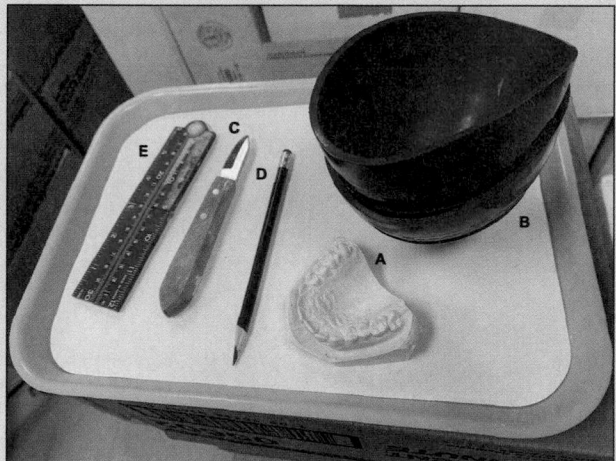

FIGURE 33-40
Equipment for trimming study models.

Procedure Steps
1. Soak the bases of the models in rubber mixing bowls for 5 minutes prior to trimming (if the models are dry). The trimming wheel on the model trimmer is more effective if the models are wet prior to trimming.

2. Don safety glasses and mask and adjust the model trimmer so that the water runs freely over the grinding wheel when the trimmer is on.

3. Invert the models so that the teeth are resting on the counter. Evaluate whether the base is parallel to the counter (Figure 33-41). Keep in mind that the art portion is ½ inch high when completed.

4. Turn on the model trimmer and trim the base so that it is parallel to the occlusal plane.

5. Rest hands on the table of the model trimmer and keep fingers away from the grinding wheel.

6. Apply light, even pressure when applying the models to the grinding wheel. Hold the model as level as possible during this procedure (Figure 33-42).

7. Return models to the counter for re-evaluation and then again to the model trimmer to achieve a parallel surface. Trim both models to this stage.

NOTE: Move the models back and forth once across the grinding surface as the model comes off the grinding wheel. This eliminates the circular grinding marks made as the wheel rotates.

8. Place the models together in occlusion (a wax bite may be necessary).

9. Evaluate again whether the objective of obtaining parallel models has been achieved. If not, grind to get the models to this stage. All other cuts will be off if this stage is not properly achieved, because this flat surface is laid on the model trimming table guide to grind the other areas.

10. Keep models in occlusion and evaluate which posterior teeth are the most distal: maxillary or mandibular. When that has been determined, take that model and draw with a pencil a line behind the retromolar area indicating where to trim (Figure 33-43).

11. Place the base surface of that model on the model trimmer table guide and cut the posterior area at a right angle with the base up to the indicated lines (Figure 33-44).

12. Put the two models back into occlusion and place the cut model (whether maxillary or mandibular) on the top.

(Continues)

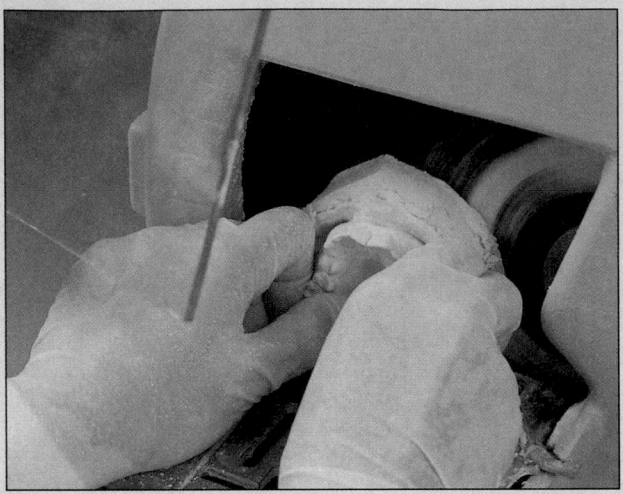

FIGURE 33-42
Study model base is trimmed as the operator maintains even pressure on the trimming wheel.

13. Place the opposite base on the model trimmer table guide while holding the models together and trim the posterior at a right angle to the base (Figure 33-45). The trimmed model acts as a guide to follow while trimming. When small particles of plaster are trimmed off the first base, it indicates that they are trimmed to the same plane.

14. Take the models off grinding wheel and place on their backs (Figure 33-46). The occlusal plane is at a right angle to the counter. If the models stay in occlusion, the objective has been met. If they fall apart and out of occlusion, then place them back onto the grinding wheel until they stay in the correct position.

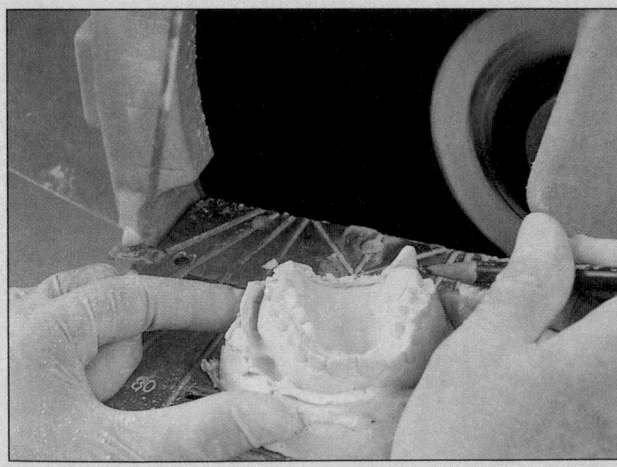

FIGURE 33-43
Pencil line is drawn from 2 mm distal from the last molar to 2 mm distal from the molar on the opposite side of the arch. This establishes a cutting line for back cut.

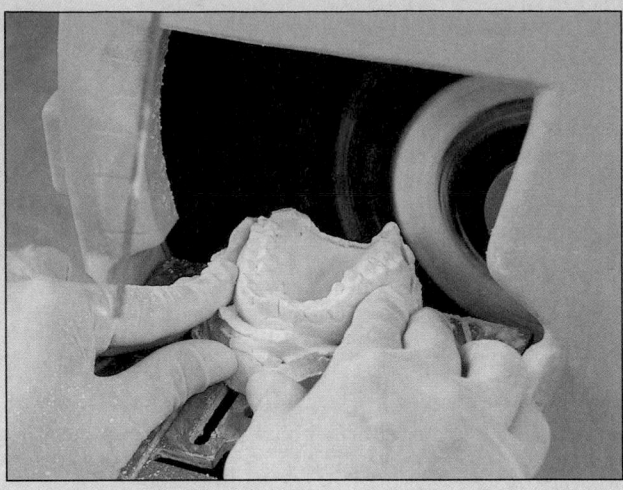

FIGURE 33-44
Posterior of model base is cut at right angle to base.

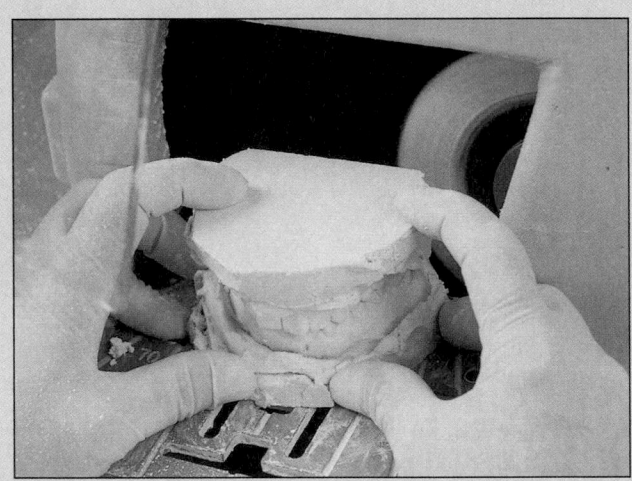

FIGURE 33-45
Models are placed together to trim back cut.

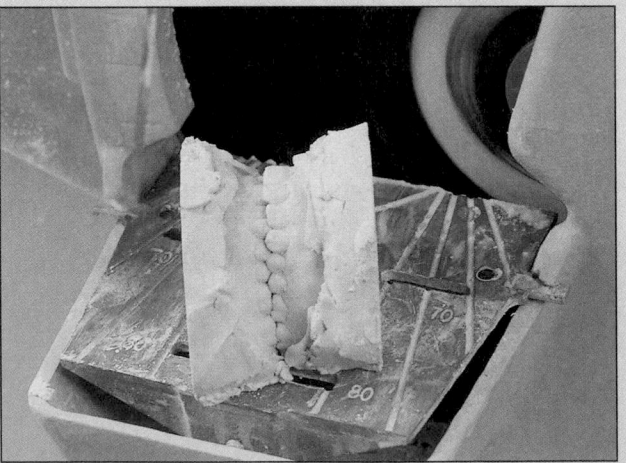

FIGURE 33-46
Models are placed on their backs on a hard, flat surface in occlusion to verify whether back cuts are correct.

15. Cut the side angles of the model next. Take the pencil and mark the following areas: outward from the middle of the mandibular premolars to the edge of the model and the maxillary cuspids in the same manner. Draw a line running parallel to the teeth at the greatest depth of the buccal vestibule, from the molars to the premolars. This line will be about 5 mm from the buccal surface of the teeth. Mark both sides of the maxillary and the mandibular models in this manner.

16. Place the model base back on the model trimmer table guide and trim the model to the pencil lines on both sides (Figure 33-47). Repeat this procedure with both models.

17. Draw a line from the middle of the central incisors to the canine/cuspid line on each quadrant using the straight edge of the measuring device on the maxillary cast (Figure 33-48). Make both anterior cuts, forming a pointed area at the midline and center of both cuspids.

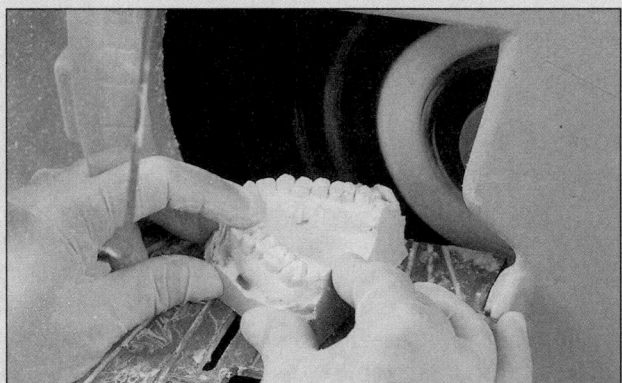

FIGURE 33-47
Vestibule or side area is cut at deepest area. A line can be drawn to establish a proper cut line.

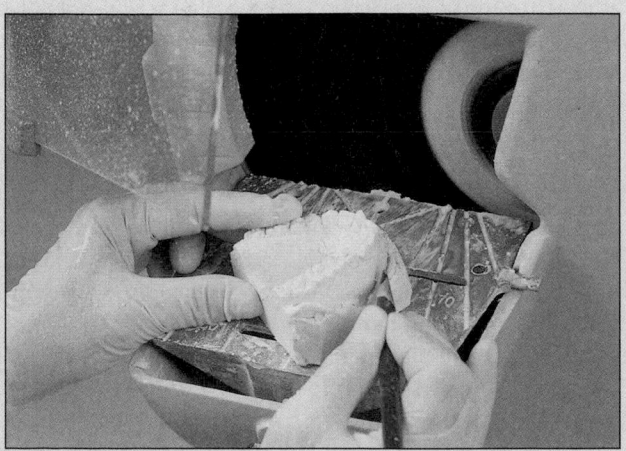

FIGURE 33-48
Line is drawn from midline of central incisors to middle of cuspid to establish a cut line for anterior.

18. Draw a rounded line from canine to canine and make the cut for the mandibular cast. If the teeth are highly irregular, adjustments may have to be done. After the lines are drawn, make sure that the cuts will not trim away the protruding teeth. If it appears that this may happen, move the lines out on each side to accommodate this. The model should appear symmetrical (Figure 33-49).

19. Draw a pencil line at the depth of the anterior vestibule as a guide for trimming if necessary (Figure 33-50).

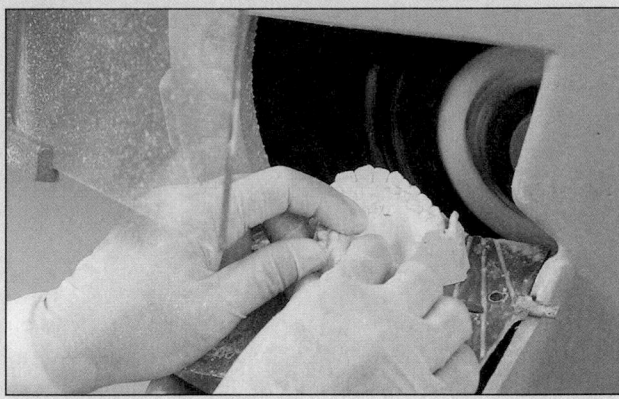

FIGURE 33-49
Maxillary anterior area is cut to a point, bringing both cuspid cuts to midline between maxillary central incisors.

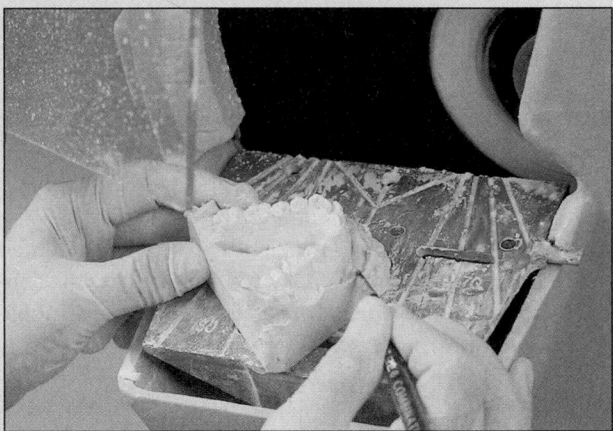

FIGURE 33-50
A rounded line is drawn on mandibular from cuspid to cuspid to indicate where the cut should be made.

20. Trim the heel cuts at a 90° angle of an imaginary line from the midpoint of the canine on the opposite side. The heel cuts are small cuts on both the maxillary and the mandibular models that finish the trimming of the models (Figure 33-51).

21. Use a laboratory knife to trim the tongue area flat and smooth other areas on the art portion. Take care not to destroy the anatomy of the diagnostic casts.

(Continues)

22. Fill any air bubbles with plaster by using dry plaster on the finger, and push it into the wet model.

23. Use a fine wet/dry sandpaper under water if necessary to complete the smoothing of the flat surfaces. Any small beads of plaster can be removed carefully from the surfaces of the teeth.

24. Place the models in a model gloss for 10 minutes or spray with gloss to provide a professional appearance and add strength.

25. Polish models with a dry cloth to buff the surface in order to achieve the desired high gloss.

26. Label both models with the patient's name and the date the models were taken. In an orthodontic office, the patient's age may also be identified on the models.

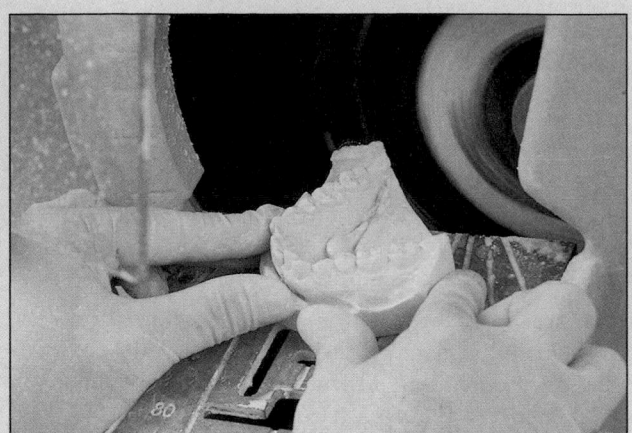

FIGURE 33-51
Heel cuts are established on models and cut.

of the patient's teeth in order to maintain the patient's occlusion and represent his or her jaws. Articulators can be simple, such as hinges that only duplicate the up-and-down motions, or they can be complex, where they are adjustable and can duplicate the side-to-side motions as well as the up-and-down motions.

Articulators can be used to study malocclusion, to wax and carve teeth for crowns and bridges, and to demonstrate to the patient the action that is of concern. They also have a number of other desired uses. The dental assistant may perform the task of mounting models or assist the dentist in this task.

Facebows and Articulators
Dental offices will use a facebow and an articulator to duplicate the function of the tempormandibular joint. The facebow allows the operator to obtain the records about the placement of the maxillary arch and its location to the joint. From this the mandibular arch can be mounted and the biting function can be duplicated. This provides the dentist the information for diagnosis or for constructing dental appliances such as crowns, bridges, veneers, partials, and dentures.

Facebow Transfer
Dental assistants will need to prepare the patient and the parts of the facebow (Figure 33-52) for the facebow transfer. This skill is allowed for trained and qualified dental assistants to complete under general supervision in some states. Following all aseptic techniques and informing the patient, the operator will use the reference plane marker and locator to mark the anterior reference point on the patient's right side according to the manufacturer's directions. (See Procedure 33-12, "Performing a Facebow Transfer.") The bite registration material or baseplate wax is then placed on the top side of the bitefork, which is then inserted into the patient's mouth where they close on it to secure it in place while the material sets. The facebow is secured to the bitefork, and the earbow assembly is attached. The finger screws are tightened to obtain the needed records; then the release screws are

loosened, the patient opens, and the entire facebow and bitefork assembly is removed from the patient. It is disinfected, and either it is sent to the laboratory or the dentist or auxiliary mounts it to an articulator (see Procedure 33-13).

Articulator
An articulator (refer to Figure 33-53) is used to replicate the up-and-down motion and lateral movement of the joint. Many articulators are on the market and used for specific reasons with enhanced functions. They have two support bows: one to stabilize the maxillary and one to stabilize the mandibular.

The hinge represents the temporomandibular joints. The first step in using this articulator is to trim the models so that they fit within the two bows easily. The top portion of the bases can then be scored. To score a model is to make cut marks in the smooth surface so that the added gypsum can adhere. The models are placed within the bows in the correct bite. Normally, the wax bite is used to establish the correct occlusion. The models are then attached to the bows using impression plaster, which flows into the scored area and around the bow. After the plaster has set, the models remain fastened to the articulator and can be opened and the wax bite removed.

Dental Waxes

Waxes are among the oldest materials used in dentistry. Over 200 years ago, impressions were taken of specific areas in the mouth with wax. The waxes are derived from a number of sources, including bees, plants, and minerals. Beeswax has to be refined and bleached to obtain uniformity of color and character. Differences in color and texture may take place if the bee has been feeding on something unusual, for example, plants all yellow in color. Certain plants in South America and Brazil bring to dentistry a hard wax that is gathered from the fronds of a tree. This wax also is used for polishing automobiles to a high gloss shine. From minerals come petroleum

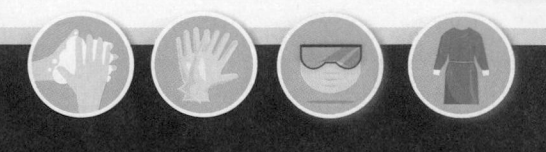

Procedure 33-12
Performing a Facebow Transfer

This procedure is completed to replicate and transfer both esthetic and functional components from the patient's mouth.

Steps written in **blue** font are performed by the operator (dentist or qualified dental assistant), and the chairside assistant's steps are written in black.

Equipment and Supplies

Patient Seating Setup (refer to Procedure 18-4)

Facebow Transfer Setup (refer to Figure 33-52)
- earbow (A)
- bitefork and transfer jig assembly (B)
- reference plane marker (C)
- reference plane locator (D)
- firm cotton roll (E)
- bite registration material or baseplate wax (F)

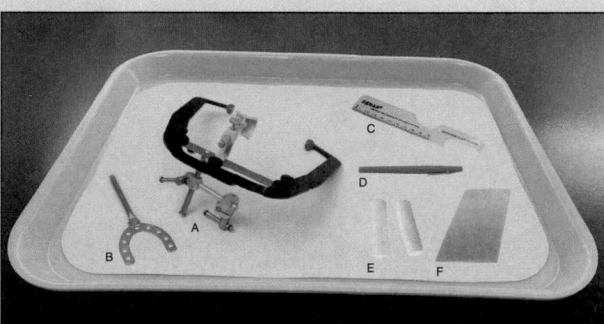

FIGURE 33-52
Facebow transfer setup.

Procedure Steps

1. Escort and seat patient (refer to Procedure 18-4).

   Marks the anterior reference point on the patient's right side using the reference plane marker and locater, according to the manufacturer's directions.

2. Apply the bite registration material or baseplate wax on the top of the bitefork in three areas, normally the anterior and both posterior sides. Evaluate the arch to ensure that there are three points of reference.

3. Transfer to operator.

   Inserts the bitefork into the mouth.

   Aligns the patient's midline with the index notch; ensures that it is parallel with the patient's horizontal and coronal planes. Moves the bitefork with the material into place on the maxillary arch (Figure 33-53).

Attaches the vertical shaft of the transfer jig assembly to the facebow frame with the clamp and tightens the screw. This should hold the facebow onto the shaft.

Loosens the side finger screws as well as the center wheel so that the earbow assembly on the facebow will open.

4. Have the patient place the bow earpieces in the ears (Figure 33-54). Have them slide the earpieces forward to ensure they are in the ears snugly.

   Tightens the finger side screws.

   Uses the nasion assembly to push against the nasion.

   Raises or lowers the bow so that the pointer aligns precisely with the anterior reference point.

   Tightens the clamps when it is aligned (Figure 33-55). Makes sure not to alter the bow when tightening all of the screws.

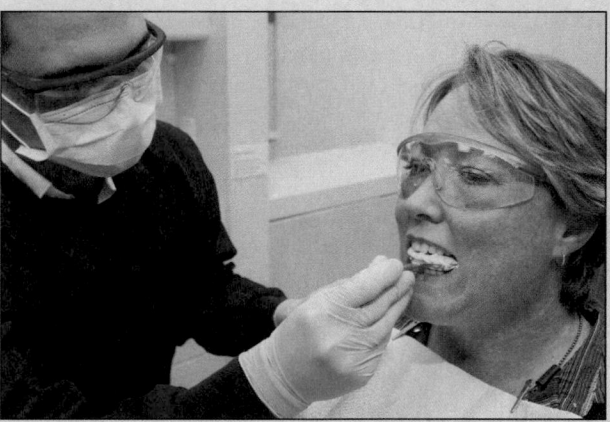

FIGURE 33-53
Move the bitefork with the material into place on the maxillary arch.

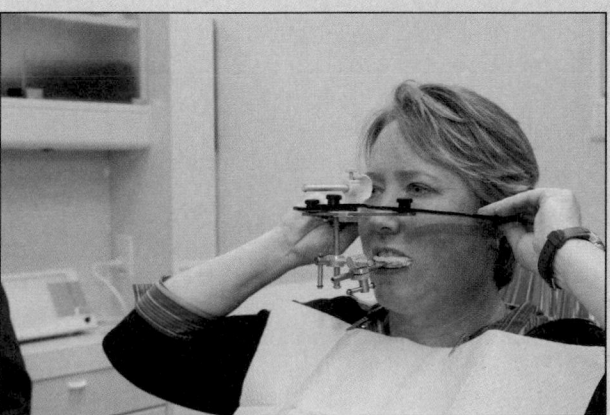

FIGURE 33-54
Have the patient place the bow earpiece into the ears.

(Continues)

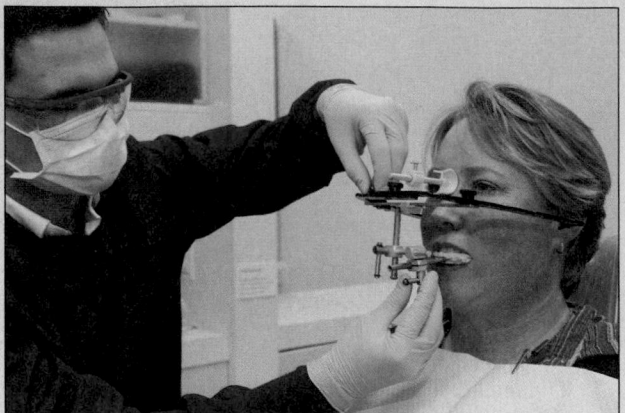

FIGURE 33-55
Retighten side finger screws to accommodate changes.

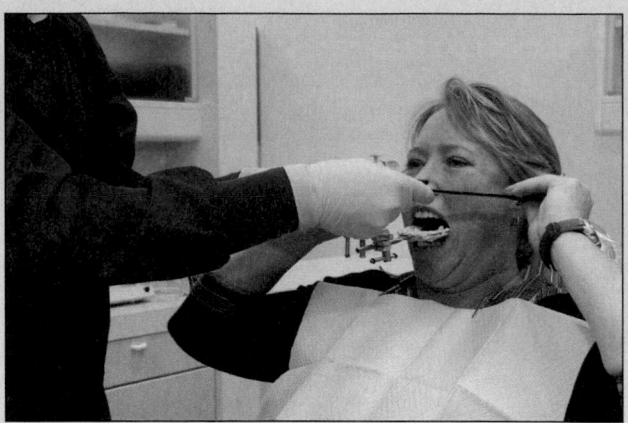

FIGURE 33-56
Removing the bitefork from the patient's mouth.

Connects transfer assembly on the facebow to the bitefork in patient's oral cavity.

Loosens the anterior finger grip and screws on the measuring bow, moves the measuring bow away from the patient's face, instructs the patient to open while holding the bow and removing it and the bitefork from the patient's mouth (Figure 33-56).

5. The bitefork is to be disinfected prior to sending to the laboratory or mounting it to the articulator.

6. Write up procedure in Services Rendered.

Date	Services Rendered
02/18/XX	Reviewed medical and dental history, BP = 120/80
	Completed Facebow transfer for fixed bridge #2–5
	RTC: Insert fixed bridge Assistant's initials

7. Dismiss and escort patient to reception area (refer to Procedure 18-5).

Procedure 33-13
Mounting Models on an Articulator after Facebow Records Have Been Completed

This procedure is performed after the facebow is disinfected and ready to be mounted. It is done in the office dental laboratory or at a commercial dental laboratory.

Steps written in blue font are performed by the operator (dentist or qualified dental assistant), and the chairside assistant's steps are written in black.

Equipment and Supplies
- PPE: examination gloves, mask, protective glasses, and protective clothing
- handwashing soap or hand sanitizer

Articulator Mounting Setup
- facebow and bitefork assembled (Figure 33-57A)
- semiadjustable articulator (Figure 33-57B)
- two mounting rings (Figure 33-57C)
- trimmed models (Figure 33-57D)
- type I plaster and water (see Figure 33-33)
- mixing bowl and spatula (see Figure 33-33)

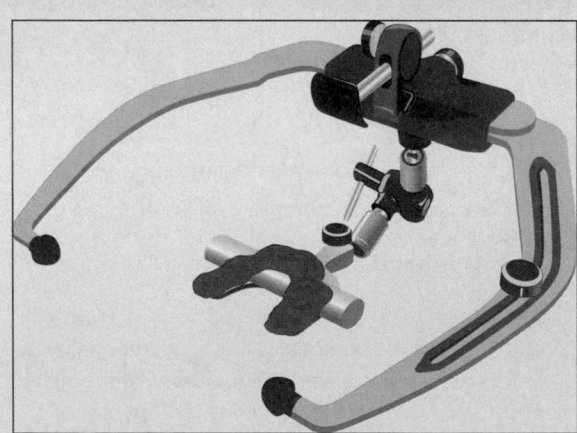

FIGURE 33-57A
Facebow and bitefork assembled.

Procedure Steps
1. Trim models so that they fit within the two bows easily. (Refer to Procedure 33-11.)

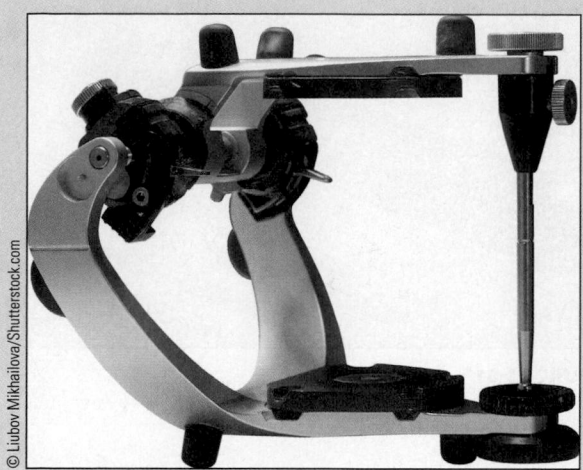

FIGURE 33-57B
Semiadjustable articulator.

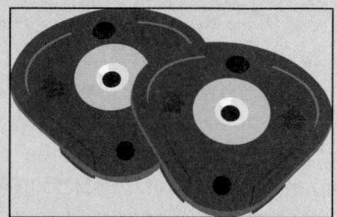

FIGURE 33-57C
Two mounting rings.

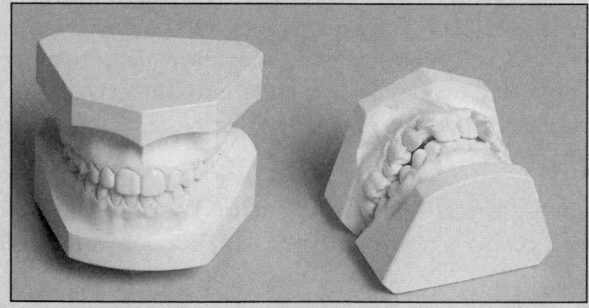

FIGURE 33-57D
Trimmed models.

2. Score the models with a knife.

Attaches the facebow to the articulator according to the manufacturer's directions.

Places the maxillary model into the bite registration material or baseplate wax that was used on the patient. Makes sure that it is seated into the impression that was established.

Lifts the articulator arm up to expose the scored area on the maxillary model.

3. Mix Type I plaster to a thick consistency. Pass to operator.

Places plaster on the model. Fills the entire space between the model and the top of the articulator, then brings the top arm with the articulator ring down onto the plaster (Figure 33-58). Makes sure some of the plaster goes through the open areas of the ring. Removes excess plaster and smooths the plaster around the ring and the model.

Removes the facebow and bitefork after the maxillary model is set. The maxillary model is now attached to the articulator.

Mounts the mandibular model using the bite registrations that were obtained during the appointment.

Holds the models together in correct bite.

4. Mix additional plaster. Pass to operator.

Mounds the plaster on the lower articulator ring until the space is filled and then allows the area of the mandibular scored model to be placed into the plaster (Figure 33-59).

Cleans any excess plaster and smooths the plaster that has been added after initial set. Models remain in the articulator and then can be opened and closed as if biting. They also allow for side-to-side excursions to be accomplished so that the dental appliance can be made properly.

Adds pin to the articulator. Centric relationship has been established for the models. The centric relationship is where the teeth are positioned when the joints are aligned. Patients often rest in this centric relationship.

Fabricates fixed or removable prosthesis.

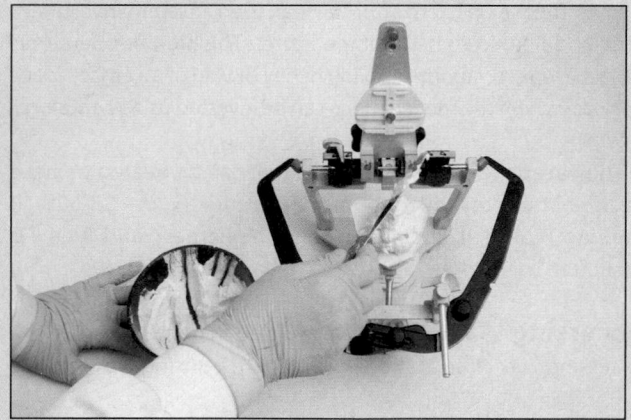

FIGURE 33-58
Fill the entire space between the model and the top of the articulator, and then bring the top arm with the articulator ring down onto the plaster.

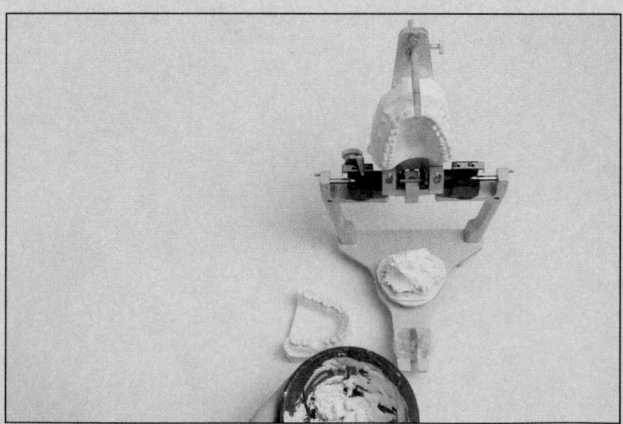

FIGURE 33-59
Mound the plaster on the lower articulating ring until the space is filled.

products, such as paraffin wax. In dentistry, only the highest grade of wax is used. It must be uniform and provide consistent results when used.

Wax Groups

Waxes are classified into three broad groups: pattern, processing, and impression. Pattern waxes are hard waxes used in crown and bridge casting (inlay wax) and the construction of the baseplate tray (baseplate wax). Processing and impression waxes have many uses in dentistry.

Pattern Wax Pattern, or inlay, wax normally is supplied in dark-colored sticks (Figure 33-60A). It is used on a die, a positive replica of the prepared tooth made from stone. The wax is melted and applied to the die, making a wax pattern that is used to create the metal and/or porcelain restoration. The composition varies from manufacturer to manufacturer, but most waxes have a certain degree of hardness, toughness, resistance to flaking, and ability to achieve a smooth surface. Desirable properties of inlay wax are that it flows at a temperature slightly above the mouth temperature, it achieves complete burnout at temperatures above 482° C, and it carves away easily without chipping or cracking. These properties are essential in using the *lost wax* technique of casting. The lost wax technique refers to the wax pattern after the wax is enclosed in investment stone and heated to high temperatures. The high temperatures cause the wax to vaporize, leaving behind a void or an empty space (lost wax) where the melted metal can be invested using centrifugal force.

The baseplate wax is a hard wax that can be heated to make the initial base on which to form a denture (Figure 33-60B). It comes in Types I, II, and III. Type III is the hardest, and Type II is most often used in the **fabrication** of baseplates.

Processing Wax Several waxes used in dentistry are in the processing wax classification (Figure 33-61). Boxing wax is a soft,

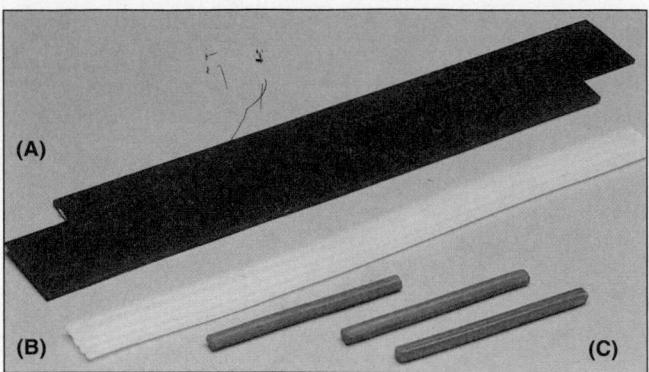

FIGURE 33-61
Processing waxes. (A) Boxing wax. (B) Utility wax. (C) Sticky wax.

pliable wax that is used to form a wax box around an impression prior to pouring it with gypsum. It comes in wax strips 1 inch wide and can be reused for the purpose of making a ring around the impression to hold the runny gypsum in place until it sets.

Sticky wax is another type of processing wax. It is brittle at room temperature but when melted with a flame source becomes soft and sticky. It adheres to a number of surfaces, such as metal, gypsum, and porcelain. It is used to hold two fractured pieces together until they can be repaired.

Utility wax, also called periphery or bending wax, is a soft wax that is adhesive and pliable. It does not require additional heat and can be molded to most surfaces. This is the wax used to bead around trays to extend them and assist in patient comfort. This wax is also used for orthodontic patients to cover the brackets and uncomfortable areas until the cheeks and lips can adjust. It is supplied in long ropes or strips and in a number of colors.

Impression or Bite Registration Waxes Normally containing copper or aluminum particles, impression waxes are used

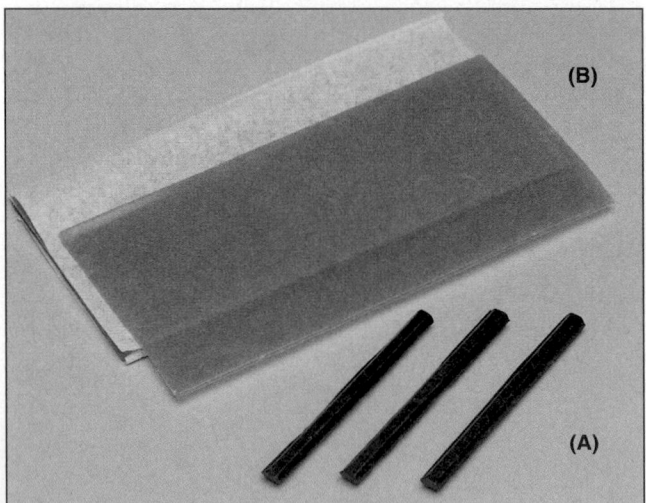

FIGURE 33-60
Pattern waxes. (A) Inlay wax. (B) Baseplate wax.

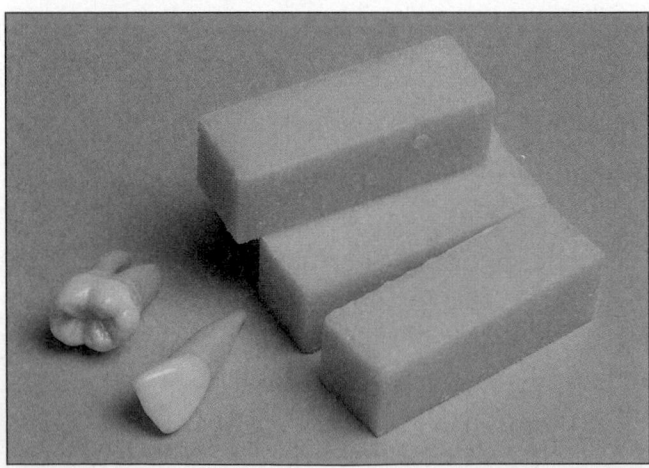

FIGURE 33-62
Study wax blocks.

to take bite registrations. They are supplied in horseshoe shapes for obtaining the maxillary and mandibular biting surfaces.

Additional Waxes Other waxes used in dentistry that are not in the three primary classifications are the study wax and the undercut wax. The study wax is hard wax supplied in blocks used for carving teeth and anatomy (Figure 33-62). Undercut wax is a putty-type wax used to fill in the undercuts prior to the impression being taken.

Custom Trays

The dentist may ask for a **custom-made impression tray** for the patient in order to obtain an accurate impression. This may be because a regular stock tray does not fit. The stock tray will not allow a minimum amount of space for the material to flow around the prepared area, or it may require that an overabundance of impression material be used to obtain the impression, therefore risking an inferior outcome. In any case, a custom tray can be fabricated to meet the need. Several materials are available to make a custom tray. It can be constructed from self- or light-curing acrylic resin, a vacuum resin, or a **thermoplastic** material. All materials must be rigid enough to provide subsistence for the material as it is inserted into and removed from the mouth. It is important that the material adapts well during the construction so that the final tray meets the required criteria. See Table 33-7 for required criteria for a custom tray.

Self-Curing Acrylic Tray Resin Custom Trays

The most common material used to make custom trays is the self-curing acrylic tray resin (Procedure 33-14). It consists of a liquid catalyst (**monomer**) that mixes with a powder (polymer) to start the process of curing (polymerization). Polymerization occurs when material changes from a plastic pliable state to a rigid state. Once this process starts, it continues until the material is set completely. The material goes through several stages as it is cured. The first stage is after the liquid and the powder are mixed together. This initial set is when the material appears sticky and, if pulled apart, appears to have spiderweb strands from particle to particle. The second stage is where the material

can be gathered into a ball, kneaded, and contoured to the model. The third stage is where the material goes through an exothermic reaction, giving off a great deal of heat while setting. When the heat has diminished and the material can no longer be shaped, the final set stage is completed. A custom tray should be allowed to set for 24 hours prior to use because it is still dimensionally unstable.

Light-Cured Acrylic Tray Resin Custom Trays

Acrylic tray resin is supplied in light-cured custom trays. The primary difference between this material and the self-curing material is that the setting time is operator controlled. The material stays pliable and workable until a light source initiates polymerization. The polymerization process happens quickly. This technique requires special equipment: an oven-like appliance with a special curing light in it (Figure 33-63). The custom tray is designed and placed in the oven for a quick setting and then is ready for use.

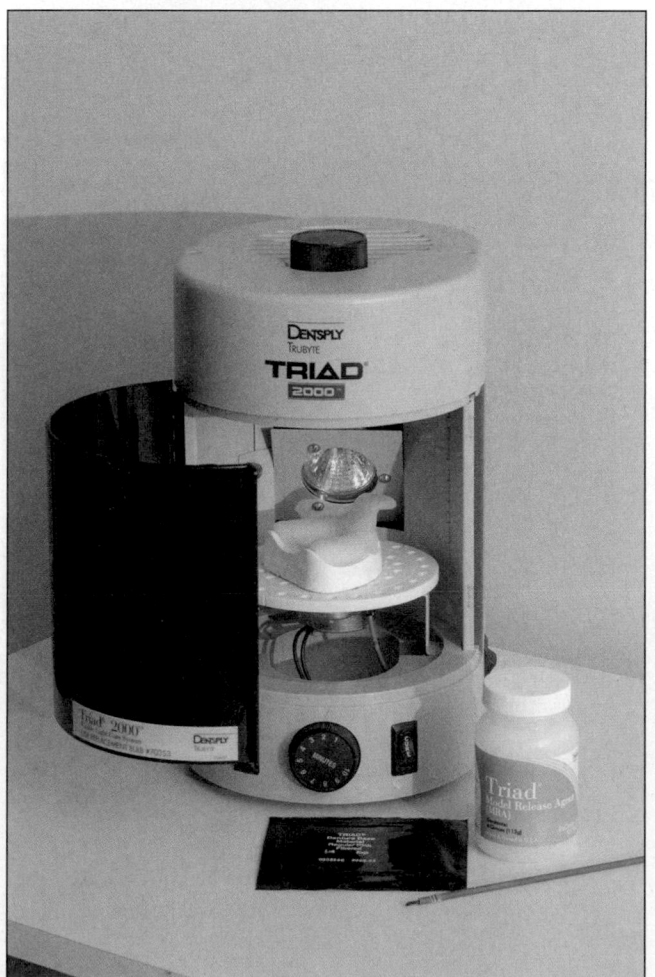

FIGURE 33-63
Triad® Visible Light Cure unit.

TABLE 33-7 Required Criteria for a Custom Tray

Stable enough to hold the material rigid during placement and removal.
Can be smoothed and contoured to the arch.
Can be adapted to an edentulous, a partially edentulous, and a full dentition.
Can be adapted to allow uniform thickness of impression material in all areas of the arch.
Can be altered and contoured to any irregular area.
Can be designed so that stops are in the spacer, therefore holding the material in a stable, specifically determined area, providing a more accurate impression.

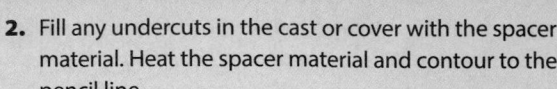

Procedure 33-14
Constructing a Self-Curing Acrylic Resin Custom Tray

This procedure is performed by the trained and qualified dental assistant in the dental laboratory on a working cast.

Equipment and Supplies
- PPE: examination gloves, mask, protective glasses, and protective clothing
- handwashing soap or hand sanitizer

Self-Curing Acrylic Resin Custom Tray Setup (Figure 33-64)
- maxillary and/or mandibular casts (A)
- laboratory knife (B)
- pencil (plain or red and blue) (C)
- wax spatula (D)
- baseplate wax (E)
- heating source (warm water or laboratory torch) (F)
- tray resin with measuring devices (not shown)
- separating medium with brush (not shown)
- wooden tongue blade and wax-lined paper cup (G)
- petroleum jelly (H)
- tray adhesive (see Figure 33-71)

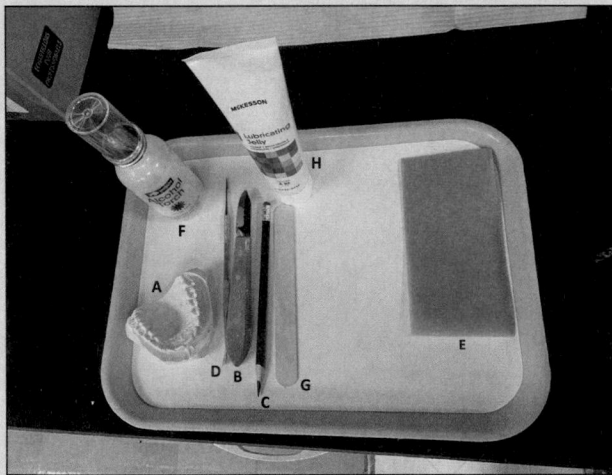

FIGURE 33-64
Self-curing acrylic resin custom tray setup.

Preparing the Cast

Procedure Steps
1. Outline the area of the cast for the spacer to be placed (Figure 33-65). This is 2 to 3 mm below the margin of the prepared tooth or 2 to 3 mm above the lowest point in the vestibule if the arch is edentulous.

2. Fill any undercuts in the cast or cover with the spacer material. Heat the spacer material and contour to the pencil line.

3. Trim the wax or spacer to the line using an angled cut instead of a blunt cut with a laboratory knife (Figure 33-66).

4. Cut the appropriate stops in the spacer (Figure 33-67).

5. Cover the spacer with aluminum foil or paint it with separating medium.

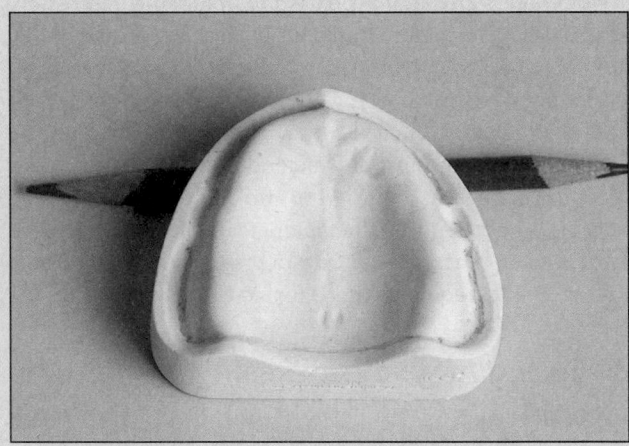

FIGURE 33-65
Tray margin is outlined on plaster or stone cast. The deepest area is marked in blue; 1 or 2 mm above this point, a red line indicating where the wax spacer is to be located can be drawn.

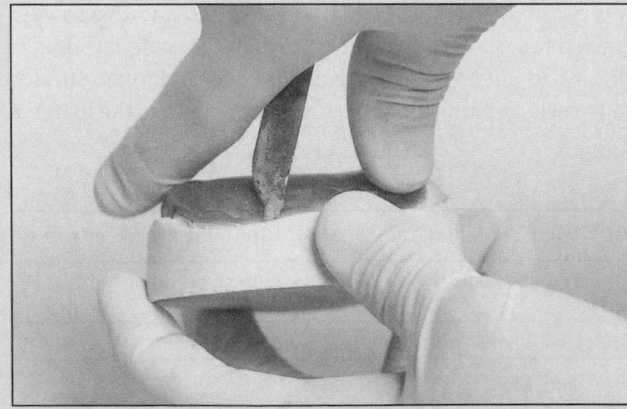

FIGURE 33-66
Wax spacer is trimmed to line on working cast.

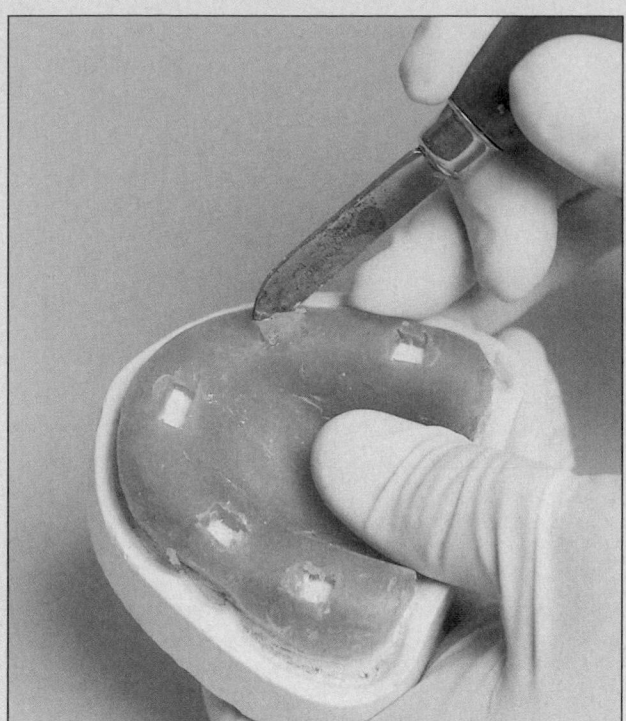

FIGURE 33-67
Stops cut into wax spacer allow room for impression material.

Mixing Custom Tray Acrylic Self-Curing Resin

Procedure Steps

1. Measure the powder and the liquid to the correct calibrations on the measuring devices according to the manufacturer's directions.

2. Mix the powder and liquid together in the wax-lined paper cup with the wooden tongue blade until the mixture is homogeneous (uniformly mixed).

3. Allow the mixture to go through initial polymerization for 2 to 3 minutes. Some manufacturers indicate that a cover be placed over the material during the polymerization.

4. Place petroleum jelly over the cast and on the palms of your hands while waiting for initial polymerization.

Contouring Custom Tray Acrylic Self-Curing Resin

The material is ready to conform to the tray after the initial set when the material is no longer sticky and can be gathered into a ball.

Procedure Steps

1. Knead the material to further mix the material and set a small amount aside for the handle (Figure 33-68). This doughy stage allows the material to be formed into a patty for the maxillary arch or a roll for the mandibular arch.

2. Place the dough-like patty for the maxillary cast, covering the wax spacer.

3. Contour and adapt it to extend 1 to 2 mm over the wax spacer (Figure 33-69A). Try to complete the adaptation with a rolled edge at the designated area. If unable to accomplish this, a laboratory knife can be used to trim the material back. (Doing this causes rough edges that need to be smoothed back later.)

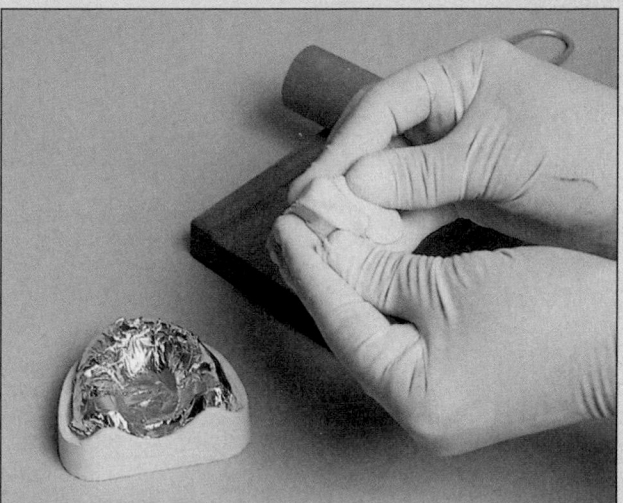

FIGURE 33-68
Custom tray material is kneaded for use.

4. Shape the material set aside for the handle.

5. Place a drop of the monomer liquid on the tray where the handle is to be adapted and then on the handle where it will be placed on the custom tray. This allows the materials to join together for a better outcome.

6. Place the handle in the midline area of the arch (Figure 33-69B). If making an edentulous custom tray, the handle should come up from the ridge and then outward. A custom tray handle that is made for an area that has teeth can come directly outward.

7. Place the handle and hold it in the proper position until the material becomes firm.

Finishing Custom Tray Acrylic Self-Curing Resin

Procedure Steps

1. Allow to set about 8 to 10 minutes. Remove the custom tray from the cast and take out the spacer material.

2. Melt wax and use a wax spatula to remove it, along with hot water and a toothbrush. If foil has been used, the cleaning will not take a great deal of time.

3. Trim the edges of the custom tray using an acrylic bur (Figure 33-70) or an arbor band after the final set (30 minutes minimum).

(Continues)

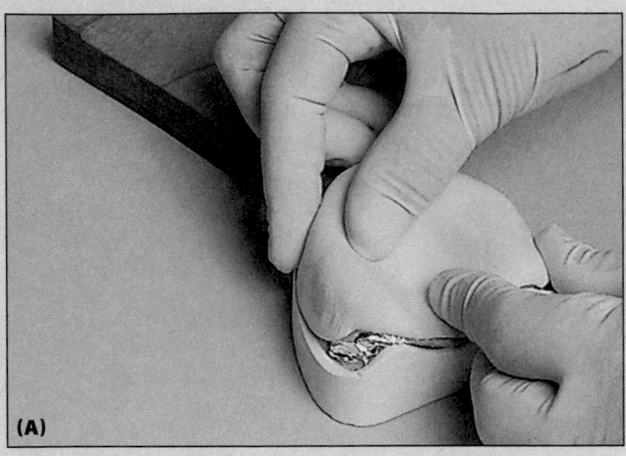
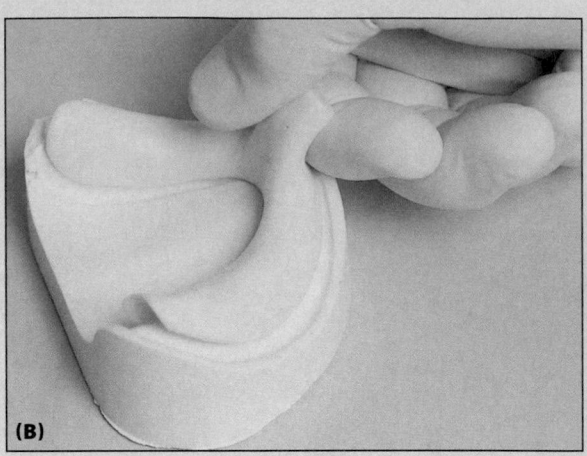

FIGURE 33-69
(A) Custom tray material is adapted to model over wax spacer. (B) Handle is attached to adapted custom tray.

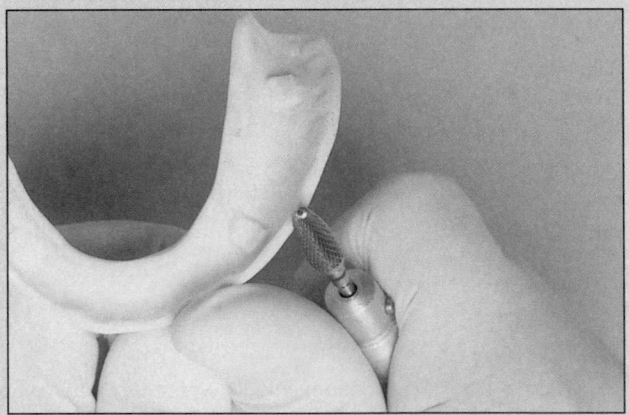

FIGURE 33-70
Custom tray is trimmed with an acrylic bur.

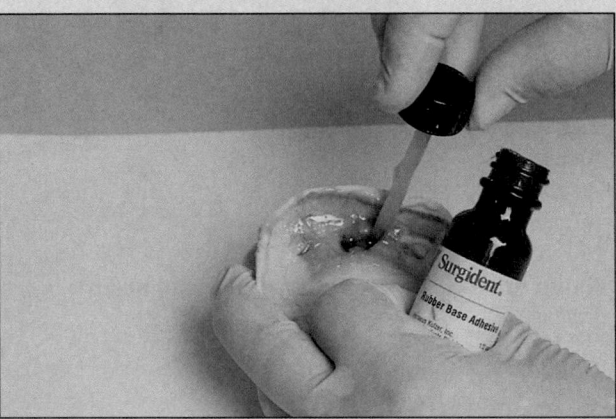

FIGURE 33-71
Adhesive is applied to custom tray in a thin coat and allowed to dry.

4. Clean and disinfect the custom tray according to the manufacturer's directions.

5. Write the patient's name on the tray.

6. Apply the adhesive provided by the manufacturer of the impression material to the inside of the custom tray and along the margins (Figure 33-71).

Vacuum-Formed Custom Trays

Like the acrylic tray resin that is light cured, the vacuum-formed custom trays require additional equipment (Figure 33-72). This unit has a frame that holds the sheets directly under a heating element and, when they are softened, the frame drops the sheet onto the cast as vacuum pressure draws the material to the model. The vacuum-forming unit has other applications in dentistry. Acrylic resin sheets are supplied in several gauges for different applications. The custom tray requires the use of a rigid, heavy, plastic resin.

Trays that are vacuum formed can be used for a number of applications in the field of dentistry. Most often they are used for custom trays, bleaching trays, night guards, mouth guards, and matrices for provisional restorations. The material comes in several gauges and thicknesses for specific applications (Figure 33-73). Custom tray material is much more thick and rigid

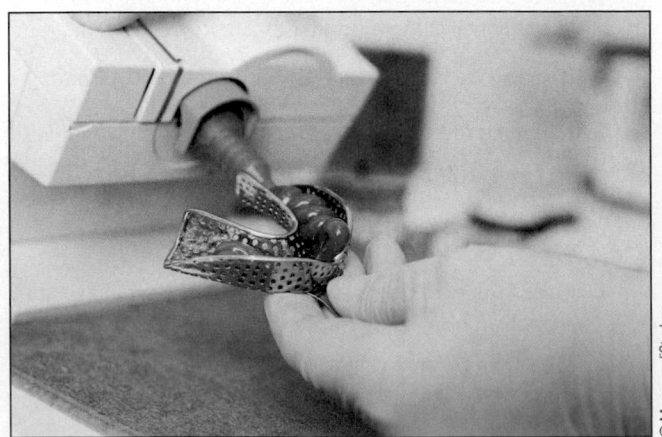

© M_a_y_a /iStock.com

FIGURE 33-72
Dispensing using a large volume mixing unit.

than the other applications. All use a **vacu-former** with a heating element, a cast, and material that can be heated and adapted through vacuum pressure.

Thermoplastic Tray Material Custom Trays

Other materials used for making custom trays are the thermoplastic beads and buttons. When these small, round beads or buttons are placed in warm water, the thermoplastic reaction takes place. Thermoplastic means that the material becomes soft and pliable when exposed to heat. Once the material is soft, it can be conformed to the model in the desired shape. As the heat dissipates, the material hardens. It is easy to identify when the material is soft enough because it appears clear and then becomes dense when it hardens.

Constructing a Custom Tray

Regardless of the material type used, the custom tray model is prepared in the same manner.

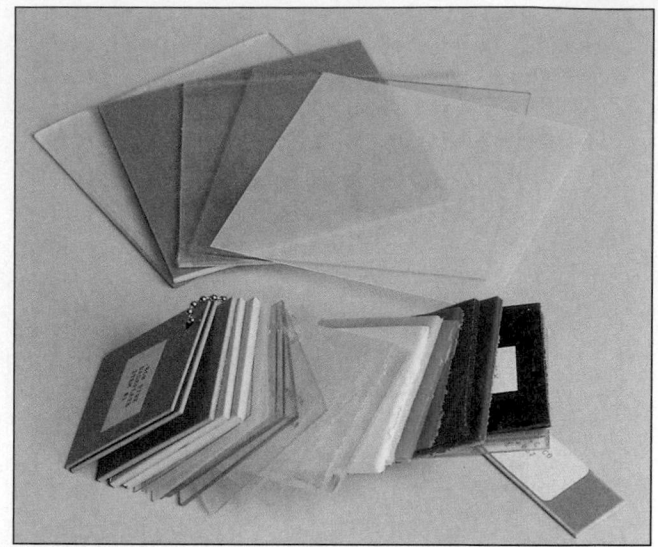

FIGURE 33-73
Various vacuum-formed materials.

Procedure 33-15
Constructing a Vacuum-Formed Acrylic Resin Custom Tray

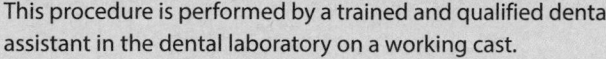

This procedure is performed by a trained and qualified dental assistant in the dental laboratory on a working cast.

Equipment and Supplies
- PPE: examination gloves, mask, protective glasses, and protective clothing
- handwashing soap or hand sanitizer

Vacuum-Formed Acrylic Resin Custom Tray Setup (Figure 33-74)
- maxillary and/or mandibular casts (A)
- laboratory knife (B)

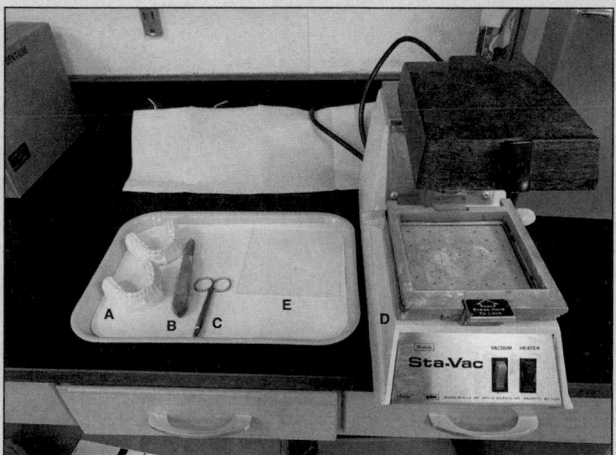

FIGURE 33-74
Vacuum-formed acrylic resin custom tray setup.

- laboratory scissors (C)
- vacu-former with heating element (D)
- acrylic sheets (E)

Preparing the Cast
Procedure Steps
1. Soak cast in warm water for up to 30 minutes prior to forming a custom tray on it. This eliminates small air bubbles. (These air bubbles coming to the surface [percolating] will cause small spaces between the cast and the acrylic sheet. Then, the custom tray would not have the accuracy desired.)

2. Place the spacer, if indicated. (A wax spacer will melt under the heating element, if used.)

3. Mark the desired outer margin of the custom tray.

4. Place the cast on the platform of the vacuum-forming unit.

Contouring Acrylic Resin Sheets during Vacuum-Forming Process
Procedure Steps
1. Select the appropriate acrylic resin sheets to be used for the procedure.

2. Place the acrylic resin sheets between the heater frame and the gasket frame and tighten the anterior knob to secure the material in place. Place the cast on the platform (Figure 33-75).

3. Make sure the heating element is in the correct place above the acrylic resin sheet and turn it on.

(Continues)

4. Watch the resin as it heats. It will begin to sag downward (Figure 33-76). Allow this to continue until the resin droops downward about 1 inch. (Overheating causes air bubbles to form on the surface of the acrylic resin.)

5. After the material is heated properly, take both handles on the frame and pull the frame downward, over the cast. Only touch the handles because the entire area is extremely hot.

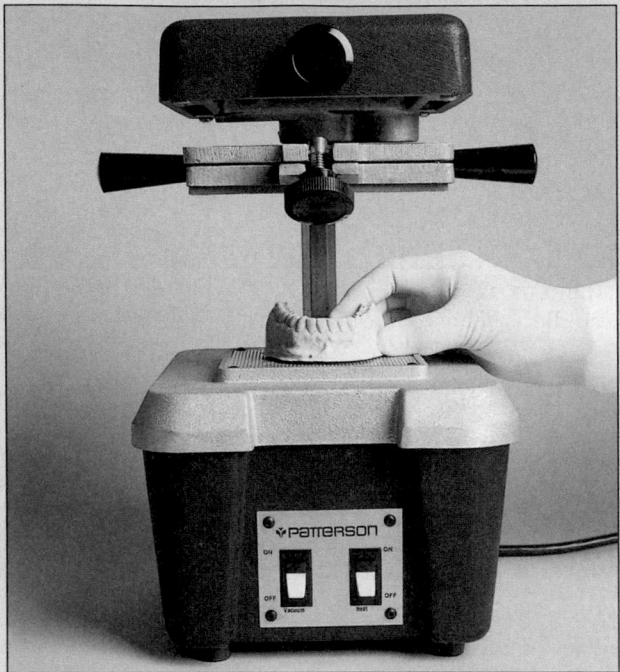

FIGURE 33-75
Resin sheets are secured in place, and the cast is placed on the platform of a vacuum-forming unit.

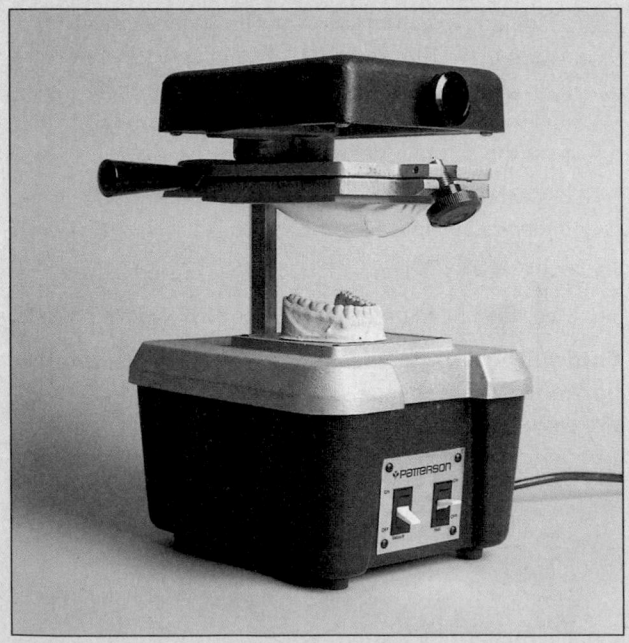

FIGURE 33-76
Resin sheet begins sagging as material is heated.

6. Turn on the vacuum immediately after the resin sheet is entirely over the cast (Figure 33-77).

7. Turn off the heating unit.

8. Allow the vacuum to continue for 1 to 2 minutes in order to cool the resin so it becomes firm again.

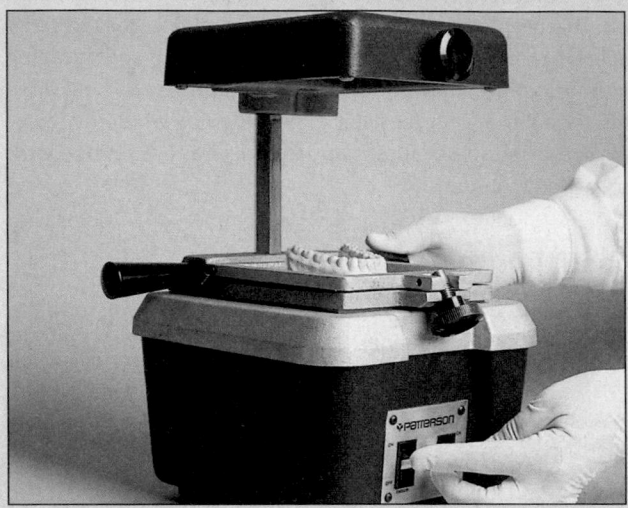

FIGURE 33-77
When resin material has sagged 1 inch below the holding ring, it is ready to be dropped into position over cast. The unit is held by handles to ensure that the operator is not burned.

Finishing Vacuum-Formed Acrylic Resin Custom Tray
Procedure Steps

1. Remove the resin material from the vacuum form after it is cooled.

2. Separate the resin-formed custom tray from the cast and, using laboratory scissors, trim to the desired form (Figure 33-78).

3. Use a torch to heat and apply a cutout handle section to the custom tray.

4. Clean and disinfect the custom tray according to the manufacturer's directions and write the patient's name on it.

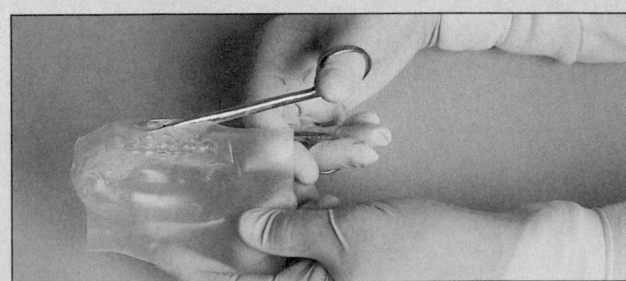

FIGURE 33-78
Vacuum form can be trimmed with scissors.

Outlining Tray Margins If a full custom tray is desired on an edentulous arch, draw a blue line at the bottom of the vestibule area around the facial surface, across the palate area on the maxillary model, around the posterior retromolar area, along the bottom of the vestibule area, and across the opposite posterior retromolar area on the mandibular model (see Figure 33-65). From that first marking, make a red line 2 mm upward (toward the ridge). This gives a definite line to follow when adapting the spacer. A spacer is placed on the model to allow room in the tray for the impression material. This spacer normally is made of pink baseplate wax, but a commercial nonstick molding material may be used (especially when using the vacuum-formed custom tray because of the heating element) or a moist paper towel can be used. When the spacer is placed, the undercuts are filled in. Undercuts are recessed areas in the model that make it impossible to seat or remove the custom tray properly. Undercuts are caused by bubbles in the plaster, cavities, or the shape of the arch or dentition. If using baseplate wax for the spacer, it can be heated with warm water or butane torch (Figure 33-79) and conformed to the model. Cut it back to the red line in an angle-forming manner (see Procedure 39-14, "Constructing Self-Curing Acrylic Resin Custom Tray"). This provides a smoother tissue side to the custom tray and is more comfortable to the patients than a blunt-edge cut. After the spacer is in place, take a warm plastic instrument to lute (secure) the edges of the wax to the cast. After the securing is accomplished, cut into the crest of the wax with a laboratory knife, making small rectangular or round holes. These stops (holes on the spacer that allow bumps to be formed on the tissue side of the tray) allow the tray to be seated 2 to 3 mm from the teeth or tissue and to prevent it from seating too deeply. This allows an adequate amount of impression material to flow around the prepared teeth or the tissue. There should be a minimum of four stops on an edentulous model, two on each first molar and cuspid area. When making a custom tray for crowns and bridges, the stops should be placed one tooth distal and mesial from the prepared tooth.

The self-curing material is exothermic. It heats up and causes the wax to melt slightly. It is advisable to place a layer of aluminum foil over the wax spacer and into the stops. The foil makes it easier to remove the wax from the tissue side of the tray after the custom tray is made. If foil is not used, a toothbrush and hot water will aid in getting the wax out of the inside (tissue side) of the custom tray.

After the cast is prepared, the custom tray material is mixed according to the manufacturer's directions and formed to the cast. In the doughy stage, the maxillary material can be shaped into a patty and the mandibular material can be rolled into a log shape prior to placing the materials on the cast. A handle can be made from the remaining material. It is placed on the anterior of the tray near the midline of the arch. It is secured by wiping the anterior area and the handle area that is to be attached with the resin liquid and then placing it on the custom tray. Because the handle is still soft when it is applied to the cast, it must be held in place until initially set up. Make sure the handle is large and strong enough to allow for leverage in placing and removing the custom tray from the mouth. Remember that the dentist will have his or her fingers and thumb on the handle while performing the procedure, so make sure it can be held easily. When working on edentulous custom trays, the handles should extend upward and outward from the model. If this is not done, the handle is placed so that it protrudes directly through the lip of the patient.

When the exothermic reaction has been completed and the model has cooled (about 10 minutes), remove the spacer and evaluate the tray. The inside of the tray does not need to be smooth because the impression material covers this area. Any rough areas on the margins and on the outside of the tray can be smoothed for patient comfort. This can be accomplished by using an acrylic bur in a straight handpiece or with an arbor band on the laboratory lathe. Wear protective glasses when performing either of these trimming procedures. When completed, clean and disinfect the custom tray according to the manufacturer's directions and place it in a barrier ready for patient use.

An adhesive is painted on the tissue side of the tray prior to taking the impression. It is normally applied in two coats. The first is allowed to dry, and the second is placed 10 minutes or so before the impression is taken. This secures the material to the custom tray. Some dentists may want holes placed in the custom tray to further lock the impression material into the tray. This can be accomplished by wearing protective glasses and using a straight handpiece with a round bur to penetrate the custom tray. Either or both techniques will secure the material into the custom tray.

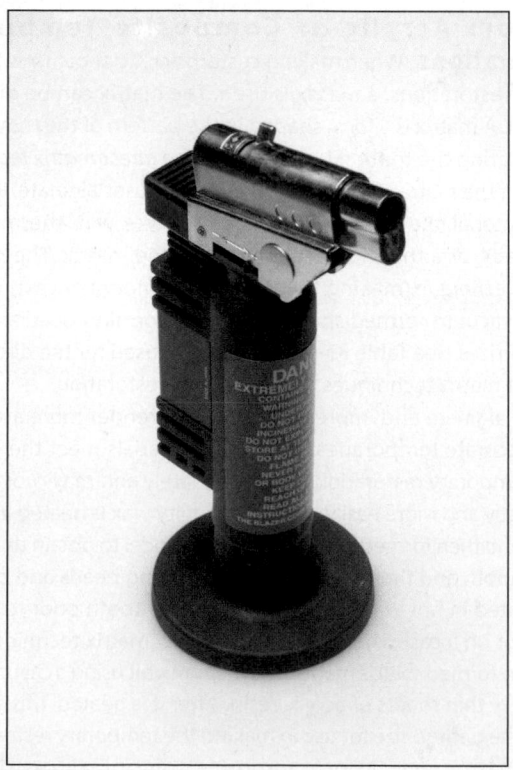

FIGURE 33-79
Butane torch.

Temporary (Provisional) Restorations

After a tooth has been prepared for a crown and prior to the seating of the crown, a temporary restoration must be adapted and temporarily cemented on the tooth to protect it in the interim. These temporary restorations stabilize and protect the tooth for the 2 days to 2 weeks it takes to make the crown(s) or bridge(s). It is important to note that these temporary restorations are not a precise fit and not intended for long-term use. Table 33-8 lists the criteria for a temporary restoration.

Types of Temporary Restorations

Temporary restorations, also known as provisional restorations, can be made of a number of materials, both custom and preformed. In many states, the function of fabricating and placing a temporary restoration is delegated to the dental assistant under the supervision of the dentist. Most offices use the preformed aluminum and acrylic crowns, along with the custom acrylic or composite crowns.

Preformed Aluminum Temporary Crowns Preformed aluminum temporary crowns are supplied in different sizes and anatomic features. They are used on the posterior teeth because they lack esthetic value. Some are made without any anatomy and resemble thimbles with parallel straight sides and flat, occlusal surfaces. More contouring is necessary to adapt this model to the tooth. Others have anatomies similar to the natural teeth and are contoured much like stainless steel crowns. Both the crowns without anatomic features and the ones with anatomic features can be filled with acrylic or composite material to obtain a more custom fit prior to setting the temporary restorations in place over the prepared teeth (see Procedures 39-16 and 39-17).

Preformed Acrylic Temporary Crowns Preformed acrylic or plastic temporary crowns are available in different sizes, shapes, and shades (Figure 33-80). The advantage of this type of crown is that it is more esthetically pleasing for anterior use. The plastic temporary crown is a form used to match the appropriate shape and contour of the tooth. It is filled with acrylic material and then removed. The preformed acrylic crowns have tabs on the incisal edge for easy placement. These tabs are removed prior to cementation. The preformed acrylic crowns are used more

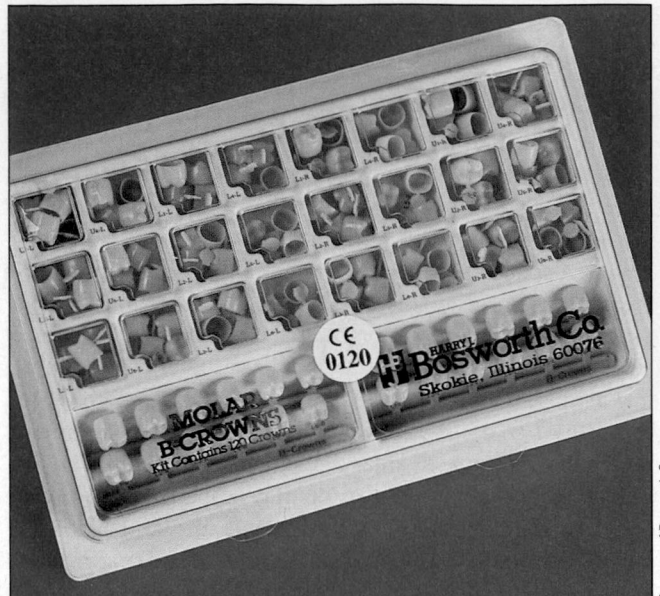

Courtesy of Bosworth Co.

FIGURE 33-80
Preformed acrylic temporary crowns.

easily because they require little adjustment and can be seated immediately. One disadvantage is that they are shorter in length, or more closely trimmed to the optimum margin length of the prepared tooth. If a patient has had periodontal disease and the crown must be lengthened to cover any areas of recession, the clear-plastic crowns adapt better. They are supplied with longer necks on the crown for this purpose. See Procedure 39-18.

Custom Acrylic or Composite Temporary Restorations When making custom acrylic or composite temporary restorations, a matrix is used. The matrix can be direct or indirect. A matrix is a form shaped in the pattern of the tooth prior to preparing the tooth (Figure 33-81). The *direct matrix technique* (making the matrix directly from the tooth) uses alginate, impression material, the freehand (block) technique, wax, thermoforming beads, or a thermoplastic button in the matrix. The *indirect matrix technique* (making the matrix on a model or cast) utilizes wax, a vacuum-formed shell, and thermoforming bead and button matrices. See Table 33-9 for the matrix used for the direct and indirect matrix techniques of a temporary restoration.

The alginate and impression materials render more anatomically accurate temporaries. The other materials meet the criteria for a temporary restoration form adequately and may prove to be less costly and more easily made. The utility wax is heated in warm water and then formed over the tooth or model to obtain the shape of the tooth and then cooled. Thermoforming beads and buttons are heated in hot water and formed on the tooth prior to preparation or on a cast when using the indirect matrix technique. The vacuum-formed shell is made on a vacuum unit using a cast covered with very thin sheets of acrylic resin. After it is heated, this sheet is cut to the desired size for use in making the temporary restoration.

A custom acrylic or composite temporary restoration (Procedure 39-19) must have good proximal contacts, good occlusal contacts, good food deflection, and good marginal

TABLE 33-8 Temporary Restoration Criteria

Comfortable and esthetically acceptable to patient.
Remains stable, with proper mesial and distal contacts and occlusal alignment, until permanent crown is cemented.
Easily removed, without damaging tooth, when the permanent restoration is ready for placement.
Fits snugly and accurately along prepared margin of the tooth. There is less than 0.05 mm of space between the temporary restoration and finish line of the margin.
Contoured in a similar fashion to original tooth, therefore protecting gingiva from irritation and interproximal areas from food impaction.

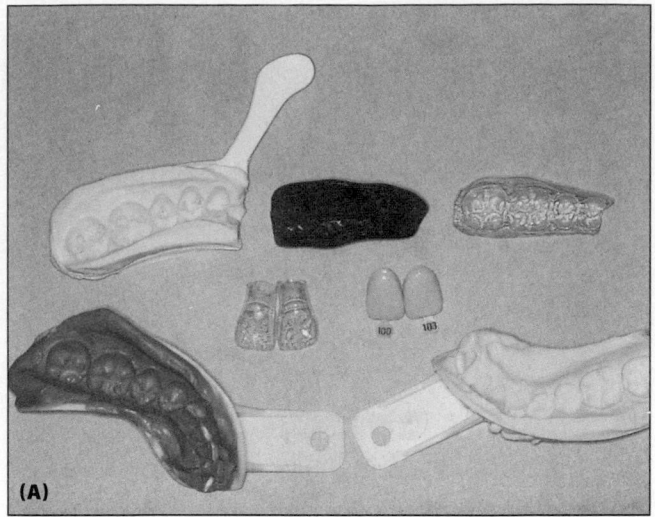

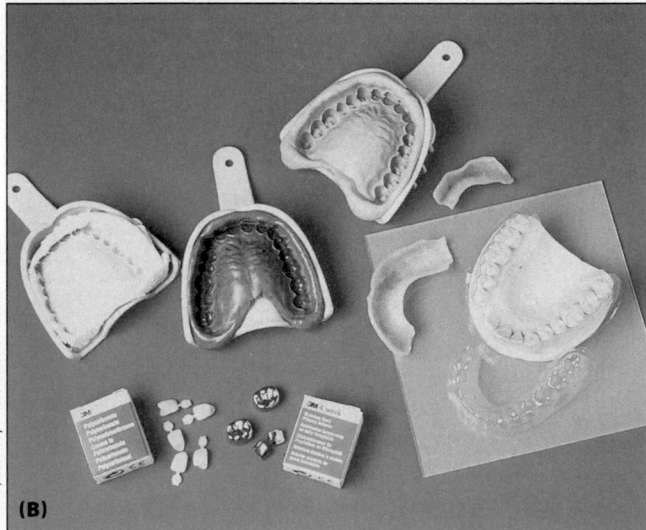

(A and B) Courtesy of 3M Dental Products Division

FIGURE 33-81
(A) and (B) various types of temporary/provisional matrices.

TABLE 33-9 Matrix Used for Both Direct and Indirect Technique

Matrix Used for Direct Technique in Making Temporary Restorations
• Alginate impression
• Impression material
• Freehand (making a block of the material and covering the prepared tooth)
• Wax
• Thermoforming beads or buttons
Matrix Used for Indirect Technique in Making Temporary Restorations
• Wax
• Thermoforming beads or buttons
• Vacuum-formed shell

contours (Figures 33-82A through D). Using the correct burs when making a temporary is essential. For making proper margins and contacts, use burs and discs (Figure 33-83) that have been developed specifically for this purpose, as the outcome of the temporary will be much more accurate.

Self-Curing Methyl Methacrylate There are several categories of materials that achieve the desired outcome of a custom temporary restoration. Each material has advantages and disadvantages. One of the routinely used older materials is methyl methacrylate. The advantages of this material are that it has good physical properties, good esthetics, better color stability than the R9 methacrylates, and a lower cost. The disadvantages are the strong odor, high shrinkage, and high exothermic heat given off during the self-cure chemical setting.

Self-Curing R9 Methacrylate The R9 (resin) methacrylates have one of the active ingredients, such as vinyl, ethyl, or isobutyl, in place of the methyl. In comparison to the methyl methacrylates, they have lower shrinkage and a lower level of exothermic heat given off during the self-cure chemical setting. They are similar in price per temporary, but they are the weakest of the methacrylates, they have poor color stability, and they have the same strong odor that the methyl methacrylates have.

Both the methyl and the R9 methacrylates come in powder and liquid forms that are mixed together to form a creamy mix. After mixing, they are allowed to condition for approximately 30 seconds and then are placed in the matrix. A dull surface appears on the top of the material, and it is placed in the mouth over the prepared tooth and held in place for the initial set. It has a rubber appearance at this time. Most manufacturers suggest that the material be taken off and on the prepared tooth during the time of 4 to 6 minutes. This is when the exothermic heat is the greatest. The excess can be trimmed off easily with scissors during this time. The final set is from 6 to 8 minutes, and the material becomes hard plastic. The range of setting time from start to finish is from 8 to 10 minutes for the materials in these two groups. Many of the newer materials are completed in half the time. The temporary restorations are removed from the matrix and trimmed with an acrylic bur to the desired shape and size.

After the temporary has been trimmed, it is polished with pumice and a rag wheel. Some of the materials in this category come with glazes. This glaze is applied after the polishing and allowed to dry for 5 minutes before the temporary is cemented.

Self-Curing Composite Material Materials in the category of self-curing composite are double the price of the methacrylates. They are much stronger materials because they are made as composites and not plastics. They do not have the odor, the shrinkage, or the exothermic reaction during setting, and they have excellent color stability.

Materials in this category come in two pastes. They are supplied in either two tubes or in a cartridge that fits into extruding guns with auto mixing tips. Both the tubes and the cartridge tips must remain clean and flowing to obtain the correct dispensed amount of the material. If they become clogged with old material,

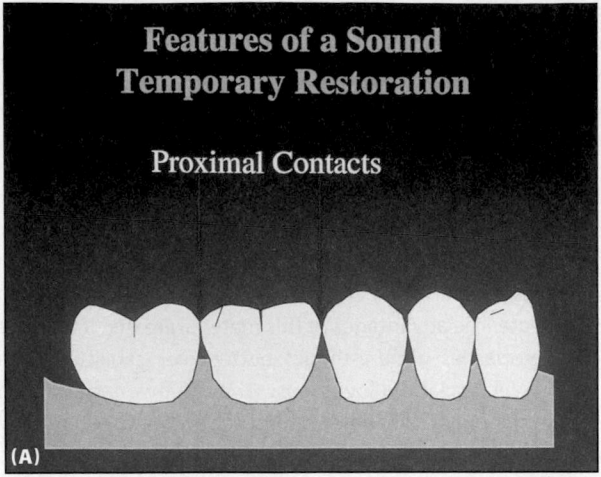

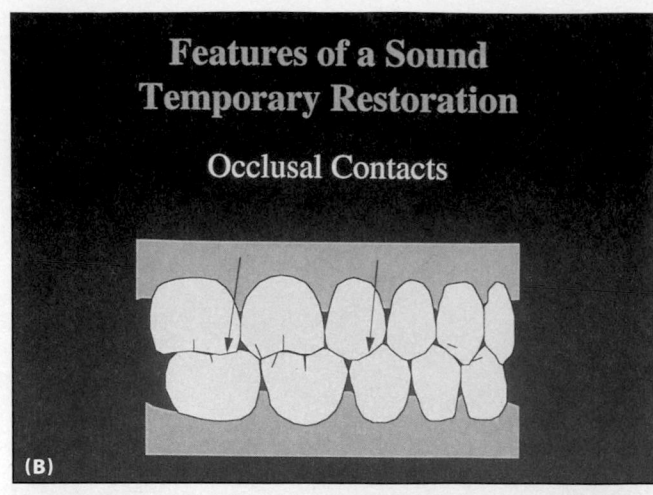

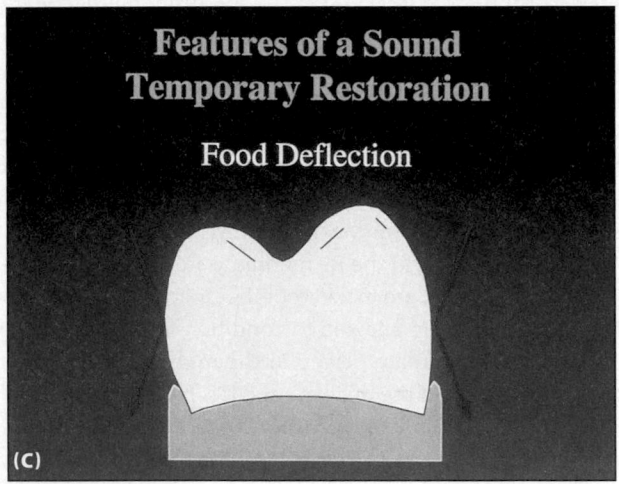

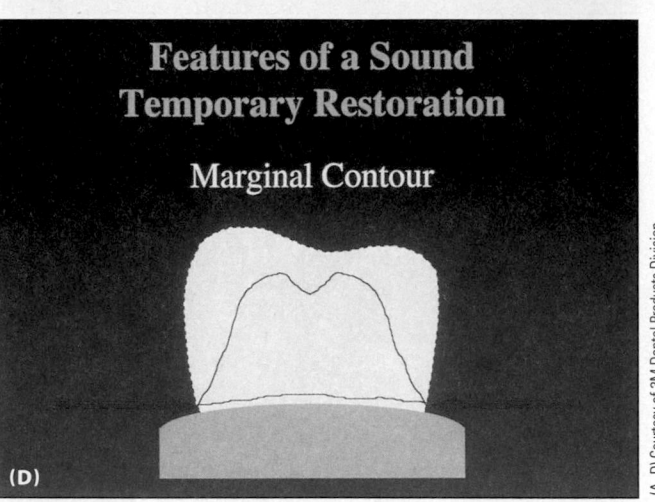

FIGURE 33-82A–D
Criteria for custom acrylic or a composite temporary restoration. (A) Good proximal contacts. (B) Good food deflection. (C) Good occlusal contacts. (D) Good marginal contours.

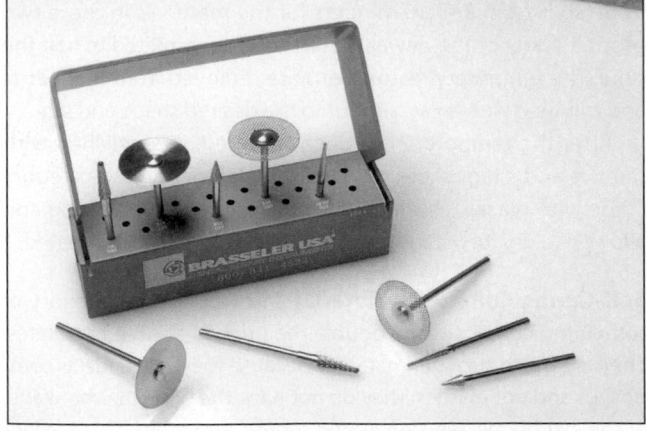

FIGURE 33-83
Provisional bur kit used when trimming temporary restorations.

use an explorer to clear the old material out. Dispense a small, pea-shaped amount on the pad before beginning, to ensure that everything is working properly.

The material is placed in the matrix and over the prepared tooth for up to 2 minutes. During the rubber stage (from 4 to 6 minutes), it is removed from the mouth to complete curing. The total time from start to finish for this material classification is up to 7 minutes. After the material is set, the surface has a greasy layer due to the oxygen in the air, which can be removed with alcohol or any other organic solvent. The trimming is done with a diamond bur, and no polish is necessary. If additional material is required on the temporary, then light-cured composite or flowable resin repair can be used and trimmed accordingly.

Multicured Temporary Materials Several multicured temporary materials are on the market. They have extended working time in the rubbery stage and improved operator control because they can be light cured on demand. They have good strength and are higher in cost. Some of the materials in this group are methacrylates, and some are composites having the characteristics of the self-curing materials. The biggest advantage of this group is light-curing control, which allows for a quicker set and unlimited setting time.

Procedure 33-16
Sizing, Adapting, and Seating Aluminum Temporary Crown

This procedure is performed at the dental unit after tooth has been prepared for a crown.

Steps written in **blue** font are performed by the operator (dentist or qualified dental assistant), and the chairside assistant's steps are written in black.

Equipment and Supplies

Patient Seating Setup (refer to Procedure 18-4)

Aluminum Temporary Crown Setup (Figure 33-84)
- maxillary and/or mandibular selection of aluminum temporary crowns (Figure 33-85)
- millimeter ruler (A)
- basic setup: mouth mirror, cotton pliers, and explorer (B)
- crown and collar scissors (C)
- contouring pliers (D)
- acrylic or composite temporary material (optional)
- sandpaper discs, rubber wheel, and mandrel (E)
- articulating paper (F)
- dental floss (G)

Procedure Steps

1. Escort and seat patient (refer to Procedure 18-4).

   Measures the available space for the temporary crown from the mesial to distal with the millimeter ruler. This aids in the selection of a preformed crown having the appropriate mesial and distal contact.

   Chooses the size of the crown according to the measurement taken with the millimeter ruler. (Prevent cross-contamination while taking the crown from the container.

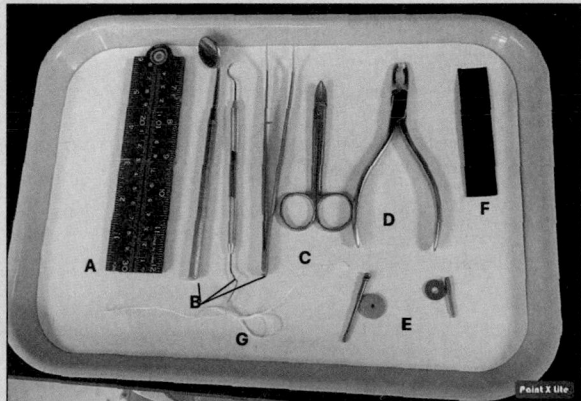

FIGURE 33-84
Aluminum temporary crown setup.

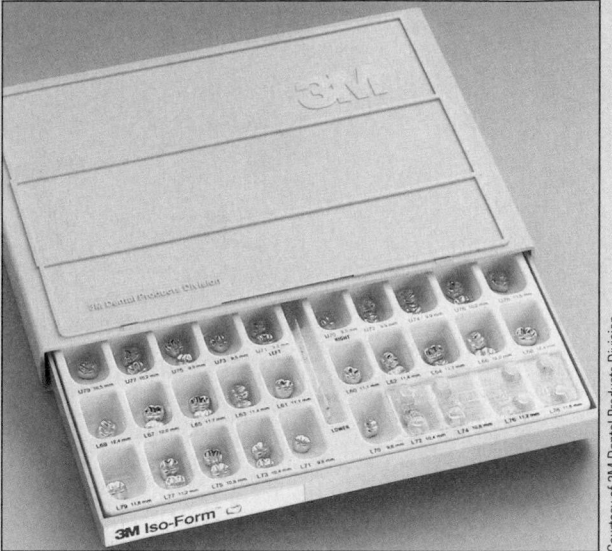

Courtesy of 3M Dental Products Division

FIGURE 33-85
Selection of Iso-form temporary crowns.

Do not use contaminated instruments.) Any crown tried that does not fit must be sterilized before replacing it in the selection tray.

2. Pass chosen crown to operator.

   Tries the selected crown on and checks for mesial and distal width. The crown will be above the occlusal plane at this time.

   Determines the length of the crown by placing the aluminum crown over the prepared tooth and using an explorer to mark the height (Figure 33-86). Another way to accomplish this is to scribe the tooth at the occlusal surface with an instrument where it aligns with the other teeth on the arch and then take that same amount off the gingival area. Either method shows that the margin of the gingival needs to be trimmed in order to fit.

   Trims the gingival margin using a crown and collar scissors (with curved blades). Crowns are never straight across the surface but are longer on the buccal and lingual margins. Use the rounded edges of the scissors to trim.

NOTE: Trimming a small amount at first allows refitting to further check the desired result (Figure 33-87). Taking too much off renders the crown useless. Making several trims to get the desired effect is a better method. Using the scissors in a continuous cutting action gives a much smoother surface. Avoid sharp, uneven edges that cause the patient discomfort around the gingival surface.

(Continues)

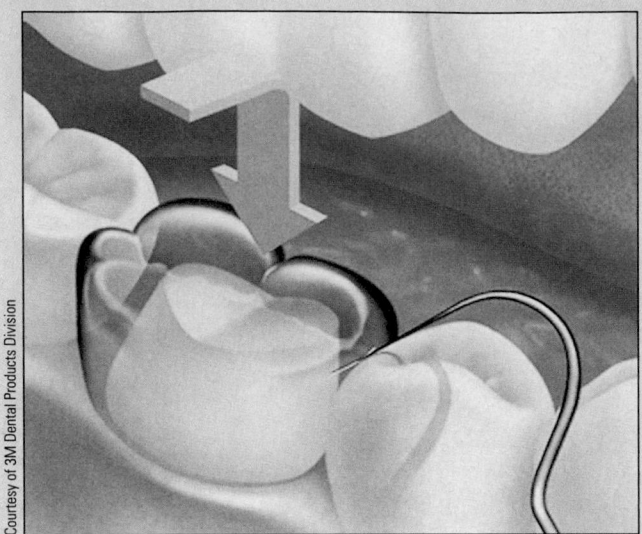

FIGURE 33-86
Explorer used to establish height of temporary aluminum crown.

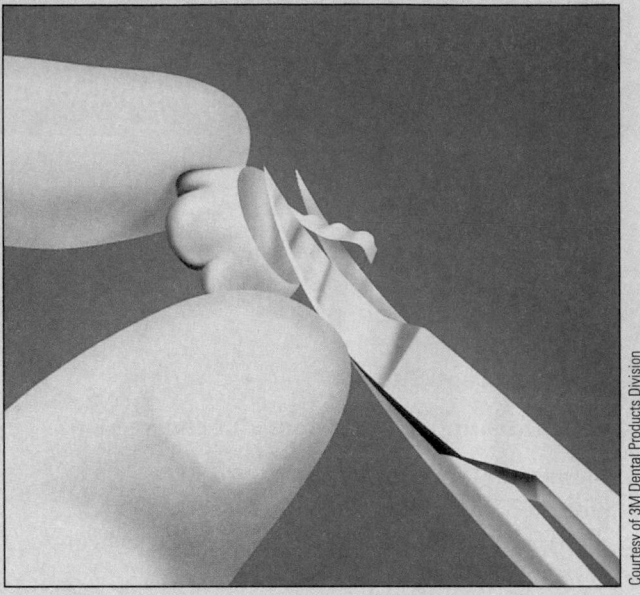

FIGURE 33-87
Trimming aluminum crown with crown and collar scissors.

Uses contouring pliers to invert the gingival edge in an inward manner after the desired length is achieved. This crimping aids in the adaptation of the circumference edge of the aluminum crown to the finish line of the preparation.

Smooths the rough and jagged edges through use of sandpaper discs and a rubber wheel. Checks that all edges are smooth and polished (Figure 33-88).

Places the aluminum crown on the prepared tooth and checks the occlusion with the articulating paper and the contacts with dental floss.

NOTE:

- If the contacts are weak, use a burnisher on the inside to extend the crown outward to get a better contact.

Fills the crown with acrylic or composite and places it on the prepared tooth. If an acrylic or a composite lining is used, the crown is filled with the material and placed on the prepared tooth.

Has patient bite into normal occlusion.

Lubricates tooth with petroleum jelly to avoid retention of the material.

Allows the material to set according to the manufacturer's directions.

Removes crown.

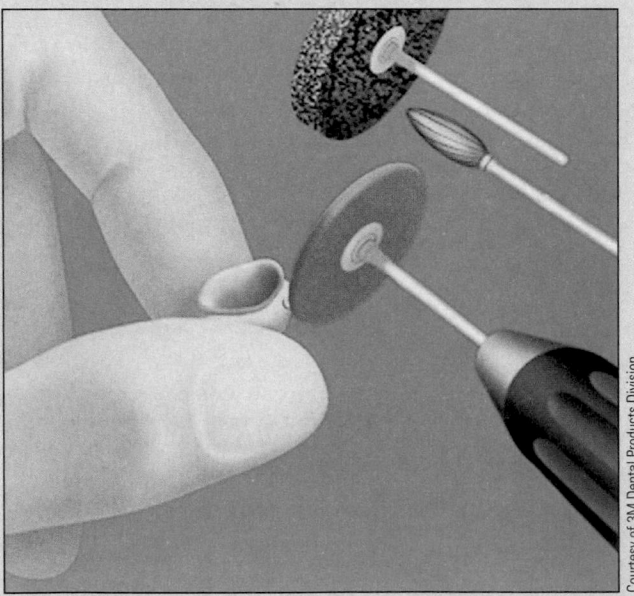

FIGURE 33-88
Smooth rough and jagged edges of temporary with rubber wheel.

Polishes away any excess material.

Checks for marginal fit, contour, and occlusion before cementation takes place.

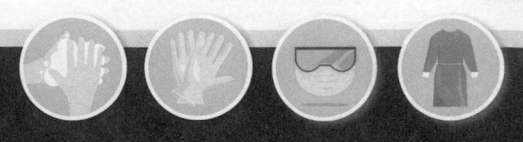

Procedure 33-17
Cementing the Aluminum Crown

This procedure is performed at the dental unit after the aluminum crown provisional restoration has been prepared, sized, and contoured to the prepared tooth.

Steps written in blue font are performed by the operator (dentist or qualified dental assistant), and the chairside assistant's steps are written in black.

Equipment and Supplies

Patient Seating Setup (refer to Procedure 18-4)

Cementing an Aluminum Crown Setup (Figure 33-89)
- cotton rolls (A)
- temporary cementation material (B)
- mixing pad (C)
- plastic filling instrument (D)
- basic setup: mouth mirror, explorer, and cotton pliers (E)
- fitted aluminum temporary (see Figure 33-85)

Procedure Steps

1. Rinse and dry the prepared tooth with cotton rolls in place.

2. Mix the temporary cementation material, such as zinc oxide eugenol, with a spatula and place in the aluminum crown. (Refer to Procedure 30-2.)

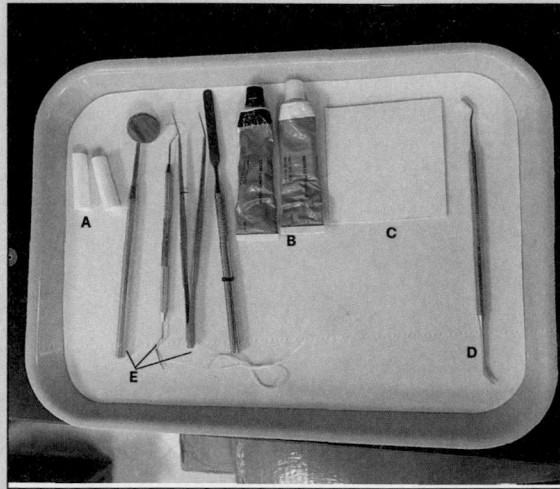

FIGURE 33-89
Cementing aluminum crown setup.

Places the aluminum crown in position over the prepared tooth and asks the patient to bite in occlusion until the cement is set.

NOTE: Some operators like the patient to bite on a cotton roll over the aluminum crown while the cement sets.

3. Pass explorer to operator.

   Removes excess cement with an explorer after the cement has set.

4. Retrieve explorer from operator.

5. Pass floss to operator.

   Checks the contacts with floss and inspects the margins to determine whether all excess cement has been removed and the crown fits correctly.

6. Pass articulating paper to operator.

   Checks occlusion with articulating paper. Adjusts if necessary.

7. Give instructions to the patient for care of the temporary aluminum crown.

8. Write up procedure in Services Rendered.

Date	Services Rendered	
02/18/XX	Reviewed medical and dental history, BP = 120/80	
	Temporary cemented preformed aluminum crown with ZOE cement #14	
	RTC: Insert PFM crown #14	Assistant's initials

9. Dismiss and escort patient to reception area (refer to Procedure 18-5).

Procedure 33-18

Sizing, Adapting, and Seating a Preformed Acrylic Crown

This procedure is performed at the dental unit after the preformed acrylic provisional restoration has been prepared, sized, and contoured to the prepared tooth.

Steps written in **blue** font are performed by the operator (dentist or qualified dental assistant), and the chairside assistant's steps are written in black.

Equipment and Supplies

Patient Seating Setup (refer to Procedure 18-4)

Preformed Acrylic Crown Setup (Figure 33-90)
- mirror, explorer, and cotton pliers (A)
- acrylic or composite temporary material (optional)
- temporary cement, pad, and spatula (B)
- articulating paper (C)
- dental floss (D)
- acrylic bur (see Figure 33-70)
- preformed acrylic temporary crown (Figure 33-91)

Preparing a Preformed Acrylic Temporary Restoration

Procedure Steps

Chooses a crown that has enough width to contact on the adjacent teeth, is long enough to be in proper occlusion, and is the correct shade.

1. Retrieve crown without cross-contaminating the other acrylic crowns. The tab at the incisal edge allows the operator to try the crown over the prepared tooth (Figure 33-91).

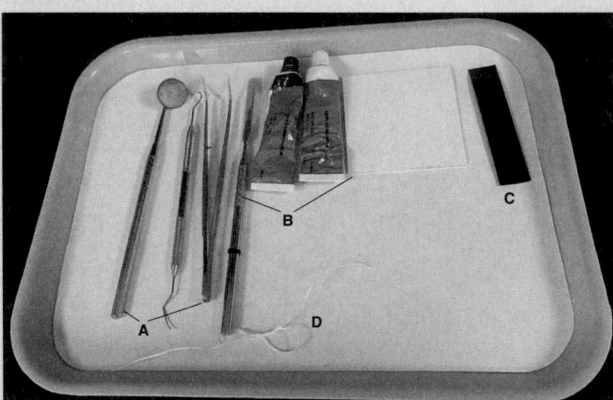

FIGURE 33-90
Preformed acrylic crown setup.

2. Pass crown to operator.

   Tries in crown.

   Takes off the tag, places the crown, and checks the occlusion with articulating paper.

   Makes adjustments, if necessary, and polishes the adjustment areas for a smooth surface for patient comfort with a rag wheel and pumice.

Cementing Acrylic Provisional Crown

1. Rinse and dry the prepared tooth and put the cotton rolls in place.

2. Mix the temporary cementation material, such as zinc oxide eugenol, with a spatula and place it in the preformed acrylic crown. (Refer to Procedure 30-2.)

   Places the preformed acrylic crown in position over the prepared tooth and asks patient to bite in occlusion or hold the crown in place until the cement is set.

NOTE: Some operators like the patient to bite on a cotton roll over the preformed acrylic crown while the cement sets.

3. Pass explorer to the operator after the cement is set.

   Removes the excess with an explorer.

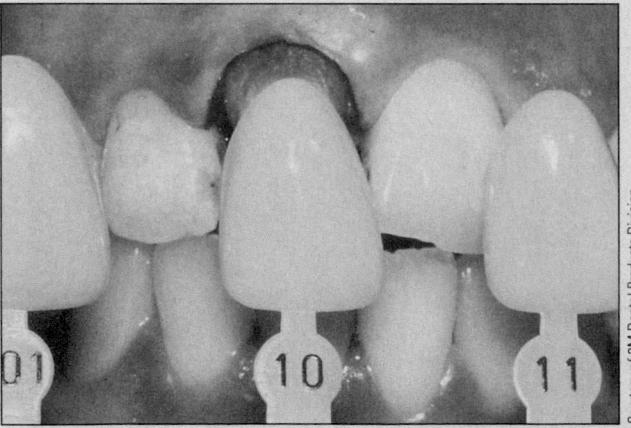

Courtesy of 3M Dental Products Division

FIGURE 33-91
Acrylic crown is tried over prepared tooth, holding onto incisal tab.

4. Retrieve the explorer from the operator.
5. Pass floss to the operator.

Checks the contacts with floss and inspects the margins to determine whether all excess cement has been removed and whether the crown fits correctly.

6. Pass articulating paper to the operator.

7. Check occlusion with articulating paper.

8. Make any adjustments if necessary.

9. Give instructions to the patient for care of the temporary preformed acrylic crown.

10. Write up procedure in Services Rendered.

Date	Services Rendered
02/18/XX	Reviewed medical and dental history, BP = 120/80
	temporary cemented preformed acrylic crown with ZOE cement #14
	RTC: Insert PFM crown #14 Assistant's initials

11. Dismiss and escort patient to reception area (refer to Procedure 18-5).

Procedure 33-19
Develop or Place a Pontic in a Model for a Three-Unit Bridge on a Dental Model; Adapt a Matrix; Make, Trim, and Fit the Three-Unit Provisional Bridge

This procedure is performed at the dental unit after tooth has been prepared for a three-unit bridge.

Steps written in blue font are performed by the operator (dentist or qualified dental assistant), and the chairside assistant's steps are written in black.

Equipment and Supplies

Patient Seating Setup (refer to Procedure 18-4)

Three-Unit Provisional Bridge Setup (Figure 33-92)
- basic setup: mouth mirror, explorer, and cotton pliers (A)
- thermoplastic buttons (one possible option for use in making a matrix, not shown)
- hot water (B)
- diamond bur and disc (C)
- temporary cement, pad, and spatula (D)
- articulating paper (E)
- dental floss (F)
- dental model with missing tooth (G)
- composite temporary material (see Figure 33-100)

Developing or Placing a Pontic on the Model Where the Tooth Is Missing

Procedure Steps

Manipulates block-out putty can to fit into the space. Ensures that the material is not wider than the other teeth in the arch (Figure 33-93).

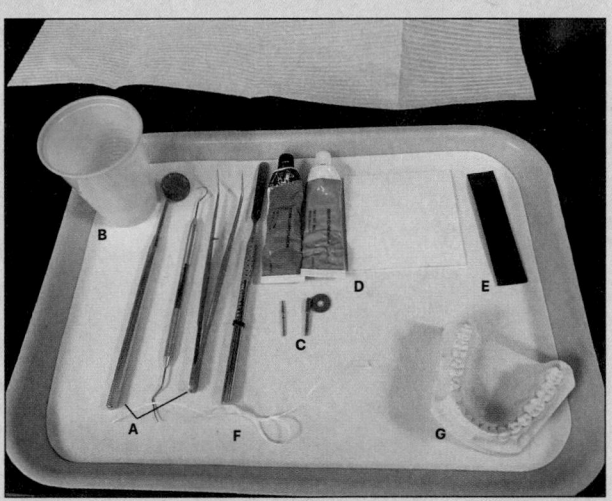

FIGURE 33-92
Three-unit provisional bridge setup.

Places a multicure provisional material into the space and light cures in place prior to making a matrix (second option).

Making Thermoforming Matrix before Tooth Preparation

Places the thermoforming matrix buttons in hot water (one button per prepared tooth).

(Continues)

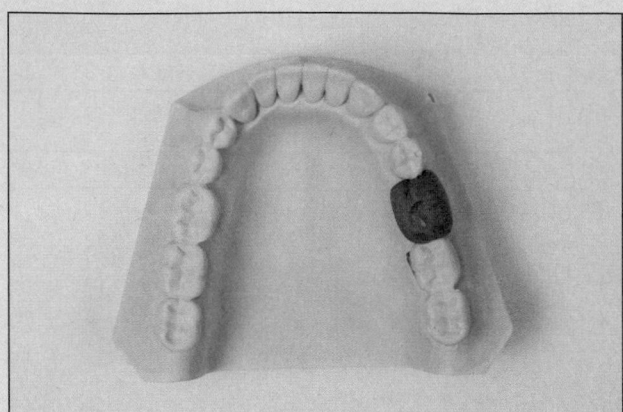

FIGURE 33-93
Developing a pontic out of block-out.

Allows the white color of the button to become clear. When that takes place, the material is pliable and able to be adapted.

Adapts the material over the teeth and tightly conforms it to the teeth area and slightly below the gingival. Ensures that the matrix covers all teeth that will be in the bridge. They should cover about one half of an extra tooth on each side of the matrix.

Removes matrix from the area when the material cools (air can be used to make this more rapid) and sets aside. The matrix will appear white and firm (Figure 33-94).

Preparing Custom Bridge Temporary Restoration

Coats the teeth on the model with a light application of petroleum jelly after the teeth have been prepared for a bridge (Figure 33-95).

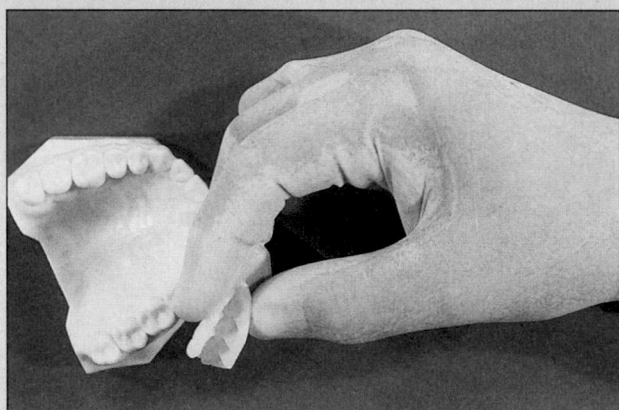

FIGURE 33-94
Matrix is removed.

1. Dispense composite self-curing temporary material on the paper pad by holding tubes at a 45 degree angle.

2. Rotate the end-dispensing handle of the base until a click is heard. (The base is the larger of the two tubes. The smaller of the two holds the catalyst and has two

dispensing ends.) Rotate the end-dispensing handle of the catalyst. Two small amounts are expelled. Each click of the dispensing handle is enough material for one temporary.

3. Mix shade with the base if being used. If a mottled effect is desired, mix the shade after the base and catalyst are mixed together.

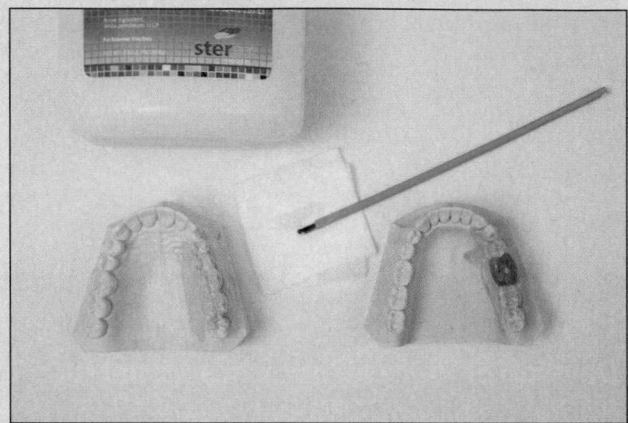

FIGURE 33-95
Place the lubricant on the model so the material will not stick to the gypsum.

4. Mix the material together to obtain a creamy substance (about 30 seconds).

5. Pass material to operator.

Places the material in the matrix.

Places the matrix over the prepared tooth (manipulation time is about 1½ minutes).

Holds it in place in the mouth for 2 minutes.

Removes it from the mouth and sets it aside for 2 minutes.

Removes the crown or bridge from the matrix (Figure 33-96). The additional curing time takes 1 minute. There are 7 minutes total time from start to finish of the set.

Removes the greasy layer with alcohol or any other organic solvent.

Marks the contact areas (Figure 33-97).

Trims with scissors, a diamond, or an acrylic bur.

Trims and smooths all areas (Figure 33-98), making sure that the area that was marked as the contact point is not trimmed away.

Cuts the embrasure area using a disc (Figure 33-99). Always uses a fulcrum when trimming provisional restorations.

Evaluates temporary restoration. Places a flowable temporary (provisional) material with a tip and dispenser

(Figure 33-100) and then light cures it (Figure 33-101), if too much material was trimmed away.

Trims material again to get the desired finished products if necessary.

Checks the contacts and occlusion (Figure 33-102).

If desired, places a glaze on the provisional (Figure 33-103) and light cures it to give it a smoother surface.

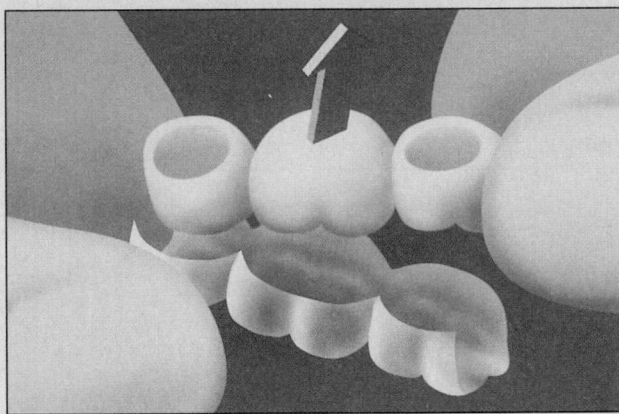

FIGURE 33-96
Remove acrylic bridge from matrix.

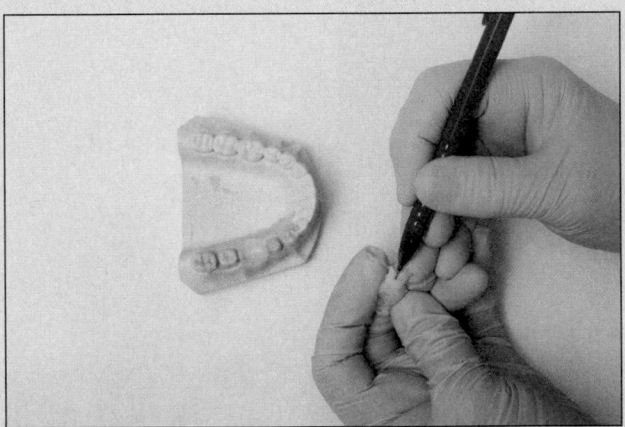

FIGURE 33-97
Mark the contact areas.

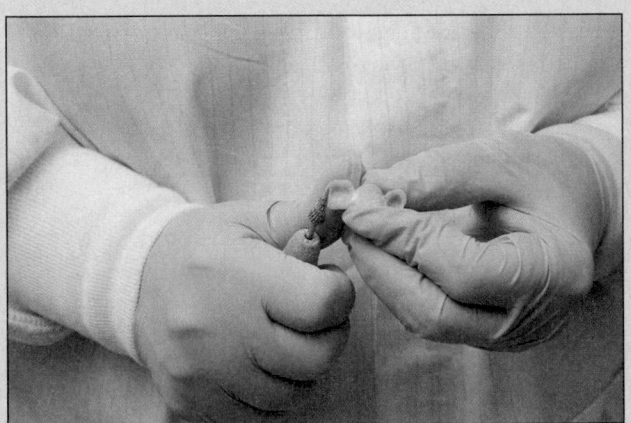

FIGURE 33-98
Trim and smooth entire provisional bridge.

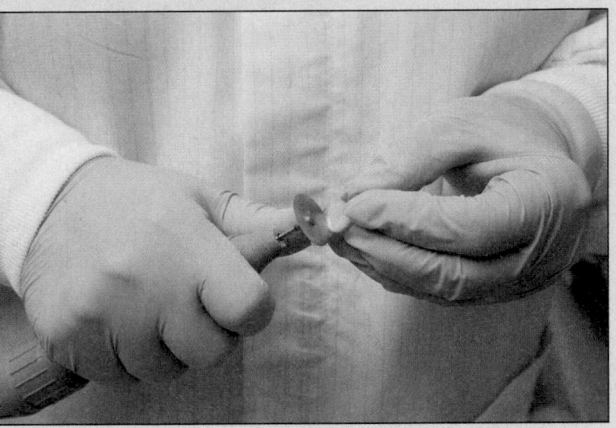

FIGURE 33-99
Use a disc to cut the embrasure area.

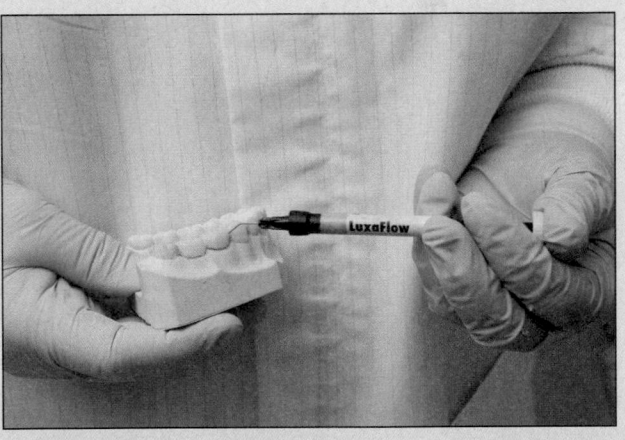

FIGURE 33-100
Place flowable temporary material on areas in need.

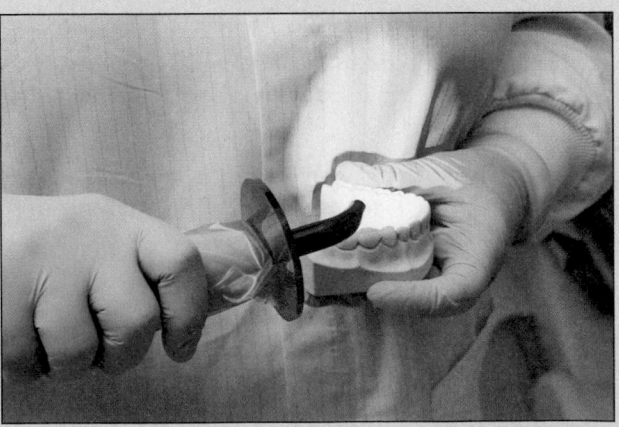

FIGURE 33-101
Light cure flowable provisional material.

(Continues)

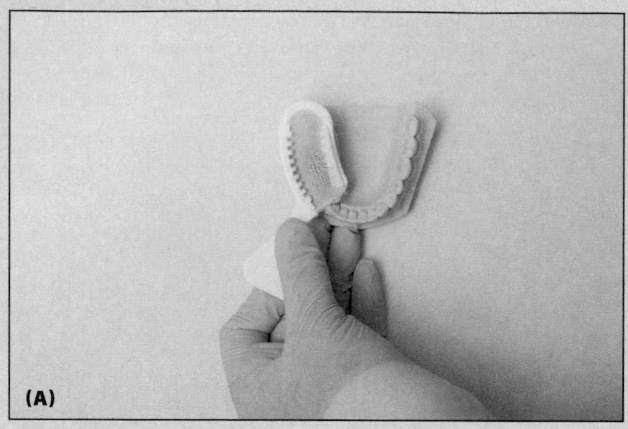

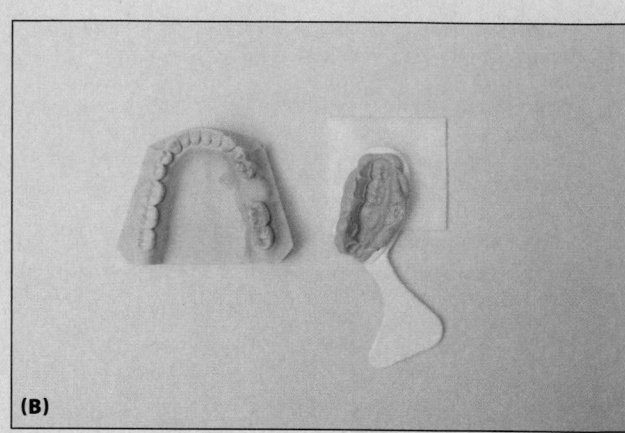

FIGURE 33-102
Check the contacts and occlusion.

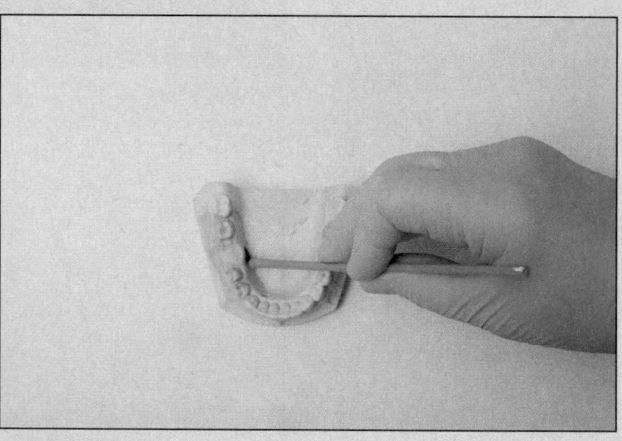

FIGURE 33-103
Place a glaze on the provisional if desired.

Procedure 33-20
Preparing a Full Crown Provisional on a Lower Left Molar on a Patient

This procedure is performed at the dental unit after tooth has been prepared for a crown. Use the impression material and triple tray to make a matrix for the provisional prior to the tooth being prepared.

Steps written in blue font are performed by the operator (dentist or qualified dental assistant), and the chairside assistant's steps are written in black.

Equipment and Supplies

Patient Seating Setup (refer to Procedure 18-4)

Preparing a Full Crown Provisional Setup (Figure 33-104)

- basic setup: mouth mirror, explorer, and cotton pliers (A)
- impression material for matrix (B)
- triple tray for matrix (C)
- composite temporary (provision) material (D)
- diamond bur (E)
- articulating paper (F)
- dental floss (G)

Procedure Steps

1. Turn off the operatory light.

   Obtains a shade for the crown.

2. Pass composite material to the operator.

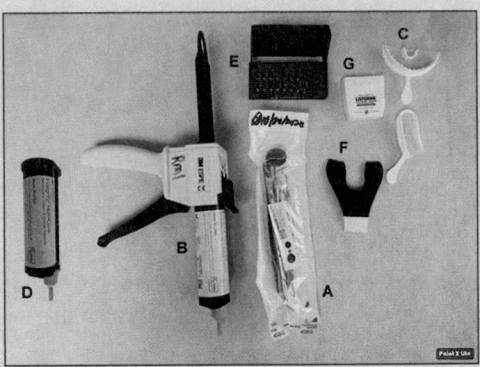

FIGURE 33-104
Preparing a full crown provisional setup.

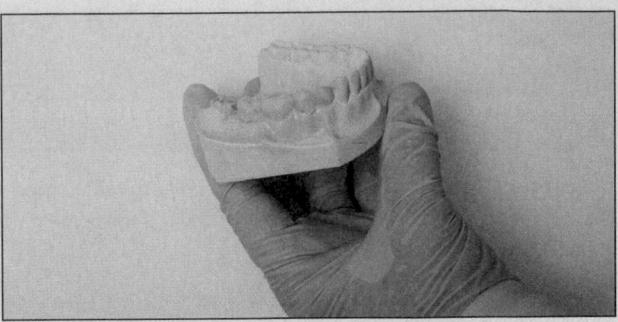

FIGURE 33-106
Evaluate the initial temporary/provisional.

Fills the impression matrix that was prepared earlier two-thirds full of composite temporary material (Figure 33-105).

Places matrix in the same position that it was when the matrix was obtained. Follows the manufacturer's directions as the material sets. It may have to be removed and replaced several times until set. Composite or multicured provisional materials take 1 to 3 minutes to set up. The multicured material sets with a curing light immediately.

Removes material from the patient's mouth or the matrix once material is set.

Evaluates the temporary (Figure 33-106). This temporary needs to have the additional flash around the edges cut off and some trimming done. It also appears thin on the occlusal surface.

Removes the greasy layer with alcohol or any other organic solvent.

Marks the contact point with a pencil if operator is just learning to do temporaries. This indicates that this area should not be removed.

Trims this full crown with a diamond bur (Figure 33-107).

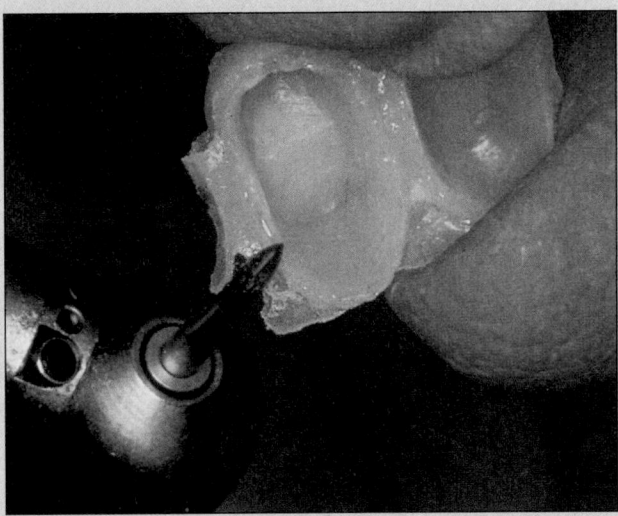

FIGURE 33-107
Trim temporary restoration.

Evaluates temporary. Uses a flowable temporary (provisional) material if too much material was trimmed away. Places on the restoration with a tip and dispenser and then light cures it. The material can then be trimmed again to get the desired finished product.

Checks the contacts and occlusion. Evaluates the provisional. This completed provisional appears to have the correct occlusion on the mesial side because it is the same height as the crown in front of it. It also appears to have a good contact. It appears to be covering the entire prepped area and smooth. Most temporaries do not have the same occlusion as the final crown. It is trimmed in a fluted figure eight pattern as the mandibular molar should have. It appears to be a good temporary.

Places a glaze on the provisional if desired, and light cures it to give it a smoother surface.

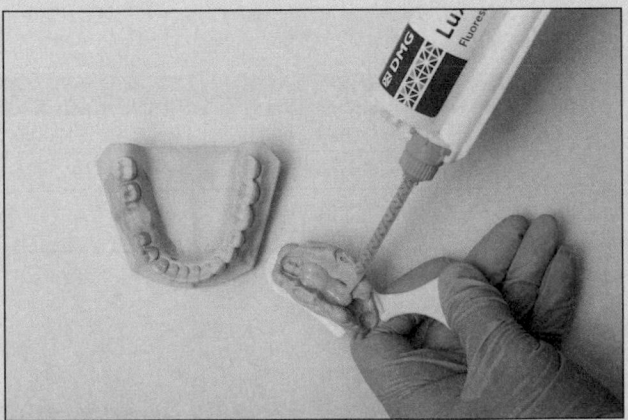

FIGURE 33-105
Filling the dental matrix with composite temporary/provisional material.

Procedure 33-21
Cementing Custom Self-Curing Composite Temporary Crown

This procedure is performed at the dental unit after the temporary restoration has been prepared and is ready to be cemented in place over the prepared tooth.

Steps written in **blue** font are performed by the operator (dentist or qualified dental assistant), and the chairside assistant's steps are written in black.

Equipment and Supplies

Patient Seating Setup (refer to Procedure 18-4)

Cementing Composite Temporary Crown Setup (Figure 33-108)

- basic setup: mouth mirror, explorer, and cotton pliers (A)
- cotton rolls (B)
- temporary luting cement (C)
- paper pad (D)
- mixing spatula (E)
- plastic filling instrument (F)
- dental floss (G)

Procedure Steps

1. Rinse the prepared tooth and dry.

2. Place cotton rolls in place.

3. Mix temporary cement material with a spatula and place in the custom composite temporary crown (refer to Procedure 30-2).

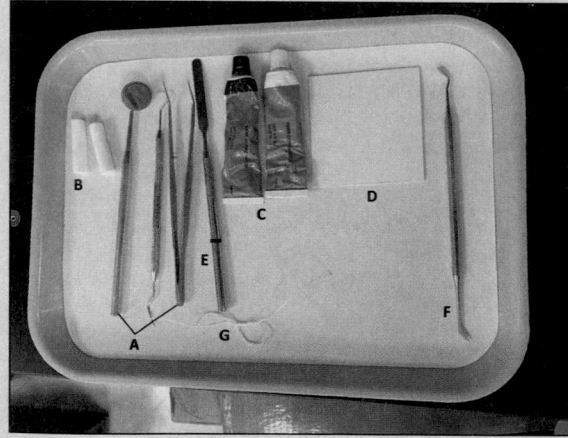

FIGURE 33-108
Cementing composite temporary crown setup.

4. Pass to operator.

   Places cement into provisional crown and inserts.

   Places temporary crown in position over the prepared tooth and asks the patient to bite in occlusion, or holds the crown in place until the cement is set.

NOTE: Some operators like the patient to bite on a cotton roll over the preformed acrylic crown while the cement sets.

5. Pass explorer to operator.

   Cleans off excess cement with explorer (Figure 33-109).

   Inspects the margins to determine whether all excess cement has been removed and whether the crown fits correctly.

6. Exchange explorer for floss.

   Checks the contacts with floss.

7. Pass articulating paper.

   Checks occlusion with the articulating paper.

8. Write up procedure in Services Rendered.

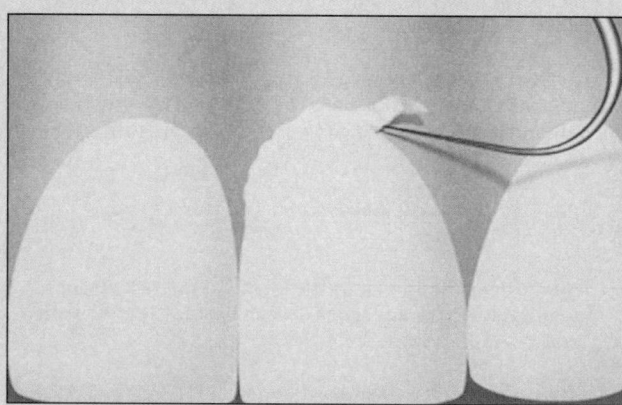

FIGURE 33-109
Temporary is placed and excess cement is removed.

Date	Services Rendered
02/18/XX	Reviewed medical and dental history, BP = 120/80
	Composite provisional placed with ZOE #19
	RTC: Insert permanent PFM crown #19 Assistant's initials

9. Dismisses and escort patient to reception area (refer to Procedure 18-5).

Chapter Summary

A number of basic functions in the dental laboratory are routinely performed by the dental assistant, such as pouring and trimming study models, fabricating custom trays, and fabricating temporaries. Many newer technologies are completed by dental assistants today such as mounting models on the articulator, taking digital impressions, and designing and fabricating crowns through computer-aided manufacturing. To accomplish these procedures, the dental assistant must understand the materials that are used, the properties of each material, and the steps in each procedure, and seek ongoing education and training on new technologies introduced in the field. Any dental assistant who has skills in performing laboratory duties is an asset to his or her employer. The better crossed-trained the dental team members are, the better the dental office functions.

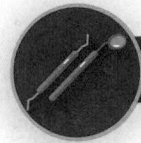

CASE STUDY

Patrick Norman came into the dental office and wanted to talk to the doctor about a space in the anterior region of his maxillary teeth. After Dr. Young completed a clinical examination, she asked the dental assistant to make diagnostic casts for further study. After talking to Patrick, the dental assistant found that Patrick has difficulty when anything is placed in his mouth and that gagging is a problem.

Case Study Review

1. What can the dental assistant do to help Patrick with the gagging problem while taking impressions for the diagnostic casts?

2. What material is used routinely for obtaining preliminary impressions?

3. Would the fast or regular set be more beneficial in this case?

4. Which arch would be taken first? Why?

Review Questions

Multiple Choice

1. Alginate substitute impression materials are silicone based. They can come in a cartridge with a mixing tip and a gun for dispensing.
   a. Both statements are true.
   b. Both statements are false.
   c. The first statement is true; the second statement is false.
   d. The first statement is false; the second statement is true.

2. If a lower water-to-powder ratio is used when mixing alginate, which of the following could result?
   a. decreased flexibility
   b. increased setting time
   c. decreased strength
   d. decreased tissue displacement

3. The final impression material that smells like sulfur is:
   a. polysulfide.
   b. polyether.
   c. polysiloxane.
   d. silicone.

4. Trays used for irreversible hydrocolloid are:
   a. water cooled.
   b. perforated.
   c. rim locked.
   d. Both b and c

5. If an impression loses water content due to heat, dryness, or exposure to air, the condition is known as:
   a. imbibition.
   b. syneresis.
   c. distortion.
   d. acceleration.

6. The final impression material that smells like sulfur is:
   a. polysulfide.
   b. polyether.
   c. polysiloxane.
   d. silicone.

7. Which of the following elastomeric materials has advantages that include high accuracy, no shrinkage, no taste, and no odor?
   a. Polysulfide
   b. Polysiloxane
   c. Polyether
   d. Alginate

8. The highest-strength type of gypsum material is:
   a. Type I.
   b. Type II.
   c. Type III.
   d. Type IV.

9. The Alginator II device makes mixing easier for mixing alginate as it rotates the bowl _____ times per minute.
   a. 100
   b. 200
   c. 300
   d. 400

10. When performing a double-pour mix for gypsum, adding more water to the base will make the base:
    a. stronger.
    b. weaker.
    c. set faster.
    d. thicker.

11. _____ of the cast is the art form, and _____ of the cast is anatomy form.
    a. ⅓, ⅔
    b. ⅔, ⅓
    c. ¾, ¼
    d. ¼, ¾

12. The _____ allows the operator to obtain the records about the placement of the maxillary arch and its location to the joint.
    a. facebow
    b. articulator
    c. amalgamator
    d. study model

13. When performing a facebow transfer, which of the following is performed first?
    a. Have patient insert the bow earpieces into their ear.
    b. Tighten finger side screws.
    c. Connect transfer assembly on the facebow to the bitefork.
    d. Apply bite registration material to the bitefork.

14. Which processing wax is used around trays to extend them and assist in patient comfort?
    a. study wax
    b. beading wax
    c. sticky wax
    d. boxing wax

15. The broad group title that encompasses the hard waxes used in crown and bridge casting (inlay wax) is:
    a. pattern.
    b. processing.
    c. impression.
    d. study wax.

16. The liquid catalyst for the self-curing acrylic tray resin is a:
    a. polymer.
    b. thermoplastic.
    c. monomer.
    d. spacer.

17. When trimming an aluminum provisional crown:
    a. the mesial and distal surfaces remain longer.
    b. the buccal and lingual surfaces remain longer.
    c. all surfaces are trimmed equally.
    d. trimming is not necessary.

18. When using a matrix to prepare a full provisional crown, fill matrix _____ with composite material before placing in the patient's mouth.
    a. ⅓
    b. ½
    c. ⅔
    d. ¾

19. Provisional restorations can be which of the following?
    a. preformed
    b. processed
    c. boxed
    d. None of these

20. The strongest temporary (provisional) restoration is the:
    a. aluminum shell temporary.
    b. self-curing methyl methacrylate temporary.
    c. self-curing R9 (resin) methacrylate temporary.
    d. self-curing composite temporary.

Critical Thinking

1. What are the effects of a lower water-to-powder ratio in a mixture of irreversible hydrocolloid? What are the effects of a higher ratio?

2. What are some of the advantages of polyether impression material?

Key Terms

Term and Pronunciation	Meaning of Root and Word Parts	Definition
accuracy (**ak**-yer-uh-see)	**accurate** = being true, correct or exact **-acy** = the condition or quality of	ability of impression to reproduce exact dimensions of the oral tissues
alginate impression (al-**juh-neyt**) (im-**presh**-uhn)	**algin** = substance obtained from seaweed/algae; used for thickening, stabilizing, and suspending agents in products **impression** = imprint, indentation produced by pressure in a material	type of impression material used for study models

Term and Pronunciation	Meaning of Root and Word Parts	Definition
articulator (ahr-**tik**-yuh-ley-ter)	**articulate** = precise relation to other parts **-or** = something that does what is expressed	mechanical device to which cast are attached to represent the jaw and teeth relationship
base (beys)	**base** = the main ingredient of a mixture	paste portion of elastomeric impression material that reacts with the catalyst paste
beading (**bee**-ding)	**bead** = to form **ing** = expressing the action of a verb	an elevation made of wax around the border of a tissue surface of a tray
bite registration (bahyt) (rej-uh-**strey**-shuh n)	**bite** = to close teeth together **register** = a permanent record **-tion** = the act of	to press teeth into a material that makes a record of how the teeth meet
calcination (kăl′sə-nā′shən)	**calcine** = to convert by heating **-tion** = the act of	to heat the gypsum to dehydrate it
cast (kast)	**cast** = to receive form in a mold; impression	replica of oral tissues made from an impression
catalyst (kat-**l-ist**)	**catalyst** = a substance that causes or accelerates a chemical reaction without being affected	paste portion of elastomeric impression material that reacts with the base paste
custom-made impression trays (kuhs-**tuhm**-meyd) (**im**-presh-uhn) (trey)	**custom** = made to the specifications of an individual **made** = to bring into existence by shaping or changing material **impression** = imprint, indentation produced by pressure in a material **tray** = a shallow receptacle for holding impression materials	impression tray made from acrylic material formed on a study model to provide a better fit to patient's oral tissues
dimensional change (dih-**men**-shuhn-uhl) (cheynj)	**dimension** = measurement in length, width and thickness **-al** = pertaining to **changes** = to make different from what it is or would be	measurement used to determine accuracy of impression material
elastomeric (ih-**las-tuh**-mer-**ik**)	**elastic** = capable to return to original length, shape after being stretched **mer** = part, segment **-ic** = of, relating to, or characterized by	impression material that has the ability to return to original dimensions when removed from the mouth
fabrication (**fab**-ri-key-**shuhn**)	**fabricate** = to make by art or skill and labor **-tion** = expressing action	making of a tray
facebow (Feys-boh)	**face** = to place in front **bow** = to bend or incline	a device used to determine the location of the maxilla in relationship to the mandible
flexibility (**flek**-suh-buhl-	**flexible** = being bent without breaking; adaptable **-ility** = capable of	ability of impression to bend or compression without breaking
gelatin time (**jel**-uh-tn tahym)	**gelatin** = to thicken **time** = to measure the amount of	the amount of time it take for the material to solidify
gypsum (**jip**-suhm)	**gypsum** = a common mineral rock used to make plaster of Paris	type of model material prepared from calcium sulfate
homogeneous (hoh-muh-**jee**-nee-uhs)	**homo** = same **gene** = nature or kind **-ous** = possessing	of uniform nature; constant property
imbibition (im-buh-**bish**-uhn)	**imbibe** = to absorb or soak up **-tion** = the act of	ability of alginate impression to absorb water if stored in water
impression (im-**presh**-uhn)	**impression** = imprint, indentation produced by pressure in a material	material that produces accurate image of oral tissues
invert (in-**vurt**)	**in** = in **vert** = to turn	inverted pour method refers to pouring both the anatomic and the art portions of the model in one step

(Continues)

Term and Pronunciation	Meaning of Root and Word Parts	Definition
irreversible hydrocolloid (ir-i-**vur**-suh-buhl) (hahy-druh-**kol**-oid)	**ir** = not **reversible** = capable of being changed; return to original form **hydro** = water **colloid** = particles dispersed within a medium	material that forms a gel that cannot be reused
monomer (mon-uh-**mer**)	**mono-** = one, single **-mer** = denoting a substance of a particular part or segment	a compound whose molecules can join together to form a polymer
pigment (**pig**-muhnt)	**pigment** = a coloring matter or substance	coloring material used to indicate when alginate impression is set and can be removed from the mouth
polyether (pol-ee-ee-**ther**)	**poly** = many **ether** = organic compounds used as a solvent	type of impression material that has hydrophilic properties
polymer (pol-**uh-mer**)	**poly** = many **mer** = part, segment	material that is a component of elastomeric impression material
polymerization (puh-lim-er-uh-**zey**-shuhn)	**poly** = many **mer** = part, segment **-ize** = the act or process of forming **-ation** = indicating a result	method by which elastomeric impression material sets
polysulfide (pol-ee-suhl-**fahyd**)	**poly** = many **sulfide** = a chemical compound containing sulfur	material used in taking final impressions; composed of a base and lead peroxide accelerator, resulting in good stability, accuracy, sharpness of detail, and a relatively long shelf life
preliminary impression (pri-**lim**-uh-ner-ee) (im-**presh**-uhn)	**preliminary** = preceding and leading up the main part or procedure **impression** = imprint, indentation produced by pressure in a material	initial image of oral tissues
provisional restoration (pruh-vizh-**uh-nl**)	**provision** = providing beforehand; serving for time being **-al** = pertaining to	short-term restoration
reversible hydrocolloid (ri-**vur**-suh-buhl) (hahy-druh-**kol**-oid)	**reversible** = capable of being changed; return to original form **hydro** = water **colloid** = particles dispersed within a medium	material that forms a gel that can be reused
silicone (**sil**-i-kohn)	**silica** = natural compound **-on** = suspended form	an elastic material used for impressions
spacer (speys-uhr)	**space** = to set some distance apart **-er** = denoting action or process	a piece of material used to create or maintain a space between two things
stock (stok)	**stock** = a supply of goods kept on hand for sale	stock trays are made in metal (reusable) or plastic (disposable) available in a many of sizes
study model (**stuhd**-ee) (**mod**-l)	**study** = examine and research detail **model** = an image in gypsum to be reproduced in a more durable material	image of oral tissues made from gypsum material
syneresis (si-**ner**-uh-sis)	**syneresis** = process of gel losing liquid and contracting	loss of liquid from alginate impression during storage that results in loss of accuracy
thermoplastic (thur-muh-**plas**-tik)	**therm** = caused by heat or temperature **al** = pertaining to **plastic** = group of synthetic or natural organic materials that may be shaped when soft and then harden	soft and pliable plastic material when heated
vacu-former (**vak**-yoo-**fawr**-mer)	**vacuum** = producing a suction pressure **form** = something that gives or determines shape **-er** = something that performs a specified action	equipment used to form a thermoplastic tray

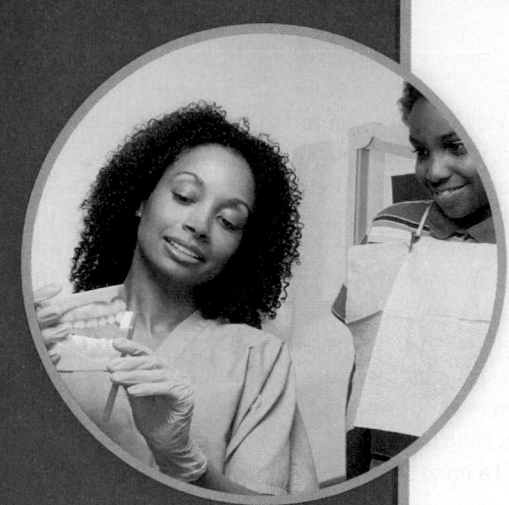

Pediatric Dentistry

Specific Instructional Objectives

At the completion of this chapter, you will be able to meet these objectives:

1. Use terms presented in this chapter.
2. Discuss need for pediatrics as a specialty and the pediatric environment.
3. Describe differences in pediatric dental caries.
4. Summarize what occurs during a pediatric oral exam.
5. Outline a good pediatric preventive program.
6. Explain special behavior management techniques for various stages of child development and patients with special needs.
7. Summarize special procedures performed in a pediatric practice.
8. Compare and contrast pulpotomy and pulpectomy procedures.
9. Defend the need for pediatric orthodontic treatment.
10. Describe common traumatic injuries and related treatment.

Introduction

Like a pediatrician, the **pediatric** dentist limits their dental practice to children. According to the American Dental Association, "pediatric dentistry is an age-defined specialty that provides both primary and comprehensive preventive and therapeutic oral health care for infants and children through adolescence, including those with special health care needs." After the required four years of dental school, pediatric dentists complete two to three years of additional specialized training to prepare for treating a wide variety of children's dental problems. The pediatric dentist also counsels caregivers on good oral health habits, dietary instructions, growth and development of the child's dentition, and preventing injuries to the mouth and teeth.

The pediatric dentist will receive referrals from general dentists and pediatricians who feel that the pediatric dentist is best suited to treat an anxious or uncooperative child who presents in their office. Children with **rampant** or severe decay or oral developmental problems may also be referred to the pediatric dentist.

The Pediatric Office

The décor in most pediatric dental offices is designed to help children feel comfortable, with activities, books, movies, and perhaps video games to entertain patients prior to or during the appointments. It is important that there is a safe, clean environment with easy to clean toys and no sharp edges on tables. The office décor is usually bright and cheerful with the doctor and office staff wearing colorful scrubs. Many offices have a "theme" throughout the office with the décor and logo (Figure 34-1).

The Concept of a Dental Home

In the twenty-first century, dental caries is still the number one childhood disease according to the U.S. Surgeon General's Report 2000. Pediatric dentists recommend the first dental visit shortly after the first tooth erupts and no later than age one to begin preventive oral health care and establish a "dental home" for the child. By starting the oral examinations early, many problems may be detected in the beginning stages that can be treated more easily.

The dental home is the ongoing relationship between the dentist and the patient, inclusive of all aspect of oral health care delivered in a comprehensive, continuously accessible, coordinated, and family centered way. Establishment of a dental home begins not later than 12 months of age and includes referral to dental specialists when appropriate.

Children who have a "dental home" are more likely to receive regular preventive oral health care. Establishing the dental home gives the child an environment in which to grow and develop into adolescence and the pediatric dentist can provide information on sealants, orthodontics, oral piercings, wisdom teeth, missing teeth, and preventing injuries during sports as the child matures.

The Pediatric Dental Team

The dental team in a pediatric office consists of the dentist, assistant, child patient, and caregiver (parent/guardian). It is vital to include the caregiver in every aspect of the child's treatment. It is the role of the dental professionals to educate the caregiver about the child's needs and to teach them child dental care techniques. Do not take it for granted that caregivers are aware of the importance of treating "baby" or primary teeth. Some may be reluctant to treat teeth that they think are just going to "fall out of the mouth" in a short while. It is the responsibility of the dental staff to explain the importance of treating primary teeth. The dental assistant can explain that the primary teeth help the child to chew food and to talk fluently, and they save a place for the permanent teeth to erupt later. Most caregivers do not realize that many primary teeth are not lost until age 12 or 13. Teaching caregivers about how to brush and clean their child's mouth, proper nursing habits, diet, and early fluoride treatments can give the child a great start to a lifetime of good oral health.

Importance of Treating Primary Teeth

Many caregivers do not know the importance of baby teeth. The caregiver will often ask the pediatric assistant, "Why should we worry about cavities in baby teeth when these teeth will just fall out?"

Following are good responses the assistant can give to this question:

The baby teeth serve very important functions.

- *Mastication*: The first stage of digestion takes place in the mouth. Chewing helps breakup food into digestible size. Without proper chewing, the digestion process may be prolonged.
- *Nutrition*: Chewing allows for better digestion and digestion allows for better nutrition. A child with decay, sore gums, and missing teeth may have difficulty chewing and may not be able to eat a well-balanced diet.
- *Speech*: Teeth are vital in forming words and speaking clearly. Anterior teeth missing at the time that the child is developing speech may result in tongue thrust and speech impediments (lisp).
- *Appearance*: Healthy and nice looking teeth are critical in building self-esteem. Children can be cruel and tease other children about "black, broken teeth and bad breath."

Neglect of baby teeth can cause severe problems.

- *Pain*: Caries pain is first triggered by sweet, hot and cold. As the caries progress toward and involve the pulp, pain is more severe and throbbing.
- *Infection*: If caries are left untreated, infection may spread to the apex and cause an abscess. The patient will feel intense pain with any biting pressure. Infection that spreads periapically can damage the development of the permanent tooth. Infection can spread to other areas in the body.
- *Malocclusion*: The primary teeth maintain space for the permanent teeth. As the primary tooth exfoliates, the permanent tooth is guided into proper alignment.

Prevention and early treatment of dental problems is a financial investment.

- *Cost*: Restoring a decayed tooth with a restoration is less expensive than pulp and endodontic treatment.
- Treating and keeping the primary teeth as natural space maintainers to guide the permanent teeth into position is less costly than corrective orthodontics.

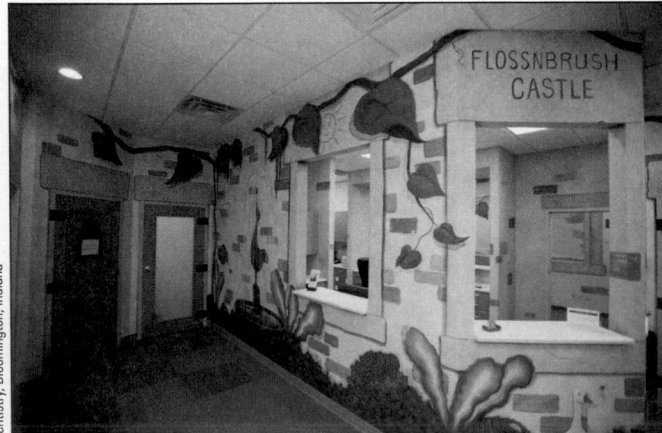

Courtesy of Dr. Keith Roberts, Bloomington Pediatric Dentistry, Bloomington, Indiana

FIGURE 34-1
Pediatric office environment; reception room.

The Pediatric Patient

The pediatric patient is different from the adult patient due to the child's special developmental needs and the relationship with the caregiver. Every child patient has at least one parent or guardian that becomes part of the appointment. The family's attitude toward dentistry and the need for the appointment influences the child's attitude. Many children are fearful or anxious about visiting the dentist or doctor. Some children are fearful due to past experiences with a medical visit or dental visit, and some due to fears transferred by the family.

How a child behaves at any dental appointment varies based on many factors, both emotional and environmental. The pediatric dental team should evaluate each child individually and not based on **chronological age** or physical development. Children also develop at different rates in their **maturity age** and **emotional age**. There are some age characteristics that can be used as guidelines by the dental team in evaluating the child and providing treatment (Table 34-1).

Children with Special Needs Pediatric dentists also are trained to provide dental treatment for children with special needs such as learning disabilities, attention deficient hyperactivity disorder (ADHD), **Down syndrome**, **autism**, **cerebral palsy**, **spina bifida**, asthma, **cystic fibrosis**, and **congenital heart disease** or related problems. A complete medical history is important to prepare for any special needs the patient may have and to be prepared to address those needs with treatment.

The Pediatric Dental Assistant

A dental assistant who works in a pediatric dental office should enjoy working with children, adolescents, and patients with special needs to be successful. Most of the procedures performed in the pediatric practice are similar to those for an adult patient. Pediatric dental assistants are trained in ways to engage the child during the appointment and in communication techniques to

TABLE 34-1 General Behavioral Characteristics of Children at Various Ages

Age	Behavior
2 to 6 years overall	Likes to be with family
	Likes to play (e.g., having a "ride" in the dental chair, seeing the "squirt gun")
	Can respond to dentist's instructions and understands simple explanations
	Transitional time from infantile behavior patterns to the more independent preschool child
2 to 4 years	Short attention span
	Wide variety of interests
	Parallel play without bothering other children
	Responds to fantasy
4 to 6 years	Shows feelings with facial expression
	Parents/guardians are very influential
	Greatest number of management problems
	Needs constant reassurance
	Moves toward integrated play
	Shows some tolerance with dislikes
6 to 12 years overall	Period of socializing
	Asserts independence
	Differences between boys and girls are more noticeable
6 to 9 years	Learning to get along with people and the regulations of society
	Friendships are important
	Usually prefers to come in for treatment without a parent/guardian
	Likes to collect things
	Aware of their place in society and likes to belong to a group
	Likes to be spoken to directly
9 to 12 years	Usually not difficult to manage
	May respond passively
	Will respond when things are explained
	Likes to be treated as an adult

help to coach and praise the child during treatment. Making the child feel good about visiting the dentist while establishing trust and confidence is a primary goal.

The pediatric dental assistant can help communicate with the child on their level but should never talk down or be demeaning. Speaking directly to the child and making eye contact will help build trust. The pediatric assistant needs to be compassionate and have patience when working with children who are uncooperative. It is important for the assistant to practice being friendly, but firm, when handling patient behavior. The pediatric assistant will stay with the child during treatment and will monitor the child's movement and behavior. The child should not be left alone while in the dental chair. The pediatric dental assistant can be a good liaison between the child and the caregiver.

Child Abuse and Dental Neglect

Child abuse is a subject no one wants to discuss, but the number of children abused or neglected continues to grow. Health care providers are legally mandated in all 50 states to report any suspected child abuse or neglect. The pediatric dentist and dental assistant are in a position to observe conditions that might be child abuse. The oral cavity is often the focus of abuse, or the injury to the mouth may be accompanied by facial bruises or jaw fractures.

It is important for the dentist and dental assistant to document any suspicious signs or conditions that might possibly indicate child abuse. The assistant should know the office protocol for reporting any abuse. If a health care provider suspects child abuse, it can be confidentially reported, and the proper authorities will handle the investigation.

The Academy of Pediatric Dentistry defines dental neglect as "willful failure of parent or guardian to seek and follow through with treatment necessary to ensure a level of oral health essential for adequate function and freedom from pain and infection". Many caregivers simply don't understand the need for dental care or due to lack of dental insurance or finances feel they cannot afford dental care. Once the caregiver is aware of the needed dental treatment, it is their responsibility to follow through with the treatment for the child. It is the responsibility of the dental staff to educate the caregiver.

Etiology of Dental Caries

According to McDonald and Avery, most experts in dental caries agree that dental decay is an infectious and communicable disease with multiple factors influencing the progression of the disease. They also recognize that dental caries is a preventable disease. Some studies suggest that early transmission of *S. mutans* from mother to child via saliva transfer is a factor in early caries. Reducing the *S. mutans* in the caregiver with xylitol gum and minimizing saliva transfer between caregiver and the child may reduce the transmission to the child. Studies suggest that there is a "window of infectivity" where the infant obtains the *S. mutans*. Having the mouth cleaned plus reducing sweets and sucrose in the infant's diet can delay the decay process. The dental assistant can reinforce the need for good oral health and dietary habits as well as continued check-ups.

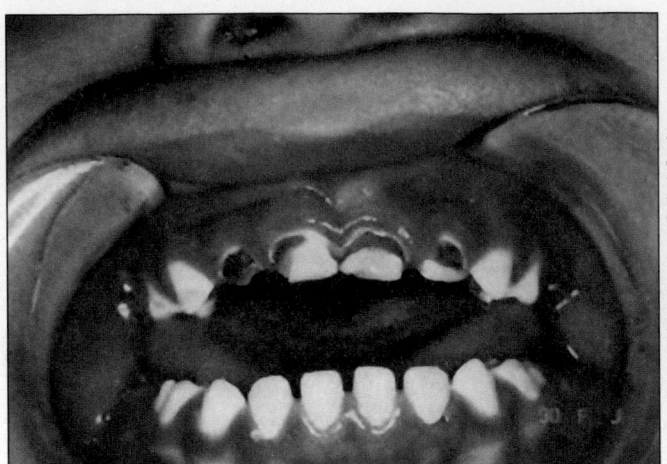

Courtesy of Dr. Keith Roberts, Bloomington Pediatric Dentistry, Bloomington, Indiana

FIGURE 34-2
Early childhood caries.

Lack of early oral hygiene and sugary liquid contribute to the rapid decay of the newly erupting teeth. Left untreated, early childhood caries can lead to abscessed, infected teeth which require extraction.

Early Childhood Caries

The Academy of Pediatric Dentistry defines early childhood caries (ECC) as the presence of one or more decayed, missing, or filled tooth surfaces in a child 71 months of age or younger. In the early 1970s and 1980s, it was known as "baby bottle tooth decay" because of prolonged or frequent nursing habits with a baby bottle or sippy cup filled with milk, juice, or other sugary liquid. The front teeth are usually affected first with some decay in the posterior teeth depending on the age of the child (Figure 34-2).

Infant Oral Exam

Pediatric dentists recommend seeing the child when the first teeth erupt by the first birthday, prior to any caries process to begin counseling caregivers on the need for early oral hygiene habits and early dietary habits.

When the caregiver and the patient arrive at the appointment, the dental assistant gathers the needed information from the caregiver on how they care for the infant's teeth and the feeding habits of the infant. The assistant can gather the past dental history of the family as well. The dentist examines the infant's mouth with a mirror and explorer and the assistant charts existing teeth and any abnormalities if present.

Pediatric Charting

Children normally develop 20 primary teeth which, using the universal numbering system, are lettered A through T. When charting, start on the upper right second primary molar or tooth A and proceed through the upper arch to the upper left second primary molar or tooth J. Then move to the lower left second primary molar or tooth K and proceed through the lower arch to the lower right second primary molar or tooth T.

The 20 primary teeth are replaced by 20 permanent teeth also called succedaneous teeth. Usually the first teeth exfoliated are the primary lower central incisors or teeth #O and #P replaced by permanent lower centrals #24 and #25, followed by the upper two primary central incisors, teeth #E and #F replaced by permanent upper centrals #8 and #9. The first permanent molars erupt posterior to the second primary molars, not replacing primary teeth, and are called nonsuccedaneous teeth. The second and third permanent molars are also nonsuccedaneous. The permanent teeth are numbered 1–32 in the universal numbering system.

Charting Present and Missing Teeth

Charting mixed dentition can be challenging since some primary teeth can be large and difficult to tell from permanent teeth. However, the primary teeth have some unique characteristics, including size and shape, enamel composition, shallow pulp chamber, and root resorption on radiographs that helps in identifying teeth (Table 34-2). When charting mixed dentition, the permanent tooth number will be used when the primary tooth has been replaced by the permanent tooth.

Charting Pediatric Conditions and Abnormalities

As the pediatric dentist performs the oral exam, they will look for conditions with the developing dentition both clinically and radiographically. In the young primary dentition, primate spacing is normal and is essential to allow space for the larger permanent teeth to replace the smaller primary teeth. Crowding of primary teeth in the anterior segments usually indicates that interceptive orthodontic treatment may be a treatment option (Figure 34-3).

The pediatric dentist will also examine the oral cavity for any abnormalities or problems that might be present. Many children suck their thumbs or pacifiers, and the upper maxillary teeth start to protrude into an open bite and the tongue can come forward into a **tongue thrust**. The pediatric dentist will note the oral habits of the young child, and if the thumb habit or pacifier habit is

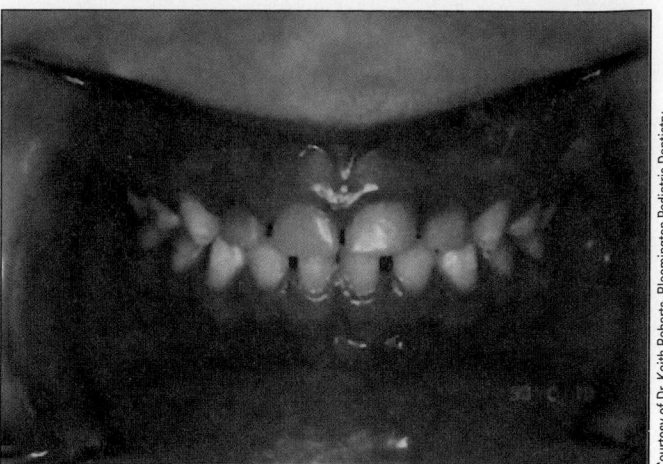

FIGURE 34-3
Primate spacing in pediatric dentition.

causing skeletal problems, the dentist will recommend ways to discontinue the oral habit.

Other abnormalities can include short frenum attachments on the lips or tongue that can interfere with normal tooth eruption, tongue thrust, and speech development. Enamel hypoplasia can result in brown or mottled enamel. Supernumerary teeth, both primary and permanent, and congenitally missing teeth, both primary and permanent, result in inadequate spacing for tooth eruption and normal occlusion. Over retained and early loss of primary teeth will also affect tooth eruption and occlusion development. Cysts and impacted teeth may cause damage to tissue and need for surgical intervention. The developmental problems of primary teeth will affect the child's developing permanent dentition and will be noted in the chart as necessary.

Prevention

A good preventive program should include five major points: oral hygiene, dietary instructions, fluoride, sealants, and routine dental checkups. As the child grows, the dental team will adapt the program to the child's age and needs.

TABLE 34-2 Comparison of Primary and Permanent Dentition

Primary Teeth	Permanent Teeth
Clinical Examination	*Clinical Examination*
Smaller crown with wider cervix	Larger crown with tapered cervix
Whiter teeth (milk teeth)	Not nearly as white
Not as distinct anatomy; molars have scallops instead of well-developed pointed cusps; shallow grooves, fossae, and pits	Well-developed anatomy; molars distinct and pointed; deep grooves and pits; well-defined fossae; appearance of mamelons
Radiographic Examination	*Radiographic Examination*
Wide flared roots beyond the width of the crown; may see absorption of roots and developing permanent tooth on radiograph	Roots are within the width of the crown; may see apex still developing and/or beginning to close
Thinner enamel with pulp closer to the enamel surface	Thicker enamel with more distance from pulp to the enamel surface

Oral Hygiene Instructions

The pediatric dentist or assistant will demonstrate techniques for cleaning the infant's mouth and erupting teeth. It is important for the caregiver to clean the mouth every day to reduce biofilm, and massaging the gums will help with tooth eruption discomfort. Before the teeth erupt, the gums of infants can be cleaned with a soft washcloth or gauze moistened in water.

Infant Tooth Brushing Instructions

Every day, when the infant is given a body bath, the caregiver can give their teeth a "bath" as well. Since an infant only has a few teeth, the caregiver can use a clean, wet wash cloth on their index finger and gently massage their gums and teeth. This will help with the teething and toughen up their gums for the teeth to erupt. This also keeps their mouth clean. As more teeth erupt, the caregiver can introduce a small soft tooth-brush to clean the teeth. At this age, no toothpaste is necessary to clean the teeth.

As more teeth erupt, a toothbrush can be used to clean the teeth and massage the gums daily. A soft toothbrush can be introduced as the teeth first begin to erupt. When brushing an infant or toddler, the caregiver can sit on the floor or bed with the child in their lap or in front of them. The child's head can be tilted back so the caregiver can see the child's mouth. Holding the child's head with one arm and using the other to brush, the caregiver can stabilize the child and clean the entire mouth. Until a child can cut meat with a knife and fork, the caregiver should continue to brush the child's teeth at least once a day. Children can then also brush to improve their dexterity and brushing technique.

Dietary Guidelines

Diet is always the hardest behavior to change. The American Academy of Pediatric Dentistry states that "caries and its **sequelae** are among the most prevalent health problems facing American infants, children and adolescents." The frequent ingestion of sugars and other carbohydrates (e.g., fruit juices, acidic beverages) and prolonged contact of these substances with teeth are particular risk factors in the development of caries." The AAPD recommends that no liquids other than milk or water be placed in a baby bottle and that the infant be weaned from the breast or bottle by age 1. Never use fruit juice or carbonated beverages in a sippy cup, and avoid sugary snacks and sugar coated cereals. A balanced diet including milk, meat, vegetables, fruit, and grain should be recommended for all patients.

Once the infant is over 1 year of age, it is important to wean them off the bottle or breast and introduce only milk or water in a sippy cup. The assistant can review with the caregiver the need to introduce healthy foods such as carrot pieces and slices of melon, apple, or papaya, in order to help baby learn on how to chew and to stimulate their dentition. It is also important to instruct the caregiver to only give the child a bottle or sippy cup

Child Tooth Brushing Instructions

The dental assistant should discuss the oral hygiene instructions with the caregiver. As the child matures, the child patient should become more involved. A disclosing agent can be used to show where biofilm remains on the teeth after brushing. A biofilm score card can be completed to show the caregiver and child areas where biofilm remains after brushing. The dental assistant can show them the areas where biofilm remains on the child's teeth and demonstrate better brushing techniques to remove all the biofilm. The biofilm score record can be used to show the caregiver and child progress in removing the biofilm over time. As the child continues to grow and develop, the assistant will continue to provide age appropriate oral hygiene instruction. The assistant can recommend a toothbrush size appropriate for the child and show the caregiver and child how to brush the teeth and gums as the teeth erupt. The caregiver and child should be taught how to floss between the areas where the contacts are closed as the situation dictates. There are special puppets designed for keeping the child's interest while being taught to brush and floss their teeth (Figure 34-4).

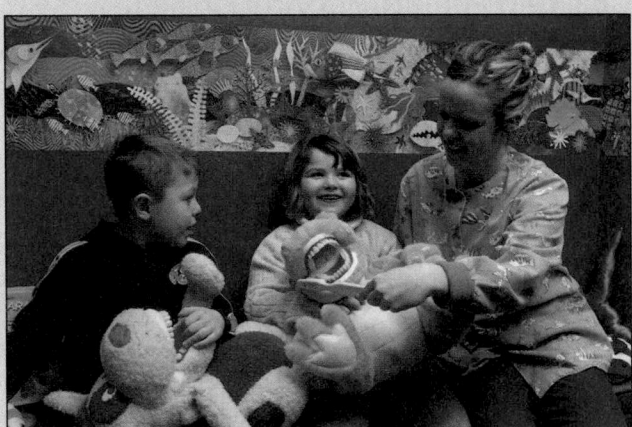

FIGURE 34-4
The assistant motivates children to brush and floss, demonstrating on puppets.

at meal time and not let the child sleep with a bottle. When an infant falls asleep with a bottle, the milk pools around the teeth, and the sugar in the milk forms the acid that causes tooth decay. Stopping the use of a bottle in bed and removing the biofilm every day helps to reduce the chance of early childhood caries.

Fluoride Application

Fluoride is one of the most important tools available for the control and prevention of dental caries in children. Both systemic and topical fluorides are extremely beneficial to developing primary and permanent dentition in the right dose. Most children receive systemic fluoride through the community water supply. Topical fluoride is delivered in many forms including fluoridated toothpaste and professionally applied fluoride. According to the American Academy of Pediatric Dentistry guidelines, parents and caregivers should be cautioned to use a "smear" of toothpaste to brush the teeth of a child under two years of age. For age 2–5 year olds, caregivers should only use a small, pea-sized amount of fluoride toothpaste and assist or perform the child's tooth brushing to prevent potential enamel **fluorosis** from excess ingestion of fluoride.

Professionally applied topical fluoride is recommended for all children and adolescents and consists of more concentrated fluoride solutions, gels, foams, and varnishes. Sodium fluoride and acidulated phosphate fluoride gel or foam delivered in a tray placed in the mouth for 4 minutes are the most common in office fluoride treatments. However, many studies are being conducted concerning the amount of fluoride swallowed during the treatment. Fluoride varnish is recommended for preschool children and high risk caries patients. Fluoride varnish is an application of 5% sodium fluoride with a resin base that causes the varnish to be sticky and remain on the teeth until brushed away the next day. It is usually clear or white or can be a light yellow color. Fluoride varnish is easy to apply and can be used on children of all ages, including infants. Since it sticks to the enamel surface, it is less likely to be swallowed, reducing stomach upset from other fluoride applications. Fluoride varnish can be applied every three to four months for best results. In adolescents, fluoride varnish can reduce the effects of acidic beverages and demineralization of enamel.

Safety

If a child likes the taste of their toothpaste, they may eat the toothpaste from the tube when their caregiver is not looking. Minor cases of excessive ingestion of toothpaste causes an upset stomach. More serious cases may result in nausea, vomiting and diarrhea. Giving the child milk or yogurt will help with their stomach upset. In rare cases, there can be more serious problems and the Poison Control should be called right away or use the web POISON-CONTROL tool for online guidance. The toothpaste should be kept out of the reach of the child to prevent potential enamel fluorosis.

Dental Sealants

According to the *2000 Oral Health in America: A Report of the Surgeon General*, up to 90% of all dental caries in children's teeth occur in pits and fissures. Even the best brushing techniques cannot reach the deep pits and fissures to remove the biofilm and food debris to avoid caries production. With this information, all dental providers should routinely be placing sealants on molars. Dental sealant is a thin coating of unfilled resin applied to the pits and fissures of the posterior permanent molars and premolars. They seal out germs and food particles from the fissures in the chewing surface of the tooth. According to the CDC, sealants can last from 5 to 10 years and should be monitored at regular dental checkups. The sealant can be reapplied or added to as needed.

The American Dental Association states that as long as the sealant remains intact, the occlusal surface of the tooth is protected from decay. How well the sealant remains on the tooth is dependent on the sealant application with a dry field. Since the application of sealants is technique sensitive, closely follow manufacturer's direction for the proper sealant application technique. (Refer to Chapter 26, "Dental Sealants," for more detail.)

Regular Checkups

The dental assistant can reinforce the need for good oral health and dietary habits as well as continued checkups. From the eruption of the first tooth until adulthood, the child's mouth is constantly changing. Regular checkups are extremely important to monitor the growth and development of the primary and permanent dentition. Dental decay is a progressive disease, and early **intervention** when decay is minor saves extensive restorative procedures if the decay is allowed to progress. Taking routine radiographs and panoramic films can assist the dentist with the diagnosis of interproximal decay and any abnormalities in tooth development.

Behavior Management

According to *Dentistry for the Child and Adolescent*, behavior management is defined as follows: "Behavior management is the means by which the dental health team effectively and efficiently performs treatment for a child and, at the same time, instills a positive dental attitude." One of the greatest challenges in pediatric dentistry is predicting how the child will react in the dental office. Since each child is an individual, even siblings behave differently in different settings. The caregiver's attitude about dentistry and their child can also influence the child's behavior. Each pediatric dentist will decide the best way to manage a child during the treatment. One way to classify a child's behavior is the Frankl Behavioral Rating Scale. The scale uses four categories for the observed behavior, ranging from definitely positive to definitely negative (Table 34-3).

Communication

Communication is the number one tool that the pediatric dental team can use with both the caregiver and child during the dental appointment. Being clear and direct in communication with the caregiver about the treatment and how the child's behavior may be handled sets the stage for the appointment.

It is imperative that the dentist has an informed consent signed by the caregiver of the child being treated. The informed consent should outline all methods of behavior management that might be used by the pediatric dentist and each method explained to the caregiver.

In dealing with the child, the entire dental team should take a positive approach and expect the child to cooperate with the dental treatment. Something as simple as a smile can communicate warmth and caring to the child. Being truthful with the child helps to build trust and rapport, and making eye contact with the child conveys sincerity. It is important to use short, positive directions and maintain control while talking with the child. Praising the child for their help and cooperation also helps reinforce the

TABLE 34-3 Frankl Scale for Pediatric Dental Patient Behavior

Patient Behavior	Definition	Rating
Good rapport with dentist; interested in dental procedures; laughing and enjoying the situation	Definitely positive	4
Acceptance of treatment; cautious at times; willingness to comply, at times with reservation, but follows directions	Positive	3
Reluctance to accept treatment, uncooperative; some evidence of negative attitude but not pronounced, that is, no sudden withdrawal	Negative	2
Refusal of treatment; crying forcefully; fearful; other evidence of extreme negativism	Definitely negative	1

child's ability to cope with the dental appointment. Sometimes, just holding the child's hand makes them feel calmer.

Nonpharmacological Behavior Management

There are generally two types of behavior management: nonpharmacological and **pharmacological**. Nonpharmacological behavior management methods include show-tell-do, voice control, distraction, modeling, and protective stabilization.

Show-Tell-Do
Show-tell-do is a technique where the doctor and/or the assistant uses a calm, clear voice and explain what is going to happen during the appointment. Showing the various items that will be used and explaining how they are used helps to familiarize the child with the procedure and alleviate fears. After the explanation and demonstration, the doctor performs the procedure. While explaining the procedure and instruments used, it is important to use words that convey the message but are not scary (Table 34-4).

Voice Control
While explaining the procedure, it is important to keep the child's attention and explain listening skills. A fearful child mostly likely is crying and not listening. Another

method for obtaining the attention of the child is voice control. The doctor will slightly raise their voice above the crying of the child so they can be heard, and say in a calm but firm voice that the child needs to listen to the instructions and help with the procedure to complete the appointment. It is important to maintain eye contact and assure the child that if they will listen, they will not be scared.

Distraction and Modeling
Distraction is another technique that works for many children. Videos playing in TVs on the ceiling or music played via earphones can help eliminate some of the noise associated with the dental treatment. **Modeling** behavior with another patient or sibling can help a reluctant child see how they should behave.

Protective Stabilization
For the very defiant or angry child or a child with special needs, **protective stabilization** may be necessary. A papoose board or pedi wrap can be used to help stabilize a child in the dental chair and prevent the child from injuring themselves or the dental staff. The protective stabilization does not hurt the child and can help calm the child during the procedure. The pedi wrap may also be used with Pharmacological Behavior Management Techniques as well to maintain the safety of the patient (Figure 34-5).

Pharmacological Behavior Management

Pharmacological behavior management includes the use of analgesics and various medications to sedate the child during

TABLE 34-4 Preferred Pediatric Wording

These are some words that can be used instead of the more technical words.

Common Wording	Preferred Wording
Shot	Pinch, sleepy juice, injection
Drill	Whistle, air blower, handpiece
Low-speed handpiece	Mr. Bumpy, shaker, smoother
Dental dam	Raincoat, umbrella
Dental dam clamp	Button
Explorer	Tooth checker
Impression material	Play doh, silly putty
Curing light	Blue flashlight
Sealant	Fingernail polish
Anesthetic	Sleepy juice
Nitrous oxide	Space mask
Numbness	Sleepy feeling, tingling
Extraction	Wiggle the tooth
Decay	Sugar bugs
Pedi wrap	Safety blanket

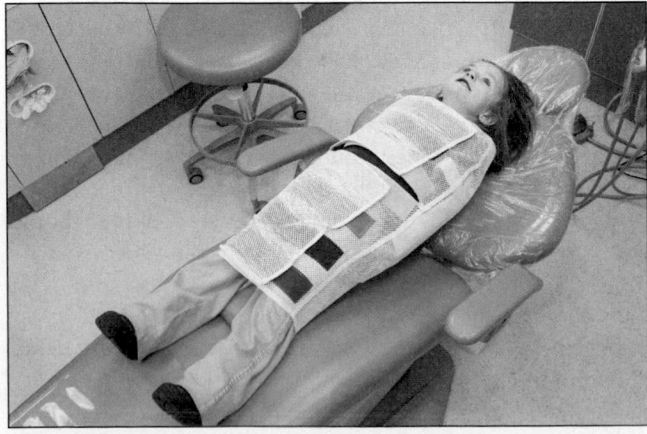

FIGURE 34-5
A child positioned in a papoose board with pedi wrap.

the dental treatment. These include nitrous oxide and oxygen, conscious sedation, and general anesthesia.

Nitrous Oxide Nitrous oxide/oxygen inhalation is a safe and effective technique to reduce anxiety and enhance effective communication, according to the American Academy of Pediatric Dentistry. Because it has a rapid onset and the effects are easily controlled and reversible, it can be used with most children with few contraindications. The child should be able to breathe easily through the nose and tolerate the nasal mask for the nitrous oxide/oxygen inhalation to be effective. Check for any leaks around the nasal mask and be sure there is a good fit for the child's face (Figure 34-6). Most children respond well to nitrous oxide/oxygen, but some do not. If the child cannot breathe through their nose due to a cold or nasal obstruction or if the child is crying and vocal, nitrous oxide can be contraindicated.

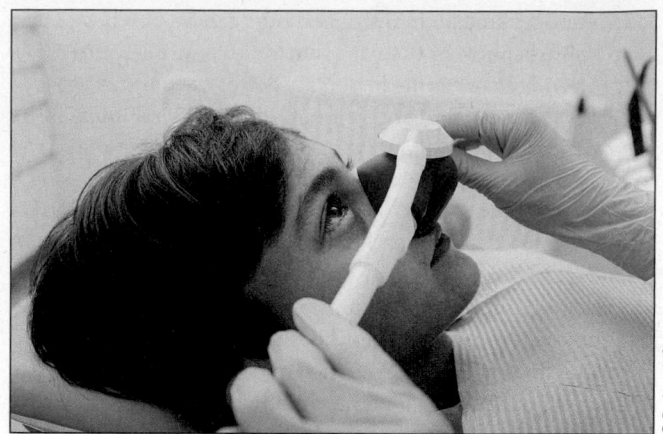

FIGURE 34-6
Nitrous mask being placed on child prior to treatment.

Conscious Sedation

Conscious sedation involves using medication such as chloral hydrate, Demerol, or Vistraril that can be administered orally or intramuscularly to control anxiety and movement in patients who are unable to have treatment due to age or a physical or mental condition. Very young children under the age of three, children unable to modify behavior or who have no self-control, and mentally or physically impaired children are classified according to the American Society of Anesthesiologists Physical Status Classification System. The pediatric dentist will make a decision on the type of sedation based on the medical history of the child. Informed consent is necessary prior to any type of sedation with pre and post instructions, for the caregiver, such as no milk or solids for 6 hours for children 6–36 months and for 6 to 8 hours for children 36 months and older plus clear liquids up to 3 hours before the procedure for children 6 months and older. The dental office must have medical equipment such as a pulse oximeter and blood pressure cuff, to monitor the child's respiration and blood pressure during the procedure. Many pediatric dentists work with a pediatric anesthesiologist to provide sedation for the patient in the dental office. All treatment procedures and patient vital statistics must be documented throughout the treatment.

General Anesthesia General anesthesia involves sedating the patient with medications delivered via an IV and can be performed in a hospital or outpatient hospital setting. Many state laws and codes require the pediatric dentist to have additional permits for the use of general anesthesia. Some states or hospitals require the dental assistant to have additional hospital training to assist with general anesthesia.

All procedures performed on the child should be thoroughly explained to the caregiver. Written caregiver consent must be given for use of protective stabilization and administration of any pharmaceuticals.

Pediatric Restorative Procedures

Pediatric dental restorations and procedures are very similar to adult restorations. However, the primary teeth have some unique characteristics—thinner enamel, shallow pulp chamber, and exfoliation. These differences make the need for some instruments and steps in the procedure to be adapted. The amalgam, composite resins, and glass ionomers restorations can be used in both primary and permanent teeth.

Pediatric Instruments and Equipment

Most instruments for pediatric patients are the same as for adult patients. The differences will be with the size of the instrument. High-speed handpieces are available with smaller heads to

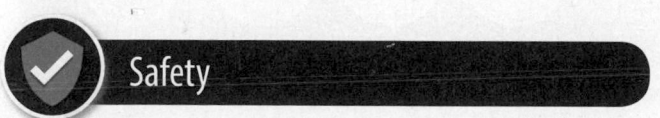

N₂O Safety
Periodically check all the hoses and connections on the nitrous unit to check for leaks or loose connections. Always be sure the scavenger system is working as well.

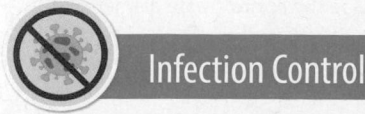

Be sure to use a nitrous mask that is disposable or autoclavable. Make sure to disinfect the nitrous unit and all hoses after each use.

accommodate smaller mouths, and burs can be purchased that have a short shank so they are shorter in length (Figure 34-7). **Extraction forceps** come in pediatric sizes so that the beaks of the forceps are smaller and fit the primary teeth (Figure 34-8). The pediatric dentist may use a mouth prop more to help the child patient to keep their mouth open if needed.

When placing a Class II restoration in a primary tooth, a T-band can be used instead of the larger adult matrix band. A T-band is a matrix that can be custom fitted to the primary tooth (Figure 34-9). Often made of brass strips that are crossed at one end, they are available in various designs and sizes. T-bands are a preformed matrix that when looped into a circle and secured can be adjusted to the smaller primary tooth. They are secured on the tooth and do not require a retainer (Procedure 34-1). Pediatric orthodontic molar bands are also designed for primary teeth for the fabrication of space maintainers.

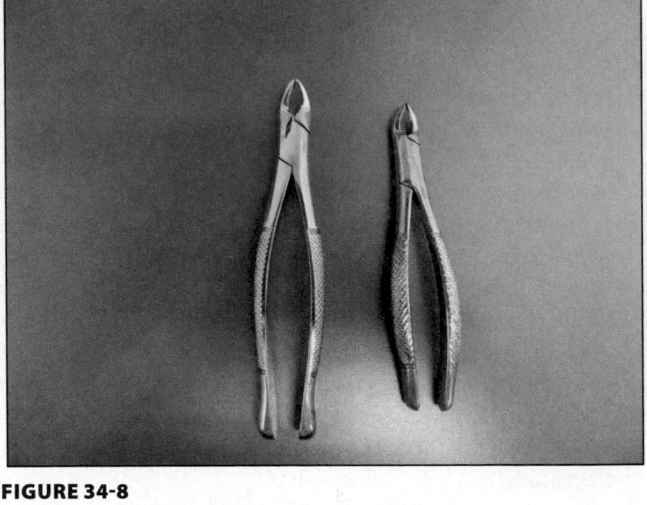

Courtesy of Dr. Keith Roberts, Bloomington Pediatric Dentistry, Bloomington, Indiana

FIGURE 34-8
Adult extraction forceps next to pediatric forceps.

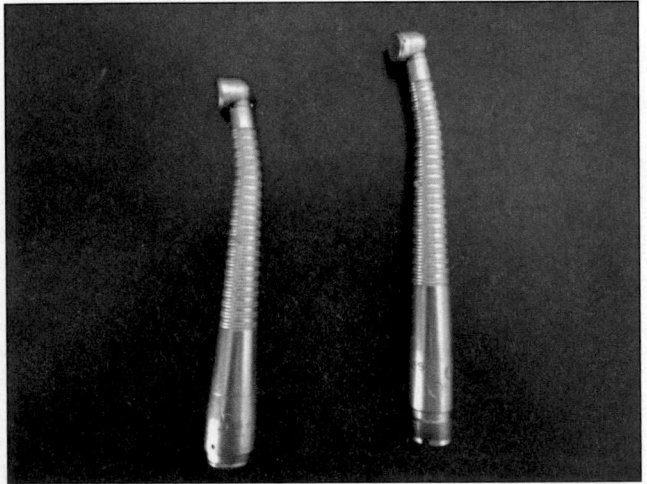

Courtesy of Dr. Keith Roberts, Bloomington Pediatric Dentistry, Bloomington, Indiana

FIGURE 34-7
Pediatric handpiece placed next to the adult handpiece.

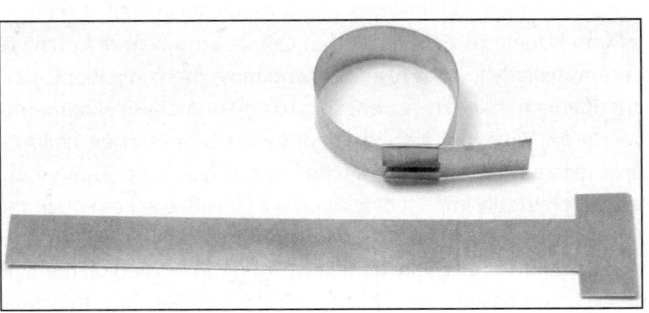

FIGURE 34-9
T-band used as matrix for primary teeth.

Procedure 34-1
T-Band Placement

For this procedure, the tooth has been prepared. The assistant assembles the matrix. The dentist places the T-band unless the state's Dental Practice Act allows a qualified dental assistant to perform this skill.

Equipment and Supplies (Figure 34-10)
- T-band assortment (A)
- T-band matrix strips (B)
- prepared matrix strip (C)
- burnisher (D)
- hemostat (E)

- cotton pliers (F)
- crown and collar scissors (G)
- wooden wedges (H)

Procedure Steps (*Follow aseptic procedures*)
1. Prepare the T-band ahead of time by selecting the appropriate band size.
   - ❑ Loop the band to shape the approximate diameter of the tooth.
   - ❑ Fold the "T" ends over the band loop, leaving a circle with a long tail or end.

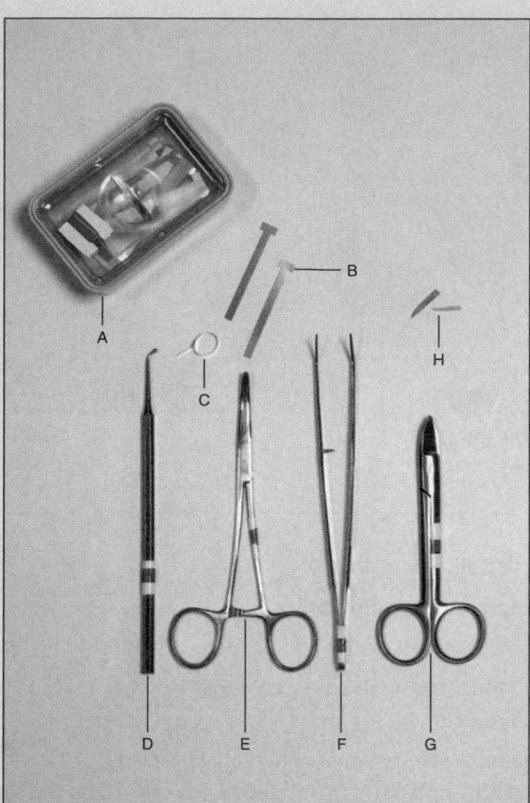

FIGURE 34-10
A tray setup for T-band placement.

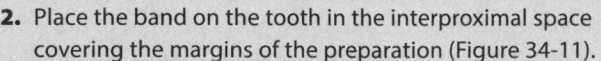

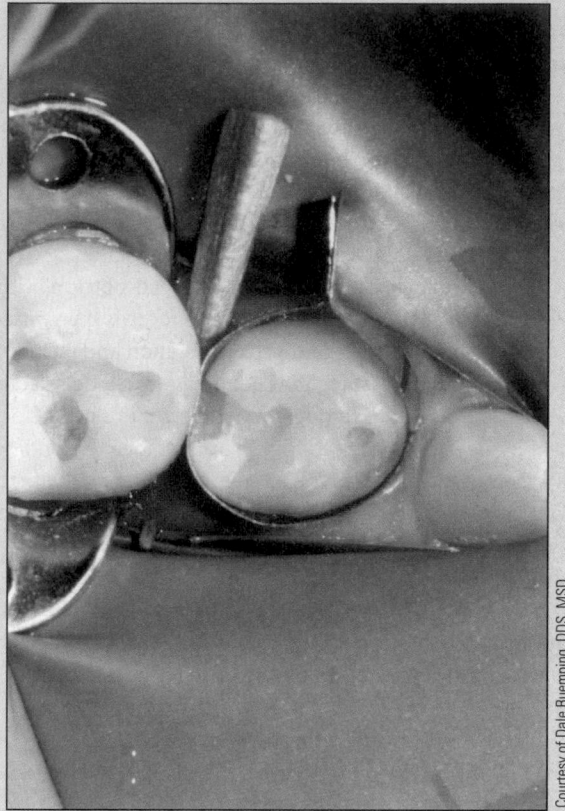

FIGURE 34-11
T-band placement on a tooth.

Courtesy of Dale Ruemping, DDS, MSD

2. Place the band on the tooth in the interproximal space covering the margins of the preparation (Figure 34-11).

3. Place the portion of the band where the "T" is folded on the buccal surface, away from the margins of the preparation.

4. Tighten the band by pulling on the free end (tail) until the band is tight around the tooth.

5. Bend the free end back toward the "T" to secure the band.

6. Remove any excess band with scissors.

7. Burnish the band and place a wedge as needed.

8. Remove the T-band.
   ❑ Fold back the overlapping section of the band to loosen the band.
   ❑ Use cotton pliers or hemostat to remove the band from the tooth.

Anesthetic Syringe Pass

Children do not understand the consequences of sudden movement or grabbing the anesthetic syringe. The pediatric dentist may request the anesthetic to be passed over the child's left shoulder or may prefer accepting the syringe behind the dental chair. The pediatric assistant is instructed to gently hold the child's upper arms and head to prevent the child from moving and reaching toward the syringe during injection or suddenly turning their head to the side.

Dental Dam

A dental dam should be used the majority of the time when placing restorations in children's teeth. The dental dam prevents debris from being aspirated by the patient and keeps the child's tongue and saliva out of the cavity preparation. It serves as protection for the child as well as allowing the operator a dry, clear field. The smaller 5 × 5 dental dam material is used for the smaller children.

Preventive Resin Restoration

Permanent teeth often develop with very deep grooves that are difficult to clean and are prone to decay. Some of these grooves form incompletely and dental caries begins. With present decay the preventive sealant would not be the best choice. Incipient caries barely into the enamel doesn't warrant a traditional resin restoration requiring a larger preparation. The preventive resin restoration is a better alternative for these early detected caries and most often does not require an anesthetic injection.

The dentist removes only the small decayed portion of the tooth with very small rotary instruments. The tooth is then rinsed, dried, and etched slightly beyond the preparation and including any remaining pits and fissures that generally would be selected for a sealant. The etchant is removed by sufficient rinsing and drying. The surface should have a "frosty" appearance. A bonding/adhesive material is applied to the etched surface and set with the resin light. The flowable resin is placed into the small preparation with a syringe and small tip and set with the resin light. The sealant resin is applied over the exposed pits, fissures, and flowable resin and set with the resin light. The sealant protects the resin, pits, and fissures from future caries, and the child is provided the long-term preventive benefit of a preventive resin restoration.

Pediatric Crowns

Since the primary teeth are going to be exfoliated at some point, the pediatric dentist uses a stainless steel crown (SSC) when full coverage of the crown is required. When placing a crown on a permanent tooth that has not fully developed or erupted, the dentist often chooses to use the stainless steel crown instead of the higher fee and multiple visits required of a gold or porcelain crown. A stainless steel crown can restore the tooth to function and keep the tooth until it is exfoliated or until a gold or porcelain crown can be placed (Figure 34-12).

The indications for use of a SSC include the following:

- Extensive multisurface caries
- Tooth fractures
- Hypoplastic and/or hypocalcified carious teeth

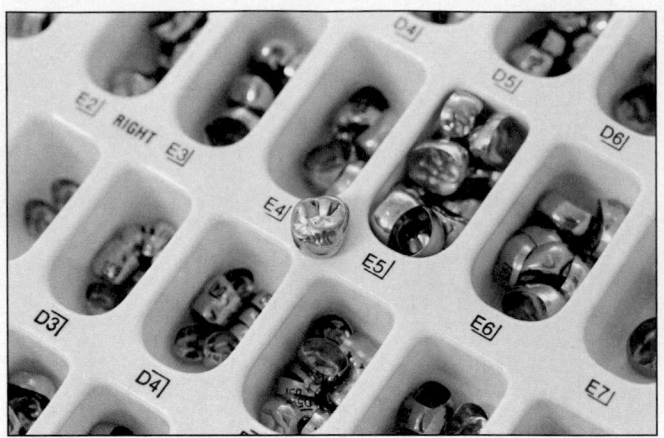

FIGURE 34-12
Stainless steel crown kit. Palmer numbering used to identify crowns' names and size.

- Failed alloy or resin restoration
- Pulpopotomy/pulpectomy
- High caries risk patient
- Primary tooth used as an **abutment** tooth for a space maintainer

Stainless steel crowns are available in a variety of sizes for both the primary and permanent teeth. Each crown has the symbol of the tooth and the crown size stamped on the crown. There are pretrimmed crowns and precontoured crowns. The pretrimmed crowns have a straight gingival margin and require trimming and contouring to fit the tooth. The length of the crown is marked by a sharp instrument, like a scaler, and the crown scissor cuts the crown to length. The contouring pliers are used to taper the cervical portion of the crown for a tight fit. The precontoured crowns are trimmed and contoured more to the natural curvature of the tooth and require minimal adjustment.

The dentist will reduce the tooth to allow for the crown to fit over the tooth. The assistant will select a crown from the crown kit to trial fit. The crown should fit to the gingival margin mesially and distally, with no open contacts and with the teeth in proper occlusion (Procedure 34-2).

Procedure 34-2
Stainless Steel Crown Placement

This procedure is performed by the dentist with the help of the dental assistant. The assistant maintains the operating field, mixes materials, and assists in preparation of the stainless steel crown. The operator (dentist, dental hygienist, or qualified assistant) places the topical anesthetic and dental dam.

Steps written in blue font are performed by the operator (dentist or qualified dental assistant), and the chairside assistant's steps are written in black.

Equipment and Supplies (Figure 34-13)

Patient Seating Setup (refer to Procedure 18-4)

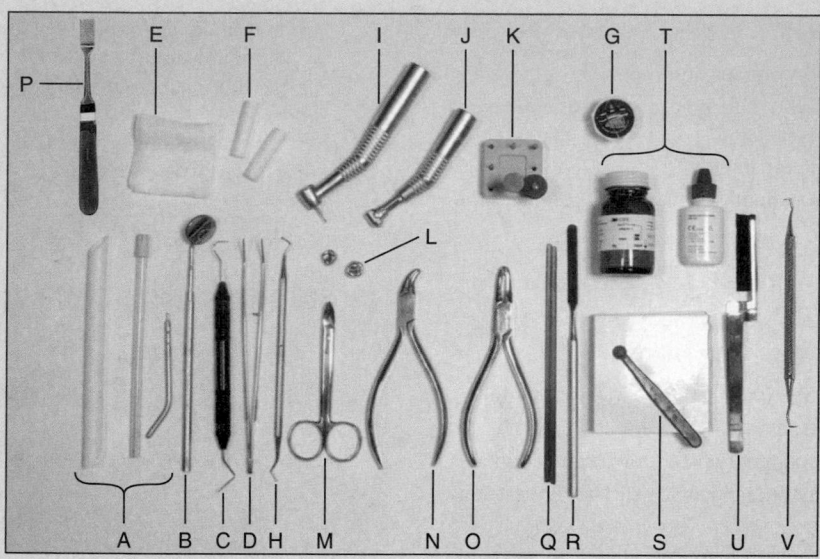

FIGURE 34-13
SSC tray setup.

Basic Setup
- saliva ejector, evacuator (HVE), and air/water syringe tips (A)
- mouth mirror (B)
- explorer (C)
- cotton pliers (D)

Expendables
- gauze squares (E)
- cotton rolls (F)
- dental floss (G)

Local Anesthetic Setup (not shown; refer to Procedure 23-2)

Dental Dam Setup (not shown; refer to Procedure 21-2)

Cavity Preparation Setup
- spoon excavator (H)
- high-speed handpiece (I)
- low-speed handpiece (J)
- bur block with assorted burs and green stone and rubber abrasive wheel (K)

SSC Tray Setup
- selection of stainless steel crowns (L)
- crown and collar scissors (M)
- contouring plier #137 (N)
- contouring plier #112 (O)
- band rocker (P)
- orangewood stick (Q)
- mixing spatula (R)
- paper pad and measurer (S)
- permanent cement (polycarboxylate or glass ionomer) (T)
- articulating forceps and paper (U)
- scaler (V)

Procedure Steps (*Follow aseptic procedures*)

1. Escort and seat patient (refer to Procedure 18-4).

2. Prepare in advance for steps in cavity preparation procedure.
   - ❏ Open patient's chart in dental software.
   - ❏ Navigate to the dental charting screen.
   - ❏ Open patient's latest radiographic history on the computer monitor, or place on view box.
   - ❏ Attach handpieces to dental unit.
   - ❏ Insert burs into handpieces.
   - ❏ Inform dentist that the patient is ready.
   - ❏ Introduce dentist as they enter the treatment area.

   Dentist greets the patient and takes position at the dental chair.
   - ❏ **Signals for the procedure to begin (refer to Procedure 20-1).**

3. Pass mouth mirror and explorer at operator's signal.

   Dentist examines tooth or teeth with mirror and explorer.

   Dentist administers local anesthetic.

4. Assist in administration of local anesthetic (refer to Procedure 23-2).

   Operator places dental dam.

5. Assist in placement of dental dam (refer to Procedure 21-3).

   Dentist prepares the tooth for the placement of the SSC.

(Continues)

❑ Reduces circumference and height of the tooth.

6. Assist in cavity/crown preparation.
   ❑ Pass handpiece with bur and excavators alternately until the tooth is prepared.
   ❑ Aspirate during preparation.
   ❑ Assist in removing dental dam as dentist prepares the gingival margin.

Dentist selects appropriate crown and adjusts sizing.

   ❑ Estimates size of SSC or measures mesiodistal diameter of edentulous space.

7. Assist in sizing the SSC (some states allow the dental assistant to fit the crown).
   ❑ Pass crown to operator to place onto preparation.
   ❑ Pass band rocker or orangewood stick as requested by dentist.
   ❑ Pass scaler to operator to examine the fit, mark extensions of the crown that blanch the gingiva and to remove the crown.
   ❑ Pass the crown scissor to cut crown extensions as needed (Figure 34-14).

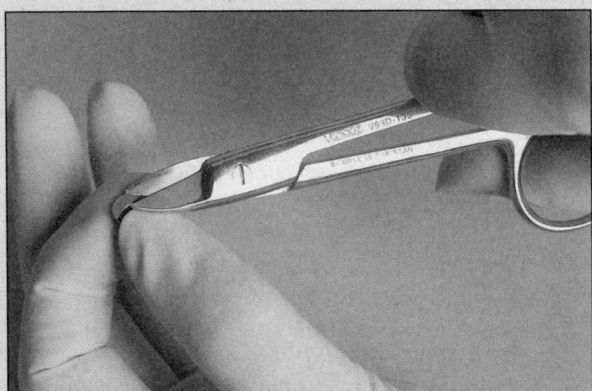

FIGURE 34-14
SSC selected and trimmed with color scissors.

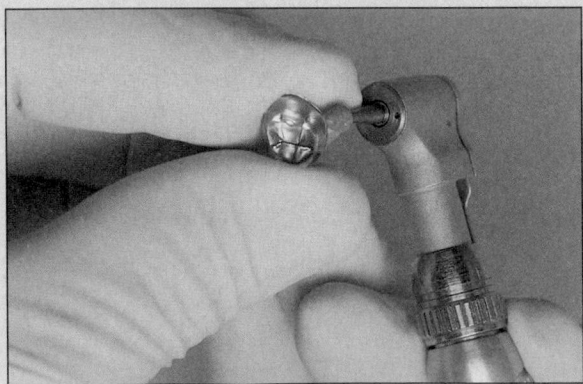

FIGURE 34-15
Crown margins smoothed with green stone.

❑ Pass handpiece with green stone for operator to smooth the rough edges of the crown (Figure 34-15).
❑ Pass rubber abrasive wheel to polish the edges of the crown.

Operator contours the gingival margins for a better fit as needed (Figure 34-16).

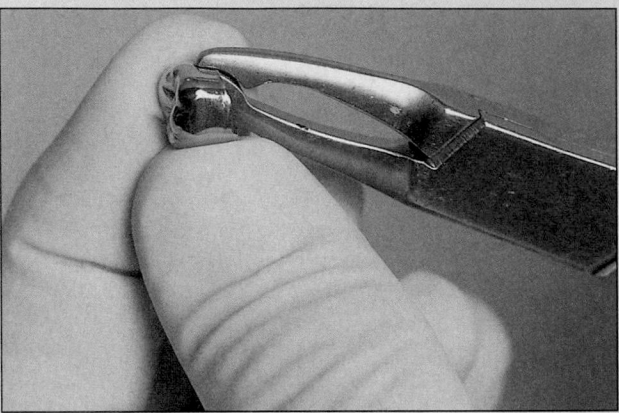

FIGURE 34-16
Crown contoured with contouring pliers; margins are then crimped with 112 pliers.

8. Pass contouring pliers.

   Dentist checks the fit of adjusted SSC.

9. Assist in checking the fit.
   ❑ Pass band rocker or orangewood stick to try-on crown.
   ❑ Pass articulating paper to check for occlusion.
   ❑ Pass dental floss to check the contacts.

10. Prepare for SSC for cementing if it fits.
    ❑ Clean the SSC in the ultrasonic cleaner and disinfect.
    ❑ Rinse and dry crown thoroughly.

    Dentist seats the crown.

11. Assist in seating the crown.
    ❑ Mix dentist's preference of cement to luting consistency.
    ❑ Fill crown 2/3 full and pass to dentist.
    ❑ Pass band rocker or orangewood stick to seat the crown.
    ❑ Pass cotton roll for patient to bite on until the cement sets.
    ❑ Pass scaler to remove excess cement.
    ❑ Pass floss to check contact and remove excess cement interproximally.
    ❑ Pass articulating paper to check the occlusion.
    ❑ Rinse patient's mouth (Figure 34-17).

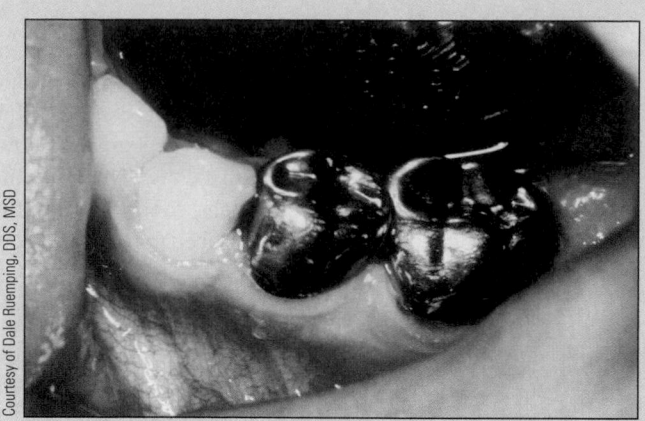

FIGURE 34-17
Stainless steel crown placed on a tooth.

Courtesy of Dale Ruempping, DDS, MSD

12. Provide patient with postoperative instructions orally and in written form.

13. Write up procedure in Services Rendered.

14. Dismiss and escort patient to reception area (refer to Procedure 18–5).

Date	Services Rendered
02/18/XX	Updated medical and dental history, no changes noted. BP = 120/80; T = 98.6F, P = 80, R = 18
	Placed 20% benzocaine gel to injection sites for 2 minutes. Administered 2 cartridges (3.6 ml) of 2% lidocaine with 1:100,000 epi to mandibular left. No reaction
#L #K	(D3 SSC), (E6 SSC) cemented with glass ionomer
	POI do not bite on lip, no eating/drinking until numbness wears off, eat only on opposite side until numbness has worn off, call office if crown feels high or if there is discomfort or pain
	Assistant's initials

Anterior Esthetic Crowns

Since anterior teeth are readily visible, an aesthetic, anterior crown may be preferred. Anterior crowns can be stainless steel, **veneered** steel, or resin strip crowns. Stainless steel crowns can be used and the facial area removed and a resin material placed in a "window" to make the steel crown more aesthetic.

More pediatric dentists use veneered steel crowns, which have a resin bonded onto the facial surface of the steel crown. However, the veneered steel crowns are more opaque, and over time the veneer can chip or crack.

The strip crowns are clear crown forms with a composite resin placed inside the crown form and then placed over the prepared tooth (Figure 34-18). The composite resin is then light cured from the facial and then the lingual surface. The crown form is then removed and the resin crown is smoothed and contoured as needed.

Pediatric Pulp Treatment

The pulp treatment for children's teeth is different from the endodontic treatment performed on fully developed, erupted permanent teeth. Permanent root canal filling material will interfere with the natural absorption of the roots of the primary roots. This will prevent the natural exfoliation of the primary tooth and eruption of the permanent tooth. Permanent root canal filling material cannot be placed in a permanent tooth that does not have the apex fully developed. The dentist will

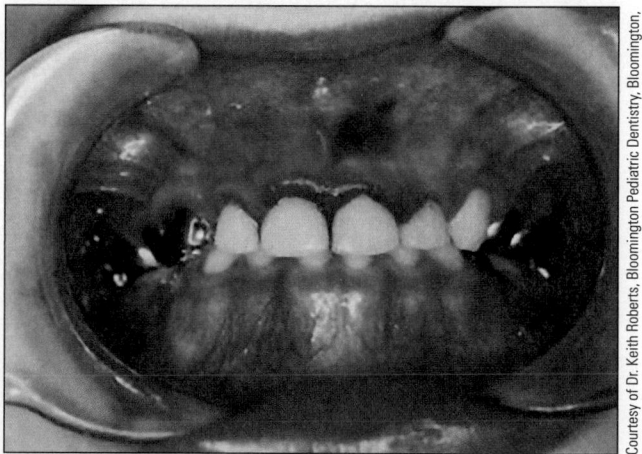

FIGURE 34-18
Strip crown.

Courtesy of Dr. Keith Roberts, Bloomington Pediatric Dentistry, Bloomington, Indiana

treat the pulp of the tooth, and once the permanent tooth has completely developed and erupted, root canal therapy will be completed.

Pulpotomy Procedure

When a primary tooth or a permanent tooth that is not fully developed is decayed/injured and the nerve is involved, the tooth may require a **pulpotomy**. A pulpotomy is the removal of the coronal portion of the pulp. A medicament is placed into the pulp chamber against the pulp canals to **cauterize** the tissue. The most common medicament used for vital pulpotomies is **formocresol**, which is placed on a sterile cotton pellet carefully expressed so that the cotton is virtually dry and placed in the pulp chamber. After 5 minutes, the pulp tissue should be adequately cauterized and bleeding has stopped. The cotton pellet is removed, and a thick mixture of zinc oxide and eugenol or IRM is placed into the pulp chamber and allowed to set. A stainless steel crown should be placed to protect the tooth until the primary

tooth is lost, or if it is a permanent tooth, a permanent crown can be placed.

More recently, a material called mineral trioxide aggregate or MTA has been approved by the FDA and is showing promising results in primary teeth. MTA is a powder composed of tricalcium silicate, bismuth oxide, dicalcium silicate, tricalcium aluminate, terracalcium aluminoferrite, and calcium sulfate dehydrate. The MTA powder is mixed with sterile saline and condensed into the pulp chamber. A stainless steel crown is placed to protect the primary tooth (Procedure 34-3).

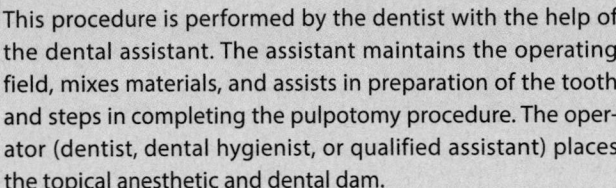

Procedure 34-3
Assisting with a Pulpotomy

This procedure is performed by the dentist with the help of the dental assistant. The assistant maintains the operating field, mixes materials, and assists in preparation of the tooth and steps in completing the pulpotomy procedure. The operator (dentist, dental hygienist, or qualified assistant) places the topical anesthetic and dental dam.

Steps written in blue font are performed by the operator (dentist or qualified dental assistant), and the chairside assistant's steps are written in black.

Equipment and Supplies (Figure 34-19)
Patient Seating Setup (refer to Procedure 18-4)
Basic Setup
- saliva ejector, evacuator (HVE), and sterile air/water syringe tips (A)
- mouth mirror (B)
- explorer (C)
- cotton pliers (D)

Expendables
- gauze squares (E)
- cotton rolls (F)

Local Anesthetic Setup (G)

Dental Dam Setup (H)

Cavity Preparation Setup
- spoon excavator (I)
- high-speed handpiece (not shown)
- low-speed handpiece (not shown)
- bur block with assorted burs (J)

Pulpotomy Setup
- formocresol (K) or mineral trioxide aggregate (MTA)
- sterile dappen dish (L)
- sterile cotton pellets (M)

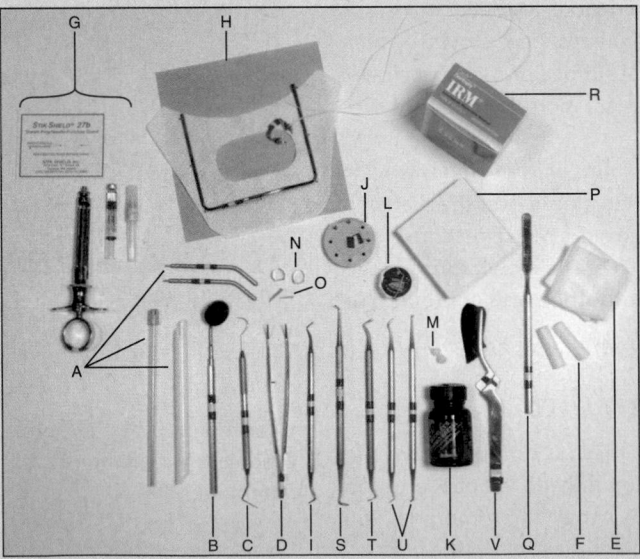

FIGURE 34-19
Formocresol pulpotomy tray setup.

Matrix Setup (as needed)

- T-bands (N)
- wooden wedges (O)

Temporary Cement Restoration Setup

- sterile glass slab (P)
- sterile cement spatula (Q)
- ZOE or IRM cement liquid and powder (R)
- plastic instrument (S)
- amalgam condenser (T)
- carvers (dentist preference) (U)
- articulating forceps and paper (V)

Procedure Steps (*Follow aseptic procedures*)

1. Escort and seat patient (refer to Procedure 18-4).

2. Prepare in advance for steps in cavity preparation procedure.
   - ❏ Open patient's chart in dental software.
   - ❏ Navigate to the dental charting screen.
   - ❏ Open patient's latest radiographic history on the computer monitor, or place on view box.
   - ❏ Attach handpieces to dental unit.
   - ❏ Insert burs into handpieces.
   - ❏ Inform dentist that the patient is ready.
   - ❏ Introduce dentist as they enter the treatment area.

   Dentist greets the patient and takes position at the dental chair.
   - ❏ **Signals for the procedure to begin (refer to Procedure 20-1).**

3. Pass mouth mirror and explorer at operator's signal.

   Dentist examines tooth or teeth with mirror and explorer.

   Dentist administers local anesthetic.

4. Assist in administration of local anesthetic (refer to Procedure 23-2).

   Operator places dental dam.

5. Assist in placement of dental dam (refer to Procedure 21-3).

   Dentist prepares the tooth.
   - ❏ **Cuts cavity prep (Figure 34-20A).**
   - ❏ **Removes coronal pulp (Figure 34-20B).**

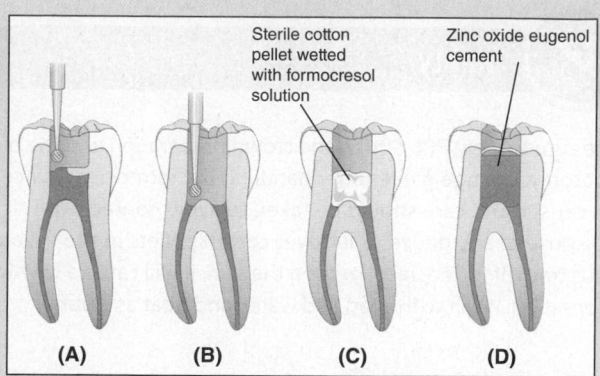

FIGURE 34-20
A pulpotomy procedure showing direct pulp exposure.

6. Assist in cavity preparation.
   - ❏ Pass handpiece with bur and excavators alternately until the tooth is prepared.
   - ❏ Aspirate during preparation.

7. Assist in placing formocresol (or MTA).
   - ❏ Apply formocresol to sterile cotton pellet with dropper.
   - ❏ Squeeze pellet in gauze square until almost dry.
   - ❏ Pass pellet with cotton pliers.

   Dentist places formocresol pellet into pulp chamber (Figure 34-20C).

8. Time for 5 minutes or until bleeding stops.
   - ❏ Do not rinse after bleeding stops.

   Dentist places pulpotomy paste or MTA (Figure 34-20D).

9. Assist in placing paste.
   - ❏ Mix dentist's preference of paste.
   - ❏ Pass plastic filling instrument.
   - ❏ Hold cement on slab at patient's chin level.
   - ❏ Pass condenser with cavity is filled.
   - ❏ Pass dentist's choice of carvers.

   Dentist prepares and places SSC at the same appointment (refer to Procedure 34-2).

10. Provide patient with postoperative instructions orally and in written form.

11. Write up procedure in Services Rendered.

12. Dismiss and escort patient to reception area (refer to Procedure 18-5).

Date	Services Rendered
02/18/XX	Updated medical and dental history, no changes noted. BP = 120/80; T = 98.6F, P = 80, R = 18
	Placed 20% benzocaine gel to injection sites for 2 minutes. Administered 2 cartridges (3.6 ml) of 2% lidocaine with 1:100,000 epi to mandibular left. No reaction
#L and #K	Formocresol pulpotomy; placed pulptomy paste (D3 SSC), (E6 SSC) cemented with glass ionomer
	POI do not bite on lip, no eating/drinking until numbness wears off, eat only on opposite side until numbness has worn off, call office if crown feels high or if there is discomfort or pain
	Assistant's initials

Safety

Be sure to wear PPE during the crown preparation and the pulpotomy. Change gloves after handling the formocresol since it is caustic and care should be taken to avoid contact with skin. Dispose of any gauze or leftover cotton pellets in the hazardous trash. If formocresol gets on the skin, it will cause a burning sensation. Wash with soap and water, and treat as a burn.

Pulpectomy Procedure

A **pulpectomy** is similar to the pulpotomy except that the nerve is removed from the pulp canal with a **barbed broach** and the canals are filed as with a root canal. After the canals are clean and filed, a thin mixture of zinc oxide and eugenol is placed in the canals with a **Lentulo bur**. The final restoration is then placed, which is usually a stainless steel crown or anterior esthetic crown.

Pediatric Orthodontic Treatment

When a child is seen early by the pediatric dentist, the child's oral development and growth can be evaluated and monitored for any future malocclusion. The size of teeth and jaws and the timing of development and eruption is genetically determined. The size of the teeth and the jaws are genetically independent of each other. The teeth may be too large for the jaws causing overcrowding and rotating teeth. The teeth may be too small for the jaws causing drifting, tipping, and rotating. A child's mouth with good occlusion will have primate spacing, a Class I occlusion with normal overjet and overbite, the teeth will be aligned with the alveolar bone, and the maxillary and mandibular teeth will meet with maximum contact. If the child does not have normal occlusion, it is called malocclusion. The child may need treatment to correct the malocclusion. The pediatric dentist has received specialty training in preventive and **interceptive** orthodontics that can eliminate the need for corrective orthodontics or more extensive treatment later.

Preventive Orthodontic Treatment

There are many conditions in the mouth that can affect the child's occlusion that the pediatric dentist can treat to prevent or minimize malocclusion. Approximately 50% of children have primate spacing. Primate spacing is genetically acquired and is the natural spacing of primary teeth that allows adequate space for the eruption of primary and permanent teeth. There are distinct diastemas between the maxillary lateral and maxillary canines and mandibular canines and mandibular first molars that accommodates larger primary and permanent teeth eruption. A child with inadequate primate spacing may have interproximal contacts, overcrowding, and rotating of teeth (Figure 34-21). With early detection, the dentist can help guide the teeth into the proper position with dental appliances.

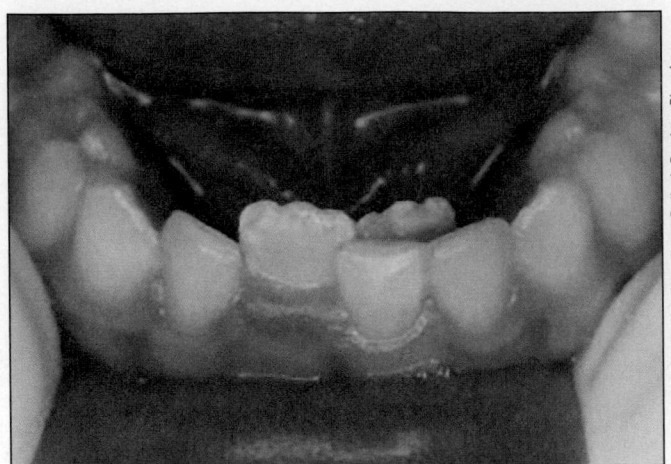

FIGURE 34-21
Inadequate primary spacing.

Courtesy of Dr. Keith Roberts, Bloomington Pediatric Dentistry, Bloomington, Indiana

There are many factors that can affect the development of the teeth. Dental caries, serious illness, nutritional deficiencies, and trauma can all impact the development of the teeth. If dental caries are allowed to progress, the carious tooth will lose tooth structure, allowing for adjacent teeth to begin drifting and a shifting of the teeth within the arches. With regular dental visits, the dentist can recognize decay and quickly restore the tooth to prevent any change in occlusion. The arrangement of the teeth can also be affected by muscle pressure. Patients who are thumb sucking, have a tongue thrust, or have strong frenum attachments can forcefully move the teeth. The pediatric dentist has many options for correcting the thumb sucking habit and tongue thrust including behavior modification and dental appliances. With early detection, the pediatric dentist can refer the child patient to a specialist to surgically correct frenum attachments before the occlusion is affected.

What happens to the primary dentition directly affects the health and eruption of the permanent dentition. The primary tooth acts as a natural space saver for the permanent teeth. The exfoliation and eruption of the teeth has a direct effect on the spacing of the teeth. Retained primary teeth causing late loss of the teeth would prevent the permanent tooth from erupting, causing the permanent tooth to erupt **ectopically**. Early loss of the primary teeth would allow for the present teeth to drift and close the edentulous space, preventing the permanent tooth from erupting into its proper position in occlusion. The pediatric dentist can closely monitor the natural exfoliation process and eruption pattern of the patient. Over-retained teeth can be extracted and spaces left from early loss of a tooth can be treated with the placement of space maintainers.

Space Maintainers When a primary tooth is lost prematurely, a space maintainer is required to hold the space for the permanent tooth. There are several different types of fixed space maintainers that can be used on the maxillary or mandibular teeth.

A band and loop or unilateral space maintainer is where a band is placed around the tooth behind the extraction site. A loop is soldered to an orthodontic band that extends from the buccal surface of the band and touches the tooth on the other side of the edentulous space to the lingual of the band. Once the tooth begins to erupt, the band and loop are removed (Figure 34-22).

Another type of space maintainer is a bilateral lingual arch. This type of space maintainer is needed when there is a space on both sides of the arch that requires two bands. An orthodontic band is placed on the teeth posterior to the edentulous space, and a soldered wire extends from the lingual surface of one band to the lingual surface of the band on the opposite side. The bilateral lingual arch can also help straighten and keep the anterior teeth in position (Figure 34-23).

A distal shoe is a space maintainer that is used when the primary second molar is extracted and the permanent molar has not erupted. It is similar to the band and loop space maintainer. The band is placed on the primary first molar and the loop with an intragingival blade that extends back to where the permanent molar will be erupting (Figure 34-24). An x-ray is required to determine how long the distal shoe should extend to the erupting permanent molar. It may be necessary to anesthetize the gingival area around the erupting permanent molar to deliver the distal shoe.

Interceptive Orthodontics

Pediatric dentists know the importance of guidance and management of the developing occlusion in the growing child using interceptive orthodontics. The skeletal support of the teeth and size of the maxillary and mandibular arch are genetically determined. The size of the teeth and the size of the arch do not always match. Due to the size of the teeth, the arch may not be large enough for all the teeth to erupt. This is called arch length inadequacy. When the pediatric dentist is examining the child's occlusion, the arch length is measured from the distal surface of the second primary molar on one side of the arch to the distal surface of the second primary molar on the opposite side. The dentist determines if all the teeth will be able to fit in the arch. If the dentist finds that there is an inadequacy, the arch can be made larger using arch expanders and palatal expanders, or teeth can be extracted to allow space for the remaining teeth to erupt (Figures 34-25 and 34-26).

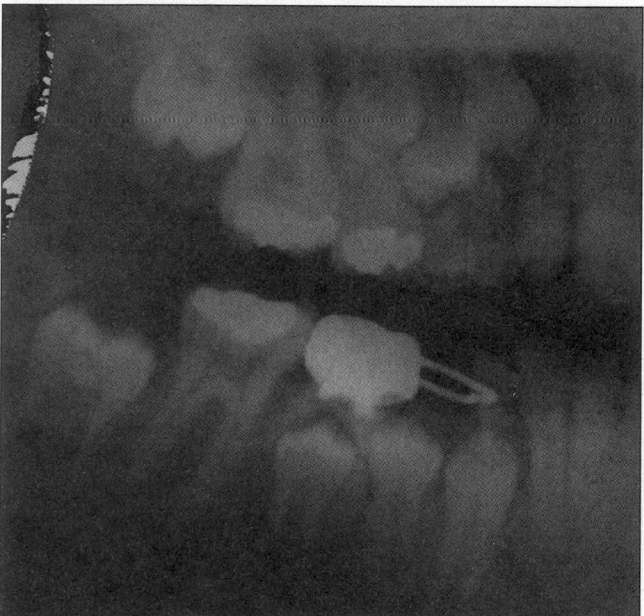

FIGURE 34-22
A radiograph of a patient with a fixed unilateral space maintainer (band and loop).

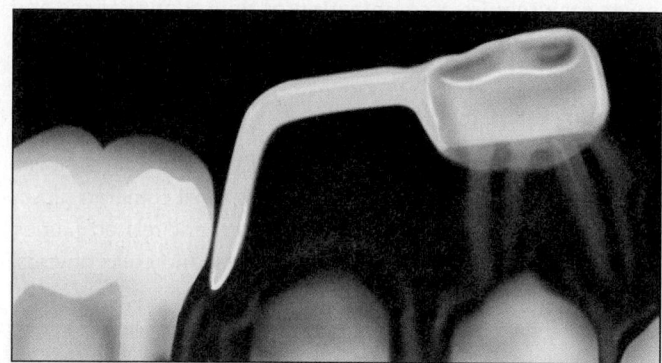

FIGURE 34-24
Distal shoe space maintainer.

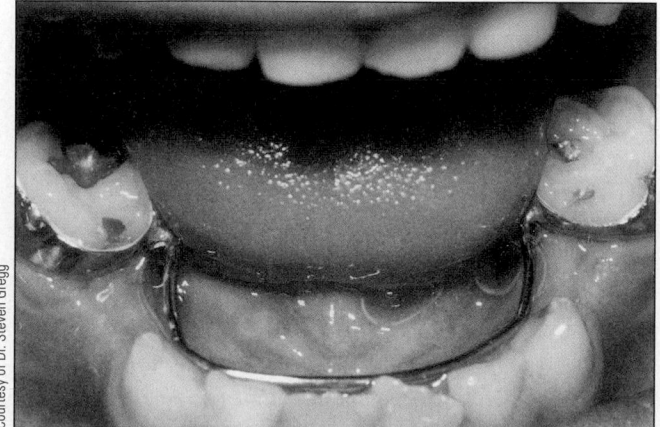

Courtesy of Dr. Steven Gregg

FIGURE 34-23
Fixed bilateral space maintainer (bilateral lingual arch).

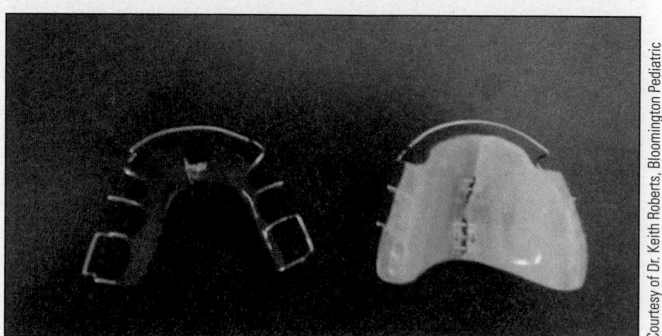

Courtesy of Dr. Keith Roberts, Bloomington Pediatric Dentistry, Bloomington, Indiana

FIGURE 34-25
Removable arch expander.

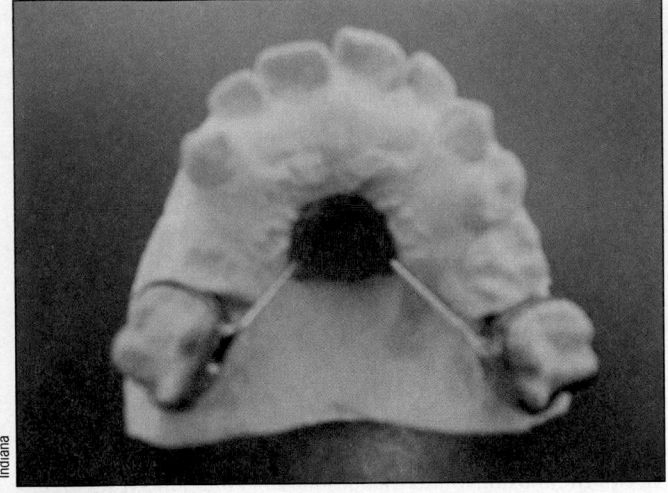

FIGURE 34-26
Fixed palatal expander.

How the maxillary and mandibular arches relate is also important for the development of occlusion. The maxillary arch should be larger, and the maxillary teeth should extend one cusp facial to the mandibular teeth. If the mandibular teeth are facial to the maxillary, this is a crossbite. A crossbite can happen with just one maxillary and one mandibular tooth in crossbite or posterior segments in crossbite; in more serious cases, the crossbite may involve the entire arch. One example of this is a Class III occlusion. Crossbites that involve just a few teeth can be corrected with dental appliances or full braces (Figure 34-27). Some Class III cases may require a combination of dental appliances and surgical correction of the jaw size relationship.

Pediatric Emergency Treatment

Traumatic injury to primary teeth and the orofacial area is a common occurrence in the pediatric office. Most common causes of child injuries include falls in infancy; sports and related injuries, collisions, and falls; automobile accidents; and child physical

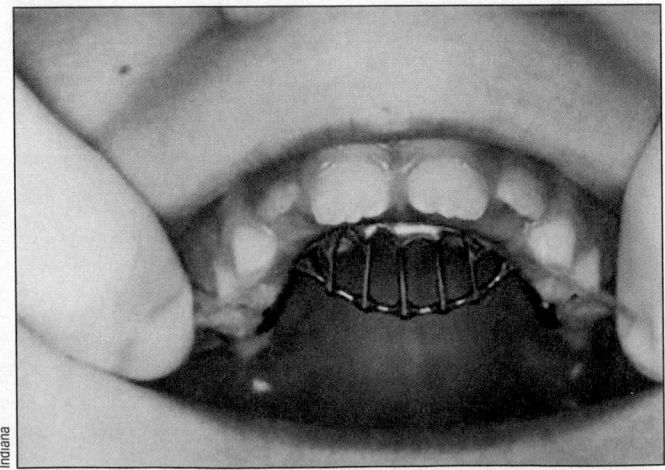

FIGURE 34-27
Crossbite appliance (can also be used as tongue/thumb habit appliance).

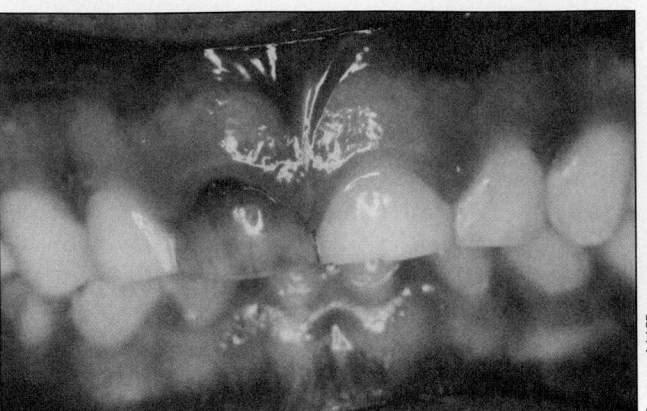

FIGURE 34-28
Color changes of injured primary teeth.

abuse (50% of injuries are to the face and orofacial areas). Injuries are seasonal with most happening in the summer when children have more outside activities. Anterior teeth rank the highest with 71% of the cases involving the maxillary central incisors. The most common age of injury is 1.5 to 2.5 years old when the child is learning to walk.

Primary Teeth Traumatic Injury

Diagnosis and complete documentation of the accident and injury are the first steps in treatment of any traumatic injury even when the injury is asymptomatic. Sometimes the teeth may become symptomatic in a few months or years later. The injured tooth may change in tooth color due to pulpal hemorrhage (reddish-brown or pink), pulp necrosis (bluish-black), and root canal obliteration (grayish-yellow) over time (Figure 34-28). The injured tooth and surrounding area should be examined at regular checkups.

Two common injuries to primary teeth are called a concussion and subluxation. A concussion is when there is injury to the tooth supporting structure without abnormal loosening or displacement of the tooth. The patient will react to percussion. Pressure from the accident may affect blood supply entering the tooth through the apical foramen. Nerve and blood vessels may become damaged or detached, which may result in pulp necrosis. Injury to the tooth supporting structure that causes an abnormal loosening without displacement of the tooth is called subluxation. In most cases, the tooth is allowed to naturally stabilize.

Primary Teeth Displacement Trauma

Displacement injuries of the maxillary anterior teeth are most common. The treatment for primary teeth is different than for permanent teeth. Some displacements seen in the pediatric office are as follows:

● Intrusive luxation: The displacement of the tooth is into the alveolar bone. In severe injuries, it may appear as the tooth has been lost (Figure 34-29). Most dentists will allow the primary tooth to spontaneously re-erupt. If the tooth is displaced into permanent tooth, the primary tooth is extracted.

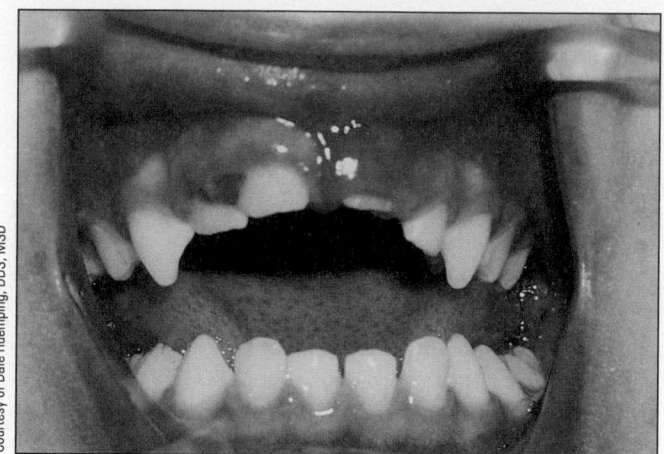

Courtesy of Dale Ruemping, DDS, MSD

FIGURE 34-29
A traumatic intrusion.

- **Extrusive** luxation: The tooth is partially displaced out of its socket. Clinically the tooth looks longer. If the primary tooth is intact and there is no sign of damaging the permanent tooth, the dentist may manually guide the tooth back into the socket. If it prematurely contacts the opposing tooth and potentially may damage the permanent tooth, the primary tooth is extracted.

- Lateral luxation: Occurs when the displacement of the tooth is in a mesial, distal, lingual, or labial direction (Figure 34-30). This injury is usually accompanied by fracture to alveolar components.

- **Avulsion**: This is when there is complete displacement of the tooth out of its socket. Due to possible injury to the permanent tooth or **ankylosis** of the tooth, the primary tooth is not reimplanted as with a permanent tooth.

Treatment for traumatized primary teeth varies greatly. Pediatric dentists consider the type and severity of the trauma, whether an alveolar fracture has occurred, and the potential effect on the developing permanent tooth. Most displacement and luxation injuries will heal spontaneously. The dentist will often give the injury time to heal, monitor only, and re-examine the tooth

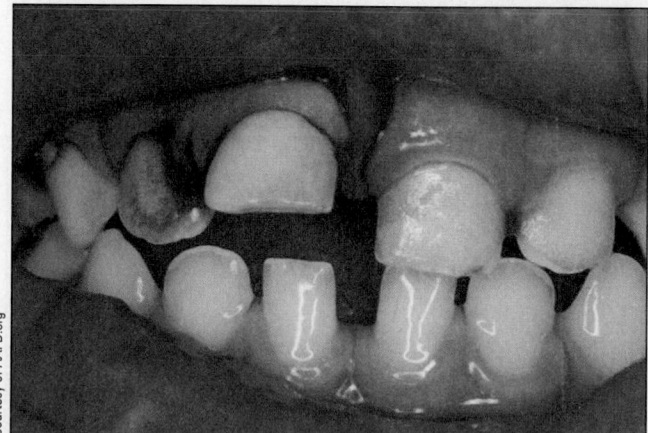

Courtesy of AAPD.org

FIGURE 34-30
A traumatic luxated tooth.

within a few days. Stabilization treatment is generally not performed on primary teeth as is used with permanent teeth. The exception would be when the loss of the primary tooth would result in a space for a period of time and when the permanent tooth has not erupted into the injury area. When there is the possibility that a very loose tooth may fall out and cause the child to choke, the tooth is extracted. Displaced teeth that interfere with occlusion are also extracted.

Effects on Permanent Tooth

The area should be radiographed whenever possible to check for the condition of the permanent tooth, fracturing of the tooth and root and alveolar bone injury. The injury may have also damaged a developing permanent tooth bud or an erupting permanent tooth lying below the injured primary tooth. Physical trauma to the primary tooth can disturb enamel formation (enamel hypoplasia) of the permanent tooth bud. Undetected periapical infection can interfere with tooth calcification (hypercalcification) of the underlying, developing permanent tooth.

Fractured Anterior Primary or Permanent Teeth

A common emergency with children is a fracture of the anterior tooth. Since children are very active, many children fall or hit their front teeth on the floor or other objects or are hit in the mouth with a ball or other objects. The fractures are usually classified as Class I, Class II, or Class III fractures depending on the size of the fracture and whether the pulp is involved or not.

When a patient presents with a fractured anterior tooth, the dentist will determine the extent of the injury and the classification of the fracture. The assistant will take an x-ray to determine if there are any root fractures or other injuries. Primary teeth with root fractures will be extracted. A fracture resulting in a pulp exposure on a primary tooth will require pulpotomy or pulpectomy treatment. A fracture of the permanent anterior tooth with a pulp exposure will require a root canal. If the fracture does not expose the pulp in a permanent tooth, then a sedative restoration may be placed to allow the tooth to heal before a final restoration is placed. If the tooth has a simple fracture of the enamel of the crown, sometimes the dentist will smooth the sharp edges, monitor, and re-examine the tooth within a few days. The caregiver should be instructed to rinse the child's mouth with warm water, keep the area clean, and apply cold compresses on the face to reduce swelling.

Orofacial Soft Tissue Trauma

Soft tissue injuries refer to injuries to the lip, tongue, frenulum, buccomucosa, floor of mouth, palate, and pharynx. These injuries may bleed a lot and are scary, but they rarely need suturing. Most small cuts and scrapes inside the mouth generally heal in three to four days with proper treatment. The most common mouth injury is from biting the tongue and oral mucosa. Cuts and bruises to the upper lip may also tear the frenum. The patient must be instructed to avoid pulling the lip out. Cuts of the lower lip are usually due to the child catching the lip between upper and lower teeth. The only injury that generally needs sutures is when the outer lip is gaping. Serious mouth injuries are to the tonsils, soft palate, and back of the pharynx. These typically are caused from the child falling with objects in their mouth. These children should be taken to the emergency room to make certain underlying tissue has not been damaged.

The treatment for most soft tissue trauma is the same:

- The first step is to stop bleeding with direct pressure against the site for 10 minutes.
- Try not to move injured area.
- Apply cold on area for 20 minutes: ice or a popsicle.
- Administer pain medication as needed: acetaminophen or ibuprofen.
- Keep on soft diet until injury closes. It is important to encourage the child to drink their favorite fluid to prevent dehydration; cold drinks and popsicles are especially good.
- Avoid salty or citrus foods that might sting.
- Rinse wound with warm water immediately after meals.

Prevention of Orofacial Injury

The best way to prevent trauma of primary teeth is to watch out for situations that can lead to dental injury. The home should be made childproof before the infant becomes mobile. Infants usually become mobile around 12–16 months, which often results in trips and falls. When children are first learning to stand, they use furniture to pull up and maintain balance. They have a tendency to fall down and hit their mouth on the furniture or pull items on the furniture down on them. It is important that there is a safe, clean environment with no sharp edges on tables, items positioned so children cannot pull items onto themselves, and furniture arranged to eliminate obstructions. Baby walkers tend to tip and cause falls. Care should be taken when using a walker, or avoid their use. Caution should be taken to never allow children to walk with any objects in their mouth, including a toothbrush. Falling with items in the mouth, including using a straw or eating food on a stick, are the most serious injuries.

Each year thousands of young children are killed or injured in car crashes. One of the most important ways of keeping children safe is the proper use of safety seats. The American Academy of Pediatrics recommends that all infants ride in rear-facing safety seats from their first ride home from the hospital until they are 2 years old. Children from 2 until school age use forward-facing safety seats with a harness, and school-aged children use a belt-positioning booster seat. Eating food on a stick and drinking with a straw can also lead to injuries with sudden stops and especially if the child is in a seat where an airbag deploys.

Teach children safe playing. Do not push or tackle when playing. Stay seated on the swing and do not jump off when the swing is in motion. When involved in any activity that may cause potential facial trauma, make sure the child uses a helmet and mouth protector. These activities include roller skating, skate boarding, bicycling, contact sports, and sports involving a ball or swinging an object. The American Dental Association and the Academy for Sports Dentistry recommend properly fitted mouth guards for recreational activities and sports that place participants at risk for oral injury. Studies show that mouth guards can significantly reduce the risk of mouth injuries and the incidence of concussion and jaw fractures in athletes.

Mouth guards are mainly worn on the maxillary teeth and are designed to stay in place while allowing the child to talk and breathe normally.

There are various types of mouth guards, including the following:

- Custom-fitted mouth guards are made by the dentist specifically for the patient. They involve taking impressions of the patient for a study model. The impressions are poured to make study models that are then used to fabricate a mouth guard. Once the mouth guard material is vacuum formed over the model, it is trimmed and finished for the patient (see Chapter 33, "Dental Laboratory Materials"; Figure 34-31). These mouth guards are more expensive but offer a better fit and the most protection to the mouth.

- Mouth-formed, or "boil and bite," mouth guards are mouth protectors that are usually purchased in sporting goods or athletic stores. These mouth guards are softened in heated water, inserted into the mouth, and then molded to fit the individual's arch (Figure 34-32). With this type of mouth guard, directions must be followed carefully to ensure that the mouth guard fits properly.

- Stock or ready-made mouth guards are preformed and ready to wear. They are inexpensive and do not fit as well as the other two types of mouth guards.

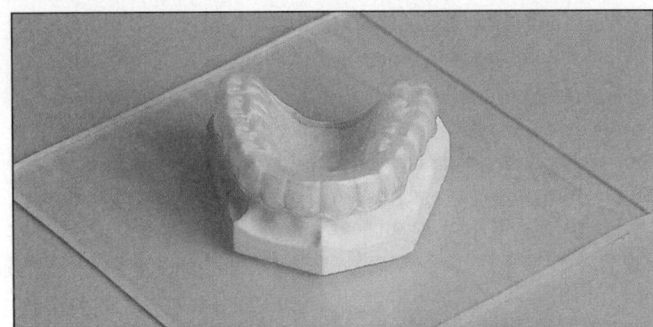

FIGURE 34-31
An example of mouth guard material and a formed mouth guard.

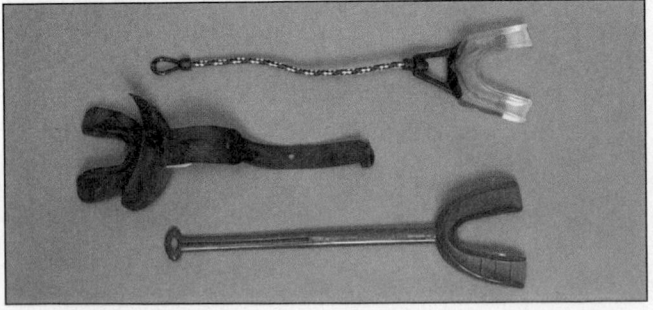

FIGURE 34-32
Various mouth guards used in athletics.

Chapter Summary

The scope of pediatric treatment includes restoring and maintaining the primary, mixed, and permanent dentition, and applying preventive measures for dental caries, periodontal disease, and malocclusion. The primary focus of the pediatric dental practice is preventive treatment and dealing with the compromised child patient. The whole staff needs to enjoy working with children and be sincere and honest in their actions and feelings. To be effective in the management of children, the dental team must be upbeat, motivated, and aware.

The role of the dental assistant in the pediatric practice will vary according to areas of responsibility. One part that the assistant is involved in is managing the child. Another part is the tasks that the assistant performs at chairside. Depending on the state, when assistants work independently, they assume the authority role and must maintain control of the child. The dental assistant is also an educator of the child and caregivers.

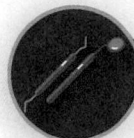

CASE STUDY

On Friday afternoon, Mr. Johnson brought his 4-year-old daughter, Shantel, to Dr. Bryan's office for emergency treatment. Shantel had fallen and hit her face. Her maxillary left central incisor was pushed into the alveolus so that only the incisal third of the tooth was exposed. Shantel had seen Dr. Bryan for an exam when she was 3-years-old.

Case Study Review

1. What is the condition of Shantel's teeth called? How will the dentist treat it?

2. At what stage of tooth eruption is Shantel likely to be? Are the permanent teeth affected? What treatment may need to be done if the permanent tooth is affected?

3. Because Shantel had only been in the office for one visit when she was 3 years, would behavior management be a consideration?

Review Questions

Multiple Choice

1. At what age does the pediatric dentist recommend the child's first dental visit occur?
   a. shortly after birth
   b. by their first birthday
   c. before preschool
   d. there is no specific recommendation.

2. Why is there a need for a child to visit a pediatric dentist?
   a. They are trained in behavior management of children.
   b. Children have different dental needs than adults.
   c. They monitor, prevent, and minimize malocclusion.
   d. All of these

3. What reason(s) can the dental assistant provide to a reluctant caregiver to have their child's teeth treated when they are going to fall out anyway?
   a. Some primary teeth remain in the mouth until age 12.
   b. They help in the development of speech.
   c. They are place holders for the permanent teeth.
   d. All of these

4. Which of these can contribute to pediatric dental caries?
   a. Caregiver saliva factors in early caries.
   b. Prolonged use of bottle may lead to ECC.
   c. Thinner enamel and higher pulp.
   d. All of these

5. What can the caregiver do to help reduce the transfer of *S. mutans* to the child?
   a. Improve their oral hygiene.
   b. Remove sugars from diet.
   c. Chew xylitol gum.
   d. Nothing can be done.

6. Charting mixed dentition is a challenge. All of these are ways to differentiate between primary and permanent teeth EXCEPT:
   a. primary teeth have thinner enamel.
   b. primary teeth have more distinct anatomy.
   c. primary teeth are whiter.
   d. primary teeth are smaller.

7. All of these are a part of the infant oral exam EXCEPT:
   a. charting mixed dentition.
   b. evaluating relationship of size of teeth and jaws.
   c. noting developments problems.
   d. coronal polishing.

8. What is the greatest dietary risk for dental health?
   a. deficiency of vitamins in diet
   b. sugar containing drinks in bottle and sippy cup
   c. absence of vegetables in diet
   d. abundance of fruits in diet

9. At what age should a child be weaned from the bottle?
   a. 6 months
   b. 1 year
   c. 1 ½ years
   d. 2 years

10. What type of topical professional application is recommended for preschool children and high risk caries patients?
    a. solutions
    b. gels
    c. foams
    d. varnishes

11. What rating would a child be given on the Frankl scale if they are uncooperative and reluctant to accept treatment?
    a. 4
    b. 3
    c. 2
    d. 1

12. What is the number one tool used in behavior management?
    a. communication
    b. modeling
    c. protective stabilization
    d. nitrous oxide

13. When would protective stabilization be used for child behavior management?
    a. a very defiant child
    b. child with special needs
    c. maintain safety of child during sedation
    d. All of these

14. When is a stainless steel crown used?
    a. after a pulpotomy
    b. tooth fracture
    c. hypoplastic carious tooth
    d. All of these

15. Which crown is made using crown forms and composite resin and is preferred for an anterior tooth?
    a. veneered steel crown
    b. strip crown
    c. ceramic crown
    d. porcelain crown

16. A _____ procedure is the removal of only the coronal portion of the pulp.
    a. pulpectomy
    b. pulpotomy
    c. direct pulp capping
    d. RCT

17. What medicament is used to cauterize the tissue during a pulpotomy procedure?
    a. eugenol
    b. etchant
    c. formocresol
    d. MTA

18. What is the name of the procedure where all the pulp is removed from the tooth and is not filled?
    a. pulpectomy
    b. pulpotomy
    c. direct pulp capping
    d. RCT

19. Which of these can forcefully move the teeth?
    a. thumb sucking
    b. tongue thrust
    c. strong frenum attachments
    d. All of these

20. What appliance is used when there is an edentulous space between two teeth to maintain the space until the permanent tooth erupts?
    a. lingual arch
    b. distal shoe
    c. band and loop
    d. arch expander

Critical Thinking

1. How does the child's chronological, maturity, and emotional age affect dental care?

2. At the child's first dental visit, the dental assistant notices the child has a lot of old and new facial bruises and a split lip. When they ask the child if he fell to get those bruises, the child tells them that his mommy hit him when he was bad. During the oral exam, they notice rampant caries and many chipped teeth. What should the assistant and dentist do?

3. Why is it contraindicated to perform a root canal on a primary and developing permanent tooth?

4. What is the function of primary teeth in the proper eruption of the permanent teeth? What happens if a primary tooth is lost early? Or retained?

5. What oral conditions and factors cause malocclusion in the pediatric patient?

Key Terms

Term and Pronunciation	Meaning of Root and Word Parts	Definition
abuse (*uh*-**byooz**)	**ab-** = away from **use** = to treat or behave toward	to treat in harmful, injurious or offensive way
abutment (*uh*-**buht**-m*uh*nt)	**abut** = join at the border **-ment** = resulting state	a tooth or tooth root that supports a prosthetic appliance like bridge or denture
ankylosis (ang-*kuh*-**loh**-sis)	**ankylose** = to unite or grow together **-osis** = abnormal condition	abnormal adhesion of bones of a joint; consolidation of two or more bones or other hard tissues into one
autism (**aw**-tiz-*uh*m)	**auto** = self **-ism** = indicating a state or condition	a tendency to view life in terms of one's own needs and desires; developmental disorder with deficits in communication and social interaction
avulsion (*uh*-**vuhl**-sh*uh*n)	**avulse** = a tearing away, a part torn off **-sion** = expressing action	a forcible tearing away or separation of a bodily structure or part; result of injury or as surgical procedure
barbed broach (bahrbd) (brohch)	**barb** = a sharp pointed part **-ed** = indicating a condition **broach** = tool for shaping and enlarging	thin, flexible endodontic instrument with sharply pointed barbs used to remove the dental pulp from root canal or pulp chamber
cauterize (**kaw**-t*uh*-rahyz)	**cautery** = electric current and lasers used to cut or destroy tissue	to burn or cut tissue with electric current and laser in surgical procedures
cerebral palsy (s*uh*-**ree**-br*uh*l) (**pawl**-zee)	**cerebrum** = largest part of brain **-al** = of or pertaining to **palsy** = paralysis; atonal muscular condition with tremors of body parts	a form of paralysis; thought to be caused by prenatal brain defect or by brain injury during birth
chronological age (kron-l-**oj**-i-k*uh*l) (eyj)	**chron** = arranged in order of time **-ology** = branch of knowledge **-ical** = pertaining to **age** = a period of human life	number of years a person has lived; used as a psychometrics standard to measure behavior, intelligence, and development and growth
concussion (k*uh*n-**kuhsh**-*uh*n)	**concuss** = to injure by a violent blow, fall **-tion** = indicating condition	an injury to a structure produced by a violent blow; temporary or prolonged loss of function
congenital heart disease (k*uh*n-**jen**-i-tl) (hahrt) (dih-**zeez**)	**congenital** = existing at birth **heart** = hollow muscular organ that pumps blood through circulatory system **disease** = a disordered or incorrectly functioning organ, part, or system	born with heart disease that affects mechanisms of the heart; heart may not work correctly or a problem in the structure of the heart
crossbite (**kraws**-bahyt)	**cross** = to move, pass, or extend from one side or place to another **bite** = contact between the upper and lower teeth when the mouth is closed naturally	deviation of tooth position or abnormal jaw position; the mandibular tooth is facial to the maxillary
cystic fibrosis (sist-**ik**) (fahy-**broh**-sis)	**cyst** = abnormal membranous sac containing fluid; develops in response to adverse conditions **-ic** = nature of **fiber** = elongated threadlike cell **-osis** = a state of disease **fibrosis** = formation excess fibrous connective tissue	hereditary chronic disease of exocrine glands producing abnormally thick mucus; impaired pancreas, chronic respiratory infections, and sweat glands infections
demeaning (dih-**mee**-ning)	**demean** = downgrade **-ing** = expressing the action	to lower in dignity, degrade, humiliate
distraction (dih-**strak**-sh*uh*n)	**distract** = to draw away or divert the mind or attention **-tion** = the act of	a condition or state of mind when the attention is diverted from the original focus or interest
Down syndrome (doun) (**sin**-drohm)	**Down** = British physician; discoverer **syndrome** = a group of symptoms that together are characteristic of a disorder, disease	congenital condition caused by abnormality in chromosomes; moderate to severe intellectual retardation and changes in certain physical features (short stature and flat facial profile)

(Continues)

Term and Pronunciation	Meaning of Root and Word Parts	Definition
early childhood caries (**ur**-lee) (**chahyld**-hood) (**kair**-eez)	**early** = before the usual or appointed time **child** = a person between birth and puberty **hood** = body of persons of a particular character or class **caries** = progressive decay of a bone or a tooth	the presence of one or more decayed, missing, or filled tooth surfaces in a child 71 months of age or younger; previously referred to as nursing bottle syndrome
ectopic (ek-**top**-ik)	**ectopia** = out of place **-ic** = relating to	occurring in an abnormal position or place, occurs congenitally or displaced by injury
emotional age (ih-**moh**-shuh-nl) (eyj)	**emotion** = any of the feelings of joy, sorrow, fear, hate, love, hate **-al** = pertaining to **age** = a period of human life	a measure of emotional maturity by comparison with average emotional development
extraction forceps (ik-**strak**-shuhn) (**fawr**-suh ps)	**extract** = to pull out with force **-ion** = denoting action **forceps** = instrument for seizing or holding objects	instrument used to remove teeth
extrusive (ik-**stroo**-siv)	**extrude** = to thrust outward **-ive** = tending to	to be forced out to a protruded position
fluorosis (floo-**roh**-sis)	**fluorine** = nonmetallic poisonous gas element; in fluoride form prevents tooth decay **-osis** = condition; especially disorders or abnormal states of formation or development	abnormal condition caused by excessive intake of fluoride; discolors and pits teeth and pathological bone changes; also called mottled enamel
formocresol (fawrm-oh-**kree**-sawl)	**form** = formaldehyde; disinfectant and preservative **cresol** = disinfectant	used in vital primary teeth needing coronal pulpotomy; it preserves the remaining pulp in the canal for the root to continue development
interceptive (in-ter-**sept**-tiv)	**intercept** = to take between; to stop, deflect on the way from one place to another **-ive** = tending to	to stop or interrupt the course or progress from one place to another
intervention (in-ter-**ven**-shuhn)	**intervene** = to occur or happen between other events or periods in time **-tion** =act or fact of	to interrupt or modify a situation
Lentulo bur (len-**tyu**-luh) (bur)	**lentus** = flexible, pliant **bur** = rotary cutting tool	motorized, flexible, spiral instrument used to apply paste filling material into root canal
luxation (**luhk**-sey-shuhn)	**luxate** = to put out of joint, dislocate **-tion** = indicating action	to loosen tooth from tooth socket
mandate (**man**-deyt)	**mandate** = to order or require	a command or authorization to act in a particular way
maturity age (muh-**choor**-i-tee) (eyj)	**mature** = fully developed in mind and body	a measure of maturity by comparison with average maturational development
modeling (**mod**-l-ing)	**model** = a standard or example for imitation or comparison **-ing** = the act	representing behavior or technique that is the standard or desired behavior
necrosis (nuh-**kroh**-sis)	**necro** = dead tissue, the dead, corpse **-osis** = denoting state	death of one or more cells in the body through injury or disease
neglect (ni-**glekt**)	**neglect** = to pay no or little attention; ignore	to be remiss in the care or treatment of
obliteration (uh-blit-uh-**rey**-shuhn)	**obliterate** = to remove or destroy all traces of; do away with, destroy completely **-tion** = the act of or the state of being	the removal of a part as a result of disease or surgery
pediatrics (pee-dee-**a**-triks)	**pedo** = child **-iatrics** = healing, medical practice	the branch of dentistry and medicine concerned with the development, care, and diseases of infants, children and patients with special needs
pharmacological (fahr-muh-**kol**-uh-jee-kuhl)	**pharmaceutical** = substance used in diagnosis, treatment, or prevention of disease **ology** = branch of knowledge, science	the science dealing with the preparation, uses, and especially the effects of drugs in treatment of disease

Term and Pronunciation	Meaning of Root and Word Parts	Definition
protective stabilization (pr*uh*-**tek**-tiv) (stey-b*uh*-li-**zey**-sh*uh*n)	**protect** = to defend or guard from injury or loss **-ive** = having the quality or function **stable** = not likely to fall or give way; able to continue or last **-tion** = the act or process of	purpose to ensure the safety of the patient; used when management techniques are insufficient; previously referred to as restraint (board/wrap)
pulpectomy (puhl-**pek**-t*uh*-mee)	**pulp** = inner substance of the tooth; contains arteries, vein, lymphatic, and nerve tissue **-ectomy** = excision, complete surgical removal	the removal of all the pulp tissue in a tooth in the course of endodontic therapy
pulpotomy (puhl-**pot**-*uh*-mee)	**pulp** = inner substance of the tooth; contains arteries, vein, lymphatic, and nerve tissue **-tomy** = cutting, incision; partial removal of a specified part, section or tissue	the removal of infected portions of the pulp tissue in a tooth; used as therapeutic measure to avoid pulpectomy
pulse oximeter (puhls) (ok-**sim**-i-ter)	**pulse** = regular throbbing of the arteries **ox(i)-** = containing oxygen **meter** = measure	measure proportion of oxygenated hemoglobin in the blood in pulsating vessels; esp. capillaries of finger or ear
rampant (**ram**-p*uh*nt)	**rampant** = widespread, unrestrained	disease growing or developing unchecked
sedate (si-**deyt**)	**sedate** = to calm or relieve anxiety	to treat with medications to calm and quiet an anxious patient
sequelae (si-**kwee**-l*uh*)	**sequel** = a consequence or result; anything that follows from something else	an abnormal condition resulting from a previous disease
spina bifida (**spahy**-n*uh*) (**bif**-i-d*uh*)	**spine** = backbone **bifida** = split spine	a congenital defect in which the spinal column is imperfectly closed so that part of the spinal cord may protrude; often resulting in neurological disorders
subluxation (suhb-luhk-**sey**-sh*uh*n)	**sub** = slightly, under **luxate** = to put out of joint, dislocate **-tion** = indicating action	an incomplete or partial dislocation of a tooth from the tooth socket
tongue thrust (tuhng) (thruhst)	**tongue** = muscular tissue attached to the floor of the mouth; aid in mastication and swallowing **thrust** = to push with force	infantile pattern of the suckle-swallow movement; tongue is placed between the incisor teeth or between the alveolar ridges during the initial stage of swallowing
veneer (vuh-**neer**)	**veneer** = any facing material that is applied to a different backing for a pleasing appearance	a layer of tooth-colored material, porcelain, or acrylic resin, attached to the surface of a natural tooth or metal crown

CHAPTER 35
Orthodontics

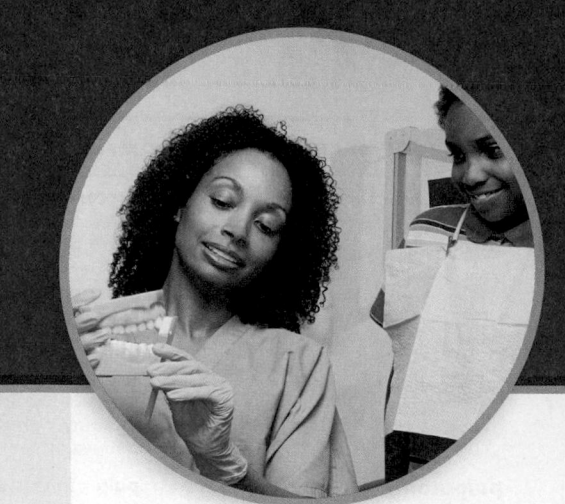

Specific Instructional Objectives

At the completion of this chapter, you will be able to meet these objectives:

1. Use terms presented in this chapter.
2. Describe the role and responsibilities of each member of the orthodontic team.
3. Discuss the purpose of each section of an orthodontic new patient exam.
4. Explain the four planes of space when evaluating the occlusion and skeletal patterns.
5. Describe three etiological factors in the cause of a malocclusion.
6. Summarize the process of developing a diagnosis and an orthodontic treatment plan by the orthodontist.
7. List each orthodontic diagnostic record that is needed for diagnosis and orthodontic treatment planning.
8. Describe the steps in conducting a treatment plan consultation with a patient.
9. Describe the types of orthodontic treatment provided to young children.
10. Describe the types of orthodontic treatment of adolescents including the use of growth appliances.
11. Describe the types of orthodontic treatment of adults including clear aligner therapy and orthognathic surgery.
12. Discuss the purpose and types of orthodontic retention of the final result.
13. Sequence comprehensive orthodontic treatment appointments.

Introduction

Most think of **orthodontics** as braces for kids, but it is much more. Orthodontics is the dental specialty that deals with the recognition, prevention, and treatment of malalignment and irregularities of the teeth, jaws, and facial profile. Patients are of all ages, ranging from young children to teenagers, adults, and seniors. Comprehensive orthodontic treatment provides a beautiful smile that brings teeth, lips, and jaws into proper alignment, and it has been shown to improve the self-esteem of the patient. Alignment of the teeth and jaws enhances dental and periodontal health by easier cleaning and improves mastication due to a more effective occlusion, with long-lasting results (Figure 35-1).

Focus of Orthodontic Treatment

Orthodontics is focused on the alignment of the teeth and the maxillary and mandibular jaws to establish a functional **occlusion** that will enhance mastication, and to create an esthetic facial appearance as well as a beautiful smile. When the teeth do not fit together properly, the relationship is then called

a **malocclusion**. Often a malocclusion is not just confined to the dental relationships, but there may be a separate skeletal problem of an abnormal jaw relationship between the maxilla and the mandible. These dental and jaw relationship problems may contribute to poor oral hygiene, which can lead to dental caries, gingivitis, and periodontal disease. Malocclusion can worsen chewing function, digestion, and overall nutritional well-being.

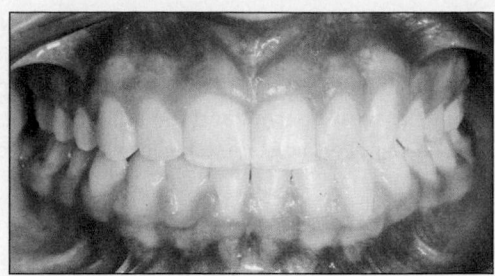

FIGURE 35-1
A healthy mouth.

Some types of malocclusion can trigger temporomandibular joint pain. A malocclusion may bring on bruxing and clenching habits that could worsen tooth wear and cause tooth fractures, dental abfractions with gingival recession, and tooth sensitivity.

Most forms of orthodontic problems have been shown to negatively affect an individual's self-esteem and psychosocial development. Children who have an imperfect smile are teased and bullied more than children who have a "normal" smile. Adults who have crooked teeth or missing teeth are less likely to be selected for employment that involves interaction with the general public.

The practitioner providing orthodontic treatment has to evaluate all of the needs of the potential orthodontic patient and determine which type of orthodontic care will satisfy those needs. If this comprehensive evaluation is done, and patients are then informed so that they have realistic expectations, the practice can anticipate having satisfaction for helping others feel good about their smile.

The Orthodontic Team

The orthodontic team has several members, each with a very specific role and responsibilities. Each member is described in detail below.

Orthodontist

The orthodontist is a licensed dentist who has two to three years of additional orthodontic residency training beyond the typical four years of dental school. The orthodontist must then pass the American Board of Orthodontics written exam to graduate and practice as an orthodontist. In many states, the orthodontist must obtain a specialty license to be listed as having a practice limited to orthodontics. Orthodontists focus on the function of the occlusion (the bite) as well as optimal facial and smile esthetics. They learn in orthodontic residency training to also use growth in children to align the maxillary and mandibular jaws for improved facial esthetics and a functional occlusion. They also learn how to prepare adult patients for orthognathic surgical alignment of the jaws, which is performed by an oral surgeon.

General dentists may provide some orthodontic care such as limited clear aligner therapy that focuses on the esthetics of the smile. Dentists receive limited orthodontic training in dental school since it is a complex specialty. They may not list themselves as orthodontic specialists unless they have completed an orthodontic residency training program. At this time dentists are not trained in dental school in the examination of an orthodontic patient or in orthodontic diagnosis and treatment planning using orthodontic records. They have to obtain this training after graduation from dental school.

The orthodontist is responsible for examining and diagnosing patients, planning the treatment for each patient, and then delivering and monitoring that treatment. Often the orthodontist may delegate the performance of procedures to a qualified team member. Even if the orthodontist delegates procedures to other team members, the orthodontist is ultimately responsible for all of the treatment that is delivered to patients.

Orthodontic Scheduling Coordinator

This individual is responsible for scheduling all orthodontic patients. Scheduling for orthodontics is different than that for general dentistry in that orthodontists often see many patients per day for short adjustment appointments. The schedule is usually computerized and organized by treatment procedure. The scheduling coordinator schedules appointments based on patient convenience. The appointment is also scheduled based on how it fits in with the practice daily plan. For children, the appointments are scheduled after school as much as possible.

The coordinator schedules all new patients, orthodontic records, treatment consults, and financial arrangements, and then sets up the appointments to start orthodontic treatment. During treatment, this member may also coordinate appointments with other specialists such as oral surgeons or periodontists. The coordinator must understand the delivery of orthodontic treatment and be able to communicate well with patients and the caregiver (parents or guardians).

Orthodontic Treatment and Financial Coordinator

The orthodontic treatment coordinator is responsible for conducting with the orthodontist the orthodontic new patient exam and all follow up with the patient, for conducting the treatment consultation and all interactions with other practitioners, and conducting the post-treatment consultation. Essentially, the treatment coordinator is the patient's go-to person if the patient or other individuals involved with the patient have any questions or concerns. This individual may also be the financial coordinator.

The financial coordinator is responsible for all of the financial interactions with patients. Orthodontic practices usually offer payment plans for financing orthodontic treatment. A financial coordinator knows how to work with insurance companies to file and track payment of claims, to set up financial contracts for monthly payments with the patient or caregivers, and to monitor payments monthly. Essentially, the financial coordinator is responsible for keeping the financial health of the practice in order.

Orthodontic Records Coordinator

In an orthodontic practice, "diagnostic records" are taken on each patient for the orthodontist to use in order to diagnose the orthodontic problems and plan treatment to correct those problems. The records coordinator produces:

1. An orthodontic series of photographs and evaluates them for diagnostic quality

2. Alginate or PVS (vinyl polysiloxane) dental impressions and bite registration, or a digital intraoral scan of the teeth and occlusion

3. Study models from the impressions or create digital models from the intraoral scan and analyzes the models for specific measurements

4. Cephalometric headfilm radiographic image to determine skeletal and dental relationships, digitizes the image, and produces an analysis of the image for the orthodontist

5. Panoramic radiographic image and reviews the image for diagnostic quality

6. Periapical radiographic images as needed to evaluate dental and bone integrity

For many of these procedures, the records coordinator must complete certification courses allowing them to perform these procedures in the state. These state regulations are spelled out in the state Dental Practice Act. Every member of the team should be knowledgeable about the state's regulations of dental personnel to be certain they are in compliance and are not in violation and subject to legal consequences.

Orthodontic Chairside Assistants or Certified Orthodontic Assistant (COA)

Orthodontic assistants perform many important chairside and nonchairside functions. If trained and licensed, they may:

1. Prepare the patient's teeth for orthodontic bonding of brackets (braces) and assist in the positioning of brackets for approval by the orthodontist before the bonding adhesive is cured that will hold the brackets in place.

2. Place and remove separators that make space between the teeth for orthodontic bands to be cemented to the teeth.

3. Fit and cement orthodontic bands to the teeth.

4. Insert an initial alignment orthodontic wire after bonding the brackets, tie it in, and give the patient oral hygiene and post-bonding instructions.

5. Select orthodontic wires depending upon the phase of orthodontic treatment and approval by the orthodontist.

6. Conduct a retie orthodontic adjustment appointment reviewing patient progress, checking orthodontic wires, summarizing patient status to the doctor, receiving and performing instructions from the doctor, and making treatment record notes.

7. Remove the orthodontic brackets and bands at the completion of treatment.

8. Place bonded or removable retainers.

Credentialing is available through the Dental Assistant National Board to become a certified orthodontic assistant (COA). In some states, dental assistants may receive board-approved training for the orthodontic assistant permit and then qualify to sit for the Orthodontic Assistant Permit Exam to be licensed to perform the duties of the orthodontic assistant.

Infection Control Coordinator

Since an orthodontic practice treats a high number of patients per day, most practices have an infection control coordinator who is responsible for sterilization of all instruments, preparing and cleaning chairs between patients, maintaining an inventory control system, ordering clinical supplies, and conducting OSHA training following the Infection Control Plan for the practice.

Orthodontic New Patient Exam

The process of orthodontic treatment has many components that are combined to provide all necessary data to the team members in the office. This will allow the best possible treatment plan to be formulated by the orthodontist for the patient.

The orthodontist will examine the occlusion and skeletal relationships of the new patient, identify the causes of problems, and determine what treatment should be provided. Understanding what the orthodontist evaluates will help the dental team to carry out the objectives of treatment and achieve the desired outcomes of various orthodontic treatment options.

Orthodontic treatment begins with the patient recognizing that they would like to improve their smile and chewing function. Patients may be referred to the orthodontist by their dentist, a friend, or a neighbor. Usually the new patient orthodontic exam is the patient's first encounter with the orthodontist and the team. The purpose of the exam is for the orthodontist to get to know the patient, understand the patient's concerns, conduct a thorough examination, note causes of malocclusion, and then propose treatment that will address those concerns. Together, the patient and the orthodontist will determine if they can achieve the desired result.

Patient Information

If the office has a new patient coordinator, this team member will obtain the basic information such as age, birthdate, and work or school attendance. In the event that the orthodontic office does not have a new patient coordinator, the dental assistant will obtain this information.

Medical and Dental History

Once the medical history is obtained, the orthodontist will determine whether or not the patient may have growth potential that could be used to align the jaws. Girls usually have a growth spurt at ages 10 years to 14 years. Boys have their growth spurt at ages 13 years to 17 years. Questions are asked to determine if the patient is about to undergo this growth spurt (Figure 35-2).

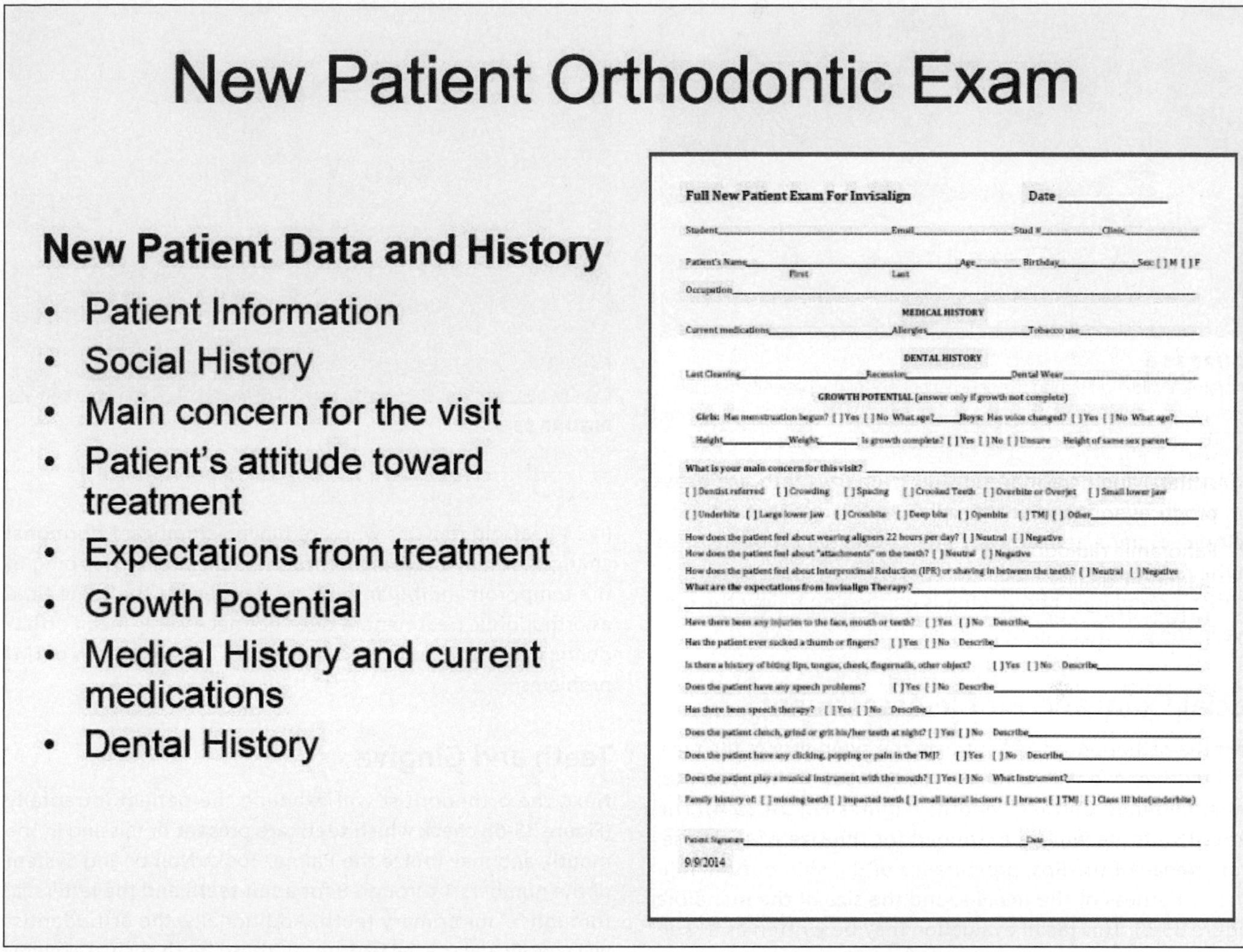

New Patient Orthodontic Exam

New Patient Data and History

- Patient Information
- Social History
- Main concern for the visit
- Patient's attitude toward treatment
- Expectations from treatment
- Growth Potential
- Medical History and current medications
- Dental History

Full New Patient Exam For Invisalign   Date _____

Student_____Email_____Stud #_____Clinic_____

Patient's Name_____Age_____Birthday_____Sex: [ ] M [ ] F
                    First   Last

Occupation_____

MEDICAL HISTORY

Current medications_____Allergies_____Tobacco use_____

DENTAL HISTORY

Last Cleaning_____Recession_____Dental Wear_____

GROWTH POTENTIAL (answer only if growth not complete)

Girls: Has menstruation begun? [ ] Yes [ ] No What age?_____ Boys: Has voice changed? [ ] Yes [ ] No What age?_____

Height_____Weight_____ Is growth complete? [ ] Yes [ ] No [ ] Unsure   Height of same sex parent_____

What is your main concern for this visit?

[ ] Dentist referred   [ ] Crowding   [ ] Spacing   [ ] Crooked Teeth   [ ] Overbite or Overjet   [ ] Small lower jaw

[ ] Underbite   [ ] Large lower jaw   [ ] Crossbite   [ ] Deep bite   [ ] Openbite   [ ] TMJ [ ] Other_____

How does the patient feel about wearing aligners 22 hours per day? [ ] Neutral [ ] Negative

How does the patient feel about "attachments" on the teeth? [ ] Neutral [ ] Negative

How does the patient feel about Interproximal Reduction (IPR) or shaving in between the teeth? [ ] Neutral [ ] Negative

What are the expectations from Invisalign Therapy?_____

Have there been any injuries to the face, mouth or teeth? [ ] Yes [ ] No Describe_____

Has the patient ever sucked a thumb or fingers? [ ] Yes [ ] No Describe_____

Is there a history of biting lips, tongue, cheek, fingernails, other object? [ ] Yes [ ] No Describe_____

Does the patient have any speech problems? [ ] Yes [ ] No Describe_____

Has there been speech therapy? [ ] Yes [ ] No Describe_____

Does the patient clench, grind or grit his/her teeth at night? [ ] Yes [ ] No Describe_____

Does the patient have any clicking, popping or pain in the TMJ? [ ] Yes [ ] No Describe_____

Does the patient play a musical instrument with the mouth? [ ] Yes [ ] No What Instrument?_____

Family history of: [ ] missing teeth [ ] impacted teeth [ ] small lateral incisors [ ] braces [ ] TMJ [ ] Class III bite(underbite)

Patient Signature_____Date_____

9/9/2014

Courtesy of Dr. Rebecca Poling

FIGURE 35-2
Medical and dental history, growth potential, habits, concerns, expectations, questions.

The orthodontist or dental assistant will also obtain the patient's dental history such as present restorations, previous trauma to the teeth or jaws, presence of pain in the teeth or jaws, oral hygiene habits, and nutrition habits. If a patient has poor oral hygiene, consumes sugary drinks such as soda, or consumes large amounts of sugary snacks, the patient may not be a good candidate for orthodontic treatment due to the high risk for dental decay and gingivitis if orthodontic appliances are worn.

The orthodontist or dental assistant asks questions about oral habits the patient has such as thumb sucking, finger sucking, lip biting, bruxism or grinding of the teeth, clenching the teeth together, and other dental habits that the patient may have that can affect the teeth.

Chief Complaint

The most important part of the new patient exam is determining the concerns of the patient (and caregiver if the patient is a minor) about the patient's smile (Figure 35-2). It is critical that the orthodontist address this concern right from the beginning. Patients want to know that they have been heard and that the practice wants the patient to be happy by having their concerns met. It is important to understand the expectations of the patient.

It is also important for the orthodontist to assess the attitude of the patient about orthodontic treatment. For example, 10-year-old children often are very excited about getting braces because it is a status symbol in fifth grade. By the time they are 13 years old, however, braces are the last thing they want! When boys are at the best age for growth and treatment (age 14), they are at the worst age socially for braces. Braces should not be placed on patients who do not want them! Patients who do not desire braces will not be compliant with oral hygiene or regularly scheduled visits to monitor and adjust the wires. As a result, treatment may not be successful.

Panoramic Evaluation

Ideally, a recent panoramic radiograph (Figure 35-3) is available so that the orthodontist may determine what teeth are present in the maxilla and mandible. The orthodontist can dictate to the assistant who is recording in the patient's chart

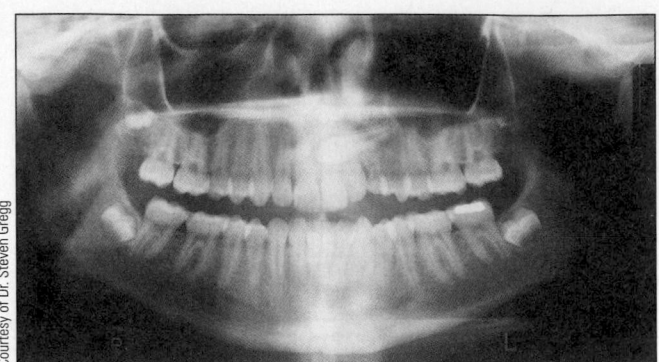

Courtesy of Dr. Steven Gregg

FIGURE 35-3
Panoramic evaluation during the new patient exam. The patient's maxillary left canine is ectopic and positioned horizontally.

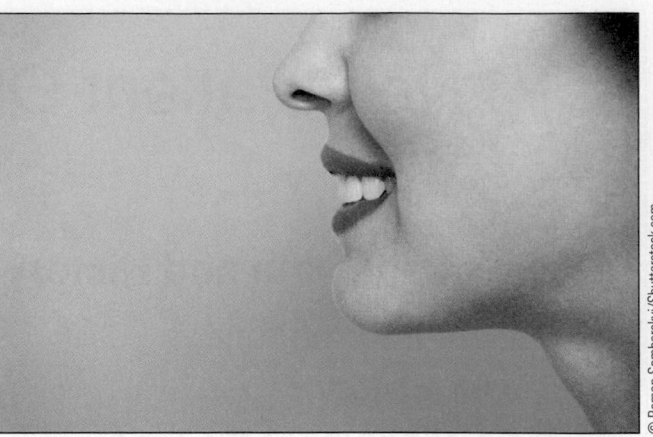

© Roman Samborskyi/Shutterstock.com

FIGURE 35-5
Normal profile.

regarding which permanent and primary teeth are present, which teeth are missing, which teeth are out of position (ectopic) or impacted, and any other potential problems seen on the radiograph. This panoramic evaluation gives the orthodontist a good idea about what is happening below the gingiva in the patient's mouth.

Facial Exam and Profile Assessment

Next the orthodontist will evaluate the symmetry of the face, the length of the face, and any unevenness of the eyes, lips, smile, midlines, and jaw lengths (Figures Figure 35-4). The patient's profile will be examined for the size of the nose, prominence of the lips, prominence of the chin button, fullness or flatness of the maxilla, and the size of the mandible (Figure 35-5). This facial evaluation may be written as a skeletal evaluation that summarizes the relationships of the jaws to each other and may later be confirmed and quantified through cephalometric analysis.

TMJ and Functional Evaluation

The function of the temporomandibular joint (TMJ) is evaluated for trauma, clicking, popping, and symptoms of pain.

In 13-year-old females who are having significant hormonal changes, it may be coincidental that clicking or popping in the temporomandibular joint may appear at the same time as orthodontic treatment. It does not necessarily mean orthodontic treatment has caused these signs and symptoms of TMJ problems.

Teeth and Gingiva

Next, the orthodontist will examine the patient intraorally (Figure 35-6), check which teeth are present or missing in the mouth, and may utilize the Palmer Tooth Numbering System of the numbers 1 through 8 for adult teeth and the letters "a" through "e" for primary teeth. Additionally, the orthodontist will specify any special features of those teeth such as crowns, unusual shapes or sizes, decay, and **hypocalcifications**. The orthodontist will note any decayed teeth that must be restored before orthodontic treatment. The current number of restored teeth may be used as an indication of oral hygiene history and tendency to develop decay.

The periodontium is evaluated for health and other factors. Usually it is more difficult for a patient to brush and floss with braces in place. If the patient has gingivitis before orthodontic treatment then the gingival condition may worsen after the braces are placed. In most cases, braces should not be placed in patients who have poor oral hygiene, poor nutritional habits, decay, and gingival disease. Oral health should be optimized before initiating any orthodontic treatment.

Often patients want to have a gap or **diastema** (Figure 35-7A) closed between the maxillary central incisors. Frequently in adults this diastema is partly due to a strong muscle pull or frenum that is deeply embedded in the bone between the teeth (Figure 35-7B). If the gap is closed but the frenum is not removed, the gap may simply reopen due to the muscle fibers embedded in the bone. It is best to close the gap, correct any tongue positioning in the gap, and then have minor surgery done by a periodontist to remove the frenum from the bone. The gap will usually heal with the space closed and it generally will not reopen.

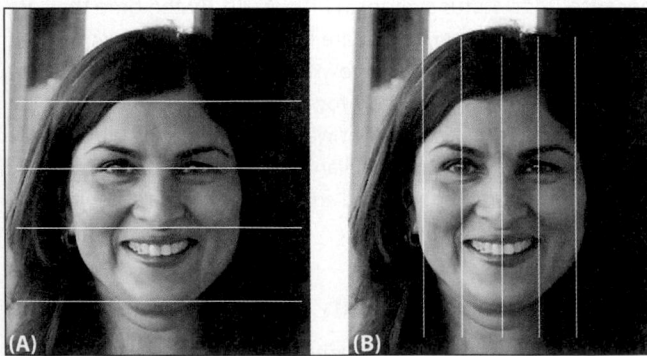

FIGURE 35-4
Facial analysis. (A) Evaluating facial horizontal proportions and (B) Evaluating facial vertical proportions.

Full New Patient Exam

Exam

1. Radiographic
2. Facial
3. Smile
4. Profile
5. Dentition
6. Perio
7. A-P
8. Transverse
9. Vertical
10. Perimeter

Name_____ Chart_____
CC_____
Date_____ Birthdate_____ Age_____

FACIAL:
Face Symm: Yes No _____
Facial shape: Oval ———WNL———Square
Interpupillary line horizontal? Yes No
Commissural line horizontal? Yes No
Cant of the Occlusal Plane? No Yes
  Skeletal?
  Mx incisors canted? (draw)
  Md incisors canted? (draw)
Is the facial midline vertical? Yes No What is off?
Nose? right left Philtrum? right left Chin? right left

SMILE EVALUATION:
Smile Line (mx incisal edges/ superior border of the lo -smile arc):
  Convex (normal) Straight across Reverse (arches up)
Mx teeth show w/ a full smile: 6 8 10 12
Buccal corridor: Deficient ————WNL————Full
Lip Line-Incisor display at rest: ____mm ____%
  Low————WNL————High
Incisor display with smiling? ____mm OK
  Excess gummy smile? _____mm of gingiva
Mx Incisors/Lower Lip: Touching Not Touching Slightly covered

PROFILE A-P:
-Maxilla: Retrognathic———WNL———Prognathic
-Dentoalveolar: Retrusive———WNL———Protrusive
-Mandible: Retrognathic———WNL———Prognathic
-Nose: Small———WNL———Large
-Lips: Thin———WNL———Large
-Chin Button: Flat or Small———WNL———Large
-Nasolabial Angle: Acute<100°———WNL———obtuse>110°
-Lower Face/Throat Angle: Acute———WNL———Obtuse
-Mentalis tension with lip closure: None Tension
-Lip Posture: Closed Open
-Lip Tone: Loose———WNL———Tight
-Lower Face Height: Short———WNL———Long
-Mandibular Plane:
  Hypodivergent-Low———WNL———Hyperdivergent-High

RADIOGRAPHIC Date: _____
1 16 17 32
Root Resorption Potential_____
Root Morph_____
Leeway Space: None Some Lots Second Molars: _____
Years to complete: _____ TMJ: _____
Other_____

OCCLUSION:

ANTERIOR-POSTERIOR:	TRANSVERSE:	VERTICAL:	PERIMETER:
Class Rt M: I II III	Midlines:	Curve of Spee:	Arch Length:
Rt C: I II III	Arch Width:	Mx: Reverse_Flat_Mod_Severe	Mx: ____mm
Lft M: I II III	Mx: Nar———WNL———Wide	Md: Reverse_Flat_Mod_Severe	Md: ____mm
Lft C: I II III	Md: Nar———WNL———Wide	Overbite: ____mm ____%	Bolton Pb:
OJ:	Xbite:	Openbite: ____	Anterior:
U inc: Retro_UR_OK_Proc		____vert	Overall:
L inc: Retro_UR_OK_Proc	Arch Shape:	____gap	Other:
Other:	Mx: V U Md: V U	TT:	
	Curve of Wilson:	Deep bite on Palate:	
	Md: Flat———WNL———Curved	Wear: Mild Mod Severe	

HABITS:
___ Mouth breathing
___ Nose breathing
___ Bruxism
___ Clenching
___ Lip entrapment
___ Thumb or finger sucking
___ Tongue thrusting/posturing
Other_____

TMJ SCREENING:
Opening ____mm NROM____
Sounds _____
Pain _____
R L L History:
  Trauma_____
  Locking open_____
  Locking closed_____
  Tenderness_____
  HA_____
  Other _____

ORAL HEALTH AND PERIODONTIUM:
OH_____ Caries_____ #Rest_____
Ging Biotype: Thin ———WNL———Thick
Attached tissue: Width: Narrow ———WNL———Wide
  Thickness: Thin ———WNL———Thick
Cortical Plate: Thin ———WNL———Thick
Gingivitis: None Mild Moderate Severe
Recession: None Mild Moderate Severe
Frenum: U La___ L La___ Ung___
Excess Gingiva:_____

Approved:
___ Case Type I-Predoc
___ Case Type II-Predoc Inv+Esth
___ PG Case Type III
_____
_____

9/10/2014

FIGURE 35-6
New patient clinical exam.

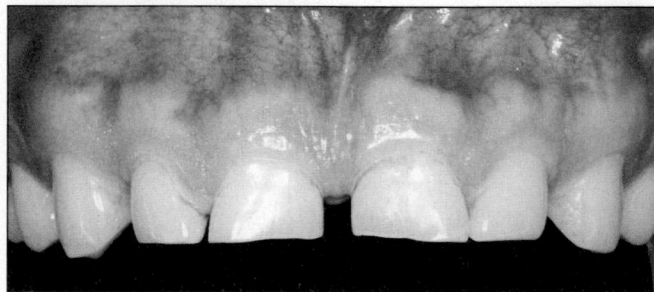

FIGURE 35-7A
Diastema and embedded frenum.

The orthodontist evaluates thin gingival tissue and areas of gingival recession that may be due to another type of abnormal frenum pull (Figure 35-8). Sometimes, patients will have severe generalized recession. These patients may not be good candidates for orthodontic treatment since the teeth may not have enough alveolar bone support. Occasionally, a patient will have isolated areas of recession that may improve or worsen with orthodontic treatment. All adult patients should have a complete periodontal exam by a dentist, a dental hygienist, or the orthodontist before initiating orthodontics so that unexpected responses to treatment may be minimized.

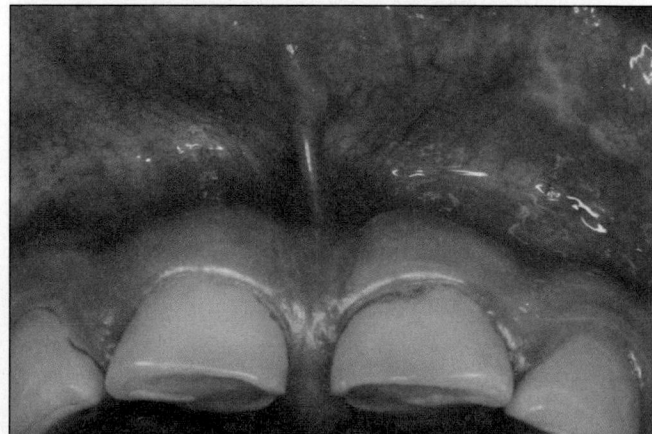

FIGURE 35-7B
Diastema and embedded frenum.

Evaluation of Occlusion and Skeletal Patterns

Orthodontists evaluate a patient's occlusion in different "planes of space." The planes are from the front to the back (anterior–posterior), side to side (transverse), up and down

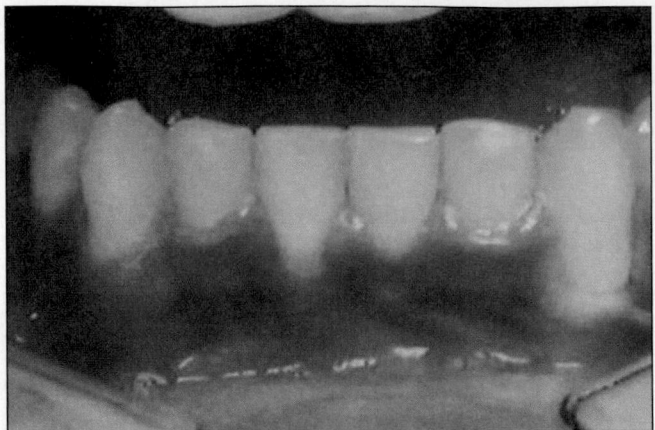

FIGURE 35-8
Illustrates thin gingival tissue, slight recession at lower right incisor, gingivitis at lower left lateral incisor, and tight frenum pull causing recession at lower left canine.

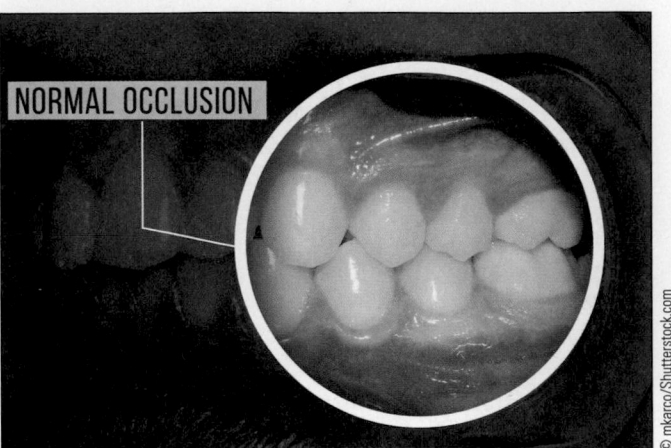

FIGURE 35-9
Normal occlusion, an Angle Class I dental relationship.

(vertical), and around each arch (perimeter). The orthodontist separately evaluates the patient's skeletal jaw relationships in the anterior–posterior plane and in the vertical plane using a cephalometric headfilm image.

Anterior–Posterior Plane of Occlusion and Related Skeletal Patterns

Imagine that the patient's head is a box. The depth of the box is measured from the front of the box to the back of the box. This plane of space is called the anterior–posterior (AP) plane or front to back. Another term that is used to describe the same plane is the sagittal plane, again just meaning front to back. The orthodontist looks at how the teeth fit together in the anterior–posterior plane of space when evaluating the occlusion.

Angle Classification Molar and Canine Edward H.
Angle was a famous dentist who started the practice of orthodontics in the latter part of the 1800s and is known as the "Father of Orthodontics." He wrote books and papers about the occlusion of patients he saw. He found basic patterns repeating in his patients and described the dental relationships between the upper and lower teeth in the anterior–posterior plane.

The most ideal dental occlusal relationship, an Angle Class I dental relationship, is when the mesiobuccal cusp of the maxillary first molar fits into the buccal groove of the mandibular first molar. Also, in an Angle Class I dental relationship, the cusp of the maxillary canine occludes between the distal of the mandibular canine and mesial of the mandibular first premolar. Dr. Angle identified these dental relationships between the maxillary and mandibular molars (and canines) as "normal" relationships, a normal occlusion, or an Angle Class I dental relationship (Figure 35-9). This terminology is used today to classify patients' dental occlusal relationships. These patients with an Angle Class I occlusal relationship usually also have a normal skeletal relationship of the maxilla and mandible in alignment with each other and acceptable profile esthetics.

Dr. Angle then labeled a malocclusion as being a dental Class I, dental Class II, or dental Class III occlusion. Class I has the first molar and canine relationships as described previously by Dr. Angle, but with malposed individual teeth or groups of teeth (Figure 35-10).

Illustration	Facial Profile
Class I	Mesognathic
Class II, Division 1	Retrognathic
Class II, Division 2	
Class III	Prognathic

FIGURE 35-10
Angle dental classifications.

In an Angle Class II dental relationship, the maxillary first molar is forward of the mandibular first molar. The cusp of the maxillary canine occludes in a forward position between the mandibular lateral incisor and the mandibular canine. The maxillary teeth are forward of the mandibular teeth, and there usually is excessive overjet. There are two types of Angle Class II, Division I and Division 2. In an Angle Class II Division 1 malocclusion, the maxillary anterior incisors are **proclined** and lean outward so that there is increased jetting out of the upper front teeth (overjet) and a chance of trauma knocking them out of the mouth. Patients who have a Class II Division 1 dental relationship with proclined maxillary incisors that stick out usually also have a Skeletal Class II jaw relationship where the maxilla may be in a normal position with the head, but the mandible is smaller and underdeveloped compared to the maxilla (Figure 35-11). The squarer shape of this patient's mandible will probably have forward growth and align with the maxilla which will correct the dental and skeletal Class II relationships. Orthodontic treatment in adolescents involves growth appliances to achieve a skeletal correction combined with bringing back the maxillary incisors with braces (Figures 35-12A and B).

Another type of dental Angle Class II Division 1 patient is one who has a different skeletal pattern where the shape of the mandible results in downward growth of the mandible, not forward, so that the mandible will not align with the maxilla (Figure 35-13). These patients often have an oval face shape. Growth appliances

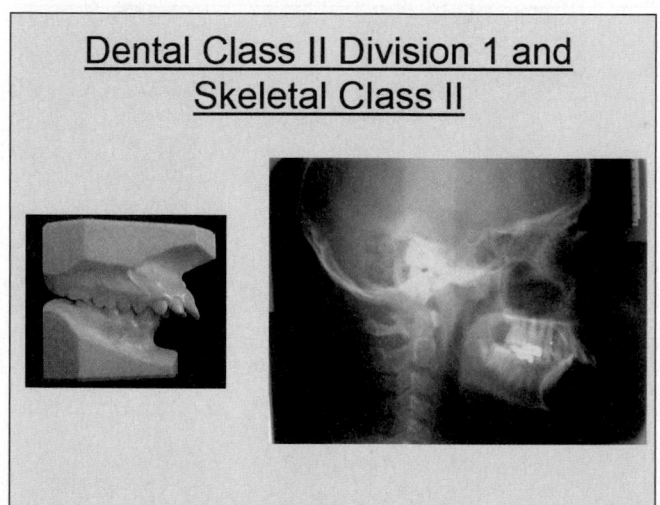

Dental Class II Division 1 and Skeletal Class II

FIGURE 35-11
Orthodontic records before orthodontic treatment. Mandible was expected to grow forward.

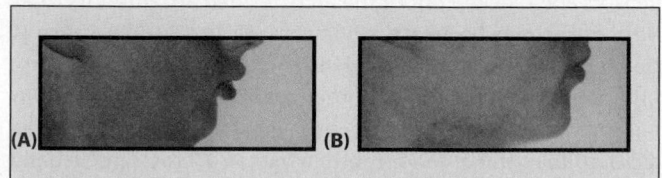

FIGURE 35-12
(A) Before orthodontic treatment and (B) after treatment with braces and growth appliances.

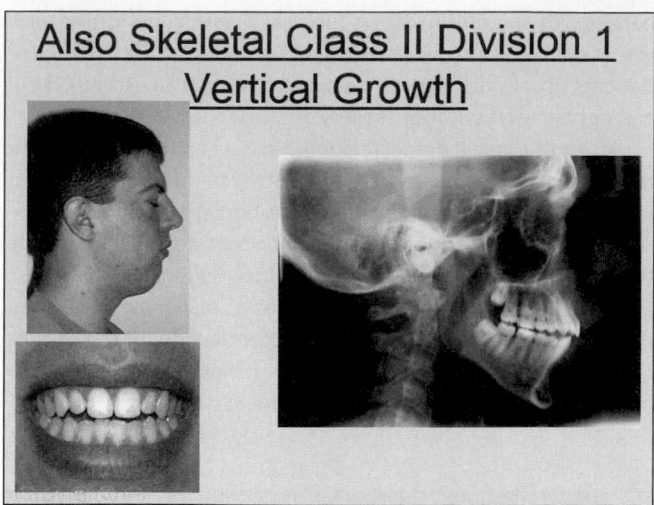

Also Skeletal Class II Division 1 Vertical Growth

FIGURE 35-13
Orthodontic records before orthodontic treatment. Mandible was expected to grow downward.

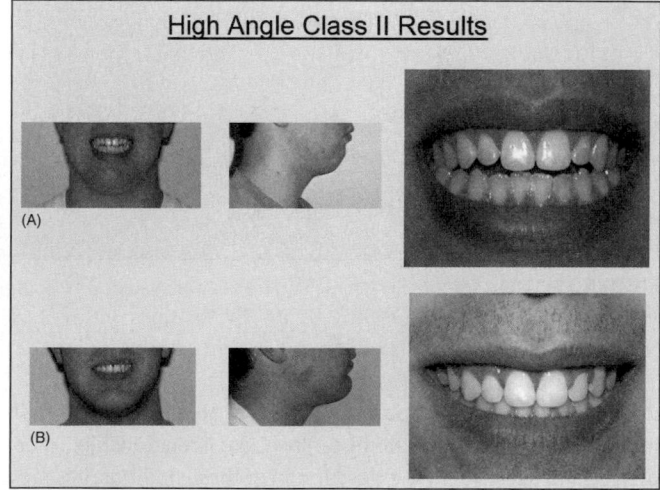

High Angle Class II Results

FIGURE 35-14
(A) Before orthodontic treatment and (B) after treatment with braces and orthognathic surgery.

do not change this downward genetic growth pattern. Usually, these patients undergo orthognathic surgical correction of the dental and skeletal relationships (Figures 35-14A and B). In some cases, adult patients with this Class II skeletal pattern can be corrected with clear aligner therapy.

In the other type of Class II malocclusion, the Angle Class II Division 2 dental malocclusion, the maxillary molars and canines are forward of the mandibular molars and canines, but the maxillary central incisors are tilted inward so that there is a small amount of overjet. These patients often have the same dental Class II relationship of a forward positioning of the maxillary dentition but differ in their skeletal patterns. The facial growth pattern and shape of the mandible in an Angle Class II Division 2 patient is one where there is forward growth of the mandible. These patients have a square facial shape. In growing young patients, the mandible grows forward, eventually aligning with the maxilla correcting the dental and skeletal Class II. These patients usually are easy to treat and to obtain an esthetic facial and dental result without surgery.

An Angle Class III dental relationship is when the maxillary first molar is positioned posteriorly and distally to the mandibular first molar, the maxillary canine may be positioned between the mandibular premolars, and the maxillary incisors are behind or inside the mandibular incisors in an **underbite** (Figure 35-15). Often, an Angle Class III patient skeletally has a small maxilla. Usually, orthodontic treatment will focus on "protraction" of the maxilla or encouraging forward growth of the maxilla using protraction headgear in a very young patient (Figure 35-16 A and B).

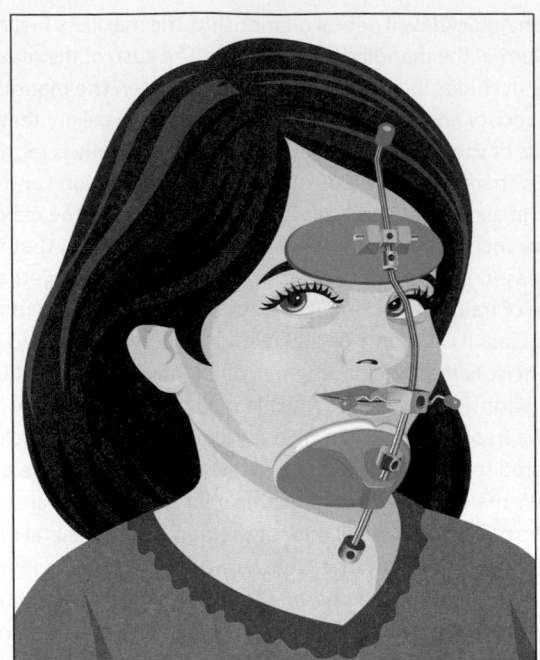

FIGURE 35-16A
Reverse pull headgear.

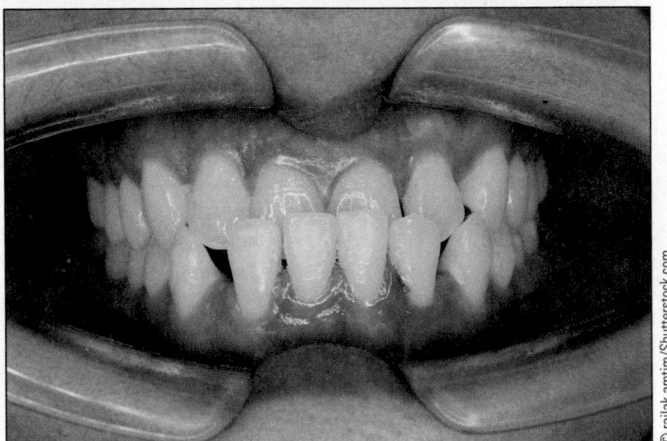

FIGURE 35-15
Dental Angle Class III malocclusion with an underbite.

In clinical practice a patient may have an exact Class I first molar relationship and a slight canine Class II relationship. To be precise and accurate in the description of these findings, it is recommended that the clinician measure, in millimeters, the severity of the dental malocclusion for a Class II or Class III (Figures 35-17A and B).

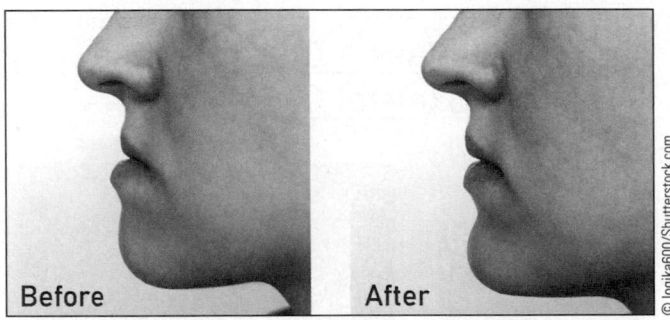

FIGURE 35-16B
(A) Before orthodontic treatment and (B) after treatment with braces and orthognathic surgery.

Overjet, Negative Overjet (Underbite), Anterior Crossbite
The next relationship that is evaluated in the anterior–posterior plane is how far the maxillary incisors stick out in front of the mandibular incisors. This is called **overjet**. Overjet is measured in millimeters from the labial surface of the mandibular incisors to the labial surface of the maxillary incisors (Figure 35-18).

Patients with a Class III molar and canine relationship will often have a negative overjet or underbite where the four maxillary incisors are behind the four mandibular incisors (Figure 35-15). The measurement of an underbite is from the labial of the maxillary incisors to the labial of the mandibular incisors. Often, a patient may only have an "edge-to-edge" bite where the incisal edges of the maxillary and mandibular incisors can touch, but then the patient will move the mandible forward to "slip" into a more comfortable Class III underbite occlusion.

An "anterior **crossbite**" may be present in some patients who have a Class I molar and canine relationship but demonstrate crowding of the maxillary incisors. In this case, the maxillary lateral incisors may be lingual to the mandibular lateral incisors and blocked out of the arch, termed an "anterior crossbite" of the maxillary lateral incisors (Figure 35-19). Space is opened to position the lateral incisors anteriorly out of crossbite, aligning them with the other maxillary anterior teeth. An anterior crossbite is in the anterior–posterior plane since it is a crossbite of the *anterior* teeth, whereas a "crossbite" usually describes *posterior* premolar and molar teeth that are malposed in the transverse plane (the next plane to be discussed; see "Transverse Plane").

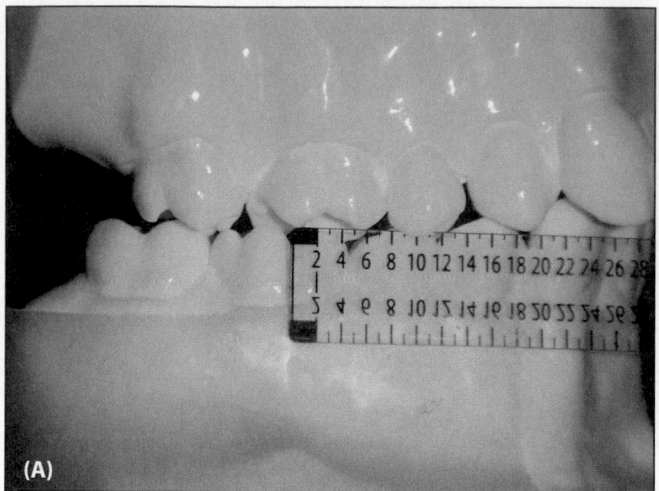 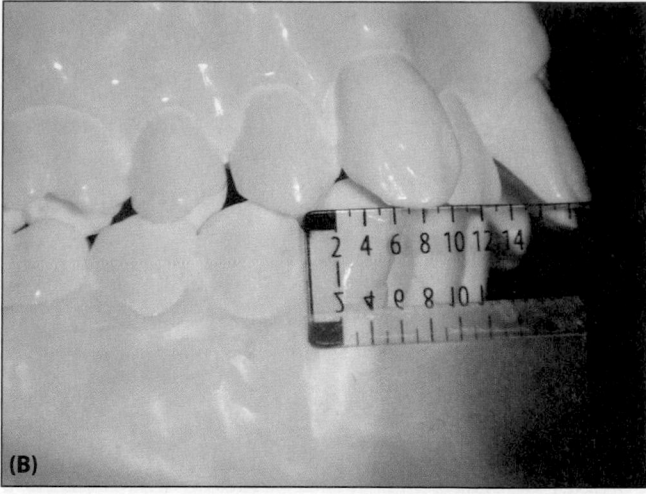

FIGURE 35-17
Measuring how many millimeters molars and canines are deviated from Class I relationship. (A) Measuring right molar Class II by 6 mm and (B) Measuring right canine Class II by 8 mm.

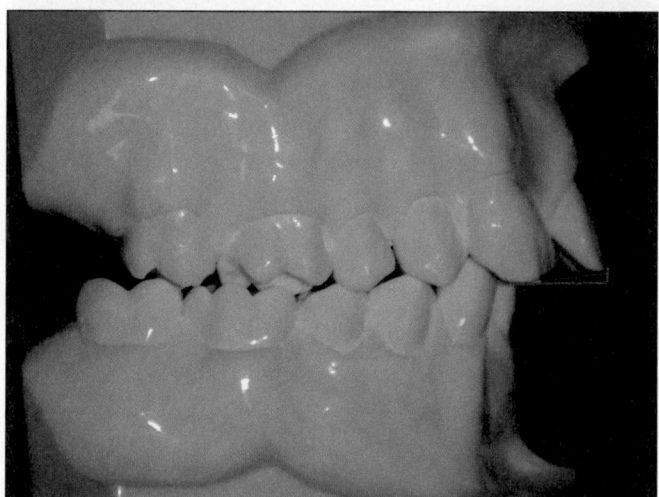

FIGURE 35-18
Measuring overjet.

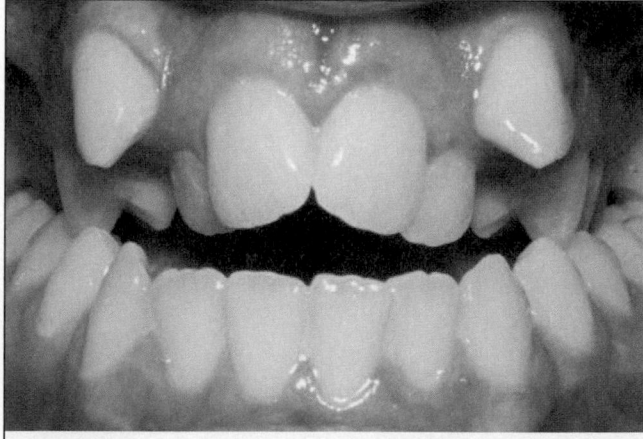

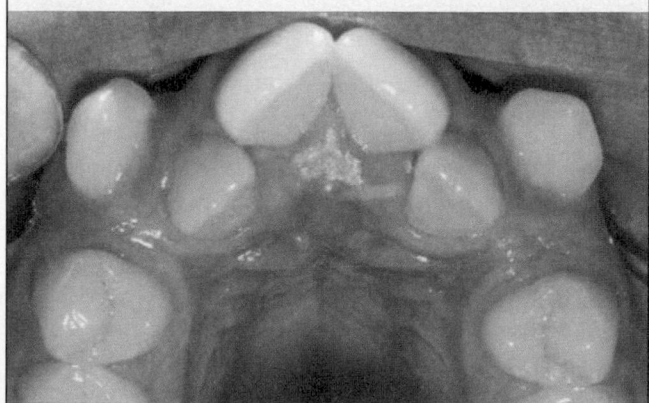

FIGURE 35-19
Anterior crossbite of maxillary lateral incisors. An anterior crossbite such as that which occurs with a palatally positioned lateral incisor is in the anterior–posterior plane of space.

Incisor Proclination or Retroclination Another
description in the anterior–posterior plane is the proclination or **retroclination** of the maxillary and mandibular incisors. When the incisors are leaning out, they are proclined (Figure 35-20).

When the incisors are leaning inward, they are described as being retroclined. When the maxillary central incisors are tipped back (as in an Angle Class II Division 2 malocclusion), the incisors are also described as being retroclined (Figure 35-21; both the maxillary and mandibular incisors are retroclined).

Transverse Plane of Occlusion

The next dimension that must be examined is the **transverse plane**. This is the horizontal, width, or side-to-side dimension.

Facial Midline and the Dental Midlines The first
relationships that are evaluated in the transverse plane are the relationships of the dental midlines to the facial midline. The facial midline is the center of the philtrum of the upper lip

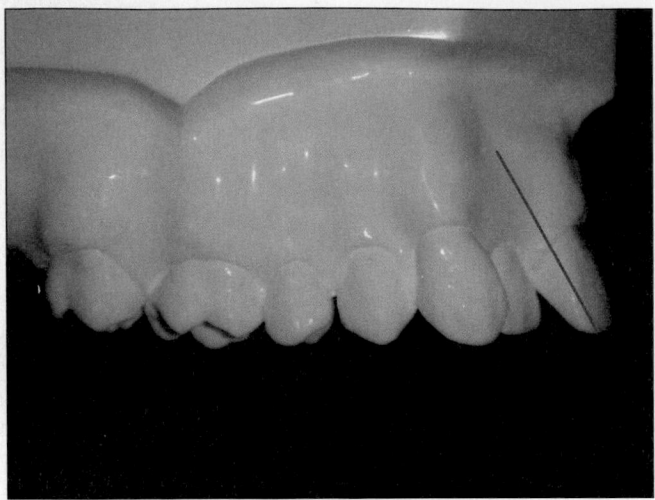

FIGURE 35-20
Proclination of the maxillary incisors.

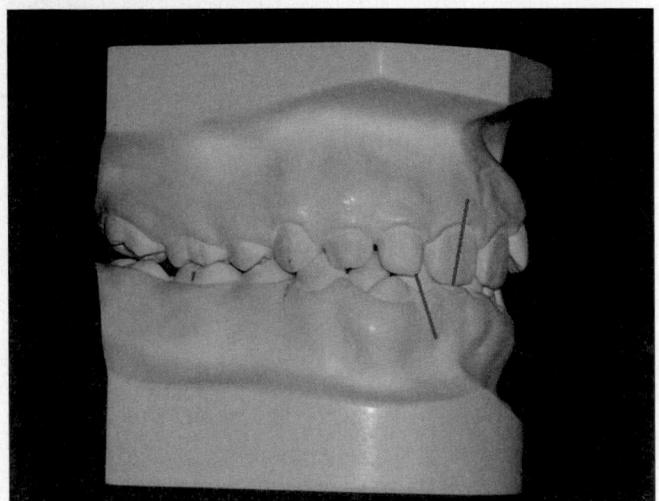

FIGURE 35-21
Retroclination of the maxillary incisors.

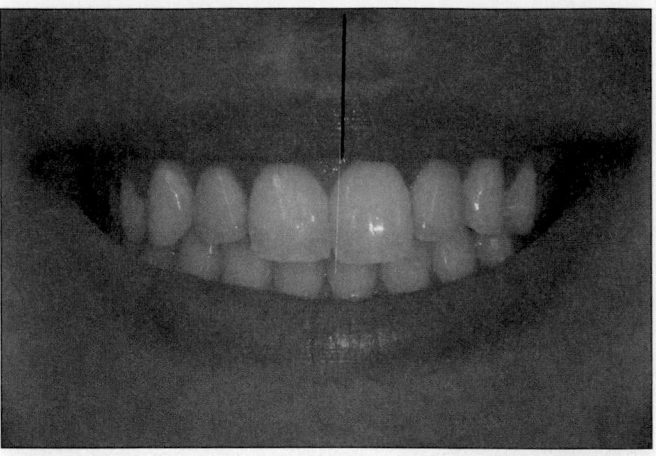

FIGURE 35-22
Facial midline at the center of the philtrum and cupid's bow.

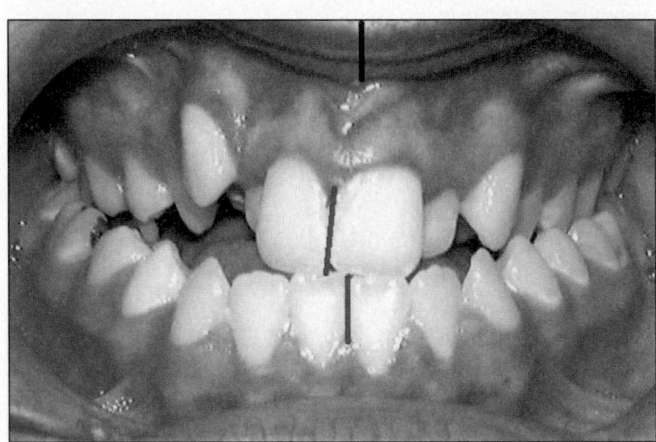

FIGURE 35-23
Deviated maxillary dental midline and bilateral posterior crossbite.

where the "cupid's bow" of the lip is located (Figure 35-22). The maxillary facial midline is assumed to be in a stable position and not easily changed, whereas the upper and lower dental midlines are easily affected by crowding and shifting of the teeth to the right or left.

The dental midlines are described relative to the facial midline. To evaluate the maxillary dental midline position relative to the facial midline, look at the dental midline with the lips in a relaxed position. Sometimes you need to use a straight vertical line extended down from the center of the philtrum to the area where the maxillary dental midline would be and measure how many millimeters it is off to the right or left from the facial midline. The mandibular dental midline is also measured in millimeters off from the stable facial midline (Figure 35-23).

Posterior Crossbites Posterior crossbites of the teeth are also evaluated in the transverse plane. There are many types of crossbites, which are due to different problems.

Full posterior lingual crossbite (bilateral) occurs when all of the back upper teeth on both sides are positioned toward the inside of the mouth as compared to the lower teeth. The upper jaw looks smaller and narrower than the lower jaw. Usually this is a skeletal problem of the maxilla being too narrow to fit over the wider mandibular jaw (Figure 35-23). In growing patients this is corrected by expanding or widening the maxilla with a maxillary expander device with cemented bands attached to the upper teeth (Figure 35-24).

Unilateral posterior lingual crossbite with a functional shift occurs when there is a posterior lingual crossbite of just one side of the arch. In children, this is often a slight narrowness of both sides of the upper jaw so that the child has to shift the mandible to one side in order to bite together completely. This is called a functional shift of the mandible to one side and shows up as a lingual crossbite on one side with the mandibular midline also shifted to one side. Research has shown that if this type of crossbite is not corrected when the child is still growing, the anatomy of the temporomandibular joint may be permanently deformed accommodating the abnormal functional shift.

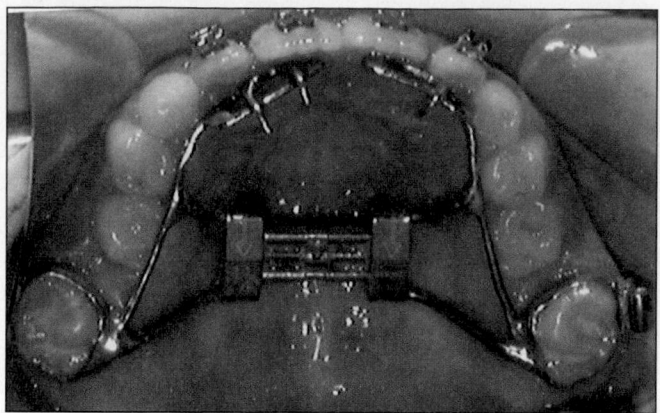

FIGURE 35-24
Palatal expander is used to widen a narrow arch. The caregiver is generally provided a key that fits in center of the device. When turned, the device expands. The caregiver is given instructions on how many times or how far the key should be turned.

Unilateral full posterior lingual crossbite occurs when the upper back teeth are all shifted as a group inside toward the palate. In this case there is full unilateral crossbite on one side, but the dental midlines are aligned with the facial midline, implying that there is no functional shift of the mandible.

Single tooth posterior lingual crossbite. Occasionally just one or two posterior teeth will be in a lingual crossbite. This is due to maxillary posterior teeth being positioned more palatally and the mandibular posterior teeth positioned more buccally.

Bilateral posterior buccal crossbite occurs when the posterior maxilla is much wider than the mandibular posterior dental area and the maxillary posterior teeth are completely on the outside of the buccal surfaces of the mandibular teeth. Often, this is called a scissor bite because the teeth pass by each other like blades on scissors.

Single tooth posterior buccal crossbite occurs when a single maxillary tooth is in buccal crossbite with a single mandibular tooth. The problem with this tooth relationship if left untreated is that the maxillary teeth will continue to erupt and become supererupted, or extruded, because they have no lower tooth to stop them. Maxillary posterior teeth can supererupt so much that they eventually need to be removed.

Arch Width and Arch Shape Other relationships that must be evaluated in the transverse plane are maxillary and mandibular arch width and arch shape. Are both arches narrow, normal, or wide? It is important when there is a crossbite to identify where the problem is so the treatment will be directed to correct the underlying root problem.

The shape of the arch also must be checked. Most normal arches are U shaped (Figures 35-25A and B). Some maxillary arches are V shaped and may appear to have more overjet than ideal (Figure 35-26).

Apical Base Widths and Related Skeletal Issues The apical base is the point where the alveolar bone at the apices of the teeth attach to the maxilla or the mandible. The width of this

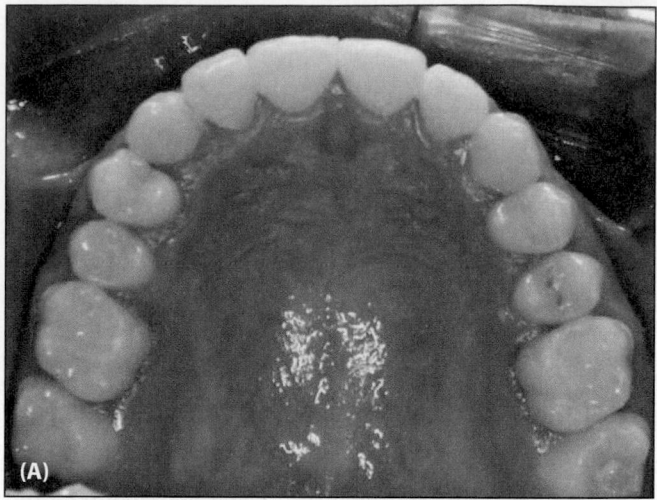

(A)

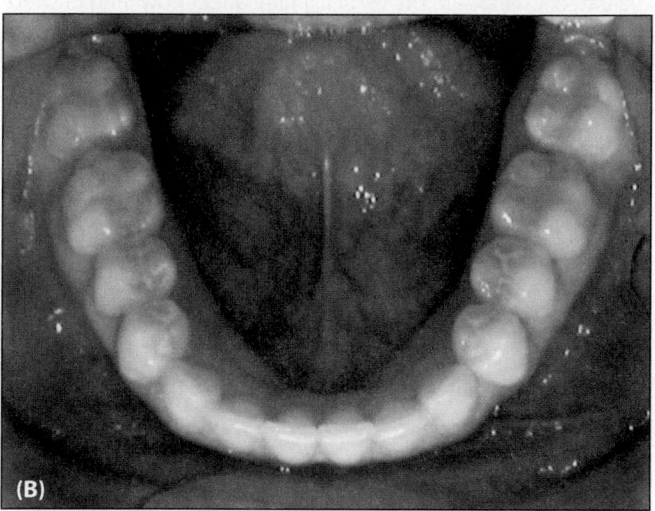

(B)

FIGURE 35-25
Normal (A) maxillary and (B) mandibular arches that are U shaped.

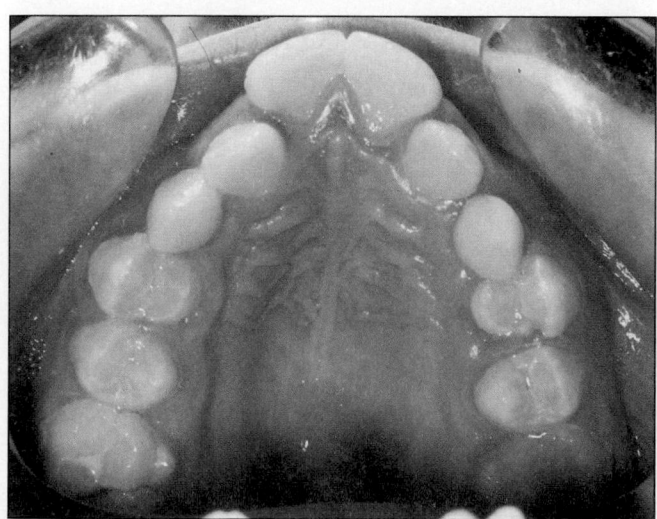

FIGURE 35-26
V shaped maxillary arch.

apical base area of the maxilla is used to assess the width or narrowness of the maxilla. If the apical base of the maxilla is very narrow or very wide, then the patient usually has a skeletal problem and may not be treated with movement of the teeth alone. The maxilla may need to be widened with a palatal expander at the palatal suture in a growing patient or via orthognathic surgery of the palate in nongrowing patients.

If the mandible apical base is very narrow, sometimes it can be widened with distraction osteogenesis, a type of skeletal expansion. If the mandibular apical base is very wide, sometimes it can be narrowed with mandibular midline surgery in the front of the jaw.

Vertical Plane of Occlusion and Related Skeletal Patterns

The vertical plane of occlusion and the anterior length of the maxilla and mandible and the alveolar bone of both must also be evaluated. Changes in the vertical plane affect how long or short the face appears to be and how open or deep the bite is.

Overbite or Openbite with a Tongue Thrust   The main vertical relationship that the orthodontist evaluates in the vertical plane is overbite or the vertical overlap of the maxillary and mandibular anterior teeth (Figure 35-27). Overbite is measured in millimeters of overlap and in percentage that the maxillary incisors are overlapping the length of the mandibular incisors. Ideally the overbite is about 2 millimeters and 20% of overlap. Moderate overbite may be 3 millimeters (30%) to 6 millimeters (60%). Severe overbite is often called a deep bite and may be 7 millimeters of overlap and more than 100% so that the mandibular incisors are not visible when the patient is biting together (Figure 35-28).

When the anterior teeth of both jaws meet along their incisal edges it is referred to as an edge-to-edge bite and has zero overbite. The patient may have an "open bite" where there is a gap between the incisal edges of the upper teeth and the incisal edges of the lower teeth. The patient may just have an "open bite

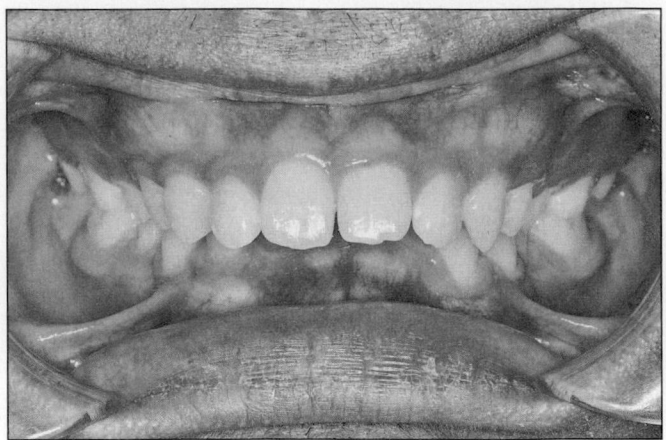

FIGURE 35-28
Severe overbite or "deep bite" where mandibular incisors are not visible.

tendency" where there is a small gap between the upper and lower front teeth. Usually, chart where the open bite is located by noting the teeth that are apart and measure the size of the gap in millimeters.

If a patient has a severe open bite, they also may have a pathological tongue thrust. This means that the patient has developed the habit of closing off the open bite gap by putting the tongue into the gap so that food will go to the back of the mouth and can be swallowed. Otherwise, food would come out of the front of the mouth. Often, an open bite is closed with orthodontic treatment and jaw surgery, but the tongue thrust habit remains, and it pushes the bite open again. The open bite cannot be corrected permanently until this tongue thrust is also eliminated. Some orthodontists have had success closing open bites and correction of the tongue thrust habit using clear aligner therapy since the aligners may close off the open bite gap so that the tongue thrust habit is no longer needed to swallow food.

Another form of open bite occurs in children who suck their thumb or fingers. The teeth do not erupt normally. The maxillary incisors may be severely proclined, and the mandibular incisors may be severely retroclined. A pathological tongue thrust also develops. A rake or barrier device can be inserted to prevent the tongue from coming forward so that the bite can close without further orthodontic treatment (Figure 35-29).

Curve of Spee   The mandibular teeth often have a curve in the bite called the "curve of Spee," named after the dentist who first identified it (Figure 35-30). This curve is ideally flat but may be slightly curved, moderately curved, or severely curved. If it is severely curved, the patient will usually have a very deep bite or overlap vertically of the maxillary and mandibular anterior teeth. The teeth function best if there is a flat curve of Spee, so orthodontists usually level or flatten out the curve of Spee.

Skeletal Deep Bite and Skeletal Open Bite   The orthodontist also evaluates the patient's vertical skeletal relationships from a cephalometric headfilm image. The patient's skeletal pattern impacts the success of comprehensive orthodontic

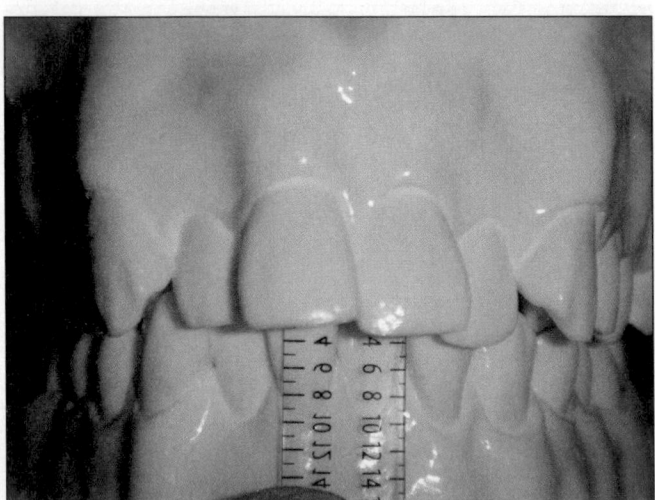

FIGURE 35-27
Measuring mild to moderate 3–4 mm overbite.

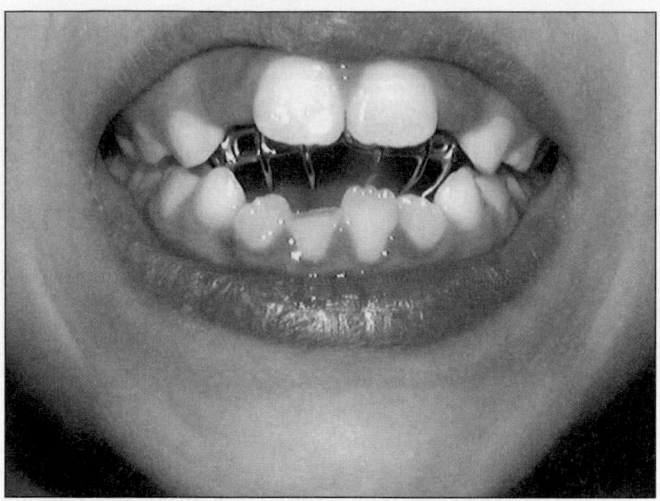

FIGURE 35-29
Open bite in a young child due to thumb sucking habit with rake appliance in place.

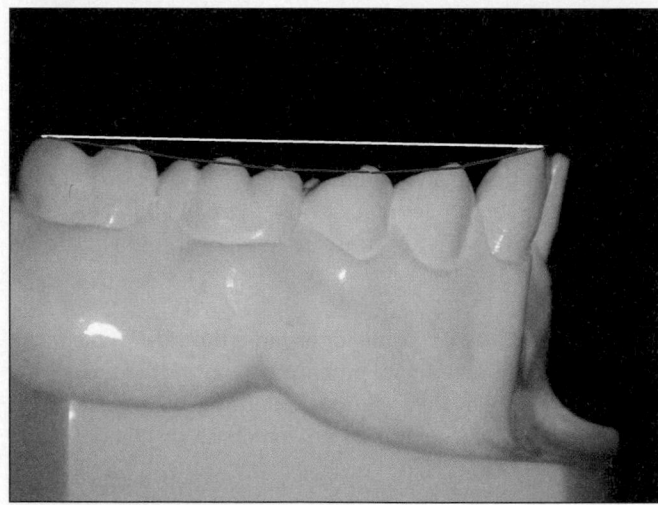

FIGURE 35-30
Mandibular model with moderate curve of Spee (red line).

treatment. Changes in the skeletal vertical dimension affect facial esthetics and bite depth in the occlusion.

For instance, the male, 13 years of age, in Figure 35-31 presents initially with a severe dental Class II Division 1, a skeletal Class II, and a deep bite occlusal relationship. The shape of the mandible indicates that this patient's mandible will grow forward and catch up with the maxillary jaw and teeth. In Figure 35-32, the results at age 15 indicate that, in fact, his mandible did grow forward, resulting in an excellent occlusion and facial esthetics.

In the second case, the male, 16 years of age, in Figure 35-33 presents initially with a dental Class II Division 1, a different type of skeletal Class II, and an open bite occlusal relationship. The patient has a long lower face and chin area, a dental open bite, and a more vertical shape of the mandible that indicates his mandible would grow downward, worsening his facial and dental esthetics, and not catch up with the maxillary jaw. In Figure 35-34, his results at age 17 required braces and orthognathic jaw surgery to achieve an excellent occlusion and facial esthetics. This type of treatment requires a collaboration of the patient, the orthodontist, and the oral surgeon.

Perimeter Plane

The **perimeter plane** includes details about the teeth and their positions. A perimeter is a border around everything else, so this plane includes everything else about the teeth that was not included in the other dimensions.

Arch Length Excess (Spacing) or Arch Length Deficiency (Crowding)
The orthodontist must evaluate if the teeth are spaced with an arch length excess (ALE, or spacing) evaluation or measuring too much arch for smaller teeth. The orthodontist must also determine if the teeth show an arch length deficiency (ALD or crowding) where the teeth are crowded because there is a small arch and large wide teeth.

In the case of an arch length excess or spacing, the amount of space in the front (from the first premolar to the other first

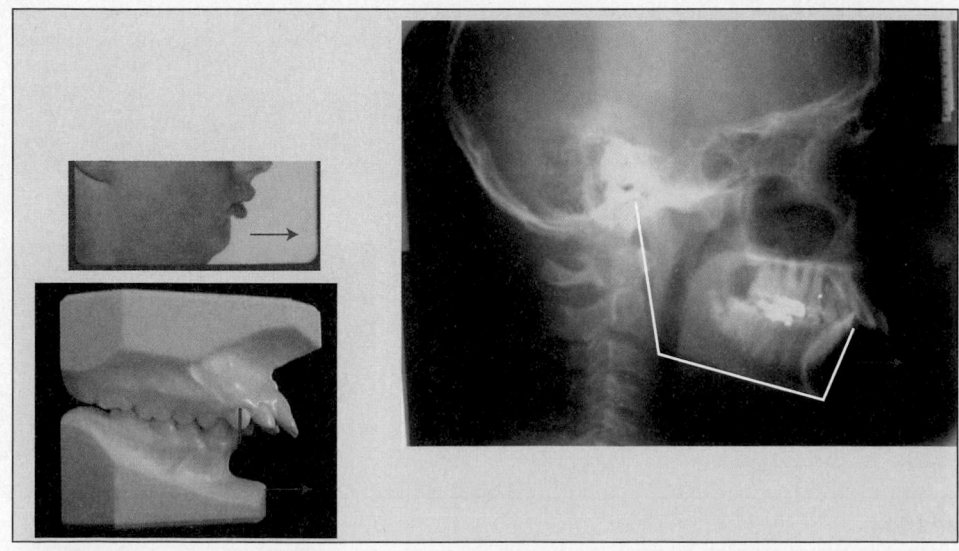

FIGURE 35-31
Class II Division 1 deep bite, skeletal Class II with expected forward growth of the mandible.

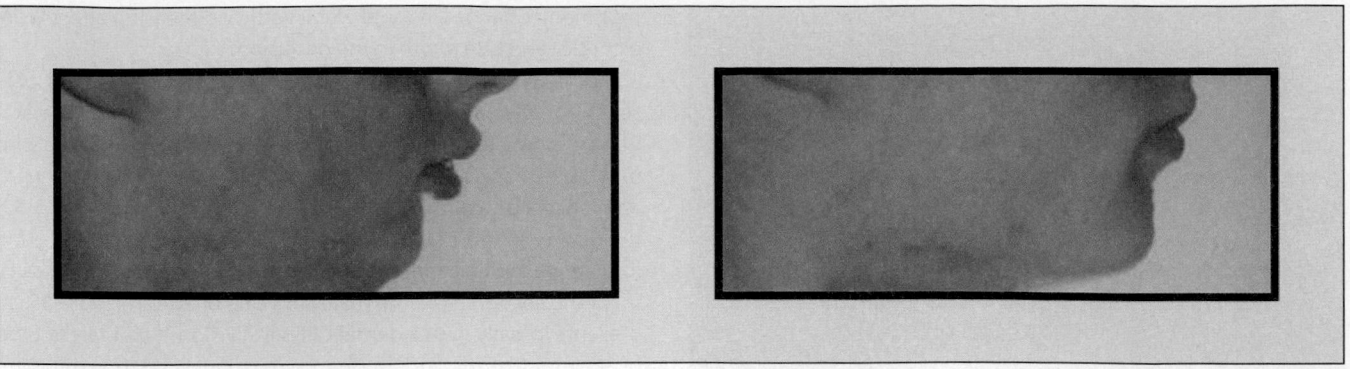

FIGURE 35-32
Skeletal deep bite orthodontic results treated with growth appliances and braces.

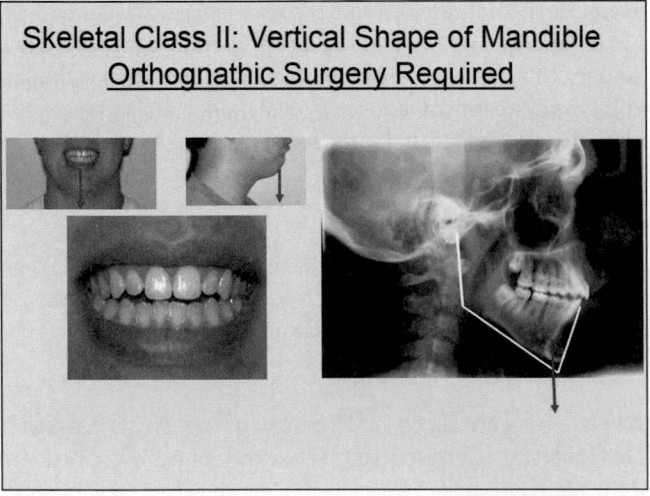

Skeletal Class II: Vertical Shape of Mandible
Orthognathic Surgery Required

FIGURE 35-33
Dental Class II Division 1 open bite, Skeletal Class II open bite with expected downward growth of the mandible.

premolar on the other side) is added and noted as a positive number of millimeters (Figure 35-35).

In the case of an arch length deficiency or crowding, the amount of crowding of the teeth from first molar to first molar is estimated as if all of the teeth were lined up, and this amount is noted as a negative number in millimeters (Figure 35-36).

Severe Rotations Regardless of spacing or crowding, some teeth may be severely rotated, which may require longer treatment and special procedures to align the teeth and then special retention procedures to hold them in alignment after orthodontic treatment. These severe rotations should be noted (Figure 35-37).

Bolton Problem Wayne Bolton, an orthodontist, examined the widths of the teeth and determined the width ratios of the maxillary teeth that would fit together ideally with the mandibular teeth. When the widths do not match up, this ratio is called

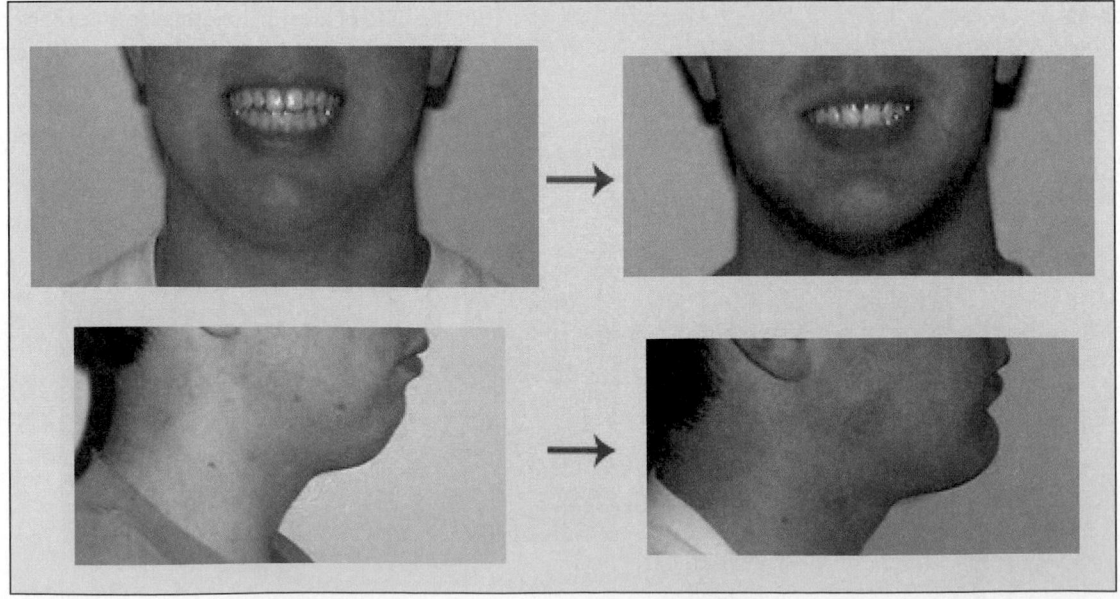

FIGURE 35-34
Skeletal open bite before treatment and after treatment with braces and orthognathic surgery.

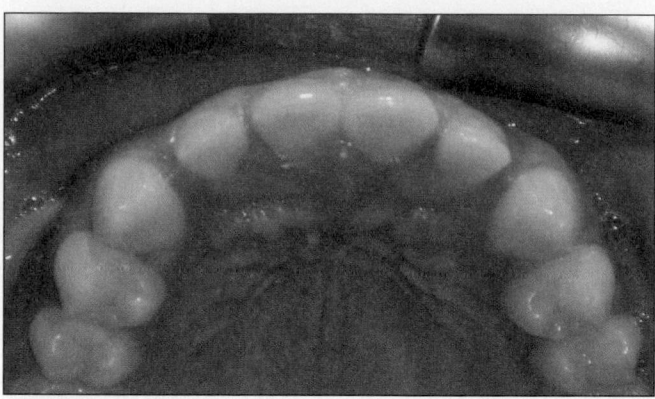

FIGURE 35-35
Spacing in the maxillary arch.

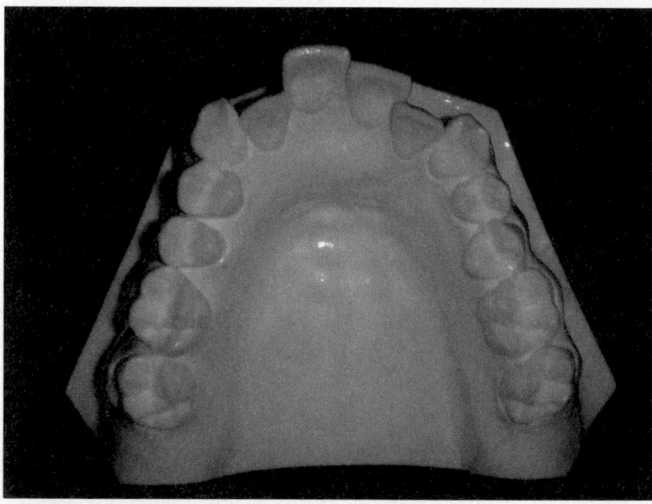

FIGURE 35-36
Moderate crowding in the maxillary arch.

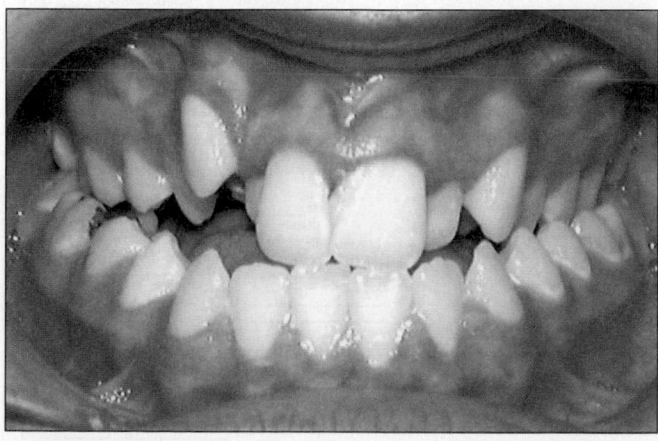

FIGURE 35-37
Severe maxillary rotations.

a Bolton problem or tooth size discrepancy. For instance, if the canines are in a perfect Class I relationship, but the patient has wide maxillary lateral incisors and normal mandibular incisors, the upper teeth will be wider than what will ideally fit with the lower teeth. The patient suffers from an "anterior Bolton" problem so that when treatment is completed there will be overjet remaining. Similarly, if the patient has maxillary **peg lateral** incisors and all spaces are closed in the upper arch, but has normal mandibular incisor widths, then the patient will have an "anterior Bolton" problem and might end up with an edge-to-edge bite, negative overjet, or underbite.

There can also be an "overall Bolton" problem. This happens when the patient is missing a mandibular second premolar but has retained the primary second molar. This primary second molar is usually 2 to 3 millimeters wider mesiodistally than the mandibular second premolar (Figure 35-38). If both premolars are present on the same side in the maxillary arch, then there will be an overall Bolton problem in that there is excess tooth structure in the lower arch due to the retained primary molar. If the patient has a perfect Class I molar relationship on that side, the excess lower tooth structure will cause a Class III canine relationship by 2 to 3 millimeters on that side. Consequently, the bite will not line up. Treatment is required to make the retained primary first molar smaller mesiodistally to allow both the molar and canines to have a Class I relationship.

Dental Wear Severe dental (tooth) wear alters the shape, size, and esthetics of the teeth and may affect the occlusion (Figure 35-39). When planning the treatment of a patient with severe wear, the dentist and the orthodontist should work together so that restorations placed for the severe wear may provide the best function and esthetics for a lifetime. Areas of severe wear that will require this type of multidisciplinary treatment should be noted and planned before orthodontic treatment is initiated.

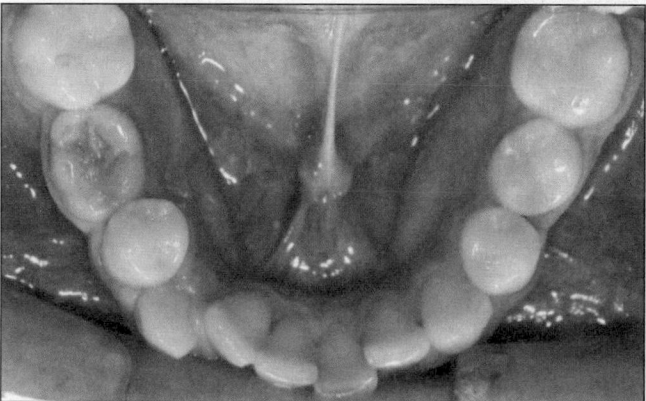

FIGURE 35-38
Retained mandibular primary second molar causing an overall Bolton problem.

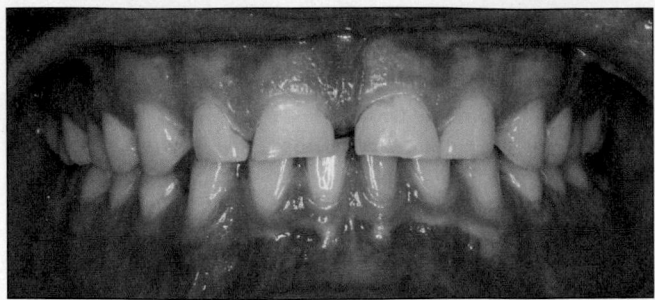

FIGURE 35-39
Severe wear of the maxillary incisors.

Etiology of Malocclusion To determine the etiology (root cause) of the problem, the orthodontist will examine the occlusion and skeletal relationships of the new patient. The etiology falls into one of three categories:

1. Genetic or heredity factors may be responsible for deviations such as supernumerary teeth, facial and palatal clefts, abnormal jaw relationships, abnormal teeth-to-jaw relationships, and congenitally missing teeth. For example, some patients may have a tooth-size-to-arch-size problem where the teeth may be too wide to fit on the narrow size of the arches, resulting in crowding. Conversely, if the teeth are too small for the large arch size, there may be gaps or spaces present between the teeth.

2. Systemic factors include systemic diseases and nutritional disturbances that upset the normal schedule of dentition development during infancy and early childhood. Dietary deficiencies impair the growth and development of the facial bones, jaws, and teeth and also causing dental crowding.

3. Local factors include trauma and habits such as thumb sucking, tongue thrusting, tongue sucking, mouth breathing, bruxism, and nail biting. Early loss of a primary tooth can cause a loss of space and overcrowding of the erupting permanent teeth. Any retained primary teeth may cause a permanent tooth to erupt ectopically due to lack of sufficient space to erupt because of retention of the primary tooth.

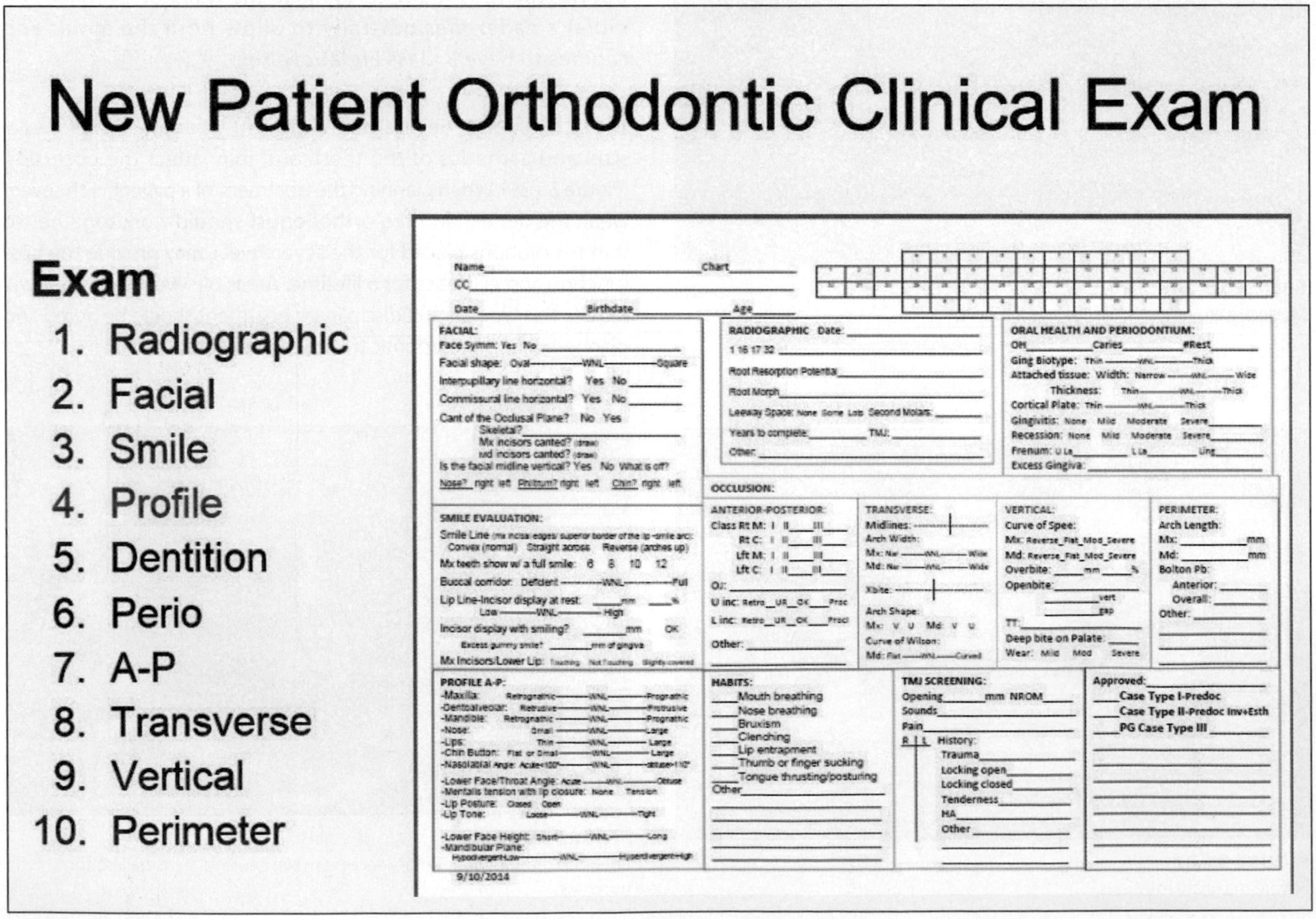

New Patient Orthodontic Clinical Exam

Exam

1. Radiographic
2. Facial
3. Smile
4. Profile
5. Dentition
6. Perio
7. A-P
8. Transverse
9. Vertical
10. Perimeter

FIGURE 35-40
Recording new patient orthodontic exam findings in patient's record.

New Patient Exam Summary

The dental assistant or new patient treatment coordinator will chart the orthodontist's findings during the new patient orthodontic examination (Figure 35-40). When the new patient exam is completed, the orthodontist or treatment coordinator will summarize what can be done to treat the patient's chief concern, identify other problems that were detected, and discuss what the overall treatment would involve, the length of time treatment would take, and the cost. Usually, if treatment is recommended, the next step is for the patient to have orthodontic records taken, from which the orthodontist will diagnose the problems and make a detailed plan for treatment.

Orthodontic Diagnostic Records and Analysis

Clinical photographs, study models or digital intraoral scans, and radiographs are necessary diagnostic records and documentation. Diagnostic records are used by the orthodontist to analyze the patient's case, make a proper diagnosis, and develop a comprehensive treatment plan that meets the needs of the patient.

Clinical Photographs

A series of photographs of the patient are taken for orthodontic records. Most orthodontists take eight photographs in this series,

but some take nine, one of which shows an extra view of the closeup of the smile (Figure 35-41).

Each image has specific criteria for the best documentation and diagnosis. If the photos are not of high quality, then a thorough diagnosis cannot be made. Also, if acceptable photos are not captured initially, they will not be a reliable reference of how things were before treatment when comparing before and after treatment photos.

Many large orthodontic practices have an imaging center where photographs and radiographs are taken along with digital intraoral scans of the teeth. Such centers have a specific background and lighting for extraoral photographs, as well as special mirrors, retractors, cameras, and computer programs to process images quickly.

Study Models or Digital Intraoral Scans of the Teeth and Analysis

To properly document and diagnose the condition and needs of the patient, a digital intraoral scan of the teeth or impressions are done to produce diagnostic study models (Figure 35-42) and include a bite registration. Usually, these impressions are taken with alginate impression material (Figure 35-43), poured in stone or plaster, and then trimmed to an exact shape. Impressions may also be taken with polyvinyl silicone material (Figure 35-44) and scanned into a computer for electronic study models. Digital intraoral scans can be done directly in the patient's mouth by using a scanning wand to capture images of the patient's teeth.

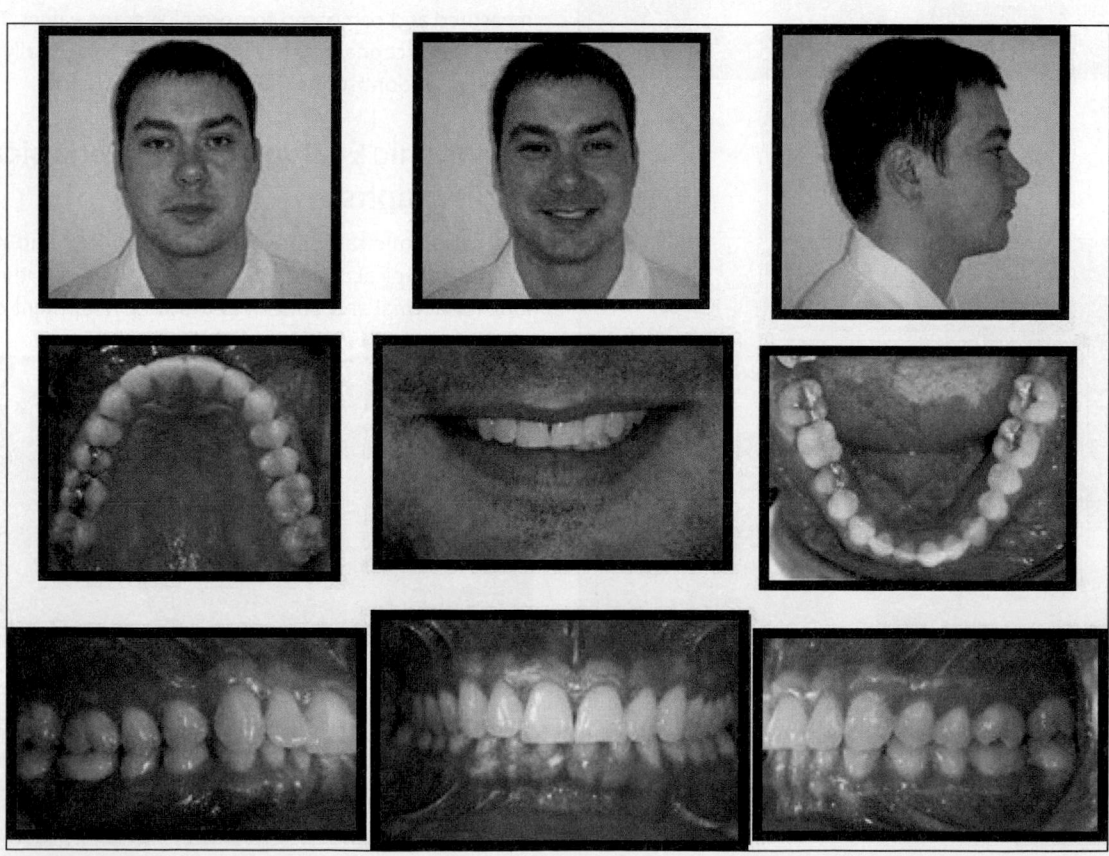

FIGURE 35-41
Photographic series.

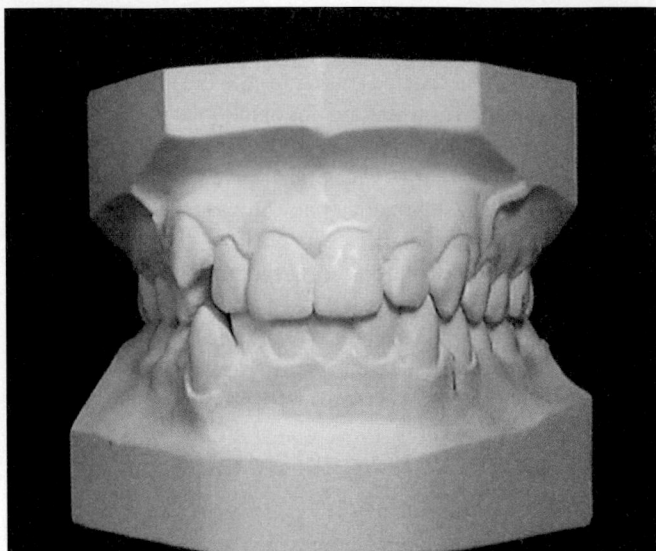

FIGURE 35-42
Diagnostic models.

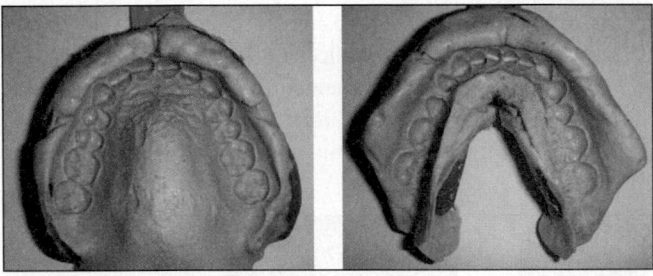

FIGURE 35-43
Alginate impressions.

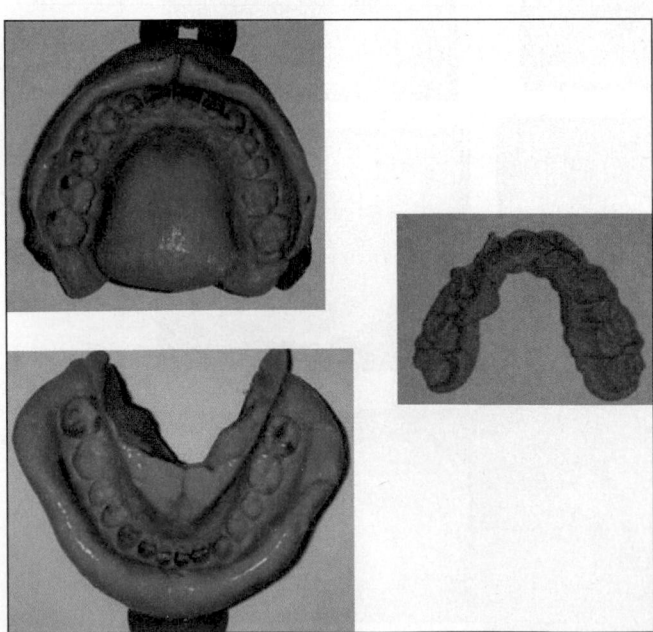

FIGURE 35-44
PVS impressions and bite.

Electronic models then are made and sent to the orthodontist over the Internet to be analyzed for the diagnosis. The advantage of electronic models is that they are stored on a computer rather than in a storage facility as with plaster and stone models.

Study models must be accurate for a proper diagnosis, and to be accurate, the impressions, scans, and pour ups must not have any distortions. Precision is critical for producing accurate records. Study models are examined to confirm evaluation of the patient's occlusion in different planes of space that were noted during the new patient examination.

After treatment, final models may be taken to compare with models taken before orthodontics. Often, orthodontists will use the before and after records to learn from what was done in treatment, what worked, and what could have been done differently.

Cephalometric Radiographs and Analysis

A cephalometric radiograph or digital image is another orthodontic record that is produced for diagnosis (Figure 35-45). This radiograph is taken from the side of the head to examine tooth and jaw relationships in the anterior–posterior and vertical planes and for analysis.

Typically, bony and soft tissue structures on a cephalometric radiograph image are digitized into a computer program and then analyzed. In the past, cephalometric headfilms were traced or drawn with pencil onto a clear sheet of acetate placed on top of the radiograph (Figure 35-46). Then analysis lines were drawn on the tracing between different landmarks, and relationships were measured and compared to normal average values. This process was called a cephalometric analysis and was usually completed by the orthodontist or a trained records assistant.

Panoramic Evaluation and Periapical Radiographs

The panoramic radiograph of the maxillary and mandibular arches is a typical radiograph or image used by orthodontists to look for normal and abnormal tooth development or concerns

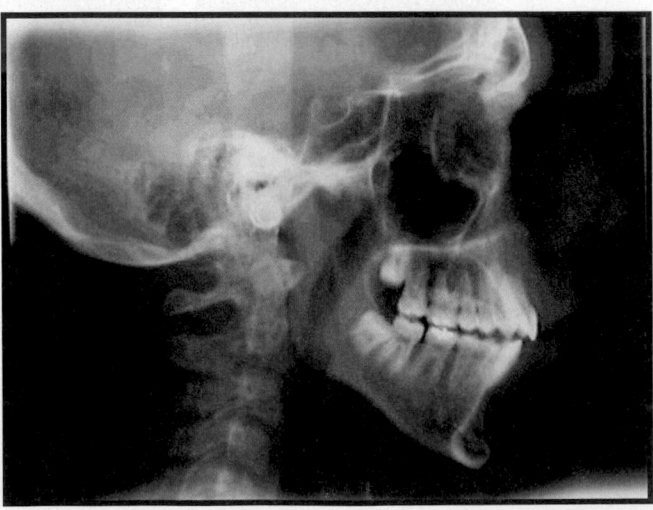

FIGURE 35-45
Cephalometric radiograph.

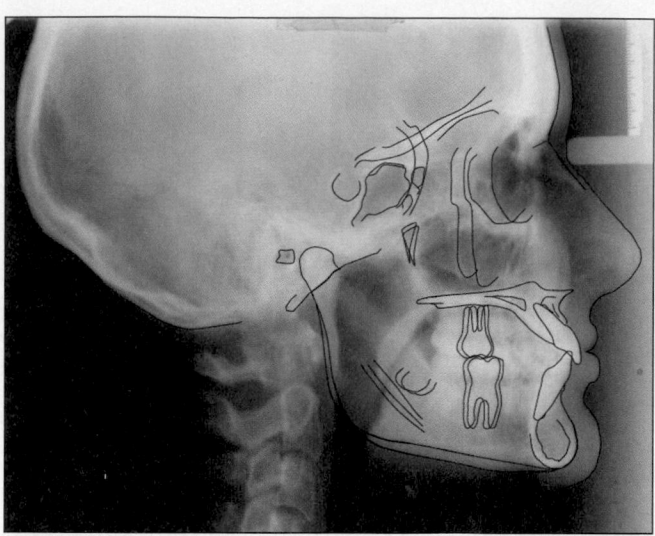

FIGURE 35-46
Cephalometric composite tracing by hand.

(Figure 35-47). If the panoramic radiograph does not provide enough detail about tooth structures, it is supplemented by periapical radiographs as needed so that these combined records provide accurate detail about the teeth and the tissues around the teeth.

Cone Beam/CAT Scan/3D Radiography

Occasionally, a patient will have a dental issue that requires a 3D scan to accurately diagnose what is going on. Cone beam imaging, which is similar to a CAT scan or 3D radiography, may be used to show a movie of the structure. This is especially useful when a patient has an impacted maxillary canine that has not erupted or come into the mouth. A 3D image will show the canine in all dimensions so accurate treatment may be planned.

Periodontal Exam

All adults 18 years or older should have a thorough periodontal exam before orthodontic treatment to rule out unseen

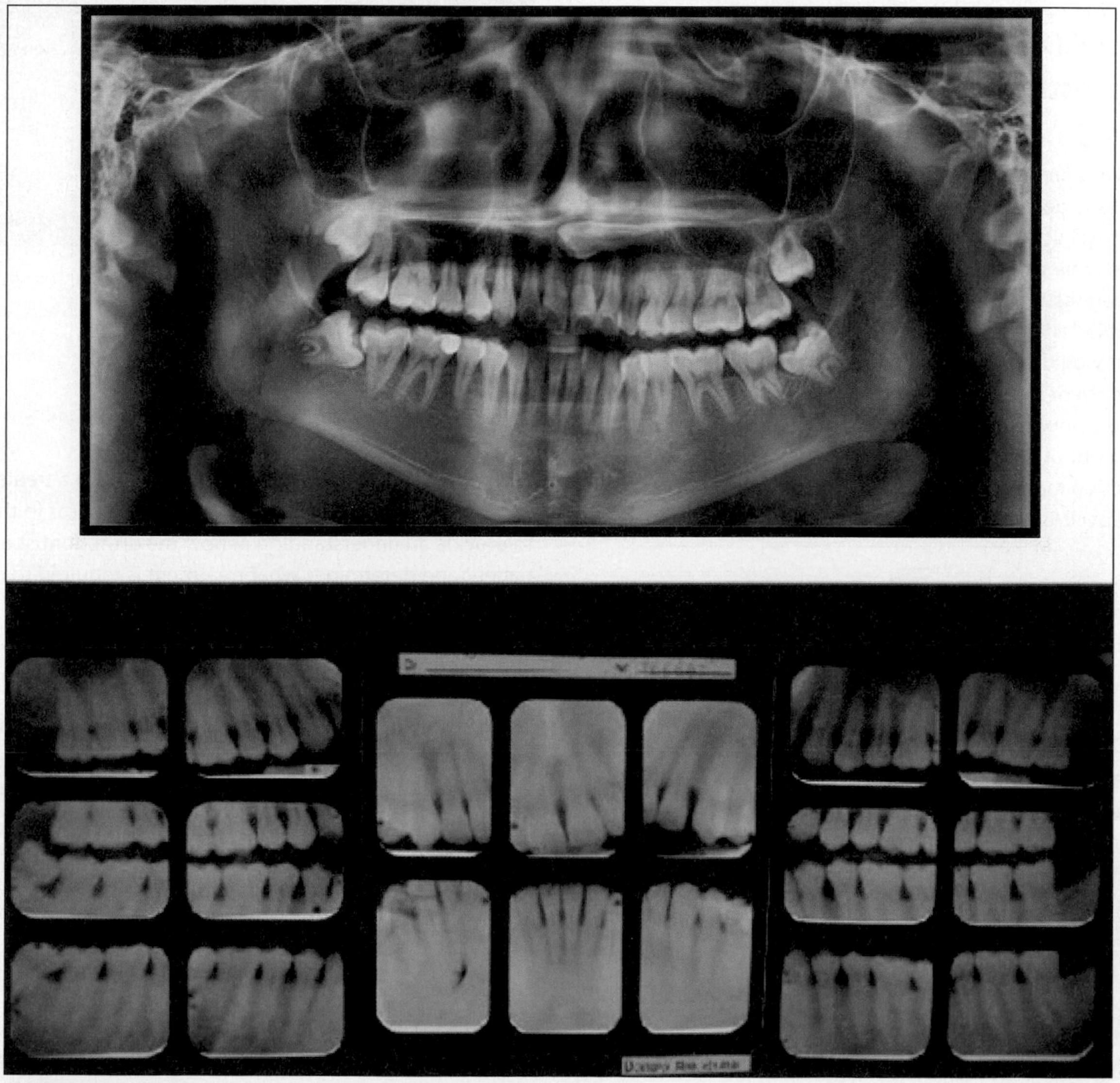

FIGURE 35-47
Panorex or FM series.

© Rames Khusakul/Shutterstock.com

periodontal problems that might worsen during orthodontic treatment. Adults may delay tooth movement until active periodontal disease is resolved to avoid future periodontal problems. Some periodontal therapy such as frenectomies and gingival recontouring should be postponed until orthodontic therapy is nearly complete for the best and most stable result.

Supplemental Diagnostic Records

Some patients will require supplemental records (Figure 35-48) for greater precision in diagnosis or for a special procedure such as orthognathic surgery. An oral surgeon working together with the orthodontist performs this surgery to move the maxilla or mandible into the correct positions. Usually, these patients have a presurgical exam and a prediction cephalometric tracing done to explore the expected surgical treatment outcomes. Also, additional photographs are often taken to document facial asymmetries that might be changed with orthognathic surgery.

Mounted Diagnostic Study Models and a Diagnostic Setup or Digital Diagnostic Planning

Patients who present with complex multidisciplinary needs and require many dental specialists to coordinate and deliver team treatment will usually benefit from a set of mounted study models that may be used for a diagnostic setup (Figure 35-49). This type of diagnostic setup is made by cutting out the teeth on the plaster model and then positioning them in wax as desired when treatment would be completed. This helps the orthodontist predict the patient's outcome more precisely and facilitates communication among the specialists and with the patient. With the advancement of computer programming, this diagnostic planning function may be completed by computer and then shared with the specialists and the patient.

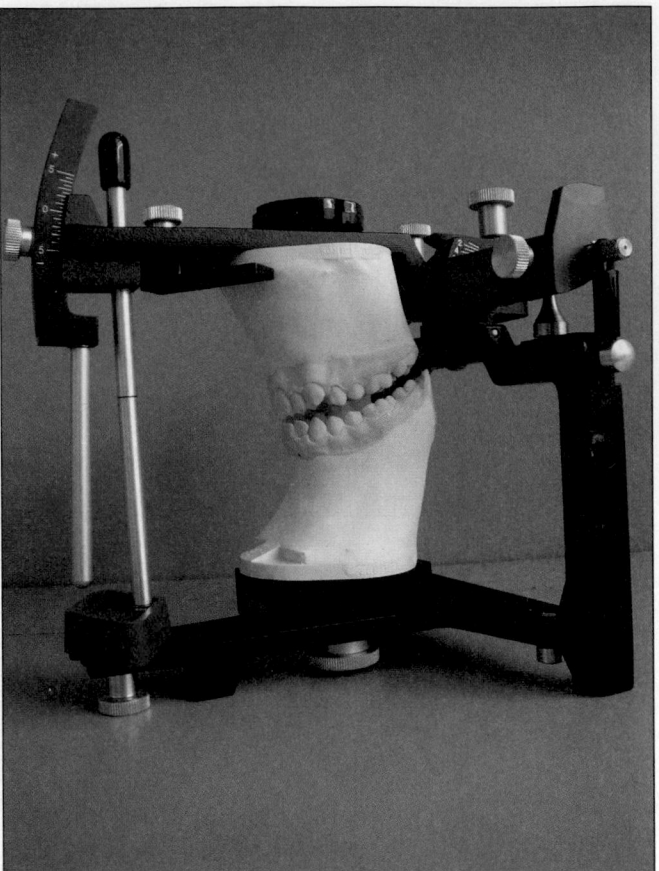

FIGURE 35-49
Study models mounted on an articulator.

Process of Diagnosis and Treatment Planning

Each orthodontist has a procedure for creating a treatment plan for a patient. Following is a summary of the steps in the process to provide an understanding of how the orthodontist evaluates a patient and determines what treatment is required to obtain the desired results.

The Problem List

The first step in the diagnostic process is to address patient concerns. Because orthodontic patients may have multiple problems, it is best to organize the problems in the same sequence as the new patient exam and then in the planes of space. First, problems should be noted in the medical and dental history, growth, social history, chief complaint, attitude and expectations, habits, facial exam and profile, and TMJ screening, then the planes of space, perimeter and finally radiographic.

Objectives of Treatment

The orthodontist will then decide the desired outcome of orthodontic treatment for each problem. For example, in the transverse plane, the mandibular dental midline may be two millimeters to the patient's right side from the patient's facial midline. The objective of

Supplemental Records

- Medical Concerns Follow-up
- Hand-Wrist Film or Vertebral Growth Analysis
- Supplemental TMJ Imaging Procedures
- Supplemental Oral Images-3D Volumetric Imaging or Cone Beam Imaging
- Occlusal Radiographs
- Periapical Shift Radiographs
- Mounted Models
- Facebow Transfer or Special Mounting
- Presurgical Photographs and Exam
- Orthodontic Diagnostic Wax-up Models

FIGURE 35-48
Supplemental orthodontic records.

treatment would be to move the mandibular midline two millimeters to the left so that the mandibular dental midline is **coincident** with the facial midline. The orthodontist will determine how to treat this problem and discuss treatment options with the patient.

Potential Treatment

Using the previous example, the orthodontist might do an extraction of a tooth on the lower left in order to have space to shift the mandibular dental midline to the left. Or the orthodontist might recommend shaving off some of the tooth enamel between the posterior teeth on the left side to shift the mandibular dental midline to the left. This diagnostic process can aid the orthodontist in choosing the best possible solutions to address the problems that were determined during the exam, from the records, and in this diagnostic phase.

Treatment Options

If there are several treatment plan options that will work, the orthodontist will list the different options along with their advantages and disadvantages. This list will be presented to the patient to facilitate the discussion about which plan will best meet the patient's needs. Once a treatment plan is selected, it is written up in detail so it may be a guide for the orthodontic team to complete all procedures listed in the plan.

Orthodontic Treatment Consultation

The final step in the diagnosis and treatment planning process is to present the records and the treatment plan to the patient and caregivers. At the treatment consultation the orthodontist will present the orthodontic records and briefly highlight the concerns. The treatment plan will be reviewed including the time treatment will take and the cost of treatment. Financial arrangements will be made so that the treatment may be paid for over the treatment period. Usually patient instructions are reviewed so that everyone is aware of the steps that will make treatment go smoothly and quickly.

Patients who understand what is planned for them and why are more likely to comply with the plan. Patients and caregivers should know the consequences of noncompliance such as missing appointments. A missed appointment will delay treatment. Additionally, if the patient does not see the orthodontist as scheduled and the pressure on a tooth is prolonged, it may shift more than desired. Additional time in treatment would then be required to move it back to the desired location. Some offices increase fees for extended time due to patient noncompliance. Additionally, patients must be made aware that if an appliance breaks or a bracket becomes dislodged, the patient must return immediately to the office so treatment can progress as scheduled.

Not only are the treatment procedures determined by what treatment is required to obtain the desired results, but also the patient's age and growth and development of their teeth and skeleton have an impact on treatment time and results. Treatment procedures are divided into treatment of young children, adolescents, and adults.

Orthodontic Treatment of Young Children

The American Association of Orthodontists recommends that all children be seen by an orthodontist at age 7 years. Usually no treatment is needed at this age, but it is a good idea to have an orthodontic checkup to be certain there are no problems developing that could be easily prevented.

Observation and Counseling

Young children under the age of 6 years usually just have their primary teeth present in the oral cavity. At the age of 6 years the first permanent molars start to erupt. This stage of tooth development is called the early mixed dentition stage, where both the primary teeth and the secondary teeth are present. At this age, children are usually monitored by the orthodontist for any habits or problems that may be present. Such issues, if resolved early, may prevent complex orthodontic problems in the future, resulting in a reduced need for orthodontic intervention.

Interceptive

Children at this phase are monitored for growth and development of the jaws and dentition as well as for habits that can affect the oral cavity and the teeth. For example, a child may have an active thumb sucking habit, even in school. The orthodontist can counsel the child with ideas about discontinuing the habit or suggest ways the caregiver can help the child stop. The child who sucks a thumb day and night will cause a narrowing of the maxillary arch from the sucking pressure and develop a posterior **crossbite**. To correct a posterior crossbite, an orthodontist may place a palatal expander on the maxillary molars and have the caregiver turn it slowly to widen the arch expanding the palate and correcting the crossbite (Figure 35-50). If the habit

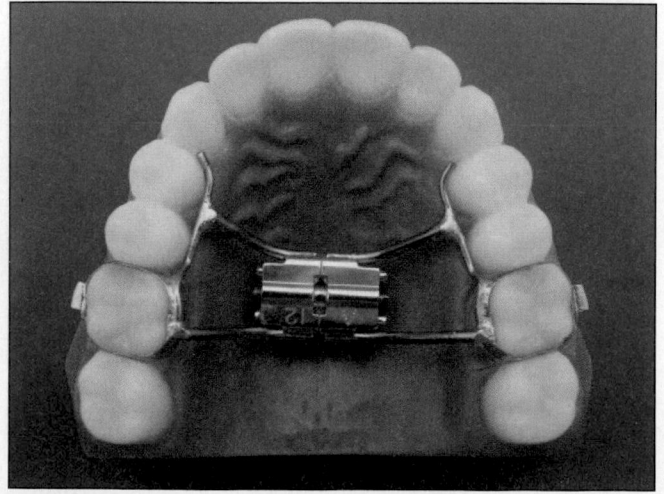

FIGURE 35-50
Palatal expander.

is continued long after the upper permanent front teeth have erupted, either excessive overjet or an open bite gap between the maxillary and mandibular anterior teeth when the child is biting together may result. Occasionally, the child is not able to stop the habit and a tongue crib appliance may be cemented to the upper first molars to act as a barrier to insertion of the thumb (see Figure 35-29).

Placement of a palatal expander also may be considered **interceptive** treatment; however, it may be removed early, as these habit problems may resolve on their own without orthodontic treatment. Additionally, a pathological tongue thrust swallowing habit can occur that the child cannot consciously stop. This tongue thrust will cause the bite to remain open and may make the open bite difficult to close permanently. Sometimes an orthodontist will insert a rake appliance that will poke the tongue when it thrusts forward to help the patient be aware of the habit. Some practitioners have success with **myofunctional therapy**, tongue swallowing training, by a myofunctional therapist or speech pathologist.

Orthodontic intervention treatment that may be recommended to create space for secondary teeth to erupt is the extraction of certain primary teeth. Usually, the family general dentist will extract the teeth as requested by the orthodontist. This allows guidance of the eruption of permanent teeth that might be blocked without primary tooth extractions. Severe decay can cause early loss of the primary teeth, which then may cause shifting of the primary teeth and blockage of the eruption of the permanent teeth. In this case, the orthodontist may suggest the removal of additional primary teeth and placement of a space maintainer (Figure 35-51) or a lingual arch (Figure 35-52) to hold the eruption space for the adult teeth. Unfortunately, the space maintainer in the photograph has shifted down into the soft tissue. It should have been made with a stop on the crown of the primary canine.

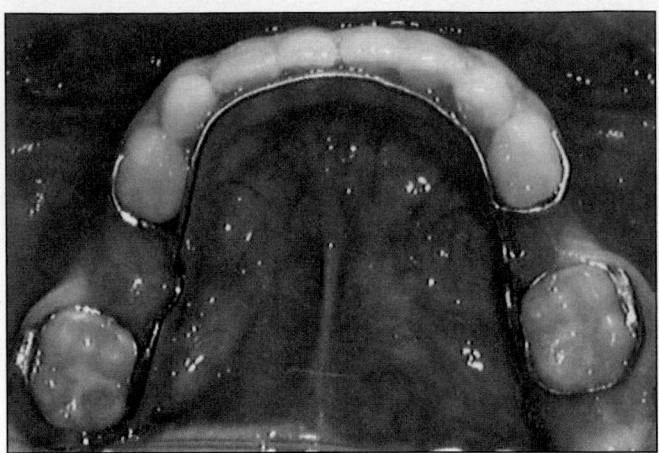

FIGURE 35-52
Lingual bar preserves space for erupting teeth bilaterally.

Phase I Early Treatment with Limited Braces, Growth Appliances, Expansion, and Extractions

As a child matures and the permanent teeth erupt, problems such as crowding, overjet due to proclination and protrusion of the maxillary incisors, and other problems become more evident. An orthodontist may recommend Phase I early treatment with some braces on just the maxillary teeth or in both arches to correct these developing problems so the child is not teased in school.

Additionally, in some young children, the maxilla does not grow properly, and these children develop what may appear as an overgrowth of the mandible, resulting in a dental and skeletal Class III underbite. In many cases, an orthodontist places a plastic splint in the upper arch and the child wears "reverse pull" headgear or "**protraction** headgear" at night to encourage forward growth of the maxilla and correct the skeletal and dental Class III relationships including the dental underbite (see Figure 35-16). This treatment will usually take about a year. The best results with this type of headgear occur when the patient is treated at a young age, often around 5 years of age.

A child also may need a growth appliance to help the growth of the lower jaw "catch up" with that of the upper jaw. Traditionally, this growth appliance has been headgear or neckgear. The wire **facebow** of the headgear (Figure 35-53) has wire ends that fit into the round headgear tubes on orthodontic bands (Figure 35-54) that are cemented to the upper first molars inside the mouth. A strap is then attached to the outer arms of the facebow (Figure 35-55), exerting backward pressure on the maxilla so that the mandible can grow forward and align with the upper jaw and upper teeth. There are three types of headgear that work with patients of differing skeletal types. Of course, for headgear to work it must be worn by the patient each night for the prescribed period of time. One way to check if the headgear is being worn is to check for looseness of the upper first molars, which is normal.

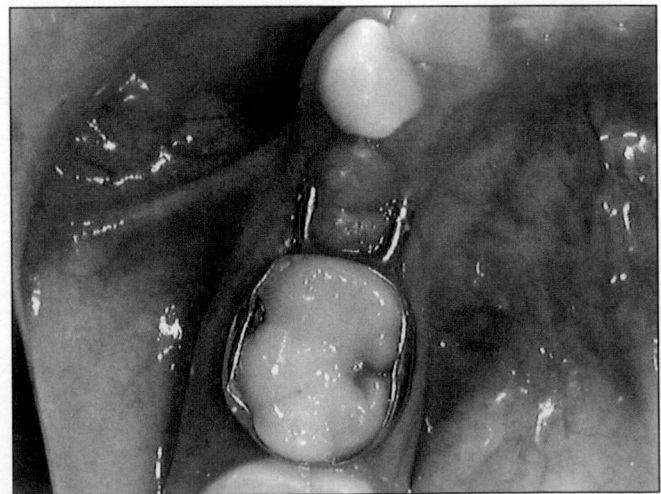

FIGURE 35-51
Space maintainer (digging into tissue) preserves space for an erupting tooth unilaterally.

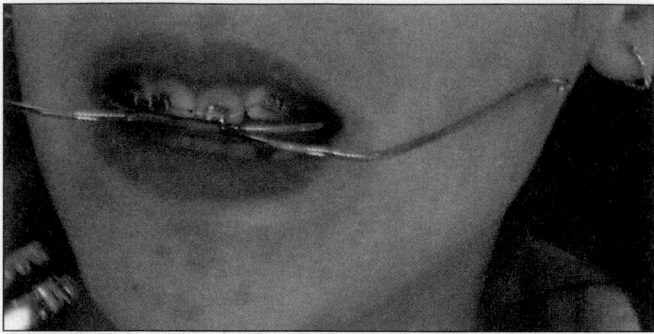

FIGURE 35-53
Cervical headgear facebow in mouth worn with a "neck strap" by the patient at night. Used with a patient with a deep bite and a square jaw and expected forward growth of the mandible.

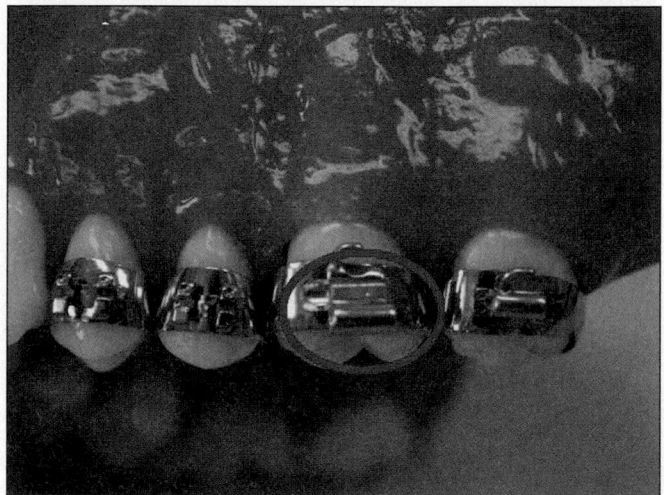

FIGURE 35-54
Ortho bands with tubes attached to allow for the insertion of the headgear bow.

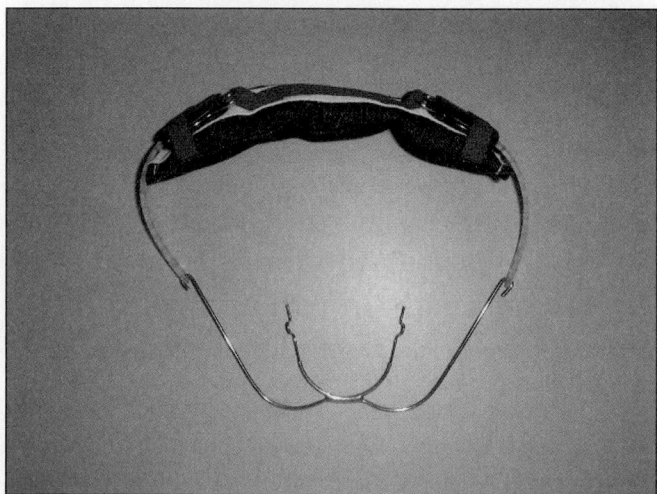

FIGURE 35-55
A "neck strap" is connected to the facebow for retraction exerting a posterior force on the maxillary teeth to correct excessive overjet.

Treatment of dental crowding may also be done during Phase I early treatment. There are essentially five orthodontic treatment methods of creating arch space to align crowded teeth: (1) Extract primary teeth using leeway space and guiding eruption, (2) extract permanent teeth, (3) expand the arches, (4) try to push back the molars (Figures 35-56A, B, and C), and (5) shave the surfaces between the teeth in the area of crowding, also known as IPR or interproximal reduction (Figure 35-57).

After Phase I early treatment is completed, the orthodontist will observe and monitor the patient to determine whether Phase II treatment with full braces is necessary as the child matures into adolescence.

Orthodontic Treatment of Adolescents

In most orthodontic practices the majority of patients are adolescents. They may be in the late mixed dentition stage or have all of their adult teeth erupted. The levels of treatment range from simple observation to full multidisciplinary complex treatment. As previously discussed, an adolescent may have no real concerns or problems but simply need observation to ensure that all of the teeth will align properly and that the skeletal relationship will be harmonious with the face.

Observation and Counseling

Most adolescents have discontinued thumb sucking and finger sucking habits and do not need counseling. However, due to stress and certain genetic factors, adolescents may start bruxing or clenching habits, especially at night. If these habits are severe, the adolescent is at risk of tooth wear. This should be discussed and the patient should be given a night guard to prevent wearing down the teeth.

Adolescents should be made aware of other **deleterious** habits they might have such as drinking acidic sugary soda, which contributes to diabetes, obesity, and tooth decay. Teenagers are very self-conscious about their appearance. A nice smile is critical for attractiveness and development of optimum self-esteem.

Since most adolescents have most or all of their teeth erupted, there typically is little need for tooth guidance. However, it is very common for adolescents to have maxillary impacted canines that will not erupt on their own (Figure 35-58). These impacted canines are often associated with maxillary peg lateral incisors. Researchers think that peg-shaped maxillary lateral incisors do not provide sufficient root guidance for the maxillary canines, so a canine then becomes impacted. A panoramic radiograph or even a cone beam image is excellent for diagnosing the position of impacted canines and the probability of orthodontic treatment bringing them into the arch. If they can be treated, the canine is surgically exposed and a special orthodontic bracket is placed on it with a little gold chain. Braces or some other fixed appliance (such as a palatal holding arch) are then placed, and a nylon elastic string is tied from the appliance to the chain bonded to the canine. This tie is tightened weekly, slowly pulling the tooth down and into the arch. Sometimes the canine is so close to the

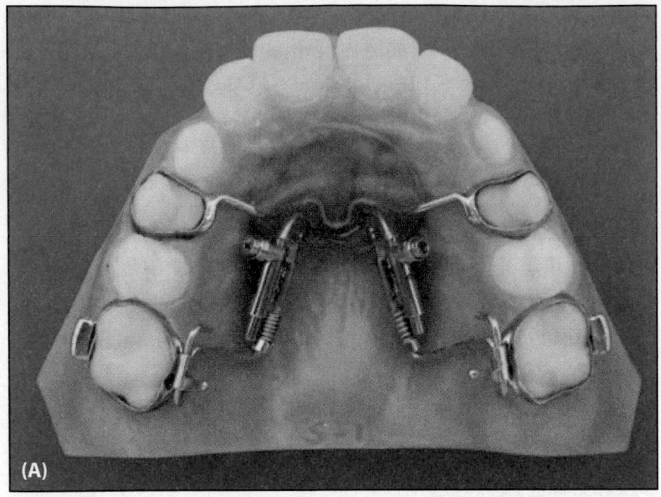

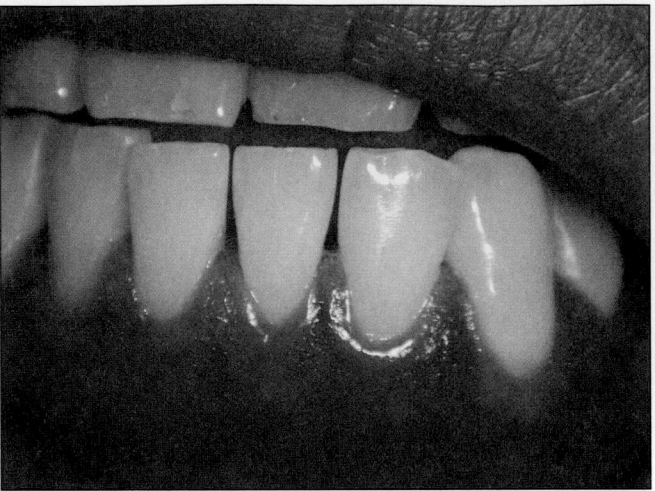

FIGURE 35-57
Interproximal reduction (IPR) has been performed on the incisors to allow space for retracting incisors to correct an underbite of the teeth.

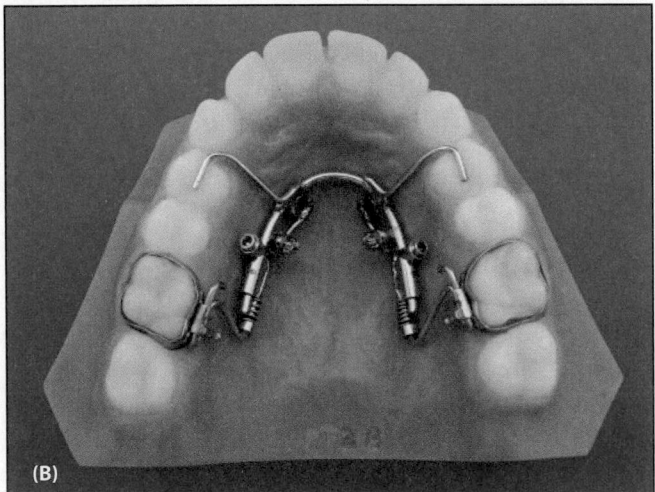

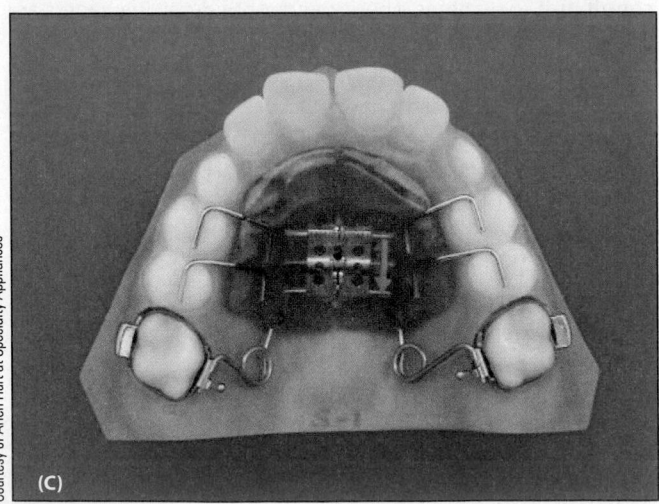

Courtesy of Arlen Hurt at Specialty Appliances

FIGURE 35-56
Fixed appliances to push back molars. (A) Distal jet appliance pushes molars back more posteriorly. (B) Horseshoe jet pushes molars back. (C) Pendex appliance pushes molars back.

lateral incisor that moving it will cause resorption to the root of the lateral incisor tooth, and the lateral may be lost. Occasionally, mandibular teeth will be impacted, and the orthodontist and patient must discuss the advantages and disadvantages of various treatment alternatives.

Phase II Treatment (Comprehensive Orthodontic Treatment) of Adolescents Following Phase I

Many adolescents will already have had Phase I treatment, and the orthodontist must determine if they need to go into Phase II or a short period of comprehensive orthodontic treatment. This involves placing braces on all teeth (Figure 35-59) and using some growth appliance as needed. Braces are the main mechanism orthodontists use to attach to the teeth in order to move them. Occasionally, clear aligner therapy is used instead of braces, but this treatment is completely controlled by compliance of the patient.

Comprehensive orthodontic treatment may take less than 12 months or as long as 3 years, depending upon the complexity of treatment and the cooperation of the patient.

Comprehensive Orthodontic Treatment of Adolescents with Growth Appliances

Often adolescent orthodontic patients will have a dental malocclusion as well as a skeletal problem that is located in the maxilla or the mandible. If the patient has growth remaining in the jaws and is willing to wear growth appliances, then some of the skeletal problem may be corrected during orthodontic treatment. If the patient is an adult with no growth remaining, skeletal problems must be corrected with orthognathic surgery.

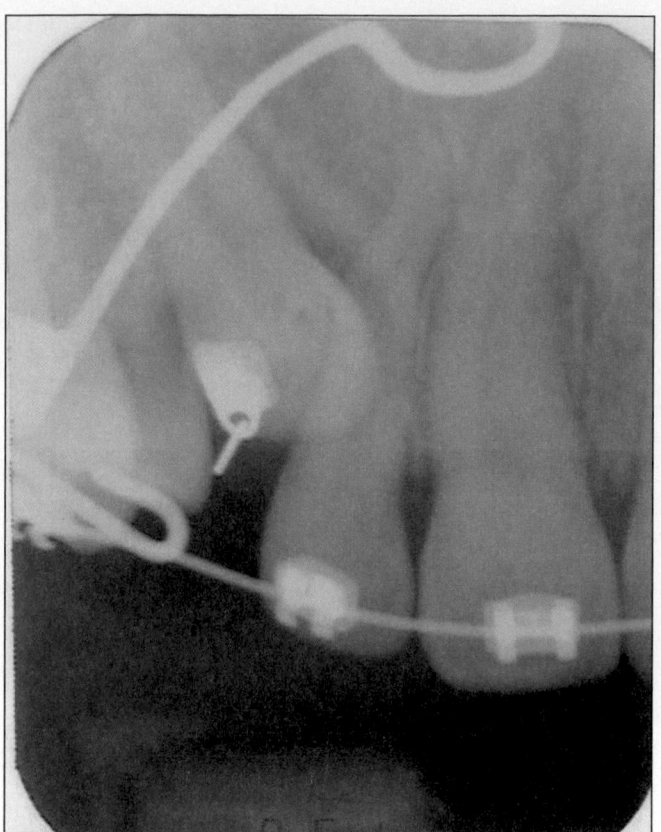

FIGURE 35-58
Radiograph shows an impacted canine with a surgically placed bracket used to pull the canine into position.

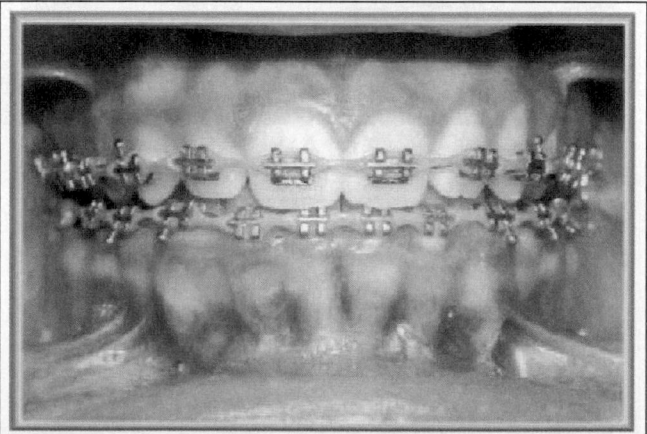

FIGURE 35-59
Orthodontic brackets on all teeth and arch wires tied in slot of bracket with gray closing chains.

Some growth appliances guide newly erupting teeth into position, others change the direction of cranial-facial skeletal growth, and still others inhibit the growth rate of one arch. As mentioned earlier in this chapter, growth appliances include different types of headgears. Other growth appliances include the removable twin block appliance, an activator, a bionator, a Frankl

appliance, and a fixed or removable Herbst appliance. All of these appliances are designed to work with the patient's jaw growth to align the jaws. The goal is to align the jaws completely and improve the occlusal relationships to allow optimal function and esthetics.

The "activator" is the original removable acrylic functional jaw orthopedic appliance designed to position the mandible anteriorly, and it has been modified many times. The activator is used to slightly expand the width of the maxillary arch, to correct minor tooth movement, to make changes in skeletal growth patterns in growing patients, and to reduce overjet. The bionator appliance (Figure 35-60A) is an acrylic removable appliance which fits on the upper and lower teeth and positions the lower jaw forward. It is used to encourage lower jaw growth in growing patients and decrease the overjet. The Frankel appliance was originally designed to have a "headgear effect" slowing the forward growth of the maxilla while encouraging the mandible to advance and grow forward to align the jaws. However, Frankel appliance use may cause the maxillary anterior teeth to become retroclined. This may result in flattening of the profile by reducing incisor proclination instead of the more esthetic change by jaw alignment (Figure 35-60B). The Herbst appliance may be a fixed appliance or removable appliance. It is used to correct a skeletal Class II relationship due to a **retrognathic** mandible. The fixed Herbst appliance holds the mandible in a forward position, encouraging horizontal growth of the mandibular condyles. The fixed Herbst appliance may also distalize the maxillary molars and, combined with forward growth of the mandible, improve the Class II dental relationship and reduce overjet (Figure 35-60C).

The fixed Mara device is another fixed cemented device that is used to correct Class II dental relationships (Figure 35-61). This device is attached to the maxillary and mandibular first molars so that when the patient bites together the patient's mandible is forced forward, encouraging habitual forward positioning of the mandible.

Bite plates are fixed or removable growth appliances used to open the bite. When the patient wears the bite plate the posterior teeth are held apart and then can erupt vertically by growth of the alveolar bone (Figure 35-62).

Comprehensive Orthodontic Treatment of Adolescents Combined with Multidisciplinary Care

A few adolescent patients have complex needs and require multidisciplinary treatment that may involve the orthodontist, the dentist, a periodontist, an oral surgeon, and a restorative specialist. Such a patient might have multiple congenitally missing teeth such as maxillary lateral incisors that need to be replaced with implants after growth of the alveolus is complete (Figure 35-63). There may have been a traumatic injury that avulsed several teeth, or the patient may have a cleft lip and palate. Usually such treatment is provided by a team of expert professionals who have experience working well together.

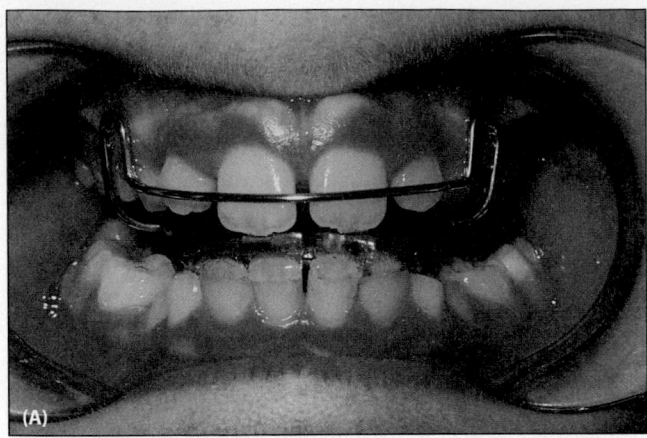

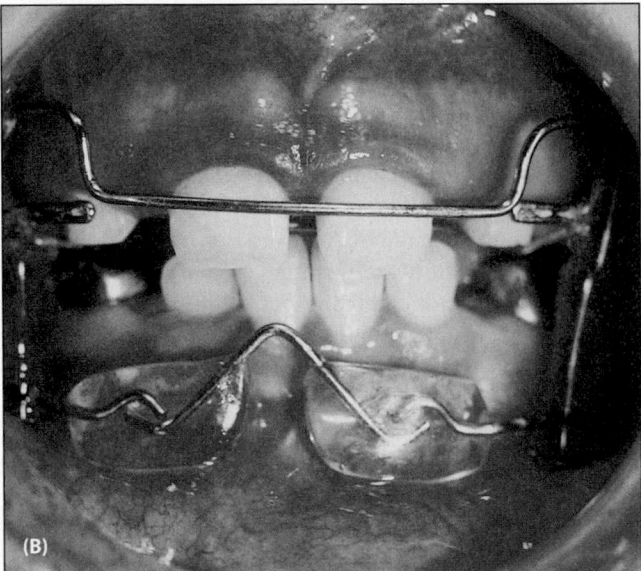

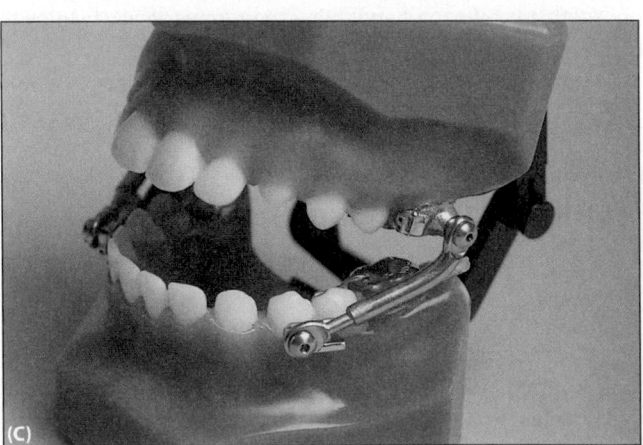

FIGURE 35-60
Removable growth appliances. (A) The bionator appliance. (B) Frankel appliance. (C) Herbst appliance.

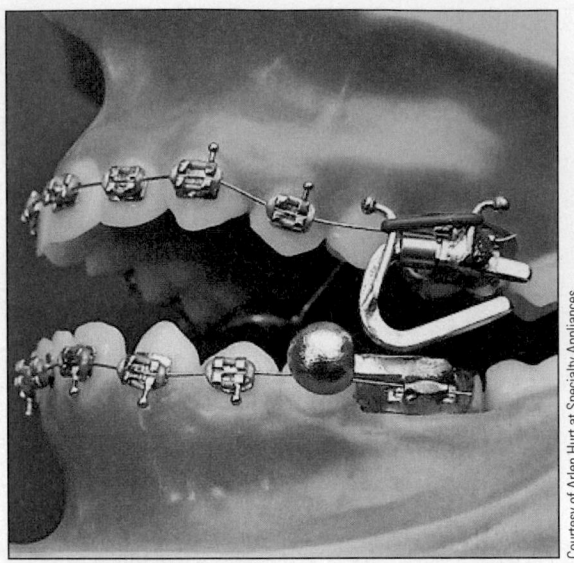

FIGURE 35-61
Fixed mara device forces jaw forward when patient bites.

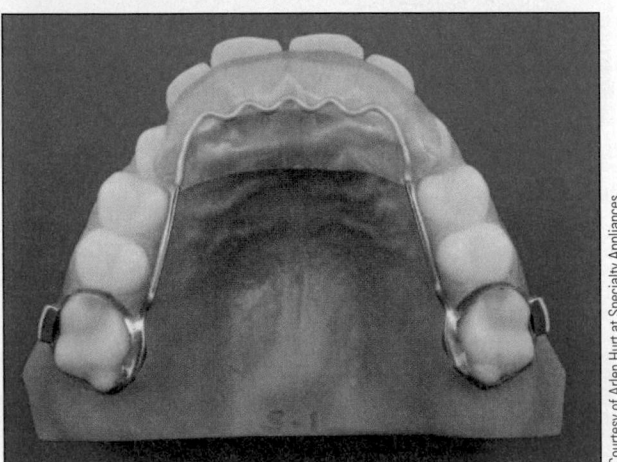

FIGURE 35-62
Bite plane used to open bite.

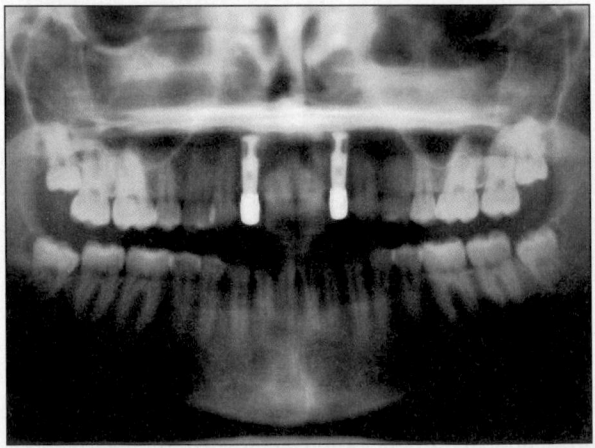

FIGURE 35-63
Panoramic radiograph shows congenitally missing lateral incisors with implant replacements.

Clear Aligner Therapy for Adolescents

Often, children in early adolescence are very self-conscious about their appearance. This focus on appearance may start to occur in girls as young as 11 years of age and in boys as young as 12 years of age. These children want to have a "perfect" smile. Otherwise, they may be teased or bullied by other children. Braces used to be a status symbol for younger children, but now may be another cause of being teased as they enter middle school. Adolescents may request teen clear aligner therapy to correct the concerns they have about their smiles since *maxillary and mandibular aligners* are clear and are much less visible than braces. Clear aligners, when worn properly, can correct a simple malocclusion and create a more esthetic smile. However, clear aligner therapy requires that the patient wear each set of custom-made removable aligners for 22 hours per day for a period of at least 7 days and then move on to the next set. Treatment may require 20 to 30 sets of aligners requiring 3 to 6 months of treatment. Clear aligner therapy cannot impact a patient's growth pattern, so aligner treatment should not be recommended to correct a skeletal problem in a growing patient (Figure 35-64). Also, removable clear aligners will not correct any severe orthodontic problems such as very crowded or spaced teeth, a deep bite, or a narrow maxillary arch with significant posterior crossbites. Adolescents who qualify for clear aligner therapy should be exceptionally responsible and willing to wear the aligners as prescribed. Teenagers who are self-conscience about removing their aligners in front of others, such as when taking them out to eat or brush their teeth, will have more difficulty complying with treatment. Finally, orthodontic treatment requires long-term retention to hold and retain the final result. Removable retainers will have to be worn nightly indefinitely to maintain the alignment of the teeth. Another option may be the placement of a "bonded" wire chain retainer that is attached to the inside of the anterior teeth in the upper and lower arches. These factors should be considered by the patient before committing to this type of treatment.

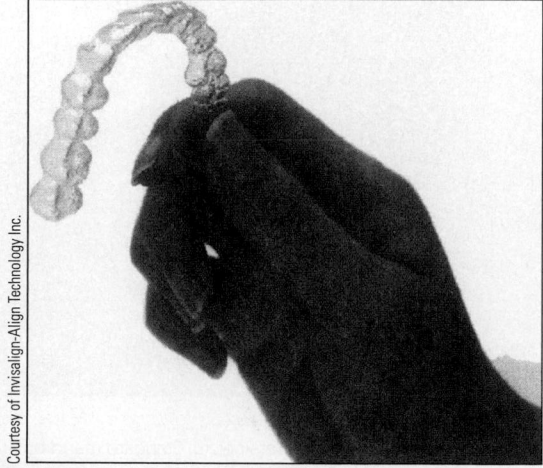

Courtesy of Invisalign-Align Technology Inc.

FIGURE 35-64
Invisalign esthetic orthodontic aligner.

Orthodontic Treatment of Adults

Adults usually have comprehensive orthodontic treatment and may be treated orthodontically at any age. In some cases, if the problems are minor such as in the case of an anterior single tooth crossbite, limited orthodontics, or esthetic orthodontic aligners may be able to correct the concern.

Comprehensive Orthodontic Treatment Combined with Multidisciplinary Treatment

Adult patients may need comprehensive orthodontic treatment that is combined with multidisciplinary treatment from a team of specialists to fully restore an adult's dentition, achieving an esthetic and functional result.

Comprehensive Orthodontic Treatment with Orthognathic Surgery

Since adults have no growth, orthognathic surgery is recommended for skeletal changes that would otherwise be corrected with growth appliances when the individual is an adolescent.

Clear Aligner Therapy

In some adult cases, if the orthodontic problems are minor such as in the case of an anterior single tooth crossbite, esthetic orthodontic aligners, also referred to as clear aligner therapy, may be recommended to correct the concerns. *Maxillary and mandibular aligners* are an esthetic orthodontic appliance that can correct a malocclusion using a series of custom-made, nearly invisible, removable aligners (Figure 35-64). The adult patient who qualifies for this type of orthodontic treatment will undergo the same process of a new patient exam, orthodontic records, and diagnosis and treatment plan by the orthodontist or dentist, and then start aligner therapy by wearing custom-made aligners that slowly move the teeth into position.

Patients wear each aligner for a minimum of 7 days until the aligner has moved the teeth the prescribed amount, which usually requires wearing them about 22 hours per day. Treatment generally lasts from 6 months to 1 year. Aligners are only removed for eating, brushing, and flossing. Teeth are moved gradually as each aligner is replaced with the next set, until the desired results are achieved.

The aligners are similar to whitening or fluoride trays in that they are custom made, but are thinner, more precisely designed, and fabricated from a more rigid **proprietary material**. The number of aligners and length of treatment depend on the complexity of the case and compliance of the patient in wearing the aligners. As with traditional braces, patients experience a brief period of adjustment as they transition to each new set of aligners. Since the aligners are removable, oral hygiene is easy to maintain while patients eat, brush, and floss as they normally would. Aligners may not produce a "perfect" result or a functional occlusion since there is less control of the orthodontic movement of each tooth than with braces.

Orthodontists and dentists who provide orthodontic treatment using aligners should know how to examine a potential orthodontic patient, take and analyze orthodontic records, and diagnose and plan each step of aligner treatment. Then the entire team must be trained in monitoring treatment progress in all patients undergoing therapy to produce the desired patient outcomes.

Practitioners must also complete a training/certification program offered through the manufacturer in order to treat patients with their product. Dental auxiliaries attending the certification program will learn the submission process, which includes PVS impressions or digital scanning impressions and bite, panoramic, and cephalometric radiographs for complex cases; an orthodontic series of diagnostic photographs; and the practitioner's tooth-movement treatment plan. Additionally, the dental team needs to know case management and practice management procedures to deliver clear aligner therapy successfully.

Orthodontic Retention

At the completion of orthodontic treatment, the orthodontist and dentist will place fixed bonded **retainers** or deliver removable acrylic retainers for the patient to wear to hold the teeth in their final position. Retainers need to be worn indefinitely. Orthodontists used to believe that, once straightened, the teeth would stay aligned if the orthodontist did a good job. Research has shown, however, that most patients will have relapse to crooked teeth unless retainers are worn to hold their teeth straight. Just as teeth can be straightened, they can and will move out of position again after treatment.

Removable retainers can be easily removed from the mouth. They have been used most frequently for orthodontic retention. There are many styles of removable retainers depending upon the preference of the orthodontist and what the patient wants to wear (Figures 35-65A, B, and C). Also, full coverage clear retainers are frequently used for retention.

Bonded lingual fixed retainers are now used by orthodontists since lifetime retention is recommended. They are bonded on the palatal or lingual surfaces (Figures 35-66A and B) of the anterior teeth. The wires of these retainers are first adapted to a model of the teeth and then bonded to each tooth for the best retention. When they are placed, the patient should be instructed in proper sulcular flossing under the retainer to prevent gingivitis and periodontal disease.

Appointments for Comprehensive Orthodontic Treatment with Braces

Delivering comprehensive orthodontic treatment with braces involves many types of appointments involving the entire practice team. All members of the team must understand the tasks performed by others so that the best care can be given to each patient efficiently. It is ideal if the orthodontist has written a detailed treatment plan that the patient has accepted at the treatment consultation with the treatment coordinator. Then the financial arrangements are set up with the patient and the first appointment is scheduled. If the treatment plan includes placement of orthodontic bands on the patient's molars, then separators may be placed immediately after the treatment consultation.

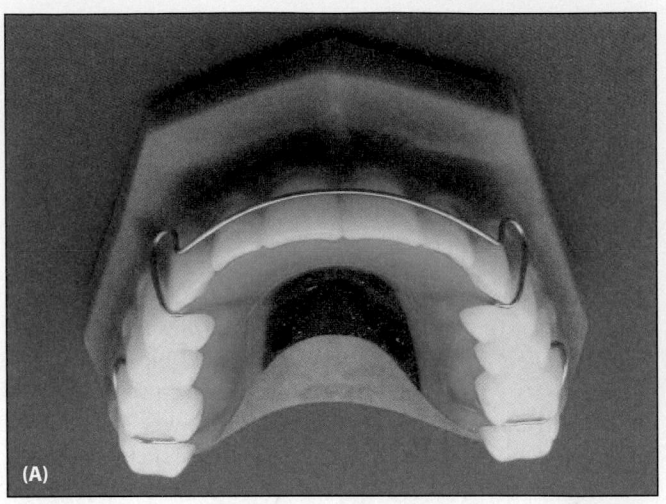

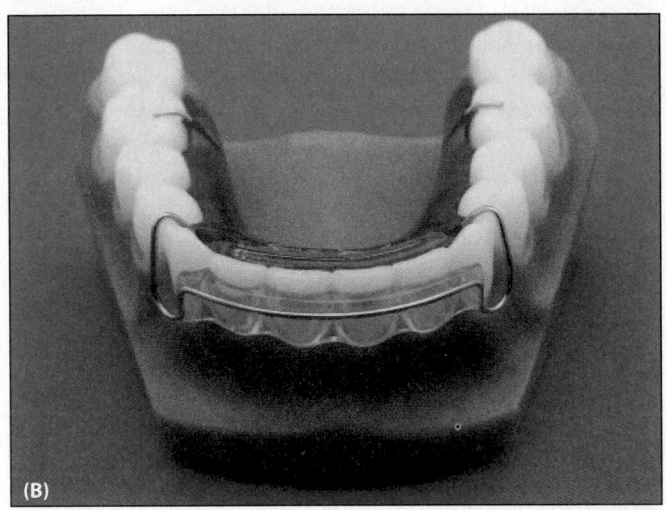

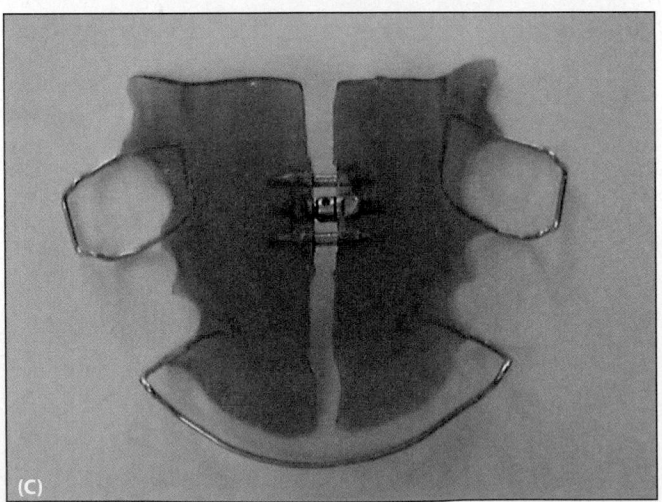

FIGURE 35-65
Hawley retainers. (A) Maxillary Hawley retainer. (B) Standard mandibular Hawley retainer. (C) Removable sagittal Hawley retainer to expand during retention.

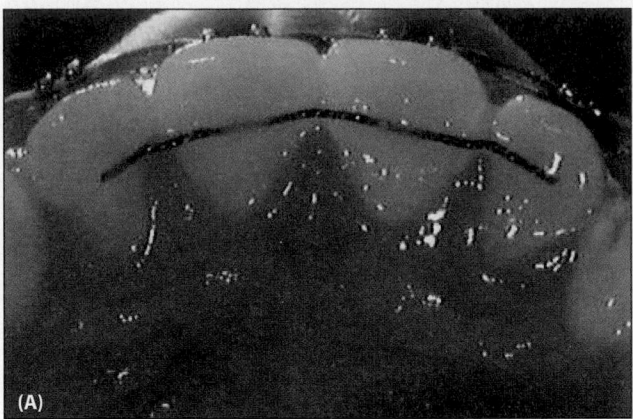
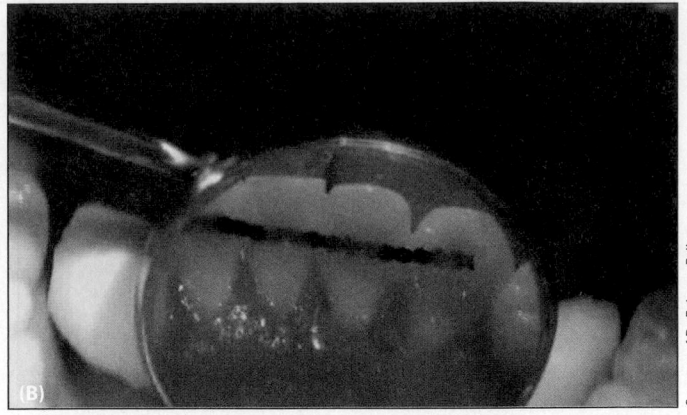

FIGURE 35-66
Bonded fixed retainers. (A) Maxillary fixed retainer. (B) Newly placed bonded mandibular chain retainer.

Orthodontic Separators

Orthodontic **separators** are placed between the posterior teeth that will have orthodontic bands fitted and cemented to those teeth (Figure 35-67). There are different types of separators that work best in certain situations (Figure 35-68). The operator who places separators should have formal training in this procedure by an individual who is trained and experienced in placing and removing separators (Procedure 35-1).

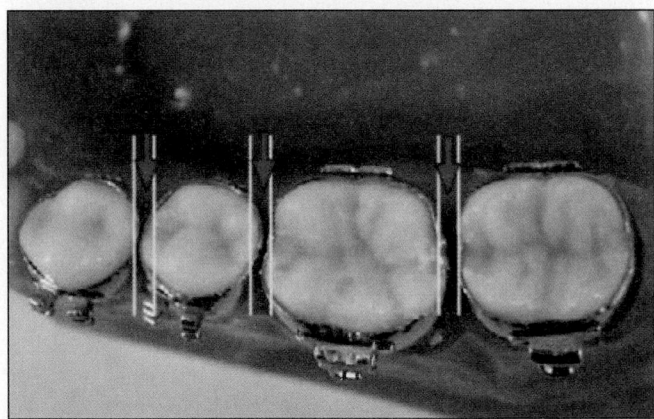

FIGURE 35-67
Separators placed to provide space between two teeth.

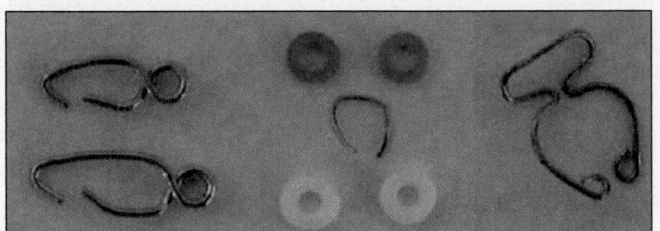

FIGURE 35-68
Types of separators.

Fitting and Cementing Orthodontic Bands

Fitting and cementing orthodontic **bands** on certain posterior teeth are often necessary to carry out the instructions of a comprehensive orthodontic treatment plan. For instance, orthodontic bands may be placed on maxillary first permanent molars because they are required for the use of a maxillary expander or headgear appliance. Usually, fitting and cementing orthodontic bands are performed by an orthodontic assistant who has been formally trained in this procedure. This individual needs to know the components of bands, band identification, band selection and fitting procedures, band cementing agents, and band positioning criteria for proper orthodontic movement of the teeth (Figure 35-69). Glass ionomer cement has greater adhesion to enamel due to ionic bonding and is often preferred to cement orthodontic bands (Table 35-1). Refer to Procedure 35-2, "Assisting with Cementation of Orthodontic Bands."

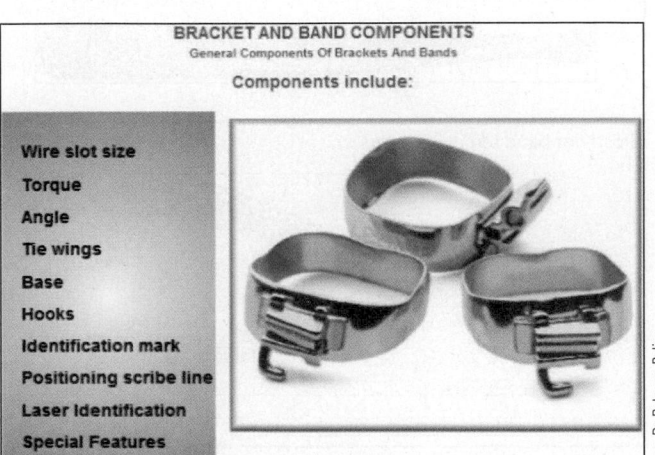

FIGURE 35-69
Components of bands.

TABLE 35-1 Banding Appointment Orthodontic Instruments

Instrument	Function
Band contouring pliers (#112) 	Stretches and shapes the posterior bands to adapt to the tooth
Band contouring pliers (#137) 	Crimps and reforms bands to adapt more tightly to the tooth
Band pusher (seater) 	Seats posterior metal bands
Band rocker 	Gently rocks band with back-and-forth motion
Bite stick with band seater 	Uses force of occlusion to seat the band
Posterior band removing pliers 	Removes posterior bands

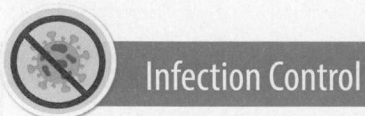

Infection Control

Instruments that are used intraorally or that come in contact with saliva or blood need to be sterilized, preferably in an autoclave. Orthodontic bands that have been tried on in the mouth must be sterilized before returning to the band kit.

Orthodontic Bonding of Brackets to the Teeth

Orthodontic bonding of **brackets** (braces) to the teeth is a complex, detailed task and should only be performed by a formally trained orthodontic assistant under the direct supervision of an orthodontist (Figure 35-70). The orthodontic assistant must know the components of orthodontic brackets, preparation of the teeth for bonding brackets, materials used in bonding, precise steps in placing and positioning brackets on the teeth, removal of flash, having the orthodontist check positioning, curing bonding adhesive, bonding difficult areas, solving problems associated with bonding, bonding to special surfaces, and bonding second molar to second molar in one appointment (Table 35-2). Refer to Procedure 35-3, "Assisting with Direct Bonding of Brackets."

Orthodontic Wires Used in the Five Phases of Orthodontic Treatment

The trained orthodontic assistant is the team member who will select and insert each orthodontic wire so it will move the teeth properly. Ideally, the orthodontist specifies on the patient's treatment plan the type of orthodontic wire that should be used during each phase of treatment. For most patients there are five phases of orthodontic treatment and five types of wires:

1. Alignment phase to straighten the teeth using alignment wires (Figure 35-71).

2. Leveling phase to open or close the bite using leveling wires (Figure 35-72).

3. Arch coordination phase to make the maxillary arch fit and occlude properly with the mandibular arch using arch coordination wires (Figure 35-73).

4. Space closure phase to close excessive spaces (arch length excess) between the teeth or, if adult teeth are extracted due to crowding (arch length deficiency), and extraction space needs to be closed, space closure wires are used (Figure 35-74).

5. Finishing phase is done to align the teeth to establish excellent esthetics, create a functional occlusion, facilitate long-term health of the teeth and periodontium, and provide stability to hold the orthodontic result indefinitely. Finishing wires are used to achieve these final results (Figure 35-75).

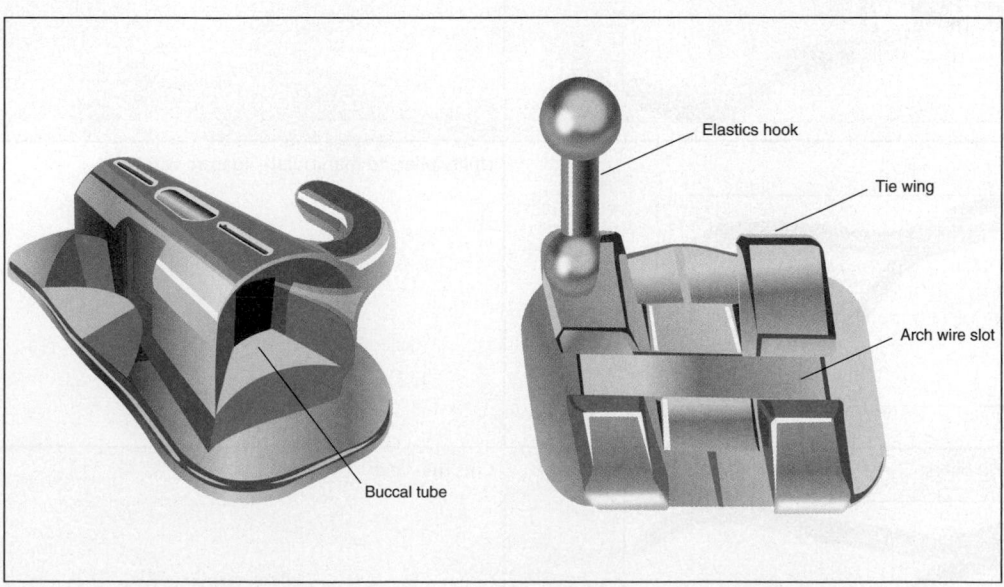

FIGURE 35-70
Orthodontic bracket components. The buccal tube is a small cylinder for the placement of the arch wire that is a part of the most posterior bracket. The hook provides for the attachment of rubber bands. Elastic tie or ligature wire is placed around the wing to secure the arch wire. The slot holds the arch wire.

TABLE 35-2 Bonding Appointment Orthodontic Instruments

Instrument	Function
Bird-beak pliers (wire bending pliers)	Contours wires and forms springs
Bracket forceps	Holds brackets for placement and positioning
Distal end cutting pliers	Used intraorally, cuts the distal ends of the arch wire and have a mechanism that grasps the cut piece of the arch wire to prevent falling into patient's throat
Elastic-separating pliers	Places elastics on brackets
Howe pliers	Utility pliers to manipulate ligature wire
Ligature wire cutting pliers	Cuts thin ligature wire

TABLE 35-2 *(Continued)*

Instrument	Function
Ligature director 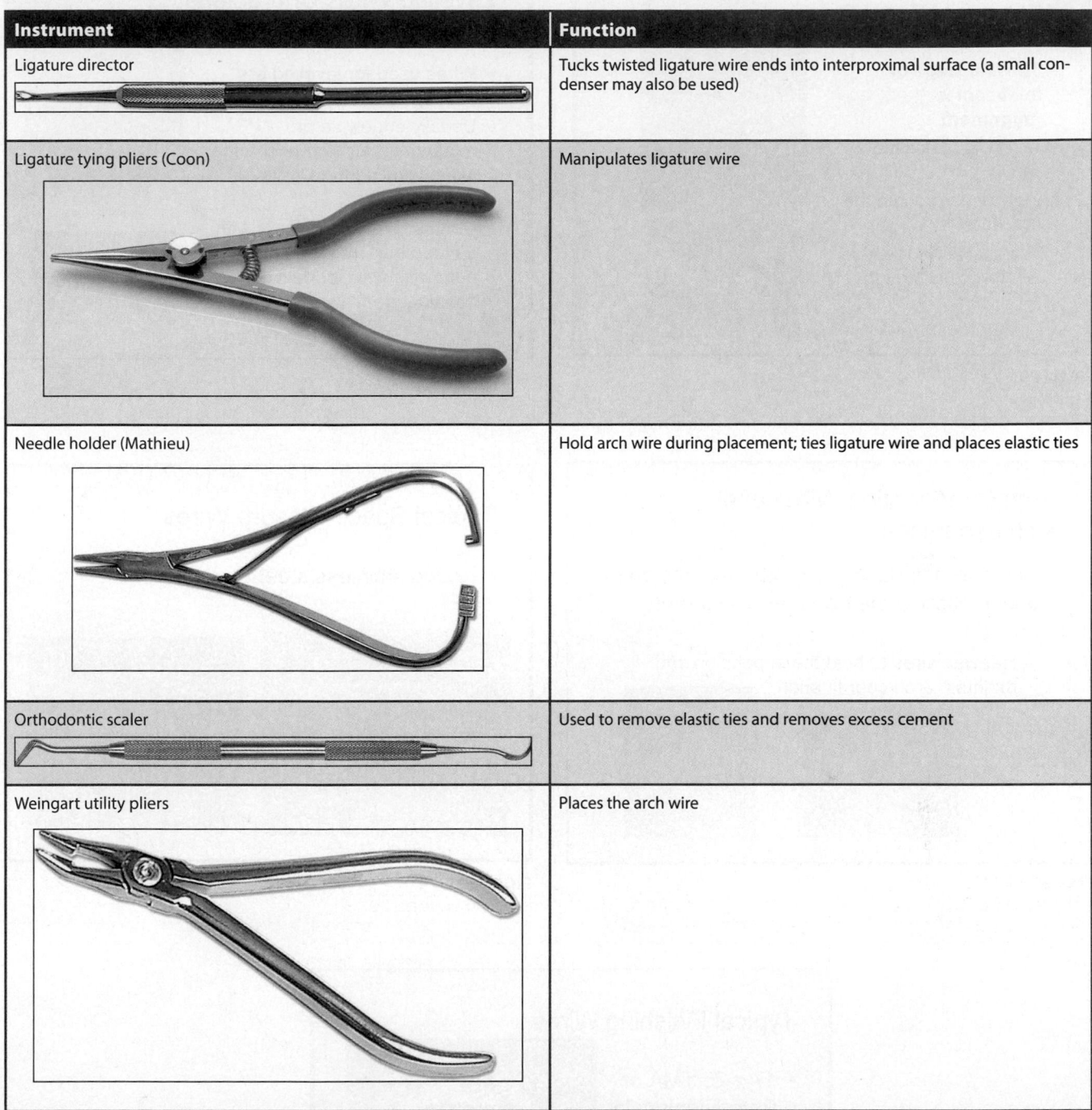	Tucks twisted ligature wire ends into interproximal surface (a small condenser may also be used)
Ligature tying pliers (Coon)	Manipulates ligature wire
Needle holder (Mathieu)	Hold arch wire during placement; ties ligature wire and places elastic ties
Orthodontic scaler	Used to remove elastic ties and removes excess cement
Weingart utility pliers	Places the arch wire

Insertion of the First Orthodontic Wire

The trained orthodontic assistant is usually the team member who selects, inserts, and ties in an initial wire in a newly bonded patient. There are several key concepts that must be followed by the orthodontic assistant so that this procedure is expertly performed. The orthodontic assistant keeps in mind that the initial wire must be fully engaged into each bracket and then firmly tied into the wire slot of the bracket using **elastic ties** or **ligature wire** ties. The initial wire must be centered at the midline so that each arch is shaped so it will fit and coordinate with the opposite arch. Refer to Procedure 35-4, "Assisting in Insertion of First Orthodontic Wire."

Alignment Wires- Basics

- The first stage of treatment is **"alignment"**
- A very light flexible wire
- Fully engaged into the brackets
- Used until the teeth are basically straight

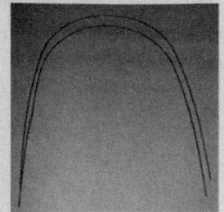
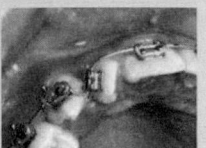

Source: Dr. Rebecca Poling

FIGURE 35-71
Alignment wires.

Leveling Wires Characteristics and Types

- Wires used for leveling are usually heavier
- Usually edgewise or rectangular for torque changes when leveling the Curve of Wilson
- Can use "memory" wires with a curve built into the flexible edgewise wire for delivery of constant gentle leveling forces

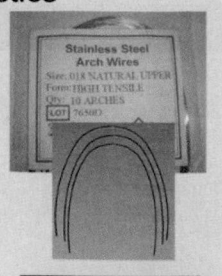
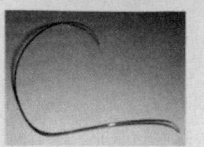

Source: Dr. Rebecca Poling

FIGURE 35-72
Leveling wires.

Arch Coordination Wires after arch expansion

- Wires to use during and after expansion or constriction in the transverse plane of space
  - Heavier wires to hold the expansion and maintain arch coordination

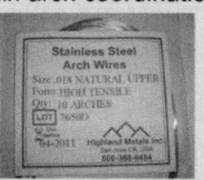
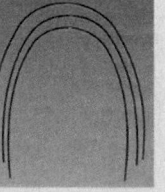

Source: Dr. Rebecca Poling

FIGURE 35-73
Arch coordination wires.

Typical Space Closure Wires

- Round stainless steel

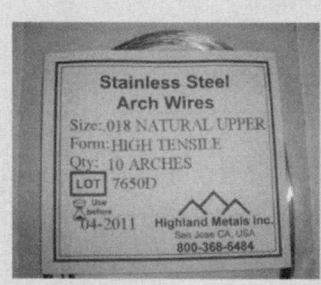
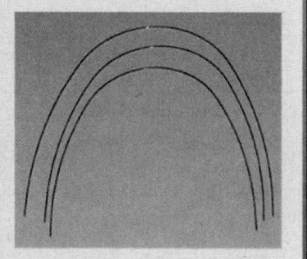

Source: Dr. Rebecca Poling

FIGURE 35-74
Space closure wires.

Typical Finishing Wires

- 17 x 25 TMA or Beta Titanium in an .018 slot
- 19 x 25 TMA or Beta Titanium in an .022 slot

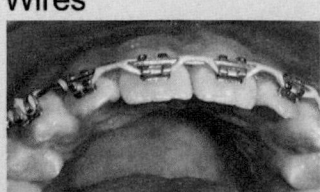

Above, wire not engaged in centrals. See how they are torqued inward? Below, wire fully engaged and wire tied.

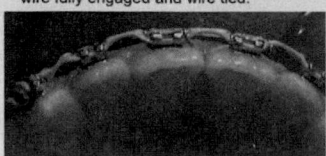

Source: Dr. Rebecca Poling

FIGURE 35-75
Finishing wires.

Safety

Ligature wires are very sharp and can pierce biohazard bags. Used and cut ligature wires must be disposed in the sharp's container to prevent any potential puncture wounds.

Orthodontic Retie Adjustment Appointment

The orthodontic adjustment appointment traditionally has been a time when the patient comes into the office for a quick check of the patient's braces and the progress of treatment. A longer appointment might include removal of the old wire and insertion of a new, more advanced wire. Today, with all of the changes in treatment with clear aligner therapy, digital messaging and telemedicine appointments, a viral pandemic, social media influencers, online quick answers to questions, and a fast-paced busy society, the orthodontic adjustment appointment is a reflection of the attitude of the orthodontist and the community that is served by the practice. For the best care of patients and practice efficiency, most orthodontists prefer to delegate most procedures to a well-trained, capable team that is trusted by the orthodontist. In this type of orthodontic practice, the formally trained orthodontic assistant is an extra set of eyes, ears, and hands for the orthodontist and the team. They are a special link between the doctor and the patient so the practice can be most efficient yet not appear to be rushed or impersonal. The orthodontic assistant should be thoroughly trained in the retie appointment procedures (Table 35-3). Refer to Procedure 35-5, "Assisting in Retie of Arch Wire."

TABLE 35-3 Arch Wire Adjustment Orthodontic Instruments

Instrument	Function
Arch bending pliers	Bends arch wire
Bird-beak pliers	Contours wire and forms springs
Three prong pliers	Adjusts headgear facebows
Tweed loop pliers	Forms headgear facebows

Orthodontic Debanding/Debonding Appointment for Removal of the Braces

The orthodontic debanding/debonding appointment to remove the braces is the final appointment concluding active comprehensive orthodontic treatment with braces. It must be followed by placement of retainers that will hold the teeth in this final position indefinitely. If retainers are not placed and worn, the teeth will immediately start moving back to their original position or even worse. Refer to Procedure 35-6, "Assisting with Debanding/Debonding Appointment."

Procedure 35-1
Assisting in the Placement and Removal of Separators

Placing the separators is generally completed during the bonding appointment or at an appointment 2 weeks prior to placement of orthodontic bands. The separators are removed and the bands placed several days following this procedure.

Steps written in **blue** font are performed by the operator (dentist or qualified dental assistant), and the chairside assistant's steps are written in black.

Equipment and Supplies

Treatment Room Preparation Setup (placed on counter)

- PPE: examination gloves, mask, protective glasses, and protective clothing
- handwashing soap or hand sanitizer
- sanitized dental treatment area and barriers placed over equipment
- dental records on computer

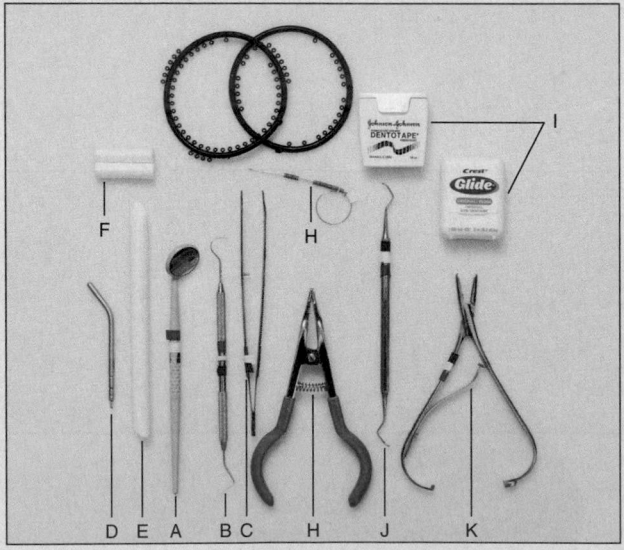

FIGURE 35-76
Placement and removal of separators setup.

Patient Seating Setup (refer to Procedure 18-4) (Figure 35-76)

- Patient napkin and napkin clip
- Patient protective glasses
- Mouth rinse in disposable cup
- Basic setup:
  - ❏ mouth mirror (A)
  - ❏ explorer (B)
  - ❏ cotton pliers (C)
  - ❏ air/water syringe tip (D)
  - ❏ HVE tip (E)
  - ❏ 2 inch cotton rolls (F)

Placement and Removal of Separators Setup (Figure 35-76)

- elastic separating pliers (G)
- separators (elastic and steel spring) (H)
- dental floss or tape (optional technique) (I)
- scaler (J)
- Mathieu needle holder (K)

Procedure Steps *(Follow aseptic procedures)*

1. Escort and seat patient (refer to Procedure 18-4).

   Operator greets the patient and takes position at the dental chair.

   ❏ **Signals for the procedure to begin (refer to Procedure 20-1).**

Placement of Elastic Separators with Separating Pliers

Operator examines the patient's mouth.

1. Pass mouth mirror.

2. Place elastic separator over the beaks of the separating pliers. Squeeze the pliers to secure the elastic on the pliers.

3. Retrieve mouth mirror and pass separating pliers.

   Places elastic separator.

   ❏ **Squeezes the pliers to stretch the elastic separator.**

❏ Places separator between two teeth that receive a band in a back-and-forth motion similar to the motion used when flossing.

❏ Inserts one side of the elastic separator below the contact in the interproximal space.

❏ Releases the tension on the separating pliers and removes the pliers.

❏ Repeats this process on all interproximal spaces around the teeth that will receive bands.

4. Continue passing elastic separators until all separators have been placed.

5. Retrieve separating pliers once the last separator has been placed.

Placement of Elastic Separators with Dental Floss

1. Place two lengths of dental floss through an elastic separator.

2. Fold over each floss length until the ends meet.

3. Pass elastic separator with dental floss.

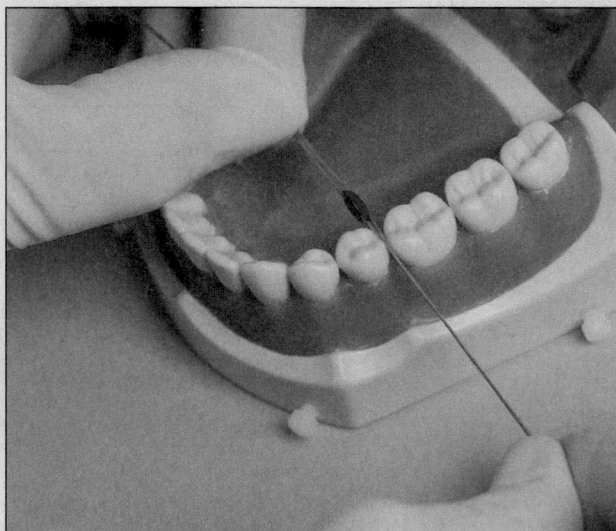

FIGURE 35-77
Dental floss stretches elastic separator for placement.

Places elastic separator with dental floss (Figure 35-77).

❏ Pulls each piece of floss by the ends to stretch the elastic.

❏ Uses a back-and-forth motion and inserts the separator into place.

❏ Releases the floss and pull free once the separator is in place.

4. Retrieve floss and dispose of in biohazard container.

Removal of Elastic Separators

1. Pass operator's preference of scaler or explorer.

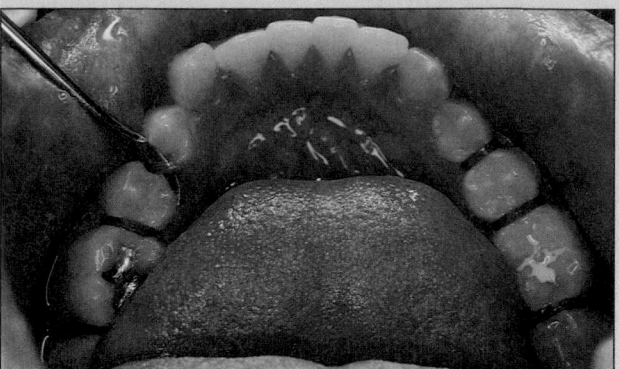

FIGURE 35-78
Removal of elastic separators.

Removes elastic separator (Figure 35-78).

❏ Inserts one end of scaler or explorer into the ring of the elastic separator.

❏ Places a finger over the top of the separator to prevent the separator from snapping and injuring the patient.

❏ Pulls gently on the instrument toward the occlusal until the elastic is free of the contact.

2. Retrieve scaler or explorer.

Placement of Steel Spring Separators

1. Pass needle holder and steel spring separator (Figure 35-79).

Places steel spring separator.

❏ Grasps the short end of the steel spring close to the coiled end with needle holder.

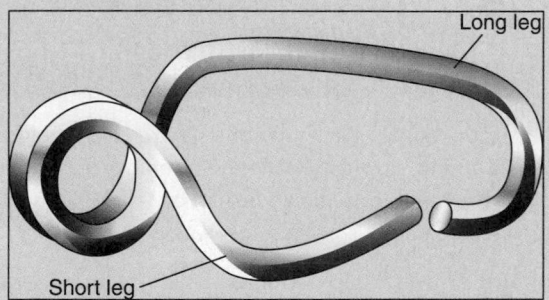

FIGURE 35-79
Steel spring separator.

❏ Hooks and engages the long arm of the separator over the occlusal surface of the tooth.

❏ Engages the hook of the separator into the lingual contact.

❏ Places finger over the occlusal arm (long leg) while stretching the gingival (short leg) arm out and then releases the short side of the spring separator and slides it in under the contact.

(Continues)

Examines the placement of the spring separator:
- ❏ Coil is on the buccal/facial side.
- ❏ Long arm is resting over the contact on the occlusal surface.
- ❏ Short arm under the contact on the gingival side.
- ❏ Spring is close to the tooth.

Gently presses the spring separator to test that it is securely in place.

2. Continue passing spring separators until all separators have been placed.

3. Retrieve needle holder once the last separator has been placed.

Removal of Steel Spring Separators

1. Pass scaler.

Removes spring separators.

- ❏ Places the finger of one hand over the spring to prevent injury to the patient.
- ❏ Places one end of a scaler in the coil and lifts upward.
- ❏ Pulls the coil toward the facial aspect once the longest side of the spring is free of the lingual embrasure.

2. Retrieve scaler.

Tells patient good bye and what a pleasure it was to see them.

3. Provide patient with postoperative instructions.
   - ❏ The patient is instructed to call the office if any of the separators fall out.

4. Write up procedure in Services Rendered.

5. Dismiss and escort patient to reception area (refer to Procedure 18-5).

Date	Services Rendered
02/18/XX	Placed spring separators between mandibular first molars and second premolar and elastic separators between maxillary first molars and second premolar
	PO do not chew ice or hard, chewy candy and follow up with all scheduled appts
	Reinforced need for good oral hygiene and calling office immediately if a separator becomes loose or falls off
	RTC: Banding appointment Assistant's initials

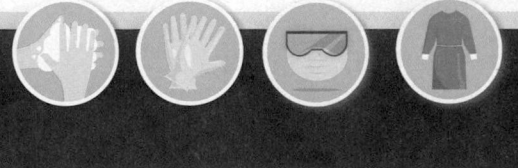

Procedure 35-2
Assisting with Cementation of Orthodontic Bands

The chairside dental assistant prepares material and transfers materials and instruments while the operator cements the bands to the teeth. This procedure can be legally performed by a trained dental assistant in some states.

Steps written in blue font are performed by the operator (dentist or qualified dental assistant), and the chairside assistant's steps are written in black.

Equipment and Supplies

Treatment Room Preparation Setup (placed on counter)
- PPE: examination gloves, mask, protective glasses, and protective clothing
- handwashing soap or hand sanitizer
- sanitized dental treatment area and barriers placed over equipment
- patient's medical and dental records

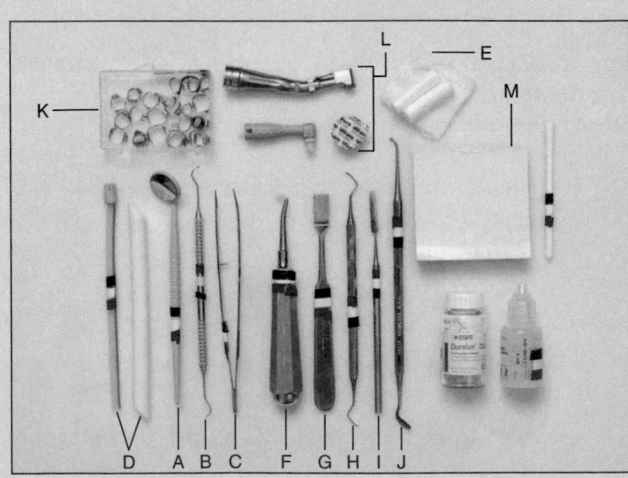

FIGURE 35-80
Cementation of orthodontic bands setup.

Patient Seating Setup (refer to Procedure 18-4) (Figure 35-80)

- Patient napkin and napkin clip
- Patient protective glasses
- Mouth rinse in disposable cup
- Basic setup:
  - ❏ mouth mirror (A)
  - ❏ explorer (B)
  - ❏ cotton pliers (C)
  - ❏ saliva ejector and evacuator (HVE) (D)
  - ❏ cotton rolls (2 inch) and 2 × 2 gauze squares (E)

Cementation of Orthodontic Bands Setup (Figure 35-80)

- band pusher (F)
- band rocker (G)
- scaler (H)
- cement spatula (I)
- plastic filling instrument (J)
- selected and prepared bands (K)
- disposable prophy angle with rubber cup and prophy paste (L)
- cement of choice and paper pad or glass slab (M)

Procedure Steps (*Follow aseptic procedures*)

1. Escort and seat patient (refer to Procedure 18-4).

   Operator greets the patient and takes position at the dental chair.

   ❏ **Signals for the procedure to begin (refer to Procedure 20-1).**

   Removes separators and polishes teeth that are to be banded (refer to Procedure 35-1).

2. Place prophy paste in rubber cup and pass disposable prophy angle.

3. Rinse and dry patient's mouth thoroughly.

   Selects bands from orthodontic band kit (Figure 35-81).

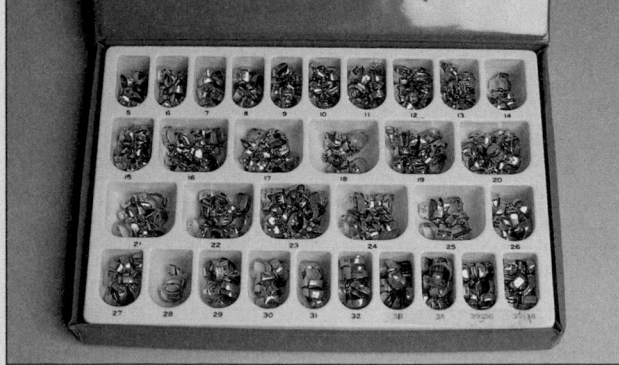

FIGURE 35-81
Selection of bands.

4. Pass operator's choice of band pusher or rocker.

   Operator trys-on selected bands.

   ❏ **Places the band over the occlusal and applies pressure with a finger.**

   ❏ **Pushes the band onto the tooth so that the margins of the band are beyond the occlusion (Figure 35-82).**

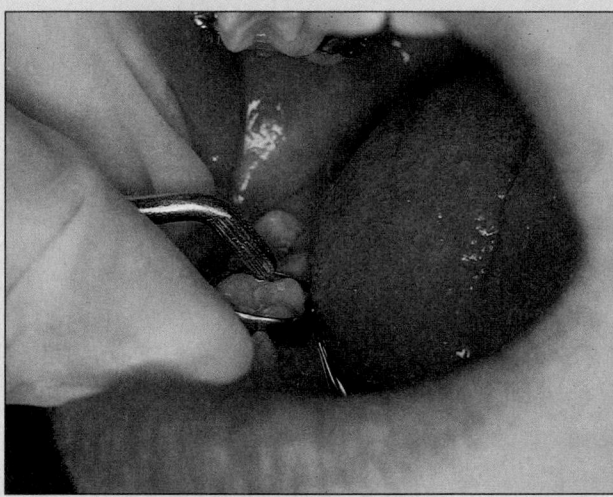

FIGURE 35-82
Band pusher is used to seat the band on the tooth.

5. Retrieve band pusher and pass scaler (or band removing pliers).

   Removes band using scaler.

   ❏ **Shapes bands using contouring pliers as needed.**

6. Retrieve scaler and rinse and dry the teeth.

   Isolates the areas where the bands are to be placed to maintain moisture control.

7. Pass cotton rolls.

8. Mix the cement according to manufacturer's directions and load the first band.

9. Wipe wax on buccal tubes/attachments, place cement from the gingival edge, and cover the inside of the band.

10. Transfer band to the orthodontist using their preferred method once the cement has been placed in the band. Transferring the band needs to be made as easy as possible. There are many methods to transfer the bands:

    ❏ Place bands on the mixing slab or pad in order to be seated.

    ❏ Pass bands on the end of the spatula or place band with gingival side up on a piece of wax or masking tape (Figure 35-83).

    Seats the band on the tooth.

(Continues)

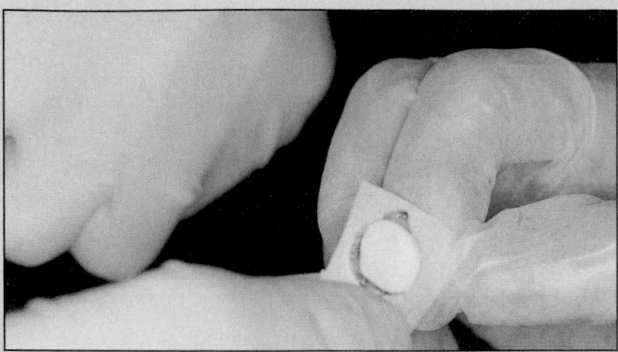

FIGURE 35-83
Assistant passes band filled with cement on tape.

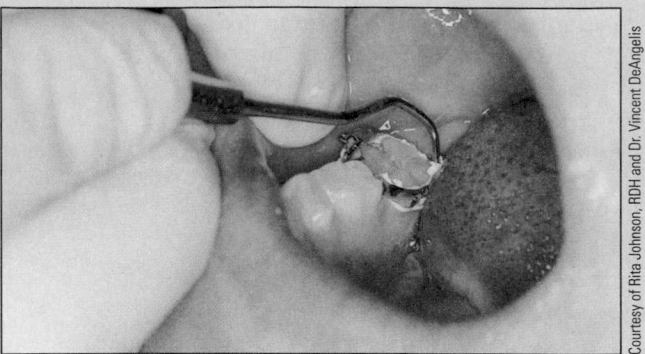

FIGURE 35-85
Excess cement is removed from around the band.

11. Transfer the operator's choice of instrument: band rocker, band pusher, or bite stick.

   Places band rocker evenly over the band and gently presses the band into the interproximal space.

   Places working end of band pusher to apply pressure to seat the band (Figure 35-84).

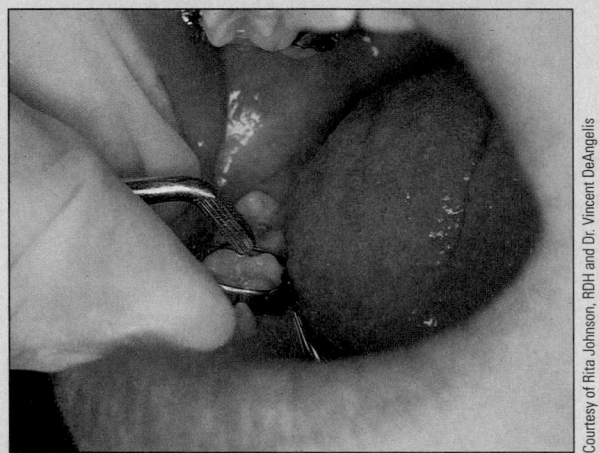

FIGURE 35-84
Seating band with band pusher.

   Positions the edge of the bite stick on the band precisely for the desired movement and asks patient to bite on the stick.

12. Continue to fill the bands and transfer them to the operator until all bands have been cemented or until the cement becomes too thick and a new mix is required.
   ❏ If a new mix is required, clean the instruments with wet gauze or an alcohol wipe and mix additional cement.

13. Allow cement to set once all bands are seated.
   ❏ Clean the cement off all used instruments during this time.

14. Remove the excess cement from around the band with a scaler after the cement is set (Figure 35-85).

15. Rinse and dry patient's mouth.

   Tells patient good bye and what a pleasure it was to see them.

16. Provide patient with postoperative instructions.
   ❏ Explain how chewing on ice and hard, chewy candy can damage the orthodontic appliance.
   ❏ Educate patient or primary caregiver about need for re-evaluation of appliances on follow-up visits.

17. Write up procedure in Services Rendered.

18. Dismiss and escort patient to reception area (refer to Procedure 18-5).

Date	Services Rendered
02/18/XX	Bands placed on all first molars
	PO do not chew ice or hard, chewy candy and follow up with all scheduled appts
	Reinforced need for good oral hygiene. Explained need to call office immediately if a bracket/band becomes loose or falls off
	RTC: Bonding appointment Assistant's initials

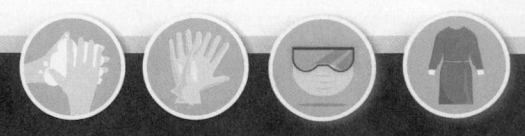

Procedure 35-3
Assisting with Direct Bonding of Brackets

The chairside dental assistant prepares material and transfers materials and instruments while the operator bonds the brackets to the teeth. This procedure can be legally performed by a trained dental assistant in some states.

Steps written in blue font are performed by the operator (dentist or qualified dental assistant), and the chairside assistant's steps are written in black.

Equipment and Supplies

Treatment Room Preparation Setup (placed on counter)
- PPE: examination gloves, mask, protective glasses, and protective clothing
- handwashing soap or hand sanitizer
- sanitized dental treatment area and barriers placed over equipment
- patient's medical and dental records

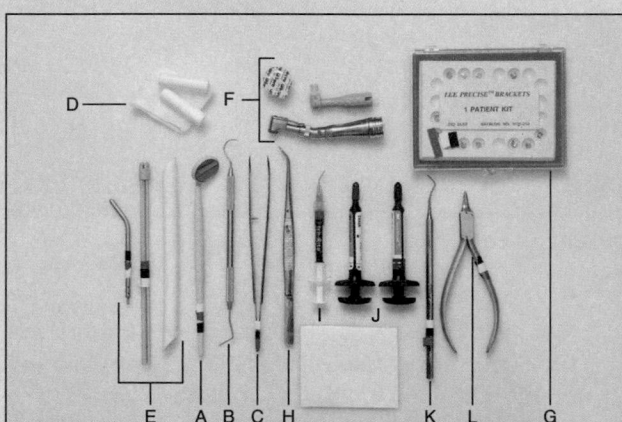

FIGURE 35-86
Direct bonding of brackets setup.

Patient Seating Setup (refer to Procedure 18-4) (Figure 35-86)
- Patient napkin and napkin clip
- Patient protective glasses
- Mouth rinse in disposable cup
- Basic setup:
  - ❏ mouth mirror (A)
  - ❏ explorer (B)
  - ❏ cotton pliers (C)
  - ❏ cotton rolls (2 inch) and 2 × 2 gauze squares (D)
  - ❏ air/water syringe tip, saliva ejector, and evacuator (HVE) (E)

Direct Bonding of Brackets Setup (Figure 35-86)
- disposable prophy angle with rubber cup and pumice in dappen dish (F)
- bracket kit (G)
- locking cotton pliers or bracket forceps (H)
- acid etchant (I)
- bonding agent (J)
- scaler (K)
- bird-beak pliers (L)
- retractors for cheeks and lips (Figure 35-88)
- resin light and protective glasses (not shown)

Procedure Steps (*Follow aseptic procedures*)

1. Escort and seat patient (refer to Procedure 18-4).

   Operator greets the patient and takes position at the dental chair.

   ❏ Signals for the procedure to begin (refer to Procedure 20-1).

2. Assistant passes mouth mirror and explorer at operator's signal.

   Examines tooth or teeth to be bonded with mirror and explorer.

   Isolates area with cotton rolls or retractors.

   Polishes teeth that are to receive brackets (Figure 35-87).

3. Retrieve mirror and explorer and make a pumice slurry at a 1:4 ratio of pumice and water.

4. Pass disposable prophy angle with slurry of pumice in rubber cup. (Polishing paste with fluoride is not used because some of the ingredients will interfere with the bonding process.)

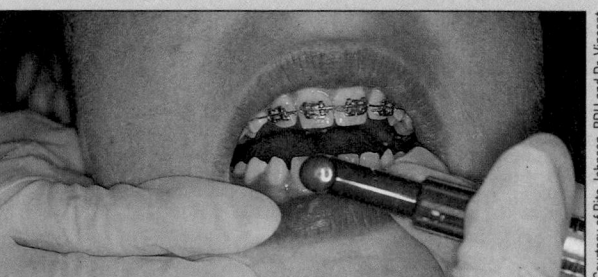

Courtesy of Rita Johnson, RDH and Dr. Vincent DeAngelis

FIGURE 35-87
Clean tooth surface.

(Continues)

5. Retrieve disposable prophy angle.

6. Rinse and dry the patient's mouth once the teeth are polished.

    Isolates the area where brackets are to be bonded.

7. Pass retractors (Figure 35-88).

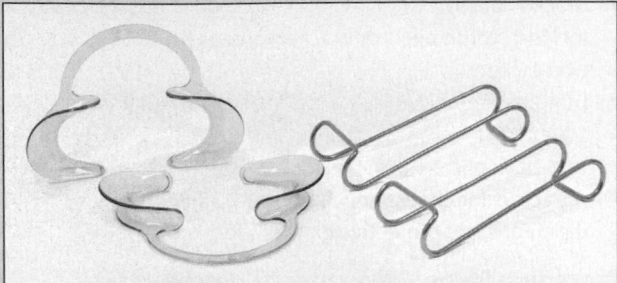

FIGURE 35-88
Retractors.

8. Pass cotton rolls after the retractors are positioned.

    Places acid etchant on the enamel facial surface of the anterior teeth receiving brackets.

9. Prepare the etchant and transfer it to the operator.

10. Set the timer for the specific amount of time, as per the manufacturer's directions.

11. Maintain the operating field to be sure it stays dry.

12. Rinse the patient's mouth long enough to ensure that all the etchant is removed from the tooth surface (approximately 30 seconds) and then dry the tooth or teeth. The teeth will have a chalky appearance.

13. Retrieve etchant syringe.

    Places the bonding agent on the etched tooth surfaces.

14. Prepare the bonding agent according to the manufacturer's directions.

15. Transfer the agent to the dentist for placement on the tooth.

    Positions the bracket on the tooth.

16. Hold selected bracket with locked cotton pliers or bracket forceps and apply bonding agent to the back of the bracket (Figure 35-89).

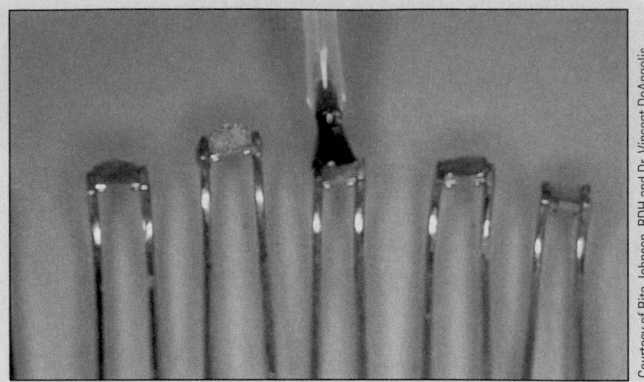

FIGURE 35-89
Bonding agent applied to bracket.

17. Retrieve bonding agent and pass the bracket with the forceps.

    Places brackets onto anterior teeth (Figure 35-90).

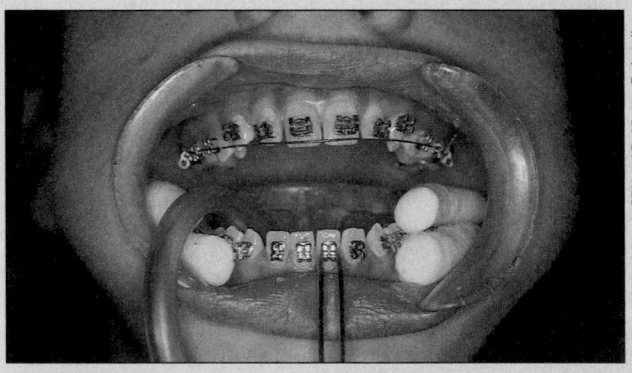

FIGURE 35-90
Place bracket on tooth and light cure.

Removes excess bonding agent from around the bracket. Care is taken to prevent removing any bonding agent from between the bracket and the tooth; this would weaken the seal and could lead to decalcification and decay.

18. Retrieve forceps and pass the scaler or explorer.

    Removes adhesive paste flash.

    Holds the bracket in position and sets the bonding agent until it is chemically set.

19. Retrieve explorer/scaler and pass resin light.

20. Retrieve resin light and pass mirror.

    Places acid etchant on the enamel facial surface of the posterior teeth receiving brackets.

21. Prepare the etchant and transfer it to the operator.

22. Set the timer for the specific amount of time, as per the manufacturer's directions.

23. Maintain the operating field to be sure it stays dry.

24. Rinse the patient's mouth long enough to ensure that all the etchant is removed from the tooth surface (approximately 30 seconds) and then dry the tooth or teeth. The teeth will have a chalky appearance.

25. Retrieve etchant syringe.

    Places the bonding agent on the etched tooth surfaces.

26. Prepare the bonding agent according to the manufacturer's directions.

27. Transfer the agent to the dentist for placement on the tooth.

28. Hold selected bracket with locked cotton pliers or bracket forceps and apply bonding agent to the back of the bracket.

    Positions the bracket on the tooth.

29. Remove retractors from the patient's mouth.

    Tells patient good bye and what a pleasure it was to see them.

30. Provide patient with postoperative instructions.
    - ❏ Explain how chewing on ice and hard, chewy candy can damage the sealant.
    - ❏ Educate patient or primary caregiver about need for re-evaluation of sealants on follow-up visits.

31. Write up procedure in Services Rendered.

32. Dismiss and escort patient to reception area (refer to Procedure 18-5).

Date	Services Rendered
02/18/XX	Brackets bonded from second premolar to second premolar in both arches
	PO do not chew ice or hard, chewy candy and follow up with all scheduled appts
	Reinforced need for good oral hygiene. Explained need to call office immediately if a bracket becomes loose or falls off
	RTC: Retie appointment Assistant's initials

Procedure 35-4
Assisting in Insertion of First Orthodontic Wire

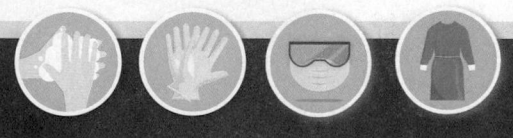

Placing the arch wire and ligature ties is generally completed during the bonding appointment. This procedure can be legally performed by a trained dental assistant in some states.

Steps written in blue font are performed by the operator (dentist or qualified dental assistant), and the chairside assistant's steps are written in black.

Equipment and Supplies

Treatment Room Preparation Setup (placed on counter)
- PPE: examination gloves, mask, protective glasses, and protective clothing
- handwashing soap or hand sanitizer
- sanitized dental treatment area and barriers placed over equipment
- patient's medical and dental records

Patient Seating Setup (refer to Procedure 18-4) (Figure 35-91)
- Patient napkin and napkin clip
- Patient protective glasses
- Mouth rinse in disposable cup
- Basic setup:
    - ❏ mouth mirror and explorer (A)
    - ❏ cotton pliers (B)
    - ❏ cotton rolls (2 inch) and 2 × 2 gauze squares (C)
    - ❏ HVE and saliva ejector (D)

Placement of Arch Wire and Ligature Ties Setup (Figure 35-91)
- selected arch wire (E)
- Weingart pliers (F)
- bird-beak pliers (G)
- elastics or ligature wire (H)

(Continues)

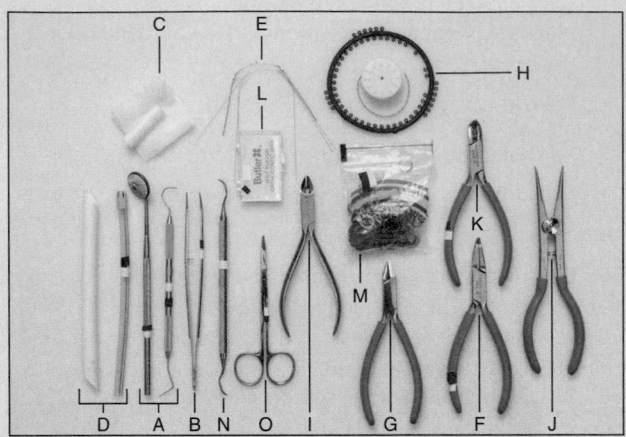

FIGURE 35-91
Insertion of orthodontic wire setup.

- ligature-cutting pliers (I)
- ligature-tying pliers (J)
- distal end-cutting pliers (K)
- orthodontic wax (L)
- rubber bands (M)
- orthodontic scaler/condenser (N)
- scissors (O)
- Mathieu needle pliers (not shown; see Table 35-2)

Procedure Steps

Operator selects the wire from the treatment plan.

❑ Marks center of wire with marker (Figure 35-92).

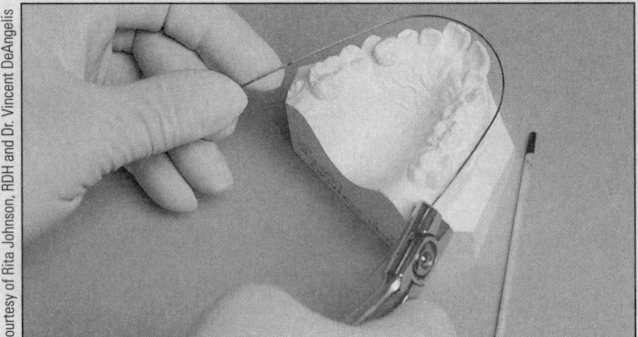

FIGURE 35-92
Arch wire center is marked and cut to size by distal end-cutting pliers.

1. Pass the Weingart pliers.

   Inserts the arch wire into the buccal tubes on the molar bands.

   Cuts off the ends of the arch wire if the wire is too long.

2. Retrieve the Weingart pliers.

   Places the arch wire in the horizontal slot of each bracket (Figure 35-93).

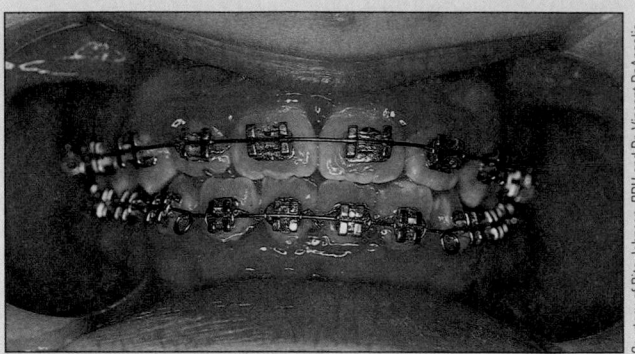

FIGURE 35-93
Arch wire placed in buccal tubes.

Centers the wire and pushes it back on both sides so the center is exactly at the dental midline.

3. Pass operator's choice of plastic rings/elastic ties and needle holder.

   Removes elastic ring.

   ❑ Positions the tips of the needle holder over the rim of the ring but not inside the lumen, which will make placement onto the tie wings difficult.

   Places elastic ties over the bracket to secure the arch wire.

   ❑ Holds the instrument near the tips.

   ❑ Places the ring of the tie over one upper wing of the bracket (Figure 35-94).

   ❑ Uses a wrist movement to stretch the tie down over the lower wing.

   ❑ Places ring in a figure 8 or butterfly tie.

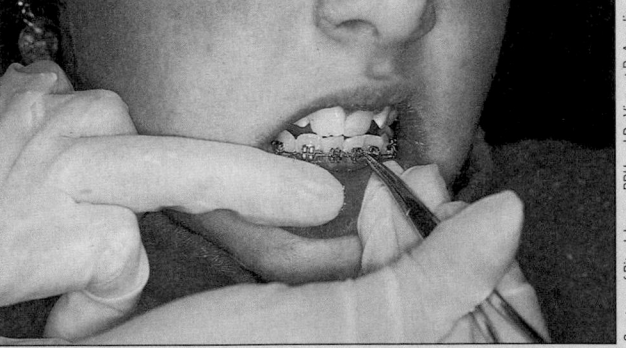

FIGURE 35-94
Elastic rings being placed on anterior bracket using a hemostat.

4. Hold elastic ties for the operator to remove as needed until all needed ties are placed. Retrieve needle holder after the last tie is secured.

5. Pass ligature wire tie.

Places ligature wire ties over the portion of alignment wire in slot that needs most engagement (Figure 35-95).

❏ Holds the ligature wire between the thumb and the index finger.

❏ Wraps the wire around the occlusal and gingival wings of the bracket in a distal–mesial direction and crosses the ends of the wire together.

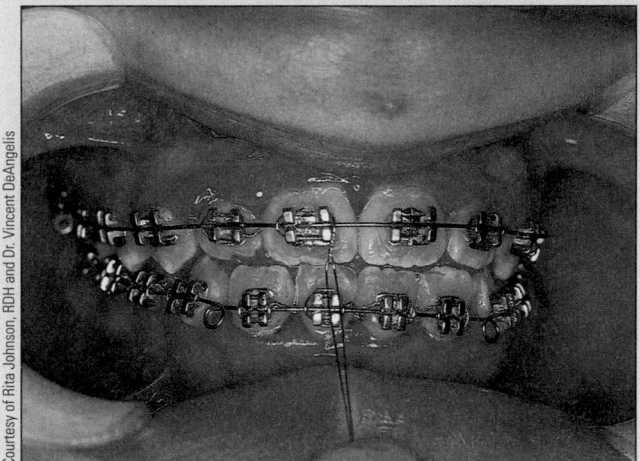

FIGURE 35-95
Ligature wire being looped around bracket.

6. Pass operator's choice of ligature-typing pliers or needle holder.

Twists the ends of the wire together for several rotations (Figure 35-96).

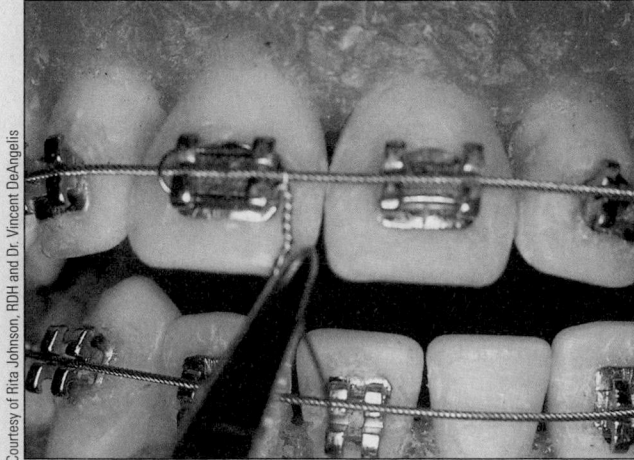

FIGURE 35-96
Ligature wire is twisted.

7. Pass ligature wire ties as needed until all needed ties are placed. Retrieve needle holder after the last tie is secured.

Cuts the twisted ends of the ligature wire, called the pigtail, to a length of 3 to 4 millimeters (Figure 35-97).

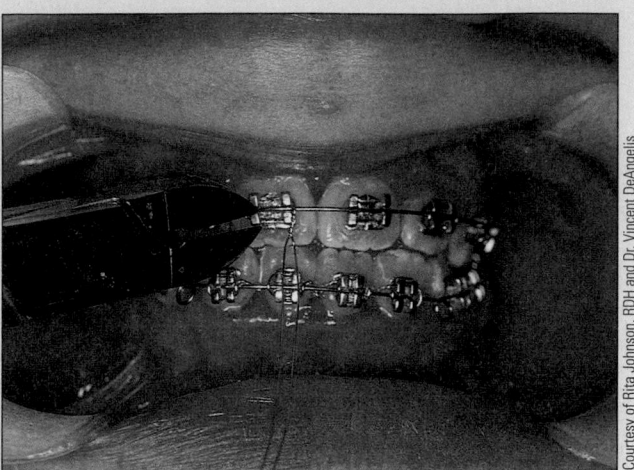

FIGURE 35-97
Ligature wire is cut with cutting wire.

8. Pass ligature-wire cutting pliers.

Bends pigtail into the embrasure space (Figure 35-98).

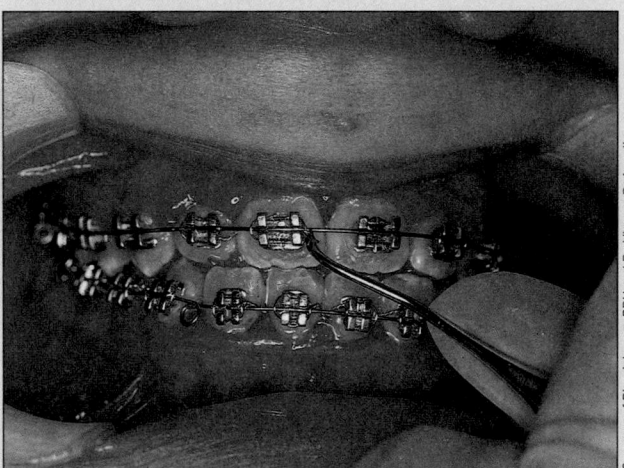

FIGURE 35-98
Ligature wire is tucked into embrasure space.

9. Pass orthodontic scaler/condenser.

Runs a finger over the area to check for sharp ends after all the pigtail ends have been tucked into place.

Checks the distal ends of the arch wire and cuts any excess.

❏ Places a cotton roll behind the cutter.

❏ Clips the end and checks for wire clipping held in the plier.

❏ Takes care not to crush the end of the bracket tube with the wire cutter.

(Continues)

10. Retrieve orthodontic scaler/condenser and pass distal end-cutting pliers.

Places rubber elastic bands at this appointment if they are on the patient's treatment plan (Figure 35-99).

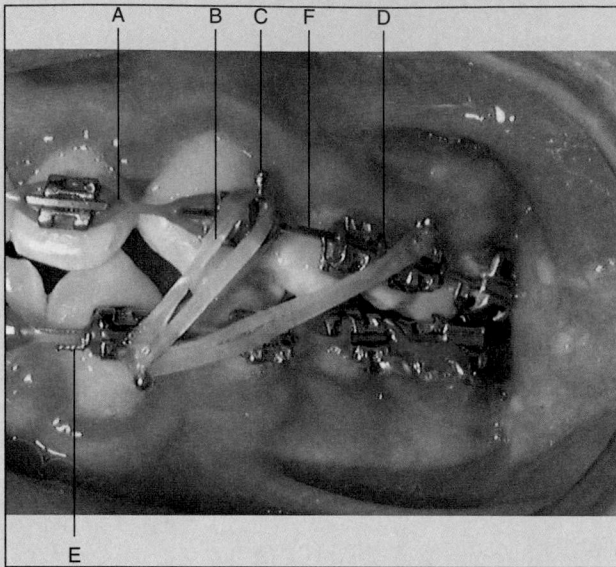

FIGURE 35-99
Placement of elastic ties and bands. (A) chain ligature tie. (B) elastic band. (C) elastic hook. (D) elastic ligature tie. (E) chain ligature tie.

11. Demonstrate how to place and remove the rubber bands.
  ❑ Place the rubber band around the index finger.
  ❑ Slide it over a hook or loop in the mandibular posterior first.
  ❑ Pull the maxillary anterior hook or loop and remove from finger.
  ❑ Explain that the rubber bands stretch over time and the patient will need to change them accordingly.

12. Have the patient practice until they are comfortable with the task.

13. Provide patient with postoperative instructions.
  ❑ The patient is given a sufficient number of elastics with instructions to call the office for more, if needed.

14. Write up procedure in Services Rendered.

15. Dismiss and escort patient to reception area (refer to Procedure 18-5).

Date	Services Rendered
02/18/XX	Arch wire secured in both arches; placement of rubber bands demonstrated and supply of bands sent home with patient
	PO do not chew ice or hard, chewy candy and follow up with all scheduled appts
	Reinforced need for good oral hygiene and calling office immediately if a bracket becomes loose or falls off
	RTC: Retie appointment Assistant's initials

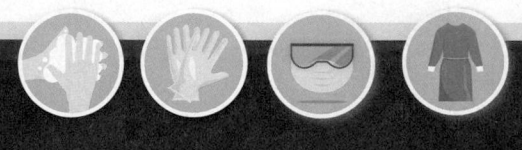

Procedure 35-5
Retie Appointment

Assisting in Retie of Arch Wire

The progress of the treatment is assessed and the arch wire and ligature ties may be replaced during the retie appointment. This procedure can be legally performed by a trained dental assistant in some states.

Steps written in **blue** font are performed by the operator (dentist or qualified dental assistant), and the chairside assistant's steps are written in black.

Equipment and Supplies

Treatment Room Preparation Setup (placed on counter)
- PPE: examination gloves, mask, protective glasses, and protective clothing
- handwashing soap or hand sanitizer
- sanitized dental treatment area and barriers placed over equipment
- patient's medical and dental records

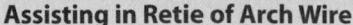

Patient Seating Setup (refer to Procedure 18-4)

- Patient napkin and napkin clip
- Patient protective glasses
- Mouth rinse in disposable cup
- Basic setup:
    - ❏ mouth mirror
    - ❏ explorer
    - ❏ cotton pliers
    - ❏ 2 × 2 gauze squares
    - ❏ HVE and saliva ejector

Retie Setup

- thin bladed snub-nose plier
- distal end cutter plier
- Weingart plier
- elastic placer or hemostat or Mathiau plier
- wire ligature cutter

Procedure Steps (*Follow aseptic procedures*)

1. Escort and seat patient (refer to Procedure 18-4).
2. Assess the patient's status.
    - ❏ Are there any problems or concerns that you have with your braces?
    - ❏ Have you been in good health?
    - ❏ Is there anything you want to ask the doctor?
    - ❏ Is there anything loose, broke, or poking?
3. Assess compliance with growth appliances.
    - ❏ How many hours out of 24 would you estimate you are wearing the headgear?
    - ❏ How many days per week out of 7 days per week do you wear the headgear?
    - ❏ With the headgear on, check:
        - The ease of putting the headgear on
        - Tightness of straps
        - Bow position when it is active
4. Assess compliance with elastic wear.
    - ❏ How many hours out of 24 are you wearing the elastics?
    - ❏ How many days out of 7 days per week are you wearing elastics?
    - ❏ Is the patient wearing the elastics correctly? If not, review the proper insertion of the elastics.
    - ❏ Is the patient wearing the correct size of elastics for the correct number of hours?
5. Examine patient's intraoral health, nutritional habits, and brushing/flossing grade (Figures 35-100 and 35-101).
    - "A"—no biofilm at the marginal gingiva, not interproximal biofilm and not gingivitis
    - "B"—slight biofilm and/or gingivitis
    - "C"—a lot of visible biofilm and significant gingivitis
    - "D"—or lower: give oral hygiene instructions (OHI) or schedule an appoint for OHI

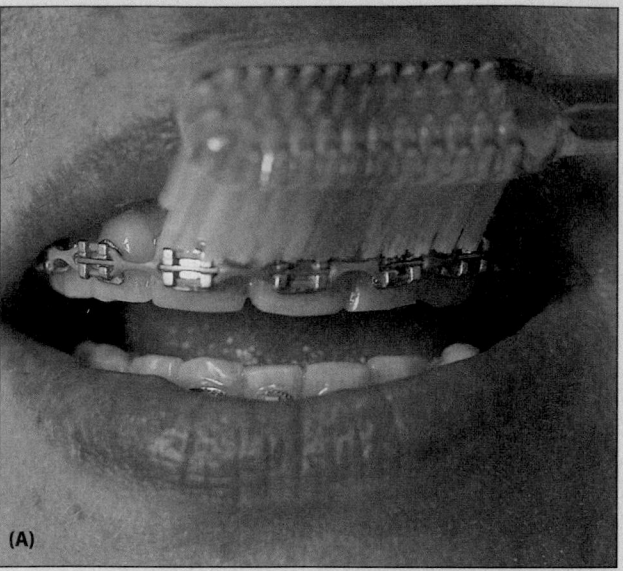

(A)

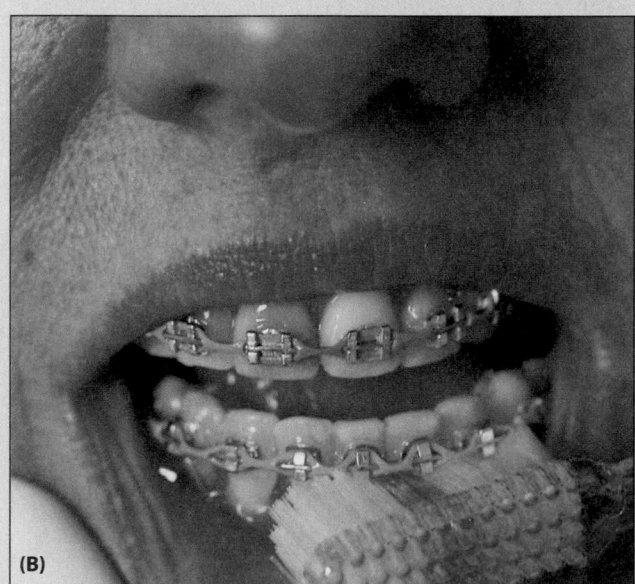

(B)

FIGURE 35-100
Tooth brushing reviewed for brushing (A) mandibular and (B) maxillary teeth with fixed orthodontic appliances.

Operator greets the patient and takes position at the dental chair.

❏ Signals for the procedure to begin (refer to Procedure 20-1).

Evaluates the occlusion and periodontium.

❏ Examines overjet, midlines, bite depth, molar and canine classification, crossbites, open bites, curve of Spee, space, crowding, rotations, eruption, and gingival health.

(Continues)

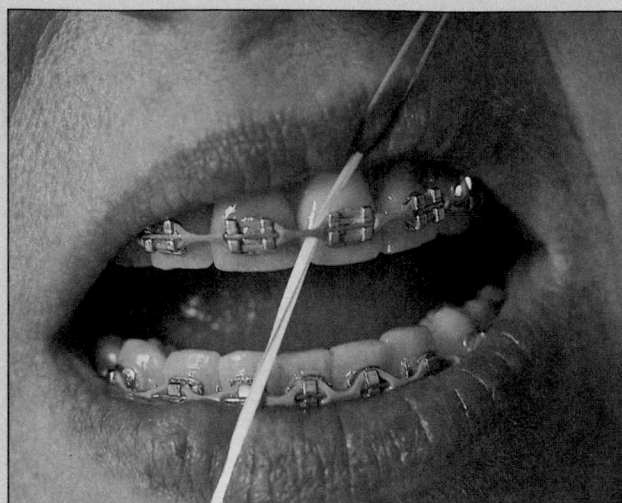

FIGURE 35-101
Floss being threaded under arch wire.

Checks the current wire.
- ❏ Checks the size of wire on the treatment card.
- ❏ Checks engagement into the brackets.
  - Fully engaged?
  - Fully expressed?
  - Acting as a holding wire?
- ❏ Notes on the tray cover how the wire was tied in previously.
  - Wire ties
  - Closing chains
  - Molars converted and wire tied?

6. Pass explorer.

Removes the elastic tie holding in the mandibular wire.
- ❏ Places explorer into the lumen of the elastic and removes it.

7. Retrieve explorer and pass marker.

Dries, marks, and removes wire ties in each arch wire if indicated.

Gives a summary of patient's status to the doctor.
- ❏ Reviews the treatment card
- ❏ Treatment phase
- ❏ Estimated target date for completion
- ❏ Maxillary wire size
- ❏ Mandibular wire size

Receives instructions from the doctor.
- ❏ Wire changes
- ❏ Retie changes
- ❏ Headgear changes
- ❏ Oral hygiene changes
- ❏ Next appointment type, interval, length, specifics

Inserts new wires to achieve the desired tooth movement.

Ties in arch wire with elastics and wire ligatures (refer to Procedure 35-4).

Completes a final check.
- ❏ Wire tie ends smooth and smooth them as needed.
- ❏ Clips arch wire ends as needed.
- ❏ Smooths sharp hooks or band edges.
- ❏ Examines for need for stops.
- ❏ Asks patient if anything is sharp.
- ❏ Gives patient supplies of wax, elastics, or other items.

8. Make complete notations in the patient's Treatment Record.

9. Release the patient, properly communicating patient instructions with the caregiver and scheduling coordinator.

Procedure 35-6
Assist with Debanding/Debonding Appointment for Removal of the Braces

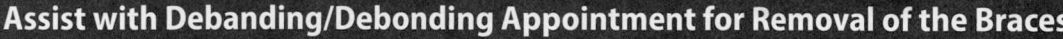

The chairside dental assistant prepares material, transfers materials and instruments while the operator removes orthodontic appliances, polishes the teeth, and takes impression for fabrication of the retainer. This procedure can be legally performed by a trained dental assistant in some states.

Steps written in blue font are performed by the operator (dentist, hygienist, or qualified dental assistant), and the chairside assistant's steps are written in black.

Equipment and Supplies

Treatment Preparation Setup (placed on counter)

- PPE: examination gloves, mask, protective glasses, and protective clothing
- handwashing soap or hand sanitizer
- sanitized dental treatment area and barriers placed over equipment
- patient's medical and dental records

Patient Seating Setup (refer to Procedure 18-4) (Figure 35-102)

- Patient napkin and napkin clip
- Patient protective glasses
- Mouth rinse in disposable cup
- Basic setup:
  - ❏ mouth mirror (A)
  - ❏ explorer (B)
  - ❏ cotton pliers (C)
  - ❏ cotton rolls (2 inch) and 2 × 2 gauze squares (D)
  - ❏ air/water syringe tip and evacuator (HVE) (E)

Debanding/Debonding Setup (Figure 35-102)

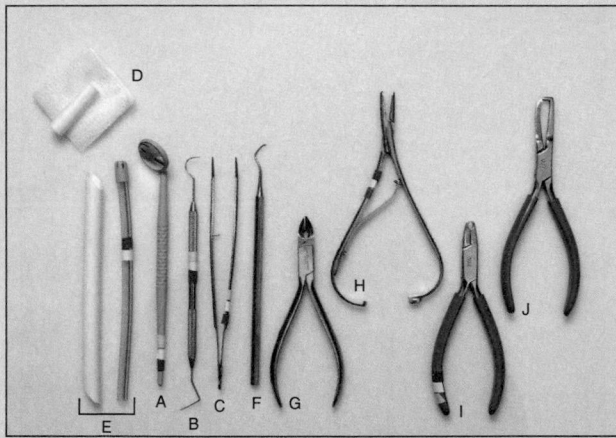

FIGURE 35-102
Debanding/debonding setup.

- orthodontic scaler (F)
- ligature wire cutting pliers (G)
- Mathieu needle holder (H)
- bracket remover and adhesive removing pliers (I)
- posterior band remover (J)
- prophy angle with rubber cup and prophy paste (not shown)
- ultrasonic scaler (optional)
- alginate impression material and selected tray (refer to Chapter 33)

Procedure Steps (*Follow aseptic procedures*)

1. Escort and seat patient (refer to Procedure 18-4).

    Asks about any patient concerns.

    Evaluates the occlusion and other potential issues that would interfere with debanding/debonding.

Has doctor check, evaluate concerns, and give approval to proceed.

2. Pass operator's preference scaler or explorer.

    Operator loosens ligature ties.

    ❏ Places tip of the explorer or scaler under the elastic and rolls over the bracket wings until the elastic is released (Figure 35-103).

    ❏ Repeats on each tooth until all elastics are removed.

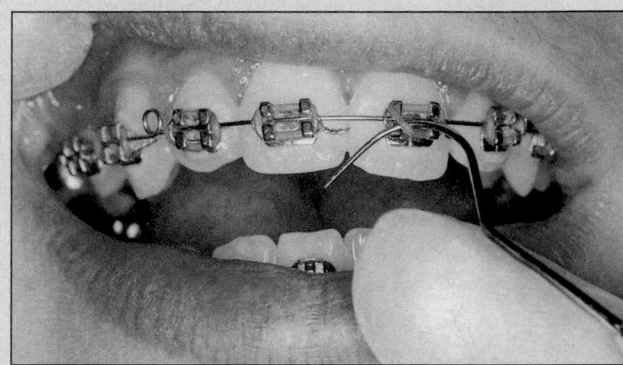

FIGURE 35-103
Insert end of scaler or explorer under the elastic and roll elastic rings over wings of bracket for removal of the elastic rings.

3. Retrieve scaler/explorer and pass ligature wire cutting pliers.

    Cuts ligature ties where the wire is exposed.

    Removes the wire from the wings of the bracket. Repeats on each tooth until all ligature wires are removed (Figure 35-104).

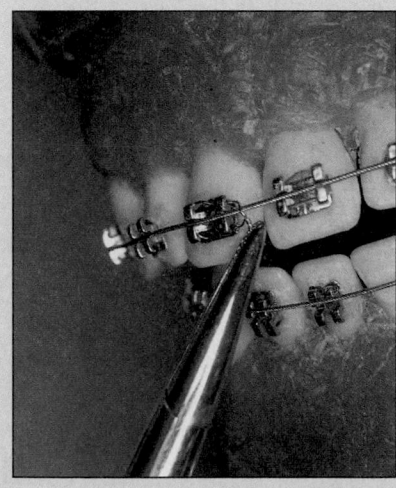

FIGURE 35-104
Pull twisted "pigtail" wire from embrasure.

(Continues)

4. Pass needle holder.

Removes the arch wire from the brackets.
- ❏ **Pulls the arch wire from the buccal tube on one side.**
- ❏ **Holds the arch wire securely to prevent injury to the patient while removing the opposite end.**

5. Retrieve needle holder and pass bracket and adhesive removing pliers.

Removes the anterior bracket using the bracket and adhesive removing pliers (Figure 35-105).
- ❏ **Places the lower beak of the pliers, with a very sharp edge on the gingival edge of the bracket.**
- ❏ **Places the upper beak, with a nylon tip, on the occlusal edge of the bracket.**
- ❏ **Squeezes the pliers together; the sharp lower beak breaks the bond and removes some adhesive.**

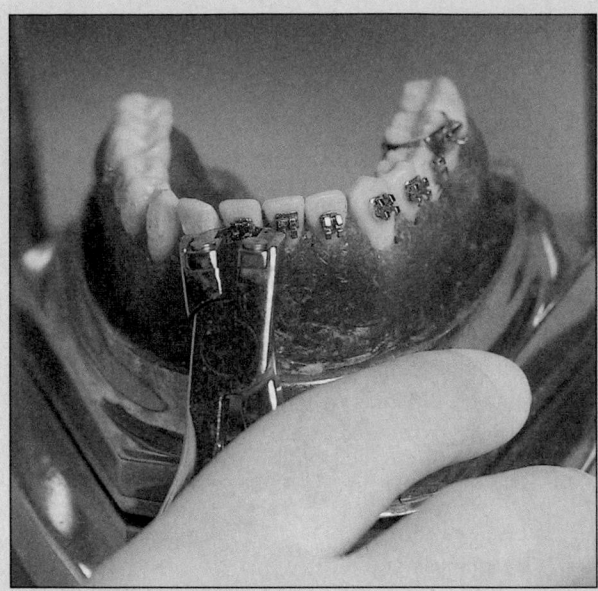

FIGURE 35-106
Bracket removal with bracket removing pliers.

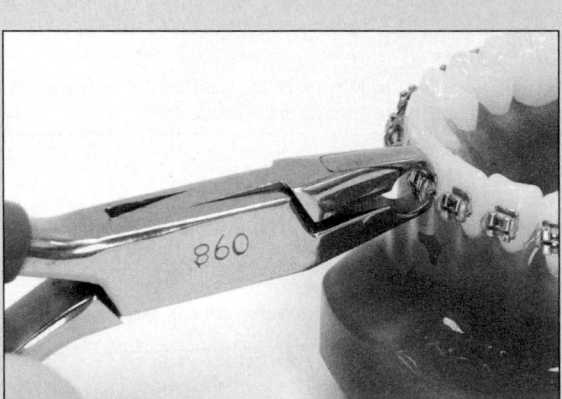

FIGURE 35-105
Adhesive removing pliers are used to break the adhesive bond holding the bracket.

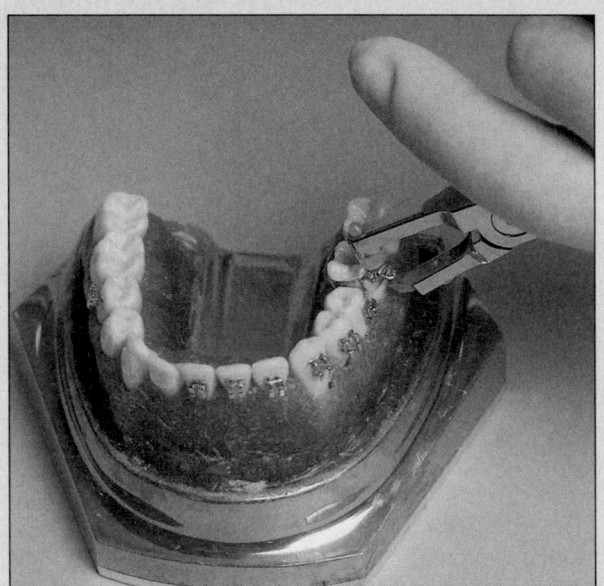

FIGURE 35-107
Band removal with band-removal pliers.

6. Retrieve bracket removing pliers and pass band removing pliers (Figure 35-106).

Removes the posterior bands (Figure 35-107).
- ❏ **Places the cushioned end of the band removing pliers on the buccal cusp.**
- ❏ **Places the end with the blade against the gingival edge of the band.**
- ❏ **Gently lifts the band toward the occlusal surface.**

- ❏ **Repeats this process on the lingual surfaces until the band is free.**

7. Retrieve band removing pliers and pass scaler.

8. Ask the doctor to check and complete finishing procedures such as occlusal and esthetic finishing.

Operator removes cement and direct bonding materials from the tooth surface with a scaler.

❏ Requests an ultrasonic scaler and/or a finishing bur to remove stubborn cement and bonding material.

Polishes tooth with rubber points.

9. Place prophy paste in rubber cup of disposable prophy angle.

10. Pass disposable prophy angle.

Polishes areas on tooth where cement or adhesive has been removed.

11. Rinse and evacuate while teeth are being polished.

Takes photographs.

Takes alginate impression of both arches to be used in construction of the retainer (refer to Chapter 33).

12. Send impressions to the lab.

Tells patient goodbye and what a pleasure it was to see them.

13. Provide patient with postoperative instructions.
  ❏ Explain how chewing on ice and hard, chewy candy can damage the sealant.
  ❏ Educate patient or primary caregiver about need for re-evaluation of sealants on follow-up visits.

14. Write up procedure in Services Rendered.

15. Dismiss and escort patient to reception area (refer to Procedure 18-5).

Date	Services Rendered
02/18/XX	Debonding/debanding appointment. Removed orthodontic appliances
	Removed cement and adhesive and polished teeth
	PO: Schedule appointment with family dentist for coronal polishing and fluoride application
	RTC: Deliver retainer/positioner appointment Assistant's initials

Chapter Summary

Orthodontics is an exciting specialty that provides many opportunities for the dental assistant as a member of the team. A trained dental assistant may be a valuable member of a general dental practice that provides clear aligner therapy to their patients for improved esthetics. Or a trained orthodontic assistant may be an essential member of the team in an orthodontic practice. Depending on the size of the orthodontic practice and the training of the team members, the responsibilities are very diverse. Trained individuals may assist with the new patient orthodontic exam, produce orthodontic records, work with the doctor to do case presentations and consultations, perform many chairside procedures independently, help patients be engaged in their treatment, provide oral hygiene instruction, and encourage patients to achieve their goals. It is a positive and rewarding role to be a member of an orthodontic team that has a powerful influence on patients' lives and attitudes.

To summarize, this chapter covered:

1. The members of an orthodontic team and the tasks that each member performs for the team.
2. Each step of conducting a new patient orthodontic exam to familiarize the reader with the anatomy of a potential patient and the conditions that may be addressed during treatment.
3. Producing orthodontic diagnostic records and preparation of those records for the doctor to analyze them.
4. The diagnosis and treatment planning process the doctor does to develop a diagnosis of the problems, develop treatment options, and review those options with the patient to finalize the treatment plan.
5. Orthodontic treatment of young children, adolescents, and adults including some appliances that may be used during treatment.
6. Orthodontic retention procedures after removal of the braces to hold the teeth in their new final position indefinitely after treatment.
7. The typical appointment sequence for comprehensive orthodontic treatment with braces.

Each state regulates the required education and list of procedures the dental assistant or orthodontic assistant may perform directly and indirectly on the orthodontic patient. In addition to assisting with orthodontic bonding and banding procedures, orthodontic assistants with the appropriate education and licensure may bond brackets, fit and cement bands, and place and remove ligatures and arch wires. To become a certified orthodontic assistant, the assistant must pass a specialty examination administered by the Dental Assistant National Board and/or the individual state board of dentistry. Again, this field of dentistry is exciting and rewarding.

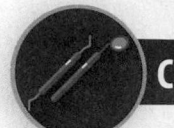

CASE STUDY

Chaz Danton, a 12-year-old male, was examined for need for orthodontic treatment by Dr. Snyder, an orthodontist. Chaz presents with a severe overjet of 10 millimeters, a deep overbite of 8 mm, and a receded mandible. When he eats toast or pizza crust, his palate becomes sore and irritated. Chaz is also congenitally missing his mandibular second premolars on both sides.

Case Study Review

1. Is Chaz's age a factor in the orthodontist's diagnosis? Explain why or why not.

2. What stage of tooth eruption should the dental assistant expect Chaz to be in? Which primary teeth are normally present?

3. Which of Dr. Angle's classes of malocclusion do you expect to see and record?

4. What is causing the irritation of Chaz's palate after eating toast or pizza crust?

Review Questions

Multiple Choice

1. Which orthodontic team member is responsible for examining, diagnosing, and planning what treatment should be provided for the patient?
   a. orthodontist
   b. scheduling coordinator
   c. certified orthodontic assistant
   d. financial coordinator

2. Which orthodontic team member places and removes bracket, bands, elastic ties, and ligature wire ties?
   a. orthodontist
   b. scheduling coordinator
   c. certified orthodontic assistant
   d. financial coordinator

3. Which occurs during the orthodontic new patient exam?
   a. thorough examination
   b. notation of cause of malocclusion
   c. discussion of patient's concern
   d. All of these

4. Which of the following may cause the patient to be a poor candidate for orthodontic treatment?
   a. consumption of large amount of sugary snacks
   b. high risk for gingivitis and dental caries
   c. dental habits
   d. All of these

5. Which classification has the same molar and canine relationship as normal occlusion?
   a. Class I
   b. Class II
   c. Class III
   d. Class IV

6. Which classification has the maxillary first molar forward of the lower first molar with the front teeth protruded?
   a. Class I
   b. Class II
   c. Class III
   d. Class IV

7. _____ factors can affect patient's abnormal jaw relationship and abnormal teeth-to-jaw relationship and may cause malocclusion.
   a. Genetic
   b. Systemic
   c. Local
   d. All of these

8. _____ factors that can cause malocclusion includes oral habits, trauma, and early and late loss of primary teeth.
   a. Genetic
   b. Systemic
   c. Local
   d. All of these

9. Which diagnostic records are generally a part of the orthodontic new patient examination?
   a. cephalometric radiograph
   b. study models
   c. clinical photographs
   d. All of these

10. Orthodontic tracings are made using which of the following types of radiographs?
   a. bitewing
   b. periapical
   c. cephalometric
   d. panoramic

11. During the consultation appointment, which of the following is discussed?
   a. cost of treatment
   b. patient's responsibility
   c. duration of treatment
   d. All of these

12. Which statement(s) is true about what causes the tooth to move during orthodontic treatment?
   a. force applied by orthodontic appliance
   b. process of resorption
   c. bone breakdown by osteoclasts
   d. All of these

13. The orthodontic treatment of oral habits that may lead to cause malocclusion are treated during which phase of treatment?
   a. observation and counseling
   b. interceptive
   c. phase I early treatment with braces
   d. phase II comprehensive treatment

14. Which provides force for tooth movement?
   a. ligature wire ties
   b. elastic ties
   c. elastic rubber bands
   d. All of these

15. What is placed in the contact areas between teeth to force the teeth apart before the placement of orthodontic bands?
   a. elastic ties
   b. elastic rubber bands
   c. separators
   d. ligature wire ties

16. Which statement(s) describe Phase II orthodontic treatment?
   a. full orthodontic treatment
   b. placement of braces
   c. takes 1 to 3 years
   d. All of these

17. Which orthodontic appliance holds the arch wire in place and transmits force to move teeth?
   a. band
   b. bracket
   c. buccal tube
   d. coil springs

18. When is the Mathieu needle holder used?
   a. holds arch wire during placement
   b. ties ligature wire
   c. places elastic ties
   d. All of these

19. Which is an acrylic appliance that fits on the upper and lower teeth to improve the overbite by positioning the jaw forward?
   a. Frankel appliance
   b. Herbst appliance
   c. bionator
   d. Hawley appliance

20. What esthetic orthodontic appliance may be used to correct minor adult orthodontic problems?
   a. retainer
   b. positioner
   c. aligner
   d. All of these

Critical Thinking

1. Do you have teeth that are out of alignment? Using orthodontic terms, identify your classification, describe the deviations, and identify the malpositioned teeth.

2. Why it is important for the patient's concerns to be addressed and to have them be an active part in goal setting and treatment planning?

3. What should be explained to the patient about holding the teeth in their new position after movement during orthodontic treatment?

Key Terms

Term and Pronunciation	Meaning of Root and Word Parts	Definition
abfractions (ab-**frak**-shun)	**ab-** = opposite to **fraction** = break into sections	loss of tooth structure not caused by tooth decay; noncarious cervical lesion; causes may be forces placed on teeth during biting, eating, chewing, and grinding
arch wire (ahrch) (wah*yuhr*)	**arch** = a curved structure **wire** = a slender, rod of metal	a wire conforming to the alveolar arch used as a source of force in correcting the positions of the teeth

(Continues)

Term and Pronunciation	Meaning of Root and Word Parts	Definition
asymmetry (ey-**sim**-i-tree)	**a-** = not, without **sym-** = same, similar **-metry** = the process of measuring	two parts of something that are not exactly the same; lack of equality or equivalence between parts or aspects of something
band (band)	**band** = a thin strip of material that encircles an object	a thin metal ring that is cemented to the teeth and secures orthodontic appliances to the teeth
bracket (**brak**-it)	**bracket** = a metal support	small metal or ceramic support bonded to teeth or bands to keep arch wires in place and help guide movement of teeth
coincident (koh-**in**-si-d*uh*nt)	**co-** = together **incident** = occurrence or event	happening at the same time
crossbite (kraws- bahyt)	**cross** = to move, pass, or extend from one side to the other side of **bite** = to grip or hold with the teeth	an abnormal relation of one or more teeth of one arch to the opposing tooth or teeth of the other arch, caused by deviation of tooth position or abnormal jaw position
deleterious (del-i-**teer**-ee-*uh* s)	**deleterious** = destroyer, destructive	harmful, injurious to health
diastema (dahy-*uh*-**stee**-m*uh*)	**diastema** = an abnormal space, fissure, or cleft in a bodily organ or part	a space between two teeth, especially a space between the maxillary central incisors
elastic tie (ih-**las**-tik) (tahy)	**elastic** = flexible, stretchable **tie** = to fasten, to draw together parts	flexible ring of rubber that fits around the bracket to secure an arch wire; a type of ligature
facebow (**feys**-bou)	**face** = the front part of the head **bow** = curved outward at the center	in orthodontics, a metal bar of a headgear appliance with an inner bow that inserts to special metal headgear tubes that are soldered to orthodontic bands placed on the maxillary first molars. The outer bow attaches to a neck strap that places a restraining force on the forward growth of the maxilla
frenectomy (fre-**nek**-t*uh*-mee)	**frenum** = a fold of membrane that restrains the motion of a part **ec-** = out from, away from **-tomy** = cutting, incision	a surgical procedure for excising a frenum or frenulum, such as the excision of the lingual frenum from its attachment into the mucoperiosteal covering of the alveolar process to correct ankyloglossia
hypocalcifications (hahy-poh- kal-s*uh*-fi-**key**-sh*uh* n)	**hypo-** = under, deficient **calcify** = to make or become hard by depositing of calcium salts	deficient calcification of bone or teeth; a defect of tooth enamel in which normal amounts of enamel are produced but are hypomineralized; in this defect the enamel is softer than normal
interceptive (in-ter-**sep**-tiv)	**intercept** = to stop or interrupt the course **-ive** = expressing function	the phase of orthodontics concerned with elimination of conditions spacing inadequacies that might lead to the development of malocclusion
ligature wire (**lig**-*uh*-cher) (wahy*uh*r)	**ligate** = tie up **-ure** = denoting action **wire** = slender flexible metal	strong flexible wire that ties the arch wire in place
malocclusion (mal-*uh*-**kloo**-zh*uh* n)	**mal-** = bad, faulty, ill **occlude** = to close, shut **-ion** = denoting action or condition	problem in the way the upper and lower teeth fit together in biting or chewing
myofunctional therapy (mahy-oh- **fuhngk**-sh*uh*-nl) (**ther**-*uh*-pee)	**myo-** = muscle **function** = to perform a specified action **-al** = pertaining to **therapy** = treatment of disease or disorders by rehabilitating process	treatment of malocclusion and speech disorders; uses muscular exercises of the tongue and lips; most often intended to alter a tongue thrust swallowing pattern
occlusion (*uh*-**kloo**-zh*uh* n)	**occlude** = to close, shut **-ion** = denoting action or condition	the relation of the teeth of both jaws when in functional contact during activity of the mandible

Term and Pronunciation	Meaning of Root and Word Parts	Definition
orthodontics (awr-thuh-**don**-tiks)	**orth(o)** = correct, straight **-odont** = having teeth **-ics** = denoting a body of facts, knowledge, principles	the branch of dentistry concerned with the correction and prevention of irregularities and malocclusion of the teeth
orthognathic (awr-**thog**-nuh-thik)	**ortho-** = straight, correct **gnath** = jaw **-ic** = having some characteristics of	having a normal relationship of the jaws; straight-jawed; having the profile of the face vertical or nearly so
overbite (oh-ver-bahyt)	**over** = above in place or position **bite** = close teeth together	occlusion where the upper incisor teeth overlap the lower incisors
overjet (oh-ver-jet)	**over** = above in place or position **jet** = jut, to extend beyond the main body or line	the measurement in millimeters from the labial surfaces of the mandibular central incisors to the labial surfaces of the maxillary central incisors
peg lateral (peg) (**lat**-er-uhl)	**peg** = object tapered toward the bottom **lateral** = lateral incisor; second tooth from the midline	lateral incisor tooth that has a conic deformity by which the tooth surfaces taper toward the incisal edge
perimeter plane (puh-**rim**-i-ter) (pleyn)	**peri-** = around, about **meter** = measure, measuring quantity **plane** = a flat surface in which is a straight line joining any two points on that surface	the boundary of a two-dimensional figure (closed occlusion)
proclination (proh-kluh-**ney**-shuh n)	**pro-** = projecting forward or outward **incline** = slant, to lean **-ate** = having appearance **-ion** = denoting action or condition	anterior-posterior tipping of the maxillary or mandibular incisors (remove mention of protrusion which is bodily positioning of a tooth anteriorly)
proprietary material (pruh-**prahy**-i-ter-ee) (muh-**teer**-ee-uhl)	**propriety** = quality of being appropriate **-ary** = for the purpose of **matter** = substance of which any physical object consists **-al** = pertaining to	belonging to a person/business who have the exclusive right; materials that one party (provider) furnishes to the other party (recipient)
protraction (proh-**trak**-shuh n)	**protract** = to extend or protrude **-ion** = denoting action or condition	extension of teeth or other maxillary or mandibular structures into a position anterior to the normal position
retainers (ri-**tey**-ner)	**retain** = to continue to hold in place or position **-ers** = designating either persons or things	appliances or devices that hold the teeth in an exact position after orthodontic tooth movement
retroclination (re-troh- kluh-**ney**-shuh n)	**retro-** = backward **incline** = slant, to lean **-ate** = having appearance **-ion** = denoting action or condition	posterior tipping of the crowns of the maxillary or mandibular incisors toward the tongue, (remove retrusion which is bodily repositioning of teeth)
retrognathism (re-truh-nuh-**thiz**-uhm)	**retro-** = backward direction **-gnath** = jaw **-ism** = denoting condition	when one or both jaws are posterior to their normal positions
separators (**sep**-uh-rey-ter)	**separate** = force apart **-or** = denoting person or thing	also known as spacers, rubber ring separators, or metal staple separators that are placed between teeth to create space for the seating of an orthodontic band
transverse plane (trans-**vurs**) (pleyn)	**trans-** = across **verse** = extending **plane** = a flat surface in which is a straight line joining any two points on that surface	extending from side to side; at a right angle horizontally to the long axis
underbite (**uhn**-der-bahyt)	**under** = below or beneath something **bite** = close teeth together	occlusion in which the lower incisor teeth overlap the upper incisors

## CHAPTER 36

Oral and Maxillofacial Surgery

Specific Instructional Objectives

At the completion of this chapter, you will be able to meet these objectives:

1. Use terms presented in this chapter.
2. Describe the duties of the surgery team.
3. Discuss the importance of the consultation appointment.
4. Discuss various surgical settings.
5. State preoperative instructions that should be provided to the patient.
6. Discuss methods used to control pain and anxiety during surgical procedures.
7. Describe oral surgery procedures.
8. Explain surgical asepsis steps.
9. Provide patient with appropriate postoperative instructions.
10. Describe how to remove sutures.
11. Describe potential postoperative complications.

Introduction

Oral surgery, also known as oral and maxillofacial surgery (OMS), is one of the nine recognized dental specialties by the American Dental Association. OMS focuses on the diagnosis and surgical and **adjunctive** treatment of diseases, injuries, and deformities of the oral and **maxillofacial** region. The specialty of oral surgery addresses tooth **extractions**, treatment of oral facial region trauma injuries and **congenital craniofacial** deformities, diagnosis and treatment of benign or malignant pathology of the head and neck, temporomandibular joint pathology, reconstructive, implant and emergency surgeries, and many more. Oral surgery can be performed in a private practice setting, or for more complicated and involved instances, in an outpatient clinic, hospital, or emergency room.

Although the general dentist studies surgical procedures, the number of surgical procedures performed in the general dentist's office depends on preference and training. General dentists refer surgical cases that go beyond their scope of training to oral surgeons.

The Oral and Maxillofacial Surgery Team

The OMS team has several members, each with a very specific role. The oral surgery office team varies according to the surgeon's goals for the practice. In addition to the oral and maxillofacial surgeon, the team usually consists of the receptionist, the business office staff, the surgical dental assistants, and, in some offices, a nurse anesthetist or an anesthesiologist. Each member is described in detail below.

Oral and Maxillofacial Surgeon

An oral and maxillofacial surgeon is a dentist who has undergone 4 to 6 years of subsequent postgraduate education and training in oral and maxillofacial surgery beyond the four years of dental school. Some oral and maxillofacial training programs incorporate a medical degree (MD) as part of the surgeon's training. Oral and maxillofacial surgery is also available as a hospital-based residency through some medical schools. Many oral and maxillofacial surgeons choose to obtain an additional medical degree in order to ensure practicing privileges in hospital operating rooms and facilities. The American Board of Oral and Maxillofacial Surgeons (ABOMS) is responsible for certifying surgeons via a series of examinations.

Receptionist and Business Staff

The receptionist and the business staff perform many of the same duties in the oral surgery office as they would in the general dental office. Because most of the oral surgeon's patients are referred by other dental and medical offices, communication and record-keeping responsibilities increase. The patient's x-rays and written information must be received in the surgeon's office before the patient's appointment. When patients first arrive at the office, they are given forms to fill out. Appointments for treatment are scheduled and insurance preauthorization claims and financial arrangements are completed before the day of the surgery.

Surgical Dental Assistant

Being a surgical dental assistant is a very demanding but rewarding profession. It requires advanced knowledge of infection control and sterile environment guidelines, excellent manual dexterity, knowledge of a highly specialized armamentarium, and tolerance to viewing and assisting during some extreme surgical situations. On the other hand, a surgical assistant has the privilege to be exposed to a variety of complicated and unusual procedures, from extraction of soft and hard tissue impacted teeth, to sinus lifts and cleft lip and palate surgeries. A surgical dental assistant has the opportunity to assist and observe procedures performed not only in an office environment but also in a sterile, outpatient, and hospital based environment.

It is common practice that during procedures performed in a sterile environment, two surgical assistants are on duty. One focuses on maintaining sterile conditions for the procedure and directly assists, while the other acts as a circulating assistant, removing and delivering instruments to and from the treatment area without disrupting the procedure or the sterile conditions present.

Even though special training is not required to become a surgical dental assistant, DANB offers a national certification exam demonstrating knowledge based competency in oral and maxillofacial dental assisting. Upon successful completion, the assistant becomes a Certified Oral and Maxillofacial Surgery Assistant (COMSA). The American Association of Oral and Maxillofacial Surgeons offers advanced training programs and certifications in areas such as advanced life support and administration of intravenous medications. Dental health care workers may take the Dental Anesthesia Assistant National Certification Examination (DAANCE) to become a Dental Anesthesia Assistant (DAA).

Nurse Anesthetist or Anesthesiologist

The oral surgeon makes the decision to have a nurse anesthetist or anesthesiologist as part of the surgical team. The nurse anesthetist may be a full- or part-time member of the surgical team, while an anesthesiologist is generally only in the office part time

and works with the oral surgeon with every patient in the hospital setting.

The responsibility of the nurse anesthetist varies but may include administering the anesthesia and maintaining the patient during the procedure, continuously monitoring the patient's vital signs, managing fluid therapy, providing or supervising postoperative recovery, conducting postoperative follow-up and patient evaluation, and maintaining records.

The anesthesiologist is hired to perform preoperative evaluations and preparations, administer anesthetics, monitor patient reactions to the anesthetic and surgery, and advise the oral surgeon of adverse reactions. The oral surgeon communicates very closely with the anesthesiologist to make certain that both have all the information they need to ensure the safety of the patient and to enable the oral surgeon to successfully accomplish the procedure. The anesthesiologist relieves the oral surgeon of anesthetizing the patient so that the surgeon can concentrate on the procedure to be performed.

Consultation Appointment

A general dentist may refer a patient to the oral surgeon when they feel the procedure is beyond their scope of expertise. During the initial consultation with the oral surgeon, the patient will be evaluated and examined thoroughly. The oral surgeon will make a diagnosis and present a plan of treatment. A series of x-rays is usually sent from the referring office; however, additional radiographs may be necessary for a complete assessment and evaluation. Periapical and extraoral radiographs such as panoramic and cephalometric films may be necessary to provide more details for accurate diagnosis and treatment planning. A three-dimensional image exposed with the use of a cone beam radiographic machine may also be necessary.

Certain fundamental principles must be followed and documented for every oral surgery evaluation. The chief complaint is the patient's report of symptoms and duration, which helps the surgeon to form an initial assessment of the situation. Present illness is the patient's description of the illness. Many times it gives valuable information and clues as to onset time, location, and symptoms. It is important to remember that information reported by the patient may be confusing and subjective. Past history and family history are two other categories that offer valuable information as to past injuries and family systemic diseases that may affect the outcome of the surgery. Finally, habits offer information on patient's sleep, diet, prescribed or over-the-counter medications, allergies, and personal habits such as tobacco and alcohol use.

Some patients may need special considerations or modifications for treatment based on their current medical condition. Treatment of diabetic patients, for example, should be performed in the morning, when blood sugar levels are more controlled, and appointments should be kept as short as possible. Such patients should also be informed of possible slower healing time. Additionally, the physician may need to be consulted regarding medication changes for the patient. For patients with other systemic diseases, such as cardiovascular disease, or for patients who use medications such as blood thinners (Coumadin, Warfarin, Plavix, etc.), a written permission for surgery must be obtained from the primary physician, since the medication regimen may need to be altered. The patient's vital signs are also recorded during the initial assessment, and all information is meticulously documented. The oral surgeon and the surgical assistant perform a series of clinical evaluation procedures in order to determine the cause of illness as well as the overall condition of the patient's oral cavity and related head and neck area.

The patient is informed of the diagnosis, the treatment and oral surgery setting options, and the forms of anesthesia available, which may include local anesthesia, nitrous oxide–oxygen minimal sedation, intravenous sedation, or even general anesthesia. If the patient is extremely anxious, medications for stress and anxiety may be prescribed. Antibiotic prescriptions are also written as needed.

Oral Surgery Settings

Oral surgery procedures can be performed in a variety of settings depending on the patient's medical condition and the complexity of the proposed treatment. Routine extractions as well as removal of impacted teeth, implant placement, and biopsies can be performed in a private dental office setting. The oral surgeon's office includes much the same equipment as a general dental office, with the addition of the recovery area and, in many offices, a room or rooms that are equipped comparable to hospital operating rooms. The recovery area is usually a separate area with large reclining chairs or beds for the patient to recover from the general anesthetic. Many private OMS offices are equipped for nitrous oxide and intravenous sedation and have all the necessary monitoring equipment for the patient's safety.

Many oral surgery procedures can be performed following the same infection control guidelines as in a general dentistry office.

Even though all instruments are sterilized, surfaces are disinfected, and proper barriers have been applied, the treatment area is not considered a sterile environment. A sterile environment is an environment that lacks any living organisms. By this definition, a dental office setting logistically cannot be considered a sterile environment. Some oral surgeon's offices may have surgical suites that are maintained sterile.

Most procedures are performed in the oral maxillofacial surgeon's office, but some cases require an outpatient or hospital setting. More complicated procedures such as cleft lip and palate surgeries, jaw reconstruction following trauma, extensive surgical procedures such as TMJ surgery or **orthognathic surgery**, or procedures on medically or physically compromised patients are often performed in a hospital operating room setting. The surgeon follows the protocol of the hospital to meet scheduling, staffing, and credentialing standards. Some hospitals allow dental assistants to assist oral surgeons after the dental assistants meet hospital standards on asepsis and operating room protocol.

For procedures done in hospital operating rooms, the personal hygiene and health of the doctors and staff is extremely important. All operating room personnel should report to their supervisor any open lesions or sores on their hands and arms, and signs or symptoms of cold, flu, or any other systemic infection.

Informed Consent

Once the diagnosis is complete and the setting for surgery is determined, the treatment options and postoperative instructions are discussed with the patient. The patient must carefully read and sign an informed consent form prior to the procedure. The informed consent identifies and explains the surgery the patient is to receive and acknowledges any risks of the treatment (Figure 36-1).

Patient Name _____
The oral surgery procedure to be performed: _____ has been explained to me to my satisfaction and I fully understand the explanation. I consent to this surgical procedure as well as to any other surgery that is necessary or advisable in the judgment of Dr. _____. I agree to the use of local anesthesia and nitrous oxide sedation for this procedure when such sedation is deemed to be appropriate and necessary. Additionally, I agree to the use of oral, intravenous sedation or general anesthesia for this procedure when such sedation or anesthesia is judged to be more appropriate and necessary by Dr. _____.
I understand that complications can arise during surgery and with the use of drugs and anesthesia. The most common complications from oral surgical procedures are pain, infection, swelling, bleeding, and bruising. In the case of grafting or implant procedures, a significant complication is non-healing or rejection. I understand that occasionally more serious complications can occur such as temporary or permanent numbness, paralysis of facial muscles, changes in the occlusion or temporomandibular joint, possible injury to adjacent teeth and tissues, bone fractures, sinus complications, referred pain to the head and neck, nausea, vomiting, allergic reactions, and delayed healing. Although life-threatening complications from the outlines surgery are extremely rare, there are inherent risks with any sedation, anesthetic, and surgical procedure.
Sedatives, anesthetics, and postoperative prescriptions can cause drowsiness, lack of awareness and coordination. These side effects could be aggravated by the use of alcohol or other drugs. I understand and agree NOT to operate any vehicle or hazardous device or to work while taking such medications until fully recovered from their effects.
I have received postoperative instructions and I fully understand them. Furthermore, it has been explained to me and I fully understand that there is no warranty or guarantee as to any result and/or cure. I acknowledge that I have asked for a full recital if any and all possible risks and alternatives to this procedure.
We invite your questions concerning this or related procedures and their risks. By signing below you acknowledge that you have read this document, understand the information presented, and have had all your questions answered satisfactorily.
Signatures:

_____   _____   _____
Patient or Guardian   Doctor   Date

FIGURE 36-1
Sample informed consent for oral surgery.

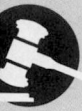

The informed consent form is a legal document that verifies that the patient has given consent to the oral surgeon to perform the surgical procedure; this is a necessary document above and beyond the general informed consent that a patient signs at a general dentist's office. The patient must acknowledge in writing that they have been informed and understand all potential risks and complications involved with the proposed procedure.

In many instances patients with congenital heart disease, prosthetic joints, artificial heart valves, or history of bacterial endocarditis require an antibiotic regimen prior to any surgical procedure. The American Heart Association (AHA) has recommended guidelines for such instances. Antibiotic premedication rationales as well as dosages are covered in detail in Chapter 14.

The AHA has also revised and implemented new guidelines for the types and dosage of antibiotic for premedication purposes. These guidelines are the result of new and updated biomedical data that reveals that some conditions previously thought to require premedication actually do not. The fact is that oral bacteria are introduced into the blood stream daily via chewing or even brushing and flossing. Often, prior to oral surgery the surgeon contacts the patient's physician to discuss concerns in regards to premedication needs and other medical clearance issues.

Preoperative Instructions

Prior to any surgical procedure, it is extremely important that a list of preoperative instructions be explained verbally and given in written form to the patient (Table 36-1). These instructions must be thoroughly documented in the patient's record.

 Documentation

05/31/XX—Ms. Jenkins was referred by Dr. Jameson, her general dentist, and presents today with swelling in the mandibular 3rd molar region. Ms. Jenkins is a 19-year-old female, currently a college student home for summer vacation. She states that she has had pain and swelling in the areas of 17 and 32 on and off for several months. She has brought PA images from her general dentist that shows impacted mandibular 3rd molars. The general dentist suggests extraction. Patient was examined and provided with amoxicillin 500 mg tablets to be taken three times per day until complete to help reduce the swelling. Patient was also provided with an order for a cone beam image at Lakeside Imaging Center. Digital panoramic image taken today. Patient provided with preoperative instructions in order to prepare her for the surgical extraction visit. Patient offered local anesthesia only, local anesthesia plus nitrous oxide sedation, or local anesthesia and IV sedation. Patient advised that all four 3rd molars should be extracted. Patient agreed and signed the surgical informed consent. Determined to perform procedure with local anesthesia and IV sedation in office setting.

TABLE 36-1 Preoperative Instructions for the Surgical Patient

DOs	DON'TS
Inform the surgeon if you are taking ANY medication.	If you are to receive intravenous sedation or general anesthesia, DO NOT eat or drink ANYTHING AFTER MIDNIGHT on the night prior to your surgery unless advised by your surgeon. This includes water, gum, breath mints, etc.
Follow instructions from your surgeon regarding any medications to be taken prior to surgery.	
Contact the oral surgeon's office prior to surgery if you have ANY CHANGE in your health status: i.e., cold, chest congestion, flu, etc.	
Brush your teeth prior to surgery. Rinse well but do not swallow any water.	DO NOT wear make-up or earrings. Keep other jewelry to a minimum.
If you have long hair, please pull it back.	DO NOT wear contact lenses.
Come to your surgery appointment with a responsible adult who can drive you home. We require that your escort remain in the waiting room during surgery. After surgery, the escort will be brought back to the recovery area to sit with you and receive postoperative instructions.	If you are a smoker—NO SMOKING before surgery (at least 12 hours) and for at least 24 hours after the surgery.
Try to be as rested and relaxed as possible.	
Wear loose fitting, comfortable clothing, shirt short or easy to roll up, low-heeled shoes.	
If surgery is in the afternoon, drink only water, juice, tea, or coffee prior to 6 am. After 6 am, take absolutely nothing by mouth.	
Inform us if you cannot keep your appointment.	

Methods to Control Pain and Anxiety

Due to the invasive nature of oral surgery procedures, the oral surgeon employs many methods to control the patient's pain and anxiety. Oral and maxillofacial surgeons have extensive knowledge and training in a variety of methods used to prevent pain and reduce anxiety. The surgeon evaluates the needs and concerns of the patient and chooses medications specifically for each individual patient and procedure. A surgeon may use local anesthesia, sedation, general anesthesia, nitrous oxide, or a combination of these. Because of the potential for medical emergencies while utilizing pain control medication, oral and maxillofacial surgeons receive specialized training in advanced life support and maintain advanced life support equipment and devices for monitoring blood pressure, heart rate and rhythm, and lung function. In the rare occasion that a medical emergency occurs, crash carts and defibrillators are available.

Local Anesthesia

A patient's medical history and the type of surgery to be performed as well as the anxiety and fears that a patient may have are the primary factors that determine the type of anesthesia the patient will receive. Topical and local anesthetics are routinely used during surgery. Local anesthetics are injections given to the area for surgery to produce a local anesthetic affect that will allow the dentist to perform procedures without discomfort to the patient. Local anesthetics are used to temporarily eliminate pain from a small area and are usually administered via injection. During local anesthesia the patient remains conscious.

Sedation

Sedation is primarily used to reduce the patient's nervous activity and anxiety and help them to remain calm. Based on the dosage and method of administration, the sedation can be minimal, moderate, or deep.

Minimal sedation or **anxiolysis** is a state in which the patient is able to respond to verbal stimuli and maintain a patent airway, yet may have some diminished cognitive function. Nitrous oxide, discussed below, has the ability to induce minimal sedation. Minimal sedation may not always be drug induced. A patient is able to self-induce a state of minimal sedation through nonpharmacological methods such as acupuncture, acupressure, or hypnosis.

Moderate sedation, also known as conscious sedation, is a drug induced state during which a patient remains conscious and is able to maintain a patent airway. Although the patient can respond to commands, consciousness is depressed. Cardiovascular function and ventilation are maintained. Moderate sedation can be induced with nitrous oxide or an intravenous sedative.

Deep sedation is a drug induced state between consciousness and unconsciousness. Patients are difficult to arouse and may respond after a painful stimulus. Patients may need assistance with ventilation though cardiovascular function is usually maintained.

General Anesthesia

General anesthesia is a drug induced state of unconsciousness. Patients are unable to be aroused even with a painful stimulus and need equipment in order to maintain ventilation. Cardiovascular function is usually impaired as well.

General anesthesia consists of four stages; each stage causes changes in breathing, muscle tone, and reflexes. Stage IV is an overdose and can lead to respiratory arrest. During administration of the general anesthetic prior to surgery, the patient proceeds into and is maintained in Stage III where surgery is performed. (Refer to Chapter 14 for details.) Many of the drugs used to induce anesthesia can be given in a lesser amount to produce sedation; greater amounts can induce a state of deep sedation or even general anesthesia. Only a skilled and trained clinician with the necessary equipment for maintenance and emergency management should administer sedatives. Additionally, state laws may vary, and each practitioner should be aware of the laws regarding scope of practice for their state.

Nitrous Oxide

Nitrous oxide (N_2O) is a colorless gas used in medicine and dentistry for its analgesic, amnestic, and anesthetic properties. Nitrous oxide has some anesthetic properties, especially in soft tissue (gingiva, cheeks), but by itself it is not capable of suppressing pain caused by dental procedures. Today, N_2O is used in dentistry as an adjunct to local anesthesia, mostly to reduce patient anxiety. In hospitals, N_2O is used in conjunction with other more powerful inhalation general anesthetics as it has the ability to enhance the effects of the other anesthetics. This allows the anesthesiologist to use less of the more potent general anesthetics, increasing patient safety. (Refer to Chapter 23 for the administration and safety in using nitrous oxide.)

The role of the surgical assistant is to monitor vital signs throughout the procedure and ensure safe and complete recovery prior to patient dismissal.

Safety

During the entire administration of nitrous oxide and oxygen, the dentist and the assistant should pay close attention to the patient's behavior and watch for signs of oversedation. These include the patient feeling hot or nauseous, stating that they feel as if they cannot move their legs, or responding only after being asked the same questions a couple of times. In this case the nitrous oxide should be decreased and the oxygen concentration increased. If necessary, put patient on 100% oxygen and allow to recover.

Oral Surgery Procedures

Oral surgery procedures require rigid adherence to infection control, knowledge of specialized instruments, and diligent patient management.

Surgical Asepsis

The oral surgery office is a higher risk area because of the increased possibility of blood contact. Since surgical procedures have tissues open and exposed to the environment with bleeding, the dentist and the dental assistant must also take aseptic procedures a step further to prevent organisms from entering the open wound. All asepsis steps discussed in Chapter 11 must be closely followed. Surgical asepsis includes the use of the surgical hand scrub and donning of sterile gloves, sterile isolation gowns, and surgical caps. Surgical personal protective equipment (PPE) must be used for all surgical procedures. A full-length drape is placed on the patient with a sterile towel placed over the patient's chest. Patients may also wear surgical caps (Figure 36-2).

Extraordinary care of surgical equipment and supplies is necessary to prevent accidental exposure. Instruments must remain sterile in bags or packs until use and should be placed on a sterile tray and sterile towel. Once the bags are open, the instruments should be covered by a sterile towel. It is critical that the chain of asepsis be maintained to prevent cross-contamination. The surgical team must avoid contact with nonsterile items or surfaces once the chain of asepsis has been established. A circulating assistant should be asked to obtain an item if needed to maintain the sterile field.

Routine Extractions

Routine extractions, also called forceps extractions, are performed more often than other surgeries. The tooth to be removed has a crown portion that can be grasped by the extraction forceps (Procedure 36-1). The main goal of a routine extraction is to cause minimum trauma to the soft and hard tissues. Unless excessive bleeding occurs, sutures are rarely used.

The basic oral surgery instruments, such as the surgical aspirating tips, retractors, mouth props, periosteal elevator, straight elevator, extraction forceps, and surgical curette, are the only surgical instruments needed for routine extractions (Table 36-2). Irrigation of the surgical site must be accomplished using an irrigating syringe and sterile saline solution. The surgical assistant's skill in assisting with an extraction procedure is critical for the smooth operation of the procedure. The dental assistant prepares the tray setup and selects extraction forceps for the specific tooth to be extracted (Tables 36-3 and 36-4). The surgical assistant's instrument transfer, oral evacuation, tissue retraction, and patient management skills are important to ensure a smooth procedure.

The extraction forceps are used to remove teeth from the alveolar bone. They are hinged instruments with various handles and beak styles. Specific forceps are used on certain teeth or in certain areas of the mouth. Dental assistants should be able to identify which forceps their dentists routinely use. One way to learn forceps is by manufacturer's numbers. Each instrument has a number imprinted on the handle and is labeled with an "L" or "R" for left or right. For example, #88R is used on the maxillary right first and second molars.

Another way to identify forceps is to learn how the design of the forceps applies to tooth morphology. Careful study of the various shapes of the beaks will allow determination of forceps for:

- Maxillary or mandibular teeth
- Right or left quadrant
- Anterior or posterior teeth
- Accommodation of teeth anatomy

For example, on #53R for the maxillary molars, one beak is pointed for placement in the bifurcated buccal root. On #88L for the maxillary molars, there is a pointed single beak on the buccal to be placed between the two buccal roots and a split beak on the lingual to engage the single lingual root.

The curve of the shank of the forceps indicates whether the forceps should be used on the maxillary or the mandibular. Mandibular forceps are often at more of a right angle, and the maxillary forceps are straight, slightly curved, or have two angles (like bayonets). For example, #17 forceps are used on the mandibular first and second molars; the beaks form an angle with the handle. The forceps for the maxillary first and second molars have two angles in the working end.

Some forceps are universal forceps and can be used on any of the four quadrants. Another example is #101 forceps, which can be used for premolars and primary teeth in either arch. Other forceps can be used on the left or right side in the same arch. For example, the #150 forceps can be used for maxillary incisors, premolars, and roots on both the left and right quadrants.

Forceps used on the anterior or posterior teeth can be distinguished by beak width. For example, on mandibular forceps #151, the beaks are smaller to fit the incisors, premolars, and roots, while mandibular molar forceps #17 are wider to accommodate the width of the molars.

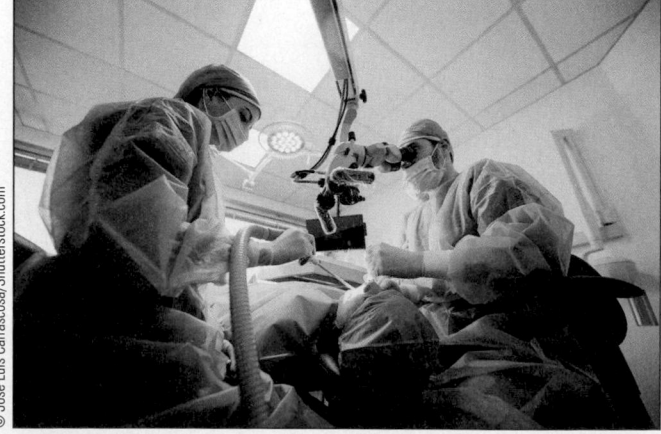

FIGURE 36-2
PPE for both the dental team and patient during oral surgery procedures.

© Jose Luis Carrascosa/Shutterstock.com

TABLE 36-2 Basic Oral Surgery Instruments

Instrument	Function
surgical aspirating tips 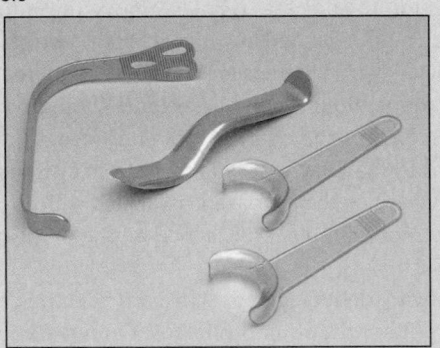	Aspirate blood and debris from the surgical site and back of the oral cavity for sedated patients. Metal tips are sterilizable, and plastic tips are single use.
retractors 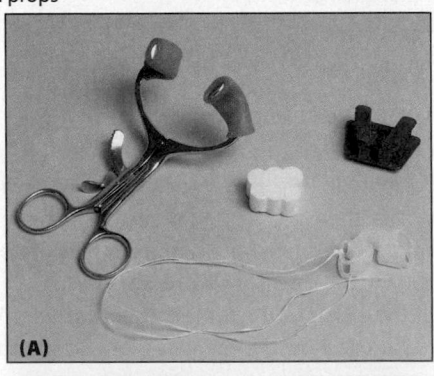	Hold lip, tongue, and cheeks so operator can view site during procedure.
mouth props 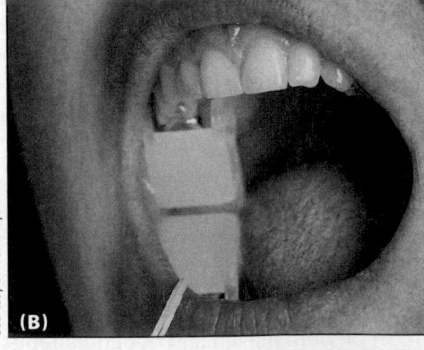 (A) (B)	Prevent patient's mouth from closing during procedure. Molt and rubber props are sterilizable, and plastic and Styrofoam props are single use. (A) Types of mouth props from left to right: molt scissors mouth prop, Styrofoam mouth prop, rubber and plastic mouth props. (B) Plastic mouth prop in a patient's mouth.

Courtesy of Isolite Systems

Instrument	Function
periosteal elevator 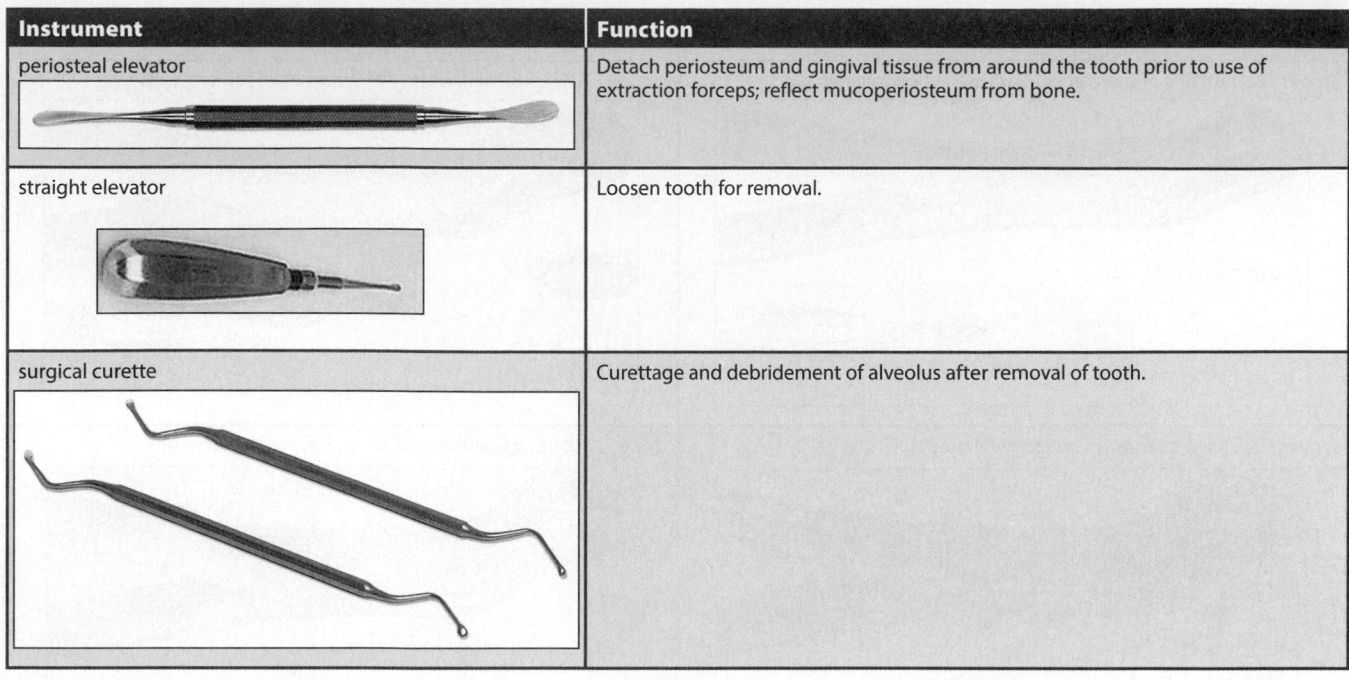	Detach periosteum and gingival tissue from around the tooth prior to use of extraction forceps; reflect mucoperiosteum from bone.
straight elevator	Loosen tooth for removal.
surgical curette	Curettage and debridement of alveolus after removal of tooth.

TABLE 36-3 Maxillary Extraction Forceps

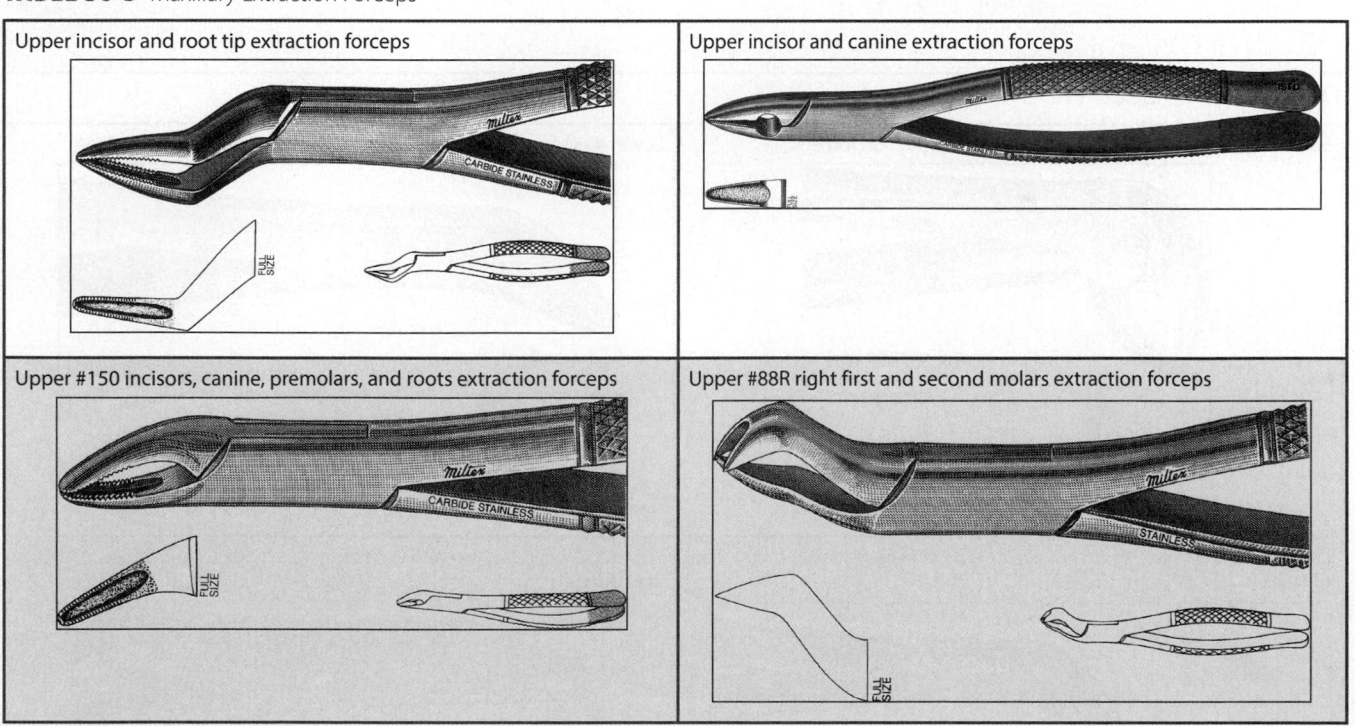

Upper incisor and root tip extraction forceps	Upper incisor and canine extraction forceps
Upper #150 incisors, canine, premolars, and roots extraction forceps	Upper #88R right first and second molars extraction forceps

(Continues)

TABLE 36-3 (*Continued*)

Upper #88L left first and second molars extraction forceps 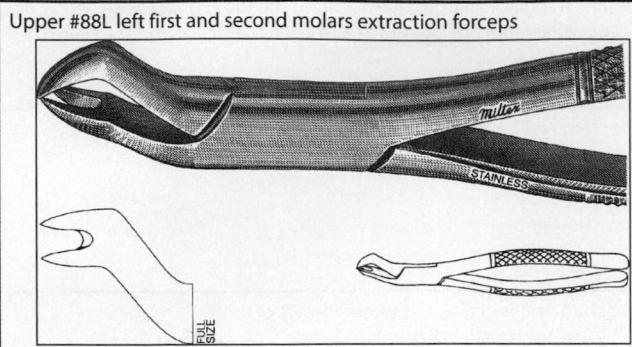	Upper #53R right first and second molars extraction forceps 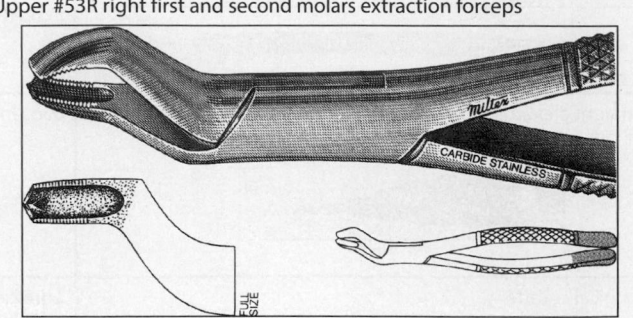
Upper #53L left first and second molars extraction forceps	Upper #210 universal third molar extraction forceps 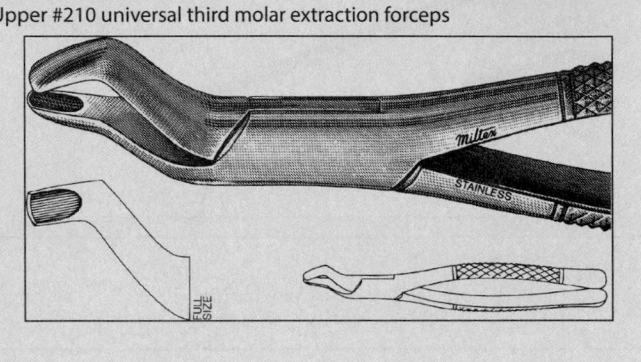

TABLE 36-4 Mandibular Extraction Forceps

Lower incisor, canine, premolars, and roots extraction forceps 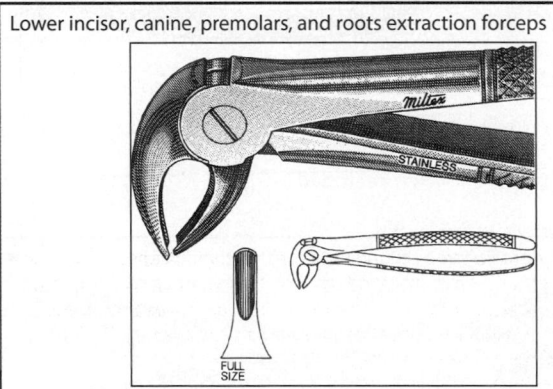	Lower #151 universal incisors, canine, and roots extraction forceps 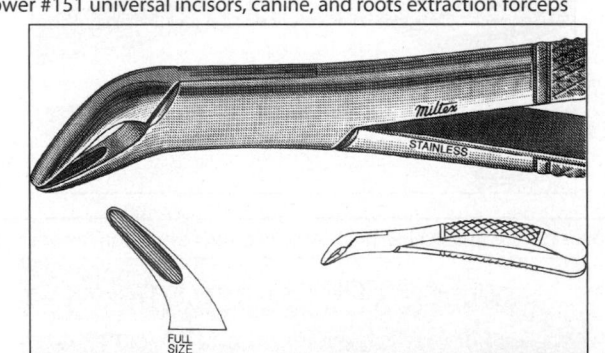
Lower #203 mandibular incisors, canines, premolars, and roots extraction forceps 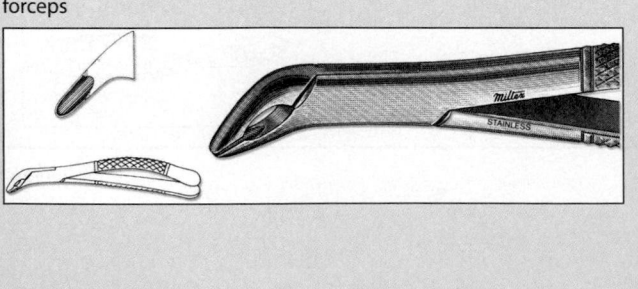	Lower #23 universal first and second molars extraction forceps "cow horns" 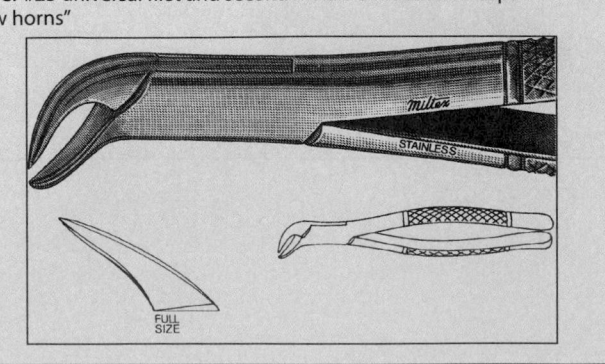

Lower #15 universal first and second molars extraction forceps with ring on handle

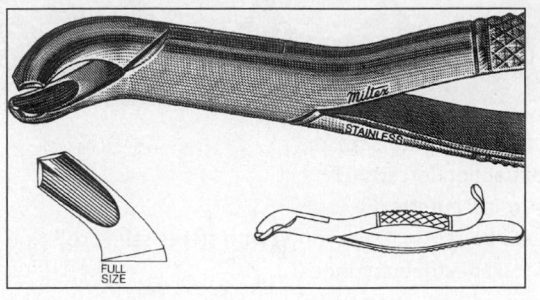

Lower #222 universal third molars extraction forceps

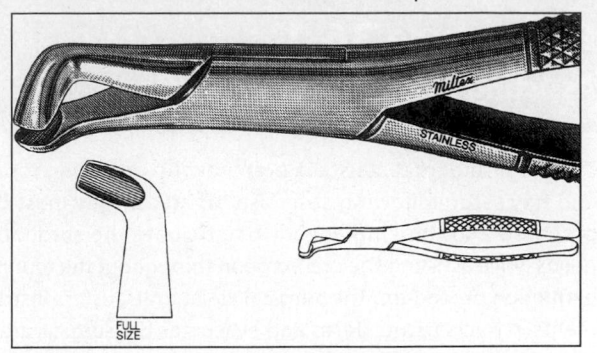

The shapes of forceps beaks are designed to accommodate the anatomy of specific teeth. For example, mandibular first and second molar forceps have narrow, pointed beaks to engage the bifurcated roots of these molars. These forceps are sometimes called the "cow horns" because of their shape.

Extraction forceps are held in a palm grasp by the operator. Some handles are straight, while others have "finger rings" or hooks on the handles (Figure 36-3). The selection is the preference of the dentist. To better visualize and learn forceps, divide them into the arches and teeth they are used on.

Postoperative Instructions After any type of oral surgical procedure, instructions are given to the patient—both verbally and in writing—to facilitate healing and minimize the risk of potential complications. (See Table 36-5 for sample

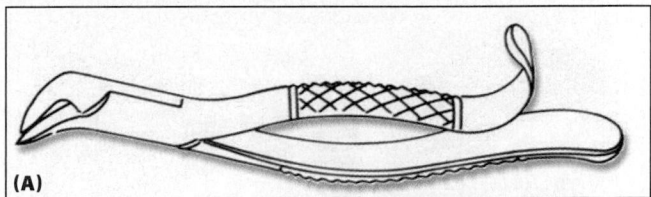

(A)

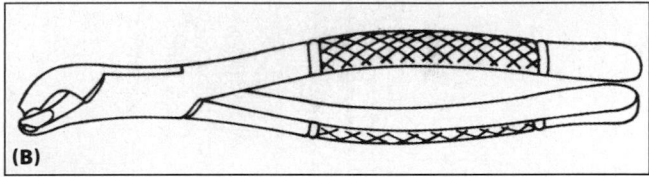

(B)

FIGURE 36-3
Extraction forceps (A) Hook handle and (B) Straight handle.

TABLE 36-5 Sample Postoperative Instruction

- Immediately following surgery, you should bite on a gauze pack for at least 30 minutes.
- Do not overexert yourself for the first 24 to 48 hours following surgery. If you must do something strenuous, place a piece of gauze on the surgical site and bite down to help protect the blood clot that has formed.
- Adequate food and especially fluid intake after surgery is essential for healing. Avoid hard or spicy food items, and avoid drinking from a straw for the first 24 hours.
- Do not consume alcohol for 48 hours, and do not miss a meal because you will feel better and heal faster.
- After surgical procedures, the pain level usually lessens by the second or third day. Take the pain medications as prescribed with a full glass of water.
- Immediately following surgery, *do not* rinse. After 24 hours, you can rinse your mouth four to six times each day using lukewarm salt water for one week. You should also start to brush your teeth gently because it will reduce the bacteria population and food debris in your mouth and promote healing. For a faster and complication-free recovery you must let the blood form a clot and leave it undisturbed. Some bleeding is expected for the first 24 to 48 hours. Use a piece of gauze or a moist tea bag, and bite down with moderate pressure. Avoid drinking from a straw or creating negative pressure in your mouth, which can dislodge the clot and cause renewed bleeding.
- Some swelling is expected for the few days following a surgical procedure. The degree varies depending on the individual and the magnitude of the procedure. For the first 24 hours, apply an ice pack to the outside of the face for 20 minutes on and 10 minutes off.
- It is normal to observe discoloration of the skin (bruising) or of the tissue around the surgery area. It should not alarm you and usually resolves within 7 to 14 days.
- Due to the lower jaw being open for an extended period of time, you may experience some stiffness. Likewise, the arm that was used for the IV medicine may have some soreness. Warm moist compresses and limited exercise will eliminate this problem.
- If a muscle relaxant was given as part of the anesthetic, sore neck, shoulder, and chest muscles are common.
- It is common following general anesthesia for the patient to experience nausea. This is related to the anesthetic but may also be a side effect of antibiotics and pain medications.
- Avoid smoking for at least 24 hours as it will increase the chance for a painful postoperative complication known as a dry socket.
- Elevated body temperature is expected following surgery for the first 24–48 hours. If the fever persists and is higher than 100°F (37°C), you should contact your physician.
- If a postoperative prescription for antibiotics has been given to you, fill it immediately and take as directed until it is finished. *Note for female patients:* Some antibiotics may inhibit the action of the birth control pills; you may want to consult with your physician for alternative methods of contraception.
- If you have undergone conscious sedation or general anesthesia, you must not operate a motor vehicle or any other heavy machinery for 24 hours.
- If absorbable sutures have been used, they will dissolve within seven days. If nonabsorbable sutures have been used, a postoperative visit is necessary to remove them.
- **Attention**: If the bleeding has not stopped after 48 hours or the swelling has not subsided and the site has become hot, hard, and painful to touch, you should contact our office immediately.

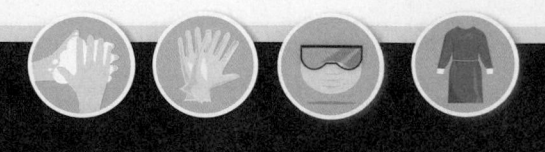

Procedure 36-1
Assisting with Routine Extraction

The surgical dental assistant prepares the operating room and tray setup following strict aseptic steps. They must be prepared and thinking ahead to anticipate the surgeon's needs while assisting the oral surgeon throughout the routine extraction procedure. The surgical assistant transfers instruments, retracts tissue, rinses and evacuates the surgical area, and maintains a sterile field at all times.

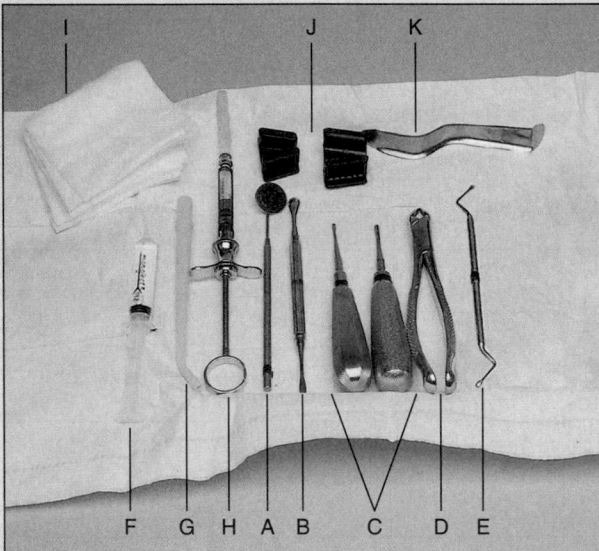

FIGURE 36-4
Routine extraction setup.

Equipment and Supplies

Patient Seating Setup

- PPE: surgical gloves, mask, protective glasses, and sterile isolation gown (sterile cap optional in office setting)
- Sterile handwashing soap and brush
- Sanitized dental treatment area and barriers placed over equipment
- Patient's medical and dental records
- Preparation of patient
  - ❏ full length drape
  - ❏ sterile towel
  - ❏ sterile cap
  - ❏ patient protective glasses
  - ❏ mouth rinse in disposable cup
- Blood pressure equipment

Local Anesthetic Setup (refer to Procedure 23-2)

Routine Extraction Setup (Figure 36-4)

- mouth mirror (A)
- periosteal elevator (B)

- straight elevators (C)
- extraction forceps (D)
- surgical curette (E)
- Leur Lock irrigating syringe with sterile saline solution (F)
- local anesthetic syringe (G)
- surgical aspirating tip (H)
- 4 × 4 sterile gauze squares (I)
- bite block mouth props (small and large) (J)
- Minnesota cheek and tongue retractor (K)
- pain/anxiety medication setup (optional)

Procedure Steps

1. Escort and seat patient (refer to Procedure 18-4).

2. Prepare in advance for extraction procedure.
    - ❏ Place instrument sterile pack on sterile surgical tray covered with sterile towel.
    - ❏ Open patient's chart in dental software.
    - ❏ Navigate to the dental charting screen.
    - ❏ Open patient's latest radiographic history on the computer monitor, or place on view box.
    - ❏ Inform dentist that the patient is ready.
    - ❏ Introduce dentist as they enter the treatment area.

    Dentist greets the patient.

    Performs surgical scrub and dons surgical gloves.

3. Doff examination gloves and perform surgical scrub; don surgical gloves.

4. Open instrument pack and organize instruments on instrument tray covered with sterile towel.

    Takes position at the dental chair.
    - ❏ *Signals for the procedure to begin (refer to Procedure 20-1).*

5. Pass mouth mirror.

    Examines the site of extraction.

    Administers local anesthetic.

6. Assist in administration of local anesthetic (refer to Procedure 23-2).

7. Transfer the periosteal elevator.

    Tests whether the patient is adequately numb by touching sharp end to tissue.

    Loosens the soft tissue surrounding the tooth and separates epithelial tissue from around the tooth using periosteal elevator.

8. Exchange the periosteal elevator and straight elevator.

❑ Have gauze ready to remove blood and debris from instrument.

Loosens the tooth within its socket using straight elevator.

9. Aspirate blood and debris from the area.

10. Maintain the operating field, adjust the light, and retract tissues as needed.

11. Exchange the straight elevator and extraction forceps.
    ❑ Observe the patient for signs of anxiety or syncope.

    Places extraction forceps beaks securely on the tooth with a firm grasp to remove the tooth (Figure 36-5).

    ❑ **Luxates the tooth; dislocates and removes the tooth from the alveolus for easy extraction.**

    ❑ **Subluxates, rotates, and lifts the tooth several times before the bone around the tooth is spread enough to remove the tooth from the alveolus for more difficult extraction.**

    ❑ **Repeats use of straight elevator as needed to further loosen the tooth.**

12. Hold gauze square in palm and receive extraction forceps in the palm with tooth being held in the beaks (Figure 36-6).
    ❑ Place gauze with tooth on the tray.
    ❑ Irrigate with saline solution in irrigating syringe as requested by surgeon.

    Examines tooth for fractured roots.

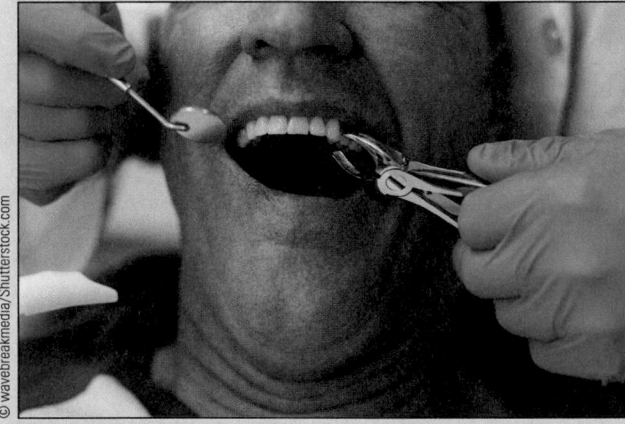

© wavebreakmedia/Shutterstock.com

FIGURE 36-5
Grasp tooth with beaks of the forceps.

13. Evacuate alveolus using surgical aspirator and pass surgical curette.

    Removes any bone chips, granulation tissue, and abscesses or cysts using surgical curette.

14. Hold gauze close to the patient's chin to remove debris from the curette.

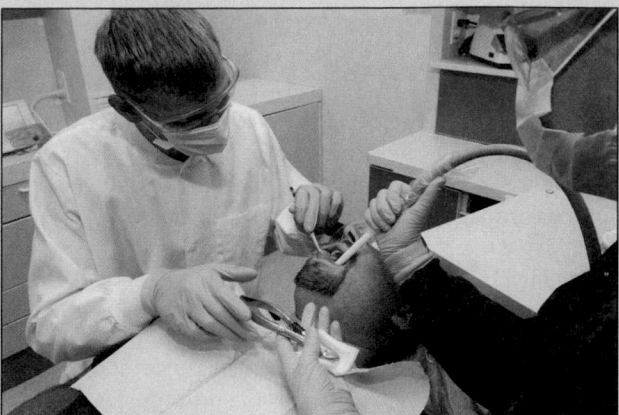

FIGURE 36-6
Dental assistant receiving extraction forceps with tooth in beaks.

15. Fold several pieces of gauze and moisten with saline solution.

16. Retrieve curette and pass folded gauze to surgeon.

    Places gauze on the top of the socket and instructs the patient to bite down firmly.

17. Return patient to upright position.
    ❑ Check and clean the patient's face.
    ❑ Allow a few minutes before giving oral postoperative instructions.
    ❑ Provide patient with written postoperative instructions and sterile gauze in container to change as needed.

18. Remove gauze after 5 minutes and check that bleeding has ceased.
    ❑ Change gauze and have patient bite on it for an additional 5 minutes if there is still bleeding.
    ❑ Have patient stay in recovery room as needed after being medicated.

19. Write up procedure in Services Rendered.

Date	Services Rendered
12/04/XX	Updated medical and dental history, no changes noted. BP = 120/80; T = 98.6F, P = 80, R = 18
	Placed 20% benzocaine gel to injection sites for 2 minutes. Administered 2 cartridges (3.6 ml) of 2% lidocaine with 1:100,000 epi to mandibular left. No reaction
#12	Ext
	POI provided oral and written postoperative instruction with patient and adult escort
	Assistant's initials

20. Dismiss and escort patient to reception area to meet person responsible for taking the patient home (refer to Procedure 18-5).

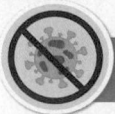

Infection Control

Extracted teeth are subject to the provisions of the OSHA Bloodborne Pathogens Standards. OSHA considers extracted teeth as OPIM, and they must be disposed of in medical waste containers labeled with the biohazard symbol. An extracted tooth containing amalgam cannot be incinerated or heat sterilized due to possible mercury vaporization and exposure. State and local regulations must be consulted regarding disposal of amalgam.

Extracted teeth can be returned to the patient upon request. They are not subject to provisions of the OSHA Bloodborne Pathogens Standards when returned to the patient.

postoperative instructions.) If the patient has undergone general anesthesia or conscious sedation for the procedure, they must recover before the instructions are given, and even then, the presence of an escorting adult or guardian is preferred.

Multiple Extractions

Multiple extractions are needed when the patient is going to have implants or a full or partial denture. When several teeth are going to be extracted, the patient may request general anesthesia. The surgical assistant prepares for intravenous sedation. The extraction process is similar for one tooth or for several teeth, but after several teeth have been removed, the bone and soft tissue must be contoured and smoothed. The alveolar ridge must be free of any sharp edges or points in order to achieve the most comfort and function for the patient. If both the maxillary and the mandibular teeth are to be extracted at one appointment, the maxillary teeth are extracted first. This prevents hemorrhage

and debris from contaminating the mandibular extraction site during surgery. Routinely, the dentist starts at the most posterior tooth and moves anteriorly.

When multiple extractions are performed significant changes occur to the patient's alveolar process. Even when extractions are routine ones, implant placement may require bone replacement (known as **grafting**). Preparation for denture insertion requires bone reshaping and recontouring known as **alveoplasty** or even alveolar bone reduction, known as **alveolectomy**. The surgeon makes an incision, and the soft tissue is retracted, exposing the underlying alveolar bone. With the use of rotary instruments and surgical handpiece as well as bone files and rongeurs, the oral surgeon shapes the alveolar ridge (Table 36-6). The soft tissue is contoured (**gingivoplasty**), and sutures are placed for faster and smoother healing. Ridge maintenance and smoothness are vital considerations for removable appliances.

The patient may choose the option of having an immediate denture placed after all the teeth in an arch are removed.

TABLE 36-6 Alveoloplasty and Gingivoplasty Instrumentation

Instrument	Function
scalpel blade	Precisely incise and excise soft tissue; disposable blades supplied in sterile package.
scalpel handle	Holds detachable scalpel blades; acts as a surgical knife.

Instrument	Function
single use scalpel handles and blades #11 #12 #10	Used once and disposed of in sharps container.
hemostat Courtesy of Integra LifeSciences Corporation [through Integra Miltex.] FULL SIZE 8-42 FULL SIZE 8-44	Retract tissue, remove small root tips, and clamp blood vessels. Multiple uses. Can be used to place scalpel blade into scalpel handle.
tissue retractors Courtesy of Integra LifeSciences Corporation [through Integra Miltex.] FULL SIZE 16-6 FULL SIZE 16-20 FULL SIZE 16-8 FULL SIZE 16-22	Holds tissue from the surgical site so operator view is unobstructed.
surgical handpiece	Used to trim alveolar and section teeth; tubing attached to saline water source; low and high speed available; rotary instruments generally have longer shanks to reach the surgical site.

(Continues)

TABLE 36-6 (*Continued*)

Instrument	Function
Rongeurs	Trim and shape alveolar bone after extractions; hinged forceps with springs in handle allow for tight grasp for ease in cutting.
surgical chisel and mallet	Surgical mallet used with chisel to gently tap the end of the chisel. Chisel used to remove and shape bone and split tooth into section.
Cryer's elevator	Loosen and remove tooth; pointed working end is placed between bifurcated roots; paired for right and left placement; bulbous handle allows for firm grip. Also referred to as flag elevators.
apical elevator	Loosen and remove retained roots; paired right and left placement.
T-bar elevator (Potts)	Loosen and remove tooth; paired for right and left placement.

Instrument	Function
root tip picks 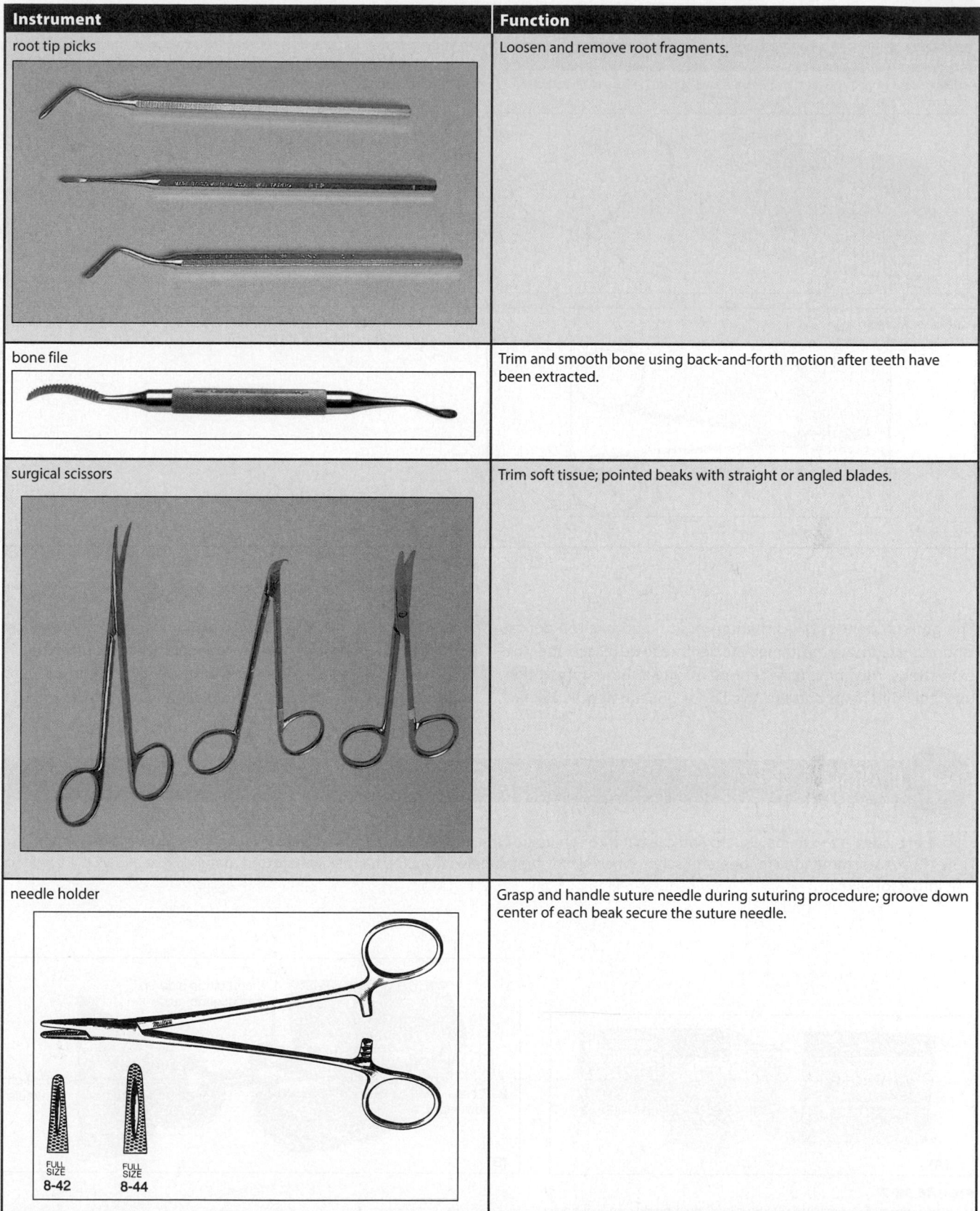	Loosen and remove root fragments.
bone file	Trim and smooth bone using back-and-forth motion after teeth have been extracted.
surgical scissors	Trim soft tissue; pointed beaks with straight or angled blades.
needle holder	Grasp and handle suture needle during suturing procedure; groove down center of each beak secure the suture needle.

(Continues)

TABLE 36-6 *(Continued)*

Instrument	Function
suture sterile package (suture needles and suture needle with attached suture thread) 	Closes up the surgical site. Available with reusable suture needles and single use suture needle with suture thread. Nonresorbable sutures made of silk, nylon, or polyester, and resorbable made of chromic gut, gut plain, and polyglycolic.
suture scissors	Allows for easy cutting of suture thread. C-shaped notch is slid under the suture and holds in place while cutting.

The general dentist takes the impression and has the dental laboratory fabricate the immediate denture to be placed after the extractions. The immediate denture is a great temporary option until the arch heals and the swelling is gone. It acts as a splint and allows the patient to have a functional mouth and walk out with teeth the same day as the extractions. The materials used in immediate dentures are the same as those used in conventional dentures. (Refer to Chapter 42 for details about dentures.)

Safety

Scalpel blades are extremely sharp and can cut through tissue with minimal pressure. Blade removal devices (Figures 36-7A and 36-7B) are recommended for operator safety when removing the blade from the handle. The slotted metal device allows the blade to fit into it for safety.

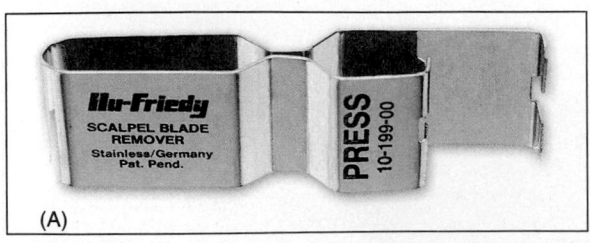
(A)

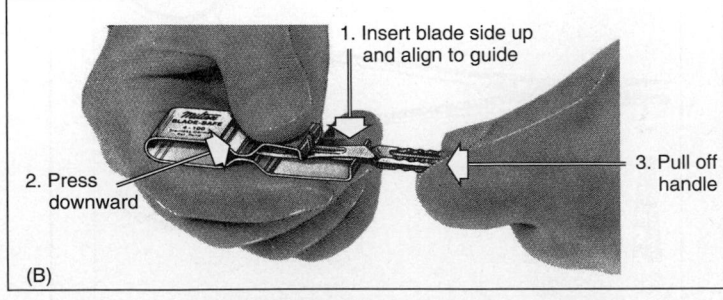
(B)

FIGURE 36-7
(A) Blade removal device and (B) Steps in using a blade removal device.

When a blade removal device is not available, a hemostat or Howe plier can be used to insert and remove the blade from the handle (Figures 36-7C through 36-7H).

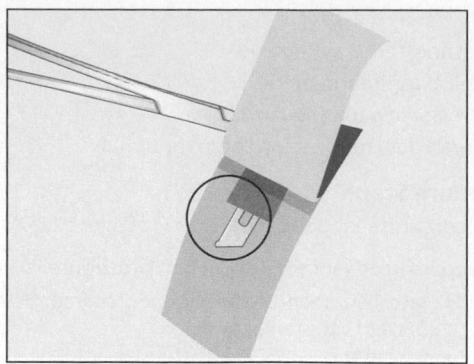

FIGURE 36-7C
Hold the blade within the packet with hemostat and open the packet to expose the slot of the scalpel blade.

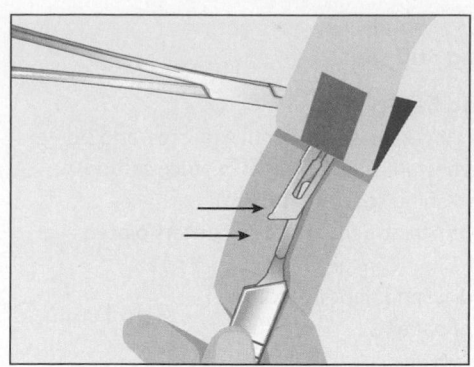

FIGURE 36-7D
Hold the scalpel handle with the diagonal of the blade and handle parallel.

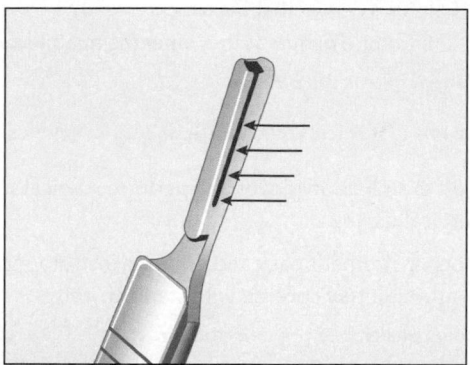

FIGURE 36-7E
Place the blade into the groove around the top of the scalpel.

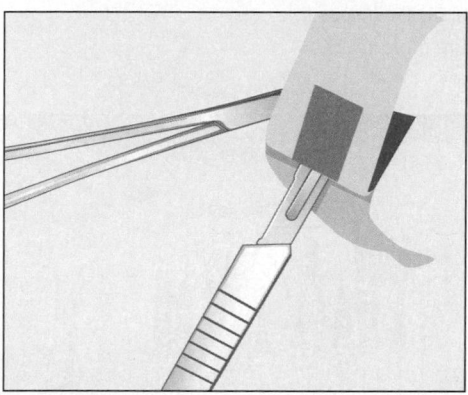

FIGURE 36-7F
Slide the blade into place.

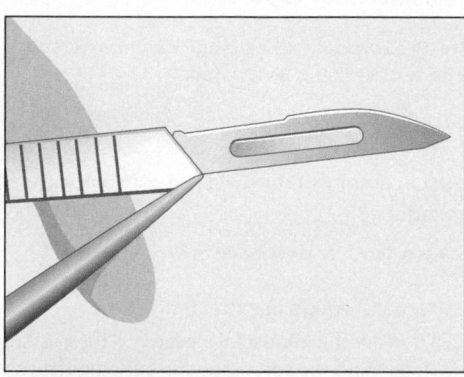

FIGURE 36-7G
To remove the blade, hold blade with the hemostat just above the diagonal of the blade.

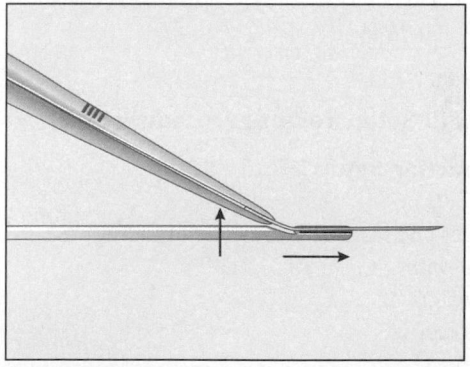

FIGURE 36-7H
Lift up on the blade while moving the blade from the notch of the handle.

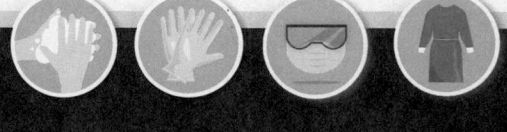

Procedure 36-2
Assisting with Multiple Extractions

The surgical dental assistant prepares the operating room and tray setup following strict aseptic steps. They must be prepared and thinking ahead to anticipate the surgeon's needs while assisting the oral surgeon throughout the multiple extraction procedure. The surgical assistant transfers instruments, retracts tissue, rinses and evacuates the surgical area, and maintains a sterile field at all times.

(Continues)

Equipment and Supplies

Patient Seating Setup
- PPE: surgical gloves, mask, protective glasses, and sterile isolation gown (sterile cap optional in office setting)
- Sterile handwashing soap and brush
- Sanitized dental treatment area and barriers placed over equipment
- Patient's medical and dental records
- Preparation of patient
  - ❏ full length drape
  - ❏ sterile towel
  - ❏ sterile cap
  - ❏ patient protective glasses
  - ❏ mouth rinse in disposable cup
- Blood pressure equipment

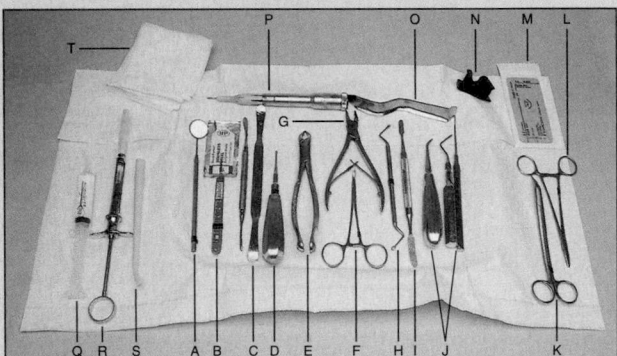

FIGURE 36-8
Multiple extraction tray setup.

Local Anesthetic Setup (refer to Procedure 23-2)

Multiple Extraction Setup (Figure 36-8)
- mouth mirror (A)
- scalpel handle and scalpel blade in sterile package (B)
- periosteal elevators (C)
- straight elevators (D)
- extraction forceps (E)
- hemostat (F)
- Rongeurs (G)
- surgical curette (H)
- bone file (I)
- Cryer elevator, apical elevator, and root tip pick (J)
- surgical scissors (K)
- needle holder (L)
- sterile package of suture needle and suture thread (M)
- bite block (N)
- Minnesota cheek and tongue retractor (O)
- surgical handpiece and surgery rotary instruments (P)
- Leur Lock irrigating syringe with sterile saline solution (Q)

- local anesthetic syringe (R)
- surgical aspirating tip (S)
- 4 × 4 sterile gauze squares (T)
- pain/anxiety medication setup (optional)

Procedure Steps

1. Escort and seat patient (refer to Procedure 18-4).

2. Prepare in advance for extraction procedure.
   - ❏ Place instrument sterile pack on sterile surgical tray covered with sterile towel.
   - ❏ Open patient's chart in dental software.
   - ❏ Navigate to the dental charting screen.
   - ❏ Open patient's latest radiographic history on the computer monitor, or place on view box.
   - ❏ Inform dentist that the patient is ready.
   - ❏ Introduce dentist as they enter the treatment area.

   Dentist greets the patient.

   Performs surgical scrub and dons surgical gloves.

3. Doff examination gloves and perform surgical scrub; don surgical gloves.

4. Open instrument pack and organize instruments on instrument tray covered with sterile towel.

   Takes position at the dental chair.
   - ❏ **Signals for the procedure to begin (refer to Procedure 20-1).**

5. Pass mouth mirror.

   Examines the site of extraction.

   Anesthetist or anesthesiologist administers IV sedation or general anesthesia as needed.

   Administers local anesthetic.

6. Assist in administration of local anesthetic (refer to Procedure 23-2).

   Extracts teeth as described in Procedure 36-1.

7. Assist oral surgeon in extracting teeth.
   - ❏ Transfer the periosteal elevator to the oral surgeon for loosening the soft tissue surrounding the tooth.
   - ❏ Transfer the straight elevator for loosening the tooth within its socket, aspirating blood and debris from the area.
   - ❏ Once the tooth is loosened transfer the forceps for the extraction of the tooth.
   - ❏ Transfer the surgical curette for debridement of the socket while aspirating following the extraction.
   - ❏ Repeat steps above as many times as teeth to be extracted.
   - ❏ Aspirate blood and debris from the area as needed.
   - ❏ Maintain the operating field, adjust the light, and retract tissues as needed.

❏ Hold gauze close to the patient's chin to remove debris from the curette.

Removes any root tips or debris after the teeth have been extracted.

8. Transfer surgeon's preference of apical elevators and root tip picks.
   ❏ Have sterile gauze to remove debris from surgical instruments.

Begins alveoplasty procedure (Figure 36-9).

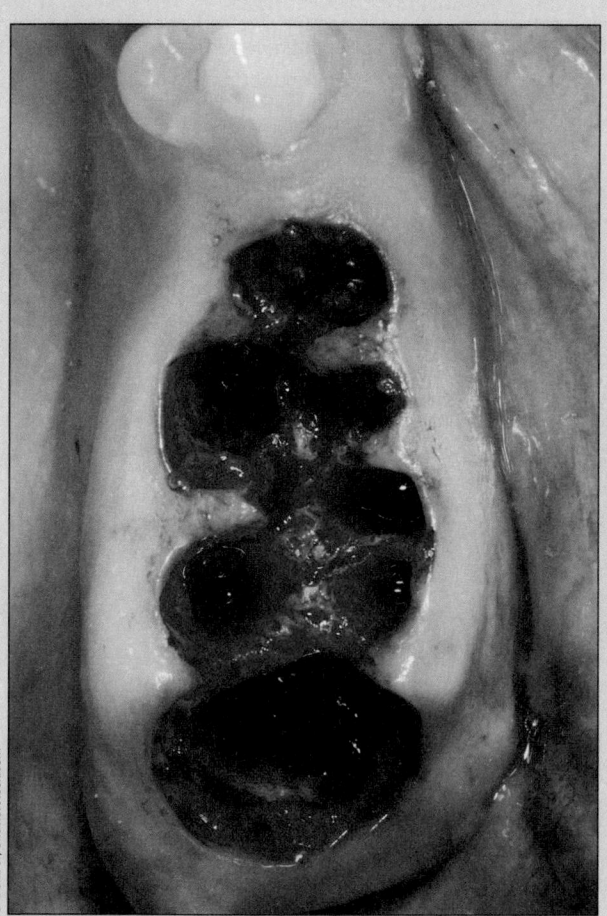

FIGURE 36-9
Surgical site after teeth were extracted, exposing uneven remaining bone structure needing alveoplasty.

9. Transfer scalpel blade to the surgeon for opening a flap and exposing the alveolar process.

Makes an incision of the buccal and lingual surface to remove interdental papillae and to expose crest of the alveolar bone.

10. Exchange scalpel and periosteal elevator.
    ❏ Rinse area with saline solution using irrigating syringe when requested.

❏ Evacuate area as necessary.

Reflects soft tissue for clear vision.

11. Exchange periosteal elevator and tissue retractor.

Retracts the flap of tissue to maintain vision; may ask the assistant to hold the retractor.

Begins initial trimming and recontouring of the alveolar bone.

12. Transfer surgeon's preference of Rongeurs and/or surgical burs.
    ❏ Keep instruments free of debris.
    ❏ Intermittently use the HVE and the irrigation syringe with sterile saline solution to maintain the operating field.

Completes final contouring and smoothing of the alveolar bone.

13. Transfer bone file.
    ❏ Rinse area with sterile saline solution.

Repositions buccal and lingual flaps and sutures in place.

14. Clasp suture needle at upper third with needle holder.
    ❏ Pass suture needle and thread in needle holder.
    ❏ Assist in holding the tissue as the surgeon places the sutures (Figure 36-10).
    ❏ Retrieve needle holder and pass suture scissors.

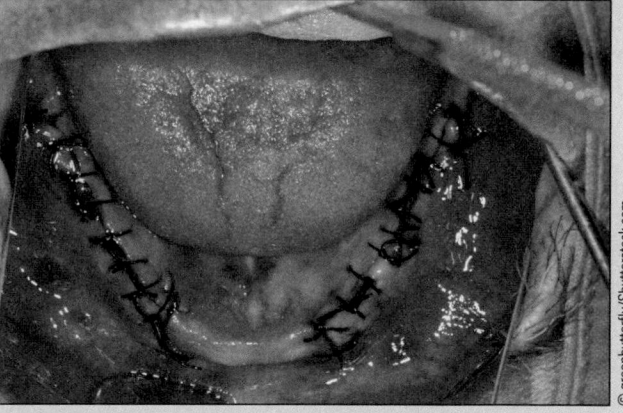

FIGURE 36-10
All mandibular teeth have been removed with sutures in place.

15. Fold several pieces of gauze moistened with saline solution and pass to surgeon.

Places gauze on the top of the surgical site and instructs the patient to bite down firmly.

16. Return patient to upright position.
    ❏ Check and clean the patient's face.
    ❏ Allow a few minutes to recover before giving oral postoperative instructions to patient and adult escort.

❏ Provide patient with written postoperative instructions and sterile gauze in container to change as needed.

17. Remove gauze after 5 minutes and check that bleeding has ceased.

❏ Change gauze and have patient bite on it for an additional 5 minutes if there is still bleeding.

❏ Have patient stay in recovery room as needed after being medicated.

18. Write up procedure in Services Rendered.

Date	Services Rendered
02/25/XX	Updated medical and dental history, no changes noted. BP = 120/80; T = 98.6F, P = 80, R = 18
	Anesthetist administered Midazolam IV sedation Placed 20% benzocaine gel to injection sites for 2 minutes. Administered 2 cartridges (3.6 ml) of 2% lidocaine with 1:100,000 epi to mandibular left. No reaction
#17–#32	Ext, alveoplasty with 10 absorbable sutures
	POI provided oral and written postoperative instruction with patient and adult escort
	RTC: Suture removal and check in 1 week Assistant's initials

19. Dismiss and escort patient to reception area person responsible for taking the patient home (refer to Procedure 18-5).

Extraction of Impacted Teeth

Extracting impacted teeth is one of the most common procedures the oral surgeon performs, especially third molar extractions. Third molars usually erupt between the late teens and early twenties. In some cases, the patient's jaw does not grow long enough to allow the third molars to erupt, or these teeth do not erupt because of blockage by other teeth. These molars then stay trapped within the jaw. Teeth may be impacted horizontally in a mesial or distal direction or vertically crowding against an erupted tooth (Figure 36-11). Many problems can arise when the impacted tooth is not extracted, such as pain, inflammation, infection, cyst development, destruction of neighboring teeth, destruction of the bone, or movement of the permanent teeth out of proper alignment.

Many factors determine the difficulty of the impacted tooth extraction, including the depth, position, or angulation of the tooth in the bone. If the third molars are partially erupted through the bone and into the soft tissues, this is called a soft tissue impaction. A hard tissue impaction occurs if the teeth are impacted in bone and not through the gingival tissues. When the tooth is impacted in the bone, dental handpieces and surgical burs are required to gain access. Additional surgical instruments

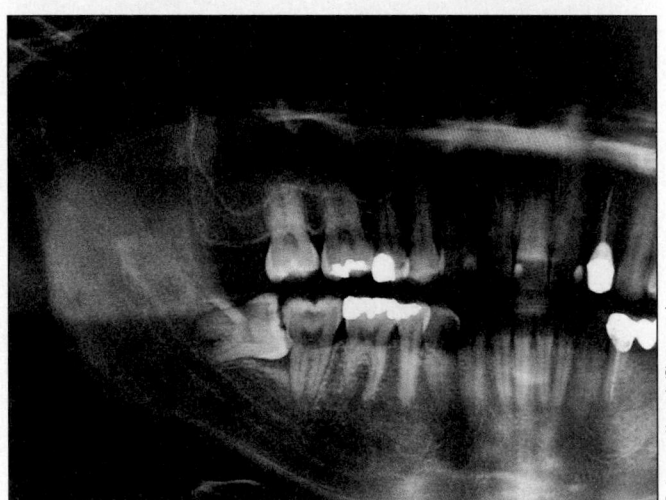

© Jatuporn Kuptasin/Shutterstock.com

FIGURE 36-11
Maxillary third molar has been extracted, and mandibular third is horizontally impacted.

are used to facilitate the removal of the tooth from the bone, such as various elevators (Procedure 36-3). Often, all impacted third molars are removed at one appointment.

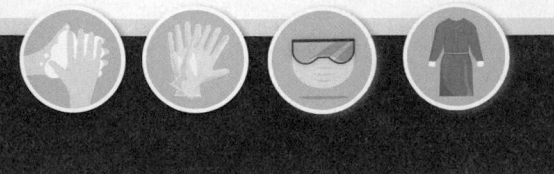

Procedure 36-3
Assisting with Extraction of Impacted Tooth

The surgical dental assistant prepares the operating room and tray setup following strict aseptic steps. They must be prepared and thinking ahead to anticipate the surgeon's needs while assisting the oral surgeon throughout the multiple extraction procedure. The surgical assistant transfers instruments, retracts tissue, rinses and evacuates the surgical area, and maintains a sterile field at all times.

Equipment and Supplies

Patient Seating Setup

- PPE: surgical gloves, mask, protective glasses, and sterile isolation gown (sterile cap optional in office setting)
- Sterile handwashing soap and brush
- Sanitized dental treatment area and barriers placed over equipment

- Patient's medical and dental records
- Preparation of patient
  - ❏ full length drape
  - ❏ sterile towel
  - ❏ sterile cap
  - ❏ patient protective glasses
  - ❏ mouth rinse in disposable cup
- Blood pressure equipment

Local Anesthetic Setup (refer to Procedure 23-2)

Extraction of Impacted Teeth Setup

Procedure Steps

1. Escort and seat patient (refer to Procedure 18-4).

2. Prepare in advance for extraction procedure.
   - ❏ Place instrument sterile pack on sterile surgical tray covered with sterile towel.
   - ❏ Open patient's chart in dental software.
   - ❏ Navigate to the dental charting screen.
   - ❏ Open patient's latest radiographic history on the computer monitor, or place on view box.
   - ❏ Inform dentist that the patient is ready.
   - ❏ Introduce dentist as they enter the treatment area.

   Dentist greets the patient.

   Performs surgical scrub and dons surgical gloves.

3. Doff examination gloves and perform surgical scrub; don surgical gloves.

4. Open instrument pack and organize instruments on instrument tray covered with sterile towel.

   Takes position at the dental chair.
   - ❏ **Signals for the procedure to begin (refer to Procedure 20-1).**

5. Pass mouth mirror.

   Examines the site of extraction.

   Anesthetist or anesthesiologist administers IV sedation or general anesthesia as needed.

   Administers local anesthetic.

6. Assist in administration of local anesthetic (refer to Procedure 23-2).

7. Pass scalpel handle with loaded scalpel blade.

   Makes incision along the ridge distal to the second molar (Figure 36-12A).

   Makes flap incision as needed for vision.

8. Maintain operating field with surgical aspirating tip.

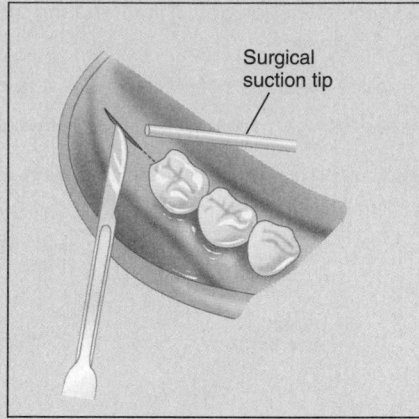

FIGURE 36-12A
Flap incision.

9. Retrieve scalpel handle and pass periosteal elevator.

   Retracts the tissue from the alveolar bone (Figure 36-12B).

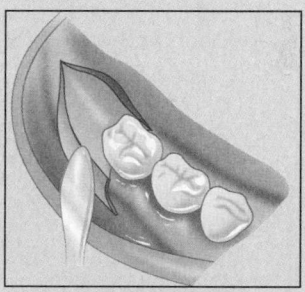

FIGURE 36-12B
Periosteal elevator used to retract tissue.

10. Evacuate and retract tissue.

11. Retrieve periosteal elevator and pass surgeon's preference of surgical bur and handpiece or chisel and mallet.

   Removes the bone over the tooth (Figure 36-12C).

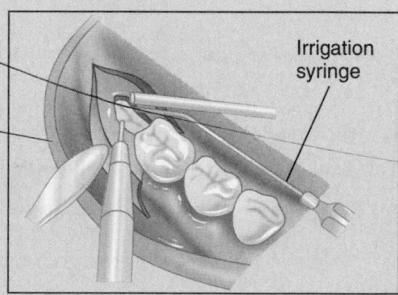

FIGURE 36-12C
Surgical bur used to to remove overlying bone.

(Continues)

12. Irrigate sterile saline solution using irrigating syringe and evacuate as needed.

13. Pass surgeon's preference of elevator and/or forceps.

Luxates and lifts tooth from socket (Figure 36-12D).

Sections tooth using burs or chisels if entire tooth cannot be removed with forceps.

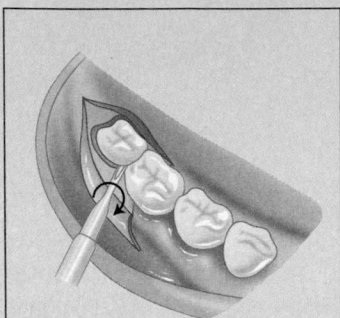

FIGURE 36-12D
Elevator used to luxate tooth.

14. Pass handpiece and burs or chisels as needed.

15. Maintain clear area with aspirating tip.

16. Transfer surgeon new gauze as needed to control bleeding and maintain clear area.

Places extracted tooth or tooth sections on a gauze square and examines that the entire tooth has been removed.

17. Pass surgical curette.

Removes the follicle (sac of thickened membrane) and debrides the tooth socket.

18. Exchange curette and surgeon's preference of Rongeurs, bone files, or burs.
   ❏ Transfers these various instruments and removes debris from working ends with gauze squares.

Contours the bone margins.

19. Irrigate with sterile saline water and evacuate area thoroughly.

Replaces the tissue flap to its normal position over the wound.

20. Clasp suture needle at upper third with needle holder.
   ❏ Pass suture needle and suture thread with needle holder.

Sutures the tissue over the wound (Figure 36-12E).

21. Retract cheek and tongue as needed to provide better access for suturing.

22. Retrieve needle holder and pass suture scissors.

23. Retrieve suture scissors and pass folded gauze moistened in saline solution.

Places gauze when suturing is completed (Figure 36-12F).

24. Return patient to upright position.

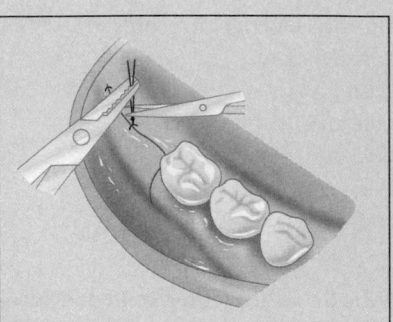

FIGURE 36-12E
Close wound with sutures.

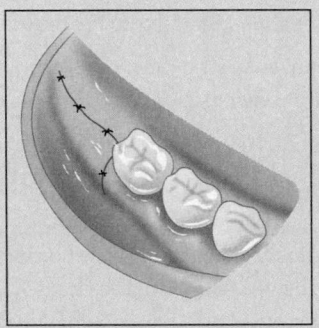

FIGURE 36-12F
Suturing completed.

   ❏ Check and clean the patient's face.
   ❏ Place ice pack on patient cheek.
   ❏ Allow a few minutes to recover before giving oral postoperative instructions to patient and adult escort.
   ❏ Provide patient with written postoperative instructions and sterile gauze in container to change as needed.

25. Remove gauze after 5 minutes and check that bleeding has ceased.
   ❏ Change gauze and have patient bite on it for an additional 5 minutes if there is still bleeding.
   ❏ Send ice pack with patient.
   ❏ Have patient stay in recovery room as needed after being medicated.

26. Write up procedure in Services Rendered.

Date	Services Rendered
07/21/XX	Updated medical and dental history, no changes noted. BP = 120/80; T = 98.6F, P = 80, R = 18
	Anesthetist administered Midazolam IV sedation Placed 20% benzocaine gel to injection sites for 2 minutes. Administered 2 cartridges (3.6 ml) of 2% lidocaine with 1:100,000 epi to mandibular left. No reaction
#32	Ext, placed 3 black silk sutures
	POI provided oral and written postoperative instruction with patient and adult escort; provided patient with prescription for pain medication
	RTC: 5–7 days for suture removal and check Assistant's initials

27. Dismiss and escort patient to reception area to meet person responsible for taking the patient home (refer to Procedure 18-5).

Biopsy

Oral cancer is one of the most aggressive types of cancer in humans, and early detection is vital in improving the prognosis and the outcome. As part of the oral examination process, general dentists perform intraoral and extraoral cancer screenings. After the oral inspection (performed with a white light and palpation) is completed, the dental professional can use other screening techniques to inspect for disease including precancerous and cancerous areas. One system uses a blue-spectrum light that causes the healthy soft tissue of the mouth and diseased or traumatized tissue fluoresce differently. Another system uses a prerinse solution and a light stick that exposes lesions as distinctly white.

If suspicious lesions are noticed, the dentist may perform a biopsy or refer the patient to an oral surgeon to perform a biopsy. There are three types of tissue biopsies depending on the method used to remove the sample. Incisional biopsy removes a portion of the questionable tissue along with a portion of normal surrounding tissue; excisional biopsy removes the entire lesion along with a sample of normal tissue, and exfoliative biopsy removes a cell layer of the lesion via surface scraping. The tissue is placed in a collection vial and sent along with the biopsy data sheet containing necessary information such as a description that includes color, shape, size, consistency, and location of the lesion. The specimen and description is sent to an oral pathologist for diagnosis.

Cleft Lip and Palate Surgery

During prenatal development, occasionally tissues of the palate or lip do not join properly. As a result, a cleft lip or cleft palate can occur. With a cleft lip there is physical separation of the upper lip on one side (unilateral) or both sides (bilateral) of the philtrum (Figure 36-13). In many cases, the separation can extend to the nose and involve the bones of the maxilla. A cleft palate is a nonjoining of the right and left sides of the palatal shelves of the maxilla and can involve the hard and/or the soft palate. There is an opening between the mouth and the nose.

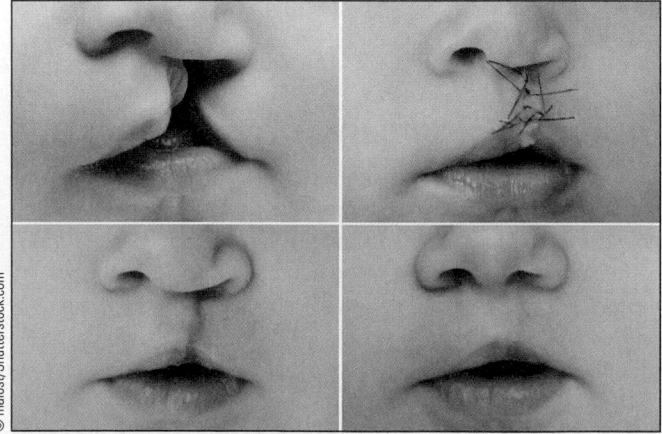

FIGURE 36-13
Images showing before and after photos of unilateral cleft lip treated by a cleft palate team.

When a child is born with a cleft lip or palate, the family is referred immediately to a cleft palate team for advice and treatment. The cleft palate team includes specialists such as the oral and maxillofacial surgeon, cosmetic surgeon, speech pathologist, and possibly occupational or physical therapists who work together to provide care for the child. With the advanced technologies now available, prenatal diagnosis of clefts is sometimes possible. This allows for the family to meet with the cleft palate team and plan for optimal care before the child is born. If these malformations are not corrected, speech problems as well as eating difficulties may occur in these patients. Occupational therapists meet with the parents and teach them how to use cleft palate nursers, which are specially designed nipples to be used with the bottle that covers the palate and prevents formula from exiting the nose. Cleft lip repairs are generally performed between 3 and 6 months old. When a baby is 10–12 months old, the cleft palate is repaired with surgery called palatoplasty. The surgeon closes the opening between the nose and mouth to create a palate that works well for speech and prevents food and liquid from leaking out of the nose.

Temporomandibular Joint Disorder

When the structures of the temporomandibular joint (TMJ) do not work together correctly, temporomandibular disorder (TMD) may be the cause. Signs include limited mandibular movement when opening the mouth (trismus) and popping and clicking when opening and closing. Patient symptoms include discomfort and difficulty in chewing, speaking, and swallowing; **tinnitus** and pain around the ear; and tenderness of masticatory muscles along with headaches and neck aches.

The general dentist treatment involves several phases of noninvasive procedures including application of ice and heat to TMJ area, relaxation techniques for the jaw, medications (pain reliever, muscle relaxant, antibiotics, anti-inflammatory agents, and anti-anxiety medications), physical therapy, occlusal splints, and orthodontic appliances. If the patient is unresponsive to treatment options, surgery may be advised. The surgeon may perform **arthroscopy** that involves inserting a tiny instrument through a small incision to remove adhesions and place anti-inflammatory agents. The irrigation of the joint, known as **arthrocentesis**, may be used to treat TMD. The surgeon injects the joint with local anesthesia and fluid to flush out inflamed fluids around the joint. Steroids may also be injected to combat inflammation. **Arthroplasty** surgery is completed to relieve pain and restore range of motion by realigning or restructuring the joint. If a joint is badly damaged and cannot be repaired, it may need to be removed and replaced. This is done only after other treatment options have been done and failed, or if this is the only course of treatment. The patient may need a partial or total joint replacement. These surgeries have become more common, and the prosthetic TMJ joints have improved.

Orofacial Trauma Patients

The oral maxillofacial surgeon is called on for the treatment of orofacial trauma patients. The surgeon sees the patient in the

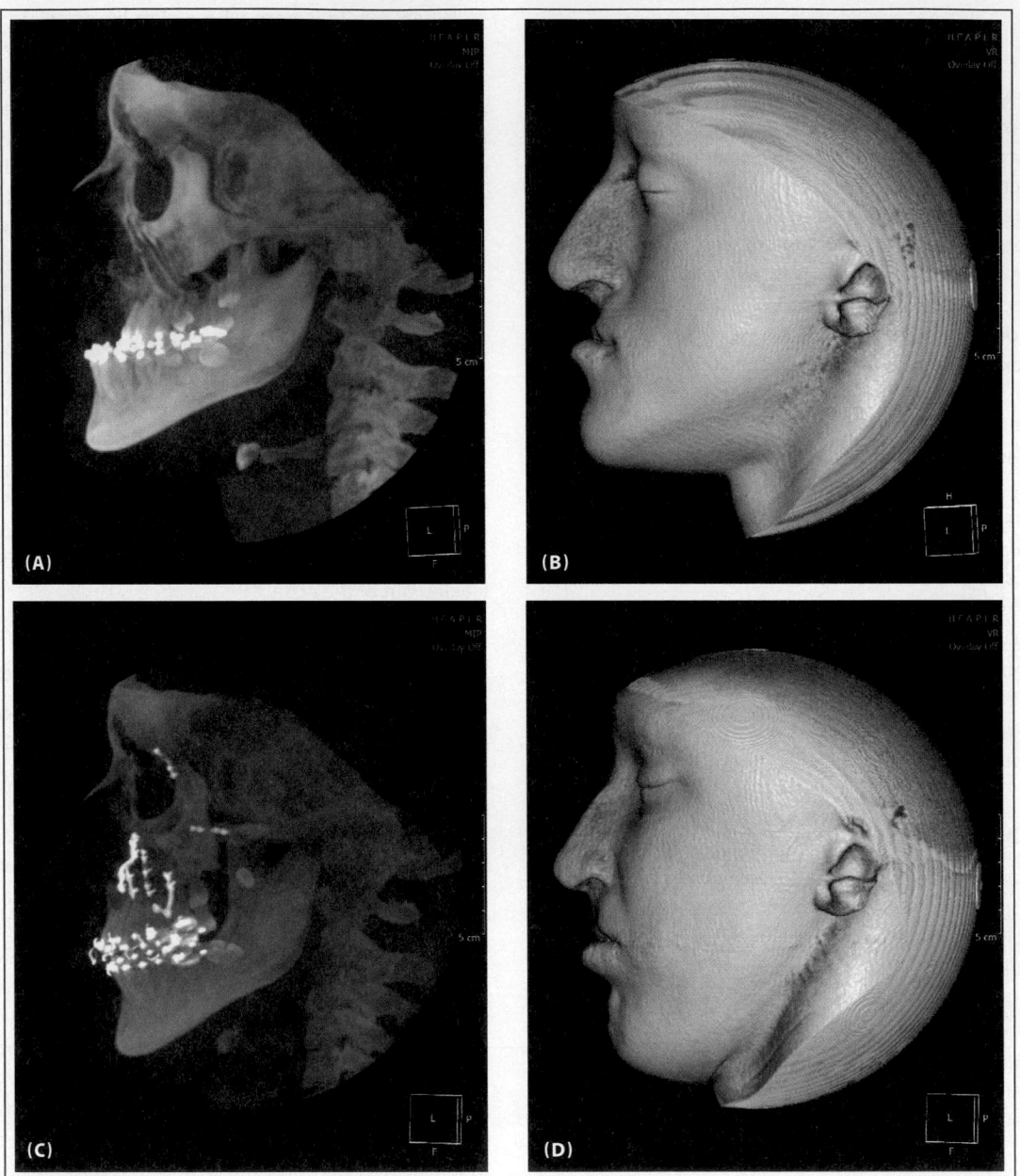

FIGURE 36-14
(A and B) Patient with collapsed maxilla and Class III due to trauma. (C and D) Repair of collapsed maxilla.

hospital to begin treatment. At first the primary role of the sur-geon is to manage any orofacial hemorrhaging and pain, and to prevent infection. With some patients treatment is given and they are sent home; however, patients with major trauma are admitted to the hospital and prepared for surgery. Diagnosis is facilitated and enhanced with advances in three-dimensional cone beam and CAD/CAM technologies. With this technology, the skull can be rotated and aligned to see the minutest details of the patient's anatomical structure. This allows surgical guides to be fabricated or robot-produced arch wires to be placed. See Figure 36-14 for examples of before and after photographs, x-rays, and skeletal views of a patient with a collapsed maxilla and a Class III due to trauma.

Orthognathic Surgery

Orthognathic surgery involves corrective surgical procedures on the maxilla, mandible, and chin to improve form and function. It improves how the teeth fit together and corrects facial proportions. Orthog-nathic surgery may be a part of the treatment plan when the patient has jaw problems that cannot be resolved with orthodontics alone.

Postoperative Procedures

A week after the surgery, the sutures are removed and the surgi-cal site is examined. The dental assistant should be aware of the possible complications that can arise after surgical procedures. Some of the most common include alveolitis and paresthesia.

Suture Removal

After oral surgery procedures and depending on the healing time required, absorbable or nonabsorbable sutures are used. For instances when nonabsorbable sutures are used, the patient is required to return to the office for suture removal. In some states, dental assistants are qualified to remove sutures.

During the suture removal appointment, the dental assistant first gently cleans and rinses the area to remove food debris and dried blood. The oral surgeon's input is then requested to determine if the tissue has healed and the sutures are ready to be removed. If so, the assistant should consult the dental chart as to the location and number of sutures that were placed. The assistant then uses sterile cotton pliers or hemostats to pull one side of the tail of the suture gently to elevate the knot (Procedure 36-4). A portion of the suture that was beneath the gingiva is now visible and should be cut with the sterile suture scissors close to but not through the knot. Using the cotton pliers, the knot portion is held and can now be pulled to remove the suture from the tissue. (This avoids pulling the knot through the tissues.) After the sutures are removed, the area is evaluated and irrigated. The patient is then instructed to rinse and can be dismissed. Suture removal is a relatively painless process and rarely requires local anesthesia.

Procedure 36-4
Assisting with Suture Removal

The surgical dental assistant prepares the operating room and tray setup following strict aseptic steps and transfer instruments while the operator removes the sutures. This procedure can be legally performed by a trained dental assistant in some states.

Steps written in **blue** font are performed by the operator (dentist, hygienist, or qualified dental assistant), and the chairside assistant's steps are written in black.

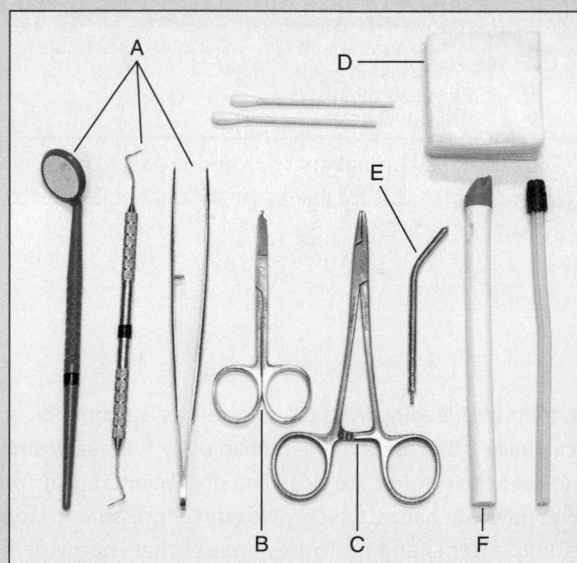

FIGURE 36-15
Suture removal tray setup.

Equipment and Supplies

Patient Seating Setup
- PPE: examination gloves, mask, protective glasses, and protective clothing
- Sterile handwashing soap and brush
- Sanitized dental treatment area and barriers placed over equipment
- Patient's medical and dental records
- Preparation of patient
  - ❏ Patient napkin and napkin clip
  - ❏ Patient protective glasses
  - ❏ Mouth rinse in disposable cup
- Blood pressure equipment

Suture Removal Setup (Figure 36-15)
- basic setup: mouth mirror, explorer, cotton pliers (A)
- suture scissors (B)
- hemostat (C)
- sterile gauze squares and cotton tip applicator (D)
- air/water syringe tips (E)
- HVE tip and/or saliva ejector (F)
- antiseptic solution (not shown)

Procedure Steps
1. Escort and seat patient (refer to Procedure 18-4).
2. Gently rinse area to remove food debris and dried blood.
   - ❏ Swab the site to remove any debris.

   Dentist greets the patient.

(Continues)

Takes position at the dental chair.
- ❑ Signals for the procedure to begin (refer to Procedure 20-1).

3. Pass mouth mirror.

Examines the site of extraction to determine if tissue has healed and is ready to remove sutures.

4. Pass hemostat.

Operator gently lifts the suture away from the tissue (Figure 36-16).

5. Exchange hemostat and suture scissors.

Cuts the suture thread below the knot, close to the tissue.
- ❑ Cuts each suture and removes individually for continuous simple sutures.
- ❑ Begins with one end and then proceeds with each suture stitch.

6. Exchange suture scissor and hemostat.

Secures the knot with hemostat and gently pulls, lifting the suture out of the tissue.

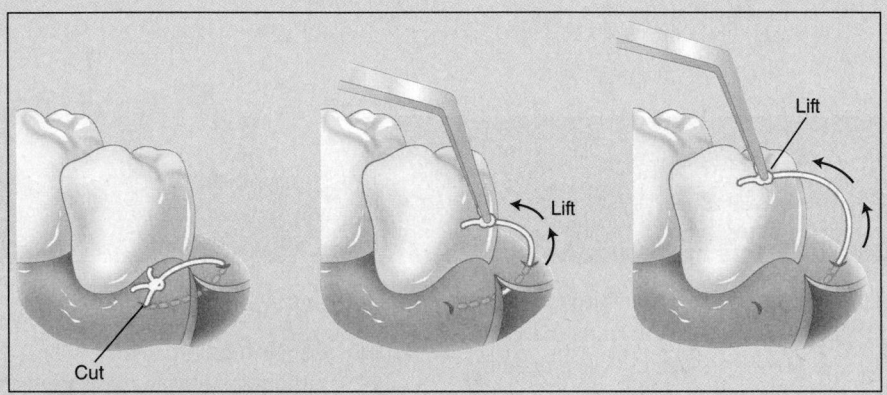

FIGURE 36-16
Removal of simple sutures.

7. Hold gauze square near the patient's chin.

Places the suture on the gauze square.

8. Irrigate surgical site with antiseptic solution if bleeding occurs.
- ❑ Instruct patient to bite on folded gauze squares to stop bleeding.

9. Count the number of sutures on the gauze square and compare to number noted on the patient's surgery service rendered.

10. Write up procedure in Services Rendered.

Date	Services Rendered
09/24/XX	Post-op appt: suture removal of 3 black silk suture Healing within normal limits No complications Assistant's initials

11. Dismiss and escort patient to reception area to meet person responsible for taking the patient home (refer to Procedure 18-5).

Postoperative Complications

After a surgical procedure, some patients do not heal as expected and experience complications. The most common postoperative complications are continued pain, swelling, bleeding, or reactions to medications. To manage pain, the oral surgeon will prescribe pain medication that is strong enough to mask the pain expected during the normal healing process. If the patient is not comfortable after taking the medication or has an unexpected reaction, they should notify the office at once.

Postoperative swelling is managed by the application of cold icepacks as directed. If the swelling does not decrease within 48 hours or if the swollen area becomes hot, hard, and painful to touch, the patient should notify the office at once.

Continued bleeding from the surgical site is a common occurrence. Unlike other areas of the human body, it is nearly impossible to keep the surgical site clean and dry. Patients are instructed to bite down on gauze, which yields direct pressure to stop the bleeding. After changing to fresh gauze that is provided, the patient should notice less and less bleeding until it stops. It has been shown that biting on a tea bag can be effective in reducing bleeding due to the tannins in the tea. It is important the patient contact the office if the bleeding has not stopped within 48 hours after the procedure.

Many of these complications are easily understood by the patient. Unique to oral surgery, however, is the complication named **alveolitis**, commonly known as "dry socket."

Alveolitis After any type of surgical procedure, the possibility for postoperative complications exists. While only 2% to 5% of people who have a tooth extracted will experience alveolitis, this is a painful complication. After an extraction, an empty socket is left in the bone. During normal healing, blood forms a clot in the socket and protects the bone and the nerves underneath. If for some reason the blood clot becomes dislodged, food debris and fluids occupy the socket, causing irritation and potential infection of the bone accompanied by severe pain. The mandibular third molars are the most frequent sites for dry socket.

The surgical dental assistant should be aware that individuals who smoke, have had excessive trauma during surgery, surgical extraction of wisdom teeth, are taking birth control pills, or have a history of previous dry sockets are more prone to this condition.

A dry socket usually becomes evident three to five days after an extraction. If a patient calls the office complaining of continued pain that radiates to the ear, increases rather than decreases over time, and is accompanied by a bad taste or odor, chances are they are experiencing a dry socket. Treatment of dry socket includes the administration of local anesthetic to the area by the oral surgeon, who then cleans the socket of any debris and examines the area for infection. The extraction site is then packed with a medicated dressing, which may need to be replaced every day for five to seven days. Some oral surgeons use a dry socket paste that dissolves in the socket over several days. Additional pain medication and antibiotics are usually prescribed as well. The pain will begin to subside after the first treatment. Treatments may have to be repeated for a few days until the patient is completely comfortable.

Procedure 36-5
Assisting with Treatment of Alveolitis

The surgical dental assistant prepares the operating room and tray setup following strict aseptic steps and transfers instruments while the surgeon treats alveolitis. Some states allow trained and qualified dental assistants to place post extraction dressings.

Steps written in **blue** font are performed by the dentist, and the surgical assistant's steps are written in black.

Equipment and Supplies

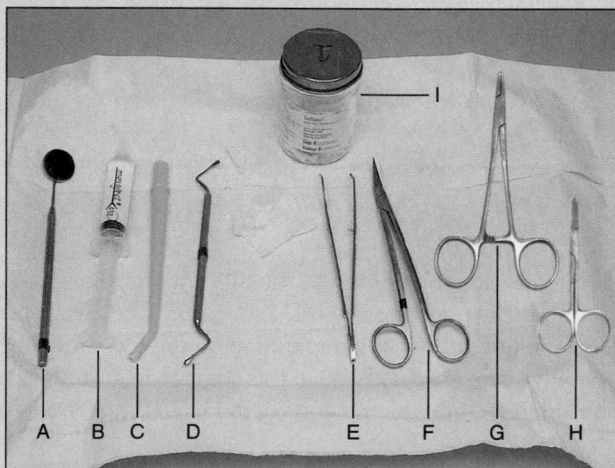

FIGURE 36-17
Trays setup for alveolitis treatment.

Patient Seating Setup
- PPE: examination gloves, mask, protective glasses, and protective clothing
- Sterile handwashing soap and brush
- Sanitized dental treatment area and barriers placed over equipment
- Patient's medical and dental records
- Preparation of patient
  - ❏ Patient napkin and napkin clip
  - ❏ Patient protective glasses
  - ❏ Mouth rinse in disposable cup

Local Anesthetic Setup (refer to Procedure 23-2)

Alveolitis Treatment Setup (Figure 36-17)
- mouth mirror (A)
- irrigating syringe and warm sterile saline solution (B)
- surgical aspirating tip (C)
- surgical curette (D)
- cotton pliers (E)
- surgical scissors (F)
- hemostat (G)
- suture scissors (H)
- iodoform sponge material (I)

Procedure Steps

1. Escort and seat patient (refer to Procedure 18-4).

   Dentist greets the patient.

   Takes position at the dental chair.

(Continues)

❑ Signals for the procedure to begin (refer to Procedure 20-1).

2. Pass mouth mirror.

Examines the site.

3. Pass irrigating syringe and warm sterile saline solution.

Irrigates the surgical site.

4. Evacuate as surgeon irrigates the surgical site.

Surgeon administers local anesthetic.

5. Assist in administration of local anesthetic (refer to Procedure 23-2).

Removes sutures.

6. Pass hemostat and suture scissors as needed.

7. Pass surgical curette.

Surgeon may gently curettage the area inside the socket to stimulate the formation of a new blood clot.

8. Pass irrigating syringe and warm sterile saline solution.

Irrigates the surgical site.

9. Evacuate while surgeon irrigates the surgical site.

10. Exchange irrigating solution for medicated dressing (iodoform sponge or iodoform gauze) held with cotton pliers (Figure 36-18).

Packs the socket with medicated dressing.

Prescribes medication for pain control.

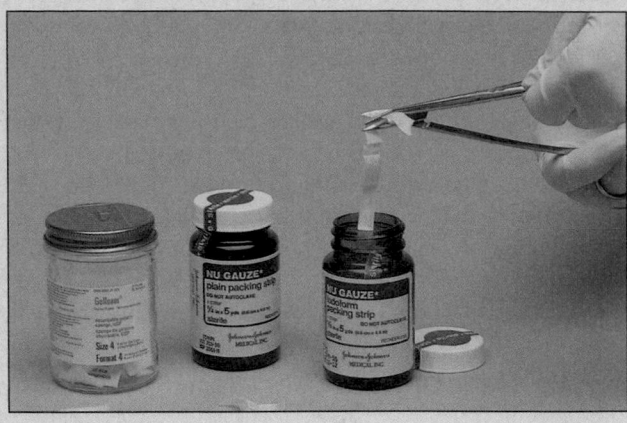

FIGURE 36-18
Examples of iodoform gauze and sponge packaging materials. The assistant is preparing to pass the gauze packing.

11. Write up procedure in Services Rendered.

Date	Services Rendered
12/30/XX	Post-op appt: patient presented with alveolitis Suture removal of 3 black silk suture Irrigated extraction site with warm sterile saline solution Packed socket with iodoform gauze Prescribed pain medication RTC: return in 1 to 2 days to treat alveolitis Assistant's initials

12. Dismiss and escort patient to reception area to meet person responsible for taking the patient home (refer to Procedure 18-5).

Paresthesia Another postsurgical complication that sometimes occurs is paresthesia. In some procedures, such as hard tissue impactions, the teeth are close to the nerves. If the nerve is bruised or damaged during the surgical procedure the patient may experience numbness of the tongue, lip, or chin that may last a few days, weeks, or months, or in extreme cases may be permanent.

Chapter Summary

The oral surgery team may vary according to the surgeon's goals for the practice. In addition to the oral and maxillofacial surgeon, the team usually consists of the receptionist, the business office staff, the dental assistants, and, in some offices, a nurse anesthetist or an anesthesiologist. The surgical dental assistant's responsibilities often vary depending on the size of the practice. Surgical asepsis, patient preparation for oral surgery, and postoperative care are discussed in this chapter. Instruments and equipment and the procedures used in oral surgery are explained. Suture removal, which is considered to be an expanded or advanced function, is explained and demonstrated.

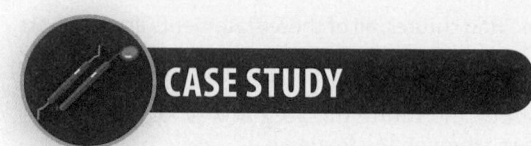

CASE STUDY

Twenty-year-old Josiah Scott's periapical radiograph taken during his recare appointment showed that his mandibular third molars have not erupted and are mesially inclined and entrapped under the second molars. The dentist explained the findings of the radiograph and told Josiah he was being referred to an oral surgeon to have the teeth removed. Josiah, when told about these findings, said that the teeth weren't bothering him, he didn't have any pain, and he didn't see a need to have them removed until they bothered him.

Case Study Review

1. What is the condition of the third molars called?

2. Will it be all right for the third molars to remain in this position? Why or why not?

3. How can the dental assistant encourage Josiah to follow through with getting the third molars extracted?

Review Questions

Multiple Choice

1. What is the education and training for an oral and maxillofacial surgeon?
   a. 4 to 6 years beyond dental school
   b. hospital-based residency in a medical school
   c. additional medical degree to receive practicing privileges in hospital facilities
   d. All of these are options.

2. Which surgery team member controls surgical asepsis, prepares for surgical procedures, and assists the surgeon during surgery?
   a. receptionist
   b. business staff
   c. surgical dental assistant
   d. anesthetist

3. All of these occur during the oral surgery consultation appointment EXCEPT:
   a. cone beam radiography may be necessary.
   b. discussion of patient's current medical condition.
   c. selection of pain and anxiety methods.
   d. impressions for immediate denture.

4. When would a hospital setting be recommended to the patient by the surgeon?
   a. medically compromised patient
   b. physically compromised patient
   c. complicated surgical procedure
   d. All of these

5. Before the surgery is scheduled but after the patient's records and examination are completed, the patient must:
   a. sign an informed consent.
   b. sign a waiver from the patient's general dentist.
   c. register with the oral surgeon's office.
   d. bring proof of identification to the oral surgeon's office.

6. Which are common preoperative instructions?
   a. antibiotic premedication
   b. determination of adult escort
   c. diet prior to surgery
   d. All of these

7. What type of drug produces a state where the patient can respond to verbal stimuli, maintain an airway, and may be between conscious and unconsciousness?
   a. local anesthetic
   b. sedation
   c. general anesthetic
   d. nitrous oxide

8. Which may be administered that will induce a state of unconsciousness and may impair cardiovascular function?
   a. local anesthetic
   b. sedation
   c. general anesthetic
   d. nitrous oxide

9. When is a routine extraction scheduled?
   a. tooth is embedded under alveolar bone
   b. tooth is embedded under gingival tissue
   c. crown portion of tooth is exposed
   d. teeth extracted for full denture

10. The mandibular forceps can be identified by the _____ curve of the shank.
    a. straight
    b. slightly curved
    c. right angle
    d. two angles

11. An incisional biopsy involves the removal of _____.
    a. all of the lesion and some normal tissue
    b. part of the lesion and some normal tissue
    c. the cell layer of the lesion
    d. All of these

12. What is it called when the surgeon treats TMD by injecting the joint with local anesthesia and flushing out inflamed joint fluid?
  a. arthroscopy
  b. arthrocentesis
  c. arthroplasty
  d. partial joint replacement

13. Which of the following instruments is used to retract tissue, remove small root tips, and clamp off blood vessels?
  a. needle holder
  b. hemostat
  c. tissue retractor
  d. surgical curette

14. An infant born with cleft lip and palate will have multiple surgeries in order to correct the tissue separation of the palate and lip. These surgeries generally begin at _____ to repair the cleft lip.
  a. birth
  b. 1 to 2 months
  c. 3 to 6 months
  d. 10 to 12 months

15. Why is surgical asepsis so critical during surgical procedures?
  a. surgical teams' increased blood contact
  b. patient tissues are open
  c. increased chance of cross-contamination
  d. All of these

16. All of these statements are postoperative instructions after the extraction of an impacted tooth EXCEPT:
  a. bite on gauze for 30 minutes.
  b. no strenuous exercise for 24 to 48 hours.
  c. drink fluids through a straw.
  d. rinse mouth with lukewarm salt water after 24 hours.

17. When removing sutures, all of these statements are followed EXCEPT:
  a. do not cut the suture knot.
  b. do not pull the suture thread that was exposed in the oral cavity through the tissues.
  c. cut the suture thread and knot.
  d. as the sutures are removed, place them on gauze.

18. The patient should call the surgical team for all of the following EXCEPT:
  a. swelling becomes hot, hard, and painful to the touch.
  b. bleeding has not stopped by the next morning.
  c. has an unexpected reaction for medication.
  d. cannot tolerate the pain.

19. What is the primary cause of alveolitis?
  a. excessive trauma during extraction
  b. abnormal postsurgery swelling
  c. dislodged clot
  d. medication reaction

20. What is the primary cause of paresthesia?
  a. patient smoked immediately following surgery
  b. dislodged clot
  c. medication reaction
  d. bruised or damaged nerves

Critical Thinking

1. If a patient has had multiple extractions in preparation for a full denture, how long does the patient have to be without teeth? Does the patient have any options?

2. During a surgical procedure, an instrument is dropped on the floor. What should the surgical dental assistant do?

3. Explain how asepsis is different when assisting a dentist during an operative procedure as opposed to assisting a surgeon during a surgical procedure.

Key Terms

Term and Pronunciation	Meaning of Root and Word Parts	Definition
adjunctive (uh-**juhngk**-tiv)	**ad-** = add **join** = put together **-ive** = expressing function	an addition to the principal procedure, as a supplement
alveolectomy (al-vee-uh-**lek**-tuh-mee)	**alveol** = tooth socket; part of jawbone containing the alveolus and roots of the teeth **-ectomy** = surgical removal, excision	surgical removal of part or the entire alveolar process of the maxilla or mandible
alveolitis (al-**vee**-uh-luhs)	**alveolus** = tooth socket **-tis** = inflammation or disease	inflammation or infection of the tooth socket; commonly known as a dry socket

Term and Pronunciation	Meaning of Root and Word Parts	Definition
alveoloplasty (al-**vee**-uh-loh-plas-tee)	**alveolus** = tooth socket **plasty** = surgical shaping	surgical reconstruction of the alveolus
anxiolysis (ang-zee-uh-**lit**-ik)	**anxiety** = distress or uneasiness of mind **lysis** = gradual reduction of severity of symptoms **-ic** = characterized by	any of a class of drugs that reduce anxiety
arthrocentesis (ahr-thruh-sen-**tee**-sis)	**arthro-** = joint **centesis** = a puncture into a body cavity; usually to remove fluid	the surgical puncture and aspiration of a joint
arthroplasty (ahr-thruh-plas-tee)	**arthro-** = joint **-plasty** = surgical repair; plastic surgery	surgical repair of a joint; patient's own tissue or artificial replacement
arthroscopy (ahr-**thros**-kuh-pee)	**arthro-** = joint **-scopy** = indicating a viewing or observation	scope used to diagnose injury or disease of a joint, or to perform minor surgery of a joint
congenital craniofacial (kuhn-**jen**-i-tl) (krey-nee-oh-**fey**-shuhl)	**con-** = with **gen** = to be born **-al** = pertaining to **cranio-** = cranium; part of skull enclosing brain **faci-** = face **-al** = pertaining to	caused by abnormal growth and development of the head and facial soft-tissue structures or bones
extraction (ik-**strak**-shuhn)	**ex-** = out **tract** = to pull or draw out **-tion** = indicating process	removal of a tooth
gingivoplasty (**jin**-jahy-voh- plas-tee)	**gingiv-** = gums **-plasty** = surgical repair; plastic surgery	surgical reshaping and recontouring of the gum tissue
grafting (**graf**-ting)	**graft** = living tissue surgically transplanted **-ing** = expressing action	surgical procedure to move tissue from one site on the body; or from another donor
maxillofacial (mak-sil-oh-**fey**-shuhl)	**maxilla** = jawbone **faci** = face **-al** = pertaining to	related to the maxilla and face
orthognathic surgery (awr-thoh-**nath**-ik) (**sur**-juh-ree)	**ortho** = straight, correct **gnath** = jaw **-ic** = relating to **surgery** = treat injuries, disease and deformities often by cutting into the body	surgery to correct conditions of the jaw and face related to structure, TMD, sleep apnea, malocclusion, and orthodontic problems
paresthesia (par-uhs-**thee**-zhuh)	**par** = condition **esthesia** = sensation or feeling	abnormal sensation (tingling, pricking, numbness) caused by pressure on or damage to nerves
tinnitus (ti-**nahy**-tuhs)	**tinnitus** = buzzing, ringing sound in one or both ears	ringing or similar sensation of sounds in the ears; symptom of underlying conditions such as age-related hearing loss, TMD, ear injury, or circulatory system disorder

CHAPTER 37
Endodontics

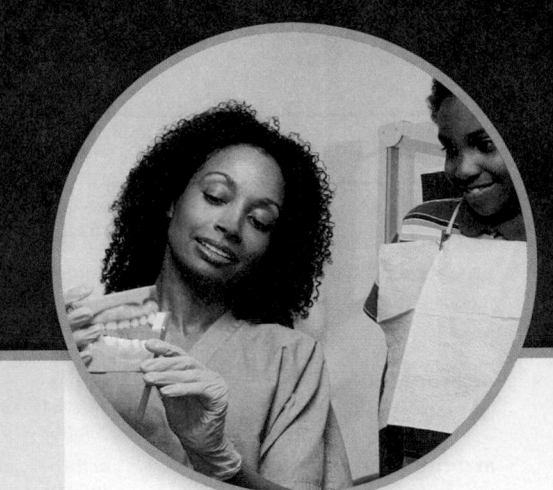

Specific Instructional Objectives

At the completion of this chapter, you will be able to meet these objectives:

1. Use terms presented in this chapter.
2. Recognize the anatomy of the pulpal tissues.
3. Describe the progression of pulpal disease.
4. Discuss periradicular and pulpal involvement conditions.
5. Describe diagnostic procedures relating to the treatment of pulpal disease.
6. Explain the difference between a tooth needing a nonsurgical endodontic procedure versus a surgical endodontic procedure.
7. Summarize the steps in completing root canal therapy.
8. Describe the appearance of intracanal instruments.
9. Explain the use of intracanal instruments.
10. Indicate the necessary postoperative instructions that should be given to the patient immediately following the root canal therapy appointment.
11. Discuss surgical endodontic procedures.

Introduction

Injury and advanced caries may expose the pulp to microorganisms, which may lead to pulpal disease. **Endodontics** is the specialty that diagnoses and treats injuries to the pulp and periapical tissues. Nonsurgical endodontic procedures are often performed by the general dentist; however; the patient is often referred to an endodontist for cases that involve endodontic surgical procedures or for cases in which the root canal(s) of the tooth is/are difficult to access for endodontic treatment. The general dentist sends written instructions and radiographs to the endodontist to prevent miscommunication. The endodontist also often communicates with the referring dentist concerning the patient's treatment and prognosis. The patient may return to the general dentist for the final restoration after the endodontic treatment is completed by the endodontist.

An endodontist has two to three years' additional study in an endodontic program that focuses on the dental pulp and periapical tissues, researching pulp therapy, and developing clinical skills in treating pulpal and periapical disease.

As an endodontic assistant, it is also important to have knowledge of pulp anatomy, pulp disease, and the progression of the disease to assist the endodontist in treating a patient's tooth, requiring root canal therapy. A thorough discussion of dental anatomy is presented in Chapter 7. In this chapter the pulp tissue anatomy will be reviewed along with the progression of pulpal disease, steps in the assistance of diagnosing pulpal and periapical disease, and root canal therapy and periapical surgery.

Pulp Tissue Anatomy

Pulp tissue, often referred to as the nerve of the tooth, is made up of blood, nerve, and connective tissues. The blood tissue provides nutrients to keep the tooth vital. In addition, the blood tissue is responsible for waste exchange for the pulp and tooth tissues. Nerve tissue contains nerve fibers which transmit pain impulses through the dentinal tubules. This pain sensation stimulates the pulp's defense mechanisms against bacterial invasion and signals sensation that can be felt by the patient. The connective tissue,

1218

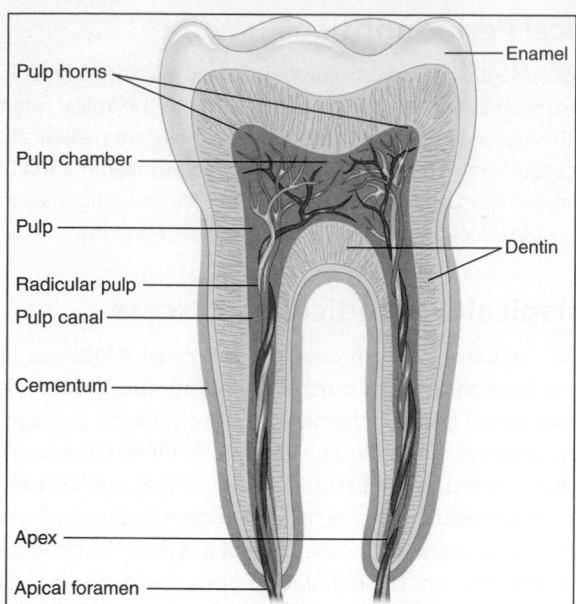

Pulp horns

Pulp chamber

Pulp

Radicular pulp

Pulp canal

Cementum

Apex

Apical foramen

Enamel

Dentin

FIGURE 37-1
Pulp tissue anatomy.

found within the pulp tissue, manufactures and maintains the extracellular material and provides cohesion and internal support of the healthy pulp.

The parts of the pulp are the pulp chamber or coronal pulp, pulp horns, pulp canal(s), radicular pulp, apex, and apical foramen (Figure 37-1). The pulp chamber is located in the coronal portion of the tooth. The pulp horns are the highest portions of the pulp chamber, extending toward, or close to, the occlusal/incisal surface. The pulp canal(s) occupy(ies) the root(s) of the tooth. The radicular pulp is the portion of the pulp located apically within the pulp canal. The apex is the tapered end of each root tip. Residing within the apex is the apical foramen. The apical foramen is the opening at the end of the root(s). Blood vessels and nerves enter the root canal(s) of the tooth via the apical foramen.

The pulp chamber is lined with specialized cells, called **odontoblasts**, which form dentin. These odontoblasts line the walls of the pulp cavity and make secondary (reparative) dentin in response to injury, stress, and possible bacterial invasion. As the pulp recedes, the secondary dentin builds to protect the pulp from damage. With age, the pulp chamber decreases in size, due to the formation of secondary dentin. Should the tooth have been under any type of stress in response to irritation or injury, tertiary dentin, also known as reparative dentin, is formed. The formation of this type of dentin within the pulp chamber and root canals of the tooth causes a gradual narrowing of the pulp chamber and pulp canal. The aging process also causes this to occur.

Progression of Pulpal Disease

A healthy pulp is said to be a **vital pulp**. Pulpitis is an inflammation of the pulpal tissue that is caused by an irritant such as an area of decay that is causing injury to the pulp. Should the injury

to the pulp occur without any means of healing itself via the **tertiary dentin**, a reversible **chronic pulpitis** may result; if bacteria have reached the pulp, an irreversible **acute pulpitis** may occur.

Once the pulp is approached by an irritant, it is very susceptible to inflammation and infection. Pulp disease progresses through many stages until the pulp ultimately dies (**nonvital pulp**) if there is not an intervention. Pulpitis may be reversible or irreversible depending on whether or not the irritant has reached the pulp of the tooth.

Reversible Pulpitis

Pulpitis begins as an inflammatory reaction to an irritant. Major causes of inflamed pulpitis are caries, impact trauma/tooth fractures, **occlusal attrition**, and **iatrogenic** trauma. Iatrogenic pulpitis may be caused by drilling the tooth with a handpiece or the use of a dental material placed near the pulp that is caustic and injures the pulp. Pulpitis is a defensive reaction which works to eliminate bacterial invaders that may cause harm to the pulp. As with any infection, inflammation begins the healing process, thus, pulpitis is associated with the first phase of healing the inflamed pulp. The symptoms of inflammation are redness, swelling, heat, pain, and impairment of function. In reversible pulpitis, the patient may state that the tooth is sensitive to cold and sometimes to sweets or to biting forces.

When there is a mild irritant and the irritant is removed early, the inflammation may subside and the pulp may return to a healthy state. For example, if there is a carious lesion which is irritating the pulp, if the decay is removed and a restoration is placed, the pulp may no longer be sensitive.

Irreversible Pulpitis

Generally irreversible chronic pulpitis occurs when there is a strong and/or persistent irritant, resulting in an **anti-inflammatory reaction** that is also more severe and persistent. Symptoms include pain to the patient that may be short and sharp or dull and continual. A true **odontalgia** occurs that literally keeps the patient up all night, with very little ability to find relief. This is because the pain from the swelling decreases in a sitting up position and increases in the lying down position. **Root canal therapy** (RCT) needs to be performed to alleviate the pressure that has been chronically building in intensity. When performing root canal therapy, the primary objective is to remove the pulpal tissue residing in both the coronal portion of the tooth and the root canal(s). When possible, the empty canals of the root are sealed.

Without the nutrients supplied by the pulp, the tooth's hard structures become brittle and may fracture. A post and core and crown may be needed in order to prevent the tooth from fracturing.

Untreated inflamed pulpitis will continue to progress into various stages. The stages of pulpal disease may include pulp **necrosis**, apical and periodontal involvement, **neoplasms**, and cellulitis. Often, if the pulpitis is not treated, many of these stages progress into affecting not only the pulp but also the adjacent tissues. Signs and symptoms of pulpitis include:

- Redness—blood flow is increased to the area, bringing in leukocytes to help fight the bacteria.
- Swelling—occurs from the increased blood flow and tissue fluid.
- Heat—occurs with the increased blood flow and activity in the area.
- Pain—occurs as the swelling presses against nerve endings. This is especially intensified as the pulp is surrounded by hard tissue that will not give to the swelling. The result is increased pressure in a centralized, small area, which results in the intensification of the pressure placed on the nerve endings.
- Impairment of function—the inflamed tissue is not able to function normally due to the swelling, pain, and effects on the nervous system. The inflammation spreads to the periodontal ligament. In turn, the periodontal ligament also responds with the presentation of inflammation. The patient begins to feel pain to the pressure of touch or percussion, and also that of mastication.

Asymptomatic Irreversible Pulpitis

The diagnosis of asymptomatic irreversible pulpitis is based on a subjective finding combined with objective clinical findings. In this case, the patient will not have symptoms, yet there is a large lesion present that may lead to pulpal exposure when removed, necessitating endodontic therapy. When thermal testing is performed, the tooth responds normally in most cases.

Necrotic Pulp

If the irritant is allowed to remain and the inflammation is not treated, infection may occur that results in the pulp tissue destruction and/or death. True pulpal **necrosis** denotes pulpal death. Teeth with total pulpal necrosis are usually asymptomatic unless inflammation has progressed to the periradicular tissues. The necrotic pulp will discolor the tooth, and the tooth's hard structure will become brittle. Discoloration of the tooth is caused by remnants of biologically decomposed pulp tissue and blood clot. Initial discoloration of the tooth crown is a sign of internal damage but not necessarily irreparable damage. Pulp necrosis is a likely diagnosis if the tooth shows gray/blue or red crown discoloration in combination with an apical radiolucency. Treatment will require RCT and possibly a post and core plus full-crown coverage.

Periapical (Periradicular) Involvement

As the pulp canal becomes infected, the infection travels through the apical foramen and begins to infect the periapical and periradicular area surrounding the apex of the tooth.

Apical Periodontitis

The periodontal ligament becomes inflamed and the alveolar bone is destroyed as the infection spreads through the apical foramen into the root area. Infection appears as a radiolucent periapical area on the radiograph (Figure 37-2). With the acute inflammation there is pain, pus formation, sensitivity to touch, and swelling. Treatment of the pulp infection will resolve the apical periodontitis.

Periapical (Periradicular) Abscess

As the infection spreads through the pulp canal, it localizes at the apex. A sac containing a **purulent exudate** (pus) accumulates from the apical foramen drainage. Initially, a natural passageway for the drainage of the exudate from the confined bone area may develop, referred to as a **fistula**. The patient feels a relief from the pain as the pressure of the pus drains. A chronic abscess is generally asymptomatic and the discharge of pus from the periodontal sulcus is unnoticed. The radiolucent destruction of surrounding bone is visible on a radiograph. The endodontist will generally prescribe an antibiotic and treatment of the pulpitis will allow for drainage of the exudate. Occasionally, in the event that a patient has a large fistula present that is filled with exudate, the endodontist can initiate the disruption of the localized infection by performing a procedure called an "I&D," or incision and drainage.

A long-standing chronic periapical infection can become acute. With an acute periradicular abscess, pus and swelling occur. The patient will suddenly notice pain to pressure, and a **parulis** may form on the gingiva along the root perimeter (Figure 37-3). The bone destruction in the periradicular area is usually not visible in an acute abscess. The patient may experience fever and feel a rapid onset of severe pain, particularly to percussion.

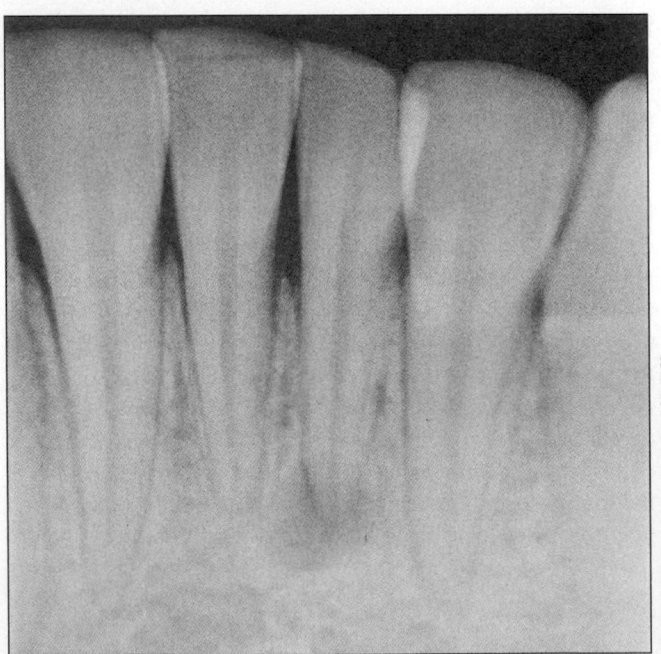

FIGURE 37-2
Radiograph of tooth with apical abscess (dark shadow at the apex).

Courtesy of Clifton O. Caldwell, Jr., DDS, FICD, FACD

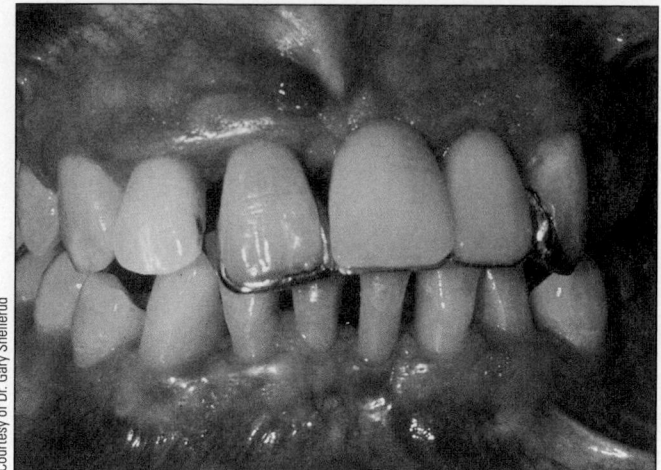

Courtesy of Dr. Gary Shellerud

FIGURE 37-3
Patient with gingival abscess (red area above tooth #8 near frenum).

If the exudate has already traveled through the bone to the soft tissue beneath, a boil filled with pus may have developed (gum boil/ parulis) near the apex of the root. The pain will be less than it was prior to the drainage of the periapical abscess. The patient will notice the abscess on the gingiva. The endodontist will prescribe an antibiotic until the infection decreases. The endodontist may lance the abscess to release some of the exudate until it is advisable to treat the pulpitis. Treatment, when there is infection present, may increase the chance of spreading the infection to other areas of the body and result in cellulitis. Treatment for this abscess is endodontic therapy.

Periapical Granuloma

A periapical **granuloma** is a mass of necrotic tissue around the apex of a nonvital tooth. A periapical granuloma usually results from pulpal necrosis. Treatment would be endodontic therapy or extraction of the tooth.

Periapical Neoplasm

If a granuloma is left untreated and the irritation continues, a **cyst** forms. A periapical cyst is a small radiolucency (typically less than 1 cm). They are usually of odontogenic origin in response to an infection of the pulp. In most cases, a large carious lesion will be visible on the tooth that exhibits the periapical cyst. Treatment is endodontic therapy or extraction of the tooth. If the cyst persists after the tooth is extracted, it is known as a residual cyst. If the periapical irritation persists, a granuloma may develop as an inflammatory response to the periapical infection. **Neoplasms** would grow and destroy more alveolar bone. Surgical removal of the neoplasm would be inevitable.

Osteomyelitis

Osteomyelitis is an infection of the bone. It is difficult to diagnose as radiographs may not detect the present infection.

Osteomyelitis may be caused by periodontal disease. Symptoms of osteomyelitis such as fatigue and trismus also make diagnosis more complicated. Once diagnosed, antibiotics can alleviate osteomyelitis.

Cellulitis

Severe infection can spread to other soft tissues (skin and connective tissue) causing **cellulitis**. When infection enters the tissue space of the skin, cheeks, jaw, and neck, these visible areas of the head and neck may become swollen. This condition potentially can become a serious skin infection and can spread to the blood or lymph nodes, resulting in severe debility or even death if untreated. Most cases of cellulitis will disappear in less than a week with antibiotic therapy. More serious cases may require IV antibiotics and analgesics. If the tissue begins to necrotize, surgery may be indicated.

Pulpal Disease Diagnosis

A crucial step in treating pulpal disease is an accurate diagnosis. The patient will usually call the office complaining of pain. Sometimes the pain will feel like it is coming from a tooth that is not infected; this is known as referred pain. The dentist uses several methods to determine the exact tooth causing the pain. The endodontic diagnostic procedures will also allow the dentist to determine the stage of pulpal disease. The endodontist uses the patient's medical and dental history, clinical examination, radiographic surveys, and diagnostic tests in diagnosis and determination of appropriate treatment of the pulpal disease.

Medical and Dental History

The first step for endodontic treatment is for the patient to fill out a medical history. Once completed, the history is reviewed and clarified to ensure that accurate and complete information is gathered.

The dental history provides the endodontist dental experiences and the signs and symptoms of the current concern. It may reveal information that relates to previous treatment of the tooth pulp to be used in diagnosis. The dental history opens the way for subjective examination (the patient's symptoms explained in their own words). The patient should be allowed to describe the type of pain, sensitivity to heat and cold, duration of the condition, and any other symptoms.

Documentation of the patient's symptoms is imperative in diagnosing pulpal disease stages.

- If the patient has a history of brief pain when they eat or drink something cold, and pain ends when the cold (stimulant) is removed, this usually indicates reversible pulpitis.

- If the pain persists after the stimulant (cold, hot, air, pressure) is removed, and there also is throbbing pain without a stimulus, this usually indicates irreversible pulpitis.

- Compression pressure is generally due to some periapical or periradicular involvement.

Noting patient symptoms often begins with the patient's call into the office complaining about a toothache.

Clinical Examination

The clinical examination uncovers signs of pulpal disease. An extraoral examination evaluates the extraoral tissue, facial asymmetry, swelling, redness, and external fistulas. The intraoral visual exam may show a large carious lesion, fractured tooth, parulis, or cellulitis. The endodontist palpates the soft tissues, the mucosa above the apex of the root, and along the root, noting any sensitivity or swelling. Normally, one or more additional teeth are palpated for comparison. Around the indicated tooth, the area may be soft and raised (pus filled).

Radiographic Survey

The endodontist generally prescribes a periapical radiograph of the tooth exhibiting the pain. The dentist can see the depth of the caries, widening of the periodontal ligament indicating apical involvement, and radiolucency of the alveolar bone, showing areas of tissue breakdown on the periapical radiographs.

The dentist needs a clear, concise periapical radiograph that shows at least 5 mm beyond the apex in order to have an adequate view of the periapical area. It needs to be an image of equal size as the tooth being radiographed. This initial radiograph is used to determine the root length for the setting of endodontic instruments. Radiographs are taken at several stages during the root canal procedure, including the initial radiograph, upon opening a canal to determine the length, upon placement of the final size files in the canals, and a final radiograph once the root canal procedure is completed (Figure 37-4).

Diagnostic Tests

There are **endodontia** tests used to determine whether the tooth has pulpal disease, the stage of the pulpal disease, and what endodontic treatment is indicated. The tests are more objective than the patient's reporting of symptoms and should be carefully

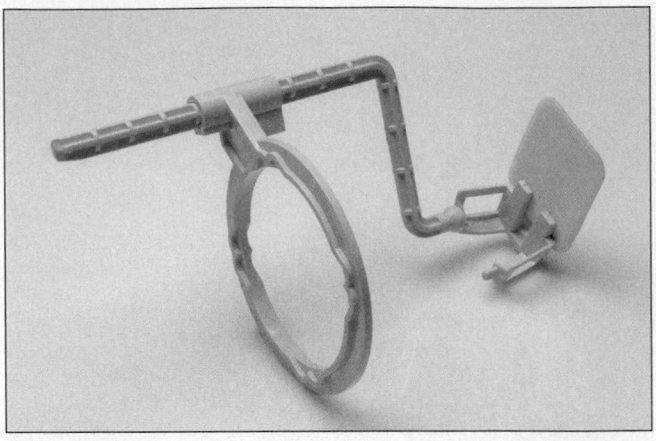

FIGURE 37-4
Endodontic x-ray film holder designed to fit over dental dam clamp and intracanal instrument. Allows for an x-ray to be exposed with an intracanal instrument in place.

recorded in the services rendered. Vitality tests are performed to assess the condition of the pulp. Many procedures are used to test for hypersensitivity and necrosis of the pulp. A tooth that is known to be healthy is tested as a point of reference called the control tooth. A tooth of the same type in the arch is the best choice. For example, if tooth #3 is in question, the best reference tooth is tooth #14. When the suspected tooth responds more severely and immediately to a stimulus test than the control tooth, the pulp is hypersensitive. If the suspected tooth responds much later or not at all, the pulp is dying or is already necrotic (Table 37-1).

Electric Pulp Test Electric pulp testers are used to conduct a mild electrical current to the pulp to test the vitality of the pulp. The tester has a dial that controls the amount of electrical current (Figure 37-5). There is no current when the dial is set at 0 and the maximum current is at 10. Because saliva conducts the electrical

TABLE 37-1 Diagnostic Chart of Pulp and Periapical Diseases

Condition	Complaint History	Radiographic Findings	Electronic Pulp Test	Thermal Testing	Treatment
Reversible pulpitis	Hot and/or cold sensitivity; sensitivity to cold most common	None; large caries or restoration; approaching pulp; cracks; signs of trauma	Normal response	Sensitivity nonlingering on removal of stimulus	Pulp capping
Irreversible pulpitis	Lingering hot or cold sensitivity to spontaneous pain; severe toothache	Irritant exposing pulp; periradicular radiolucency or widened PDL	Exaggerated response	Lingering sensitivity	RCT
Necrotic pulp	Past history of pain to no pain; may complain of discoloration	Pulp exposed; periradicular radiolucency or widened PDL	No response	No response	RCT
Acute periradicular involvement	Biting/chewing discomfort; recent restoration	Normal; periradicular radiolucency or widened PDL	Variable; moderately sensitive or not sensitive	Not usually sensitive	Adjustment of occlusion; RCT may be necessary
Acute periradicular abscess	Biting/chewing discomfort to pain; slight to large amount of swelling; gum bump	Periradicular radiolucency or widened PDL	Normal	Normal	I&D, RCT

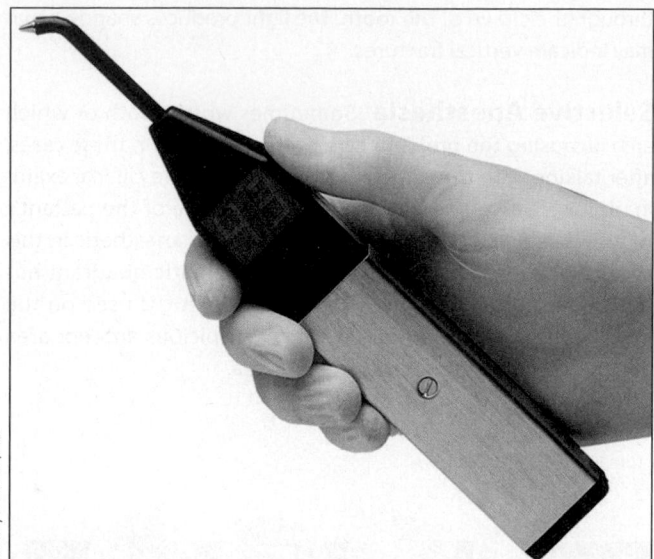

FIGURE 37-5
Electric pulp tester.

Courtesy of Parkell, Inc.

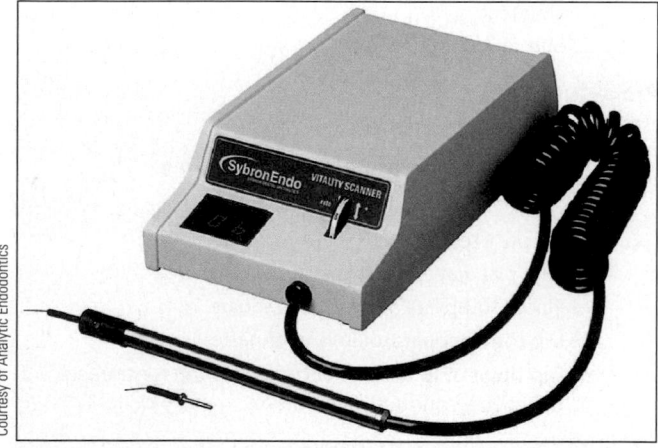

FIGURE 37-6
Vitality scanner.

Courtesy of Analytic Endodontics

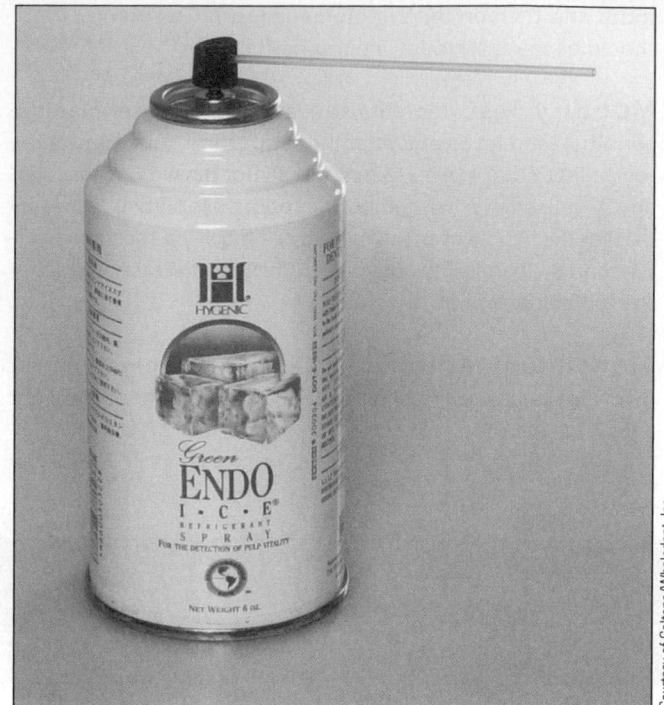

FIGURE 37-7
Endo ice used to test the vitality of a tooth.

Courtesy of Coltene/Whaledent, Inc.

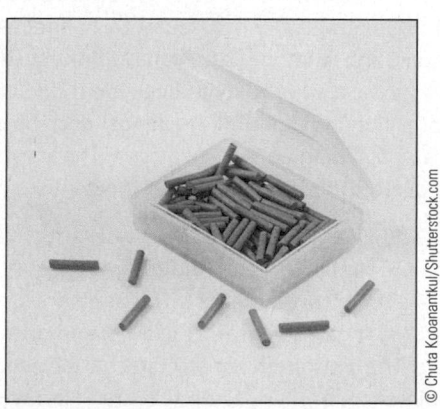

FIGURE 37-8
Gutta-percha sticks are used for heat testing and sealing canal opening after obturation.

© Chuta Kooanantkul/Shutterstock.com

current, the tooth is dried and toothpaste is applied before the tester electrode is placed on the tooth. If the patient first feels the current in the control tooth at setting 5 but feels current below setting 5 on the tooth in question, that tooth is hypersensitive. If the control tooth feels current at 5 and the tooth being tested only feels current above 5, the tooth is losing sensitivity and is possibly necrotic.

A vitality scanner allows the dentist to scan each tooth in minutes (Figure 37-6). The scanner indicates endodontic problems in the early stages. The probe on the scanner records a reading and then automatically resets for the next tooth.

Thermal Test Thermal tests are used to evaluate the pulp's response to hot and cold. The dentist uses ice (usually water that is frozen in a sterilized, anesthetic carpule), dry ice, frozen ethyl chloride, or carbon dioxide (Figure 37-7) for the cold test. A heated **gutta-percha** stick is generally used for the heat test (Figure 37-8). The teeth are dried and the control tooth is tested and compared to the tooth in question. The patient has an early and violent response to cold and heat when the pulp is infected, and no response if the pulp is necrotic. However, if the patient arrives with a symptomatic tooth, the heat test is often not used, as an immediate response can entice a severe thermal reaction.

Percussion Test Pain to **percussion** indicates that the surrounding periapical or periradicular tissue is involved. The dentist taps the occlusal or incisal surface of the tooth with the blunted end of an instrument (mouth mirror) or has the patient bite on a burlew disc or bite stick. The tapping is first done on a control tooth and then on the symptomatic tooth. The control tooth should be the same tooth in the opposite arch.

Mobility Test Mobility is evaluated to determine the condition and involvement of the supporting structures of the tooth. Teeth that move 2–3 mm should not have root canal therapy because they lack sufficient support. Mobility is tested by placing the handle of an instrument or a finger on the lingual surface and the handle of another instrument on the facial surface of the tooth and applying pressure.

Transillumination Test The transillumination test involves the use of a strong fiber optic light that transmits light

through the crown of the tooth. The light produces shadows that may indicate vertical fractures.

Selective Anesthesia Sometimes which tooth or which arch is causing the problem cannot be identified. In these cases, after talking with the patient and completing the clinical examination, selective anesthesia is used. One area of the patient's mouth is selected and an injection is given. If anesthetic in this area alleviates the discomfort, the problematic quadrant has been determined. Usually, selective anesthetic is used on the maxillary teeth beginning in the most suspicious anterior area and then progressing to the posterior area.

Procedure 37-1
Assist in Pulpal Disease Diagnosis

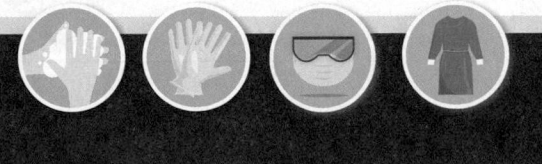

The assistant prepares the treatment area for patient seating and assembles the diagnostic tray setup. After the patient is seated, the assistant needs to review and document the patient's health history first, followed by the history of the tooth pain and what the patient may think caused the problem. Once the area of pain has been identified, the assistant discusses the findings with the dentist and the dentist prescribes what radiographs are necessary. The assistant exposes and processes the radiograph(s) for the dentist's viewing.

During the clinical examination, the assistant prepares instruments and materials needed during the examination and transfers them to the dentist. The assistant uses the HVE and A/W syringe and rinses, evacuates, and dries the area as needed. The assistant must pay direct attention to the dentist's direction, as many teeth that are experiencing pulpal disease can be hypersensitive to air and water. The assistant also records findings in the services rendered.

Steps written in blue font are performed by the operator (dentist or qualified dental assistant), and the chairside assistant's steps are written in black.

Equipment and Supplies
- Basic setup: mouth mirror, explorer, and cotton pliers
- Electric pulp tester and electrodes
   - ❏ cotton rolls
   - ❏ toothpaste
   - ❏ cotton tip applicator
   - ❏ gauze squares
- Dry ice spray
   - ❏ cotton pellets
- Gutta-percha sticks
   - ❏ heat source

- Percussion test
   - ❏ bite stick or burlew disc

Procedure Steps
1. Pass cotton rolls to dentist.

   Dentist isolates area before use of pulp testing.
   - ❏ **Places cotton roll into the vestibule.**

2. Prepare pulp tester.
   - ❏ Turn dial that controls current level to zero.
   - ❏ Place toothpaste onto a gauze square.
   - ❏ Dip cotton applicator into toothpaste.
   - ❏ Dip tip of pulp tester electrode into the toothpaste to act as a conducting medium.

3. Pass a gauze for dentist to dry the teeth before using the tester; air on sensitive teeth may be very painful.

4. Retrieve gauze square and pass pulp tester.

   Dentist tests the control tooth first.
   - ❏ **Asks patient to signal when they notice a sensation which is usually a tingling or hot feeling.**
   - ❏ **Places the tip on the facial surface of the tooth and gradually increases the power. Takes caution to not place the electrode on a metal restoration, wet surface, gingiva, or artificial crowns.**
   - ❏ **Informs assistant of readings.**

5. Record tooth number and readings for each tooth tested.

6. Prepare for cold test.
   - ❏ Grasp cotton pellet with cotton pliers.
   - ❏ Spray frozen ice onto the cotton pellet.

7. Retrieve pulp tester and pass cotton pliers.

   Dentist places cotton pellet on tooth surface.

8. Record tooth number and findings of ice test.

9. Prepare for heat test.
   - ❏ Place one end of the gutta-percha stick into the heat source.

10. Retrieve cotton pliers and pass heated gutta-percha stick.

    Dentist places gutta-percha stick on tooth surface.

11. Record tooth number and finding of the heat test.

12. Retrieve gutta-percha stick and pass dentist's preference of burlew disc or bite stick.

    Dentist places the disc or stick against the tooth in question and asks the patient to close.

13. Write up procedure in Services Rendered.

Date	Services Rendered
10/06/XX	EMG appt: presented with pain and swelling in area of #7 Clinical examination reveals a carious lesion on the mesiolingual aspect of #7. Periapical radiograph reveals pathology at the apex of #7.
#7	Completed pulpal diagnostics on tooth
	Patient responded 3 on pulp testing on #7 and 5 on control tooth #10. Patient claims tooth is sensitive to percussion and cold.
	Patient prescribed amoxicillin after confirming no allergies. Rx amoxicillin 500 mg tab, pharmacy to dispense 21 tabs. Patient instructed to take one tab three times per day. Patient advised to take ibuprofen for pain as needed. Confirmed medical history and there are no contraindications to ibuprofen.
	RTC: Patient will return in 7 days for endodontic therapy on #7.
	Assistant's initials

Treatment Plan

Once all the information has been gathered and the dentist has made a diagnosis, the patient is informed of the necessary endodontic treatment. The patient must sign a consent form and make appointments and financial arrangements before treatment begins. To minimize anxiety and answer questions about the upcoming procedure, endodontic pamphlets or videos may be provided.

Classification of Endodontic Treatment

Endodontic treatment is divided into two classifications: nonsurgical and surgical. Nonsurgical procedures can be performed by the general dentist who is knowledgeable about the procedure needed while surgical procedures are performed almost exclusively by the endodontist.

Nonsurgical Endodontic Procedures

These are procedures that are performed to prevent further damage to the pulp, interrupt the progress of pulpal infection, and maintain the vitality of the tooth. If these procedures are successful, removal of the pulp tissue and root canal therapy may be avoided.

Pulp Capping

There are two pulp capping procedures: indirect and direct pulp capping. Indirect pulp capping is performed when an irritant or caries is approaching the pulp, but the pulp has not been directly exposed. When there is a mild irritant and the irritant is removed early, the inflammation may subside and the pulp may return to a healthy state, after restorative treatment. Reversible chronic pulpitis is generally treated with an **indirect pulp cap** when the pulp has not been exposed. It is important to note that an indirect pulp cap procedure is applied to the thin layer of affected dentin that is covering the pulp. Removal of this affected dentin would result in pulpal exposure. This procedure should be performed only on teeth that have no signs of irreversible damage such as an apical infection.

A sedative, temporary restoration is placed for approximately 4–6 weeks to allow time for secondary dentin to form. If successful, a thicker layer of dentin will be stimulated by the medicated liner/base placed to cover the affected pulp. After 4–6 weeks, radiographs may be taken to confirm the healthy state of the newly formed dentin surrounding the pulpal area. If the radiograph confirms the health of the pulp to be responding favorably to the previous indirect pulp capping procedure, a permanent restoration is then placed.

Reversible chronic pulpitis is generally treated with a **direct pulp cap** when the pulp has been exposed. The pulp exposure may occur as the caries process enters the pulp chamber or from the removal of the caries during the cavity preparation procedure. Pulpal exposures caused by the removal or excavation of such caries can be referred to as being iatrogenic. A palliative liner/base is placed directly over the exposed pulp followed by a temporary restoration for 4–6 weeks. After the 4–6 weeks, the tooth is radiographed. Hopefully the level of dentin has grown over the exposed pulp area and a permanent restoration can be placed.

Direct and indirect pulp capping are two nonsurgical procedures that a dentist can perform to promote the vitality of the tooth, even in the event of pulpal exposure. Both procedures are acts of preservation of the vital pulp rather than the decision to begin root canal therapy. By medicating the tissue surrounding the pulp affected by gross caries, it is the intent of the dentist to exhaust all means of saving a vital tooth. In any event, these procedures do not always achieve what the dental team's expectations are of them, and the tooth is unable to remain vital. If poor results are seen during the 4–6-week period that the dental patient has the temporary restoration in the tooth, the root canal treatment must be initiated to avoid extraction.

The success rate for the indirect pulp capping treatment is much higher than direct pulp capping. Most treatment for pulpitis also includes being prescribed antibiotics to systemically rid the area of bacteria. In addition, anti-inflammatory medications can be prescribed to reduce and assist with inflammation of the affected area. Dental patients are encouraged to comply with the dentist's orders in the regiment of length of time and frequency that the antibiotic and anti-inflammatory agents are prescribed.

Pulpotomy
A **pulpotomy** is performed when the pulp has been exposed due to deep carious lesions, tooth fractures or irreversible pulpitis has been diagnosed, and the possibility of retaining the vitality cannot be achieved through the placement of a direct pulp cap. All the pulp is removed from within the coronal pulp chamber. Medicaments are placed to stop the bleeding and to preserve the remaining pulp tissue in the pulp canal. By leaving healthy pulp tissue in the canal(s) of a developing permanent tooth, the apices will be able to complete formation referred to as **apexogenesis**. A medicated base and temporary restoration are placed.

Pulpectomy
A **pulpectomy** is the complete removal of the pulp from the chamber and the canal(s). A pulpectomy is the first phase of root canal therapy in which all of the diseased or necrotic pulp tissue is **extirpated** and the entire pulp cavity is cleansed. This process is known as **debridement**. Once all vitality of the tooth is removed, the canals of the tooth are mechanically shaped using **intracanal** instruments. In addition to the intracanal instruments, chemicals may be used to help dissolve **sclerotic** dentin and to kill bacteria.

The pulpectomy procedure is performed on primary teeth and the roots of the primary teeth are not **obturated** to allow for the resorption of the roots as the permanent teeth erupt. Allowing for the primary roots to remain is beneficial, as these roots guide or direct the permanent teeth to erupt into the intended position of the tooth.

The pulpectomy procedure without filling the canals is also performed on young, permanent teeth when the apices are not fully developed. When the pulp tissue is removed, the remaining tooth structure is no longer supplied with nutrients. Without nutrients, the tooth is essentially necrotic, and it becomes brittle. A temporary crown is placed to protect the weakened hard tissue of the tooth. Most endodontically treated teeth will require permanent, full-crown coverage as the optimum long-term treatment.

Root Canal Therapy
When there is an infection of the pulp tissue of a tooth that cannot be reversed, there are often basically two treatment options: the extraction of the tooth or root canal therapy. Should the patient elect to have the tooth removed, the space remaining at the extraction site needs to be replaced with either a permanent or a removable prosthesis. A prosthesis is recommended to avoid continued bone loss of the edentulous ridge, drifting of adjacent teeth, and the possible eventual loss of more teeth. The retention of the natural tooth, if possible, is always better than the placement of an artificial tooth.

The primary difference between pulpectomy and root canal therapy is that in root canal therapy, the root canals are shaped, decontaminated, and filled using gutta-percha, silver points, a filling paste, or a combination of the filling materials. Root canal therapy (RCT) is the most common endodontic procedure and is also referred to as root canal, root canal treatment, endodontic treatment, and conventional endodontic treatment.

RCT Preoperative Procedures
Root canal procedures have the reputation of being painful. Although, in reality, the root canal procedure is relatively painless, it remains the most feared dental procedure. For the average patient, having an RCT is reported by patients as being no more painful than having a routine filling placed. Most apprehension is thought to be due to the painful events leading up to the actual treatment. Sedation along with local anesthetic administration may be used to reduce the pain and help the patient relax.

In some cases, achieving adequate pain control is difficult. When there is an abscessed tooth, the area is swollen, and there may be a parulis. The high amount of pus in the infected area contains acids that inactivate local anesthetic agents, making it very difficult to anesthetize the area. The dentist may need to drain the abscess and release the pressure of the pus to obtain adequate anesthesia. With the presence of infection and pus, the dentist may opt to prescribe a week of antibiotics prior to the RCT. This will help reduce the infection and allow the local anesthetic to work more effectively when the patient returns for the endodontic procedure. If the tooth is hypersensitive or symptomatic, it may require injection of additional anesthetic directly into the pulp or pulp tissue.

It is critical to use only sterile items such as sterile gloves and to isolate the tooth that is receiving endodontic treatment from the oral cavity and oral microorganisms found within the mouth. Using the dental dam during the root canal therapy is considered standard of care by the American Association of Endodontics. One of the main goals of RCT is removing bacteria and contaminants from within the tooth. The dental dam:

- Allows for isolation and protection of the interior of the tooth from being recontaminated by indigenous bacteria of the oral cavity during the procedure.

- Isolates the infected tooth from the other teeth, providing a contrast between the tooth and the surrounding area and allowing for greater visibility by the operator.

- Prevents debris and dental materials from entering the patient's oral cavity and oropharynx.

- Prevents ingestion of files and other small instruments that are necessary in RCT procedures.
- Retracts the patient's lips and tongue from the immediate area being worked in allowing for better access, visually and instrumentally.

The dentist or assistant may punch one hole in the dental dam for single isolation, to expose only the tooth being treated. A plastic dental dam frame is often preferred by dentists as it enables them to expose radiographs through the radiolucent plastic frame during the procedure (Figure 37-9). The dentist may request that the tooth and surrounding area be swabbed with a sterile cotton pellet soaked in antiseptic solution.

Access Root Canals Obtaining access into the pulp chamber is the initial step in RCT. The dentist removes all caries if present and enters the pulp chamber using a high-speed and low-speed handpiece and preference of rotary instruments as used in the cavity preparation setup. The dentist usually uses the diamond or tungsten carbide fissure burs and a high-speed handpiece to make initial access into the affected tooth. The anterior teeth are accessed from the lingual surface and the posterior teeth are accessed from the occlusal surface.

Once access to the pulp chamber is made, longer shanked round burs are used to remove the infected pulp tissue from the chamber. In addition, the long shanked burs are used to assist in the removal of the infected dentin to the pulpal floor until the orifice of the pulp canals is visible. A dentist may use a side-cutting Gates–Glidden drill, held in the low-speed handpiece, to open and flare the coronal portion of the canal orifice (Figure 37-10). These drills have a safe-ended tip and are available in sizes 1 through 6. The number of bands at the base of the drill indicates its size.

Sometimes the canals are not easily viewed, and the dentist may need to use an endodontic explorer to locate canals (Figure 37-11). The dentist continues to prepare the opening to make it wide enough to obtain straight access to each canal without sacrificing the tooth structure. An endodontic spoon excavator

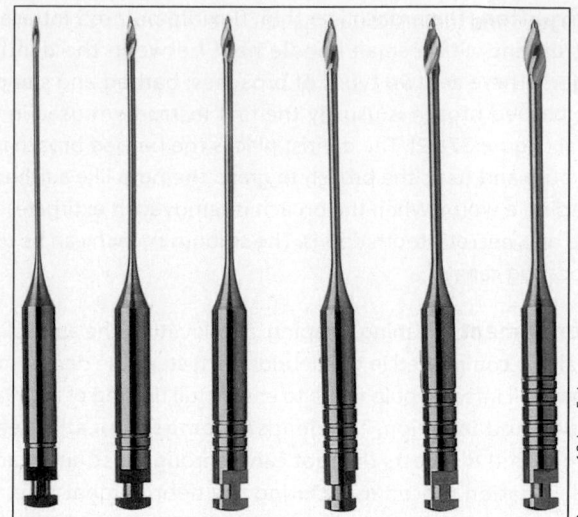

FIGURE 37-10
Gates–Glidden drills. The tip of the drill is elliptically shaped and has a noncutting end.

may be used to reach the bottom of the pulp chamber and to remove deep caries and pulp tissue. The access opening prepared in the tooth allows entrance to the pulp canal for removal of the pulp tissue in the canal.

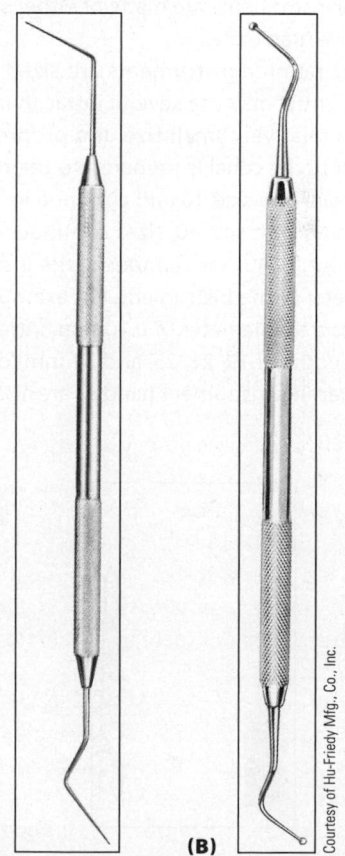

(A) **(B)**
FIGURE 37-11
(A) Endodontic explorer. (B) Endodontic spoon excavator.

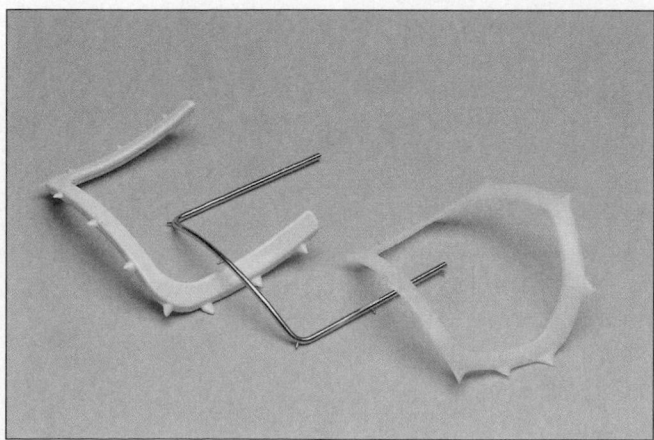

FIGURE 37-9
Plastic dental dam frames (lower right frame, also referred to as an Otsby frame).

Extirpation The broach is a thin, flexible pointed intracanal instrument with a small handle held between the dentist's fingers. There are two types of broaches: barbed and smooth. The barbed broach is usually the first instrument used in the canal (Figure 37-12). The dentist places the barbed broach into the pulp and turns the broach to grasp the pulp like a fishhook grasping a worm. When the broach is removed, it extirpates the pulp and necrotic tooth debris. The smooth broach can be used in locating canals.

Debridement Cleaning, shaping, and locating the apex of the canal is accomplished in the debridement step. The dentist must remove all infected pulp tissue to ensure full healing of all inflammation and infection. The dentist **biomechanically** cleans, shapes, and disinfects the root canal through instrumentation and irrigation procedures. During the debridement step, the root canal(s) is/are cleaned and shaped using intracanal instruments. The dentist uses endodontic hand **reamers** and **files** and intracanal rotary instruments to remove vital and necrotic tissue and infected dentin. The primary objective in shaping the canal is to form a smooth, tapered canal to facilitate in proper irrigation, disinfection, and obturation.

Intracanal Instruments Hand intracanal instruments (reamers and files), power-assisted instruments, and intracanal solutions are used in debridement of the pulp canals. The dentist holds the small handle of the intracanal hand instruments between their fingers. Intracanal instruments are made of either stainless steel or a more expensive titanium alloy.

These tapered, pointed instruments are sized by diameter and length. The dentist may use several intracanal instruments beginning with a relatively small size and progressing to the next larger size until the canal is prepared to the desired diameter. The sizes begin with size 10 and continue in intervals of 5 to size 60. Beginning with size 60, sizes continue in intervals of 10 to sizes 70 through 140. The number of the instrument represents the diameter of the instrument. For example, a number 10 instrument has a tip diameter of 0.10 mm. Intracanal instruments come in lengths of 19, 21, 25, and 31 mm for the various canal lengths. Intracanal instrument handles are also color coded

for quick recognition of the file. For example, purple is the color for the number 10 intracanal instrument. Generally the handles are colored and have the file number on the instrument handle.

The reamer is a hand file with the working end as a spiral with a few, large cutting blades (flutes) (Figure 37-13). It is used to make a rougher and quicker cut to remove dentin and enlarge the root canals in diameter. The dentist holds the small handle between their fingers and uses this instrument with a reaming action (rotary cutting motion).

The Hedstrom file has sharp flutes that cut aggressively and are finer and closer together, and spiral grooves that are cut into the shank (Figure 37-14). The dentist uses the file to make

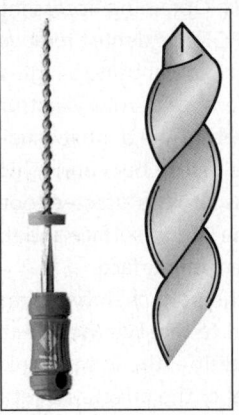

FIGURE 37-13
Reamer is used to clean, enlarge, and smooth the canal walls. Handles are color coded and numbered according to diameter. Also supplied with notched end used with an endodontic handpiece.

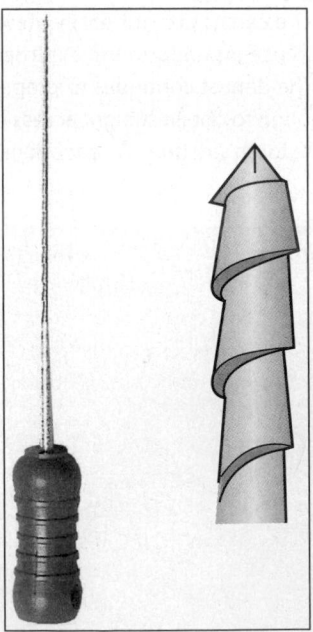

FIGURE 37-14
Hedstrom file removes necrotic tissue, scrapes, widens, and smooths the wall of the canal. Also supplied with notched end used with an endodontic handpiece.

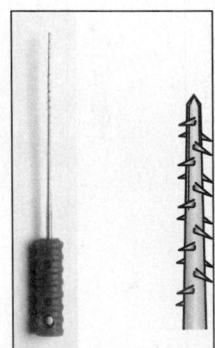

FIGURE 37-12
Barbed broach used to remove soft tissue from the pulp canal. Supplied in various diameters.

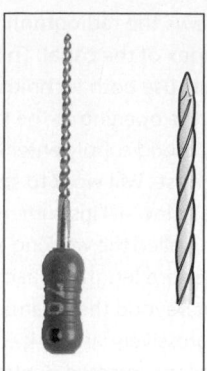

FIGURE 37-15
K-type file removes necrotic tissue and scrapes and widens the wall of the canal. Also supplied with notched end used with an endodontic handpiece.

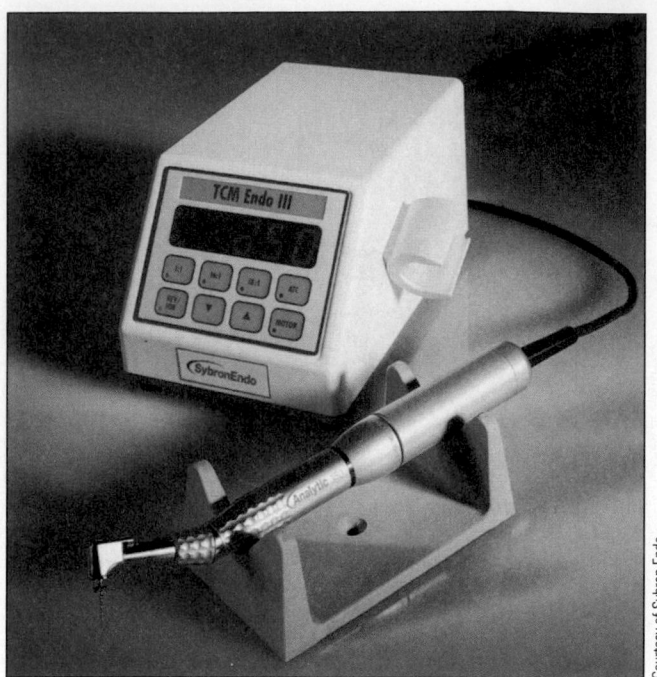

Courtesy of Sybron Endo

a smoother, finer cut of the dentin and to shape the root canal. The canal structure is cut using a filing action (scraping or pulling stroke). The color-coded handle of the Hedstrom file has the identification symbol of a circle for easy recognition as well as the file number. The Hedstrom files are also referred to as H-type files.

The K-type file has a working-end shank that is more flexible with near right-angle flutes with a tightly twisted design. The dentist can ream or file the canals with these files using a twisting motion. The K-type files, reamers, and Hedstrom files all have corresponding sizes. The identification symbol for the K-type file is a square for easy recognition. The size of the file is also written on the color-coded handle (Figure 37-15).

Flex files are another group of files that are crafted for optimal flexibility, strength, and sharpness. They are used to negotiate curved and narrow canals. The identification symbol for the flex file is a square. They are supplied with a notched end to be used with an endodontic handpiece.

Power-assisted instruments provide mechanical movement of root canal cutting instruments using an endodontic handpiece (Figure 37-16). The various intracanal instruments are available for use in a low-speed handpiece; a shank that is inserted into the handpiece allows these intracanal instruments to be used as rotary instruments in the canal of a tooth. The dentist uses sonic and ultrasonically activated endodontic low-speed handpieces in conjunction with the intracanal instruments.

An endodontic bender can be used to carefully bend the intracanal instruments, pluggers, and spreaders to conform to the shape of the root canal.

An endodontic organizer is used for the arrangement of reamers and files according to size and length (Figure 37-17). The organizer generally has holes to hold the intracanal instruments vertically in a sponge saturated in a disinfectant. When the intracanal hand files are moved in and out of the sponge, the debris from within the root canal(s) is removed and caught within the sponge.

Determining Working Length   The location of the end of the canal and the final working length are also determined during the debridement step. Finding the length of the canal is an important

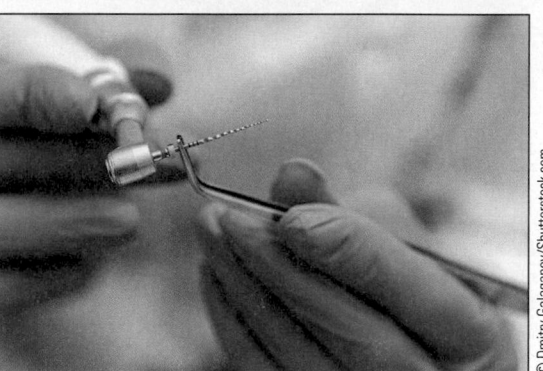

© Dmitry Galaganov/Shutterstock.com

FIGURE 37-16
Endodontic handpiece used with reamers and files to clean and enlarge the root canal. Intracanal instruments should be inserted using endodontic locking pliers to prevent contamination.

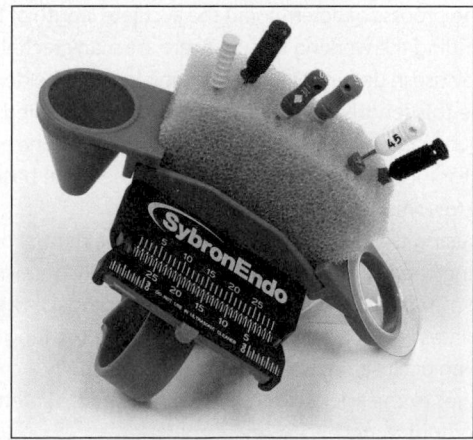

FIGURE 37-17
Endodontic organizer stores and organizes reamers and files. Many organizers have disposable sponges in order to use a new sponge with each patient.

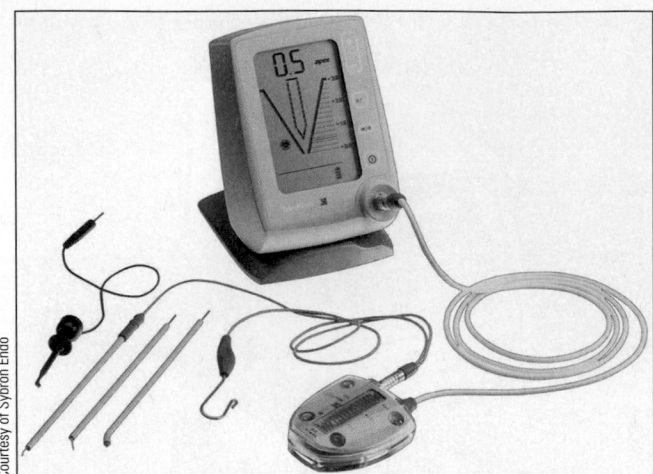

Courtesy of Sybron Endo

FIGURE 37-18
Apex locator used to locate the apex of the tooth and display the information on a digital readout.

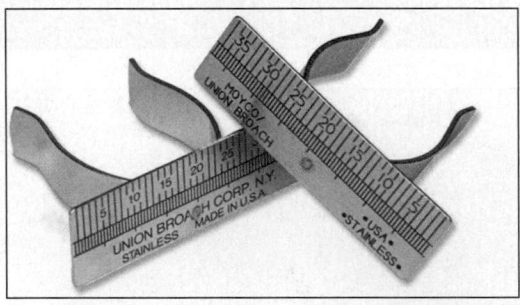

FIGURE 37-19
Millimeter ruler marked in 0.5 mm with a finger clip for ease in measuring the estimated length on the radiograph.

step to ensure that the canal is ultimately not obturated too short or too long. If the canal is filled too short of the anatomical apex, the bacteria-infected tissue may be left in the canal. In contrast, using a file that is too long may penetrate the apex and push bacteria into the surrounding periapical tissues and cause more irritation for the patient. The process of determining the accurate length of the canal is called finding the working length. There are many techniques the dentist may use in determining the working length. The dentist may determine this length by using an electric device called an apex locator or the radiographic technique (Figure 37-18). The electronic apex locator locates the apex or bottom of the canal based on its resistance to a small electric current.

When using the radiographic technique, the dentist begins by establishing the estimated length. This is usually determined by using the initial radiograph taken during diagnosis. The dentist uses a stainless steel metal ruler and measures the length of the root from an occlusal/incisal reference point (usually a cusp tip or incisal edge) to the apex (Figure 37-19). This is also referred to as the radiographic length.

A smaller sized hand file is set to this estimated length using a rubber stopper referred to as the test file (Figure 37-20). The dentist places the test file in the canal with the stopper at the reference point and takes a second radiograph with the file in place in

the canal. The dentist views the radiograph to make certain the end of the file is at the apex of the canal. This is the "true length" of the canal. Many dentists use both techniques.

The apical foramen is the opening at the location of the tips of the root where nerve and blood supply enter the tooth and supply the dental pulp. Most dentists will work to shape the canal 1 mm short of this point. All the intracanal instruments used in the procedure are set to this length, called the working length (Figure 37-21). It is important that the entire length of each of the tooth's root canals is cleaned, but not beyond the foramen opening. The dentist continues to use progressively larger sized files to increase the diameter of the canal until the infected dentin is removed and the canal is shaped. The last file used is the "master file."

The assistant needs to record the final file size and length for each canal receiving root canal therapy. Teeth generally have one main canal per root, but the number of individual canals can vary. Some roots will have a second root canal, referred to as an **accessory** canal. The principal canal is given number 1, and additional canals start with number 2. For example, one of the maxillary molar roots is the mesiobuccal root (MBR). If it has two canals, it is recorded as MBR1 and MBR2. This information is also important for determining the cost of the RCT procedure. The fee for an RCT can be expensive as it is determined not only by the

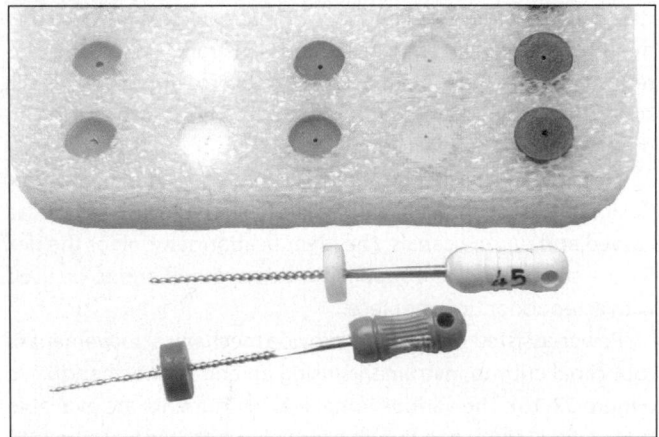

FIGURE 37-20
Endodontic measuring stops (rubber stoppers) are round or square pieces of rubber placed on reamers and files to mark the length of the root canal.

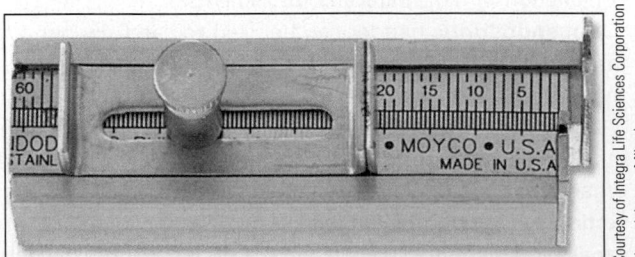

Courtesy of Integra Life Sciences Corporation (through Integra Miltex)

FIGURE 37-21
Millimeter-measuring device for the placement of rubber stoppers on intracanal instruments. The measurement can be locked in, the rubber stopper is placed in the device, and the intracanal instrument is inserted through the rubber stopper until the tip of the instrument touches the preset measurement.

treatment but also by the number of canals and difficulty of the procedure.

The dentist shapes the canal using a reaming and filing motion up to the predetermined working length. Reaming is a continuous clockwise rotation of the instruments to enlarge and shape the canal. When filing, the dentist moves the instrument in and out to refine and shape the canal. Intracanal hand files are manipulated in the dentist's fingers, and rotary instruments are placed in a low-speed handpiece. Endodontic handpieces hold the root canal instrument and vibrate vigorously.

Intracanal Solutions Intracanal solutions (sodium hypochlorite, EDTA, and sterile/distilled water) and irrigating syringes are used to rinse, remove debris, and disinfect the root canals (Figure 37-22). After the tooth is opened for endodontic treatment, only sterile solutions should be used to rinse or irrigate the tooth. The air/water syringe can only be used to rinse and dry the working area when the canals are still closed at the beginning of the RCT procedure and after the canals have been sealed at the end of the procedure.

A syringe is used to carry and place irrigating solutions into the root canal. The syringe tip is flat to place the solutions against the canal walls and not out the apical foramen. The dentist generally irrigates the canals:

- Before the use of intracanal instruments once pulp tissue is removed.
- At intervals during instrumentation, usually after each file size is used.
- At the completion of canal instrumentation and before placement of medication or prior to obturation.

While the dentist is shaping the canal, irrigating solutions are used to reduce the heat from the friction of the instruments against the dentin and to remove debris collecting in the canal. The dentist will need to periodically flush out (irrigate) the canal to help wash away accumulated debris and contaminants. Rotary files are rarely used in dry canals. The dentist irrigates the canal using a sterile syringe, or the dentist may choose to use an ultrasonic irrigating device. Care needs to be taken to not apply too much pressure when irrigating the canal. Too much pressure may cause solutions to exit the foramen, which may cause irritation and inflammation. Irrigation has an important role in preparing the canal, reducing the heat from the friction of instrumentation and making the treatment less traumatic for the patient and less stressful for the dentist during endodontic treatment. The main goal is to get the cleanest canal possible.

Irrigating solutions remove debris created during instrumentation and dissolve and/or flush out remnants of the pulp, dentin, bacteria, and bacterial by-products not removed by mechanical instrumentation. Diluted sodium hypochlorite is the solution most commonly used to remove as many contaminates as possible from the tooth's nerve space. It is an excellent disinfectant, tissue solvent, and lubricant.

Many of the irrigating solutions used in root canal therapy cannot come in contact with the oral mucosa as they are irritating to soft tissue. This can be prevented with a correctly placed dental dam, and also with the assistant using a surgical tip for suctioning during the irrigating procedure. A smaller surgical aspirating tip is preferred by many endodontists while irrigating canals. The slender size of the surgical tip allows for the dental assistant to remain in the pulp chamber while the endodontist is irrigating in the canal(s).

After the canals are irrigated, they are dried with sterile absorbent paper points shaped like the root canal (Figure 37-23). Paper points are held using endodontic cotton pliers and placed one at a time until the canal is dried. Several points are used to ensure the canal is dry. Endodontic cotton pliers resemble standard cotton pliers (Figure 37-24). They are available in locking and nonlocking designs. They have a grooved tip and allow for easy grasping of paper points as well as filling materials necessary

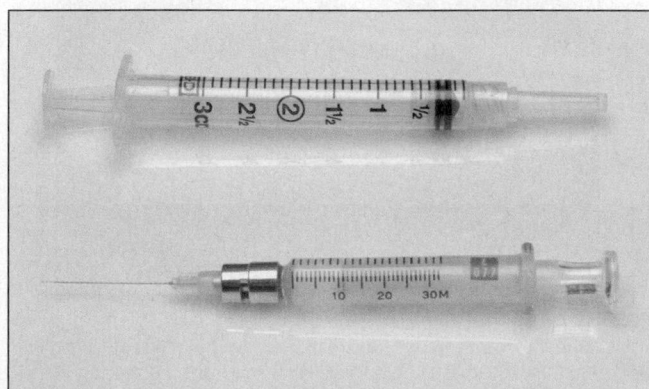

FIGURE 37-22
Endodontic irrigation syringe (Luer Lock syringe) is supplied as a disposable plastic syringe and as an autoclavable glass nonsterile syringe with disposable tips. The syringe is filled with an intracanal solution used to irrigate the root canal.

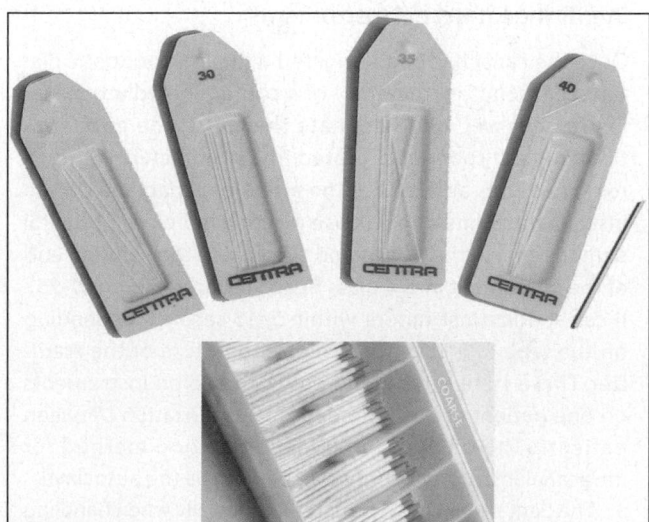

FIGURE 37-23
Absorbent paper points are supplied as sterile and nonsterile points in various sizes from x-fine to coarse to match the length and width of the canal. Some points are colored coded to match intracanal instruments.

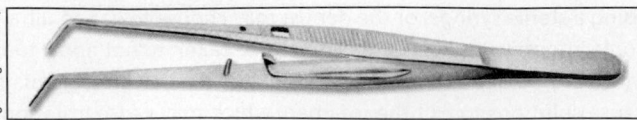

Courtesy of Integra Life Sciences Corporation (through Integra Miltex)

FIGURE 37-24
Endodontic locking pliers with grooved tips to better grasp absorbent paper points and endodontic intracanal instruments and material.

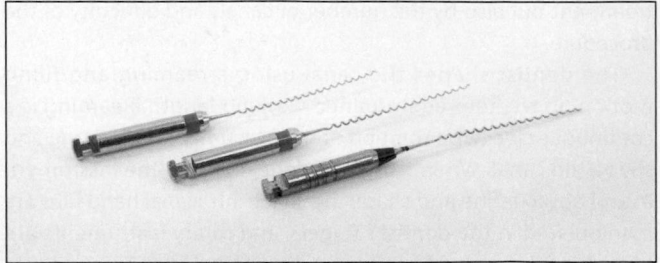

FIGURE 37-26
Lentulo spirals are used with low-speed handpieces and contra-angle attachments.

to complete the root canal. The locked design allows grasping of materials without the need for continuous finger pressure to keep the beaks closed. Most dentists have two pliers on the tray to allow multiple passing of instruments.

The dentist may trim the paper points with scissors to adjust the size to fit the canal. Sterile paper points and cotton pellets may also be used in placing medicaments into the root canals.

Intracanal Medication Once the canal is dry, most dentists prepare and fill the canal in one appointment. In some cases, however, the dentist temporarily seals the tooth to finish the procedure on another appointment. Whether the canals are obturated after a single-visit or multivisit treatment depends on the degree to which the tooth's root canal system harbors infection, the patient's pain level, the presence of swelling, and the number of canals involved. When the tooth is necrotic and has an active infection, multiple appointments may be necessary to place intracanal medications before the infection subsides and the dentist is able to fill the canals.

Intracanal medications are used to help reduce the presence of bacteria, preventing further infection and inflammation. If the infection is severe enough, dentists may require that the patient be placed on a course of antibiotics prior to obturation. This antibiotic therapy allows the concentration of the infection to be minimized and assists in reducing the inflammation. After access into the canals is made, an interim antimicrobial intracanal medication can be placed into the canal with a spiral filler, called a Lentulo spiral, attached to the low-speed handpiece (Figure 37-26). A sterile paper point or cotton pellet can be coated with the medication and placed into the canal as an alternative to using the rotary equipment. Intracanal medicaments include calcium hydroxide to reduce bacterial growth, corticosteroids to reduce inflammation and pain, and most recently chlorhexidine gel.

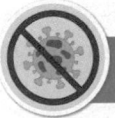 ## Infection Control

Sterilizing Intracanal Instruments

Once the canal has been irrigated with an endodontic disinfection solution, the entry of a contaminated intracanal instrument will recontaminate the canal. The endodontic organizer sponge saturated in a disinfectant helps to remove debris and reduce the amount of bacteria on the instrument. Some dentists use a quartered piece of dental dam to remove the debris and then place the working end of the instrument into a glass bead sterilizer (Figure 37-25). It can sterilize instrument within 5–15 seconds depending on the type of instrument and temperature of the sterilizer. These sterilizers should only be used on instruments on one patient and is not adequate sterilization between patients. The only acceptable sterilization method for intracanal instruments between patients is the autoclave.

The dental team must be careful especially when handling the very small and very sharp intracanal instruments. They should be transferred using the endodontic locking pliers and avoid transferring using your hands alone.

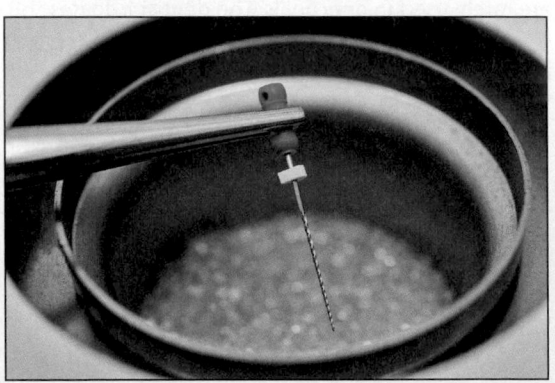

FIGURE 37-25
The chamber of the sterilizer is filled with glass beads 1 cm in size that heats up to 250°C (482°F) to 350°C (662°F). All intracanal instruments must be held with endodontic locking pliers to make certain hands do not come in contact with the chamber. Instruments should be free of loose debris before being placed into the beads. The beads should be replaced periodically (manufacturer's directions) and are supplied in bags.

© al7/Shutterstock.com

Endodontic Microscope The number of endodontists using an advanced endodontic microscope is increasing, and these tools are becoming an integral part of endodontic treatment (Figure 37-27). With these microscopes there is a variety of high levels of magnification, ranging from 23 to 203. There is also high-intensity illumination that adds brightness in a concentrated area and is designed to be shadow free. The microscopes come in many designs to meet the needs of different offices. They can be mounted on the wall or ceiling or can be on a base or stand.

The benefits for the dentist include the increased capability to find canals in teeth with difficult anatomies; the ability to see problems at an earlier stage; easier identification of tooth fractures; greater precision in techniques and thus fewer failures and need for retreatment; and greater success in completing more complex treatments, thus avoiding the need for surgery. The microscopes are ergonomically designed to allow the dentist to sit more upright and thus reduce neck and back strain. They are flexible and easy for the dentist to adjust. They are expensive and fragile, and care should be taken to follow manufacturer's directions closely.

Obturation of Root Canal After debridement, the pulp cavity is free of debris and ready to fill. The obturation procedure seals the dentinal tubules and fills the cavity. Obturation prevents contaminants from seeping back into the tooth from the periradicular area and recontaminating the canals. Even after the most diligent efforts at debridement, it is likely that some debris remains in the canal. The sealing process helps to ensure that contaminants still contained in the canal do not seep out to inflame the periradicular tissues.

During the obturation procedure, the dentist fills the canal with a permanent filling material to avoid bacterial growth and provide strength for the remaining tooth structure. The dentist uses materials and techniques capable of densely filling the entire root canal(s) and providing a tight seal from the apex to the floor of the pulp chamber, preventing reinfection.

The filling of the canal is primarily completed with gutta-percha, though **silver points** are sometimes used. Gutta-percha is a firm, rubberlike material that is able to precisely conform to the shape of the canal (Figure 37-28). It is made from a dried resin of the Taban tree and exists in two forms. Gutta-percha points are made in sizes corresponding to the endodontic files for filling

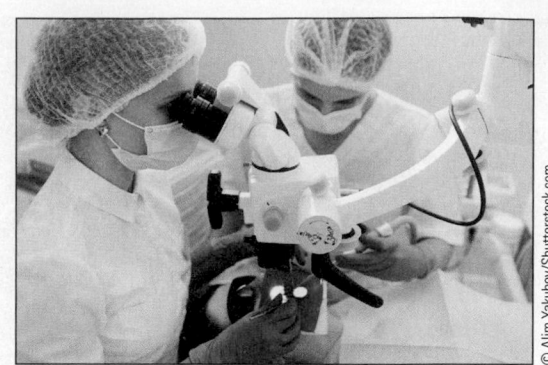

FIGURE 37-27
Endodontic microscope.

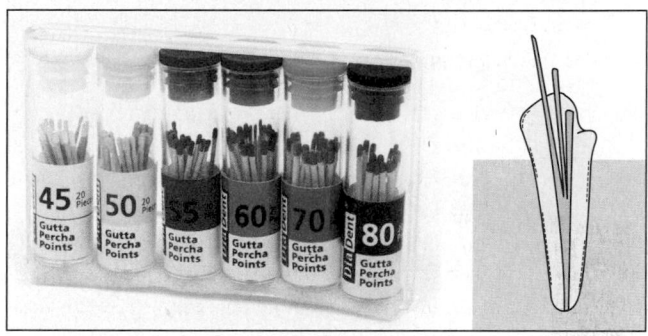

FIGURE 37-28
Gutta-percha points are cone shaped and are supplied in graduated sizes to match endodontic files. They are used to fill the root canal. The smallest sized gutta-percha are used as accessory points.

the root canal and gutta-percha sticks that are used in thermal testing and sealing the root canal openings.

Sealers are also required during the obturation process. There are three types of root canal sealers used in the obturation procedure: the eugenol, noneugenol, and medicated canal sealers. Sealers are used to seal the dentinal tubules, help the gutta-percha to adhere to the dentin, and make the gutta-percha cohesive with the surrounding auxiliary gutta-percha during the filling of the root canal. Sealers are available in paste, powder, and liquid form (Figure 37-29). The paste form is supplied as a base and catalyst in tubes. Equal amounts of the materials are placed on a supplied mixing pad and mixed to the manufacturer's directions.

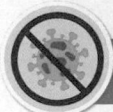 **Infection Control**

Periodontic maintenance and cleaning are required to produce high-contrast images. It is important to closely follow the microscope manufacturer's directions. Manufactured barriers for specific microscope types are available to protect from airborne contaminates. Debris can be removed using a small vacuum cleaner or by dabbing with a moist paper towel or gauze square. Several manufacturers supply oil-free compressed air cylinders for dusting the glass surfaces. Never blow off debris with air from the air/water syringe (most have moisture in the air), and do not attempt to blow off dust with a strong breath as saliva droplets will mix with dirt and produce an abrasive slurry. Use only cleaning solvents and disinfectants recommended by the microscope manufacturer, and never use facial tissues as they leave a residue.

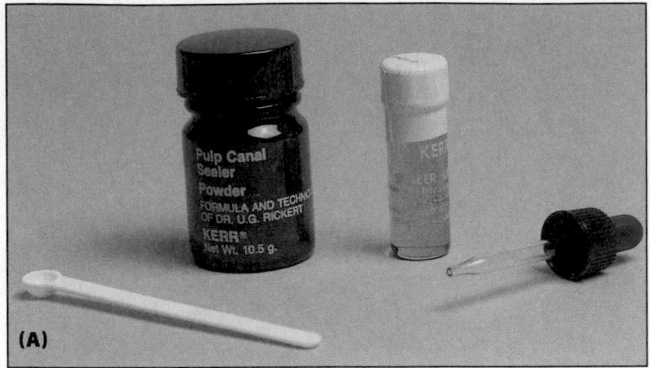

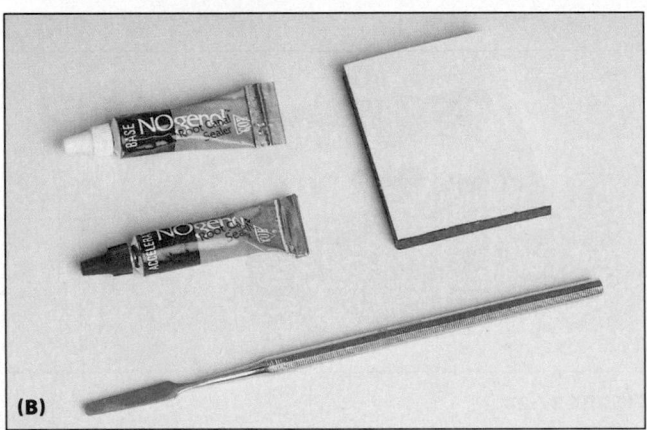

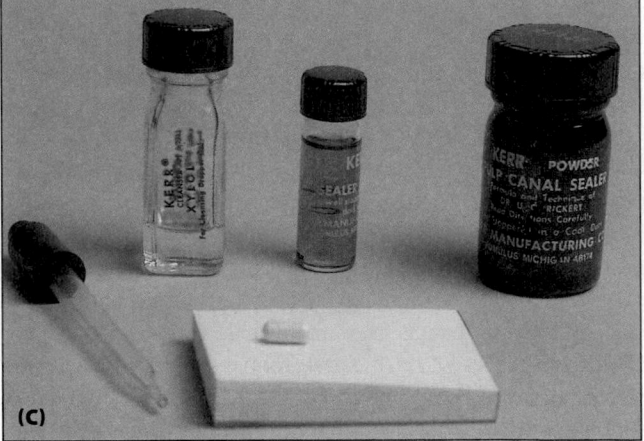

FIGURE 37-29
Root canal sealers. (A) Powder/liquid sealer. (B) Two-paste system.
(C) Capsules of powder and liquid sealer.

The paste form sealer is also manufactured as a paste, with no requirement of mixing by the assistant. The powder/liquid form is mixed on a sterile glass slab with a sterile spatula according to manufacturer's directions. Sealers are mixed to a homogeneous, thick, creamy consistency. The Lentulo spiral can be used in the low-speed handpiece to transport and place the sealer into the root canal before placement of the gutta-percha points.

Obturation Techniques   There are two common techniques used in placing the gutta-percha into the canals: cold lateral condensation and warm vertical condensation. Both of these techniques and their specific instruments are discussed in detail below.

Cold Lateral Condensation Technique   The dentist selects the master gutta-percha point which is the core-filling material and takes a radiograph with the point in the canal to verify the length as being correct. The master gutta-percha point is usually the same size as the master file (Figure 37-30). The master gutta-percha point is indicated as the gutta-percha point that is able to obtain the largest diameter of the canal; however, it also must be able to reach the apex of the tooth but not go past the apex.

Upon reading the radiograph, the master point can be cut to the working length of the master file to prevent overextension of filling material into the periapical tissues. With the proper sized master gutta-percha point in place, three or more **auxiliary** (accessory) points are cut to length and set aside for obturation. The accessory points are generally the smallest sized gutta-percha points. These points will be placed adjacent to the master gutta-percha point and laterally condensed into the canal.

Once all the gutta-percha points have been set aside, root canal sealer, usually available as a creamy paste material, is placed in the canal by the tip of the master gutta-percha point. The sealer is often placed on a disposable paper pad for use during the endodontic root canal therapy procedure. When a sufficient amount of sealer has been gathered on the master gutta-percha point by rolling the point in the sealer, the point is carefully placed into the canal using the endodontic locking pliers.

Once the master gutta-percha and the sealer are in place, the addition of the auxiliary points is continued until no other auxiliary points can fit into the canal. After each individual auxiliary gutta-percha point is placed, long handled or finger spreaders are used to laterally compact the cold gutta-percha points. The spreader is a long, tapered, pointed instrument that is used to compress gutta-percha into the prepared canals (Figure 37-31). There are several sizes available for the dentist to use corresponding to the canal size and the size of the gutta-percha points. The finger spreader has a short handle designed for insertion in posterior teeth. The spreaders condense the gutta-percha against the walls of the root canal to make space for the accessory points.

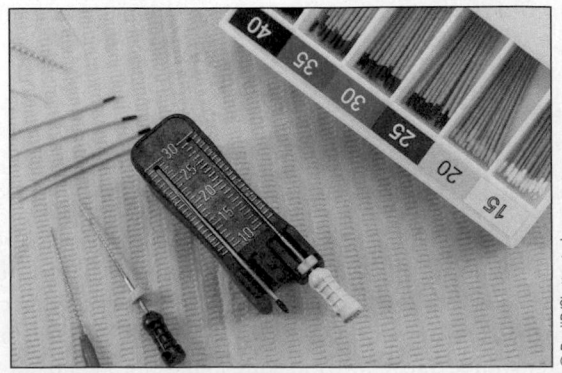

FIGURE 37-30
The master gutta-percha point is the same size and length as the master file.

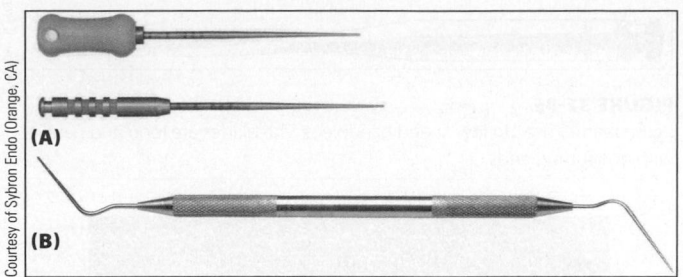

FIGURE 37-31
Endodontic spreaders. (A) Finger spreaders and low-speed attached spreader. (B) Long handle spreader.

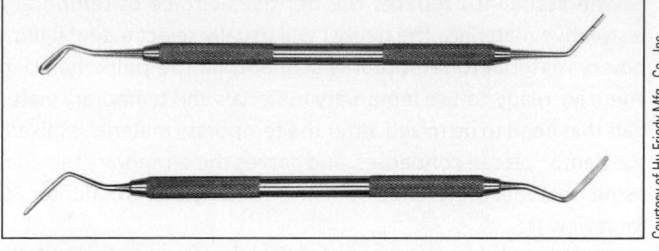

FIGURE 37-33
Glick endodontic instrument used to remove excess gutta-percha and condense gutta-percha in the canal opening.

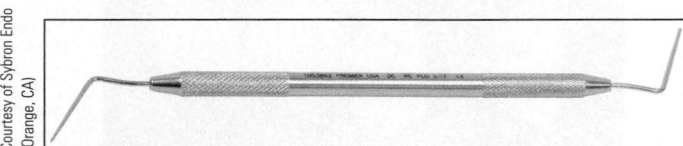

FIGURE 37-32
Endodontic pluggers available in various sizes to fit into the canals.

Endodontic pluggers (condensers) are used to condense the gutta-percha to provide space for additional gutta-percha points (Figure 34-32). This process forces the master gutta-percha point and the auxiliary points to be condensed as one complete unit of gutta-percha filling material, which in turn completely fills the root canal.

Once the canal has been completely filled, the dentist may take a radiograph to verify that the canal is completely filled and contains no voids. Once the sealed canal is verified by viewing the processed radiograph, the dentist removes the excess gutta-percha to the level of the canal orifice. This portion of the procedure is accomplished by the dentist using the heated paddle end of an instrument, generally a Glick endodontic instrument, to melt the gutta-percha (Figure 37-33). The portion of the gutta-percha extending into the area of the pulp chamber is melted and adheres to the heated end of the instrument. The dental assistant can be readied with wet cotton gauze 2 × 2 pad to assist in the removal of this excess gutta-percha from the dentist's instrument. Care must be taken in doing so, as the end of the instrument can be very hot. Using the condensing end of the Glick instrument, the remaining gutta-percha is condensed in the canal opening.

The accesses at the apex and crown must be well sealed to prevent recontamination of the canal. However, the gutta-percha should not extend beyond the apex of the root(s) as this can result in complications such as pain and infection post-procedure. The dentist takes a final periapical radiograph of the filled canal for the patient's records.

Warm Vertical Condensation Technique A source is needed to apply heat to the gutta-percha filling material. A special unit designed to heat the gutta-percha also has an applicator to deliver the heated gutta-percha directly into the root canal

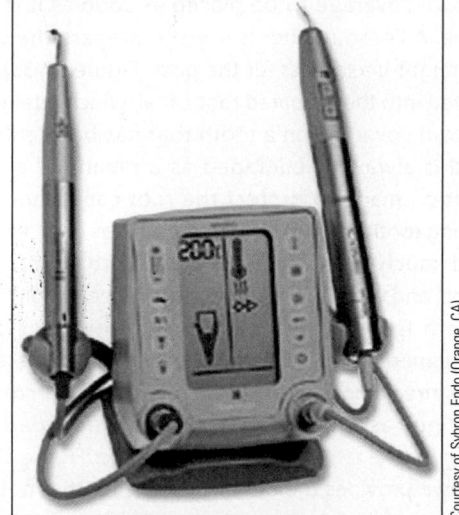

FIGURE 37-34
Gutta-percha obturation system softens the gutta-percha before placing it in the canal. It has temperature control to adjust the viscosity of the gutta-percha.

(Figure 37-34). Special heat carriers/pluggers are designed with one end pointed to allow the dentist to use lateral condensation and a flat tip for vertical compaction.

When using this technique, gutta-percha material is preheated and injected directly into the root canal(s). The root canal sealer is placed in the canal before the injection of the gutta-percha. This can be accomplished by the use of a Lentulo spiral attached to a low-speed handpiece. With the working length established, heat source systems are used to preheat the gutta-percha prior to its injection. The gutta-percha is vertically pressed into the root canal using heat carrier/pluggers for warm lateral and vertical condensation.

Temporary Restoration A temporary restoration is placed to restore the tooth to its original form and function until a permanent restoration is placed. An adequate coronal filling or restoration must be placed to prevent oral bacterial microleakage. The patient must be cautioned to protect against breaking the temporary and come into the office immediately if the temporary is compromised.

The assistant prepares the dentist's choice of temporary restorative materials. The dentist will usually select a dental temporary material to temporarily seal and fill the pulp chamber. There are ready-to-use temporary materials and temporary materials that need to be mixed. After the temporary material is mixed, the dentist places, condenses, and carves the temporary material using personal preference of instruments. (Refer to Chapter 30 for review.)

The dental dam is removed and the occlusion is carefully examined by the dentist to make certain there is no pressure against the newly endodontically treated tooth.

Permanent Restoration The endodontist will refer the patient back to the general dentist for a post and core and full-crown coverage to be placed as soon as it is reasonably possible. A Peeso reamer is used to prepare the canal orifice for a straight-line access for the post (Figure 37-35). The post is cemented into the prepared root canal, which retains the crown. Full-crown coverage on a tooth that has been endodontically treated is always encouraged as a means of a final dental restoration made to protect the root canal therapy and the remaining tooth structure. After a tooth has been endodontically treated, much of the inner, coronal tooth structure has been removed, and it is in a weakened state. Once the pulp is removed, the tooth is left without a source of nutrient or moisture replenishment. The remaining tooth structure becomes brittle and will break more easily. Placement of a full-crown or cusp-protecting cast gold covering is recommended to provide strength for the remaining tooth structure (Figure 37-36). A full-cast crown provides the best seal. If the tooth is not adequately

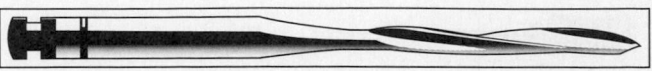

Courtesy of Premier Dental Products Company

FIGURE 37-35
Peeso reamer used in low-speed handpiece. The blades are long and parallel with noncutting ends.

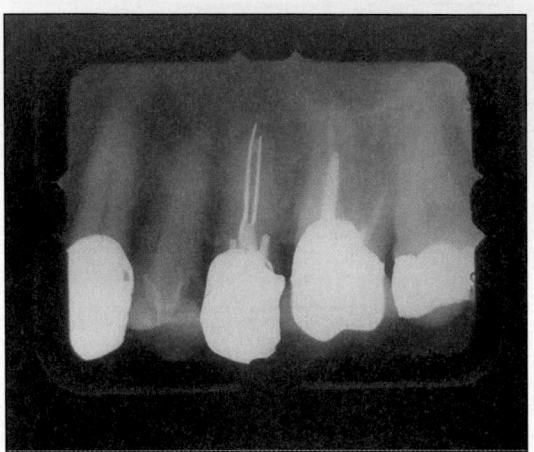

FIGURE 37-36
Radiograph of completed RCT, pins, and full-crown coverage.

sealed, microleakage may occur, causing eventual root canal therapy failure and requiring retreatment, an apicoectomy, and **retrograde** filling or an extraction. Although the tooth without pulp no longer feels pain, the tooth structure can still decay. Proper home care and regularly scheduled dental visits are vital to the longevity of the tooth that has received root canal therapy.

Procedure 37-2
Assist in Root Canal Therapy (Cold Lateral Condensation Technique)

Root canal treatment is usually completed in one appointment, but this varies depending on the degree of infection and the dentist's judgment. The dentist may decide to postpone filling the canal to allow more time to treat the infection. When this occurs, the canal is irrigated and sometimes medicated, and a temporary filling is placed in the coronal portion of the tooth at the first appointment. The patient is rescheduled for a continuation of the procedure at a second appointment. Procedure 37-2 is presented with the RCT being completed at one appointment, but the procedure is divided into two phases, debridement and obturation, which also mirrors how the two appointment RCTs would be performed.

Debridement Phase of RCT

During the RCT procedure, the assistant anticipates and transfers instruments and materials to the dentist, as indicated by the dentist. Smaller items are passed with the locking cotton pliers, for example, paper points, gutta-percha points, and cotton pellets. The assistant rinses and evacuates the area to keep a clear view of the oral cavity in which the assistant and dentist are working, and to prevent recontamination of the open pulp canals during the debridement phase of treatment. It is important that the assistant keep all irrigating syringes filled and ready for the dentist as needed. Radiographs, as required by the dentist, should also be taken by the assistant.

These may include radiographs to obtain a working length for the canal(s).

Steps written in **blue** font are performed by the operator (dentist or qualified dental assistant), and the chairside assistant's steps are written in black.

Equipment and Supplies

Patient Seating Setup (refer to Procedure 18-4)

RCT Debridement Tray Setup (Figure 37-37)

- mouth mirror (A)
- explorer (B)
- cotton pliers (C)
- endodontic explorer (D)
- endodontic spoon excavator (E)
- endodontic locking pliers (F)
- millimeter ruler (G)
- Glick endodontic instrument (H)
- anesthetic setup (I)
- sterile cotton supplies: cotton rolls, cotton pellets, and gauze squares (J)
- dental dam setup (K)
- high-speed handpiece (L)
- low-speed handpiece (M)
- bur block with assortment of burs (N)
- barbed broach, reamers, files with rubber stops in endodontic organizer (O)
- irrigating syringe and solution (P)
- sterile paper points package (Q)
- Gates-Glidden drills (R)
- temporary cement (S)

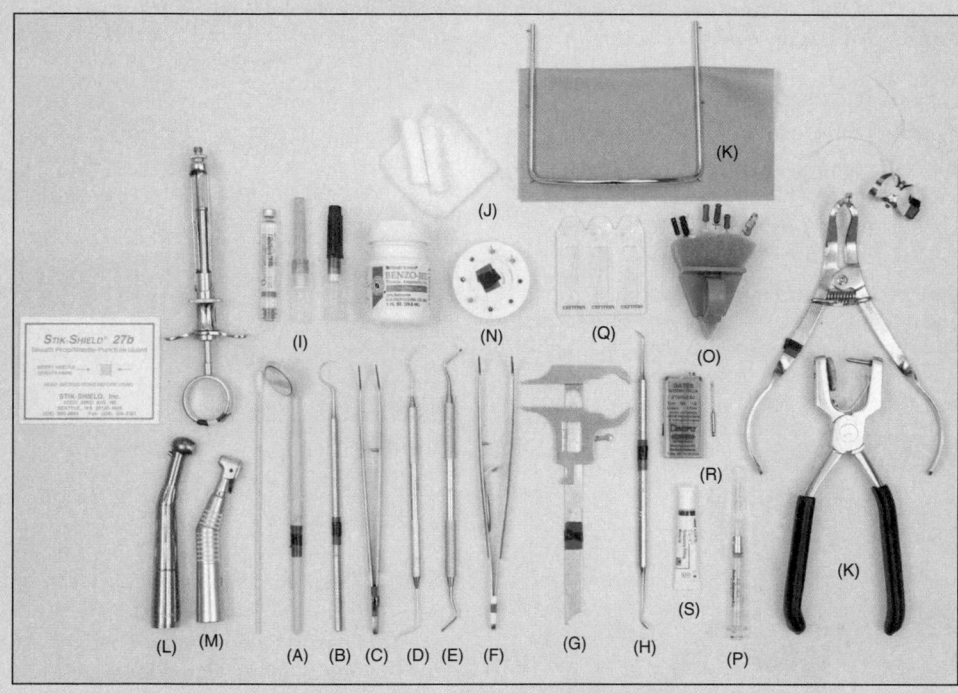

FIGURE 37-37
RCT debridement tray setup.

Procedure Steps

1. Escort and seat patient (refer to Procedure 18-4).

2. Prepare in advance for steps in cavity preparation procedure.
   - ❏ Open patient's chart in dental software.
   - ❏ Navigate to the dental charting screen.
   - ❏ Open patient's latest radiographic history on the computer monitor, or place on view box.
   - ❏ Attach handpieces to dental unit.
   - ❏ Insert burs into handpieces.
   - ❏ Inform dentist that the patient is ready.
   - ❏ Introduce dentist as they enter the treatment area.

   Dentist greets the patient and takes position at the dental chair.
   - ❏ **Signals for the procedure to begin (refer to Procedure 20-1).**

3. Pass mouth mirror and explorer at operator's signal.

   Dentist examines tooth or teeth with mirror and explorer.

   Dentist administers local anesthetic.

4. Assist in administration of local anesthetic (refer to Procedure 23-2).

   Operator places dental dam.

5. Assist in placement of dental dam (refer to Procedure 21-3).

(Continues)

6. Place disinfectant onto cotton tip applicator and wipe area to remove bacterial contaminants.

   Dentist gains access to root canals.

7. Assist with cavity preparation.
   - ❏ Prepare handpieces with dentist's choice of burs.
   - ❏ Use high-speed evacuation to remove water spray from high-speed handpiece.
   - ❏ Transfer endodontic explorer once pulp cavity has been accessed.
   - ❏ Pass Gates-Glidden drills in low-speed handpiece if dentist needs to open and flare the orifice to make better access to the root canal orifice.
   - ❏ Pass endodontic spoon excavator per dentist request to remove deep caries and pulp tissue.

   Dentist extirpates the pulp and necrotic tooth debris.

8. Assist in extirpation.
   - ❏ Transfer barbed broach.
   - ❏ Receive broach in gauze once pulp has been extirpated.
   - ❏ Dispose of broach in sharps container.
   - ❏ Transfer endo explorer to locate canals if needed.
   - ❏ Transfer irrigating syringe loaded with irrigating solution as needed and use high-speed evacuation while tooth is being irrigated. (Note: Air/water syringe cannot be used once the canals are open.)

   Dentist determines estimated length of canal using radiograph and millimeter ruler or electronic apex locator (Figure 37-38). (This procedure presents the radiographic technique.)

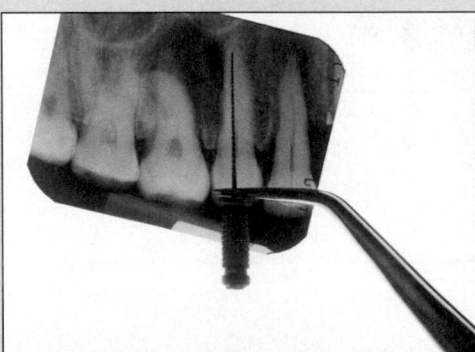

FIGURE 37-38
Measuring length of the root using a radiograph and test file.

9. Assist in determining working length of file.
   - ❏ Set small file to estimated length (referred to as test file).
   - ❏ Transfer test file for dentist to place into canal.
   - ❏ Prepare patient for dental x-ray; place lead apron on patient.
   - ❏ Expose radiograph and bring up on computer for dentist's viewing.
   - ❏ Place rubber stoppers on progressive sizes of reamers and files at determined working length.

   Dentist completes debridement of the pulp canals.

10. Assist in debridement.
    - ❏ Transfer reamers and files in progressive sizes until the canal is properly enlarged and refined.
    - ❏ Keep the files and reamers in order and free of debris; the dental dam is often used to remove debris from intracanal instruments as gauze squares will become entangled.
    - ❏ Record tooth number, canal name (as needed), file size, and file length, for example, #9 35 at 20 mm.
    - ❏ Assist in irrigating canals to remove debris (Figure 37-39).
    - ❏ Pass loaded syringe and suction while irrigating.
    - ❏ Pass small endodontic file per dentist request to rub irrigating solution against walls of canal to biochemically clean the root canals.

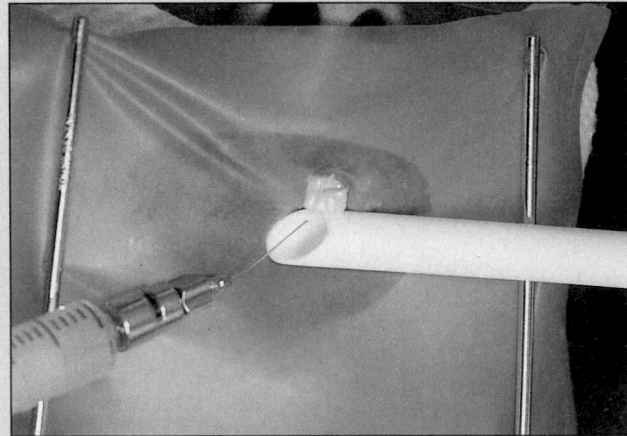

FIGURE 37-39
Irrigating the root canal.

- ❏ Pass absorbent points engaged in endodontic pliers to dry canal once debrided.
- ❏ Prepare for obturation when the canal is open and free of debris (Figure 37-40).

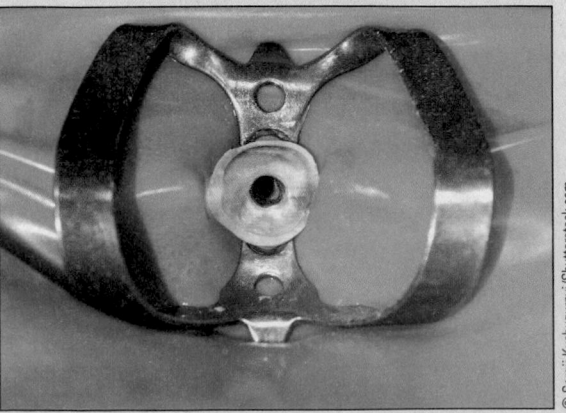

FIGURE 37-40
Tooth accessed exposing the pulp canal.

© Sergii Kuchugurnyi/Shutterstock.com

Note at this point in the RCT, the dentist may decide a second appointment needs to be scheduled.

❏ Assist in placement of intracanal medication as needed.

❏ Prepare the temporary restorative materials.

❏ Assist the dentist in placement of temporary.

❏ Remove the dental dam and dismiss the patient.

Obturation Phase of RCT

Radiographs are taken periodically throughout the procedure for the dentist to evaluate the progress. Once the canal is adequately enlarged and free of disease, it is permanently filled to prevent debris, fluids, and bacteria from entering the canal. There are many materials and techniques available to fill the canal, but gutta-percha materials are most common.

If the obturation phase is being performed at a second appointment, the temporary is removed and the canal is flushed with irrigating solution to remove debris.

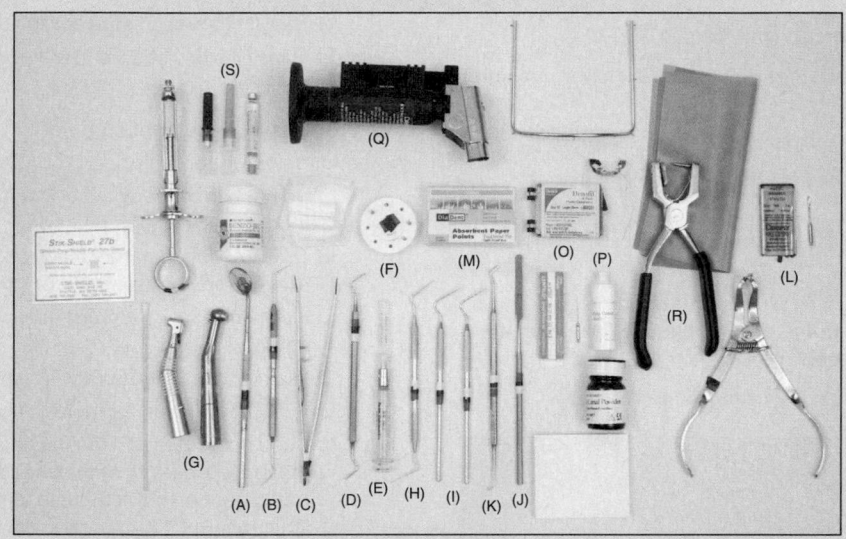

FIGURE 37-41
RCT obturation tray setup.

Equipment and Supplies

RCT Obturation Setup (Figure 37-41)

- mouth mirror (A)
- endodontic explorer (B)
- endodontic locking pliers (C)
- endodontic spoon excavator (D)
- irrigating syringe (E)
- bur block with assortment of burs (F)
- high-speed and low-speed handpieces (G)
- spreaders (H)
- pluggers (I)
- spatula (J)
- Glick instrument (K)
- Peeso reamers (L)
- absorbent sterile paper points (M)
- Lentulo spiral (N)
- gutta-percha (O)
- root canal sealer (P)
- heat source (Q)
- dental dam setup (R)
- anesthetic setup (S)
- temporary cement restoration setup (refer to Procedure 29-6)
    ❏ IRM powder (or dentist's choice of material), liquid, measurers, and manufacturer's directions

❏ cement spatula

❏ mixing paper pad or glass slab

❏ gauze squares

❏ IRM capsules and manufacturer's directions

❏ amalgamator

❏ plastic filling instrument

❏ assortment of carvers

❏ articulating paper in holder

❏ cotton pellets

Procedure Steps

Dentist selects a gutta-percha point as the master point.

1. Assist dentist in selection of master gutta-percha point.
    ❏ Pass gutta-percha point the same size as the master file and blunt the end.
    ❏ Trim point to last length of master file.
    ❏ Pass point with endodontic locking pliers.

Dentist places gutta–percha point into canal.

2. Expose and process radiograph with master point in the canal(s) to verify size and length.

Dentist places master point and auxiliary points.

(Continues)

3. Assist in placement of master point and auxiliary points.
- ❑ Mix intracanal sealing material.
- ❑ Roll master point in intracanal sealing material.
- ❑ Transfer master point in the direction of the working area, with endodontic forceps.
- ❑ Transfer spreader to condense points.
- ❑ Roll auxiliary gutta-percha points (usually smallest points) in sealing material.
- ❑ Pass one auxiliary gutta-percha point at a time, as needed, until the canal(s) is/are obturated.
- ❑ Follow each auxiliary gutta-percha point with the spreader to condense the material.

4. Expose final radiograph with filled RCT.

Dentist seals gutta-percha points over the canal opening once the canal is completely filled.

5. Assist in sealing the canal.
- ❑ Heat paddled end of Glick instrument or plugger in heat source.
- ❑ Pass heated plastic instrument to cut and seal gutta-percha points over the canal opening (Figure 37-42).
- ❑ Prepare to collect the cut excess gutta-percha from the heated instrument, using two 2 × 2 gauze squares, damp with alcohol.

Dentist places temporary restoration.

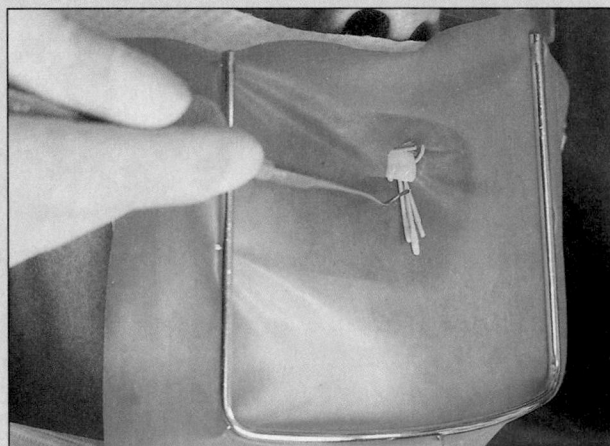

FIGURE 37-42
Root canal filled with gutta-percha points. The excess is being removed by the heated tip of the instrument.

6. Assist in placing temporary.
- ❑ Pass cotton pliers containing a large cotton pellet to be placed in the coronal portion of the tooth.
- ❑ Mix temporary material on glass slab.
- ❑ Pass plastic instrument.
- ❑ Hold glass slightly below patient's chin level.
- ❑ Hold gauze square to clean the instrument from excess while dentist places the temporary.
- ❑ Transfer condensers for dentist to condense material into cavity preparation.
- ❑ Transfer carvers for dentist to shape temporary restoration.
- ❑ Transfer dam clamp forceps to remove the dental dam.
- ❑ Transfer articulation paper in forceps to check occlusion.

7. Provide patient with postoperative instructions orally and in written form.
- ❑ Do not bite tongue or cheek or have very hot or hard food until anesthetic wears off.
- ❑ Take anti-inflammatory medication patient normally uses (ibuprofen, aspirin) prior to numbness wearing off.
- ❑ If pain increases, prescribe analgesic provided by dentist.
- ❑ Restrict to only light physical activity.
- ❑ Avoid chewing on temporary; chew on opposite side.
- ❑ Good home care and regular dental visits are important to the longevity of the endodontically treated tooth; decay can still occur in remaining tooth structure.
- ❑ Call office immediately if temporary filling feels high, disrupted, or lost; fever over 100°F (37°C); or pain and swelling increases.
- ❑ Return to the general dentist for the final restoration of the tooth.
- ❑ Follow-up radiographs may be taken at 6-month and 1-year intervals.

8. Write up procedure in Services Rendered.

9. Dismiss and escort patient to reception area (refer to Procedure 18-5).

Date	Services Rendered
02/18/XX	Updated medical and dental history, no changes noted. BP 120/80; T=98.6F, P=80, R=18, endodontic consent form signed
	Placed 20% benzocaine gel to injection sites for 2 minutes. Administered two cartridges (3.6 ml) of 2% lidocaine with 1:100,000 epi. No reaction
	POI do not bite on lip, no eating/drinking until numbness wears off, eat only on opposite side until numbness has worn off, take OTC anti-inflammatory meds and prescribed medications as directed, restrict to light physical activity first 24 hours, call office if restoration feels high, disrupted, or lost; if there is fever 100F +; or if pain or swelling increases.
#9	RCT cold lateral condensation technique; canal filed to a size file 35 at 20 mm, WL, MF, MP, and final radiograph exposed, IRM temporary placed
	Assistant's initials

Routine RCT Series of Radiographs

Assistant exposes multiple radiographs during root canal therapy. Below are radiographs included in a routine RCT series of radiographs:

1. Diagnostic periapical radiograph: Used to diagnose pulpal and periapical disease at initial appointment. Radiograph needs to show the entire periapical area. Also used to find the estimated length of the root canal.

2. Trial working length (TL) periapical radiograph: Trial (test) file is set at the estimated length and placed into the canal. The (TL) periapical radiograph is used to determine the true length of the root canal.

3. Working length (WL) periapical radiograph: Endodontic file is set 0.5–1.0 mm short of the major foramen to determine the length of file used to prevent penetration of apical foramen.

4. Master file periapical radiograph (MF): Shows the largest file used at WL to complete the root canal preparation. Final file size and length used.

5. Master gutta-percha point periapical radiograph (MP): Used to evaluate fit and length of gutta-percha point prior to placement. Point is final file size and length.

6. Initial condensation periapical radiograph: Evaluate fit and length after sealer is placed and two accessory gutta-percha points are placed. Also used with injection technique to evaluate the fill of apical portion of the canal.

7. Final periapical radiograph: Evaluate gutta-percha condensation of the root canal.

Endodontic Retreatment In most cases, teeth that have been treated endodontically will last as long as natural teeth. However, patients may continue to experience sensitivity to heat and pain in some teeth. This can happen immediately after treatment or years later. If the tooth fails to heal and the disease process continues or starts again, it can be retreated and have a second chance to heal.

Root canal treatment may fail for a variety of reasons:

● Abscess did not heal.

● Narrow or curved canals were not treated during first treatment.

● New decay forms along the filling material.

● Complicated canal anatomy, such as supplemental canals, went undetected.

● Restoration was not placed soon enough after treatment.

● Restoration became loose, cracked, or broken, and exposed the tooth to new infection.

If the patient feels pain and discomfort with a tooth that has had root canal treatment, they should return to the endodontist and discuss treatment options. The endodontist will reopen the tooth to gain access to the root canal. Since the entire pulp has been removed, the patient may not require a local anesthetic. This can be difficult to accomplish because the tooth may have a crown, post, and core material, and all of these have to be removed to permit access.

After removing the restorative materials, the endodontist can clean the canal and carefully examine the inside of the canal. After cleaning, the canal will be filled and sealed, and a temporary filling will be placed. The patient will then return to their general dentist for the final restoration, which may include a new post, core buildup, and crown.

Sometimes the endodontist may believe that the problem is at the apex of the tooth and will recommend an apicoectomy (a surgical endodontic procedure discussed later in this chapter).

Surgical Endodontic Procedures

An endodontic procedure is usually classified as surgical when the coronal entrance to the pulp is difficult to access. In addition, surgical endodontic procedures may be required when access to the necrotic pulp is not possible. Other reasons for resorting to a surgical endodontic procedure may be if the passage from the pulp to the canal(s) is blocked. This may occur due to sclerotic dentin, internal resorption, dilacerated roots, fractured roots, or extensive periapical involvement. Some surgical endodontic procedures may be necessary if decay is extensive and the diseased portion of the tooth needs to be removed, allowing the healthy portion to remain in place.

Apicoectomy and Retrograde Filling One of the most common endodontic surgical procedures is the **apicoectomy**. An apicoectomy is usually done when a root canal procedure has not been successful and an infection remains present at the apex of the previously endodontically treated root. If retreatment of the root canal procedure is not possible, an apicoectomy may be performed in order to remove the infection. A surgical opening into the gingiva (gingiva **flap**) is made, and the dentist drills through the alveolar bone to gain access to the root's apex (Figure 37-43). The apex of the root is surgically removed, and an **apical curettage** may be performed. This is where the diseased tissues are removed from the area by scraping with a **surgical curette**.

Retrograde surgery is a surgical procedure that is necessary when the apex, or root end, of a tooth is not sealed. The objective of root canal therapy is to place a filling material in the canals of the tooth, paying special attention to affirm that this material has met the junction of the apical foramen, or apex. In doing so, the endodontist can be assured that the very end of the root canal(s) has been sealed. Sealing of this area prevents bacteria, infection, and their nutrients from invading the remaining nonvital tooth.

Retrograde surgery is performed after a root canal has been completed, only if the apex of the tooth has been diagnosed as having pathology or can be seen on a dental radiograph as not being sealed and other more conservative treatment options may not be possible. Once the endodontist has gained access to the infected area via the surgical flap and removal of bone over the infected apex, the infection is removed. However, if for any reason the apical portion of the tooth being treated must be removed, an apicoectomy has been performed. In this case, an amalgam filling material is usually placed to seal the apical end of the root being treated. In many cases, the patient may not present with symptoms because the tooth has already received root canal therapy.

Additionally, a retrograde surgery may sometimes be necessary when the canal leading to the apex is blocked, preventing the intracanal instruments from reaching the apex. The dentist must then gain access through the apex.

Apical pulp extirpation and apical canal debridement are performed with instruments, with access through the alveolar bone, and into the apex. Occasionally, an apicoectomy is also performed and the area is filled with a dental material (often amalgam). Note: In most situations involving a tooth that has been endodontically treated, the retrograde procedure allows for the

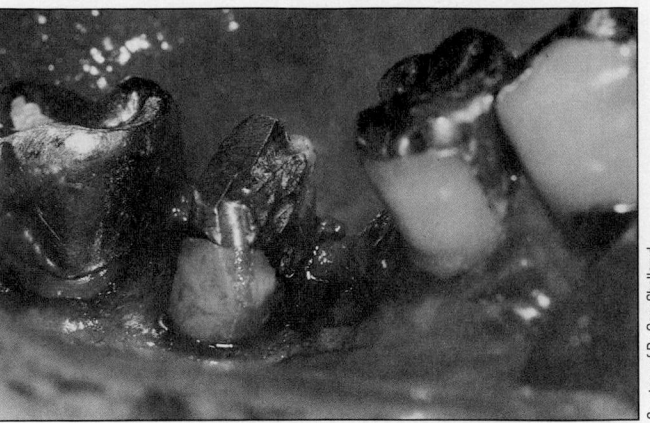

FIGURE 37-44
Hemisection on a mandibular first molar. One root and half the crown over the root are removed.

apical infection of the root canal treated tooth to be treated and sealed, in hopes of the tooth no longer being a source of infection. The retrograde procedure is primarily used to seal the apex, where it had not been sealed previously.

Apical Abscess Curettage The dentist must gain entrance to infected periapical tissues using the flap procedure when there is an apical abscess. The infected periapical tissues and exudate are removed using surgical curettes. The infection may require that an incision and drainage (I&D) be performed. This procedure is most often completed after other attempts of clearing up the infection have failed.

Tooth Hemisection Hemisection means "to cut in half." Therefore, a hemisection is completed when one-half of a tooth is removed. This usually refers to teeth that have two roots such as maxillary premolars or mandibular molars. The remaining half is restored as a single-rooted tooth and may be anchored to the adjacent teeth in order to provide greater stability (Figure 37-44).

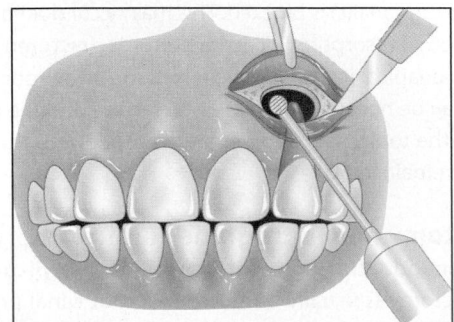

FIGURE 37-43
Apicoectomy.

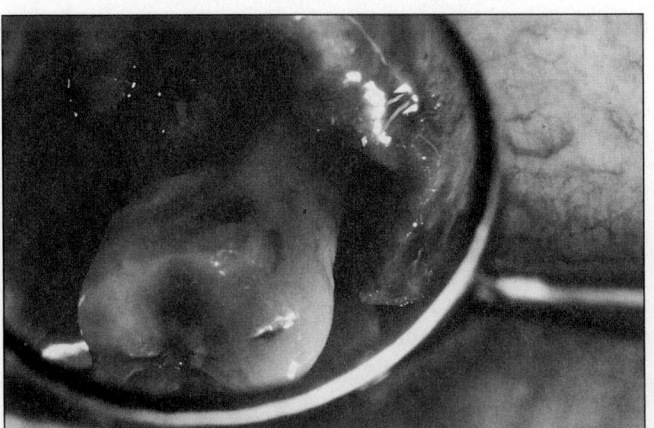

FIGURE 37-45
Root amputation on a mandibular first molar. The crown is saved, but the diseased root is surgically removed.

A hemisection may be performed when decay is affecting the **furcation** of a tooth or periodontal disease is affecting the furcation of a tooth. Multirooted teeth may also require root removal; this procedure is known as root amputation or root resection

Root Amputation (Resection) When a root of a multi-rooted tooth, generally the molar, cannot be debrided or obturated, this root may need to be **amputated**. Root amputation, also known as root **resection**, is completed on those teeth that have already been treated with root canal therapy; however, because of the inability to access one or more of the roots, the root canal therapy cannot be completed entirely. In order to be successful in the overall health of the tooth, removal of the unobturated root itself results in the removal of the source of infection present. One

key factor is the overall health condition of the tooth. The tooth should be solid with healthy bone support.

During a root amputation procedure, a flap procedure is initially performed, and the specified root is revealed and removed (Figure 37-45). The surgical field is cleansed, and the flap is surgically closed. Patients may need to be placed on a preventative antibiotic prescription to prevent infection of the area. The endodontist will require periodic visits to radiograph the healed area to confirm the establishment of ossification.

Traumatic Injuries Injuries including intrusions, extrusions, and avulsions may need to be referred to an endodontist for treatment to save the tooth or teeth. The description and treatment for these injuries are discussed in Chapter 30.

Chapter Summary

Endodontics comprises the diagnosis and treatment of pulp and periapical tissue diseases. Procedures include diagnosis, root canal treatment, and periapical surgery. The endodontist is assisted by dental assistants who perform traditional assisting responsibilities in addition to expanded duties specific to endodontics as allowed by state dental practice acts. Endodontic diagnosis includes patient medical and dental history; clinical examination, including pulp testing; and review of communication if the patient is sent from a referring dentist.

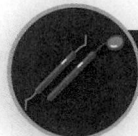

CASE STUDY

Gerald Frank, age 67, had an appointment with Dr. Chu for examination of his mandibular right side. He has been experiencing sharp, continual pain, and it often keeps him up at night. Upon examination, Dr. Chu suspects that the mandibular first molar is causing Mr. Frank's problem.

Case Study Review

1. What are the key indications for treatment?

2. What diagnostic tests may be performed?

3. Identify a possible diagnosis and treatment.

4. What are the basic steps in completing this procedure?

Review Questions

Multiple Choice

1. Which part of the tooth is the opening at the end of the root?
   a. radicular pulp
   b. apex
   c. apical foramen
   d. pulp horn

2. The portion of the pulp located in the apical third for the root is the _____.
   a. pulp chamber
   b. pulp canal
   c. radicular pulp
   d. pulp horns

3. If pulpitis is caused by accidently touching the pulp with a rotary instrument, it is referred to as what?
   a. impact trauma
   b. occlusal attrition
   c. tertiary
   d. iatrogenic

4. Which pulpal disease can return to a healthy state after the removal of an irritant?
   a. pulpal necrosis
   b. reversible pulpitis
   c. irreversible pulpitis
   d. acute pulpitis

5. Which pulpal disease is a true odontalgia with short, sharp, continual pain requiring RCT?
   a. pulpal necrosis
   b. reversible pulpitis
   c. irreversible pulpitis
   d. acute pulpitis

6. Which of the following diseases is a localized destruction of tissue and accumulation of exudates at the end of an infected tooth?
   a. periodontitis
   b. apical periodontitis
   c. osteomyelitis
   d. periapical abscess

7. What may occur when severe infection enters the tissue space, causing swelling?
   a. osteomyelitis
   b. periodontitis
   c. granuloma
   d. cellulitis

8. What is indicated when the patient experiences throbbing pain that persists after the removal of cold and hot stimulis?
   a. reversible pulpitis
   b. irreversible pulpitis
   c. necrotic pulp
   d. periradicular involvement

9. What can be used to test the vitality of the pulp by conducting a mild electrical current?
   a. gutta-percha stick heat test
   b. ethyl chloride cold test
   c. transillumination test
   d. electric pulp test

10. Nonsurgical procedures are performed in order to:
    a. stop the pulpal infection.
    b. maintain tooth vitality.
    c. prevent further pulp damage.
    d. All of these

11. What procedure is performed on permanent teeth to treat irreversible pulpitis when the apices are not fully developed?
    a. direct pulp cap
    b. indirect pulp cap
    c. pulpotomy
    d. pulpectomy

12. During which step of the RCT procedure is the pulp tissue removed?
    a. access root canals
    b. extirpation
    c. debridement
    d. obturation

13. The root canals are filled during which step of the RCT procedure?
    a. access root canals
    b. extirpation
    c. debridement
    d. obturation

14. Which instrument grasps the pulp and removes it from the canal?
    a. barbed broach
    b. endodontic reamer
    c. endodontic file
    d. Peeso reamer

15. Which instrument has spiral grooves used to enlarge and smooth the root canals?
    a. barbed broach
    b. endodontic reamer
    c. endodontic file
    d. Peeso reamer

16. All of the following statements are true about endodontic retreatment EXCEPT:
    a. the patient does not feel pain and discomfort.
    b. the need for retreatment can occur immediately or years later.
    c. the endodontist will reopen the tooth to gain access to the root canal.
    d. the problem could be supplemental canals and/or unusual anatomy of the canal.

17. All of these are postoperative instructions provided the patient after RCT EXCEPT:
    a. takes anti-inflammatory medication.
    b. resumes normal physical activity.
    c. calls office if temporary is lost.
    d. avoids hot and hard food until anesthetic wears off.

18. In which of the following procedures are one root and the overlying crown surgically removed?
    a. hemisection
    b. root amputation
    c. pulpotomy
    d. apicoectomy

19. Which procedure is performed to gain access to the apex of the root canal?
    a. pulpotomy
    b. root canal treatment
    c. apicoectomy
    d. root amputation

20. What procedure is performed to fill the root canal when the root end cannot be sealed with the filling material?
    a. root resection
    b. apical curettage
    c. indirect pulp capping
    d. retrograde surgery

Critical Thinking

1. How would an assistant explain pulpotomy, pulpectomy, and root canal treatment to a patient?
2. Is anesthetic always administered for root canal treatment? Explain.
3. What is the difference between K-type files and Hedstrom files?

Key Terms

Term and Pronunciation	Meaning of Root and Word Parts	Definition
accessory (ak-**ses**-*uh*-ree)	**access** = a way or means of approach or entry **-ory** = something having a specified use	a relatively narrow tubular passage or channel
acute pulpitis (*uh*-**kyoot**) (puhlp-**ahy**-tis)	**acute** = sudden in nature and severe in intensity **pulp** = located in the center portion of a tooth, made up of living connective tissue and cells called odontoblasts **-itis** – inflammation of	the inflammation of the pulp that is sudden and severe in intensity
amputate (**am**-py*oo*-teyt)	**amputate** = to cut off	surgery to remove all or part of a structure
anti-inflammatory reaction (an-tee-in-**flam**-*uh*-tawr-ee) (ree-**ak**-sh*uh* n)	**anti-** = against **inflammation** = reaction of tissues to injurious agents **-ory** = something having a specified use **re-** = again, back **action** = something done or performed	defense mechanism of organism to protect from infection and injury
apexogenesis (ey-peks-oh-**jen**-*uh*-sis)	**apex(o)** = referring to the root tip **gen-** = origin, source **-esis** = action or process	procedure with reversible pulpitis leaving pulp in root to stimulate the process of development of the root end (apex)
apical curettage (**ey**-pi-k*uh* l) (ky*oo*r-i-**tahzh**)	**apex** = tip of root **-al** = pertaining to **curette** = scoop-shaped surgical instrument used to remove tissue **-age** = physical effort	endodontic surgical procedures for removing contents present inside a surgical cavity
apicoectomy (ey-pi-koh-**ek**-t*uh*-mee)	**apic/o-** = apex **-ectomy** = surgical incision	the surgical incision at the apex
auxiliary (awg-**zil**-yuh-ree)	**auxiliary** = additional, supplementary	used to supplement in function; for example, auxiliary points are used to supplement filling in the gaps in the root canal
biomechanically (bahy-oh-mi-**kan**-i-k*uh*l-ee)	**bio-** = biology, life **mechanical** = performed by use of machine/device **-ly** = having the quality of	applying mechanical laws to living structures; relationship between the biology of the structure and the physical influence of the dental restoration
cellulitis (sel-y*uh*-**lahy**-tis)	**cellul/o** = cell **-itis** = inflammation of	inflammation of cellular or connective tissue
chronic pulpitis (**kron**-ik) (puhlp-**ahy**-tis)	**chron/o** = time **-ic** = pertaining to **pulp** = located in the center portion of a tooth, made up of living connective tissue and cells called odontoblasts **-itis** – inflammation of	inflammation of the pulp chamber over an extended period of time which causes irreversible changes in the quality of the pulp tissue
cyst (sist)	**cyst** = a bladder, sac	abnormal lesion that is a closed, bladderlike sac of a thick-walled membrane formed in tissues containing semifluid matter

(Continues)

Term and Pronunciation	Meaning of Root and Word Parts	Definition
debridement (dih-**breed**-m*uh* nt)	**debride** =removal of dead/unhealthy tissue **-ment** = the action of	the medical removal of dead/unhealthy/defective tissue to improve the healing potential of the remaining healthy tissue
direct pulp cap (dih-**rekt**) (puhlp) (kap)	**direct** = immediate **pulp** = located in the center portion of a tooth **cap** = a covering	the process by which a dental material is placed immediately over an area of pulpal exposure, in hopes of the pulpal tissue being able to heal itself with the assistance of the medicated, direct pulp cap material
endodontia (en-doh-**don**-shee-*uh*)	**end(o)** = innermost, within **dont** = tooth **-ia** = a thing, condition	a term pertaining to the inner part of a tooth
endodontics (en-doh-**don**-tiks)	**end(o)-** = within **-odont** = having teeth **-ics** = indicating a science relating to a particular subject	the branch of dentistry which deals with the study and treatment of the dental pulp and periradicular area
extirpate (**ek**-ster-peyt)	**extirpate** = to remove or destroy totally	to remove by surgery; to remove or destroy completely
file (fahyl)	**file** = narrow tool of steel with ridges for reducing and smoothing surfaces	endodontic files are surgical instruments used to clean and shape the root canal
fistula (**fis**-choo-luh)	**fistula** = narrow passage or duct	a tract or passage between the periapical area of a tooth and the soft tissue or bone of the mouth, formed when abscess forces a path through the bone and gum into the mouth to allow pus to escape
flap (flap)	**flap** = to swing or sway back and forth loosely	a flat, thin piece of tissue, usually attached on one side, incised to open to underlying tissue
furcation (**fur**-keyt-sh*uh* n)	**furcate** = forked, branching **-ion** = denoting action or condition	the anatomical area where the roots divide on a multirooted tooth
granuloma (gran-yuh-**loh**-muh)	**grain** = a cellular or cytoplasmic particle **-ule** = denoting capsule **-oma** = tumor	a form of localized nodular of inflammatory cells found in tissues; abnormal formation of newly growing capillaries formed early in wound healing and repair
gutta-percha (**guht**-uh) (**purch**-ah)	**gutta** = a drop, form of a cone **gutta percha** = rubbery substance derived from milky sap of trees	plastic, rubber type of filling material used in endodontics
hemisection (hem-i-**sek-** sh*uh* n)	**hem/o-** =one half **sect/o-** = to cut **-tion** = a process	a surgical procedure of cutting a tooth with two roots in half
iatrogenic (ahy-a-tr*uh*-**jen**-ik)	**iatri/o** = physician/ medical treatment **gen/o** = produced by **-ic** = pertaining to	caused by medicine or treatment that was given to the patient
indirect pulp cap (in-d*uh*-**rekt**) (puhlp) (kap)	**indirect** = not immediate **pulp** = located in the center portion of a tooth **cap** = a covering	the process by which a dental material is placed in the prepared tooth cavity, even though the pulpal tissue has not been exposed; used to assist in the healing process of the dentin and to reduce possible sensitivity from the placement of a final restoration
intracanal (in-tr*uh*-kuh-**nal**)	**intra-** = within **canal** = channels through which nerves and blood vessels pass	instruments, solutions, or medicaments used inside the root canal
necrosis (n*uh*-**kroh**-sis)	**necr/o** = dead cells **-osis** = condition	pertaining to dead cells or tissues within the body
neoplasm (**nee**-*uh*-plaz-*uh* m)	**ne/o** – new **-plasm** = growth; formed substance	also known as tumors; neoplasms are either malignant (cancerous) or benign (not cancerous)
nonvital pulp (non-**vahyt**-l) (puhlp)	**non-** = not **vital** = relating to life **pulp** = innermost soft, fleshy part of the tooth	dead pulp; does not respond to electronic pulp testing or thermal testing
obturate (**ob**-t*uh*-reyt)	**obturate** = to stop up, close	to block the passage of; to close

Term and Pronunciation	Meaning of Root and Word Parts	Definition
occlusal attrition (*uh*-**kloo**-zh*uhl*) (*uh*-**trish**-uhn)	**occlude** = fitting together of teeth of the lower jaw with the corresponding teeth of the upper jaw **-al** = pertaining to **attrite** = worn by rubbing/friction **-ion** = denoting action or condition	the mechanical wearing away of the occlusal surfaces due to function or nonfunctional tooth-to-tooth contact; may result in pulpal disease
odontalgia (oh-don-**tal**-j*uh*)	**odont** = tooth **-algia** = pain	pain within a tooth; a true toothache
odontoblasts (oh-**don**-t*uh*-blast)	**odont** = tooth **blast** = an immature, embryonic stage in the development of cells of tissue	one of a layer of specialized cells lining the pulp cavity of a tooth; forms dentin
orifice (**awr**-uh-fis)	**orifice** = an opening; a mouthlike opening	an opening to a cavity or passage of the body
osteomyelitis (os-tee-oh-mahy-*uh*-**lahy**-tis)	**osteo** = bone **myel** = bone marrow **-itis** = inflammation	an inflammation of the bone and bone marrow, usually caused by bacterial infection
parulis (p*uh*-**roo**-lis)	**parulis** = gumboil	a small abscess on the gum; originating in an abscess in the pulp of a tooth
percussion (per-**kuhsh**-*uh*n)	**percuss/o** = tapping **-ion** = action; condition	an examination technique that involves tapping on the incisal or occlusal surface of a tooth to assess vitality
pulpectomy (puhl-**pek**-t*uh*-mee)	**pulp** = the soft tissue found within a tooth **-ectomy** = surgical excision	the removal of all or part of the pulp of a tooth
pulpitis (puhl-**pahy**-tis)	**pulp** = the soft tissue found within a tooth **-itis** = inflammation	inflammation of the dental pulp due to deep caries and trauma or during removal of caries
pulpotomy (puhl-**pot**-*uh*-mee)	**pulp** = the soft tissue within a tooth **-otomy** = process of cutting or making an incision	surgical removal of the coronal portion of the tooth
purulent exudate (**py**oo **r**-*uh*-luh nt) (**eks**-yoo-deyt)	**purul/o** = pus **-ent** = pertaining to **exud/o** = oozing fluid composed of pus **-ate** = composed of	an oozing fluid composed of pus
reamer (**ree**-mer)	**ream** = to enlarge to desired size **-er** = denoting action or process	an intracanal instrument with cutting edges nearly parallel to long axis of a twisting shaft; rotating reamer scrapes and enlarges the canal wall
resection (ri-**sek**-shuhn)	**resect** = surgery to cut out part of an organ or structure **-ion** = denoting action or condition	surgical removal of part or all of a tissue, structure, or organ; another term for root amputation
root canal therapy (root) (kuh-**nal**) (**ther**-*uh*-pee)	**root** = embedded portion of a tooth into bone **canal** = tubular passage or duct **therapy** = treatment of a disease	removal of the dental pulp and filling of the canal with a filling material
retrograde (**re**-truh-greyd)	**retro** = backward; behind **grade** = to change or blend something gradually; merge	in dentistry, the action of creating a small preparation at the end of the apex to be sealed with a restoration
sclerotic (skli-**rot**-ik)	**sclera** = hard membrane **-ic** = relating to	a hardening of a tissue or part from chronic inflammation and abnormal growth of fibrous tissue; an increase of connective tissue
silver point (**sil**-ver) (point)	**silver** = a very ductile malleable brilliant grayish-white element having the highest electrical and thermal conductivity of any metal **point** = a sharp or tapering end	a silver point may be used in place of a gutta-percha point in filling canals that have extreme bending

(Continues)

Term and Pronunciation	Meaning of Root and Word Parts	Definition
surgical curette (**sur**-ji-kuhl) (ky*oo*-**ret**)	**surg-** = surgeon or surgery **-ical** = having characteristics of **cure** = means of healing or restoring to health **-ette** = small	surgical instrument with a small scoop end for scraping or debriding tissue or debris
tertiary dentin (**tur**-shee-er-ee) (**den**-tn)	**tert-** = third, being one of three stages or parts **-ary** = pertaining to **dentin** = hard tissue forming the major portion of the tissue surrounding the pulp cavity	forms as a reaction to caries, wear, and fractures; protects pulp chamber against infection; includes reparative dentin or sclerotic dentin
transillumination (trans-i-**loo**-muh-ney-sh*uh*n)	**trans** = through, beyond **illumine** = light up **-ate** = denotes function	use of fiber-optic light transmission through tooth for diagnosis of tooth condition; primarily associated with caries and fracture diagnosis
vital pulp (**vahyt**-l) (puhlp)	**vital** = relating to life **pulp** = innermost soft, fleshy part of the tooth	an alive and healthy pulp

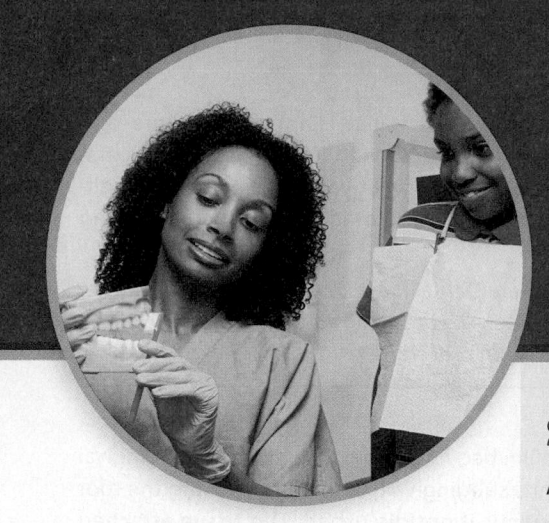

Periodontics

Specific Instructional Objectives

At the completion of this chapter, you will be able to meet these objectives:

1. Use terms presented in this chapter.
2. Discuss the role of the members of the periodontal team.
3. Define periodontal disease.
4. Identify the causes of periodontal disease.
5. Discuss the American Association of Periodontology (AAP) classifications of periodontal disease.
6. Describe the components of the periodontal examination.
7. Describe sharpening for periodontal instruments.
8. Describe the instruments used in periodontal treatment.
9. Discuss nonsurgical methods of periodontal surgery.
10. Compare and contrast the adjunctive therapies used in periodontal treatment.
11. Discuss the healing process related to nonsurgical periodontal procedures.
12. Compare and contrast the surgical periodontal methods.
13. Outline the postoperative instructions related to periodontal therapy.
14. State the purpose of periodontal dressings.
15. Compare and contrast the types of periodontal dressings.
16. Define periodontal maintenance.
17. Describe the role of the dental assistant in periodontal procedures.

Introduction

Periodontal disease is the inflammation of the soft and hard structures that support the teeth, known as the periodontium. Periodontal disease, if not managed and allowed to progress, can lead to tooth mobility and eventually tooth loss. The signs and symptoms of periodontal disease will be discussed later in this chapter.

Periodontics is a specialty that treats the supporting tissues of the teeth and the placement, maintenance, and treatment of dental implants. Nonsurgical periodontal therapy (NSPT) is often treated in a general dentistry practice. Periodontal patients who are medically compromised or in the advanced stages of the disease are often referred to a periodontist for therapy. A *periodontist* is a dentist who receives an extensive three years of specialty training in periodontics after completion of dental school. In many cases, the periodontist works closely with the patient's general dentist in collaborating treatment.

Management of the periodontal patient is a team effort. The periodontal team includes the periodontist, general dentist, dental assistants, dental hygienists, and business office staff.

- The periodontist coordinates treatment with the general dentist in the overall care of the patient. The periodontist screens the patient, performs the surgical care, and provides continual care according to the patient's needs.

- The dental assistant performs chairside assisting duties and expanded functions allowed by state dental practice acts, including placing and removing periodontal dressing, removing sutures, and performing coronal polishes. The dental assistant takes radiographs, takes impressions for study models, places sealants, and administers fluoride treatments. The dental assistant also gives pre- and postoperative instructions and prepares the treatment room for surgery. These functions are in addition to treatment room preparation and maintenance and sterilization procedures. The dental assistant is involved in educating and motivating the patient throughout the treatment. In some offices, the dental assistant may also perform laboratory tasks, such as pouring study models or making periodontal splints.

- The dental hygienist performs traditional hygiene procedures and, depending on the state Dental Practice Act, may also administer local anesthetic or perform gingival curettage. In a periodontal practice, the hygienist often sees patients who have more advanced periodontal disease; therefore, responsibilities include root planing and clinical examination procedures.

Periodontal Disease

Ancient human skulls demonstrate evidence of bone destruction associated with periodontal disease, and early civilizations had treatment methods such as using wire to tie loose teeth together. Periodontal diseases are the most common reason for tooth loss in adults. Periodontal disease occurs in children and adolescents with marginal gingivitis and gingival recession, which are the most prevalent conditions (Figure 38-1). The AAP has reported that approximately three out of four adults will experience some form of periodontal problem in their lifetime. Research demonstrates that there is a possible connection between periodontal disease and other systemic diseases such as cardiovascular disease. Periodontal disease involves the *periodontium,* which represents the tissues that support the teeth. The anatomy of the periodontium was discussed in Chapter 7. It is important to understand the anatomy of the periodontium in order to understand periodontal disease and its treatment.

Causes of Periodontal Disease

The most significant local irritant causing periodontal disease is dental plaque or biofilm. There are many different organisms in the oral cavity, with some having the ability to invade the periodontium and cause disease. These microorganisms adhere to the **pellicle** on a tooth and over time produce an extracellular slime layer that protects the multiplying microorganisms. The microcolonies that are produced are called biofilm or dental plaque. Dental biofilm begins forming around the supragingival margin and expands subgingivally and apically along the root surface into the sulcus if not disturbed. The tissue attached biofilm irritates the sulcus lining and causes ulcerations and inflammation (Figure 38-2). These ulcerations allow the bacteria in the biofilm to invade the blood vessels in the underlying connective tissue. The invasion of the bacteria into the body makes this tissue-attached biofilm the most detrimental. As the biofilm matures on the tooth, it can mineralize and appears as a yellow or brown deposit on the teeth called calculus (Figure 38-3). If the biofilm and calculus are not removed, then supragingival and subgingival accumulation of biofilm and calculus will develop on the teeth. Poor oral hygiene results in the buildup of biofilm and calculus. Failure to brush and floss daily can lead to plaque formation and debris buildup on the teeth and appliances. Proper brushing and flossing techniques are discussed in Chapter 16. Dental plaque or biofilm can be easily removed with proper brushing and flossing, but calculus (Figure 38-3) has to be removed professionally with hand and ultrasonic instruments.

Before 1985, researchers believed it was either biofilm or calculus that caused periodontal disease. In 1985, researchers discovered that it was an individual's (host) immune response to the biofilm accumulation around the periodontal tissues that causes periodontal disease. Currently, researchers believe that the main risk factor for periodontal disease is the host bacterial response. There are also contributory risk factors for periodontal disease.

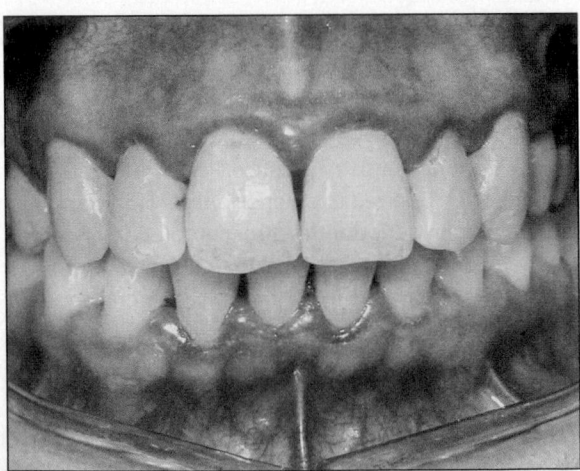

FIGURE 38-1
View of patient with mild gingivitis.

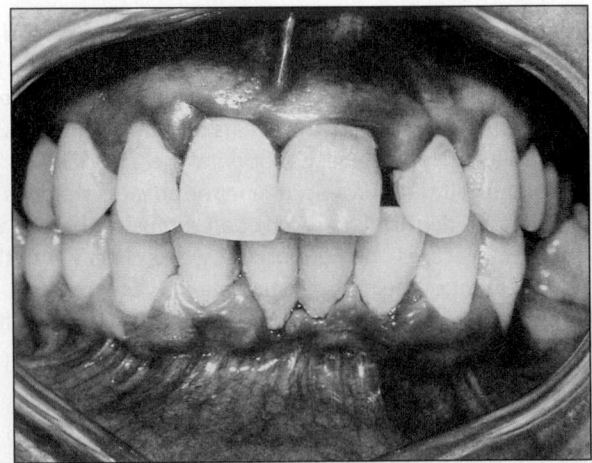

FIGURE 38-2
Unhealthy gingiva with inflammation.

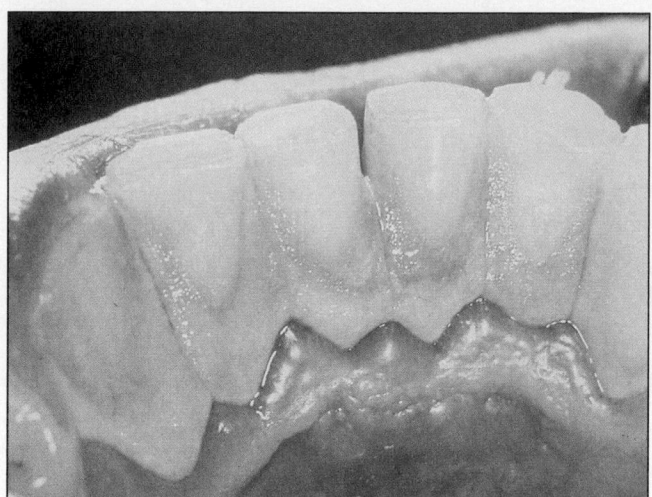

FIGURE 38-3
Unhealthy gingival tissues and lingual calculus.

Table 38-1 provides risk factors that can contribute to a person's susceptibility to periodontal disease and its progression.

Progression of Periodontal Disease

Periodontal disease begins as an inflammatory reaction to the accumulation of biofilm at the gingival margin if left undisturbed. Inflammation begins as the body's first line of defense to eliminate the bacteria to protect the body. The body's first line of defense is the white blood cells that seek to engulf the bacteria

in the sulcus. If the inflammation is not reduced by these white blood cells, the immune system uses additional systems against bacterial invaders to destroy the bacteria in order to protect the body.

Inflammation of the periodontium is divided into two categories: gingivitis and periodontitis. *Gingivitis* is inflammation of the gingival tissues (Figure 38-3). Gingivitis is usually caused by accumulation of biofilm along the gingival margin and the patient's response. *Periodontitis* is inflammation of the supporting structures of the periodontium, which includes the gingival tissues, periodontal ligament, bone, and cementum. The signs and symptoms of periodontal disease include swollen and bleeding gingiva, receding gingiva, mobile teeth that begin to have gaps between them, exudate between gingiva and teeth, ulcerations in the oral cavity, persistent bad breath, a change in the alignment of the teeth, or change in the way dentures and/or partials fit. Any of these symptoms can lead to further complications and eventual tooth loss if left untreated (Figure 38-4). Gingivitis does not always progress to periodontitis, but periodontitis always starts with gingivitis. Gingivitis is reversible with compliance in home care, but periodontitis is irreversible.

Classifications of Periodontal Disease

In 2018, the AAP revised the previous 1999 classification system. The AAP classification system now has four categories for periodontal disease. Each category also includes grading criteria such as direct evidence of bone loss and contributing risk factors. Table 38-2 provides the AAP classification of periodontal disease. Based on the AAP criteria, the quadrant or

TABLE 38-1 Risk Factors for Periodontal Disease

Risk Factor	Rationale
diabetes mellitus	Diabetic patients have a three times greater risk of periodontal disease because they have an altered healing response. These patients can have an increase in attachment and bone loss.
HIV/AIDS	HIV/AIDS patients have a reduced immune response, thereby making them at risk for periodontal disease.
local factors	Faulty restorations or crown margins, removable appliances, and orthodontic appliances can be risk factors for biofilm accumulation and periodontal disease.
malocclusion	Improper tooth alignment and occlusion can lead to biofilm and calculus formation in areas where food and debris are not removed easily.
medications	Some medications can cause xerostomia or gingival hyperplasia, which can cause an individual to be more prone to periodontal disease.
improper nutrition	A balanced diet is important in maintaining health, including oral health.
osteoporosis	Patients with osteoporosis have a greater risk of alveolar bone resorption, attachment loss, and tooth loss.
poor oral hygiene	Patients who exhibit poor oral hygiene are at greater risk for periodontal disease because their immune response may not be able to keep the bacteria from invading the body.
smoking	Smokers have a two times greater risk for periodontal disease because of the changes in the oral tissues that are produced. Smokers exhibit more bone loss, deeper pockets, host alterations, and alterations in the vascular system (constricted blood vessels). Because of this, a smoker's gingiva may appear pink and healthy because of the constriction of the blood vessels.
stress	Stress puts a person at risk for periodontal disease because it reduces the immune response in an individual.

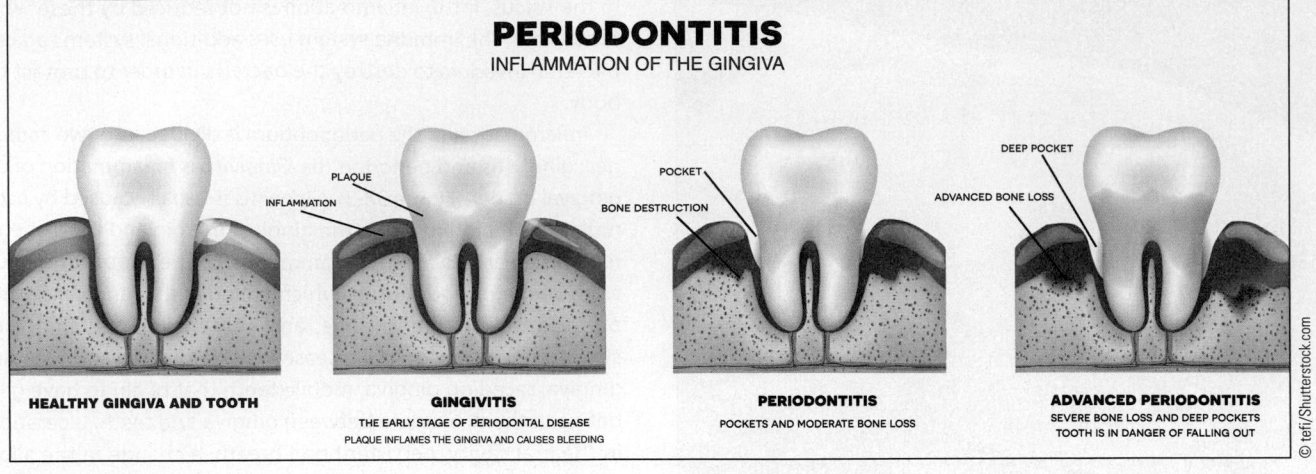

FIGURE 38-4
Progression of periodontitis.

TABLE 38-2 American Association of Periodontology Classification for Periodontal Disease

stage I (mild) periodontal disease	Probing depths of less than or equal to 4 mm, and a clinical attachment loss (CAL) of less than or equal to 2 mm. Good prognosis; no surgical therapies are needed.
stage II (moderate) periodontal disease	Probing depths of less than or equal to 5 mm, and CAL of less than or equal to 3–4 mm. Horizontal bone loss is present. Nonsurgical and surgical therapies are needed. Good prognosis; no tooth loss is expected. Patient will require maintenance follow-up care.
stage III (severe) periodontal disease	Probing depths of greater than or equal to 6 mm, and CAL of greater than or equal to 6 mm. Vertical bone loss may present along with class II or II furcation involvement. Surgical therapies will be needed. Possibility of loss of less than or equal to four teeth. Fair prognosis with maintenance therapy.
stage IV periodontal disease	Probing depths of greater than or equal to 6 mm, and CAL of greater than or equal to 6 mm. Less than 20 natural teeth may be remaining in the dentition. Possibility of loss of greater than or equal to five teeth. Prognosis is questionable with maintenance therapy. Patient will require care from multiple specialists.

sextant with the most severe condition determines the condition for the entire oral cavity. Table 29-9 provides information regarding radiographic appearance of bone loss in each stage of periodontal disease.

In addition to the staging criteria, there are grading criteria. Grading provides the possibility of progression of periodontal disease after treatment is completed. These include A (no or slow progression), B (moderate progression), or C (rapid progression). Risk factors such as current smoking status or a systemic disease such as diabetes are considered when grading. Only one grade is assigned to a patient.

Periodontal Examination

The first appointment with the periodontist is often an information-gathering appointment. After completing the medical and dental history, the patient is seated in the treatment room for an extraoral and intraoral examination. Radiographs and impressions are taken and a periodontal exam is completed. The exam includes biofilm and calculus deposit assessment, gingival examination,

periodontal probing, recession, bleeding assessment, discharge of pus or *suppuration*, tooth mobility, furcation involvement, and occlusal analysis. All these assessments are completed and used to determine a diagnosis and formulate an individualized periodontal treatment plan. Each of these will be discussed in this section.

Medical and Dental History

The medical and dental history gives the operator and the patient the opportunity to learn about each other. The operator gains information about why the patient is seeking treatment; if there is a systemic condition such as tuberculosis, HIV, AIDS, or diabetes; how the patient feels about their teeth; previous dental treatment; and if the patient has any oral habits that have contributed to the present condition. The patient has the opportunity to ask questions to the dental healthcare provider and gain an understanding of what is involved with periodontal treatment. The patient's history must be accurate and complete. A history checklist should open the way for significant conversation between the patient and the dental assistant, and dentist.

Sample Medical History Form The following types of questions should be answered by the patient:

1. Chief complaints

   ● Why did you come to the periodontist?

   ● Specifically, what area(s) of your mouth is (are) causing you concern?

   ● Do you currently have pain in or near your ears?

   ● Does any part of your mouth hurt when clenched?

   ● Are there any areas in your mouth that have unhealed or inflamed sores?

2. Medical history

   ● Are you ill at this time? If so, what is (are) your ailment(s)?

   ● Are you currently undergoing any medical treatment(s)? If so, what kind(s)?

   ● Are you taking any medication(s)? If so, what kind(s)?

   ● Have you ever had adverse responses to any type(s) of antibiotic? If so, what type(s)?

   ● Have you ever had adverse responses to any type(s) of anesthetic? If so, what type(s)?

   ● Are you pregnant?

   ● Are you allergic to anything?

   ● Do you have any of the following?

     · rheumatic fever

     · heart murmur

     · cardiovascular disease

     · hepatitis

     · kidney infection

     · tuberculosis

     · diabetes

     · AIDS

     · HIV

   ● Do you have, or have you ever had, problems with any of the following?

     · prolonged bleeding

     · allergies

     · oral symptoms related to pregnancy, menstruation, or menopause

   ● Do you have any oral conditions present? If so, how long have they been present, and has there been any treatment for them?

3. Oral history

   ● Have you had any extractions? Have you had any restorations?

   ● Do you have any problems after dental treatment, such as bleeding, pain, or swelling?

   ● Do you have any problems with your teeth, such as bleeding gums, pain, mobility, or sensitivity?

   ● Do you have difficulty with your joints when eating or opening and closing your mouth?

4. Oral habits

   ● Do you have any habits such as grinding, clenching, or mouth breathing?

   ● Do you smoke?

   ● Do you use alcohol or drugs?

5. Family history

   ● Does anyone in your family have a history of periodontal disease?

6. Oral hygiene

   ● Which brushing technique do you use?

   ● Do you floss? If so, how often?

   ● What type of toothbrush and toothpaste do you use?

   ● Do you use any other oral hygiene aids? If so, what kinds?

Clinical Examination

The clinical examination includes an extraoral examination of the face and neck; an intraoral examination of the tongue, palate, buccal mucosa, the teeth, and the oropharynx area; and the periodontal examination. Refer to Chapters 9 and 22 regarding completion of a clinical examination.

Periodontal Examination

The periodontal examination is a thorough examination of the periodontium using periodontal charts. The periodontal charts depict the condition of the patient's periodontal tissues. The charting is completed either manually or on a computer. The oral cavity is examined, and information is gathered by the dentist or hygienist while the dental assistant records the information on the periodontal chart (Figure 38-5). The periodontal exam includes several components.

Periodontal Risk Assessment In addition to the assessments mentioned discussed later in this section, a *periodontal risk assessment* may be prescribed to see if there is any additional information needed to aid in the periodontal treatment plan. The American Academy of Periodontology has an online questionnaire for periodontal risk assessment that can be completed with a patient during the initial visit. The results of the questionnaire can be printed and explained to the patient to help them better understand periodontal disease and aid in their successful treatment outcome.

Periodontal Screening and Recording (PSR) System Another method that is used to evaluate the periodontal health of a patient is the *periodontal screening and recording (PSR)* system. It was developed by the American Dental Association and

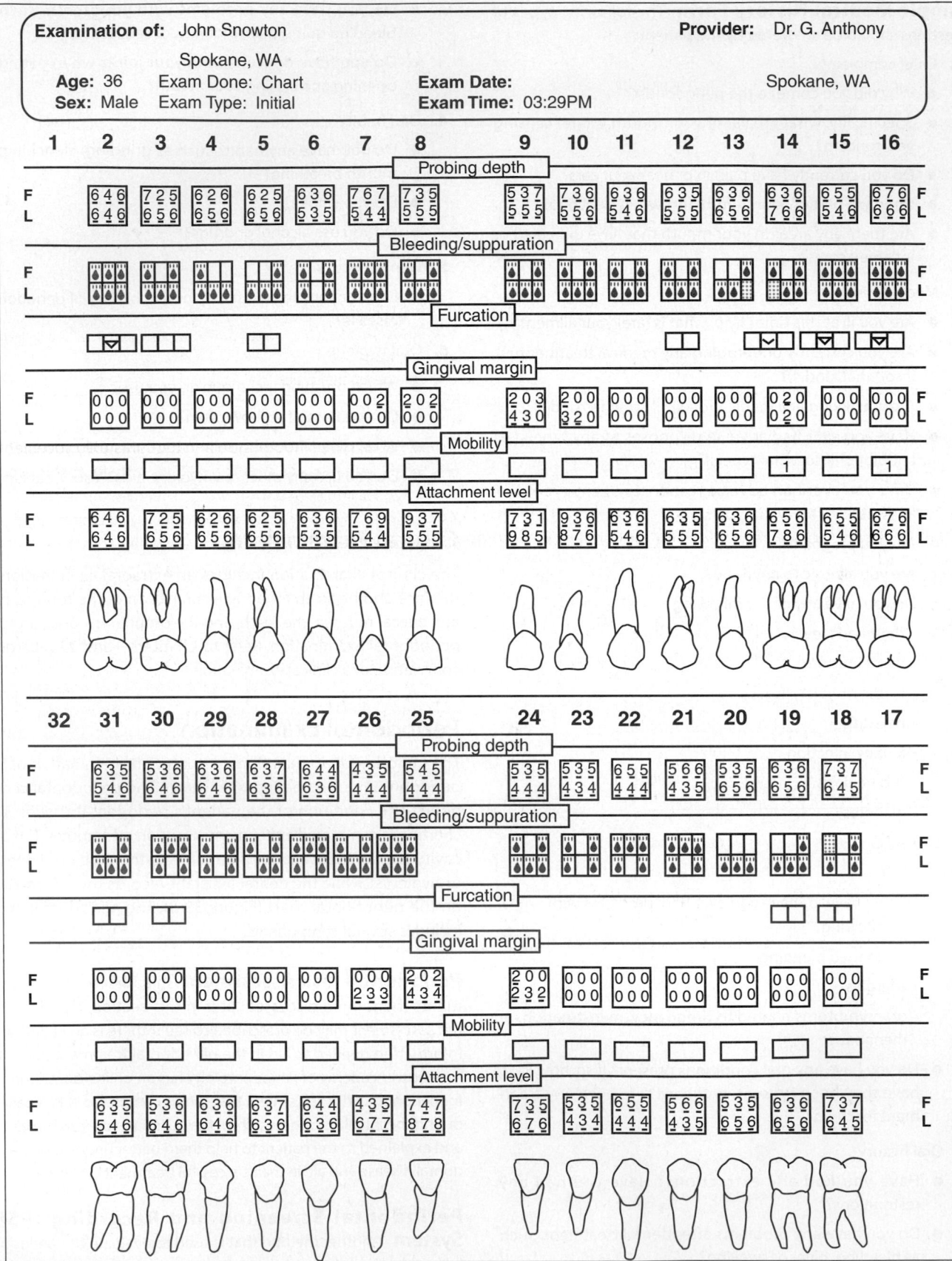

FIGURE 38-5

Periodontal chart includes probing depth, bleeding index, notation for any furcation involvement, level of gingival margin, tooth mobility, and the attachment level for both arches.

the American Academy of Periodontology. This system was designed to provide a simple, standardized system to effectively screen and provide for detection of periodontal disease. It allows the clinician to determine if a greater comprehensive evaluation is necessary. It is not meant to replace the traditional periodontal examination, but it does indicate when a partial or full periodontal evaluation is needed. It should be completed on every patient over the age of 18 annually.

The periodontal screening procedure involves dividing the mouth into sextant sections (three maxillary sections and three mandibular sections). The three sections include one anterior section and left and right posterior sections. A specially designed probe, which has a rounded tip and color-coded bands that extend from 3.5 to 5.5 mm on the shank of the probe, is used for this assessment (Figure 38-6). All six areas on each tooth are probed, but only the highest screening score in each sextant is recorded. The probe is used to assess the relationship of the gingival margin and the colored band.

Plaque and Calculus Assessment

The patient's oral hygiene is evaluated, and the amount of biofilm and calculus present is determined. Dental biofilm is invisible and requires a disclosing solution to reveal the amount of dental biofilm on the surfaces of the teeth. The plaque is documented on the surfaces of teeth, and the total teeth and surfaces are divided, giving a score known as a plaque index or plaque score. This evaluation includes both supragingival and subgingival deposits. These assessments help the dentist in designing and implementing personal home care instruction.

Periodontal Probing

The process of *periodontal probing* measures the depth of the *periodontal pocket* with a periodontal probe. A normal sulcus is 3 mm deep or less. When the depth is greater than 3 mm, it is termed a periodontal pocket. To determine the sulcus depth, six sites are probed and recorded on each tooth. There are three sites on the facial, including mesiofacial, midfacial, and distofacial, and three sites on the lingual, including mesiolingual, midlingual, and distolingual. The periodontal probe is inserted into the sulcus until the operator feels resistance (Figure 38-7). Tactile sensation indicates the level of the epithelium attachment. The calibrations on the probe measure the depth of the pocket. These are recorded on the chart.

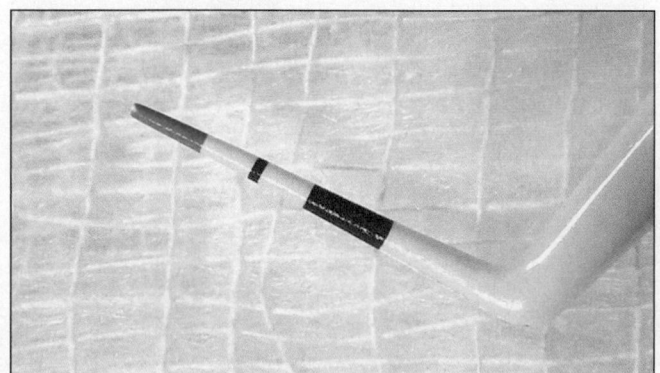

FIGURE 38-6
PSR color-coded probe.

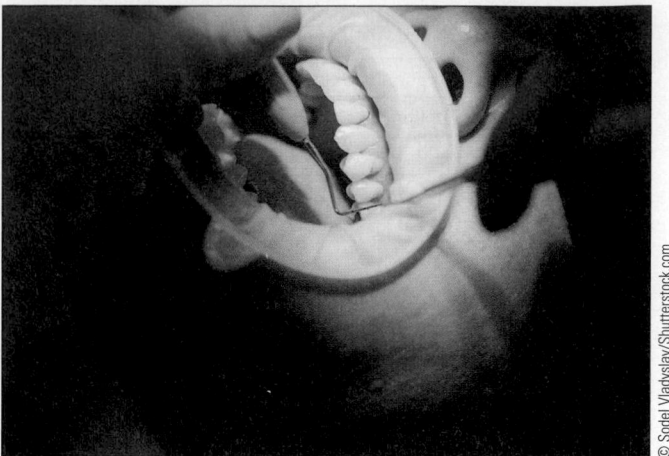

FIGURE 38-7
Using the periodontal probe.

Tooth Mobility

Tooth mobility measures the movement of the tooth within the alveolar bone. The mobility test is accomplished by pushing the tooth in a buccolingual direction using the handle ends of two instruments or by using the automatic device for assessing mobility. The amount of movement is measured in millimeters (mm) using the following scale: 0 (0 mm) is normal, 1 (1 mm) is slight, 2 (2 mm) is moderate, and 3 (3 mm) is severe.

Furcation

Molar teeth and some premolars have multiple roots and furcations between the roots. If the epithelial attachment detaches and migrates apically and/or recession occurs, the furcation of a tooth is exposed. Furcation involvement is noted on the periodontal chart in four different classifications according to their extent. Furcation is measured with a special periodontal probe called the Nabers probe. Each periodontal chart or computerized software system has a symbol for each of the four furcation classifications. Table 38-3 provides the furcation involvement classifications.

Gingival Evaluation

The appearance of the gingiva is evaluated in terms of color, consistency, contour/shape, and size. Gingival appearance is documented in order to determine the presence or absence of infection. Table 38-4 compares the description of gingival appearance between healthy and diseased gingiva.

Bleeding on Probing

The *bleeding index* involves recording the bleeding or suppuration, which is the amount of blood or fluid present during probing (Figure 38-8). It is a major indicator of inflamed gingiva.

Gingival Recession

Gingival recession can be a normal part of aging and should be assessed and documented at each appointment. Whenever recession is present, there is attachment loss of the junctional epithelium with resulting bone loss and exposure of the cementum of the roots (Figure 38-8). Recession can also occur with occlusal trauma, toothbrush abrasion, and oral habits. Recession is measured with a periodontal probe from the gingival margin to the CEJ.

TABLE 38-3 Glickman's Classification of Furcation Involvement

class I	Pocket formation into the beginning of the furcation, but the bone is intact in the furcation.
class II	Early loss of bone in the furcation; the explorer can reach the furcation but cannot pass through to the other side.
class III	Advanced loss of bone in the furcation; an explorer can pass completely through to the other side, but the gingiva is not receded.
class IV	Complete loss of bone in the furcation; the explorer passes through the furcation to the other side and can be seen clinically because of gingival recession

TABLE 38-4 Terms to Describe Gingival Appearance

	Healthy Gingiva	**Unhealthy Gingiva**
color	pink, light pink, pale pink	red, bright red, bluish red
consistency	firm, resilient	edematous, spongy, fibrotic
contour/shape	fills embrasures, follows contour of the teeth, knife-edged, pyramidal	blunted, recessed, punched out, swollen, rolled, cratered
size	fits snugly around the tooth	enlarged

Gingival Cleft The gingival cleft is a fissure or elongated opening that extends toward the root of the tooth. The margin of the gingival tissue forms a "V" instead of the smooth, rounded border, exposing the cementum covering the root (Figure 38-9).

Occlusal Evaluation A thorough *occlusal analysis* is performed by the dentist to determine if there are any occlusal discrepancies that are impacting the periodontium. Impressions are taken of the maxillary and mandibular teeth; models are poured and mounted on an articulator. The dentist obtains additional measurements so the models on the articulator mimic the occlusal relationship of the patient's teeth when closed. In doing this, the dentist is able to determine if the patient will need an occlusal adjustment in order to allow for proper dental occlusion.

Suppuration *Suppuration* or pus in the gingival sulcus assessed during periodontal probing is a clinical sign that infection is chronic. Suppuration indicates that the white blood cells have been fighting off the bacteria in the gingival sulcus for an extended period of time. Suppuration is indicated on the periodontal chart (see Figure 38-5).

Radiographic Survey A full mouth series of radiographs is taken at the initial periodontal examination (refer to Figure 28-36). Radiographs help the dentist assess the patient's periodontal health. They can determine the height of alveolar bone around the teeth. Bone levels are important to evaluate because in health the crest of the alveolar bone is about 1–1.5 mm apical to the CEJ (refer to Figure 28-36). In periodontal disease, bone loss or reduced bone levels are visible on a radiograph. The level of horizontal bone should be parallel to an imaginary line drawn from the CEJ on one tooth to the adjacent tooth. When a patient develops periodontal disease, there may be a loss of either horizontal or vertical bone or both. Refer to Chapter 29 regarding radiographic appearance of bone loss.

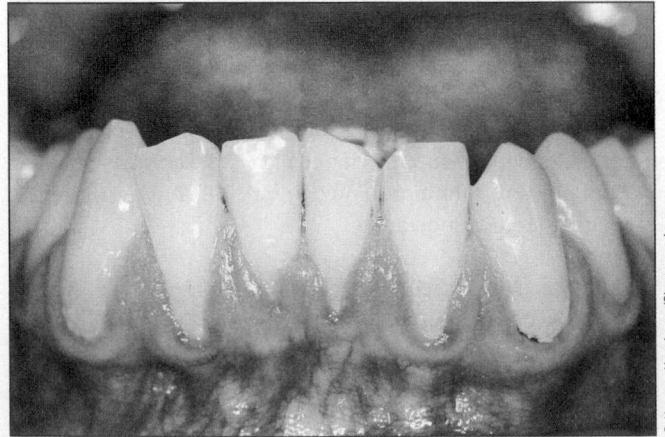

© Kasama Kanpittaya/Shutterstock.com

FIGURE 38-8
Bleeding on probing and gingival recession.

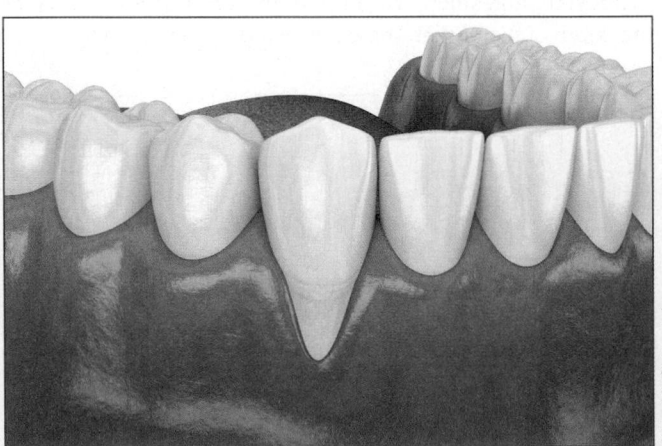

© Alex Mit/Shutterstock.com

FIGURE 38-9
Gingival cleft.

Presentation of Treatment Plan

After gathering all the periodontal diagnostic information, the periodontist determines the appropriate treatment plan for the patient. The patient is then scheduled for a consultation appointment. During this appointment, the prognosis (anticipated outcome) of the patient's condition and the treatment sequence are explained. Charts, radiographs, study models, and photographs are used to educate the patient. The patient's role in the treatment is discussed. The patient must be actively involved in the treatment and motivated to follow the home care plan and keep treatment appointments. The treatment may include nonsurgical and surgical methods. Once all questions are answered and the treatment plan is understood, appointments and financial arrangements are completed.

Chemotherapeutic Agents

In the treatment of periodontal disease, the periodontist mechanically removes dental biofilm and calculus from the tooth root surface. Most patients have an excellent response to this treatment, but for those patients who do not respond to the removal of dental deposits, or for those patients who have aggressive forms of periodontitis, the periodontist may also prescribe therapeutic agents, including antibiotics and nonsteroidal anti-inflammatory agents.

Some of the antibiotics commonly prescribed are penicillin or amoxicillin, tetracycline, erythromycin, and clindamycin. These are commonly administered between 5 and 14 days prior to surgical procedures. In nonsurgical periodontal therapy, which is normally from two to four appointments, at 1- or 2-week intervals, antibiotic therapy is provided during and after the periodontal treatments.

The anti-inflammatory drugs reduce the level of inflammation and are effective adjuncts in periodontal therapy. A few examples of the drugs administered include ibuprofen and acetylsalicylic acid (aspirin).

Periodontal Instruments

Periodontal instruments are designed to probe, scrape, file, and cut the hard surfaces of the teeth, alveolar bone, and soft tissues of the gingiva. These instruments must be kept sharp. Usually, the hygienist or a specially trained assistant is responsible for maintaining periodontal hand instruments.

Instrument Sharpening

There are many benefits of using properly sharpened instruments. Sharp edges make the operator's work easier and faster, improve the quality of procedures, and enhance patient comfort. After repeated use, the cutting edges of instruments become dull and rounded, making the blades less effective and more difficult to use. At this point, the operator applies more pressure and becomes fatigued more easily. The patient may feel the added pressure and discomfort.

There are manual and mechanical methods for sharpening periodontal instruments. Mechanical devices are more expensive, but they are effective and easy to use, and provide consistent, precision sharpening (Figure 38-10). These devices usually have sharpening guides that adjust for various instruments and mechanically rotating discs. Manually sharpening instruments involve using handheld sharpening stones (Figures 38-11A, B, and C). Sharpening stones are frequently used and are available in various shapes, sizes, and hardness (grits). Finer grits are often used to sharpen dental instruments because the finer grit (smaller particles) abrades metal slowly. There are several types of stones, including Arkansas stones, India oil stones, and ceramic stones.

Water is used with some of the stones as a lubricant; with some others, honing oil is used. Other types of oil are not used, because they may leave a residue that cannot be removed. The lubricant serves as a means for moving the metal particles of the instrument away from the blade and preventing them from becoming embedded in the stone. After use, the stones are thoroughly cleaned by scrubbing with a stiff brush, soap, and water, or they are cleaned ultrasonically. The stones are then sterilized properly.

There are many techniques for sharpening dental instruments; some use geometric concepts and terms, while others use the "telling time" approach. The latter technique uses the face of a clock for orientation and positioning. With this method, the instrument is held stationary and the stone moves. The elbow is positioned on a stable surface with the hand upright. The end of the instrument to be sharpened is held downward in one hand, toward the wrist; the other hand holds and moves the sharpening stone against the instrument (Figure 38-11C). The positioning and technique of sharpening dental instruments requires additional information and training. It is a skill that takes time and practice, but it is extremely valuable to dentists and hygienists using these instruments.

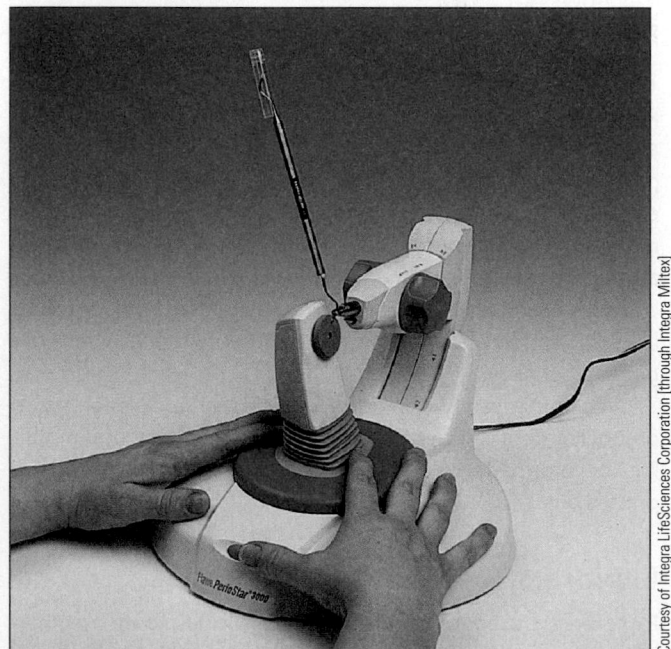

FIGURE 38-10
Mechanical sharpening device.

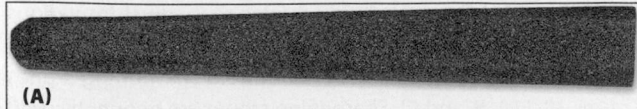

(A)

(B)

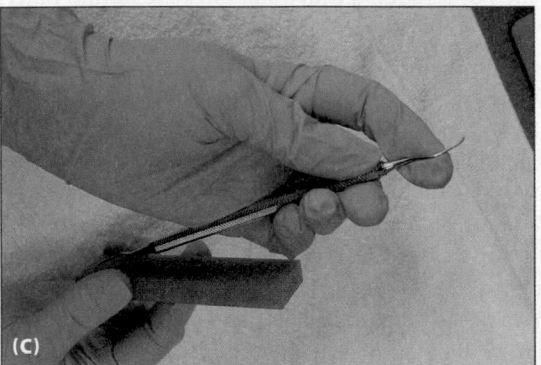

(C)

FIGURE 38-11
(A) Arkansas cylindrical dental instrument sharpening stone. (B) Arkansas thick wedge dental instrument sharpening stone. (C) Correct grasp and position when sharpening a dental instrument using the Arkansas stone.

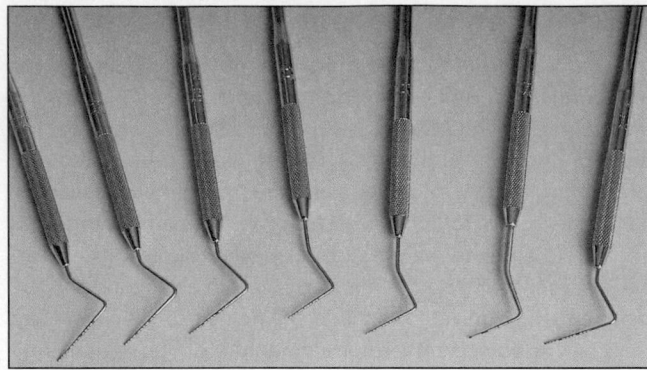

FIGURE 38-12
Varied periodontal probes.

Periodontal Probes

The *periodontal probe* is the primary instrument used in the periodontal examination (Figure 38-12). This is a calibrated instrument used to measure the depth of periodontal pockets. The probe is also used to measure areas of recession, bleeding, or exudate. The calibrations on the periodontal probe are in millimeters and vary depending on the manufacturer and the operator's preference. These markings may be indentations or color coded for easy reading. The probe may be flat, oval, or round in cross section but must be thin enough to fit easily into the gingival sulcus.

A computerized probe system detects and stores information on pocket depth, recession, furcation involvement, and mobility. The information is shown on a computer screen and can be printed out.

Explorers

Explorers are used to detect and locate calculus, tooth irregularities, faulty margins on restorations, and furcation involvement. The explorer gives the operator the best tactile information for assessment. The explorers used in periodontics are supplied in a variety of shapes, similar to those also used in general dental procedures (Figure 38-13). The working ends are thin and sharp. They may be curved or at near right angles to adapt to the curves of the tooth surfaces.

Curettes

The *curette* is a hand instrument used for removing subgingival calculus, smoothing the root surface, and removing the soft tissue lining of the periodontal pocket (Figure 38-14). The working end has a cutting edge on one or both sides of the blade, and the end is rounded, not pointed like the scaler (Figure 38-15). The curette is an instrument that is designed to adapt to the curves of the root surfaces (Figure 38-15). There are two basic curettes: *universal curettes*, which are used throughout the oral cavity, and *Gracey curettes*, which are supplied in a set of several instruments that are designed and angled to be used in specific areas. The curette handles are similar to those on the scalers.

Scalers

A *scaler* is a sharp hand instrument that is used to remove hard deposits such as *supragingival* (above the gingiva) and *subgingival* (below the gingiva) calculus from the teeth. Scalers are supplied in a variety of shapes and angulations to access all surfaces of the teeth. The working end of a scaler has two sharp edges that come to a point (Figure 38-16). The handles are often large and are ribbed, serrated, or knurled. Sometimes, the metal handles are covered with color-coded rubber grips to prevent muscle fatigue and for better control of the instrument.

Sickle Scalers *Sickle scalers* are designed to remove supragingival calculus. These scalers have two cutting edges along the margins of the curved blade (Figures 38-16A and B).

Jacquette Scalers Jacquette scalers, like sickle scalers, are designed to remove supragingival deposits. They have straight blades with cutting edges on both the sides. The Jacquette scaler has three angles in the shank of the instrument (Figures 38-16A and C).

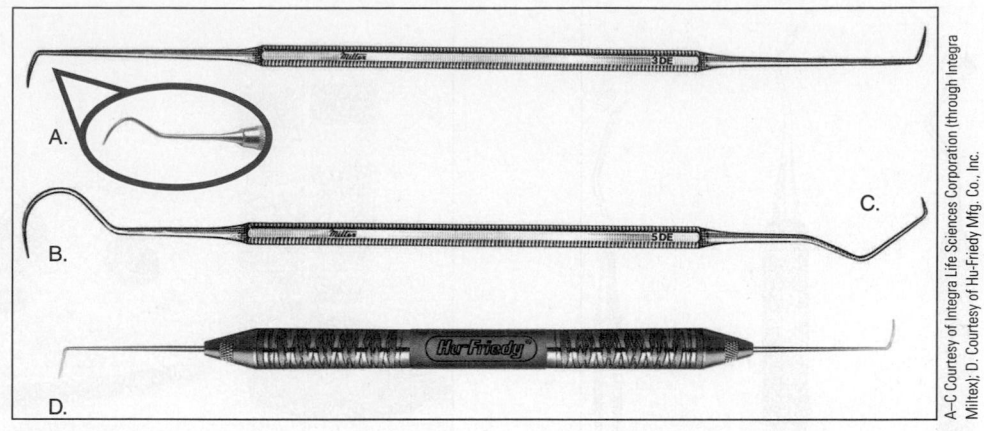

FIGURE 38-13
Types of explorers.

A–C Courtesy of Integra Life Sciences Corporation (through Integra Miltex); D. Courtesy of Hu-Friedy Mfg. Co., Inc.

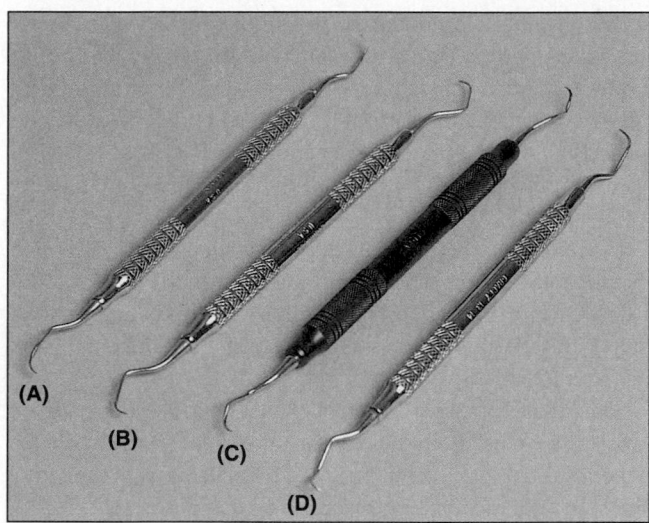

FIGURE 38-14
Gracey periodontal curettes. (A) No. 5–6; (B) No. 7–8; (C) No. 9–10; (D) No. 13–14.

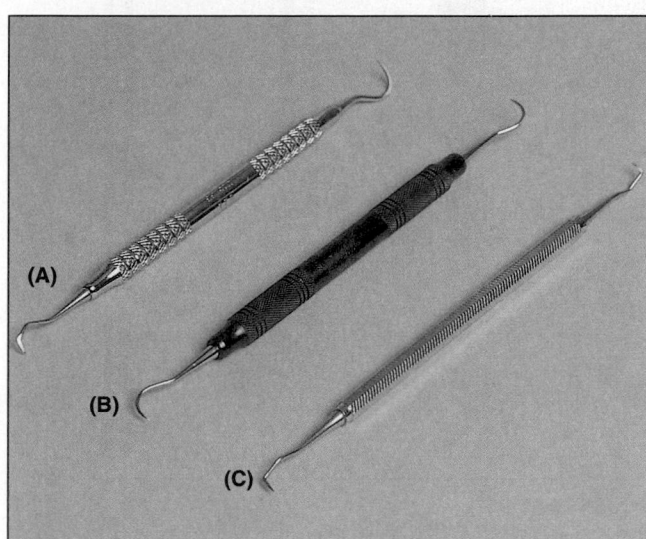

FIGURE 38-16
Types of periodontal scalers. (A) Combination instrument with a sickle scaler on one end and a Jacquette scaler on the other. (B) Sickle scaler. (C) Jacquette scaler.

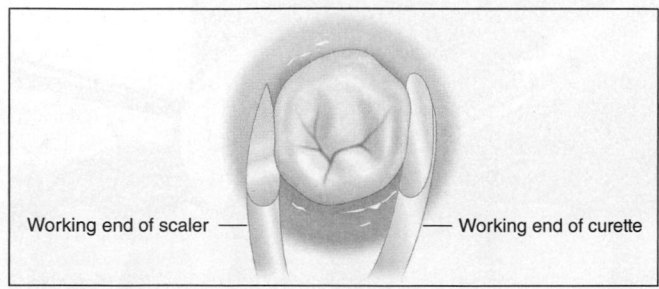

FIGURE 38-15
The working ends of a scaler and a curette showing how they are positioned on a tooth.

Working end of scaler — Working end of curette

Chisel Scalers A *chisel scaler* is used most often in the anterior of the oral cavity. The blade of the chisel is slightly curved, and the cutting edge is beveled (Figure 38-17A).

Hoe Scalers The *hoe scaler* has a blade bent at a 90° angle at the end of the working end. This cutting edge is beveled and sharp. The hoe scaler is placed in the periodontal pocket to the base and then pulled toward the crown of the tooth with even pressure to plane and smooth the root surface (Figure 38-17B).

Files

Periodontal files are supplied in a variety of blade shapes and shank angulations (Figure 38-17C). They are used in a pulling motion interproximally to remove calculus and for root planing. Files are also used to remove overhanging margins of dental restorations.

Ultrasonic Instruments

The *ultrasonic instruments* are used to remove hard deposits, stains, and debris during scaling, curettage, and root-planing

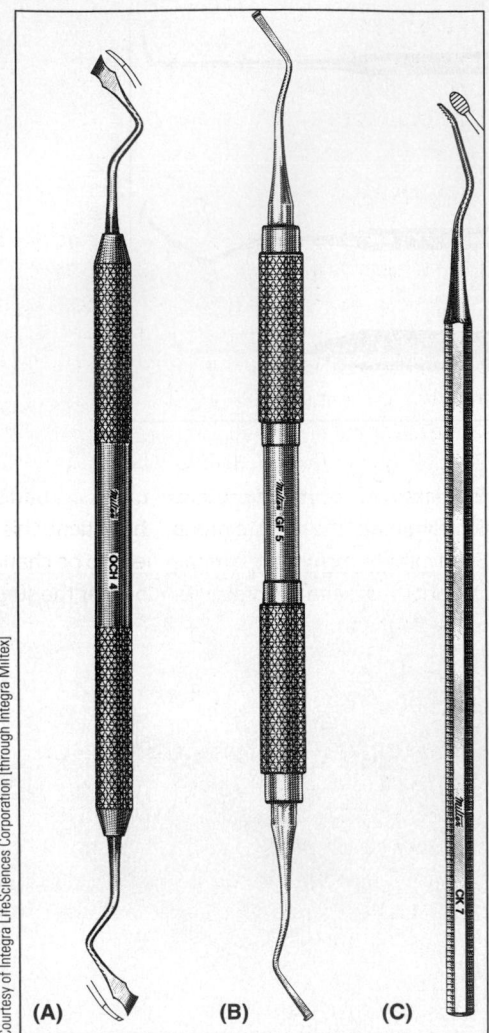

FIGURE 38-17
Periodontal (A) chisel, (B) hoe, and (C) file.

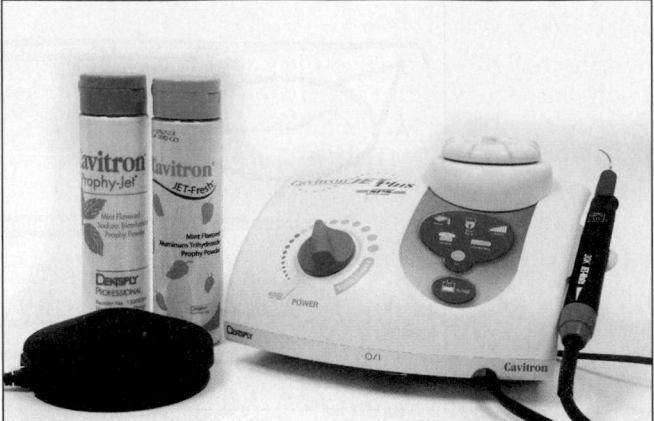

FIGURE 38-18
Ultrasonic unit.

procedures (Figure 38-18). Typically, they are used as an adjunct to manual scaling procedures. Ultrasonic units generate high-power vibrations to a handpiece with a variety of tips. These vibrations cause the calculus to fracture and be dislodged. Because ultrasonic vibrations cause heat, the units have cooling systems that circulate water through the handpieces and out openings near the tips (Figure 38-19). The water spray cools and also flushes the area. It is beneficial for a dental assistant to be present to evacuate the volume of water and debris. Although the ultrasonic units are effective and fast, care must be taken to prevent injury to the tissues and the teeth.

Air Polishing Systems

An *air polishing system* is sometimes called air-powder polishing or jet polishing. This is another method used by the dentist or the hygienist to polish the teeth following scaling and root planing. The primary objective of polishing is to remove extrinsic stain, supragingival biofilm, and soft debris while polishing the tooth surface.

Polishing is also used to clean the tooth prior to sealant placement and bonding procedures and is used on exposed tooth surfaces of patients in orthodontic treatment. This method uses a fine powder abrasive, air that is delivered under pressure, and water through the nozzle of the handpiece. The abrasive is usually finely powdered sodium bicarbonate or nonsodium powder as the slurry.

The removal of biofilm and extrinsic stain is accomplished in a reasonable amount of time, and there is minimal loss of tooth structure when the air polishing system is used as directed by the manufacturer. This system is used to polish both the crown and the root surface.

Some disadvantages of the air polishing systems include significant aerosol spray; possible mild stinging in other areas of the mouth due to the deflected spray; contraindicated for patients with respiratory illness; and not recommended for use on composite restorations, demineralized enamel, or the margins of porcelain or cast restorations. When using the air-powder polisher, the handpiece tip is held 4–5 mm away from the tooth surface and is kept in constant motion.

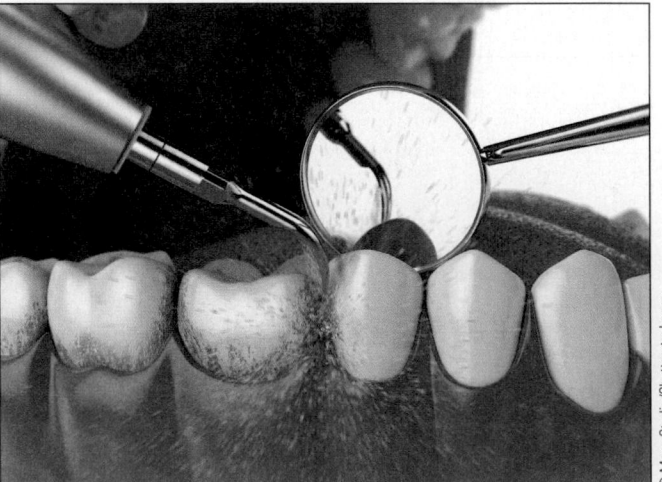

FIGURE 38-19
Ultrasonic unit in use.

Periodontal Knives

A *periodontal knife* or gingivectomy knife is used to remove gingival tissue during periodontal surgery (Figure 38-20). The knives most commonly used are the broad-bladed Kirkland knives (Figure 38-20A). These knives are kidney shaped and sharp around the entire periphery of the blade. They are supplied as either single- or double-ended instruments.

Interdental Knives

A periodontal knife that is used to remove soft tissue interproximally is called an *interdental knife*. The Orban Nos. 1 and 2 are popular interdental knives. These spear-shaped knives have long, narrow blades with cutting edges on both sides of the blade (Figure 38-20B).

Periotomes

A *periotome* is a fairly new instrument that is used to sever the periodontal ligament (PDL) prior to a traumatic extraction as well as to prepare the tissue for dental implants. These instruments are available in a variety of shapes, including narrow, angled, and wide. Some are designed for use on anterior teeth and others on posterior teeth. Periotome blades are thin, flexible, and sharp enough to cause minimal damage to periodontal ligaments. Periotomes may be single ended or double ended, and are made of stainless steel (Figure 38-21).

Surgical Scalpel

A *surgical scalpel* is used for periodontal surgical procedures to remove gingival tissue (Figure 38-22). The surgical scalpel is also

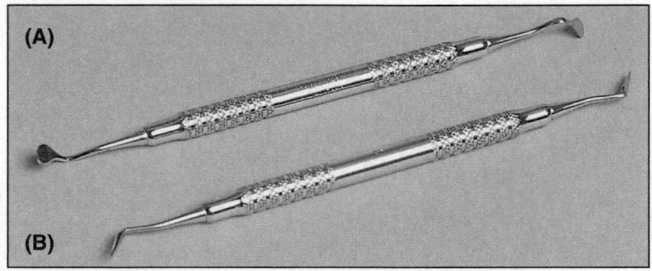

FIGURE 38-20
Gingivectomy knives. (A) Kirkland broad-blade knife. (B) Orban interdental knife.

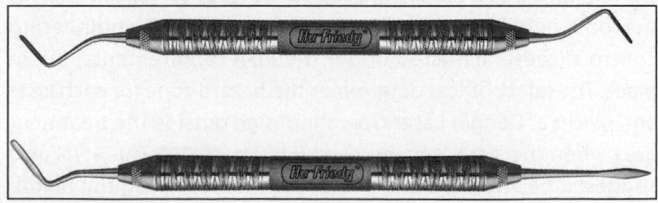

FIGURE 38-21
Periotomes.

known as the Bard–Parker scalpel. The scalpel has two components: a sterilizable metal or plastic handle and a disposable blade. The blades come in different shapes and sizes (Figure 38-23). Disposable scalpels are also available (Figure 38-22).

Electrosurgery

An *electrosurgery* cauterizes the tissues during many periodontal surgeries. The electrosurgery unit uses tiny electrical currents to remove or contour soft tissues and lesions and also coagulates (provides hemostasis) the blood during the procedure (Figure 38-24). The electrosurgery unit consists of a control box, foot-operated on/off controls, a terminal plate that is placed behind the patient's back or shoulders, and another terminal that is a probe with various cutting tips that the dentist uses for the surgery. There is also a cordless electrosurgical cauterizer that is DC battery powered, which eliminates the need to ground the patient; this unit will run for 35–40 minutes before the batteries need to be changed. The dental assistant must keep the oral evacuator near the surgical site to remove the debris and odors.

Pocket Marking Pliers

The *pocket marking plier* is used to transfer the measurement of the pocket to the outside of the tissue so that the operator can see the depth level of the pocket. The pocket marking pliers have one straight, thin beak placed in the pocket, and another bent at a right angle at the tip. When the beaks are pinched together, the gingival tissue is perforated, leaving small, pinpoint markings (Figure 38-25).

Periosteal Elevators

A *periosteal elevator* is used to reflect soft tissue away from the bone. The elevators are usually double ended, with a long, tapered end, and a round, bladed end (Figure 38-26).

Periodontal Scissors, Rongeurs, and Forceps

The *periodontal scissors* are used during periodontal surgery, mainly to remove tags of tissue and to trim margins (Figure 38-27). There are other uses and many varieties, but most often the blades are long and very thin.

A *soft tissue rongeur* or nipper is a hinged plier used to shape the soft tissue (Figure 38-28A). *Tissue forceps* are used to retract tissue or to hold the tissue in place. They are designed similarly to hemostats, except that the beaks are curved near the end at right angles to each other (Figure 38-28B).

Lasers

A dental laser is a medical device that generates a precise beam of concentrated light energy. "Laser" is an acronym for *Light Amplificiation by Stimulated Emission of Radiation*. The efficiency of the laser is based on the peak absorption rates of unique laser wavelengths by hard or soft tissues and other dental materials

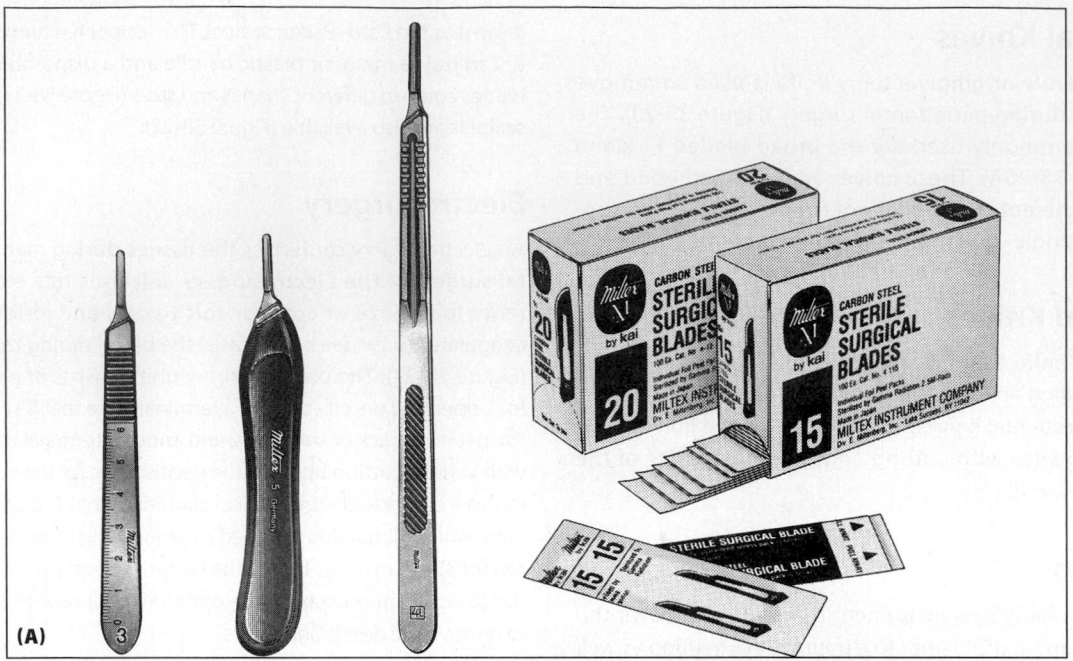

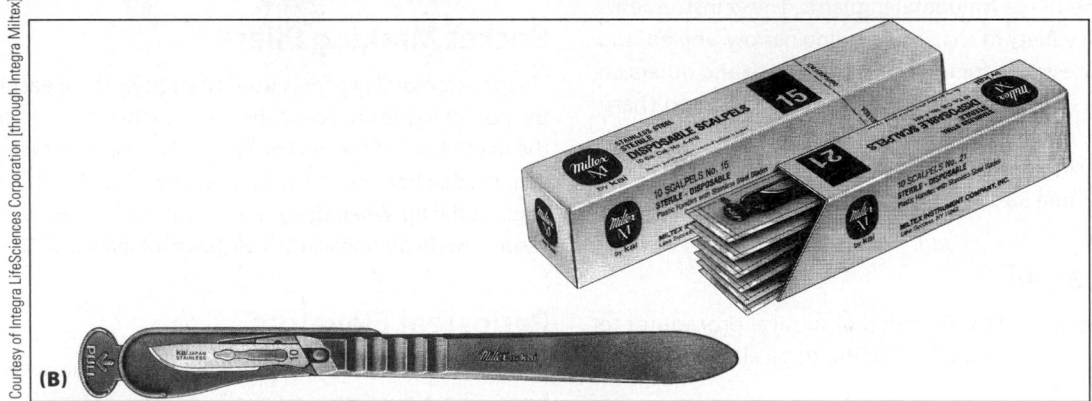

Courtesy of Integra LifeSciences Corporation [through Integra Miltex]

FIGURE 38-22
(A) Surgical blade, Bard–Parker scalpel, and blades. (B) Disposable scalpels.

(e.g., composites or whitening solutions). There are many types of dental laser wavelengths to meet the needs of the dentist. Some standard dental laser wavelengths include erbium (Er:YAG), Nd:YAG, argon, CO_2, and diode laser wavelengths. There is also a water-using device called the YSGG hydrokinetic system, which has similar uses and benefits.

The dentist must complete training to become qualified to use lasers. There are many courses available, and the companies that sell dental lasers offer comprehensive training and support packages. When the dental laser is used in the office, there is training for dental assistants and hygienists as well. For more information, visit the Institute for Laser Dentistry (ILD) website at *http://www.laserdentistry.ca*.

Who Regulates Lasers in Dentistry? The Food and Drug Administration (FDA) regulates lasers as medical devices. They control the following:

● Engineering controls such as on/off key or password

● Emergency stop button

● Foot control cover guard

● Safety interlock on paneling and housing

● Software diagnostics

● Five-second delay in standby mode

● System time-out

● Visible and auditory sounds when laser is being used

The American National Standards Institute (ANSI) also provides recommendations when using dental lasers. The office should have a person designated as the laser safety officer. This person would be responsible for making sure all engineering controls (these are listed under the FDA requirements) are in place. The safety officer determines the hazard zone for each laser and places a "Danger Laser Operating" sign outside the treatment area when the laser is being used (Figure 38-29). The ANSI also suggests the importance of reviewing and following the manufacturer's instructions for each laser used in the office. The safety officer selects and makes sure appropriate protective eyewear is available. They should check with the manufacturer to find the

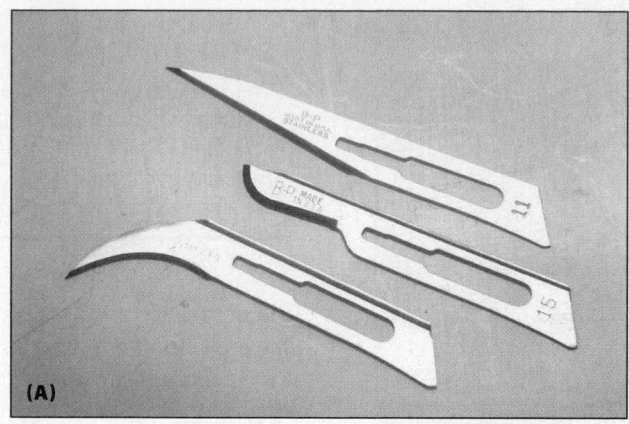

(A)

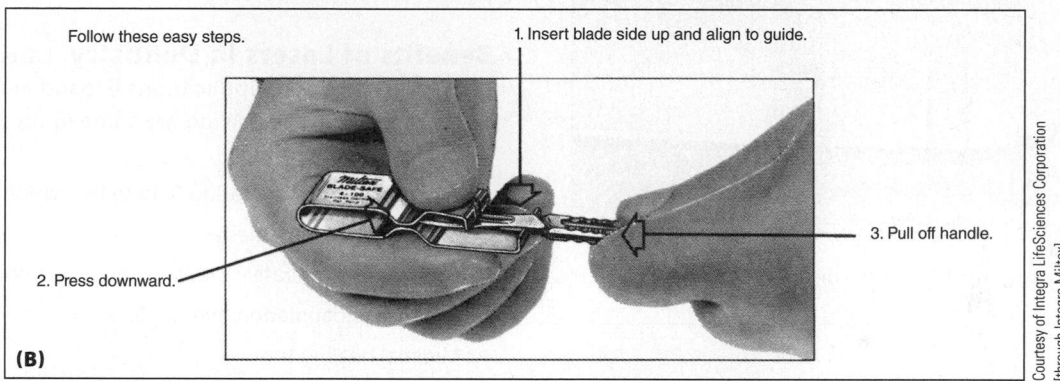

Follow these easy steps.

1. Insert blade side up and align to guide.

2. Press downward.

3. Pull off handle.

(B)

Courtesy of Integra LifeSciences Corporation (through Integra Miltex)

FIGURE 38-23
(A) Various surgical blades. (B) Blade remover.

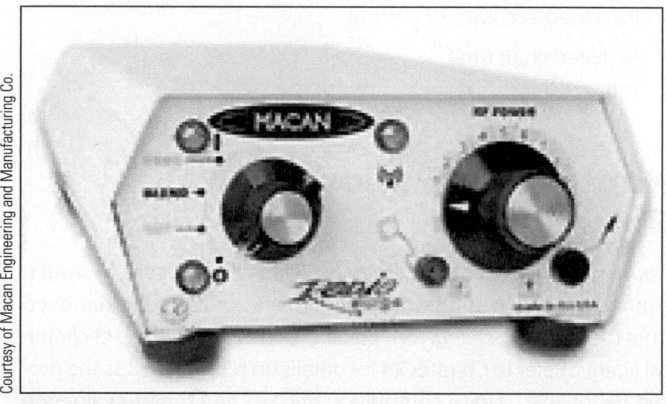

Courtesy of Macan Engineering and Manufacturing Co.

FIGURE 38-24
Electrosurgical unit with various electrodes.

kind of specially filtered eyewear that is needed with the brand or type of laser in use.

Uses of the Dental Laser
Dental laser uses include procedures on hard and soft tissues. In periodontal practice, laser uses include the following:

- Sulcular debridement and laser curettage
- Gingivectomy, gingivoplasty, and frenectomy (Figure 38-30)

- Removal of fibromas and other tumors and lesions
- Excisional new attachment procedure (ENAP)
- Implant exposure
- Treatment for aphthous ulcers
- Tissue fusion, which eliminates the need for sutures
- Elimination of granulation tissue
- Biopsy
- Crown lengthening
- Bleeding control
- Osseous procedures

Other uses of the dental laser include tissue retraction for crown impressions, some cavity preparation and caries removal, transillumination for detection of caries microfracture, laser etching, composite curing, endodontic therapy, pulpotomy treatment, and in-office whitening.

Safety When Using Lasers The primary required safety measure is protective eyewear to be worn by the dentist, staff, and patient when the laser is being used (Figure 38-31). When using high-powered lasers such as diodes, Nd:YAG, or erbium, special filtered protective eyewear must be worn. Additionally the tissues surrounding the area being worked on should be covered or shielded during the procedure with wet gauze.

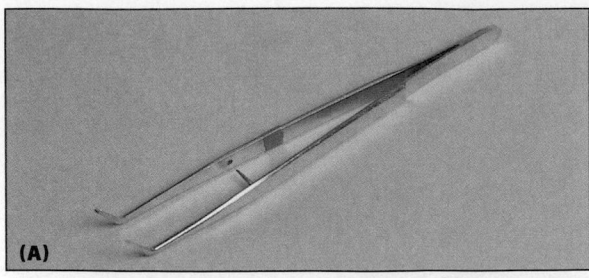

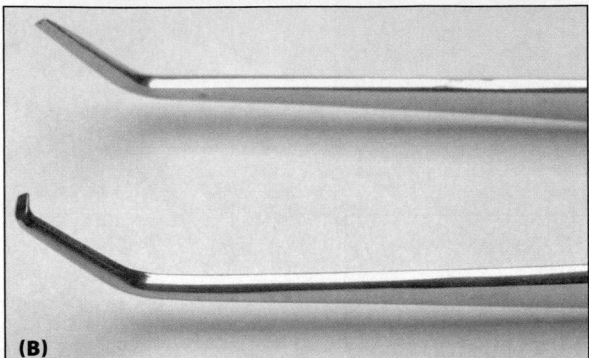

FIGURE 38-25
(A) Pocket marking pliers. (B) Close-up of the working ends of the pocket marking pliers.

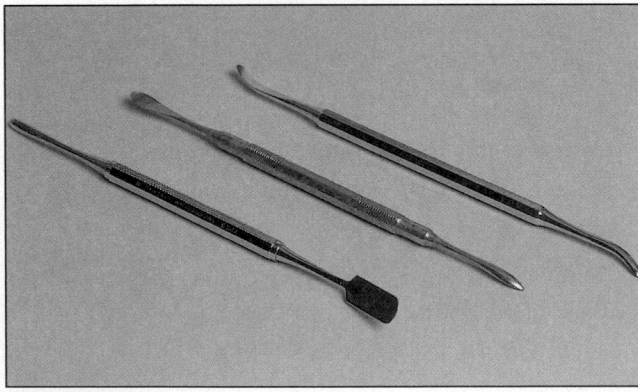

FIGURE 38-26
Various periosteal elevators.

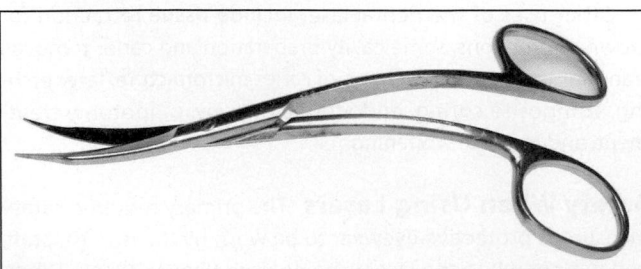

FIGURE 38-27
Periodontal scissor.

The dental assistant should use high-volume evacuation to draw the cloud or plume as well as other debris once the tissue is vaporized. Instruments that may be used when using the laser are matte coated to prevent any laser reflection during a procedure.

Benefits of Lasers in Dentistry Laser technology is rapidly advancing as applications expand and awareness of benefits increases. Following are some of the benefits of this technology:

- A near-bloodless operating field so that vision is improved
- Minimal or no anesthesia
- Minimal postoperative swelling and discomfort
- Enhanced coagulation (hemostasis)
- Minimal healing time
- Reduced damage to surrounding healthy tissues
- Decreased risk of infection, because areas are sterilized by the laser during procedure
- Decreased need for sutures at the surgical site
- Increased accuracy of cutting
- Reduced chair time
- Decreased fear and anxiety for the patient

Nonsurgical Periodontal Procedures

Nonsurgical periodontal therapy (NSPT) is the process by which supragingival and subgingival biofilm and calculus are removed from the teeth by scaling, root planing, and adjunctive use of chemical agents. Refer to Chapter 24 for details on NSPT as well as the procedure for NSPT. Upon completion of NSPT and the re-evaluation appointment to assess gingival healing, reduction in inflammation, and bleeding, adjunctive therapies may be implemented if needed. Adjunctive therapies will be discussed later in this chapter. The patient is closely monitored on a 3–4-month recall or periodontal maintenance schedule if healing of tissues has occurred.

Occlusal Adjustment

Occlusal adjustment is the process of stabilizing a patient's occlusal relationship (Procedure 38-1). A patient's periodontal health can be compromised if there are any discrepancies in the patient's

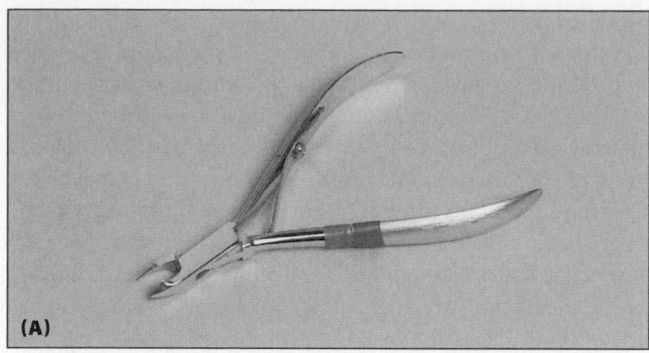

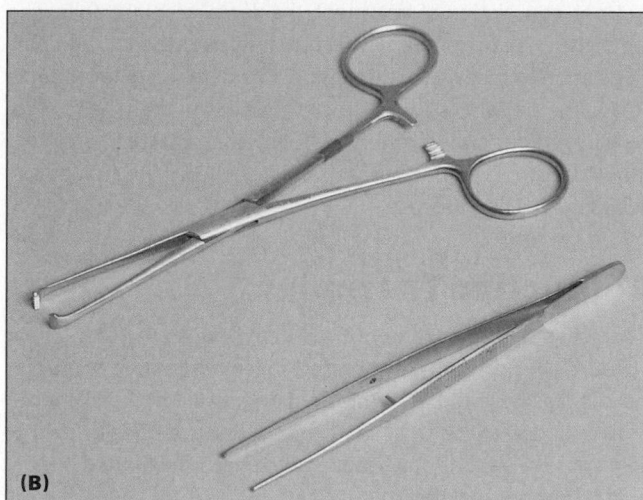

FIGURE 38-28
(A) Soft tissue rongeur. (B) Tissue forceps.

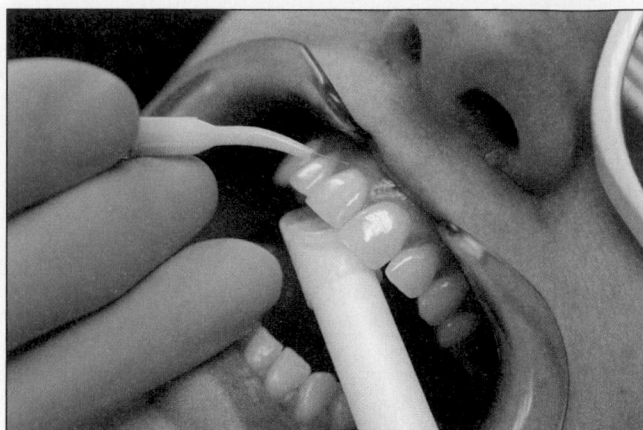

FIGURE 38-30
Dental laser in use.

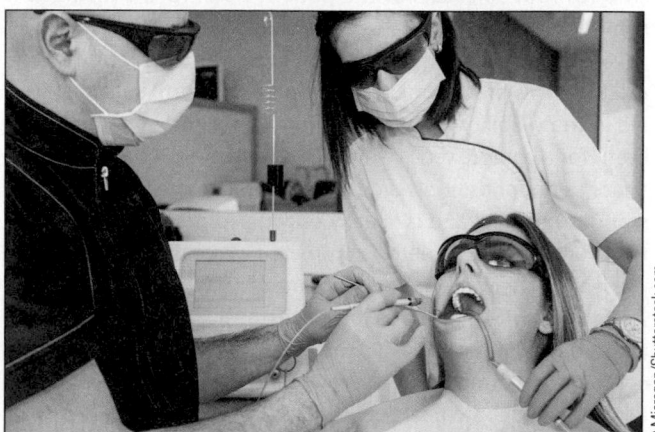

FIGURE 38-31
Dental laser safety: dentist, assistant, and patient wearing safety glasses.

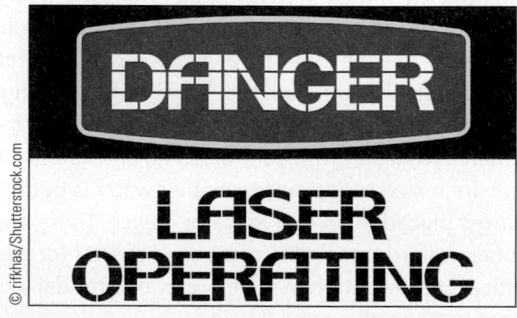

FIGURE 38-29
Warning signs must be posted in areas where lasers are being used to prevent injury to the eyes of others who may come into the area and are not wearing the filtered eyewear.

occlusal relationship. The procedure may take more than one appointment, and a patient may be prescribed an occlusal guard at night. An occlusal guard or mouth guard is prescribed when the discrepancies cannot be completely adjusted or the patient has a habit of clenching or grinding. The occlusal guard is prescribed for use at night to keep the TMJ, teeth, and periodontal tissues from traumatic biting forces caused by the occlusal discrepancies.

In a routine prophylaxis, deposits from above and just slightly below the gingival margins are removed. In a periodontal scaling, the subgingival deposits are more extensive and involve removal of irritants from deep pockets and smoothing of the root surface (Figure 38-32).

Root Planing

After the biofilm and calculus are removed from the periodontal pocket and the root surface, the cementum is often rough and irregular. This provides a surface ideal for accumulation of biofilm and calculus formation. The roughness is removed by *root planing*. This is a process of planing or shaving the root surface

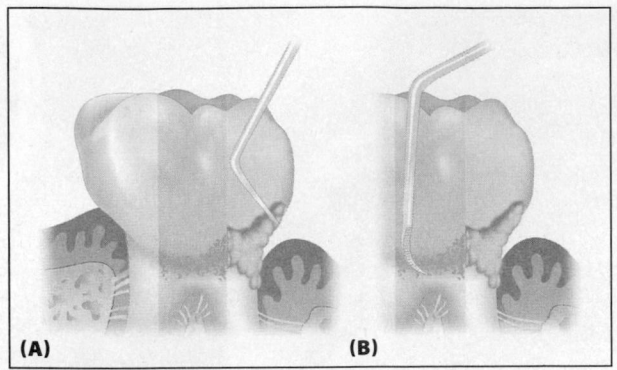

FIGURE 38-32
Placement of instruments for scaling. (A) Supragingival scaling.
(B) Subgingival scaling.

with curettes and other periodontal instruments to leave a smooth root surface. For the patient's comfort, anesthetic is sometimes given during this procedure.

Gross debridement refers to the gross removal of biofilm and calculus. This pretreatment procedure is performed primarily to aid in the visibility of the teeth used to facilitate an exam of the teeth for a comprehensive evaluation and diagnosis by the dentist or periodontist. However, this is not recommended, is not the standard of care, and is usually only performed when the dentist is unable to adequately complete a clinical exam due to the presence of heavy calculus. Quadrant or sextant scaling is usually performed with the use of local anesthesia, and the time allotted can range from 60 to 90 minutes. Quadrant and/or sextant scaling appointments are usually scheduled on different days to allow the patient to heal between visits.

When all quadrants and sextants have been completely scaled and root planed, the patient is scheduled for a reevaluation appointment. The reevaluation appointment is scheduled from 4 to 6 weeks after the last quadrant or sextant scaling to allow for complete healing of all gingival tissues. The reevaluation appointment allows for reassessing of the gingival tissues to determine success of the nonsurgical periodontal therapy. If needed, additional scaling and polishing is completed on the patient and the patient is scheduled for either periodontal maintenance or surgery depending on the success of gingival healing. Periodontal maintenance and periodontal surgeries are discussed later in this chapter.

Gingival Curettage

Gingival curettage, also known as soft tissue curettage, is a procedure that involves scraping the inner gingival walls of the periodontal pockets to remove inflamed tissue and debris. This is accomplished with curettes and is ideally performed after the scaling and root planing of the teeth.

This procedure is performed with local anesthetic and is performed deliberately to promote healing of the gingival tissues after root planing is performed. The newest research suggests that there is no significant therapeutic benefit, and therefore, the AAP and the ADA do not list gingival curettage as a method of treatment. Laser periodontal therapy is considered to be a curettage type of procedure because it removes the diseased lining of the sulcus as the laser passes over and removes the diseased tissue. This form of laser curettage promotes a blood clot to form, causing a different type of healing mechanism in the pocket wall, and therefore is the preferred method of curettage. Care must be taken as sometimes subgingival scaling can inadvertently cause removal of the inside lining of the gingival sulcus.

Upon completion of treatment, the dental assistant, following the dentist's instructions, may recommend over-the-counter pain medication to relieve any discomfort. The dental assistant should advise the patient to avoid spicy foods, citrus fruits, and alcoholic beverages and to otherwise follow a normal diet. Smoking should be stopped, because the smoke irritates the tissues and delays the healing process.

Adjunctive Therapies

Adjunctive therapies refer to treatment that is used along with nonsurgical periodontal therapy. These adjunctive therapies include oral irrigation, systemic drug delivery, and locally applied drug delivery. These treatment therapies have been shown to help improve periodontal healing outcomes when added to nonsurgical periodontal therapy.

Oral Irrigation

Oral irrigation is the process of loosening food and loosely adherent biofilm from tooth surfaces at the gingival margin to promote health at the gingival margin. There are many pulsating water devices on the market that can be purchased over the counter to supplement oral hygiene self-care (refer to Chapter 40). Research has shown that some of the oral irrigation devices on the market can help to reduce bleeding and inflammation when used along with daily brushing and flossing. However, there are mixed results as to whether water is better than mouth rinses placed in an oral irrigator device. There are also professional oral irrigators that can be purchased for use in a dental office. Oral irrigation may be prescribed for daily use to supplement toothbrushing and flossing.

Systemic Antibiotic Therapy

Systemic antibiotic therapy is the oral administration of antibiotics along with NSPT. Patients who exhibit aggressive periodontal disease may benefit from daily systemic antibiotic therapy. It is also important to take a thorough medical history to reveal medications that a patient is taking and any allergies before prescribing systemic antibiotics. Research has suggested the idea of culturing the bacteria in the periodontal pocket to see what type of bacteria is present before prescribing a systemic antibiotic. Some dental offices are using a variety of mail order services to culture bacteria and prescribe antibiotic treatment.

Locally Applied Drug Delivery

Locally applied drug delivery is the process of placing a site-specific and sustained releasing antimicrobial drug in the periodontal pocket. There are several locally applied antimicrobial drug delivery agents on the market that are applied professionally. These drug delivery agents can be applied directly (locally) into the periodontal pocket following scaling and root planing or at the reevaluation appointment. Evidence has shown that there is enhanced improvement in periodontal health when using locally applied antimicrobial agents along with nonsurgical periodontal therapy. Table 38-5 provides information about locally applied antimicrobial agents.

Peridex®

Peridex® or chlorhexidine gluconate 0.12% is an oral rinse that is classified as an antibiotic. It is used to manage the symptoms of gingivitis. One of the side effects of Peridex® is staining of the teeth or removable dental appliances. The patient should be advised about this side effect. Though rare, Peridex® can also result in allergic reactions.

Enzyme Suppression Therapy

Scientists have found that some patients with chronic periodontitis produce too much of the enzyme collagenase, which predisposes them for periodontal disease. A therapy called *enzyme suppression therapy* can produce attachment-level gain and reduction in pocket depths in some periodontal patients. The enzyme suppression therapeutic daily regimented dose of 20 mg of doxycycline is prescribed for some patients with chronic periodontitis along with traditional NSPT.

Precautions/Contraindications

There are precautions and contraindications to any of the adjunctive therapies used in nonsurgical periodontal therapy. Allergies to any of the medications found in the locally applied medications need to be assessed in the medical history. Many of the antimicrobial therapies contain the antibiotic tetracycline. Also, it is important to evaluate patients who have a predisposition to

oral candidiasis because many of these medications suppress the growth of or kill bacteria and allow growth of fungi.

Healing

In order to determine healing following nonsurgical periodontal therapy, the reevaluation appointment is scheduled to evaluate the gingival tissue. Based on the outcome, the course for continued periodontal therapy, restorative therapy, and/or surgery is determined. The following procedures are performed at the reevaluation appointment prior to any additional scaling and root planing or polishing: periodontal probing, determining the amount of biofilm and calculus, and, in some instances, additional radiographs may be obtained.

Healing occurs as repair of existing tissues rather than regeneration of tissues lost to periodontal disease. The bacteria present at the reevaluation appointment are less pathogenic and more similar to the bacteria present in health. Recession may occur in some cases due to the reduction of inflammation and healing of gingival tissues. New connective tissue may reattach to the cementum, and new bone may populate around the teeth. It usually takes 4 weeks for the junctional epithelium and the underlying connective tissue to completely heal. After 4 weeks, it is safe to probe teeth and get accurate periodontal probe readings. Bleeding on probing at the reevaluation appointment indicates that there is need for additional scaling and root planing. Along with additional scaling and root planing, local delivery agents may be placed in the pockets that have BOP and/or periodontal probing readings of 5 mm or more. If a patient presents with BOP and periodontal pockets of 5 mm or more, they may be scheduled for further nonsurgical periodontal therapy or periodontal surgery depending on the patient and risk factors. In some cases, nonsurgical periodontal therapy is completely successful and the patient is placed on a 3–4-month periodontal maintenance appointment regimen. Periodontal maintenance is discussed later in this chapter.

Surgical Periodontal Procedures

Periodontal surgery is scheduled for high-risk patients and those patients who don't respond favorably to nonsurgical periodontal therapy. There are different types of periodontal surgeries performed to correct gingival, connective tissue, and bony defects. The reasons for periodontal surgery include to reduce or eliminate periodontal pockets, create or improve root access, treat bone

TABLE 38-5 Locally Applied Antimicrobial Agents

Agent	Medication
PerioChip®	chlorhexidine gluconate chip that is absorbed by the body (Perio Products, Ltd.); biodegradable
Arestin®	minocycline HCl powdered microspheres (OraPharma, Inc.); biodegradable
Atridox®	doxycycline hyclate gel (Atrix Laboratories); biodegradable

defects, correct mucogingival defects, promote new tissue attachment, and improve the ability to perform oral home care.

Preoperative Instructions

Before the procedure, the dental assistant, following the dentist's instructions, should complete the following:

- Confirm that the patient understands what procedure they are in the office for that day.
- Explain the procedure and answer any questions.
- Confirm the patient has prepared as instructed—instructions will vary depending on the type of anesthetic the patient is receiving and the procedure being completed.
- Provide instructions verbally and in writing prior to the start of the procedure if the patient is to receive intravenous sedation.

Gingivectomy

A *gingivectomy* is the surgical removal of diseased gingival tissue that forms the periodontal pocket. The pocket must be eliminated to prevent the accumulation of debris and bacteria. This surgical procedure reduces the height of the gingival tissue, which provides visibility and access in order to remove irritants and smooth the root surface (Procedure 38-2). This promotes the healing process and makes it easier for the patient to access the area during cleaning. The gingivectomy procedure is common for patients who exhibit gingival overgrowth because of certain medications, such as phenytoin, cyclosporine, and calcium channel blockers. Having the excess gingival tissue removed enhances a patient's appearance and improves home care (Figure 38-33). If a patient continues on the medication, however, then the gingiva may continue to overgrow and the need for additional surgery in the future is increased.

The gingivectomy procedure involves marking the pocket depths with pocket marking pliers and then excising the gingival tissue with periodontal knives, a scalpel, surgical scissors, or electrosurgery. After the tissue is excised, calculus and necrotic root tissue are removed and smoothed with scalers and curettes. The area is rinsed gently and covered with a gauze sponge until the hemorrhage is controlled. Once the blood clots have formed, a periodontal dressing is placed to promote healing, reduce the chance of infection, and prevent disturbance to the area.

Gingivoplasty

A *gingivoplasty* is reshaping the gingival tissue to remove deformities such as clefts, craters, and enlargements. A gingivoplasty does not involve the removal of periodontal pockets; it is completed to recontour the gingiva and often immediately follows a gingivectomy (Figure 38-33). A gingivoplasty is performed with periodontal knives, a scalpel, rongeurs, rotary diamonds, curettes, and surgical scissors. The gingival margin is tapered and thinned, creating a scalloped edge. Interdental grooves are contoured. A periodontal dressing is placed over the wound to promote healing of the gingival tissue and removed in 7–14 days.

Postoperative Treatment Following Surgery

Upon completion of a surgical procedure, the dental assistant, following the dentist's directions, gives the patient postoperative instructions. These instructions are given to the patient (and also to the support person) both verbally and in written form to take home with them. The instructions include office phone numbers in case the patient has questions or problems with the surgery, and also include the following information:

- **Medications and pain management.** The patient can expect mild to moderate discomfort after surgery. Analgesic tablets (i.e., Tylenol, Motrin, or nonaspirin analgesics) can be taken as needed or as directed by the periodontist. Prescription medications should be taken for 2–3 days after surgery or as directed. Antibiotics may also be prescribed; the patient should carefully follow the instructions and take the antibiotics as directed until they are finished.
- **Activity.** The patient should limit their activity for 24 hours following surgery because increased activity can lead to increased bleeding.
- **Smoking.** The patient should not smoke or chew tobacco for 12–72 hours depending on the surgery and the periodontist instructions. Tobacco interferes with and slows the healing process.
- **Oral hygiene.** Normal brushing and flossing should be completed by the patient in areas not involved in the surgery. Brush only the biting surfaces of the teeth involved in surgery. Gently rinse the mouth with warm salt water after 24 hours.
- **Diet.** The patient should avoid hot, spicy foods and citrus foods; eat soft foods; and chew on the healthy side of the mouth so that the periodontal dressing is not disturbed.
- **Swelling and bleeding.** Some swelling may occur. The patient should place an ice pack over the area for 10 minutes and then remove for 10 minutes, repeating as needed. Some seepage and bleeding may occur and is normal; however, if it persists, the patient should call the dentist.

Periodontal Flap Surgery

A *periodontal flap surgery* involves surgically separating the gingiva from the underlying tissue. The gingiva is incised with a scalpel and then separated with a periosteal elevator. Once the tissue is retracted, the periodontist has good visibility and access to bone, tooth, and tooth roots (Figures 38-34 and 38-35).

The design of the flap depends on the objectives of the surgery and the periodontist. The amount of exposure necessary for the surgery and the repositioning of the flap are important considerations. The periodontist exposes an area large enough to remove the irritants completely with the periodontal instruments. The appearance of the gingiva after the surgery depends

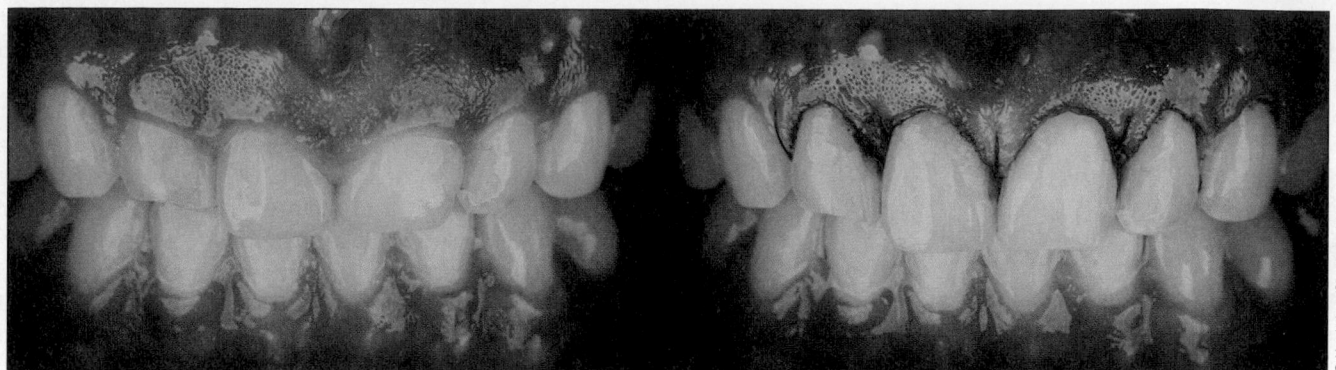

FIGURE 38-33
Gingivectomy and gingivoplasty.

on the proper repositioning of the flap. The tissue is positioned to heal in a manner that leaves as little evidence of the surgery as possible.

When the flap is retracted, the diseased tissue and debris are removed, the roots are planed, and the alveolar bone is trimmed and contoured. The area is rinsed with a saline solution, and the flap is repositioned and sutured. A *periodontal dressing* may be applied to protect the surgical site (Figure 38-36).

Osseous Surgery

An *osseous surgery* removes defects and deformities in the bone caused by periodontal disease and other related conditions (Procedure 38-4). Two types of bone surgeries that correct the deformities are *osteoplasty*, reshaping the bone, and *ostectomy*, removal of bone.

Osseous surgery can be either additive or subtractive. During additive osseous surgery (sometimes called *bone augmentation*), bone grafting is completed to fill in areas.

Bone Grafting   A bone graft is performed to promote bone growth by adding bone or a bone substitute to the alveolar bone (refer to Figure 39-9). There are several types of bone replacement grafts. Refer to Chapter 39 regarding the types of bone grafts available.

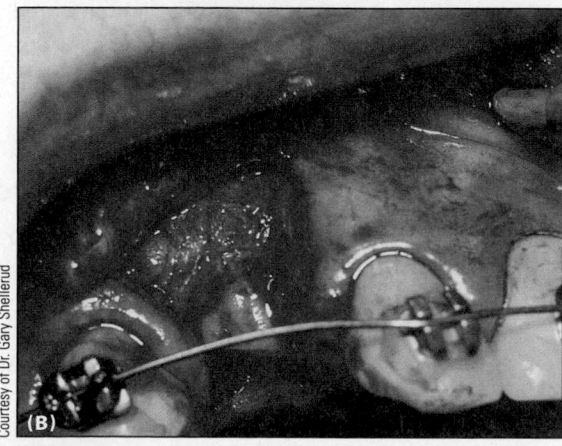

FIGURE 38-34
Flap surgery to expose an impacted tooth. (A) Making incision. (B) Retracting tissue.

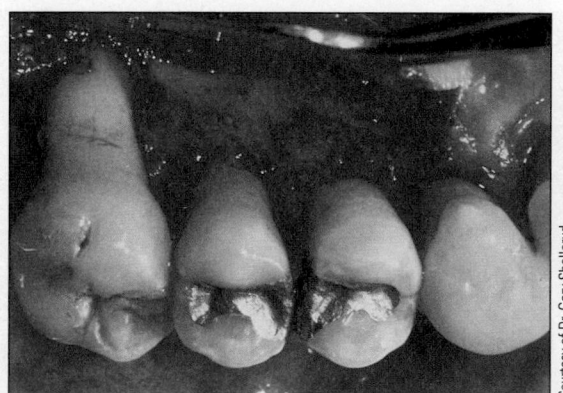

FIGURE 38-35
Periodontal flap and osseous surgery. A flap is laid and alveolar bone exposed.

When the bone is harvested from a different site on the patient to perform a graft elsewhere, the bone from the donor site is removed with chisels, rongeurs, files, diamond burs, and stones. After the bone has been grafted or removed and contoured, the flap is repositioned and sutures are placed. A periodontal dressing is then placed.

Mucogingival Surgery

A *mucogingival surgery* is reconstructive surgery on the gingiva and/or mucosa tissues. The surgeries may involve covering exposed roots, increasing the width of the gingival tissue, and reducing frenum or muscle attachments. Periodontal disease can cause negative changes in the gingiva, and mucogingival surgery improves these areas. Some of the mucogingival surgeries include gingival grafts, connective tissue grafts, frenectomy, and guided tissue regeneration.

Gingival Graft   A *gingival graft* is a procedure where tissue is taken from a site in the patient's mouth and placed on another site. This type of gingival graft is done when the amount of attached gingiva is inadequate and there is recession. The patient's palatal tissue is the most frequent site that is harvested. The palatal tissue is sutured after harvesting. The area where the palatal tissue is placed to provide tissue coverage is positioned and sutured in place (Figure 38-37). A periodontal dressing is placed over the sutures to keep the tissue in close contact to the tooth and promote healing of the gingival tissues for the next 7–14 days.

Connective Tissue Graft   A *connective tissue graft* is a procedure like the gingival graft, but the difference is that connective tissue (requiring a deeper excision) is harvested from the hard palate. The patient's palatal tissue is sutured after harvesting. This procedure requires a small flap at the receptor site, and when connective tissue is placed over the recession, the gingival tissue is sutured over the palatal connective tissue, and a periodontal

dressing is placed for the next 7–14 days. This type of tissue graft is more predictable due to the fact that tissue adaptation and color blend are more predictable.

Frenectomy   The frenectomy is a complete removal of the frenum, including the attachment to the underlying bone. The frenum may be removed if it is attached too close to the marginal gingiva. The procedure involves incising the frenum and removing a triangular section. The periodontal fibers are separated and cut to the bone. The labial mucosa is then sutured to the apical periosteum. The periodontal dressing is prepared and placed over the suture site.

Guided Tissue Regeneration   A *guided tissue regeneration (GTR)*, or selective cell reproduction, uses barrier membranes to maintain a space between the gingival flap and the root surface of the tooth in order for tissues to regenerate in a periodontal defect. Cells capable of forming new cementum, periodontal ligament, and supporting alveolar bone must move into the surgical site to produce these tissues, but they must not be interfered with. Therefore, apical epithelial migration must be delayed and gingival connective tissue from the flap must be kept away from the surgical area for regeneration to take place.

The membranes used as a barrier are classified as nonabsorbable or absorbable. Both have proven to be successful techniques. The technique involving nonabsorbable membranes has been on the market longer and requires a second appointment in about 3–4 weeks to remove the barrier. Selection of the type of membrane to be used is determined by the dentist's preference and the type of periodontal defect.

Crown Lengthening Procedure

Gingival tissue and bone may need to be contoured to promote a normal level of gingival tissue around a crown, bridge, or veneer. This procedure is called *crown lengthening* and requires a periodontal flap to expose the bone and gingival tissue prior to the procedure. After the bone and connective tissue are contoured, the periodontal flap is sutured, and a periodontal dressing is placed for the next 7–14 days. The goal of this surgery is to promote a healthy gingival height around a crown, bridge, or veneer.

Periodontal Dressings and Sutures

Sutures are usually attached to a needle and are chosen for the type of surgery and area to be placed. Sutures are either removable (nonabsorbable) or nonremovable (absorbable). The number of sutures needed depends on the type of surgery and tissue involved. Sutures are placed to keep tissue together to promote healing and reduce bleeding. Sutures may or may not be covered by a periodontal dressing after a periodontal surgical procedure.

Periodontal dressings or packs are placed after periodontal surgical procedures and after sutures are placed. The dressings do not have any medicinal qualities; they are bandages used to protect the tissue during the healing process. A periodontal dressing should be comfortable, smooth, and nonirritating.

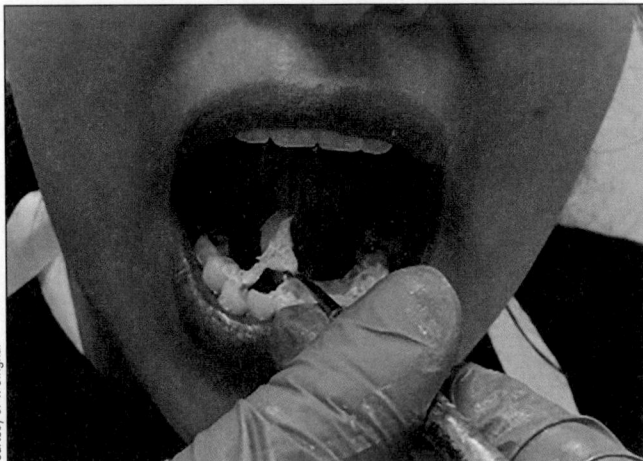

Courtesy of V. Singhal

FIGURE 38-36
Placement of periodontal dressing.

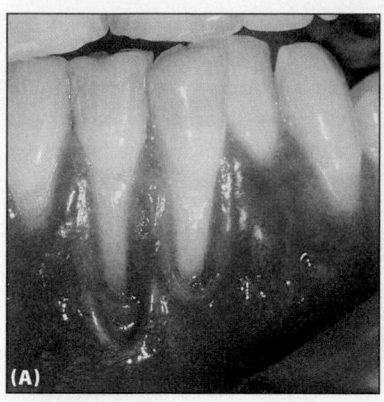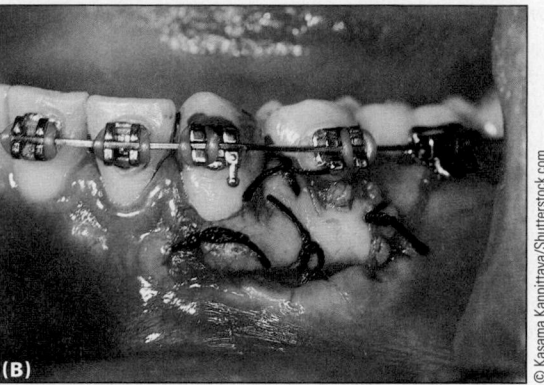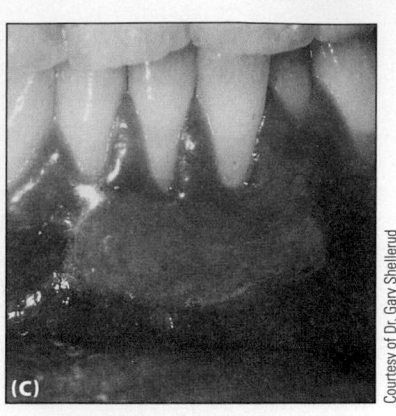

FIGURE 38-37
Gingival graft. (A) Gingival recession shows need for graft. (B) Palatal tissue graft is positioned over area of recession and then sutured in place. (C) Graft after healing period.

The following are objectives of the periodontal dressing:

- Minimize postoperative infection and hemorrhage.
- Protect the tissues during mastication.
- Cover the surgical site in order to reduce pain due to trauma or irritation.
- Provide support for the teeth that are mobile.
- Aid in holding the gingival flaps in position.

Types of Periodontal Dressings

The most common types of materials used as periodontal dressings are zinc oxide–eugenol materials, noneugenol materials, light-cured dressings, and gelatin-based materials.

Zinc Oxide–Eugenol Materials   Zinc oxide–eugenol materials are supplied in a powder (zinc oxide) or liquid (eugenol or oil of cloves) form that can be mixed before the procedure and stored for later use. The presence of eugenol in this dressing can cause an allergic reaction. The area becomes red, and a burning sensation is experienced by the patient. Some periodontal dressings can be mixed prior to placement, prepared ahead of time, and kept in the refrigerator until ready for use. The surgical site dictates the best type of periodontal dressing to use, and many practitioners do not place periodontal dressings over sutures based on personal preference. Patients are instructed by the assistant on the best way to care for their mouths so as not to disturb the sutures while they help the tissue heal. If a periodontal dressing is placed, the patient is scheduled to return to the office in 7–14 days to have it removed along with sutures. Periodontal dressings can be placed and removed by a dental assistant in most states. Sutures can be removed by dental assistants in most states as well. The dental assistant should be aware of the functions delegated by their state regulations.

Noneugenol Materials   The noneugenol materials come in a two-paste system: one tube of base material and one tube of accelerator. The two pastes are dispensed in equal portions on a paper pad and mixed together prior to placement (Procedure 38-4). The noneugenol dressings do not cause sensitivity problems, and some noneugenol dressing materials have bacteriostatic agents added.

Light-Cured Periodontal Dressings   Light-cured periodontal dressing material comes in syringes. It can be placed directly on the surgical site or placed on a mixing pad. If it is placed directly on the tissues, it can be contoured into the desired position and then light cured. The material may also be dispensed onto a paper pad, manipulated to the required shape and size, placed over the tissues, and then light cured (Figure 38-38).

Gelatin-Base Dressings   Gelatin-base dressings offer good stability and dissolve in 24–48 hours. They are excellent for use after soft-tissue augmentation.

Patient Healing

Healing after periodontal surgery is complex and requires the patient to be evaluated postsurgery at different intervals to measure and document their periodontal status. Successful periodontal

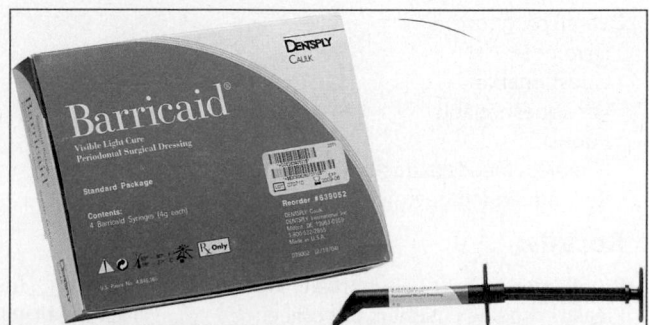

FIGURE 38-38
Light-cured periodontal dressing.

surgery may have one or more of the following possible outcomes: stimulation of alveolar bone growth, formation of a long junctional epithelium, resolution of inflammation and reduction of periodontal pocket, regeneration, and stimulation formation of new connective tissue attachment. Radiographs are taken at various intervals to determine the amount of alveolar bone that is present. Periodontal probing may be documented along with gingival recession except in the case of certain procedures that do not allow this because of interference with blood clot and healing. Mobility, furcation, accumulation of biofilm and calculus, and occlusion are evaluated as well as tissue health after periodontal surgery. Home care and nutritional status are monitored at each postsurgery interval visit to ensure healing and to prevent infection. Postsurgery periodontal therapy may require a patient to be evaluated up to one year after the initial surgery. Each patient is evaluated at intervals according to the type of surgery performed, systemic health of patient, and risk factors.

Periodontal Maintenance

Periodontal maintenance is an ongoing program designed to prevent periodontal disease from recurring for patients who have undergone nonsurgical or surgical periodontal therapy.

BOX 38-2 Supportive Periodontal Care Report

(Name and address of Dental Office)

Date: _____   PREMEDICATION TAKEN: _____

To Dr. _____   Allergies: _____

Patient/DOB: _____

Medical Update   **PLAQUE FREE SCORE:** _____

History:
Medications:
Changes:

Clinical Examination Reveals:

Diagnosis:
Risk factors:
  Smoking
  Diabetes
  Family History
  Other
Gingival tissue tone:
Cancer screening:
Parafunctional habits: yes/no
Wears nightguard: yes/no
Wears removable appliance: yes/no

Evaluation of Findings

No appreciable change since last visit:
Periodontium essentially healthy and stable:
Surgical history:
Areas of recent surgery:
Additional surgical needs:

Restorative needs:

Overall prognosis:
  Favorable
  Questionable
  Very questionable
  Poor
  Hopeless (needs extraction)
  Recommended treatment

Recalls:

Recall interval: _____ alt./non-alt. Date of last recall: _____ (dentist or periodontist)
Please schedule patient in our office: _____ Next recall in this office: _____
( ) Please Have Your Receptionist Call Patient   ( ) Patient Will Call You
Comments:

The American Academy of Periodontology renamed supportive periodontal therapy (SPT) as periodontal maintenance because it is a more inclusive term. Other names for periodontal maintenance include continuing care and periodontal recall. Periodontal maintenance is scheduled after active therapy at different intervals from 3 to 4 months according to the health and risk factors of each patient. Periodontal maintenance continues at varying levels for the life of the dentition or its implant replacements.

The periodontal maintenance visits are scheduled for 60–90 minutes and include a through clinical assessment, radiographs if necessary, assessment of home care, and scaling and polishing. Patients are also evaluated for any additional dental treatment needs. Patients may alternate their 3–4-month periodontal maintenance visits with a general dental office prophylaxis after the initial periodontal maintenance visit with the periodontist. The periodontist and general dental office exchange clinical findings and radiographs with one another. A periodontal patient may move from active therapy to periodontal maintenance and back to active care if the disease recurs. Research has shown that it is vital for patients to complete their periodontal maintenance visits at the intervals prescribed by the dental office in order to prevent further periodontal destruction. Box 38-2 provides an example of a clinical report exchanged by dentist and periodontist.

The Role of the Dental Assistant

As part of periodontal procedures, the dental assistant prepares the treatment area for patient seating and assembles the periodontal tray setup based on the procedure scheduled. After the patient is seated, the assistant should first review and document the patient's health history. After careful review of the health and dental history information, the periodontist completes the procedure scheduled, and the dental assistant assists. The dental assistant also takes and necessary prescribed radiographs, obtains impressions, and provides oral hygiene instructions. The dental assistant records the findings on the patient's chart. It is important to maintain sharp periodontal hand instruments available for the root planing procedures. Depending on the state practice act, the scaling of supragingival deposits and coronal polishing may be performed by the dental assistant. It is always important for the dental assistant to keep the patient comfortable throughout each procedure. For surgical procedures, the patient is given time to recover, and vital signs may continue to be monitored. When the patient has recovered fully, the patient's escort is called to review the postsurgical instructions. The assistant will remain with the patient until it is time to dismiss them to the waiting area or car. The assistant ensures the patient is cleared to ride home with their escort, if necessary, before dismissal.

Procedure 38-1
Occlusal Adjustment

The procedure is performed by the general dentist or the periodontist. It involves marking the patient's bite and adjusting the occlusal surfaces of the teeth. The dental assistant prepares the articulating paper or wax; maintains the operating field; and changes burs, discs, and stones in the handpiece.

Steps written in blue font are performed by the operator (dentist or qualified dental assistant), and the chairside assistant's steps are written in black.

Equipment and Supplies

Patient Seating Setup (refer to Procedure 18-4)

Occlusal Adjustment Setup (Figure 38-39)
- Cotton rolls and 2 × 2-inch gauze sponges (not shown)
- Articulation forceps and articulating paper and/or occlusal wax
- Low-speed handpiece
- Diamond burs, various discs, and stones
- Polishing wheels and discs

Procedure Steps (*Follow aseptic procedures*)

1. Escort and seat patient (refer to Procedure 18-4).

Dentist greets the patient and takes position at the dental chair.

❑ **Signals for the occlusal adjustment procedure to begin (refer to Procedure 20-1).**

2. Transfer mouth mirror and explorer.

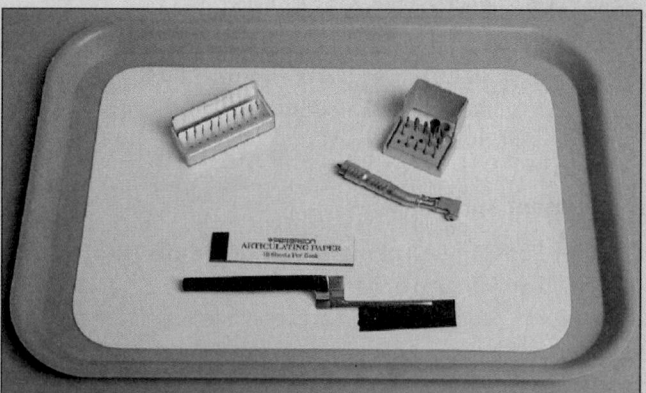

FIGURE 38-39
Occlusal adjustment setup.

Dentist/periodontist examines the oral cavity including the teeth.

3. Retrieve explorer.

4. Assist in preparation for occlusal adjustment procedure.
   - ❏ Dry the quadrant with the air syringe or a gauze sponge.
   - ❏ Exchange explorer for articulating paper.

   Dentist places articulating paper over the occlusal surfaces and instructs the patient to bite down and grind the teeth side to side.

   Dentist removes articulating paper and evaluates the marks left by the articulating paper (the markings indicate how teeth in the maxillary and mandibular arches occlude).

5. Assist in completing occlusal adjustment procedure.
   - ❏ Change burs, discs, and stones as requested by the dentist/periodontist.
   - ❏ Transfer the handpiece to the dentist/periodontist.

- ❏ Use the air/water syringe and the evacuator to maintain the field.

6. Write up procedure in Services Rendered.

7. Dismiss and escort patient to reception area (refer to Procedure 18-5).

Note: This process is repeated until the teeth occlude evenly over the quadrant. Each quadrant is evaluated and adjusted.

Date	Services Rendered
02/18/XX	Updated medical and dental history, no changes noted. BP = 120/80; T = 98.6F, P = 80, R = 18
	Occlusal adjustment completed
	RTC: Assistant's initials

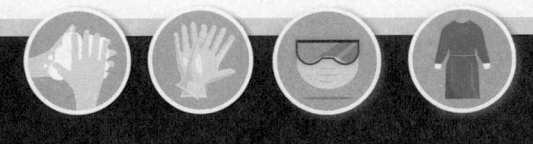

Procedure 38-2
Gingivectomy

This procedure is performed by the periodontist in order to remove diseased gingiva and clean the periodontal pockets. The dental assistant prepares the instruments and materials, prepares the patient, and performs assisting responsibilities during the procedure. Depending on the state Dental Practice Act, the dental assistant may place and remove the periodontal dressing (Refer to Procedures 38-4 and 38-5.).

Steps written in blue font are performed by the operator (dentist or qualified dental assistant), and the chairside assistant's steps are written in black.

Equipment and Supplies

Patient Seating Setup (refer to Procedure 18-4)
- Handwashing soap or hand sanitizer
- Sanitized dental treatment area and barriers placed over equipment
- Patient's medical and dental records
- Patient seating setup (refer to Procedure 18-4)
  - ❏ Patient napkin and napkin clip

- ❏ Patient protective glasses
- ❏ Saliva ejector, evacuator (HVE), and air/water syringe tips and surgical aspiration tip
- ❏ Basic setup: mouth mirror, explorer, and cotton forceps
- ❏ Mouth rinse in disposable cup
- Blood pressure equipment
- Patient

Gingivectomy Setup (Figure 38-40)
- Anesthetic setup (not shown; refer to Procedure 23-2)
- Pocket marker (not shown; refer to Figure 38-41)
- Periodontal dressing material (refer to Figure 38-38 and Procedure 38-4)

Procedure Steps (*Follow aseptic procedures*)

1. Escort and seat patient (refer to Procedure 18-4).

   Periodontist greets the patient and takes position at the dental chair.
   - ❏ Signals for the procedure to begin (refer to Procedure 20-1).

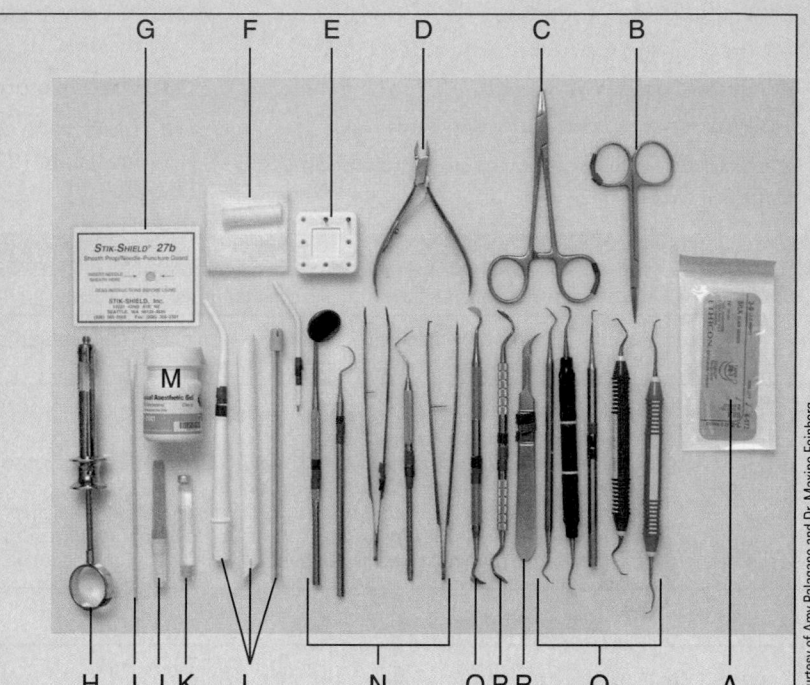

A. Suture
B. Suture scissors
C. Needle holder
D. Rongeur
E. Bur block
F. Gauze and cotton roll
G. Needle recapping device
H. Syringe
I. Cotton tip applicator
J. Needle
K. Local anesthetic cartridge
L. Suction tips
M. Topical anesthetic
N. Basic set up
O. Kirkland knife
P. Interproximal knife
Q. Assorted scalers
R. Scalpel handle and blade

Courtesy of Amy Palagano and Dr. Maxine Feinberg

FIGURE 38-40
Gingivectomy tray setup.

2. Assist with preparing patient for gingivectomy.

   Periodontist examines the area needing gingivectomy.

3. Pass mouth mirror and explorer at operator's signal.

   Periodontist examines patient's periodontal probing record.

   ❏ Exchanges explorer for probe.

4. Retrieve probe.

   Periodontist administers local anesthetic.

5. Assist in administration of local anesthetic (refer to Procedure 23-2).

   Periodontist marks pocket depths with pocket markers (Figure 38-41).

6. Pass pocket markers.

   Periodontist performs gingivectomy.

7. Assist with gingivectomy.
   ❏ Pass interdental knives and retrieve pocket markers.
   ❏ Maintain operating field.

❏ Transfer scissors, Rongeurs, and handpiece with burs as requested by dentist.
❏ Use gauze to clear debris from operating field.

Periodontist completes gingival curettage and scales and planes root surfaces to remove irritants and promote healing.

8. Assist with curettage and root planning.
   ❏ Transfer scalers.
   ❏ Irrigate with sterile saline and evacuate the area.

   Periodontist places sutures.

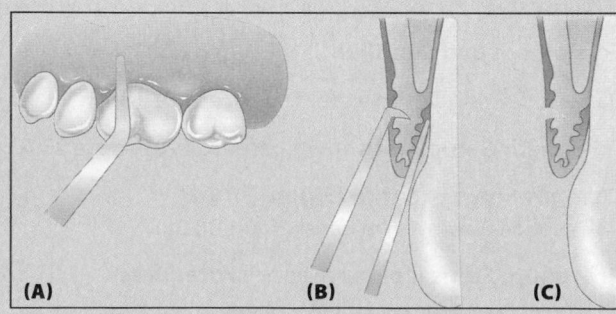

(A)   **(B)**   **(C)**

FIGURE 38-41
Gingivectomy procedure. (A, B) Marking pocket depth with pocket marker. (C) Incising marked tissues with periodontal knives.

(Continues)

9. Assist in suturing procedure.

❑ **Prepare and transfer needle and suture.**

❑ **Retract tissues as needed.**

❑ **Pass scissors to cut suture thread.**

Operator prepares and places periodontal dressing (refer to Procedure 38-4).

10. Assist with preparation and placement of periodontal dressing.

11. Write up procedure in Services Rendered.

12. Dismiss and escort patient to reception area (refer to Procedure 18-5).

Date	Services Rendered
02/18/XX	Updated medical and dental history, no changes noted. BP = 120/80; T = 98.6F, P = 80, R = 18
	Placed 20% benzocaine gel to injection sites for 2 minutes. Administered two cartridges (3.6 ml) of 2% lidocaine with 1:100,000 epinephrine to mandibular left. No reaction
	Mandibular right quadrant gingivectomy teeth #28-30. Noneugenol dressing placed Postoperative instructions provided—Take prescribed medications as instructed for post-op discomfort, limit activity for 24 hours to minimize bleeding, no smoking for 48 hours, normal oral home care in the nonsurgical area should be performed, brush only the biting surfaces of the teeth in the surgical area. Rinse with warm salt water after 2 hours. Avoid hot spicy foods and acidic foods, chew on side opposite to surgery, place an ice pack for 10 minutes on and then 10 minutes off to minimize swelling and repeat as needed. Some seepage may occur—call office if it persists.
	RTC: remove dressing Assistant's initials

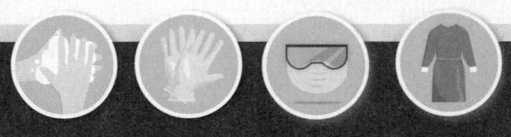

Procedure 38-3
Osseous Surgery

This procedure is performed by the periodontist. It involves removing and recontouring diseased and defective bone tissue. The extent of the periodontal disease process determines the amount and type of surgery performed. Depending on the state Dental Practice Act, the qualified dental assistant may place and remove the periodontal dressing (Refer to Procedures 38-4 and 38-5.)

Steps written in blue font are performed by the operator (dentist or qualified dental assistant), and the chairside assistant's steps are written in black.

Equipment and Supplies

Patient Seating Setup (refer to Procedure 18-4)

Anesthetic Setup (not shown; refer to Procedure 23-2)

Osseous Surgery Setup (Figure 38-42)
• Periodontal dressing material (Figure 38-38)

Procedure Steps (*Follow aseptic procedures*)

1. Escort and seat patient (refer to Procedure 18-4).

Periodontist greets the patient and takes position at the dental chair.

❑ *Signals for the procedure to begin (refer to Procedure 20-1).*

2. Pass mouth mirror and explorer at operator's signal.

Periodontist examines the area needing osseous surgery.

Dentist administers local anesthetic.

3. Assist in administration of local anesthetic (refer to Procedure 23-2).

Periodontist makes tissue flap.

❑ *Reflects tissue flap, stabilizes with tissue retractors, and exposes bone.*

4. Assist with flap procedure.

❑ Pass scalpel with blades.

❑ Exchange scalpel and retractors.

❑ Irrigate the area with sterile saline solution and evacuate area as needed.

A. Suture
B. Suture scissors
C. Needle holder
D. Rongeur
E. Bur block
F. Gauze and cotton roll
G. Needle recapping device
H. Syringe
I. Cotton tip applicator
J. Needle
K. Local anesthetic cartridge
L. Suction tips
M. Topical anesthetic
N. Basic set up
O. Kirkland knife
P. Buck knife
Q. Hemostat
R. Bone file
S. Chisel scaler
T. Hoe scaler
U. Assorted scalers
V. Tissue forceps
W. Scalpel handle and blade

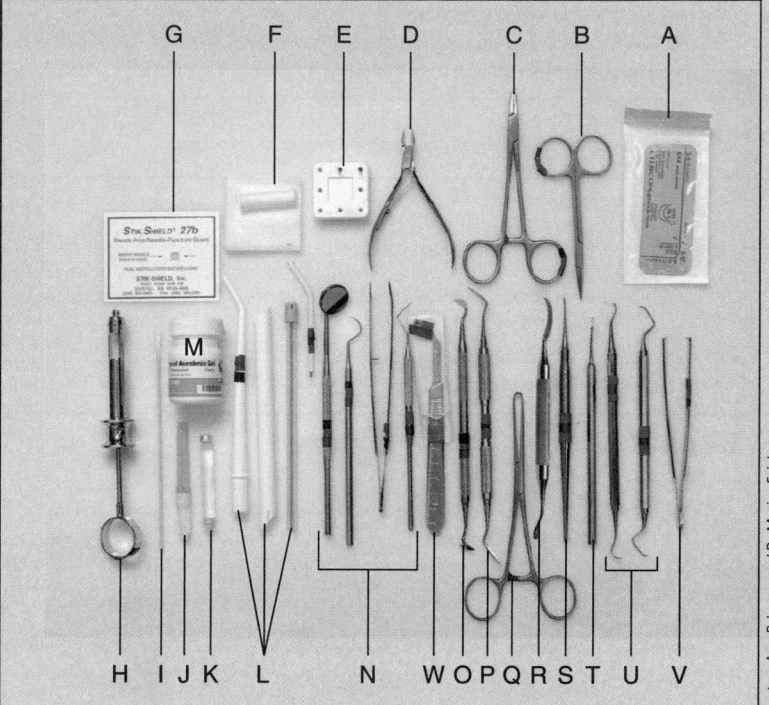

Courtesy Amy Palagano and Dr. Maxine Feinberg

FIGURE 38-42
Osseous surgery tray setup.

Periodontist performs osseous surgery.
❏ **Removes diseased bone and completes gingival curettage.**
❏ **Scales and planes root surfaces to remove irritants and promote healing.**

5. Assist with surgery.
❏ Transfer scissors, Rongeurs, and handpiece with burs as requested by dentist.
❏ Irrigate the area with sterile saline solution and evacuate area as needed.

Periodontist shapes bone with burs, stones, Rongeurs, chisels, and files.

6. Assist with shaping bone.
❏ Pass surgical instruments as requested.
❏ Irrigate the area with sterile saline solution and evacuate area as needed.

❏ Keep instruments clean by removing debris from instruments with the gauze sponge.
❏ Maintain operating field.

Periodontist places tissue flap in position for suturing.

7. Assist with suturing.
❏ Prepare needle and suture.
❏ Transfer needle and suture.
❏ Stabilize tissues with tissue forceps during suturing.

Operator prepares and places periodontal dressing (refer to Procedure 38-4).

8. Assist with periodontal dressing.
❏ Remove debris from patient's face.
9. Write up procedure in Services Rendered.
10. Dismiss and escort patient to reception area (refer to Procedure 18-5).

(Continues)

Date	Services Rendered
02/18/XX	Updated medical and dental history, no changes noted. BP = 120/80; T = 98.6F, P = 80, R = 18
	Placed 20% benzocaine gel to injection sites for 2 minutes. Administered two cartridges (3.6 ml) of 2% lidocaine with 1:100,000 epinephrine to mandibular left. No reaction
	Mandibular right quadrant osseous surgery teeth #28–30. Noneugenol dressing placed Postoperative instructions provided—Take prescribed medications as instructed for post-op discomfort, limit activity for 24 hours to minimize bleeding, no smoking for 48 hours, normal oral home care in the nonsurgical area should be performed, brush only the biting surfaces of the teeth in the surgical area. Rinse with warm salt water after 2 hours. Avoid hot spicy foods and acidic foods, chew on side opposite to surgery, place an ice pack for 10 minutes on and then 10 minutes off to minimize swelling and repeat as needed. Some seepage may occur—call office if it persists.
	RTC: remove dressing Assistant's initials

Procedure 38-4
Preparation and Placement of Noneugenol Periodontal Dressing

This procedure immediately follows a periodontal surgical procedure such as flap surgery or gingivectomy. The periodontist routinely places the dressing, but in some states the qualified dental assistant is allowed to place and remove the periodontal dressing. The dressing is placed after the surgery to protect the tissues and promote the healing process. The periodontal dressing should be placed once the bleeding is controlled.

Steps written in blue font are performed by the operator (dentist or qualified dental assistant), and the chairside assistant's steps are written in black.

Equipment and Supplies

Periodontal Dressing Setup
- Cotton rolls and 2 × 2-inch gauze sponges
- Noneugenol periodontal dressing material (base and accelerator) (Figure 38-43A)
- Paper pad and tongue depressor (Figure 38-43A)
- Approved lubricant (Figure 38-43A)
- Spoon excavator and sickle scaler to contour dressing (Figure 38-43D)

Procedure Steps (*Follow aseptic procedures*)

1. Prepare dressing placement (Figures 38-43A and B).
   - ❏ Coat patient's lips lightly with approved lubricant.
   - ❏ Dispense base and accelerator of dressing material onto paper pad in equal lengths.
   - ❏ Mix material until homogeneous.

   Operator places dressing.

   - ❏ Allows material to set for 2–3 minutes so it is less tacky.
   - ❏ Lubricates gloved fingers with approved lubricant for easier handling of material.
   - ❏ Molds dressing material into a thin strip slightly longer than the length of the surgical site.
   - ❏ Divides the strip into two strips, one for the buccal/facial aspect and one for the lingual/palatal aspect of the surgical site.
   - ❏ Forms a hook on end of one of the strips and places this around the most posterior tooth (Figure 38-43C).
   - ❏ Adapts the rest of the strip along the facial/buccal surface, gently pressing the material into the interproximal areas (Figure 38-43D).
   - ❏ Applies the second strip in the same manner on the lingual/palatal surface.
   - ❏ Ensures the pack covers the gingiva evenly without interfering with occlusion, tongue movements, or frenum attachments.

2. Pass spoon excavator or scaler as requested.

   Operator checks dressing for overextensions.

   - ❏ Removes overextensions with a spoon excavator or scaler.
   - ❏ Gently presses the instrument onto the dressing to detach the extra material.
   - ❏ Smooths the pack and evaluates it for even thickness.
   - ❏ Asks the patient how the dressing feels.

❑ Instructs the patient to move their tongue, cheeks, and lips to mold the pack.

❑ Makes any adjustments to ensure the dressing is securely in place, trimmed, and contoured.

3. Write up procedure in Services Rendered.

4. Dismiss and escort patient to reception area (refer to Procedure 18-5).

Date	Services Rendered
02/18/XX	Noneugenol dressing placed after osseous surgery was completed and hemorrhaging controlled. Postoperative instructions provided. The pack is kept on for 1 week after surgery. The pack will harden in a few hours and then withstand normal chewing stresses. The pack may chip and break off during the week but should remain intact as long as possible. If there is pain when pieces of the pack come off or the pack becomes rough, the patient should call the office. The patient should brush the occlusal surface of the teeth involved in the surgery and continue to brush and floss the rest of the teeth as normal.
	RTC: remove dressing Assistant's initials

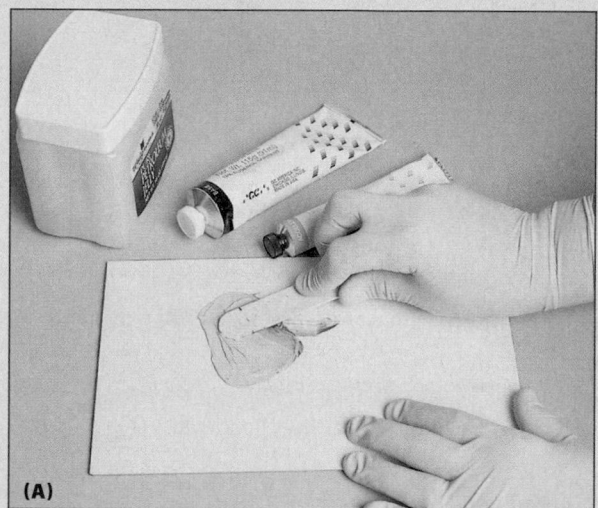
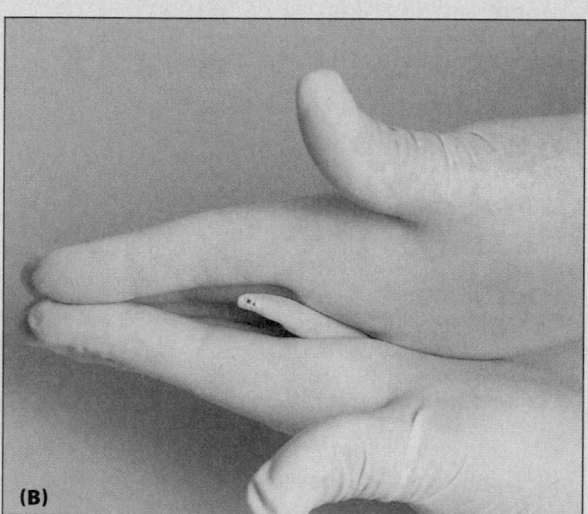
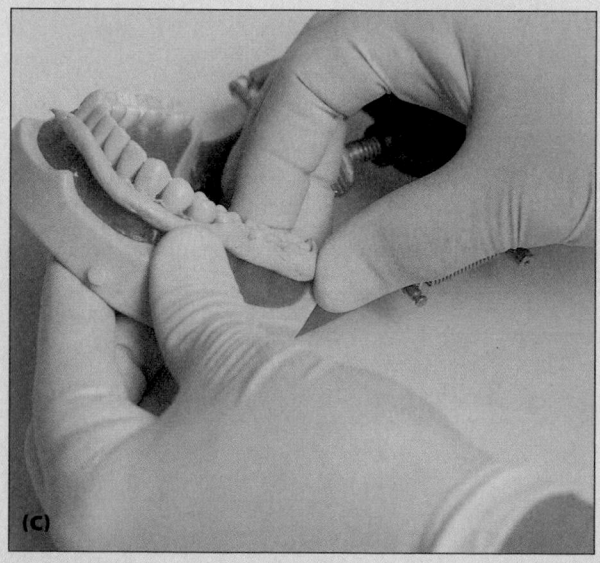
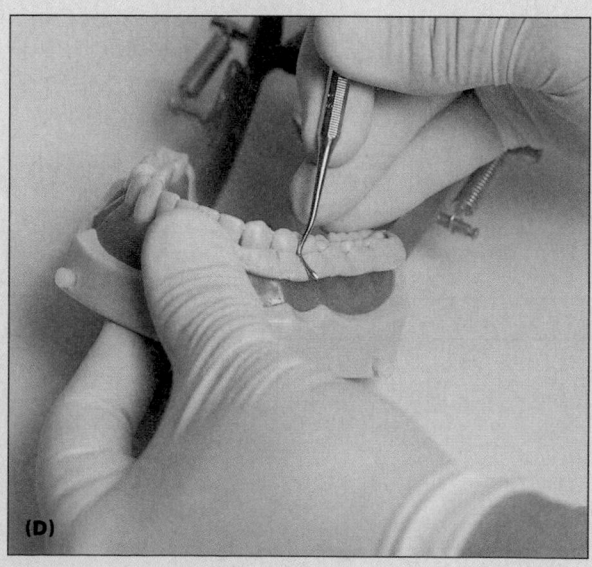

FIGURE 38-43
Preparation and placement of periodontal dressing. (A) Mixing the materials. (B) Preparing the materials for placement. (C) Placing the dressing on tissue. (D) Contouring dressing.

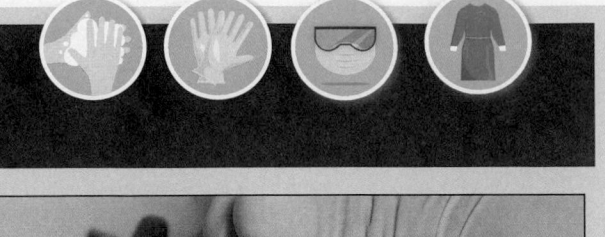

Procedure 38-5
Removal of Periodontal Dressing

This procedure is performed by the periodontist or the qualified dental assistant, depending on the state Dental Practice Act. The patient has worn the dressing for 7–10 days. The patient's oral cavity is examined before removing the dressing to check for areas where the dressing may have loosened or come off completely.

Steps written in **blue** font are performed by the operator (dentist or qualified dental assistant), and the chairside assistant's steps are written in black.

Equipment and Supplies

Patient Seating Setup (refer to Procedure 18-4)

Periodontal Dressing Removal Setup
- 2 × 2-inch gauze sponges
- Periodontal probes
- Spoon excavator or surgical hoe or sickle scaler to remove the dressing (Figure 38-44)
- cotton pliers

Procedure Steps (*Follow aseptic procedures*)

1. Escort and seat patient (refer to Procedure 18-4).

   Examines the dressing.

   Inserts instrument of preference along the margin and applies lateral pressure to remove the dressing away from the tissues (Figure 38-44).

   ❏ Note the pack may come off in large pieces and then the particles can be removed with scalers and cotton pliers.

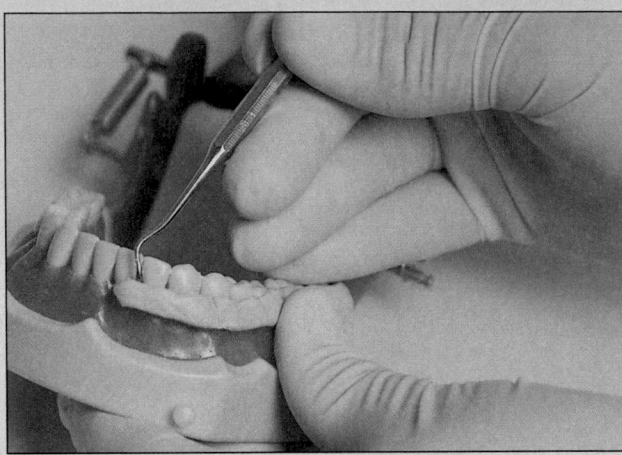

FIGURE 38-44
Removing periodontal dressing.

2. Pass instrument preference as requested.

3. Rinse the area with warm water to remove remaining debris.
   ❏ Use air/water syringe carefully.

4. Write up procedure in Services Rendered.

5. Dismiss and escort patient to reception area (refer to Procedure 18-5).

Date	Services Rendered	
02/18/XX	Updated medical and dental history, no changes noted. BP = 120/80; T = 98.6F, P = 80, R = 18	
	Mandibular right quadrant osseous surgery teeth #28–30. Noneugenol dressing removed from mandibular right quadrant osseous surgery teeth #28–30.	
	RTC:	Assistant's initials

Chapter Summary

According to the American Academy of Periodontology, three out of four adults will experience, to some degree, periodontal problems at some time in their lives. In children and adolescents, marginal gingivitis and gingival recession are the most prevalent conditions.

In this chapter the dental assistant student learns the symptoms, causes, and classifications of periodontal disease. Diagnostic procedures including the medical and dental history, clinical examination, periodontal screening and recording system, types of x-rays taken, and how the treatment plan is put together and presented to the patient are described. The student learns the instruments and equipment used as well as the nonsurgical and surgical procedures routinely completed in a periodontal office. There is also information on the use, benefits, and safety of dental lasers. The dental assistant performs chairside assisting duties and the expanded functions allowed by the state Dental Practice Act, including placing and removing periodontal dressing, removing sutures, and performing coronal polishes.

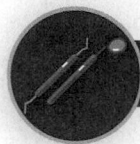

CASE STUDY

Melissa Moore is 42 years old. She has been Dr. Sanchez's patient for 14 years. Melissa has her teeth examined and cleaned every 6 months. Over the years, she has developed several teeth with pocket readings of between six and eight. At Melissa's last cleaning appointment, the hygienist explained that she found over 10 areas with periodontal probing readings of over six and areas where the tissues bleed easily. Melissa is in good general health but has been taking medication to reduce anxiety for the past 6 months.

Case Study Review

1. Are Melissa's periodontal readings within the normal range?

2. What questions should be asked in reference to the change in her condition over such a short period of time?

3. What should the patient be advised regarding her periodontal condition?

Review Questions

Multiple Choice

1. Which periodontal team member places and removes the periodontal dressing, takes impressions for splints, and provides pre- and postoperative instructions?
   a. periodontist
   b. dental assistant
   c. dental hygienist
   d. lab technician

2. Which statements are true regarding periodontal disease?
   a. It involves inflammation of soft and hard structures supporting the teeth.
   b. It may cause tooth mobility.
   c. It may result in tooth loss.
   d. All of these are true.

3. What do current researchers believe is the primary cause of periodontal disease?
   a. biofilm
   b. calculus
   c. host bacterial response
   d. host viral response

4. Using the AAP classification, which grade represents rapid progression of periodontal disease?
   a. A
   b. B
   c. C
   d. D

5. How many sites are probed to determine the sulcus depth?
   a. 5
   b. 6
   c. 10
   d. 12

6. At what sulcus depth is it considered a periodontal pocket?
   a. 2 mm
   b. 3 mm
   c. 4 mm
   d. All of these

7. Suppuration during periodontal probing is indicated by _____ in the gingival sulcus.
   a. biofilm
   b. blood
   c. pus
   d. calculus

8. Which instrument is used to remove subgingival calculus?
   a. sickle scaler
   b. Jacquette scaler
   c. curette
   d. probe

9. The working end of the periodontal instrument used to remove supragingival calculus has sharp cutting edges on both sides of the blade. This instrument is a:
   a. hoe.
   b. file.
   c. scaler.
   d. curette.

10. What is used to manually sharpening periodontal instruments?
    a. finer grit Arkansas stone
    b. coarse grit ceramic stone
    c. rotating disc
    d. rotating stone

11. Which nonsurgical method shaves the root surface with curettes to leave a smooth root surface?
    a. root planing
    b. gingival curettage
    c. oral irrigation
    d. scaling

12. Which adjunctive therapy will subdue collagenase and help reduce pocket depths?
    a. locally applied antimicrobial agent
    b. systemic antibiotic treatment
    c. oral irrigation
    d. enzyme suppression therapy

13. All of these are signs of healing at the reevaluation appointment EXCEPT:
    a. regeneration of tissue.
    b. presence of less pathogenic bacteria.
    c. new bone around the teeth.
    d. less bleeding on probing.

14. Which surgical procedure is performed to remove diseased soft tissue and eliminate periodontal pockets?
    a. ostectomy
    b. flap surgery
    c. gingivoplasty
    d. gingivectomy

15. All of the following are safety measures to be in place when using dental lasers EXCEPT:
    a. special protective eyewear should be worn by the dentist only.
    b. a warning sign should be posted by the treatment room when lasers are in use.
    c. a moist gauze should cover tissues not being treated with the laser.
    d. matte coated instruments should be used.

16. Periodontal surgery that involves recontouring of the alveolar bone is called:
    a. mucogingival surgery.
    b. gingival grafting.
    c. osteoplasty.
    d. ostectomy.

17. All of these are postoperative instructions provided the patient after periodontal therapy EXCEPT:
    a. take all medications as directed by periodontist.
    b. return to normal activity after surgery.
    c. chew on opposite side of surgery.
    d. use ice pack for swelling.

18. Which periodontal dressing is an excellent choice after soft-tissue augmentation?
    a. zinc oxide–eugenol materials
    b. noneugenol materials
    c. light-cured periodontal dressing
    d. gelatin-base dressings

19. All of these statements are true about periodontal maintenance EXCEPT:
    a. it is designed to prevent recurrence of periodontal disease.
    b. appointments are scheduled 12 months after periodontal therapy.
    c. it includes assessment of home care.
    d. scaling and polishing are performed as needed.

20. Which procedure(s) may be performed by a periodontal dental assistant depending on the state practice act?
    a. scaling supragingival deposits
    b. coronal polishing
    c. sharpening periodontal hand instruments
    d. All of these

Critical Thinking

1. What are the signs and symptoms of periodontal disease?

2. Lasers are being used more and more for dental treatments. Discuss the benefits of using lasers in the periodontal office.

3. Discuss the purpose of placing periodontal dressing and which type of periodontal dressing might cause an allergic reaction to the patient.

Key Terms

Term and Pronunciation	Meaning of Root and Word Parts	Definition
pellicle (**pel**-i-*kuh* l)	**pellicle** = a thin skin or membrane; film; scum	dental pellicle is a protein film that forms on the surface; it forms in seconds after a tooth is cleaned or after chewing; it protects the tooth from the acids produced by oral microorganisms after consuming carbohydrates

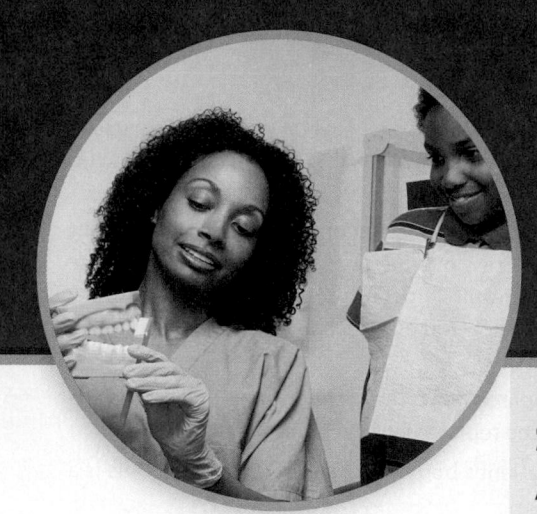

## CHAPTER 39

Dental Implants

Specific Instructional Objectives

At the completion of this chapter, you will be able to meet these objectives:

1. Use terms presented in this chapter.
2. State the advantages of dental implants.
3. State the disadvantages of dental implants.
4. Describe the differences in implant success rate based on location.
5. Describe the parts of an implant.
6. List the considerations for dental implants.
7. Identify the contraindications for dental implants.
8. Describe the patient selection factors for implants.
9. Describe the process for patient preparation for implant placement.
10. Compare and contrast the types of implants.
11. Describe the purpose of immediate load implants.
12. Compare and contrast the steps in the single-surgery and the two-surgery techniques.
13. Outline the postoperative home care instructions.
14. Define the implant-retained prosthesis.
15. Describe the role of the dental assistant in an implant procedure.

Introduction

A *dental implant* is an artificial tooth root that is surgically placed within the alveolar bone. Dental implants are one of the biggest advancements in dental treatment over the past 40 years. Implants first became available in the 1970s and evolved into the implants of today. Since the 1970s the design of implants has improved. Titanium roots were implanted in a patient for the first time in 1965.

The insertion of dental implants provides a long-term option for the replacement of teeth compared with more traditional choices, such as bridges or partial dentures. Implants have become an effective and popular treatment for people who are missing teeth or who have lost a tooth or teeth due to advanced dental decay, periodontal disease, or injury. Once the implant is secure and stable, it then holds the replacement crown, bridge, partial, or denture.

Advantages of Dental Implants

There are many advantages to dental implants versus removable appliances, including the following:

- **Better esthetics.** Since dental implants osseointegrate with bone to become permanent, they look and feel like the natural teeth.

- **Better speech.** Speech may be affected by removable oral prosthesis that do not fit well. Dental implants improve the speech of the patient as compared to poorly fitting dentures.

- **Increased comfort.** Since implants become permanent, they are more comfortable than a removable appliance.

- **Better chewing ability.** Patients who have poorly fitting dentures have difficulty with mastication. Dental implants allow the patient to eat in a manner that is similar to their natural teeth.

- **Increased self-esteem.** Implants restore the look of the dentition and improve self-confidence.

- **Improvement in oral health.** Bridges require reduction of the abutment teeth. Since tooth reduction is not required with an implant, the natural tooth structure of the surrounding teeth is maintained. It is easier to access the area around an implant for oral home care.

- **Longevity.** With good oral home care, implants can last a lifetime.

- **Convenience.** Dental implants do not need adhesives to keep them in place and do not need to be removed at night. As a result, they are more convenient than a removable oral prosthesis.

- **Reduced alveolar bone resorption.** The alveolar bone resorbs when a person loses a tooth. Dental implants can prevent bone resorption related to tooth loss. With the loss of multiple teeth, the face starts to get a "caved-in" appearance (Figure 39-1). Implants can restore the natural appearance of the face.

Disadvantages of Implants

Though implants have many advantages, there are disadvantages as well. These include the following:

- **Cost**. The average cost of an implant plus crown is about $3,500. The cost to replace one tooth with an implant and crown is higher than the cost of a removable prosthesis which can replace multiple teeth.

- **Healing after surgical placement.** The healing time depends on the location of implant placement as well as the quantity and quality of the bone in the area. Overall treatment time can range from 3 to 12 months. The general health of the dental implant patient and whether or not there is a need for bone grafting determines healing time as well. Sinus lifts will be discussed later in this chapter.

- **Complications related to surgery.** Placing implants requires surgery. As a result, discomfort, swelling, and bleeding are not uncommon.

- **Bone loss.** Slight bone loss over several years is not unusual. If extensive bone loss takes place, the implant may need to be replaced.

- **Excellent oral hygiene.** Excellent oral home care is important for long-term success of a implant. Dexterity issues or poor oral hygiene can result in loss of supporting bone over time. Additionally, infection and eventual loss of the dental implant may take place.

- **Accessories replacement.** The crown which is placed on the implant may need replacement over time.

- **Failure.** The patient's body may reject the implant. This is a rare occurrence.

Dental Implant Success Rate

Dental implants have a great success rate, with variances depending on where the implants are placed and what they do. For example, the anterior teeth success rate ranges from 90% to 100%, while the posterior teeth success rate ranges from 85% to 95%. One determining factor for implant success is the quality and the quantity of the bone where the implant is to be placed. Due to the presence of the sinus and insufficient bone, the maxillary posterior area is one of the most difficult locations for implant placement. Bone augmentation can help correct this problem by lifting the sinus floor and providing bone for the placement of the dental implants (Figure 39-2). The sinus lift procedure is performed by the oral maxillofacial surgeon.

There may be inadequate bone at the dental implant sites based on the anatomy of the maxilla or the mandible (Figure 39-3). The deficiency is filled with bone or bone substitute to enhance the bony ridge (Figure 39-4). Modifying the ridge can improve appearance and also increase the success rate of implants (Figure 39-5). This procedure requires a gingival flap to be opened to expose the bone. This procedure is performed by the periodontist or oral maxillofacial surgeon.

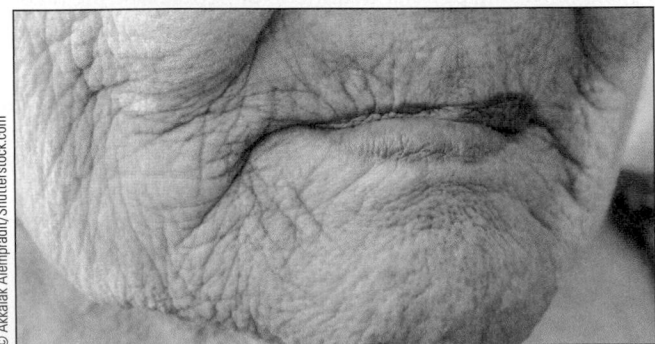

FIGURE 39-1
Edentulous patient.

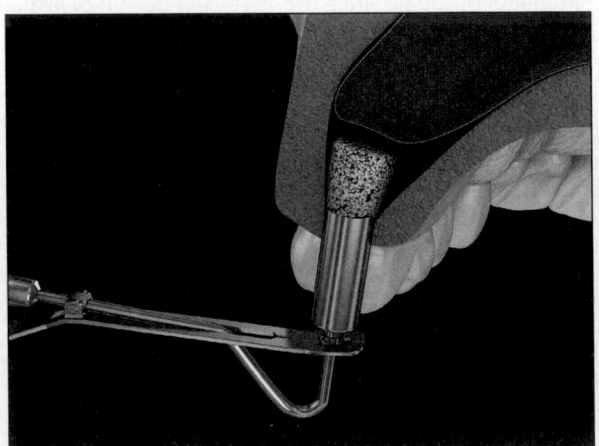

FIGURE 39-2
Sinus lift and adding bone.

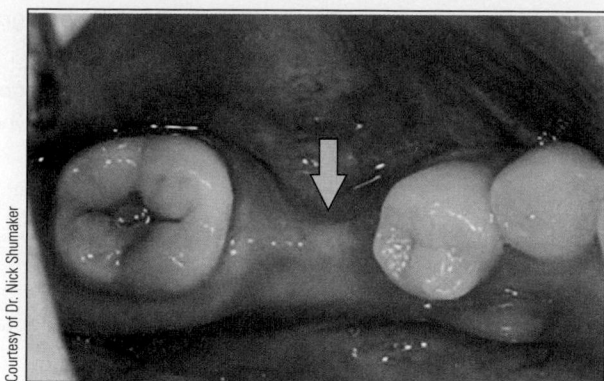

FIGURE 39-3
Before ridge augmentation bone graft and dental implant.

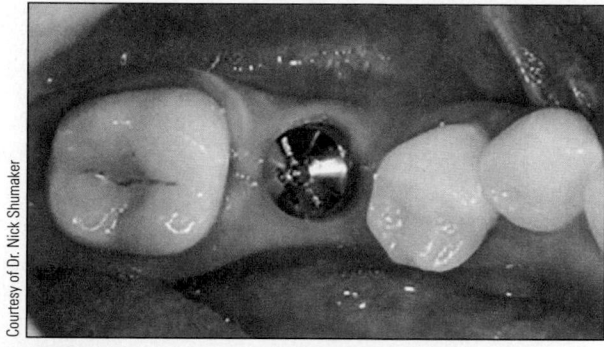

FIGURE 39-4
After ridge augmentation bone graft and dental implant, prior to restoration.

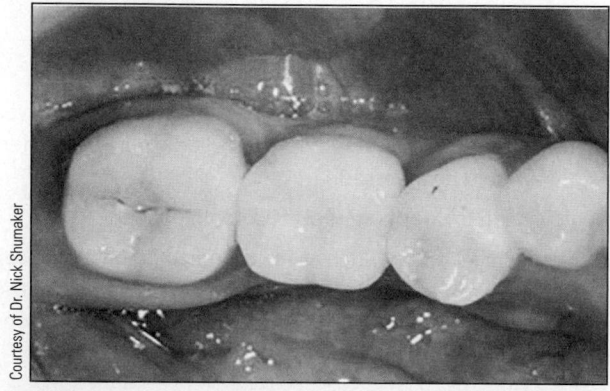

FIGURE 39-5
After ridge augmentation bone graft, dental implant placement, and final crown restoration

Implant success also depends on the load that the implant has to bear; for example, an implant that has to support a partial denture will experience greater stress than one that supports a crown.

Parts of an Implant

The dental implant bodies are usually made of titanium alloys, as titanium enhances the process of osseointegration. The dental implant surface can vary. The surface of dental implants affects the long-term integration and stability of treatment. A porous surface contributes to more bone contact than a machined titanium surface.

Implant Body or Fixture

The implant body or fixture is placed during the first stage of implant surgery. It functions as the foundation for the restoration and becomes a permanent part of the alveolar bone. The implant body can be threaded (Figure 39-6) or nonthreaded. When the natural teeth are lost, bone loss is common. But when the implant is placed, the bone tissue tends to grow around it. The commercially available implant bodies are made of either commercially pure titanium or titanium alloys. Some implant bodies contain hydroxyapatite crystals. The hydroxyapatite crystals may enhance osseointegration.

Abutment

The abutment is the part of the implant which is screwed to the body of the implant and resembles a prepared tooth (Figure 39-6). It is the part that provides support to the artificial crown and lies between the crown and the implant body. The abutment provides retention to the prosthesis.

Healing Screw and Healing Cap

The *healing screw* is a nonpermanent part of the implant, used while the soft tissue over the implant body is healing. The healing screw facilitates the suturing of the soft tissue, and it also prevents the growth of gingival soft tissues over the edge of the implant.

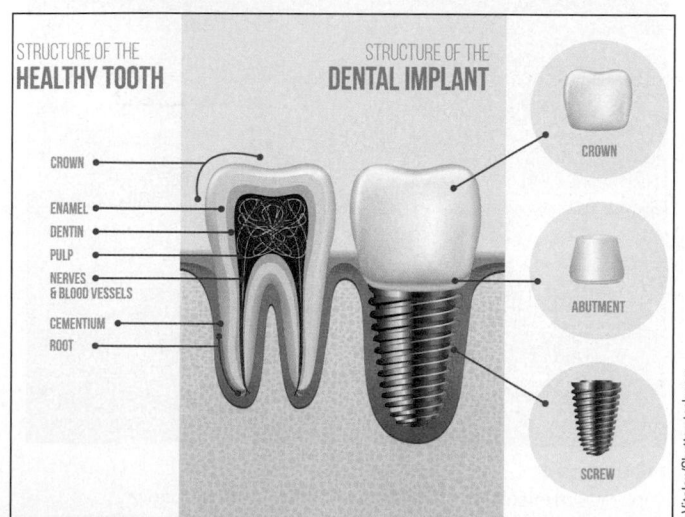

FIGURE 39-6
Structure of implant compared to structure of natural tooth.

Healing caps are the dome-shaped caps placed over the healing screws. They project through the soft tissue into the oral cavity (Figure 39-7) and range from 2 to 10 mm in length. They prevent the overgrowth of the soft tissues over the implant body. They also function as a guide for the placement of the permanent restoration after the second stage of the surgery.

Dental Implant Connectors

All dental implants require the restoration and abutment to be connected to the implant head (Figure 39-8). For this purpose, there are three main connector types:

- **Internal hex connectors.** These connectors are shaped like hexagons. An internal hex connector is an opening in the dental implant head. This opening is where the restoration or abutment is screwed into.

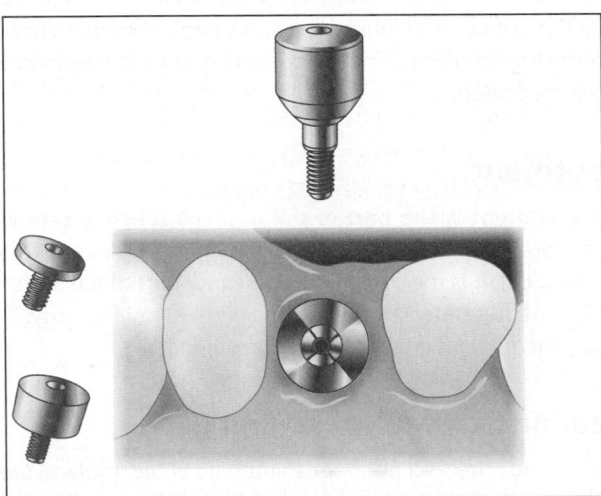

FIGURE 39-7
Healing cap on the dental implant.

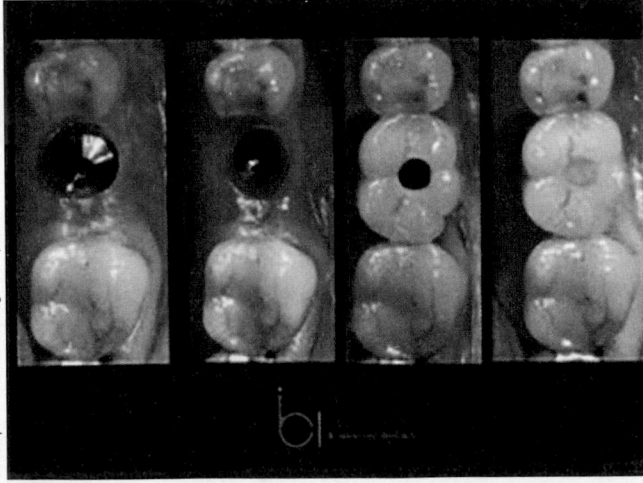

FIGURE 39-8
Implant with internal hex connector and finished implant crown.

- **External hex connectors.** These connectors are also hexagonal in shape. They sit on top of the dental implant head.
- **Internal octagon connectors.** These connectors are octagonal in shape. The restoration or abutment is screwed into the opening of the internal octagonal connector.

Considerations for Dental Implants

Among the most common indications for undergoing the dental implant procedures are the following:

- Fixed replacement of a missing tooth or teeth
- Support for a full denture or a removable partial denture
- An implant-supported bridge to replace multiple missing teeth
- Prevention of alveolar bone resorption that may follow tooth loss
- Positive and cooperative attitude of the patient
- Patient's good overall health
- Adequate quantity and quality of alveolar bone

Crown/Bridge

The crown or bridge is an artificial replacement that restores the missing tooth structure by surrounding part or all of the remaining structure with a material such as cast metal, porcelain, or a combination of materials such as metal and porcelain. It is the top part of the restoration, which is visible in the oral cavity (Figure 39-6). The crowns are fabricated by a dental technician and aid in esthetics, mastication, and balancing of the occlusion.

Contraindications for the Placement of Implants

There are a few contraindications to implant dentistry. However, there are some systemic, behavioral, and anatomic considerations that should be assessed.

- Negative and uncooperative attitude of the patient
- Medical considerations such as uncontrolled diabetes, cancer, or hormone replacement therapy, which may decrease the chance of success of the dental implant; certain medications such as oral bisphosphonate
- Patient with a bruxism habit
- Poor quality or quantity of alveolar bone
- Anatomical locations of nerves or sinus that may prevent appropriate implant placement
- Allergies to materials used in dental implants
- Inability to pay for implants

Patient Selection for Implants

The clinical standard of care involves routine consideration of dental implant placement in any missing area of the oral cavity. All dental professionals must become thoroughly aware of these valuable procedures involved in careful patient selection. Implant success is dependent on the following predictors:

- Quantity and quality of alveolar bone
- Clinician experience
- Masticatory forces
- Patient commitment to regular postoperative recalls
- Good oral hygiene home care

Implant failures are rare and usually can be corrected. Reasons why implants may fail include the following:

- The soft and/or hard tissues may have an infection that did not heal.
- The implant fails to integrate.
- The implant fractures or breaks.
- There is damage to the nerve in the mandible due to implant placement.
- There is damage to the maxillary sinus or nasal cavity due to implant placement.

Medical History The treatment planning process for implants begins with the patient meeting with the general dentist. After an initial consultation, the dentist may refer the patient to a specialist such as an oral surgeon, a prosthodontist, or a periodontist. Some general dentists have undergone extensive training in dental implant placement and are able to perform all dental implant procedures in their own offices.

In the initial appointment, the patient's medical history is reviewed to determine if there are any contraindications to treatment. For example, uncontrolled type I diabetes can delay healing due to poor quality of circulating blood. This may lead to implant failure. Cardiovascular disease may also impact success due to poor quantity of blood circulating to the implant site. The patient's attitude toward the procedure should also be determined. Osteoporosis, which often affects postmenopausal women, may affect osseointegration by impairing bone metabolism.

A history of radiation therapy to the area where an implant is to be placed may be a risk factor for late implant failure due to diminished salivary production and blood supply to the alveolar bone and soft tissues. Osteonecrosis is also a risk factor. Active chemotherapy is a contraindication to dental implant placement. Age is not considered a significant risk factor on its own; however, implants should only be placed after maxillary and mandibular growth has been completed in the young adult.

People who smoke have a statistically greater risk of early implant failure compared to people who do not smoke. While smoking is not an absolute contraindication to implant therapy, the patient who smokes should be advised that there is an increased risk of implant complications and should be offered smoking cessation methods.

Dental History The dentist evaluates the condition of the existing teeth and gingival soft tissues as well as the height and width of the edentulous alveolar ridge. People with poor oral home care, active infection, or uncontrolled dental decay are poor candidates for dental implants. Periodontal disease is one of the most common causes of tooth loss. The same pathogens responsible for periodontal disease are believed to be involved in infections related to implants and implant failure. A comprehensive periodontal evaluation and periodontal treatment should be completed prior to implant placement to ensure the patient has optimal periodontal health before treatment begins.

The quantity and quality of alveolar bone is an important consideration. An ancillary procedure such as a bone graft (Figure 39-9) or sinus augmentation (Figure 39-2) may be needed to provide sufficient bone for successful implant placement in the maxilla. For mandibular implants, there must be sufficient alveolar bone present superior to the inferior alveolar canal. There are generally four types of bone grafts used:

- *Autografts* are those where the bone to be grafted is harvested from the patient's own body. Thus, this graft is very compatible with the body. Autografts are generally the best graft technique and usually result in the greatest regeneration of missing alveolar bone.
- *Allografts* are taken from other human donors. The bone is tested and sterilized. The patient's body converts the donor

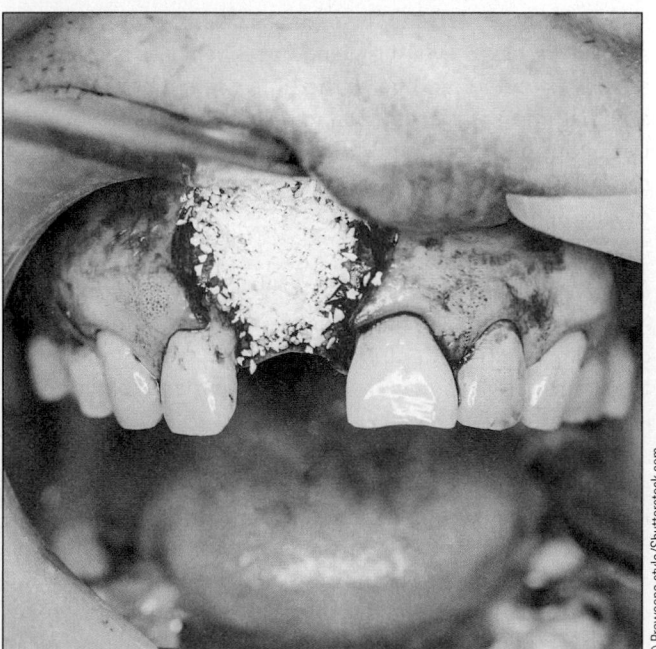

FIGURE 39-9
Bone graft for future implant placement.

bone into their own bone to rebuild the alveolar bone in the needed area.

- *Xenografts* have an animal source such as cattle. The bone is specially processed to ensure it is biocompatible and sterile. The body uses this bone as a replacement for the patient's natural bone. Once this process is complete, dental implants may be placed in this area.

- *Alloplastic* grafts are synthetic materials. For bone replacement, a man-made material such as calcium phosphate is used.

Bruxism may reduce the success of dental implants. The forces generated during bruxism have a particularly negative impact on an implant while the alveolar bone is healing. Natural teeth have a periodontal ligament that allows each tooth to have slight movement and absorb forces related to biting. The dental implant does not have this periodontal ligament, and the implant is anchored directly into the alveolar bone. The implant does not have the ability to move and absorb forces. As a result, the dentist may prescribe wearing a custom mouthguard at night to reduce the forces that the implant may experience.

Psychological Evaluation

The dentist evaluates the patient's attitude toward dental implants as well as the ability to cooperate during the procedure. The dentist also assesses the overall outlook for dental treatment. Psychological evaluation of the implant candidate includes abstract factors that may affect the outcome of the treatment. The patient must have realistic expectations of the restoration in regard to its function and esthetics. The dentist also considers the expectations of the implant patient. How the expectations will be met should be discussed with the patient. The procedures involved are also discussed with the client. The patient also should have a realistic understanding of the time commitment involved and that implant placement and restoration involves a number of appointments and phases. Additionally, the patient should be made aware that osseointegration and healing require time.

Clinical Evaluation

Part of the clinical evaluation is the implant location. Research has shown that the failure rate of implants in the edentulous maxilla may be higher than in the mandible. This may be a factor in patient selection for implants.

The oral examination includes evaluation of the radiographs. The patient must have sufficient bone width and height for implant placement and successful osseointegration of the implant. The partially edentulous patient must also have adequate space for the implant. The patient's gingival tissues are examined for health. Panoramic and cephalometric radiographs, as well as tomographic images (refer to Chapter 29), are needed to evaluate the height, width, and quality of bone.

Radiographic Evaluation

By considering the implant site, the practitioner determines the types of images needed. The dental assistant obtains all the prescribed radiographs. A periapical radiograph shows the location of tooth roots and opaque foreign bodies that can affect the implant site but does not indicate the width or depth of the bone in a buccal lingual direction (refer to Chapter 29).

Panoramic radiographs provide the location of anatomical landmarks that can impact placement. These include the maxillary sinus or inferior alveolar canal. Panoramic radiographs also can provide bone height (refer to Chapter 29). However, with the periapical radiograph, the panoramic image is inadequate for the examination of bone width. It is usually used in the initial treatment planning phase for implants.

Computer axial tomography, also known as computed tomography (CT) provides the greatest detail with 3D views of the mandible or maxilla (refer to Chapter 29). The CT scan can provide bone volume and density as well as accurate positions of anatomical landmarks.

Patient Preparation

To prepare the patient for implant surgery, a thorough evaluation is performed by the dentist. This includes a comprehensive dental exam, radiographs, and models of the patient's maxilla and mandible. The dentist consults with the patient's physician regarding any existing medical condition and may prescribe antibiotics before performing the surgery.

The dental assistant or the dental implant coordinator explains the dental implant procedure to the patient and answers any questions the patient may have. The dental assistant or the dental implant coordinator also explains and obtains the signed informed consent from the patient. The patient is advised to stop the use of tobacco products and alcohol as both can lead to the dental implant failure. The patient is advised to avoid eating and drinking for at least 6–8 hours before the dental implant surgery. The dental assistant verifies all the above mentioned steps before the patient gets ready for the implant surgery. The patient is also instructed not to drive for 24 hours after the dental implant surgery. Thus, a family member or a friend is needed to drive the patient to and from the dental office.

Treatment Sequence

The dental implant procedure requires a team effort between the patient and the dental team. Depending on the type of implant chosen, the dentist develops a treatment plan. If the patient is missing one tooth, then one implant and a crown are placed (Figure 39-10). If the patient is missing multiple teeth, then an implant-supported bridge may be part of the treatment plan (Figure 39-11). If the person is missing all the

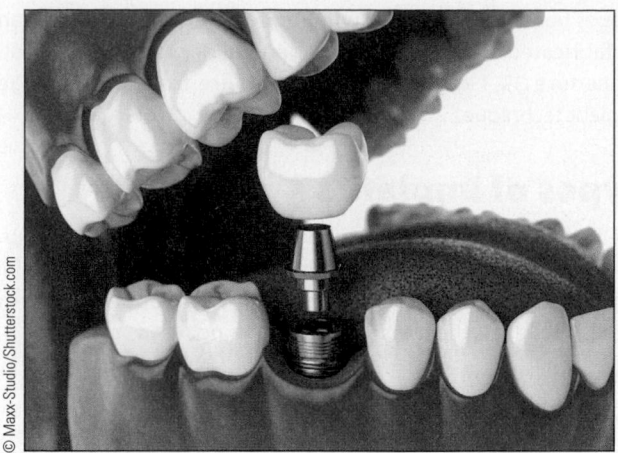

FIGURE 39-10
Single-tooth implant with crown.

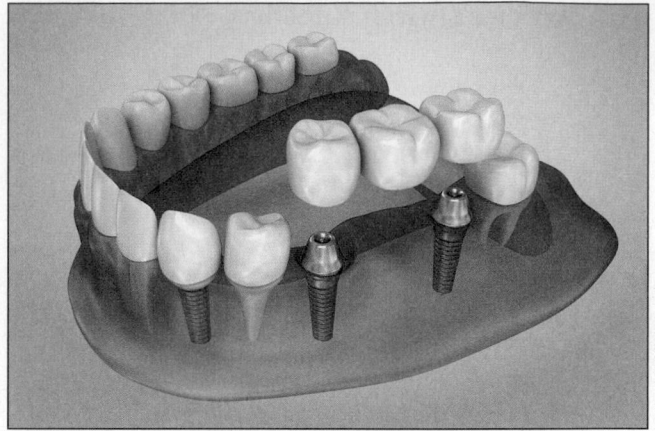

FIGURE 39-11
Implant-supported bridge.

teeth in the dentition, then an implant-supported full bridge (Figure 39-12) or full denture may be part of the treatment plan (Figure 39-13). It can take several months to complete all phases of the dental implant process prior to actual placement of the implant. The process begins with the patient meeting with the restorative dentist. After a preliminary consultation, the restorative dentist refers the patient to the oral surgeon or periodontist. Some general dentists complete additional training to be able to do dental implants in their office. A diagnostic consultation is then scheduled. Included in this appointment are panoramic and cephalometric radiographs as well as 3D images, a medical and dental history review, an oral examination, and study casts. Study casts may also be used to fabricate a *surgical stent* (Figure 39-14). This stent or *template* is placed over the tissues during surgery to guide the dentist in placing the implant. The stent is made of clear acrylic and is sometimes called a template.

Like any surgery, dental implant surgery poses some health risks. Problems are rare, though, and when they do occur, they are usually minor and easily treated. Risks include the following:

● Infection at the implant site

● Injury or damage to surrounding anatomical structures

● Damage to a nerve which can cause pain, paresthesia, or *dysesthesia*

● Damage to the nasal cavity

● Sinus problems if an implant inadvertently protrudes into the sinus cavity

● Allergic reaction to materials used in dental implants

● Rejection of the implant

● Failure of osseointegration

After the diagnosis is complete and the patient accepts the treatment plan, the necessary consent forms are signed

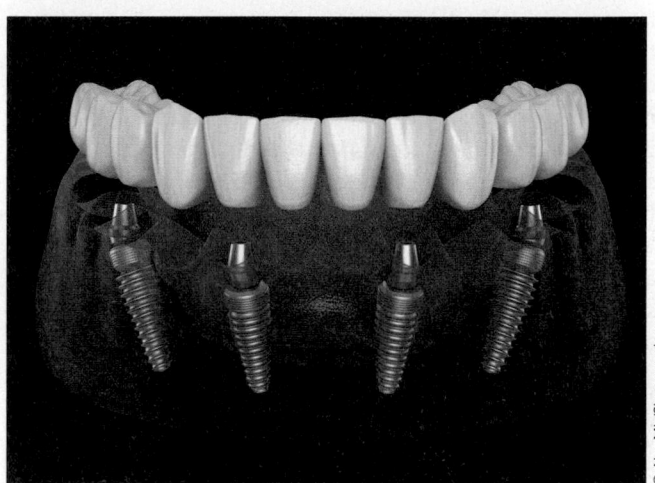

FIGURE 39-12
Implant-supported full-arch bridge.

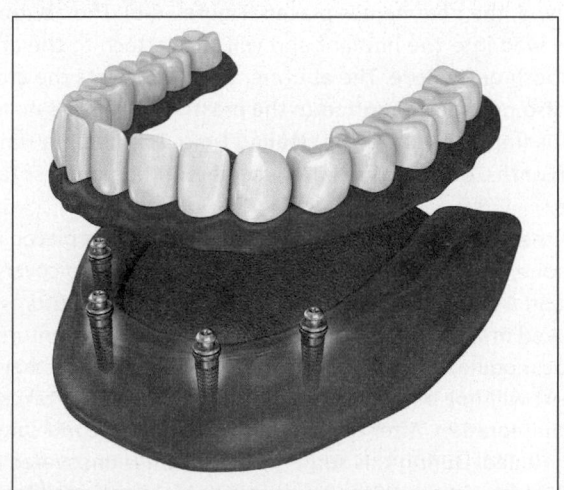

FIGURE 39-13
Implant-supported overdenture.

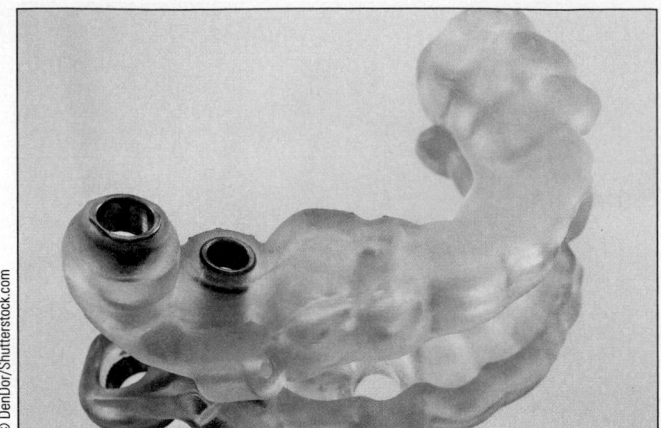

FIGURE 39-14
Surgical stent for implant placement.

by the patient, the financial arrangements are completed, and treatment appointments are scheduled. There are several techniques used to place dental implants. Often, one of the factors in selecting the technique is the amount of *load* the implant can tolerate and still be successful. The load is the amount of pressure or strain put on the implant once placed in the bone. Other factors include the dentist's preference and skill level.

There are usually two phases of treatment: surgical and restorative. The surgical phase can be accomplished with either a one-stage or a two-stage technique. Implant-supported restorations are discussed in Chapters 40 and 42.

In the *one-stage implant technique*, the implant is inserted into the bone, but the extruding end is not covered with gingival tissue. A stent may be used to guide the process of implant placement. The implant protrudes through the tissue and a healing cap is placed. The *healing cap* is a metal cap or screw that fits on the dental implant and keeps tissue and debris from getting into the implant (Figure 39-7). When the healing cap is removed, the *abutment* is placed (Figure 39-6). The abutment is screwed into the implant and will later attach to the artificial tooth or denture. The abutment post supports the crown and also provides retention to the prosthesis. There is no load on this implant during the healing time. The healing time is 2–6 months, during which the osseointegration process takes place.

In the *two-stage implant technique*, the implant is placed into the bone, and gingival tissue is sutured into place to cover the implant. A stent may be used to guide the process. Sutures are removed in 7–10 days. If there is an old prosthesis (denture), it can be modified or relined by the restorative dentist so that the patient will not be without teeth during the time it takes for osseointegration. After the osseointegration, a second surgery is scheduled. During this surgery the implant is uncovered and checked for stability. If the implant is stable, a cap or abutment is placed. The cap protrudes out of the tissue. Once the soft

tissues have healed, the crown, bridge, or other prosthesis can be fabricated and placed by the general or prosthetic dentist. Procedure 39-1 discusses the procedure for the two-stage implant technique.

Types of Implants

The two most common types of dental implants include the subperiosteal and the endosteal. A third type of implant, called a mini dental implant (MDI), is also becoming very popular. A fourth type of implant is the transosteal, which is not used very often.

Subperiosteal Implants

The *subperiosteal implant* is often used on patients whose dentures no longer fit well because the alveolar bone has resorbed and there is not enough bone available for traditional implants. Subperiosteal implants are most commonly placed on the mandible. The titanium implant rests on top of the alveolar bone with abutment posts or bars above the mucoperiosteum in the cuspid and first molar area. The denture connects to this structure for support and retention (Figure 39-15). The subperiosteal implant requires one or two surgeries, depending on the technique.

Endosteal Implant

The *endosteal implant* is also known as an endosseous implant and is made of titanium. The alveolar bone must be sufficient in height, width, and length for a successful placement. Endosteal implants are available in various widths, lengths, and designs, including cylinders, screws, and combinations of the two. There is also a blade design that is used when the bone is too thin to support a screw-type implant without grafting (Figure 39-16). It has a post that extends into the oral cavity through the mucoperiosteum. Endosteal implants can function as an abutment for dentures or orthodontic appliances. The term is derived from the Greek words *endon*, meaning "within," and *osteon*, meaning "bone". A root form tooth implant creates a root and structure that is similar to the natural root and tooth. This type of implant can be placed on a bone structure that is wide enough to support the implant. The implant is imbedded into the bone and left for several months to heal. Once the alveolar bone heals around the implant, a tooth extension is added to complete the process. The techniques for endosteal implants include either a one- or a two-stage insertion (refer to Procedure 39-1). Both of these will be discussed later in this chapter.

Mini Dental Implants

The *mini dental implant (MDI)* is smaller in diameter (less than 3 mm) and narrower than other dental implants (Figure 39-17). It is made of biocompatible titanium alloy, which can be placed

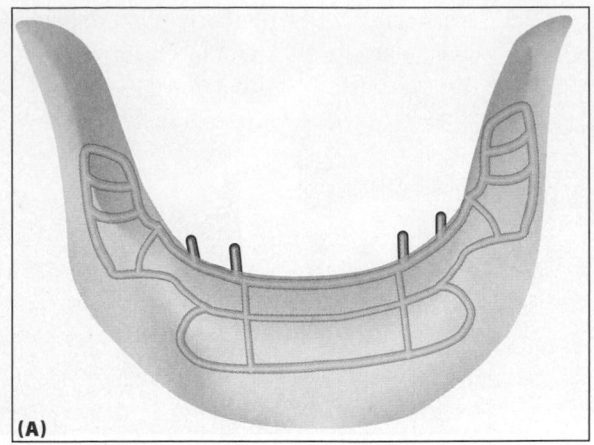

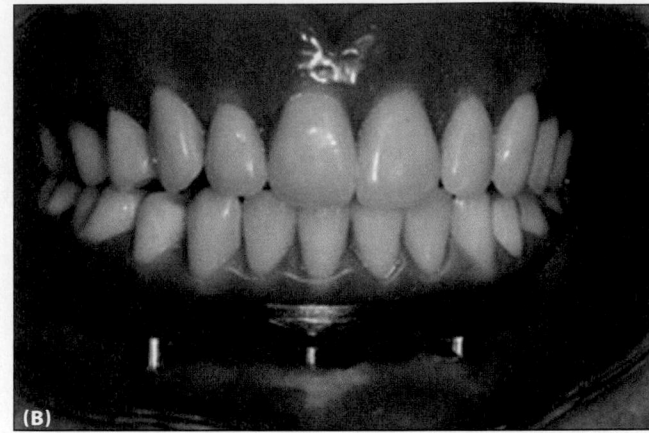

FIGURE 39-15
(A) Subperiosteal implant. (B) Subperiosteal implants in place.

directly through the mucosal tissue and into the bone. The MDIs are used for retention of a full or partial dentures (Figure 39-18), especially in the mandible; for crowns in small spaces; and for retention in orthodontic procedures.

MDIs consist of various designed heads, a threaded body with assorted styled tips that are sharp or slightly blunted, and

the metal housing. There is a ball-shaped extension on top of the implant. This extension is what a denture of partial denture will fit over. The denture usually has an O-ring that fits over the ball-shaped extension of the implant.

Some of the benefits of MDIs include the following:

- A minimally invasive procedure
- Much faster healing than traditional implants and in some cases can be used immediately
- Less time for the procedure than traditional dental implants
- Lower cost for the patient as compared to traditional implants

With the procedure for placing the MDIs, the dentist does not incise the tissue and lay a flap; instead, the dentist uses specially

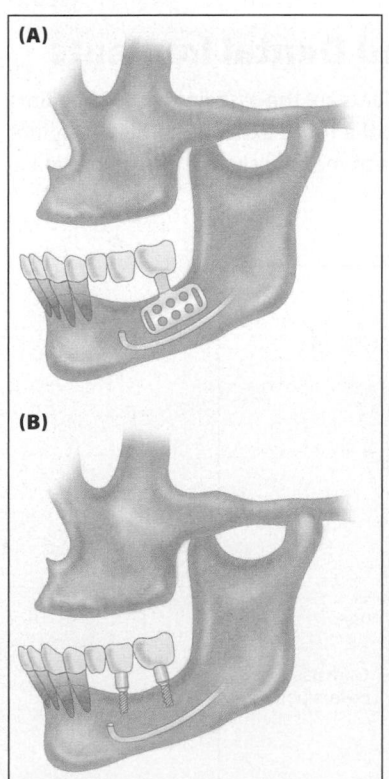

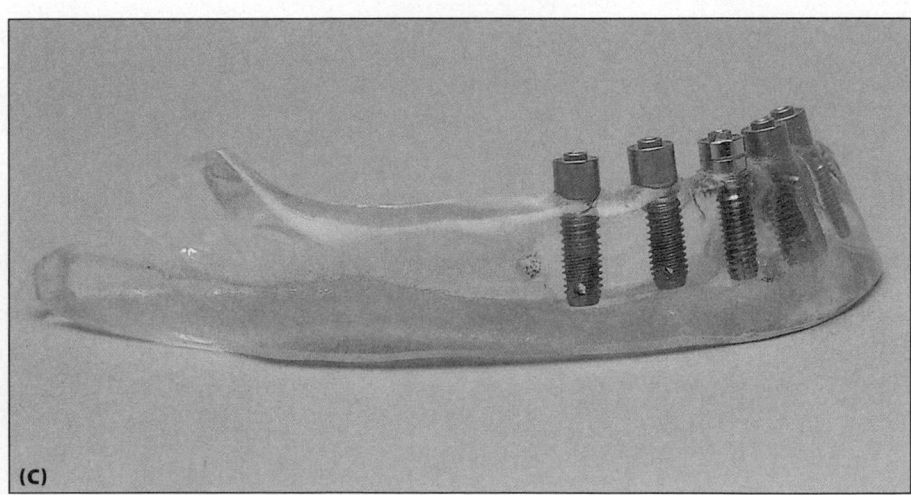

FIGURE 39-16
Sample of endosteal implants. (A) The blade implant. (B) The screw or cylinder implant. (C) A model showing the screw or cylinder implant.

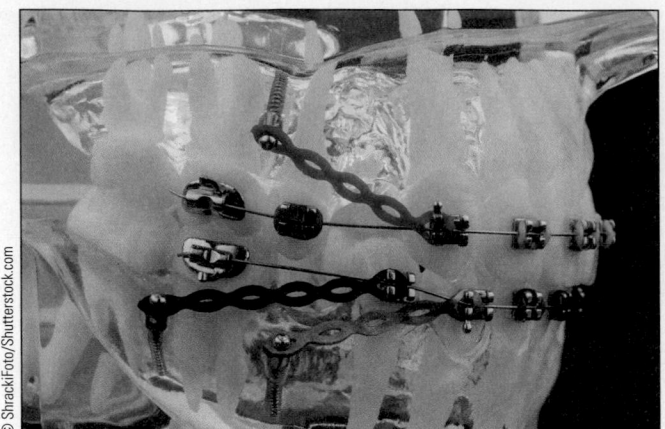

FIGURE 39-17
Mini dental implant in an orthodontic case.

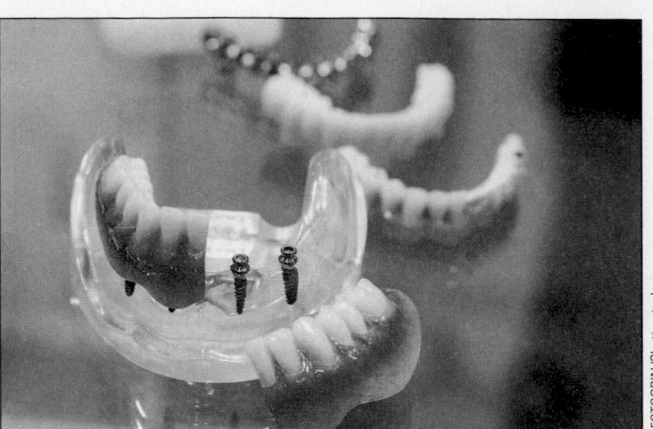

FIGURE 39-18
Mini dental implant for support of denture.

designed burs and drills a small pilot hole through the tissue and into the bone. The dentist places the MDI in the pilot hole and then uses a handheld driving device and a torque wrench to seat the implant. Postinsertion pain and irritation are much less than with standard dental implants. MDIs systems are successfully used for retention in specific cases but are not designed to replace osseointegrated dental implants.

Transosteal Implant

The *transosteal implant* is used in an edentulous area of the mandible and passes through the cortical plate and the alveolar bone (Figure 39-19). Usually this type of implant is only used with patients who have severely resorbed alveolar ridges that will

not support the other types of implants. These implants are also known as *staple* or *transosseous implants*. They consist of screws, nuts, and a pressure plate. The screws are inserted through the bone, penetrating the entire jaw and attaching to the pressure plate on the border of the mandible. The denture is secured to the screws that protrude through the gingival tissue. These implants are also made of titanium and will fuse to the bone through osseointegration.

Immediate Load Dental Implants

Immediate load dental implants are the osseointegrated implants that are placed at the time of a tooth extraction. This procedure cuts down the healing time tremendously. The dental implant is

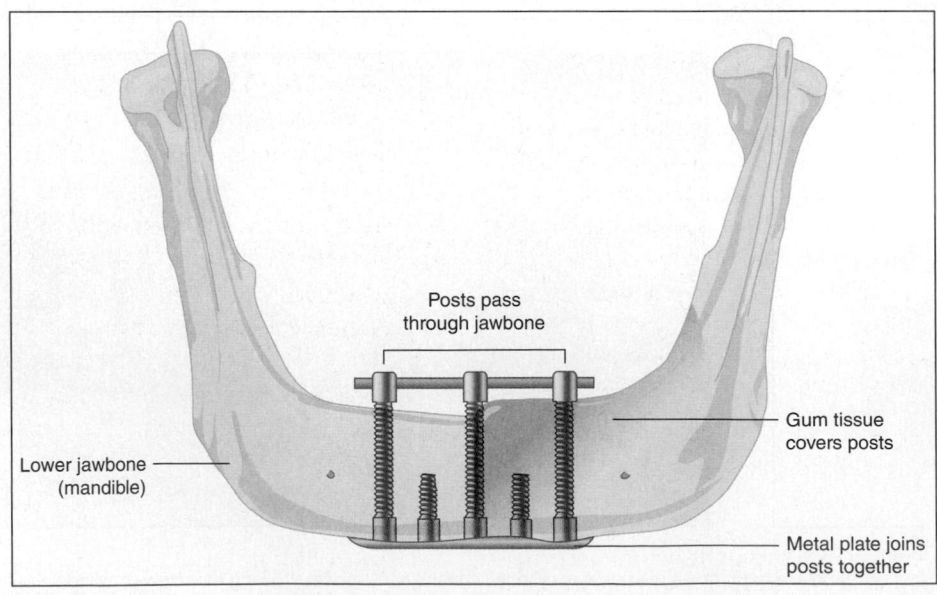

Posts pass
through jawbone

Lower jawbone
(mandible)

Gum tissue
covers posts

Metal plate joins
posts together

FIGURE 39-19
Placement of a transosteal dental implant.

surgically placed right after the tooth extraction, and the crown is immediately attached to the implant. Immediate loading has been defined as a restoration placed in occlusion with the opposing dentition within 48 hours of implant placement. Loading an implant involves any device or attachment (e.g., healing abutment, temporary crown) that puts the implant into connection with the oral cavity. This is a fairly new procedure, and not all implant dentists offer it. To be a candidate for this procedure the patient must have sufficient bone to stabilize the implant, and the implant must be secure enough to withstand the force of attaching the crown. There also must not be any history of infection at the implant placement site.

Surgical Techniques for Implant Placement

There are two techniques for implant placement. One requires a single-surgery, and the other requires two separate surgical steps. Both are discussed in this section.

Single-Surgery Technique

The *Single-surgery technique* involves fabricating the impression for the implant on a model. The model is constructed by using computed tomography (CT) scans. Some clinicians may prefer to use a stent to guide implant placement. After the implant is fabricated on the model, surgery is performed to incise the tissue via a flap and expose the alveolar bone. The implant is seated in the bone, and the tissue is sutured back into place. A healing cap is placed at the same time. The tissue is sutured back in place. Healing is allowed to take place for several months, and the healing cap is then removed. The connector is screwed into the implant, and the crown is then either cemented or screwed onto the connector.

Two-Surgery Technique

When using the *two-surgery technique*, during the first surgery the tissue is incised and the alveolar bone is exposed. The *osteotomy* or removal of bone is completed and the implant is seated in place. A stent may be used to guide implant placement. A cover screw which covers the top of the implant is placed and the flap is sutured back. Once healing takes place, the flap is opened, the cover screw is removed and the healing cap is placed. The flap is then positioned around the healing cap. Once healing is completed, the healing cap is removed and the crown is placed onto the implant. Procedure 39-1 discusses the two-surgery technique.

Postoperative Care and Home Care Instructions

Once the second surgery is completed in the two-surgery technique, the exposed portion of the dental implant must be kept clean. The patient must perform daily hygiene maintenance on the implant and prosthesis. The instruments and techniques for implant hygiene are discussed in Chapters 16 and 40,

Postoperative Instructions after Implant Placement

- Plan to have someone drive you home after the dental implant surgery.
- Only clear liquids should be taken during the first two days after surgery. Milk may be taken with medication. Blended or mashed food may be added after the second day. Smoking and alcoholic beverages should be avoided.
- Local anesthesia wears off about three or four hours after the procedure, so over-the-counter or prescribed pain medication may be required.
- Softly biting on a gauze pad for 15–30 minutes may control slight bleeding. If bleeding persists, contact the office.
- Sedation is effective for 24 hours after administration. During this time, please do not drive a vehicle or operate machinery.
- While you are still numb, avoid chewing and drinking hot drinks so that you don't accidentally bite or burn your mouth or tongue.
- Rest with your head elevated for the first few days.
- Avoid strenuous exercise for at least 24 hours following surgery.
- Eat soft and mild foods such as yogurt, soup, and pudding for the first few days after the surgery.
- The dentist will place a surgical dressing over the implant site after the surgery. The surgical dressing should remain in for about two weeks until your follow-up appointment. Apply an ice pack to the implant area for the first few days after dental implant surgery to help alleviate swelling.
- If your doctor prescribes antibiotics, finish the course as directed to minimize your risk of infection. Avoid trauma to the dental implant site.
- Don't push against the implant with your tongue, use a toothpick in the area of the implant, or brush the implant site until cleared by your dentist.
- For a few weeks, you will not be able to eat very chewy, hard, or sticky foods, such as tough meat or crusty bread.
- Avoid spicy or acidic foods like chili or orange juice for the first few weeks. Do not drink alcohol or smoke for at least two weeks after dental implant surgery.
- Your dentist may schedule three or four checkups in the first year after your dental implant surgery to check your bone and the fit and health of the implant.
- After the first year, see your doctor for follow-up treatments, maintenance visits, and examinations on a regular basis as recommended.
- Maintain your oral home care by brushing and flossing regularly once cleared by your dentist.
- Contact the dental office if you have any pain after the procedure.
- Gently rinse your mouth with warm saltwater solution after each meal. Avoid over-the-counter mouth rinses.

and are also touched on later in this chapter. The patient should also have routine dental examinations to evaluate the implants along with the rest of the oral cavity.

Dental Implant Maintenance

Dental implants require maintenance just like natural teeth. Plaque and calculus build up on the implant and need to be removed routinely. The patient should be informed of their role and responsibility in maintaining their dental implant and should be scheduled for continuous support and care of the tissues that surround the implant, known as peri-implant tissues, as well as the implant. This support should include a clinical assessment of the condition of the soft tissues, a plaque index, depth and bleeding on probing, and a check of mobility and occlusion. Radiographs are also often taken. Some patients are at a higher risk for *peri-implantitis* or inflammation of the tissues surrounding the implant due to chronic periodontitis, diabetes, poor oral hygiene, or smoking. The patient should be advised of the aids available, and a home care regimen should be recommended. The student should refer to Chapter 16 for a detailed discussion regarding oral home care aids. The toothbrushes selected, either automatic or manual, should be a soft, multitufted nylon brush. There are also numerous aids for use as adjuncts to the toothbrush, including the following:

- Threading systems (Figure 39-20)
- Dental floss, including dental implant floss (Figure 39-21)
- Interproximal brushes, end-tufted brushes (Figure 39-22)
- Water irrigators (refer to Figure 40-54)
- Antimicrobial rinses (refer to Figure 40-55)

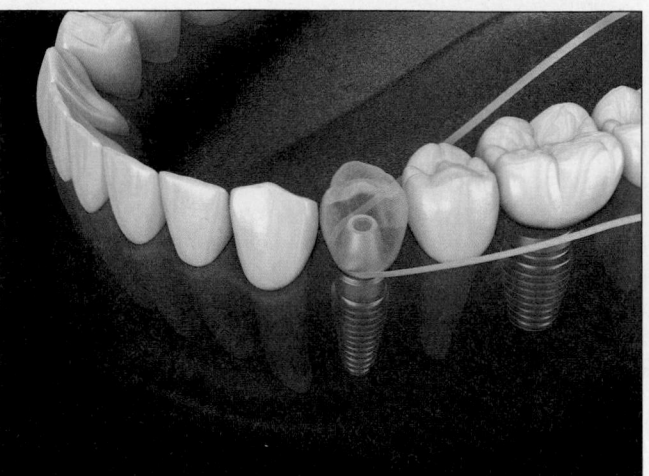

FIGURE 39-21
Use of dental floss to clean around implant.

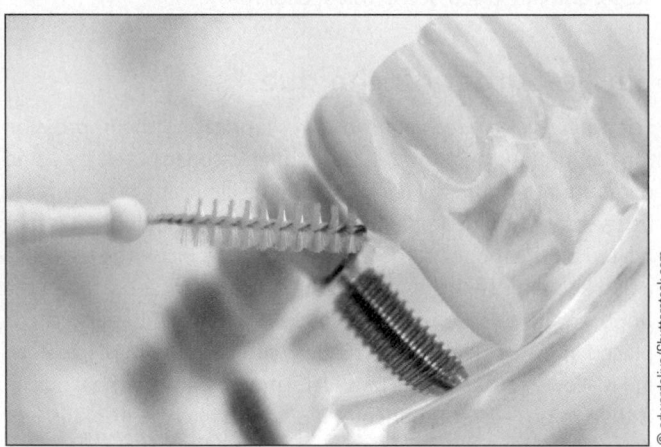

FIGURE 39-22
End-tufted brush to clean around implant.

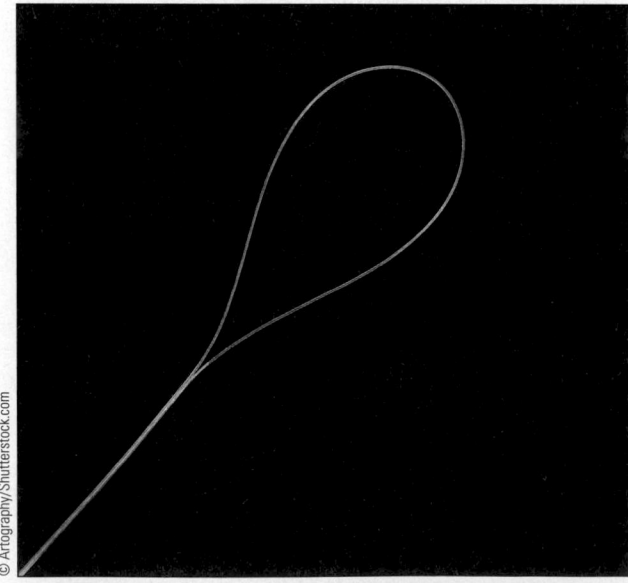

FIGURE 39-20
Floss threader.

Some types of dental floss works well on dental implants, or are designed specifically for implants. The floss for dental implants is a wider band of ribbon that wraps around the implant and is moved in a back-and-forth motion (shoeshine motion) (Figure 39-21).

Interproximal brushes provide easy access around the implant due to their small heads (Figure 39-22). The brushes remove plaque and stimulate the gingival tissues to increase the blood flow in the surrounding areas. The interproximal brush and instruments are inserted interdentally and are angled toward the occlusal or incisal surface. A gently rotating motion of the brush is suggested for use around the implant and near the gingival margin.

In the dental office, special instruments which are available in plastic, nylon, or graphite are used as they prevent damage to the titanium surface of the implant (Figure 39-23). During scaling and root planing procedures, plastic or plastic-coated scalers and curettes, and a soft polishing agent are used to prevent the scratching or damaging of the implant.

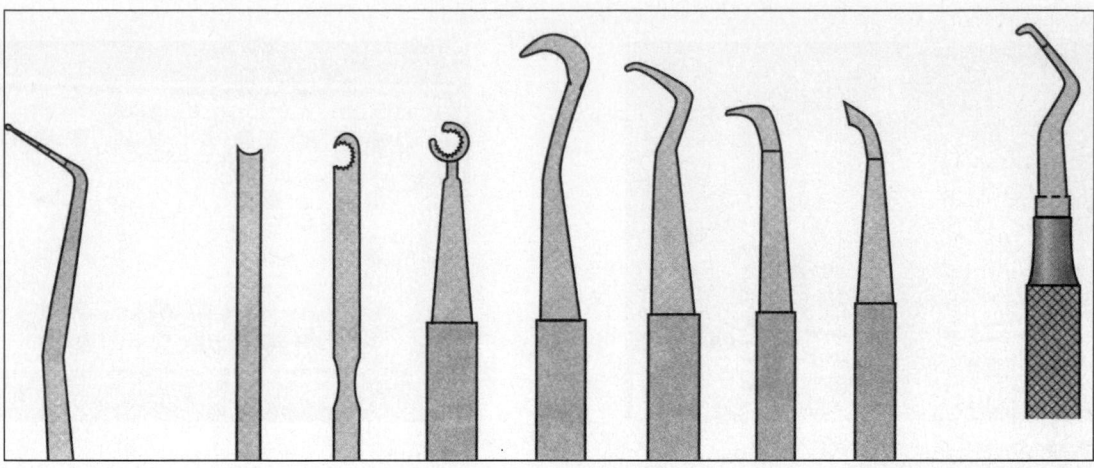

FIGURE 39-23
Plastic instruments used to clean and maintain dental implants.

Procedure 39-1

Two-Stage Implant Technique

This procedure is completed by the dentist. Steps written in **blue** font are performed by the operator (dentist or qualified dental assistant), and the chairside assistant's steps are written in black.

Equipment and Supplies

Patient Seating Setup (refer to Procedure 18-4)

Anesthetic Setup (refer to Procedure 23-2)

Implant Surgery Setup for First Appointment in Two-Stage Technique (Figure 39-24)

- intravenous sedation setup (not shown)
- surgical HVE tip (not shown)
- sterile gauze and cotton pellets (not shown)
- sterile template (see Figure 39-14)
- scalpel holders (A)
- bone file (B)
- scalpel blades (C)
- Rongeurs (D)
- needle holder (E)
- sutures (F)
- surgical curette (G)
- mouth mirror (H)
- explorer (I)
- cotton pliers (J)
- surgical scissors (K)
- tissue forceps (L)
- bite block (M)

- Buck 5 6 periodontal knives (N)
- Kirkland knife (O)
- periosteal elevator (P)
- assorted Gracey scalers and jacquette scalers (Q)
- implant kit (Figures 39-25A and B)
- tongue and cheek retractors (Figure 39-26)
- Osseocision® surgical drill system with irrigation (Figure 39-27)
- surgical barriers (Figure 39-28)
- surgical gloves (see Figure 11-26)

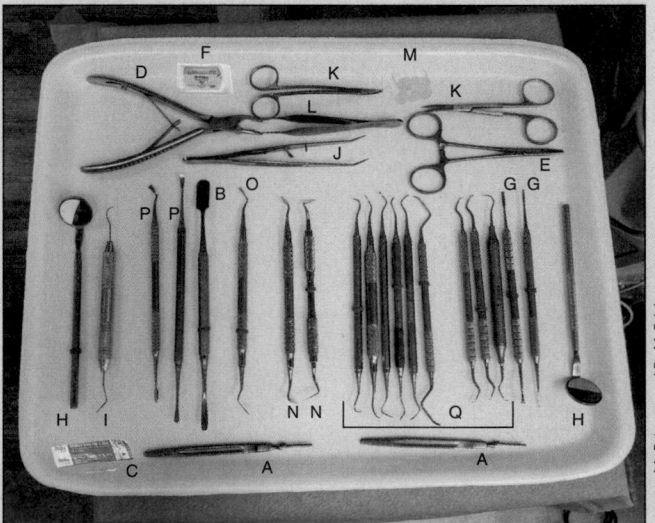

Courtesy of A. Palagano and Dr. M. Feinberg

FIGURE 39-24
Implant tray setup.

(Continues)

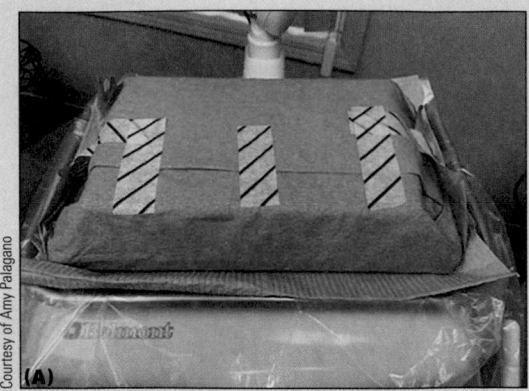
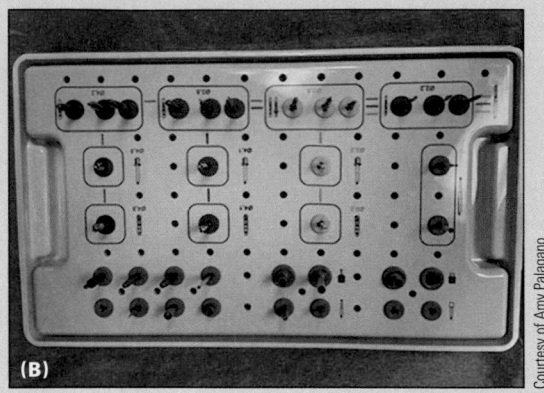

FIGURE 39-25

(A) Implant drill kit in sterile wrapping placed on bracket tray. (B) Implant drill kit opened for use.

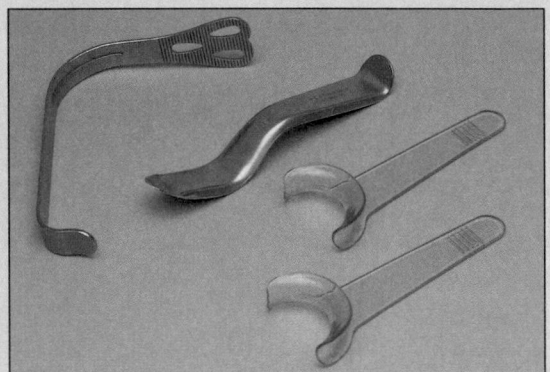

FIGURE 39-26

Tongue and lip and cheek retractors.

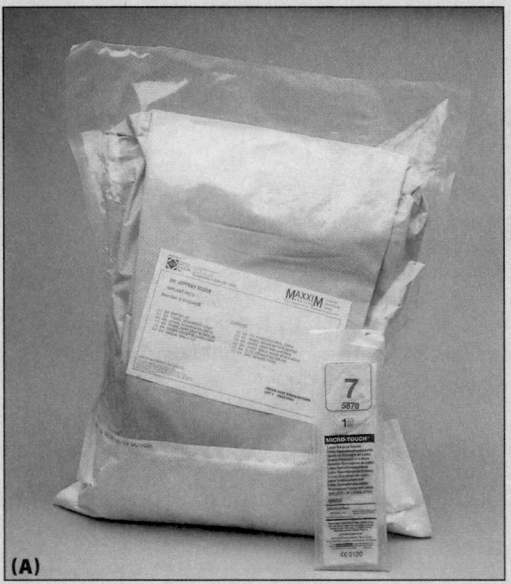

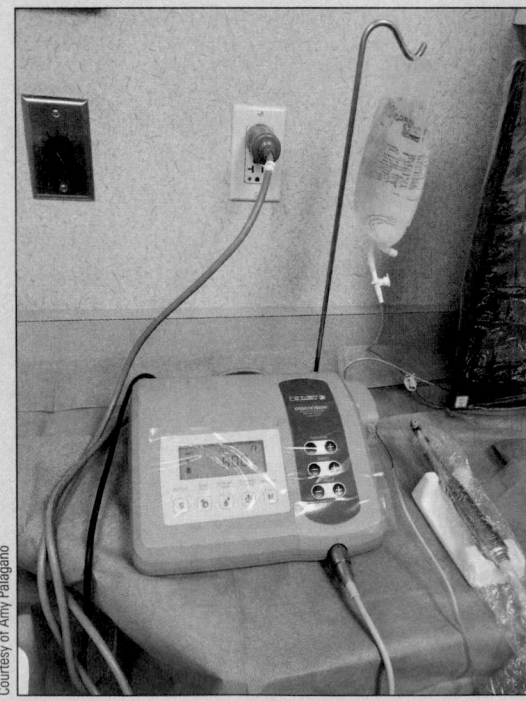

FIGURE 39-27

Osseocision® implant drilling system with coolant.

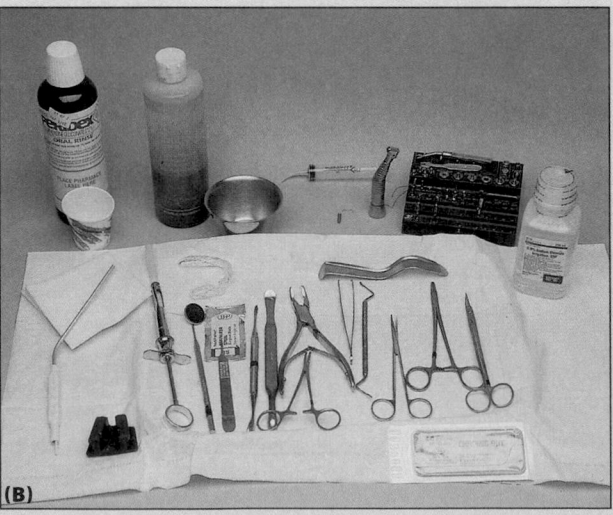

FIGURE 39-28

(A) Surgical barrier kit. (B) Tray setup for implant surgery.

Courtesy of Amy Palagano

Procedure Steps

1. Escort and seat patient (refer to Procedure 18-4).

Dentist greets the patient and takes position at the dental chair.

❑ Signals for the procedure to begin (refer to Procedure 20-1).

2. Pass mouth mirror and explorer at operator's signal.

Dentist examines area with mirror and explorer for implant placement.

3. Transfer instruments to assist in implant placement.

Dentist administers intravenous sedation.

❑ Operator assists with the administration of local anesthesia (refer to Procedure 23-2).
❑ Operator passes surgical template.

Dentist seats surgical template in the oral cavity and marks target through the template onto the soft tissues.

❑ Operator retrieves template.
❑ Operator passes scalpel with attached blade while maintaining the operating field.

Dentist incises tissues to ridge of bone.

❑ Operator passes periosteal elevator and retrieves scalpel with attached blade while maintaining operating field.

Dentist reflects incised tissues with periosteal elevator.

❑ Operator passes Osseocision® surgical drill and changes implant bur sizes as needed.
❑ Operator suctions irrigation fluid and maintains operating field.
❑ Operator passes implant and either mallet to tap into place or ratchet wrench.

Dentist places implant into position.

❑ Operator prepares the healing screw for placement.

Dentist fixes the healing screw onto implant.

Dentist places soft tissue flaps in position.

❑ Operator transfers suture with needle holder.

Dentist sutures tissue.

❑ Operator cuts suture where required with surgical scissors.
❑ Operator retrieves suture needle.

Operator provides patient with post-operative instructions orally and in written form once patient is recovered.

4. Inform the patient that the soft tissues will be tender due to surgery.

Dentist provides prescriptions for pain management.

5. Write up procedure in Services Rendered.

Date	Services Rendered
02/18/XX	Updated medical and dental history, no changes noted. BP = 120/80; T = 98.6F, P = 80, R = 18
	Intravenous sedation administered with valium. Placed 20% benzocaine gel to injection sites for 2 minutes. Administered two cartridges (3.6 ml) of 2% lidocaine with 1:100,000 epi to mandibular left. No reaction
	#19 Endosteal implant placed (cylinder, 3.5mm)
	POI provided Rx for Tylenol #3 provided, 10 tablets, take three times daily as needed.
	RTC: place implant abutment Assistant's initials

6. Dismiss and escort patient to reception area (refer to Procedure 18-5).

Second Surgical Procedure

The second appointment should be scheduled 3–4 months after the first appointment to allow for osseointegration.

Equipment and Supplies

Patient Seating Setup (refer to Procedure 18-4)

Anesthetic Setup (refer to Procedure 23-2)

Implant Abutment Placement Setup

- surgical HVE tip
- sterile gauze and cotton pellets
- cotton pliers (Figure 39-24J)
- sterile template (see Figure 39-14)
- hydrogen peroxide
- scalpel holders (Figure 39-24A)
- scalpel blades (Figure 39-24C)
- needle holder (Figure 39-24E)
- sutures (Figure 39-24F)

Procedure Steps

1. Escort and seat patient (refer to Procedure 18-4).

(Continues)

Greets the patient and takes position at the dental chair.

❑ Signals for the procedure to begin (refer to Procedure 20-1).

2. Pass mouth mirror and explorer at operator's signal.

Examines surgical site with mirror and explorer.

Operator assists in transferring instruments during the placement of the abutment.

❑ Operator assists with the administration of local anesthesia (refer to Procedure 23-2).
❑ Operator passes template.

Dentist positions template over osseointegrated implant, and the site is marked with a sharp instrument.

❑ Operator retrieves template and passes holder with attached scalpel.

Dentist opens soft tissue to reveal healing screw.

❑ Operator retrieves scalpel and attached blade while maintaining operating field.

Dentist removes healing screw.

❑ Operator retrieves healing cap and passes sterile cotton pellet in cotton pliers.

Operator cleans inside of implant with sterile cotton pellet.

❑ Prepares abutment.
❑ Passes abutment.

Dentist places abutment.

❑ Operator passes needle and suture on needle holder.

Dentist sutures tissues around the abutment.

❑ Operator cuts end of suture with surgical scissors and retrieves needle.

Operator provides patient with postoperative instructions orally and in written form.

3. Write up procedure in Services Rendered.

Date	Services Rendered
02/18/XX	Updated medical and dental history, no changes noted. BP = 120/80; T = 98.6F, P = 80, R = 18
	Placed #19 abutment after removal of healing screw
	POI provided and appointment scheduled with dentist for final implant crown
	Assistant's initials

4. Dismiss and escort patient to reception area (refer to Procedure 18-5).

Water irrigators are available to remove debris and plaque from around the dental implant. The patient should be advised, however, to use the irrigators at the lowest pressure setting in order to prevent damage to the tissues. The gentle spray should be directed interproximally and kept at a horizontal level along the gingival margin. The spray should not be directed into the gingival sulcus.

Antimicrobial rinses, such as chlorhexidine gluconate and phenolic compounds, are recommended for many dental implant patients. The rinses are used once or twice daily depending on the type. The chlorhexidine gluconate rinses are safe and aid in fibroblast attachment to the implant surface.

Implant-Retained Prostheses

The fixed prosthesis stage usually begins approximately 6 months after the surgery. The dental implants have been in place long enough for substantial osseointegration to take place and are ready for the last step of the implant procedures. The dentist takes impressions and designs the retainers that will cover the implant. The retainer may be a crown or part of a bridge. The abutments are fabricated in the dental laboratory and are either screw retained or cement retained (Figure 39-29). The screw-retained prosthesis uses one screw to attach the abutment to the implant and a second screw to attach the abutment to the prosthesis.

The cement-retained prosthesis uses transitional cement to attach the prosthesis to the abutment. Transitional cement is used so that, in case of problems with the implant, the entire system can be retrieved. Figure 39-30A shows a radiographic image of an implant. Figure 39-30B shows a clinical photograph of an implant with a final prosthesis on #7.

Role of the Dental Assistant

Implant dentistry is the fastest growing area of dentistry and therefore an increased need for trained and qualified dental assistants who can assist the dentist in sharing the quality treatment tasks.

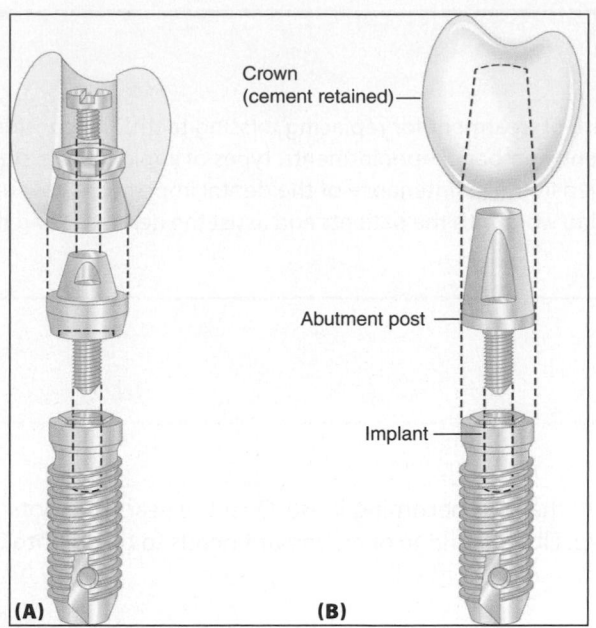

FIGURE 39-29
(A) Screw-retained implant prosthesis. (B) Cement-retained implant prosthesis.

Implant Coordinator

An implant coordinator is an expanded functions dental auxiliary position. The job duties of this position include the following:

- Participating in the initial implant consultation visit
- Discussing each step of the procedure including the fees
- Listening to the expectations of the patient
- Educating the patient about implants through models and other visual aids
- Explaining the risk, benefit, and alternatives, and obtaining the informed consent
- Documenting refusal of care if the patient chooses not to proceed with treatment

- Discussing insurance coverage
- Explaining the interdisciplinary process of care to the patient and coordinating all appointments
- Setting up the treatment room for each appointment and assisting during the procedure
- Assisting updating the treatment plan sheet
- Performing or assisting with CBT scans and other diagnostic tools
- Engaging the implant team
- Assisting with communication between the patient and all health care providers and the dental laboratory
- Coordinating with the dental insurance
- Collecting the medical narratives
- Monitoring follow-up appointments
- Communicating with appointment schedulers to track lab cases
- Marketing the practice for implants and organizing a marketing plan

Implant Supply Company Representative

Implant supply company representative jobs are one of the highest paying positions within the medical device sales industry. They are generally filled by the top 10% of the medical sales representatives. To qualify for this position, the applicants usually spend five or more years in medical or dental equipment sales. This position requires a challenging combination of skills, including the following:

- Qualification and ability to provide technical advice to the practitioner during the implant process
- Ability to build strong professional relationships with the dental team
- Excellent verbal and written communication skills

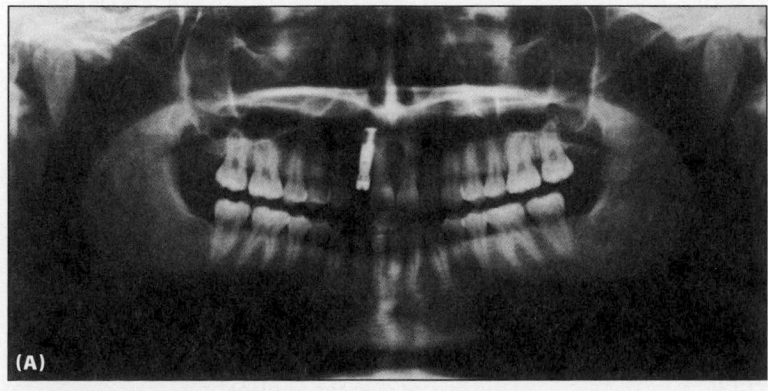
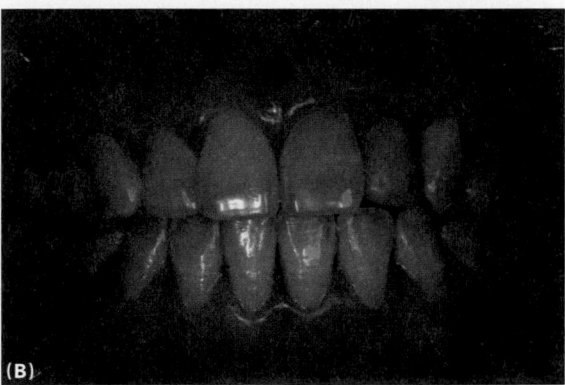

FIGURE 39-30
(A) A panoramic radiograph of the dental implant. (B) A patient's smile after the crown has been seated on the dental implant.

Chapter Summary

This chapter covers dental implants, which have become the standard of treatment for replacing missing teeth. The considerations for the patient are discussed, including preparation of the patient, number of appointments, types of implants, and steps of the procedure. Postoperative instructions as well as what is involved in the maintenance of the dental implant are covered. This chapter gives the dental assistants the information they will need to work with the patients and assist the dentist during the dental implant procedure.

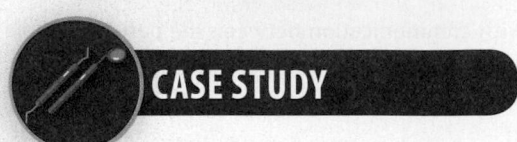

CASE STUDY

Lucas Smart, 46 years old, had a retained primary tooth that was becoming loose. Over the years the roots had resorbed, and now the tooth needs to be removed. Either a bridge or an implant needs to be put into its place.

Case Study Review

1. What information would Lucas need to know about both options?

2. How many appointments would be needed for the dental implant?

3. Discuss which dental professionals would be involved with this procedure.

4. What does the maintenance of dental implants include?

Review Questions

Multiple Choice

1. Which of the following is an advantage of dental implants?
   a. cost
   b. better esthetics
   c. healing time
   d. surgical complications

2. Which of the following is a disadvantage of dental implants?
   a. improved speech
   b. improved comfort
   c. implant failure
   d. better chewing ability

3. Dental implants have differences in success rates depending on where the implants are placed. Success in the anterior areas ranges from 85% to 95%, while the posterior teeth success rate ranges from 90% to 100%.
   Select the correct response based on the statements above.
   a. Both statements are true.
   b. Both statements are false.
   c. The first statement is true; the second statement is false.
   d. The first statement is false; the second statement is true.

4. Which of the following is not correct regarding implant placement?
   a. The maxillary posterior areas usually have a very high success rate due to proximity of the maxillary sinus.
   b. Bone augmentation in the area of the maxillary sinus may be beneficial in providing bone prior to implant placement.
   c. Bone deformities in the maxilla or the mandible can lead to insufficient bone for implant placement.
   d. Implant success after placement is also determined by the load the implant bears.

5. Match each part of the implant with the correct description
   a. implant body
   b. abutment
   c. healing cap
   d. connector
   e. crown
      1. artificial replacement that restores the missing tooth structure
      2. placed during the first stage of the implant surgery and is fixed in the alveolar bone
      3. dome-shaped caps which project through the soft tissue into the oral cavity to prevent the overgrowth of the tissues over the implant body
      4. part which provides support to the artificial crown
      5. allows attachment of restoration to implant

6. Which of the following is not an indication for dental implants?
   a. Patient unwilling to cooperate with pre- and postoperative instructions
   b. Support for removable oral prosthesis
   c. Patient has good overall health
   d. Prevention of resorption of alveolar bone after tooth loss

7. Which of the following is a contraindication for dental implants?
   a. sufficient bone of good quality
   b. ability to pay
   c. allergies to materials used in implants
   d. cooperative patient attitude

8. One reason implants may fail is due to good healing of the bone and tissues after implant placement. Another reason implants fail is due to fracture of the implant.
   Select the correct response based on the statements above.
   a. Both statements are true.
   b. Both statements are false.
   c. The first statement is true; the second statement is false.
   d. The first statement is false; the second statement is true.

9. Which of the following statements regarding implant considerations is not correct?
   a. Osteoporosis may affect osseointegration by impairing the bone metabolism.
   b. Uncontrolled type II diabetes is a contraindication as healing after implant placement may be delayed.
   c. The presence of cardiac disease does not impact the success of a dental implant.
   d. Active chemotherapy is not a contraindication for dental implant placement.

10. The same pathogens responsible for periodontitis have been implicated in implant infections and implant loss. A comprehensive periodontal evaluation and appropriate treatment are provided to ensure people have optimal periodontal health possible prior to implant placement.
    Select the correct response based on the statements above.
    a. Both statements are true.
    b. Both statements are false.
    c. The first statement is true; the second statement is false.
    d. The first statement is false; the second statement is true.

11. Which of the following is correct regarding patient selection factors for implants?
    a. Bruxism is not a consideration since implants are made of a strong titanium alloy.
    b. Patient cooperation is not a factor since implants are metal and do not need maintenance.
    c. Radiographs to determine bone height and width are an important part of the clinical evaluation.
    d. Since implants are not impacted by periodontal disease, poor oral home care is not a factor that needs consideration.

12. Match the type of bone graft with the correct description
    a. allograft
    b. xenograft
    c. autograft
    d. alloplastic
       1. harvested from animals
       2. harvested from the patient's own body
       3. harvested from the other human donors
       4. man-made, synthetic materials

13. The subperiosteal implant is used on patients whose dentures no longer fit well. It is most commonly placed in the maxilla.
    Select the correct response based on the statements above.
    a. Both statements are true.
    b. Both statements are false.
    c. The first statement is true; the second statement is false.
    d. The first statement is false; the second statement is true.

14. Endosteal implants are available in various sizes. Bone must be of sufficient height, width, and length for successful placement.
    Select the correct response based on the statements above.
    a. Both statements are true.
    b. Both statements are false.
    c. The firstfirst statement is true; the second statement is false.
    d. The firstfirst statement is false; the second statement is true.

15. Which of the following is correct regarding mini dental implants (MDIs)?
    a. A gingival flap is not required for placement of the MDI.
    b. Healing time is longer with an MDI as compared to an endosteal implant.
    c. MDIs are more expensive than other types of implants.
    d. MDI placement procedure takes more time than placement of other implants.

16. The transosteal implant is used in an edentulous area of the mandible and passes through the cortical plate and the alveolar bone. This type of implant is reserved for use in patients who have severely resorbed alveolar ridges that will not support other types of implants.
    Select the correct response based on the statements above.
    a. Both statements are true.
    b. Both statements are false.
    c. The first statement is true; the second statement is false.
    d. The first statement is false; the second statement is true.

17. An immediate load dental implant is placed 48 hours after the tooth is extracted from the oral cavity. The restoration is placed on the immediate load dental implant after osseointegration takes place.
    Select the correct response based on the statements above.
    a. Both statements are true.
    b. Both statements are false.
    c. The first statement is true; the second statement is false.
    d. The first statement is false; the second statement is true.

18. In the one-stage implant technique, the implant is inserted into the bone, but the extruding end is not covered with gingival tissue. In the two-stage implant technique, the implant is placed into the bone and gingival tissue is sutured into place to cover the implant.

Select the correct response based on the statements above.
a. Both statements are true.
b. Both statements are false.
c. The first statement is true; the second statement is false.
d. The first statement is false; the second statement is true.

Critical Thinking

1. A patient presents to the periodontist office you are working in as a dental assistant. You assist the periodontist with the exam and development of a treatment plan. The patient then asks you what is required after the surgery for implant placement. What do you tell the patient?

2. The patient then asks you about how the implant should be maintained long term. What do you tell them about home care in addition to brushing?

3. You have recently taken a position as a dental assistant in a periodontist practice. The practice does a significant number of implant procedures. You are available to assist the periodontist during implant procedures but also have been assigned to the role of implant coordinator. What is your role as the implant coordinator?

4. Why would a patient choose dental implants over other possible treatments?

5. Explain what information needs to be gathered for the consultation appointment when a patient decides on an implant as a possible treatment.

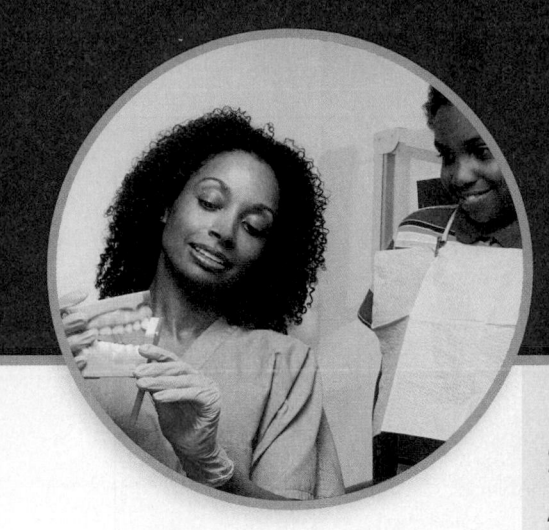

## CHAPTER 40

Fixed Prosthodontics

Specific Instructional Objectives

At the completion of this chapter, you will be able to meet these objectives:

1. Use terms presented in this chapter.
2. State the objectives of fixed prosthodontics.
3. Differentiate among the types of fixed prosthodontic restorations.
4. Explain patient factors considered in a fixed prosthodontic procedure.
5. Discuss the components of the preparation appointment.
6. Paraphrase the steps in the first appointment for a fixed dental prosthesis.
7. Describe the importance of gingival retraction cord.
8. Identify the different methods of gingival retraction.
9. Discuss the process for taking an impression.
10. List the steps that take place at the lab when fabricating a fixed prosthesis.
11. Describe the communication tools available for use for communicating with the dental lab.
12. Outline the steps of the second treatment appointment for a fixed dental prosthesis.
13. Discuss the concerns related to a fixed dental prosthesis.
14. Discriminate methods of oral hygiene care for a fixed dental prosthesis.
15. Examine the changing trends related to an increase in fixed dental prosthetics.
16. Describe the components of the informed consent for fixed dental prosthodontics.
17. Identify charting symbols for a fixed prosthesis.

Fixed Prosthodontics

Prosthodontics is one of the nine dental specialties recognized by the American Dental Association (ADA). After graduating from an accredited dental school, the new dentist may choose to complete a 3-year post graduate program in prosthodontics. Specializing in prosthodontics includes restoring missing teeth through the use of removable dental appliances, or fixed dental appliances or a combination of the two. This chapter will focus on fixed dental appliances. Fixed prosthodontics involves the replacement of missing teeth with a cast prosthesis, which is permanently cemented in place. A fixed dental restoration is also known as an *indirect restoration*. This is because the tooth is prepared in the office by the dentist; an impression is obtained and then sent to the lab. The dental lab fabricates a model with a removable die, and a dental technician fabricates the restoration indirectly from the model (Figure 40-1).

Fixed prosthodontics can be used to restore a single tooth or restore multiple teeth. When deciding on the type of fixed prosthodontic replacement, there are several things that the dentist must consider. These include the amount of natural tooth structure that will remain after the tooth is prepared, the location of the tooth or edentulous area, the condition of the surrounding natural teeth, and the type of restorative material that will be used.

The dentist discusses the options with the patient, and together they decide about the type of the fixed prosthesis and the material to be used. Several factors are considered when making this decision. These factors include patient age, patient gender, ability of patient to pay for treatment, number of visits needed to complete treatment, and also the motivation and ability for oral home care.

Fixed prosthodontic fabrication requires collaboration with a dental laboratory. The dental lab and the dentist should have good communication between them. The dentist should provide clear and detailed instructions to the lab technician regarding the design and materials of each restoration.

The Objectives of Fixed Prosthodontics

Fixed prostheses replace missing teeth and tooth structures in order to:

- Protect a tooth that has lost tooth structure due to decay or fracture
- Restore function to the dentition
- Support a bridge to replace a missing tooth in an edentulous area
- Restore an implant
- Restore esthetics
- Improve speech
- Enhance oral hygiene
- Restore occlusion

The fixed prosthesis becomes part of the natural dentition and is maintained with routine brushing and flossing techniques. The main disadvantages are the expense of the prosthesis and the time involved in preparing the tooth, taking the impression, fabricating the restoration, and permanently cementing it in place. Restorations routinely take at least two appointments to complete. Dental insurance may cover some of the expense of prosthetic restorations.

There are several advantages of having a permanent restoration. The restoration is secure in the oral cavity, is esthetic, and restores function for many years. These advantages outweigh the initial monetary expense and time commitment.

General dentists normally include fixed prosthodontic procedures in their practice; however, cases that are beyond their level of expertise are referred to a specialist known as a *prosthodontist*. A prosthodontist usually specializes in fixed and removable dental prosthetic appliances. Removable appliance will be discussed in detail in Chapter 42.

Types of Fixed Prosthodontics

The dentist and patient have a variety of fixed prostheses as well as materials to select from depending on which will suit the function, appearance, and finances to meet all their objectives. Each type of fixed prosthesis is discussed in this section.

Full Crown A *full crown* is an indirect restoration that completely covers the anatomic crown of an individual tooth (Figure 40-1A and B). It completely encircles a prepared tooth or is placed on an implant as the final restoration. This type of crown is indicated in cases of extensive caries, fracture of a crown, amelogenesis imperfecta, or tetracycline staining. Full crowns are usually indicated when significant tooth structure has been lost and a simple restoration is not possible to protect the tooth from further deterioration. A full coverage crown will be permanently cemented onto the tooth to protect the

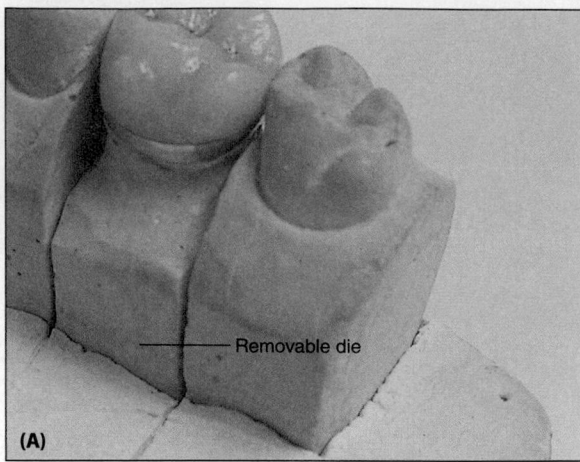

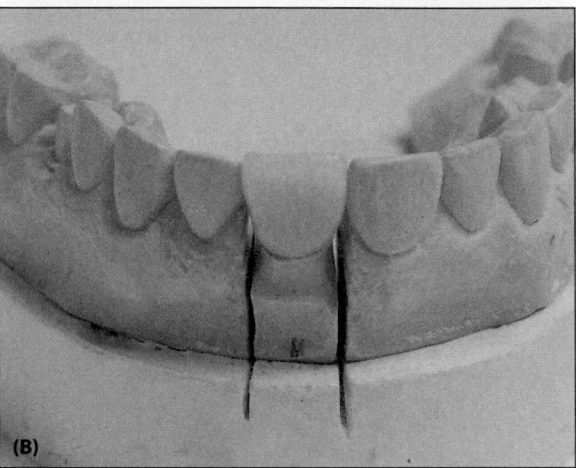

FIGURE 40-1
(A) Prosthodontic model with removable die and porcelain fused to metal crown. (B) Prosthodontic model with removable die and porcelain crown.

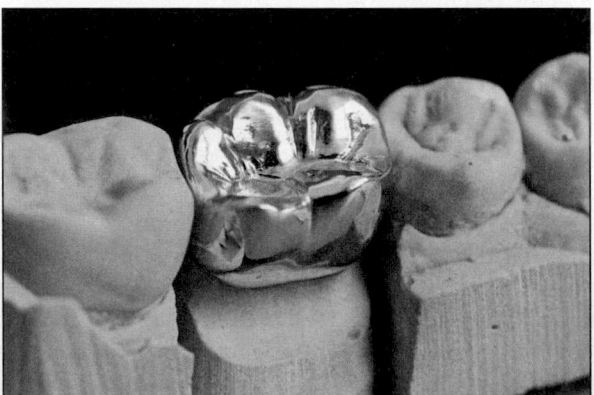

FIGURE 40-2
Full gold crown on a prosthodontic model.

remaining tooth structure from further deterioration due to biting forces. Full crowns may be all porcelain and are also known as all porcelain jacket crowns (Figure 40-1B), all metal such as gold (Figure 40-2) or porcelain fused to metal crowns also known as PFM (Figure 40-1A). Recently a material known as zirconia has become available for crowns (Figure 40-3). This material will be discussed later in this chapter.

Porcelain Fused to Metal Crowns The *porcelain fused to metal* (PFM) crown has a metal shell that can be precious or semiprecious metal covered by porcelain for esthetics. The metal shell gives the crown strength as compared to an all porcelain crown. Some patients may have a sensitivity to some of the semiprecious metals used. An allergy test can be performed by the patient's physician to confirm that there are no allergies to the metals that may be used in a crown. If the patient does have an allergy, then a gold crown or a porcelain fused to gold crown may be used.

All Porcelain or All Ceramic Crowns Porcelain crowns are an option as well (Figure 40-1B). All porcelain crowns are usually used in the anterior as they are more esthetic. They reflect light in a manner similar to natural tooth structure and also have a translucency that is similar to natural tooth structure. All porcelain crowns are more fragile than a PFM as they do not have a metal shell underneath for support (Figure 40-1A). All porcelain crowns do not have a metal collar that may be visible at the margin like with a PFM crown. Porcelain jacket crowns today are also made of *zirconia*, which is a highly translucent crystalline material with porcelain placed on top of it.

All Metal Crowns Metal crowns are made of palladium alloy, gold alloy (Full Gold Crown, FGC), or a base-metal alloy such as chromium or nickel (Figure 40-4). These crowns are stronger than the full porcelain crown and can last longer than the full porcelain crown but may not meet the esthetic requirements of a patient. Gold crowns are usually used to restore molars and possibly premolars if esthetics is not a concern.

Gold is a material that is gentle to the tissues and does not result in allergic reactions. Gold crowns have been used in dentistry for a long time. The hardness of gold is close to natural tooth hardness. As a result, gold crowns do not cause wear in the opposing tooth. Gold crowns require less reduction of tooth structure during the preparation appointment (see Procedure 40-3). This results in more tooth structure remaining, which results in a stronger tooth. Gold crowns do not chip or break so they last for a long

time. If a tooth with a gold crown breaks, it is usually because the underlying tooth structure has fractured or decayed. Nonprecious alloys are much less expensive than gold and may be used when finances are a consideration. Nonprecious alloys are also used when esthetics are not a concern and when strength is desired in the restoration. Some nonprecious alloys may contain nickel. Nickel, beryllium, cobalt, chromium, and palladium may cause immune problems or toxicity. The dentist and patient together decide what material is best for the patient. This decision is based on patient medical and dental history as well as financial concerns that the patient may have.

Partial Crown The 3/4 crown (Figure 40-5) and 7/8 crown are restorations that are in between a traditional inlay and a gold crown. These are also known as *onlays* (Figure 40-6).

Onlay An onlay covers the anatomic crown of the tooth with the exception of the facial surface. In a traditional crown, all walls and the occlusal surface of the tooth are reduced. An onlay requires minimal reduction and allows for conservation of the

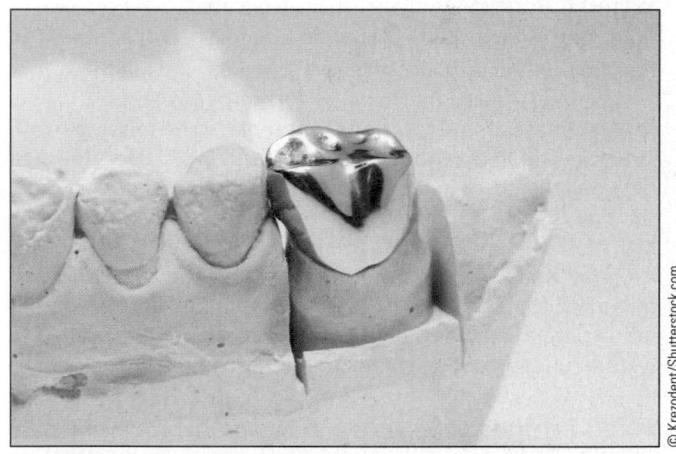

FIGURE 40-4
Metal crown.

© Krezodent/Shutterstock.com

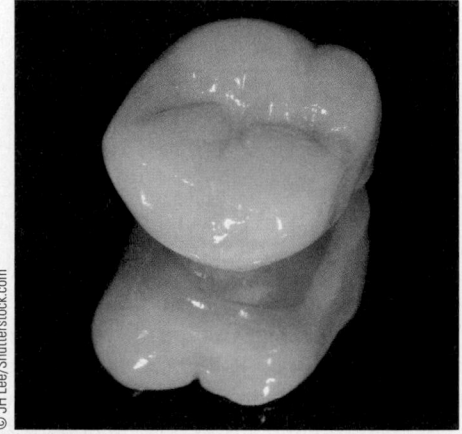

FIGURE 40-3
Zirconia crown.

© JH Lee/Shutterstock.com

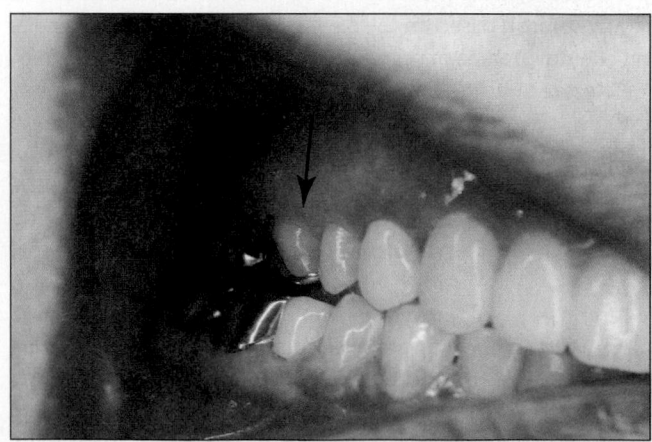

FIGURE 40-5
Three-quarter crown.

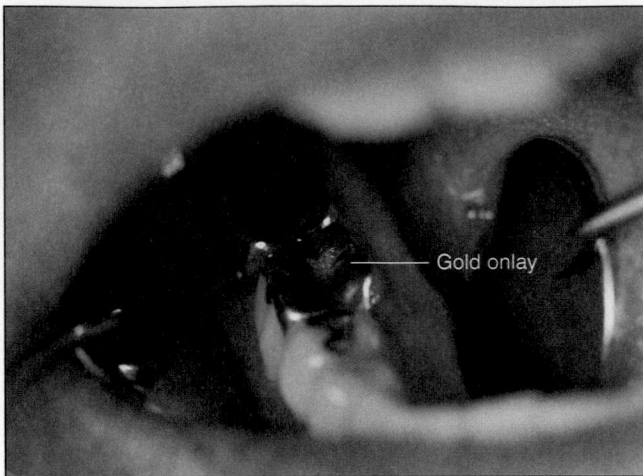

FIGURE 40-6
Gold onlay restoration on a mandibular first molar.

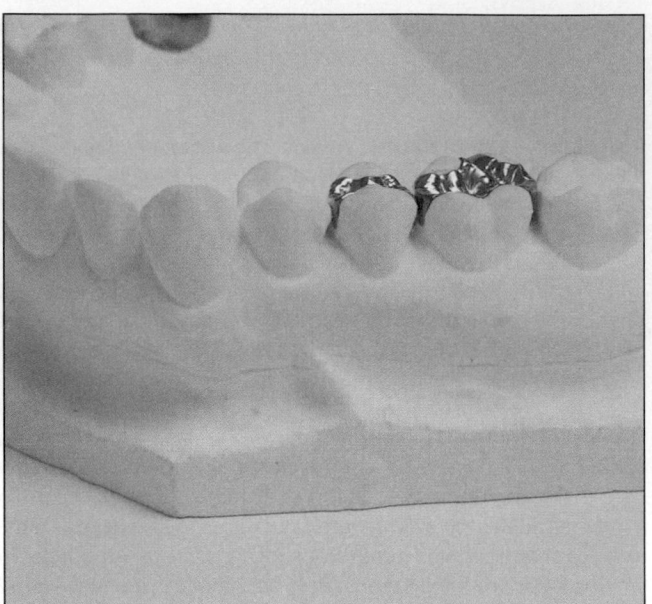

FIGURE 40-7
Gold inlay restorations.

natural tooth structure. An onlay may be treatment planned if tooth structure is remaining but a cusp has fractured. Onlays are indirect restorations and are usually fabricated from porcelain or gold. Onlays are usually placed on premolars, and at times the first molar when esthetics may be a concern.

Inlays Inlays are restorations that replace the missing tooth structure within the tooth (Figure 40-7). An *inlay* covers the area between the cusps in the middle of the tooth and the proximal surfaces that are involved. Inlays are MOD (mesio-occluso-distal), MO (mesio-occlusal), DO (disto-occlusal), or O (occlusal). An inlay is also cast restorations that is made of a variety of materials. The extent of the lost tooth structure and the preparation determine which type of cast restoration is best suited to restore function and preserve the strength of the tooth.

Fixed Bridges A bridge is a restoration that spans the space of a missing tooth or teeth. The bridge is divided into units, and each unit of a bridge represents a tooth. A bridge may replace one or more adjacent teeth in the same arch. The missing tooth is replaced by a *pontic* (Figure 40-8), which can be designed in a variety of forms based on the contact with the mucosal surface of the edentulous area of the ridge.

The teeth adjacent to the pontic are called *abutments*. Crowns, inlays, or onlays may be placed on the abutment teeth to support and stabilize the pontic. The cast restorations on the abutment teeth are also known as retainers (Figures 40-8 and 40-9). A bridge can be supported by only natural teeth, only implants, or a combination of natural teeth and implants (Figure 40-10). A bridge with several units is more prone to failure. As a result, implants combined with natural teeth to support the bridge or an implant supported bridge may be a better option. Bridges are usually fabricated by the dental laboratory and then cemented in the oral cavity. Acrylic bridges can be fabricated directly in the oral cavity. Bridges are made of a variety of materials to meet the patient's esthetic and functional needs.

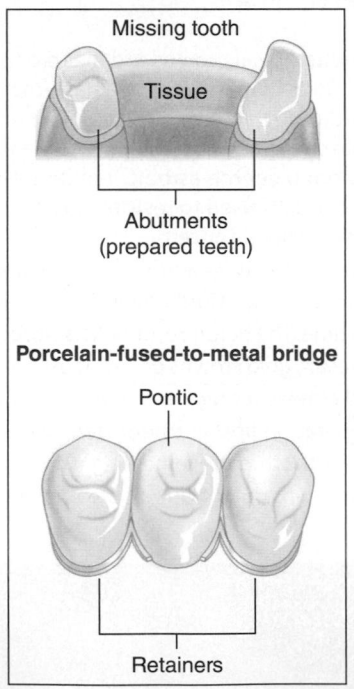

FIGURE 40-8
Three-unit bridge abutments, pontics, and retainers.

Cantilever Bridge Bridges can also be retained by one or two teeth on the same side. This type of bridge is known as a *cantilever bridge* (Figure 40-11). The cantilever bridge is used in areas of the oral cavity that are under less stress, such as the anterior teeth. This procedure involves anchoring the false tooth to one side over one or more natural and adjacent teeth. Cantilevered bridges are not preferred because there is no supporting

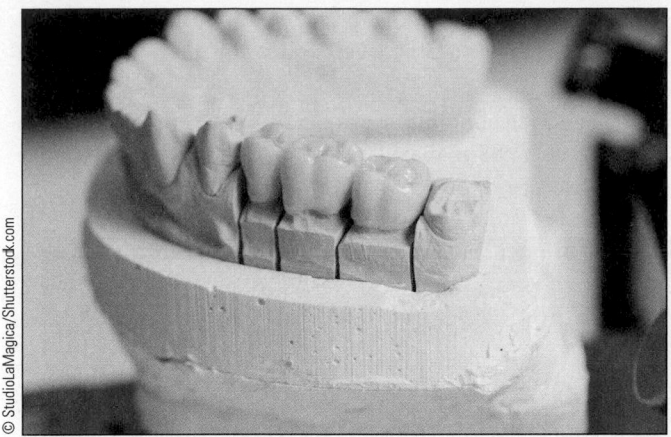

FIGURE 40-9
Three-unit bridge abutments, pontics, and retainers.

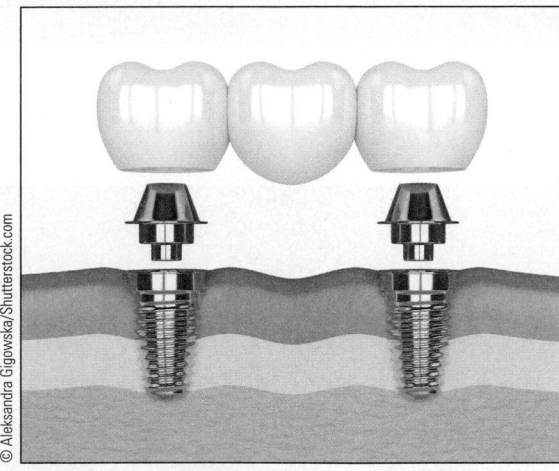

FIGURE 40-10
Implant supported three-unit bridge.

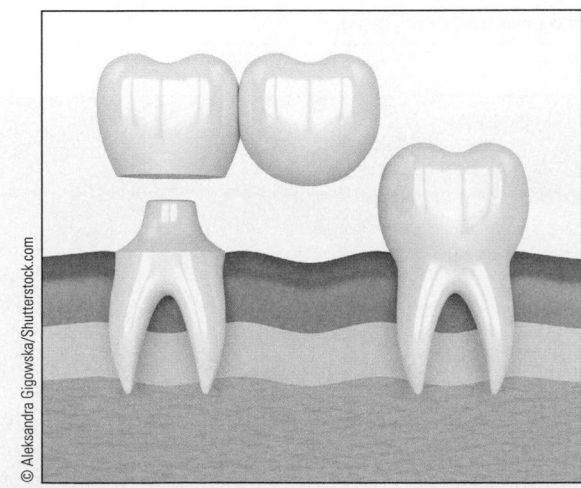

FIGURE 40-11
Cantilever bridge.

abutment on one side of the edentulous space. This results in excess force on the pontic and the supporting abutments. As a result of the excess forces, the bridge can dislodge.

Resin Bonded Maryland Bridge A *Maryland bridge*, or resin-retained fixed bridge, is used to replace one tooth. Abutment teeth have very little tooth structure removed during preparation. The bridge consists of a pontic with extensions (retainers) of varying shapes (Figure 40-12). The extensions are designed to attach to the abutment teeth, on or toward the lingual surface. The retainers of the Maryland bridge are roughened by electrolytic etching to increase their bonding to the natural tooth structure. Although these restorations have an esthetic advantage, they have minimal retention. As a result, they are more likely to dislodge. The patient should be made aware of this, and the patient should be advised to be careful while biting into foods.

Veneers A *veneer* (also known as lumineer or laminate) is a thin layer of tooth-colored material such as resin or porcelain that covers much of the facial surface (Figure 40-13). Veneers are used on anterior teeth to cover teeth that are intrinsically stained; teeth affected by abrasion, erosion, and enamel hypoplasia; or to

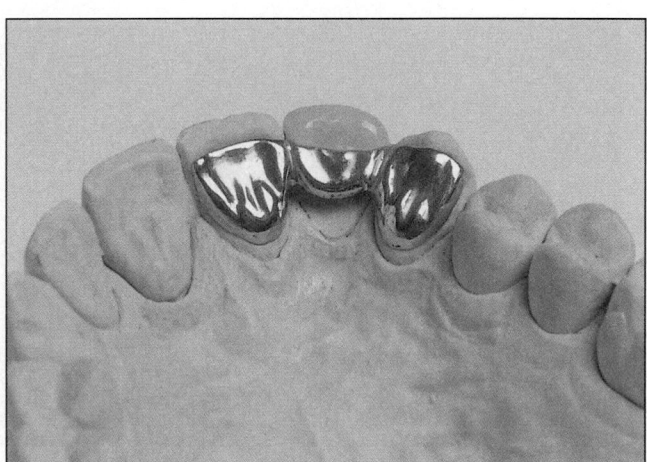

FIGURE 40-12
Maryland bridge.

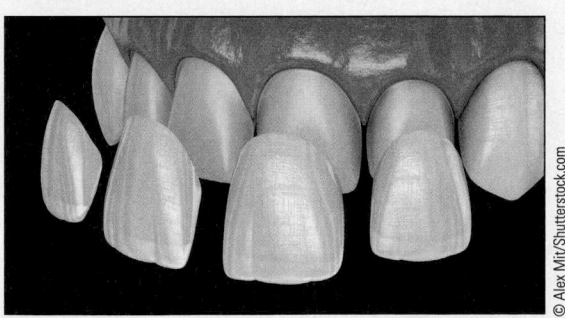

FIGURE 40-13
Porcelain veneers.

reshape the anatomy of the teeth. Veneers are cemented to the prepared tooth with a special resin cement such as Panavia™. Veneers improve appearance with very little removal of the tooth structure. Examples include the following:

- Full facial coverage on anterior maxillary teeth—covered with veneers for a natural appearance (Figures 40-14A and B).

- Tetracycline stains on the maxillary anterior teeth—veneers cover the stain for improved appearance (Figures 40-15A and B).

- Diastema (an abnormal space between two adjacent teeth in the same arch) on maxillary central incisors—veneers close the space (Figures 40-16A and B).

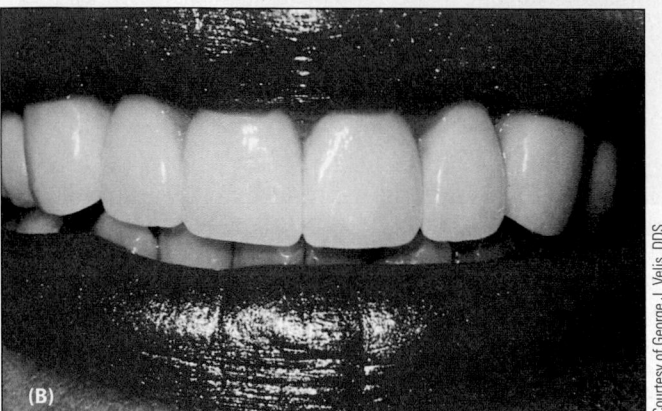

FIGURE 40-14

Veneers on anterior teeth. (A) Before placement. (B) After placement of veneers.

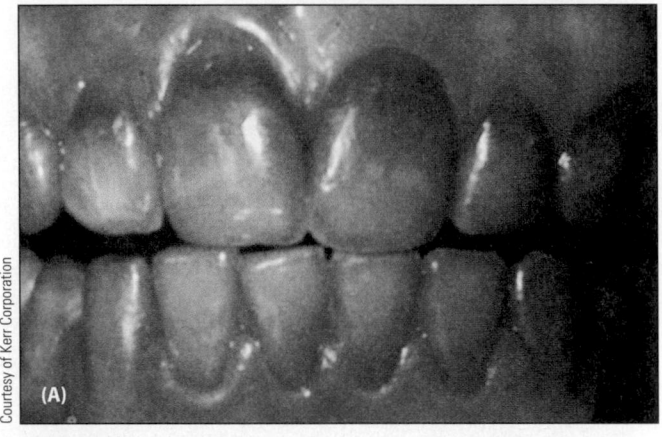
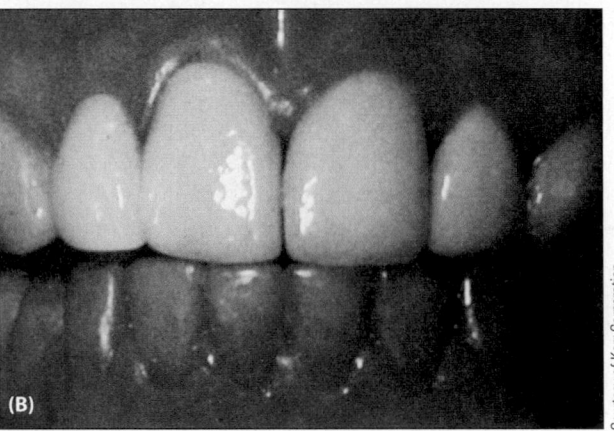

FIGURE 40-15

(A) Patient with tetracycline staining. (B) Patient with tetracycline staining after direct resin veneers have been placed.

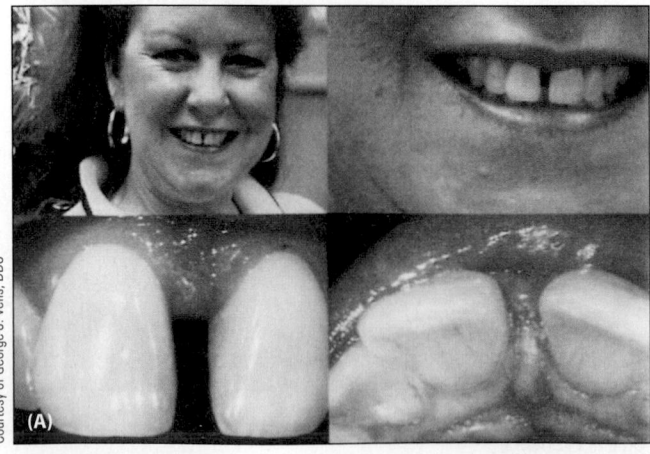
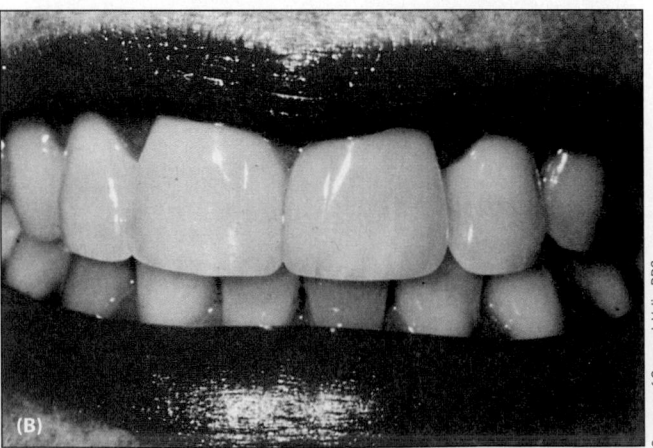

FIGURE 40-16

(A) Patient with diastema between two central incisors. (B) Same patient with diastema after indirect resin veneers have been placed.

Veneer procedures are changing constantly as technology progresses. There are many types of veneers, materials used, and techniques. Direct resin veneers, indirect resin veneers, and porcelain veneers are the three types that are discussed in the following sections.

Porcelain Veneers A porcelain veneer requires two appointments and is fabricated in the dental laboratory. Porcelain veneers are natural in appearance and are durable. The technique for the porcelain veneer is sensitive to shade selection and gingival margin adaptation if the veneer is to look natural and adapt well. Procedure 40-2 outlines the steps involved in placing porcelain veneers.

Direct Resin Veneers A *direct resin veneer* is made in the dental office directly on the patient's tooth. This procedure requires one appointment. In preparation for the veneer procedure, little if any tooth structure is removed. The tooth is etched, adhesive is applied, and opaque resin as well as body shade are placed. The incisal shade follows. The shade can be varied between the incisal edge and body of the veneer. The veneers are contoured and finished. Generally, these materials are light cured and require routine polishing and periodic maintenance.

Indirect Resin Veneers An *indirect resin veneer* requires two appointments. At the first appointment, the tooth is prepared and an impression is taken. The impression is sent to the laboratory for fabrication of the veneer. During the second appointment, the veneer is bonded in place. These veneers do not bond well to resin cement. They lack strength and wear at a faster rate than porcelain veneers.

Patient Factors

The dentist performs a comprehensive medical and dental examination of the prospective prosthodontic patient and verifies motivation of the patient toward receiving an appliance to determine whether or not the patient is a good candidate. Factors to be considered are those that are outlined in Box 40-1. Clinical information obtained during treatment planning can play a critical role in the success of a fixed prosthodontics appliance.

Patients with uncontrolled diabetes experience a higher rate of infection and periodontal disease. These patients may be a better candidate for a removable dental prosthetic appliance.

Xerostomia reduces the ability of the oral cavity to wash away food particles from the teeth. Xerostomia also results in increased acidity of the oral cavity, leading to an increase in dental decay. Oral home care maintenance is more difficult in the presence of xerostomia; this may lead to a failure of dental work, including a fixed dental prosthesis.

Preparation Appointment

The initial appointment is usually a preparation appointment. At this visit, prior to the start of treatment, radiographs will be obtained as needed and an oral exam will be competed. Preliminary impressions are obtained and study casts are fabricated in preparation for treatment.

Occlusal Exam

All active disease processes such as caries or periodontal disease must be treated prior to the fabrication of any fixed prosthetic appliances. Occlusion is also evaluated, and the *smile line* of the patient is recorded as well. This allows the dentist to consider esthetics (Figure 40-17).

Radiographs

The full mouth series of radiographs (FMX) and panoramic images (refer to Chapter 28) are beneficial when treatment planning for a fixed dental prosthesis. If implants are required as part of the treatment plan, three dimensional cone beam images may be necessary. Refer to Chapters 27–29 regarding information obtained from dental radiographs.

BOX 40-1 Clinical Factors that Can Determine the Success of a Fixed Dental Prosthesis

- Medical and dental history
- Chief complaint
- Finances
- Intraoral and extraoral exam
- Radiographs and diagnostic models and photographs
  - Age
  - Periodontal status
  - Existing natural teeth
  - History of decay
  - Attrition of the dentition
  - Patient expectation of outcomes
  - Emotional status of the patient
  - Esthetic concerns
  - Xerostomia
  - Previous dental prosthesis

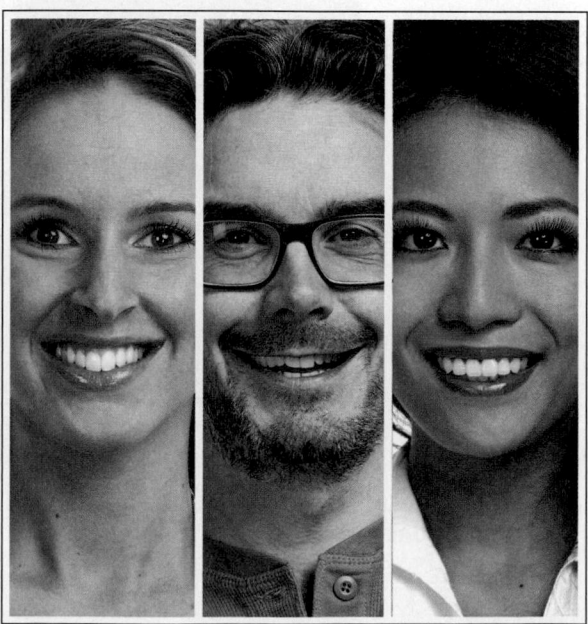

FIGURE 40-17
High, low, and moderate smile lines.

© kurhan/Shutterstock.com

Preliminary Impression and Study Casts

Study casts are important when treatment planning for a fixed prosthetic appliance. After the exam and treatment planning is completed, the dental assistant obtains preliminary alginate impressions and pours the study models. This preliminary impression may be used to fabricate the *provisional* or temporary crown. Some practitioners may prefer to use an acrylic or stainless steel prefabricated provisional crown. Acrylic provisional crowns are used in the anterior areas, and the stainless steel provisional crowns are used in the posterior areas (Figure 40-18A). The study models aid in the evaluation of occlusion, fabrication of provisional crowns, and preparation of the diagnostic wax-up if needed as well as the assessment of the final appearance of the prosthetic appliance (Figure 40-18B).

Selecting a Shade

Shade selection is important, especially if esthetics of a prosthesis is a factor. Selecting a shade can be subjective as color perception varies between people.

Selection of the shade can vary based on the person selecting the shade, the object, and the source of light. Ideally, the shade should be obtained under a natural light source.

Hue, *chroma*, *value*, and translucency of the color are important when selecting a shade. Hue is the quality that differentiates colors. In a standard shade guide these are usually grouped as the reds or yellow–reds or yellows or grays (Figure 40-19). Chroma is the intensity of the color, and value is the brightness or lightness of the color. Value is a little more difficult to determine with a manual shade guide than hue and chroma.

The patient should not be wearing lipstick or face makeup or large jewelry or eye glasses during the shade selection process. The teeth should be clean at this time as well. The patient should be at eye level, and the dental professional should be positioned between the light source and the patient. Shade selection is accomplished by placing the manual shade guide tabs on either side of the tooth to be restored or on either side of the edentulous area (Figure 40-20). The operator

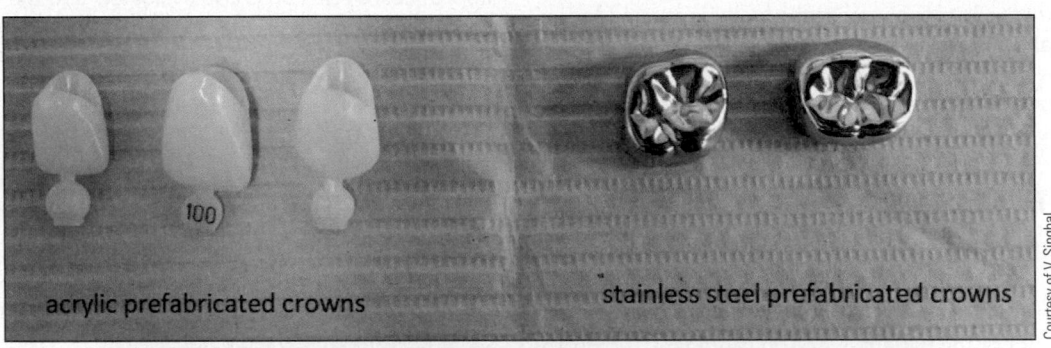

acrylic prefabricated crowns   stainless steel prefabricated crowns

Courtesy of V. Singhal

(A)

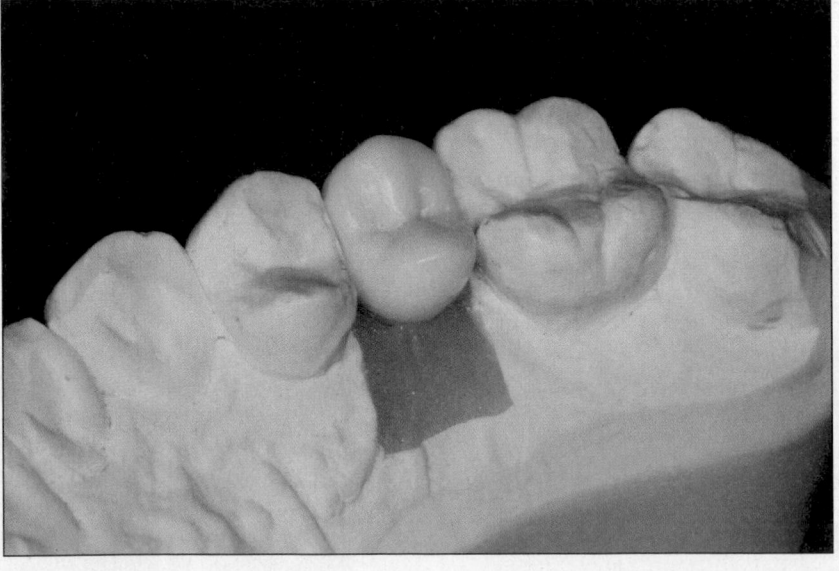

© JH Lee/Shutterstock.com

(B)

FIGURE 40-18
(A) Prefabricated provisional crowns. (B) Diagnostic wax up of a second premolar on a study model.

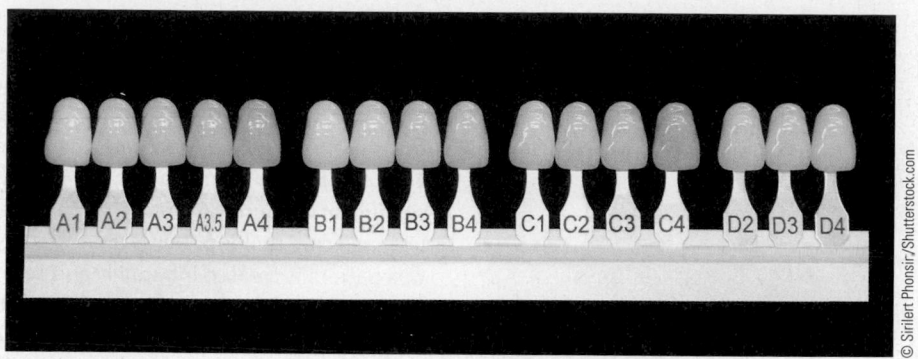

FIGURE 40-19
Dental shade guide.

records the gingival and incisal shades. These shades should also be noted on the lab prescription. Some offices may use digital shade guides.

The patient should be involved in the shade selection for the final fixed dental prosthesis. Some patients may opt to whiten their teeth prior to the fabrication of the permanent fixed prosthesis. Many dental offices will schedule patients for a shade match of anterior teeth once the whitening process has been completed. This will allow for an accurate shade selection.

Case Presentation

During an appointment for a simple fixed prosthodontic case, the case presentation may take place at the initial visit. In a more complicated case, the case presentation may take place after the initial visit so the dentist has time to study the preliminary models and the radiographs and develop a treatment plan.

During case presentation the dentist discusses the type of prosthesis and the series of appointments that would be needed for each treatment plan option. A member of the office team would discuss the financial aspect and insurance coverage. The patient should be allowed to ask questions. These questions may be answered through the use of visual aids such as models and

radiographs. The patient then decides which treatment is the best option for them. This is an important aspect of informed consent.

First Treatment Appointment

Multiple appointments may be required in a fixed prosthodontics case. During the first treatment appointment the teeth are prepared for the prosthesis. At this visit, a bite registration (Figure 40-21) is obtained before the local anesthetic is administered. The tooth is then reduced in order to accommodate the fixed dental prosthesis (Figure 40-22).

Once the final impression of the prepared tooth is obtained, a provisional crown is placed. The provisional crown is important as it protects the prepared tooth until the final prosthesis is cemented. The shade selection, bite registration, final impression, and written laboratory prescription are sent to the dental laboratory. The lab usually needs 7 to 10 days to fabricate the fixed dental appliance. Depending on the distance between the dental

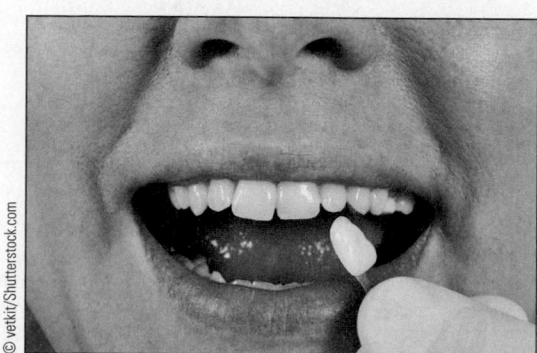

FIGURE 40-20
Selecting a shade.

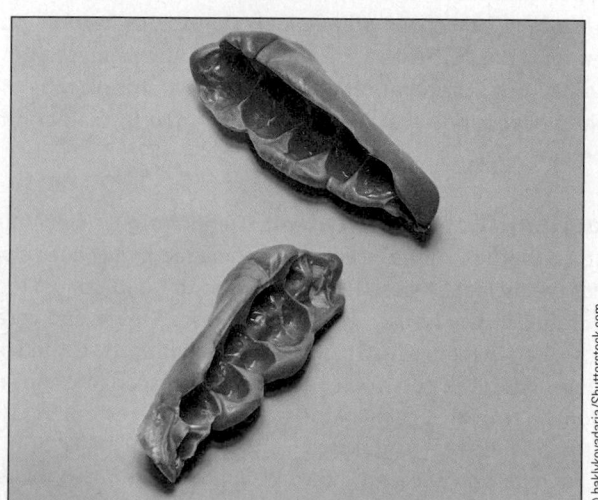

FIGURE 40-21
Bite registration.

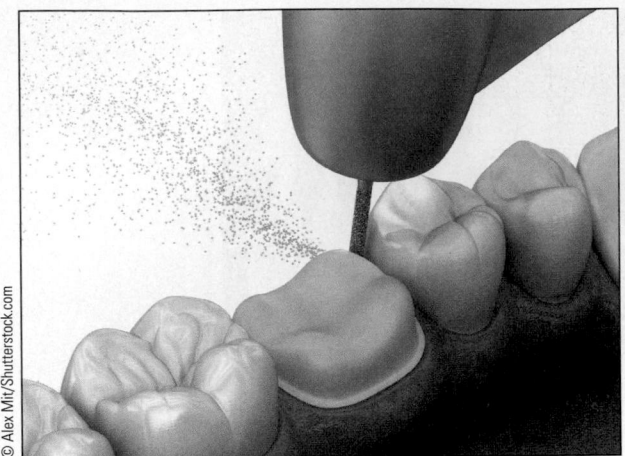

FIGURE 40-22
Crown preparation on maxillary second molar.

office and laboratory, the dental office should also allow for shipping time of the case to the lab and from the lab back to the dental office.

Anesthetic Application

Local anesthetic is administered at the start of the preparation visit after the bite registration has been obtained. Refer to Chapter 23 for steps in assisting with local anesthesia administration.

Tooth Preparation

After the teeth to be prepared have been anesthetized, the dentist uses selected burs in a high-speed handpiece to reduce the teeth circumferentially and to also shape the teeth. Diseased tooth structure will be removed along with some healthy tooth structure. Diamond burs are commonly used to prepare the teeth for a fixed dental prosthesis (Figure 40-23). These may be kept in a bur block along with carbide burs. Diamond burs provide a smooth finish to the prepared tooth. During tooth preparation, the dental assistant uses the high speed evacuation and the air/water syringe to maintain the operating field.

Post and Core Fabrication Depending on how much natural tooth structure is remaining, some teeth may need a *post and core buildup*. A post and core is used to build up lost tooth structure so the new crown has retention. A post and core is completed in teeth which have been endodontically treated previously. After the post and core have been placed into the endodontically treated canal of the tooth, the final restoration such as the crown is then completed.

For retention, the post should be approximately two-thirds of the length of the root. Posts are usually serrated for added retention and are also held in place by cement. After the post is cemented in

place, a core is built up around it. The buildup may be amalgam or composite (Figure 40-24).

There are prefabricated posts available as a kit. The kit contains posts of different diameters and length. These types of posts are usually used on teeth that have retained a sufficient amount of tooth structure (Figure 40-25). Teeth that have lost a significant amount of tooth structure may need a custom cast post and core buildup. This is fabricated by the dental lab after a wax pattern is created intraorally and sent to the lab. The lab will then use this pattern to cast the final cast post and core, which will then be cemented into the patient's tooth (Figure 40-26). In teeth that have lost minimum tooth structure, retention pins may be sufficient to support the restorative material and then the final cast restoration (Figure 40-27).

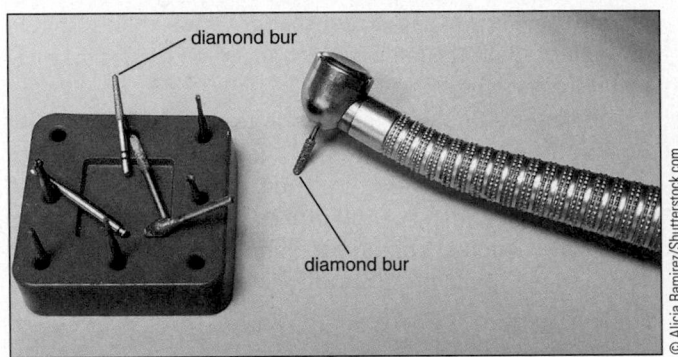

FIGURE 40-23
Diamond burs.

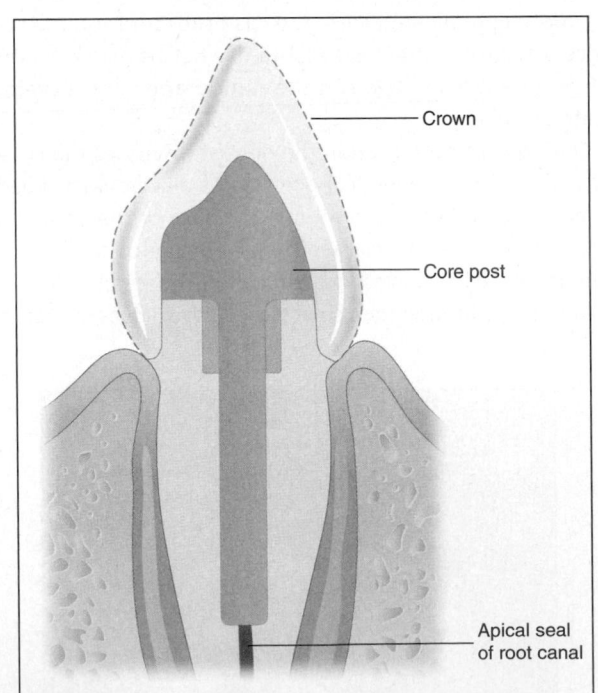

FIGURE 40-24
Core post in a nonvital tooth.

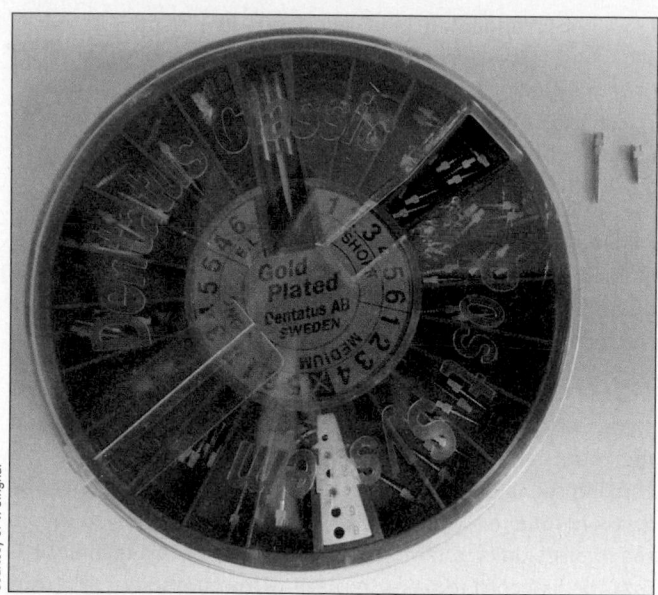

FIGURE 40-25
Prefabricated post kit.

Courtesy of V. Singhal

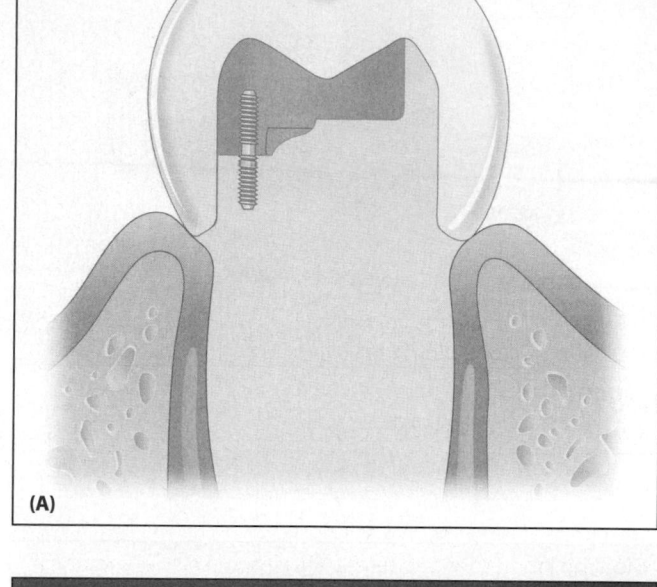

(A)

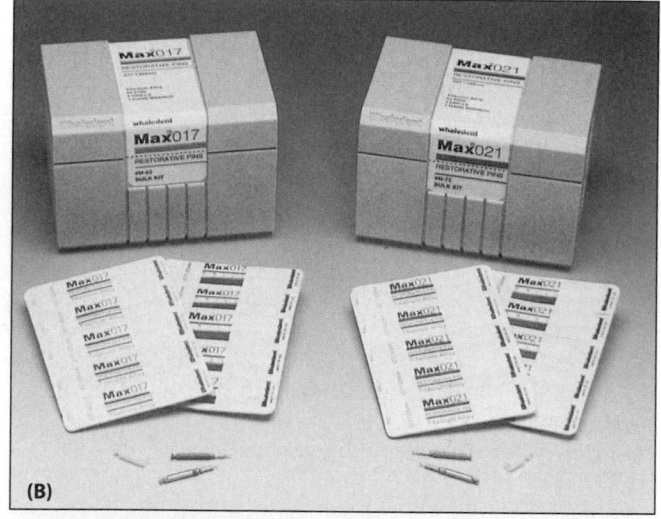

(B)

Gingival Cord Packing The margins of the prepared tooth may be subgingival. In anterior teeth it may be intentional for esthetic reasons. Subgingival margins may be because the presence of extensive decay. A good impression of the margin is needed for a proper fitting prosthesis, which prevents leakage under the crown. Thus, the impression material must be able to flow under the soft gingival tissue.

There are various methods available for tissue management in order to obtain a good impression of the prepared tooth, the most common being the use of a retraction cord (Figure 40-28). Retraction cords may be twisted or braided. They are available in different sizes to accommodate a variety of sulcus depths. The dental assistant can use a Balshi packer (Figure 40-29) or

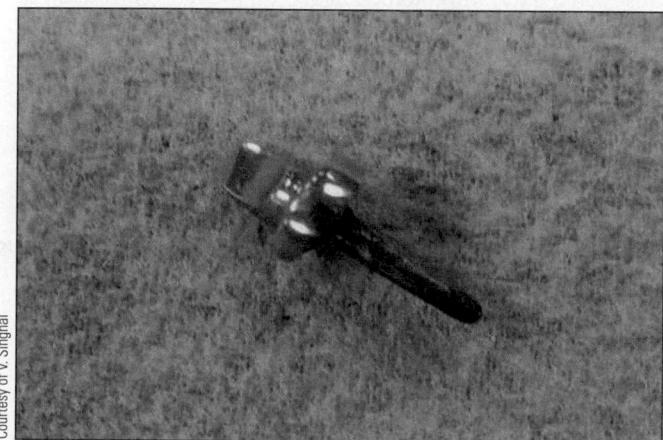

Courtesy of V. Singhal

FIGURE 40-26
Cast post and core.

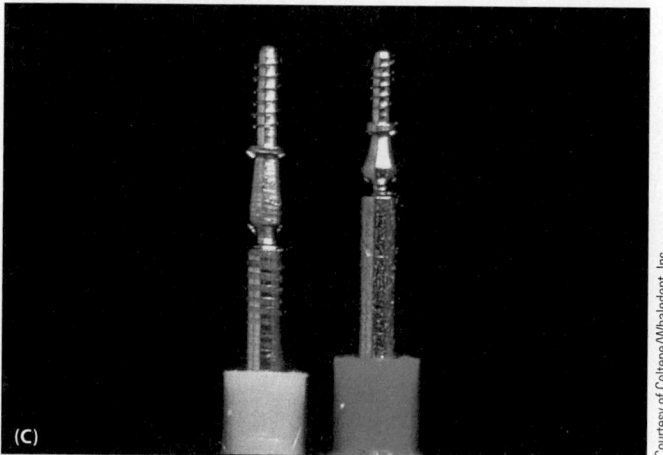

(C)

Courtesy of Coltene/Whaledent, Inc.

FIGURE 40-27
(A) Pins placed in a prepared tooth for support and retention. (B) Retention pin kit. (C) Close-up of pins (maxillary restorative pins).

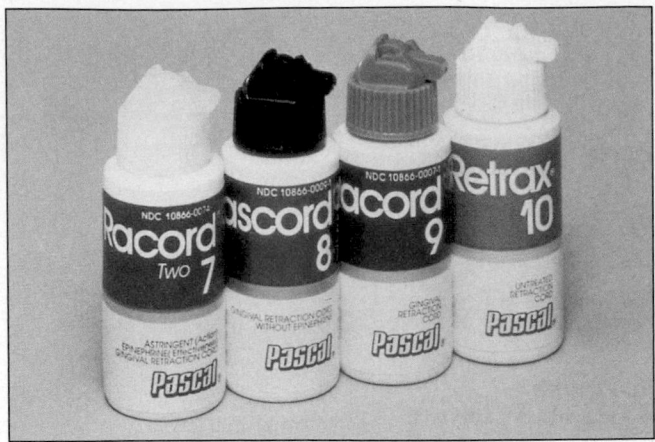

FIGURE 40-28
Various types of retraction cords.

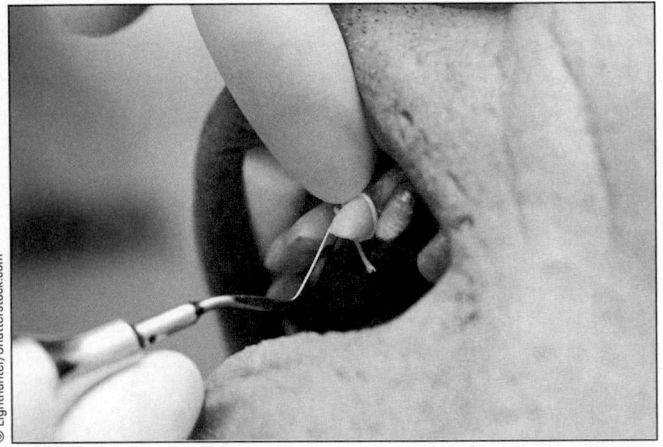

© Lighthunter/Shutterstock.com

FIGURE 40-29
Packing of retraction cord subgingivally around a prepared tooth.

another cord-packing instrument to gently push the gingival retraction cord under the free gingival soft tissue. The assistant should start at one end and place the cord under the soft tissue around the tooth until the other end is reached. A small piece of the end is left above the soft tissue for removal prior to injecting the light body final impression material (Figure 40-30A). The retraction cord should not be placed too deep or too shallow in the sulcus (Figures 40-30B and 40-30C). In these instances the gingiva will not be retracted from the margin of the preparation, impacting the quality of the final impression. Once the retraction cord is in place, a folded piece of gauze or a cotton roll should be placed between the prepared teeth, and the patient should be requested to bite on the gauze. This helps to keep the prepared site free of moisture.

Some retraction cords are treated with a chemical agent such as Hemodent® to minimize bleeding. The gingival retraction cord is left in place for 5 to 7 minutes if chemically treated and up to 15 minutes if untreated. Mechanical retraction of the soft tissues allows the impression material to reach the subgingival margin of the prepared tooth.

Gingival retraction cord with epinephrine should not be used as epinephrine can lead to palpitations and hypertension in those who are sensitive to the effects of epinephrine.

Other Methods of Gingival Retraction There are many other methods available to prepare the soft tissue for an impression of the preparation and surrounding soft tissue. Some other more commonly used methods are discussed in this section.

Double Cord Technique This method involves two retraction cords, one is placed on top of the other (Figure 40-30D). A size 00 thin retraction cord is first placed subgingivally. A second larger cord impregnated with a hemostatic agent is placed above the first cord for a minimum of 5 to 7 minutes and removed before the impression is obtained. The advantage of this technique is that the first cord remains in place within the sulcus and thus reduces the tendency of the gingival margin to recoil and displace the impression material. The first cord helps to control the hemorrhaging in the area of the tissues.

Electrosurgery and Laser If the gingival tissues are bulbous and esthetics is not a concern, the dentist can use electrosurgery to create a trough around the preparation. Lasers can be used as well. Both lasers and electrosurgery combined with other methods work well when there is significant gingival bleeding.

Final Impression and Bite Registration

After the tissues have been managed appropriately, the final impression material, selected by the dentist, is prepared by the dental assistant. Various types of final impression materials are used including polyvinyl siloxane, polysulfide, polyether, and reversible hydrocolloid. Many dentists prefer to use a triple tray (Figure 40-31). This is a double sided quadrant/posterior or anterior tray that captures the maxillary and mandibular quadrant on the side of the prepared tooth at the same time when the patient closes on the tray. This method allows for the bite registration to be captured at the same time the impression is taken. This allows the lab to fabricate the crown in the patient's correct occlusion. When using a triple tray, a light body final impression material is injected around the prepared tooth and the adjacent teeth with a plastic disposable syringe once the gingival packing cord has been removed. At the same time, the triple tray is filled on both sides with a heavy body material and seated in the patient's oral cavity. The patient is asked to bite completely and remain closed until the material sets.

Once the impression material has set, the final impression is removed from the oral cavity. The impression is then disinfected and examined by the dentist to ensure the entire margin was captured and that the impression is free of bubbles (Figure 40-32A). The dental laboratory technician must be able to see the margins on the **dies** produced from the impression to fabricate a dental prosthesis that fits well and seals the margins of the tooth.

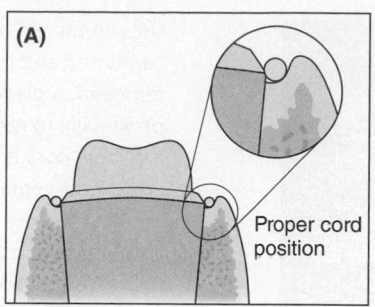

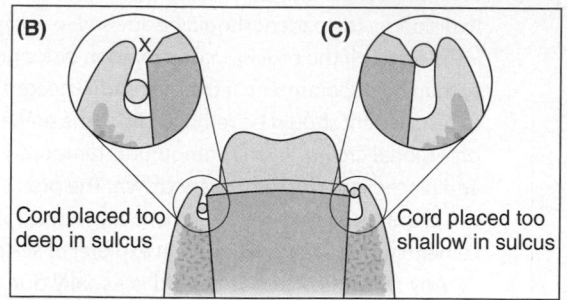

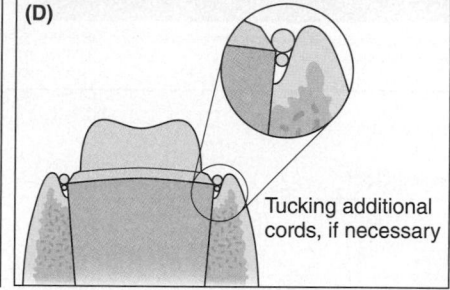

FIGURE 40-30

(A) Retraction cord placed correctly. (B) Retraction cord placement at root depth. (C) Retraction cord placed too shallow. (D) Double retraction cords placed correctly.

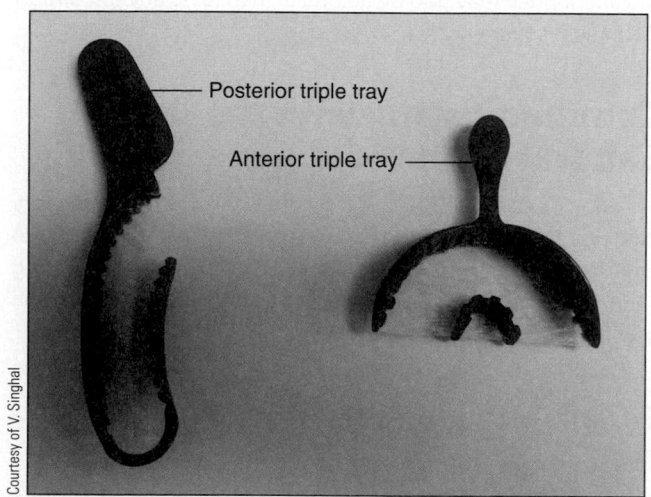

Courtesy of V. Singhal

FIGURE 40-31

Triple tray.

If the triple tray method is not used, then an impression must be taken of the arch with the prepared tooth using the crown and bridge impression material of choice; an alginate impression of the opposing arch is also needed. A separate bite registration must be obtained as well. All three of these items are evaluated for accuracy and are disinfected. They are then sent to the dental lab. At the dental lab, there are several steps that take place before the fixed prosthesis is sent back to the dental office:

1. Pour the final impression to make the master model and die (replica of prepared tooth) (see Figure 40-1).

2. Create a wax pattern on the die, which is then removed from the master model.

3. Prepare the wax pattern for casting by placing the wax pattern on a sprue pin and placing the pin on the mold base in the ring mold (Figure 40-32B). The sprue pin will later provide a passage for the molten metal to flow into the investment mold.

4. Mix the *investment material*, pour it into the mold, and let it set. The ring of investment material, with the wax pattern and sprue pin in the middle, is heated to the desired temperature. At the same time the metal is heated. Once the investment material has been heated enough to "burn out" the wax pattern/sprue pin, leaving a negative pattern and passage, and the metal has reached the desired temperature, a centrifuge-casting machine is used to complete the casting procedure.

5. The casting ring is then cooled by placing it in water to aid in the removal of the investment material. The excess casting metal from the sprue channel and base is removed from the casting with laboratory burs and discs. The casting is then polished.

6. Prepare the gold casting for adding the porcelain veneer layer.

7. Paint the porcelain on the crown in layers, and then cure it in an oven at high temperatures.

8. Finish and polish the porcelain-fused-to-metal crown.

Provisional Coverage

After the final impression has been obtained, the provisional restoration is fabricated and then cemented on the prepared tooth with temporary cement such as zinc oxide eugenol (ZOE)

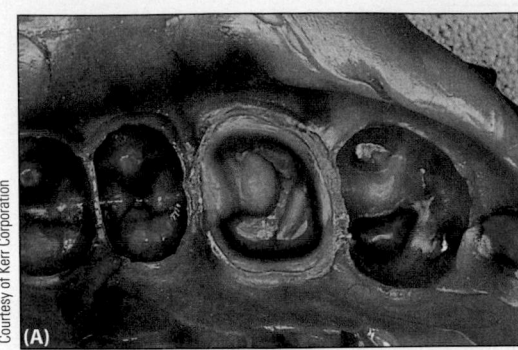

Courtesy of Kerr Corporation

(A)

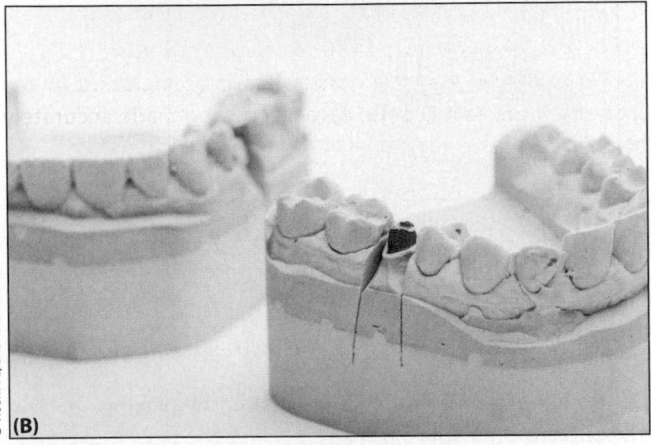

© Room 76/Shutterstock.com

(B)

FIGURE 40-32

(A) Final impression for crown with heavy body orange colored material and light body blue material. (B) A drawing of the wax pattern placed on a sprue pin.

or Temp-Bond®. The provisional or temporary crown protects the preparation from fracture or shifting while the laboratory is fabricating the final restoration. The occlusion and interproximal contacts should also be checked for accuracy. Provisional restorations can be made chairside or can be fabricated by the dental laboratory from the preliminary model. A laboratory fabricated restoration adds to the expense of the treatment case but saves chairside time. This type of restoration may be beneficial if the provisional restorations will be work for an extended period of time. Chairside restorations take some time to fabricate and are less costly to make.

A provisional that fits well needs a minimal amount of temporary cement. The temporary cement can be mixed by

the dental assistant. Once the provisional restoration has been cemented and the once the cement has set, the excess cement is removed. A piece of knotted dental floss is carefully passed interproximally to remove residual cement. If the provisional includes a bridge, floss is passed under the pontic areas as well to remove any excess cement from that area.

After the provisional is cemented in place, the patient should receive instructions about the importance of oral home care. Patients should be instructed not to floss around the provisional and to refrain from eating sticky foods as these may cause the provisional to dislodge. The patient should be advised to notify the dental office immediately if the provisional restoration dislodges before the next scheduled appointment. If the provisional needs to be recemented, excess cement should be removed from the prepared tooth and the provisional crown. A small amount of temporary cement is mixed and placed into the temporary crown. The provisional is placed on the prepared tooth and the cement allowed to fully set. Any excess cement must be removed with an explorer or scaler.

Any sensitivity to hot or cold is usually due to pulpal inflammation caused by tooth preparation. This will usually diminish within 7 to 10 days after the preparation appointment.

Desensitizing toothpaste such as Sensodyne® may aid in reducing the sensitivity where the provisional restoration was placed. Over-the-counter pain medications such as ibuprofen or acetaminophen may also be helpful in managing any discomfort the patient experiences.

Communicating with the Dental Laboratory

Two-way open communication through the use of preliminary models and other communication tools between the dental lab and the dentist is critical for a successful outcome regarding patient treatment. The lab and the dentist should have a common goal for successful patient treatment.

Communication Tools

Some communication tools are important to convey information accurately between the dental office and the dental lab. Today, many modern dental laboratories have clients from all over the world. In order for the dental technicians to satisfy demanding patients and clients with high expectations, facebow recordings, lab prescriptions, and digital communication methods are important tools.

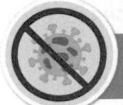 **Infection Control**

Cleaning and Disinfection of Dental Laboratory Materials

Impression materials as well as bite registrations are sources for cross-contamination. They should be disinfected with an EPA registered disinfectant before they are sent to the lab. The dental health care worker should provide the type of disinfectant as well as the exposure time to the disinfectant to the lab. This prevents duplication of disinfection as well as overexposure of the materials to the disinfectant.

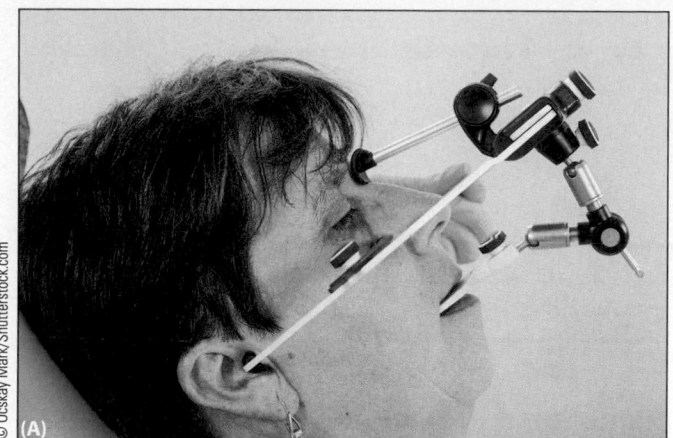

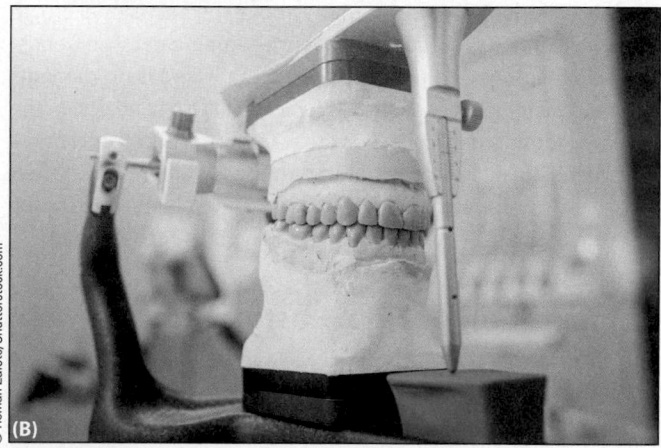

FIGURE 40-33
(A) Facebow to obtain relationship between TMJ and maxillary arch. (B) Dental articulator with relationship of patient's TMJ and maxilla on mounted casts.

Facebow The facebow system is used in prosthodontics to transfer the relationship between the maxillary arch and temporomandibular joint to the casts that are mounted in the articulator (Figure 40-33). Refer to Chapter 33 for the facebow procedure and mounting of models onto an articulator.

Lab Prescription The blank lab prescription forms are generally provided to the dental office by the lab. Specific case related information should be included on the lab prescription form (Figure 40-34). This may include the type of prosthesis as well as the type of metal and shade for porcelain. The lab technician is responsible for interpreting what is written and following the dentist's requests.

The written lab prescription also includes the name and contact information about the dentist as well as the patient's name, age, and gender; the date the lab prescription was written; and the date that the dentist would like the case returned (Figure 40-34). Some prescriptions may include diagrams. The prescription should be signed by the dentist, and the dentist's license number should be written on the prescription as well (Figure 40-34). If the lab

needs clarification, the technician may call before completing the case and returning it to the dental office. The dental lab and the dentist must keep a copy of the lab prescription as per state law specifications.

Digital Communication

Technology has advanced rapidly over the past few years, and digital methods of communication allow rapid transmission of information between the dental office and the dental lab. This rapid transmission of information also allows a more effective method of addressing any questions or concerns.

Digital Camera Digital images are extremely advanced today and allow the laboratory technician to work from an accurate image. A shade guide should be included in the image though, as it is difficult to interpret a shade accurately from a picture.

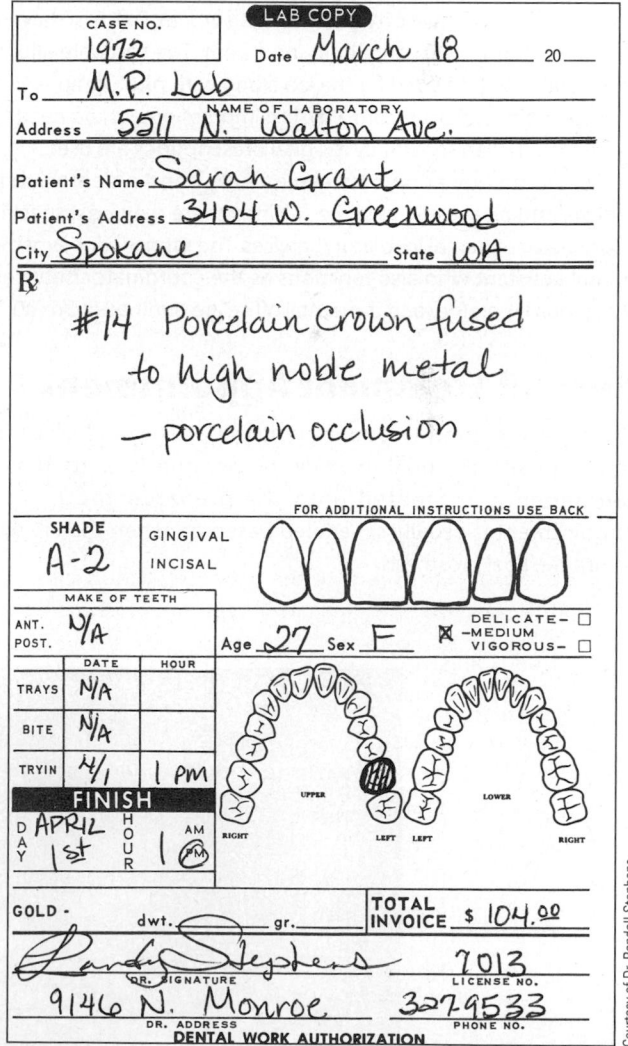

FIGURE 40-34
Dental lab prescription.

Digital Shade Electronic shade-guide systems allow for exact shade measurement so the restoration exactly matches the existing shade of the proximal teeth or the desired shade for the restoration. Precise shade matching for a single anterior restoration to the existing proximal teeth is very difficult. A slight variation in shade can be very noticeable in such instances. A digital shade guide allows for an exact match. Vita Easyshade® and Shofu ShadeEye NCC are just two examples of systems. These systems are expensive and start at $3,500. They can greatly enhance communication with the lab.

Video Communication The Internet has allowed for effective communication between the dental office team and the dental laboratory technician. Through the use of a computer camera and the Internet and services such as Skype or Zoom, a live video session can take place. This mode of communication can also allow the patient to be involved to discuss the restorative case and what they desire as an outcome.

Digital Laboratory Slips Dental laboratories today are transitioning to digital lab prescriptions, which can be emailed to the lab. Some dental software systems such as Dentrix® have a digital prescription feature built into them. The software allows instructions to be added for the lab along with photographs that may be in the patient record. Physical impressions would need to be sent to the lab separately if digital prescriptions are used.

The communication between a dentist and a dental lab is critical, and as a result, in some settings there may be a specific coordinator of dental laboratory services. The primary duties of the dental assistant who also functions as the coordinator between the dental laboratory and the dental office are outlined in Box 40-2.

Second Treatment Appointment

During the second treatment visit the provisional crown is removed and the final fixed dental prosthesis is fitted and permanently cemented onto the prepared tooth. This appointment is usually scheduled based on when the lab will return the final prosthesis.

BOX 40-2 Responsibilities of the Dental Lab Coordinator

- Clinical support
- Maintaining financial and laboratory records
- Laboratory support and communication
- Preparing models and articulators for dental laboratories
- Managing inventory for on-premise dental laboratory materials

---

Removal of Provisional Restoration

When the patient arrives for the second appointment, the dentist examines the oral cavity to ensure that the provisional crown is in place. The dental assistant may remove the provisional crown by using a crown removal instrument or a hemostat. The dentist inspects the prepared tooth to ensure that there is no damage. Any residual temporary cement is removed with a hand scaler. The prepared tooth is gently rinsed with warm water and gently dried. Anesthetic is usually not required for this visit unless the tooth is sensitive. If local anesthetic has not been administered, care should be taken to not use cold water when rinsing the prepared tooth.

Cementation of Final Restoration

The dentist now begins to seat the permanent restoration to check fit. The dentist also checks the seal around the margins and that the restoration is esthetically pleasing as well as functional. The fixed prosthesis may need to be adjusted to ensure a good fit. Once the dentist and patient are satisfied with the fit and esthetics of the final fixed appliance, it is cemented with the permanent cement (Figure 40-35). If a porcelain or PFM crown is the restoration of choice, the lab sends the restoration back after the porcelain has been glazed in an oven. If the porcelain needs to be adjusted, the appliance must go back to the lab again for glazing of the porcelain before it is cemented with permanent cement. The permanent cementation task is completed by the dentist. After isolating the preparation

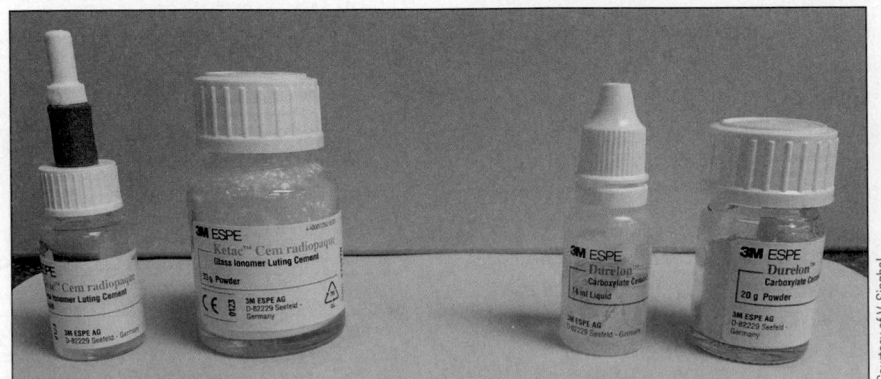

FIGURE 40-35
Permanent cements for fixed prosthesis.

Courtesy of V. Singhal

with cotton rolls, the dental assistant mixes the permanent cement according to the manufacturer's directions and then applies the cement to the tooth surface of the prosthesis. The prosthesis is seated onto the prepared tooth by the dentist. The patient is asked to bite down on a cotton roll or on an orange stick until the cement is fully set. Once the cement is set, the dental assistant can remove any excess cement with a hand scaler or an explorer.

The patient is provided with the home care instruction verbally and is provided written instructions at the time of the cementation appointment. The instruction includes guidelines on how to properly maintain the new fixed prosthesis. Home care instructions are discussed later in this chapter.

Procedure 40-1
Placing and Removing Retraction Cord—Advanced Chairside Function

This procedure is performed by the dentist or the expanded-function dental assistant. After the tooth has been prepared, the retraction cord is placed. The equipment and supplies are included as part of the veneer or crown/bridge tray setup, and this procedure is part of a veneer or crown/bridge preparation treatment session (Procedures 40-2 and 40-3). The specific items needed to place and remove the retraction cord are listed.

Steps written in **blue** font are performed by the operator (dentist or qualified dental assistant), and the chairside assistant's steps are written in black.

Patient Seating Setup (refer to Procedure 18-4)

Retraction Cord Setup (Figure 40-36)
- cotton rolls and 2 × 2 inch gauze
- HVE tip and air/water syringe tip and saliva ejector
- scissors
- hemostat
- retraction cord(s)
- cord packing instrument such as a Balshi packer
- cotton pliers

Procedure Steps

1. **Dentist prepares tooth.**

2. **Operator places cotton rolls for isolation on the facial/buccal surface. If the preparation is on a mandibular tooth, places cotton roll on lingual as well.**
   - ❏ **Dries the area.**
   - ❏ **Selects the cord to be placed around the tooth.**
   - ❏ **Twists the cord ends to tighten the fibers together.**
   - ❏ **Places the cord in a hemostat or cotton pliers.**
   - ❏ **Loops cord around the tooth and tightens slightly (Figure 40-37). The ends should be towards the buccal/facial surface for easy access.**
   - ❏ **Releases the hemostat or cotton pliers, leaving cord in place.**
   - ❏ **Packs the retraction cord into place using the packing instrument. Cord should be apical to the preparation around the cervical area of the tooth.**

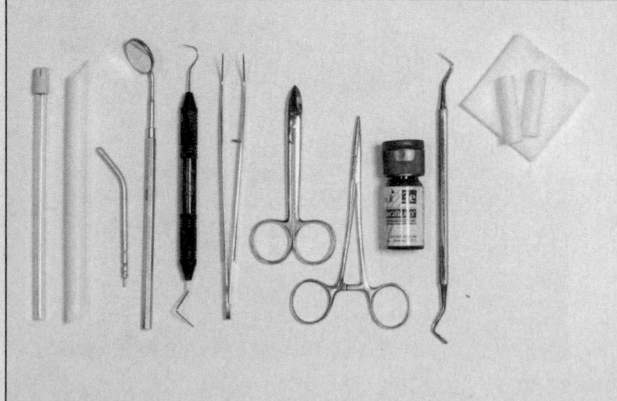

FIGURE 40-36
Placing and removing the retraction cord tray setup.

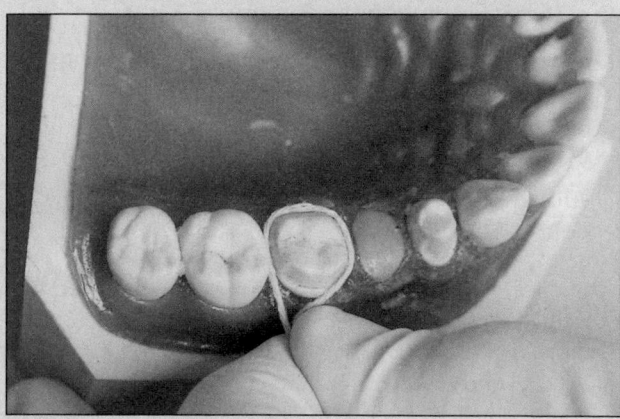

FIGURE 40-37
A retraction cord looped around a prepared tooth for placement in the gingival sulcus.

(Continues)

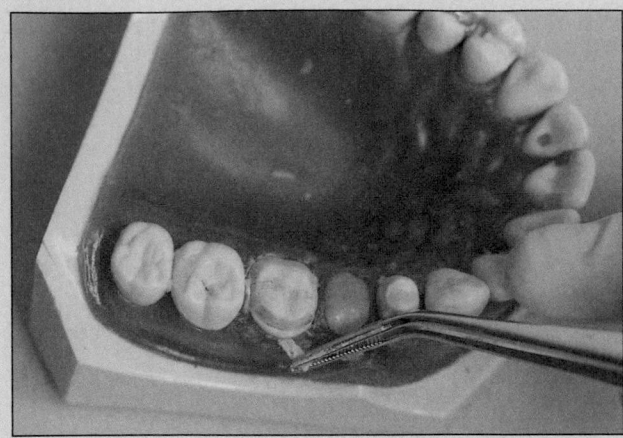

FIGURE 40-38
A retraction cord looped around a prepared tooth with a tag left out for easy removal.

❑ Leaves the tip of the cord out slightly for easy removal just before taking the impression (Figure 40-38).

❑ Leaves cord in place for 10–15 minutes for mechanical retraction.

❑ Grasps end and removes cord before taking the impression.

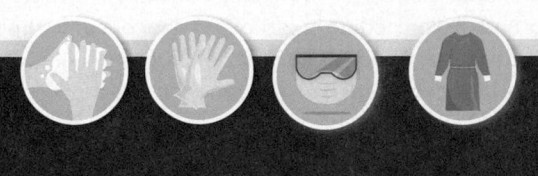

Procedure 40-2
Porcelain Veneers

This procedure is performed by the dentist and is completed in two appointments. During the first appointment, the tooth is prepared and impressions are taken; at the second appointment, the porcelain veneer is applied. Between appointments, the impressions are sent to a dental laboratory, where the porcelain veneer is fabricated.

Steps written in **blue** font are performed by the operator (dentist or qualified dental assistant), and the chairside assistant's steps are written in black.

Patient Seating Setup (refer to Procedure 18-4)

Anesthetic Setup (refer to Procedure 23-2)

Veneer Preparation Appointment Setup (Figure 40-39)
- cotton rolls and 2 × 2 inch gauze
- high-speed handpiece and assorted burs
- shade guide
- articulating paper in articulating paper holder
- spoon excavator
- low-speed handpiece with prophy angle, rubber cup, and pumice
- retraction cord and placement instrument
- bite registration materials
- alginate impression materials for model of opposing arch
- final impression materials (polyvinyl siloxane or polyether) including impression trays, syringes
- provisional veneer and temporary cement
- laboratory prescription form

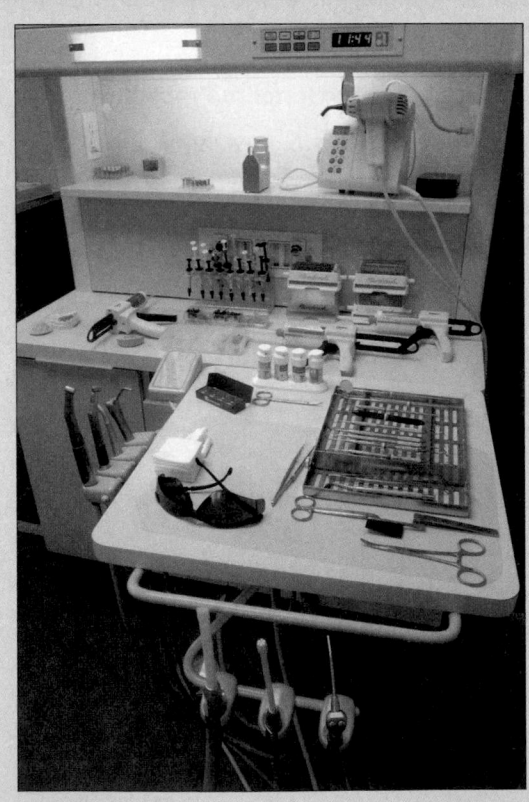

FIGURE 40-39
Porcelain veneers tray set up for preparation appointment, including the impression materials, bite registration materials, curing light, shade guide, and provisional materials.

Dental Laboratory Setup (refer to Chapter 33)

- light cured temporary cement and cement spatula and mixing pad
- curing light

Procedure Steps

1. Escort and seat patient (refer to Procedure 18-4).

   Dentist greets the patient and takes position at the dental chair.

   ❏ **Signals for the procedure to begin (refer to Procedure 20-1).**

2. Pass mouth mirror and explorer at operator's signal.

   Dentist examines tooth or teeth for veneer preparation with mirror and explorer.

3. Assist in taking bite registration and impressions.
   ❏ Mix materials and transfer instruments.

   Dentist obtains bite registration (refer to Chapter 33).

   Operator obtains opposing arch impression (refer to Chapter 33).

4. Pour model with stone (refer to Chapter 33).

   Dentist administers local anesthetic.

5. Assist in administration of local anesthetic (refer to Procedure 23-2).

   Operator pumices teeth to be prepared with rubber cup.

6. Assist in pumicing teeth.
   ❏ Pass disposable prophy angle with pumice in rubber cup in low-speed handpiece.
   ❏ Use high-speed evacuation to suction and air/water syringe to rinse and dry tooth for better visibility.

   Dentist selects shade.

7. Assist in determining shade.
   ❏ Retrieve disposable prophy angle and pass shade guide.
   ❏ Turn dental lamp off.
   ❏ Record shade on patient's chart.

   Dentist prepares teeth according to the design of the veneer.

   ❏ **Prepares the incisal edge and the cervical margin carefully so that the finished veneer is even with the gingival crest, or just slightly subgingival (Figure 40-40).**

8. Assist in preparing the teeth.
   ❏ Exchange shade guide for high-speed handpiece with appropriate diamond bur.

   ❏ Use high-speed evacuation to suction and air/water syringe to rinse and dry tooth for better visibility.

   Dentist examines the prepared tooth.

9. Exchange high-speed handpiece for mirror and explorer.
   ❏ Retrieve mirror and explorer after examination is completed.

   Operator isolates the area for placement of retraction cord.

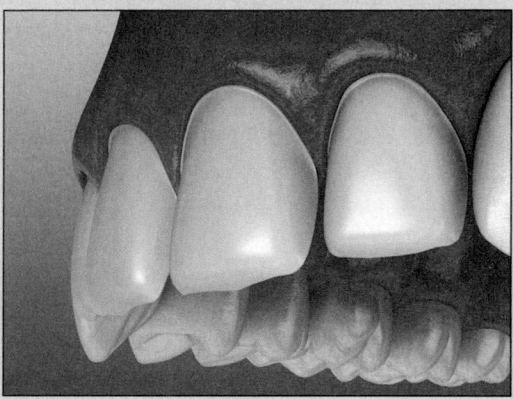

FIGURE 40-40
Teeth prepared for porcelain veneers.

10. Pass cotton rolls.

    Operator places subgingival retraction cord.

11. Pass retraction cord and placement instrument.

    Dentist takes impression of prepared teeth.

12. Assist in taking impression.
    ❏ Prepare for impression with polyvinylsiloxane or polyether (refer to Chapter 33).
    ❏ Retrieve placement instrument and pass mirror and light body injectable impression material to dentist upon signaling.
    ❏ Pass cotton pliers to remove retraction cord.
    ❏ Retrieve pliers and cord and retract soft tissue while light body impression material is being syringed around prepared tooth.
    ❏ Prepare and pass tray with heavy body impression material and retrieve light body material syringe.
    ❏ **Operator obtains final impression.**
    ❏ **Operator removes tray once material is set.**

(Continues)

Dentist inspects the impression to ensure that all margins are clearly visible and impression is without bubbles.

13. Mix dental materials and transfer instruments, including curing light, during provisional veneer fabrication and cementation procedure.

    Operator fabricates provisional veneers.
    - ❏ **Uses the stone model and stock tray to obtain an impression with putty and polyvinyl siloxane using the two-step method (refer to Chapter 33).**
    - ❏ **Places the methyl methacrylate material into the area for the provisional veneers in the impression.**
    - ❏ **Places the impression with the methyl methacrylate material into the patient's oral cavity and seats. Allows material to set.**
    - ❏ **Removes tray and teases out the acrylic provisional from the impression.**

- ❏ **Finishes the provisional veneers with rotary instruments in low-speed handpiece.**
- ❏ **Dentist checks occlusion with articulating paper and adjusts as needed with rotary instruments.**
- ❏ **Cements provisional veneers with temporary cement.**

Dentist makes a final check of all work of an expanded assistant. In some states the dentist must perform a final examination of a placed restoration.

14. Assist in final evaluation of veneer.
    - ❏ Pass mirror and explorer.

15. Provide patient with postoperative instructions orally and in written form.
    - ❏ Inform the patient that the soft tissues will be tender for several days because of the retraction cord placement.

16. Write up procedure in Services Rendered.

Date	Services Rendered
02/18/XX	Updated medical and dental history, no changes noted. BP = 120/80; T = 98.6F, P = 80, R = 18
	Placed 20% benzocaine gel to injection sites for 2 minutes. Administered two cartridges (3.6 ml) of 2% lidocaine with 1:100,000 epi to mandibular left. No reaction.
	#8 and #9 prepared for veneers, (shade #), placed provisional veneers
	POI do not bite on lip, no eating/drinking until numbness wears off, eat only on opposite side until numbness has worn off, do not chew or bite with provisional veneers, call office if provisional veneer feels high or if there is discomfort or pain.
	RTC: deliver fabricated veneer Assistant's initials

17. Dismiss and escort patient to reception area (refer to Procedure 18-5).

18. Complete lab prescription and send impression to dental laboratory.

Cementation Appointment (Second Appointment)

The second appointment should be scheduled as soon as possible after the first appointment. The laboratory should be scheduled ahead of time so the turnaround time is minimal.

Patient Seating Setup (refer to Procedure 18-4)

Veneer Cementation Appointment Setup (Figure 40-41)
- cotton rolls and 2 × 2 inch gauze
- cheek and lip retractors
- porcelain veneer from laboratory
- high-speed handpiece and assorted burs
- low-speed handpiece with prophy angle, rubber cup, and pumice

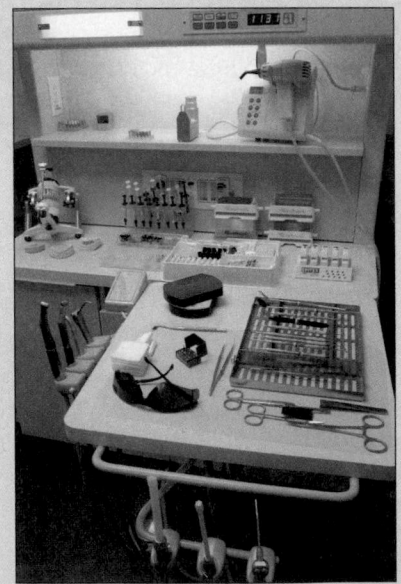

FIGURE 40-41
Porcelain veneers tray setup for cementation appointment, including veneers back from the lab, curing light, and permanent cement/bonding agent.

- small spoon excavator or other hand instrument
- scaler
- Panavia® cement
- etchant and applicator
- curing light
- assorted diamond finishing burs

Procedure Steps

1. Escort and seat patient (refer to Procedure 18-4).

   Dentist greets the patient and takes position at the dental chair.

   ❏ Signals for the procedure to begin (refer to Procedure 20-1).

2. Pass mouth mirror and explorer at operator's signal.

   Dentist examines tooth or teeth for veneer final cementation with mirror and explorer.

3. Retrieve mouth mirror and explorer at operator's signal.

4. Assist with preparing veneer and cementation procedure.
   ❏ Clean and disinfect the inside of the veneer with an acid etchant from the Panavia® system as per manufacturer's instructions.
   ❏ Apply primer to inside of veneer and dry as per manufacturer's instructions.
   ❏ Apply cement to veneer.

   Dentist proceeds with veneer cementation.
   ❏ Removes the provisional veneers with a hand instrument.
   ❏ Removes residual temporary cement from the prepared teeth.
   ❏ Operator cleans the teeth disposable prophy angle with a rubber cup and pumice.

❏ Tries veneers on teeth.

❏ Makes adjustments on veneers with finishing diamond.

❏ Places veneer on prepared tooth and cures cement with curing light.

❏ Operator removes excess cement with explorer or scaler.

❏ Finishes margins of veneer with diamond finishing bur (Figure 40-42).

❏ Polishes veneers with rubber wheels, cups, and polishing paste.

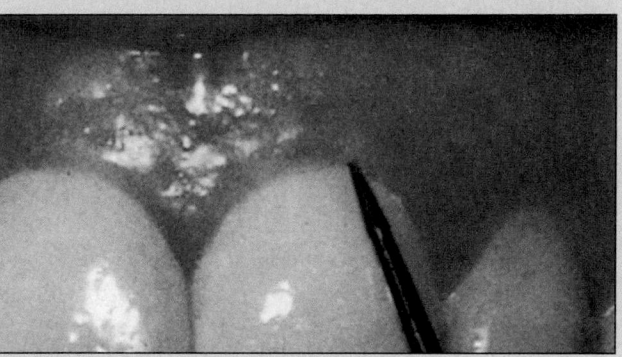

FIGURE 40-42
Finishing porcelain veneer margins with diamond bur.

Courtesy of Kerr Corporation

5. Provide patient with postoperative instructions orally and in written form.

6. Write up procedure in Services Rendered.

7. Dismiss and escort patient to reception area (refer to Procedure 18-5).

Date	Services Rendered
02/18/XX	Updated medical and dental history, no changes noted. BP = 120/80; T = 98.6F, P = 80, R = 18
	Delivered #9 veneer and cemented with Panavia™
	POI call office if veneer feels high or if there is discomfort or pain; chewing on ice and hard, chewy candy can damage restorations
	Assistant's initials

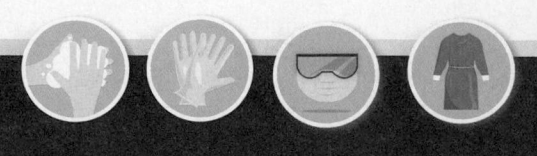

Procedure 40-3
Gold Crown Preparation

This procedure is performed by the dentist and is completed in two appointments. During the first appointment, the tooth is prepared and impressions are taken; at the second appointment, the gold crown is cemented. Between appointments, the impressions are sent to a dental laboratory, where the gold crown is cast.

Steps written in **blue** font are performed by the operator (dentist or qualified dental assistant), and the chairside assistant's steps are written in black.

Patient Seating Setup (refer to Procedure 18-4)

Anesthetic Setup (refer to Procedure 23-2)

Gold Crown Preparation Appointment Setup (Figure 40-43)

- cotton rolls and 2 × 2 inch gauze, dental floss
- HVE tip and air/water syringe tip and saliva ejector and three-way syringe tip
- high-speed handpiece and assorted diamond burs, fissure burs, and discs
- low-speed handpiece with burs, discs, and stones
- dental dam setup
- spoon excavator, scaler, plastic filling instrument, cement spatula, and glass slab or mixing pad
- retraction cord placement setup (refer to Procedure 40-1)
- bite registration materials (not shown)
- alginate impression materials for model of opposing arch (not shown)
- final impression materials (polyvinyl siloxane or polyether) and stock tray or custom tray

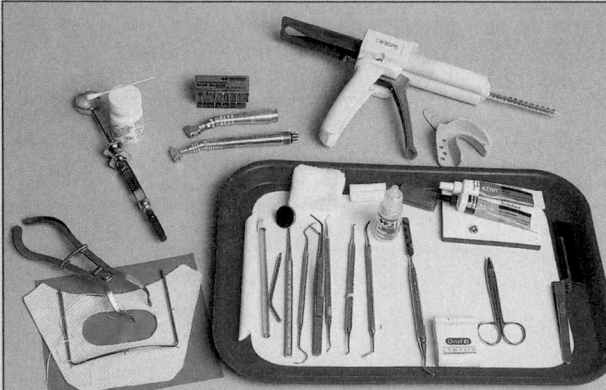

FIGURE 40-43
Tray setup for the preparation appointment.

- crown and bridge scissors
- provisional crown materials (not shown) and temporary cement (refer to Chapter 33)
- laboratory prescription form and packaging for impressions (not shown)

Procedure Steps

1. Escort and seat patient (refer to Procedure 18-4).

   Dentist greets the patient and takes position at the dental chair.
      ❏ **Operator signals for the procedure to begin.**

2. Pass mouth mirror and explorer at operator's signal.

   Dentist examines tooth or teeth for crown preparation with mirror and explorer.

3. Assist in gold crown preparation.
      ❏ Retrieve explorer.

   Dentist administers local anesthetic.

4. Assist in administration of local anesthetic (refer to Procedure 23-2).

5. Mix materials and transfer instruments to assist in tooth preparation and taking impressions.
      ❏ Opposing arch impression model is poured with stone (refer to Chapter 33).

   Dentist selects shade.

6. Pass shade guide and note shade selected.

   Dentist completes crown preparation.

      ❏ **The tooth must be reduced to accommodate the thickness of the metal.**

      ❏ **The margins of the preparation are either finished in a chamfer or shoulder preparation. The chamfer provides adequate bulk and extends easily into the gingival sulcus. The shoulder provides a ledge that is sometimes beveled (Figure 40-44). A bevel is an angled or slanted, instead of horizontal, surface. For a gold crown usually a chamfer is preferred.**

7. Assist with crown preparation.
      ❏ Exchange shade guide for high-speed handpiece with appropriate diamond bur.
      ❏ Use high-speed evacuation to suction and air/water syringe to rinse and dry tooth for better visibility.

❑ Exchange high-speed handpiece for mirror and explorer.

Dentist examines the prepared tooth.

8. Pass mirror and explorer.

Operator places subginglval retraction cord (refer to Procedure 40-1 and Figure 40-45).

9. Assist in placing retraction cord.
   ❑ Isolate the area with cotton rolls.
   ❑ Pass retraction cord and placement instrument.
   ❑ Prepare for final impression with polyvinylsiloxane or polyether.
   ❑ Retrieve cord placement instrument and pass mirror and light body injectable impression material to dentist upon signaling.

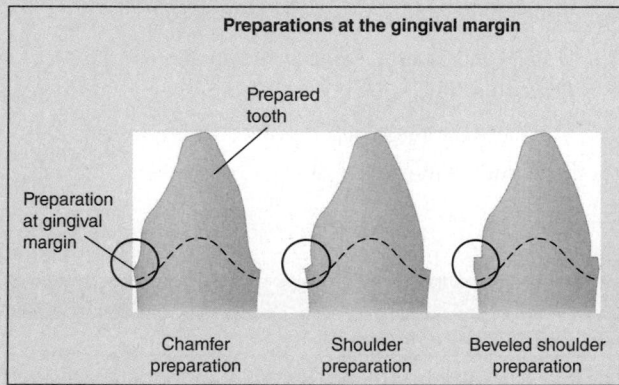

FIGURE 40-44
Preparations at the gingival margin.

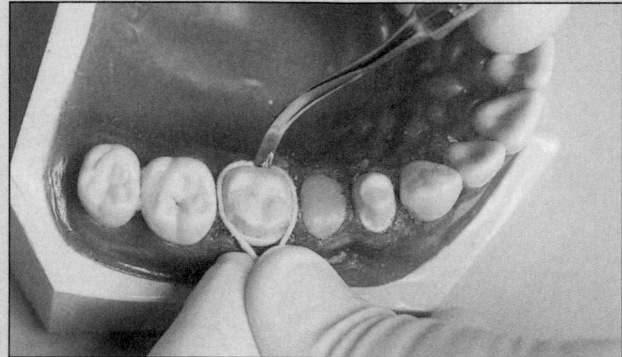

FIGURE 40-45
Placing the retraction cord around a prepared tooth.

Operator removes subgingival retraction cord (refer to Procedure 40-1).

Dentist takes soft tissue impression.

10. Assist in taking impression.

❑ Retract soft tissue while light body impression material is being syringed around prepared tooth.
❑ Prepare to pass tray with heavy body impression material to operator and retrieve light body material syringe (Figure 40-46).

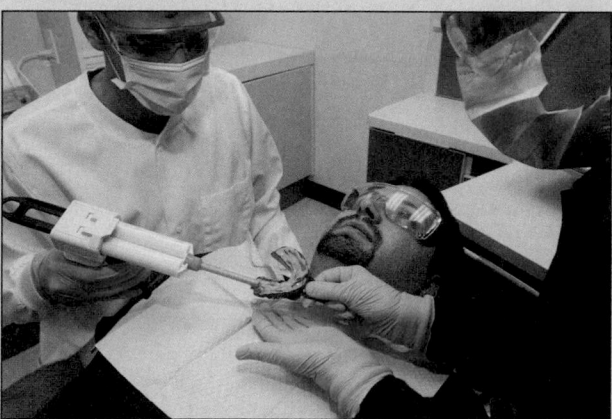

FIGURE 40-46
A dental assistant receives a syringe with light-body impression material and transfers the tray with medium to heavy-bodied impression material to the dentist.

Operator places tray with heavy body impression material in oral cavity.

❑ **Holds tray in place according to manufacturer's recommended time.**
❑ **Removes tray once material is set.**
❑ **Dentist inspects the impression to ensure that all margins are clearly visible and impression is without bubbles (Figures 40-47 and 40-48).**

11. Mix dental materials and transfer instruments during provisional veneer fabrication procedure.

In states that allow the dental assistant to fabricate and temporarily cement the provisional crown, the dental assistant may perform this function. In states that do not allow the dental assistant to fabricate and/or place temporary restorations, these steps would be completed by the dentist.

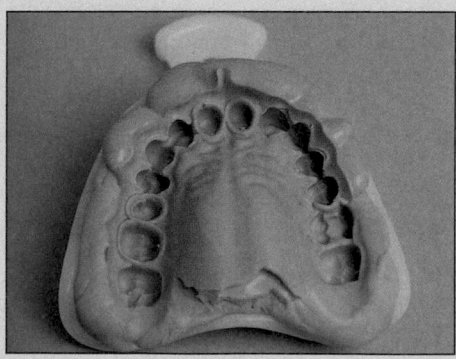

FIGURE 40-47
Final impression.

(Continues)

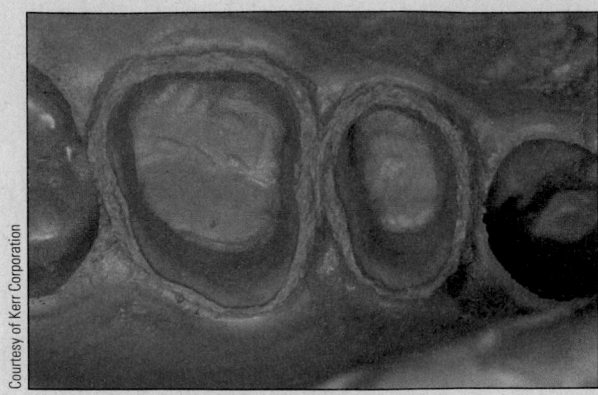

Courtesy of Kerr Corporation

FIGURE 40-48
A close-up of the preparation margins in the final impression.

Operator fabricates and cements the prefabricated provisional crowns.

❑ **Trims and contours the provisional crown with crown and bridge scissors or crimping and contouring pliers.**

❑ **Holds articulating paper in articulating forceps for the patient to bite on to check occlusion.**

❑ **Adjusts as needed.**

❑ **Polishes the provisional crown.**

❑ **Mixes the temporary cement.**

❑ **Places temporary cement inside the provisional crown.**

❑ **Seats the provisional crown and asks patient to bite on bite stick.**

❑ **Removes excess cement once fully set.**

❑ **Uses dental floss to check the interproximal contacts.**

12. Rinse and evacuate the patient's oral cavity before the patient is dismissed.

13. Provide patient with postoperative instructions orally and in written form. Inform the patient that the soft tissues will be tender for several days because of the retraction cord placement.

14. Write up procedure in Services Rendered.

15. Dismiss and escort patient to reception area (refer to Procedure 18-5).

16. Complete laboratory slip, disinfect the impression, and send both to the dental lab.

Date	Services Rendered
02/18/XX	Updated medical and dental history, no changes noted. BP = 120/80; T = 98.6F, P = 80, R = 18
	Placed 20% benzocaine gel to injection sites for 2 minutes. Administered 2 cartridges (3.6 ml) of 2% lidocaine with 1:100,000 epi to mandibular left. No reaction.
	#30 gold crown preparation. Maxillary alginate impression obtained for counter model. Gingival retraction cord placed around #30 for 7 minutes. Impression obtained with polyvinyl siloxane. Acrylic temporary fabricated and cemented with Tempbond.
	POI do not bite on lip, no eating/drinking until numbness wears off, eat only on opposite side until numbness has worn off, call office if restoration feels high or if there is discomfort or pain; chewing on ice and hard, chewy candy can cause temporary to loosen and fall off.
	Assistant's initials

Cementation Appointment (Second Appointment)

The second appointment should be scheduled as soon as possible after the first appointment. The laboratory should be scheduled ahead of time so the turnaround time is minimal. This procedure is performed by the dentist. The dental assistant prepares the instruments and materials, prepares the patient, and performs assisting responsibilities during the procedure.

Patient Seating Setup (refer to Procedure 18-4)

Gold Crown Cementation Setup (Figure 40-49)

- cotton rolls, floss, and 2 × 2 inch gauze
- cheek and lip retractors (not shown)
- HVE tip and air/water syringe tip and saliva ejector
- gold crown from laboratory (not shown)

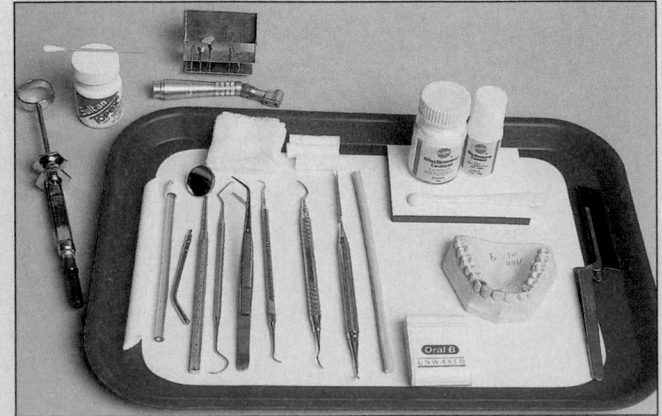

FIGURE 40-49
Tray setup for cementation appointment.

- high-speed handpiece and assorted burs
- low-speed handpiece with finishing burs, discs, and stones
- spoon excavator and scaler
- permanent cement such as glass ionomer, polycarboxylate, resin, or zinc phosphate (not shown)
- orangewood bitestick
- plastic filling instrument and cement spatula
- anesthetic setup (if required) for vital teeth (not shown)

Procedure Steps

1. Escort and seat patient (refer to Procedure 18-4).

   Dentist greets the patient and takes position at the dental chair.

   ❏ **Signals for the procedure to begin (refer to Procedure 20-1).**

2. Pass mouth mirror and explorer at operator's signal.

   Dentist examines tooth and provisional crown.

   Dentist removes the provisional crown.

3. Retrieve explorer and transfer instruments for removal of provisional crown.
   ❏ Transfer preferred hand instrument such as scaler or spoon excavator.

   Dentist removes any residual temporary cement from the prepared tooth.

4. Rinse and gently dry the area.

   Dentist tries crown on tooth.

   ❏ **Seats the cast crown on prepared tooth and checks the margins.**

   ❏ **Adjusts the proximal surfaces until the crown fully seats and margins are sealed.**

5. Assist during try-in.
   ❏ Transfer high-speed handpiece as needed.

   Dentist places crown on prepared tooth and asks patient to bite down on bite stick.

6. Assist in mixing materials and transferring instruments during cementation of the final fixed prosthesis.
   ❏ Keep the area clean and dry.
   ❏ Isolate the area with cotton rolls.
   ❏ Mix cement as per manufacturer's instruction and place inside of crown with plastic filling instrument when signaled.
   ❏ Transfer crown and bite stick (Figure 40-50).

   Dentist examines the occlusion of the crown and adjusts as needed.

7. Assist in examining occlusion of crown.
   ❏ Transfer the articulating paper to check occlusion.

   ❏ Transfer dental floss to check proximal contacts.
   ❏ Transfer the low-speed handpiece with finishing burs and discs and stones as needed.

   Operator removes excess cement once cement sets with scaler or explorer (Figure 40-51).

   ❏ **Uses dental floss to remove excess cement interproximally.**

8. Assist in removing cement.
   ❏ Pass scaler/explorer and floss as needed.
   ❏ Rinse and evacuate.

9. Provide patient with postoperative instructions orally and in written form.

10. Write up procedure in Services Rendered.

11. Dismiss and escort patient to reception area (refer to Procedure 18-5).

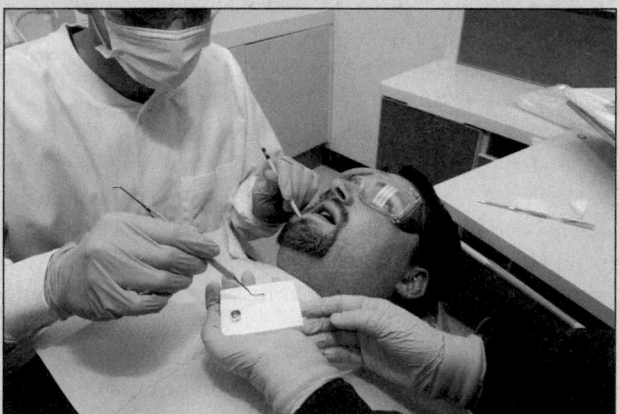

FIGURE 40-50
The dental assistant passes the final cement and crown for cementation.

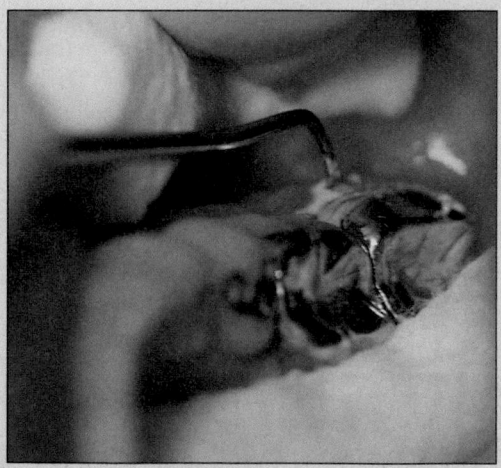

FIGURE 40-51
After the crown is cemented permanently, excess cement is removed from the margins of the crown.

(Continues)

Date	Services Rendered
02/18/XX	Updated medical and dental history, no changes noted. BP = 120/80; T = 98.6F, P = 80, R = 18
	Delivered #30 porcelain fused to metal crown
	POI call office if veneer feels high or if there is discomfort or pain; chewing on ice and hard, chewy candy can damage restorations
	Assistant's initials

Concerns Regarding Fixed Dental Prosthesis

Oral home care and maintenance is an important part of fixed prosthodontics. Dental prosthodontic treatment may have potential complications such as pulpal infection, periodontal infection, or discomfort or pain after final cementation of the appliance. If the patient does not have good home care of if the patient does not return to the dental office for maintenance visits, decay may also occur. Proper maintenance and home care are discussed in this lesson.

The dental professional should be able to effectively evaluate a problem the patient is experiencing and then provide appropriate treatment. Over-the-counter and prescription medications may be needed to ensure success of the fixed dental appliance. Use of fluorides, dentifrices, mouthwash, flossing aids, analgesics, and **chemotherapeutic** agents may be beneficial for long-term success of the fixed dental appliance.

One problem that can occur is a space between the gingiva and the pontic of a fixed bridge. This problem may be present at the time the prosthesis was fabricated, or it may occur sometime after cementation due to gingival recession. The gap allows food to collect under the pontic (Figure 40-52). If the food particles are not removed, they may cause inflammation of the gingiva as well as decay on the adjacent abutment teeth. Another problem that may occur is the fracture of a fixed bridge. Ceramic bridges are more fragile than

a porcelain fused to metal (PFM) prosthesis. Fractures can occur due to *masticatory* or chewing forces. A porcelain fracture can leave an opening that may allow leakage under the remaining prosthesis, leading to decay or infection. The porcelain of a PFM may also chip. In such cases the tooth is usually covered by the metal shell underneath. Patients should be advised to refrain from chewing on hard food items such as nuts or ice. A fixed appliance cannot be repaired. If the appliance does become damaged, it would need to be replaced.

A crown may also become loose or may dislodge. If this occurs, the patient should be advised to immediately contact the dental office. If there is no damage to the crown or the underlying tooth, the crown can be recemented. However, the dentist should evaluate why the crown dislodged. If the occlusion is high, the occlusal forces can cause the crown to dislodge. In that case the occlusion should be adjusted. A dark line along the margin of the crown may be visible (Figure 40-1a). This is the metal under the PFM. In posterior areas this is not an esthetic concern. However, in anterior areas, this may be unaesthetic. Gingival recession may cause the metal to become visible over time.

Oral Hygiene

Indirect dental restorations are expensive. The cost depends on a variety of factors such as the type of metal used, the number of units, the need for additional procedures such as endodontic therapy and a post and core buildup as well as the location of the practice and customary fees. Dental insurance usually covers 50% of the cost of fixed restorative care. Many dental plans have a maximum annual coverage limit of $1,000 to $1,500. As a result, the insurance may only cover one crown per year.

Good oral home care and maintenance is important in ensuring the fixed prosthesis lasts for a long time. A major reason a fixed appliance fails is because of the development of decay on the supporting teeth. Decay can occur due to poor oral home care. With proper oral hygiene, the fixed appliance will last much longer. Many patients have the false belief that a crown or bridge will allow the tooth to become resistant to decay or that the "root has been removed from under the crown." The fixed dental prosthesis is supported by natural tooth structure, so good oral care is critical. Refer to Chapter 16 regarding the use of floss threaders, tufted floss (also known as superfloss (Figure 40-53), gauze strips, interdental brushes, and end tuft brushes for performing oral care at home.

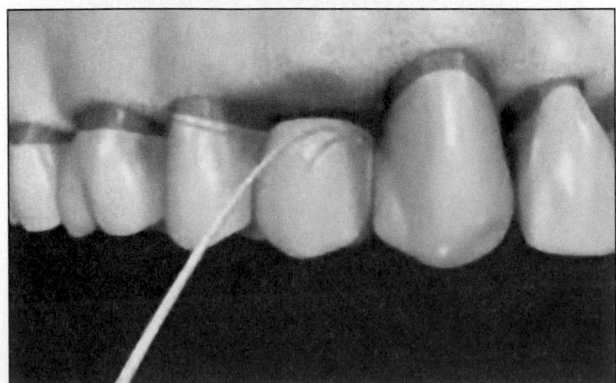

FIGURE 40-52
Gap under pontic of bridge.

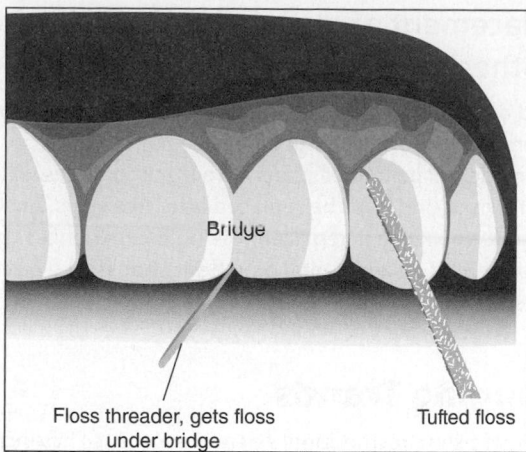

FIGURE 40-53
Tufted floss used under the pontic of a bridge.

Water Irrigation System The primary purpose of water oral irrigation in fixed prosthesis is to remove food particles from around crowns and under the pontic of a bridge. This reduces harmful bacteria in these areas and reduces the risk of decay and periodontal disease. Water irrigators should be used daily for maximum benefit and effect (Figure 40-54).

Diet The dental team may advise the patient to avoid extremely hard foods and sticky foods in the area of the permanent crown. Hard foods can cause the porcelain to fracture, and sticky foods may cause a fixed dental appliance to become loose or dislodge. Foods such as ice, popcorn, chewing gum, and nuts should be avoided. Biting on pens and pencils and fingernails can also damage a fixed dental appliance. Regular consumption of acidic foods such as lemons, limes, and oranges diminish the finish on the porcelain of a fixed dental appliance.

Oral Rinses In case there is some gingival sensitivity after the procedure, the patient can be advised to rinse with warm salt

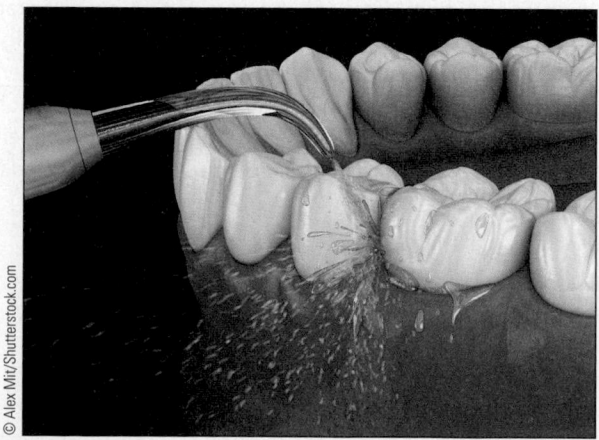

FIGURE 40-54
Dental irrigator.

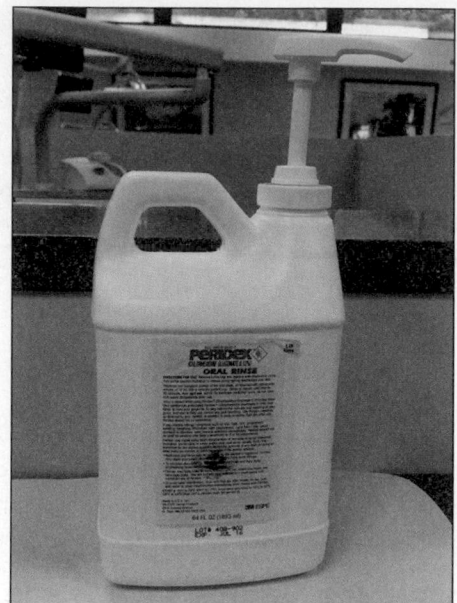

FIGURE 40-55
Peridex prescription oral rinse.

water for 2–3 days. This sensitivity can occur due to manipulation of the gingival soft tissues. The patient is advised to not to use the salt water rinses if they are on a salt-restricted diet due to medical concerns such as hypertension. When choosing an over-the-counter oral rinse, it is important to avoid alcohol containing rinses which can sometimes irritate and dry the oral cavity. Prescription oral rinses containing 0.12% chlorhexidine gluconate, such as Peridex®, are used for short-term management of periodontal conditions (Figure 40-55). Refer to Chapter 38 for more details regarding periodontal disease regarding periodontal disease.

Structural Stresses on a Fixed Appliance

If the occlusion of a fixed dental prosthesis is not correct, this can affect the TMJ causing pain and **crepitation**. The bridge may warp or may fracture or become dislodged. The dentist adjusts occlusion with the use of articulating paper (Figure 40-56). The articulating paper indicates where the dentist needs to adjust occlusion of the fixed prosthesis before permanently cementing the appliance.

Dental Sensitivity Related to Fixed Dental Prosthesis

Development of abutment teeth sensitivity to hot and cold may take place over time. This may occur due to preparation of the tooth that caused trauma to the nerve of the tooth. In such cases it is best to be conservative and monitor the tooth for 6 months as the sensitivity may diminish over time. If the sensitivity does not diminish or the area becomes painful, endodontic therapy may be necessary. The endodontic procedure is usually completed by drilling through the crown

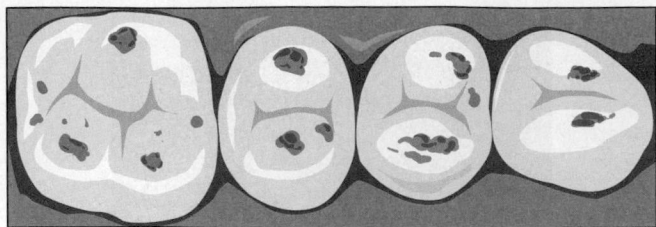

FIGURE 40-56
Marks with articulating paper on fixed prosthesis tell dentist where to adjust occlusion.

on the sensitive abutment. Amalgam or composite is placed over the opening in the crown once the endodontic therapy is completed.

Xerostomia and Sjögren's Syndrome

Some patients suffer from decreased salivary flow. This may be due to Sjögren's syndrome but can also be caused by many commonly prescribed medications such as antihypertensive agents. Sjögren's syndrome may occur as a primary form of the disease (50% of cases). In this case the disease is not associated with any other disease processes. Sjögren's syndrome can also occur as a secondary disease (50% of cases) that manifests in the presence of another **autoimmune** disease such as rheumatoid arthritis.

It is estimated that nearly four million people in the United States have Sjögren's syndrome, making it a common autoimmune disorder. More than 90% of those affected by Sjogren's syndrome are women. The disease can affect people of any race. The average age of diagnosis is around 40. Saliva functions as a natural cleanser to wash away food particles. Decreased salivary flow can lead to food particles that accumulate around teeth and fixed dental prosthetic appliances. As a result, fixed prosthodontic work may be more susceptible to decay. Fluoride use may be beneficial in preventing decay in patients who have a fixed prosthesis. Chapter 16 discusses the benefits of fluoride in detail.

Many patients who suffer from dry mouth tend to consume sugary drinks or sugary candy to stimulate salivary flow. The high sugar content in these products plus the decreased salivary flow can result in rampant decay on the natural tooth structure, including abutment teeth of a fixed dental appliance. Patients should be advised to drink water instead of sugary substances. Recommendations for the use of products such as Biotene® which aid in moisture replenishment of the oral cavity can also be provided. Patients should be educated on the effects of sugary substances on the dentition, particularly when salivary flow decreases.

Replacement of an Existing Fixed Dental Prosthesis

A fixed dental appliance should not be replaced if there are no problems such as decay or fracture.

Many dental insurance plans in the United States will allow for a crown or bridge to be replaced after five years. Anytime a prosthetic appliance is replaced, the pulp experiences trauma. Replacement of a fixed dental prosthesis should take place only if necessary.

Changing Trends

The use of fixed prosthodontics dental appliances has increased significantly in the recent years. This increase is due to a change in dental practice that now focuses on saving the natural dentition rather than extracting teeth. As a result, more people today are retaining their natural teeth, and the number of full dentures being fabricated has been decreasing over the years. Many teeth are retained because of advancements in fixed dental prosthodontic appliances and materials. More people today are aware of the importance of oral hygiene in maintaining the dentition. A significant number of the population receives fluoride in toothpaste, rinses, and the water supply. All of these factors have contributed to an increase in the retention of the natural dentition, and as a result, a greater need for fixed dental prosthodontics.

Informed Consent

The informed process was discussed in detail in Chapter 3. Informed consent for a fixed dental prosthetic appliance should contain information related to:

- Proposed fixed prosthesis treatment
- Advantages and disadvantages of the proposed treatment
- Risks and potential consequences of not performing the proposed fixed prosthesis treatment
- Alternative treatment options
- Cost of all presented treatment options and a payment plan

Whenever a patient's case may be outside the scope of practice for a dentist, the patient should be referred to a specialist. The dentist must inform the patient that the needed treatment would be better managed by a specialist. The office staff should assist the patient in finding a specialist. When referring a patient to a specialist, the following information must be documented in the patient record:

- Description of the problem
- Reasons for referral
- Name and specialty of the referring dentist

Any broken appointments or last minute cancellations should be documented in the patient's record. These actions may be negligence on the part of the patient and can have a negative impact on treatment. For example, if a patient has a provisional restoration but does not return in a timely manner for permanent cementation of the final prosthesis, the temporary crown may become loose or dislodge. This may cause the prepared tooth to shift, resulting in a poor fit of the final restoration. With proper documentation, the practice is protected against legal action should the patient decide to claim negligence against the dentist.

Documentation of Fixed Prosthodontic Treatment

Some states allow the dental assistant to make the clinical notes. The supervising dentist reviews and then initials the entry. The dental assistant should document all details of each visit from the initial consultation visit until the final cementation visit of the fixed dental prosthesis. Any follow-up visits should also be documented in the patient's record. The documentation should also include any concerns the patient may have and how the issues will be resolved by the dentist. Once resolved, the records should state the patient's level of satisfaction with the treatment.

Charting Fixed Prosthodontics

General charting is reviewed in detail in Chapter 22. However, each specialty also uses specific documentation for charting a patient's existing condition, existing restorations, and what has been decided for the treatment plan. Table 40-1 provides the commonly used dental charting abbreviations and symbols for fixed prosthesis. Figure 40-57 provides sample charting for fixed prosthetic appliances.

Documenting Patient Instructions

In addition to treatment provided and prescriptions written, documentation of preoperative and postoperative instructions related to fixed prosthodontics should be noted in the patient record. Complete documentation protects the practice from legal action and also allows the office staff to have all chronological documentation of all events at all patient appointments in the patient's record.

TABLE 40-1 Symbols and Abbreviations Used in Fixed Prosthodontics

Symbol/ Abbreviation	Meaning
"X" or "="	missing tooth or pontic
^	diastema
‖	open contact
Au	gold
BII	bridge supported with two implants
Br, brdg	bridge
C & B	crown and bridge
CL	crown lengthening
Cr	crown
fxd	fixed
Fxd, fx pros	fixed prosthodontics
IFPD	implant fixed partial denture
inl	inlay
onl	onlay
P & C	post & core
PC	porcelain crown
PLV	porcelain laminate veneer
PMC	porcelain to metal crown
pom	porcelain on metal
pon	pontic
porc	porcelain
prov	provisional
res	resin

Patient Chart

Patient Name: John Doe
Patient ID: 7623

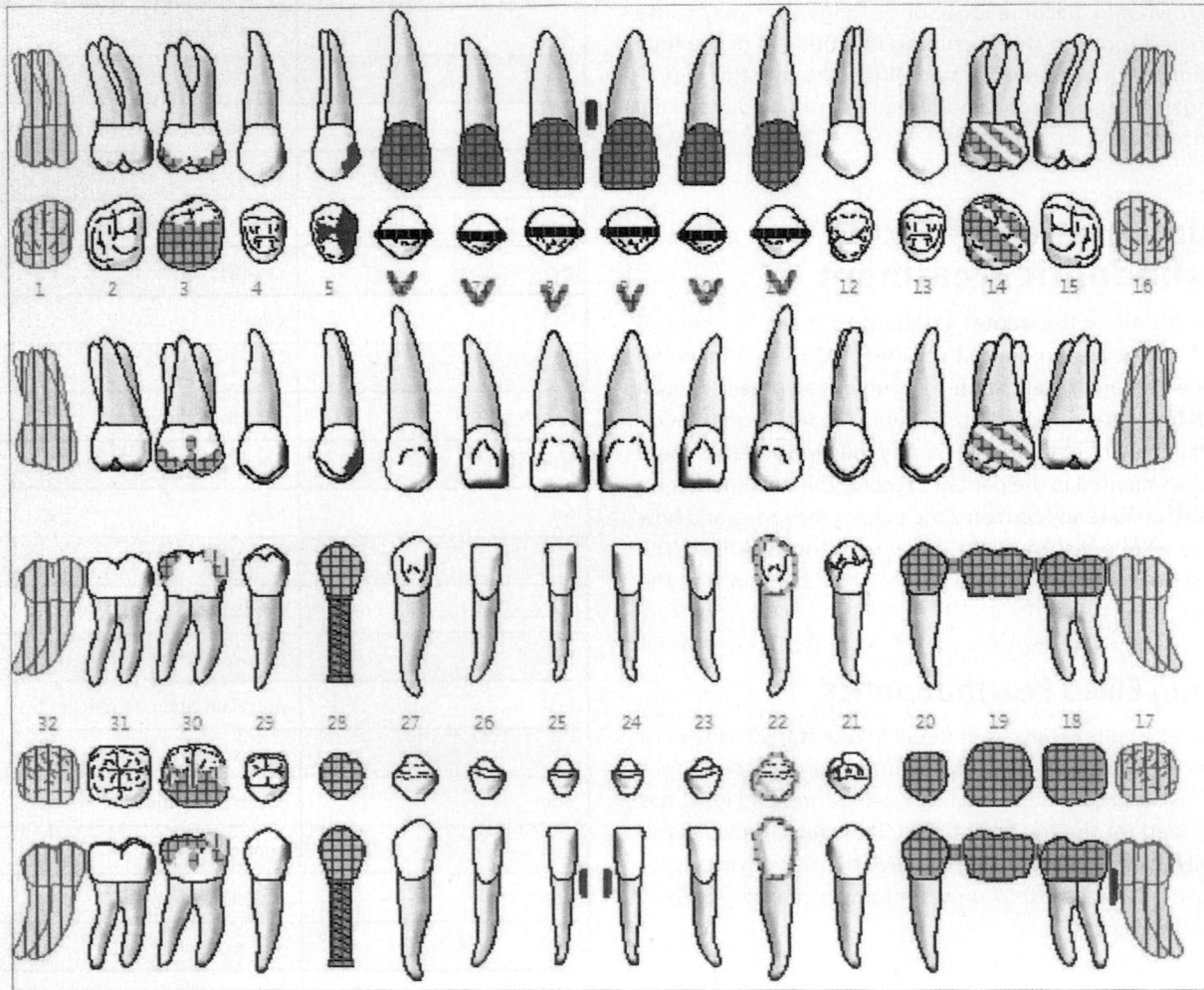

Date	Description	Tth	Surf	Status	Fee
8/14/20XX	D6210 - PONTIC-CAST HIGH NOBLE METAL	19		Proposed	$0.00
8/14/20XX	D6790 - CROWN-FULL CAST HIGH NOBLE METAL	18		Proposed	$0.00
8/14/20XX	D6790 - CROWN-FULL CAST HIGH NOBLE METAL	18		Proposed	$0.00
8/14/20XX	D6790 - CROWN-FULL CAST HIGH NOBLE METAL	20		Proposed	$0.00
8/14/20XX	D2544 - ONLAY-METALLIC-4 OR MORE SURFACES	30	MODB	Proposed	$0.00
8/14/20XX	D2544 - ONLAY-METALLIC-4 OR MORE SURFACES	3	MODL	Proposed	$0.00
8/14/20XX	D2620 - INLAY-PORCELAIN/CERAMIC-TWO SU	5	MO	Proposed	$0.00
8/14/20XX	D6010 - SURG PLACE OF IMPLANT BODY:ENDO IMPLANT	28		Proposed	$0.00
8/14/20XX	D6066 - IMPL SUPP PORC FUSED TO METAL(T,TA,HNM)	28		Proposed	$0.00
8/14/20XX	D2740 - CROWN-PORCELAIN/CERAMIC SUBST	22		Proposed	$0.00

FIGURE 40-57
Sample charting for fixed prosthetic appliances.

Chapter Summary

Fixed prosthodontics encompasses replacement of missing teeth or parts of teeth with extensive restorations. There are many types of fixed prostheses and a variety of materials used for preparation, fabrication, and cementation. The dental assistant is involved in all stages of fixed prosthodontic treatment. It is important to understand the sequence of the procedure and the various types of restorations when assisting the dentist.

The goal of this chapter was to assess the more common procedures in order to give the dental assistant the background needed to assist the dentist. Restorations routinely take at least two appointments to complete. The assistant explains the steps of the procedure to the patient, answers questions, and provides postoperative and home care instructions.

Gingival retraction is an important step when preparing the tooth for the final impression. Margins of the preparations must be exposed so that the impression will reflect an accurate image of the tooth and preparation, and thus ensure that the fixed prosthesis will fit perfectly. Learning about the various materials and techniques helps the dental assistant become more skilled when working with the dentist.

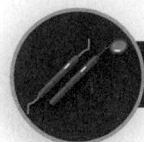

CASE STUDY

Ann Arthur is unhappy with the appearance of her anterior teeth. The maxillary and mandibular incisors are a dull, medium-yellow shade. There is a slight diastema (space) between the maxillary central incisors. Ann has considered treatment for several years and has scheduled an appointment for next week. She has dental insurance through her husband's insurance plan.

Case Study Review

1. What are the two concerns Ann has about her anterior teeth?

2. What treatment options are available?

3. Once a treatment plan is in place, how might financial information, such as insurance, be considered by the business staff?

Review Questions

Multiple Choice

1. A fixed dental prosthesis can improve esthetics but will not restore function to a tooth that has experienced fracture caused by decay.

   Select the correct response based on the statements above.

   a. Both statements are true.
   b. Both statements are false.
   c. The first statement is true; the second statement is false.
   d. The first statement is false; the second statement is true.

2. Which of the following prosthetic restorations covers only the area between the cusps on the occlusal surface of the tooth?

   a. three-quarter crown
   b. inlay restoration
   c. onlay restoration
   d. veneer restoration

3. Which of the following is a restoration that completely encircles the anatomic crown of tooth?
   a. veneer
   b. inlay
   c. onlay
   d. gold crown

4. Which of the following restorations covers the anatomic crown including any fractured cusps with the exception of the facial surface?
   a. inlay
   b. veneer
   c. onlay
   d. gold crown

5. Which of the following is not a component of the preparation and records appointment?
   a. shade selection
   b. tooth preparation
   c. radiographs
   d. occlusal exam

6. When selecting a shade for the new fixed prosthesis, hue, chroma, and value are considered. Match the definition of each to the term.
   a. Hue
   b. Chroma
   c. Value
      1. saturation of the color within each group
      2. quality which distinguishes one color from another
      3. relative amount of lightness or darkness

7. Which of the following is correct regarding obtaining a shade for a fixed dental prosthesis?
   a. The shade should be taken under artificial room lighting.
   b. Patient should be wearing make-up and jewelry when obtaining a shade.
   c. The patient should be involved in the selection of the shade.
   d. The shade guide tabs should be held next to the patient's skin when taking a shade.

8. Which of the following is not correct regarding the preparation and records appointment?
   a. The dentist checks the occlusion between the maxillary and the mandibular teeth.
   b. The smile line is not important when considering a fixed dental prosthesis.
   c. Radiographs would be obtained to evaluate the dentition.
   d. The case is presented to the patient based on findings during the appointment.

9. At the first appointment for the fixed dental prosthesis, the occlusion is obtained after the local anesthetic is administered. The shade is also obtained at this appointment.

   Select the correct response based on the statements above.

   a. Both statements are true.
   b. Both statements are false.
   c. The first statement is true; the second statement is false.
   d. The first statement is false; the second statement is true.

10. If a tooth has lost a significant amount of tooth structure, which of the following methods would not be used to provide support to the tooth and the final fixed prosthesis?
    a. glass ionomer cement base
    b. core buildup
    c. retention pins
    d. post-retained cores

11. Which type of gingival retraction is accomplished by placement of a retraction cord?
    a. mechanical
    b. chemical
    c. surgical
    d. None of these

12. Which of the following is not correct regarding the provisional crown?
    a. The provisional crown may be made chairside.
    b. The provisional crown may be made by the lab from a pretreatment model.
    c. The provisional crown protects the prepared tooth from damage.
    d. The provisional crowns are cemented with a permanent cement.

13. Which of the following is not correct regarding gingival retraction cord?
    a. The use of gingival retraction cord displaced the gingiva around the preparation so impression material can flow into that area.
    b. The gingival retraction cord is placed subgingivally with a Balshi packer or other packing instrument.
    c. Gingival retraction cords with epinephrine are beneficial as the epinephrine causes vasoconstriction and reduction in bleeding.
    d. If the cord is treated with an agent such as Hemodent® it should be left in place for 5 to 7 minutes before taking the final impression.

14. Electrosurgery and laser are beneficial with other methods of gingival retraction when gingival bleeding is difficult to control.
    a. True
    b. False

15. Which of the following materials is *not* used to take the final impression after the tooth is prepared?
    a. polyvinylsiloxane
    b. alginate
    c. reversible hydrocolloid
    d. silicone impression materials

16. Place each of the following steps that take place at the dental lab when fabricating a fixed prosthesis in the correct sequence.
    a. create a wax pattern on die
    b. burnout the wax pattern to create a negative of the wax pattern
    c. Pour final impression for model and die
    d. place wax pattern on sprue pin in casting ring
    e. place casting ring in centrifuge and melt metal to create casting
    f. mix investment material and pour into mold

17. Which of the following is not included on the dental laboratory prescription form?
    a. dentist's name
    b. date of prescription
    c. patient's signature
    d. type of prosthesis to be fabricated

18. Which of the following is NOT correct regarding the cementation visit?
    a. Local anesthesia is not usually needed on the cementation visit.
    b. The provisional may be removed with a crown removal instrument.
    c. Retraction cord should be placed in order to ensure the crown fits properly.
    d. All of these are correct.

19. Match each of the concerns related to a dental fixed prosthesis with the correct description.
    1. Dark line near gingival margin on tooth with crown
    2. Fractured porcelain on porcelain jacket crown
    3. Gap under the pontic of a bridge
    4. Loose crown
    5. Tooth reacts to hot and cold after new restoration
    6. TMJ pain and structural stress on bridge

    a. May occur due to gingival recession or due to faulty manufacturing
    b. May occur due to eating ice or nuts and can result in decay due to leakage
    c. Metal collar of porcelain fused to metal crown showing
    d. Contact dentist for evaluation and possible re-cementation
    e. Adjust occlusion
    f. Use a toothpaste designed for sensitive teeth

20. Which of the following is NOT correct regarding trends related to an increase in fixed dental prosthetics?
    a. People are retaining their natural dentition due to improvements in oral home care education.
    b. People are retaining their natural dentition due to an increased consumption of sugary foods.
    c. People are retaining their natural dentition due to availability of fluoride in water and toothpastes.
    d. People are retaining their natural dentition due to a change in philosophy to retain teeth rather than extracting.

Critical Thinking

1. What are some tools that can be used to perform oral home care on a fixed dental prosthesis?
2. Why might xerostomia lead to failure of a fixed dental prosthesis?
3. What is the role of the dental assistant as the dental lab coordinator?

Key Terms

Term and Pronunciation	Meaning of Root and Word Parts	Definition
autoimmune (aw-toh-i-**myoon**)	**auto-** = self, same **immune** = protected against a specific disease by inoculation or as the result of innate or acquired resistance	relating to the immune response of an organism against any of its own tissues, cells, or cell components
chemotherapeutic (kee-moh-ther-*uh*-**pyoo**-tiks)	**chemo-** = chemical, chemically induced, drug **therapy** = the treating or curing of disease; curative **-ic** = having to do with	relating to chemotherapy; the treatment of disease using chemical agents or drugs that are selectively toxic to the causative agent of the disease, such as a virus, bacterium, or other microorganism
crepitation (**krep**-i-tey-sh*uh* n)	**crepitus** = crackling, a rattling **-ate** = denoting function **-ion** = denoting action or condition	to make a crackling or popping sound; crackle; the noise produced by rubbing bone or irregular cartilage surfaces together, as in arthritis
die (dahy)	**die** = forming material in the construction of something	the positive reproduction of the form of a prepared tooth in any suitable hard substance, usually in metal or specially prepared artificial stone

## CHAPTER 41

Computerized Impression and Restorative Systems

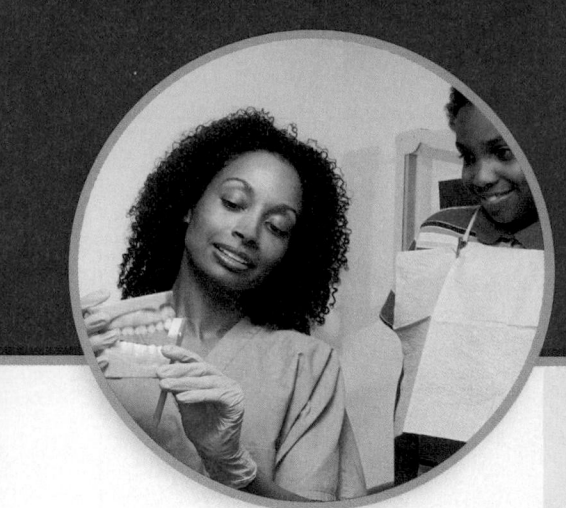

Specific Instructional Objectives

At the completion of this chapter, you will be able to meet these objectives:

1. Use terms presented in this chapter.
2. Explain the CAD/CAM restorative systems.
3. Compare and contrast the advantages and disadvantages of the CAD/CAM technology.
4. Explain the role of the dental assistant during CAD/CAM procedures.
5. Describe the considerations the patient should be made aware of when using CAD/CAM technology.
6. Describe the steps in a CAD/CAM procedure.

Introduction

Over the last 30 years, *computer-aided design* (CAD) and *computer-aided manufacturing* (CAM) technology has become increasingly popular for the fields of dentistry and prosthodontics. Techniques, software, and materials have improved, becoming easier to use and incorporate into dental practice, and this technology continues to advance. CAD/CAM technology is used in both the dental office and the dental laboratory. This technology is capable of many procedures from digital impressions and design to the production of complete restorations, surgical guides, fixed partial and full dentures, implant abutments, and orthodontic appliances. The digital impressions may be used as an alternative to or as an adjunct to traditional impressions. The system can take a digital impression of a prepared tooth or a traditional final impression of a prepared tooth.

CAD/CAM

The first CAD/CAM restorative system, called CEREC (chairside economical restorations of esthetic ceramics), was developed in Switzerland in 1980. The CEREC 3 has the ADA Seal of Acceptance (Figure 41-1). Since then there have been a number of systems on the market, each with their own technology and computer programs.

The CAD portion of the process involves the use of a scanner to create a digital model of the preparation (Figure 41-2). Once the model (Figure 41-3) has been generated on a computer workstation, the doctor, an expanded function assistant, or lab technician can design the restoration. The CAM portion of the process involves the use of a mill or special printer to fabricate what was designed during the CAD process. This could be a **coping**, the final restoration, or a working physical model.

With a CAD/CAM system, the tooth can be prepared and the restoration fabricated right in the office. CEREC AC with Bluecam (Sirona Dental Systems) and Planmeca Fit (Planmeca) are examples of two chairside CAD/CAM systems. After the tooth is prepared for the prosthesis, a computer program is used to design the fixed prosthesis. This digital design is sent to the milling machine for fabrication (Figure 41-4). Materials used to fabricate the restoration include all-ceramic or ceramic-resin blocks (Figure 41-5). The milling machine is usually located in the lab area of the office. A block of ceramic material matching the patient's tooth color is selected and placed in the milling chamber. The milling chamber also contains an attachment for a block of ceramic material, two diamond burs, and water. The CAM software uses the transferred information on the restoration and begins the milling process (Figure 41-6). Within a determined amount of time, the restoration is milled.

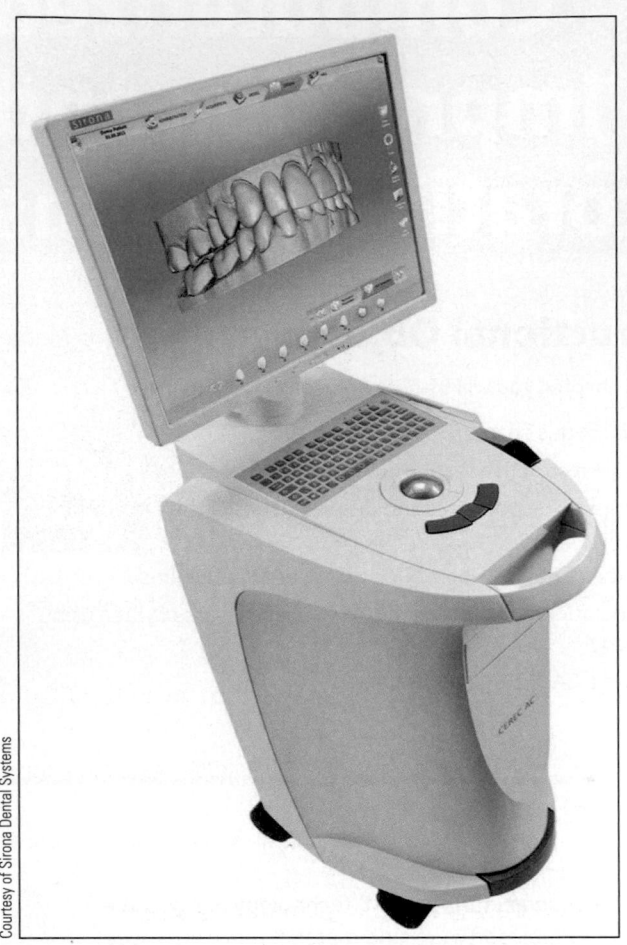

Courtesy of Sirona Dental Systems

FIGURE 41-1
The CEREC CAD machine.

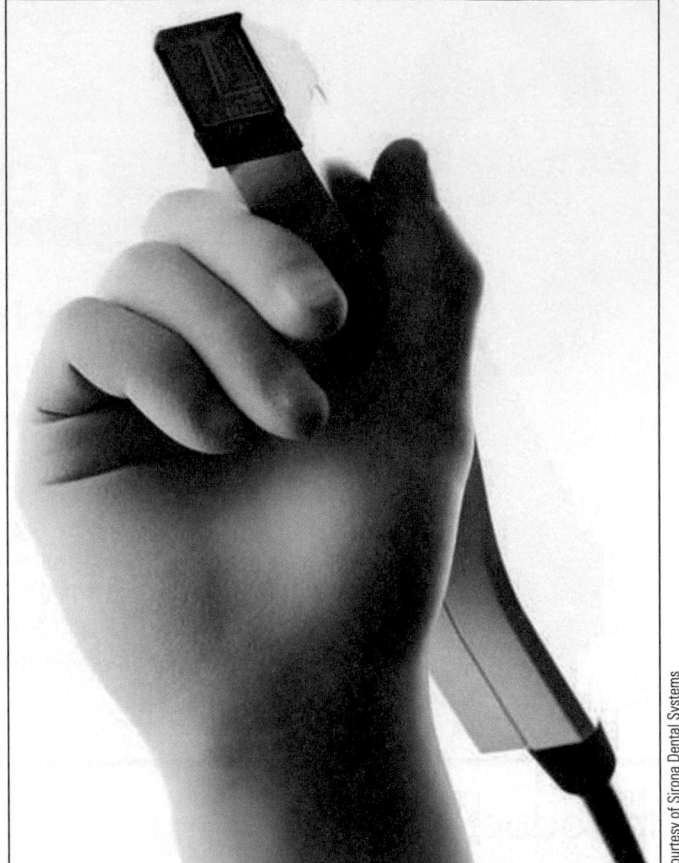

Courtesy of Sirona Dental Systems

FIGURE 41-2
CAD/CAM scanner used to scan an image of the teeth into the computer.

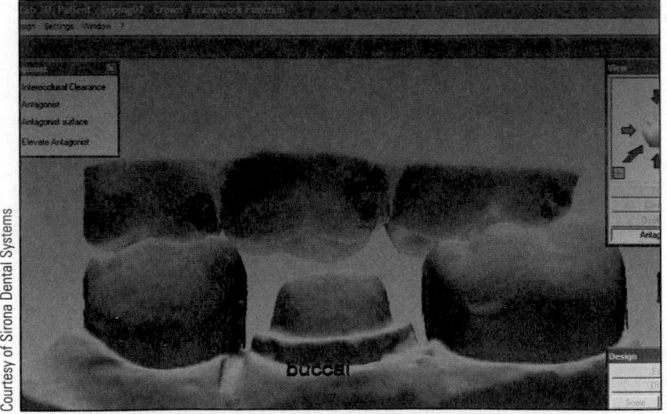

Courtesy of Sirona Dental Systems

FIGURE 41-3
A computerized image of a prepared tooth that is ready for a crown to be designed.

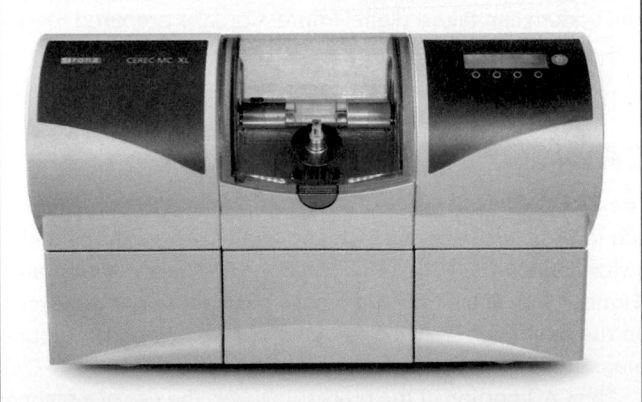

Courtesy of Sirona Dental Systems

FIGURE 41-4
A CAM system unit, which mills ceramic blocks into restorations, such as crowns.

Once completed, the finished restoration is ready to be cemented or bonded in place (Figure 41-7). The patient only needs one appointment and never has to wear a provisional restoration. Some systems have the ability to stain and glaze the restoration to obtain the exact shading desired by the patient and the dentist.

The advantages of the CAD/CAM system include the following:

- The procedure is completed in 1 day.
- Able to evaluate the impression immediately.
- Able to modify the preparation immediately if needed.

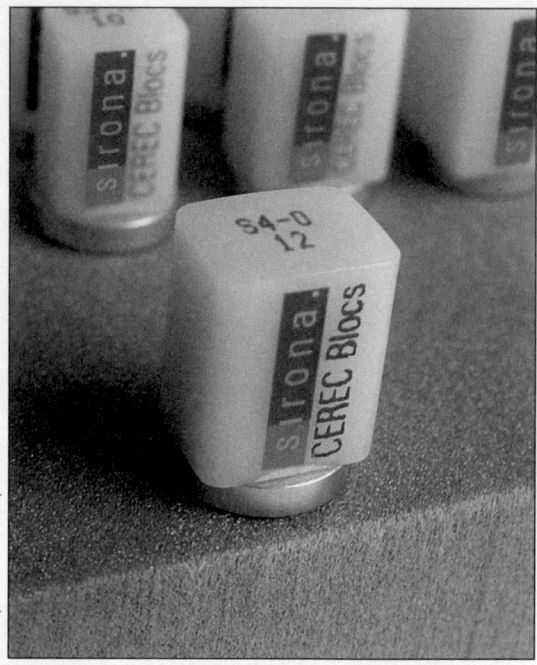

Courtesy of Sirona Dental Systems

FIGURE 41-5
Ceramic blocks for the CAM.

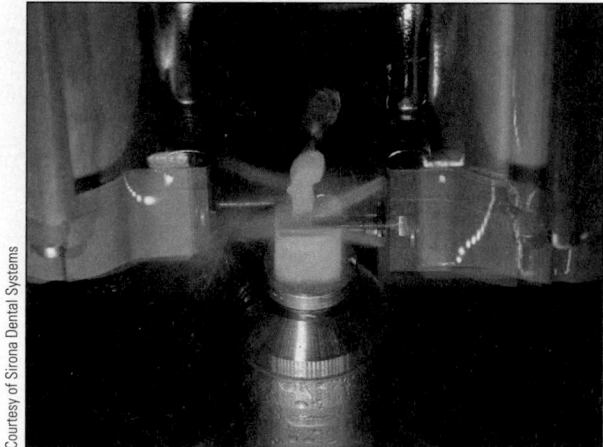

Courtesy of Sirona Dental Systems

FIGURE 41-6
A close-up of the milling process.

- Accuracy of final restoration due to elimination of shrinkage/distortion.
- No impressions are taken with a tray and traditional impression materials.
- Instant laboratory input (if applicable).
- The patient does not need to have provisional restorations.
- Without the provisional restoration, tooth sensitivity may be reduced.
- The dental laboratory is not involved in many cases reducing the waiting time for final restoration.

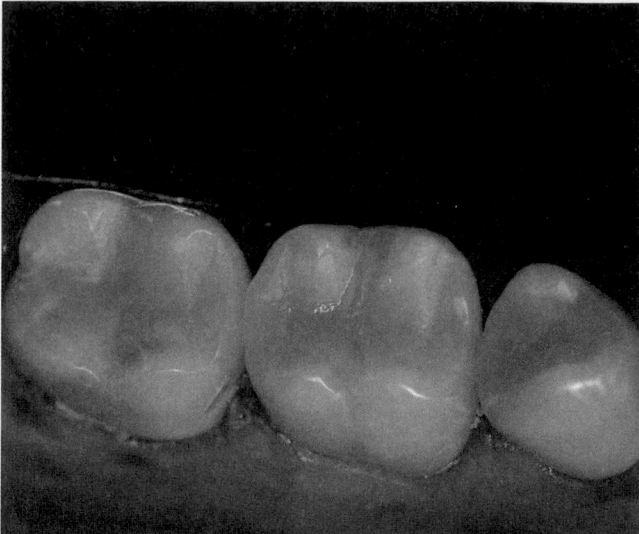

FIGURE 41-7
Teeth restored with a ceramic restoration designed and fabricated by the CEREC system.

The disadvantages of the CAD/CAM system include the following:

- The cost may be greater than traditional restoration procedures.
- The learning curve requires extra time for the dentist or dental assistant.
- May involve a longer appointment for the patient.
- Technology that is always changing.
- Lab participation, if a lab is involved with fabricating the restoration.
- Large size of intraoral scanner.

Digital Impression Systems

An office may also opt for only a digital impression system. Primescan by Dentsply Sirona and PlanScan Intraoral Scanner by Planmeca are two digital impression systems that are available for use. With this technique the patient will need two appointments to complete the procedure, just like the traditional procedure, but this eliminates the need for in-office impressions. At the first appointment, the dentist scans the preparation, views the digital impression, and in some cases designs the restoration. The digital model of the prepared tooth, the adjacent teeth, and the opposing arch are then sent electronically to the appropriate dental laboratory or milling center for fabrication of the final restoration or substructure (Figure 41-8). Many dental laboratories have an interface with dental offices. This allows for a smooth transfer of information between the office and the lab. Dental laboratories use *computer surface digitization* (CSD) to acquire a 3D record of the geometry of the preparation in order to prepare the final restoration. The dentist sends the shade and the type of material to be used. The lab mills the restoration and sends it to the dental office for the next appointment (Figure 41-9). In this scenario, the patient would need to wear a provisional restoration.

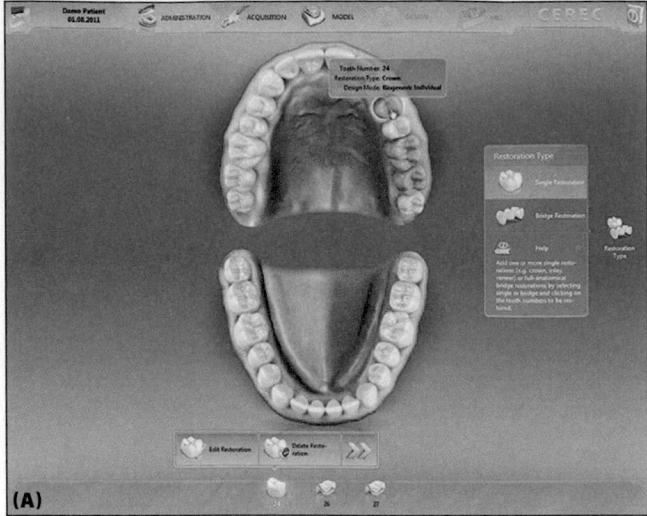

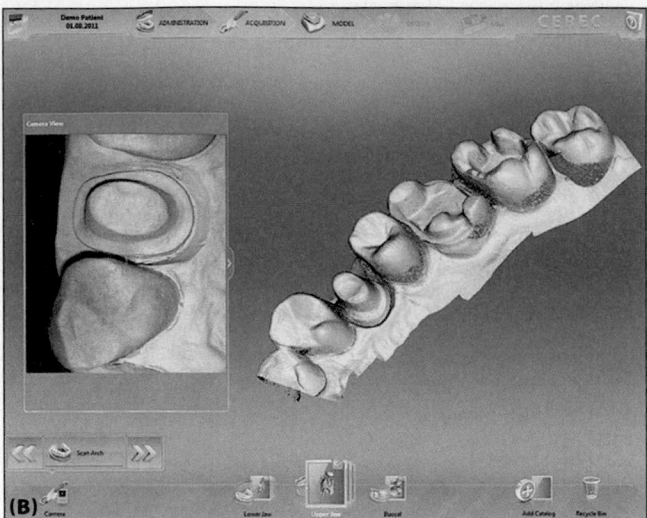

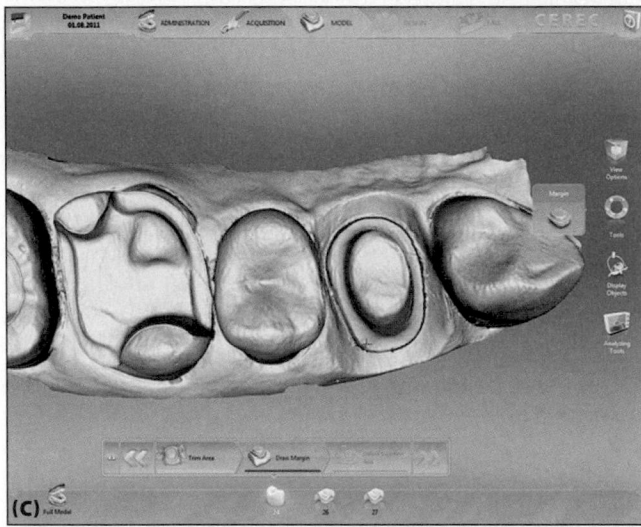

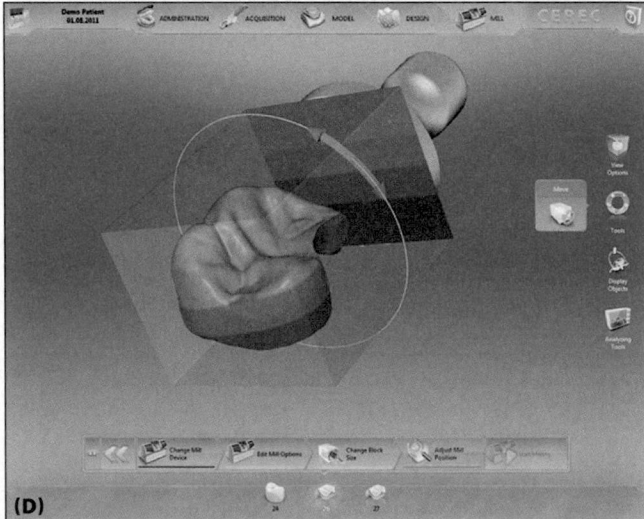

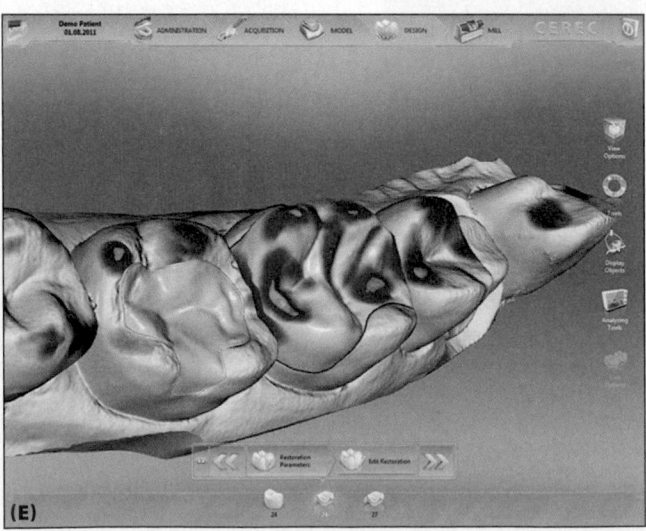

FIGURE 41-8

(A and B) CAD digital impressions. (C) CAD digital impressions. (D) A restoration milled from a ceramic block. (E) A virtually designed restoration.

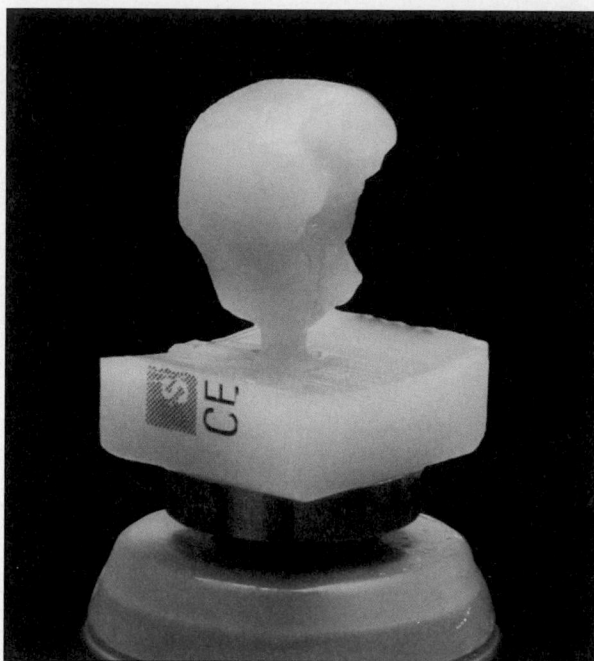

FIGURE 41-9
A finished restoration after the completion of the milling process, before being cut from the ceramic block.

Soft Tissue Management

Management of soft tissue during the preparation and digital impression taking is critical for the success of the final restoration. The accuracy of the restoration depends on the scanner's ability to visualize the margin of the preparation. The best way to accomplish this is by placing the margin above or at the gingival margin. When it is not possible to place a supragingival margin, it is important to manage the soft tissue so the margin is clearly visible during the digital impression. Gingival retraction methods are discussed in Chapter 40.

The Role of the Dental Assistant

The dental assistant's role in CAD/CAM procedures will vary from office to office following the dentist's directions and preferences. In some offices the dental assistant sets up the scanner, gets the computer software open and ready, and prepares the milling machine. During the procedure the assistant assists the dentist and ensures they have what they need to complete the procedure. In other offices the dental assistant may assist the dentist

during cavity preparation and then, depending on the assistant's training and skills, may scan the preparation to create the digital impression. The margins in the digitized impression can be enhanced with CAD/CAM software. Once the impression is approved by the dentist, a virtual restoration is designed for the dentist to evaluate and double-check, especially along the margins. When the dentist has approved the virtual restoration, the assistant sends this information to the CAM equipment for the milling of the restoration.

Upon completion of the restoration, the dental assistant assists the dentist as the restoration is tried on the tooth to ensure the margins, contacts, and occlusion are where the dentist wants them to be. This process is similar to what is outlined in Procedure 40-3, "Cementation Appointment." The assistant may then polish and glaze the restoration before assisting the dentist with the final cementation.

It requires training for the dental assistant to become proficient in using these systems. Many of the manufacturers provide training to the dentist and office team members when the units are purchased. Many schools and consultants are also training dental team members and dentists on how to integrate CAD/CAM into their offices. Continued education and training are required to keep up with the latest technology. Learning this new technology advances the dental assistant's knowledge and skills, making the dental assistant a more valued member of the dental team. Learning new technologies can also be motivating and rewarding for the dental assistant's career.

Patient Considerations

Patient considerations include providing the patient with the information needed to understand the treatment, the time commitment involved, and the cost of the procedure. Once the patient understands the need for a cast fixed prosthesis, the treatment options are explained. In many instances it is the dental assistant who will explain the CAD/CAM option. Some offices have videos, pictures, or brochures for the patient to look at. The patient should be made aware that although CAD/CAM restorations only require one appointment, it is usually a much longer appointment. The patient should be aware of the cost differences between the routine treatment and the CAD/CAM system. Once the patient understands this option, the dentist and patient together will determine if this treatment is best for them. The CAD/CAM restoration will be similar to routine fixed prosthodontic treatments, providing quality work, materials, and results.

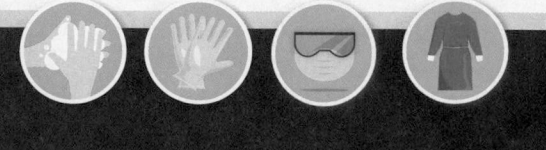

Procedure 41-1
CAD/CAM Restoration

This procedure is performed by the dentist and the dental assistant, and is completed in one appointment. In the first step the tooth is prepared. The next step is to scan the tooth

preparation and the surrounding tissues for the impression using the CAD system. The CAD system then designs the restoration and sends the information to the CAM system. The

(Continues)

CAM system then mills the restoration. After trying the restoration on the patient and making any necessary adjustments, it is ready for cementation.

Steps written in blue font are performed by the operator (dentist or qualified dental assistant), and the chairside assistant's steps are written in black.

Patient Seating Setup (refer to Procedure 18-4)

Anesthetic Setup (refer to Procedure 23-2)

Turn on and prepare the CAD system (see Figure 41-1)

Turn on and prepare the CAM system for the milling process (see Figure 41-4)

Have ceramic blocks ready for selection (see Figure 41-5)

Ceramic Crown Preparation Appointment Setup
- cotton rolls and 2 × 2 inch gauze, dental floss
- high-speed handpiece and assorted diamond burs, fissure burs, and discs
- low-speed handpiece with burs, discs, and stones
- dental dam setup
- spoon excavator, scaler, plastic filling instrument, cement spatula, and glass slab or mixing pad
- ceramic shade guide
- retraction cord and placement instrument
- Optispray (reflective powder that assists the scanner in picking up details of the preparation)
- ceramic block selection
- cementation setup (including etching materials) (refer to Chapter 30)
- curing light (if a light cured cement is used)

Procedure Steps
1. Escort and seat patient (refer to Procedure 18-4).

   Dentist greets the patient and takes position at the dental chair.

   ❏ *Signals for the procedure to begin (refer to Procedure 20-1).*

2. Pass mouth mirror and explorer at operator's signal.

   Dentist examines tooth or teeth for crown preparation with mirror and explorer.

   Dentist sprays teeth and surrounding tissues with the Optispray to enhance the occlusion and bite registration on the images before the tooth is prepared.

   Dentist obtains digital bite registration.

3. Assist in taking digital bite registration.

   Dentist administers local anesthetic.

4. Assist in administration of local anesthetic (refer to Procedure 23-2).

   Operator pumices teeth to be prepared with rubber cup (refer to Chapter 26).

5. Assist in pumicing teeth.

   Dentist selects shade.

6. Assist in determining shade (refer to Chapter 40).
   ❏ Retrieve disposable prophy angle and pass shade guide.
   ❏ Turn dental lamp off.
   ❏ Record shade on patient's chart.
   ❏ Place appropriate ceramic block in milling machine (Figure 41-10).

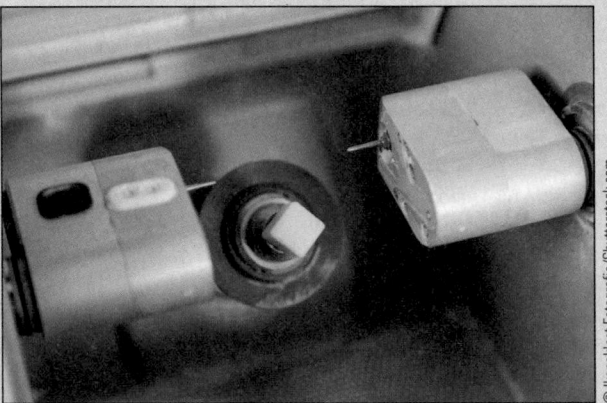

FIGURE 41-10
A ceramic block ready for milling by the CAM system.

Dentist prepares teeth according to the design of the ceramic crown.

7. Assist in preparing the teeth.
   ❏ Exchange shade guide for high-speed handpiece with appropriate diamond bur.
   ❏ Use high-speed evacuation to suction and air/water syringe to rinse and dry tooth for better visibility.

   Dentist examines the prepared tooth.

8. Exchange high-speed handpiece for mirror and explorer.
   ❏ Retrieve mirror and explorer after examination is completed

   Operator isolates the area for placement of retraction cord.

9. Pass retraction cord and placement instrument.

   Operator places subgingival retraction cord (refer to Procedure 40-1 and Figure 40-45).

Dentist coats the tooth preparation and surrounding tissues with reflective powder for the scanning of the three-dimensional impression.

Operator removes retraction cord (refer to Procedure 40-1).

Dentist obtains digital impression by positioning camera over the preparation.

Dentist designs the replacement part for the missing areas of the tooth, creating a virtual restoration using data from the proprietary software.

10. Transfer the virtual data with use of software to the milling machine, where diamond burs will work simultaneously under water coolant to mill the restoration from the ceramic block.

11. Remove the finished restoration from the milling machine.

Dentist places milled restoration on the prepared tooth and makes any needed adjustments (Figure 41-11).

Operator etches and rinses tooth and places bonding agent.

12. Mix cement per manufacturer's instructions.

13. Assist in final evaluation of fixed prosthesis.
   ❏ Pass mirror and explorer.

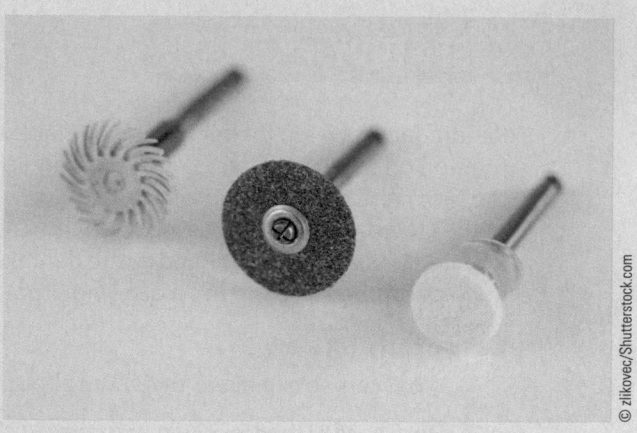

FIGURE 41-11
Discs, a rubber-polishing wheel, and ceramic stones are used to adjust and polish the restoration.

Dentist checks occlusion and contacts.

14. Provide patient with postoperative instructions orally and in written form.
   ❏ Inform the patient that the soft tissues will be tender for several days because of the retraction cord placement.

15. Write up procedure in Services Rendered.

16. Dismiss and escort patient to reception area (refer to Procedure 18-5).

Date	Services Rendered
02/18/XX	Updated medical and dental history, no changes noted. BP = 120/80; T = 98.6F, P = 80, R = 18
	Placed 20% benzocaine gel to injection sites for 2 minutes. Administered 2 cartridges (3.6 ml) of 2% lidocaine with 1:100,000 epi to mandibular left. No reaction.
	#30 ceramic crown preparation. Digital impressions of arches and occusion obtained. Gingival retraction cord placed around #30 for 7 minutes after completion of preparation. Retraction cord removed and digital impression obtained. Restoration milled. Finished ceramic crown permanently cemented with resin modified glass ionomer cement.
	POI do not bite on lip, no eating/drinking until numbness wear off, eat only on opposite side until numbness has worn off, call office if restoration feels high or if there is discomfort or pain.
	RTC: Six month recare visit Assistant's initials

Chapter Summary

This chapter covers information on the ever-growing and advancing CAD/CAM technology. CAD/CAM systems are used by the dentist in the dental office and in the dental laboratory. After reading this chapter, the student will have gained an understanding of computer-aided design (CAD) equipment and computer-aided manufacturing (CAM) systems. The components of the CAD/CAM systems are identified and explained. The steps for preparing the tooth, taking the digitized impression, designing the virtual restoration, and manufacturing the final restoration are described in detail. The technology is discussed including patient considerations and the role of the dental assistant. Also explained is how CAD/CAM systems are used with dental laboratories.

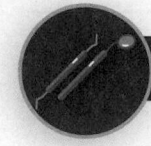

CASE STUDY

Kendra James was in for her routine dental examination, and Dr. Mendes found decay under an MOD restoration on tooth #5. After taking x-rays and completing the examination, Dr. Mendes recommended that the MOD restoration be replaced with a crown. Kendra was concerned about the time involved and the cost of the crown. Dr. Mendes has included the CAD/CAM technology in his office since Kendra's last appointment. After speaking with Kendra, the dental assistant found out that Kendra was also concerned about the impressions because she has a gagging problem.

Case Study Review

1. What can be explained to Kendra about the time and expense of a crown procedure?

2. Discuss the steps involved with the CAD/CAM technology.

3. What can the dental assistant do to help Kendra with her gagging concerns?

Review Questions

Multiple Choice

1. Which of the following does CAD stand for?
   a. computer-assisted design
   b. computer-aided draft
   c. computer-aided digital
   d. computer-aided design

2. Where is CAD/CAM used?
   a. in the dental office only
   b. in the dental laboratory only
   c. in both the dental office and the dental laboratory
   d. None of these

3. Which of the following CAD/CAM procedures is the dental assistant able to perform?
   a. Turn on the computer and ready the computer programs.
   b. Set up the scanner to create a digital impression.
   c. Prepare the ceramic block to be milled.
   d. All of these

4. With CAD/CAM training the dental assistant can complete all of the following EXCEPT:
   a. scan the cavity preparation to create a digital impression.
   b. create the digital restoration using the CAD system.
   c. send the digitized restoration to the CAM for milling *without* the dentist's evaluation and consent.
   d. place the ceramic block in the milling machine.

5. Which of the following is NOT an advantage of CAD/CAM?
   a. The fee is reduced because there is no dental laboratory involvement.
   b. No impressions are taken with routine materials and trays.
   c. The patient does not need to have provisional restorations.
   d. It saves time for the patient.

6. Which of the following is NOT a component of CAD/CAM?
   a. intraoral camera (scanner)
   b. CAD/CAM software
   c. milling machine
   d. gold or gold alloy blocks

7. Which of the following is NOT true regarding CAD/CAM?
   a. Images of the occlusion or bite registration are scanned before the tooth is prepared.
   b. No shade needs to be taken; the computer selects the shade to match the patient's teeth.
   c. The digitized impression can be modified to enhance the gingival margins of the preparation.
   d. Diamond burs and water are used during the milling process of the ceramic block.

8. Restorations using CAD/CAM technology in the dental office and laboratory are _____.
   a. completed in one appointment
   b. completed in two appointments
   c. Both a and b are correct
   d. None of these choices are correct.

9. CAD/CAM systems sometimes use a _____ to obtain an enhanced digital image.
   a. reflective powder
   b. polishing agent
   c. desensitizing agent
   d. water solution

10. The patient should be made aware of the shorter appointment time for CAD/CAM *and* the greater cost of the restoration as compared to a traditional lab fabricated cast restoration.
   Select the correct response based on the statements above.
   a. Both statements are true.
   b. Both statements are false.
   c. The first statement is true; the second statement is false.
   d. The first statement is false; the second statement is true.

Critical Thinking

1. What are the advantages of using CAD/CAM technology in the office?

2. Name the types of materials that are used to mill the restoration.

3. Explain why the dentist may choose to place a gingival retraction cord before the preparation is scanned.

Key Terms

Term and Pronunciation	Meaning of Root and Word Parts	Definition
coping (**koh**-ping)	**coping** = a protective cap or covering	portion of a restoration made of a foundation (coping) material and a veneering material

## CHAPTER 42

Removable Prosthodontics

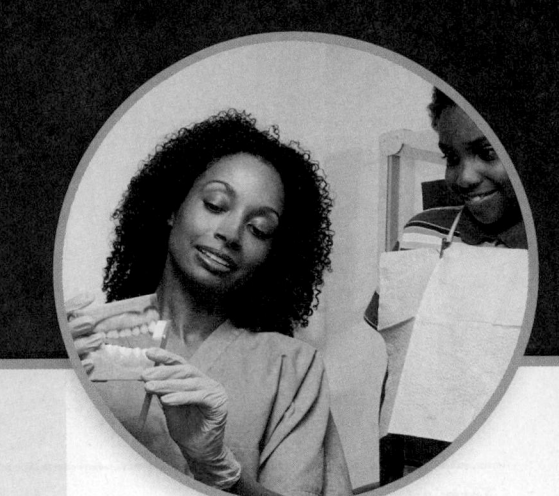

Specific Instructional Objectives

At the completion of this chapter, you will be able to meet these objectives:

1. Use terms presented in this chapter.
2. Describe the objectives of removable prosthodontic treatment.
3. List the types of partial dentures.
4. Discuss the Kennedy classifications of edentulous areas.
5. Describe the types of full dentures.
6. Discuss each component of the removable partial denture (RPD).
7. Compare and contrast the indications and contraindications of RPDs.
8. Compare and contrast the advantages and disadvantages of RPDs.
9. Describe the sequence of appointments in an RPD cases.
10. Define the role of the dental assistant in an RPD case.
11. Describe each surface of the full denture.
12. Describe each component of the complete denture.
13. Compare and contrast the indications and contraindications for full dentures.
14. Compare and contrast the advantages and disadvantages of the full denture.
15. Describe the sequence of appointments in a full denture case.
16. Discuss postdelivery care related to full dentures.
17. Define the role of the dental assistant in a full denture case.
18. Explain the impact of xerostomia and its effects on the removable prosthodontic patient.
19. Explain the function of denture adhesives.
20. Compare and contrast denture relining and denture rebasing.
21. Explain the process of denture repair.
22. State the function of denture cleaners.
23. List the common abbreviations used in removable prosthodontics charting.

Introduction

The term *prosthodontics* is a combination of the words *prosthesis* (replacement) and *dentes* (teeth). Dental removable prosthodontics includes complete dentures, which replace all of the missing teeth in an arch, and partial dentures, which replace some missing teeth in an arch. Tooth loss can occur for reasons such as dental decay or periodontal disease. Teeth may also be missing due to a genetic disorder, drug use, or trauma. Partially edentulous patients may prefer removable prosthodontics as opposed to fixed prosthodontic appliances for esthetic, financial, or functional reasons. The benefit is that the patient can insert and remove these prostheses independently for maintenance and hygiene. Additionally, a removable prosthesis can be repaired and adjusted easily and requires shorter appointments as compared to extensive fixed prosthodontic appliances. Prosthodontics is one of the nine recognized specialties of the American Dental Association (ADA). A dental school graduate completes an additional 3 years of training in a dental prosthodontic residency program.

Objectives of Removable Prosthodontic Treatment

The basic objectives of prosthodontics treatment are to restore the function of the missing natural teeth by replacing them with artificial teeth. These include improvement of several factors:

- masticatory functions
- esthetics
- speech (by improving the pronunciation of those words containing *sibilants*, or hissing sounds, or *fricatives*, such as "f" or "v" sounds)
- self-esteem

Types of Partial Dentures

Partial dentures replace some of the teeth that may be missing in a dentition and are available as transitional (acrylic base) or cast (metal framework) partials.

Transitional Partial Denture

Transitional partial dentures are also called flippers (Figures 42-1). Transitional partial dentures are the least expensive of all of the removable partial dentures (RPD).

The abutments are clasped with wrought wire clasps, which are inserted into the acrylic denture base (Figure 42-1). Flippers are mostly intended to be used only for a short period of time.

This might be while waiting for healing of tissues after implant placement or after extractions of some of the teeth in the dentition. The pink acrylic of the denture base in a flipper is the same acrylic material used to make standard full or complete dentures. One advantage to a flipper is that new teeth can easily be added. Although a flipper is a temporary solution, many people keep a flipper for a long period of time. The flipper is not as strong as the cast metal framework of a traditional partial denture. As a result, they tend to break more easily. The wrought wire clasps that allow for retention of the flipper are not as strong as the cast metal clasps found in the cast partial dentures. The denture base rests only on the soft tissue and as a result is less stable than the partial dentures that are supported by existing teeth in the dentition.

As the bone resorbs, it becomes necessary to **reline** a flipper more often. Relining will be discussed later in this chapter.

Cast Partial

Removable partial dentures with cast metal frameworks have been utilized in dentistry for a very long time (Figures 42-2).

Initially, the metal framework of an RPD was fabricated from gold. However, due to cost, gold is no longer used. The frameworks today are cast from an alloy called chrome cobalt. This metal is extremely strong and as a result can be cast very thin. These frameworks are much less likely to break as compared to a flipper partial denture. These types of partial dentures are supported by the existing teeth in the dentition. As a result, they

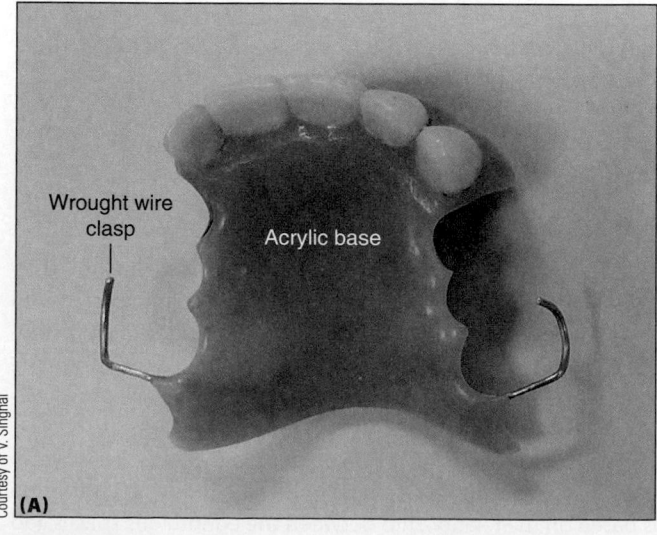

Wrought wire clasp

Acrylic base

(A)

Courtesy of V. Singhal

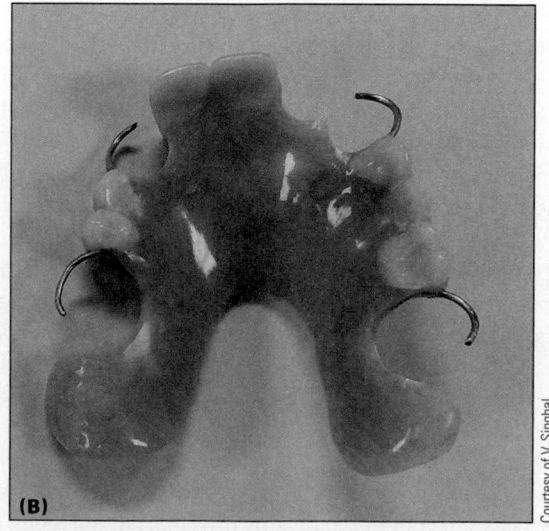

(B)

Courtesy of V. Singhal

FIGURE 42-1
Maxillary flippers.

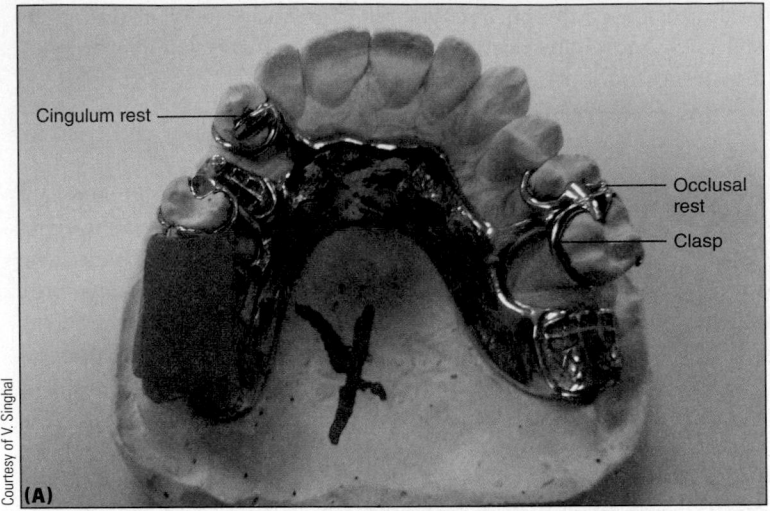

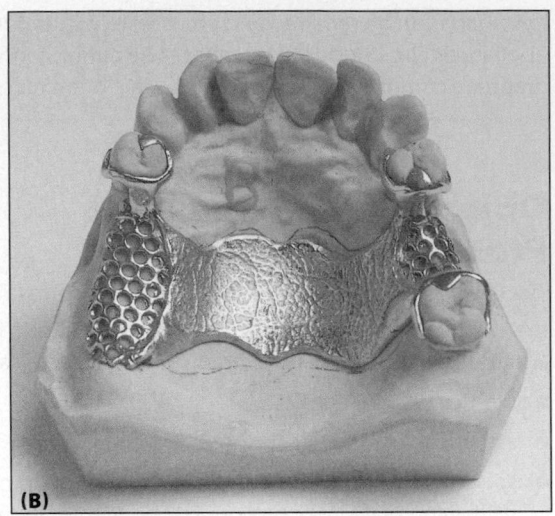

Cingulum rest

Occlusal rest

Clasp

Courtesy of V. Singhal

(A)

(B)

FIGURE 42-2
(A) Mandibular partial denture framework. (B) Maxillary partial denture framework.

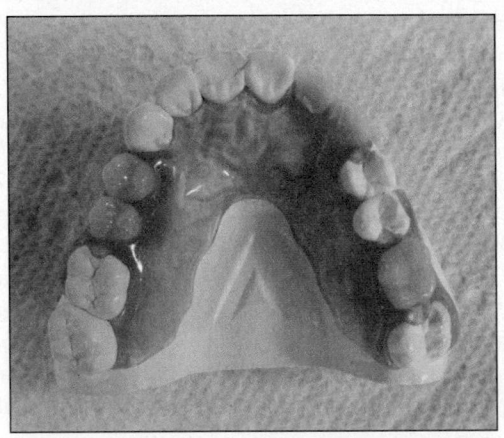

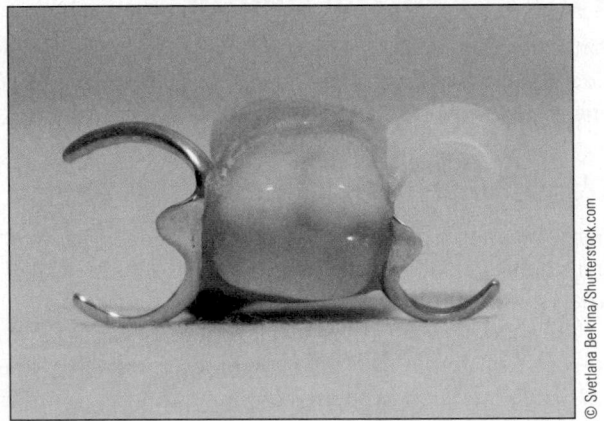

© Svetlana Belkina/Shutterstock.com

FIGURE 42-3
Flexible plastic partial denture.

FIGURE 42-4
Nesbit partial denture.

are very stable and retentive. The abutment teeth may need to be slightly prepared with a bur before taking the final impression so that the partial denture can rest on the teeth without interference from the opposing arch when the patient bites. The preparation is completed by the dentist. Since the metal framework rests on the abutment teeth, this type of partial does not need a reline as frequently as a flipper (Figure 42-2).

The most recent advance in dental materials has been the use of flexible materials for the fabrication of removable dental appliances (Figure 42-3). The flexible plastic material is used in place of the metal framework and the standard nonflexible pink acrylic material. The flexible partials can include metal clasps or flexible plastic clasps.

A Nesbit denture is a type of denture used to replace missing teeth in the posterior area of the oral cavity. Nesbit dentures use metal clasps to connect to healthy proximal natural teeth. Many dentists do not recommend Nesbit dentures because they are

very small and there is a risk of swallowing the partial denture (Figure 42-4).

Kennedy Classification of Edentulous Arches

The main purpose for creating a classification system for partially dentulous arches is to enable the dentist to communicate with the patient which missing teeth will be replaced with a prosthesis. The treatment plan of an edentulous region depends on the Kennedy classification. The design of the removable prosthesis will determine its success.

The Kennedy classification system is the most commonly used system (Figure 42-5 and Box 42-1). Kennedy's classification is based on the relationship between the edentulous spaces and the abutment teeth.

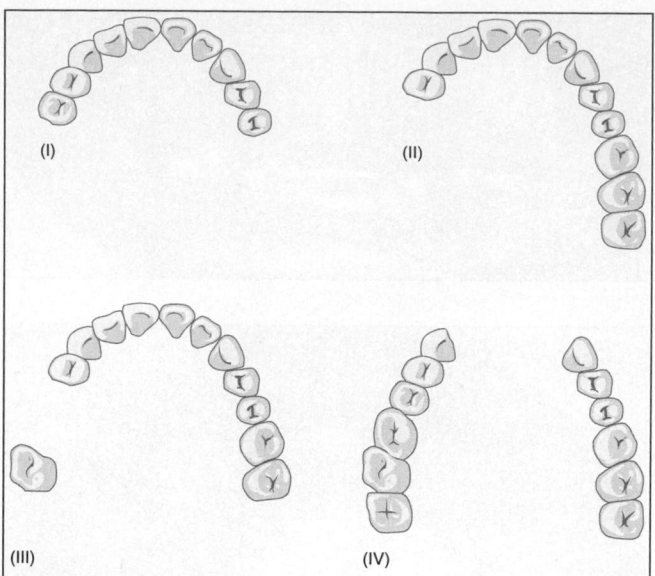

FIGURE 42-5
Kennedy classification.

BOX 42-1 Edentulous Areas Classifications

Class I: Edentulous areas are bilateral and are located posterior to the remaining natural teeth (Figure 42-5).

Class II: Edentulous area is unilateral and is located posterior to the remaining natural teeth (Figure 42-5).

Class III: Edentulous area is unilateral with natural teeth remaining anterior and posterior to it (Figure 42-5).

Class IV: A single, bilateral edentulous area that crosses the midline located anterior to the remaining natural teeth (Figure 42-5).

Types of Full Dentures

Complete dentures or full dentures are worn by patients who are missing all of the teeth in an arch or in both of the arches. Full dentures (Figure 42-6) are usually fabricated from an acrylic material. However, the base of the complete denture could be made up

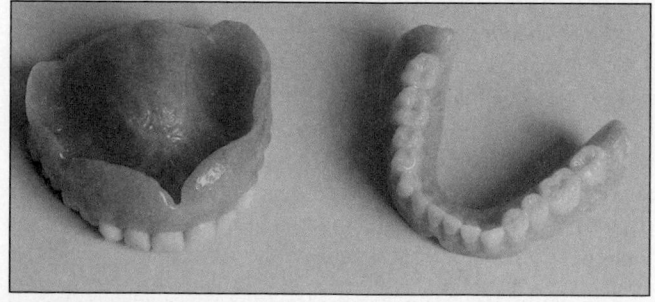

FIGURE 42-6
Full maxillary and mandibular denture: denture base, artificial teeth, tissue side of denture on the left (maxillary), and occlusal view on the right (mandibular).

of all acrylic resin, metal, or acrylic with a metal framework within. Traditional full dentures are usually fabricated after any remaining teeth have been removed and the gingival tissues have healed. These dentures are ready for insertion approximately 8–12 weeks after the teeth have been removed. The exception is an immediate partial denture, which is discussed below.

Immediate Denture

An immediate denture is a complete or partial denture inserted immediately after extractions of the anterior natural teeth. For the patients who need a complete immediate denture, the posterior teeth are often extracted six to eight weeks prior to fabrication of the immediate (if they are not missing already). This allows the extraction site to heal so a better-fitting immediate denture may be fabricated. Five to six visits may be required for the fabrication of an immediate denture. This does not include any additional visits that may be needed for surgical procedures such as an alveoloplasty.

The process of making an immediate dental prosthesis consists of impressions, centric relation, selection of denture teeth, and a try-in of the posterior teeth. After the try in and the centric relation is obtained, the dental lab technician will remove the remaining anterior teeth on the model and replace these with the acrylic denture teeth. The denture is then processed and finished and returned to the dental office. On the day of denture insertion, the anterior teeth are extracted and the denture is immediately inserted.

Immediate dentures need a future reline and as a result are usually more expensive than conventional dentures. A reline is needed because the denture becomes loose due to healing of the extraction sites following insertion of the denture. A permanent reline is needed about six months postinsertion once the soft tissues and bone at the extraction sites have healed. The bone undergoes shrinkage during the healing process. Traditional dentures fit better as they are fabricated six to eight weeks after extraction, and the tissues have had time to heal and shrink prior to denture fabrication. Relining will be discussed later in this chapter.

One significant advantage of an immediate denture is esthetics as the patient will not be without anterior teeth. Additionally, the immediate denture acts a bandage to protect the tissues and reduce bleeding and swelling. Furthermore, it is easier for a dental professional to duplicate the shape, color, and size of the natural teeth while some are still present in the oral cavity. One disadvantage is that there is no option of a full try-in for the patient to see how the denture(s) look before insertion.

Regardless of how the denture is fabricated, in general, the maxillary denture is much easier for the user to adapt to as compared to the mandibular denture. This is mostly because of the shape of the mandible, movement of the tongue muscles, and lack of suction in the mandibular arch as compared to the maxillary arch. Many dentists recommend supporting the lower denture with two to four implants (Figure 42-8). This type of denture is known as an overdenture. Overdentures are discussed in more detail later in this section. The use of implants when designing a full denture appliance increasingly has been shown to improve a patient's denture wearing experience by increasing the denture's stability, as well as preventing the resorption of the patient's bone. Implants used with full appliances have also been shown to help with appliance retention.

In the maxillary arch, the denture is more stable as it is able to adhere to the palate due to a suction effect created in the posterior palatal area. The anatomy of the mandibular arch does not allow for suction for denture adherence. The maxillary dentures are more comfortable due to the larger area of the palate, as compared to the mandibular dentures, which rest on a U-shaped mandibular ridge.

Overdentures

An overdenture is a prosthetic denture that is prepared to fit over implants (Figure 42-7) or retained roots. To fabricate this type of denture, a dentist completes endodontic therapy on certain healthy roots or places dental implants in the arch on receiving the denture (Figure 42-8). Sometimes special prefabricated attachments, such as magnets and a snap design, are used (Figure 42-8). The tissue side of the overdenture is made with the component that will align with the implant or retained root.

It is important that the overdenture user be diligent with proper oral home care and have regular dental hygiene visits. This will minimize the risk of failure of the dental implants and overdenture as well as any retained teeth or roots.

Some patients may wish to keep a second set of dentures in case one breaks or gets lost. A second set of partial or full dentures is also beneficial when denture wearers have to leave their original denture with the dentist for a repair or a reline. Despite the extra expense, a second set of dentures is an excellent investment. Patients are advised to store the spare denture in a moist and airtight container to prevent it from distorting as the plastic acrylic may warp if it becomes dry.

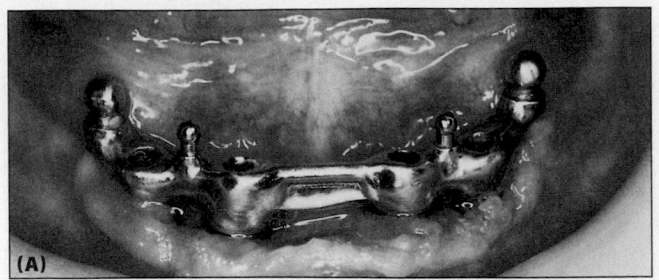

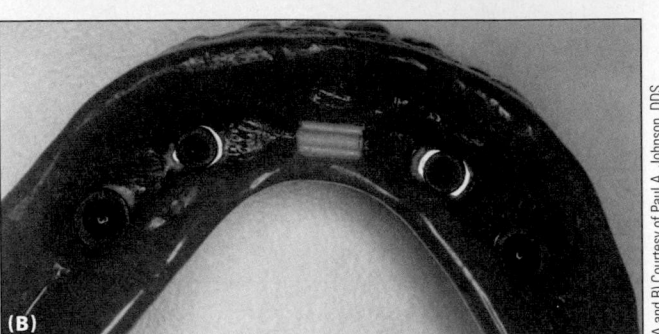

FIGURE 42-8
(A) Dental implants for a denture. (B) Denture with snap design to fit over dental implants.

(A and B) Courtesy of Paul A. Johnson, DDS

Removable Partial Dentures

Success of a removable dental prosthesis depends on good communication between the patient and the dental professional. The patient's attitude, cooperation, and motivation are important, as is good general health of the patient. Patience and understanding from the patient and the practitioner during the RPD fabrication procedure is important. This section will discuss the design and components of the removable partial denture as well as the sequence or appointments for fabrication of a removable partial denture.

Components of a Removable Partial Denture

The cast maxillary or mandibular partial denture is made up of six structural elements. Each element is important in restoring function to the oral structures. These six elements are the major connector, minor connector, rest, direct retainer (which contains a reciprocal arm, retentive arm, shoulder, and rest and clasps), indirect retainer (minor connector and rest), and denture base.

The metal framework is the base for the cast removable partial denture (see Figure 42-2). Frameworks are made of a very strong chrome cobalt alloy and come in various shapes. All other parts of the framework are connected to the framework, and the framework is composed of several parts.

Connectors Connectors are used to connect quadrants of a partial denture. Connectors hold the working components of the partial denture in the proper position and evenly distribute masticatory forces. Connectors are classified as major or minor.

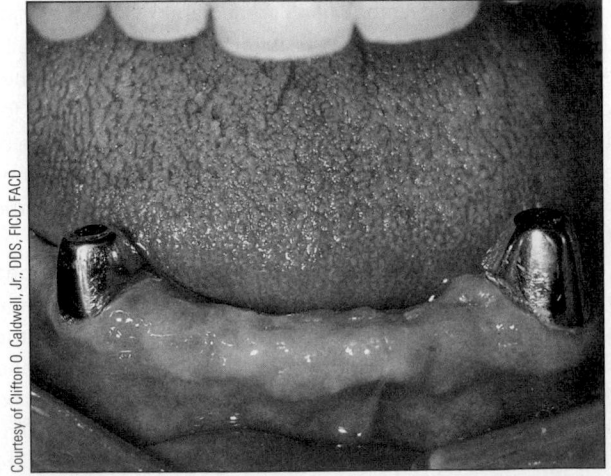

Courtesy of Clifton O. Caldwell, Jr., DDS, FICD, FACD

FIGURE 42-7
Overdenture supported with abutments (roots are restored with cast gold post and dome-shaped core combination).

Major Connectors Major connectors have different designs based on the arch the partial denture is being designed for. However, all major connectors must be rigid. They also provide support to the tissues and protect the soft tissues. Additionally, they keep the denture base in position. Some major connector designs will be discussed in this section.

Mandibular Major Connector Mandibular major connectors have six basic designs: lingual bar (Figure 42-9), lingual bar with a continuous bar indirect retainer, labial plate, cingulum bar, lingual plate (Figure 42-10), and sublingual bar. The lingual bar and lingual plate are used the most frequently.

Maxillary Major Connectors Maxillary major connector designs are as follows: palatal strap (Figure 42-2B), palatal plate, complete palatal coverage, anteroposterior type, U-shaped, and palatal bar.

Minor Connectors Minor connectors join the major connector to the remainder of the RPD. These include rests and clasps and indirect retainers. All of these will be discussed in this section. Minor connectors allow the RPD to function as a single unit.

Rest The rest is a small extension of the removable prosthesis made to fit or sit on the occlusal or incisal surface of the adjoining teeth (Figure 42-2A). The rest gives stability to the partial denture by providing support. If required, the dentist will slightly prepare the occlusal, incisal, or lingual surface on the tooth so the rest(s) can sit within the prepared area. This preparation can be performed using a round or oblong-shaped carbide bur or diamond bur. Despite efforts to maximize esthetics, rests are still slightly visible but are necessary for retention.

Retainers Retainers provide stability to a prosthesis and prevent movement of the removable partial denture away from the tissues and the teeth. Retention may be direct or indirect.

Direct Retainers Most retention of a removable partial denture is provided by direct retainers. The most common type of direct retainer is the clasp (Figure 42-2A) of the removable partial denture.

There are basically two types of clasps that provide retention, support, and stability to the partial denture:

1. **Circumferential or Akers clasps** are made up of two arms that surround the tooth on opposing sides. They are in contact with the tooth along their entire length (Figure 42-11).

2. **Vertical projection clasps or bar or Roach clasps** only contact the tooth at a certain point of the clasp. They come toward the undercut area from the gingival area (Figure 42-12).

Indirect Retainers An indirect retainer may be needed in some partial denture designs to prevent forces that may cause a partial denture to become unbalanced (Figure 42-11). An indirect retainer may be an additional occlusal or incisal rest along with a minor connector that is placed in an area that is a distance away from the edentulous area.

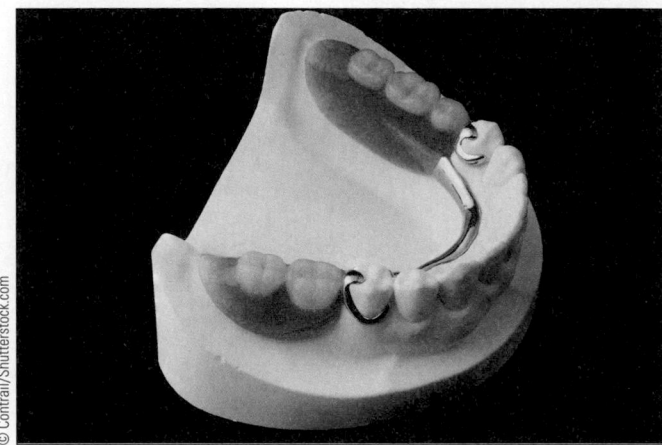

FIGURE 42-9
Lingual bar major connector.

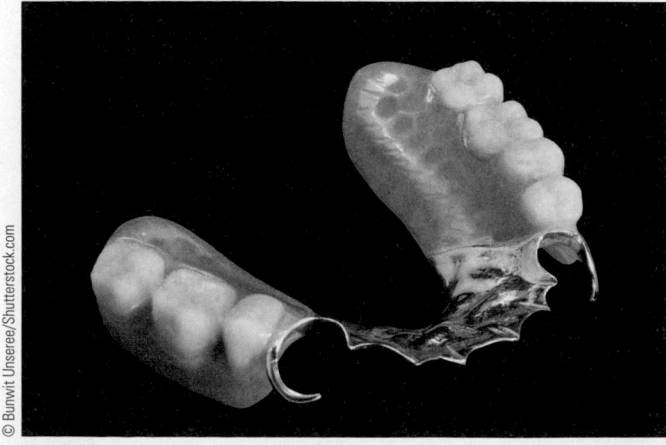

FIGURE 42-10
Lingual plate partial denture.

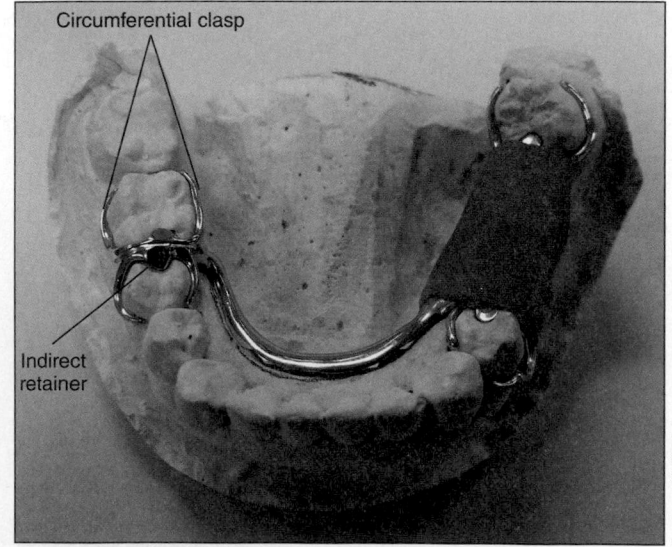

FIGURE 42-11
Mandibular lingual bar framework partial denture with circumferential clasps and occlusal rests as indirect retainers.

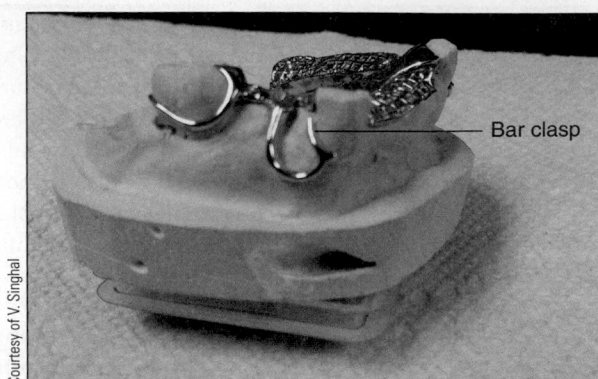

FIGURE 42-12
Mandibular framework partial denture with bar clasp.

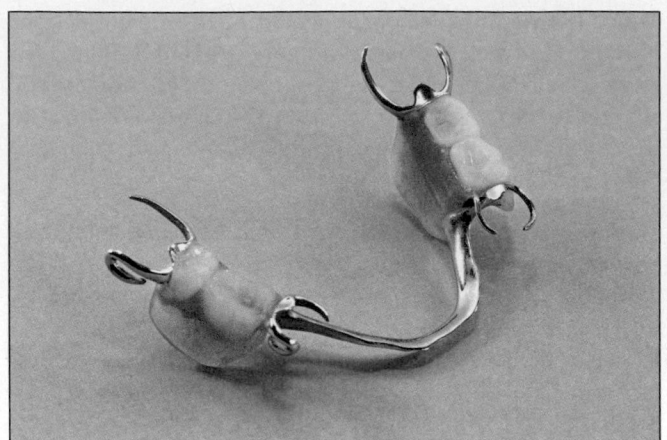

FIGURE 42-14
Partial denture with tooth borne saddles.

Denture Base The denture base is the acrylic portion of the removable appliance that replaces the gingival tissue (Figure 42-13). It often has pink lines within it that resemble tissue fibers to mimic the natural appearance of the gingival soft tissue. The artificial teeth are secured in the denture base.

Saddle The saddle is the part of the denture base that holds the acrylic or porcelain denture teeth (Figure 42-13). It can be either tooth-tissue borne (Figure 42-13) or tooth borne (Figure 42-14). The RPD design may have separate saddles in the same denture for different edentulous areas.

Artificial Teeth Artificial teeth are made of porcelain or acrylic. They are available in a number of shades and shapes. The teeth are replacements for natural teeth (Figure 42-15). If they are porcelain, they are held into the denture base with either *diatoric* holes in the posterior teeth areas or pins in the anterior areas (Figure 42-16). In the case of acrylic, they are actually bonded directly to the denture base. The prices for both types of teeth are comparable.

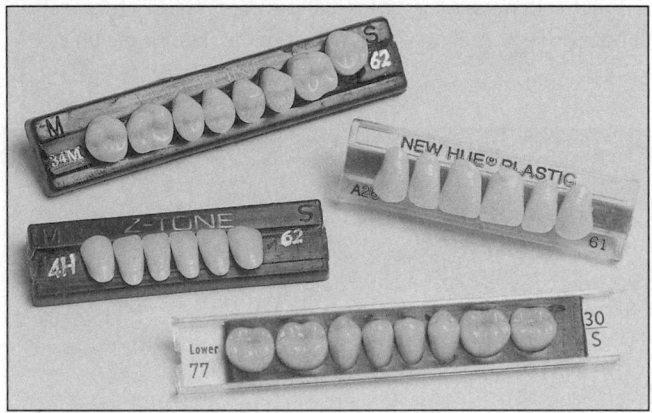

FIGURE 42-15
Sets of denture teeth showing shade and mold.

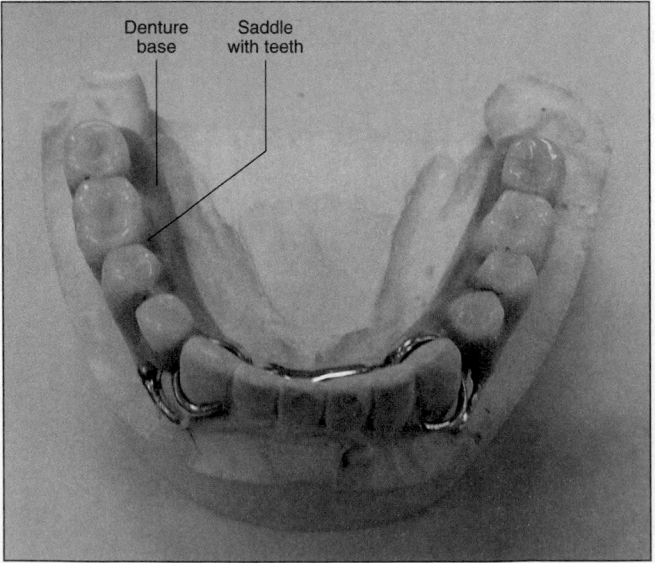

FIGURE 42-13
Partial denture with tooth-tissue borne saddles.

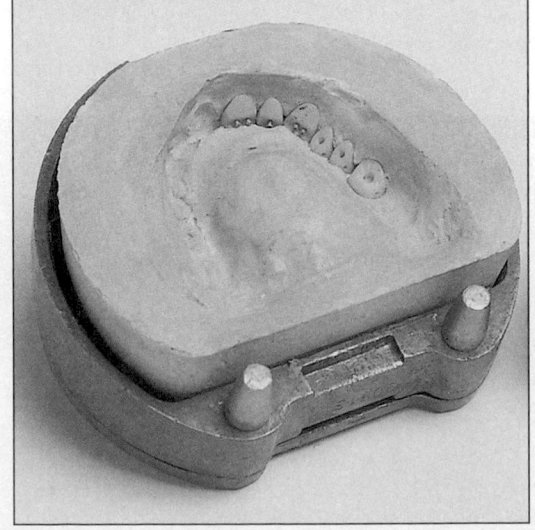

FIGURE 42-16
Porcelain teeth showing pins and diatoric holes. (Note: These teeth are in a model in a flask ready for acrylic base material to be placed over them.)

Acrylic teeth are made from poly methyl methacrylate (PMMA). They are susceptible to abrasion and wear down more easily when compared to porcelain teeth. Over time the wear may lead to a reduction in tooth length. Acrylic teeth are stain resistant, but the surface has tiny microscopic depressions that can harbor bacteria. Overnight soaking is necessary to effectively clean and remove the bacteria. Acrylic teeth have several advantages when compared to porcelain teeth. Acrylic teeth are more resistant to breakage as compared to porcelain teeth and are the best choice for people who have bone loss. Acrylic teeth absorb some of the occlusal forces, resulting in a decreased transmission of forces to the underlying alveolar bone and soft tissue. Additionally, similar to natural teeth, acrylic teeth do not make any sound when they come in contact with the natural or other acrylic opposing teeth.

Porcelain teeth are more natural looking and are harder than acrylic teeth. They are more resistant to wear than acrylic teeth. However, porcelain teeth are more likely to chip or crack. Whether the dentures have acrylic teeth or porcelain teeth, they must be handled carefully during cleaning. Dentures should be cleaned over a washbasin that is filled with water or over a towel. This will reduce the risk of breakage in case the denture is dropped. Porcelain teeth cause excessive wear of the natural teeth if they are in contact with them during occlusion. It is difficult to polish porcelain teeth due to lack of sophisticated lab equipment in a dental office; therefore, they are sent back to the lab for any readjustments.

Porcelain teeth may also cause an undesirable "clicking" sound during chewing or speaking when the denture teeth meet. This sound is noticeable by others and may be embarrassing to the patient. With dentures, regardless of the type of teeth, there is an adjustment period. The patient should have patience during this time.

Indications and Contraindications for Removable Partial Dentures

Indications for a removable partial denture are provided in Box 42-2. Contraindications for a removable partial denture are provided in Box 42-3.

BOX 42-2 Indications for a Removable Partial Denture

1. To replace several teeth in the same quadrant or in both quadrants of the same arch
2. To replace missing teeth for patients who do not wish to have a fixed bridge or implant
3. When a fixed bridge or implant may not be possible due to bone loss
4. To function as a transitional RPD in a patient who is on the path to becoming edentulous
5. As an interim prosthesis until a patient can afford fixed bridges or implants in the future
6. In patients who are considered vulnerable, such as those with physical, emotional, or mental disabilities

---

BOX 42-3 Contraindications for a Removable Partial Denture

1. Patient will not accept the RPD due to esthetics
2. Persistent poor oral hygiene
3. Patient does not have satisfactory teeth present in arch to support RPD
4. Rampant decay
5. Significant periodontal disease
6. Allergy to the acrylic denture base material

Advantages of Removable Partial Dentures

Many people feel self-conscious when speaking in public if they have missing teeth. Thus, partial dentures can improve an individual's confidence and self-esteem by providing a more esthetic and youthful look.

Since partial dentures are removable, the gingival tissues are able to rest when the patient is not wearing them. In the future, if the patient loses another natural tooth, the tooth can be added to the existing partial denture base.

Missing teeth can result in movement of the remaining teeth, resulting in a change in the occlusion and possibly a loss of function (Figure 42-17). Teeth can also supraerupt from their sockets if the occluding tooth in the opposing arch is missing (Figure 42-18). A removable partial denture helps the natural teeth retain their positions.

When posterior teeth are missing, the patient loses the "stops" in the oral cavity. The patient loses the ability to occlude. In addition, with loss of the dentition, people may have a difficult time pronouncing words, and it may be more difficult for others to understand them. An RPD can improve a person's ability to talk and to chew food. Additionally, a damaged partial denture is easier to repair as compared to a fixed dental prosthetic appliance.

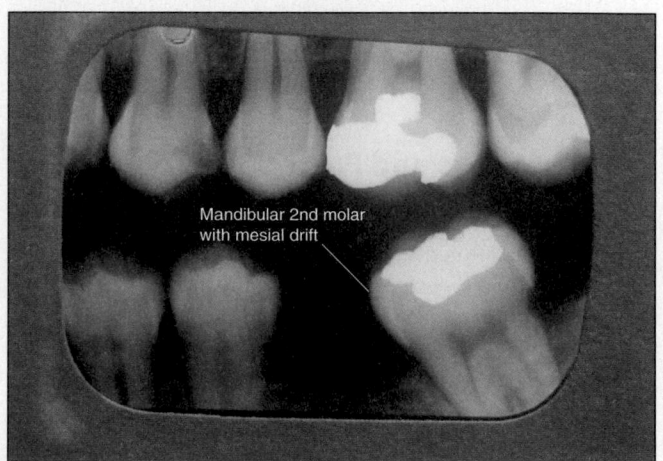

Mandibular 2nd molar with mesial drift

FIGURE 42-17
Mesial drift due to loss of proximal tooth.

Courtesy of V. Singhal

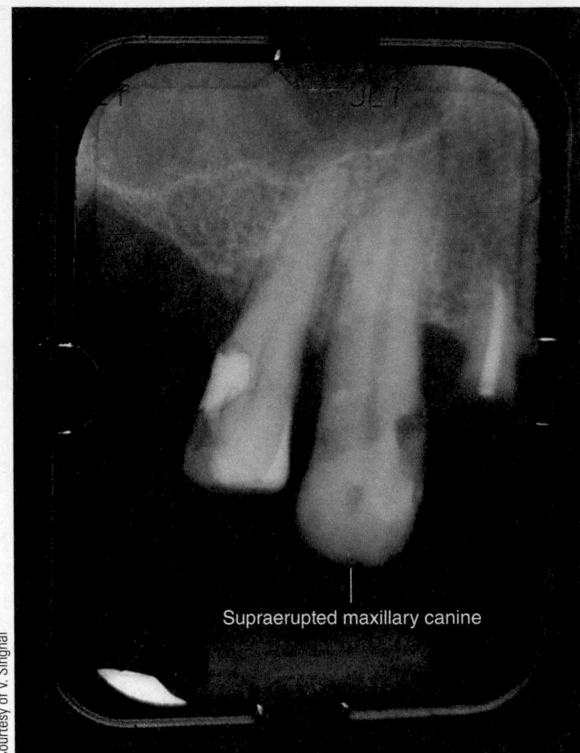

Supraerupted maxillary canine

FIGURE 42-18
Supraeruption of tooth due to loss of opposing tooth.

Disadvantages of Removable Partial Dentures

When one loses a single tooth, there are various tooth replacement options to consider such as a removable partial denture, an implant, or a fixed bridge. Most patients are not satisfied with a single tooth partial denture option due to the bulk of metal and acrylic and the unsightly clasps necessary to stabilize the prosthesis.

One disadvantage of tooth loss followed by replacement with an RPD is the bone loss that occurs due to the absence of the natural tooth root (Figure 42-19). Additionally, biting forces may cause the partial to move. Some partial denture wearers may also experience gingival irritation resulting in discomfort.

Appointments and Procedures for a Removable Partial Denture

A series of appointments is needed to fabricate a partial denture. The process usually involves minor shaping of the teeth followed by impressions. Models are then poured from the impressions. These models are then used to fabricate the partial denture framework by the dental laboratory technician. After try-in visits and adjustments, the partial denture is processed and finished and sent to the office. The dentist inserts the removable appliance, and home care instructions are provided to the patient.

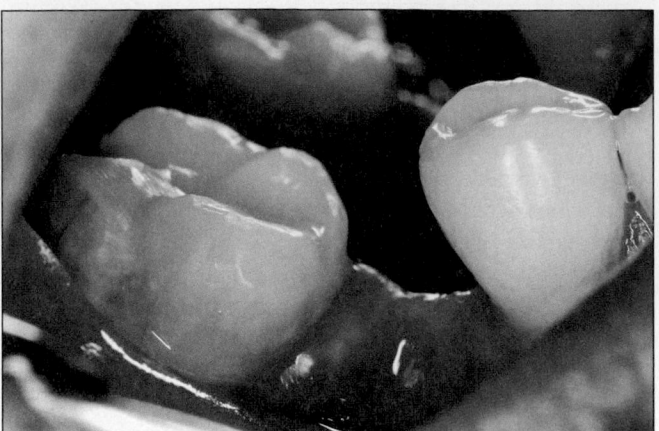

FIGURE 42-19
Resorption of alveolar bone due to tooth loss.

Prior to the initial appointment for RPD fabrication, radiographs are obtained to evaluate the health of the alveolar bone. The patient's face and oral tissue are examined to determine the shade and shape of the artificial teeth. An oral prophylaxis is performed to ensure that all remaining teeth are maintained. Any required restorative dental work would also be completed prior to fabrication of an RPD.

Consultation and Examination During the first appointment for a removable prosthesis, the patient is examined, and a detailed medical and dental history is obtained. The dentist and patient also discuss the patient's expectations of dental treatment and attitude toward an RPD. The dental assistant should also educate the patient about the removable partial denture. The indications and contraindications outlined in Boxes 42-2 and 42-3 are considered and discussed by the dentist and the patient.

Records Appointment During the first appointment for denture construction, the preliminary alginate impressions are obtained (refer to Chapter 33 for the alginate impression procedure). Prior to the start of the procedure, the patient's health and dental history is updated to note any health or oral condition changes that may impact fabrication of the RPD. The impressions are disinfected and poured immediately with dental stone. Many practitioners prefer to fabricate a custom tray for the arch in which the RPD is to be fabricated. The custom tray is fabricated on the preliminary models (Figure 42-20). The custom tray is used to obtain the final impression after the teeth are prepared for the RPD.

Preparation and Final Impression Prior to the third visit, the dentist designs the partial denture. At the third visit, the dentist performs any tooth preparations, if needed, based on the design for the RPD. The custom tray that was fabricated from the preliminary models is now used to obtain the final alginate impression. The impression is immediately poured in stone. The final model that is obtained from this impression is used to

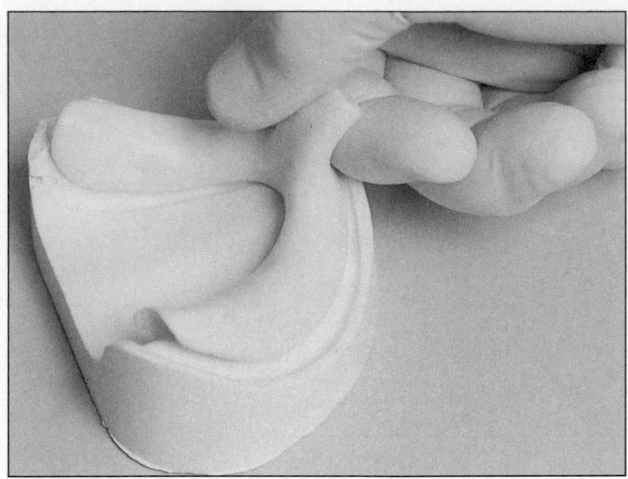

FIGURE 42-20
Mandibular custom tray for final impression.

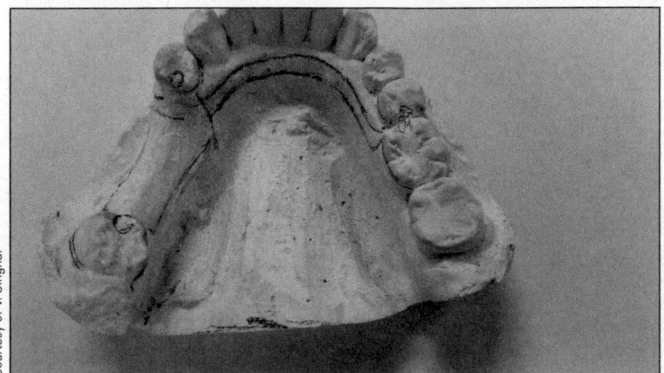

Courtesy of V. Singhal

FIGURE 42-21
Final model with design of RPD framework.

fabricate the RPD. The model obtained from the final impression provides a much more accurate replica of the patient's teeth and tissues as compared to a preliminary model obtained from a stock tray.

A bite registration is then obtained (refer to Chapter 33) and a facebow is used to obtain the relationship between the maxilla and the condyle (refer to Chapter 33). When the stone sets in the final models, the dentist draws the design of the partial denture framework on the final model (Figure 42-21). The models are then mounted on an articulator. The dental assistant, after consulting with the dentist, selects the shade and mold of the teeth and notes it in the chart. The dental assistant completes the laboratory prescription for the cast metal framework. The articulated models with pencil markings to show the design and the lab prescription are sent to the prosthetic dental lab. The lab technician constructs the denture framework based on the design provided and sends it back to the office for a try-in of the framework.

Laboratory Prescription The prescription includes the patient's name, age, gender, and the date of return of the case. It also includes dentist's name, license number, office contact information, and instructions to the technician. The dentist notes the

teeth that are missing and that will be included in the prosthesis. The dentist may mark the **height of contour** and retention areas as well as the type of clasps and rests. The prescription also includes information regarding the location of the rests and retention arms of the clasps. The prescription, with detailed instructions and articulated models, is sent to the lab.

Try-In Appointments There are usually two try-in appointments. The first is for the cast partial framework. The laboratory creates a wax model based on the design sent by the dentist (Figure 42-22A). The framework is then cast (Figure 42-22B). The cast framework will also be sent back with the wax rims in the edentulous areas (Figure 42-22C). The metal framework is the base for the teeth and the saddles. It must fit properly. If the framework does not seat properly or rocks when seated, a new final impression may need to be taken and sent to the lab. A new framework will need to be cast and a new try-in visit will be scheduled. Every step must be completed carefully to ensure that the framework fits well. For example, alginate impressions must be poured immediately. If there is a delay in pouring the model, the finished framework may not fit. The lab also must ensure that steps are taken to minimize distortion or warping of the final framework. If the framework fits well, it is sent back to the lab for addition of the teeth into wax in the edentulous areas (Figure 42-23). A new prescription with a detailed description of the mold and shade of the teeth is also included. The unfinished partial is then sent back to the office for a final try-in. At the second try-in appointment, the dentist evaluates the fit, comfort, and function of the appliance. The dentist also evaluates the setting of the teeth in the wax as well as the shade and mold of the denture teeth. Some dental offices may combine these steps into one appointment. The patient is requested to say certain words with the "f," "v," "th," and "s" sounds to verify pronunciation. If the previously obtained centric relation is found to be inaccurate at this visit, a new bite registration is recorded. The dental assistant notes any changes on the new laboratory prescription, which is sent along with the RPD back to the lab. The lab will adjust the teeth based on the new centric relation and send the case back to the office for another try-in. Once the patient and the dentist are satisfied with the occlusion, esthetics, and function of the removable partial denture during the try-in phase, the RPD is sent back to the laboratory for finishing and processing.

Delivery Appointment On the day of the final delivery of the appliance, the dentist inserts the RPD and uses articulating paper to confirm that the occlusion is accurate. Any uneven areas of occlusion are adjusted with an acrylic bur in a handpiece. The patient and dentist also check the esthetics of the appliance. The dentist also checks for pressure points on the tissue side of the denture with pressure indicating paste (PIP; Figure 42-24). This paste is placed evenly and thinly inside of the denture, and the denture is then inserted into the oral cavity. Any areas of pressure result in the paste being erased from those areas. The dentist adjusts these areas with a low-speed straight handpiece and an acrylic bur. Some states allow EFDAs to perform minor adjustments to the removable partial denture. The dentist also

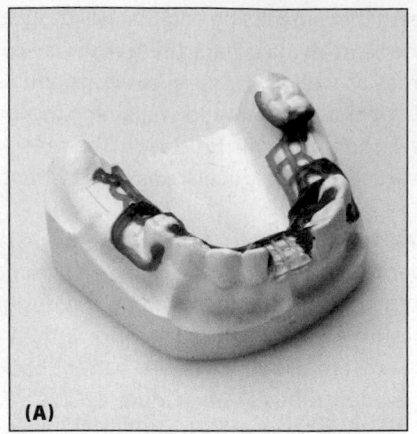

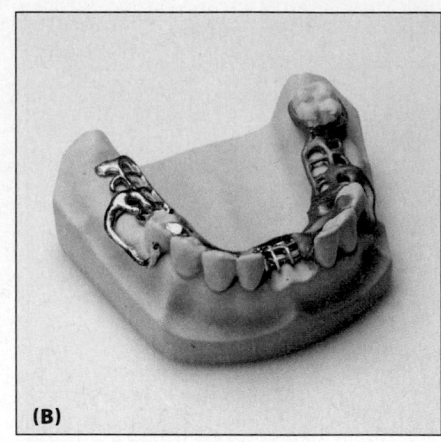

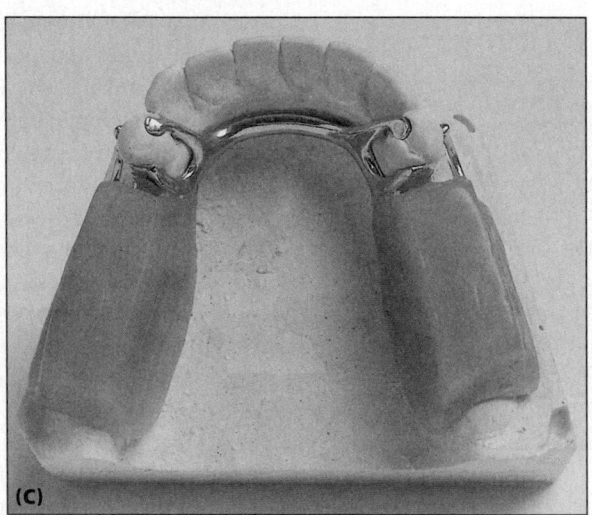

FIGURE 42-22

(A) Wax-up of a partial denture. (B) Metal framework made from wax-up of partial. (C) Metal framework with wax bite rims ready for placement of the denture teeth.

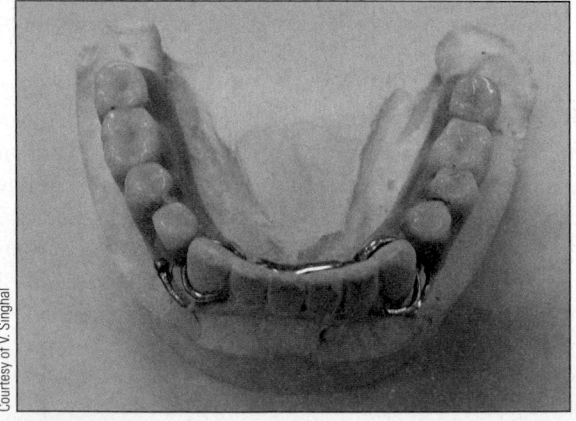

FIGURE 42-23

Partial denture framework and wax saddles with teeth for try-in.

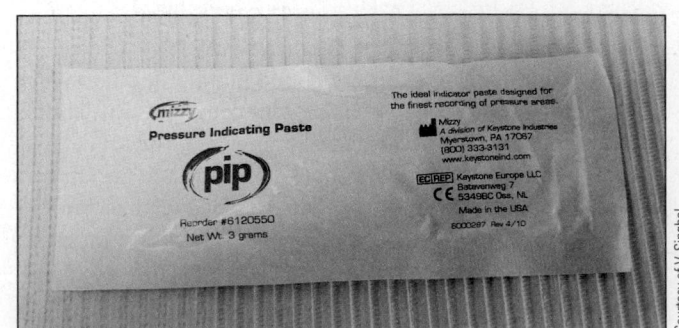

FIGURE 42-24

Pressure indicating paste.

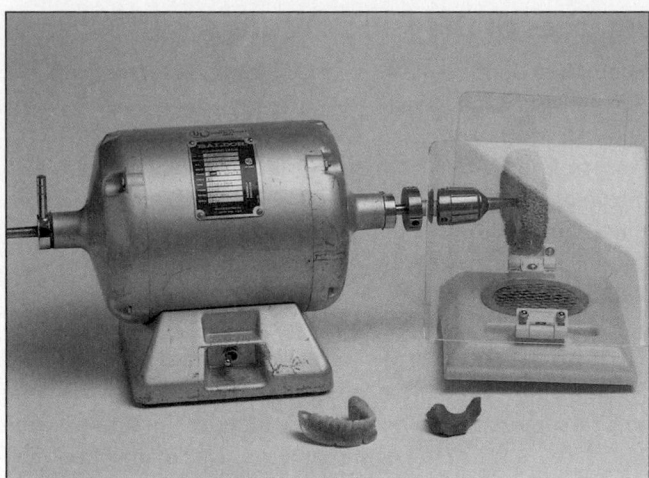

FIGURE 42-25
Dental lathe with rag wheel and Tripoli to polish prosthesis.

requests the patient to practice inserting and removing the RPD to increase the patient's confidence in using the appliance. Once all adjustments have been completed, the dental assistant polishes the partial in the nontissue side areas that were adjusted. The polishing is completed with the use of a dental lathe, a rag wheel, and Tripoli polishing compound (Figure 42-25). The dental assistant gives the patient home care instructions before the patient leaves the office.

Home Care Instructions The dental assistant provides the oral and written home care instruction. The dental assistant makes sure that the patient understands the instructions by asking the patient open-ended questions and allowing the patient to ask any questions. In areas with a significant population of bilingual patients, it is advised to have the home care instructions printed both in English and in other spoken language(s). Box 42-4 outlines sample instructions provided to patients regarding care of an RPD.

Postdelivery Care Over time the edentulous ridge will resorb, resulting in decreased retention of the partial denture. Loss of retention and movement of the partial may result in sore spots. Regular postdelivery examinations of the existing natural teeth and the edentulous ridge as well as the appliance are important in maintaining oral health. Regular postdelivery visits will allow the dentist to tighten any loose clasps and reline as needed.

Role of the Dental Assistant in Removable Partial Denture Procedures

The registered dental assistant performs many important functions during removable partial denture procedures. Some of the functions delegable by the dental assistant are dependent upon each state's scope of practice. The functions may include: preparation of the operatory and the patient, obtaining of all necessary medical and dental information, recording of vital signs, and obtaining all radiographs prescribed by the dentist. Additionally, the dental assistant can take alginate impressions, select the

BOX 42-4 Patient Instructions for Care of a Removable Partial Denture

- The denture should be handled with care when cleaning. Clean the denture while standing over a folded towel placed on a countertop or over a sink of water in case the denture is accidentally dropped.

- Food and plaque can build up on the denture, so it should be brushed daily. Ideally, a denture brush should be used. However, a standard, soft-bristled toothbrush may also be used. A brush with hard bristles can damage the denture and should be avoided.

- Purchase denture cleansers with the American Dental Association (ADA) Seal of Acceptance. These have been evaluated for safety and effectiveness. Moisten the brush and apply the denture cleaner. Be sure to brush all surfaces of the denture. Be gentle to avoid damaging the appliance. Standard household cleaners and many toothpastes are abrasive and may scratch or damage the denture. These should not be used to clean a denture.

- After eating, remove dentures from mouth and brush or rinse all parts of the appliance.

- A denture could warp if it is not kept moist. At night, the denture should be placed in an ADA-approved soaking solution or water.

- Be sure to brush and floss your natural teeth to keep them clean from food buildup and plaque. It is important to maintain your natural dentition.

- Your denture is fabricated to fit your mouth. Over time, the soft tissues and the bone that support your denture may shrink and the denture may become loose. Loose appliances can cause irritations in your mouth. Persistent irritation can result in infections. You should return to the office so we can check the appliance.

- If your denture breaks or if a denture tooth comes out, contact your dentist. Attempting to repair yourself may do more damage, and it may not be possible to repair the appliance. It is important to see your dentist annually for an exam and to check the partial denture.

- It will take time for the muscles of your mouth and face to adjust to the new appliance. Start training the muscles by eating soft food first, and then progress to your normal diet. Avoid foods that are sticky and hard.

- The muscles of your face and mouth and tongue need to learn to talk with a new appliance. Practice repeating difficult words several times. Also talk and read out loud so your muscles get used to the new appliance.

shade of the denture teeth, and perform bite registration procedures. The dental assistant can provide dietary analysis, postdelivery instructions, and clinical instruction that can promote oral health. Please refer to your state scope of practice regulations regarding delegable functions.

Full Dentures

Full or complete dentures are removable prosthetic appliances for people who are completely edentulous in one or both arches. Dentures today are not only esthetic but comfortable and functional as well. They are similar in appearance to natural teeth and aid in improving smiles and facial appearance. Dentures improve speech and mastication of food. Accurate impressions and measurements are obtained to create the custom fit dentures.

Treatment planning for full dentures requires a thorough dental examination and medical history review. Additionally, a discussion with the patient regarding their expectations for dental treatment is important in determining the success of dental treatment and full dentures. Box 42-5 provides a list of indications for full dentures. Box 42-6 provides contraindications for full dentures.

Patients receive complete or full dentures when they are edentulous in one or both the arches. The prosthesis is similar to an RPD, except that the full denture will replace all of the teeth in the edentulous arch. Generally, complete or full dentures are fabricated for geriatric patients. Some young patients who are born edentulous or who are born with congenital malformations of the dentition may also benefit from complete dentures. It is important to have a thorough knowledge about the various parts of a complete denture. A complete denture has three surfaces and four component parts.

BOX 42-5 Indications for Full Dentures

- The patient is edentulous in one or both the arches.
- The existing teeth have extensive decay or periodontal disease and cannot be restored.
- Any remaining natural teeth are in poor condition due to decay or periodontal disease and cannot support a removable partial denture.
- The patient is unable or unwilling to maintain implants or an implant supported denture.
- Patient has significant bone loss in maxilla and/or mandible.
- The patient does not have the financial resources for implants or implant supported dentures.

BOX 42-6 Contraindications for Full Dentures

- Removable partial dentures, if possible, are a better option
- Disabilities (physical, emotional, mental) that may not allow for full dentures
- Excessively large tori
- Patient would not accept the denture due to esthetic concerns
- Allergy or sensitivity to denture materials
- Patient does not have desire to replace missing teeth
- Severe gag reflex

Surfaces of the Full Denture

A complete denture has three main surfaces, each of which is different visually and functionally.

Tissue Surface The tissue surface of the denture is also known as the impression surface. The final impression determines the profile of the denture contour (Figure 42-6). This surface will be in contact with the soft tissues when the denture is seated in the oral cavity.

Polished Surface The polished surface of a denture (Figure 42-26) extends from the border of the denture toward the occlusal surface. The polished surface includes the external palatal surface (Figure 42-26) of the denture as well as the buccal and lingual surfaces of the teeth. This polished surface includes the external lingual, buccal, and labial flanges (Figure 42-26). Flanges will be discussed in detail later in this section. A well-polished, smooth surface is resistant to the collection of food debris.

Occlusal Surface The occlusal surface is the portion of the denture that contacts with the occlusal surfaces of the opposing

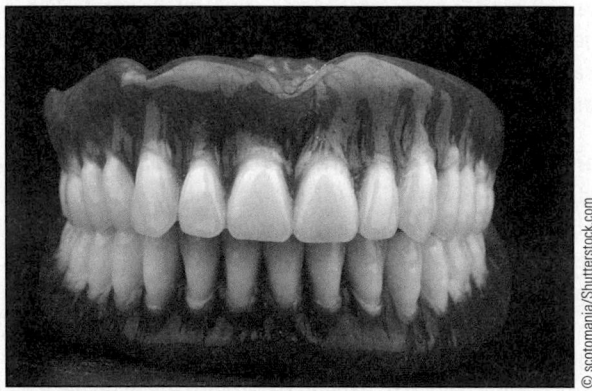

FIGURE 42-26A
Polished surface of dentures.

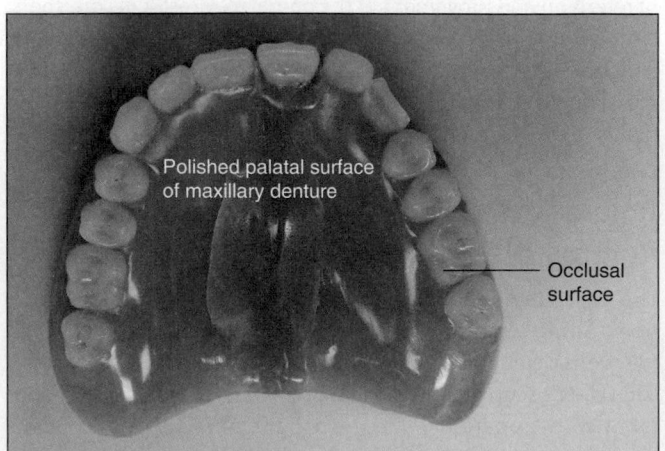

FIGURE 42-26B
Polished palatal surface and occlusal surface of a maxillary denture.

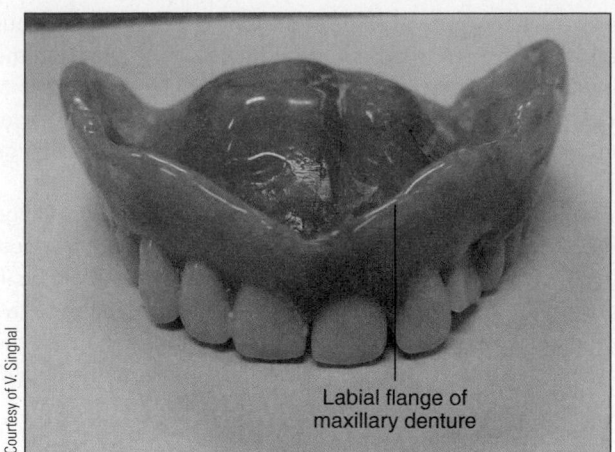

Courtesy of V. Singhal

Labial flange of maxillary denture

FIGURE 42-26C
Labial flange.

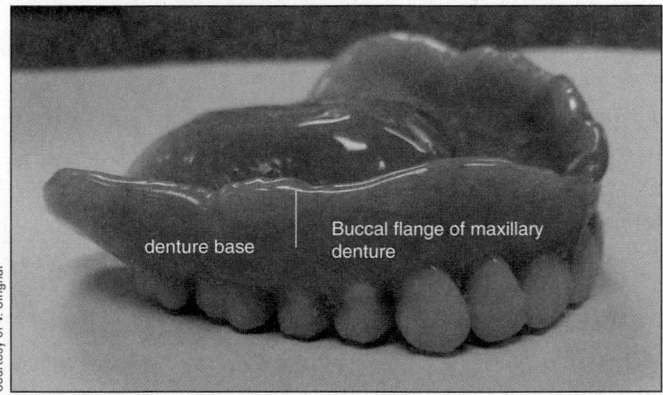

Courtesy of V. Singhal

denture base

Buccal flange of maxillary denture

FIGURE 42-26D
Denture base and buccal flange.

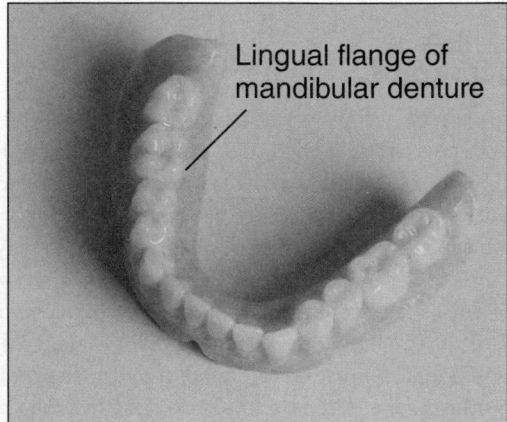

Lingual flange of mandibular denture

FIGURE 42-26E
Lingual flange.

arch (Figure 42-26B). The occlusal surface of the denture teeth resembles the natural teeth and contains sluiceways to aid in mastication.

Components of a Full Denture

The denture base is made up of several components, each of which is important to the function and/or esthetics of the denture.

Denture Base   The denture base is the acrylic portion of the denture that replaces the gingival soft tissues and the alveolar ridge (Figure 42-26D). The denture base is fabricated to fit over the residual alveolar ridge and surrounding gingival soft tissues. The acrylic material is made from a powder called polymethylmethacrylate (PMMA). The acrylic is available in different shades to match the varying shades of gingival tissue based on different skin tones. The external surface of the full denture extends over the retromolar pad on the mandibular arch and the maxillary tuberosity area on the maxillary arch (Figure 42-27).

The denture base helps to disperse the forces that act on the denture teeth to the tissues. This part of the full denture is responsible for retention and support. The denture base may be made up of all acrylic or a metal framework inserted in the acrylic for additional strength (Figure 42-28). The metal part of the denture base can be fabricated using gold or chromium alloys. Gold is rarely used today due to the high cost. The selected artificial teeth are then added to the denture base during processing.

Denture Border   The denture border is the edge of the denture base where the polished surface and the tissue surface meet (Figure 42-26C). In a maxillary denture, the border is responsible

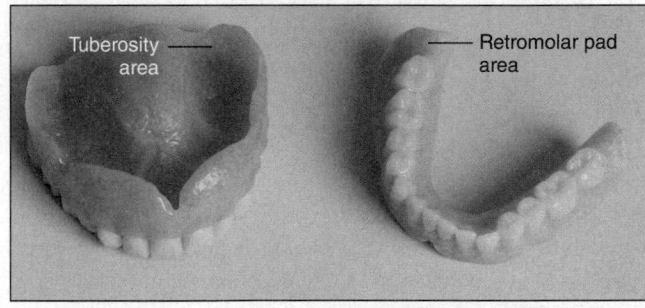

Tuberosity area

Retromolar pad area

FIGURE 42-27
Tuberosity and retromolar pad areas of a maxillary and mandibular denture respectively.

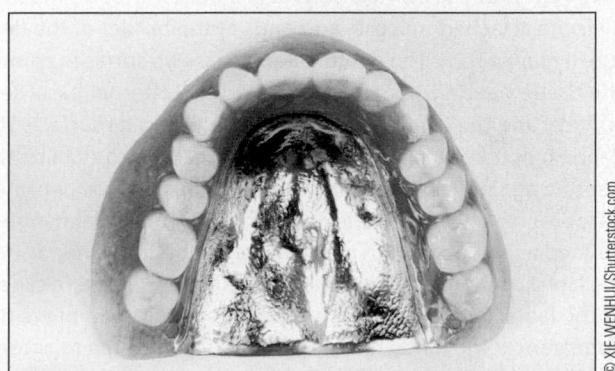

© XIE WENHUI/Shutterstock.com

FIGURE 42-28
Maxillary full denture with metal for strength.

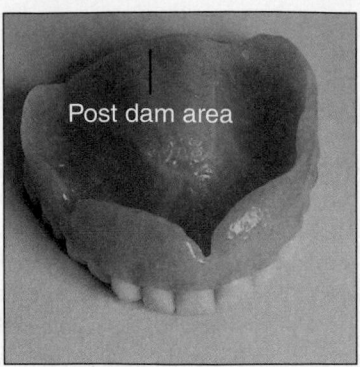

FIGURE 42-29
Post dam area of maxillary denture.

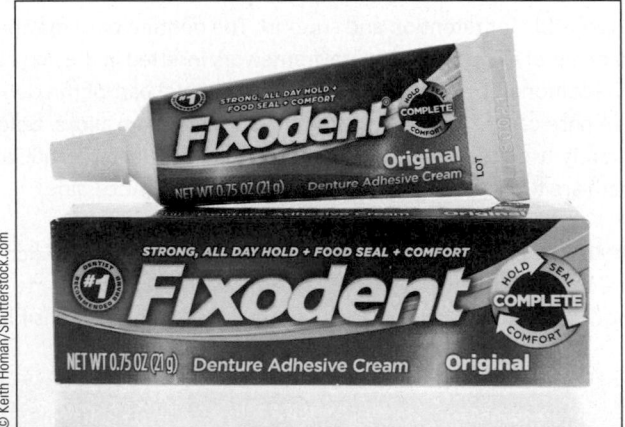

© Keith Homan/Shutterstock.com

FIGURE 42-30
Dental adhesive.

for the **peripheral seal**. The denture border should be smooth and without sharp edges to prevent trauma to the soft tissue. Denture borders that are too long or overextended can cause hyperplastic tissue changes such as epulis fissuratum (refer to Figure 9-30). However, the border should not be short or under-extended as the peripheral seal may not be adequate.

Denture Flange The flange is the vertical part of the base that begins at the cervical area of the denture teeth, expands over the attached mucosa, and ends at the border of the denture (Figure 42-26). The denture flange has two surfaces, namely the tissue bearing surface, also called the internal basal seat surface, and the external labial or external lingual surface. The flange functions to provide a peripheral seal and to stabilize the denture against horizontal movements. The flanges are named based on the vestibule they extend into. The labial flange is defined as the portion of the denture flange that extends into the labial portion of the oral cavity (Figure 42-26). The thickness of the labial flange provides support to the lip to improve the appearance. The labial flange has a V-shaped notch to accommodate the labial frenum.

The buccal flange is the portion of the denture flange that extends into the buccal vestibule of the oral cavity (Figure 42-26).

The buccal flange provides support to the cheeks in edentulous patients, thus restoring the natural fullness of the face. In the mandibular denture, the buccal flange disperses the occlusal forces to the broad flat bone buccal to the teeth in the posterior mandibular area. Relief should be provided in the buccal flange for the buccal frenum.

The lingual flange is the part of the mandibular denture flange that extends into the space between the tongue and the lingual surfaces of the mandibular teeth (Figure 42-26). It should be in contact with the floor of the mouth to provide stability to the denture. An overextended or long lingual flange can cause the mandibular denture to dislodge when the muscles of the floor of the mouth are activated.

Post Dam Retention of a maxillary denture depends on the seal with the palate. The post dam is the posterior edge of the maxillary denture (Figure 42-29). It is also known as the postpalatal seal. It helps to maintain the denture through suction. It is important to obtain this area in the final impression of the full denture. The appointment steps and impression techniques for full dentures will be discussed later in this chapter.

Artificial Teeth Artificial teeth for full dentures are similar to those for partial dentures and are the anatomical substitute for natural teeth. Refer to the information provided earlier regarding artificial teeth.

Advantages

Full dentures provide a great smile with a natural appearance. They are made of durable materials and can last for many years with proper care. Dentures typically last from 5 to 10 years, after which they need repair or replacement. Full dentures can correct several problems affecting speech and the ability to masticate.

Disadvantages

Full dentures take time to get used to. There may be initial speech concerns to overcome as the tongue and the lips have to get used to something new in the oral cavity. These speech concerns usually last only a couple of days. The patient also needs to remove and clean the denture regularly. Oral sores may occur initially, and the dentures may need to be adjusted in the areas of the sore spots. The patient should return to the office for adjustments. The patient should be reminded that the dentures must be cleaned and also must be removed at night. The oral cavity changes over the life of the dentures, so dentures may need to be relined or replaced to achieve a better fit. A person with a denture has less than 25% chewing efficiency as compared to a person who chews with their natural teeth. In the case of a full maxillary denture, the palate is covered, which can reduce taste of foods and the sensations of hot or cold. In some cases, denture wearers may need to use adhesive to keep the denture in place (Figure 42-30).

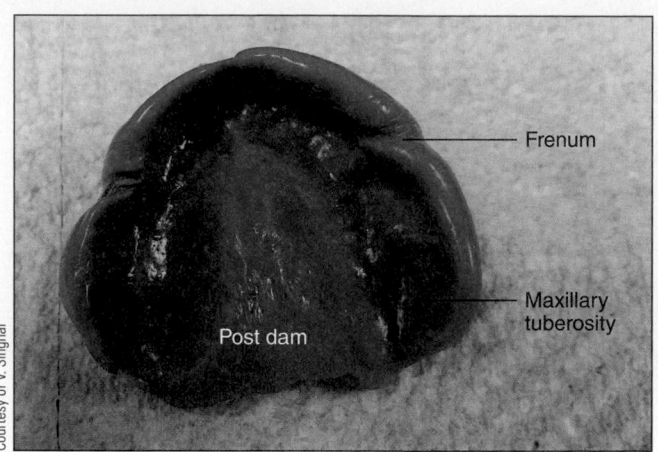

FIGURE 42-31
Maxillary denture final impression with post dam area and frenum attachments.

Courtesy of V. Singhal

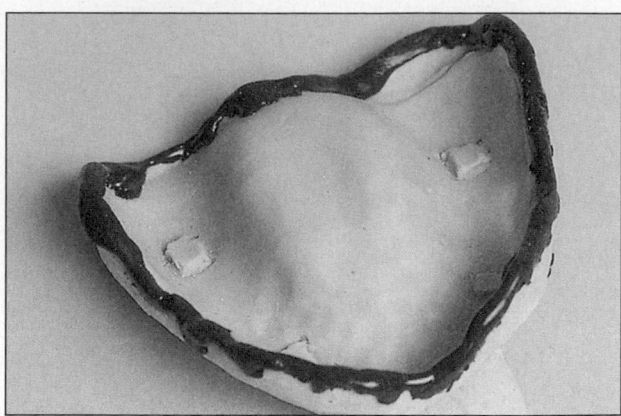

FIGURE 42-32
Custom tray that has been border molded to fit patient for the final impression.

Appointments and Procedures for Full Dentures

Similar to partial dentures, the process of making a full denture involves a series of appointments. Impressions are needed, and models are poured from the impressions; the models are then used to fabricate the full dentures by the dental technician in a dental laboratory. After try-ins and adjustments, the dentures are finished and inserted, and home care instructions are provided to the patient. Prior to the initial appointment for full denture fabrication, radiographs are obtained to check on the health of the alveolar bone. The oral tissues are also examined, and the shape of the face and skin color may be used to determine the shade and shape of the artificial teeth.

Consultation and Examinations
In the first appointment for denture fabrication, the medical and dental histories of the patient are updated. Any necessary radiographs and intraoral photographs are obtained. An intraoral and extraoral exam is completed and a treatment plan is finalized. In certain cases, oral surgery may be required prior to denture fabrication. This may be to remove any tori that may interfere with the denture or to remove any remaining teeth prior to denture placement.

The dentist must provide the patient with all the facts about the new denture. This includes the advantages and disadvantages outlined earlier so the patient knows what to expect prior to the start of treatment.

The patient may be a candidate for an immediate denture. This would be treatment planned and discussed with the patient. Regardless of the type of denture, there is a sequence of visits; each of these are outlined below.

At each visit, a step in the denture fabrication process is completed and the case is then sent to the dental laboratory. The laboratory completes the procedure requested by the office and then send the case back to the dental office for the subsequent visit.

It generally takes five visits to the dental office to complete denture fabrication from the preliminary impressions to the insertion of the appliance. This section will provide the details of each visit.

First and Second Visits
At the first visit for denture fabrication, preliminary alginate impressions are obtained for both arches. Even if a denture is going to be fabricated for only one arch, a preliminary alginate impression should be obtained of the opposing arch in order to mount the casts on an articulator based on the patient's centric relation. Refer to Chapter 33 regarding how to obtain an ideal alginate impression. The study casts are sent to the dental lab with a lab prescription for a custom tray for each arch that will be receiving a full denture.

Digital Impressions
The use of digital impressions is growing quickly. Digital impressions can be used to fabricate dentures. Refer to Chapter 41 regarding digital impressions.

Once the office has the custom trays, the final impression of the gingiva and edentulous ridges is taken by using zinc oxide eugenol paste, elastomeric impression materials or alginate (Figure 42-31). In this final impression, landmarks of the dental arches are accurately reproduced. The final impression is obtained after border molding is completed. Border molding allows the dentist to capture all of the details of the soft tissues (Figure 42-32). Maxillary impressions should include the hamular notches, the post dam area, the right and left tuberosities, and the frenum attachments (Figure 42-31). The mandibular impressions should include the right and left retromolar pads, the mylohyoid ridge on both sides, the oblique ridge on both sides, the genial tubercles in the anterior area, as well as the frena. If an alginate impression is taken, the stone model must be fabricated immediately to avoid distortion of the impression.

Post Dam Area
The post dam is at the posterior of a maxillary full denture to accomplish a complete seal between denture and tissues (Figure 42-29). The shape of the posterior palatal seal

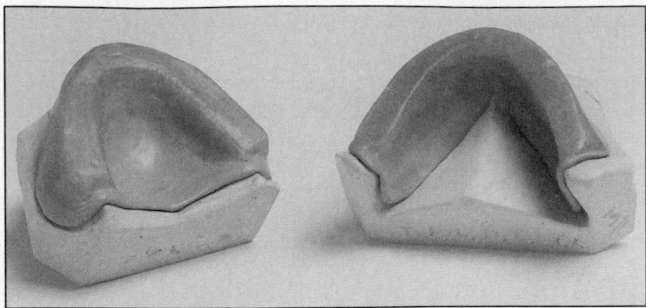

FIGURE 42-33
Baseplates and bite rims made in dental laboratory from final impressions.

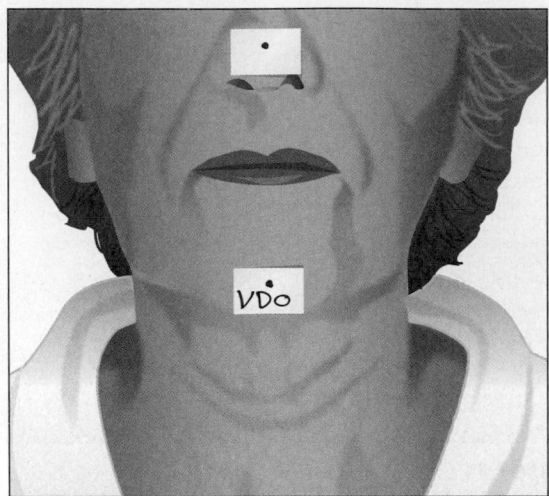

FIGURE 42-35
Patient with tape markings placed to determine vertical dimension occlusion (VDO).

varies from patient to patient. It is important to obtain the anatomy of this area in the impression to ensure that the maxillary denture has retention (Figure 42-31). Prior to the third visit, the dental laboratory fabricates a denture baseplate and wax rim (Figure 42-33) on the model fabricated from the final impression.

Third Visit The wax rims represent the teeth. At this appointment the wax rims are adjusted to the correct lip drape and so the correct amount of teeth and gingival tissue are visible when the patient smiles. At this appointment, centric relation, facebow transfer, and teeth selection are also completed. The baseplate and rim are used to obtain the centric relation for articulation of the final dental models. The rims are used by the lab for placement of denture teeth while the models are mounted on the articulator (Figure 42-34). The wax is available in the form of wax sheets or horseshoe-shaped wax rims.

The dentist inserts the baseplate and rims into the oral cavity and records the vertical dimension of occlusion (Figure 42-35). The midline is marked on the wax rim, and the centric relation is obtained. The shade and mold of teeth is also selected.

The facebow record is an important procedure designed to mount the maxillary cast on the articulator. The facebow allows the placement of the maxillary cast on the articulator in the same position as the maxilla is in the patient. Refer to Chapter 33 regarding the steps in completing a facebow transfer.

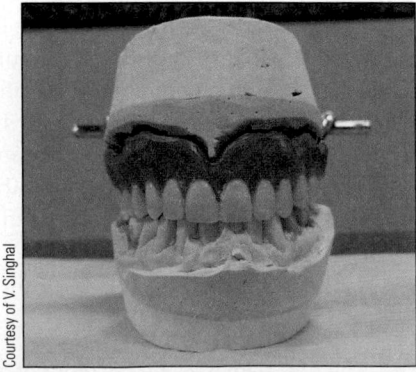

FIGURE 42-34
Maxillary denture with teeth in wax on articulator.

All of this information is sent to the lab to allow the laboratory technician to mount the final models based on the patient's centric relation and facebow transfer. In some offices, the dental assistant may use the facebow transfer and the centric relation to mount the models on the articulator. Once the models are mounted, the laboratory technician sets the teeth into the wax rims and sends the articulated models with the setup back to the office for the try-in by the patient.

Fourth Visit At the fourth visit, the patient tries the dentures while the teeth are in wax (Figure 42-34). Once the dentures are inserted in the oral cavity, the dentist checks the smile line to ensure that the edge of the maxillary anterior teeth is visible and that the maxillary midline is centered. The dentist also verifies centric relation and then asks the patient to pronounce certain words or to read a paragraph that has been provided. The dentist focuses on the "f," "v," "th," and "s" sounds. This allows the dentist to check that the patient is able to pronounce sounds correctly. Once all of the above have been confirmed and the patient is satisfied with the esthetics, the denture is returned to the lab for finishing and processing into acrylic (refer to Figure 42-16). If any adjustments need to be made to the denture, the setup should be returned to the laboratory technician with specifics on what needs to be corrected. The denture should then be returned for another try-in visit. Try-ins should be completed until the denture is correct and the patient is satisfied. Changes cannot be made once the denture is processed and teeth are in acrylic, so it is important to make any needed changes while the teeth are in wax.

Fifth Visit The fifth visit is the insertion visit. The patient presents to the office, and the finished and processed dentures (Figure 42-26A) are inserted. The dentist checks centric relation at this visit and makes minor adjustments if needed with a straight handpiece and an acrylic bur. A warm number 7 spatula may also be used to soften the wax and slightly move the teeth if needed. The patient is asked to swallow, chew, and speak, using "f," "v," "th," and "s" sounds. The dentist also checks to see that the denture extends into the mucobuccal fold and is not too long. Areas that are long can cause sore spots on the soft tissues and should be adjusted. Pressure indicator paste (PIP) is used to check the tissue side of the denture for pressure spots that may irritate the gingival soft tissue; these areas are adjusted as needed as well. After adjustments have been made, the nontissue side of the denture should be polished

<hr>

BOX 42-7 Polishing a Denture (Expanded Function)

- Pumice nontissue acrylic surfaces of dentures using pumice brushes.
- Do not polish the denture teeth.
- Use pumice and rag wheel to polish peripheries.
- Obtain a high shine with acrylic polish and dry wheel.
- If scratches are visible after high shine, go back to pumice.

<hr>

BOX 42-8 Postinsertion Home Care Instructions for Dentures

- Initially, a new denture may feel strange in your mouth. The cheeks, lips, and tongue need time to adapt to the new dentures.
- It will take a little time to learn to chew food with the new dentures. Start by slowly chewing on very small pieces of soft food. Food should be placed on both sides of the mouth at the same time. This will prevent the denture from becoming unbalanced. Once you are comfortable with small pieces of soft food, you can progress to larger pieces of soft food and then to harder foods. You may not be able to bite into foods with the front teeth as this may cause the denture to dislodge.
- Speaking will also require practice. Your tongue needs to get used to the new appliance. The adjustment period is about 2 weeks. Practice reading aloud so you can adjust to the new appliance.
- Denture adhesives are usually not needed with well-fitting dentures. The lower denture will not have the suction that the upper denture has. Keeping the lower denture balanced is important. Be sure to chew on both sides at the same time. The muscles of the cheeks and tongue also help to keep the denture in position. The lower denture may need some adhesive.
- Remember to thoroughly rinse the oral tissues at least once daily. You can also gently brush your gums.
- Thoroughly clean all surfaces of a denture with a denture brush and mild cleanser made for cleaning dentures. Clean the adhesive out of the dentures at the end of each day.
- Dentures should not be worn when sleeping.
- When dentures are not in the mouth, they must be stored in a container with water to prevent them from drying and warping.

to ensure that it is smooth. Box 42-7 provides the steps in polishing a denture.

Home Care Instructions The dental assistant provides home instructions verbally and in writing. These are outlined in Box 42-8.

Postdelivery Care The patient should be scheduled to see the dentist 24 hours after insertion of the new dentures. Several postdelivery visits may be needed to adjust the dentures if the patient is experiencing sore spots on the gingival tissue caused by the denture rubbing in some areas.

Role of the Dental Assistant in Full Denture Procedures

The registered dental assistant performs many important functions during removable partial denture procedures. Some of the functions delegable to the dental assistant depend upon each individual state's scope of practice. These functions may include preparation of the operatory and the patient, obtaining a detailed medical and dental history, and obtaining all radiographs prescribed by the dentist. Additionally, the dental assistant can take preliminary alginate impressions, select the shade of the denture teeth, perform bite registration procedures, and polish the denture after adjustments have been made. The dental assistant can also provide dietary counseling and oral home care instruction. Refer to your state's scope of practice regarding delegable functions.

Healthy Oral Environment

Success of complete and removable partial dentures requires a healthy oral cavity. Dental professionals must be aware of the signs and symptoms of denture related problems as well as how to determine the cause of the problem and how to manage the problem. The need for removable prosthodontic services is increasing with the growth of the aging population. Associated with a growing population of older individuals is the rise in the consumption of prescription medications by older patients. Many U.S. adults consume at least one medication and may take multiple drugs. Many of these medications cause oral side effects.

Xerostomic Denture Wearers

A common side effect of many common prescription medications is xerostomia. Refer to Chapter 14 for medications that cause xerostomia. Consult with the patient's physician regarding possible drug substitutions or elimination. Dental assistants play a key role in effective communication with the patient on this topic as well as with communication between the dentist and the patient's pharmacy. Denture retention is important to patient acceptance of the prosthesis and successful function. Saliva plays an important role in retention of the dental prosthesis, particularly for the maxillary full denture. For appropriate retention, the saliva layer between the mucosa and the tissue side of the denture must be thin.

- Difficulty with speech
- Upon oral examination, the mouth mirror may stick to the oral mucosa
- Cracking of vermillion border of lips
- Angular chelitis
- Tongue coated with food and plaque debris
- Irritations and sores along denture supported tissues
- Retained natural may be decayed
- Patient frequently stops to moisten lips

When considering removable prosthodontic treatment of xerostomic patients, the office should communicate with the laboratory so the denture is designed in a manner that provides excellent retention. Dentures that include metal bases provide better retention than the all acrylic dentures (Figure 42-28).

A detailed medical history can reveal the risks and causes of xerostomia. Upon clinical examination of the patients with xerostomia, the dentist may notice the findings outlined in Box 42-9. Refer to Chapters 9 and 14 for methods of managing xerostomia.

Denture Sore Spots

Sore spots from dentures may occur due to pressure or rubbing at a particular site. Sore spots can lead to discomfort, difficulty with chewing and speech, as well as excess saliva production because of the presence of the dentures. Additionally, candidiasis is a fungal infection common in denture wearers, especially those with xerostomia. Sore spots require an adjustment of the dentures by the dentist. Patients are advised to see the dentist immediately and to not stop wearing the new dentures as the sore spots show when the denture is in use. These provide a visual guide for the dentist regarding areas to be adjusted. Sore spots may also develop when dentures have become loose due to bone resorption. Loose dentures can place pressure on certain areas and may need to be relined by a dentist.

A dental assistant educates the denture patient about appropriate oral hygiene techniques. The dental assistant advises the patient to rinse the oral cavity with warm salt water as it can alleviate some of the tenderness of any sore spots present. This is contraindicated in patients who have hypertension. The patient is also advised to avoid eating foods that may irritate sore spots, such as acidic foods and spicy foods.

For controlling the discomfort related to denture sores, the dentist may prescribe topical anesthetic creams or ointments and antimicrobial mouth rinses. If candidiasis is present, the systemic antifungal treatment of choice is fluconazole (Diflucan).

Topical treatment of the soft tissues that support the denture is managed by placing an antifungal cream on the tissue surface of the denture before the patient inserts the denture. Refer to Chapter 14 for information regarding topical oral antifungal agents.

Denture Adhesives

In some cases, a denture adhesive may be needed to aid in retention (refer to Figure 42-30). With proper use, adhesives:

- allow saliva to be more adhesive.
- fill any previous voids that may have been present between the tissue surface of the denture and the soft tissues.
- decrease soft tissue irritation.
- reduce the impaction of food under the base of the denture.
- improve chewing ability.

There are several types of denture adhesives to choose from, and many of them are zinc-free. A dental professional can educate the patient about which denture cream, strip, or powder is right for them and that well-fitting dentures do not need an adhesive. The patient should be advised that a small amount of adhesive should be used. If a large or thick amount of paste is required for retention, then a reline may be indicated.

Denture Relining

Over time, the denture may need to be relined, **rebased**, or remade due to normal wear. This may be necessary due to the natural progression of aging. The edentulous ridge recedes over time, causing the dentures to become loose and make chewing and talking more difficult for the patient. The recession of the bone can even change the facial features. Both reline and rebase are discussed in this section.

A denture reline is completed by adding a thin layer of denture acrylic to the denture and placing it into the oral cavity. The patient then bites gently on the denture, and the material fills in the empty space between the denture and the soft tissues to provide a better fit once it is cured. The need for a reline varies from patient to patient, but most dentists recommend relining every 2 years. There are three main types of denture relines.

1. **Temporary reline.** This type of relining is performed using a medicated relining material to soothe and heal gingival swelling and inflammation. Once the tissues heal and the inflammation improves, a new denture can be fabricated or a hard reline can be completed.

2. **Soft reline.** This type of reline is completed using a soft material that is flexible and lasts for approximately 2 years before needing replacement. It is used in cases of oral irritations caused by the denture. It is similar to a temporary reline but lasts longer.

3. **Hard reline.** This type of reline usually is prescribed on full sets of dentures and can be completed by an indirect or direct method.

Direct Relining In the direct relining technique, a chairside acrylic material is used to take an impression of the tissues of the arch where the denture is placed. The material bonds to the tissue surface of the denture. These materials are not very durable and are only a short term solution. This procedure is completed by the dentist. In this technique, the tissue surface of the denture is cleaned and then made slightly rough with an acrylic bur. The denture flanges are slightly reduced to prevent overextension of the flanges. The reline material is then mixed and applied to the tissue surface of the denture based on manufacturer's instructions. The denture is then inserted in the oral cavity, and the patient is asked to bite gently on the denture. This ensures that the occlusion is not altered by the reline procedure. While the material is soft and not yet set, border molding is completed. The denture is kept in place for about 5 minutes, after which it is removed and carefully examined. Depending on the type of material used, the denture may need to be placed in a hydroflask to complete the curing process. The end product is a better fitting and more comfortable denture due to its new and well-adapted fitting surface. Since this type of reline is completed at chairside, the patient receives the denture back within a short period of time.

Indirect Relining In the indirect relining technique, the tissue surface is cleaned and made rough with an acrylic bur. The flanges are slightly reduced by the dentist. A wash impression is then obtained using the tissue surface of the denture as a custom tray. The impression materials may be zinc oxide eugenol paste or an elastomeric impression material, and the patient is asked to bite gently on the denture. This impression is then disinfected and sent to the dental laboratory along with a completed lab prescription. In the laboratory the lab technician replaces the impression paste with heat-cured acrylic, which lasts longer than the materials used for direct relines. Although the indirect method involves more time than the direct reline method, it provides a more durable and longer lasting reline.

At Home Relining There are some over-the-counter relining kits available with instructions so patients may reline their dentures themselves at home. These kits are inexpensive as compared to the in-office or lab relining procedures but can lead to problems. Uneven relining can cause an occlusion that is not balanced, resulting in uneven chewing forces. This can result in TMJ pain due to inconsistent pressure on the joint. If the relining performed at home is not smooth on the tissue surface of the denture, gingival sores can result.

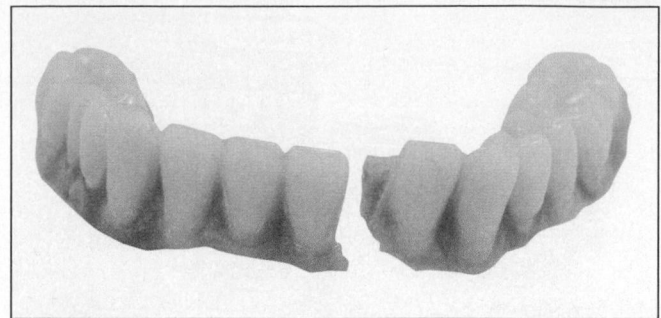

FIGURE 42-36
Mandibular denture in need of repair.

Denture Rebasing

Denture rebasing is the process of refitting a denture by replacing the denture base material without changing the occlusion of the denture teeth. Denture rebasing is a less common practice in prosthodontics as compared to relining. During rebasing the dentures have to stay with the dentist or lab for about one to three days. The technique for rebasing is similar to that of relining. The exception is that the laboratory technician will remove the palate of the maxillary denture and create a new one in wax prior to processing the denture. Over time, relines cause the palate to increase in thickness. A rebase can be performed to reduce this palatal thickness. Rebasing a denture is more complex than relining a denture. In many cases, a new denture is a better option than rebasing an existing denture.

Denture Repair

A denture repair is replacing or repairing broken, missing, or worn parts of a denture (Figure 42-36). A denture repair can be performed in a dental office by the dentist or a trained dental assistant or in a dental lab by a technician. A denture can be temporarily fixed by the patient with a store bought repair kit.

In the office, the dentist examines the broken denture and determines if any impression of the patient's oral cavity is needed. The dentist then instructs the dental assistant on what is required to complete the repair. Some dentures may break in such a way that they cannot be repaired. In that case, a new denture is recommended.

Denture Cleaners

Denture cleansers come in various formulations such as creams, pastes, gels, and tablets that are designed to clean both full dentures and removable partial dentures (RPD). Denture cleaning tablets are added into warm water to create an effervescent solution (Figure 42-37). Denture cleaning creams, pastes,

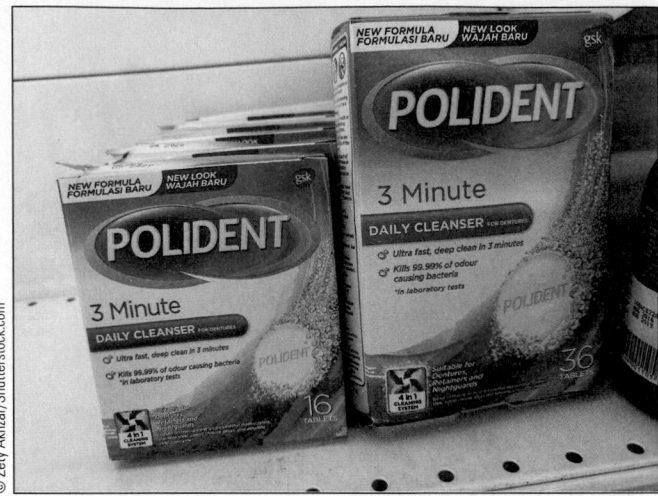

FIGURE 42-37
Effervescent denture cleaner.

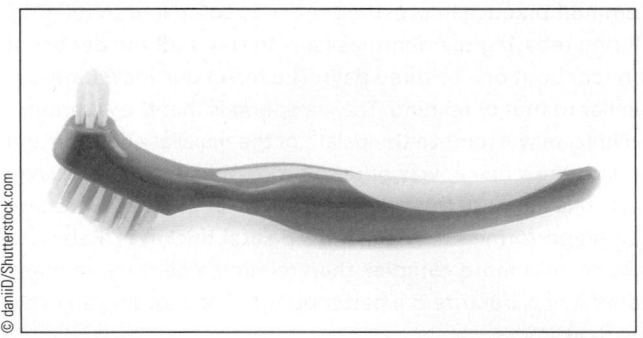

FIGURE 42-38
Denture brush.

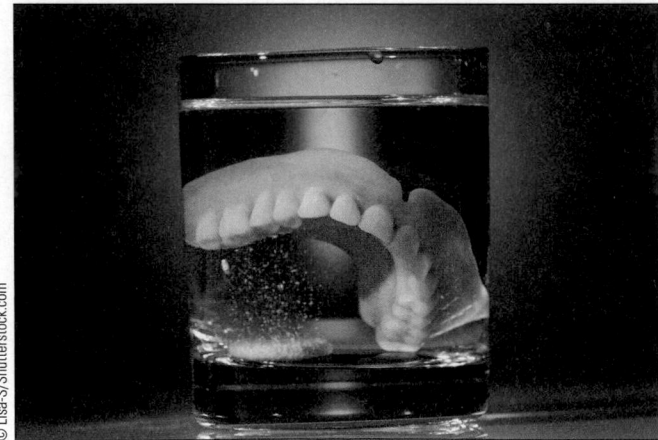

FIGURE 42-39
Denture being cleaned in water with the use of denture cleaning tablet.

or gels are brushed on the denture after it is removed from the oral cavity. The dentures are then rinsed to remove the cleaning agent. There are also mechanical denture cleaners such as

denture brushes (Figure 42-38) and ultrasonic denture cleaners for home use.

Soaking dentures in the ADA-approved denture cleaners following the manufacturer's instruction helps kill germs that can cause odor (Figure 42-39).

The dental assistant advises the patient that dentures should receive the same care as natural teeth; dentures should be brushed daily to remove food particles and bacteria. Brushing also removes stains from the denture. When cleaning dentures, the patient should be instructed to first rinse the dentures to remove any food particles. Next, residual denture adhesive should also be removed from the denture and the oral cavity. The patient is advised to moisten the brush and apply the preferred denture cleaner and the brush gently to every surface of the denture.

Patients should be warned to not use abrasive powdered household cleansers, which can damage a denture, or bleach, which may cause the pink portion of the denture to become white. After brushing the denture, it should be placed in water or a denture cleanser solution to prevent it from drying and warping when not in the patient's oral cavity. Patients are advised to not to place dentures in hot water, as this could cause them to warp.

Charting for Removable Prosthodontics

Dental charting provides a visual of the conditions in a patient's oral cavity. This includes the presence of disease such as decay, missing teeth, and periodontal disease as well as any restorations that are present. Dental charting is used by dental practitioners to determine the patient's level of dental health. Charting should be updated at each visit. Additionally, notes should be maintained related to the patient's home care.

The dentist, hygienist, expanded function dental auxiliary, or assistant can complete dental charting. Charting may be completed on paper dental charting forms or on computer software as part of the electronic dental record. Dental hygienists normally enter charting as part of the initial or periodic periodontal exam.

Charting Abbreviations

On a manual charting system, blue pencil is usually used to mark the missing teeth and existing restorations, and red pencil is usually used to mark the problem areas and the proposed treatment. The computerized system may use different colors for charting (Figure 42-40).

There are many abbreviations, acronyms, or symbols used when charting in dentistry. The Council on Dental Practice (CDP) of the American Dental Association maintains a uniform list of dental abbreviations, symbols, and acronyms. A list of commonly used prosthodontics charting symbols and abbreviations is provided in Table 42-1.

Patient Chart

Patient Name: A Dexter
Patient ID: 5671

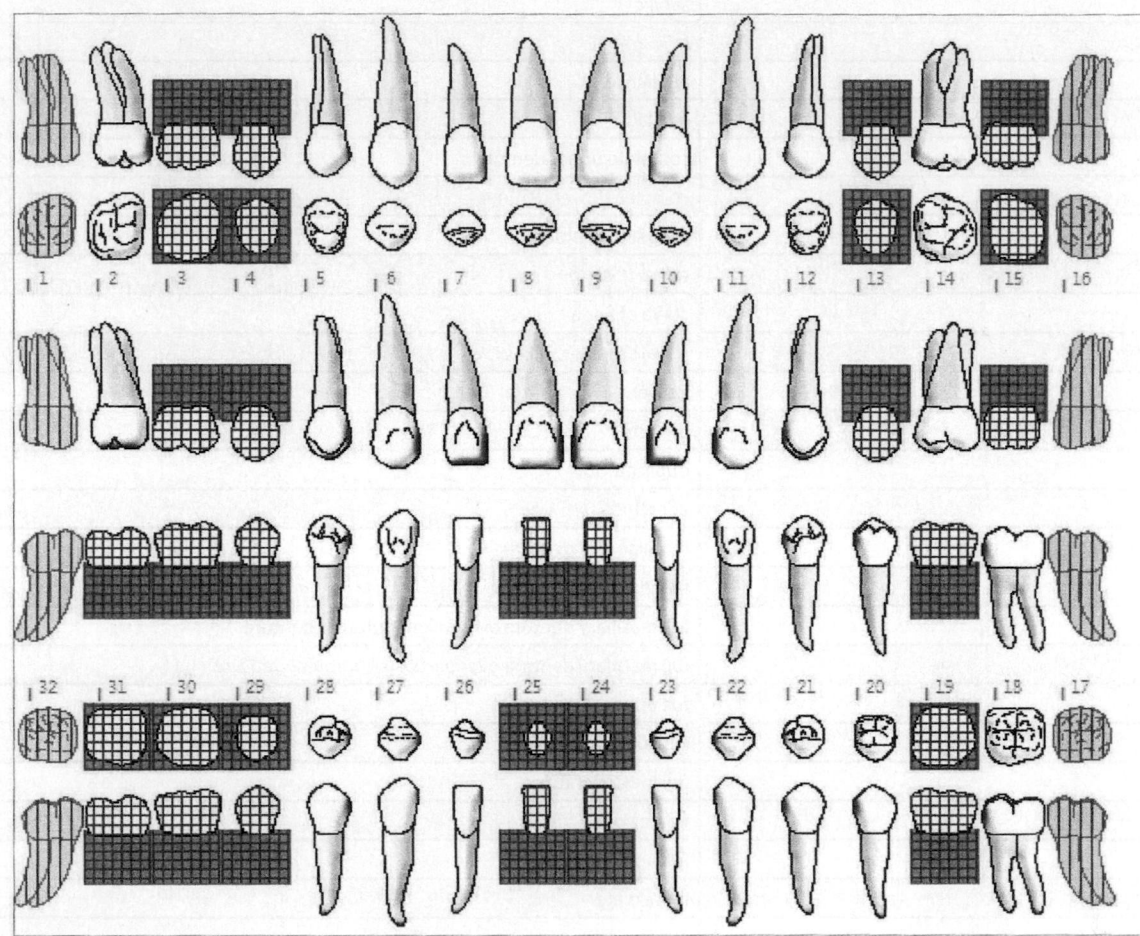

Date	Description	Tth	Surf	Status	Fee
10/19/20XX	D5213 - MAXILLARY PARTIAL-CAST METAL, RES BASE	3-4,13,15,		Proposed	$1,350.00
10/19/20XX	D5214 - MANDIBULAR PARTIAL-CAST METAL, RES BASE	19,29-31		Proposed	$1,350.00
10/19/20XX	Missing Tooth	1		Condition	
10/19/20XX	Missing Tooth	3		Condition	
10/19/20XX	Missing Tooth	4		Condition	
10/19/20XX	Missing Tooth	13		Condition	
10/19/20XX	Missing Tooth	16		Condition	
10/19/20XX	Missing Tooth	17		Condition	
10/19/20XX	Missing Tooth	19		Condition	
10/19/20XX	Missing Tooth	24		Condition	
10/19/20XX	Missing Tooth	25		Condition	
10/19/20XX	Missing Tooth	29		Condition	
10/19/20XX	Missing Tooth	30		Condition	
10/19/20XX	Missing Tooth	31		Condition	
10/19/20XX	Missing Tooth	32		Condition	

FIGURE 42-40
Computerized charting for removable prosthodontics.

TABLE 42-1 Removable Prosthodontic Abbreviations

Abbreviation/ Symbol	Meaning/Word or Term
ab	abutment
acr	acrylic
acry	acrylic
adj	adjustment
appl	appliance
alg	alginate
C/	complete upper denture
/C	complete lower denture
Co	centric occlusion
COW	curve of Wilson
COS	curve of Spee
CRO	centric relation occlusion
del	deliver
dtr	denture
dup	duplicate
edent	edentulous
F/	maxillary full denture
/F	mandibular full denture
F/F	full maxillary denture over full mandibular denture
F/P	full maxillary denture over partial mandibular denture
F/U	full upper denture
FH	Frankfurt horizontal
FLD	full lower denture
fmwk	framework
FU(D)	full upper denture
imm (or immed)	immediate
impr	impression
man	mandibular
max	maxilla
occ	occlusion
PL (or PLD)	partial lower denture
pmma	polymethylmethacrylate
prelim	preliminary
pros (or prosth)	prosthodontics
reb	rebase
rel	reline
rem	removable
rem pros	removable prosthodontics
RPD	removable partial denture
sft	soft
sh	shade
sma	study model analysis
temp	temporary
VD	vertical dimension
VDO	vertical dimension occlusion

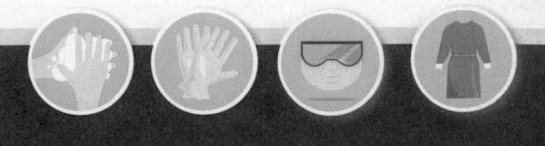

Procedure 42-1
Fabrication of Partial Dentures

Visit 3: Preparation and Final Impression

This procedure is performed by the dentist and is completed in multiple appointments. Between appointments, the lab will complete necessary steps as instructed by the dentist on the written prescription.

Steps written in **blue** font are performed by the operator (dentist or qualified dental assistant), and the chairside assistant's steps are written in black.

Patient Seating Setup (refer to Procedure 18-4)
Final Impression Setup (Figure 42-41)

- cotton rolls and 2 × 2 inch gauze, dental floss (not shown)
- high-speed handpiece, round diamond, or carbide burs (not shown)
- wax or silicone bite registration materials
- final impression materials (polyvinyl siloxane or polyether) (refer to Chapter 33)
- custom tray (refer to Chapter 33)
- laboratory prescription form
- packaging for impressions (not shown)
- shade guide for denture teeth
- tray adhesive

Procedure Steps

1. Escort and seat patient (refer to Procedure 18-4).

   Dentist greets the patient and takes position at the dental chair.

   ❑ Signals for the procedure to begin (refer to Procedure 20-1)

2. Pass mouth mirror and explorer at operator's signal.

   Dentist examines oral cavity and the teeth to be prepared as per partial denture design with mirror and explorer.

3. Retrieve explorer.

4. Assist in obtaining bite registration, preparing teeth for partial dentures and final impressions.

   Dentist obtains bite registration (refer to Chapter 33).

   Operator obtains opposing arch impression (refer to Chapter 33).

5. Pour model with stone (refer to Chapter 33).
   ❑ Transfer high-speed handpiece with appropriate round bur.

   Dentist prepares teeth according to the design of the partial.

6. Use high-speed evacuation to suction and air/water syringe to rinse and dry tooth for better visibility.

7. Exchange high-speed handpiece for explorer.

   Dentist examines the prepared teeth.

8. Prepare materials for impression with polyvinylsiloxane or polyether (refer to Chapter 33).

   Dentist inspects the impression to ensure that all areas are clearly visible and impression is without bubbles.

   Dentist obtains shade using shade guide.

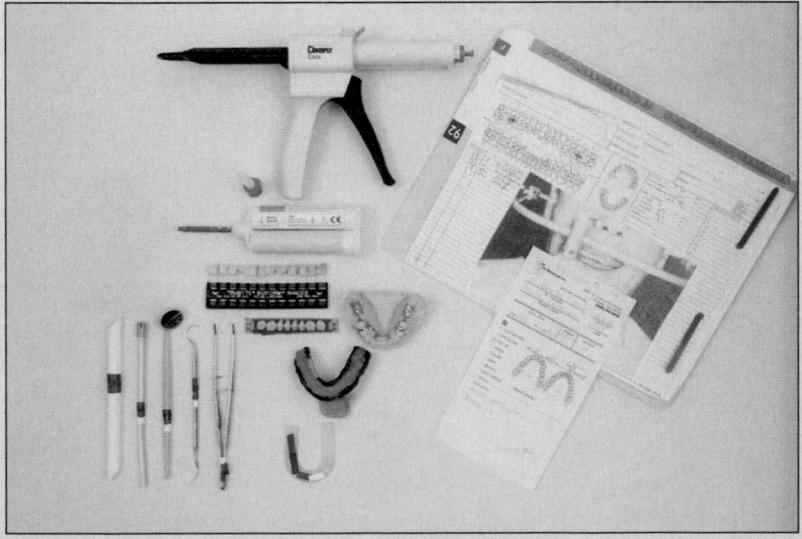

FIGURE 42-41
Tray setup for preparation and final impression visit for partial dentures.

(Continues)

9. Write up procedure in Services Rendered.

Date	Services Rendered
02/18/XX	Updated medical and dental history, no changes noted. BP = 120/80; T = 98.6F, P = 80, R = 18
	Mandibular teeth prepared for partial denture. #19distal occlusal and #31 distal occlusal prepared for rests. Maxillary #5 and #11 prepared for rests. Final impressions taken with polyvinyl siloxane in custom trays. Bite registration obtained with silicone. Selected teeth shade B2.
	RTC: framework try-in Assistant's initials

10. Dismiss and escort patient to reception area (refer to Procedure 18-5).

11. Complete laboratory slip, disinfect the impression, and send both to the dental lab.

Visit 4: Framework Try-In Appointment

Patient Seating Setup (refer to Procedure 18-4)

Framework Try-In Setup (Figure 42-42)
- partial denture framework from dental laboratory
- hand mirror for patient viewing
- contour pliers
- articulating paper in articulating paper holder

Procedure Steps
1. Escort and seat patient (refer to Procedure 18-4).

   Dentist greets the patient and takes position at the dental chair.

   ❏ *Signals for the procedure to begin (refer to Procedure 20-1).*

2. Pass mouth mirror and explorer at operator's signal.

   Dentist examines oral cavity and prepared teeth with mirror and explorer.

3. Exchange explorer for partial denture framework.

   Dentist inserts partial framework for try-in.

   Dentist removes partial denture framework for adjustment.

4. Exchange mirror for pliers for adjustment of partial denture clasps.

   Dentist adjusts clasps on partial denture and reinserts into patient's oral cavity.

5. Pass mouth mirror and articulating paper on holder.

   Dentist checks occlusion with articulating paper to ensure the rests are not interfering with occlusion.

6. Provide patient with hand mirror for viewing of framework.

7. Write up procedure in Services Rendered.

Date	Services Rendered
03/01/XX	Updated medical and dental history, no changes noted. BP = 120/80; T = 98.6F, P = 80, R = 18
	Partial denture framework try in. Framework fits well. Patient satisfied.
	RTC: final try-in Assistant's initials

8. Dismiss and escort patient to reception area (refer to Procedure 18-5).

9. Complete laboratory slip, disinfect the framework, and send both to the dental lab.

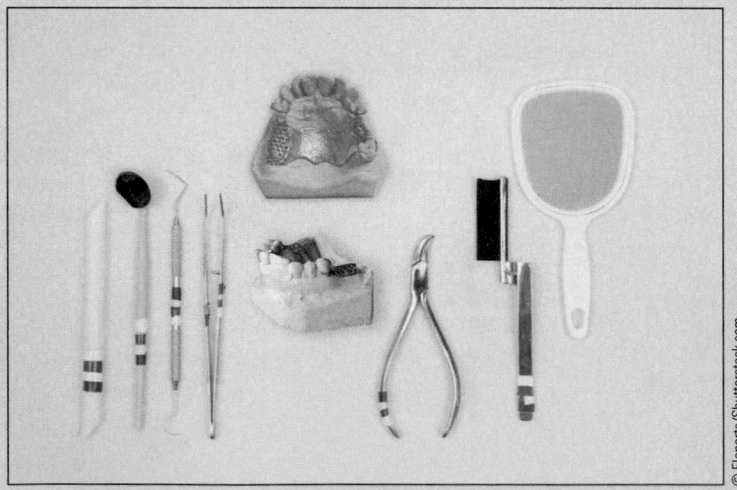

© Elenarts/Shutterstock.com

FIGURE 42-42
Tray setup for partial denture framework try-in appointment.

Visit 5: Final Try-In Appointment

Patient Seating Setup (refer to Procedure 18-4)

Framework with Teeth Set in Wax Try-In Setup
- partial denture framework with teeth set in wax (based on bite registration obtained) from dental laboratory (Figure 42-43)
- hand mirror for patient viewing
- contour pliers
- articulating paper in articulating paper holder
- #7 spatula

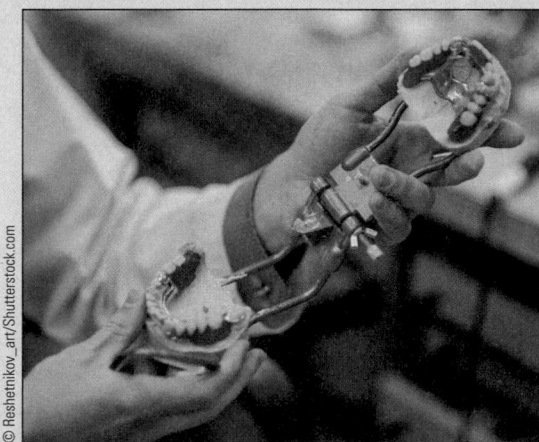

© Reshetnikov_art/Shutterstock.com

FIGURE 42-43
Partial denture setup on an articulator.

Procedure Steps
1. Escort and seat patient (refer to Procedure 18-4).

   Dentist greets the patient and takes position at the dental chair.

   ❑ **Signals for the procedure to begin (refer to Procedure 20-1).**

2. Pass mouth mirror and explorer at operator's signal.

   Dentist examines oral cavity and prepared teeth with mirror and explorer.

3. Exchange explorer for partial denture framework with teeth set in wax.

   Dentist inserts partial framework with teeth set in wax for try-in.

4. Pass articulating paper on holder.

   Dentist checks with articulating paper to ensure the occlusion is even on both sides.

5. Transfer articulating paper and handpiece as needed.

   Dentist adjusts occlusion as needed.

   Dentist removes try-in setup from oral cavity.

6. Pass warm #7 spatula for adjustment of teeth.

   Dentist adjusts teeth of partial denture with warm #7 spatula.

   ❑ **Inserts adjusted partial denture into oral cavity and checks occlusion and esthetics.**
   ❑ **Requests patient state sibilant sounds and fricative sounds.**
   ❑ **Checks smile line.**

7. Provide patient with hand mirror for viewing of framework and teeth set in wax.

8. Write up procedure in Services Rendered.

Date	Services Rendered
03/15/XX	Updated medical and dental history, no changes noted. BP = 120/80; T = 98.6F, P = 80, R = 18
	Partial denture final try-in. Occludes well. Patient satisfied with esthetics and fit. Send for finish and process.
	RTC: insertion and delivery Assistant's initials

9. Dismiss and escort patient to reception area (refer to Procedure 18-5).

10. Complete laboratory slip, disinfect the setup, and send both to the dental lab.

Visit 6: Insertion and Delivery Visit of Finished Partial Denture

Patient Seating Setup (refer to Procedure 18-4)

Partial Denture Insertion Setup
- finished partial denture from dental laboratory (Figure 42-44)
- hand mirror for patient viewing (not shown)
- contour pliers (not shown)
- low-speed handpiece with acrylic burs and finishing burs (not shown)
- pressure indicating paste (PIP; Figure 42-24)
- articulating paper in articulating paper holder

Procedure Steps
1. Escort and seat patient (refer to Procedure 18-4).

   Dentist greets the patient and takes position at the dental chair.

   ❑ **Signals for the procedure to begin (refer to Procedure 20-1).**

(Continues)

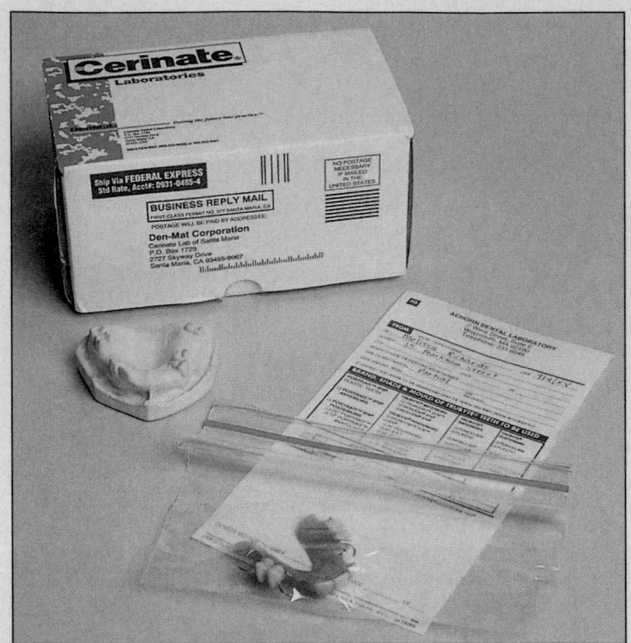

FIGURE 42-44
Complete partial denture returned from denture laboratory.

2. Pass mouth mirror and explorer at operator's signal.

   Dentist examines oral cavity and prepared teeth with mirror and explorer.

3. Exchange explorer for finished partial denture.

   Dentist inserts partial framework with teeth.

4. Pass articulating paper on holder.

   Dentist checks with articulating paper to ensure the occlusion is even on both sides.

   Dentist evaluates length of flanges.

5. Pass low-speed handpiece with acrylic bur.

   Dentist adjusts occlusion and flanges as needed (Figure 42-45).

   Dentist removes partial denture from oral cavity.

6. Retrieve partial denture and apply PIP to tissue side of partial denture.
   ❏ Transfer partial denture to dentist

   Dentist inserts adjusted partial denture with gentle pressure on occlusal surface.

Dentist removes partial denture to adjust pressure spots on tissue surface.

7. Retrieve partial denture and remove PIP from partial denture.

   Dentist inserts adjusted partial denture into oral cavity.

   Dentist requests patient state sibilant sounds and fricative sounds.

   Dentist checks smile line.

8. Polish partial denture on nontissue side and avoid teeth when polishing.

9. Provide patient with hand mirror for viewing of finished partial denture.

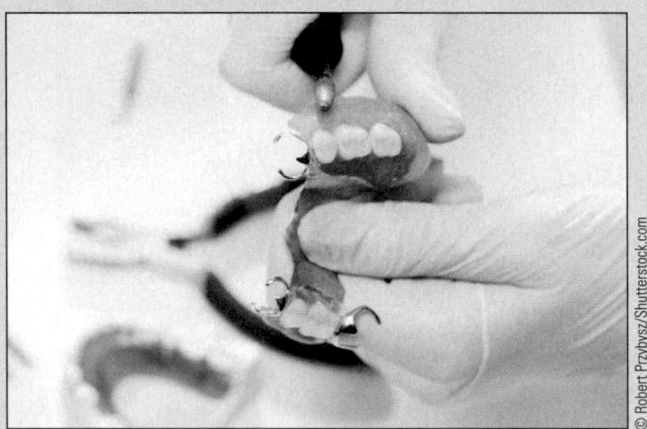

FIGURE 42-45
Partial denture being adjusted with acrylic bur.

10. Write up procedure in Services Rendered.

Date	Services Rendered
03/29/XX	Updated medical and dental history, no changes noted. BP = 120/80; T = 98.6F, P = 80, R = 18
	Partial denture insertion and delivery. Fits well. Patient satisfied. Post op instructions provided verbally and in writing.
	RTC: evaluation Assistant's initials

11. Dismiss and escort patient to reception area (refer to Procedure 18-5).

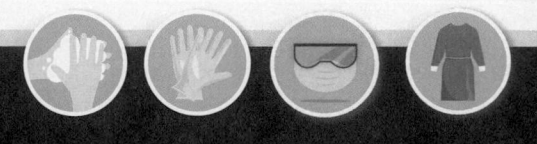

Procedure 42-2
Full Dentures Fabrication

Visit 2: Final Impression

This procedure is performed by the dentist and is completed in multiple appointments. Between appointments, the lab will complete necessary steps as instructed by the dentist on the written prescription.

Steps written in **blue** font are performed by the operator (dentist or qualified dental assistant), and the chairside assistant's steps are written in black.

Patient Seating Setup (refer to Procedure 18-4)

Final Impression Setup (Figure 42-46)
- cotton rolls and 2 × 2 inch gauze, dental floss
- high-speed handpiece round diamond of carbide burs
- final impression materials (zinc oxide eugenol paste, elastomeric impression materials, or alginate) (refer to Chapter 33)
- custom tray for each arch that will be receiving a full denture (see Figure 42-20)
- compound wax for border molding (see Figure 42-32) and Bunsen burner
- laboratory knife to trim border molding
- laboratory prescription form
- packaging for impressions (not shown)
- tray adhesive

Procedure Steps

1. Escort and seat patient (refer to Procedure 18-4).

   Dentist greets the patient and takes position at the dental chair.

   ❏ **Signals for the procedure to begin (refer to Procedure 20-1).**

2. Pass mouth mirror at operator's signal.

   Dentist examines oral cavity and edentulous ridge.

3. Mix materials and transfer instruments to assist in obtaining impressions.
   ❏ Exchange mirror for custom tray.

   Dentist checks fit of custom tray.

4. Prepare for impression with polyvinylsiloxane or polyether.
   ❏ Retrieve custom tray and warm compound wax. Place compound wax on small area of border of tray and pass tray.

   Dentist places tray with warm but pliable compound wax in oral cavity.

   ❏ **Moves soft tissues to establish accurate length for the periphery and to include adjacent tissues in the final impression.**
   ❏ **Removes tray once material is set.**

5. Add compound material to each area of the tray and pass until border molding is complete.

   Dentist completes border molding in small areas at a time and inspects the tray to ensure that all areas are clearly visible and all soft tissues have been included.

6. Prepare and pass tray with impression material of choice to operator (refer to Chapter 33).

   Dentist takes impression.

   ❏ **Places tray in oral cavity.**
   ❏ **Holds tray in place according to manufacturer's recommended time.**

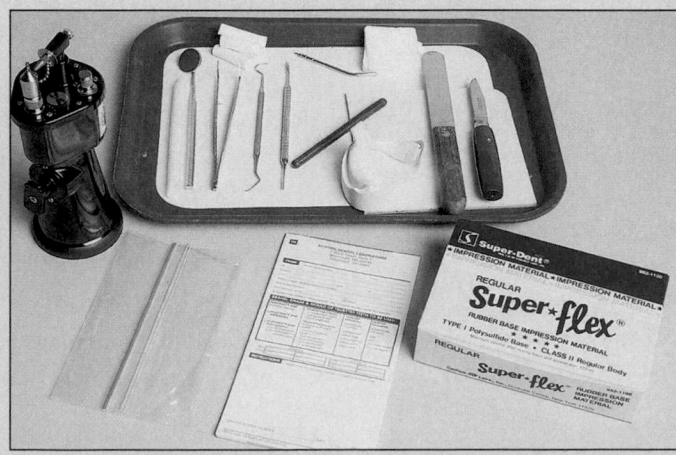

FIGURE 42-46
Tray setup for final impressions of complete denture with custom trays.

(Continues)

❏ Removes tray once material is set.

❏ Inspects the impression to ensure that all areas are clearly visible and impression is without bubbles.

7. If alginate is used, pour final model with stone immediately after disinfecting tray and impression (refer to Chapter 33).

8. Write up procedure in Services Rendered.

Date	Services Rendered
02/18/XX	Updated medical and dental history, no changes noted. BP = 120/80; T = 98.6F, P = 80, R = 18
	Completed border molding. Final impression taken with polyvinyl siloxane in custom tray. Disinfected and sent to lab for baseplate and rims
	RTC: Centric relation and facebow transfer Assistant's initials

9. Dismiss and escort patient to reception area (refer to Procedure 18-5).

10. Complete laboratory slip, disinfect the impression, and send both to the dental lab.

Visit 3: Centric Relation and Facebow Transfer

Patient Seating Setup (refer to Procedure 18-4)

Centric Relation and Facebow Transfer Setup (Figure 42-47)

- baseplates and rims from lab for each arch receiving a partial denture
- laboratory knife, #7 wax spatula, Bunsen burner
- wax sheet (not shown)
- shade guide (not shown)
- millimeter ruler and Boley gauge used to measure length, width and thickness of teeth and denture materials
- photographs of the patient showing the shapes and shades of the teeth (not shown)
- laboratory prescription form and container to send case to lab (not shown)

Procedure Steps

1. Escort and seat patient (refer to Procedure 18-4).

   Dentist greets the patient and takes position at the dental chair.

   ❏ Signals for the procedure to begin (refer to Procedure 20-1).

2. Pass mouth mirror at operator's signal.

   Dentist examines oral cavity and edentulous ridge with mirror.

3. Pass baseplate with rim.

   Dentist inserts baseplate with rim for try-in.

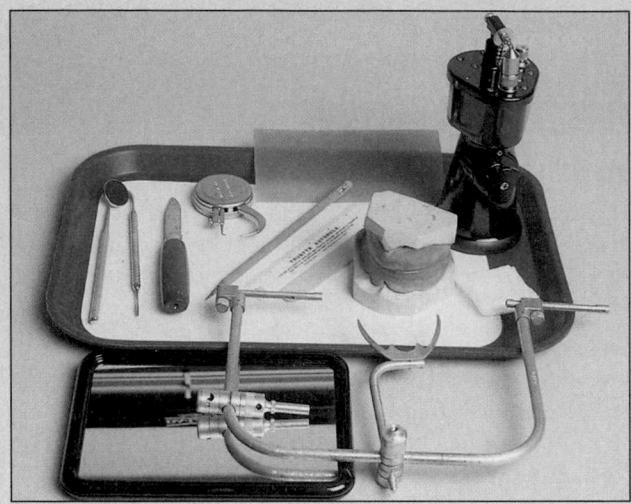

FIGURE 42-47
Tray setup for centric relation appointment.

4. Pass explorer.

   Dentist marks midline on wax rim with explorer.

5. Retrieve explorer.

   Dentist removes baseplate with rim for adjustment of width of rims using Bunsen burner and wax spatula.

6. Transfer warmed wax spatula as needed.

   Dentist inserts baseplates with wax rims and obtains vertical dimension of occlusion (Figure 42-35).

7. Transfer facebow.

   Dentist completes facebow transfer (refer to Chapter 33).

8. Retrieve facebow.

9. Retrieve baseplates with rims.

10. Prepare notch in posterior areas of maxillary rim and in mandibular rim (Figure 42-48).

11. Warm soft wax and place in notched areas.

12. Pass baseplates to operator.

    Dentist places baseplates intraorally and asks patient to swallow, place tongue on roof of mouth, and close on soft wax to obtain centric relation.

    ❏ Removes baseplates and rims.

13. Retrieve baseplates with rims.

14. Pass denture teeth shade guide.

    Dentist selects denture teeth shade and mold.

15. Retrieve shade guide.

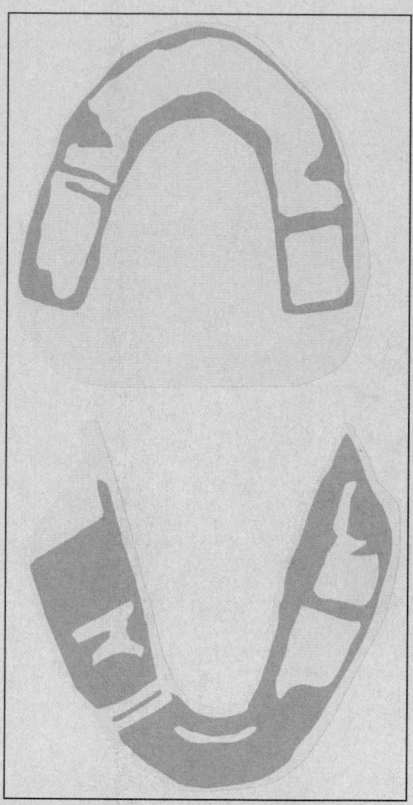

FIGURE 42-48
Notched rims for centric relation.

16. Write up procedure in Services Rendered.

Date	Services Rendered
03/01/XX	Updated medical and dental history, no changes noted. BP = 120/80; T = 98.6F, P = 80, R = 18
	Vertical dimension of occlusion obtained, facebow transfer completed, centric relation obtained, mold A32 selected. Mounted models and articulator sent to lab for setting of teeth in wax rims.
	RTC: final try in Assistant's initials

17. Dismiss and escort patient to reception area (refer to Procedure 18-5).

18. Complete laboratory slip, disinfect the baseplate and rims, and send both to the dental lab.

Visit 4: Final Try-In Appointment

Patient Seating Setup (refer to Procedure 18-4)

Final Dentures with Teeth Set in Wax for Try-In (Figure 42-49)

- full dentures with teeth in wax mounted on an articulator (Figure 42-50)

- hand mirror for patient viewing (not shown)
- laboratory knife, #7 wax spatula, and Bunsen burner
- lab prescription form (not shown)
- box for sending the case to the lab (not shown)
- articulating paper in articulating paper holder

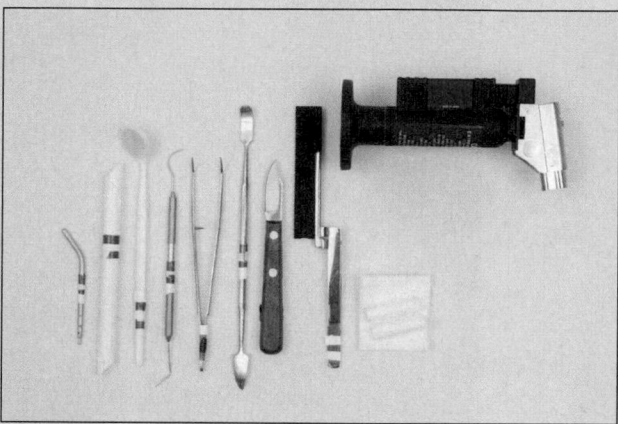

FIGURE 42-49
Tray setup for try-in appointment for full denture.

Procedure Steps

1. Escort and seat patient (refer to Procedure 18-4).

   Dentist greets the patient and takes position at the dental chair.

   ❑ **Signals for the procedure to begin (refer to Procedure 20-1).**

2. Pass mouth mirror at operator's signal.

   Dentist examines oral cavity with mirror.

3. Exchange mirror for maxillary denture baseplate with teeth.

   Dentist inserts maxillary full upper denture for try-in.

4. Pass mandibular full denture for try-in.

   Dentist inserts mandibular full denture for try-in.

   ❑ **Evaluates denture for esthetics, retention, and comfort.**
   ❑ **Requests patient to make sibilant sounds and fricative sounds.**
   ❑ **Checks smile line.**

5. Pass articulating paper on holder.

   Dentist checks occlusion with articulating paper.

   ❑ **Adjusts teeth if needed with warm #7 spatula.**

6. Retrieve articulating paper and holder.

(Continues)

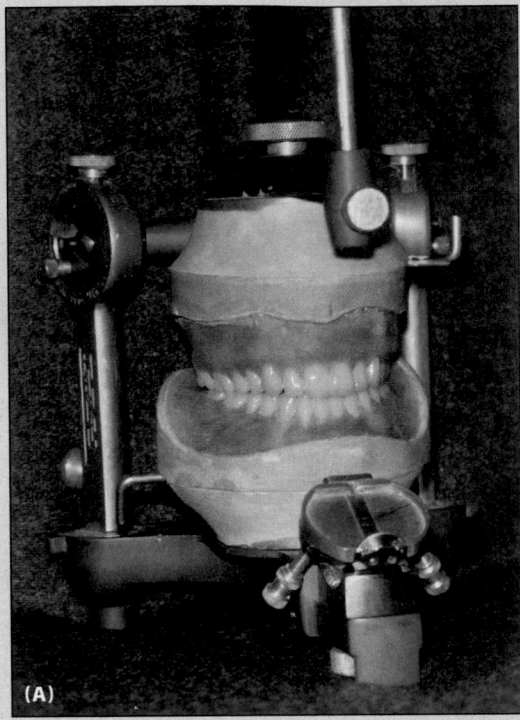
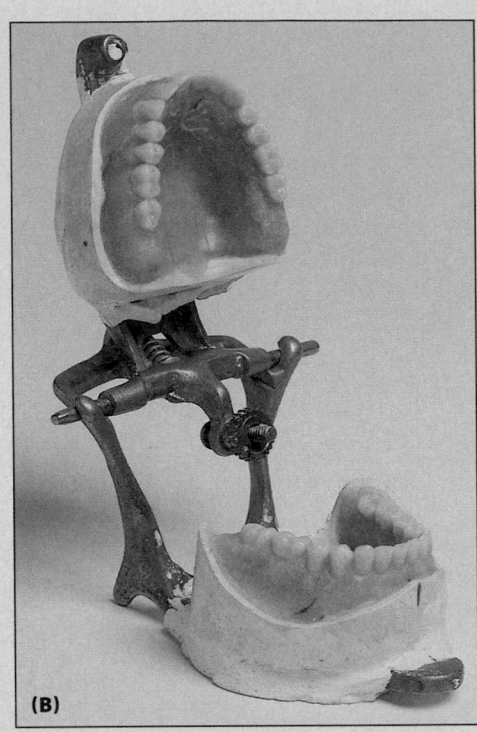

FIGURE 42-50

Wax bite rims with denture teeth on an articulator ready for try-in appointment. (A) Maxillary and mandibular dentures articulated in a closed position. (B) Maxillary and mandibular dentures articulated in an opened position.

7. Provide patient with hand mirror for viewing of framework.

   Dentist removes dentures.

8. Disinfect dentures and place them back on the articulator.

9. Write up procedure in Services Rendered.

Date	Services Rendered
03/15/XX	Updated medical and dental history, no changes noted. BP = 120/80; T = 98.6F, P = 80, R = 18
	Full dentures final try in. Fits well. Occlusion satisfactory, checked smile line and sibilant and fricative sounds. Patient satisfied. Send to lab for finish.
	RTC: insert Assistant's initials

10. Dismiss and escort patient to reception area (refer to Procedure 18-5).

11. Complete laboratory slip and send disinfected setups and slip to the dental lab.

Visit 5: Insertion and Delivery Visit of Finished Full Dentures

Patient Seating Setup (refer to Procedure 18-4)

Full Denture Delivery and Insertion Setup (Figure 42-51)

- finished full denture from dental laboratory
- hand mirror for patient viewing
- low-speed handpiece with acrylic burs and finishing burs
- pressure indicating paste (see Figure 42-24)
- home care instructions pamphlet, denture brush, denture case for placement of dentures when they are not worn by the patient
- articulating paper in articulating paper holder

Procedure Steps

1. Escort and seat patient (refer to Procedure 18-4).

Dentist greets the patient and takes position at the dental chair.

❑ **Signals for the procedure to begin (refer to Procedure 20-1).**

2. Pass mouth mirror at operator's signal.

Dentist examines oral cavity with mirror.

3. Retrieve mirror and pass maxillary denture.

Dentist inserts full maxillary denture.

4. Pass mandibular denture.

Dentist inserts full mandibular denture.

5. Pass articulating paper on holder.

Dentist checks the denture fit.

Checks with articulating paper to ensure the occlusion is even on both sides.

Checks flanges.

Requests patient to say sibilant and fricative sounds.

Removes dentures to adjust.

6. Pass low-speed handpiece with acrylic bur.

Dentist adjusts occlusion and flanges as needed and reinserts.

7. Retrieve dentures and apply PIP to tissue side of dentures.

8. Pass dentures to dentist.

Dentist inserts full dentures with gentle pressure on occlusal surfaces.

❑ **Removes full dentures and adjusts tissue surface pressure spots.**

9. Retrieve dentures and remove PIP.

10. Polish partial denture on non-tissue surfaces.

11. Provide patient with hand mirror for viewing of finished dentures.

12. Instruct patient on removal and insertion of dentures.

13. Instruct patient on home care of dentures.

14. Instruct patient to call office if sore spots occur and to return for adjustments in those areas.

15. Write up procedure in Services Rendered.

Date	Services Rendered
03/30/XX	Updated medical and dental history, no changes noted. BP = 120/80; T = 98.6F, P = 80, R = 18
	Full dentures insertion and delivery. Fits well. Patient satisfied. Post op instructions and home care instructions provided verbally and in writing.
	RTC: postoperative evaluation Assistant's initials

16. Dismiss and escort patient to reception area (refer to Procedure 18-5).

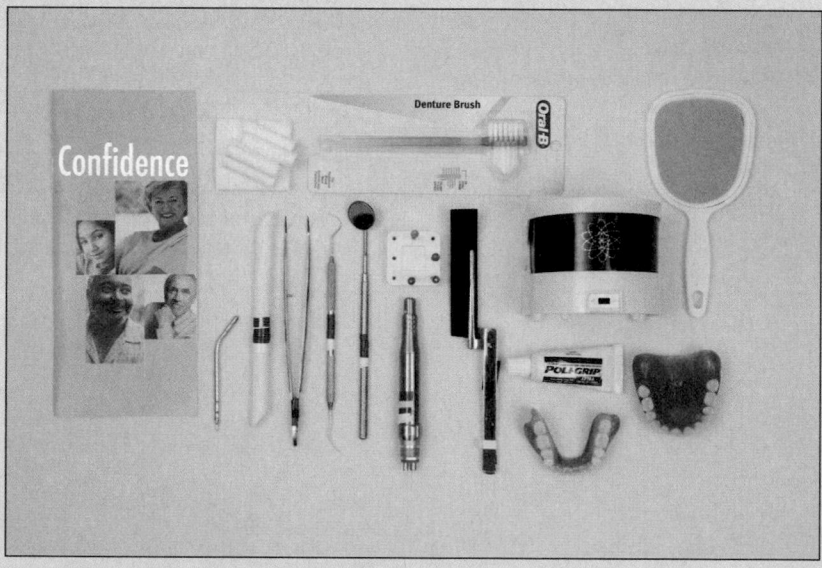

FIGURE 42-51
Tray setup for insertion and delivery of full dentures.

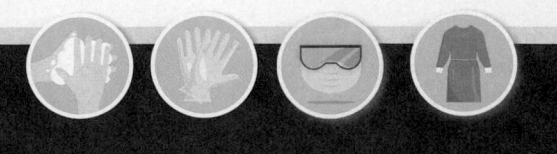

Procedure 42-3
Chairside Denture Reline

This procedure is performed by the dentist in one visit. The dental assistant prepares the materials and the patient.

Steps written in **blue** font are performed by the dentist, and the chairside assistant's steps are written in black.

Patient Seating Setup (refer to Procedure 18-4)

Chairside Reline Setup (Figure 42-52)
- cotton rolls and 2 × 2 inch gauze
- chairside reline material (hard or soft based on dentist's preference)
- pressure indicator paste (PIP) and PIP cleaner
- patient's removable prosthesis
- low-speed handpiece and acrylic bur

Procedure Steps

1. Escort and seat patient (refer to Procedure 18-4).

   Dentist greets the patient and takes position at the dental chair.

   ❏ **Signals for the procedure to begin (refer to Procedure 20-1).**

2. Pass mouth mirror at operator's signal.

   Dentist examines oral cavity and removable prosthesis.
   ❏ *Removes prosthesis from oral cavity.*

3. Prepare to assist in chairside reline.
   ❏ Retrieve oral prosthesis.
   ❏ Clean oral prosthesis by placing in ultrasonic unit for five minutes.
   ❏ Pass low-speed handpiece with acrylic bur and prosthesis to dentist.

   Dentist roughens the tissue surface of the prosthesis with a low-speed straight handpiece and an acrylic bur.

4. Mix material as per manufacturer's instructions.
   ❏ Place in the tissue side of oral prosthesis covering the entire tissue surface.
   ❏ Pass oral prosthesis to dentist.

   Dentist places oral prosthesis in patient's oral cavity and asks patient to bite until the material sets.

   ❏ **Explains to the patient that there may be a slight burning as material sets.**
   ❏ **Removes denture from oral cavity once material is set.**

5. Pass low-speed handpiece with acrylic bur to dentist.

   Dentist trims excess material with a low-speed straight handpiece and acrylic bur.

6. Retrieve prosthesis and apply PIP to tissue surface of prosthesis.
   ❏ Pass prosthesis to dentist.

   Dentist checks for pressure spots.

7. Transfer low-speed handpiece as needed.

   Dentist adjusts pressure spots and inserts.

8. Retrieve prosthesis, clean and return to patient.

9. Write up procedure in Services Rendered.

Date	Services Rendered
02/18/XX	Updated medical and dental history, no changes noted. BP = 120/80; T = 98.6F, P = 80, R = 18
	Completed chairside reline of maxillary full denture. Denture fits well, patient satisfied.
	RTC: recare visit Assistant's initials

10. Dismiss and escort patient to reception area (refer to Procedure 18-5).

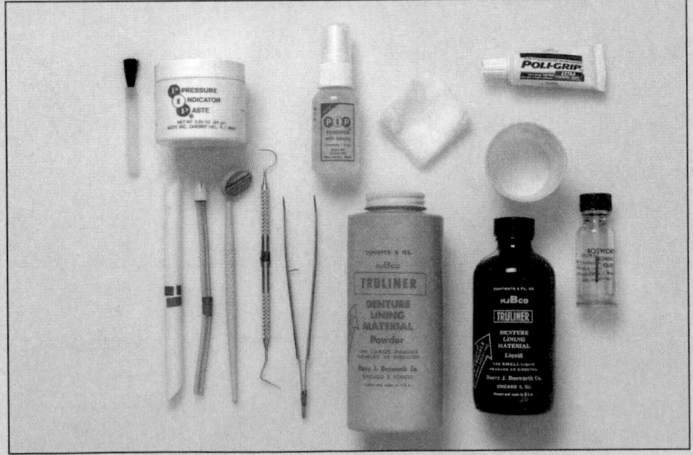

FIGURE 42-52
Chairside reline tray setup.

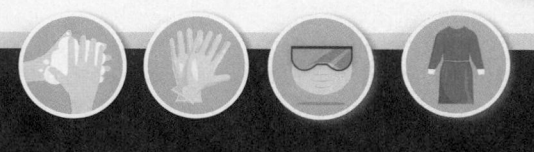

Procedure 42-4
Laboratory Denture Reline

This procedure is performed by the dentist in one visit. The dental assistant prepares the materials and the patient.

Steps written in blue font are performed by the dentist, and the chairside assistant's steps are written in black.

Patient Seating Setup (refer to Procedure 18-4)

Laboratory Reline Setup
- cotton rolls and 2 × 2 inch gauze
- polysulfide or polyether impression material
- patient's removable prosthesis
- low-speed handpiece and acrylic bur

Procedure Steps

1. Escort and seat patient (refer to Procedure 18-4).

   Dentist greets the patient and takes position at the dental chair.
   - ❑ **Signals for the procedure to begin (refer to Procedure 20-1).**

2. Pass mouth mirror and explorer at operator's signal.

   Dentist examines oral cavity and removable prosthesis.

   Dentist removes prosthesis from oral cavity.

3. Prepare to assist in laboratory reline.
   - ❑ Retrieve mirror, explorer, and oral prosthesis.
   - ❑ Clean oral prosthesis by placing in ultrasonic unit for five minutes.
   - ❑ Transfer low-speed handpiece with acrylic bur.

   Dentist roughens the tissue surface of the prosthesis with a low-speed straight handpiece and an acrylic bur.

4. Retrieve prosthesis.
   - ❑ Mix impression material as per manufacturer's instructions and place in the tissue side of denture, covering the entire tissue surface.
   - ❑ Pass prosthesis to dentist.

   Dentist places prosthesis in patient's oral cavity and asks patient to bite until the material sets.
   - ❑ **Removes dentures from oral cavity once impression material is set.**

5. Write up procedure in Services Rendered.

Date	Services Rendered
02/18/XX	Updated medical and dental history, no changes noted. BP = 120/80; T = 98.6F, P = 80, R = 18
	Impression taken with polyether impression material using the denture as a custom tray. Denture with impression sent to lab for reline. Patient scheduled for insertion.
	RTC: Denture insert Assistant's initials

6. Dismiss and escort patient to reception area (refer to Procedure 18-5).

7. Complete laboratory slip, disinfect the impression and denture, and send both to the dental lab.

Note: The insertion visit for a laboratory reline procedure is a second visit and is similar to the insertion for a new denture. The insertion visit is coordinated with the lab so the patient is not without the denture for a long period of time. The lab will complete the reline and return the denture. Follow insertion visit steps in Procedure 42-2.

Chapter Summary

Removable prosthodontics, like fixed prosthodontics, refers to the replacement of missing teeth and tissues with artificial structures, or prostheses. With removable prosthodontics, however, the prosthesis can be removed from the oral cavity of the patient. Most patients prefer to have fixed prostheses, but in some cases it may not be the treatment of choice due to existing conditions. The dental assistant's main functions are to prepare materials, record measurements and details for the fabrication of the denture, provide patient education and support, and perform some laboratory procedures. The procedures in removable prosthodontics do not require many instrument exchanges, and the assistant does not continually maintain the oral cavity throughout the appointment with the air/water syringe and the HVE. The steps in removable prosthodontics involve extraoral and intraoral procedures. The dental assistant has all the items prepared so that the dentist can explain to the patient the diagnosis, the proposed treatment plan, and the prognosis. Both full dentures and partial dentures are discussed in this chapter, including advantages, disadvantages, the components of both prostheses, and the appointment schedules. Steps of a denture reline and repairs are described, as well as how to polish a removable appliance. The overdenture procedure is explained along with the advantages and disadvantages relating to it.

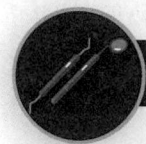

CASE STUDY

Mrs. Abbas has been told by Dr. Lim that she needs a maxillary full denture. Mrs. Abbas has had problems with her teeth over the years because of advanced periodontal disease. She is an office manager for a group of physicians and is very conscientious about her appearance and apprehensive about wearing dentures.

Case Study Review

1. What denture procedure would allow Mrs. Abbas to continue to function with her natural teeth while her maxillary denture is fabricated?

2. What types of patient information are available?

3. To prepare the patient for the denture procedure, what should the dental assistant consider?

Review Questions

Multiple Choice

1. Which of the following is the objective when replacing missing teeth with removable prosthodontic treatment?
   a. restore masticatory function
   b. improve patient speech
   c. consider esthetics
   d. All of these

2. Removable prosthodontics include all of the following procedures EXCEPT:
   a. partial denture.
   b. full denture.
   c. crown and bridge.
   d. immediate denture.

3. Which partial denture is intended for temporary use during healing phases?
   a. flipper
   b. cast framework
   c. Nesbit
   d. advanced nylon-like flexible appliance

4. Which Kennedy classification describes a unilateral edentulous area located behind the present natural teeth?
   a. Class I
   b. Class II
   c. Class III
   d. Class IV

5. Which type of denture is placed the day the anterior teeth are extracted?
   a. overdenture
   b. full acrylic
   c. immediate
   d. transitional

6. A _____ is a small extension that sits on the occlusal of a remaining tooth to provide stability for the partial denture.
   a. major connector
   b. minor connector
   c. rest
   d. retainer

7. When is removable partial denture contraindicated?
   a. when a patient cannot afford a fixed bridge
   b. when there is too much bone loss for a fixed bridge
   c. when the patient doesn't like the looks of a denture
   d. until the patient can afford a fixed bridge

8. All of these are disadvantages of a removable partial denture EXCEPT:
   a. patient complaints about discomfort.
   b. bone loss due to absence of natural tooth.
   c. patient feels it is bulky.
   d. difficulties with appearance and speech.

9. Which are sent to the laboratory for the fabrication of a removable partial denture?
   a. preliminary impressions
   b. final alginate impressions
   c. models mounted on articulator
   d. All of these

10. All of these duties are performed by the dental assistant in a removable partial denture case EXCEPT:
    a. take preliminary impressions.
    b. take final impression.
    c. pour models.
    d. provide patient with home care instructions.

11. Which surface extends from the denture border to the biting surface of the teeth?
    a. tissue surface
    b. polished surface
    c. occlusal surface
    d. surface of artificial teeth

12. What is the part of the mandibular denture that extends into the space between the tongue and lingual surface of the teeth?
    a. border
    b. flange
    c. base
    d. post dam

13. The following statements are true about postdelivery care EXCEPT:
    a. patient sees dentist the day after the denture is delivered.
    b. dentist examines if patient has sore spots.
    c. patient is provided home care.
    d. dentist makes minor adjustments for patient comfort as needed.

14. All of these duties are performed by the dental assistant in a removable full denture case EXCEPT:
    a. obtain prescribed radiographs.
    b. take final impression.
    c. take bite registration.
    d. polish denture after adjustments.

15. The dentist would recommend the use of a denture adhesive for all of these reasons EXCEPT:
    a. denture is loose.
    b. to aid in retention of the denture.
    c. to decrease irritation of the soft tissue.
    d. to reduce food impaction.

16. When would a denture be relined?
    a. to soothe and heal gingival swelling and inflammation
    b. when there are oral irritations caused by the denture
    c. prescribed every 2 years
    d. All of these

17. When are dentures rebased?
    a. to repair a broken part of a denture
    b. to soothe and heal gingival swelling and inflammation
    c. when the denture needs to be refitted
    d. prescribed every 5 years

18. The dentist will repair a denture to replace or repair broken or worn parts. Some dentures cannot be repaired and a new denture is prescribed.

    Select the correct answer based on the statements above.
    a. Both statements are true.
    b. Both statements are false.
    c. The first statement is true; the second statement is false.
    d. The first statement is false; the second statement is true.

19. Dentures must be brushed daily to remove food particles and bacteria. The patient should be instructed to remove stubborn stains with a powdered household cleaner.

    Select the correct answer based on the statements above.
    a. Both statements are true.
    b. Both statements are false.
    c. The first statement is true; the second statement is false.
    d. The first statement is false; the second statement is true.

20. Which is the abbreviation for mandibular full denture?
    a. /F
    b. FLD
    c. /C
    d. All of these

Critical Thinking

1. What types of materials can be used to take the final impression for a partial denture?

2. During which complete denture appointment must the baseplates and bite rims be ready for use?

3. What is an overdenture? When would a patient be a good candidate for an overdenture?

4. How does xerostomia effect the removable prosthodontic patient?

Key Terms

Term and Pronunciation	Meaning of Root and Word Parts	Definition
height of contour (hahyt) (**kon**-*too*r)	**height** = a high place above a level **contour** = a line that defines the bounds of an object	the highest point of a surface, especially of a curving form like a tooth structure
peripheral seal (p*uh*-**rif**-er-*uh*l) (seel)	**peri** = around **-al** = related to **seal** = close tightly	to seal the margins
rebase (ree-beys)	**re-** = again **base** = bottom support	to refit a denture by replacing the denture base material without changing the occlusal relationship of the teeth
reline (ri-**lahyn**)	**re-** = again **line** = to cover the inner side or surface	to replace the lining; to resurface the tissue side of a denture with new base material to make it fit more accurately
undercut (**uhn**-der-kuht)	**under** = removal of tooth structure near the gingival edge to provide a seat or placement area **cut** = to trim; carve	the portion of a tooth that lies between its height of contour and the gingivae, only if that portion is of less circumference than the height of contour

## CHAPTER 43

Cosmetic Dentistry and Teeth Whitening

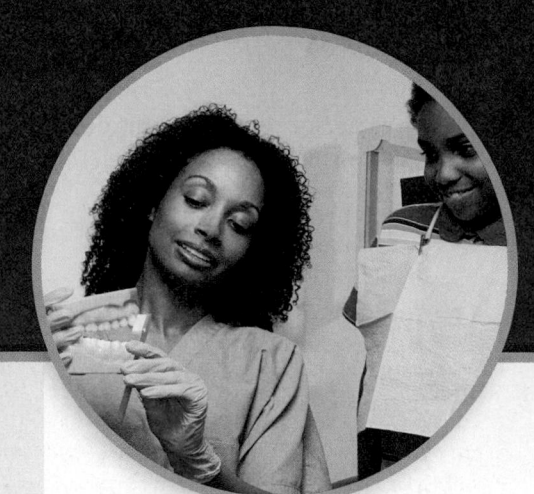

Specific Instructional Objectives

At the completion of this chapter, you will be able to meet these objectives:

1. Use terms presented in this chapter.
2. Describe the duties and credentialing of the cosmetic dental team.
3. Discuss procedures that are included in cosmetic dentistry.
4. Explain how teeth are whitened.
5. Discuss indications in selecting candidates for dental whitening.
6. Discuss contraindications in selecting candidates for dental whitening.
7. Describe the procedures for dental office whitening for vital and nonvital teeth.
8. Describe the procedures for home whitening and over-the-counter whitening materials.
9. Discuss esthetic prostheses that are used in cosmetic dentistry.
10. Discuss the role of occlusion in cosmetic dentistry.
11. Discuss the role of contouring soft tissues in cosmetic dentistry.

Introduction

Cosmetic dentistry includes treatment that generally improves the esthetic appearance and function of a person's dentition, gingival soft tissue, and occlusion. Cosmetic dentistry is not a recognized specialty of dentistry by the American Dental Association; however, many general dentists practice a variety of cosmetic dental procedures and coordinate with dental specialties to produce the patient's "smile makeover."

Cosmetic Dental Team

Most dentists do some cosmetic dentistry, but to be an actual "cosmetic dentist," the dentist needs continuing education at the postgraduate level and additional credentialing. The American Academy of Cosmetic Dentistry (AACD) is the largest international dental organization dedicated to the art and science of cosmetic dentistry. Members from all over the world include cosmetic and reconstructive dentists, dental laboratory technicians, educators, researchers, dental students, hygienists, corporations, and dental auxiliaries. To keep up to date with ongoing advancements in cosmetic dentistry, the AACD offers continued

education through workshops, lectures, and publications. Dentists and their staff may also belong to local study clubs that provide support and updated information on products and techniques.

Two advanced credentialing programs are offered through the AACD: accreditation and fellowship. To become an accredited member, the dentist must take continuing education courses and pass an examination process. This process includes a written exam and a clinical exam, in which the dentist submits clinical casework. Once the dentist successfully passes the written and clinical exams and becomes an accredited member of the AACD, they may choose to continue the pursuit of clinical education and fellowship. Fellowship is achieved when the dentist submits 50 clinical cases that exhibit competency in cosmetic dentistry.

The staff of the dentist who performs cosmetic dentistry is similar to the staff of any dental office: front office personnel, business office staff, chairside assistants, and dental hygienists. Each member of the team plays an important part in the process of enhancing the appearance of a person's smile. The assistant is available to answer the patient's questions and provide reassurance and positive support throughout the procedure. The dental assistant may also accompany the dentist in additional training seminars, courses, and workshops and, therefore, is knowledgeable about assisting with specific techniques and preparing various materials. Because they are close to both the dentist and the patient, assistants may be involved in designing the right smile for a specific person.

Many procedures are included in cosmetic or esthetic dentistry. The cosmetic dentist performs some of these, and others are completed by various specialty dentists, including the orthodontist, periodontist, oral and maxillofacial surgeon, and prosthodontist.

Procedures in Cosmetic Dentistry

Before any dental treatment begins, the dentist should thoroughly discuss with patients their expectations and esthetic desires. This discussion should include a history as well as the patient's attitude toward previous treatments. These first steps can facilitate success of the cosmetic treatment by establishing clear and open communication between the patient and the dentist and dental staff. Patients need to explain their concerns with the appearance of their teeth in as much detail as possible. The dentist may inform the patient of ways that the appearance of their teeth can be enhanced, with the use of before and after pictures, models, videos, computer programs, and pamphlets.

Most types of restorations and materials used in general dentistry are also a part of cosmetic dentistry. There is a variety of tooth restorations the patient can choose that will replace tooth structures with tooth-colored restorative materials. Composite restorations and porcelain crowns, inlays, and onlays are examples of cosmetic restorations.

Tooth Whitening

Tooth whitening is a cosmetic method for lightening dark or discolored teeth. The primary indications for tooth whitening are extrinsic stains mostly from tobacco, dark foods and beverages, aged teeth, and intrinsic staining, such as mild tetracycline or fluorosis. The process of tooth whitening has become one of the most requested services provided by the dental profession. Whitening procedures have been proven safe and effective by the ADA and the Food and Drug Administration (FDA). Research is continually being done, and dental professionals need to keep up to date on new materials and techniques.

The procedure for lightening teeth may be referred to as tooth whitening or tooth bleaching. According to the FDA, the term *whitening* refers to the restoration of a tooth's surface by removing dirt and debris. Any product that cleans (e.g., toothpaste) is considered a whitener. The FDA allows the term *bleaching* to be used only when the teeth can be whitened beyond their natural color. The term *whitening* is more commonly used because *whitening* sounds better than *bleaching*, even when describing procedures and products that contain bleach.

With all bleaching procedures, the patient needs to understand the procedure steps and the outcome possibilities. The bleaching process will lighten most teeth, and although some teeth will never be the whitest or the brightest, they will be improved. Results will vary according to composition of the tooth enamel and product used (Figure 43-1). The patient's dedication to following procedures and limiting foods and habits that stain the teeth

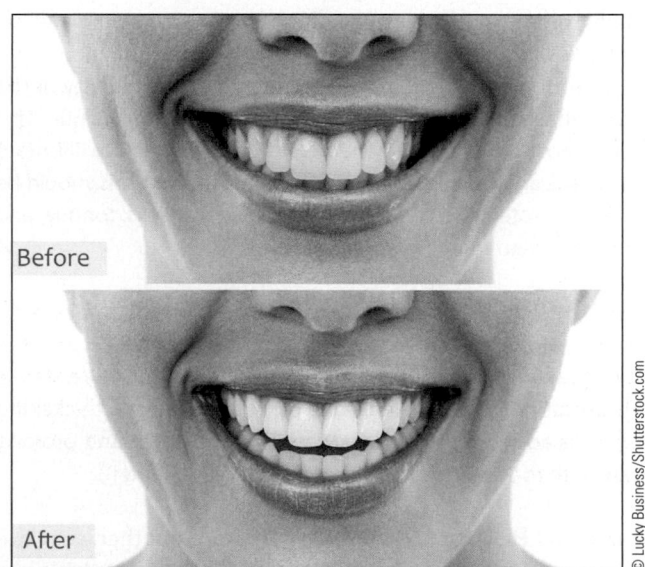

Before

After

FIGURE 43-1
Patient before and after whitening process.

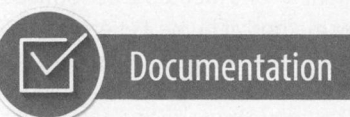 **Documentation**

All legal forms should accurately describe the treatment, the expected outcome, and the financial agreement. The patient should sign a consent form that is specifically designed for the dentist and the expected treatment. The dentist and staff must determine whether the patient realizes the limitations of dentistry and fully understands that cosmetic dentistry is more expensive and poorly covered by routine dental insurance plans. Special precautions must be taken by dentists who practice primarily cosmetic dentistry because subjective opinions about treatment results may determine whether a patient feels the treatment met with their expectations or files a lawsuit. Comments made by the patient during the case presentation or course of treatment that indicate concerns or doubts and dentist's response to patient concerns should be included.

will enhance the process and bleach the teeth faster. Examples of foods and beverages that can cause extrinsic stains are beets, licorice, coffee, or tea. The health of the gingiva and surrounding tissues must be protected by adhering to technique suggestions. Ingestion of the solutions should be kept to a minimum. The patient must realize that bleaching may be an ongoing treatment, with repeated bleaching necessary every few years.

How Teeth Are Whitened

The process of tooth whitening is achieved by applying either hydrogen peroxide or carbamide peroxide gel to the tooth structure. The teeth turn a lighter shade when hydrogen peroxide or nonperoxide whitening material penetrates the enamel and into the dentin. The tooth-whitening gel can be accelerated by a blue LED or UV light, depending on the system.

Today, the most commonly used materials are hydrogen peroxide, carbamide peroxide, and sodium perborate. Sodium perborate is a non–hydrogen peroxide system that contains sodium chloride, oxygen, and fluoride.

Hydrogen Peroxide Hydrogen peroxide breaks down into water and oxygen. When this happens, free radicals of oxygen are released and act with pigments in both intrinsic and extrinsic stains, producing a whitening effect. Available in liquid and gel forms, it varies in strength from a 5% to 35% solution.

Hydrogen peroxide may cause temporary sensitivity of the pulp when the solution penetrates the enamel and dentin. This is the most common side effect. Hydrogen peroxide will irritate the tissue and discolor clothing; therefore, precautions should be taken to protect the patient's eyes, face, lips, cheeks, tongue, and clothing when using hydrogen peroxide.

Carbamide Peroxide Carbamide peroxide, a complex form of urea and hydrogen peroxide, is used in a 10% to 20% solution. It is weaker than hydrogen peroxide solution but more stable. This solution is also available in liquid or gel form. A thickening agent is added to increase adhesion to the tooth and prolong exposure to the whitening agent (Figures 43-2A and B).

Sodium Perborate Sodium perborate, another weak oxidizing agent, is sometimes mixed with hydrogen peroxide and used to whiten nonvital teeth. This compound is the ingredient used in many household bleaching agents that are safe for colors.

Indications for Dental Whitening

Dental whitening of teeth is one of the most conservative treatment options to correct or improve the color of discolored teeth. There are a variety of reasons for the discoloration of teeth. Sometimes, the shade of the teeth is naturally toward yellow or gray, and these patients can esthetically enhance the color of their teeth with bleaching. As teeth age they also naturally change color from various yellow to brown stains.

Causes of tooth stains or discolorations are varied, and the whitening or bleaching techniques are selected based on the

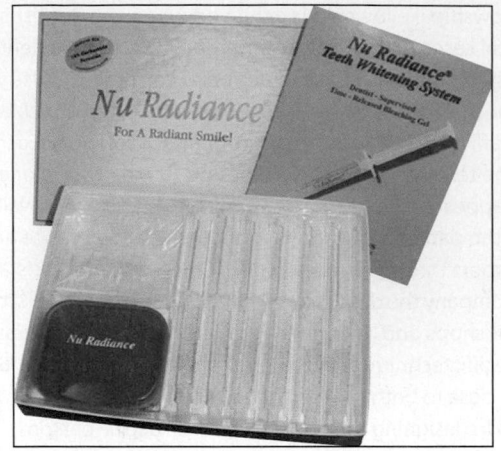

(A)

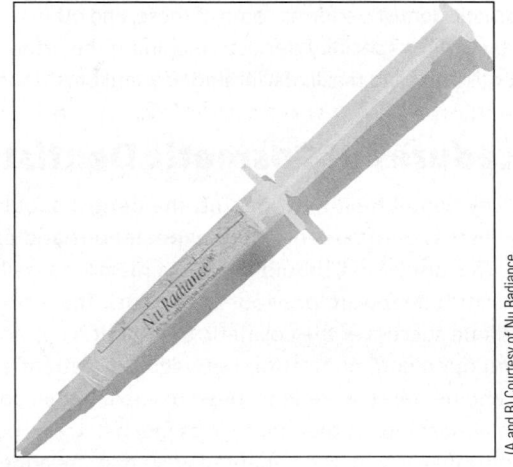

(B)

(A and B) Courtesy of Nu Radiance

FIGURE 43-2
(A) Whitening kit. (B) Whitening material supplied in syringe.

extent of the stain and its causes. The success of the bleaching process depends on the amount of stain and the patient's ability to follow postoperative instructions. Extrinsic stains include stains from diets and habits such as tobacco, tea, and coffee. Intrinsic stains include tetracycline stains, dental fluorosis, discoloration due to injury, and nonvital endodontically treated teeth. For indications and contraindications in selecting candidates for whitening, refer to Table 43-1.

Whitening Techniques

There are two methods of whitening: one method is performed in the dental office, and the other method at home. Patients can use one or the other or a combination to meet their needs. Both vital and nonvital teeth are bleached in the office. There are advantages and disadvantages to each method, and these should be presented to the patient. Considerations include the amount of stain and its origin, number of visits to the office versus the amount of time the whitening trays are worn at home, expense of in-office whitening (which is higher than in-home whitening), and the amount of instruction and guidance the patient requires (Table 43-2).

TABLE 43-1 Indications and Contraindications for Tooth Whitening and Selecting an Appropriate Candidate for Dental Whitening

Indications
• Acquired superficial stains over time
• Age-related stains
• Patients who desire conservative treatment to improve appearance
• Color change related to pulpal trauma and necrosis
• Interproximal discolorations
• Healthy gingiva and unrestored teeth

Contraindications
• Pregnancy
• Patients under the age of 16 (larger pulp chamber can cause increased sensitivity)
• Hypersensitive teeth
• Allergy to whitening materials
• Severe discoloration such as that caused by tetracycline or fluorosis
• Noncompliant patient (take-home whitening)
• Patients with unrealistic expectations
• Multiple restorations that may result in an uneven whitening effect

TABLE 43-2 Advantages and Disadvantages of Take-Home and In-Office Whitening

Take-Home	In-Office
Advantages	**Advantages**
Less in-office time	Quick and noticeable color change in short period of time
Can use trays at home for future touch-ups	Great marketing for practice
Can vary percentage and duration based on sensitivity	No patient compliance required
Technique is easy for patient to follow	
Less cost to patient	
Disadvantages	**Disadvantages**
Requires patient compliance	Higher cost
Sensitivity with higher percentages	More chair time and technique sensitive
	Some patients experience more sensitivity

When patients inquire about teeth whitening, discussing available options and understanding their perceptions about their appearance are important. Factors to consider—and that determine the ultimate success of the whitening process—are summarized as follows:

• Degree of stains or discolorations
• Cause of stains or discolorations
• Whitening technique
• Whitening solution and strength of solution
• Vital versus nonvital teeth

• Presence or absence of restorations in teeth to be whitened (existing restorations will not change color with whitening techniques)

Nonvital Whitening Endodontically treated teeth sometimes turn dark due to blood, pulpal debris, and restorative materials that are used to fill the canal. These teeth can be lightened by both internal and external bleaching. One of the most common bleaching techniques is the walking whitening technique. This technique calls for a thick paste of hydrogen peroxide, sodium perborate, or a combination of the two to be placed in the coronal portion of the nonvital tooth. With the bleach mixture temporarily sealed in place, the patient can leave the office and return for evaluation and another possible treatment as instructed by the dentist. Sometimes, heat is applied with a heated instrument or unit in order to achieve desired results.

An alternate method for whitening nonvital teeth consists of two major steps: (1) After the tooth has been treated endodontically, it is isolated with the paint-on dental dam; (2) then a whitening agent is placed in the unfilled pulp chamber of the tooth. A 30% to 35% hydrogen peroxide solution is applied with a cotton tip applicator or cotton pellets. A heated instrument is then placed in the pulp chamber to activate the peroxide. This procedure may be repeated several times to reach the desired whitening effect.

Vital Whitening in Dental Office Whitening vital teeth in the office involves the application of whitening liquids or gels, often with the application of heat, a curing light, or laser (Figure 43-3). This is sometimes called power whitening or laser whitening if a laser is used for the setting process. In-office whitening offers patients immediate results with minimal maintenance. The patient's teeth are isolated tightly, with the dental dam or a light reflective barrier, to prevent irritation to the gingiva by any chemicals, and then they are polished with a pumice or prophy paste. The actual whitening steps depend on the types of materials used and the technique. The whitening materials are cured by the laser or light, and then the excess material is removed between applications (Figure 43-4). The whitening may take several applications before the desired shade is reached.

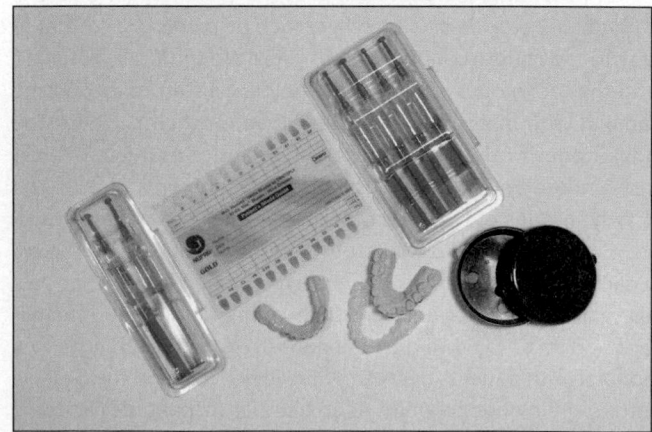

FIGURE 43-3
In-office whitening materials.

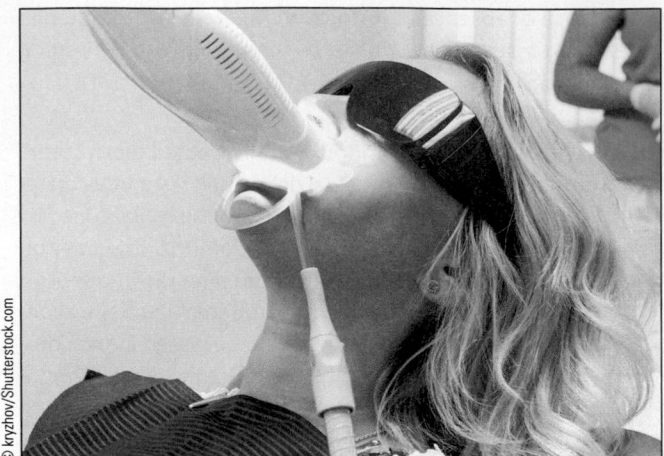

FIGURE 43-4
Laser whitening process.

When the procedure is finished, the teeth are rinsed thoroughly, the isolation is removed, and the teeth may be polished with a fluoride prophy paste.

If the patient had the laser whitening, they will be scheduled for a checkup and possible refresh treatment. When the heat treatment procedure is used, the patient is scheduled for their next whitening appointment within 1 to 2 weeks. The patient should be told that the teeth may be sensitive. This process usually takes three appointments. The patient can also use take home custom whitening trays and gel for periodic touch ups.

Dehydration during Whitening Procedures

Teeth dehydrate when they are isolated for a period of time and may temporarily appear whiter after dehydrating for several hours. Dehydration may also cause the teeth to be more sensitive during the procedure. Make certain to follow the manufacturer's directions for times.

Office Assisted Home Whitening Techniques   For home whitening, the patient applies a bleaching agent, usually carbamide peroxide or diluted hydrogen peroxide, in a custom-fit tray for specific amounts of time. There are multiple materials, and the techniques vary greatly. The dental staff must become familiar with materials being prescribed for their patients. The advantages of the home bleaching techniques include fewer visits to the dental office, less expense, and convenience. The disadvantages of these techniques are that the patients must be motivated to follow the routine, the time involved for the bleaching process can take several weeks, the bleaching materials can cause nausea and sensitivity to the gingiva, and there is lack of direct monitoring by the dentist. Home bleaching is very popular with patients because of the lower cost and the positive results when done properly. As an alternative, patients can come to the office for a startup appointment, or assisted whitening, and then complete the process with home bleaching. Usually,

two appointments are needed to prepare the patient for home bleaching. At the first appointment, the impressions for the custom trays are made. The second appointment is for delivery of the bleaching trays; instructions are also given to the patient (Figures 43-5A and B).

Whitening Shade Guides   Shade guides are used in the dental office to measure tooth shades before and after tooth whitening. Most shade guides are hand-held displays of a wide range of tooth shades (Figure 43-6). Most manufacturers provide shade guides with their specific materials, which are generally

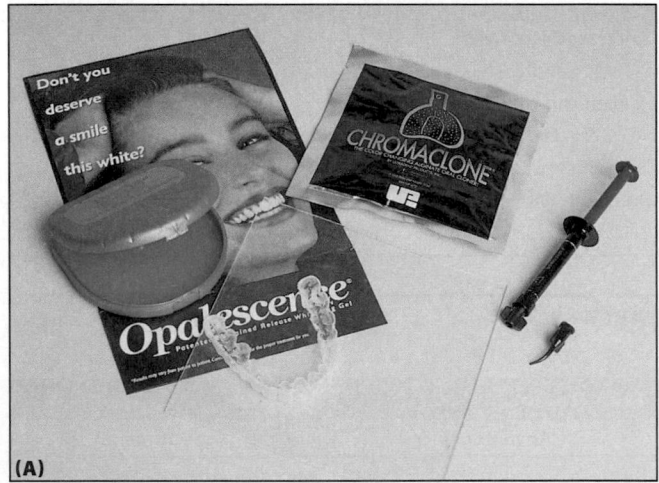

(A)

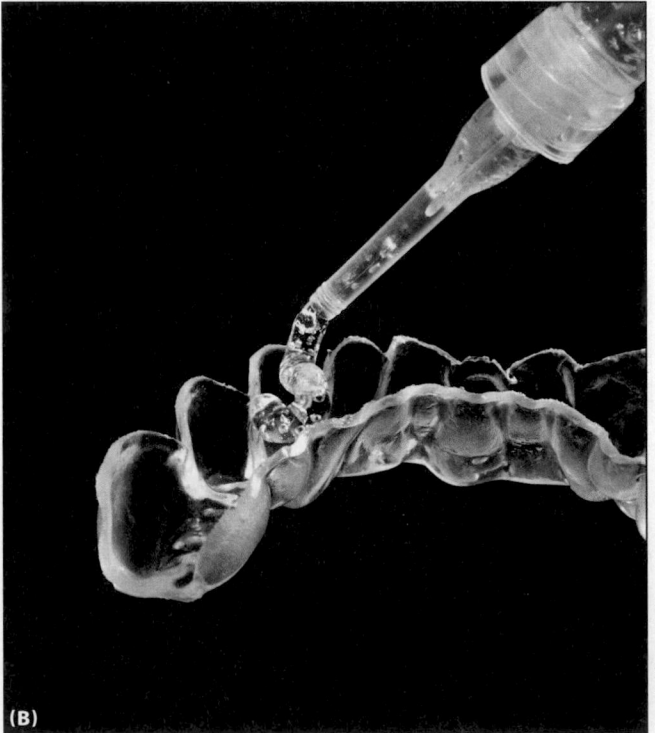

(B)

FIGURE 43-5
(A) Home whitening kit. (B) Loading custom tray with whitening gel.

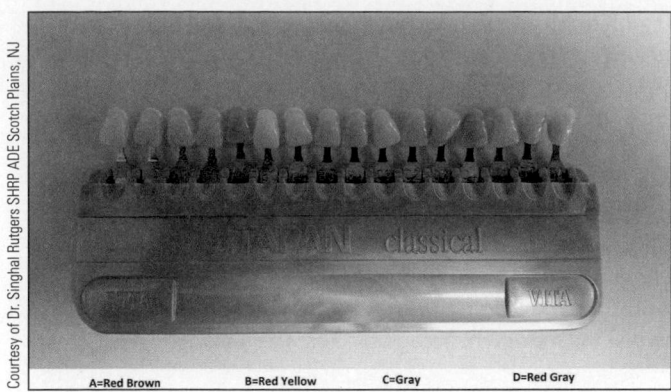

FIGURE 43-6
Shade guide.

not interchangeable. But manufacturers also cross-reference their shade guides with those of the Vitapan Classic Shade Guide. The standard shade guides usually include 16 shades. The shades are arranged on the display beginning with the light shades and progressing to the darker shades. Teeth are predominately white, with varying degrees of gray, yellow, or orange tints. The shade also varies depending on the patient's age, the thickness and translucency of the teeth, and the distribution of enamel and dentin on the tooth.

The shade of the whitening material should be selected before the teeth are subjected to any prolonged drying because dehydrated teeth become lighter in shade as they lose translucency. Also, good lighting is necessary when choosing the color. Natural light is preferred, but overhead/ceiling lights or the dental light may be used—however, keep them at a distance to decrease the intensity. The shade guide is held next to the teeth as close as possible. Some dentists have their dental assistants select or assist in the shade selection. The final shade selection is verified by the patient with use of a hand mirror (Figure 43-7).

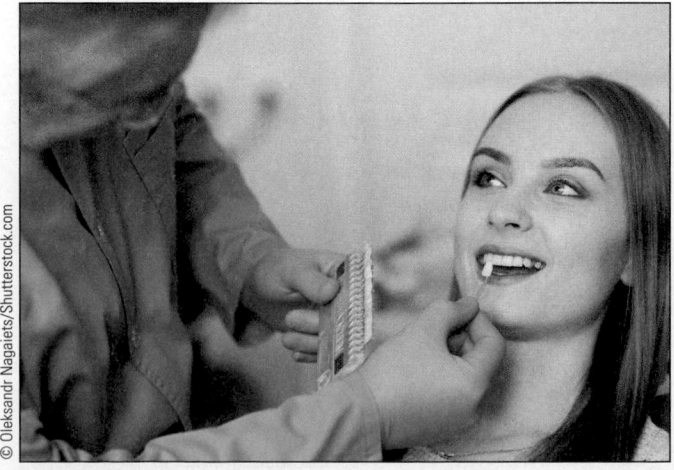

FIGURE 43-7
Shade is checked before and after the whitening process.

Precautions with Tooth Whitening Techniques

- Whitening materials may cause tooth sensitivity to hot and cold. The patient should be advised to use a toothpaste for sensitive teeth.
- Whitening may cause irritation to gingival tissues in affected areas.
- Sloughing of gingival, lip, and cheek tissues may occur.
- Patients should contact their dentist if any of these side effects occur.
- Tooth sensitivity is sometimes treated with sodium fluoride.
- Patients should be instructed to discontinue whitening procedures until sensitivity has disappeared and they have checked with their dentist.

Over-the-Counter Whitening Materials Many over-the-counter (OTC) whitening products are available, including whitening strips, gels, tray systems, toothpastes, mouth rinses, and even chewing gum. Although these methods do whiten the teeth to varying degrees, there is no professional guidance or evaluation. The ADA recommends that patients consult with their dentist to determine the most appropriate means of whitening their teeth. This is especially important if the patient has many restorations, crowns, and distinctive stains. If the patient chooses an OTC method, they must follow the manufacturer's directions carefully and proceed with caution. The most common side effects include temporary tooth and gingival sensitivity, and on rare occasions, irreversible tooth damage. These products generally contain a less-concentrated whitening agent (compared to agents used in dental practices), usually hydrogen peroxide gel or carbamide peroxide.

Whitening Strips Whitening strips are an alternative to tray-based whitening systems. Because the strips are very thin, they do not interfere with the user's normal routine. The number of strips in a kit depends on the concentration of the whitening agent. OTC products are available in a 6% hydrogen peroxide solution to be worn over a 14-day period, or a 10% solution that is worn for 7 days. The user may achieve desired results before using all kit contents and can stop at any time.

The strips are gently pressed on the facial surface of the anterior teeth to create maximum contact with the teeth. They are typically intended to be worn for 30 minutes two times a day. The initial whitening can be seen in a couple of days, and final results will last for about 4 months.

Strip users should be aware that these products do not work on existing restorations and may cause temporary tooth and gingival tissue sensitivity. Patients are encouraged to consult with their dentist when using OTC teeth-whitening products.

Whitening Gel OTC whitening gels are painted on the facial surface of the anterior teeth. Care should be taken to keep the gel on the tooth surface and away from the gingival tissues. Some gels contain 18% carbamide peroxide agent and can be used on a daily basis.

Home Tray Whitening Systems Although many tray whitening systems are delivered through the dental office, OTC systems are available as well. The trays in these systems may be preformed stock trays or thermoplastic trays that can be heated and then molded to the teeth. The trays often do not properly adapt to the teeth and are not trimmed or contoured to prevent excess whitening agent from contacting the gingival tissues. The manufacturer's instructions should be followed carefully, and a less-aggressive approach should be taken to prevent tooth and gingival sensitivity.

The tray with the whitening solution is usually worn for a couple of hours every day to every night for up to 4 weeks or longer depending on the staining and the desired level of whitening. Several white-light teeth whitening systems are now available that can be done at home. These systems are similar to the laser but use an advanced light transmitter to activate the whitening gel. The systems come with a tray that holds the gel when placed in the mouth. The light is then placed to cover the tray for 10 minutes. Once the desired shade is reached, the procedure is repeated once a month for maintenance.

Whitening Toothpastes Most toothpastes contain a whitening agent, and some toothpastes are designed specifically as whitening agents. The whitening agents used in toothpaste include hydrogen peroxide, calcium peroxide, and sodium percarbonate. These agents contribute to the whitening effect, but the primary whitening is accomplished by the mild abrasive in the toothpaste. The abrasive agent (hydrated silica, dicalcium phosphate dehydrate, and calcium carbonate) rates very low on abrasive rankings. Whitening toothpastes can lighten the shade of the tooth to one shade lighter, while in-office light activated whitening can lighten the tooth eight shades. The ADA seal on toothpaste packaging indicates that abrasive particles do not exceed the maximum acceptable abrasive ranking.

Mouth Rinses and Chewing Gum Mouth rinses and even a few chewing gum products contain whitening agents. Like whitening toothpastes, the percentage of whitening agent in these products is very low. Chewing gum contains ingredients that act like stain removers and other ingredients that coat the tooth and make it harder for stains to adhere to the tooth. The minimal whitening effects of gum are temporary, but tooth whitening gum can be helpful in maintaining the whitening obtained from professional or OTC whitening when chewed between meals.

The whitening rinses also freshen breath and reduce biofilm and gum disease. It is recommended they be swished around the mouth for 60 seconds twice a day before brushing. Results should be seen in 12 weeks according to manufacturers. Because of the short exposure time, whitening rinses are not as effective as other whitening techniques. Discontinuation of use is advised if the teeth or gingival tissues become irritated or sensitive.

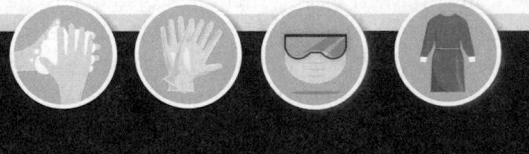

Procedure 43-1
Professional In-Office Whitening for Vital Teeth

The chairside dental assistant prepares material and transfers materials and instruments while the operator completes the whitening procedure. The operator (dentist, dental hygienist, or qualified assistant) is usually trained by a representative from the manufacturer or by video and step-by-step instructions enclosed in the initial package. The operator completes the process by following the steps provided by manufacturer's instructions. In-office whitening products differ from each other, so always read and understand instructions before use.

Steps written in blue font are performed by the operator (dentist or qualified dental assistant), and the chairside assistant's steps are written in black.

Equipment and Supplies

Patient Seating Setup (refer to Procedure 18-4)

Basic Setup
- mouth mirror
- explorer
- cotton pliers

Dental Dam Setup (refer to Procedure 21-2)

Whitening Procedure Setup
- water-based lip lubricant
- hand mirror
- shade guide
- low-speed handpiece
- prophy angle cup
- polishing paste
- LED whitening light
- UV curing light
- LED and UV protective glasses

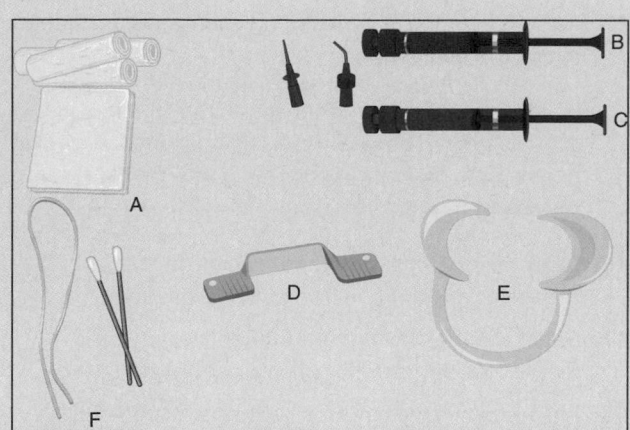

FIGURE 43-8
Whitening procedure setup.

Whitening Kit Materials (Figure 43-8)

- gauze squares and cotton rolls (A)
- hydrogen peroxide or carbamide peroxide gel, various strengths 15%–43% (syringes and tip) (B)
- protective gingival barrier gel (syringe and tip) (C)
- bite block (D)
- cheek retractor (E)
- floss and cotton tip applicators (F)

Procedure Steps (*Follow aseptic procedures*)

1. Seat patient. Record any changes to medical history (refer to Procedure 18-4).

   Operator greets the patient and takes position at the dental chair.
   ❏ Signals for the procedure to begin. (Refer to Procedure 20-1.)

2. Pass mouth mirror and explorer at operator's signal.

   Examines tooth or teeth with mirror and explorer.

3. Exchange mirror and explorer and shade guide.

   Selects shade of preselected teeth to be whitened.

4. Record shade of each tooth.

   Takes intraoral photos or digital photos with patient's permission.

5. Prepare prophy angle and prophy paste or flour of pumice.

6. Pass prophy angle.

Polishes the crowns of the teeth to remove biofilm and debris that may interfere with the whitening process.

7. Prepare and assist in placement of dental dam (refer to Procedure 21-3) or protective gingival barrier gel.

   Places dental dam or protective gingival gel as a barrier to protect the tissues from the whitening agent.
   ❏ Places lip and cheek retractor to isolate the teeth (Figure 43-9).

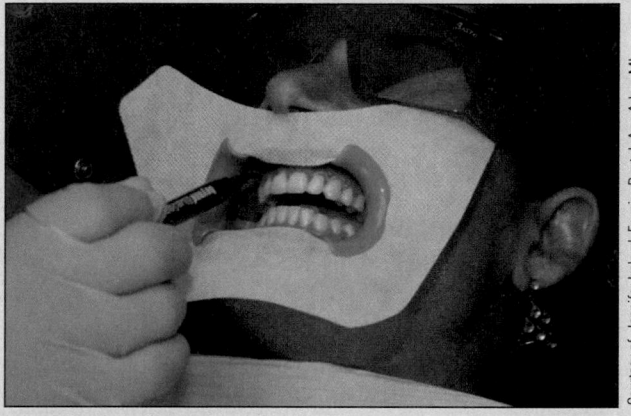

FIGURE 43-9
Example of soft tissue isolation required for in-office whitening.

Courtesy of Jennifer Ireland, Enspire Dental, Ann Arbor, MI

   ❏ Places protective barrier gel on the gingival tissues, being careful not to get any of the gel on the tooth surface. Can use a cotton tip applicator or explorer to carefully remove excess gel.

8. Pass cotton rolls.

   Places cotton rolls in vestibule and/or saliva ejector to keep the area dry.

9. Pass UV curing light.
   ❏ Patient and dental professionals must wear UV protective glasses.

   Light cures protective material until set.

10. Pass operator's preference of brush, applicator, or syringe.

(Continues)

Applies the whitening gel to the tooth surface. Follows the manufacturer's instructions for the specific steps of the materials being used.

11. Pass or place LED or UV light directly on isolated area.

Positions the light over the teeth and turns on for time specified in instructions. Intensity and length of time can be adjusted according to comfort and desired shade.

Repeats application of whitening gel until the desired shade is reached or as suggested by manufacturer's directions.

12. Ask periodically if the patient is sensitive. If the patient is uncomfortable, the patient can discontinue the procedure at any time.

13. Pass the hand mirror to the patient and ask if satisfied with shade.

14. Rinse area thoroughly and evacuate when completed.

15. Remove isolating materials with cotton pliers or assist in removal of dental dam.

If using a protective gingival barrier gel, it is easily removable with water and cotton pliers. A dental dam is removed by cutting the interseptal areas and removing it from the patient's mouth.

16. Allow the patient to rinse, and examine the patient's tissues, removing any remaining barrier with floss.

17. Select post-treatment shade from shade guide and record. Take photos with patient's permission.

18. Provide patient with postoperative instructions (POI) orally and in written form. Ask if there are any questions. Provide patient with sensitive toothpaste.

19. Enter treatment and services. Post services rendered: ADA Code D9972: external whitening per arch preformed in office.

20. Dismiss and escort patient to reception area (refer to Procedure 18-5).

Date	Services Rendered
04/14/XX	Completed in-office whitening treatment Name of product used, total time, and % strength of gel
	Record shade prior to treatment and after treatment Intraoral photos or digital photos taken before and after treatment
	Custom whitening trays impressions for patient maintenance and gel (name of product and % strength) Complications and sensitivity issues POI: avoid substances that may stain teeth; explained teeth may be sensitive following whitening procedure, sensitivity toothpaste given; whitening not permanent; will need to be refreshed periodically with trays and gel
	Next visit: Follow up appointment for delivery of whitening trays and gel Assistant's initials/operator initials

Cosmetic Prosthodontics

Fixed and removable prosthodontics procedures are an important part of cosmetic dentistry. Although cosmetic prosthodontics are more esthetic, the drawbacks are that the relative strength of the ceramic and porcelain materials versus metal is lower, the cost, and that insurance does not pay the difference in the cost of cosmetic and noncosmetic prostheses.

Fixed Prosthodontics

Crowns on anterior teeth must be considered not only in terms of function but also in terms of esthetics. For most patients the appearance of the anterior teeth is very important. As a result, the size, shape, and shade of an anterior crown must match the remaining anterior teeth. This may not always be possible due to the shade or condition of the remaining anterior teeth. In that case, the patient may be advised to consider crowns on all anterior teeth in order to ensure an exact match (Figure 43-10).

The porcelain jacket crowns are considered to be the most esthetically pleasing as they most closely resemble a natural tooth in translucency and ability to reflect light. Margins of an anterior crown are usually placed slightly subgingivally for esthetic purposes. However, if the patient experiences gingival recession in the future, the porcelain margin of a porcelain jacket crown is much less visible than the margin of porcelain fused to metal crown. A thin dark line where the metal meets the porcelain may be visible with gingival recession.

Porcelain veneers are another consideration for restoration of anterior teeth. Porcelain veneers can be used to restore shade, length, and shape of an anterior tooth or teeth. They can also be used to close diastemas.

Cosmetic fixed bridges may be composed of porcelain fused to metal units, all porcelain units, or a combination of these. If the adjacent premolar is missing, the attached pontic fabricated to fill the gap may be porcelain fused to metal.

Removable Prosthodontics

Removable prosthodontic appliances may be considered for patients based on number of teeth missing, periodontal condition, and cost.

Removable partial dentures (RPD) can replace missing teeth at a considerably lower cost than a fixed bridge can. When an RPD is the best option, esthetics as well as function and occlusion must be considered. If anterior teeth are missing, particularly maxillary

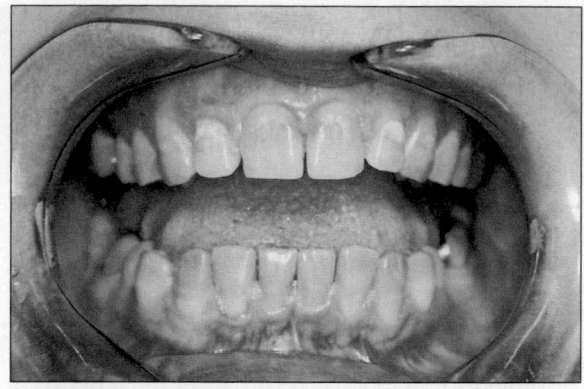

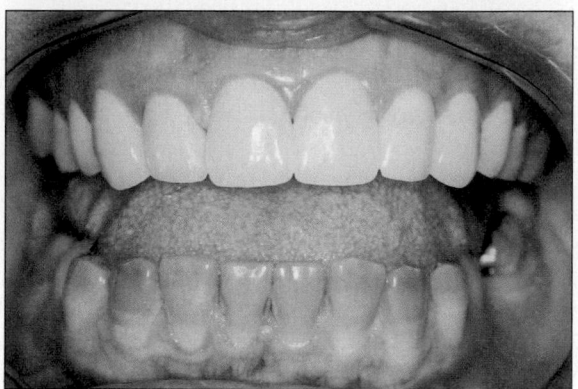

FIGURE 43-10
Before and after photographs of maxillary porcelain crowns.

anterior teeth, cosmetics become a critical factor. Today, denture teeth are available in a variety of shades that mimic natural tooth structure. Denture teeth are also available in a variety of shapes and sizes. Female teeth are usually smaller and slightly more rounded than male teeth. Male teeth are larger and slightly squarer in comparison (Figure 43-11).

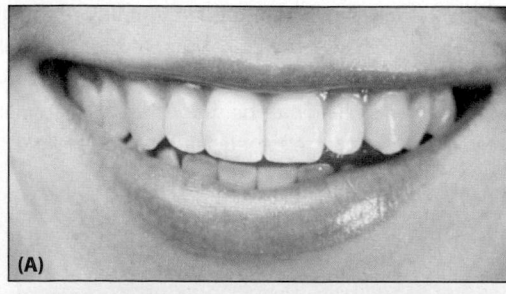

(A)

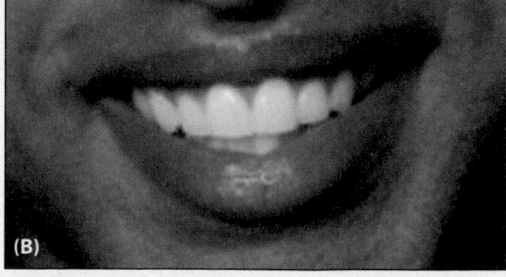

(B)

FIGURE 43-11
(A) Feminine teeth appear more rounded. (B) Masculine teeth appear more squared.

Full dentures may be necessary for patients who have lost all natural teeth in either one arch or both arches. A full denture must take into consideration function and esthetics. The natural bite that the patient has as well as the vertical dimension of the patient's arches must be factored in when fabricating full dentures. Vertical dimension of occlusion (VDO) is the distance between the maxilla and the mandible when the teeth are in full occlusion. This must be recreated in a patient who is edentulous and can be accomplished taking esthetics and phonetics into consideration.

Occlusion in Cosmetic Dentistry

Another area considered essential in successful esthetic treatment is occlusion. The cosmetic dentist will examine the patient's occlusion to determine whether any malocclusion exists. Malocclusions may result from skeletal, dental, or muscular problems. The mandible and maxilla are evaluated separately and in relationship to each other. A patient with occlusal problems involving orthodontic principles beyond the scope of the dentist should be referred to a specialist for a diagnosis. The orthodontist must consider whether restorative techniques may be a better means of treatment than extensive orthodontic therapy.

Traditionally, the dentist takes detailed, precise impressions of the patient's maxillary and mandibular arches. These impressions are poured up in stone and articulated. The dentist consults with a lab technician on the function of the patient's bite and how esthetic restorations will be affected.

Placing cosmetic restorations has a significant impact on occlusion, which is a topic in the subdiscipline of neuromuscular dentistry. The field of neuromuscular dentistry is defined as "the science of occlusion that objectively measures the physiologic functions affected by occlusion to achieve an optimal relationship between the skull and the mandible."

Occlusion is evaluated and treated so that the muscles that control the jaw position are optimal for ideal function and the patient's comfort. Several devices are used to assist in evaluating occlusion before cosmetic treatment begins. One such analysis system uses a grid-based sensor to provide vivid graphics for the dentist to use in determining and adjusting a patient's bite to achieve the perfect bite (Figures 43-12A, B, and C).

Contouring Soft Tissues in Cosmetic Dentistry

Cosmetic dental treatment may also include contouring of the soft tissues. As part of the evaluation, the dentist will examine and probe the gingival tissues and sulcus. The appearance of the gingival tissues is just as important as other elements in the mouth for achieving a pleasing smile. Most of these procedures require some surgery; some may be performed by a knowledgeable and skilled general dentist but are more commonly completed by a periodontist.

Soft Tissue Contouring

Indications for soft tissue contouring include incomplete passive eruption of one or more teeth. With this condition, the patient

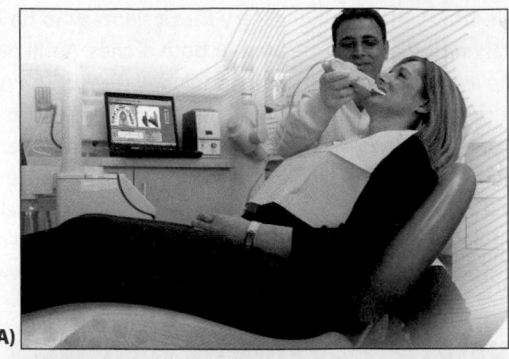

(A)

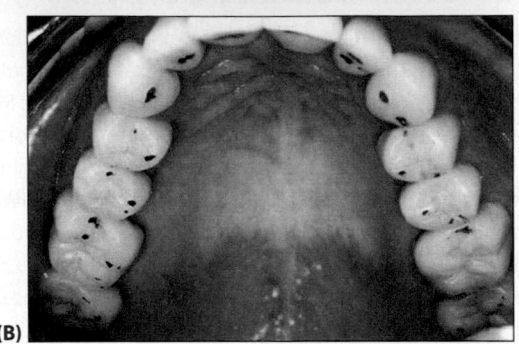

(B)

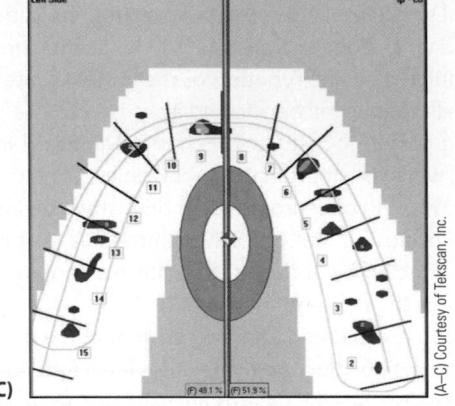

(C)

(A-C) Courtesy of Tekscan, Inc.

FIGURE 43-12
(A) Patient having occlusion scanned and evaluated. (B) Arch marked with articulating paper. (C) Graphic scan of occlusal analysis.

appears to have very short teeth with a lot of gum tissue showing, hypertrophied or malpositioned papilla, inflamed tissues as a result of orthodontic treatment, hypertrophied gingival tissue from drug therapy (such as Dilantin), or hypertrophied gingival tissue from poor oral hygiene or pathologic conditions.

In some cases, the anterior teeth appear shorter than normal. This can be caused by gingival tissue enlargement, short clinical crowns, or altered or delayed eruption. It is important for the dentist to evaluate the cause of the problem before proceeding with treatment. For example, gingival enlargement may be caused by gingival inflammation from a systemic problem such as diabetes or pregnancy, or from a hereditary problem such as gingival fibromatosis. In some cases, the tooth fails to erupt normally, and the width of the gingiva can be quite large; in others a short clinical crown may be the result of attrition due to bruxism. After the diagnosis and etiology are determined, a treatment can be selected that may include esthetic crown lengthening to improve

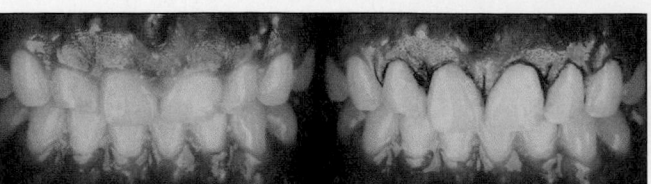

© kksakultap/Shutterstock.com

FIGURE 43-13
Gum surgery for teeth lengthening.

the patient's appearance (Figure 43-13). Esthetic crown lengthening is indicated to establish the proper relation of the gingival margin with the lip and to increase the length of the teeth for appearance and for prosthetic crown retention.

Electrosurgery or lasers are used to remove and contour the gingival tissues. Both techniques require that the dentist become familiar with the equipment and skilled in the detailed application steps.

Electrosurgery equipment and techniques have been used for many years. The equipment has improved, as have the precise techniques required for esthetic contouring. Electrosurgery equipment includes a unit that produces various current strengths, various styles of electrode tips, and a foot pedal control.

Dental lasers are becoming increasingly popular and have proven to be an ideal technology for gum contouring and reshaping. Soft tissue lasers offer degrees of precision that surpass other techniques while minimizing pain and other discomfort. The dentist will choose a dental laser among several types available based on primary intended use.

Surgical Lip Repositioning

Repositioning of the lip is another procedure that may be indicated to correct excessive gum tissue showing. In a normal smile, 1–2 mm of gingiva should be visible. Visibility of 4 mm or more is considered to be unattractive. In some cases, this may be due to overfunctioning of the lip muscles allowing for greater visibility of the gingival soft tissue. To resolve the issue, surgical intervention that will allow the lip to be repositioned so no more than 2 mm of gingival soft tissue is visible when smiling may be suggested to the patient. This procedure will result in a more esthetically pleasing smile.

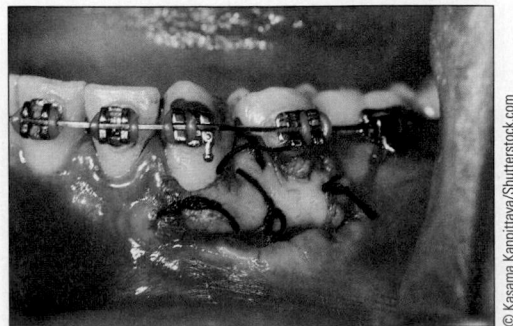

© Kasama Kanpittaya/Shutterstock.com

FIGURE 43-14
Free gingival graft (tissue graft that harvested from the palate, used to treat gingival recession and inadequate attached gingiva) suturing to donor side at gingiva of lower premolar tooth.

Tissue Grafting

Connective tissue grafting procedures may be necessary when there is gingival recession present that exposed the root surface of teeth (Figure 43-14). Root exposure can lead to sensitivity and root caries and can be esthetically unpleasing. The graft tissue is usually taken from the patient's hard palate and then attached to the area where the gingiva has receded. This will prevent further recession and future root caries. The connective tissue graft is preferred when esthetics is a consideration as this graft allows for esthetic blending of tissues.

Chapter Summary

Cosmetic dentistry can be a life-changing experience for both the patient and the dental team. These procedures involve many and varied aspects of dentistry and provide esthetic services to patients. Cosmetic dentistry involves detailed, comprehensive treatments that can involve orthodontics, oral maxillofacial surgery, occlusion adjustments, endodontic treatment, and periodontics.

Tooth whitening may also be a part of esthetic treatments desired by patients to improve the appearance of their teeth. Various materials and techniques are discussed, including nonvital and vital tooth whitening, in-office and home whitening techniques, and available OTC products.

The dental assistant plays an important role in all cosmetic and tooth-whitening procedures. The assistant must be educated and trained to assist the dentist and be actively involved in providing information to the patient.

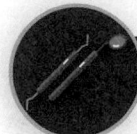 **CASE STUDY**

Chance Hall works with the public and expressed his concern about the color of his teeth during his recare visit. He cannot get off work to make several visits for whitening treatments and has a limited budget. While discussing the whitening options with Dr. Garrett, he also shared a desire to see color change as soon as possible.

Case Study Review

1. Which tooth whitening option would best suit Mr. Hall's concerns?

2. What can the dentist recommend to speed up the whitening procedure?

3. Discuss options available for Mr. Hall to achieve his goal of having whiter teeth.

Review Questions

Multiple Choice

1. Which dental organization is dedicated to the art and science of cosmetic dentistry?
   a. ADA
   b. AACD
   c. AAPD
   d. ADAA

2. All of these restorations are examples of cosmetic restorations EXCEPT:
   a. composite resin restoration.
   b. porcelain crown.
   c. amalgam restoration.
   d. ceramic inlays.

3. All of these statements describe how vital teeth are whitened EXCEPT:
   a. hydrogen peroxide or carbamide peroxide are used.
   b. whitening material penetrates the enamel and dentin.
   c. process can be accelerated by blue LED or UV light.
   d. whitening material is placed inside the tooth.

4. Which of the following agencies and organizations has proven the safety and effectiveness of whitening procedures?
   a. American Dental Association
   b. State drug administrations
   c. Food and Drug Administration
   d. Both a and c

5. All of these are indications that the patient is a good candidate for tooth whitening EXCEPT:
   a. age-related stains.
   b. acquired stains.
   c. color change due to pulpal trauma.
   d. patients with unrealistic expectations.

6. All of the following are true statements about in-office whitening EXCEPT:
   a. the teeth are polished before application of the whitening materials.
   b. the actual whitening steps depend on the type of materials applied.
   c. the barrier gel is placed around the gingival margins.
   d. the teeth are polished with a fluoride prophy paste after the whitening materials have been placed, and then the mouth is rinsed thoroughly.

7. Which of the following whitening materials is typically used in home whitening techniques?
   a. diluted hydrogen peroxide
   b. sodium hypochloride
   c. sodium fluoride
   d. phosphoric acid

8. When a tooth is endodontically treated and turns dark due to blood, pulpal debris, or restorative materials, it can be lightened by:
   a. vital whitening procedures.
   b. nonvital whitening procedures.
   c. home whitening procedures.
   d. None of these, because it cannot be lightened with any whitening procedures.

9. Which is considered the most esthetic crown for anterior teeth due to its close resemblance to the natural tooth?
   a. porcelain fused to metal
   b. ceramic fused to metal
   c. porcelain jacket crown
   d. full metal crown

10. Which describes female teeth used in dentures to provide the most natural appearance?
    a. smaller and squarer
    b. smaller and more rounded
    c. larger and squarer
    d. larger and more rounded

11. _____ is the science of occlusion that objectively measures the physiologic functions affected by occlusion to achieve an optimal relationship between the skull and the mandible.
    a. Neurological dentistry
    b. Neuromuscular dentistry
    c. Skeletal dentistry
    d. Skeletal muscular dentistry

12. Soft tissue contouring is accomplished with a:
    a. dental laser.
    b. electrosurgery unit.
    c. Both a and b
    d. None of these

13. When would crown lengthening treatment be recommended?
    a. to establish proper relation of gingival margin with lip
    b. to increase length of teeth for appearance
    c. in preparation for prosthetic crown retention
    d. All of these

14. What procedure might be necessary when there is gingival recession?
    a. crown lengthening
    b. tissue grafting
    c. veneer
    d. repositioning of the tooth

15. What is the sequence in office whitening of teeth procedure?
    a. isolation, pumice teeth, LED or UV light, application of whitening agent
    b. pumice teeth, isolation, application of whitening agent, LED or UV light
    c. pumice teeth, isolation, LED or UV light, application of whitening agent
    d. isolation, application of whitening agent, LED or UV light, pumice teeth

16. What substance should be avoided after the teeth have been whitened?
    a. beets
    b. licorice
    c. coffee
    d. tea
    e. All of these

17. What whitening agent is typically used for in-office whitening?
    1. hydrogen peroxide
    2. phosphoric acid
    3. carbamide peroxide gel
    4. bleach
       a. 1, 2
       b. 1, 3
       c. 2, 3, 4
       d. 1, 2, 3, 4

18. What negative results may occur from whitening procedures?
    a. irritation to the gingival tissue
    b. sloughing of soft tissue
    c. sensitivity to hot and cold
    d. All of these

19. What are the drawbacks in placing cosmetic prosthodontics versus noncosmetic prosthodontics?
    1. lower strength
    2. higher cost
    3. poor insurance coverage
    4. greater esthetics
       a. 1, 2
       b. 1, 3
       c. 1, 2, 3
       d. 1, 2, 3, 4

20. What should be recommended for a patient feeling tooth sensitivity after their first whitening treatment?
    a. toothpaste for sensitive teeth
    b. sodium fluoride
    c. discontinue whitening until sensitivity disappears
    d. All of these

Critical Thinking

1. Explain why formal informed consent must be part of the patient's records.

2. When patients mention that they are interested in teeth whitening, what options could the dental assistant tell them about?

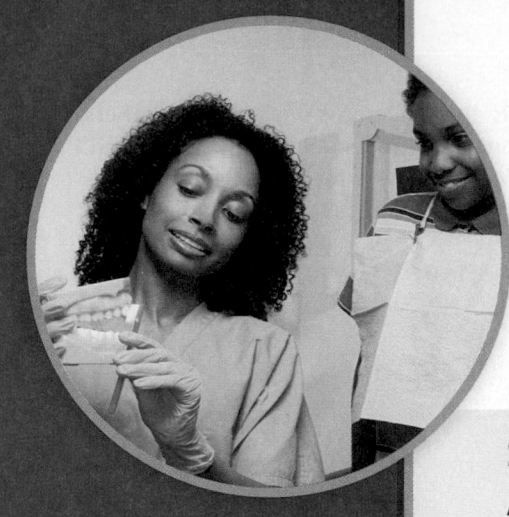

Dental Practice Management

SECTION IX
Dentral Practice Management

Specific Instructional Objectives

At the completion of this chapter, you will be able to meet these objectives:

1. Use terms presented in this chapter.
2. Explain the appropriate format of a welcome letter.
3. Identify marketing ideas for dentistry.
4. Identify the components of a reception area.
5. Identify the dental office staff and their areas of responsibility.
6. Outline the proper procedure for answering an incoming call.
7. Describe proper phone messaging etiquette.
8. Describe telephone and business office technology and its uses.
9. Discuss the presentation of a patient care plan.
10. Explain the different elements that go into appointment scheduling.
11. Compare and contrast a computerized recare system to a manual recare system.
12. Give examples of the ways in which computers are used in the dental office.
13. Differentiate between expendable and nonexpendable supplies.
14. Explain why ergonomics is important at a computer workstation.
15. Describe the use of a computerized inventory management system.
16. Identify computerized and manual systems for the management of patient accounts.
17. Discuss the different aspects of managing office finances.
18. Explain dental insurance as it applies to the dental office.
19. List common examples of insurance fraud made by dental practices.
20. Explain common dental benefit and claim terminology.
21. Discuss common avenues of teledentistry.

Introduction

Dental practice management includes the administration organization of the dental practice, the general patient flow, staff assignments, financial responsibilities, and record keeping. It is the place where all business activities transpire. A well put together practice management team ensures the practice functions ethically, efficiently, and safely while being productive and making a profit. A dental practice consists of many team members, who can include the dentist, dental assistant, dental hygienist, administrative assistant, and other administrative staff. While the leader of the dental practice remains the dentist, it is the role of the **administrative assistant** to manage the practice. This is the person who has a primary responsibility for the business activities of the practice and oversees other staff members in the business office.

Good practice management requires organization, good communication skills, the willingness of all team members, and a welcoming environment. The dental health profession is a people-oriented one and will remain that way even with the ever-changing world of technology. After all, the most important asset in a dental practice is the patients. Effective use of resources, comprehensive knowledge of computer technology, maintaining a consistent sound culture in the office, and meeting the mission are all contributions to running a successful practice.

Dental practice management successfully orchestrates the vitality of a dental office in the following ways:

- Office compliance with the practicing state
- Profits and financial success
- Patient and staff relations
- Electronic equipment operations
- Records management
- Retention and growth

An effective practice management team leads the dentist and staff into a successful, profitable business, enabling patient satisfaction and the ability to continue providing dental services to the community.

Welcome Letter

A **welcome letter** is often used as a powerful marketing tool for the practice. The welcome letter and other successful internal and external marketing ideas are used as a vehicle to introduce a new practice, new associates, and new staff and for various other announcements pertaining to the dental office. Because a welcome letter is the first established communication to the patient, its components are relied upon to ensure a good first impression. Creating a positive image that shows your practice will provide the best quality care possible is the goal. In order for the welcome letter to deliver its purpose, it must use a warm, hospitable approach to fortify interpersonal relationships between the dentist and these potential patients. It should speak of the commitments the office makes to the patient as well as any other unique qualities the practice possesses. Direct the patient to visit the office website to further get to know the practice and staff.

Welcome letters can be sent to various audiences:

- New members of the community
- New patients who have scheduled appointments
- Potential patients in the area through a mailer
- Potential patients through clubs or organizations

Format

When composing a welcome letter, first determine who the letter is intended to reach and what the objectives of the letter are. For instance, the practice could be looking to welcome a new patient to the practice, or it could be trying to establish name recognition as a marketing tool. In any event, it should be sincere and express the practice's enthusiasm about the services they could provide to the patient. Office letterhead and high-quality paper should be used, which displays the effort put into the letter. Some offices may send out brochures in place of a letter; however, this may lose personal value and could mean the difference setting your practice apart from the next. Grammar and spelling should be thoroughly checked. Sending out correspondence to a patient or potential patient with grammatical and spelling errors can portray that the office does not care about quality. This can then be associated with

the care patients can expect to be received in the office. When typing the letter, do not use any fancy font. Acceptable fonts are Times New Roman or Arial, size 12. Always remember who you are writing the letter to, and choose your font accordingly. To help with formatting, you can utilize the Letter Wizard available in some word processing programs. You can then choose which letter format best suits your style. Common and acceptable options include full block and semiblock styles. **Full block format** letters are most common and are left justified and single spaced, with the exception of a double space between paragraphs. **Semiblock format** letters, which are less common, are similar to the full block; however, each paragraph is indented, and the date and closing portions are to the right of the page. Figure 44-1 shows examples of full and semiblock format letters.

In addition to the letter format, it is important in identifying the standard components of a letter, which will ensure you have included all necessary information to your recipient. Table 44-1 lists the common components of a letter.

Marketing a Dental Practice

While the overall goal of the dental practice is to provide quality care to the patients, it is important to understand that the practice is a business. Commitment to patient care and meeting the needs of the community are the objectives of every dental office. However, if a practice is to be successful in meeting the needs of the community, it must approach dentistry from a business idealism, as well. The practice cannot provide care to the community if it does not remain sustainable. Marketing is a means of attracting and retaining patients who are satisfied with the practice. All members of the dental team need to be involved in marketing the practice. It can be rewarding for dental assistants to attract patients to the practice, whether through external or internal methods.

Even during off hours, a dental assistant is still associated with the dental practice where they are employed. When people ask what your occupation is, it provides an opportunity to do **external marketing** for the practice. Other planned external activities can be done, such as dental health education in the community at schools and senior centers. Professionalism and enthusiasm enhance any marketing attempts.

Bruno M. Santos, DDS
100 East Main Street-Suite 120
Yourtown, US 98765-4321

August 15, 20XX **(DATELINE)**

Kulus B. Nazari. DMD
50 North Broad Street
Mytown, US 43200 **(INSIDE ADDRESS)**

Dear Dr. Nazari: **(SALUTATION)**

RE: Emma P. Golubeva **(REFERENCE)**

I am referring Ms. Golubeva, age 18, to your office for an oral surgery evaluation of impacted wisdom teeth #'s 1 and 16. Ms. Golubeva was seen in our office today and presented with pain and pressure. Radiograph evaluation showed full bony impaction of the maxillary third molars. Please evaluate for removal.

Enclosed is a copy of the most recent panoramic radiograph, dated 8/15/20XX.

Ms. Golubeva will call your office for an appointment. I would appreciate a report of your findings.

Sincerely yours, **(COMPLIMENTARY CLOSE)**

(SIGNATURE OF SENDER)

Bruno M. Santos, DDS **(NAME TYPED)**

lk **(REFERENCE INITIALS)**

(ENCLOSURE, IF ANY)

(A)

Bruno M. Santos, DDS Yourtown, US 98765-4321
100 East Main Street-Suite 120

August 15, 20XX **(DATELINE)**

Kulus B. Nazari. DMD
50 North Broad Street
Mytown, US 43200 **(INSIDE ADDRESS)**

Dear Dr. Nazari: **(SALUTATION)**

RE: Emma P. Golubeva **(REFERENCE)**

I am referring Ms. Golubeva, age 18, to your office for an oral surgery evaluation of impacted wisdom teeth #'s 1 and 16. Ms. Golubeva was seen in our office today and presented with pain and pressure. Radiograph evaluation showed full bony impaction of the maxillary third molars. Please evaluate for removal.

Enclosed is a copy of the most recent panoramic radiograph, dated 8/15/20XX.

Ms. Golubeva will call your office for an appointment. I would appreciate a report of your findings.

Sincerely yours,
(COMPLIMENTARY CLOSE)
(SIGNATURE OF SENDER)
Bruno M. Santos, DDS **(NAME TYPED)**

lk **(REFERENCE INITIALS)**

(ENCLOSURE, IF ANY)

(B)

FIGURE 44-1
Examples of (A) full and (B) semiblock format letters.

TABLE 44-1 Components of a Letter

Sender's address	This section can be omitted if included in the office letterhead. Include the street address, city, and zip code.
Date	The date should be written in the American date format (placing the month before the day) and placed 2 inches from the top of the page.
Inside address	This is the recipient's address. Include a personal title such as *Ms., Mr.,* or *Dr.* When writing the address, use the USPS. format and place it below the sender's address, or 1 inch below the date.
Salutation	This is to whom you are addressing the letter. Use the proper personal title as you used in the inside address.
Body	Includes the introduction to the letter. This is where you state your main point and discuss your purpose of the letter. Remember to be friendly and concise.
Closing	Choose the formal closing you wish and capitalize the first letter only, such as "Thank you" or "Warm regards." Leave four spaces between the closing and your name and title.
Signature	Sign your name above your name and title.
Name and title	Include your name and title.
Enclosures	If you are including any enclosures in your letter, such as patient registration forms, discounts, or brochures, include the word "Enclosures" one line below your name and title.

In addition to the welcome letter (discussed previously), **internal marketing** can be accomplished in a number of ways. One person or the whole staff can participate. The ideas are limitless, but Table 44-2 lists some popular possibilities.

Online Marketing

Marketing using the Internet is increasingly popular with dental offices. It allows them to reach large numbers of existing and potential patients for a relatively small cost. Search engines process searches numbering in the billions daily, so one could say with confidence that a prospective patient will be searching for a dentist online. In addition, the cost of online marketing is less than direct mail, as it eliminates the cost of postage and printing.

Website An office website is an example of both internal and external marketing. It serves as a way for existing patients to contact the practice or learn about new dental techniques being offered by the practice. Some offices set up secured websites, or patient portals, that allow patients to make or check appointments, review their accounts, and make payments online. Websites also attract new patients to the practice by providing information about the dentist and staff, practice philosophy, location details, and the hours that the practice sees patients. The office website provides a way for the office to introduce the dentist and staff. Each individual can have a photo accompanied by a biography including their professional qualifications and a brief personal fact that patients can relate to, such as favorite hobbies or pets.

A dental practice can set up a website using one of the many templates available. Often, offices will use a professional website developer to assist them in the design to create a more unique appearance (Figure 44-2). Once the website is online, it must be maintained. Someone in the office needs to check to make sure that the links work so that patients and future patients can obtain information. New and updated material needs to be added to keep the website current. Finding fun facts and news can involve everyone in the practice. Often when a website developer or marketing team is in control, they offer periodic maintenance and update options.

Remember that the practice's online presence must be Health Information Portability and Accountability Act (HIPAA) compliant (see Chapter 3, "Ethics, Jurisprudence, and the Health Information Portability and Accountability Act"). Having a photo release form ready for all patients to sign at the new patient visit will save time later. Even if your practice is posting smile transformation photos that don't show the patient's entire face, ask and receive their written permission.

TABLE 44-2 Internal Marketing Ideas

Monthly newsletters or blogs with tips for dental health
Patient reactivation programs
Offering entry into a raffle for liking or following social media pages
Referral contests for patients allowing them the chance to win prizes for recommending the office to friends and family
Flowers sent to patients as a referral thank you
Birthday greetings or cards for special occasions, such as a new baby, an anniversary, or a graduation
Special dental services coupons, such as discounts on services like whitening
Refrigerator magnets, lip balm, pens, and toothbrushes noting the dental office and phone number

Social Media Social media, such as Facebook, Twitter, and Instagram, can also be used to attract patients and stay in contact with existing patients. This type of marketing seems simple, but it takes time and must be monitored closely. The practice should have a plan for the types of things the practice would like to post and follow. Remember that posts on social media create a personality for the practice! Think about how the patients see a post as compared to how the office staff may see it. For example, Dr. Smith gets a new boat and tweets out photos. Some patients may see it as a sign they are paying too much for their dental care, rather than Dr. Smith's reward for working hard. However, if Dr. Smith tweets out photos of his new baby, patients may feel like part of the family. You want to update frequently enough to keep patients engaged but not overwhelm them with content. It is often more effective to have one person in the office in charge of doing all the social media postings.

Reviews Positive reviews can be extremely helpful in building a dental practice, but if you have negative reviews patients and

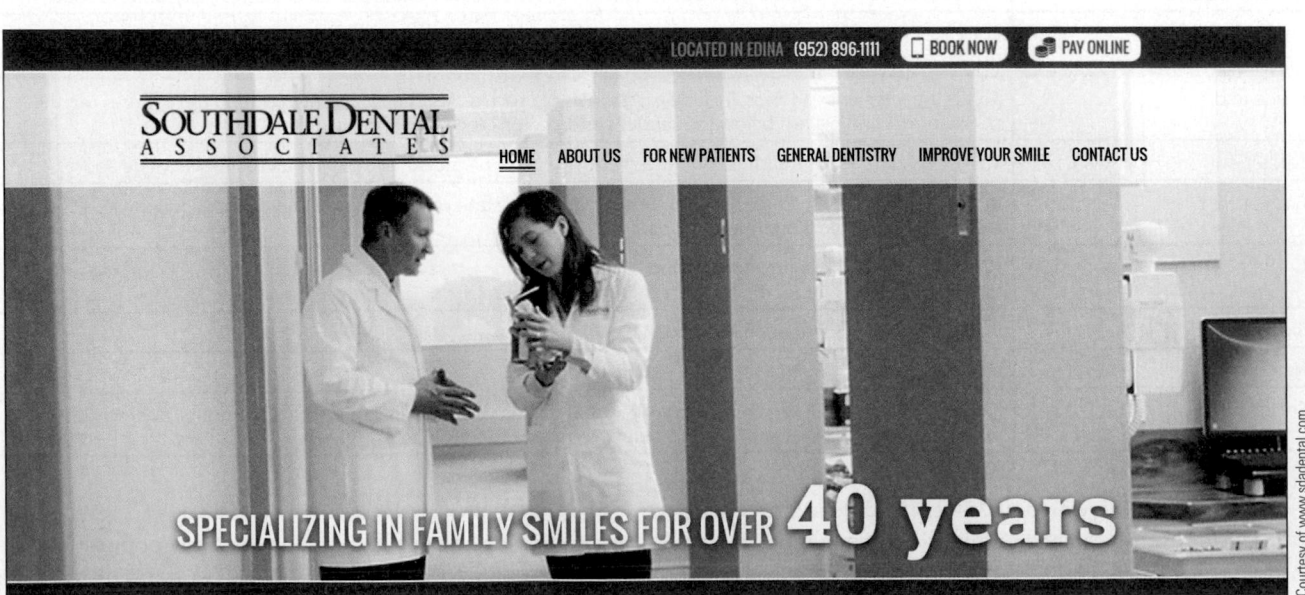

FIGURE 44-2
The office website should be visually appealing and functional.

prospective patients see those too. There is nothing wrong with asking patients who have had a good experience in your office to write a review.

While it is always disappointing to receive a poor review, it can be constructive. Sometimes the person is right, and by letting you know, they have given the practice an opportunity to correct the problem. To avoid this happening on a public forum, the office can choose to have an anonymous patient satisfaction survey available to the patient. The practice may also receive a poor review that is unjustified. If this happens it is best not to argue about its validity online since it draws attention to the comment. Simply contact the person privately to discuss their concerns.

The goal of marketing is to attract new patients to the practice and retain current patients. Go that *extra mile* to make patients comfortable. Treat them with dignity every time they are in the office.

Reception Area

The reception area is a place where patients are greeted (Figure 44-3). Avoid referring to it as a waiting room as this gives it a negative connotation: patients are busy, their time is important, and they do not want to wait. The colors, design, and artwork should be relaxing and comfortable, and seating should be available so that each patient can have their own space. Keep in mind that individuals from different cultures have varying personal space requirements. The seating should be arranged in a way that allows people to cluster together or remain distant from others.

The reception area should be kept neat and clean. This may require frequent attention throughout the day. Patients looking around the reception area and seeing dust, dirty glass, or discarded trash will wonder if this is a reflection of the overall cleanliness of the practice. Special attention should be taken to keep children's toys and puzzles clean. Patients are also acutely aware of dental office smells, so efforts should be made to eliminate them as much as possible.

Provide magazines containing short stories so that patients can read them if they are waiting. The magazines should be current. An office that has out-of-date magazines shows indifference to the patient, and it reflects negatively on overall care. Many dentists have brochures and pamphlets related to the procedures

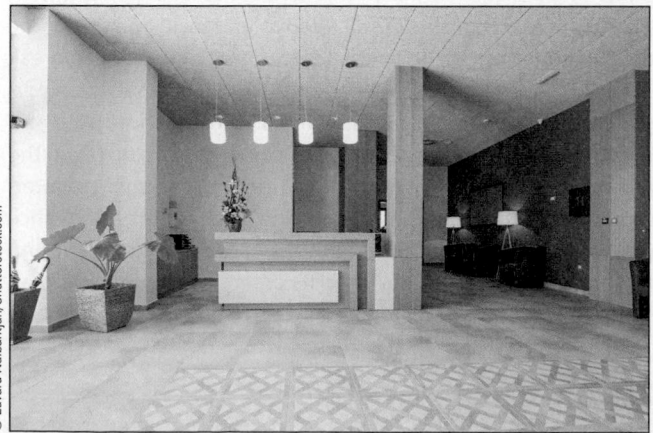

FIGURE 44-3
Neat and organized reception area.

performed in the office. This is also an area in which to display marketing materials. Having a digital photo album on display showing before and after cosmetic procedures or giving a visual aid showing restorative and preventative procedures could motivate patients to complete treatment.

Some offices have photos of staff members. Patients like to feel that they can get to know the staff members who are taking care of them. Consider providing coffee bar areas where patients can relax with a beverage (coffee and juice), or areas with toys and games for children and teens. Providing Internet access for patients in the reception area is also a growing trend.

Reception areas must be comfortable for everyone regardless of ability. In 1990, Congress originally passed the Americans with Disabilities Act (ADA); since then it has been amended several times. It mandates that individuals with disabilities have access to health care facilities, including dental offices. Patients with sight or hearing impairments must be provided with assistance to enable them to complete forms and fully understand treatment plans. To accommodate physically disabled patients, all doors and hallways should be wide enough for wheelchair access, and a ramp should be available in areas where stairs are present and no elevator is available. Restrooms must be accessible and ADA compliant.

Front Office Staff

The front office staff, or business office staff, is an integral part of the team. They are responsible for the flow and efficiency of the business. Depending on the size and needs of the office, the front office staff can consist of an administrative assistant, also referred to as a front office assistant or receptionist, and/or a front office manager. There are times where an office will have both an assistant and a manger, while other smaller offices may just employ one front office staffer as a front office manager.

Either way, these individuals must be able to complete multiple tasks on time and pay close attention to details. They must be organized, have knowledge of dental treatments, and exhibit good communication and problem-solving skills. All individuals in the front office need to be knowledgeable in using business machines such as computers, scanners, faxes, copy machines, and high-tech phone systems. They must be able to communicate effectively, listen to and observe patients, and serve as a liaison between the patient and clinical staff. This individual must be able to respond to patients who may be upset in a calm, tactful, and appropriate manner.

These responsibilities are often viewed as "behind the scenes" activities. Without these required responsibilities being met, the practice cannot flourish, nor can it be profitable. This can be further broken down into accounts receivable and accounts payable (to be discussed later in the chapter). These finances are normally handled in two separate bookkeeping systems. This individual also submits **claims** to the patient's dental insurance and makes financial arrangements with the patients for payment of the dental service.

The front office staff is normally responsible for tasks including, but not limited to, the following:

● Greeting patients

● Assisting patients in filling out initial paperwork required for treatment

- Answering the telephone and taking messages as necessary
- Scheduling appointments
- Maintaining the patient chart system and records
- Accepting and recording patient payments
- Billing insurance claims

Telephone Techniques

The front office is in charge of a number of responsibilities that take place in the office on a day-to-day basis. How effective the administrative assistant is at carrying out the responsibilities will mean the difference between a successful dental practice and an unsuccessful dental practice. While particular responsibilities are placed on one person, there may be times where assistance is needed. For that reason it is imperative that all members of the staff be aware of the proper protocol and procedures involved in administration. This includes proper and effective communication with patients.

How you communicate over the telephone can have a positive or negative effect on the dental practice. So much time is put into how people present themselves in person-to-person contact that they often forget about the **telecommunications** aspect of the business. Dental staff should take pride in their appearances and how they present themselves to others. The same should be said of how their image is presented over the telephone. In person, the dental assistant is able to make nonverbal cues and use body language, such as smiling or showing confusion. In a telephone conversation they are only left with the use of their voice, which increases the need for learning proper phone etiquette. Regardless of who is on the other end of the phone, a patient, representative, or colleague, the person should be kept well informed and feel appreciated. How many times have you been placed on hold while trying to contact an office to make an appointment or to ask a question? We all have been on the receiving end of poor customer service. Applying what you have learned in our own lives regarding customer satisfaction into our responsibilities as dental staff will help ensure you provide professional services. This responsibility begins with professional telephone techniques. As a professional, the dental assistant needs to know proper telephone etiquette, how to manage incoming and outgoing calls, and how to create a good image.

Basic Telephone Techniques

Often, a ringing telephone can be viewed as an interruption. The reality is, the person on the other line is the reason for the office's existence. This may be a patient who is calling for the first time, and the telephone interaction can be the first impression to the patient, before they even enter the office. Answer the call promptly within the first two rings. Developing and following these skills can assist in better telephone communication, resulting in a positive effect for the practice.

1. **Speak clearly.** Remember, the person on the other end of the phone cannot see you; they can only hear you. Speak clearly and at a reasonable rate. Often dental assistants can be busy at the office and speak with a rapid nature. When answering a call, slow down and enunciate words so as to not appear mumbled.

2. **Use a normal tone.** Avoid shouting or speaking softly. If the person asks you to repeat yourself, chances are you may be speaking too softly. It may be wise to adjust your tone according to the person's reactions. Remember to speak with a smile. Talking to someone who is monotone can be quite dull. Use enthusiasm and normal voice inflections to show eagerness and interest as you speak.

3. **Identify the practice.** Most times, the office may have a specific greeting they would like you to say upon answering the phone. For example, "Good morning. This is Doctor Juma's office. This is Nicolette speaking. How may I help you?" Always be sure to identify yourself to the person calling. This will lead them to do the same, so you know how to properly address them.

4. **Address the person properly.** When the person identifies themselves, address them by their title and not their first name. Example: "Good afternoon, Mrs. Chen."

5. **Avoid slang.** When speaking to the caller, use proper verbiage, such as "yes" instead of "yeah." Instead of saying "hold on a sec," say, "May I place you on hold for one minute, Mrs. Chen?"

6. **Focus on the call.** Avoid being distracted by your environment.

Answering Calls

An administrative assistant must be prepared to answer incoming calls at any time while juggling the other responsibilities of the front desk. It is crucial that the caller feels that they have the total attention of the assistant. Good listening and communication skills help portray an image of an organized, efficient, and courteous dental office. The front office assistant must be able to listen carefully to the caller and make judgments, after gathering information, that will aid in the patient's care. It may be necessary to *screen* the calls to get the caller in touch with the right person to solve the problem. If the patient asks to speak to the dentist, the front office assistant must first try to help, identify the patient's concern, and take a telephone number where the doctor can call the patient back. If the dentist is with another patient, they should not be interrupted. This can be for a few reasons. The patient who is currently with the dentist has a set appointment that deserves the dentist's undivided attention. In addition, if the dentist is interrupted, it can cause treatment delays or can break infection control procedures. In the event it is a patient emergency, the administrative assistant can write a short note and give it to the dentist in the treatment room out of sight from the patient. This may also be the case if the dentist asks you to interrupt them in the event they are waiting for a call. Knowing office policy on when the dentist would like to be interrupted during treatment (e.g., when other dentists or family members call) can help alleviate some of the uncertain moments.

Placing Callers on Hold

In the event you need to place a caller on hold, kindly ask for their permission. Prior to placing the caller on hold, wait for their response. Try to minimize hold time to no more than a few minutes. If necessary, check in and ask whether the caller would like to continue to hold, or whether it would be more convenient to receive a call back. It is best to stick to the agreed upon time for returning the call. For example, if you tell the caller you will return their call within the hour, keep to that time frame.

Taking Messages

There are times when a call will require you to take a message, either because the person they are requesting is not available, or you need to search for further information per a request. Many offices will use a message book, or phone message book, to log calls (Figure 44-4). Table 44-3 lists the common areas filled out for a phone message.

After the message is written, repeat it to the caller to verify that it was written correctly. Also, enter your initials or name in case the person receiving the messages has questions. Do not make promises to the caller you cannot keep. If you are not completely sure you can return the call that day, do not promise it. The same goes for a caller wishing to speak to the dentist. Only promise a call back time when you are sure the dentist will be able to return the phone call. In the event the dentist will be returning a patient call, always have the proper phone message, the patient's chart (if an established patient), and any additional information they may need ready to complete the call.

TABLE 44-3 Items Needed When Taking a Phone Message

The caller's name
Date
Time of call
Message
Name of person who took message
Urgency
Call back number
Best time to reach the caller

Outgoing Calls

When telephone calls are made from the office, the same professional, positive approach should be followed. Be prepared and know the information that needs to be conveyed or sought. Most offices call the next day's patients to confirm their appointments. To avoid a repeat call to the patient, use some type of indication system to keep track of which patients have been called. Most dental **software** used today has some indicator that can be noted in the appointment book, such as a color-coded bar on the side of the appointment (Figure 44-5). This bar can tell you if the patient was confirmed, if a message was left, if there was no answer, and so on. If calling an insurance company, have all the information handy, including the patient's chart and forms, so that any questions that come up can be answered appropriately.

If calling and leaving a message, take care with any information recorded on the answering machine. Remember that all health care issues are confidential and should be discussed only with the patient. Only leave a message on a machine if the patient filled out a proper release to do so.

It is best if no personal telephone calls are made at the office. If the need arises, make them during your lunch hour, if possible. The telephone is for dental office business, and personal matters belong outside the office.

When phone calls need to be made to insurance companies and patients living or working in other parts of the country, keep in mind that there are time differences between different parts of the world.

English as a Second Language

The U.S. Census Bureau shows that as of 2013, one in five U.S. residents speaks a language at home other than English. Many of these individuals may face barriers to accessing basic dental care. It is probable to encounter many patients whose primary language is not English in the dental office. As health care workers, we are responsible to try and meet the needs of all patients, including those with such barriers. The dentist is responsible for providing an **interpreter**, if necessary, for communication. This is not always feasible, however. Some patients will bring family members who can translate. In any event, it is important that communication, either on the telephone or in the office, be

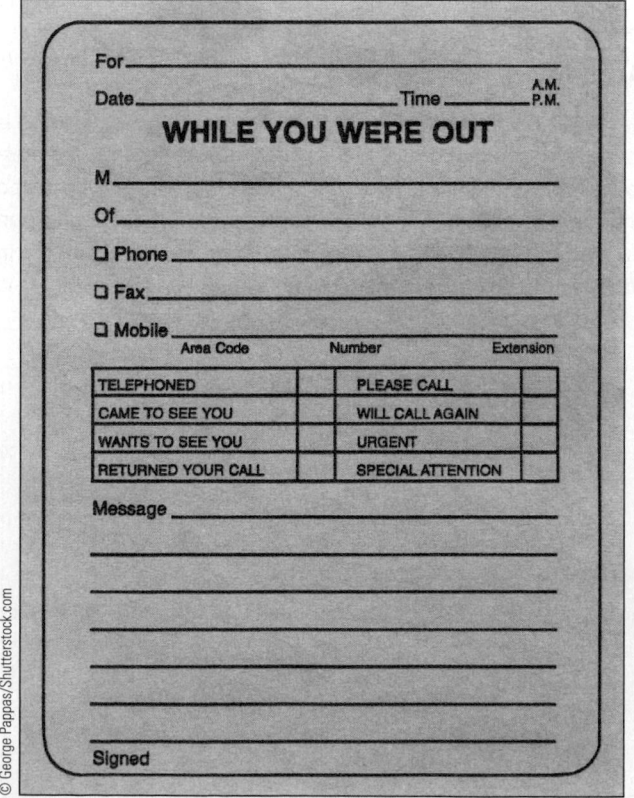

FIGURE 44-4
Paper message book.

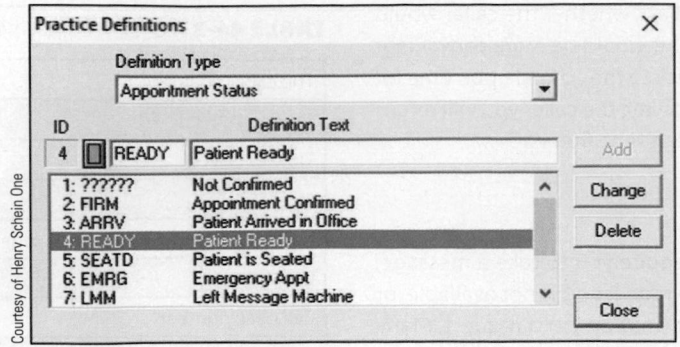

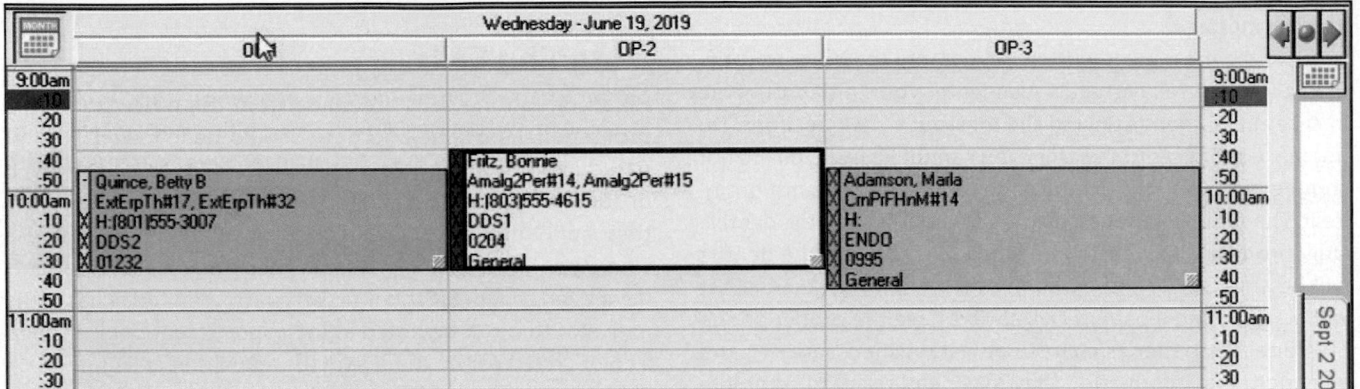

FIGURE 44-5
Color-coded appointment status in dental software.

handled in a manner that provides the patient with the pertinent and clear information. There are several things to remember when speaking to patients whose first language is not English:

● Be patient.

● Speak at a normal volume. Raising the voice does not increase the other person's ability to understand the words.

● Speak more slowly, if necessary, and avoid complicated words, metaphors, or slang terms.

● A patient who does not speak English may be able to understand English well. Do not assume that the patient does not comprehend what is being said.

● Ask the patient if clarification is needed.

● Repeat the information, if necessary, until understood.

Communication Technology

Every phone call is important. There will be times when a caller will try to reach you after office hours. Just like during office hours, your **phone messaging system** can be the first communication the caller has with your office, so it is important to depict the same skills through the message as in person. This type of messaging can be done through many avenues. Whichever messaging system is used, the purpose is to allow a caller to leave a message while the practice is closed or unavailable.

Answering Machine

An **answering machine** (Figure 44-6) records messages and is found in the dental office. Many times, offices have preset messages for typical times of the day, such as lunch and closing, and change the message to the appropriate option depending on need. In any event, the message should be clear and spoken in the same manner as you would speak in person. Table 44-4 lists

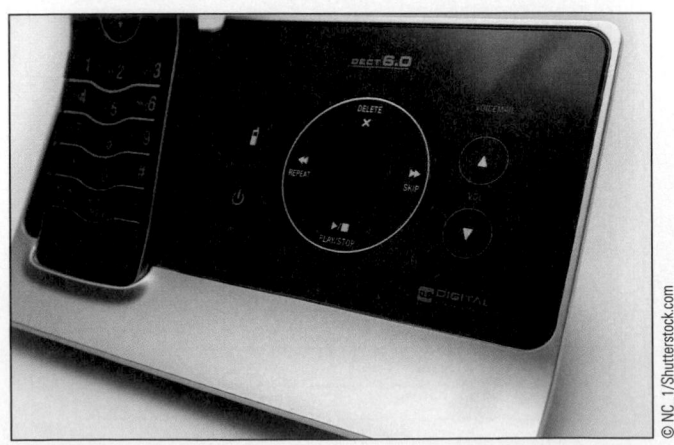

FIGURE 44-6
Answering machine.

TABLE 44-4 What Should Be Included When Recording an Away Message

A welcoming greeting that identifies the office
The reason the machine is answering (away from the desk, closed, etc.)
What time the office will reopen
Instructions on leaving a message, for example, "Please leave a brief message, date and time of your call, return phone number and the best time to reach you."
Emergency contact; this can be the dentist's cell phone number or a dentist's on call number

important factors that should be included when recording a message.

If the phone system is used to take messages during the work day, the front office assistant must remember to check for those messages. Generally, phone systems have something such as a blinking light or a special tone that can be heard when picking up the phone. When checking answering machine messages, log them into your message book and be sure to take note of all information. From there, you can sort through messages and return calls in the order of importance.

Answering with Headphones

The administrative assistant completes numerous tasks where their hands are needed, so offices may use headphones (Figure 44-7) to answer calls. These allow the person taking the calls to be able to write things down much more easily. They may also be utilized to talk to other team members throughout the office. This interactive ongoing communication will help make the office run smoothly.

Answering Services

Some offices have **answering services** that are staffed by live operators. Having a person at the other end of the line can be more reassuring to patients and other callers. Having a live person on the other end is also helpful in the event a new patient calls. A good first impression may mean the difference to a potential patient considering going elsewhere. These services also can provide flexibility in screening and routing calls, as well as offer bilingual services that would otherwise be unavailable with an in-office answering system. Most of the fees for the answering services are by the month or by the number of calls received. This service is more expensive than an in-office answering system.

Voicemail

Voicemail, which is similar to an answering machine, allows for messages to be remotely accessed. Voicemail also allow for message taking while a call is in progress, whereas an answering machine cannot. Some offices may utilize both an answering machine (for when they are out of the office) and voicemail (for when the phone is in use). Voicemail requires an access code to be used when retrieving messages, which may offer more security to access messages than an answering machine.

Fax Machines

Fax machines are common in the dental office (Figure 44-8). Fax is a facsimile transmission used to send and receive written messages through the telephone lines. It is important that it be sent to the correct address, taking care that confidential protected health information be handled conscientiously. Some ways to safeguard a fax machine include the following:

- Set user authentication—monitors who is sending a facsimile to whom and when.
- Place machine in an area where only authorized users may access.
- Do not leave any forms in machine after facsimile is transmitted.
- Train staff on proper and safe handling of patients protected health information.

FIGURE 44-7
Phone headset allowing for hands-free telephone use.

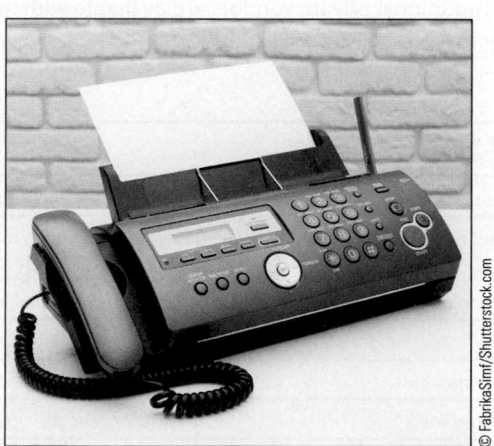

FIGURE 44-8
Fax machine.

Email

Email (electronic mail) is another common form of communication used by dental practices. It can be very convenient and saves time and money over paper mail. Email can be saved so that all the parties involved in the electronic conversation have a history of it. Multiple email addresses can be used to send the same message to a group of people, or a message can be forwarded to a third party for whom the message might be relevant.

Email can be used, with their consent, to contact patients. Patient privacy rules apply to this form of contact, so protected health information (PHI) should not be included unless the patient has approved in writing to do so and has signed any necessary releases. Refer to Table 44-5 for guidelines to follow when sending an email.

Cell Phones

Cell phones have become so common, many families no longer have traditional land lines. When updating patient records, document what the best number is to reach them at for confirmation of appointments and other communication. Today, many offices offer communication through text messages, such as confirming appointments and offering specials. Cell phone etiquette for the staff is listed in Table 44-6.

Cell phones can also be used as an alternative to an after-hours answering service. The office cell phone belongs to the office, but staff members take it home at night and weekends to answer possible emergency calls. The dental team member talks to the patient and determines if they should contact the dentist, schedule an emergency visit, or if the call can be returned during business hours. Remember that emergencies can be anything from a true dental emergency requiring immediate assistance to a problem that needs to be scheduled quickly but not immediately.

U.S. Postal Service

The U.S. Postal Service (USPS) has numerous ideas and plans for small businesses. Check their website, *www.usps.com*, under business solutions to find services that may help your dental office. Several additional private vendors are available with new ideas and services available for mail and shipping as well. If your practice

TABLE 44-5 Guidelines When Sending Emails

Use complete sentences.
Grammar and spelling should be accurate.
Be polite and remain professional.
Proofread your email before sending it.
Never send an email when you are upset, mad, or frustrated.
Capitalize appropriately. Using all CAPITAL letters is viewed as shouting.
Use the subject line to summarize the message in a few words.
Keep your message brief and to the point.
Use an appropriate salutation and closing.
Using an electronic signature can be helpful in providing additional contact information.
Do not send personal email from an office computer.
Never include credit card or other personal or office financial information.

TABLE 44-6 Cell Phone Etiquette in Health Care Settings

Turn your cell phone to vibrate when you are in the office.
Leave your phone in your purse or locker during work hours.
During lunch or break times, find a private area to make calls.
No phone calls in the restroom—anyone can be in the restroom overhearing the conversation.
If you use your cell phone to take photos, keep in mind what or who is in the background. A patient or PHI that might be visible is a violation of HIPAA.

has a need for a confirmation of delivery, use certified mail. The mailperson has the individual receiving the mail sign for it, and then a copy of the signature is given to the sender for the sender's records. Certified mail is used when the practice must prove that a patient has received a letter. If no proof is required, but the dental practice wants to track the package or letter, a tracking number can be obtained and used to track it online. Table 44-7 shows USPS services that a small business, such as a dental office, can use.

TABLE 44-7 USPS Services

Certificate of mailing	A receipt showing that an item was mailed.
Certified mail	Gives the sender a mailing receipt at the time of mailing and online access to the date and time of delivery. It also provides the recipient's signature at the delivery time.
Collect on delivery (COD)	Collect payment when the merchandise is delivered.
Delivery confirmation	An online service that verifies the delivery date, location, and time.
Insured mail	Insurance coverage that is purchased when the mailer sends the items.
Registered mail	The most secure type of mail, which ensures the protection of important mail.
Restricted delivery	Mail is delivered only to the specified individual.
Return receipt	Gives the sender proof of delivery.

Patient Care Plan

After the dentist completes a thorough examination on the patient, they then develop a treatment plan or **care plan**. The care plan is a written document that reports the options the dentist can provide for dental care and managing the patient's dental condition. Each patient who is seen in your office will have a unique and different set of needs. The care plan will be individualized to that particular patient at the time they present in the office. Depending on the individual care plan of the patient, such as financial obstacles or priority of needs (the patient's chief complaint), the care plan may have to be altered. For instance, if the care plan proposes multiple bridges, the patient may opt to get a partial denture instead of the bridges due to finances. In some cases, the dentist may develop more than one care plan to present options, which alleviates the need for altering the original plan.

The monitoring or creation of patient care plans is vital to the success of a dental practice. Patients who have been fully informed of their treatment options, time line of completion for the care plan, financial responsibilities associated with the intended care plan, and how the various dental insurance plans are applied to the intended treatment are more likely to remain with a dental practice.

Presenting the Care Plan

Presenting the care plan can vary among different offices. Proper time spent on the presentation to the patient permits the patient to understand the plan and make the appropriate decision. It is best when the care plan is presented in a designated consult area, or a private area of the office outside the operatory. All visual aids, including the patient chart, educational materials, models, and brochures should be available to assist in presenting. The dentist should present all options to the patient in terms the patient can easily understand. A good way to involve the patient in their care plan is to encourage the patient to ask questions about the different plans and be informed of the advantages and disadvantages of each. Instead of asking the patient if they have any questions, ask them which questions they have. That shows the patient you are assuming they will have a question and may open them up to ask what they are thinking. After the patient is informed of their options, the administrative assistant presents the financial estimate for each treatment option being offered. The patient then chooses the care plan that best suits their needs, the financial arrangements are made, and treatment is then scheduled. Informed consent of the treatment is at the time of acceptance; however, the office may wish to utilize a formal document for the patient, dentist, and witness to sign. This is most helpful in larger, more extensive cases. An informed consent includes the number of appointments, finances, and requires the patient's signature.

Patients who are fully informed about their proposed treatment options can develop a bond of trust between themselves, the dentist, and dental staff. A well-received line of communication between patient and provider/staff is the ideal in growing a successful practice and maintaining it.

Appointment Scheduling

Appointment scheduling is another form of communicating with patients. An efficient appointment system keeps the office running smoothly and contributes to its success. Mainly it is ideal to have one person who is in charge of scheduling; however, this may not be feasible in larger practices. In some practices, patients schedule future appointments in the operatory with the dental assistant or dental hygienist. It is important that all clinical and administrative staff are aware of and adhere to the scheduling protocol and policies the office maintains.

The goal of an efficient appointment system is to ensure patients will be seen on time, operators make appropriate use of the time given, and the day is balanced. By working as a team, the staff can complete these goals, reduce stress in the office, and allow for quality care to be given to the patient.

An appointment book can be either paper or computerized (Figure 44-9). Today, making appointments is no longer restricted to calling the office, directly speaking with someone, and scheduling. The option of scheduling online through a **patient portal** has become popular. This is unique to the practice in which you will work; however, regardless of the system being used the guidelines will be the same.

Appointment Scheduling Guidelines

The appointment book manager must first **matrix** the **appointment book**. When utilizing a paper book, most commonly the book is found on a desk surface and has a view of the week at a time. A book should be picked that allows appropriate room to write in the appointments legibly. Other considerations on choosing a book are the intervals of time for each row, printed or "fill-in" dates, and number of columns that correspond to the number of operatories available. When utilizing a software program, the appointment can be tailored to your needs for all these options and many more. This can include changing views of the appointment book from day to week to month, searching for available appointments, locating existing appointments, development of a computerized recare system, unscheduled lists (Figure 44-10), ASAP lists, use of colors for each operator or appointment type, goal tracking (Figure 44-11), and communication with the operatories on patient arrival. Regardless of which system your practice chooses, the following are considerations when developing the appointment book.

- **Columns.** Columns in the appointment book represent the operatories or treatment areas available that day. Operators are anyone who is treating the patient in the dental chair. This can be the dentist, dental hygienist, or an expanded function dental assistant. The larger the practice, the more columns will be needed. In this case, if computer software is not available, use of another book is necessary.

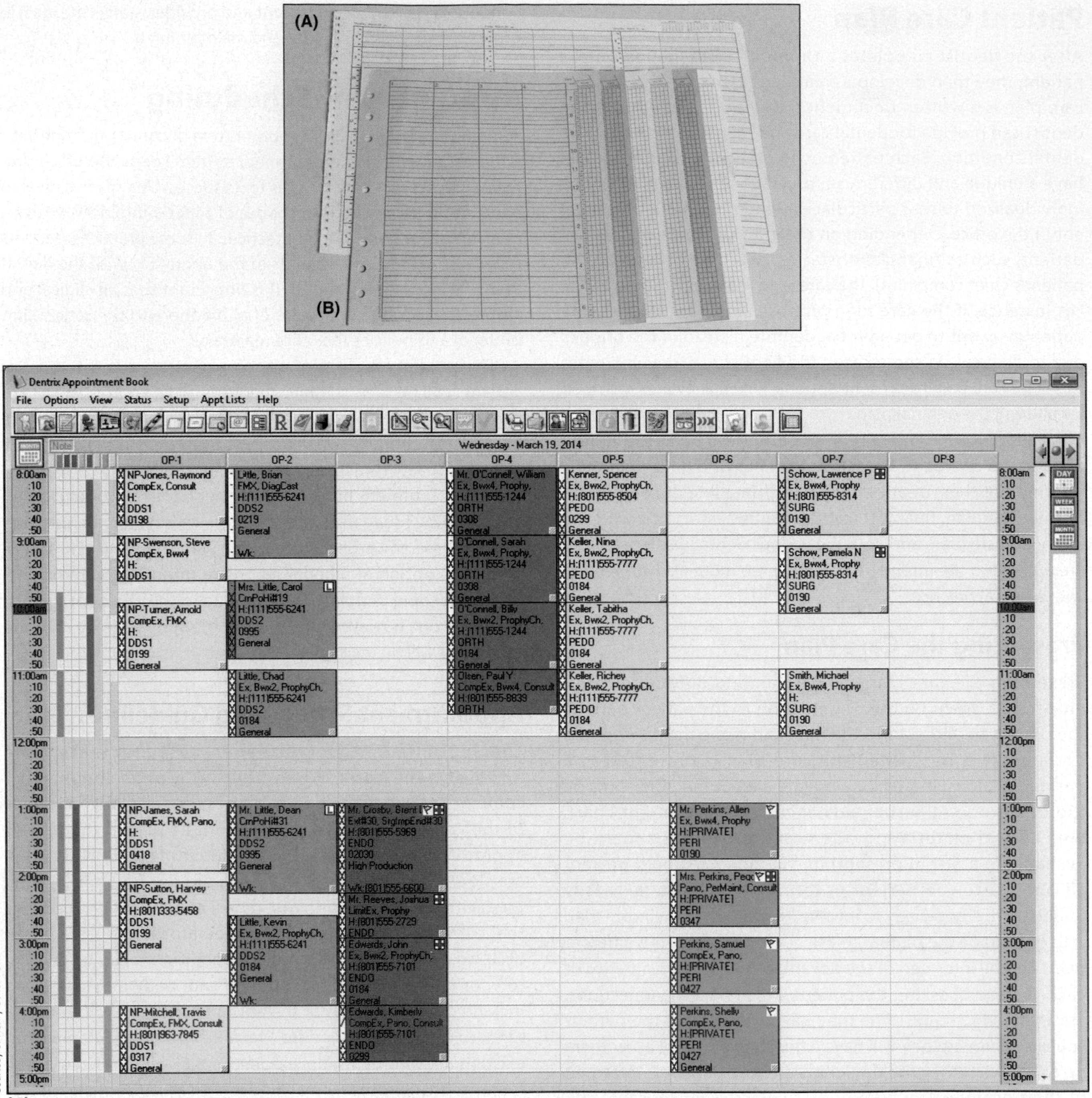

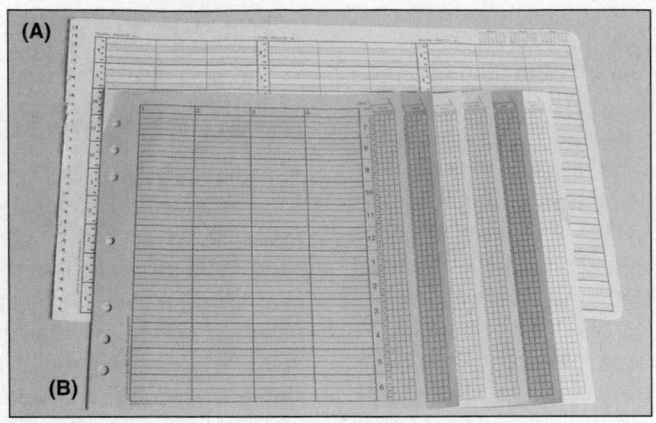

(C)

Courtesy of Henry Schein One

FIGURE 44-9

Appointment book options: (A) Showing paper appointment book pages with a 15-minute interval. (B) Showing color-coded appointment book pages allowing efficient use of the dentist's and dental auxiliaries' time. (C) Computerized appointment book page showing use of nine different operatories.

- **Units of time.** The *units of time* represent how much time each row represents. This is usually in 10-, 15-, or 30-minute intervals, referred to as units of time. This is based on the dentist's preference. For example, in a practice where the dentist prefers a 10-minute interval, an appointment requiring an hour of length would be six units. Use of a smaller interval will allow for a better advantage of production when scheduling.

If there is only a 30 minute unit and the dentist needs to schedule a 10-minute reevaluation, it could mean 20 minutes lost time.

- **Outlining the schedule.** Once the office agrees on the units of time and number of treatment areas, the next step is to outline the schedule using **time blocks**. This includes office hours, blocking out for lunch or breaks, buffer time, holidays

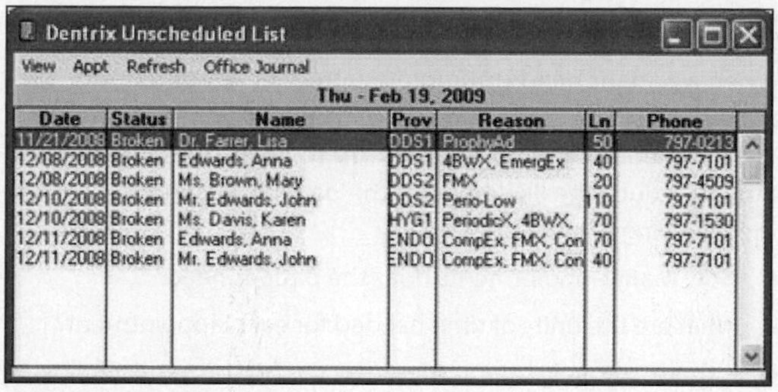

Dentrix Unscheduled List

View Appt Refresh Office Journal

Thu - Feb 19, 2009

Date	Status	Name	Prov	Reason	Ln	Phone
11/21/2008	Broken	Dr. Farrer, Lisa	DDS1	ProphyAd	50	797-0213
12/08/2008	Broken	Edwards, Anna	DDS1	4BWX, EmergEx	40	797-7101
12/08/2008	Broken	Ms. Brown, Mary	DDS2	FMX	20	797-4509
12/10/2008	Broken	Mr. Edwards, John	DDS2	Perio-Low	110	797-7101
12/10/2008	Broken	Ms. Davis, Karen	HYG1	PeriodicX, 4BWX,	70	797-1530
12/11/2008	Broken	Edwards, Anna	ENDO	CompEx, FMX, Con	70	797-7101
12/11/2008	Broken	Mr. Edwards, John	ENDO	CompEx, FMX, Con	40	797-7101

Courtesy of Dentrix

FIGURE 44-10
Unscheduled list using dental software.

or any other day the office is closed, as well as scheduled office meetings. Office hours are the hours in which a patient can be treated. This does not include break, lunch, or time closed.

Buffer times are the times set aside to allow for emergencies. Usually it is beneficial to allow for one in the morning and one in the afternoon or evening. The length depends on the preference of the doctor but should be one to two units, depending on the unit time your office chooses. If this appointment is not needed, it can be filled last minute with a smaller appointment, such as an appliance insert or postoperative appointment.

When closing the office for holidays, it is important to take note of holidays the office will be open and closed. These days might be more desirable to patients if they do not have work and school is closed. Make a note in the appointment book in advance to be prepared for the day.

Elements in Appointment Scheduling

When it is time to schedule the patient's appointment, there are different aspects that should be considered by the administrative assistant or the dental staff personnel who are in charge of scheduling. When scheduling, the staff needs to consider the treatment to be completed, the needs of the patient, and following proper appointment scheduling protocol. A well scheduled book takes into consideration the dentist's down time, such as when they are waiting for an impression to set or a patient's anesthetic to take effect. This would be an appropriate time for the dentist to check in on a hygiene patient or to do another quick procedure such as removing sutures. Coming up with strategies to follow for common occurrences is important for any dental practice.

Scheduling of Dental Hygiene

Scheduling units of time for dental hygiene patients is usually discussed and agreed upon by the dentist and the dental hygienist. The dental hygienist should discuss with the administrative assistant appropriate units of time for typical procedures scheduled. This can be for a new patient adult and child, recare patient adult and child, pit and fissure sealants, or root planing and scaling. Each appointment will need a specific time to treat the patient appropriately.

Scheduling of New Patients

Patients generally do not like to wait too long for an appointment and may choose to find an office that can take

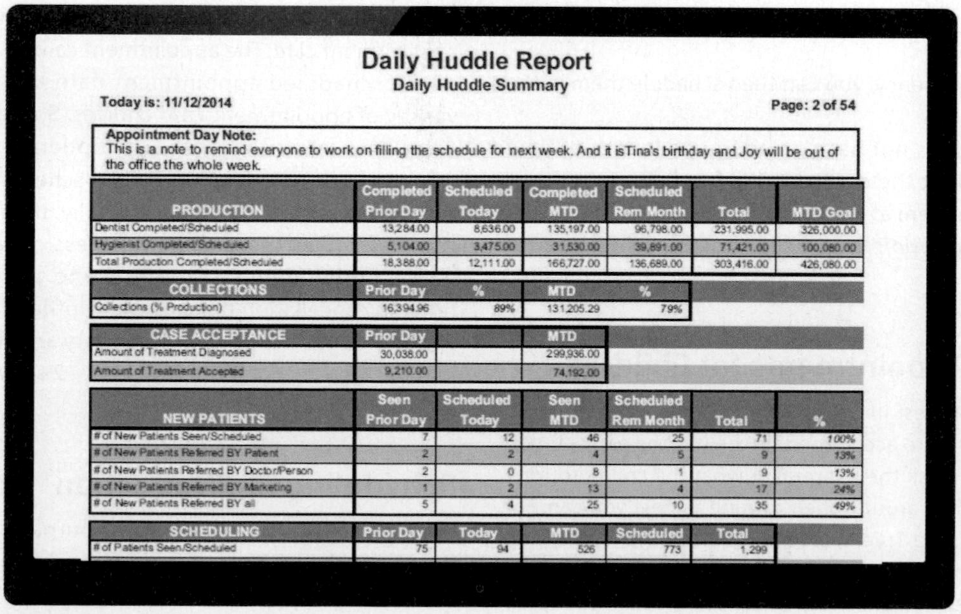

Daily Huddle Report

Daily Huddle Summary

Today is: 11/12/2014

Page: 2 of 54

Appointment Day Note:
This is a note to remind everyone to work on filling the schedule for next week. And it isTina's birthday and Joy will be out of the office the whole week.

PRODUCTION	Completed Prior Day	Scheduled Today	Completed MTD	Scheduled Rem Month	Total	MTD Goal
Dentist Completed/Scheduled	13,284.00	8,636.00	135,197.00	96,798.00	231,995.00	326,000.00
Hygienist Completed/Scheduled	5,104.00	3,475.00	31,530.00	39,891.00	71,421.00	100,080.00
Total Production Completed/Scheduled	18,388.00	12,111.00	166,727.00	136,689.00	303,416.00	426,080.00

COLLECTIONS	Prior Day	%	MTD	%
Collections (% Production)	16,394.96	89%	131,205.29	79%

CASE ACCEPTANCE	Prior Day		MTD
Amount of Treatment Diagnosed	30,038.00		299,936.00
Amount of Treatment Accepted	9,210.00		74,192.00

NEW PATIENTS	Seen Prior Day	Scheduled Today	Seen MTD	Scheduled Rem Month	Total	%
# of New Patients Seen/Scheduled	7	12	46	25	71	100%
# of New Patients Referred BY Patient	2	2	4	5	9	13%
# of New Patients Referred BY Doctor/Person	2	0	8	1	9	13%
# of New Patients Referred BY Marketing	1	2	13	4	17	24%
# of New Patients Referred BY all	5	4	25	10	35	49%

SCHEDULING	Prior Day	Today	MTD	Scheduled	Total
# of Patients Seen/Scheduled	75	94	526	773	1,299

Courtesy of Dentrix

FIGURE 44-11
Using a dental software huddle report to track the progress of the offices monthly goal.

them sooner. When a new patient calls, thank the patient for choosing this office. New patients should be seen soon after they call for an appointment. It may be beneficial to set aside a time each day to allow for new patients. Most front office new patient protocol involves completing the personal information of the registration form, including who referred them to the office. Ask the patient if a particular day each week is best and if they prefer mornings or afternoon. Offer the patient two different scheduling options to allow for flexibility. Ask the patient for their email to send them any necessary forms to fill out ahead of time and bring with them the day of the appointment. If they do not fill out the necessary forms online, ask the patient to arrive 15 minutes prior to the appointment so they may fill out these necessary forms. At the end of the call, send a welcome packet to the patient before the time of their appointment. This packet can include the welcome letter, any informational material about the office, directions to the office, date and time of appointment, and any forms you wish to have the patient complete (patient registration, health history, etc.). Many offices send a thank you note to persons referring patient to the office.

Scheduling of an Emergency

This is when the buffer time previously decided will be used. When a patient calls for an emergency, it is important to decide whether or not it is a true emergency. You can decide this by asking the following questions:

- How long has the tooth been troubling you?
- What type of pain is it? A dull ache, pressure, or sharp pain?
- Is it sensitive to hot or cold? Or both?
- Which tooth is it?
- Is there any swelling?
- Do you have a fever?

If it is a true emergency, you can then schedule them in the buffer time set aside.

If the dentist does not have an adequate length of time open, tell the patient the dentist is full for the day, but they will be able to see them at a specific time to relieve the tooth from pain. A later appointment can then be scheduled for treatment.

Scheduling Appointments for Children

Children are at their best in the morning. The younger the child is, the better it may be to accommodate them in the earlier times. It may be helpful to ask their caretaker what the child's routine is like. Try to schedule around their routine as best you can. For example, scheduling a 3-year-old right before their usual nap time may not be the best idea. Older children who are in school may need to be seen after school hours or on their scheduled days off. Having these days noted in the appointment book will help in scheduling.

Scheduling Multiple Appointments

When a patient needs multiple treatments appointments, they may want to schedule a series of appointments at one time. When scheduling appointments, try to keep the same day and time to reduce the likelihood of the patient forgetting. Consider the following:

- How many appointments does the patient need?
- What are the units of time needed for each appointment?
- Is there a cross in operatories (e.g., seeing the dentist followed by the hygienist)?
- Is there a lab case? Allow for fabrication and delivery time.

Scheduling Appointments for the Expanded-Function Practice

Depending on the state, dental assistants may have an expanded-function license that allows them a larger scope of practice. When an office employs an expanded-function assistant, appointments may be made in a separate column for effective use of time. For instance, if a patient is coming in for a treatment of a crown, they can first be scheduled with the expanded-function assistant for an alginate impression, which is needed to create a cast for the provisional crown needed later in the appointment. This can assist in making the day more productive and the staff feeling more relaxed in the services they are providing. In order for appropriate scheduling to take place, the administrative assistant must be aware of state law and understand which duties the expanded-function assistant can perform and were agreed upon by the dentist.

Appointment Card

After the appointment is made, the patient is given the appointment card. The appointment card is written notification of the scheduled appointment date and time. There are a variety of appointment card choices. Some are in the form of a business card; others have the option to have a removable sticker so the patient can place the scheduled time directly to their own calendar at home. Typically, the information on the card resembles that on the business card (practice/dentist name, phone number, address) and also includes a short note on cancellation policies. Many offices are matching their appointment cards to their stationary and including the office logo for easy recognition. Figure 44-12 shows an option for an appointment card available for use.

Scheduling for Production

While the dental office and staff's purpose is to provide quality care to the patients, it is also a business. Having a well put together schedule can help maximize production and contribute to the overall profitability of the office. Often, the schedule is set at the opening of the practice and is rarely redesigned after. This

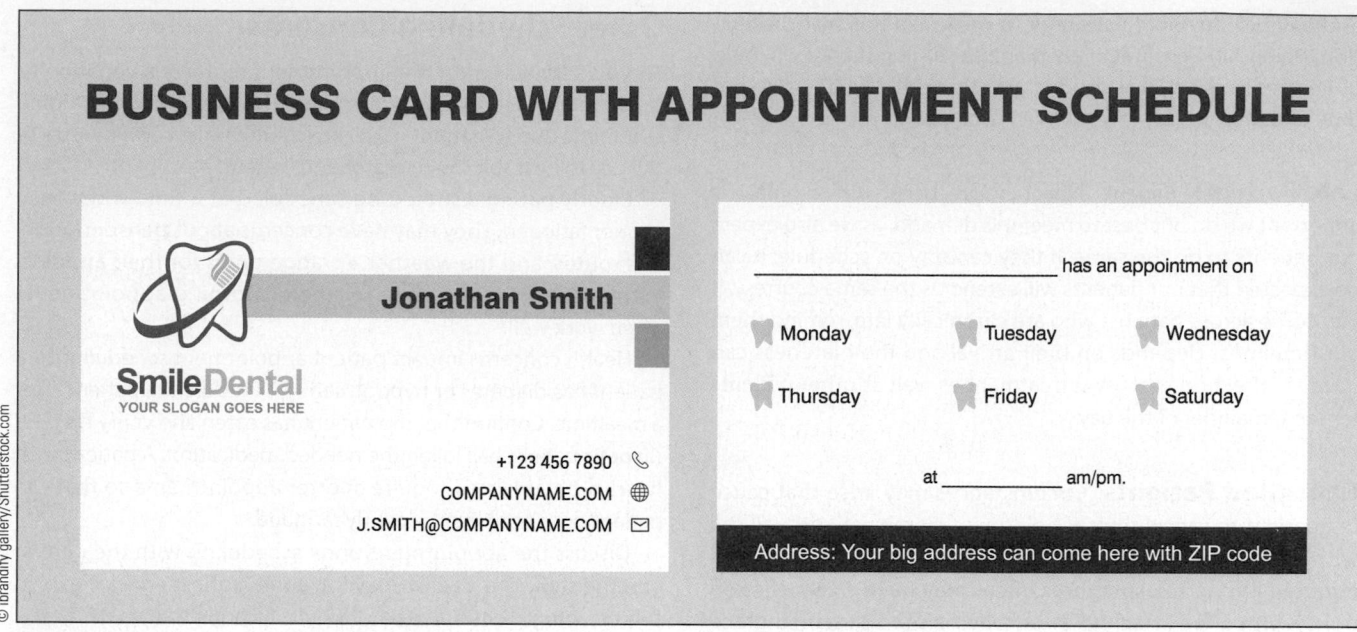

FIGURE 44-12
Appointment card.

can lead to a stagnant production, causing misery to the dentist. The truth of the matter is, there are ways to help maximize production and allow for the practice to reach its highest potential. When setting up the schedule, have production goals in mind and consider the following:

● **Establish the ideal production per day.** When setting the goals, find a reasonable production for the month and span it over the days in that month. For instance, if the practice monthly goal is $60,000, and the office is open for 20 business days that month, set the daily goal of $4,000. While this may not be exactly achieved every day, it gives a starting point on where you want production to be. You can then build the schedule around this goal so as to not have an overly busy day followed by a slow day. Keeping a pace will help reduce tension and stress in the office.

● **Higher production first.** When designing the schedule, block out times for higher production, and only fill these blocks with the appropriate treatments. About 60% of your production should be completed in the morning.

● **Schedule on a per chair basis.** The dentist ideally should be working two chairs simultaneously, with one chair left open for nonproductive procedures or emergencies. This allows for flexibility in the office and will contribute to an increase in production.

While these concepts might seem difficult at first, when followed appropriately they will become second nature over time. It is easy for someone to book a higher production, such as a crown and bridge procedure, rather than fear that it will not get filled. Any break in scheduling these higher production blocks should be avoided, and in the event a block is not filled 24 hours before the day, another appointment may be placed there.

Confirmation of Appointments

At times missed appointments are unavoidable, and they can be expected. Inclement weather, accidents, illnesses, and simply forgetting are all reasons a patient may cancel or not show for their scheduled appointment. Confirmation of appointments will help catch these cancellations in advance to allow enough time in advance to fill the schedule and effectively use that time. The way the office confirms appointments can vary greatly from practice to practice. Some may give a courtesy call the day before the appointment, while others may call a week in advance. Some may send reminder calls a few weeks prior to the appointment, while others may choose to email the patients. Today with the development of new technologies, many have added text messaging as a means of confirmation. A simple text a few days before, and then the day of the appointment, can remind a patient of their appointment time. The patient can then reply with a confirmation or a cancellation by a press of a button. There are many different options when it comes to an appointment reminder or confirmation. This is up to the office which method they feel is best, and it can be revisited if the current method is not effective.

Conditions Affecting Patient Scheduling

There will be patients who are habitually late, do not show, or cancel appointments. Most offices have this type of patient and have to develop a strategy to minimize this lost production. Being able to effectively manage these patients will help us keep the schedule as productive as possible while using our time effectively.

Late Patients Patients expect the practice to run on time. It is important we do our best to meet this demand, as we also expect our patients to do the same. If they can stay on schedule, it can be expected that our patients will extend us the same courtesy. If you come across patients who are chronically late, remind them our timeliness depends on their arrival and their lateness can have an effect on their own treatment as well as other patients for the remainder of the day.

Cancelled Patients Circumstances may arise that cause the patient to cancel their appointment. Some patients will call with an apology for a legitimate excuse. Others may call last minute with no explanation. Offices may have a cancellation policy with a fee attached if cancelled after a specified grace period. If you notice a patient makes a habit out of cancelling appointments, it is best not to offer prime time appointments, as these times should be saved for patients who are consistent with keeping their appointments. Patients may reconsider breaking their appointment if they find out there is a fee, or if they have to wait 3 months out to schedule another one. In the event a patient fails to show for their scheduled appointment, this is called a broken appointment. The administrative assistant should wait 10 minutes into the scheduled appointment and then call the patient on their preferred phone line. The patient may be able to come right in and salvage the remaining time of the appointment. If this is not possible, you may then offer another time for the patient to come in. In any case, all broken or cancelled appointments must be noted in the patient chart for future reference.

Call Lists

A **call list** is a list that is kept for last minute cancellations. Patients who have to wait a lengthier period of time for their appointment may wish to be placed on a call list. The call list is also used to call patients who request or are seeking certain times of the day. This can be kept manually or on the practice's dental software program. When kept manually, note the patient's name, units needed, the best phone number to reach them, the treatment needed, and the provider. For call lists kept in the computer, there is an option to place the patient on a call list when scheduling the appointment with any notes attached (needs a 6 pm or after, Saturdays only, available last minute, etc.). Figure 44-13 shows a computer software call list, where you can select an option of the type of call list desired to view. The administrative assistant can then upload the call list in the event of a cancellation and allow for effective use of the potentially lost time.

Other Scheduling Concerns

There are times when the appointment requires a variation to the normal procedures of scheduling. This can include providing extra time due to patient need, or scheduling at certain times of the day to best suit the operator and patient.

Elderly patients should be scheduled at a time when they are not fatigued. They may have concerns about transportation, bus routes, and the weather. Arrange times for their appointments that are convenient for them. Morning appointments often work well.

Health concerns impact patient appointment scheduling. If a patient has diabetes or hypoglycemia, schedule the patient after a mealtime. Confirm that the patient has eaten and verify that the diabetic patient has taken the needed medication. A patient with heart problems may require shorter appointments so that the patient does not become overly fatigued.

Discuss the appointment book scheduling with the dentist and the staff. The dentist may have the highest energy level in the morning. Scheduling a difficult, tedious treatment at the end of the day may be overtaxing. Also, scheduling the same procedure repeatedly may make it difficult on the dental team members. Staggering the types of treatment allows the dental team to be prepared for the procedures and makes the day go smoother and faster. Also, scheduling the same procedure several times in a row may make it difficult to accomplish the sterilization procedures when only a limited number of specific instruments are available for the specific procedure. During staff meetings, talk over appointment scheduling that works well, and define the best policy approach.

Recare Systems

A recare system is one of the most important aspects in ensuring patients return for their preventative care as recommended. The administrative assistant is responsible for knowing which recare schedule the patient is on and schedule accordingly. In addition to scheduling in advance, patients may want to be notified at a later time to schedule an appointment. In this event, there are different ways to guarantee the patient is notified promptly of their expected return. Regardless of which system is used, the goal is to make sure that every patient in the dental office is either under regular treatment or on a recall system.

Computerized Recare System

With increased computer use in dental offices, most current recare systems are done from a computer-generated printout. It may also be sent to the patient via email or text message. Patient preferences can be preset in certain software systems. Information is placed in the computer after the regular appointment is completed. The program allows a date for the recare appointment to be indicated. At the end

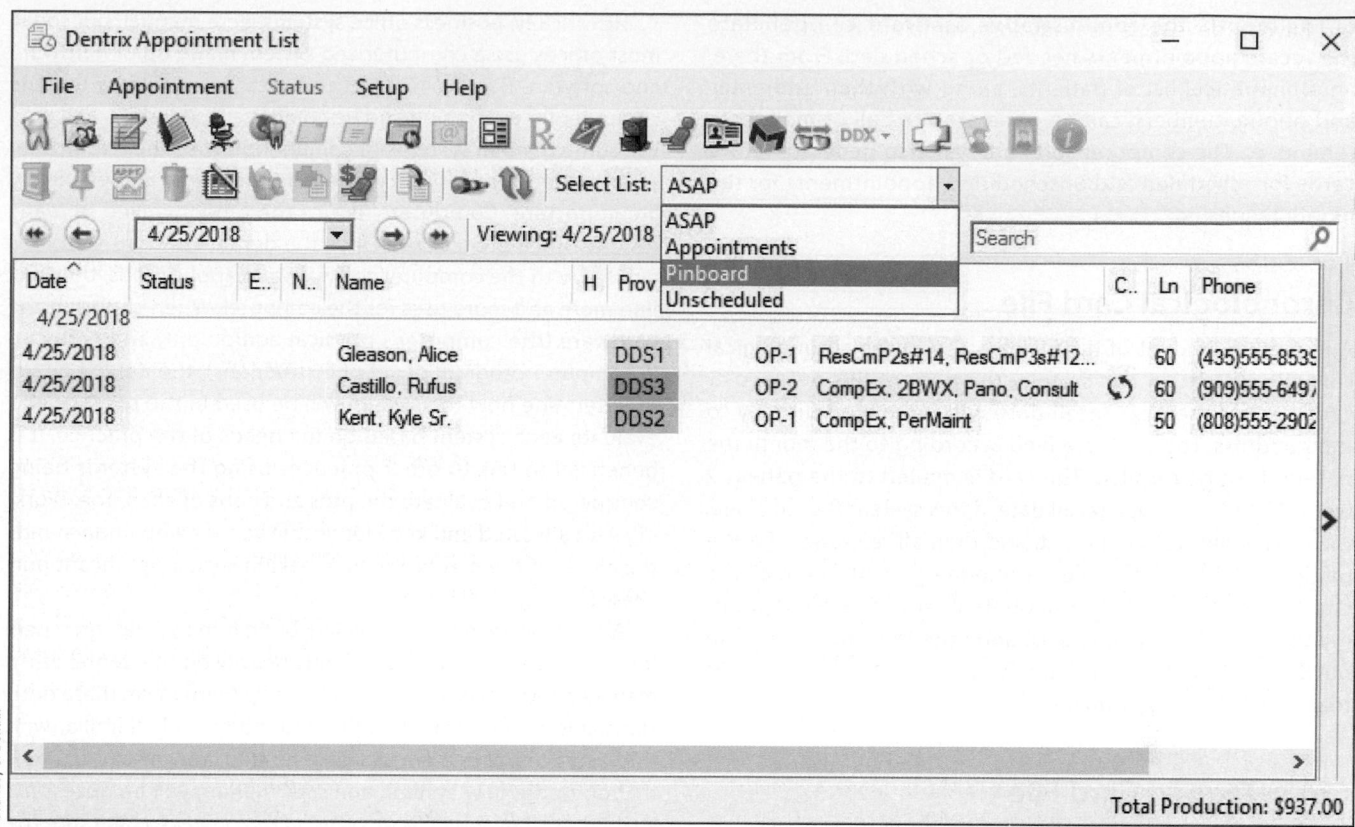

FIGURE 44-13
Computer software call list.

Procedure 44-1
Preparing for the Day's Appointments

Preparing for the upcoming day is important to ensure that optimal care is provided to patients in a calm, efficient environment.

Equipment and Supplies
- access to computer dental software:
  - ❏ patient's charts
  - ❏ day's schedule
- phone or automated confirmation system
- printer

Procedure Steps

Day before Appointment
1. Review schedule.
2. Review patient charts for any special concerns or notes.
3. If laboratory inserts are scheduled, check to ensure it is ready and on premises.
4. Review account balances.
5. Identify any health concerns (i.e., patient needs premedication, medical clearance, etc.).
6. Confirm patient appointments.
7. Print daily schedule.
8. Give schedules to the dental team.

Day of the Appointment
1. Review answering service.
2. Make any necessary changes to the schedule if needed (patient cancels, emergency, etc.).
3. Office staff meets in the morning to review the daily schedule. Review any messages if necessary. This brief meeting allows staff to discuss any patient concerns and create a plan to make the day run smoothly.
4. Create and print new daily schedule if necessary.
5. Provide clinical team with patient information.
6. Greet patients and seat them in the treatment rooms.

of the month, the administrative assistant can generate the recare appointments needed or scheduled. From there, an alphabetical list of patients, along with their addresses and phone numbers, can be generated to call or mail them reminders. The computer software can also generate recare cards for scheduled and unscheduled appointments for the month requested.

Chronological Card File

A minimum amount of time is invested in the chronological card file system. In this system, the patient fills out a postcard so that the next recall date will be mailed directly to their address. The cards are filed according to the month the patient is to be recalled. The card is mailed to the patient 2 weeks before the given recall date. If this system is used alone, the card is sent to the patient, and then all references for the patient recall are lost, unless someone goes through all the charts and makes a list of patients needing recall appointments. It is better to make a list and note the patients who do not schedule appointments and follow up with telephone calls to schedule the appointment.

Color-Tagged Card File

Another type of recall system is the color-tagged card file. In this system, every patient has an index card with their name, address, telephone number, and any other special notations printed on it. The cards are filed alphabetically, and a colored tag is clipped to each card indicating in which month the patient requires a recall appointment. For example, a yellow tag is clipped to a card if the patient needs a recall appointment in January. The tagged file cards are reviewed each month, and calls are made to schedule the patients needing continued care. If they do not schedule, they can be moved up to the next month or later, if requested. After the patient is scheduled, the card is attached to the chart and updated at the time of the patient's appointment. A new color-coded tag is then attached to the card and filed in the index system. The advantage of this system is that the cards are available with information on them about prior appointments. Disadvantages are the time it takes to complete a card for each patient and the possibility of the tag falling off.

Business Office Systems

While the overall goal of the dental practice is to provide quality care to the patients, it is important to understand that the practice is a business. The commitment to patient care and meeting the needs of the community are objectives of every dental office. However, if a practice is to be successful in meeting the needs of the community, we must approach dentistry from a business idealism, as well. The practice cannot provide care to the community if it does not remain sustainable.

Historically, business office systems were manual, but today most offices use a computerized system made up of hardware and software (Figure 44-14). The dental practice may use the computer for everything and be completely paperless, or it may use some manual systems in conjunction with their computer system. In today's fast-paced dental office, time and efficiency are important. Computers reduce the time involved in many routine office procedures. Once the dental assistant becomes familiar with the computer software and applications, they will find more and more uses for the computer. When choosing the hardware (the computer's physical equipment) and software (a computer program or set of instructions), the dentist needs to determine how the system will be used in the practice and evaluate each system based on the needs of the practice. It is beneficial to talk to other practices using the systems being considered and evaluate the pros and cons of each one. Working with a trusted and knowledgeable vendor who understands the needs of the practice before making such a significant purchase is always advisable.

After the research is completed, bring it to the staff members for their input. The dentist may rely heavily on the dental office manager and business office staff to help them make these decisions. It is important that all the staff members be familiar with the system. It takes a great deal of time to convert all the information to the new system, and staff training will be necessary, so it is best if everyone is involved in the process. Make sure the system that is purchased meets not only current needs but allows for future growth within the practice.

Word Processing

Word processing has largely replaced typewriters. It allows the dental team member to use a computer keyboard to type memos, letters, and reports, and to make corrections easily. Word processing software allows for spelling checks, deletions, cutting and pasting information, and much more. The documents can be saved, stored, and retrieved for use at a later time. If needed, it can be changed or updated and used again without having to create a whole new document. Typing a letter has been made much easier via computer and word processing software. Dental management software often contains prewritten letters as part of its word processing function. They can be used as is, customized, or even integrated with a patient database to send personally addressed letters to a large number of patients.

Graphics

Graphics software is a program or a collection of programs. With the use of graphic software, numeric information can be transformed for various uses. Graphics are used to develop the office's webpage, create the log, create or edit digital images, diagrams, and graphs (Figure 44-15). This allows information to be summarized in a graphic format for easy visualization. Dental software

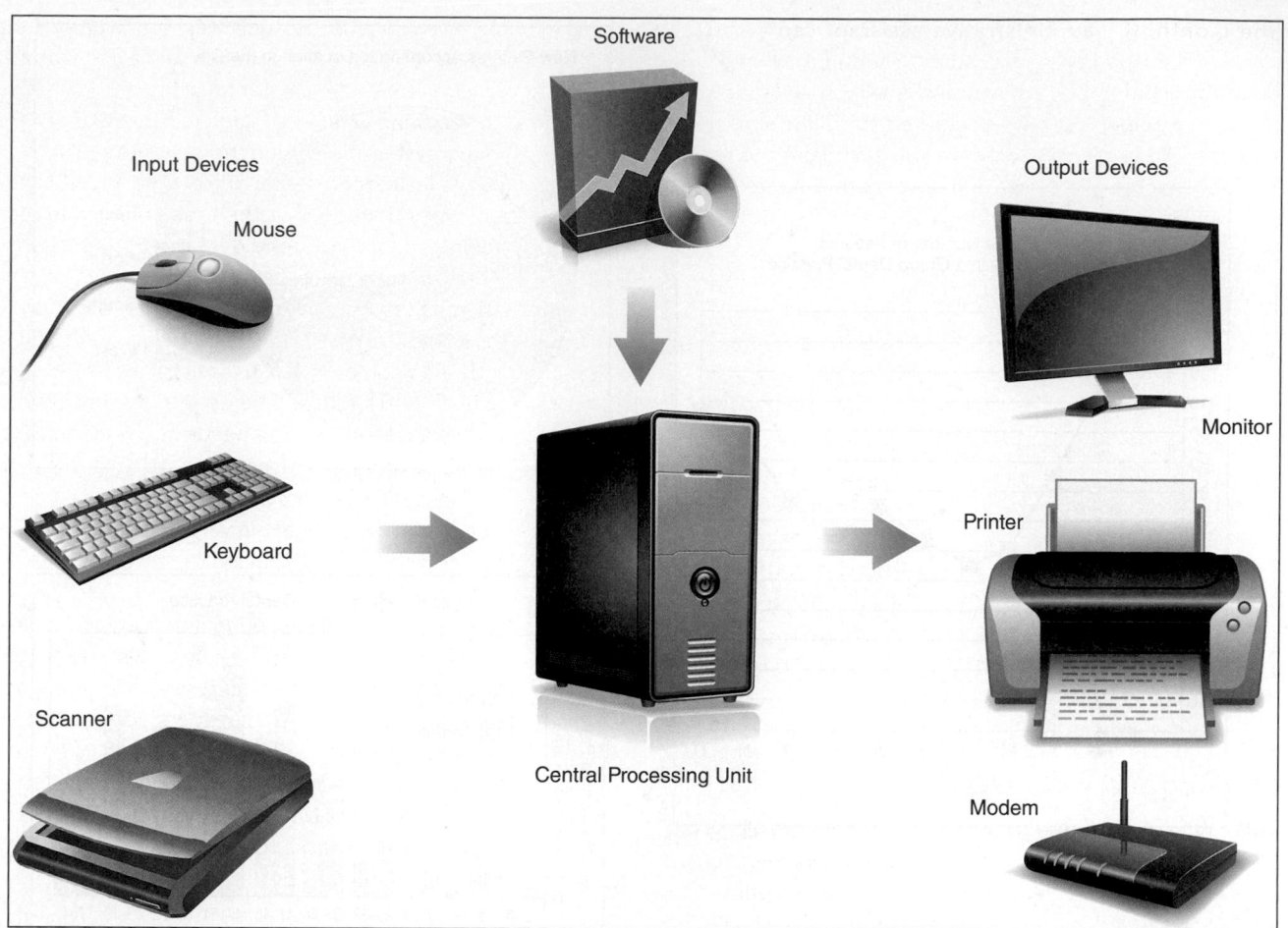

FIGURE 44-14
Components of a computer system in a dental office.

uses a practice's data to allow the practice to create graphs that track trends and evaluate possible changes.

Spreadsheets

Spreadsheets are a computerized worksheet that allows for programmed calculations. Spreadsheets electronically calculate the numerical data to be analyzed. This calculation and recalculation, which used to take hours, is completed in seconds with spreadsheet software. Spreadsheets are used in the dental office to prepare monthly and yearly financial statements and accounts payable, along with other uses. The data from a spreadsheet can be converted into a graph or chart, presenting information that can be interpreted at a glance.

The software used in dentistry can track the practice's success in many ways. The office can view office totals according to specified criteria and through any time frame. It can also be viewed in a graphic display (Figure 44-16). Many patient groups can be identified, and a report generated. For instance, if the office wanted to see how many patients had porcelain crowns in the past year, it can be easily found. This would allow the office to assess whether there is a need to purchase

a machine (CAD/CAM) for designing and manufacturing crowns. All types of information are available and can be readily accessed.

Dental Office Software

A large variety of dental office software programs are available. Choose the software that best meets the office's needs. It should have general-purpose functions that include database management, word processing, graphics, spreadsheets, bookkeeping, insurance, and online communication.

There are numerous types of dental practice management software that cover the clinical aspect of the practice as well as general functions. These software programs can be **cloud based**, **server based**, **proprietary**, or hybrid. Before choosing software, the practice must think about **scalability** and how much storage they may need in the foreseeable future. For instance, if the practice chooses to purchase cloud-based software, they want to consider the amount of storage included. As the practice grows, more data storage may need to be purchased. This can add to the overall cost of the software in the long run.

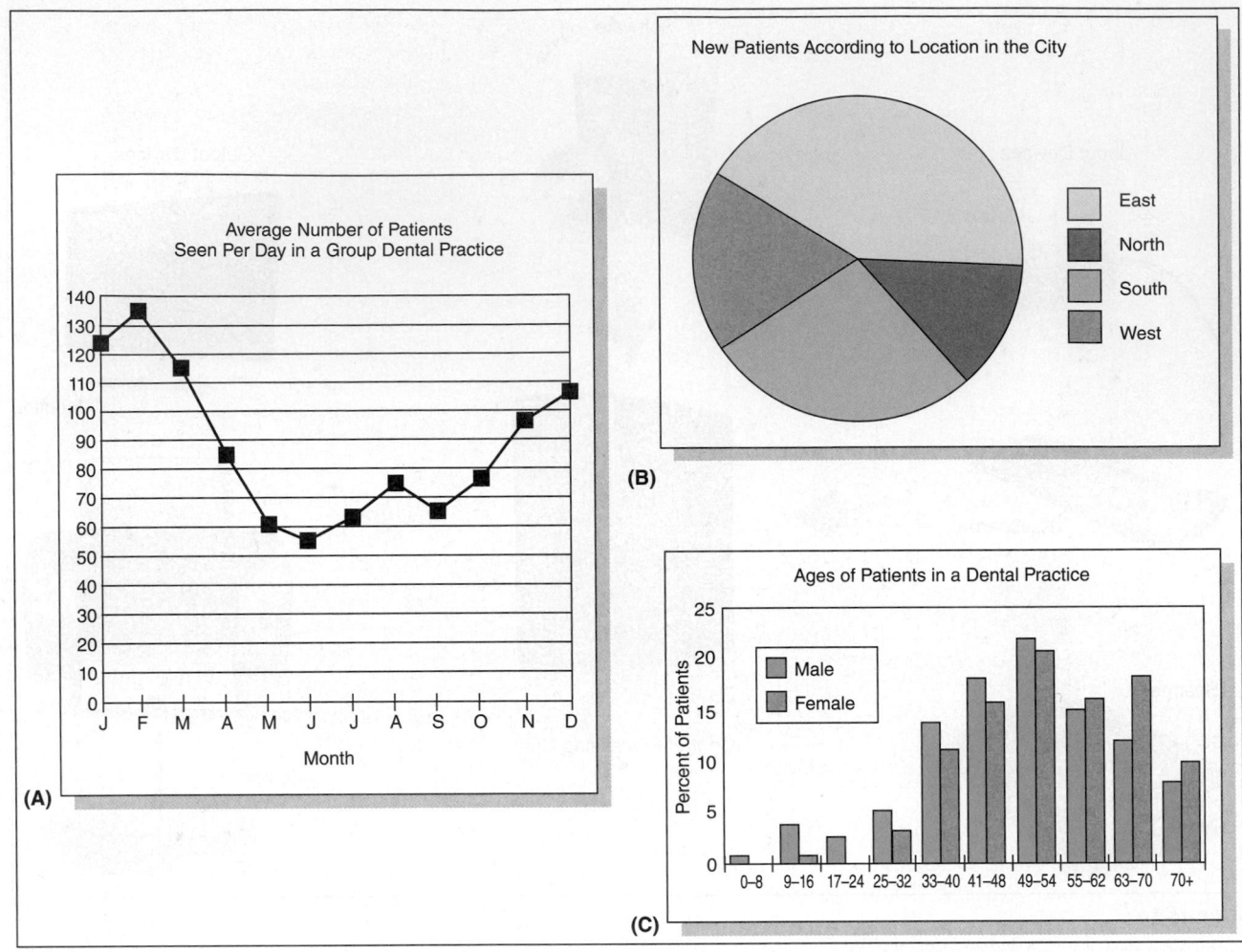

FIGURE 44-15
Graphs and charts make information easier to interpret: (A) Line graph. (B) Pie chart. (C) Bar graph.

Another consideration **integration**. Different software companies offer different options. Choose the best software that matches the needs of the practice. Adding on items later could be an issue if the add-on is not compatible with the current software. For instance, if digital images are an important factor, choosing a software system that is compatible with the digital imaging software is necessary.

Two software programs that are commonly used within dental offices are the Dentrix system available from Henry Schein Inc. and Eaglesoft available from Patterson Dental. Both software programs have a wide range of applications and training. This training may be provided by the manufacturers of the software, online webinars, or alternate training sites. Both programs are updated often to provide the newest services available to the dental team.

Employee Records

As important as it is to keep accurate patient records, it is just as important to keep accurate employee records. This includes the employee's resume, training records, documentation of injuries at work, payroll, and taxes. If the employee provides patient care, all licenses, registrations, and certifications required by the state should be kept on file. To ensure safety and security, if the person is handling money or has access to credit card payments, it is recommended they have a background check. All positive as well as negative occurrences should be recorded. This includes absences, tardiness, and incident reports as well as positives such as efforts made in team work and positive feedback. Form I-9 for all employees should be kept on file, which ensures employment eligibility.

Some states may require yearly education for infection control and hazard communications. These records should be kept for proof of all employees' completion. This includes evidence following the state rules and regulations as well as OSHA compliance records and handbook. By law, a practice must keep employee records for the duration of employment plus 30 years thereafter. If the practice is sold, the records become owned by the new practice owner.

Inventory Management

Inventory management refers to overseeing and organizing of ordering all office materials and supplies. This applies to both

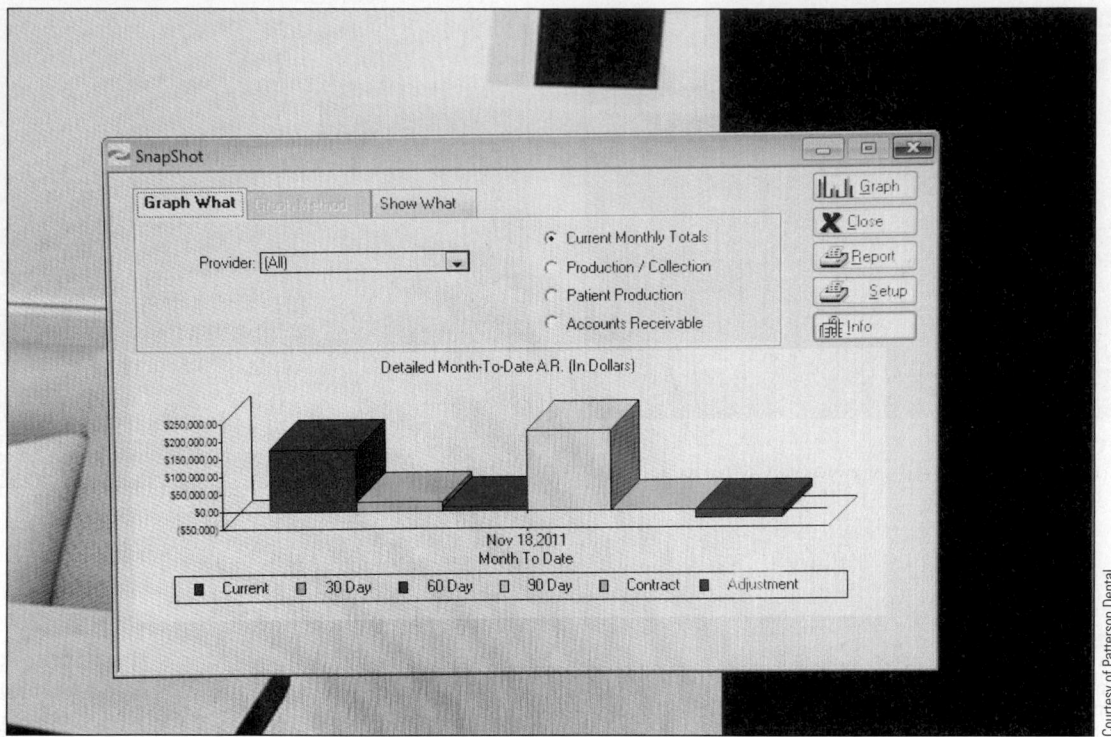

FIGURE 44-16
Computer software graph showing dental office production.

the clinical and business aspects. Routinely there is one person in charge of inventory and ordering; however, all staff must be knowledgeable about the products they routinely use as well as aware of the procedures the office uses to maintain inventory. The clinical assistant is responsible for ordering clinical supplies, and the administrative assistant is responsible for the business supplies. Employing an organized and well thought out management system can help eliminate waste, save money, and reduce overstocking.

When looking around the dental office, the number of supplies and materials can be quite overwhelming. A solid inventory management system helps reduce the stress that can come along with taking inventory and ordering supplies, and the fear of running out of a product. An inventory management system can be done either by hand or electronically.

A paper inventory control template is an example of how to catalogue the office products used in the office. Once a routine is established and the correct quantity of a product is determined, a monthly assessment of products on hand can be easily determined. One system that can be used is the red flag inventory system. These red flag cards can be purchased and contain information about the product on them, such as the price, name, where ordered, and date ordered.

If the office decides, they can utilize an electronic inventory management system. This computerized system can track the inventory in the office and offers an automated replenishment order. Use of a mini bar code scanner (Figure 44-17) allows for

easy scanning and electronic ordering at the time the product is removed from inventory. The computerized system also allows you to check on orders, view invoices, and track packages.

Research has shown that the optimal amount of purchasing fees to operate a dental practice should be between 6% and 12% of the total operating costs. In most dental practices, this percentage is often doubled, drawing away from the overall production calculations of the practice.

The following recommendations can be applied to the management of dental inventory in any dental office:

- Maintain a 30 day supply of most items used.

- Determine if a sales representative would be an advantageous asset to the office's inventory management. Often, this can reduce the purchasing costs of many products.

- Determine shelf life, cost, and ordering time frame of all products used.

- Establish an inventory order target total per month.

- Request free samples of a new product before purchasing.

- Maintain a monthly log of overused products and underused products.

A reduction in the amount of revenue spent on supplies and the ordering of such takes time to implement successfully. Strategic calculations of the past spending allocations can be useful in creating realistic projections for reducing the cost of supplies.

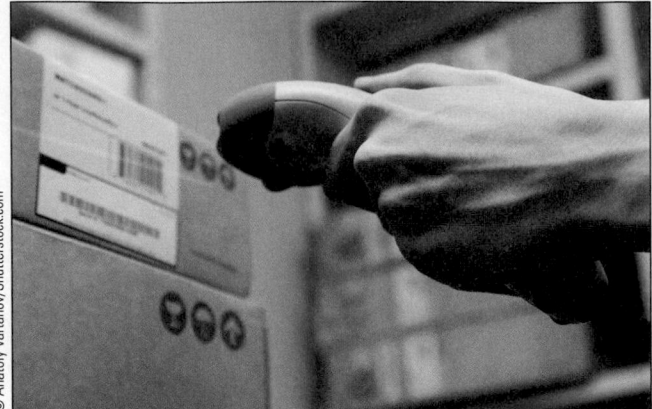

FIGURE 44-17
Mini barcode scanner for use with electronic inventory systems.

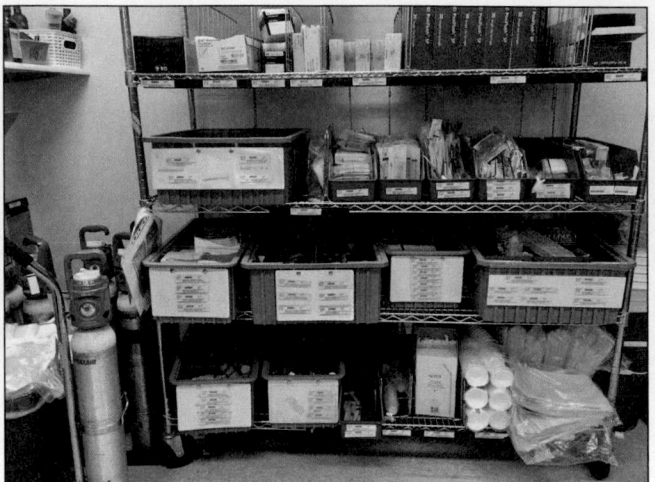

FIGURE 44-18
Storage area neatly organized.

Ordering Supplies

Setting up an ordering system is one way to help the office run smoothly, and it ensures excellent communication between all team members. All items should be assessed once a year, catalogued, and included in this very important system's manual. Dental products change, as do the needs of the dental provider. With the ever-changing technology, there are current materials and products coming out each year. It is imperative that a master inventory list be created for the current products that are being used in the office and updated as products change. Some common information found on an inventory master list includes the following:

- Name of the product and any descriptive information needed, such as fast-set, quantity, and size
- Reorder quantity and reorder point
- Shelf life of the product
- Supplier name and contact person to order from
- Catalog numbers if applicable

Most offices have a storage room or area to stock products the office uses. If this area is not organized, the items can be shoved around and misplaced, causing an unnecessary reorder or shortage of the product when needed. Figure 44-18 shows a neat and organized storage area.

Supplies can be considered consumable or disposable. **Consumable supplies** are used up a little at a time, such as composite and impression materials. **Disposable supplies** are supplies that are used and then discarded, such as gauze, saliva ejectors, and bibs. If the item is low cost, it is considered **expendable**. When the item is a piece of equipment that will eventually need to be replaced, such as an instrument, it is considered **nonexpendable**. The larger, more costly equipment, such as a dental unit or x-ray unit, is considered major equipment.

Another reason for inventory assessment is to check for expired products. As we assume that the manufacturer will send us the freshest product available, we may have a short time usage for particular products. Use of products that will expire first is essential to eliminating product waste. Knowing the **shelf life** of all products will help in the ordering process. If you know a particular product only has a 6-month shelf life, you would order that product accordingly. This also helps eliminate waste.

When it is time to order supplies, make sure you have approval for ordering before you contact the supplier. When you contact the supplier, have all necessary information, including the catalog number and page number where the product can be found. Always check for specials and sales as suppliers will often have promotions for certain products.

The rate of use should be noted as well as how long the product usually takes to receive. For example, if a product is used daily but is sent in 7 days, you want to make sure you have enough on hand. If the product is used monthly and the time to receive is next day, it may be alright to order this product with less expectancy time.

Suppliers will offer a lower price if products are ordered in larger quantities. This is considered a **quantity purchase rate**. If there is a longer shelf life, or if the product is used often, taking advantage of this quantity purchase rate can assist in greater savings to the dentist when ordered by quantity.

In the event a product is not available from the supplier, the order is considered to be on **backorder**. When items are placed on backorder, it will usually ship as soon as the supplier receives the item. If there is not enough product in the office, ordering elsewhere may need to be considered. If the item needs to be ordered through another supplier, be sure to cancel the backordered item to avoid duplication of a product.

Sometimes after we receive the product, the need to return or exchange may arise. This can happen due to the wrong item being sent or the item being damaged or broken. If this happens, contact the supplier immediately to rectify the situation. Follow-up is important until the supplier provides the appropriate credit or sends the appropriate product.

Procedure 44-2
Reordering Supplies

The front office assistant may be assigned specifically to order supplies, or this task may be shared by several dental assistants.

Equipment and Supplies

Red Flag Reorder Tag System
- red flag reorder tags that have surfaced for reordering
- telephone
- indicator tabs

Electronic Bar Code System
- bar code wand
- telephone
- access to the computer

Procedure Steps

Red Flag Reorder Tag System
1. Gather the red flags indicating the items that require reordering.
2. Obtain the ordering information for each item on the card.
3. Place an indicator in the upper-right corner to indicate that this item is to be ordered immediately.
4. After the item is ordered, place the indicator in the upper-left corner until the product arrives.
5. When the item arrives, remove the indicator from the tag, place the most recently received items to the back of the supply (using the older materials first), and place the red flag ordering tag on the minimum quantity needed in stock before reordering must be accomplished again.

Electronic Bar Code System
1. Identify the items that require reordering. This system is used for commonly ordered items.
2. Obtain the book that has the product information and bar codes identified.
3. Use the bar code wand to input the items needed. Run the wand over the bar codes of the items needing to be ordered. Indicate on the transmitter the number of items needed. The order is then transmitted directly to the dental supply company for ordering.
4. Place a date on the listed items, and indicate the number that have been ordered on the forms provided with the electronic bar code system.

Computer Safety

Use computer virus software to protect the office system if there is any chance that the office may download information from the Internet or accept files from other computer systems. Everything could be lost if unprotected. Most offices back up their files daily to make sure that a copy of the information is available if the system crashes due to an Internet virus, fire, or water damage. Most dental software offers the option to have a daily backup to a cloud that is encrypted for the highest level of safety. Even if the possibility of losing the data is remote, it takes a great deal of time to reconstruct the system if this happens. Always have a backup of critical information.

Computer Ergonomics and Eye Care For those individuals who spend a great deal of time on the computer, it is important to practice recommended computer ergonomics (see Figure 44-19). For instance, posture is critical for preventing injury. Choose a comfortable cushioned chair with back support and four to five casters forming a stable base. The height of the chair should allow the feet to be flat on the floor with the desk surface slightly lower than elbow level. Keep items used frequently close at hand.

Other recommended aids include an ergonomic keyboard, which allows the wrists to remain in a flat position. A wrist rest for the mouse is used to keep the wrist in a level position. Screen glare protectors can be used to deflect and reduce monitor glare. Eye care professionals advise that, for every 20 minutes of computer use, look 20 feet away for 20 seconds to allow the eyes to rest. If the eyes are dry, use artificial tears, or blink more often.

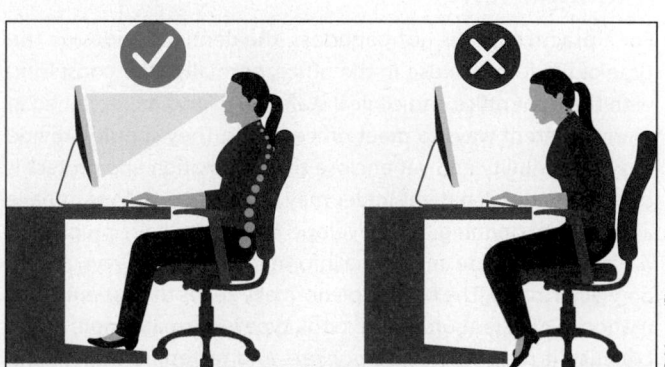

FIGURE 44-19
Correct posture while working on a computer.

© Maanas/Shutterstock.com

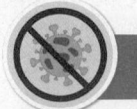

Infection Control

Keyboards

Infection control for keyboards in the dental office has long been a concern. Aerosol spray from handpieces during treatment can land on computer keyboards, and using the keyboard with gloved hands causes cross-contamination. Keyboards are difficult or nearly impossible to clean, and microorganisms multiply and are spread and transferred throughout the office. Many dental offices are covering keyboards and the mouse with a barrier during treatment. This barrier or keyboard overlay is acceptable, but it is still difficult to clean, and keying in patient procedure data is cumbersome. There are keyboards available that act like a typical spring-key keyboard but have a flat surface that can be disinfected with surface disinfectant (Figure 44-20), or removed and placed in the dishwasher. Some offices have incorporated voice to text technology using a microphone, eliminating some of the need for keyboards.

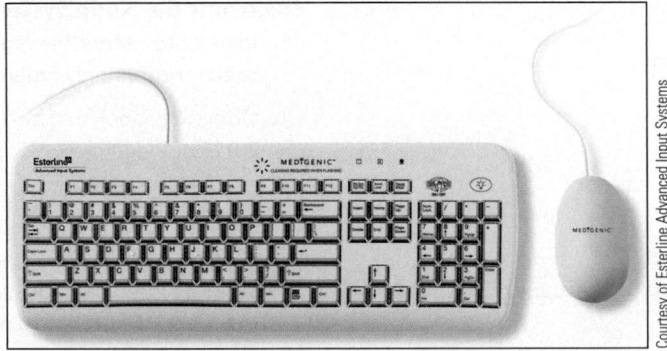

Courtesy of Esterline Advanced Input Systems

FIGURE 44-20
Flat keyboard design and mouse allow for easy disinfection, with timed alert for users to become aware that disinfection has not occurred.

Dental Records Management

Accurate dental records management is essential for quality patient care at any dental office. It is also necessary because of the legal issues that every dental office must face today. The records must be filled out completely, reflecting all pertinent information.

Equipment and Supplies for Record Management

For a practice that is not paperless, the dentist decides on the type of file folder to use in the office, normally after consulting with the front office and clinical staff. File folders are designed in many different ways to meet office needs. They should provide easy accessibility and yet enclose the information and protect it during storage. A patient folder may be like an envelope or have a book-type opening. The envelope folder may have preprinted data on the outside and all the information sheets, x-rays, and so on placed inside. The book type normally keeps the patient information in constant order. The book type is normally more costly because it requires added pockets and fasteners to hold the information sheets secure.

File cabinets are also available in several primary types, such as vertical, open-shelf lateral, and movable. The vertical file cabinet is widely used in home filing (Figure 44-21A). The files are retrieved by lifting the appropriate file upward and outward. Open-shelf file cabinets seem to be the most widely used in the dental office, normally with a color-coding system that allows for easy chart identification (Figure 44-21B). The records from the open-shelf lateral files are retrieved by pulling them out laterally from the shelf. Some large offices may have movable file units that are powered electrically or physically by easy handles. Patient names are typed on the labels and attached to the file for quick identification.

Patient Chart Filing

Most filing systems used are organized alphabetically. These systems index the individual names. The patient name is divided into three units: the last name, first name, and middle name or initial. File all the charts according to the last name; if two patients have the same last name, such as Smith, then file by the first names. For example, if the office has a John Smith and a Jim Smith, Jim is filed before John in the file cabinet. Occasionally, two patients with the same first and last name become patients. Use their middle names or initials to file properly. Alphabetical filing requires accuracy during the removal and replacement of the chart. These tasks must be done correctly, or a lot of time can be wasted trying to find a chart.

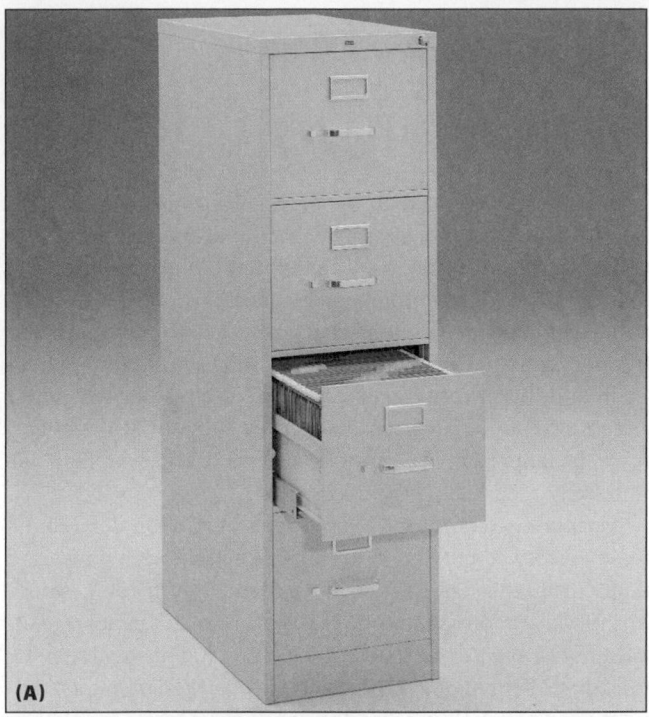

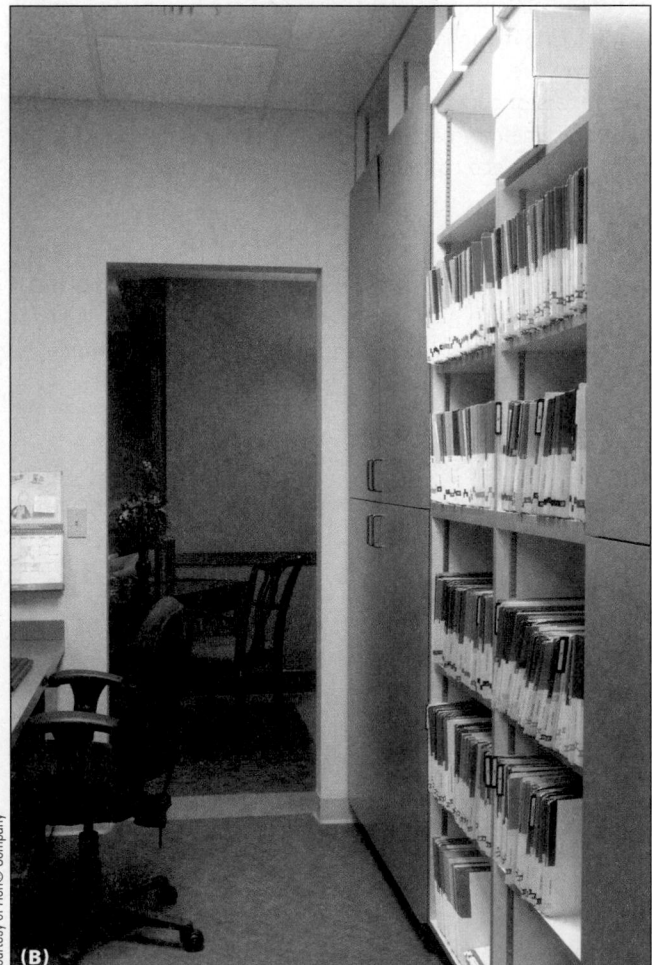

Most dental offices use some form of color coding for their patient filing (Figure 44-22). The file folder may be color coded so that all the patients with a last name beginning in A or S have yellow charts, and all the patients with B or T have blue charts. Other charts may have colored tabs that are placed on either plain or colored charts to make the filing and retrieval of files more efficient. The larger the practice, the more tabs are required to break down the charts into smaller groupings. This makes filing easier and reduces the number of errors and lost charts that may occur, because any visible color differences are quickly identified. Color coding by adding date stickers helps clinical assistants and front office assistants track active and inactive accounts.

Tickler File A well-organized office has a tickler file that serves as a reminder of any action that needs to be taken in the future. Most offices use sticky notes (reminder notes that have adhesive strips on one side) to remind office personnel of things that need to be taken care of immediately. Sticky notes can often become lost or get misplaced as the adhesive on the back can wear off. A tickler file normally uses index cards in an index box marked with approximate dates by which certain tasks should be completed (Figure 44-23). Many computer software programs have tickler files available so that information can be stored and retrieved when necessary.

Record Confidentiality

The patient has the right to confidential treatment and records (see Chapter 3, "Ethics, Jurisprudence, and the Health Information Portability and Accountability Act"). The patient chart contains private information that must be kept confidential. With the usage of computers and fax machines, great care must be used when placing anything where others can see it. Place computer

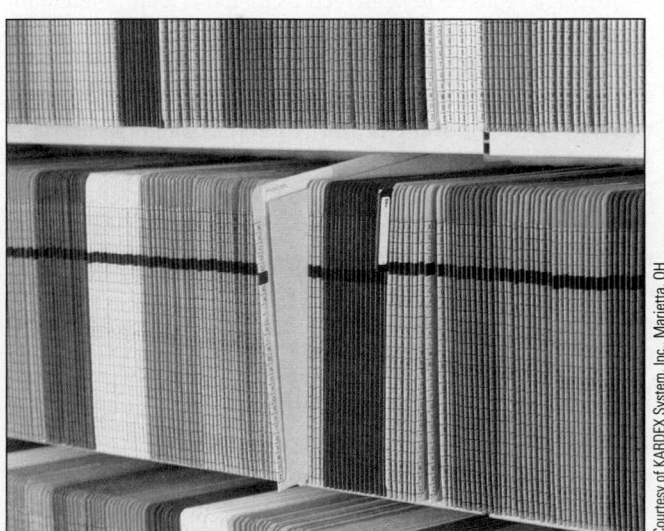

FIGURE 44-22
Color-coded patient files. Yellow file selected for "Carl." "F" side tab selected for "Friend."

FIGURE 44-21
(A) Vertical file cabinet. (B) Open-shelf lateral file cabinet.

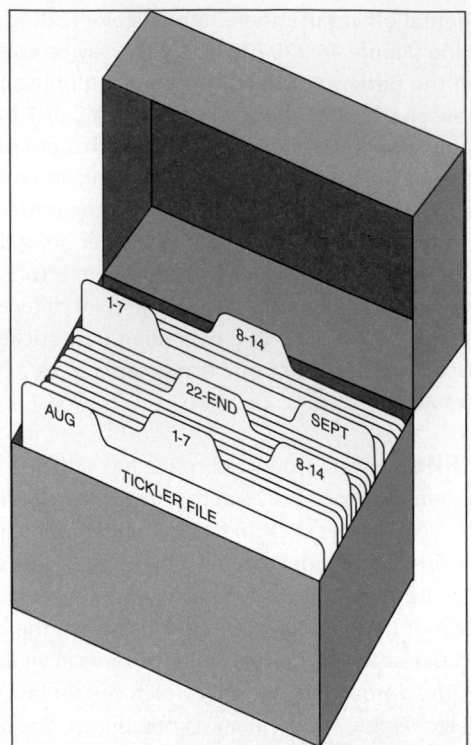

FIGURE 44-23
Tickler file for daily review and follow-up actions in patient management.

monitors out of the view of other patients. When sending a fax, attach a cover sheet that advises the receiver of the confidential nature of the material, and make sure that the fax machine that is receiving the material is located in an area where only the appropriate individuals can access it.

Archival Storage

Dentists are required to keep records for a predetermined number of years. These laws are determined by the state in which the practice is located. It can be as little as 2 years or upward of 10 years. This can create storage concerns for the practice when there are older paper charts. The contents of older paper charts can be scanned and stored electronically in an archive file. Computer systems allow a practice to archive charts of patients that move from the area, change practices, or pass away. Even though the patient's chart is archived, the electronic record is still available quickly and easily within inactive or archive records, but it is not cluttering the active records.

Electronic Record Keeping

The federal government mandated that all medical records be electronic by 2014. This piece of legislation is called the American Recovery and Reinvestment Act of 2009, or ARRA. While this legislation does not specifically require dental practices to have electronic records, dental practices have used this date as a goal.

Incentives have been made available to ease the financial burden of moving toward electronic record keeping.

Paperless Dental Practice

With current dental software, it is possible for a dental practice to be paperless. This is the goal of the electronic records mandate: to eliminate physical patient charts that must be stored and retrieved. The advantages are that patient information can be accessed by the dentist from multiple locations, and dental office staff never has to search for a chart, saving time and improving efficiency. Another advantage is the ease of transferring patient records for interprofessional care. The disadvantage is that if there is a computer problem, it affects everything. If the server is down, patients' records will not be accessible and treatment will most likely need to be postponed.

A paperless (computerized) patient chart should contain a health history completed in the software itself or on paper and scanned into the computer. All the patient's information, including insurance information, a clinical chart with radiographs, treatment notes, and dental charting, will be included. Any letters or additional information can be scanned and linked from the treatment or administrative notes. Insurance claim forms are already part of the patient computer ledger and can be viewed without printing. Everything is available with a few clicks on a keyboard from anywhere.

The process of converting from paper to paperless charts can seem overwhelming at first, but the convenience of accessible legible patient records soon outweighs the problems.

Managing Office Finances

There are various features of the business management team of any dental practice. All dental practices have the responsibility of financial management. The primary focus of financial management is related to the following objectives:

- Patient account management
- The processing of accounts receivable for services rendered
- The processing of accounts payable, related to the function of the dental practice
- Billing procedures

Patient Account Management

Patient accounts can be managed through either a computerized bookkeeping system or a manual system, such as the pegboard system. Most dental offices have converted from a manual bookkeeping system to a computerized system because it offers great versatility and the ability to quickly analyze the finances of the practice.

Computerized Account Management Systems Computerized management systems are much quicker and allow offices to gather information more rapidly. Computerized patient

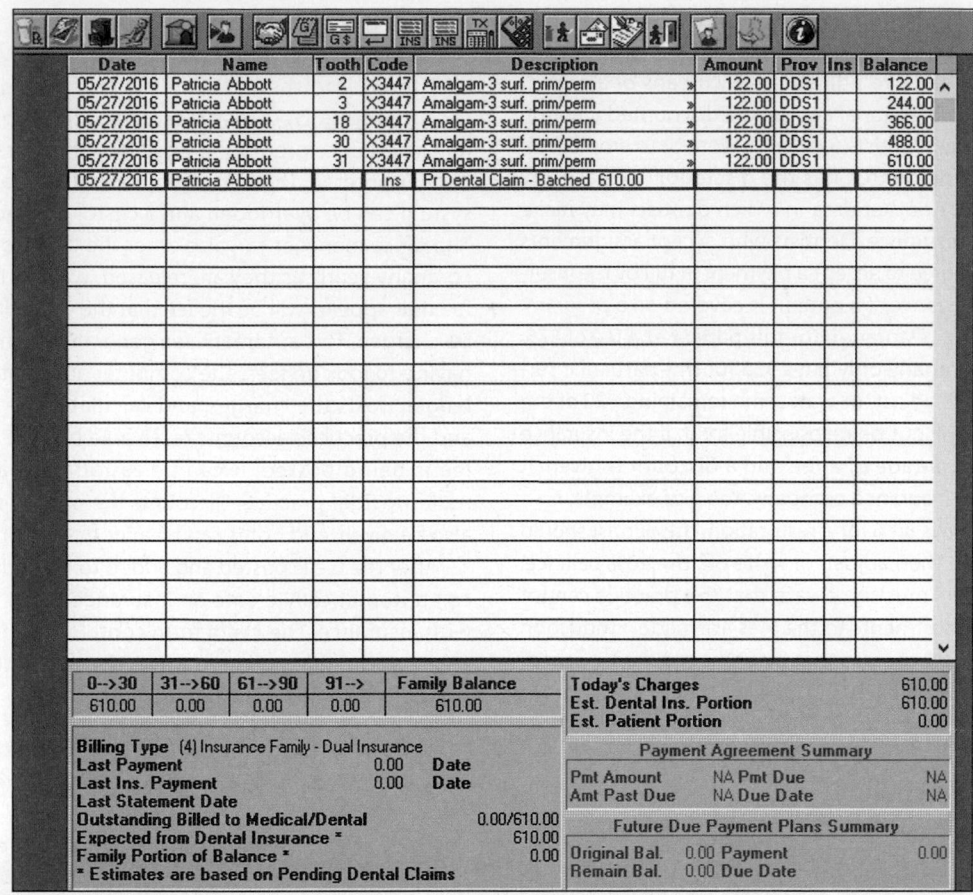

FIGURE 44-24
Computer patient ledgers provide a summary of all fees, payments, and insurance.

ledgers contain information about each patient, including name, address, telephone number, insurance coverage, and the person responsible for the account (Figure 44-24). This ledger also lists office visits, the services provided, and procedure codes. Dental software is very user friendly and, with some practice, managing financial accounts is easy. Many software programs use icons (small pictures) to direct the user to the exact function needed.

Accounts Receivable

As discussed, the primary concern of the dental office is patient care, but without sound financial management, the office will not thrive and the patients will ultimately suffer. With the high cost of materials and equipment, profit management is critical. The accounts receivable of the dental office encompasses the money owed to the practice. The bookkeeping in this area must be accurate and carries with it a great responsibility. This position may be occupied by the front office assistant or the dental office manager. Like the information in the patient's records, the financial information must remain confidential. All transactions, payments,

adjustments, and charges must be handled in a safe and professional manner. Any employee engaging in unlawful activities may be prosecuted under the law and required to repay the employer for any theft. Insurance fraud also brings with it prosecution and possible imprisonment.

Fee for Service In the dental office, a fee schedule is used to define what patients are charged for each service. Insurance companies set what is called a **usual, customary, and reasonable (UCR) fee**. The UCR is the average fee up to the 90th percentile that the dentists in the area charge for the same procedure. Often, the office fee for a procedure will not reflect the UCR for certain insurance companies. If a dentist feels that they would like to charge a greater amount for a service, insurance companies will not pay above the UCR fee schedule. Therefore, the patient will be billed for the overage unless the dentist is contracted with the insurance company and has agreed to accept their payment as payment in full. To avoid the patient becoming upset with an unexpected cost, the administrative assistant or office manager should discuss out-of-pocket costs expected at the time of the consultation appointment. The UCR fee schedule is reviewed annually and adjusted as necessary.

Dentists have the right to adjust fees by means of a professional courtesy. This professional courtesy, a discounted amount, may be offered to other dentists for dental work or to employees, family, and friends. The dentist has the discretion to make any adjustments desired. Another area in which dentists may make adjustments is with insurance. Dentists who accept assignments in specific programs agree to accept a payment in full by the insurance company. For instance, if a patient is covered on a program, and the dentist does a restoration for this patient at a fee of $75, but the insurance company only pays $55 for this particular service, the dentist has to adjust, or waive, the remaining $20 of the fee, and the patient will not be responsible for it. If the insurance company pays a percentage of a fee and a discount is given, it must be given to the insurance company, too. For example, if an insurance company pays 80% for a restoration, the dentist should not take the 80% and then adjust, or write off, the 20% balance. Dental team members must be aware that the practice cannot survive if constant adjustments to the fees are made. Production must be balanced by other cases that meet the regular fee schedule to maintain a viable practice.

Posting Patient Fees Each time the patient is in the office, information about the treatment received by the patient is entered into the computer system using **current dental terminology** (CDT) codes. Most computer programs have the fees for the practice preprogrammed into the system. Once the CDT code is entered, the fee automatically appears. Of course, the system can be overridden and a custom fee added if necessary. The office manager can also enter the UCR from each insurance company yearly as they are released. With all these options, the fee that appears will be the fee that the individual patient should be charged. This automatic fee generation eliminates errors and having to look up fees. The computer automatically updates the ledger, posts the charges, and calculates the patient's balance and the practice's accounts receivable balance. As the treatment fee is being posted, it can be assigned to any provider in a multiprovider practice. Discounts the patient might receive can also be given, and notes can be added regarding the treatment.

After the fee is posted and added to the ledger, the computer can automatically create an insurance claim form for patients with insurance. The claim form contains the patient and insurance information and uses the CDT code so that the insurance company recognizes the procedure.

Procedure 44-3
Posting Patient Charges

The front office assistant performs this task during or at the end of the day.

Equipment and Supplies
- access to the computer
- confirmation of treatment completed
- CDT codes
- financial agreement, if one was made
- printer
- appointment cards

Procedure Steps
1. Escort patient to the front desk.

2. Post the treatment in the computer using CDT codes (can be completed by the clinical team or the administrative assistant).

3. If there are discounts that the patient will be receiving, deduct them according to the category, such as courtesy or professional discounts. If multiple dentists are in the practice, make sure the production is credited to the correct dentist.

4. Using the financial agreement, ask the patient to pay all or part of the treatment fee, depending on insurance coverage.

5. Discuss any new treatment plan.

6. Agree upon any new financial arrangements, if necessary.

7. Schedule the next appointment. This could be continued treatment or their next recare. Every patient should leave knowing when they should return and why!

8. Give the patient a walkout statement that includes the day's charges, any payments posted, insurance information, any outstanding balance, and when their next appointment is scheduled.

9. Give the patient an appointment card.

Procedure 44-4
Balancing Day Sheets

The front office assistant balances the day sheets at the end of each day.

Equipment and Supplies
- access to the computer
- printer
- the day's schedule

Procedure Steps

End of Day

1. In the office manager of the dental software, choose "Day Sheet Report."

2. Select provider range. Select "All" for all providers.

3. Select billing type "All."

4. Select the date range.

5. Options to include are as follows:
   - ❑ **MTD and YTD Totals**. Includes balances for month and year
   - ❑ **Extended MTD**. Includes the average production and average charge per patient
   - ❑ **Provider Totals**. Shows the production and collection for each provider individually
   - ❑ **Compare to Fee Schedule**. Compares the transaction charges to a specified fee schedule

6. Select the report type, based on preference. To show the charges posted in order they were completed for the day, choose "chronological."

7. Click OK.

8. Print out an end of day sheet following your software instructions. **Hint:** Some dental office managers in practices that take in lots of payments do a test close earlier in the day so that mistakes are discovered before they are ready to leave for the day.

9. Total the payments you collected and make sure they equal the amount on the day sheet.

10. Prepare a deposit slip. Directions are in Procedure 44-5.

11. When your accounts balance, close the day and back up the computer. Once the day is closed, the next work date will automatically appear and you will no longer be able to make changes on the day you just closed.

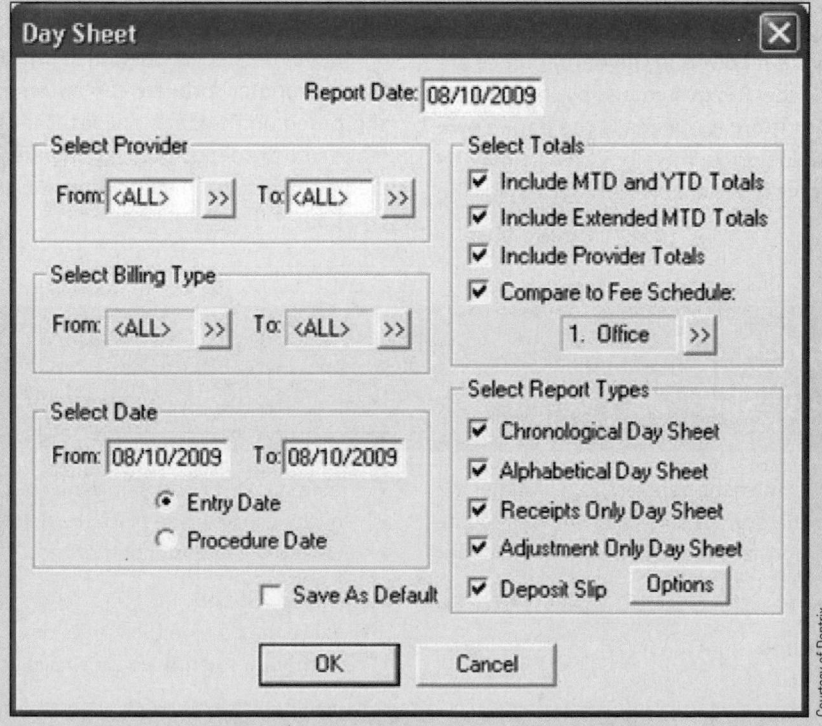

Courtesy of Dentrix

Posting Patient Payments Ideally, every patient should make a payment for the dental treatment that they receive on the day of service, either in full or the estimated portion that is their responsibility after insurance. Every time a patient makes a payment, or an insurance company makes a payment on behalf of a patient, it must be entered into the patient's ledger. Once you are in the ledger, select the patient. This is done by adding a payment. Once you access the payment screen, either by selecting it by name or by its icon, it is as simple as filling in the blanks. It is important to designate how the payment was made so at the end of the day you can balance your accounts. If a patient makes a payment with a credit card, then this option is selected. If the payment was by check, then the assistant enters the check number as well as the amount. Cash payments are designated as cash. If payment is from an insurance company, it will be either by check or by an electronic transfer of funds, and the option of payment by an insurance company must be specified.

Cash Payments It is important to keep enough cash in the office to make change if the need arises. Some dental offices offer a discount to patients who pay cash in advance (checks included) for the entire treatment the patient is to receive. If a patient pays in cash, it is important to give a written receipt showing the payment on the account. This can be done easily by printing a walk-out statement.

Check Payments Some offices require that the patient use a driver's license number on the check or another form of identification for the check. If there is a fee associated with a check that does not clear, the patient should be told of the fee or the policy should be posted visible to the patient.

Other checks that may be received in the dental office are cashier's checks. A cashier's check is guaranteed by the bank for the amount in which it is written. It is actually the bank's own check that the patient has paid for. Traveler's checks may be used by out-of-town patients. They are safer than cash for the

user. They are written in specific denominations ($20, $50, etc.) and require a signature from the user that matches the one on the check at the time of use. A certified check could be used by a patient as well. A certified check is one that the bank has verified as good for the amount indicated.

Credit Card Payments Patients may use credit cards to pay for services. The office takes the card, uses a card reader to enter the amount, and swipes the card or inserts a chipped card. The patient signs electronically or on a printout of the transaction. The payment is entered into the computer as a credit card payment, and the patient is given a receipt. Credit card vendors charge a processing fee to the practice. For this reason, some offices may only prefer to take certain credit cards over others. Usually a sign is posted with accepted credit cards in the office.

With practice, the front office assistant can accomplish these tasks quickly and accurately. After posting a fee that the patient owes or a payment that the patient has made, the patient account can be viewed on the computer monitor or printed out if the patient desires a copy. This copy is often called a walk-out statement (Figure 44-25).

Bank Deposits

Patient and insurance payments need to be deposited into the bank. How often the deposits are made depends on the practice. The cash is noted separately, and all the checks are endorsed with the office endorsement stamp, which indicates the specific bank that is utilized. Most offices have restrictive endorsement stamps that state "for deposit only." This protects the office if the check is stolen or lost. A deposit slip with the date, practice name, account number, listed currency and checks, and the total amount of the deposit identified on it is written for each deposit. Most computer software can automatically generate a deposit slip based on the day's entries. The front office assistant must make sure the deposit slip is generated and the cash, checks, and credit card receipts match before making the deposit.

Procedure 44-5
Preparing a Deposit Slip

The front office assistant creates the deposit slip, and either the front office assistant or the dentist takes it to the bank to be deposited. Deposits are normally made in person or placed in a night deposit box.

Equipment and Supplies
- deposit slip
- copy of the day's schedule
- cash and checks received for that day

- office stamp for endorsing the check
- envelope in which to place the deposit slip, checks, and cash
- access to a computer and printer

Procedure Steps
1. Place the date on the bank's deposit slip, or use the computer to print a deposit slip.

2. Separate the currency (coin and paper money) from the checks.

Inner City Dental Care
222 S. First Avenue
Carlton, MI 11666
(814) 555-7155

DEPOSIT SLIP

—————————— 19 ——

First Bank
5411 Brown Rd.
Carlton, MI 11666   ⑆ 1 2 20 14 9 3 2⑆

Front

CURRENCY	
COIN	
CHECKS	
TOTAL FROM OTHER SIDE	
TOTAL	

List all items separately

Total
Enter on front side

Back

Sample deposit slip.

3. Tally the coins and place or confirm the total sum in the designated space on the deposit slip.

4. Tally the paper money and place or confirm the total sum in the designated space on the deposit slip.

5. On the back of the deposit slip, list each check separately, listing the patient's last name and the amount of the check in the space provided in the right-hand column. With a computerized system, if you have entered the information correctly throughout the day, the checks will be listed for you. Double-check for errors using the day's schedule.

6. Total the list amounts from the checks on the back of the deposit slip and place this sum in the area on the front of the deposit slip in the space identified as checks.

7. Total the currency (both coins and paper money) and the check amount, and place this sum at the bottom of the deposit slip under "Total." This amount should match the total identified on the payments column on the day sheet. One way to check that the total is accurate is to add up the coins, paper money, and each check. This verifies that the sum is correct.

Procedure 44-6
Reconciling a Bank Statement

The administrative assistant or dental office manager reconciles the bank statement each month. This can be done manually or with the help of a computer, but, regardless of the method, the process remains the same.

Equipment and Supplies
- bank statement (shown below)
- checkbook
- calculator
- access to a computer

Procedure Steps

1. Make sure that all checks and deposits have been added to or subtracted from the checkbook.

2. Subtract any bank service charge from the last balance listed in the checkbook.

(Continues)

3. Check off each listed check in the bank statement against the checkbook and verify the amount listed.

4. Check off each deposit listed in the bank statement against the checkbook and verify the amount listed.

5. On the back of the bank statement, place the ending balance from the front of the statement in the ending balance space on the worksheet.

6. List all checks from the checkbook that have not cleared the bank in the section provided on the back worksheet.

7. List all deposits from the checkbook that have not been received by the bank on the space provided on the worksheet on the back of the statement.

8. Total the checks not cleared and the deposits not received. Subtract the checks not received from the ending balance on the bank statement, and add the deposits not received to the ending balance on the bank statement. This balance should agree with the checkbook balance. If there are any bank charges on the statement, make the corresponding adjustments to the checkbook balance.

Front

Summary of Account Balance   Closing Date 1/15/XX

Account # 1257-164013   Ending Balance $8,347.62

Beginning Balance	$ 7,152.18
Total Deposits and Additions	$ 8,643.86
Total Withdrawals	$ 7,433.21
Service Charge	$ 15.24

Number	Date	Amount	Number	Date	Amount
201	12/18/XX	173.82	234	1/4/XX	96.31
223*	12/18/XX	44.12	235	1/4/XX	73.48
224	12/20/XX	586.00	236	1/6/XX	325.40
225	12/21/XX	24.15	237	1/7/XX	40.00
226	12/22/XX	33.90	238	1/8/XX	66.77
228*	12/23/XX	1250.00	241*	1/9/XX	15.55
229	12/24/XX	11.75	242	1/10/XX	12.45
230	12/24/XX	19.02	243	1/10/XX	4441.64
231	1/2/XX	43.80	244	1/10/XX	64.55
232	1/3/XX	39.00			
233	1/4/XX	71.50			

*Denotes gap in check sequence

Date	Deposit Amount	Date	Deposit Amount
18-Dec	361.75	4-Jan	825.00
19-Dec	586.00	5-Jan	1286.71
20-Dec	918.21	7-Jan	608.00
21-Dec	201.00	8-Jan	811.15
2-Jan	475.00	9-Jan	1092.68
3-Dec	1478.36		

Back

1. Enter ending balance from the front of this statement

$ 8,347.62

2. Enter deposits not shown on this statement.

$ 3,162.50

3. Subtotal (add 1 and 2)

$ 11,510.12

4. List outstanding checks or other withdrawals here

Check #	Amount
222	37.89
227	161.15
239	11.50
240	92.12
245	835.17
246	21.75
247	586.00

5. Total outstanding checks.

$ 1,745.58

Balance (subtract 5 from 3)

$ 9,764.54

This should equal your checkbook balance

Monthly Billing

Sending monthly billing statements is expensive and time consuming, so, ideally, patients pay at the time of services in order to avoid having to print and mail statements; but sometimes, statements do need to be sent.

The computer generates monthly statements from the ledger in the database with an age analysis of the balance. Many offices include return stamped envelopes to aid the patient in sending a payment. Reviewing the statements before sending them is a good idea so that statements for very small amounts are not sent. If your cost of sending a statement is $3, sending out a statement asking for a payment of $1 would be inefficient. Keep in mind if a patient has insurance, often those accounts are not sent statements until the insurance has paid and any remaining balance is actually owed by the patient. A statement should be sent out only when necessary and not for informational purposes.

Payment Plans For more expensive dental treatment, offering several payment options after the treatment plan is discussed helps the practice remain healthy and productive. When treatment is diagnosed, the front desk assistant or dental office manager may set up financial arrangements. Often, an initial down payment is requested when treatment is done. The balance is then divided, and this fixed amount is paid over an arranged time frame. For instance, a patient may have $1,000 worth of dentistry to complete. The office may request 20% as a down payment, with the additional $800 being paid in $200 increments over the next 4 months. The patient signs the payment plan along with the dental office manager or dentist. If payments extend over 4 months, and finance charges are added to the unpaid balance, the patient must be notified in advance under the federal **Truth in Lending Act (TILA)**. This law, which is designed to protect consumers in

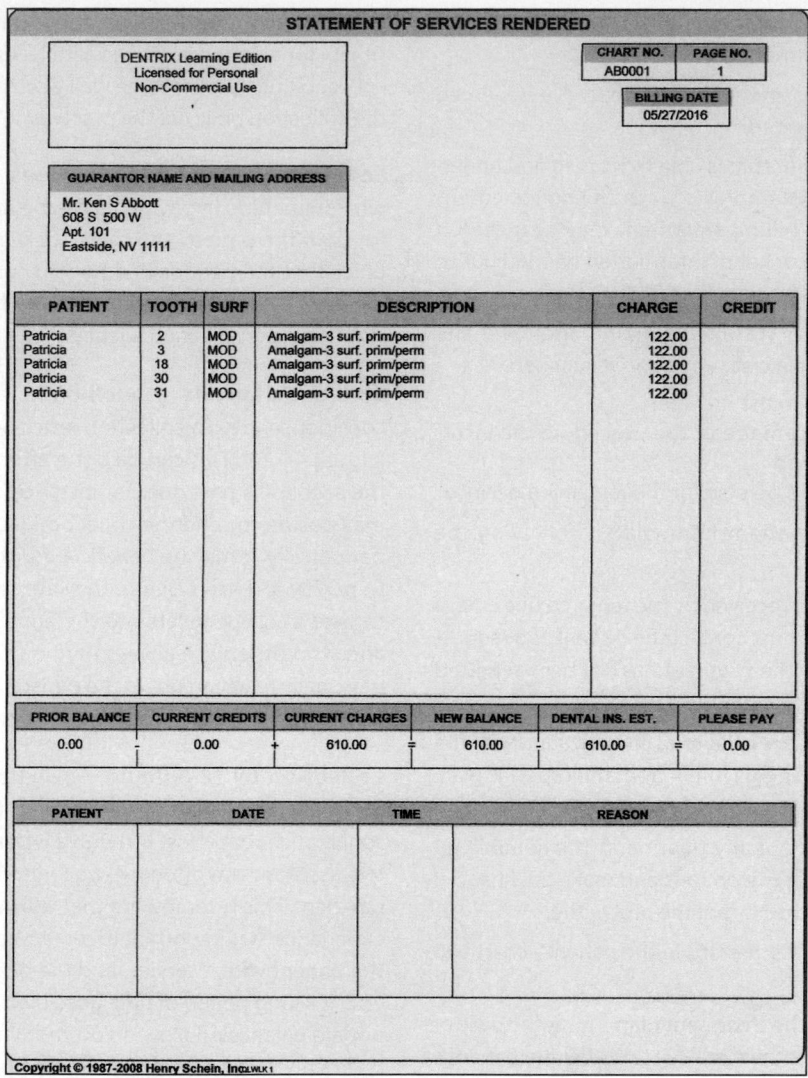

STATEMENT OF SERVICES RENDERED

DENTRIX Learning Edition
Licensed for Personal
Non-Commercial Use

CHART NO.	PAGE NO.
AB0001	1

BILLING DATE
05/27/2016

GUARANTOR NAME AND MAILING ADDRESS

Mr. Ken S Abbott
608 S 500 W
Apt. 101
Eastside, NV 11111

PATIENT	TOOTH	SURF	DESCRIPTION	CHARGE	CREDIT
Patricia	2	MOD	Amalgam-3 surf. prim/perm	122.00	
Patricia	3	MOD	Amalgam-3 surf. prim/perm	122.00	
Patricia	18	MOD	Amalgam-3 surf. prim/perm	122.00	
Patricia	30	MOD	Amalgam-3 surf. prim/perm	122.00	
Patricia	31	MOD	Amalgam-3 surf. prim/perm	122.00	

PRIOR BALANCE	CURRENT CREDITS	CURRENT CHARGES	NEW BALANCE	DENTAL INS. EST.	PLEASE PAY
0.00 −	0.00 +	610.00 =	610.00 −	610.00 =	0.00

PATIENT	DATE	TIME	REASON

FIGURE 44-25
Patients should receive a walkout statement when they leave the office.

credit transactions, requires that clear disclosure of contract terms and any associated costs be given to the consumer. The dental office should use a truth-in-lending form, which can be custom designed from a computer-generated template, to notify the consumer of financial arrangements. The patient is given one copy of the payment plan and the original is kept in the patient's record. This information may also be noted on the ledger to remind the patient of the arrangements when the statement is sent out.

Loans An additional payment option is a loan. These dental/medical loans are becoming very popular and often have no interest payments for 12–18 months if paid in full during that time period. Many dental offices provide this information to patients and assist them in completing the paperwork. Some patients may have their own loan sources and use a bank they work with already. To receive loans, patients must complete the appropriate paperwork. Some loan agencies can quickly verify that patients meet requirements; others need a day or two. In this system, the patient may pay additional loan fees, but payments can be established through loan agencies over an extended period of time.

Collections In an effort to continue to receive payment for services rendered in a dental practice, care must be taken to ensure that there is a team or staffed department within the practice that consistently monitors the collections aspect of the office. Without the financial collection of outstanding debt from either the patient or insurance company, the practice cannot operate efficiently or effectively. Below are common methods to ensure that the practice's accounts receivables are established as revenue in an estimated amount of time.

1. Ensure that patients completely understands the billing process before any treatment is provided.

2. Explain to the patient payment options for services rendered before treatment is provided.

3. Create a billing statement that is able to be read and understood by the patient. Examples of your billing statement and how to read your billing statement may be included in the office welcome packet of information handed out to patients at their first visit.

4. Ensure that the billing statement plainly indicates the following information in a clear and concise manner:
   a. Total amount owed to the provider
   b. What cost and percentage of the procedure the insurance covered and paid
   c. Expected due date to be paid for the remaining balance

5. Send invoices to the patient immediately following the treatment rendered.

6. If payment has not been received by the required due date, a business staff member must contact the patient and request information about why the payment has not been remitted yet (explained later in this section).

7. Patient's responsibility as related to communicating with the dental insurance regarding payment from their specific plan.

8. Discuss financial arrangements with your emergency patients before delivery of any treatment. The administrative assistant can discuss the options and make the financial arrangements prior to the start of the procedure.

9. Document *all* financial discussions in the patient's chart and record.

10. Post all treatment into the treatment plan. This is the duty of the clinical staff, not the front office staff. Link the patient's insurance plan to their account so that the printout of the treatment plan is accurate. This takes conscientious effort to research their plan and percentages of what the intended treatment will cost the patient after the insurance has paid their portion.

11. Inform the patient that estimates of what insurance will pay are just an estimate and done as a courtesy to them. They are responsible for the full balance that insurance does not cover.

In addition to collectively monitoring the outstanding accounts receivable aspect of the office's dental patient, it is also imperative that the patient's dental insurance activity after a claim has been sent also be monitored. Patients often refuse to pay any portion of the bill until the insurance has responded to the claim. This anticipation of the dental insurance paying part of the claim prior to the patient paying for their portion of the bill is deemed a disaster. Many offices that provide many expensive dental services (crown and bridge work, cosmetic, in-house whitening, etc.) require that half of the total amount of the fee for the service be paid on the date of the initial restorative visit. This excludes the possibility of the patient not completing the treatment, as they have already paid for half of the intended procedures. Although this rule usually only attracts those patients who accept responsibility for a debt they have willfully agreed to, this implemented collection rule proves to be well worth the rigidity of the terms of the collection policy of the practice.

Contacting Patient for Collections Often contacting patients who are behind in payments can be an uncomfortable situation for both the patient and the staff. Dentists have a procedure in place for time periods and how to contact these patients ranging from collection letters, collection by telephone, and as a last result using a collection agency.

Collection Letters In addition to a statement, a dentist may consider sending a collection letter personalized to the patient (Figure 44-26). This can be done after a certain number of days the account is past due. For instance, after 60 days, the practice may decide to send the collection letter and continue to do so periodically. It may be beneficial for the administrative assistant to review all letters before they are sent out. You may not want to send a collection letter to someone who is a long-time patient and who otherwise always paid on time. In this circumstance, personally reaching out to the patient by way of a phone call may be the better option to discuss any payment options.

Collection by Telephone Collection by telephone can be a great way to reach out to the patient for payment. It adds a personal touch that is lost through a letter. However, the administrative assistant can often feel uncomfortable asking patients for a payment. This is something that will improve over time and with experience. It is important to remember that your office provided the patient with a service, and the patient must pay for that service. If a long period of time goes by, it will be less likely to collect unpaid balances. Follow up promptly when patients are to make payments. Table 44-8 reviews some tips for collection by phone.

Collection Agency It is unfortunate, but sometimes the need will arise for a third party to attempt collections. A **collection agency** is used when all other means for collections have been exhausted. The use of a reputable, professional agency is a must. Check who owns the company, who makes the collection calls, ask for references, review the policies, and ensure it aligns with what you want for your patients. Once the collection agency is chosen and a patient is sent to collections, the administrative assistant stops all collection attempts to the patient. No more statements should be sent, and no more collection letters or phone calls should be made. The patient needs to send payment to the collection agency. Make an indication in the patient record to ensure none of the previous occurs. The collection agency takes a percentage of the money recovered from the patient.

Accounts Payable

The accounts payable are the amounts that the practice owes others, such as necessary expenses. The expenses that are required to run the dental practice are called overhead. The total accounts receivable is calculated as the gross income, or profits made before taxes and office expenses are paid. Subtract

Tamara Riegel, D.D.S.
909 Central
Rockford, LA 20011

December 1, 20XX

Mr. John Cooper
41 Sandiford Drive
Locust, LA 22011

Dear Mr. Cooper:

Your account with our office
is three months past due, and
you have not responded to our
previous requests for payment.
Please pay your balance of
$152 at this time, or contact
us with an explanation of why
you cannot pay.

Please call me at 555-7823 if
you have a question about your
account. Otherwise, we expect
your payment immediately.

Sincerely,

Natalie Short
Accounts Manager

Tamara Riegel, D.D.S.
909 Central
Rockford, LA 20011

December 29, 20XX

Mr. John Cooper
41 Sandiford Drive
Locust, LA 22011

Dear Mr. Cooper:

Your son, Royce, had a
seriously infected tooth in
March when he came to Dr.
Riegel for treatment. Dr.
Riegel was pleased to use her
experience and education to
treat Royce, and it was in
this same spirit of
cooperation that we expected
you to pay your account within
a reasonable amount of time.

Four months have passed and
you have still not remitted
the $152 outstanding balance
on your account. We cannot
continue to keep your unpaid
account on our books. If you
are experiencing financial
difficulties, please call the
office so we can arrange a
payment schedule that is
agreeable to both of us.

Sincerely,

Natalie Short
Accounts Manager

Tamara Riegel, D.D.S.
909 Central
Rockford, LA 20011

February 1, 20XX

Mr. John Cooper
41 Sandiford Drive
Locust, LA 22011

Dear Mr. Cooper:

You have not replied to our
previous notices regarding
your unpaid balance of $152.
Unless we hear from you
personally within 14 days,
your account will be given to
the Rockford Medical and
Dental Collection Service.

Do not wait any longer to
contact me at 555-7823 if you
wish to maintain your previous
good credit record with Dr.
Riegel. As previously
suggested, we will cooperate
in arranging a suitable
payment schedule, if needed.

Sincerely,

Natalie Short
Accounts Manager

FIGURE 44-26
Collection letters sent to patients with delinquent accounts, drafted to encourage patients to pay their bills.

TABLE 44-8 Tips for Collections by Telephone

1.	When calling the patient, make sure you are speaking to the person responsible for the account.
2.	Ask if the time is convenient for them to talk. If not, ask for a better call back time.
3.	When leaving a message to a third party or on a machine, do not give specifics; simply state your name and the phone number and ask for the call to be returned.
4.	Typically try not to call too early in the morning or too late in the evening.
5.	Be prepared with all the account information available.
6.	Be positive and polite; do not portray that you do not expect them to pay. Remember, sometimes patients simply forget.
7.	Do not be threatening.
8.	If the patient promises to pay by a certain date, look out for the payment. If the payment is not made, follow up promptly with the patient.

the accounts payable from the gross income to identify the net income, which is the actual profit of the office after all taxes and expenses are paid. The net income is the true profit the practice makes. The practice cannot remain vital if there is no net income for the dentist. It is not advisable to operate a business in an unprofitable manner for long.

Some of the expenses are fixed (remain the same) each month. These include the mortgage, full-time salaries, and some utilities. Other expenses are variable, meaning that they fluctuate and are dependent on the needs for the month. Variable overhead expenses include dental supplies, dental laboratory costs, and equipment repairs. The front office assistant, along with the dentist, can document the monthly overhead and evaluate whether costs can be cut without decreasing patient service. One of the highest monthly variable overhead costs is in the area of dental supplies.

Petty Cash

Petty cash is the money kept in the office for minor expenses, such as for coffee supplies or postage-due letters. Most offices keep less than $100 in this account. The front office assistant oversees this cash account. Each time it is used, a voucher or receipt is placed in the cash box until the money gets low. Then the fund is replenished by writing another check to the cash fund, bringing it up to the original amount. The check is noted as petty cash and the receipts total the amount replenished to the account.

Payroll

The front office assistant or dental office manager may complete the employee payroll. Each employee fills out a W-4 form, or the employee's withholding allowance certificate, when they begin employment, which includes their name,

address, Social Security number, and the total number of **allowances** (exemptions) to be claimed. With this information, payroll is calculated using the charts provided by the Internal Revenue Service. Federal taxes are based on the amount earned, marital status, number and type of allowances claimed, and length of pay period. Most state and local taxes are calculated on the total gross earnings of the employee. A required deduction under the Federal Insurance Contributions Act (FICA), commonly called Social Security, is calculated on the basis of gross pay. The employer is required to match this deducted amount and send both contributions to the federal government quarterly. Other deductions that may be taken from the employee's paycheck are health and life insurance payments, along with retirement or savings contributions that are put in another account.

At the end of the year, the employer is required to give each employee a W-2 wage and tax statement (Figure 44-27). This statement is used by the employee to submit their federal income tax. The statement includes total wages earned and the tax deductions made for the year by that employee.

a Control number 3203	22222	Void ☐	For Official Use Only OMB No. 1545-0008	

b Employer's identification number 317 600 23	1 Wages, tips, other compensation 18,500.00	2 Federal income tax withheld 2,950.00
c Employer's name, address, and ZIP code Lewis & King, D.D.S. 2501 Center Street, Suite 23 Northborough, OH 12345	3 Social security wages 18,500.00	4 Social security taxes withheld 1200.00
	5 Medicare wages and tips 18,500.00	6 Medicare tax withheld 220.00
	7 Social security tips	8 Allocated tips
d Employee's social security number 263-58-5296	9 Advance EIC payment	10 Dependent care benefits
e Employee's name (first, middle initial, last) Ellen L. Armstrong	11 Nonqualified plans	12 Benefits included in box 1
498 Menaul Road Northborough, OH 12345	13 See Instrs. for box 13	14 Other 360.00 Dental Care

19 Statutory employee ☐	Deceased ☐	Pension plan ☐	Legal rep. ☐	Hshld. emp. ☐	Subtotal ☐	Deferred compensation ☐

f Employee's address and ZIP code

16 State OH	Employer's state I.D. No. 24	17 State wages, tips, etc. 18,500.00	18 State income tax 750.00	19 Locality name OH	20 Local wages, tips, etc. 18,500.00	21 Local income tax 63.50

Cat. No. 10134D   Department of Treasury—Internal Revenue Service

Form **W-2** **Wage and Tax Statement** **20--**

Copy A For Social Security Administration

For Paperwork Reduction Act Notice, see separate instructions

FIGURE 44-27
W-2 form, summarizing all earnings and deductions for the year. The employer prepares a yearly W-2 form for each employee by January 31.

Procedure 44-7
Writing a Business Check

The front office assistant or dental office manager writes out the office accounts payable for the dentist to review and sign.

Equipment and Supplies
- checkbook with check and stub (shown below)
- calculator
- access to a computer and printer, if checks are written electronically

Procedure Steps

1. Write or type in the date. Make sure the date is current.

2. Write or type in the name of the payee. Verify that this is the correct payee.

3. Write in the numbers for the correct amount and write out the amount in the designated area. Check that the numerical and written amounts agree and are correct.

4. Fill out the memo, indicating what the check is for.

5. Fill out the date, payee, memo information, and amount on the check stub.

6. Verify that everything is accurate, including spelling.

7. Have the dentist sign on the signature line after reviewing the account payable.

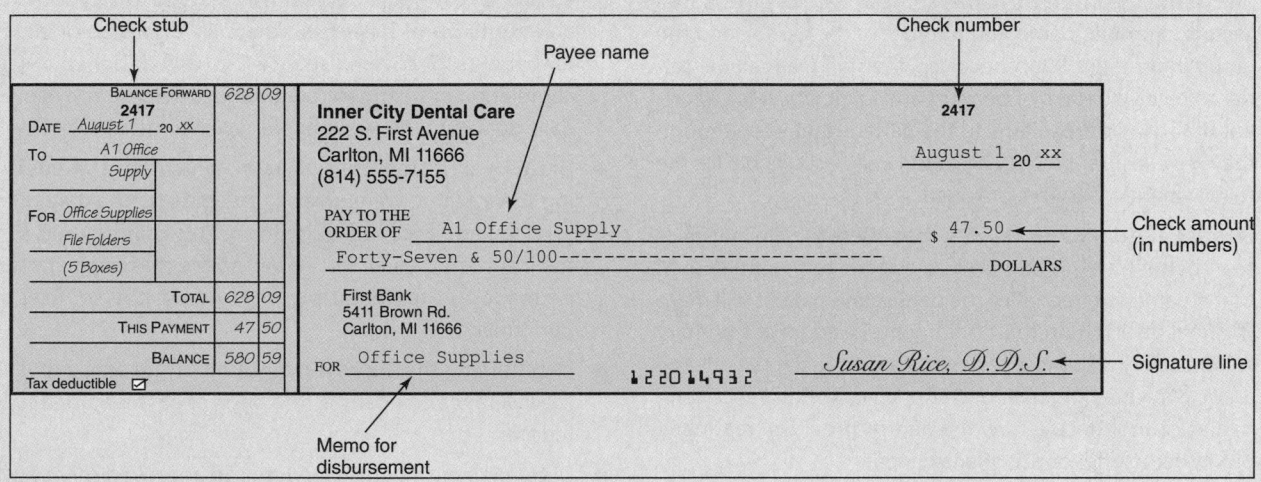

Dental Insurance

Dental insurance allows individuals the opportunity to access care while providing some benefit. As more companies offer dental insurance, more and more people are seeking care. A dental insurance plan is a highly complex area that can create confusion for many dental patients. The complexities of a dental insurance plan and the lack of sufficient information provided by some insurance companies make it almost impossible for some patients to properly understand their employer-provided dental benefits. Nearly every dental office will offer to bill insurance for their patients as a service to the patient. While insurance can remain complex for some patients to understand, it is important for the administrative assistant to gain a full understanding of the operations for benefit to the office as well as to help the patient better understand their benefits.

What Is Dental Insurance?

A **dental insurance** plan is a contract between the patient's employer and an insurance company. These are benefits that the patient, spouse, or family members, when applicable, receive in compensation for dental services. Patients are awarded specific dental insurance coverage, which is based on the terms of a contract that is negotiated between the patient's employer and the dental insurance company. The goal of most dental insurance policies is to provide basic benefits for preventative care, as well as for specific dental services. The services are based on the cost of the policy to the patient's employer and the negotiated arrangements with the insurance company. Because the benefits for the patient are decided between the patient's employer and the insurance company, there may be services that are not covered. The selection of noncovered services is not based on what the patient or family members need or want but is strictly based on the contract with the insurance company. Patients often confuse dental benefits with medical benefits. Dental benefits tend to have limited coverage with variable maximums. While dental insurance may not cover a procedure, it does not mean the treatment is not necessary and should not be completed.

Parties Involved in Insurance

There are four parties involved in the patient's dental insurance that the dental assistant needs to be familiar with in:

1. **Group.** The group is classified as the employer, union, or someone who represents the group. The group makes the contract with the insurance carrier and decides the benefit level, deductible, maximums, limitations, and any **exclusions** in the program. The patient is provided with their group number.

2. **Patient.** The patient has the responsibility to provide the office with the insured's name, address, date of birth, social security number, name and number of the carrier, and the group information. Once received, the staff may call the carrier to receive details of benefits and eligibility. It is important that the staff explains to the patient that even though they have insurance, they are ultimately responsible for the full payment of services provided.

3. **Dentist.** The dentist works with the patient to help maximize their benefits. While this is true, it needs to be understood that regardless of benefits, the dentist and patient will make the final decision on their treatment. The dentist's primary responsibility is to provide necessary care to the patient and assist in maintaining their overall oral health. Insurance companies cannot decide how the dentist provides treatment, but rather to offer or not offer a benefit.

4. **Dental carrier.** The dental carrier (insurance company) administers a plan based on the contract with the group. This includes the processing of claims and payment for services rendered.

Managing Insurance Benefits

Within the business office of a dental practice, the insurance management team is led by an insurance administrator, or an individual who manages or directs a dental benefit program on behalf of the program's sponsor. Refer to Table 44-9 for common dental insurance terms. While working with this leader, other staff members assist in numerous responsibilities associated with dental insurance. Many of these responsibilities are as follows:

- Identifying the patient's **certificate of eligibility** for their dental insurance, which includes all eligible individuals, or persons entitled to any dental benefits under a specific plan.

- Identifying who the **claimant**, or the person who is filing the claim. Note that this may be the patient but may also be the person who actually is the policy holder, or **subscriber**.

- Determining the **effective date**, or the date the coverage goes into effect and from which time benefits are afforded. It should be noted that the group effective date can be different from the patient's effective date.

- Establishing the **coordination of benefits**. Should there be more than one insurance involved (e.g., both parents in a family work and have separate dental insurances from their respective employers), a general rule when coordinating benefits is stipulating that the **primary carrier** is the member's own insurance through their employer. Dependent children's primary carrier is determined by the birthday rule. A **secondary carrier** is the plan covering the patient as a dependent when the patient is the spouse or dependent child of the parent whose birthday occurs later in the calendar year. Claims are submitted to the primary carrier first for benefits. Some insurance companies may use the gender rule. This is where the father is always considered primary. Once the primary is received, the claim is then submitted to the secondary carrier with proof of payment from the primary carrier for additional coverage. Occasionally a dental policy will include an **extension of benefits**. This is an extension of eligibility for benefits for covered services, usually designed to ensure completion of treatment commenced prior to the expiration date; duration is generally expressed in terms of days.

- Drafting and submitting a claim, which is a statement listing services that were given to the patient, the date of these services, and a signed claim form. This claim form is sent to the insurance carrier and serves notice that payment should be made to the dental provider where the services were performed.

- Determining the approved amount, or the amount used by the insurance company as the basis of payment for a submitted fee.

- Determining if a dental service is an approved service, which distinguishes if the service meets the standards maintained under the dental insurance plan.

- Determining if the dentist is considered a **participating provider** for the eligibility of the patient utilizing the dental insurance. A participating provider is any duly licensed dentist with whom the dental plan has an agreement to render care to beneficiaries under rules and regulations promulgated by a board of directors or agency.

- Determining if the dentist is considered a **nonparticipating provider**—a dentist who has not entered into an agreement with a service corporation, commercial carrier, or agency and has not agreed to rules and regulations as promulgated by a given board of director. Often, patients are referred to a dental specialist who specializes in performing a procedure that a normal dental provider does not. If the specialist is not a participating provider for the patient's dental insurance plan, this does not void the patient's request to have services provided by this specialist. However, the insurance benefits of the patient may not apply when treatment is provided by the nonparticipating dentist or specialist. Often, a percentage of the services provided are covered with out-of-network fees, which can drastically reduce the percentage of payment.

- Determining the **maximum benefit** that the dental insurance will pay, as determined by the policy. The definition of the maximum benefit is the maximum dollar amount a dental plan will pay toward the cost of dental care incurred by an individual or family in a specified period, whether a calendar year or a contract year.
- Determining the **individual deductible** amount, or that portion of the covered dental care expense that the patient must pay before the plan's benefits begin; this could be a yearly or a one-time deductible amount.
- Determining the **family deductible** amount, if applicable. This is a deductible that is satisfied by combined expenses of all covered family members; for example, a program that has a

$50 deductible may limit its application to a maximum of $125 per family, regardless of the number of family members.

- Determining the **copayment**, or the amount or percentage of the total approved amount that the subscriber is obligated to pay; this is not to be confused with the deductible amount.
- Determining if there are any exclusions present in the dental insurance plan. Exclusions are those services that are not covered by the plan.
- Determining the premiums, also known as the amount charged, by the dental benefit organization for coverage of a level of benefits for a specified time.
- Determining the table of allowances for each patient. This table is a list of specified amounts that will be paid toward the cost of dental services rendered; in most cases, the patient pays the difference between the allowance and the actual cost of service.

TABLE 44-9 Dental Insurance Terms

Assignment of benefits	The patient assigns benefits to be paid directly to the dentist or the provider.
Beneficiary	The patient who is entitled to dental insurance benefits.
Benefit-less-benefit	Refers to nonduplication of benefits pertinent to subscribers of more than one plan. Such plans allow reimbursement to be limited to the higher level allowed of the two plans.
Birthday rule	Refers to cases when both parents have coverage for a child patient: the primary carrier is held by the parent whose birthday month and day (not year) comes earliest in the calendar year.
Carrier	Usually the dental insurance company.
Coordination of benefits (COB)	Refers to provisions made by two carriers to coordinate (share) benefits between them, which are not to exceed 100% of the dental charges for an eligible subscriber.
Coverage	Benefits available to the person covered by dental insurance.
CDT codes	Codes that are published in the CDT under the ADA's jurisdiction.
Deductible	The amount paid before benefits take effect.
Dependents	Children covered under dental insurance.
Dual coverage	Two dental coverages; the primary is in first position and the balance is normally paid by the secondary insurance.
Eligibility	Determining if a patient is eligible for dental benefits.
Exclusions	Items that dental insurance does not cover.
Explanation of benefits (EOB)	A detailed description showing the payment or denial of an insurance claim.
Fee for service	A payment to providers on a service-by-service, rather than a salaried or capitated, basis.
Group plan	A plan in which several individuals are covered.
Individual plan	A plan in which an individual has a plan without a group of individuals.
Patient	A person receiving treatment.
Predetermination of benefits	Submitting the treatment plan to the carrier to determine what the insurance will pay on the dental services; this is often called the pretreatment estimate (estimate completed before treatment).
Premium	The amount the carrier charges the subscriber.
Primary insurance	The insurance of the subscriber.
Provider	The dentist who performs the dental service.
Reimbursement	A payment made by the carrier to the patient, or the dentist on behalf of the beneficiary, toward the dental fee incurred.
Secondary insurance	The insurance of the subscriber's spouse.
Subscriber	An individual with dental insurance.

Insurance Fraud

It can be frustrating to hear patients say they only want to do what the insurance will cover. As an oral health care provider, the dentist wants to provide quality care to the patient, and in a perfect world, money would be no object. Unfortunately, insurance companies make decisions about what is or is not covered regarding patient services. For example, the dentist may recommend, and the patient want to have, a bridge to replace missing teeth. The insurance responds that the patient has reached their maximum benefits for the year. Because of this, dentists may feel pressured to make unethical decisions to help the patient receive care by completing the work and postdating the insurance claim. This is a fraudulent act. As the administrative assistant, it is important to understand these fraudulent situations and the consequences that come along with them. Some other examples of fraud include:

- Billing for services not rendered
- Changing the date of service
- Billing before the date of service
- Billing the carrier for higher fees than charged to the patient
- Use of wrong codes with the intent to bill more for the service

Dental Claims

As a courtesy to patients, most dental offices submit insurance claims. The entire claim must be filled out. Dental claims can be submitted either electronically or by paper and mailed in. Each carrier has specific criteria for filing a claim, and if these are not followed, the claim is declined. It is extremely important to make sure the claim form is completely and correctly filled out to save the administrative assistant time in the event it gets declined. Once the administrative assistant becomes familiar with the different carriers, they can make note of techniques that may work with each company. In some cases, sending supporting documents such as periodontal charting, radiographs, or photographs can help approve a benefit. Knowing which procedures require this documentation can help speed up the approval process.

To submit a claim to insurance, the dentist uses the CDT codes. These codes are published in the *Current Dental Terminology* under the ADA's jurisdiction. The codes are updated every 2 years—new codes are added and obsolete codes are deleted. CDT codes follow a five-digit system for identifying dental procedures and services. The first digit of the code is the letter D for dental, which distinguishes the codes from medical ones. The second digit designates the category of service (e.g., preventative is 1). The third digit designates the class of service in the category, the fourth the subclass of service, and the fifth is open for expansion. An example of a CDT code is D1110 for adult prophylaxis. The CDT code for a child's prophylaxis is D1120. Table 44-10 lists the current CDT standard codes used.

Included on the claim form is the name and address of the carrier, as well as the patient's name, address, date of birth, ID number (this is different than the patient's Social Security number), sex, and phone numbers. In addition, the employer, the relationship to the subscriber, the subscriber ID, and the group number are

TABLE 44-10 CDT 2016—Current Dental Technology Standard Codes

Diagnostic	D0100–D0999
Preventive	D1000–D1999
Restorative	D2000–D2999
Endodontics	D3000–D3999
Periodontics	D4000–D4999
Prosthodontics, removable	D5000–D5899
Maxillofacial prosthodontics	D5900–D5999
Implant services	D6000–D6199
Prosthodontics, fixed	D6200–D6999
Oral and maxillofacial surgery	D7000–D7999
Orthodontics	D8000–D8999
Adjunctive general services	D9000–D9999

also noted on the form. Secondary insurance is also included on the form when applicable. The claim form also has two boxes for patients to sign. One of the boxes is for *release of information*. The release of information allows the dentist to release the patient's dental treatment information to the carrier (insurance company). Without this consent, the dentist cannot release this confidential information. The other box for the patient to sign is the assignment of benefits. Assignment of benefits authorizes the carrier to pay the dentist directly. If this box is unsigned, the check goes directly to the patient. When this box is unsigned, the office should arrange for payment of the entire dental treatment, because the office is not guaranteed to receive the insurance money. To facilitate electronic filing, dental offices use *signature on file*. This form is completed during patient registration and covers both the release of information and the assignment of benefits, if the patient has signed for both. When an office uses signature on file it is critical that the form is signed and is part of the patient's chart.

Paper Claims Each carrier has developed their own paper claim form. When submitting a paper claim, it is helpful to use the universal claim form provided by the American Dental Association (ADA). It is an option to use and accepted by all insurance carriers (Figure 44-28). These claim forms can be purchased through the ADA directly or through the supply vendor. The administrative assistant must review all claims to ensure their accuracy and completeness before submitting through the mail. In the event that radiographs are sent to a carrier, duplicates must be sent as the carrier is not required to return radiographs. Radiographs should be placed in a mount or envelope and properly labeled with the patient's name, date of radiographs, tooth number, and dental office name and address.

Electronic Claims Many offices are taking advantage of practice management software. This software makes submission of a claim as easy as a click of a button. The use of an electronic claim form allows for a faster and more accurate option

ADA American Dental Association® Dental Claim Form

HEADER INFORMATION

1. Type of Transaction (Mark all applicable boxes)

☐ Statement of Actual Services   ☐ Request for Predetermination/Preauthorization

☐ EPSDT / Title XIX

2. Predetermination/Preauthorization Number

DENTAL BENEFIT PLAN INFORMATION

3. Company/Plan Name, Address, City, State, Zip Code

OTHER COVERAGE (Mark applicable box and complete items 5-11. If none, leave blank.)

4. Dental? ☐   **Medical?** ☐   (If both, complete 5-11 for dental only.)

5. Name of Policyholder/Subscriber in #4 (Last, First, Middle Initial, Suffix)

6. Date of Birth (MM/DD/CCYY) | **7. Gender** ☐M ☐F ☐U | **8. Policyholder/Subscriber ID (Assigned by Plan)**

9. Plan/Group Number | **10. Patient's Relationship to Person named in #5** ☐ Self ☐ Spouse ☐ Dependent ☐ Other

11. Other Insurance Company/Dental Benefit Plan Name, Address, City, State, Zip Code

POLICYHOLDER/SUBSCRIBER INFORMATION (Assigned by Plan Named in #3)

12. Policyholder/Subscriber Name (Last, First, Middle Initial, Suffix), Address, City, State, Zip Code

13. Date of Birth (MM/DD/CCYY) | **14. Gender** ☐M ☐F ☐U | **15. Policyholder/Subscriber ID (Assigned by Plan)**

16. Plan/Group Number | **17. Employer Name**

PATIENT INFORMATION

18. Relationship to Policyholder/Subscriber in #12 Above ☐ Self ☐ Spouse ☐ Dependent Child ☐ Other | **19. Reserved For Future Use**

20. Name (Last, First, Middle Initial, Suffix), Address, City, State, Zip Code

21. Date of Birth (MM/DD/CCYY) | **22. Gender** ☐M ☐F ☐U | **23. Patient ID/Account # (Assigned by Dentist)**

RECORD OF SERVICES PROVIDED

	24. Procedure Date (MM/DD/CCYY)	25. Area of Oral Cavity	26. Tooth System	27. Tooth Number(s) or Letter(s)	28. Tooth Surface	29. Procedure Code	29a. Diag. Pointer	29b. Qty.	30. Description	31. Fee
1										
2										
3										
4										
5										
6										
7										
8										
9										
10										

33. Missing Teeth Information   (Place an "X" on each missing tooth.)

1 2 3 4 5 6 7 8 9 10 11 12 13 14 15 16

32 31 30 29 28 27 26 25 24 23 22 21 20 19 18 17

34. Diagnosis Code List Qualifier ☐ (ICD-10 = AB)

34a. Diagnosis Code(s)   A _____   C _____

(Primary diagnosis in "A")   B _____   D _____

31a. Other Fee(s)

32. Total Fee

35. Remarks

AUTHORIZATIONS

36. I have been informed of the treatment plan and associated fees. I agree to be responsible for all charges for dental services and materials not paid by my dental benefit plan, unless prohibited by law, or the treating dentist or dental practice has a contractual agreement with my plan prohibiting all or a portion of such charges. To the extent permitted by law, I consent to your use and disclosure of my protected health information to carry out payment activities in connection with this claim.

X _____

Patient/Guardian Signature   Date

37. I hereby authorize and direct payment of the dental benefits otherwise payable to me, directly to the below named dentist or dental entity.

X _____

Subscriber Signature   Date

BILLING DENTIST OR DENTAL ENTITY (Leave blank if dentist or dental entity is not submitting claim on behalf of the patient or insured/subscriber.)

48. Name, Address, City, State, Zip Code

49. NPI | **50. License Number** | **51. SSN or TIN**

52. Phone Number (   )   - | **52a. Additional Provider ID**

ANCILLARY CLAIM/TREATMENT INFORMATION

38. Place of Treatment _____ (e.g. 11=office; 22=O/P Hospital) (Use "Place of Service Codes for Professional Claims") | **39. Enclosures (Y or N)**

40. Is Treatment for Orthodontics? ☐ No (Skip 41-42) ☐ Yes (Complete 41-42) | **41. Date Appliance Placed (MM/DD/CCYY)**

42. Months of Treatment | **43. Replacement of Prosthesis** ☐ No ☐ Yes (Complete 44) | **44. Date of Prior Placement (MM/DD/CCYY)**

45. Treatment Resulting from ☐ Occupational illness/injury ☐ Auto accident ☐ Other accident

46. Date of Accident (MM/DD/CCYY) | **47. Auto Accident State**

TREATING DENTIST AND TREATMENT LOCATION INFORMATION

53. I hereby certify that the procedures as indicated by date are in progress (for procedures that require multiple visits) or have been completed.

X _____

Signed (Treating Dentist)   Date

54. NPI | **55. License Number**

56. Address, City, State, Zip Code | **56a. Provider Specialty Code**

57. Phone Number (   )   - | **58. Additional Provider ID**

©2019 American Dental Association

J430 (Same as ADA Dental Claim Form – J431, J432, J433, J434, J430D)

To reorder call 800.947.4746 or go online at ADAcatalog.org

FIGURE 44-28

American Dental Association universal claim form.

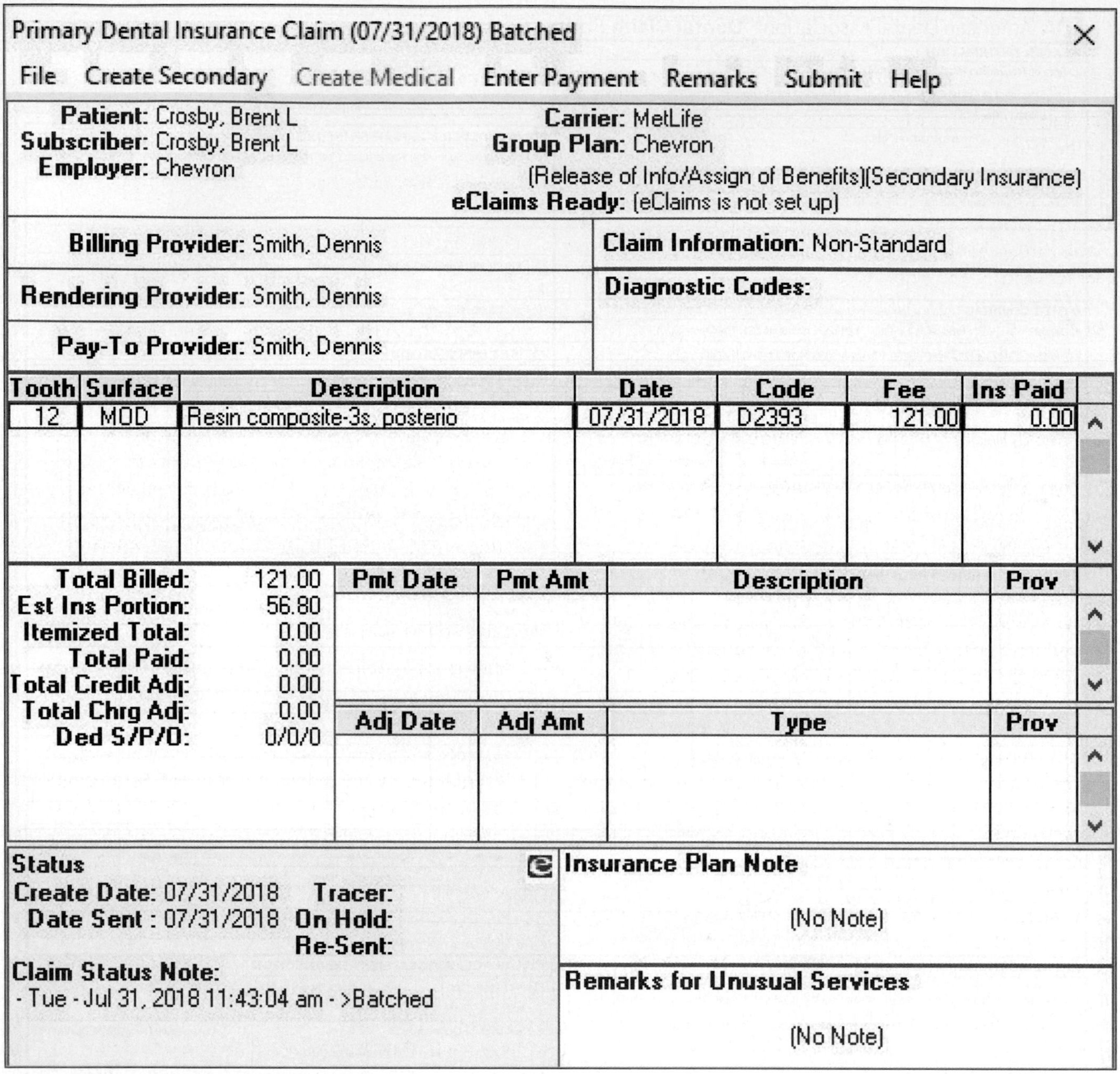

Primary Dental Insurance Claim (07/31/2018) Batched   ✕

File   Create Secondary   Create Medical   Enter Payment   Remarks   Submit   Help

Patient: Crosby, Brent L   **Carrier:** MetLife
Subscriber: Crosby, Brent L   **Group Plan:** Chevron
Employer: Chevron
(Release of Info/Assign of Benefits)(Secondary Insurance)
eClaims Ready: (eClaims is not set up)

Billing Provider: Smith, Dennis   **Claim Information:** Non-Standard

Rendering Provider: Smith, Dennis   **Diagnostic Codes:**

Pay-To Provider: Smith, Dennis

Tooth	Surface	Description	Date	Code	Fee	Ins Paid	
12	MOD	Resin composite-3s, posterio	07/31/2018	D2393	121.00	0.00	▲
							▼

		Pmt Date	Pmt Amt	Description	Prov	
Total Billed:	121.00					▲
Est Ins Portion:	56.80					
Itemized Total:	0.00					▼
Total Paid:	0.00					
Total Credit Adj:	0.00					

		Adj Date	Adj Amt	Type	Prov	
Total Chrg Adj:	0.00					▲
Ded S/P/O:	0/0/0					
						▼

Status
Create Date: 07/31/2018   **Tracer:**
Date Sent : 07/31/2018   **On Hold:**
    Re-Sent:
Claim Status Note:
- Tue - Jul 31, 2018 11:43:04 am ->Batched

Insurance Plan Note

(No Note)

Remarks for Unusual Services

(No Note)

Courtesy of Dentrix

FIGURE 44-29
American Dental Association formatted electronic claim form.

to the dental practice. In addition to saving time, monetary savings, such as envelopes and stamps, are a benefit as well. The computer software uses the information in the patient database and the information the front office assistant has entered regarding insurance coverage to generate the claim form. When submitting claims electronically, the office must abide by the regulations put forth by HIPAA. All protected health information that is transmitted must use a universal language, a standard format, and a government-assigned

identifying number, a National Provider Identifier (NPI). This is a unique 10-digit identification number issued by the Centers for Medicare and Medicaid Services. This is a HIPAA standard for anyone submitting electronic claim forms. This number does not carry any identifying information about the provider, such as the state in which they practice, and is therefore intelligence free. Claim forms in ADA format may be printed with all necessary information already completed (Figure 44-29).

Use of a Clearinghouse For a fee (minimal fee either monthly or per claim), the dental office has the option to send the claim to a clearinghouse to check for errors or missing information. In the event information is missing, the clearinghouse will send the claim back to the dental office to correct. The clearinghouse will then send the claim with all appropriate information and in the correct format to the insurance carrier.

Submitting Directly to a Carrier Submission directly to the carrier requires the use of online access, usually free of charge. Being able to submit electronically allows for a reduction in transmitting time, as it is immediate. Once the carrier receives the claim into their system, payments are released within 24 hours. This reduces the wait time for payment, which could take weeks with paper mail. Access to history of **predeterminations**, rejections, and payments for claims can be accessed by the dentist using their unique password.

Dental Claim Benefits When it comes time for the carrier to send payment for services rendered, the carrier will send a breakdown of benefits called an **explanation of benefits (EOB)**. The EOB is sent to the dentist and the patient. Sending the EOB to the patient allows for the patient to see what was paid by the carrier for the services and what is owed to the dentist, or the patient responsibility. Payment will be in the form of a paper check or electronically transferred. Payment is made to whoever benefits are assigned to, either the patient or the dentist. In order for the funds to be directly deposited into an account, the dentist needs to fill out the appropriate forms for authorization for each carrier. Electronically transferring funds can significantly cut down on the time it takes to receive payment for the rendered services. Typically it could take 23–48 hours after the carrier receives the claim.

When receiving the EOB, the administrative assistant should double check that all services were paid for correctly. In the event the patient receives the payment from the carrier accidentally, the patient can sign the check over to the dentist. This is the fastest and most efficient way to eliminate delay of payment for services your practice provided. Table 44-11 lists guidelines for successful submissions of claims.

Dental Benefit Programs

There are many plans available for patients to receive affordable dental care besides the standard dental insurance programs. These include indemnity plans, capitation, alternative benefits, and Medicaid.

Indemnity Plans

Indemnity plans pay fees for services either to the patient or the dentist (when benefits are assigned directly to the dentist). They are most often referred to as plans. This means reimbursement is based on each treatment rendered. The following are different types of indemnity plans, or fee-for-service plans:

- Preferred provider organization (PPO)
- Exclusive provider organization (EPO)
- Point-of-service plan (POS)
- Reasonable and customary plans (R&C)
- Usual, customary, and reasonable plans (UCR)

Table 44-12 highlights the different plan descriptions.

Capitation

Capitation is when a practice will receive a scheduled payment for providing services to patients who either choose or are assigned to the practice. A dental health maintenance organization (DHMO) is an example of a capitation program. A DHMO is a set group of dentists who provide broad and affordable care at a low monthly premium. The payment is usually on a monthly basis but can be quarterly too. This is a fixed payment, and the dentist receives this payment even if services were not rendered. The patient can only receive care from the assigned dentist but may be referred out for qualified services when needed. Generally, the patient has no out-of-pocket costs; however, for larger procedures a copayment may apply.

Alternative Benefits

An alternative benefit plan may be an option when traditional dental coverage is not included in a benefit package. Alternative plans can include the following:

- **Flexible spending accounts (FSA).** This is an account that is regulated by the federal government. Some employers may offer this type of medical savings account that can be used on out-of-pocket medical and dental expenses. This can include copays or noncovered services. Generally, money is placed into the account throughout the year by the employee, employer, or both. Money from an FSA must be used in that year; however, some employers may offer a grace period of 60 days. Any unused money is forfeited at the end of the determined time. An FSA saves the patient money in the long run because the money is pretaxed. When spending money from the FSA account, the patient will retain a receipt from the dentist and submit it to their employer for reimbursement. For the most part, FSA covers expenses accrued for preventative and necessary treatment, not cosmetic or whitening procedures.

- **Dental savings plan.** This is a plan that the patient signs up for to receive a reduced fee from the participating dentist. There are no claim forms to be sent, just a discount off the regular office fees.

- **Group discount.** Larger corporations may decide to join in a contract with a dental practice to provide services to employees at a discounted rate. The employee pays a monthly fee to be offered the discount. Generally these plans have no limitations or exclusions, just a discounted fee for service.

- **Voluntary plans.** This plan is similar to the employer sponsored plan, but the employee pays the full lower rate premium. There is no cost to the employer, as the plan is voluntary to the patient.

Procedure 44-8
Filing Insurance Claims

The front office assistant prepares, completes, and sends insurance claims for patients at the end of each appointment or at the completion of their treatment.

Equipment and Supplies
- access to a computer
- access to the Internet
- completed insurance claim forms

Procedure Steps

1. If you have made errors in charges, or failed to update patient and insurance information, update the information before sending insurance claims. Errors on claims delay payments. Some software offers a validation report to prevent errors and possible payment delays.

2. Create insurance claims according to your software instructions. Commonly, this is done through the patient ledger and is done daily.

3. Before sending them electronically, they are batched into a group so that they all go together at the end of the day.

4. Send the claims electronically from the batch processor. Follow the specific directions for the software being used. You do not have to send each claim to each insurance company individually. The computer software allows you to send them as a group.

5. Confirmation that the claim was sent is automatically added to the patient ledger. If the claim was not sent, "No" will appear under the Ins column on the ledger

6. If, at a later date, you want to print the claim, you can do so by selecting it from the ledger and clicking "Print."

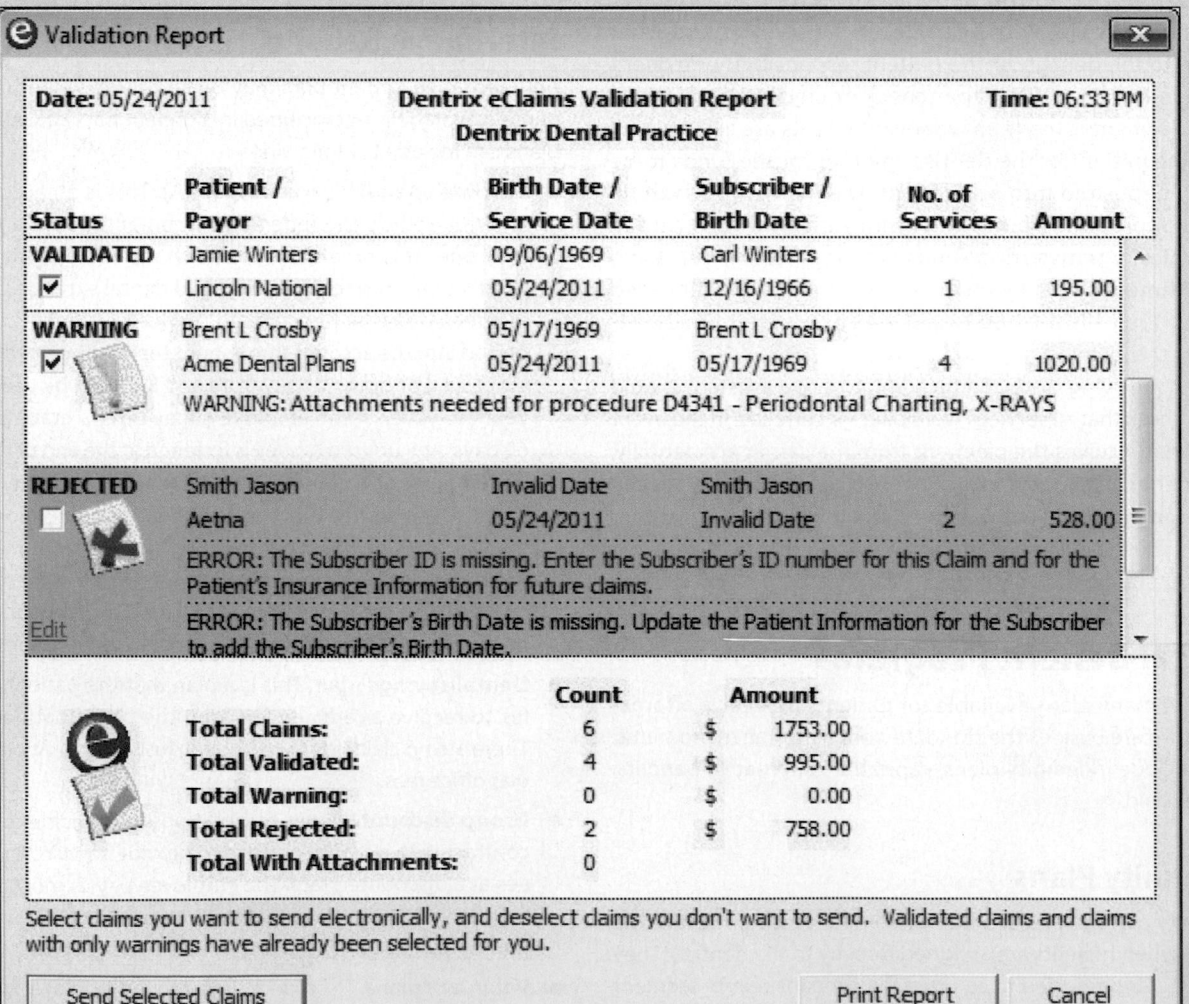

Sample validation report.

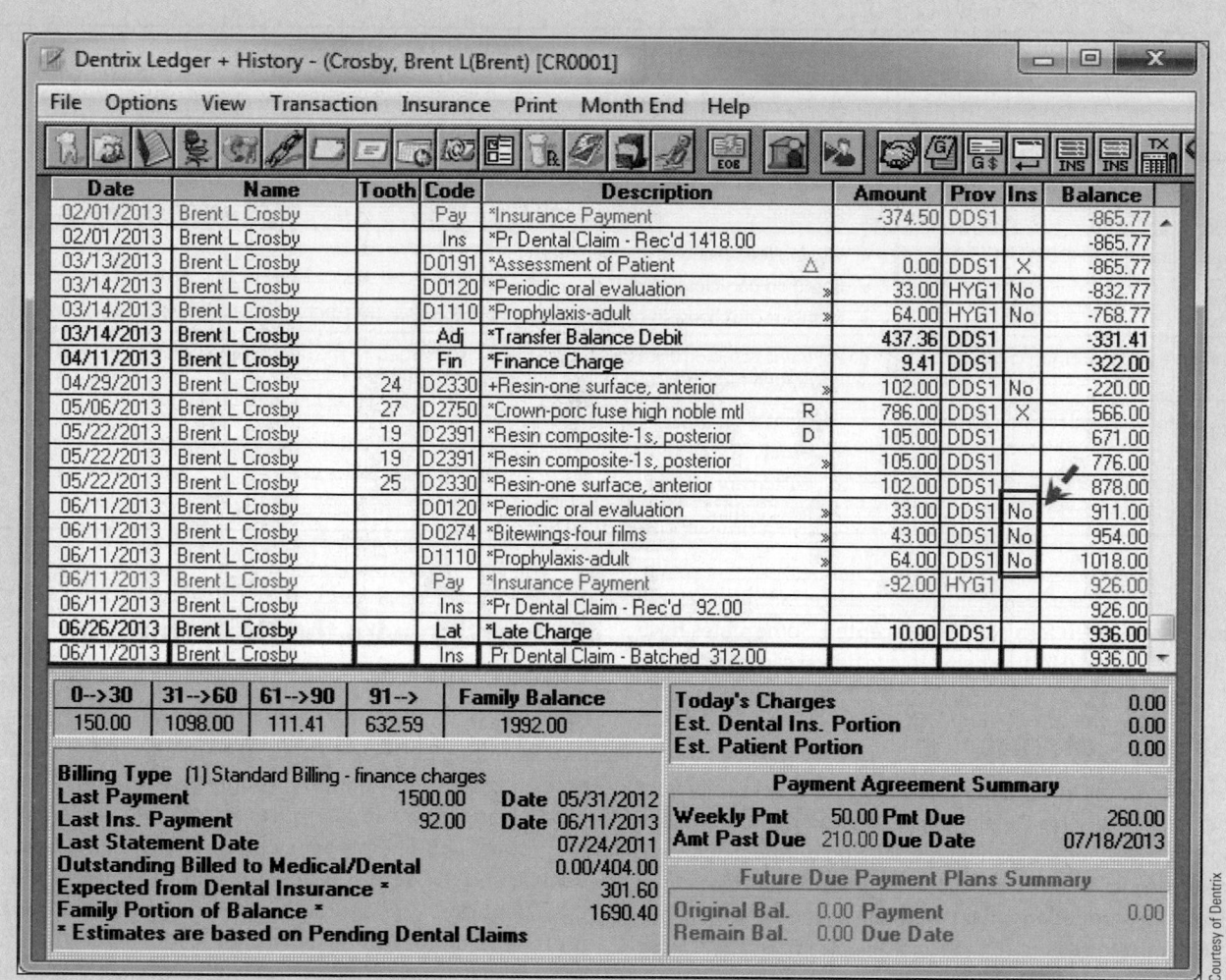

Date	Name	Tooth	Code	Description	Amount	Prov	Ins	Balance
02/01/2013	Brent L Crosby		Pay	*Insurance Payment	-374.50	DDS1		-865.77
02/01/2013	Brent L Crosby		Ins	*Pr Dental Claim - Rec'd 1418.00				-865.77
03/13/2013	Brent L Crosby		D0191	*Assessment of Patient	0.00	DDS1	X	-865.77
03/14/2013	Brent L Crosby		D0120	*Periodic oral evaluation	33.00	HYG1	No	-832.77
03/14/2013	Brent L Crosby		D1110	*Prophylaxis-adult	64.00	HYG1	No	-768.77
03/14/2013	Brent L Crosby		Adj	*Transfer Balance Debit	437.36	DDS1		-331.41
04/11/2013	Brent L Crosby		Fin	*Finance Charge	9.41	DDS1		-322.00
04/29/2013	Brent L Crosby	24	D2330	+Resin-one surface, anterior	102.00	DDS1	No	-220.00
05/06/2013	Brent L Crosby	27	D2750	*Crown-porc fuse high noble mtl	786.00	DDS1	X	566.00
05/22/2013	Brent L Crosby	19	D2391	*Resin composite-1s, posterior	105.00	DDS1		671.00
05/22/2013	Brent L Crosby	19	D2391	*Resin composite-1s, posterior	105.00	DDS1		776.00
05/22/2013	Brent L Crosby	25	D2330	*Resin-one surface, anterior	102.00	DDS1		878.00
06/11/2013	Brent L Crosby		D0120	*Periodic oral evaluation	33.00	DDS1	No	911.00
06/11/2013	Brent L Crosby		D0274	*Bitewings-four films	43.00	DDS1	No	954.00
06/11/2013	Brent L Crosby		D1110	*Prophylaxis-adult	64.00	DDS1	No	1018.00
06/11/2013	Brent L Crosby		Pay	*Insurance Payment	-92.00	HYG1		926.00
06/11/2013	Brent L Crosby		Ins	*Pr Dental Claim - Rec'd 92.00				926.00
06/26/2013	Brent L Crosby		Lat	*Late Charge	10.00	DDS1		936.00
06/11/2013	Brent L Crosby		Ins	Pr Dental Claim - Batched 312.00				936.00

0-->30	31-->60	61-->90	91-->	Family Balance
150.00	1098.00	111.41	632.59	1992.00

Today's Charges 0.00
Est. Dental Ins. Portion 0.00
Est. Patient Portion 0.00

Billing Type [1] Standard Billing - finance charges
Last Payment 1500.00 Date 05/31/2012
Last Ins. Payment 92.00 Date 06/11/2013
Last Statement Date 07/24/2011
Outstanding Billed to Medical/Dental 0.00/404.00
Expected from Dental Insurance * 301.60
Family Portion of Balance * 1690.40
* Estimates are based on Pending Dental Claims

Payment Agreement Summary
Weekly Pmt 50.00 Pmt Due 260.00
Amt Past Due 210.00 Due Date 07/18/2013

Future Due Payment Plans Summary
Original Bal. 0.00 Payment 0.00
Remain Bal. 0.00 Due Date

Courtesy of Dentrix

TABLE 44-11 Guidelines for Successful Submission of Claims

1.	Take note of any special information needed by a carrier.
2.	At each appointment, ask the patient if there has been any change in their insurance benefits.
3.	Establish a routine for gathering and submitting claims, for example, reviewing claims at the time of service and sending all claims for that day at the end of a business day.
4.	Make sure there is an adequate supply of forms needed if filing through mail.
5.	Always keep an updated CDT manual in the office for reference.
6.	Establish a filing system for outstanding claims for each month. Periodically search for unpaid claims. For example, at the first of each month, review the unpaid claims from the previous month. This allows you to call the carrier to check for an update and reconcile in a timely manner.

Medicaid

Medicaid is a federal assisted health care plan that is offered to lower income individuals and that started as Title XIX under the Social Security Act of 1965. Medicaid is offered to and provides payment to certain low-income individuals and families and those who have a need, such as the disabled, children, blind, and aged. Benefits vary from state to state. Individuals 21 years of age and younger have mandated dental coverage by federal law; however, adult coverage is limited depending on the state. Reimbursement is only paid to dentists who participate with Medicaid. When a dentist participates with Medicaid, they agree to charge only the contracted amount and do not bill a balance to the patient. In the event the patient has other coverages, that third party payer is considered primary. Generally speaking, forms must be typed or electronically submitted within 12 months from the date of

TABLE 44-12 Fee-for-Service Plans

Preferred provider organization (PPO)	• Payments based on a discounted fee schedule • Participating providers agree to fees • Do not balance: bill the patient for the difference
Exclusive provider organization (EPO)	• Benefits only payable to a participating provider • No benefits to out-of-network providers • Emergency coverage may be available
Point-of-service plan (POS)	• Varying fee schedules and benefits • Based on participation of the dentist • Members can choose in-network or out-of-network care, the latter resulting in a higher copay to the patient
Reasonable and customary plans (R&C)	• Payment based on a reasonable fee (fee most charged by the dentist) and customary fee (fee most charged for a service in a geographical area)

Usual, customary, and reasonable plans (UCR)	• Payment is based on a combination of fees:
	  o Usual
	  o Customary
	  o Reasonable

service. Handwritten forms are not accepted. Some states have Healthy Kids Dental (HKD) to help provide dental care to minors.

Staying Current

Keeping up with all the new trends in the dental office comes from attending seminars; researching on the Internet; reviewing information from numerous companies; reading dental magazines; and attending local, regional, national, and international meetings. Much of this information can be accessed via the Internet, allowing the dentist to stay up to date on available information. However, it is also helpful to go to booths at meetings and conferences where vendors allow dental team members to learn by using the instruments, seeing and hearing about equipment, and so forth.

Teledentistry

Teledentistry is a service that has been vastly growing in the past few years, especially since the development of the pandemic surrounding the COVID-19 virus. Teledentistry refers to a collection of services using a variety of technology to offer care to the patient. Third-party payers typically provide coverage for services using a virtual method. Teledentistry can be either synchronous or asynchronous.

Synchronous teledentistry uses a live interaction between the dentist and the patient. **Asynchronous** teledentistry uses a prerecorded message that is transmitted to the dentist through secure electronic means. The dentist will then use this information to evaluate the patient's needs.

All services provided through teledentistry are expected to be given with the same care that the patient would receive if they were present in the office. The site the dentist uses must be secure, and all laws and licensed scopes of practice must be followed. All services and information must be properly documented into the patient's chart.

Connecting with the Office through Mobile Devices

Dentists can now stay current with their practices by utilizing mobile dental software. This software allows the dentist to access practice information through smartphone technology via an application (or "app" for short). If a patient has an after-hours dental emergency, the patient is able to call the dentist, and the dentist is able to review the patient file over the telephone. The dentist can see if the patient has been prescribed medications, when medications and treatments were provided, and quickly scan for an available emergency appointment. The dentist can also review financial records and stay up to date on how the practice is doing.

Web Conferencing

In a busy office, taking time to attend a conference is difficult. Many practices are seeking webinars (Web-based seminars) for training and information. Offices can view a seminar, lecture, workshop, or presentation that is broadcast over the Web to the dental team members watching online. Some of the workshops are interactive and allow the participants to respond to the speaker. Brainstorming sessions can also be done through interactive webinars.

Distance Learning

Online education for health care professionals is an easy, convenient, and cost-effective way to learn. Many courses are accepted for all or part of continuing education requirements. Colleges, universities, private companies, DANB, ADA, and ADAA all have a wide variety of courses available. These courses can be taken using a computer from any location and at any time that is convenient for the dental assistant.

Chapter Summary

The dental reception area must be an environment in which all patients feel welcome and comfortable. Today, dentistry can be a positive experience, and dental treatment can be pain free. This positive image is developed when the patient first steps into the reception area. Patients may not consciously realize the message that is being received, but the dental office should present an atmosphere that relieves anxiety.

Front office staff has changed dramatically in recent years. All individuals in the front office require knowledge of business machines such as computers, fax machines, and copy machines. These individuals must be organized, have knowledge of dental treatments, and have good communication and problem-solving skills. Today most practices have moved toward a paperless system, which helps to organize and make the practice more efficient.

A dental office is a business as well as a health care facility. Dental assistants, along with all members of the dental team, need to be involved in the everyday office relations of the practice, for both the clinical side and business side.

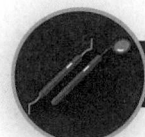

CASE STUDY

Martha Johnson is a new graduate of an accredited dental assisting program and has received her dental assisting national certification. She will be the administrative assistant in the office of Dr. Ward. Dr. Ward's practice is currently paperless and uses dental software for records and financial management.

Case Study Review

1. When submitting the dental claim, what are some important factors to help the claim be processed quickly?

2. What types of storage are available for the dental software?

3. A patient comes in for treatment and states that their insurance will not be active until the next day. They ask you to date the treatment for tomorrow. As an administrative assistant, how do you respond?

Review Questions

Multiple Choice

1. Which is true of the full block letter format?
   a. It is the least common style.
   b. There is a double space between paragraphs.
   c. Each paragraph is indented.
   d. The closing is to the right of the page.

2. Some common ways for marketing include all of the following EXCEPT:
   a. a website.
   b. social media.
   c. email.
   d. door to door.

3. In what year was the Americans with Disabilities Act passed by Congress?
   a. 1980
   b. 1990
   c. 2000
   d. 2005

4. The front office staff is an important part of the team and is responsible for the flow of the office. There is always an administrative assistant and an office manager who work together.
   a. Both statements are true.
   b. Both statements are false.
   c. The first statement is true; the second statement is false.
   d. The first statement is false; the second statement is true.

5. When a patient calls the office:
   a. speak loudly so the person can hear you.
   b. do not ask the patient's name for privacy reasons.
   c. multitask with other office duties.
   d. address the person properly.

6. If the patient calls and asks to speak to the dentist:
   a. first ask the patient if they want an appointment.
   b. ask them to hold while you see if the dentist is available.
   c. identify first what the reason for the call is.
   d. tell the patient the dentist does not take calls.

7. When presenting the patient the care plan:
   a. avoid having the patient ask questions.
   b. spend as little time as possible as the day is busy.
   c. allow the patient to choose the plan that best suits their needs.
   d. present only the best possible plan.
8. Appointment books are normally set up in _____ minute units.
   a. 10
   b. 15
   c. 60
   d. Both a and b
9. Which type of recare system is filed according to the month the patient is to be recalled?
   a. color-tagged card file
   b. computer generated
   c. chronological
   d. None of these
10. Which of these is a computerized worksheet that allows for programmed calculations?
    a. word processing
    b. graphics
    c. spreadsheet
    d. dental software
11. Eye professionals advise that for every 20 minutes of computer use, the user should relax the eyes by looking at a distant spot for how long?
    a. 10 minutes
    b. 10 seconds
    c. 20 minutes
    d. 20 seconds
12. An example of an expendable supply is:
    a. gauze.
    b. saliva ejector.
    c. dental instrument.
    d. Both a and b
13. Electronic inventory management systems offer automated replenishment. The use of a scanner is what allows the product to be ordered once it is removed from the inventory for use.
    a. Both statements are true.
    b. Both statements are false.
    c. The first statement is true; the second statement is false.
    d. The first statement is false; the second statement is true.

14. When storing patient files, the following are common cabinets used EXCEPT:
    a. vertical.
    b. open-shelf lateral.
    c. movable.
    d. stackable.
15. A check guaranteed by the bank is called a:
    a. certified check.
    b. cashier's check.
    c. voucher check.
    d. money order.
16. An example of a fixed cost is:
    a. the cost of supplies.
    b. the cost of treating dental patients.
    c. salaries.
    d. the cost of dental materials.
17. The insurance birthday rule pertains to the:
    a. primary carrier.
    b. dependent child of two parents who have dental coverage.
    c. stepchildren who have dental coverage.
    d. secondary carrier.
18. Assume that a patient had dental work totaling $60, and is eligible for benefits under two insurance carriers that have a benefit-less-benefit provision. One carrier allows $400 for this service, and the other allows $450. The second carrier would pay $450, and the other would pay:
    a. $0.
    b. $100.
    c. $450.
    d. $50.
19. A set group of dentists who provide broad and affordable care at a low monthly premium is an example of:
    a. capitation.
    b. fee for service.
    c. indemnity plans.
    d. Medicaid.
20. Live interaction between the dentist and the patient is considered:
    a. synchronous.
    b. asynchronous.
    c. recorded.
    d. hybrid.

Key Terms

Term and Pronunciation	Meaning of Root and Word Parts	Definition
administrative assistant (ad-**min**-uh-strey-tiv) (uh-**sis**-tuh nt)	**administrate** = to manage the affairs of the business **-ive** = expressing function **assist** = to give support or help **-ant** = serving in the capacity of	office employer responsible for managing the office including patient records, financial records, and appointment scheduling
allowances (uh-**lou**-uh ns)	**allow** = to give permission to or for; permit **-ance** = indicating an action, state	a sum of money allotted or granted for a particular purpose, as for expenses

Term and Pronunciation	Meaning of Root and Word Parts	Definition
answering service (**an**-ser-ing) (**sur**-vis)	**answer** = a spoken or written reply or response to a question, request **-ing** = the action of **service** = an act of helpful activity	a business that receives and answers telephone calls for its clients
appointment book (*uh*-**point**-m*uh* nt) (boo k)	**appoint** = to arrange the time of a meeting **-ment** = denoting an action or resulting state **book** = written work usually on sheets or paper fastened or bound together within covers	a book containing a calendar and space to keep a record of appointments
asynchronous (ey-**sing**-kr*uh*-n*uh*s)	**a** = another **synchronous** = to occur at the same time	communication that is prerecorded and not occurring at the same time
backorder (**bak**-awr-der)	**back** = overdue, behind **order** = to request	a retailer's order for a product that is temporarily out of stock with the supplier
buffer time (**buhf**-er) (tahym)	**buffer** = to cushion, protect **time** = limited period or interval between two successive events	an established block of time slot(s) on appointment when dentist is unavailable to patient visits; catch-up
call list (kawl) (list)	**call** = to ask or invite to come **list** = a series of names/items written together in a meaningful grouping	a list of patients who are able to come into the dental office to fill an appointment slot at short notice
capitation (kap-i-**tey**-sh*uh* n)	**capitation** = a fee or payment of a uniform amount for each person	scheduled payment for providing services to patients who either choose or are assigned to the practice
care plan (kair) (plan)	**care** = conscientious treatment for someone or something **plan** = a method of proceeding	an agreement between the patient and health professional to help the patient manage their health
certificate of eligibility (ser-**tif**-i-kit) (**el**-i-j*uh*- **bil**-i-tee)	**certify** = confirm; to attest as certain **-ate** = denoting a function **eligible** = worthy of choice; legally qualified **-ity** = expressing state or condition	an official identification care or similar document issue to program beneficiaries as evidence of entitlement to services
claim (kleym)	**claim** = demand as a right or as due	amount due for services submitted to the insurer or patient
claimant (**kley**-muh nt)	**claim** = demand as a right or as due **-ant** = characterized by or serving in the capacity of	a person who makes a claim
cloud-based (kloud) (beyst)	**cloud** = any mass that is similar **based** = to form a foundation	information stored on a remote server
copayment (koh-**pey**-m*uh* nt) (**pey**-m*uh* nt)	**co-** = jointly, indicating partnership or equality **pay** = to settle a debt; to give compensation **-ment** = denoting an action or resulting state	a contributory payment by an employer, usually matching that of an employee
collection agency (k*uh*-**lek**-sh*uh* n) (**ey**-j*uh* n-see)	**collect** = to receive payment **-ion** = denoting action **agency** = an organization or company that provides some service for another	a business that specialized in debt collections; pursues payments of debts owed; also known as debt collector
coordination of benefits (koh-awr-dn-**ey**-sh*uh* n) (**ben**-*uh*-fit)	**coordinate** = to combine in harmonious relation or action **-ation** = indicating an action, process **benefit** = a payment made by employer or insurance company to help someone	process of determining which of two or more insurance policies will have the primary responsibility of processing and paying a claim
current dental terminology (**kur**-*uh* nt) (**den**-tl) (tur-m*uh*-**nol**-*uh*-jee)	**current** = prevalent, customary, most recent **dent** = teeth **-al** = relating to **term** = a word or group of words designating something, especially in a particular field **-logy** = bodies of knowledge	a code set with descriptive terms developed and updated by the American Dental Association; reports dental services and procedures to dental benefits plans

(Continues)

Term and Pronunciation	Meaning of Root and Word Parts	Definition
deductible, family (dih-**duhk**-t*uh*-b*uh* l) (**fam**-*uh*-lee)	**deduct** = to take away from a sum **-ible** = given to **family** = basic social unit consisting of parents and their children	the amount for which the entire family covered by the insurer is liable on each loss, injury, or treatment before an insurance company will make payment
deductible, individual (dih-**duhk**-t*uh*-b*uh* l) (in-d*uh*-**vij**-oo-*uh* l)	**deduct** = to take away, as from a sum or amount **-ible** = capable of **individual** = a single human being	the amount for which the insured is liable on each loss, injury, or treatment before an insurance company will make payment
dental insurance (**den**-tl) (in-**shoo r**-*uh* ns)	**dent-** = teeth **-al** = relating to **insure** = to guarantee or protect against risk, loss, or damage **-ance** = indicating an action, state, or condition	designed to pay a portion of the costs associated with dental care
dental practice management (**den**-tl) (**prak**-tis) (**man**-ij-m*uh* nt)	**dent** = tooth or teeth **-al** = pertaining to **practice** = the business of a professional person **manage** = to take charge, or care of **-ment** = denoting an action	the business principles utilized the formation, operation, or management of a dental office
effective date (ih-**fek**-tiv) (deyt)	**effect** = something that is produced by an agency of cause **-ive** = expressing tendency, disposition **date** = a particular month, day, and year at which some event happened or will happen	a date on which a transaction is recorded or when an agreement takes effect
exclusions (ik-**skloo**-zh*uh* n)	**exclude** = to shut out from consideration; privilege **-ion** = denoting action or condition	the act or an instance of denying specific dental treatment to be covered in dental insurance plan
explanation of benefits (EOB) (ek-spl*uh*-**ney**-sh*uh* n) (**ben**-*uh*-fit)	**explain** = to make known in detail **-ion** = denoting action or condition **benefit** = something that is advantageous or good; an advantage	a notice from the insurance company which is sent explaining the coverage of the services received
extension of benefits (ik-**sten**-sh*uh* n) (**ben**-*uh*-fit)	**extend** = to stretch out; draw out to full length **-ion** = denoting action or condition **benefit** = something that is advantageous or good; an advantage	a group policy clause that allows employees not currently working to extend coverage past the expiration date of the policy; only lasts until the employee returns to work
full block format (*foo* l-blok) (**fawr**-mat)	**full** = complete **block** = kept in shape **format** = the general physical appearance of written or typed information	business letter with all information justified against the left margin
integration (in-ti-**grey**-sh*uh*n)	**integrate** = to bring together **ion** = a suffix	combining
interpreter (in-**tur**-pri-ter)	**interpret** = to understand something **er** = names of occupations	a person who translates languages
inventory management (**in**-v*uh* n-tawr-ee) (**man**-ij-m*uh* nt)	**inventory** = a complete listing of merchandise or stock on hand **manage** = to take charge or care of **-ment** = denoting an action or resulting state	the overseeing and control of the ordering, storage, and use of merchandise
marketing, external (**mahr**-ki-ting) (ik-**stur**-nl)	**market** = place that sells goods **ing** = denoting action **extern** = a person connected with an institution but not a resident **al** = suffix meaning pertaining to	advertising and promoting services outside the practice
marketing, internal (**mahr**-ki-ting) (in-**tur**-nl)	**market** = place that sells goods **ing** = denoting action **intern** = a person who works as a resident of the institution **al** = suffix meaning pertaining to	advertising and promoting services within the practice

Term and Pronunciation	Meaning of Root and Word Parts	Definition
matrix (**mey**-triks)	**matrix** = something that constitutes the place or point from which something else originates, take form, or develops	appointment matrix, also referred to as outlining, blocks off times the doctor is unavailable
maximum benefit (**mak**-suh-muh m) (**ben**-uh-fit)	**maximum** = the greatest quantity or amount possible **benefit** = something that is advantageous or good; an advantage	the maximum amount a health plan will pay in benefits to an insured individual during that individual's lifetime
patient portal (**pey**-shuhnt) (**pawr**-tl)	**pati** = to undergo **-ent** = suffix for a noun **portale** = of a gate	an online service for patients that is secure
phone message system (fohn) (**mes**-ij) (**sis**-tuh m)	**phone** = an instrument of sound transmission; telephone **message** = a communication containing information sent by telephone, email, etc. **system** = an assemblage or combination of things or parts forming a complex or unitary whole	a computer-based system that allows users and subscribers to exchange personal voice messages; to select and deliver voice information; and to process transactions relating to individuals, products, and services using an ordinary telephone
predeterminations (pre- dih-tur-muh-**ney**-shuh n)	**pre-** = before; in advance of **determine** = to settle or decide by an authoritative decision **-ation** = indicating an action, process	a review by medical staff to determine if the service being requested is appropriate for the patient's medical needs
primary carrier (**prahy**-mer-ee) (**kar**-ee-er)	**primary** = first or highest in rank or importance **carry** = to manage, conduct **-er** = names of occupations	insurance company of which the patient is a member; the insured
proprietary (pruh·**prai**·uh·teh·ree)	**proprietor** = having ownership -ry = indicates a place or a business	having ownership
provider, nonparticipating (pruh-**vahy**-der) (non-pahr-**tis**-uh-pey-ting)	**provide** = to make available **-er** = designating persons of their occupation **non-** = bit **participate** = to take or have a part as with others **-ing** = expressing action	doctor is not authorized to participate in Medicare; not yet contracted with a health plan
provider, participating (pruh-**vahy**-der) (pahr-**tis**-uh-pey-ting)	**provide** = to make available **-er** = designating persons of their occupation **participate** = to take or have a part as with others **-ing** = expressing action	doctor agrees to accept assignment for all services furnished to Medicare patients
quantity purchase rate (**kwon**-ti-tee) (**pur**-chuh s) (reyt)	**quantity** = a particular or indefinite amount of anything **purchase** = to acquire by the payment of money **rate** = the amount of a charge or payment with reference to some basis of calculation	often offered by sellers to entice buyers to purchase in larger quantities
scalability (skei·luh·**bi**·luh·tee)	**scale** = to adjust in amount **ability** = skill to do something	the ability to change in size
secondary carrier (**sek**-uh n-der-ee) (**kar**-ee-er)	**second** = next after the first **-ary** = pertaining to **carry** = to manage, conduct **-er** = names of occupations	dependent is under someone else's health insurance plan; provide reimbursement of dental expenses after exhaustion of coverage available through the primary plan
semiblock format (**sem**-ahy-blok) (**fawr**-mat)	**semi** = partially, somewhat **block** = kept in shape **format** = the general physical appearance of written or typed information	all text is left aligned, paragraphs are indented, and paragraphs are separated by double or triple spacing
server-based (**sur**-ver) (beysd)	**serve** = to be of service **er** = suffix to form a noun or verb **base** = to form a foundation **ed** = suffix for past tense	information stored on a local server

(Continues)

Term and Pronunciation	Meaning of Root and Word Parts	Definition
shelf life (shelf) (lahyf)	**shelf** = plank fixed horizontally to hold objects **life** = the period of activity or effectiveness of something inanimate	the length of time for which an item remains usable and fit for consumption
software (**sawft**-wair)	software = the programs used to direct the operation of a computer	a program that is used to direct the computer in a task
subscriber (suh b-**skrahy**-ber)	**subscribe** = to give approval to the contents of a document by signing one's name **-er** = designating person of special circumstances	a person or organization who pays the premiums, or a person whose employment makes him or her eligible for membership in the insurance plan
supplies, consumable (suh-**plahyz**) (kuh n-**soo**-muh-buh l)	**supply** = to furnish or provide with what is lacking or requisite **consume** = to destroy or expend by use; use up **-able** = capable of	products that consumers use recurrently; items which get used up
supplies, disposable (suh-**plahyz**) (dih-**spoh**-zuh-buh l)	**supply** = to furnish or provide with what is lacking or requisite **dispose** = to get rid of; discard **-able** = capable of	products designed for or capable of being thrown away or used up
supplies, expendable (suh-**plahyz**) (ik-**spen**-duh-buh l)	**supply** = to furnish or provide with what is lacking or requisite **expend** = to use up **-able** = capable of	products that are consumed in use
supplies, nonexpendable (suh-**plahyz**) (**nawn**- ik-**spen**-duh-buh l)	**supply** = to furnish or provide with what is lacking or requisite **non-** = not **expend** = to use up **-able** = capable of	products are not consumed in use that retain their original identity during the period of use
synchronous (sing-kruh-nuhs)	**syn** = together **chron** = time **os** = mouth, opening of the body	communication occurring live, at the same time
telecommunication (tel-i-kuh-myoo-ni-**key**-shuh n)	**tele** = transmission over a distance **communicate** = to give or interchange thoughts or information **-ion** = denoting action or condition	transmission of information in the form of electromagnetic signals by technology
teledentistry (**tel**-ee) (**den**-tuh-stree)	**tele** = at a distance **dent** = tooth **ist** = a person who practices something **ery** = a suffix that signifies occupation	the use of technology to virtually provide services
time block (tahym) (blok)	**time** = a particular part of the year or day **block** = to obstruct something	blocking out time of the day for use other than procedures
Truth in Lending Act (trooth) (lend-iNG) (akt)	**true** = conformity with fact or reality **lend** = to contribute to **ing** = a verbal action **act** = to do something	U.S. federal law that is designed to protect consumers in any credit transaction
unit of time (**yoo**-nit) (tahym)	**unit** = any specified amount of a quantity, by comparison with which any other quantity of the same kind is measured or estimated **time** = limited period or interval between two successive events	scheduling of patients is based on how long the patient will be in the chair; units may be in 10, 15, and 30 minutes intervals of time
usual, customary, and reasonable fee (yoo-zhoo-el) (**kuhs**-tuh-mer-ee) (**ree**-zuh-nuh-buh l) (fee)	**usual** = habitual or customary **custom** = the usual way of acting in given circumstances **-ary** = pertaining to **reason** = to form conclusions, judgments, or inferences from facts or premises **-able** = tending to **fee** = a charge or payment for professional services	amount paid for a service depending on the geographic location where those services are rendered
welcome letter (**wel**-kuh m) (let-er)	**welcome** = a word of kindly greeting, as to one whose arrival gives pleasure **letter** = a written or printed communication	a letter sent to new patients containing a welcome message

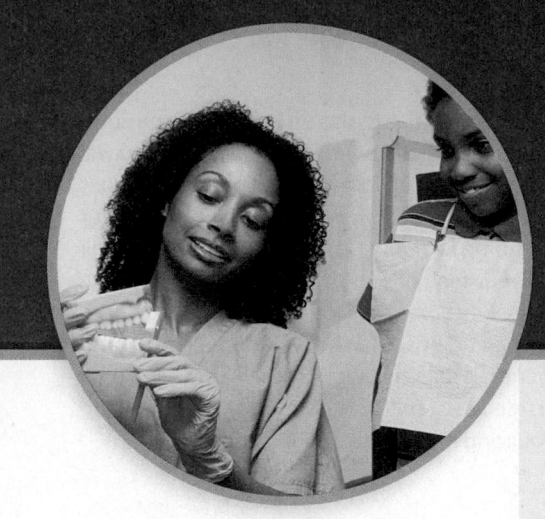

## CHAPTER 45

Career Planning

Specific Instructional Objectives

At the completion of this chapter, you will be able to meet these objectives:

1. Use terms presented in this chapter.
2. Research the state credentialing requirements.
3. Develop personal career objective.
4. Create personal career portfolio.
5. Compose master electronic cover letter and resume.
6. Request references for letter of recommendations.
7. List ways a job seeker can begin a job search.
8. Discuss arranging for an interview.
9. Complete job application accurately and thoroughly.
10. Prepare for preinterview.
11. Describe how to interview for dental assisting position.
12. Describe the goal of job orientation of a new employee.
13. Explain what the employee can do to keep their job.
14. Explain how to handle being placed on performance or professional probation and being fired.
15. Develop plan for career and job advancement.
16. Defend the need for professional development and continuing education.

Introduction

As the required formal training necessary to become a dental assistant nears completion, you can switch your goals toward becoming an employed dental assistant. The first step in this process is obtaining national certification and state registration or licensure. A dental assistant is eligible to take the dental assisting examination and can obtain national certification by the Dental Assisting National Board (DANB) through three pathways. (See box "DANB Certification Pathways.") Then, your employment search begins.

DANB Certification Pathways

Pathway I

- Graduation (or anticipated graduation) from a Commission on Dental Accreditation (CODA) accredited dental assisting or dental hygiene program, or current registered dental hygienist (RDH).
- Current cardiopulmonary resuscitation (CPR), basic life support (BLS), or advanced cardiac life support (ACLS)

Pathway II

- Minimum of 3,500 hours work experience as a dental assistant, accrued over a period of at least two years to a maximum of four years; employment must be verified by a licensed dentist

- High school graduation or equivalent
- Current cardiopulmonary resuscitation (CPR), basic life support (BLS), or advanced cardiac life support (ACLS)

Pathway III

- Former DANB CDA certificant or graduation from a D.D.S. or D.M.D. program
- Current cardiopulmonary resuscitation (CPR), basic life support (BLS), or advanced cardiac life support (ACLS)

Reprinted with permission of the Dental Assisting National Board, Inc., (DANB).

Know Your State Requirements

It is important to be aware of the state requirements in the state in which you are seeking employment. Many states have requirements, job titles, and specific allowable functions for various levels of dental assisting. Many states have some type of registration that allows dental assistants to take radiographs after some education and skill proficiency are met. This may be part of the dental assisting program. Some states have a variety of requirements for various levels of dental assisting skills. There may be an entry-level *registration*, where the dental assistant fills out a form, pays a fee, and receives a registration card. There is no examination, but the registration requires the dental assistant to know and follow the laws and rule changes of the state. In other states the registration is for dental assistants who have successfully completed a dental assisting program and have met certain criteria to perform dental assisting skills. States may also require a *license* (or registration; terms vary with each state) in order for dental assistants to perform certain expanded functions or duties. Licensed dental assistants must pass a written exam and, in some states, a clinical exam on specific skills. The DANB provides written examinations that states can use for the different levels of dental assisting skills. Go to the DANB website to find information on your state's requirements.

When conducting the search for suitable employment, it is necessary to be well prepared and goal oriented. Being knowledgeable about how to write a cover letter and prepare a resume is important. Effective cover letters and resumes lead to job interviews. Understanding the interview process and possessing the skills necessary to interview successfully lead to job offers.

A Job Search Plan

Looking for a job is a job in itself. You will find your first dental assisting job by having a plan. The steps in a well thought out plan involve establishing career objectives, creating a portfolio, and searching resources for the right position.

Establishing Career Objectives

A career objective is a statement that describes what position you want, what you want to do, and where you want to work. An effective objective includes a specific job title, skills you wish to employ, and an environment in which you want to work. Job skills in which dental assistants are generally trained include assisting in infection control, office administration, chairside assisting, expanded functions, and office management.

Now that you are near the end of your formal dental assisting training, you probably have a list of skills that you are proficient in and like to perform, and those that are not your favorites. In searching for a job, you can narrow your search to specific job titles and skills. This is a good place to start looking for your ideal job. However, if the search is too narrow, there may not be many jobs fulfilling your requirements, and you may need to widen the search.

There is a lot to consider in determining what work environment you like best. Do you prefer general dentistry or one of the dental specialties? Size of practice is also an important consideration. Do you like a small, medium, or large dental office? You will also need to discover if you like a loose and flexible environment or one that is tightly structured. Do you need a full-time job, or can you accept a part-time job? A well thought out objective will give you direction in your search.

Following is a specific career objective: "I am seeking a full-time position as a chairside assistant in a fast-paced general practice." A more general objective would read: "I am seeking a position as a chairside assistant." Too general would be: "I am seeking a position utilizing my dental assisting education."

Creating a Portfolio

A portfolio is an organized collection of evidence that allows you to put your best work forward. A well-developed portfolio showcases your best work and accomplishments to potential employers, sets you apart from the other applicants, and gives you an advantage over the competition. The presentation of the portfolio represents your organization and professionalism. The portfolio will help you with the following:

- Prepare for interviews
- Prove that you are a prepared and capable assistant
- Demonstrate your work through screen shots of your projects
- Communicate and keep focused during your interview
- Develop the habit of documenting and creating a database of your work

A career portfolio is one of your most important job hunting tools. It allows you to develop a complete picture of who you are: your education, experience, depth of skill development, accomplishments, and potential as a dental assistant. The portfolio increases the chance of getting the second interview if it is well written and coherent. Simple spelling, grammatical, and typographical errors can destroy the benefit of an otherwise strong career portfolio.

The type and content of your portfolio is up to you. You should keep all materials in a folder as you work on them (Figure 45-1). There are many types of portfolio binders, with the leather-bound, three-ring binder being the most popular. All originals should be kept in sheet protectors with everything neat and clean in your portfolio. You should continue to add to your portfolio as you grow professionally. Extra copies of the portfolio information should be kept inside a separate folder to leave with the dentist after the interview. You should also have all the information electronically available for quick response to a job lead.

Table of Contents The Table of Contents is a list of the parts of the portfolio organized in the order the parts appear. The contents contained in the portfolio may include:

- Table of contents
- Cover letter
- Resume

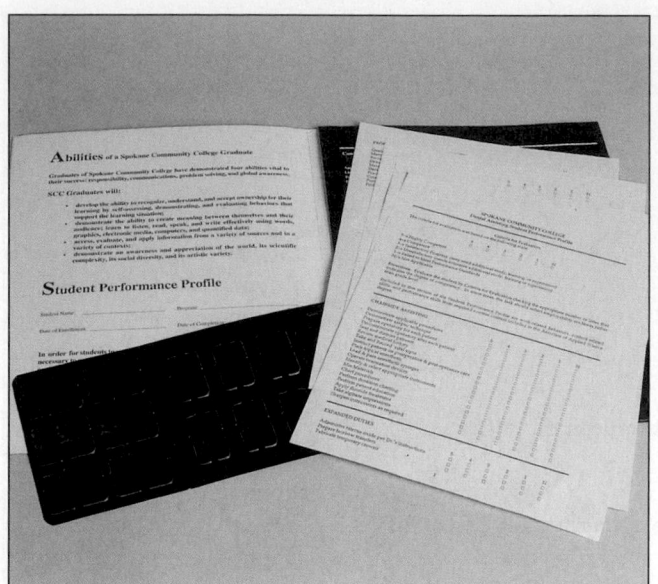

FIGURE 45-1
A personal portfolio is an effective way to share your certificates and letters of recommendation with the dental office.

- Professional requirements
- Fact sheet of skills
- Educational accomplishments
- Community participation
- Recommendations

Cover Letter A cover letter is also referred to as a letter of introduction to a prospective employer. It accompanies a resume and introduces the job seeker. If responding to an ad, you should use keywords found in the ad to customize the letter to explain your suitability for the job being advertised and why you selected this job. Include specific information about the dental office and dentist. With so much information on the Internet, this is usually easy to do.

The cover letter offers you a chance to emphasize some of your personal characteristics and skills, as well as to expand on and give examples of your accomplishments. In your cover letter, you need to show your initiative, the extra things you did above and beyond the call of duty, how you helped to improve the working environment, and your patient management skills. You can include compliments you have received from dentists and examples of situations where you made the patient feel comfortable. Assistants who are bilingual and have specific computer skills are in high demand and should highlight these skills (Figures 45-2 and 45-3).

If you address the letter to the dentist directly, it sends a positive message to the employer. It shows that you are truly interested because you took the time to write an individual letter instead of a general cover letter addressed "Dear Employer." The letter should be on quality bond paper in Times New Roman or Arial, 10–12 point font, single spaced,

with double spacing between each key component. Following are the key components of a standard cover letter expected by an employer:

Header The header highlights your personal contact information. You need to include your full name, address, telephone number, and email. You can make your name stand out by centering the header and using a bold and larger font for your name.

Recipient Information At the right margin and just below your personal information is the contact information pertaining to the recipient of your cover letter. Included in this section is their full name and address. When addressing the dentist in this section, you would write their first name followed by credentials: John Smith, D.D.S, (or D.M.D.).

Salutation It is best to address your salutation to a contact person, dentist, or person identified in the advertising. When you are addressing the dentist, you would write out the word "Doctor" (do not use the abbreviation), omit the use of credentials, and end with a colon: "Dear Doctor Smith:"

Body of Letter The primary purpose of the cover letter is to get an interview. In the first paragraph, you need to target the position you are applying for, where the posting was listed, or how you heard about the position. Identify the reasons for the interest in the position, such as the dental office having a good reputation for providing quality dental care.

In the body of the letter, you need to be persuasive and highlight your most marketable skills and accomplishments. This is where you emphasize how you feel you are qualified for this position. List the qualifications that would be assets to the employer and dental team members, for example, being a graduate of an accredited dental assisting program (with an explanation on how this academic background makes for a qualified dental assistant). Mention any relevant work experience.

At the conclusion of this section, you need to ask for an interview. Close with a statement that encourages a speedy response: "I am available for an interview at your convenience and will be calling within the next five days to confirm an interview time with you," or "I am looking forward to meeting with you and your dental team in the near future."

Closing The letter must end with a professional closing. The most commonly used closing is the word "Sincerely," followed by four spaces and your full name; for example, "Sincerely, Jane Smith." Your signature should appear between the closing and your name, signed using a black or blue pen.

Enclosures After your typed name, type two returns and then type, *Enclosure: Resume.* Any other enclosure can be listed beneath the word *resume*, such as letter of recommendations.

Resume A resume is a document that presents a summary of your relevant education, work experience, awards, and references

Student: First Name/Last Name
Street Address
City, State ZIP
Telephone, Email

Recipient: First Name /Last Name
Company
Street Address
City, State ZIP

Dear First Name /Last Name:

**Paragraph #1: Opening: Introduce yourself, why you want to observe in this office
                 and identify desire to career shadow**

I am a beginning student of the Dental Assisting program at [Name of your school]. One of the
requirements of the program is to observe in dental offices.

Why: I have also been a patient in your practice and feel that you have a very professional office.
Or

Why: Your office has been recommended to me by Sarah James who is a patient in your
       practice. She has told me that your office is an excellent example of a professional
       dental practice.

I would appreciate the opportunity to complete my career shadowing hours in your office.

Paragraph #2: Body: Your skills and knowledge to date.

I would like to give you a brief overview of my knowledge, skills, and experience to date.
- I have studied infection control, dental anatomy and chairside assisting.
- I have successfully completed bloodborne pathogen, infection control and HIPAA training.
- I have mastered the skills of performing tasks in the sterilization area, and preparing the
  treatment area and seating the patient.

Paragraph #3: Conclusion

Thank you for your time and consideration. I look forward to speaking with you about this shadowing
opportunity. I will call next week to see if career shadowing in your office is possible. Please feel free to
call at any time to discuss the requirement of this position.

Sincerely
Your signature
Your First name/Your Last Name
Enclosure

FIGURE 45-2
Example of internship/shadow cover letter.

(Figure 45-4). The purpose of the resume is to get an interview, so you need to make yours stand out in a positive way. For the job seeker, the resume is used as a personal marketing tool to get the employer's attention. Employers, on the other hand, use the resume to screen candidates for the job interview without having to meet all the applicants in person. An employer often receives several resumes, so it is your challenge to highlight your relevant qualifications on one page in a way that captures the employer's attention. You should prepare an attractive, error-free resume and use standard 10–12 point Times New Roman or Arial font

Student: First Name/Last Name
Street Address
City, State ZIP
Telephone, Email

Recipient: First Name /Last Name
Company
Street Address
City, State ZIP

Dear First Name /Last Name:

Paragraph #1: Opening: Identify position and where you found the position

I am writing in response to the classified ad seeking to fill the position of chairside dental assistant in your dental practice. *State information you know about this office.*

Paragraph #2: Body: Your needs - enter job requirement from job ad
Your qualifications - enter related skill or experience

Paraphrase statements from ad. I would like to give you a brief overview of my skills and experience. I am confident that I will be an asset to your dental practice as your chairside assistant. Here is how my qualifications meet your requirements...

- I have good chairside assisting skills and have experience working in dental clinics in all aspects of dental assisting.
- I have good people skills, am a team player, and have been praised for my excellent patient management skills.
- I have obtained certificates in CPR, and DANB certificates in ICE and RHS.
- I have the ability to learn new tasks quickly with confidence and ease.

Paragraph #3: Conclusion

My enclosed resume provides my background and skills. Thank you for your time and consideration. I look forward to speaking with you about this employment opportunity. Please feel free to call at any time to discuss the requirements of this position.

Sincerely
Your signature
Your First name/Your Last Name
Enclosure

FIGURE 45-3
Example of response to advertisement cover letter.

and bullets. Resumes need to be printed on good quality bond paper that matches your cover letter. You should prepare a master electronic resume to keep updated and to modify for specific positions.

A resume gives you an opportunity to explain what you have done and what you are capable of doing. Employers often scan resumes to look for keywords as a way to identify potential candidates. Some important keywords are in the areas of job titles, skills, credentials, affiliations, and familiarity with software programs and equipment. It is important when writing your resume to include keywords found in advertisings or postings. You can also find keywords in job descriptions used in the Occupational Outlook Handbook such as *people skills*, *initiative*, and *certified dental assistant*.

Following are the key components of a standard resume that are expected by an employer:

Identification The resume should open with your contact information—name, address, phone number, and email address. It is essential that a potential employer can easily reach you.

Procedure 45-1
Preparing a Cover Letter

The dental assistant prepares a cover letter as an introduction to a future employer when applying for employment.

Equipment and Supplies
- quality paper
- information to be included in the cover letter
- computer
- printer

Procedure Steps

1. Gather correct names and addresses.

2. Select a format for the cover letter.

3. Select the font and font size (usually 12-point size).

4. Outline the information to include in the cover letter.

5. Create the cover letter including:
   - ❏ Header
   - ❏ Recipient information
   - ❏ Salutation
   - ❏ Body of letter
   - ❏ Closing
   - ❏ Enclosures

6. Ensure that the cover letter is neat and free of errors.

Career Objective Your career objective tells the employer what position you are seeking and your top selling points, for example, "Highly motivated formally trained dental assistant seeking a full-time position as a chairside assistant in a fast-paced general practice."

Education For new graduates, or applicants with little or no work experience, education history should be the next section. Your education section should include the educational institutes attended, addresses, dates of graduation, subject studied, and any professional qualifications achieved. Your list always starts with the most recent institution you attended and proceeds in reverse chronological order (i.e., the first school you attended would be the last on the list). List certificates, registration, degrees, and continuing education courses that have been completed. Also, list any academic awards received, such as scholarships.

Work Experience If you have a lot of work experience, this section should precede the section on education. Your dental assisting work experience is critical in distinguishing you as the best candidate for the position. For the best chance of getting the job you desire, you need to get this part right. Like the education section, your work experience is listed in reverse chronological order. After each work experience, you will include tasks that you performed. Tasks should be written using action statements like, "assisted dentist during operative procedures." Whenever possible, write tasks not only as responsibilities but also as achievements and contributions to the workplace, such as, "improved chairside assisting and increased office efficiency." It is also important to include tasks related to patient management skills such as, "worked

with patients with special physical needs. Utilized behavior management techniques and restraints under the dentist's supervision."

Activities The activities section allows you to demonstrate your leadership, organization, and teamwork abilities. You can include school activities (sports, club membership), professional memberships, workshops, and community service. This section is optional and can be included if you have room on your resume.

References Listing references on a resume was once standard practice, but job skills experts now debate whether to include this section. Many experts feel that you should simply include the statement "References are available upon request" to signal the end of your resume. If you do choose to include references, you should list three to five names on a separate sheet with the header "References" (Figure 45-5). Each reference should include the individual's name, their job title or association to you, address, phone number, and email address. You must always get a person's permission before you list them as a reference.

It is helpful if your references know your key accomplishments and skills. If a reference is unaware of your more recent accomplishments, you can offer to send them a current resume to help get updated. It is important to have references who relate specifically to the desired characteristics and pertain to the employment that is sought. Some characteristics include integrity, reliability, work ethic, good communication skills, and team spirit.

You should also keep your references aware of jobs you are seeking and be sure to thank them for their help.

Jane Smith
Street Address, City, State, ZIP
(XXX) 251-5465 janesmith@dental.com

OBJECTIVE
Highly motivated dental assistant seeking a full time position as a chairside assistant in a fast-paced general practice.

EDUCATION
Dental Assisting Program, Name of School, Street Address, City, State, ZIP
- Completed HIPAA and Infection Control training
- AHA Basic Life Support certificate
- DANB ICE certificate

Home High School, Street Address, City, State, ZIP
Major: Core 40 with honors

EXPERIENCE
Dental Clinic, Name of School, Street Address, City, State, ZIP
- Sanitized and sterilized instruments; assembled instrument setups, prepared treatment room and patient seating.
- Assisted in new patient examination procedure, charted conditions and recorded services rendered.
- Provided oral hygiene instructions; recorded plaque scores, performed toothbrush prophy.
- Exposed, processed and mounted radiographs under direct supervision.
- Performed front office duties, managed patient records, scheduled appointments, greeted patients, completed correspondence, checked out patients, filed records.
- Managed records: hazard communication, infection control and inventory.

James Smith, D.D.S., Street Address, City, State, ZIP
- Shadowed staff 30 hours.
- Sanitized, sterilized and prepared setups.
- Prepared treatment area, seating and dismissed patients.
- Assisted in amalgam and resin operative procedures.
- Performed front office duties; greeting patient, answering phone and filing.

Restaurant Name, Street Address, City, State, ZIP
- Supervised other employees, operated cash register, kept track of financial obligations.
- Promoted to Team Leader within 3 months.

HONORS AND ACTIVITIES
H.O.S.A.; Health Occupations Students of America.
- Attended HOSA State Conference.
- Placed in top ten in Dental Assisting.
- Held position of Local HOSA Community Service Chairperson.

REFERENCES
References are available upon request.

FIGURE 45-4
Combination resume.

Reference List

Ms. Nicole Clark
Dental Assisting Instructor
Street Address
City, State, ZIP
email

Ms. Sally Hughes
Dental Office Manager
Street Address
City, State, ZIP
email

Mr. Jeff Davis
English Teacher
Street Address
City, State, ZIP
email

Dr. David Klein, D.D.S.
Family Dentist
Street Address
City, State ZIP
email

Pastor Frank Pointer
Family Church Pastor
Street Address
City, State, ZIP
email

FIGURE 45-5
Example of reference list.

Procedure 45-2
Preparing a Professional Resume

The dental assistant prepares a resume for a future employer when applying for employment.

Equipment and Supplies
- quality paper
- information to be included in the resume
- computer
- printer

Procedure Steps
1. Gather correct names, addresses, and dates.
2. Select a format for the resume.
3. Select the font and font size (usually 12-point size).
4. Outline the information to be included in the resume.
5. Create the resume including:
   - ❏ Personal data
   - ❏ Career objective
   - ❏ Education
   - ❏ Work experience
   - ❏ Activities
   - ❏ References
6. Ensure that the resume is neat and free of errors.

Types of Resumes There are three types of resumes: chronological, functional, and a combination chronological–functional. The chronological resume is the most common resume and is generally best suited for most job seekers. It focuses on the work experience and positions held with the most recent first and lists skills and accomplishments in the experience sections. Dates are cited throughout the resume.

A functional resume places the skills and accomplishments in a section above the employment history. This resume does not necessarily list information in chronological order. This resume is best for one who needs to build on similar skills to make a career change or focus on volunteer experience or skills developed outside of work. You need to write down all skills and accomplishments beginning with an action verb. Organize the list according to the skills and accomplishments most relevant to the job and those that are your greatest assets. Then arrange the skills and accomplishments into categories such as assisting skills, computer skills, education, and experience. Write a brief summary of these skills and accomplishments describing what you can offer to the job (positive personal characteristics, new technology skills, current certificates) in place of the standard objective found in the chronological resume. Write a brief chronological work history at the end of the resume. This can include the names of companies for which you have worked, your titles, a one-line description of the tasks and responsibilities of the job, and the dates of employment.

A resume that combines a chronological and functional format is called a combination resume. This resume allows you to emphasize your strengths, downplay skills that are no longer relevant, and show a continuous work history. This resume offers the best of both resumes and is popular with both job seekers and employers.

Professional Requirements Many states have professional requirements to obtain a position as a dental assistant. The assistant should show documentation of meeting these requirements. Requirements may include proof of completing hepatitis vaccination; TB tests; and specific certifications such as CDA, RDA, and dental radiographer licenses.

Fact Sheet of Skills A list of specific skills ratings is beneficial in documenting the assistant's proficiency. Many of the dental assisting programs provide the students with such a list, and it should be included in the portfolio (Figure 45-6).

Education Accomplishments In this section of the resume, you concentrate on what you have accomplished in dental assisting education. This may include transcripts, certificates, diplomas, and any other evidence unique to you and your education. Academic awards and honors received such as national honor society, dean's list, and scholarships are filed in this area. Professional certificates and licenses earned through AHA, DANB, and state licensure and certificates of participation from conferences and workshops you have attended should be included.

Community Participation Your portfolio should also include some focus on your participation in dental health community activities. Volunteering in a free dental clinic and internship records in a dental office should be included in this section. A summary of your experiences, written on company letterhead and signed by a supervisor, is preferred. Other activities specific to your community that you may consider including are school clubs, organizations, or sports; fund-raising events; and religious groups. Military records, awards and badges, and listing of your military service may be helpful for many positions.

Recommendations Letters of recommendations and thank you notes received for your community contributions should be filed in the last section of your portfolio. You should ask professionals to write letters of recommendation describing your strengths, abilities, and experiences. Ideally you want three to five references who have known you for a long time who will write letters of recommendations. You want to ask previous supervisors (employment and internships) and coworkers who worked closely with you and can speak highly of your work ethic, skills, and performance. You should also include an educational mentor and a personal character reference such as professionals you met

Dental Assisting Skills Assessment Student Name	
Dental Assisting Skills	
Pass/Fail	
A. Performing Sterilization Assistant Skills	
Aseptic Hand Washing	Pass
Personal Protective Equipment	Pass
Sanitize/Disinfect Instruments/Work Area	Pass
Sterilize Items Using Autoclave/Chemiclave/Statim	Pass
Biological Monitoring System Test	Pass
Maintenance of Sterilization/Sanitation Equipment	Pass
Infection Control Records	Pass
B. Performing Chairside Records Assistant Skills	
Identifying Oral Structures	Pass
Record/Assemble/Obtain Patient Information	Pass
Chart Patient Conditions/Pathology	Pass
Recognize Oral Pathology	Pass
Follow HIPAA Regulations	Pass
Write services rendered/ Provide PO instructions	Pass
C. Oral Health Management	
Perform Biofilm Index	Pass
Provide Appropriate Oral Hygiene Instruction	Pass
Perform Toothbrush Prophy	Pass
D. Performing Chairside Assistant Skills	
Test Operation of Dental Office Equipment	Pass
Demonstrate Opening and Closing Procedures	Pass
Prepare Treatment area for Patient Seating	Pass
Transfer and Exchange instruments	Pass
Aspirate during Procedures	Pass
Assist during New Patient Exam	Pass
Identify, Prepare, and Assist with Preventive Procedures: Basic, Expendable, Patient Seating, Prophylaxis, Fluoride Application	Pass
Assist with administration of local anesthetic	Pass
Assist with dental dam placement	Pass
Assist during amalgam procedure	Pass
Assist during composite procedure	Pass

FIGURE 45-6
Example of skills fact sheet.

during volunteer work, close family friends, coaches, and clergy. Avoid listing family members.

Once you have developed your list of potential references, you may want to ask them to write you a letter of recommendation for your portfolio (Figure 45-7). The best way to ask someone to write a letter of recommendation is to send a letter requesting a recommendation. In a letter you can communicate what jobs you are seeking and some of the qualifications. This will help the writers describe how your strengths and accomplishments make you fit for the job you are seeking. Again, be sure to thank people for writing you a letter of recommendation.

GENERAL GUIDELINES:

- Give the writer a properly addressed envelope.
- Indicate deadline.
- Request letter well in advance of the deadline (at least two weeks).
- Check back to see that the letter has been sent.

SELECTING A WRITER:

- Select a person who knows you well and shows interest in you. For example, counselor, teacher, employer, close family friend, community service supervisor.
- Select a person who is familiar with your potential and your achievements.
- Select at least one teacher whom you have had as an instructor in the dental assisting program.
- Ask teachers with whom you have had more than one class (when possible).
- Select a teacher who has challenged you the most.
- Select a person who could best explain your extra efforts in school or on the job.
- Select a person who can vouch for your character, ethics and citizenship.

Example of Request for letter of Rec

Your Street Address
City, State Zip
Current Date

Writer Name
Address
City, State Zip

Dear _____:

For my Dental Assisting Class, I have been given the assignment to request a letter of recommendation for entry-level employment from a person who knows my qualifications and abilities. Would you please write a letter for me?

This assignment needs to be completed prior to _____; therefore, it would be helpful if I could receive this letter from you not later than _____.
You may use the enclosed, self-addressed envelope for your convenience in mailing this letter to my instructor.

Hopefully, you will find the time to help me complete this assignment.

Sincerely,
Your Signature

Your Name
Enclosure

FIGURE 45-7
Requesting a letter of recommendation.

Employment Opportunities

Whether graduating from an accredited program or just trying to obtain a position in a dental office, there are several important tasks that must be accomplished first. Planning future employment is important. It may be necessary to obtain dental assisting national certification for the state in which employment is sought. If this is the case, reflect on the pathways available and seek the one that best suits your needs.

After obtaining the necessary credentials, the next goal is to prepare for obtaining successful employment. Research should be done to identify the type of practice that will be the most interesting, stimulating, and enjoyable. When choosing an employer, find one who has a good reputation and whose philosophy is similar to your own. A dental assistant needs to feel that they are working with the dentist and other team members to care for patients in the best manner possible. Prior to obtaining the position, do research and talk to employees who work for the dentist to make sure that this practice would be a good employment match for you. Another aspect of employment is working well with other employees. Are they team players? Is compatibility possible?

It is important to find employment that best suits the individual's needs and allows for the best possible situation for the dental assistant, the employer, and the patients. Before taking the first position offered, consider the following:

- What qualities are desired in an employer?
- What areas of growth are available in this situation?
- From an employee's position, what strengths can be brought to this position?
- What individual areas can be improved upon?
- Overall, what type of dentistry is interesting?

Solo or Partnership Practice
The majority of dentists practice in solo practices in which there is only a single dentist. A dentist may hire another dentist under a contractual agreement; this hired dentist is a dental associate. An associate relationship may turn into a partnership, in which each dentist has equal rights and duties. A partnership is developed through a legal agreement, which makes both dentists responsible for any accounts payable. However, a partner is not held responsible for malpractice suits against the other partner.

Partnerships in dental practices are increasing. This is due to the tremendous startup cost that a dentist faces upon graduation from dental school. Therefore, a newly graduated dentist may work in an established practice as a dental associate, and then, after an allotted period of time, become a partner. Another way that dentists are dealing with the costs of their practices is to share a building and/or front office employees while still maintaining solo practices.

Group Practice
Another type of dental office is the group practice. In a group practice, any number of dentists (both general and specialty) can share a building and remain independent. Positive aspects of this type of practice are the opportunities to talk over cases with each other, reduced overhead, and increased patient coverage on weekends and holidays. In addition, the total number of employees in the group practice may lend itself to offering more complete and extensive benefit packages. The more employees under the same insurance plan, the better the rates for the employer.

Dental Specialty Practice
If a dental assistant likes to assist primarily in oral surgery, endodontics, periodontics, orthodontics, prosthodontics, pathology, pediatric dentistry, or dental public health, specialty offices are available. Fewer employment opportunities are available in the areas of pathology and dental public health. Dental specialists work with general dentists to care for specific cases. The general dentist refers the patient to a specialty office to obtain a special service, and then the patient returns to the general dental office for routine care.

Public Health and Government Programs
Public health programs often include oral health care. Dental assistants can gain employment in these public health or government clinics to provide oral health information, collect data, and provide dental treatment. These programs care for patients who are eligible to receive dental care for free or at a reduced rate. They are local, state, or federally funded. Often, federal or state grants set up programs to meet the specific needs of people who cannot afford dental care. These programs may also collect data on specific diseases this group of people may have. Usually, the guidelines of the programs change or have to be renewed annually. A dental assistant is an employee hired by the overseer of the grant. This dental assistant may receive great satisfaction treating patients in this type of program.

Teaching, School Clinics, and Laboratories
Dental schools and dental assisting schools also employ dental assistants who work in the clinic with students, teach, or serve as administrators for the program. In dental schools, the dental assistants work with student dentists to simulate four-handed dentistry, or work in dental laboratories to help students perfect their skills.

Teaching in dental assisting programs or schools is a career choice some dental assistants consider after working in the field for a while. Teaching often requires additional education that varies with each state. Some require a bachelor's degree and a certificate, registration, and/or license from the state. If the school is American Dental Association accredited, a bachelor's degree for the program director and faculty is now required. This is a challenging and rewarding career path for dental assistants that find teaching an area they are interested in but still want to stay in dental assisting.

Veterans' Hospitals
Veterans' hospitals hire dental assistants to assist the dentists on staff in the clinics. Employment in this area must be obtained through the civil service office. Points are given to individuals who have worked in the service or have been employed in veterans' programs before. A list of qualifications can be obtained from the civil service office that advertises the employment position.

Dental Supply Companies
Dental supply companies hire dental assistants as sales representatives for goods and supplies. Normally, a dental assistant in this position does not utilize their chairside skills, but becomes knowledgeable about products while traveling from dental office to dental office providing product information and ordering supplies.

Insurance Companies
Dental assistants are also hired by insurance companies to process dental insurance claims. Having knowledge of and a background in dental terminology and procedures is an asset for understanding situations and processing dental insurance claims.

Contact	Thank You	Referrals	Status	Letter of Rec
contact 1	X	Dr. A	contacted	X
		Dr. B	contacted	
contact 2	X	Dr. C	contacted	X
contact 3	X	none		

Position	Posting	Sent	Follow-up	Status
Dr. A	June 3	June 5	June 15	interview 6/21 at 3 PM
Dr. B	June 10	June 12	June 22	no answer
Dr. C	June 11	June 13	June 23	filled

FIGURE 45-8
Job seeking journal.

Employment Search

After a decision is made about the desired type of dental practice, locating open positions is the next step. Many dentists advertise in daily newspapers in the classified section and on online job search websites. Other areas where employment opportunities are posted include local dental and dental assistant societies and associations. Most local societies have newsletters or other services that list job openings. If graduating from a dental assisting program, career placement services may be available at the school. Some employment agencies have listings for dental assistant jobs, and most dental supply houses know of dentists who are hiring. Leaving a cover letter and resume with some of these agencies may be a consideration.

An additional resource for an employment search is the Internet; start with a search for "employment in dental professions." This is especially helpful when planning to relocate.

Searching for the Right Position

Now that you have completed your portfolio, you are ready to begin your search for the right position. There are many ways you can begin your job search. The traditional way of searching is through job postings and advertisings. You can look through newspaper ads or go online to look through job search engines and through professional association postings. If you are a member of the American Dental Assisting Association, you have access to job postings placed in your area and in other states. One of the more effective ways to search for a job is through networking.

Networking Career networking refers to the process of using personal connections to find jobs. You stand a better chance of getting an interview if you can preface your cover letter or call by saying, "I received your name from Kevin, your dental salesperson. He told me you are looking for an enthusiastic dental assistant." If the dentist thinks highly of the salesperson, you just changed a cold call into a warm call. Developing relations for employment

purposes has become an important part of the job search. Some jobs get filled through networking before the job has even been advertised.

When you begin looking for a job, you should inform as many people as you can. The wider you cast your net, the more likely you are to be successful in your networking. Remember the Law of 250: Every person knows at least 250 other people. You can network through your internship, by volunteering and through professional association meetings, workshops, and seminars. You can also network with contacts from any part of your life: your dentist, friends, relatives, neighbors, teachers, and your holiday card list. You want to network where people frequently communicate including community groups, your hairdresser, and Facebook. Some job seekers develop their own websites advertising that they are looking for a job. Once you have your contacts you can send your resume to them by mail or email, or have a brief telephone conversation to follow-up on possible jobs. Start a journal of all the people you know, and keep a record of all your contacts, employers you have contacted, and status of all your contacts (Figure 45-8). You are well on your way to finding a position as a dental assistant.

Arranging an Interview

Now that you have completed your career portfolio, you are ready to send your cover letter and resume and arrange for an interview. There are many ways to send your cover letter and resume to potential employers, including by email, fax, mail, phone call, and walk-in. The method you use to send your application information depends on the manner in which you heard of the position and the employer's preference. Whenever possible, address the cover letter to the contact person, customize the resume to specifications of the position, include originals to reinforce your personalization of your information, and send information in a flat 8 × 10 envelope to maintain its professional appearance.

Sending resumes electronically is the most common method. When employers post an advertisement online, they often state

Date

Dear Doctor Jones:

Just a note to say thank you for giving me the opportunity to discuss your opening for a dental assistant. I appreciate our conversation and you were very helpful.

Again, thank you for your time. I am looking forward to hearing from you soon.

Best Regards,

Your Signature

FIGURE 45-9
Example of a thank you note.

that they only want to receive responses via email. Make certain you read the entire advertisement and follow the directions. Some want you to complete an application online and paste your resume into an email, while some want you to attach the resume as a text document. If you have a choice, paste your cover letter first into the email addressed to the contact person mentioned in the ad and send your resume as a word document attachment. Type the position you are applying for in the subject line. When jobs are posted online, the employer receives a large amount of replies from candidates with similar qualifications. In order to not be just another email, mail your cover letter and resume after you apply online to show the employer that you are determined and really desire the position. By using email, the employer will also not be able to see your quality paper, and mailing your originals will make you stand out and impress the employer.

Some advertisements require that the resume is faxed to their office. If you do not have a fax, you will be able to fax your information from a local printing store. When using the fax machine, the quality the employer sees on their end will not look as professional as from your end. Again, follow up by mailing your cover letter and resume.

If you hear about a position through networking, it is best to mail your application information. You should call the employer within 1–2 weeks after you mail your resume to confirm that they received it and to reiterate your continued interest in being considered for the position. Ask the dental personnel who answers the phone who you should speak to about a position in the dental office. When this person answers the phone, ask if they have a moment to answer a couple of questions about the position. Some appropriate questions are: Is the position still open? Do you know when you will be arranging interviews? Send a handwritten thank you note within a day of this informational interview. You should use a small, conservative thank you card to help you in keeping your message brief (Figure 45-9).

Although phone calls and walk-ins give you an opportunity to meet the receptionist, view the inside of the office, and allow them to make a personal connection with you, this does not always work to your advantage. Most dental office personnel are busy, and hearing from you unexpectedly may irritate them. If you feel these methods are your only options, make certain you assure them that you do not wish to interrupt them and make your contact brief. When calling, you should verify the address and to whom your letter should be addressed (Figure 45-10). In a walk-in without an appointment, again assure them that you do not wish to interrupt them and ask permission to leave your application information with them.

Job Application

The job interviewing process often starts with completing a job application that benefits the interviewer and prospective employee. Interviewers use job applications to standardize and verify information obtained from all applicants to screen for job interviews. Applications are also signed by the applicant attesting that all information you are providing is accurate. Job applications ask a wide variety of information including information that is not normally put on a resume. The employer may request the application be completed online, ask you to come into the office, or have you complete the application after you have been invited for the interview.

The application gives you the chance to sell yourself by explaining why you believe you are qualified for the job. A well completed job application is another key marketing tool for you in the job search process. Before you start completing applications for a job, you need to have your up-to-date master resume, cover letter, and fact sheet and practice filling in sample applications (Figure 45-11). Online and paper job applications typically request the same information. Make a follow-up call a week or so after you have applied to check on the status of your application.

Online Application Some jobs advertised online require that you create an account when you apply. You will need to register with a current email address to confirm your account. Your user name will either be your email address or a user name you select, and you will need to choose a password to access your account.

Receptionist: Good Morning, this is Dr. Smith's office. How may I help you?

Applicant: Hello, my name is (first and last name). Kevin, your dental supply retailer, informed me that you have an opening for a dental assistant. Could you please tell me who I can talk to about this position?

Receptionist: Yes, Jane is talking to applicants.

Applicant: Is she available to come to the phone?

Receptionist: We are just accepting resumes at this time and then she will get back with you.

Applicant: Could you please give me the full name of the person to whom I should address my letter and the mailing address?

Receptionist: You can address it to Jane Klein at 321 S Road, Hometown, State, ZIP

Applicant: Thank you. May I please repeat this information to make certain I have written it properly? (It is important to repeat information to show receptionist you are aware of the professional way in which to handle a phone call.)

Receptionist: *Confirms that the information is correct and ends the call.*

FIGURE 45-10
Example of a phone call to a potential employer.

It is best to apply directly with the employer website whenever possible, even if you find the listing in a job search engine. Before you start an online application, you should download, print, and fill it out to make certain you know exactly what information you will need and avoid making errors. Once you have completed your online application, carefully proofread and make certain you have submitted all required materials before you click the submit button. You will generally be asked to click a box to acknowledge that you are submitting complete and accurate information. The checked box also counts as your signature.

Completing the Application The employer often judges the appearance of your application as a clue to your professionalism, quality of your work, and penmanship. You need to make certain your answers are complete and legible. You need to return a neat application without any mars, wrinkles, or bends. If you are submitting your application at the office, your appearance and demeanor are also important. Greet the receptionist politely when requesting or submitting an application. The receptionist's first impressions are important as a future coworker and are often passed along. Every time you make contact with an employer, dress ready to go to work. The employer may need to have the position filled as soon as possible and want to interview you after you complete the application.

You need to be organized and bring everything needed to complete the application. You will need the fact sheet, resume,

cover letter, and two black or blue ink ball point pens (in case one stops working). It does not create a good impression when a job seeker needs to borrow the employer's pen or telephone books to complete an application.

Be prepared for all kinds of job applications. There are simple one-page applications to detailed, multipage applications. This is not a timed test, so you can take your time. Use your fact sheet for ease in completing in office applications, take your time to be accurate and complete, and use your best penmanship. Completing the application properly is your first chance to present your skills for completing patient records to the employer. A blank space may flag an interviewer that you are not thorough or that the answer would be damaging. You can write "Does Not Apply" (DNA) or "Not Applicable" (N/A) in the space when the question does not apply to you.

Job Application Components Most job applications have the following key components.

Instructions The applicant is provided instructions for completing the form. It is important that you read the entire application prior to completing it. Instructions may request that the application be completed in ink and answers printed legibly. Pay close attention to what the application is requesting; for example, in the name field, does the form ask for first or last name? You have only one chance to answer correctly. You cannot erase information, and crossing out shows lack of forethought. As you

MY FACT SHEET   *Complete and carry with you on your job search*

Applicant's Name (Last)	First	Middle Initial	Social Security Number - -
Mailing Address (Number)	Street		Work Telephone Number ( )
City	State	Zip Code	Home Telephone Number ( )

EDUCATION

Name of School	Location of School	Degree or Course of Study	Date Completed

EMPLOYMENT HISTORY – Begin with your most recent job. List each job separately.

Job Title   Dates Worked From _____ To _____   Pay $ _____ Per _____
Name of Employer   Name of Supervisor
Address:
    City   State   Zip Code
Telephone Number ( )   Reason for Leaving:
Duties Performed:
_____
_____
_____

Job Title   Dates Worked From _____ To _____   Pay $ _____ Per _____
Name of Employer   Name of Supervisor
Address:
    City   State   Zip Code
Telephone Number ( )   Reason for Leaving:
Duties Performed:
_____
_____
_____

Job Title   Dates Worked From _____ To _____   Pay $ _____ Per _____
Name of Employer   Name of Supervisor
Address:
    City   State   Zip Code
Telephone Number ( )   Reason for Leaving:
Duties Performed:
_____
_____
_____

Job Title   Dates Worked From _____ To _____   Pay $ _____ Per _____
Name of Employer   Name of Supervisor
Address:
    City   State   Zip Code
Telephone Number ( )   Reason for Leaving:
Duties Performed:
_____
_____
_____

PERSONAL REFERENCES: List the names of three references that employers may contact.

1) Name   Telephone # ( )   Relationship (Teacher etc.)
Address:
    City   State   Zip Code
2) Name   Telephone # ( )   Relationship (Teacher etc.)
Address:
    City   State   Zip Code
3) Name   Telephone # ( )   Relationship (Teacher etc.)
Address:
    City   State   Zip Code

FIGURE 45-11

Example of fact sheet. A copy of this fact sheet is included in your workbook for you to complete and take with you for your interview.

complete your answers, you should tailor your answers to the position you are applying for.

Personal Information Applications ask for the applicant's name, address, Social Security number, email address, and home and mobile telephone numbers. Try to avoid entering birth dates. Questions about being convicted of a crime, driver's history, whether you legally work in the United States, and have a work permit if under age 18 may be asked. The employer may point out that you will be tested for illegal drug use and a criminal check will be completed.

Applications may ask about health requirements. Many employers want the applicant to have a physical examination or a vaccination series as a condition of employment. The employer must pay for these requirements and can only request them after hiring.

Position Desired Applications will provide a line for "Position Desired." You need to enter a specific position. Do not respond "will do anything" or "open." It is acceptable to list more than one position that is open.

There may be a section where you can explain why you are seeking this position. Applicants are asked to summarize information that has not already been asked that will help judge qualifications.

The application may ask what salary the applicant expects if hired. It is acceptable to write "negotiable" instead of a salary figure. The employer will look at the salaries paid previously as a reference point. There is a broad range of dental assisting salaries, and in some states five different job titles. You again need to do your homework. How much you will earn as a dental assistant depends on where you work and your qualifications. You can search the Occupational Outlook Handbook, which provides national median pay. The Bureau of Labor Statistics (BLS) can provide salaries more specific to your area. Salaries vary per state as salaries are dependent on many factors like cost of living and the demand, for and supply of dentists and assistants. Even in the same state, you cannot expect to earn as much in rural areas as dental assistants in big cities or highly urbanized places.

You can also expect increased salaries by adding to your qualifications. More education and experience, and higher levels of skills and credentialing increase pay. As an entry-level assistant, you will make a lower salary because you have to become familiar with your duties, improve your skills, and get more experience. As you become more familiar with the way the dentist works and the duties you need to perform, you will receive raises and new opportunities for career growth. As you become more familiar with your duties, you will get more responsibilities, which are great to add to your resume. Earning the national certification (CDA) and expanded functions with state certification (RDA), supervisory and lead assistants are on the higher end of the salary scale.

Most applications will ask about the applicant's availability. Your response should be "immediately" if you are unemployed. If you are employed, you need to state availability after 2 weeks'

notice. It is important to always protect your job history by giving 2 weeks' notice. You are also more likely you will get good references from your employers if you treat them with respect.

Education When completing this section, you should list the most recent education first. On the application you will be asked to identify each institution by name, location, number of years attended, and degrees earned. There is generally an area for high school, college, and trade schools, and details of any special courses. You may be asked to expand on your skills, qualifications, and credentials. Whenever possible, try to avoid graduation dates and be prepared to provide transcripts at the time of employment.

Work Experience Most recent jobs should be listed first. Be prepared to identify the previous employer's name, complete mailing address, and phone number. There is generally a space for your job title, starting and ending employment date, starting and ending salary, description of duties, supervisor name, and reason you left. Try to avoid negative responses like "fired" and "quit." Some more acceptable answers include "took a job with more responsibility," "returned to school," "seasonal," "moved," "business closed," or "temporary work." Always make certain you answer truthfully and do not talk negatively about past employers. You should always answer yes if asked if the employer can be contacted.

Many have an area for office skills, use of computers, various software programs, and office equipment. Applications request information about any military service. The branch of service, specialty, and dates of entry and discharge are generally asked in this section.

References Most applications have a space for three references including the name, position, company address, and phone numbers of the references. Always ask permission to use their names, keep your references updated, and let them know when you find a job.

Application Certification You must tell the truth on an application and must sign a statement certifying that you have completed the application accurately. Inaccuracies and omitting information can be grounds for not being hired and for termination in the future for misrepresentation or lying on the job application. Following is a job certification section where you need to sign your name verifying that you have been truthful and give permission for the employer to follow up on information provided.

I hereby certify that all entries on this job application and any attachments are true and complete.

I also agree and understand that any falsification of this information may result in my forfeiture of employment.

I understand that all information on this job application is subject to verification, and I consent to criminal history and background checks.

I also agree that you may contact references and educational institutions listed on this application.

Make certain that your application is consistent with your resume. Read and check your application for completeness and any spelling errors before turning it into the receptionist.

Employment Test Along with the application, many employers are asking applicants to complete a personality test or aptitude test. The personality test provides the employer with information in these areas: general reasoning, agreeableness, assertiveness, customer service, integrity, empathy, openness to new experience, conscientiousness, emotional resilience, extroversion, nurturance, optimism, teamwork, and work drive. The aptitude test usually has specific questions about your dental assisting knowledge.

Preinterview

As soon as you send your resume and cover letter and complete the application, expect that every call could be for an interview. This is also referred to as the preinterview call. Most interviewers use this call as a part of the prescreening process. They see if you are what they are looking for and decide if you are a match for the position. The 3–10 minutes you are on the phone is your opportunity to make a good impression and get your interview.

The preinterview is as important as your actual interview because if you do not handle the call well, you will not get the interview. There are some questions you need to answer to make sure you are ready for that important call. How do you answer the phone you gave the potential employer to call? If a caller is put on hold, what is your message? What kind of music do you play during the wait time? Does this sound professional and make a good impression?

You may need to change the message and music you have recorded on the phone you will be answering for the interview. Keep your job journal and resume near you at all times. Answer every unidentified call a little more professionally, "Hello, this is your first name?" If you are not able to answer professionally or have time for the possible 10 minute call, it is better to let the call go to message. This also allows you to find a quiet area and get a mindset for the preinterview. A possible professional message you can use is, "Hello, this is (your first name). I am unable to answer your call at the moment. Please leave your name, a brief message, and a number I can reach you. I will return your call as soon as possible."

The preinterview caller generally asks a few questions, confirms details of your resume, and if you pass the screening sets up a time for your interview. Ask the caller to whom you are speaking, write down their name, and answer their questions courteously without going into too much detail. Share your personality by being honest, friendly, professional, and staying focused on what they are saying. By having your resume available, you can quickly scan your own dates and details of your resume to make certain you do not give any conflicting information. If employers ask if they can contact your previous employers and references, always say yes. Remember by law your previous employer can only answer specific questions, and have faith

they will respond appropriately. When asked when you would be available for an interview, try to get in as soon as possible. Write down the date and time of the interview and repeat the information back to the caller. Ask for specific directions if you are uncertain and if there is anything they would like you to bring to the interview. Thank them for the opportunity of an interview, and always let the caller end the conversation.

The Interview

You have successfully scheduled your interview. You may now feel a rush of anxiety. Take a deep breath and remember you have prepared your portfolio for this interview. But your work is not done. You need to prepare for the interview itself for the best opportunity to succeed and get the job. Do homework on the potential employer, visit the interview location, develop your talking points, have questions ready to ask the employer, rehearse the interview with a friend, and decide what to wear.

Research Dental Office

Your interview will go more smoothly if you know about the business where you are interviewing. Most dentists have websites describing the dentist and staff, office policy, office hours, and pictures of the office. Often on the same page is a rating on the dentist. Your interest in getting the job will show through your knowledge of the office.

Visit Location

It is important to arrive 15 minutes prior to your interview time. There is no excuse for being late. Driving by the location will allow you to make certain you will be able to find the office, check for any road delays, and time the trip. Rushing to an unknown location will help to increase anxiety, whereas visiting the location in advance will help you relax before the interview. Always go to your interview alone.

Develop Talking Points

The dentist's goal for the interview is to find the best dental assistant for the position. The interviewer is looking for the applicant who has the desired motivation and the assisting and people skills necessary for the job. Interview questions are similar. You can practice answering common questions in advance. Refer to Figure 45-12 for a list of common interview questions. Questions from the following areas are most asked:

- Why you became a dental assistant, and why you want this position
- Procedures, instruments, and materials in which you have developed proficiency
- Attributes of being a team player
- Professional characteristics: attendance, reliability, honesty, work ethic, and attentiveness.

What does team work mean to you? Are you a team player?

Can you deal with a lot of different types of people all day?

Do you work well under stress?

What do you see yourself doing in 5 years?

Why do you want to work here?

How would you describe the value of a dental treatment to a patient?

What is the most important aspect of a successful dental practice?

What do you think are the most important attributes of a dental assistant?

What are your strengths as a dental assistant?

What are your weaknesses as a dental assistant?

Explain four-handed dentistry.

What will you bring to my practice to increase productivity and revenue?

FIGURE 45-12
Common interview questions.

- Efficiency in handling and maintaining dental equipment
- Familiarity with computerized office programs
- Dental laboratory proficiency
- Knowledge of rules and regulations affecting dentistry
- Certificates and licenses held

Everybody is trying to cut costs and shop for a good deal. An employer also wants the most for their money. The best deal for a dentist is to hire an assistant who can perform multiple tasks and has all the previous attributes. You need to develop talking points that let the interviewer know that you have all these qualities and you are that special person they have been seeking. The employer wants an employee who will work above and beyond.

Have Questions Ready

Most interviewers expect the interviewee to have questions. This shows that the applicant is interested and has been focused during the interview. Make sure you do not ask a question about information covered by the interviewer unless you are asking for clarification. You should ask a couple of questions related to your responsibilities and duties. This will also help you make certain you will be doing the job you want if hired. Questions about the employer's support of continuing education both in time and reimbursement is important for a dental assistant who desires to continue growing professionally. You should ask general questions about the employer's pay structure so you can decide if you can afford this job. Specific questions can be held until your second interview or when you are offered the position. You need to remember that the interview is for you too to see if you want the job. Ask for a tour of the facility and to meet the dental staff.

Practice Interview

Anyone actively interviewing can benefit from practicing interview skills. The Society of Human Resources Management reveals that the interview performance and professionalism are more influential than the candidate's background and qualifications in being hired. Seitz and Cohen write that "through mental rehearsal, job seekers can practice interviews with a successful outcome until the unconscious mind believes it has already happened." Through practice and rehearsal of the interview, you will build your confidence and self-assurance.

After you have developed a list of common interview questions and written your answers, you are ready to practice rehearsing for your interview. Watching good examples of interviews and making notes of what you want to replicate will help you get ready for your interview. If you can recruit a friend or family member to take the role of the interviewer and simulate a real interview, you will gain important feedback about your interviewing skills in this mock interview (Figure 45-13). Research has shown that the more you interview, the more skilled and relaxed you will become. You and your mock interviewer need to develop a script for the interview.

Videotaping your mock interview will allow you to focus on your verbal and nonverbal performance. You will want to exhibit a friendly personality, relaxed demeanor, good posture, enthusiasm, and confidence. You can watch for inappropriate body language, such as nervous hand gestures, nervous rocking, awkward facial expressions, fidgeting, and brushing hair back from eyes. You can also listen more closely to the verbal aspects of your performance: poor grammar, clearing throat, use of stalling sounds "uh" and "um," and nervous giggling.

Answer interviewer questions honestly and in complete sentences to convince your potential employer that you are the

Following are suggestions for your mock review. You and your mock interviewer should discuss the details of your script. You should provide the interviewer with your list of interview questions.

Interviewer: Is sitting at the desk reviewing your resume.

Assistant: You enter the room, greeting the interviewer warmly with a smile.

Interviewer: Offers a handshake greeting,

Assistant: You look the interviewer in the eyes, extend hand to introduce yourself, "Hi, I am Anaya. It is very nice to meet you," and give a firm handshake.

Assistant: You wait for interviewer to tell you where to sit.

Interviewer: Asks you to take a seat and points to the chair you are to sit in.

Assistant: You adjust your seat so you are not sitting directly across from the interviewer with your best side towards the interviewer where you can maintain eye contact, but do not stare. (Sitting directly in front of the interviewer can be intimidating for the interviewer and the interviewee.)

Assistant: You want your body language to exhibit confidence, poise and enthusiasm. Sit slightly forward in the seat with both feet flat on the floor with your hands relaxed in your lap. Make certain that you exhibit good yet comfortable posture with your shoulders slightly back.

Assistant: Place your portfolio and copies to leave with the interviewer on floor next to you.

Interviewer: Asks you five questions from the interview list.

Assistant: You answer interviewer questions honestly and in complete sentences.

Assistant: You use your portfolio to illustrate your answers when appropriate.

Interviewer: Asks you if you have any questions.

Assistant: You ask the three questions you have developed.

Interviewer: Stands up and tells you that someone will get back with you with a final decision.

Assistant: Stand up, look interviewer in the eye, smile, and offer your handshake. Thank interviewer for the opportunity to interview. Ask when you might be hearing about their decision.

FIGURE 45-13
Sample mock interview script.

best candidate (Figure 45-14). Be yourself and, if nervous, say so, and then continue on. Make sure that the dentist's name is pronounced correctly, and always address the dentist as Dr. _____ unless asked to do otherwise. Use examples and personal work experiences to emphasize that you have already accomplished the expectations of the job. Use your portfolio to illustrate your answers. In areas that you do not have the desired experience, explain how you are willing and eager to learn. Some of the most common and harder questions are, "Tell me about yourself. Why do feel you should get this position? What assisting skills do you bring to this office?" You should rehearse answers for these questions. This is also a cue to share your portfolio and show the interviewer your fact sheet of skills. When questioned about working with patients, assure the dentist that you enjoy working with people, and give examples when possible. Be prepared to ask two to three questions when directed by the interviewer.

It may surprise you, but many interviewers are nervous about the interview too. You will be one of the most memorable

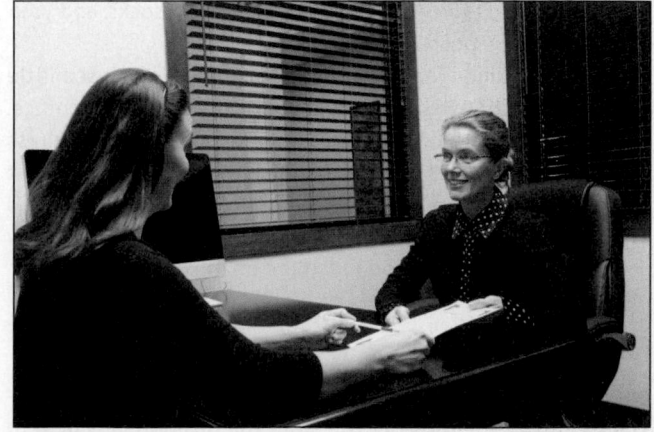

FIGURE 45-14
During the interview be prepared, and listen carefully to the interviewer before answering questions.

candidates if you do your part to make the interview a comfortable conversation. This can also be done by telling stories that will help the interviewer conclude that you are easy to talk to and would be a positive addition to the dental office.

Wait for the interviewer to indicate that the interview is over. The interviewer usually closes the session by asking if the interviewee has any further questions. This is the time to ask prepared questions. If all areas have been covered, say, "The specific questions I had prepared to ask have been answered. Can I clarify anything in regard to my background and experience?" If all questions have not been answered, show them that you are prepared and have done your research, for example, "I have reviewed your Web page and found that you are very team oriented. Do you have regular staff meetings?" As you leave the interview, smile, look them in the eye, and offer your handshake. Thank the interviewer for the opportunity and ask when you might be hearing about their decision. After the interview, make notes in your journal about what was discussed, what you learned about the job, and the names of the people you met in the office. This is especially important if you are interviewing in several offices in preparation for a second interview.

Interview Dress

There is always a concern about what to wear for an interview. Should you wear a uniform or dress in business casual? The general recommendation is that you should look the way you would if you were actually working. With this in mind, you may want to wear clinic attire. Your uniform should be clean and wrinkle-free with your clean clinic shoes. Meticulous grooming is a must. You should take out piercings, make sure your hair is clean and out of your face, check that your hands are well manicured, and brush and floss your teeth, making sure your breath smells nice. Females should wear light colored fingernail polish and lightly applied make-up and perfume. Males need to shave or have facial hair neatly trimmed and lightly apply cologne.

If you choose to wear business casual, nice pants and a shirt, or a skirt and dress shoes are good options. Solid blue or black dress pants and a button down blouse or shirt make a good interview presence (Figure 45-15). You need to wear socks, and your shoes need to be polished.

When deciding what to wear, you need to dress just a little better than the prevailing dress at the prospective dental office. You need to promote yourself as a professional and also dress like one. You need to look like someone the dentist would want to work at their office. Dressing appropriately for an interview is especially important for young people. It demonstrates maturity and that you will show good judgment on the job.

Follow-Up Letter

A follow-up letter is good business etiquette and lets the interviewer know how strongly you want the position. It is best to send the letter on the same day as the interview.

Most likely the other applicants have not had the thorough job skills training you are receiving and will fail to send a letter.

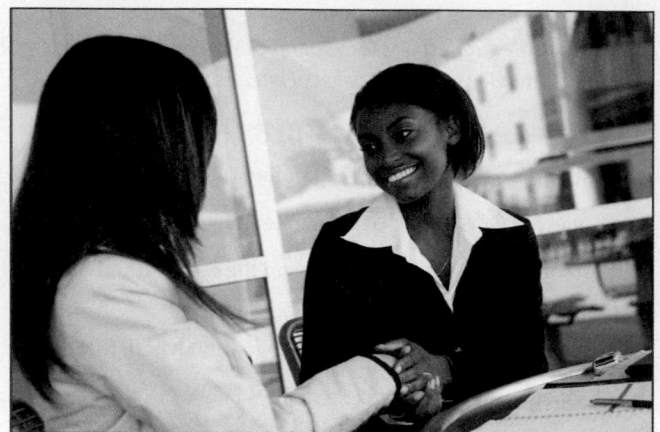

FIGURE 45-15
Appearance should be professional and neat.

This is one more opportunity for you to stand out from the other applicants. In your follow-up letter, you are able to express appreciation for the interview, recap the interview and emphasize why you are the right person for the position. Now that you know the office and what is expected of the position, you can stress specific tasks you have performed as evidence of your capability to fulfill the requirements. You can also explain how you appreciate the kindness of the staff, that you felt at home right away, and that you would be honored to work at such a respectable dental office. Refer to Figure 45-16 for a follow-up letter sample.

Second Interview

If the dentist requests a second interview with you, it is a strong indication that you are on the short list of candidates. Most dentists interview candidates a second time before making a hiring decision.

Working Interview The dentist may request a working interview where you work in the office as a dental assistant for a day. This is your chance to convince the dentist that you can bring something to that practice that will be a real asset. The dentist is aware that you need to be oriented to the practice and won't expect you to fully step into the position. The goal of the working interview is for the dentist to see your fundamental assisting skills, chairside etiquette, patient communication, initiative, and how you interact with the rest of the staff. It is important to remember that if you act like you are comfortable, you will help make the staff feel comfortable with you.

You can prepare for a working interview by reviewing instruments, tray setups, and fundamental assisting skills like instrument transfer and positions for HVE and saliva ejector. When you arrive at the office, ask the interviewer what your responsibilities are for the day and if there are any tasks they would prefer that you not perform. Be positive, complete all your responsibilities in a timely manner, ask pertinent questions as needed, and make sure you are good with the patient concerns. If there is down time between your assigned responsibilities, ask if there is anything

Date

Dear Interviewer's Name,

Introduction: Start by thanking the interviewer for the opportunity to interview for the specific position. Express appreciation for how the staff made you feel comfortable and welcomed. (2–3 sentences)

Body: Highlight points you discussed during the interview and describe why you think you are the perfect candidate. Review experiences and accomplishments that are evidence that you are a qualified for the job. Make certain not to repeat statements from your cover letter. (3–5 sentences)

Closing: Restate your appreciation for being considered for the position and that you are looking forward to their hiring decision.

Sincerely,

Your Signature

Your Name

FIGURE 45-16
Sample follow-up letter.

Procedure 45-3
Preparing a Follow-up Letter

The dental assistant prepares a follow-up letter after an interview with a future employer.

Equipment and Supplies
- quality paper
- information to be included in the follow-up letter
- computer
- printer

Procedure Steps

1. Gather correct names, addresses, and dates.

2. Select a format for the follow-up letter.

3. Select the font and font size (usually 12 points).

4. Outline the information to be included in the letter.

5. Create the follow-up letter, including the following:
   - ❏ Express appreciation for interview
   - ❏ Emphasize why you are the right person for the position
   - ❏ Reference the resume
   - ❏ Restate an interest in becoming a member of the office team.

6. Ensure that the follow-up letter is neat and free of errors.

you could help with, such as breaking down rooms, setting up trays, and fetching instruments before you are asked.

Accepting the Job

At the close of the working interview, dentists may ask to complete the second interview in their office. They generally clarify previous questions, ask how you felt about the office after your working interview, and ask you if you have any questions. At this point, it is best to ask specific questions that you had while working during the day: "Who will be your supervisor? What is

the orientation and training for this position? What would be the working schedule for this position?" Don't forget this is also a chance to see if this office is a good fit for you as well.

If you are offered the position, you need to learn more details about the pay structure. First of all, make certain you know what your pay will be before you ever accept a position. You also need to know the dentist's evaluation process, probation period, benefits packet, sick days, vacation time, and raise policy. These are all hard questions, but you need to learn how to negotiate for yourself and also shop for your best deal. Remember, if you can perform multiple tasks you are worth more to the dentist. If you are an EFDA, you save them a lot of money and can negotiate a higher salary. One of the hardest questions from the interviewer is, "What do you expect to be paid?" Dentists understand that it is not desirable to make a lateral move in pay. It is acceptable to state, "The lowest starting salary I would accept is what I am making now. But, with my additional training and skills in assisting and starting a new career I expect higher pay." You then need to explain that you will prove through your dedication, level of assisting and patient skills, and hard work that you will deserve a raise at the first evaluation.

Check the office's policies on requirements for uniforms, payment of professional dues, opportunities for continued education, sick days, holidays, and vacation time. Know what your specific responsibilities are and what the office hours will be.

Once you have negotiated the details of the job, thank the employer for the job offer and ask if you can study the benefit package and get back with them by the next day. Let them know that you are looking forward to working for them and being a part of the dental team.

Turning Down an Offer

Turning down an offer is often harder than accepting the job. You need to decline the job without causing hurt feelings, burning bridges, or making a bad reputation for yourself. Make certain that you are polite and courteous as you thank them for the offer. Take time to make it personal and explain that you have decided to decline their offer. Try to end the conversation on friendly terms.

Job Orientation

You have accepted your first dental assisting job. Your first day as a real dental assistant will be exciting and stressful. You might feel a bit nervous at being solely responsible for your patients and performing live procedures with which you may have little or no practical experience. Even if you feel comfortable with the majority of the procedures, every facility is different. You will need to figure out where supplies are located, how the operatories are organized, and the facility's routines. Hopefully, you inquired about the office's dress policies before your first day on the job. There are few things more uncomfortable than showing up dressed inappropriately.

Ideally, you will be oriented by an experienced dental assistant who closely monitors you until you are comfortable with your job and the office routines. The goal of the orientation is to smooth your transition into the dental office to establish a successful, productive working relationship for all involved. Most orientations focus on teaching you about the job you will be doing and becoming acquainted with the office personnel. You also will be introduced to the dental office philosophy, goals, policies, and rules of the dental practice.

Take an active role during your orientation. Ask lots of questions of the dental staff and observe procedures that are performed, whether on your patient or someone else's. Ask the assistants you are working with for feedback on how you are

doing. If there is an office procedure manual, you may want to ask if you can take it home to study. Request a copy of your job description as your reference point.

At some point in the orientation, you will need to complete paperwork such as the federal W-4, request for automatic deposit, and forms to initiate benefits. Most benefits such as insurance do not kick in until after a 30-day probation period. Ask if you can take the information home so you can take time to complete the forms accurately. This will also give you the opportunity to discuss the benefits and details of the position with your family

Try to go to break or lunches with coworkers. Bring snacks as well as money for meals until you are familiar with the office customs. Many offices are busy, and you might not have time to go out for lunch. If coworkers go out for lunch, ask if you can go along, even if you are not asked. During lunch breaks, ask the dental staff to share their stories about the office. Include questions about the doctor's preferences and pet peeves. Watch what you share about your personal life. Especially as a new graduate, you want to appear mature, and some personal activities can be used against you.

Be nice to everyone, and thank the people who help you. Experienced employees can give you valuable information. For example, the front office can teach you the office secrets of patient scheduling, patient records, and the phone system. During your orientation you will probably have a lighter patient load, which may leave you some down time. When you have time, you should offer to help other assistants with their duties. You will learn most about the office and show you are a team player, and they will be more willing to help you in the future. Be open and do not judge or become involved in conversations about other coworkers.

Orientation is not just a one-day program; it is an ongoing process that typically continues over a 6-month period in most dental offices. You need to closely pay attention to the office norms, customs, and traditions and try to fit in. During orientation you will learn how the office performs each procedure. Be aware that there may be slight differences in the way the office performs some of the procedures you learned during your academic training. There are about as many ways to perform a procedure as there are dentists. It is important that you are flexible and learn to perform your tasks in the manner your dentist prefers. Refrain from remarks such as, "That is not how I learned it at school." Instead, inform the trainer if they introduce something you did not learn at school or learned differently. Assure them that you are excited about learning more dental procedures and would appreciate them teaching this area more thoroughly. It is important to report back to the trainer until you master the skill to make certain you are performing the task properly.

Keeping Your Job

Keeping your job is as important as getting the job. Even though dentistry is one of the least affected professions during economic hard times, dentists still need to control their overhead to run a profitable business. Employees are the greatest overhead costs. When costs need to be cut, the dentist has to evaluate the benefit of each employee. The employees who keep their jobs are the ones that the dentist or office cannot function without.

As a new assistant, you need to come to work each day upbeat, ready to do your best, establish relationships with all the patients, be the best team player you can be, and make yourself indispensable. Are you the happy smiley face that everyone loves to see every day? Do you make your dentist's job easier and the dental practice more profitable? If you can answer yes, you will keep your job. Following are factors that will influence your success in the dental practice to help you keep your job and grow within it.

Attitude

One of the most important factors is a positive attitude toward everybody in the dental practice, your patients, and your responsibilities. Your attitude affects every other factor to becoming a successful assistant. A positive attitude is reflected in a simple smile, enthusiasm, initiative, and absence of negativism. You need to think positively about your work and dwell on the aspects of your work you like.

As a new employee, you will be expected to make some mistakes. How you handle criticism for your mistakes, and what you do about it, reflects your attitude. Accept the criticism when you make a mistake and do not blame others. If someone criticizes your work, the best way to respond is to thank the person for their help and learn how to do the task correctly. Check with your supervisor to make certain you are performing the task to their standard, and make an effort to not repeat the same mistake. It will be your attitude that will be remembered, not the mistake. Your relations with your patients, coworkers, and supervisors will be easier if you approach them positively. Workers with a positive attitude make other people around them feel good, and that attitude is reflected back to you.

Attendance

Be on time all the time. Punctuality demonstrates respect for your job and for others and their time. Arrive at work on time every day. Return from all breaks and lunch promptly. Show up for staff meetings prepared and on time every time. Employers maintain records of your attendance. Many states recognize poor attendance and chronic lateness as grounds for termination. Whenever you miss work, everybody else in the office must work much harder to fill in the void caused by your absence. This may cause stress and resentment from your coworkers and dentist. If you miss work and your job gets done in your absence, it will not take long for everybody to realize that you are not needed or that they need to replace you with an assistant who is more dependable.

Take care of all outside practical matters so that attention can be placed on fulfilling employment responsibilities. Make sure that child care is arranged (if applicable) and that backup care is available in case the primary caregiver has an emergency. Arrange for reliable transportation.

Make sure you know the policy for reporting absences before your first absence. It is also important to notify your supervisor if you are running late to work. Employers understand occasional,

unavoidable absences. We all get sick sometimes; but even if you are truly ill you need to minimize your number of absences. You are in a health care profession, and you are expected to maintain good health to be able to go to work. Make sure you eat right, exercise, and get adequate rest to function at your best every day on the job.

Appearance

You should have asked or been told what you are expected to wear to work. The dentist sets acceptable dress attire for the dental office. Most dentists will want you to wear a uniform. Many offices purchase matching uniforms for the dental staff and wash the uniforms at work. The dentist may specify that you wear nursing shoes or leather, tied shoes with a rubber sole with over-the-ankle socks. Because dentistry is a health care profession involving infection control and the requirement to meet patient care needs, dental staff attire may be prescribed by law.

As an employee, you should look as well-groomed and professional each day as the day you interviewed and were offered the job (Figure 45-17). Uniforms should be clean and well pressed, and shoes should be clean and in good condition. Unfortunately,

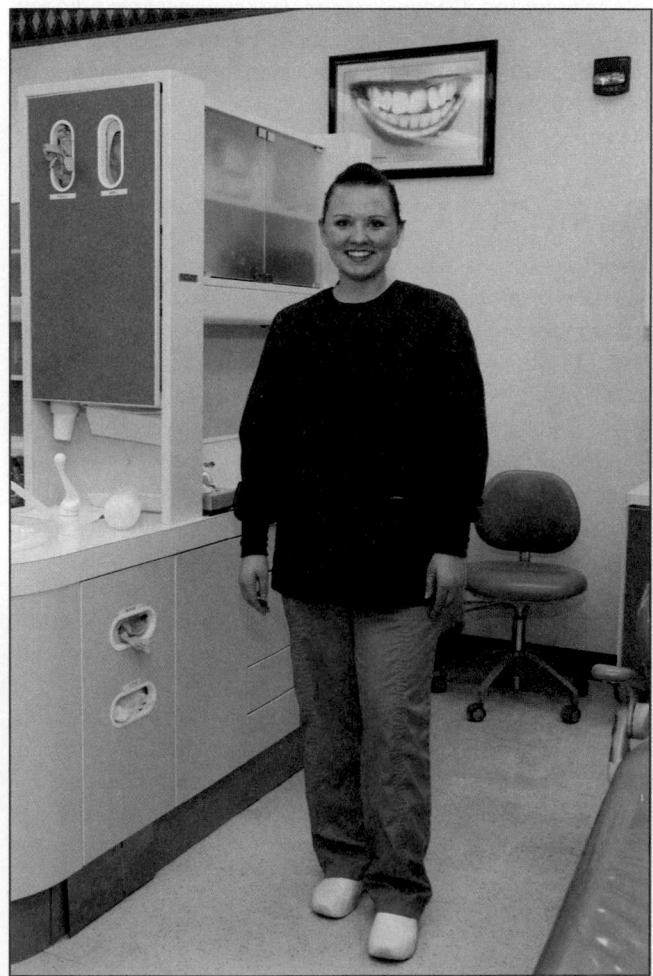

FIGURE 45-17
Maintaining a professional appearance on the job is important for the dental assistant.

an employer's perception of an employee's abilities may be influenced by the employee's appearance. Therefore, dental assistants should always look and act like professionals and be well prepared for the job every work day.

You need to maintain good personal hygiene, well-manicured nails, and have your hair away from your face. Most dental office policy prohibits body tattoos or piercings visible during patient care. Do not become lazy with your appearance as you are a representative of the dentist and the dental office.

Dependability

Make sure that the expectations of the job are identified, and then try to go above and beyond those expectations, especially if planning to advance. If expectations are unclear, talk with the office manager or employer to clarify areas of concern. A successful assistant always follows through with assignments in a timely fashion without being reminded, whether these are routine assignments or special tasks. Keep a small planner and take careful notes when you are given specific instructions. Ask questions to make sure you know what is expected of you, and write the deadline in your planner. If it looks like you may not be able to meet the deadline, inform your supervisor in advance. Often, others in the office are depending on your work. One of the most serious causes of work stress is failing to keep commitments. Work with your supervisor to set reasonable and realistic deadlines.

Patient Care

Providing personal assistance and caring for your patients are vital parts of your job. You are expected to educate your patients and to make them feel more at ease and comfortable with their dental treatment. Learning how to develop your patient care skills is key to your success as an assistant. One way to analyze how well you are doing in patient care is to ask yourself, "Would I like to be treated like I treat my patients?" Listen to what your patient is telling you and your supervisor asks of you. As an assistant, you will have the most time to talk to the patient. The patient may have new symptoms since the last time they were in the office that you need to be aware of, or they may not be feeling well the day of the appointment. By closely watching and listening to the patient, you may be able share this information with the dentist to enhance treatment or avoid an emergency.

Your patients carefully watch your behavior, skills, and professionalism. You are the dentist's office ambassador, and your actions reflect on the office. If your patients think you treat them badly, they may assume that it is the dentist's fault and seek care from a different dentist. Lost patients mean lost income for the practice.

Competence

You were hired because the dentist thought you had the skills and abilities to get the job done. You now need to prove the dentist made the right choice by remaining focused and keeping your job performance at a high level. Make sure you only perform those skills with which you are proficient, and request the help of your supervisor if you are not certain of the task. You need to develop habits that will avoid accidents for you, your patients, and fellow workers.

Besides caring for the patient, a good assistant will also care for the dentist. The dentist has a lot of pressure on them daily and only has two hands. They need a competent assistant to help them be more efficient and successful. An assistant needs to have the treatment area and patient ready for the dentist without a loss of time. You need to be next to the patient assisting the dentist throughout the procedure. While assisting the dentist, you also need to create an atmosphere in which the patient feels cared for, is relaxed, and remains calm during the treatment. If you are organized and keep your treatment area neat, you are less likely to lose time looking for things you need, or more importantly the things your employer might need. A neat treatment area is a time saver and saves your company money. You will be able to have all the instruments and materials ready to transfer instruments before the dentist even knows they need the instrument. This allows the dentist to focus on performing the procedures.

Team Player

One thing a dentist never wants to hear from an assistant is, "It isn't my job." If you say that often enough, you may not have your job much longer. An assistant's job is not done until the last patient has been dismissed and all closing routines are completed. It should not matter if it is not your patient or your treatment area. If you are not already a team player, you need to develop these skills. Begin by looking for opportunities to serve all patients and to help coworkers. Although it is important for your supervisor to know that you are performing great work, do not try to grab all the limelight. Make sure you recognize the work of others and that the team gets the credit for their contributions. Managing assistants generally earn their positions by doing the work that others did not want to do. Employers appreciate employees who help get the job done, whatever it is.

Joining in office gossip and complaining about your job may seem like an easy way to fit in with coworkers, but there may be severe consequences, including a bad reputation and losing your job. You also need to avoid the impulse to criticize the dentist and dental practice and avoid the temptation of venting on social networking sites. Remember, anyone in the world can find what you put online, and employers can take action against any employee whose online actions hurt the company. Keep your thoughts to yourself, or share with close friends and family when not in the office. Almost everyone has much more respect and trust for people who do not spread stories or backstab others.

A common reason for being dismissed from a job is an inability to get along with coworkers. The efficient assistant who is also a good team player is the one most often remembered at performance evaluation and who gets the raise at review time. You will also be happier on the job if you maintain good relationships with your coworkers and supervisors.

Honesty and Respect

Employers rank honesty and respect as qualities that impress them in new employees. Most employees know that they should not steal money, equipment, or big item materials from their employee. Less obvious is taking smaller items like toothbrushes, toothpaste, and floss home for the family without permission. But what you need to see is the bigger picture. If every employee in a large dental practice took these items whenever they wanted to, this could potentially be a large cost to the practice. Routinely taking out more materials than needed for the procedure and disposing of the unused ones is also a loss of revenue. Dentists respect assistants who treat the office as it were their own by conserving materials, keeping the office orderly, and looking for ways to make the office more profitable.

The test for employee honesty is doing what is right even if no one is looking. The dentist, coworkers, and patients have to put a lot of trust in the assistants. Lack of honesty is dangerous in a health care job because it could cause injury or infection to patients, coworkers, and yourself. For example, suppose you are responsible for the dental handpieces and you forget to complete routine maintenance, but you check it off the list anyway. What if you were rushed between patients and instead of changing the handpieces you just wiped them quickly with a spray disinfectant? What could be the result of your actions? Now you can see why honesty is such a critical quality dentists seek in assistants. Even if the assistant's supervisor is not looking, chances are another coworker is. What is that coworker's responsibility to the dentist?

Being honest also means not stealing time from your employer. The employee who comes in late, leaves early, works too slowly on purpose, or talks or plays too much is a time stealer because they get paid for work not done. You need to focus on your job, work hard, and give your employer the time you are getting paid for from the start to the end of the day. Do not take your cell phone into the treatment area, and do not accept routine personal calls unless absolutely necessary. Most employers do not mind a little time spent on employee personal matters. Just remember when it comes to raises and lay-offs, the most productive employees will get the raise and keep the job.

Show pride in yourself and respect toward others. You should never utter derogatory or minority-related slurs about yourself or others. This language disturbs others and makes others doubt your maturity and competence. The best way to get respect is to show respect toward yourself and to others.

Losing Your Job

Being called into the supervisor's office for an unscheduled meeting about your job performance is very uncomfortable. Being placed on probation or getting fired is every employee's worst nightmare.

Being Placed on Probation

Rarely does anyone get placed on probation or lose a job without warnings and notice. They have been told informally about attendance, missed deadlines, poor quality of work, or unprofessional acts. Probation is the last step to get the employee working. A formal probation will identify what the employee needs to improve, the behavior the dentist wishes to see, methods to meet expectations, and a time frame for expected changes to occur.

There are three basic types of probations. The first is triggered when the employee is not satisfactorily performing the tasks of the job. The supervisor has to decide if the employee does not have the capacity to do the job or is lacking the drive to do it properly. The second type occurs when the employee is performing the skills properly but is doing things that violate office policy or is demonstrating a poor work ethic. These include frequent absences or requests to leave early, idling or spending time on personal matters, poor interaction with patients, inappropriate dress, poor attitude, and complaints about the job and to coworkers. An employee who continues to behave inappropriately after being notified may be written up for insubordination. The third type is a combination of the two previously mentioned. This type of situation is very difficult for the employee to turn around and generally results in a short probation period and termination.

Saving Your Job

Sometimes finding out that you are not working up to expectations comes as a shock. Listen to your supervisor's feedback and do not make excuses for your poor performance. If you do not understand what is being asked of you, ask for clearer instructions. Be honest with yourself and take an objective look at your situation. Is there anything you need to learn from this experience? If you slacked off on your work or didn't get along with coworkers, you need to recognize and correct these problems.

All employers want their employees to succeed. In order to keep your job, you need to have a positive attitude toward your supervisor and keep an open line of communication. If you have problems completing your job tasks in the future, let your supervisor know before it becomes a major problem. It is easier to fix small problems along the way than to have to deal with a full-blown crisis. You should not try to bluff your way through; be honest and seek help. Your supervisor can show you how to complete the job or arrange for more training. Your output at work depends on your skills and abilities. Like many things in life, your job will depend on what you put into it. Ask for instruction on how to improve, and return to the supervisor to make certain you are performing correctly.

If you are guilty of a poor attitude toward work and others, you need to change your destructive behavior. When describing how well an employee works, it is referred to as their work habits. Like any kind of habit, it takes a lot of effort to break a habit. Some common poor work habits cited in research include procrastination, putting personal life before work while at work, being late, social media addiction, and bad body language.

Production also suffers if you are not a consistent worker. You need to ask yourself if you gave the job 100% or if you were there for a free ride. Your employer cannot afford to pay an employee who is not productive and is not a team player. You need to step back and make a self-assessment of your people skills. Are you friendly, courteous, and supportive of your coworkers? If you feel someone is unwilling to work with you or just isn't compatible with you, stay polite and focus your time on the job you were hired to do.

Leaving a Job

Sometimes an employee is unable or unwilling to meet the employer's expectations and decides it would be better to leave the job. Some employees may strongly feel that they have done their best, have shown good skills, and have been a good employee. They may even feel that the accusations are unfair. In such a situation, your best option may be to leave and look for a work environment that is more suitable.

When you are given a warning or placed on probation, remain respectful and professional. Thank the supervisor for the help they have given you and apologize for letting them down. Let the supervisor know you that you will do your best, and follow through on that promise, but start looking for another job. Review your job skills, add to your job search to be able to meet the job requirements of your potential supervisor, and request a working interview alongside this supervisor. Once you get your next job, ask for an exit interview with the dentist and give a full 2 weeks' notice. Do everything possible to leave a position on good terms with the employer. Then, if the new career does not proceed as planned, returning to the prior job when an opening is available is a possibility.

Being Fired

Even if one is fired after the probationary period, one needs to keep cool, contain one's emotions, and avoid "burning bridges" with the current employer. If the employee has not done anything too horrible, the employee may find that the supervisor will be willing to help in various ways to find a new position. Employers generally have no desire to keep an employee from being hired elsewhere. The employee should meet with the supervisor to try to agree on what the supervisor will tell potential future employers, or obtain a reference letter that states the reason for termination in a way that the employee and supervisor agree upon.

Again, the employee needs to complete a self-analysis; otherwise history may repeat itself. Some reasons the employees cited in research for poor performance and job difficulties include that they were bored with the work, didn't like getting up in the morning, didn't like the way the boss treated them, didn't think they were getting paid enough, had coworkers who didn't get along with them, and found the job cut into their social life too much.

Advancing in Your Job

If you want to advance in your position, you need to first make sure you are completing your current tasks successfully. Your supervisor will not be inclined to give you more skillful tasks if you are not getting your current jobs done accurately. You may need to ask your supervisor formally for more tasks to be added

to your responsibilities. Don't wait to be recognized as your supervisor may not realize that you are capable of doing more.

If your desire is to advance in your job, you need to find ways to expand your knowledge of the equipment, materials, and procedures used in the dental office. A valuable asset to the dentist is an assistant who is a problem solver. Instead of telling your supervisor about problems immediately as they occur, take a moment and try to find a solution. Your dentist and supervisor deal with problems all day and welcome the efforts of an assistant who provides solutions instead of problems. Dental equipment is always having minor breakdowns, and an assistant who reads the manufacturer's directions, learns how to maintain the equipment properly, decreases breakdowns, and makes minor repairs as needed is always appreciated. If it is a big problem, you should take it, as well as your solution, to the dentist before acting on it. Your ability to anticipate problems, help solve these problems, and avoid them in the future will help the dental practice to grow and will help your career grow.

You need to be aware of the necessary skills for work today, but you also need to know any additional skills you need to acquire to stay current with changes in dentistry. You should ask to attend training and for new assignments. If you take a close look at the assistants in your office, those who are moving up are the ones who have shown to be willing to do undesirable assignments and to take on new duties.

The successful assistants are those who are always seeking ways to increase their skill level, stay up with career changes, and commit to lifelong learning.

Professional Development

You are either nearing or have already taken part in the commencement ceremony that marks the end of your formal dental education. Are you aware that commencement means the beginning and the ending? As a new graduate, you are ending one phase of education and beginning the new phase of continuing education. You are entering a professional life filled with new learning and discovery and professional development.

Professional development is the lifelong process of active participation in learning activities that assist in maintaining and advancing continued competence in professional practice. Professional development is the commitment to lifelong learning that begins within the entry-level educational program and continues throughout the career of the dental professional.

With your formal education you have gained the foundational knowledge and skills that enable you to be a valued member of the dental team. However, basic knowledge is not adequate to last throughout your entire career. The American Dental Education Association (ADEA) Core Competencies for entrance into the allied dental professions states that the dental assistant must "continually perform self-assessment for lifelong learning and professional growth" (ADEA Competency C.6). This statement assumes that dental professionals accept the obligation to keep current with the knowledge that will allow them to provide the best care for their patients.

The ethical health care principles of beneficence and nonmaleficence dictate that the services dental assistants provide will not just help the patient, but above all cause no harm. What would happen if you used the wrong or outdated treatment? It is not possible to know the answer if you are unaware of the harm that outdated therapies can cause. Dentistry is always evolving; to keep pace with the dental profession it is your responsibility to yourself and your patients to periodically ask, "Am I still competent?"

Dental Care Growth The dental field is experiencing tremendous growth due to an increase of the population seeking regular dental visits. Oral health is now more widely recognized as an integral part of the overall health. Public dental health education has been actively promoting the necessity of dental care, and the scope of dental insurance has increased, making dental care more affordable. There is also an increase in the older population, making a new emphasis on geriatric dentistry and a greater demand for dental services at all age levels. The supply of dentists has not been able to keep up with the growing need for dentistry.

More dental care can be provided to the population by increasing the number of dentists educated. However, this takes time. Providing dental care to a greater population can be more quickly remedied by increasing the number and duties of the dentist's auxiliary. The number of patients a dentist may successfully treat greatly increases with the addition of a highly qualified assistant. According to the ADA Future of Dentistry report, many dentists perceive a problem in delivering quality patient care with a shortage of chairside dental assistants. The dentist is not able to see as many patients or perform as many procedures without the help of an assistant. Without an assistant the appointment times are longer, the patient's waiting times are longer, and the dentist's work days are longer.

There is also a push to have the dental auxiliary perform more duties, and duties requiring higher skills, to assist the dentist in treating more patients. As a result, the role of the dental assistant is rapidly changing, and a new career ladder is evolving. Currently, there is not a national agreement on the duties, job titles, and credentialing of dental assistants. Each state has its own State Dental Practice Act that defines the duties legally delegated to assistants within that state.

DANB has researched job titles of dental assistants throughout the United States. The general job titles range from entry level, to dental assistant, DANB certified dental assistant, registered dental assistant, and expanded functions dental assistant. Refer to http://www.dentalassisting.org/PDFs/JobTitles.pdf for job titles within the various states.

As a new assistant, you not only need to maintain your current skills and certifications but also stay abreast with future trends of the dental assisting career. Not all dentists utilize the higher skill levels assistants can achieve and do not require DANB certification. The higher level certification may not be in your state yet. To stay abreast of the changes in the dental profession, you want to be prepared to show your next employer that you are on the cutting edge in your field and be prepared in advance for any certification changes in your state.

You need to monitor legislation in your state regarding the duties and credentialing of dental assistants. Once new duties are legislated, the state board of dentistry will establish the qualifications assistants need to earn the required credentials. This includes the requirements for the dental assistant examination and standards for approval of dental assisting educational programs, courses, and continuing education.

Technology Is Changing Dentistry The continual advancement of technology has quickened the pace of our lives and has required us to update our knowledge constantly to stay current. This constant scientific and technological innovation and change has also had a profound effect on the dental field. Advances in dental technology are quickly transforming dental practices. New dental technologies are designed to make procedures easier, faster, and more ergonomic and provide more patient comfort. Dental equipment, instrumentation, materials, and procedures are ever-changing. A major challenge for the dentist is to integrate and apply the new technology in the dental office and to get all the dental staff on board. An assistant who continues to learn on an ongoing basis and who is eager to learn new procedures is an asset to the dentist and office. An important skill a successful dental assistant needs to develop is the ability to apply the right knowledge effectively. If you doubt this, ask someone who is unfamiliar with computers to find an article on the Internet.

You need to be the assistant who volunteers to learn about the latest dental material or equipment that interests the dentist. For example, you can take the initiative to study the manufacturer's directions of use and maintenance, read about new dental materials, call for additional manufacturer's assistance, attend training seminars, and help your dentist to learn how to use the materials. Dental assistants in four-handed dentistry can be more than a second pair of hands; they can also fulfill the saying that "two heads are better than one." Do not wait for your dentist to teach you. Become a partner in the learning process by not only learning your side of the chair. Learn what the dentist is doing to better assist during the procedure. If you desire to be an assistant who stays on the cutting edge of dentistry, you need to make time for learning, seek out your own opportunities, use available resources, and find new resources.

You cannot depend on your dentist to provide the necessary education. Lack of knowledge of new technology prevents your personal and professional growth, so it is important that you commit to lifelong learning as a practice for self-improvement. You need to be smart about what you are learning and plan your path of learning somewhat like your school counselor guided your studies in school. When selecting what to learn, make sure it is targeting your needs. Can what you are learning be applied to your life, your job, or your career plan? Will this increase your marketability?

One thing you can depend on is that change will always occur in the dental field. A dental assistant must adopt the concept that learning is forever if they hope for job stability and long-term growth. Nothing can grow without change. A dental assistant needs to meet change with the acquisition of knowledge and skills through continual learning.

Plethora of Learning Opportunities

There are numerous sources for learning opportunities afforded dental assistants through dental associations, dental suppliers, dental material and equipment manufacturers, study clubs and coworkers, and their own dentists.

American Dental Assistants Association

A good place to start is by continued membership in the American Dental Assistants Association (ADAA). An important function of the ADAA is to support dental assistants in achieving continued education. Whether you need to or desire credentials to be employed as a dental assistant in your state, you can gain information about credentialing and continuing education from DANB.

The ADAA is committed to the lifelong learning of its members. The ADAA identifies lifelong learning "as one of the values on which the future of dental assisting and dentistry will be built." This is reinforced in the ADAA member Statement of Commitment:

> As a professional dental assistant, I will promote the advancement of the careers of dental assistants and the dental assisting profession in matters of education, legislation, credentialing and professional activities which enhance the delivery of quality dental health care to the public.

The ADAA can assist you in achieving your lifelong learning goals. It offers something for all roles of dental assisting, as well as inspiring courses to develop you as an individual. The ADAA education library carries an extensive list of over 60 courses and continues to grow. The library serves as an essential resource to advance your clinical knowledge and skills and effective management of a dental practice. Continuing dental education (CDE) courses are offered online and in the classroom and include study in many areas including areas of radiology, infection control, medical emergencies, business management, pharmacology, oral hygiene, trends in dentistry, and much more. The ADAA official publication is *The Dental Assistant*, which also includes professional featured articles and continuing education courses. The ADAA produces an e-newsletter that is delivered to their subscribers weekly. The newsletter will keep you updated on new materials, equipment, and procedures and association notifications.

As an ADAA member there are several continuing education options. You need to research what is available for you through the national, state, and local associations. Most associations have dental assisting meetings sponsored by recognized dental groups that conduct lectures, seminars, exhibits, and even some comprehensive courses. Upon successful completion of ADAA courses, dental assistants not only gain invaluable information for their professional growth but they can also earn credits for certification and most state credentialing requirements. Dental assistants as guests of an ADA or ADHA member can also attend continuing education activities of all dental associations. It is also important to be a part of the ADAA to support your career.

The ADAA fights for your profession and lobbies for you in Congress, but in turn they need support from their members to keep the organization going strong.

DANB Professional Certification

Dentistry is on the rise and is one of the fastest growing career areas in the nation. With this growth, dentistry is also becoming more regulated, and more states are developing career ladders and beginning to require professional certification for dental assistants. Professional certification is the process by which dental assistants prove that they have the knowledge, experience, and skills to perform a specific job by passing an exam that is accredited by DANB. The dental assistant is provided a certificate as the proof of acquiring the competence. DANB develops the exam and monitors and upholds the prescribed standards of the ADAA.

The Certified Dental Assistant (CDA) is currently the only credential that has nationwide recognition and participation. The CDA is considered the standard of competence and in many states the requirement to perform specific dental assisting duties. In some states the dental assistant duties are regulated and only those certified are allowed to perform clinical duties. Assistants with the CDA credential enjoy many benefits. According to a DANB survey, certified dental assistants are trusted with more responsibilities, have better employment, earn higher pay, stay longer in the profession, and have a greater job satisfaction. Dentists report that certification demonstrates professionalism, increases practice efficiency, and enhances the overall quality of patient care and the reputation of the dental care. Certificants are lifelong learners who will continue to develop knowledge, stay on the cutting edge of dental trends and technology and elevate the dental assisting profession. A DANB certified assistant can proudly hang a framed certificate and note the credentials CDA behind their name (Figure 45-18).

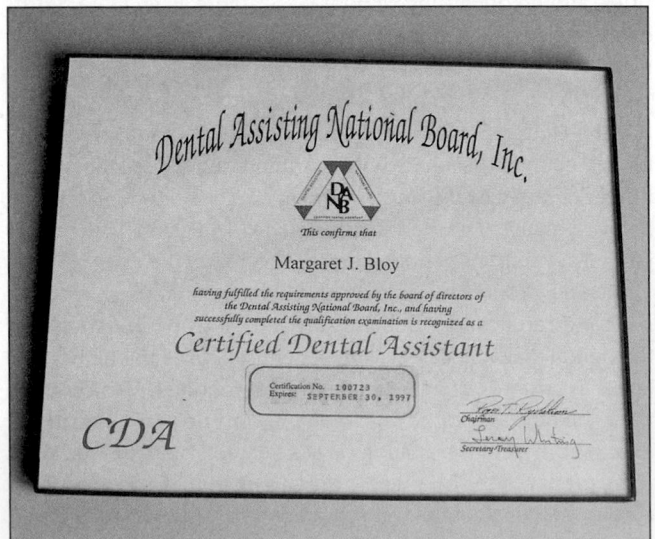

FIGURE 45-18
Dental Assisting National Board (DANB) certificate.

DANB requires its certificants to maintain their certification by earning 12 continuing dental education (CDE) credits a year. DANB follows the ADA definition of CDE and includes educational activities that review existing concepts and techniques and information beyond the basic dental assisting education. DANB has a strong belief in lifelong learning and states that its objective in CDE "is to improve the knowledge, skills and abilities of the individual to provide the highest quality of service to the public and the profession." The fact that DANB requires CDEs for renewal is one of the reasons it is recognized as the national certification agency for dental assistants, which is consistent with states that have mandatory certification and CDE requirements.

Earning CDE can be an enjoyable experience as it lends itself to professional networking, developing professional relationships, and socializing with dental colleagues. DANB offers many options to earn CDE, such as attending meetings, conventions, volunteering in free dental clinics, reading dental journals, and completing home study courses and online courses in topics that meet DANB recertification requirements. One of the roles of DANB is to evaluate and recognize activities that meet DANB recertification requirements. DANB and all the dental associations (ADA, ADHA, and ADAA) develop courses to meet these requirements. Another good source for approved DANB CDE courses is the Dental Assisting Learning and Education (DALE) Foundation.

DALE

The DANB Board of Directors has established a nonprofit educational and research foundation called the Dental Assisting Learning and Education (DALE) Foundation. The Dale Foundation's mission, "is to benefit the public, advance dental assistants and promote certification for the dental assistants by developing and providing quality education and conducting sound research to support and promote oral health." The DALE Foundation was created to provide additional resources to help the advance of the dental team. The DALE website states, "Our online dental continuing education courses and study aids help you learn the skills you need to take your career to the next level, at your own pace and on your own time." DALE adheres to the same quality and high standards of the DANB recertification requirements. This is another good resource for you to use to remain current in dentistry and dental assisting, to prepare for certification, and to maintain certification.

Professional Development Plan

You have already achieved an important goal in your life by completing your formal education. Using the job skills information presented earlier, hopefully you have some job leads or may already have a job. As you enter the dental workforce, you have a lot of choices and decisions to make. Some of you will decide to remain as chairside assistants while others will have the desire to work toward the highest level of assisting allowed in their state's dental practice act and acquire the appropriate credential. Although entry-level positions are available, many dentists prefer to hire dental assistants who have met state requirements to take on additional duties in the office.

Once you have decided on your career goal, you can reach it much more easily when you have a plan. Whether your goal is being a better employee, getting a raise or promotion, or just a personal milestone, a plan will help you succeed. You need to map out your professional development plan and commit to lifelong learning. According to the Department of Education and Sciences, lifelong learning is the "lifelong, voluntary, and self-motivated pursuit of knowledge for either personal or professional reasons." Lifelong learning will also enhance your social inclusion, active citizenship, and leadership in the dental profession. Who knows? You may become a strong advocate for one national dental assisting career ladder and national credentials and become an officer within the ADAA. Lifelong learning will also improve your competitiveness, employability, career mobility, and job satisfaction.

New graduates recite the ADAA Pledge to "Always be loyal to the welfare of the patients who come under my care." While the Pledge does not specifically mention lifelong learning, it is clearly impossible to achieve professional competence, and meet today's standards of care, without this commitment. Nothing stays stagnant, and as a dedicated professional neither should you. With a desire for learning and discovery you will keep the promise you made to society, your patients, and your profession.

Continued Success

The career of dental assisting is a very rewarding one, both professionally and personally. The work environment is a pleasant one that usually does not require evenings or night shifts. The goal of dental offices is to provide the best care possible for their patients. The patients are appreciative of the dental assistants who care for their needs. The dental assistant who provides a pleasant smile while providing care makes everything go better for the patient. Most days, dental assistants go home feeling good about the skills and knowledge they used to provide quality dental care to their patients. Continue to improve dental assisting skills and knowledge through continuing education, and stay challenged to stay knowledgeable about new techniques and materials. Be the best dental assistant possible. Good luck in your career!

Chapter Summary

It is important to find employment that will best suit individual needs and that allows for the best possible situation for the dental assistant, employer, and patients. Before taking the first position available, plan ahead. It may be essential to obtain dental assisting national certification for the state in which employment is sought. National certification for dental assistants is not mandatory in every state, but it assures patients and the dentist that the assistant has the basic knowledge and background to perform as a professional on the dental team. Make sure that the expectations of the job are identified, and then try to meet and exceed them if planning to advance. Learn how to prepare a cover letter and resume that reflect your experience and skills. The interview process is discussed, including how to prepare for the interview and then how to complete the process with a follow-up letter. Each dental assistant is responsible for maintaining a positive attitude at work. Set goals to learn new skills and stay abreast of changes in technology and materials. A dental assisting career is very rewarding, both professionally and personally. Be the best dental assistant possible.

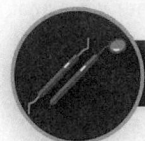

CASE STUDY

Dr. Bryan and Dr. Adebayo are hiring a dental assistant to replace Phong Ho, a dental assistant who is leaving at the end of the month. Phong has been a chairside dental assistant for 7 years for Dr. Bryan and Dr. Adebayo. Svetlana Maklavic has applied for the position and will be the first dental assistant applicant to be interviewed.

Case Study Review

1. What paperwork should Svetlana bring to the interview?

2. How should Svetlana prepare for the interview?

3. What clothes should Svetlana wear for an interview with Dr. Bryan and Dr. Adebayo? What else should the applicant consider about their appearance?

4. Why should Svetlana arrive for the interview 15 minutes early?

Review Questions

Multiple Choice

1. Which of the following is an important consideration in developing your personal career objective?
   a. the position you want
   b. what duties you want to perform
   c. in what kind of practice you would like to work
   d. All of these are important

2. Why is it important to create a personal career portfolio in a binder?
   a. to prepare for the interview
   b. to develop habit of documenting your work
   c. to stay focused during your interview
   d. All of these are important

3. A cover letter is a(n):
   a. listing of personal data for the employer.
   b. listing of education.
   c. introduction to your employer.
   d. career objective for the position being sought.

4. The document that introduces the prospective employee and presents the individual's educational background, training, and previous employment experiences is a:
   a. cover letter.
   b. resume.
   c. follow-up letter.
   d. interview.

5. All of these are good choices to ask for a letter of recommendation EXCEPT:
   a. previous supervisors.
   b. previous teachers.
   c. family members.
   d. coaches.

6. Which is one of the more effective ways to search for a job?
   a. job postings in newspapers
   b. job search engines
   c. career networking
   d. job placement agency

7. Which is true about the interview?
   a. It does not require a follow-up.
   b. It is a time for questions and answers about salary and benefits.
   c. It requires little preparation.
   d. It requires that you prepare, listen carefully, and think before answering questions asked.

8. Which of the following is one of the most frequently asked questions in the interview process?
   a. Do you have child care for your child?
   b. Do you have transportation to and from home?
   c. Do you have a background in dentistry?
   d. Why should we hire you for this position?

9. Why does an interviewer use a job application?
   a. To standardize information asked of all applicants.
   b. Applicant certifies that all information is true and accurate.
   c. It may ask information not normally found on the resume.
   d. All of these

10. All of these statements are true about the preinterview call EXCEPT:
   a. if the call is not handled well the candidate may not get the interview.
   b. the receptionist is just trying to set an interview date.
   c. it is considered a part of the prescreening process.
   d. the message and music on your phone need to be professional.

11. All of these statements are true about the interview EXCEPT:
   a. drive to the interview location before the interview date.
   b. confirm the interview the day before.
   c. rehearse for the interview.
   d. have questions ready to ask the interviewer.

12. What is the primary goal of the job orientation?
   a. To see how you function under pressure.
   b. To allow you a smooth transition into new position.
   c. To see if you are a skilled assistant.
   d. To determine if you are a team player.

13. The key to becoming an ideal employee is/are:
   a. a high standard of personal hygiene.
   b. skill and knowledge.
   c. a positive attitude.
   d. All of these

14. What can a new dental assistant do to plan for an advancement?
   a. Perform all assignments well
   b. Ask supervisor for more duties
   c. Expand knowledge of procedures used in the office
   d. All of these

15. Where can the dental assistant obtain continuing education opportunities?
   a. American Dental Assistants Association
   b. DANB Professional Certification
   c. DALE
   d. All of these

Critical Thinking

1. What are the state credentialing requirements in the state where you are applying for a dental assisting position?

2. If you are placed on probation, what can you do to save your job?

3. What are you including in your professional development plan?

4. What are the three reasons the new dental assistant needs to be involved in continuing education?

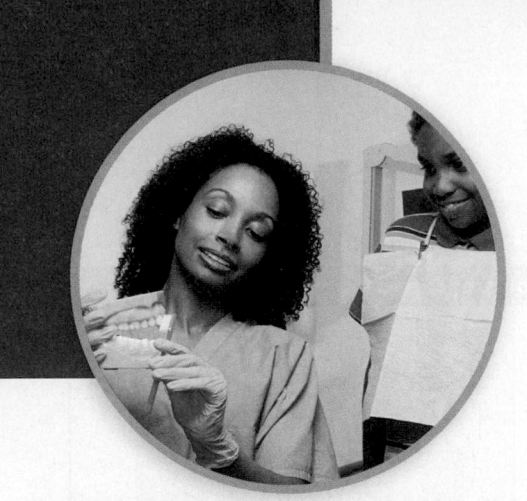

Stages of Tooth Eruption

Development of Human Dentition

Prenatal	Infancy	Early Childhood
4 months in utero	Birth	18–30 months
6 months in utero	4–8 months	2–3 years
■ Primary Dentition ■ Permanent Dentition	8–12 months	3–4 years
	9–15 months	4–5 years
	15–21 months	5–6 years

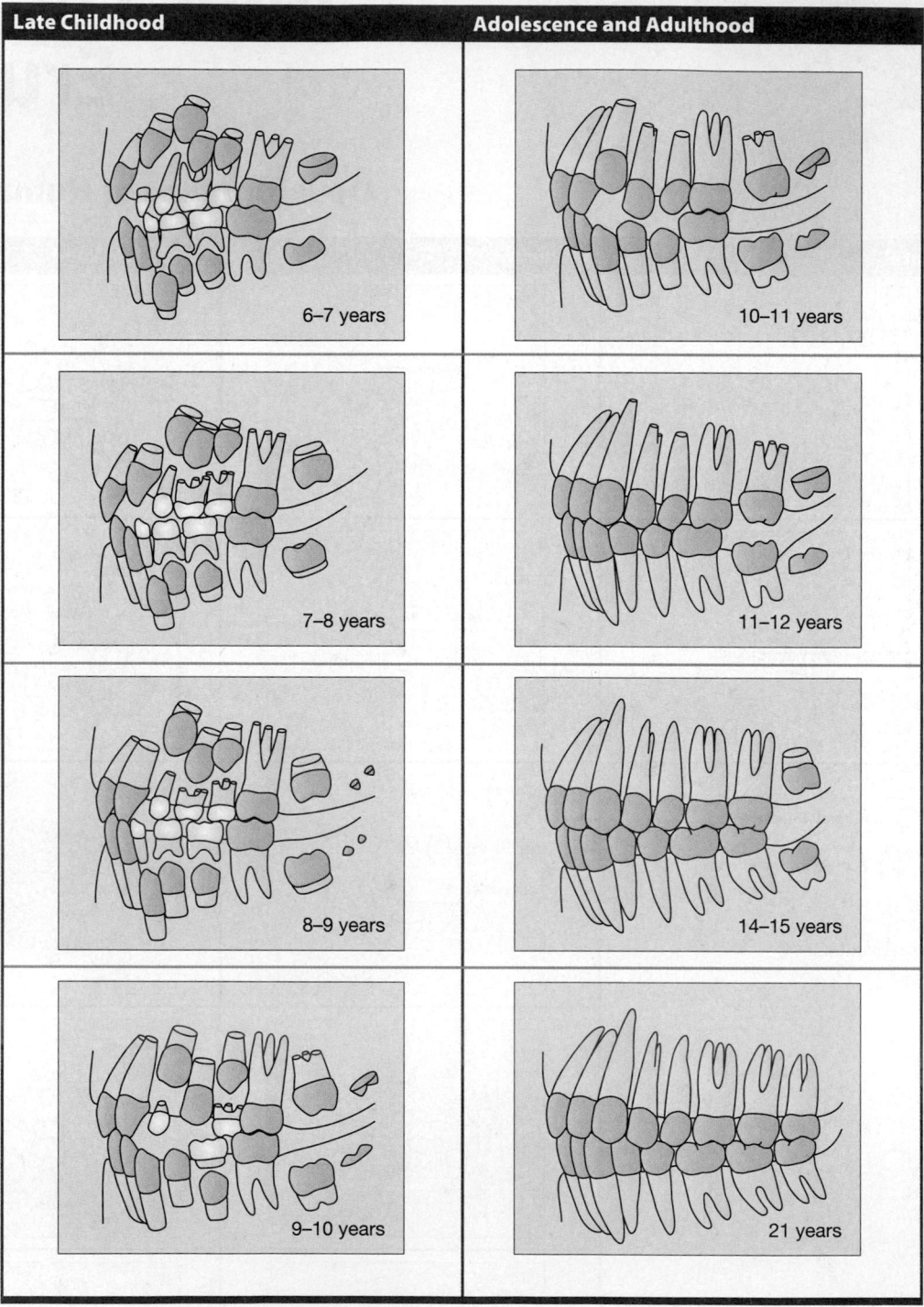

Late Childhood

6–7 years

7–8 years

8–9 years

9–10 years

Adolescence and Adulthood

10–11 years

11–12 years

14–15 years

21 years

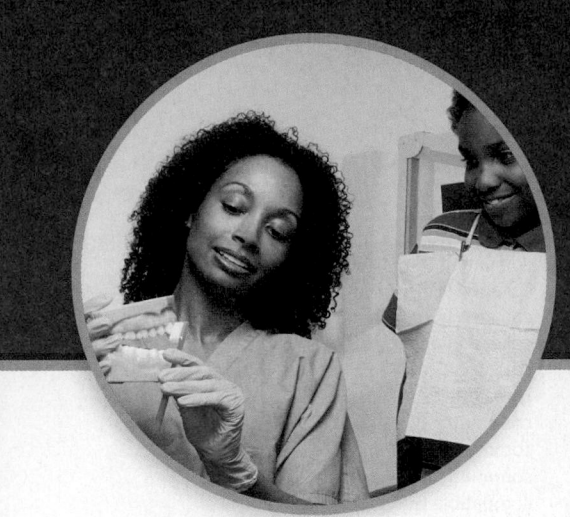

Glossary

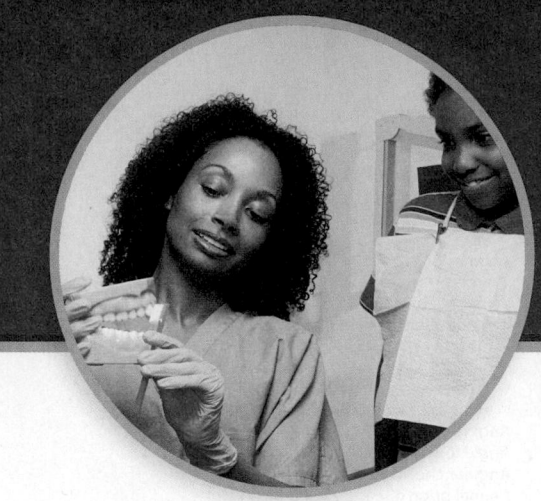

Index

columns, 1405–1406
communicating with patients, 1405
confirmation of appointments, 1409
dental hygiene, 1407
elderly patients, 1410
elements in, 1407
emergency, 1408
expanded-function practice, 1408
goal of, 1405
guidelines, 1405
health concerns, 1410
late patients, 1410
multiple appointments, 1408
new patients, 1407–1408
outlining, 1406–1407
preparation, day's appointments, 1411
scheduling for production, 1408–1409
tracking report, 1405, 1407f
units of time, 1406
unscheduled list, dental software, 1405, 1407f
Apposition, 176
Appositional stage, 178, 178f
Apthous ulcers, 963
Aqueous medium, 523
Archival storage, 1420
Area-specific curettes, 764, 764f, 765f
Argon laser technology, 809
Aristotle, 12t, 13
Armamentarium, 636
anesthetic cartridge, 735, 735f
anesthetic syringe. *See* Anesthetic syringe
bagged instruments, 760, 760f
dental hygiene, 760, 760f
dental injection needle, 735–736, 736f
high-volume evacuation (HVE), 761
lists, 760, 761t
local anesthesia, 733
needlestick prevention device, 733, 734f
sterilization wrap, 760, 761f
topical anesthesia, 733
Arrector pili muscle, 111
Arrhythmias, 381, 422
Arteries, 100, 101f
Arthritis, 521t
Articular eminence, 124, 130
Articulating forceps, 394, 395f, 585, 585f
Articulating paper, 586
Articulation, 585
Articulations joints, 82
Articulator, 1070f, 1074
Artifacts, 880
Artificial teeth, 1352–1353, 1360
ASD. *See* Autistic spectrum disorder
Asepsis, 292
Aseptic technique, 292
Aspiration techniques, saliva ejector, 655–656
Aspirin, 402, 417
Aspirin burns, 241, 241f
Assault, 61, 62f
Assessment
components of dental hygiene, 753
dental examination, 753
hard and soft deposits, 753
measuring periodontal disease, 754–756
risk factors
dental caries, 754, 755f
periodontal disease, 754, 755f
Asthma, 108, 391, 1105
attack, 445, 446t
causes, 445
chronic lung disorder, 445
dental management, 445
medical history questions, 445, 446t
medications, 445
types of, 445t
Atherosclerosis, 381
Atom
composed of, 823
electrons, 823, 824
neutrons, 823–824
Atria, 98
Atrioventricular (AV) node, 99
Atrophy, 384

Attached gingiva, 166
Attachment unit, 183, 184f
Attitude, 37
Auscultation, 699
Auspices, 64
Autism, 378, 1105
Autistic spectrum disorder (ASD), 378
Autoclave, 330–333, 331f–333f
Autografts, 1287
Autoimmune disease, 1330
Automated devices, 497–499
automated toothbrushes, 497–498
oral irrigator, 498–499
Automated external defibrillator (AED), 66
Automated toothbrushes, 497–498
Automated washing/disinfectors, 319
Automatic mixing machine, 1060, 1060t
Automatic processing
care and maintenance, 896
daylight loader, procedure, 895
infection control, 849
AutoMatrix, 1008, 1008f
Autonomic nervous system (ANS), 87, 90
Autonomy, 58
Autopolymerizing sealant system, 807–808
Auxiliary staff, 36
Avulsed tooth, 965, 965f
Avulsion, 965
Axial skeleton, 82

B

Baby boomer, 42, 42f
Backdrop, 49
Backorder, 1416
Bacteria, 266–269, 268f
Bacterial endocarditis, 102–103
Bacteria morphology, 266, 267f
Bactericidal or bacteriostatic, 420, 496
Baker, John, 13
Bank deposits, 1424
procedure, 1424–1425
reconciling bank statement, 1425–1426
Barbiturate, 416
Bartholin's duct, 137
Basal cell carcinoma, 112f, 248, 248f
Basal metabolic rate (BMR), 525
Bases, 595, 995–999
Baton technique, 641
Battery, 61, 62f
Beading, 1052
Behavior management, 1109–1111, 1110f, 1110t, 1111f
Bell's palsy, 91
Bell stage, 177–178, 177f
Belly, 133
Belt and pulley, 597
Beneficence, 58, 60
Benefit programs, dental
alternative benefits, 1437–1438
fee-for-service plans, 1439, 1440t
indemnity plans, 1437
medicaid, 1439–1440
Benign neoplasms, 246
Bent traditional film packet, 879
Benzocaine ointments, 962
Benzodiazepines, 416–417
Beriberi, 521t
Bicuspids, 103, 192
Bifid tongue, 940, 940f
Bifid uvula, 162
Bifurcated root, 183, 207
Bilaterally, 160
Bioavailability, 502
Bioburden, 312
Biofilm, 22, 327, 518
hard and soft deposits, 753
Biofilm control, 481
Biofilm control record, 489–490, 489f
Biofilm removal aids, 490–493, 493–494f
end tuft brush, 492
floss aids, 490–492, 491f
interdental brush, 492
toothpick, 492

Biological agents, oral cavity
actinomycosis, 235
aphthous ulcers, 236, 236f
candida albicans, 237–238
cellulitis, 238, 238f
herpes simplex virus, 235–236, 235f
herpes zoster (shingles), 236, 236f
syphilis, 236–237, 236f, 237f
Biological effects of radiation
daily radiation exposure, 836
damage body tissues, 835
dosimetry badges, radiation monitoring, 836f
nonlinear nonthreshold curve, 836f
occupational exposure, 836
radiosensitive cells, 835–836
somatic and genetic effects, 835
Biologic indicators (BIs), 336
Biotene, 113, 1330
Bisecting technique, 868–872
adult full mouth series, exposure sequence, 873t
angle procedure
maxillary and mandibular periapical exposures, 873
maxillary canine exposure, 873
maxillary incisor exposure, 874
factors affecting
exposure time, 868–869
head position, 868–869
horizontal angulation, 871–872
receptor position and placement, 869
vertical angulation, 869–871
paralleling technique, 852–856
Bisection of angle technique (BAT). *See* Bisecting technique
BIS-GMA, 807
Bisulfites, 415–416
Bite registration, 1052, 1057–1058, 1058f
Bite registration waxes, 1078–1079
Bitewing exposures, 876
horizontal premolar, 866
molar bitewing, 867
Black, Arthur D., 15
Black's formula, 384, 384f
Black, Greene Vardiman, 15, 16f
Black hairy tongue, 242, 243f
Bloodborne pathogens, 272
Bloodborne Pathogens Standard, 19, 339
Blood clotting, effects on, 413
Blood, components of, 100–101
Blood disorders, 386–393
cancer, 391–392, 391f
coagulation disorders, 386–387
dental management of patient with, 386
endocrine disorders, 388
kidney disease, 390
musculoskeletal disorders, 387–388
psychiatric disorders, 388–390
red blood cell disorders, 386
respiratory disease, 390–391
white blood cell disorders, 386
Blood pH, 112
Blood pressure, 100
classifications and dental management protocol, 436
diastolic, 434
procedure, 435
sphygmomanometer, 434, 434f
systolic, 434
Blood typing, 100–101, 103t
Blood vessels, 100
Blurred image, 880
BMI. *See* Body mass index
BMR. *See* Basal metabolic rate
Body cavities, 79, 80f
Body language, 38–40, 38f, 39f, 50
Body locations and directions, 79–80
anatomical position, 79, 79f
body cavities, 79, 80f
body planes, 79
directional terms of body, 79, 80t
Body mass index (BMI), 527
Body planes, 79